OXFORD TEXTBOOK OF
RHEUMATOLOGY

OXFORD MEDICAL PUBLICATIONS

OXFORD TEXTBOOK OF
RHEUMATOLOGY

SECOND EDITION

VOLUME 2
Sections 5–6 and Index

Edited by

P. J. Maddison

Consultant Rheumatologist, Gwynedd Hospitals NHS Trusts, Bangor, UK

David A. Isenberg

Professor of Rheumatology, University College London, London, UK

Patricia Woo

Professor of Paediatric Rheumatology, University College London
and Institute of Child Health, London, UK

David N. Glass

Professor of Pediatrics and Director, Division of Rheumatology,
Children's Hospital Medical Center, Cincinnati, Ohio, USA

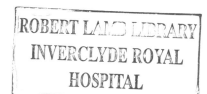
Oxford   New York   Tokyo
OXFORD UNIVERSITY PRESS
1998

Oxford University Press, Great Clarendon Street, Oxford OX2 6DP

Oxford   New York
Athens   Auckland   Bangkok   Bogota   Bombay
Buenos Aires   Calcutta   Cape Town   Dar es Salaam
Delhi   Florence   Hong Kong   Istanbul   Karachi
Kuala Lumpur   Madras   Madrid   Melbourne
Mexico City   Nairobi   Paris   Singapore
Taipei   Tokyo   Toronto   Warsaw

and associated companies in
Berlin   Ibadan

Oxford is a trade mark of Oxford University Press

Published in the United States
by Oxford University Press, Inc., New York

First edition published 1993
Second edition published 1998

A catalogue record for this book is available from the British Library

Library of Congress Cataloging in Publication Data

ISBN 0 19 262697 3 (set)
0 19 262698 1 (Vol. 1)
0 19 262699 X (Vol. 2)

Typeset by Dobbie Typesetting Limited, Tavistock, Devon

Printed in Hong Kong

Preface to the Second Edition

Four years ago, in 1993, the first edition of this textbook was published to considerable acclaim. The many rapid developments in the basic science of rheumatology, imaging of joints, bones, and soft tissues, and exciting advances in treatment for some of the previously most intractable rheumatic diseases, have persuaded us that a second edition is timely and will contain sufficient new material both to stimulate and inform the reader.

The second edition has benefited, we believe, from the rearrangement of some chapters, the expansion of many others which have been brought up to date, and the addition of several completely new chapters. Our contributors have also been asked to provide expanded reference lists to facilitate access to the original sources. This approach ensures freshness of ideas and style, which is complemented by the improved quantity and quality of the colour figures. We also wished to make this a textbook to which rheumatologists could refer as a guide to their management of both the common and more unusual rheumatic conditions. To facilitate this aim, algorithms of optimal treatment are provided in the clinical chapters with additional practical management suggestions, including a section on joint and soft tissue injection.

The textbook has been designed as an attractive and informative manual for rheumatology trainees, full-time clinicians, and academic rheumatologists. We have encouraged our authors to express their opinions freely, to bring areas of dispute into the open, and to present a balanced view overall. As in the first edition, this volume places special emphasis upon the perspective of the age of the patient when dealing with the presentation of various rheumatic conditions, and a number of chapters focus on paediatric rheumatology. Another important emphasis in this edition is on the overlap of rheumatology with other subspecialties. This is provided by a series of chapters co-authored by rheumatologists and colleagues with expertise in a wide range of related conditions.

It has been both a challenge and a pleasure for us to edit the second edition which we hope will build on the clarity and standards of production of the first.

Peter Maddison
David Isenberg
Patricia Woo
David Glass

Preface to the First Edition

These are exciting times for the study of rheumatology. Current research, incorporated in this textbook and integral to the editors' enthusiasm for their project, continuously increases our knowledge of the molecular basis of many of the rheumatic diseases. These advances more than justify a new textbook written to complement the successful *Oxford Textbook of Medicine*. As with the other volumes in this series, it is designed to be comprehensive and sufficient for both the trainee and the general physician who require up-to-date information.

The book begins with the variations in presentation of rheumatic symptoms at different ages. There follow chapters dealing with those syndromes, which are not easy to classify and which may be best considered as regional. Although the aetiology of these syndromes is still incomplete they are such a significant part of practice that they demand comprehensive cover. Special emphasis has been placed on back symptomatology both in children and in adults as this problem represents an especially large part of rheumatological practice. Chapters in the third part of Section 1 then discuss rheumatic disease in relation not only to general (internal) medicine but also to other specialties, including psychiatry, anaesthesia, obstetrics, and ophthalmology. The text provides both a comprehensive account of these extensive and pervasive interactions and more focused discussions, either on an area of particular interest to the authors or of special clinical interest; hence the variety of approaches ranges from the general view to the in-depth analysis of a specialist topic.

The next two sections, dealing primarily with basic science, include conceptual advances of relevance to rheumatology and provide an understanding of the rationale for newer therapies being introduced into clinical practice. We have not attempted to replace basic science textbooks; rather we have indicated good reviews on specific topics, concentrating in our volume on how the different areas interact within the context of rheumatic diseases. For example, genetic abnormalities of collagen are described in relation to diseases of cartilage and bone. The joint is treated as a functional unit, and its physiological and biomechanical disturbances are described in the context of a variety of diseases. Parts of the immune system currently thought to be important in the pathogenesis of chronic inflammation are highlighted in some detail. The sections finish with a review of available and innovative ways of controlling inflammation.

Volume 1 concludes with discussion of clinical laboratory practices. Considerable advances have been made in developing laboratory and imaging techniques for clinical assessment. In this section, guidance is given on the selection of appropriate investigations as well as an indication of future developments.

Volume 2 contains the necessary systematic and comprehensive review of the rheumatic diseases. We have tried to encompass rheumatic diseases met throughout the world together with their epidemiological and environmental influences. To this end, authors have been selected who have appropriate clinical experience and established reputations in teaching and research. Colour has been used in this volume to enhance the clinical descriptions while the authors provide a personal as well as an informative approach to management. The final section deals with the important aspects of surgery and rehabilitation. A comprehensive review of surgical techniques has not been attempted. Rather, the major principles have been established to enable appropriate referral as well as the early recognition of complications of surgery.

Throughout the text, considerable emphasis is placed on the age of presentation, thus ensuring that a paediatrician faced with a rheumatological problem is well catered for. Referencing has been selective rather than exhaustive; with the knowledge that computer searches are widely available, we feel that the space may be better used for clinical description.

No project of this magnitude is complete without acknowledgements. We would like to thank the staff of Oxford University Press for their unfailing help. Thanks are also due to our staff, Sheena Stewart, Carolyn Keith Haun, Louise Kittredge, Geraldine Brown, Ann Maitland, and Kate Young for their invaluable assistance in preparing the text.

Peter Maddison
David Isenberg
Patricia Woo
David Glass

Contents

Volume 1

Preface to the Second Edition		v
Preface to the First Edition		vi
Contributors		xi

1 Clinical presentation of rheumatic disease

1.1.	Clinical presentation in different age groups	3
1.1.1	The adult patient *Anthony S. Russell and John S. Percy*	3
1.1.2	Children and adolescents *Ross E. Petty*	9
1.1.3	The geriatric age group *Evan Calkins*	22
1.1.4	Principles of examination *Elisabeth Paice*	39
1.1.5	Outcomes assessment in rheumatology *Oliver Sangha, Gerold Stucki, and Matthew H. Liang*	51
1.1.6	Psychological aspects of rheumatic disease *S. P. Newman*	63
1.1.7	Growth and skeletal maturation *Daniel J. Lovell and Patricia Woo*	72
1.2	Common clinical problems	89
1.2.1	Spinal problems	89
1.2.1.1	Spinal problems in adults *Andrew O. Frank*	89
1.2.1.2	Spinal problems in children *Charles S. B. Galasko*	114
1.2.2	Regional problems	135
1.2.2.1	The upper limbs in adults *Adel G. Fam*	135
1.2.2.2	The lower limbs in adults *Robert W. Simms*	150
1.2.2.3	The arm and leg in children *Patience H. White*	162
1.2.3	Extra-articular features of rheumatic diseases *Ian D. Griffiths*	169
1.3	Views from different perspectives	181
1.3.1	Pregnancy and lactation	181
1.3.1.1	Pregnancy *W. Watson Buchanan and Walter F. Kean*	181
1.3.1.2	Antirheumatic drugs in pregnancy and lactation *W. Watson Buchanan and Walter F. Kean*	188
1.3.2	The skin *C. R. Lovell and P. J. Maddison*	199
1.3.3	Neurological complications *I. T. Ferguson and Peter Hollingworth*	216
1.3.4	The cardiovascular system *Laura F. Wexler and Michael E. Luggen*	229
1.3.5	The respiratory system *Stephen G. Spiro and David A. Isenberg*	240
1.3.6	The gastrointestinal system *Erkki Eerola and Reijo Peltonen*	255
1.3.7	The endocrine system *Chad Deal*	277
1.3.8	Oncology and haematology *Michael Ehrenfeld and Yehuda Shoenfeld*	288
1.3.9	An anaesthetic perspective *Allan I. Binder and Frances Dormon*	298
1.3.10	The eye *Elizabeth M. Graham and Alison M. Leak*	310
1.3.11	The kidney *Carolyn P. Cacho, Jay B. Wish, Frances B. Wheeler, and Gary M. Kammer*	321
1.3.12	Psychiatric issues in rheumatology *Malcolm P. Rogers and Simon Helfgott*	332

2 Pathophysiology of musculoskeletal disease

2.1	Molecular genetics and its relevance in rheumatology *Patricia Woo*	347
2.2	Molecular abnormalities of collagen and connective tissue *F. Michael Pope*	353
2.3	Articular cartilage *Tim Hardingham*	405
2.4	Bone in health and disease *Roger Smith*	421
2.5	The physiology of the joint and its disturbance in inflammation *Paul Mapp, Cliff. R. Stevens and David R. Blake*	441

2.6   Skeletal muscle damage   455
       Joan M. Round and D.A. Jones

2.7   Biomechanics of articulations and derangements
       in disease   477
       Anthony Unsworth and Andrew A. Amis

2.8   The neurophysiology of pain   487
       Hans-Georg Schaible

3   The process of inflammation

3.1   Cells and mediators   503
       Mark J. Walport and Gordon W. Duff

3.2   Lymphocyte traffic in inflammation   525
       Dorian O. Haskard

3.3   Specific immune responses   545
       B. P. Wordsworth, S. J. Bowman, and John I. Bell

3.4   Animal models of arthritis   559
       W. B. van den Berg

3.5   Modification of inflammation   575
       3.5.1   Non-steroidal anti-inflammatory drugs   575
               Peter Brooks

       3.5.2   Antirheumatic drugs   581
               A. M. Denman

       3.5.3   Therapeutic immunomodulation   608
               A. M. Denman

4   Investigation of the rheumatic
     diseases

4.1   Acute phase response   623
       *Rosamonde E. Banks, John T. Whicher, Douglas Thompson,
       and Howard A. Bird*

4.2   Haematology   633
       Charles Richardson, Bridget Griffiths, and Paul Emery

4.3   Biochemistry   647
       *Rosamonde E. Banks, Douglas Thompson,
       John T. Whicher, and Howard A. Bird*

4.4   Microbiology and diagnostic serology   657
       Geoffrey Scott

4.5   Autoantibody profile   665
       P.J. Maddison

4.6   Joint fluid   667
       J. Lawrence Houk

4.7   Gene marker analysis   687
       Rafal Ploski and Øystein Førre

4.8   Immune complex detection   703
       Bryan D. Williams

4.9   Imaging   715
       4.9.1   Imaging in adults   715
               Peter Renton

       4.9.2   Imaging in children   751
               G. H. Sebag and J.-F. Quignodon

4.10   Histopathology   775
       Patrick J. Gallagher and Janice R. Anderson

4.11   Electrophysiology   799
       Adam Young

Index   I.1

Volume 2

Preface to the Second Edition   v
Preface to the First Edition   vi
Contributors   xi

5   The scope of rheumatic disease

5.1   Epidemiology   811
       5.1.1   Epidemiology and the rheumatic diseases   811
               Alan J. Silman

       5.1.2   Epidemiology of rheumatic diseases in
               selected non-European populations   828
               Patricia A. Fraser

5.2   Nosology of the chronic inflammatory rheumatic
       diseases   843
       Patricia Woo and David N. Glass

5.3   Infections   849
       5.3.1   Pyogenic arthritis in adults   849
               Marc L. Miller

       5.3.2   Pyogenic arthritis in children   861
               Mary Anne Jackson and Komal B. Desai

       5.3.3   Osteomyelitis and associated conditions   868
               Emilio Bouza and Patricia Muñoz

       5.3.4   Lyme disease   884
               Daniel W. Rahn

       5.3.5   Viral arthritis   896
               Stanley J. Naides

       5.3.6   HIV infection   906
               Robert Winchester and Silviu Itescu

       5.3.7   Mycobacterial diseases   927
               Sanjiv N. Amin

       5.3.8   Brucellar arthritis   937
               E. Pascual

       5.3.9   Parasitic involvement   945
               Tomás S. Bocanegra

       5.3.10 Fungal arthritis   954
               Carol A. Kemper and Stanley C. Deresinski

       5.3.11 Immunodeficiency   966
               A. D. B. Webster

5.3.12   Rheumatic fever   972
Allan Gibofsky and John B. Zabriskie

5.4   Rheumatoid arthritis   983
   5.4.1   Immunopathogenesis of rheumatoid arthritis   983
         Ravinder N. Maini and Marc Feldmann

   5.4.2   Rheumatoid arthritis–the clinical picture   1004
         Frank A. Wollheim

   5.4.3   Juvenile rheumatoid arthritis (rheumatoid factor positive polyarthritis)   1031
         Barbara M. Ansell

5.5   Spondylarthropathies   1037
   5.5.1   Spondylarthropathy, undifferentiatated spondylarthritis, and overlap   1037
         Andrei Calin

   5.5.2   Spondylarthropathies in childhood   1049
         Taunton R. Southwood and Murray H. Passo

   5.5.3   Ankylosing spondylitis   1058
         Andrei Calin

   5.5.4   Psoriatic arthritis   1071
         Dafna D. Gladman

   5.5.5   Reactive arthropathy, Reiter's syndrome, and enteric arthropathy in adults   1084
         Bernard P. Amor and Antoine A. Toubert

5.6   Arthropathies primarily occurring in childhood   1099
   5.6.1   Pauciarticular-onset juvenile chronic arthritis   1099
         David D. Sherry, Elizabeth D. Mellins and Barbara S. Nepom

   5.6.2   Systemic-onset juvenile chronic arthritis   1114
         Ronald M. Laxer and Rayfel Schneider

   5.6.3   Rheumatoid factor-negative polyarthritis in children ('seronegative polyarthritis')   1131
         Anne-Marie Prieur

5.7   Systemic lupus erythematosus   1145
   5.7.1   Systemic lupus erythematosus in adults   1145
         David A. Isenberg and Angela C. Horsfall

   5.7.2   Systemic lupus erythematosus in children   1180
         Earl D. Silverman and Alison A. Eddy

   5.7.3   The antiphospholipid antibody syndrome   1202
         Munther A. Khamashta and G. R. V. Hughes

5.8   Scleroderma and related disorders in adults and children   1217
   Carol M. Black and Christopher P. Denton

5.9   Polymyositis and dermatomyositis   1249
   5.9.1   Polymyositis and dermatomyositis in adults   1249
         Ira N. Targoff

   5.9.2   Polymyositis and dermatomyositis in children   1287
         Lauren M. Pachman

5.10   Sjögren's syndrome   1301
   Athanasios G. Tzioufas, Pierre Youinou, and H. M. Moutsopoulos

5.11   Primary vasculitides   1319
   5.11.1   Classification of vasculitis   1319
         David G. I. Scott and Richard A. Watts

5.11.2   Wegener's granulomatosis   1331
         Wolfgang L. Gross

5.11.3   Classical polyarteritis nodosa, microscopic polyarteritis, and Churg-Strauss syndrome   1351
         D. Adu and Paul A. Bacon

5.11.4   Small vessel vasculitis   1366
         Clive E. H. Grattan and Victoria A. Jolliffe

5.11.5   Polymyalgia rheumatica   1373
         G. S. Panayi

5.11.6   Large vessel vasculitis   1382
         Richard A. Watts and David G. I. Scott

5.11.7   Behçet's syndrome   1394
         Hasan Yazıcı, Sebahattin Yurdakul, and Vedat Hamuryudan

5.11.8   Primary vasculitis in children   1402
         Michael J. Dillon

5.12   Overlap syndromes in adults and children   1413
   Enrique Roberto Soriano and Neil John McHugh

5.13   Miscellaneous inflammatory conditions   1433
   5.13.1   Amyloidosis   1433
         Gunnar Husby

   5.13.2   Familial Mediterranean fever   1445
         Pnina Langevitz, Avi Livneh, Deborah Zemer, and Mordechai Pras

   5.13.3   Panniculitis   1450
         Jeffrey P. Callen

   5.13.4   Neutrophilic dermatoses   1450
         Jeffrey P. Callen

   5.13.5   Sarcoidosis   1456
         Barry Bresnihan

   5.13.6   The chronic, infantile, neurological, cutaneous, and articular syndrome (CINCA)   1470
         Anne-Marie Prieur

   5.13.7   Multicentric reticulohistiocytosis   1474
         P. J. Maddison

   5.13.8   Hyperlipidaemias   1478
         Keng Hong Leong, J. Reckless, and Neil John McHugh

5.14   Soft-tissue rheumatism   1489
   Brian Hazleman

5.15   Osteoarthritis   1515
   Michael Doherty, Adrian Jones, and T. E. Cawston

5.16   Crystal arthropathies   1555
   Ann K. Rosenthal

5.17   Diseases of bone and cartilage   1583
   5.17.1   Osteoporosis and osteomalacia   1583
         A.K. Bhalla

   5.17.2   Paget's disease of bone   1610
         Adrian J. Crisp

   5.17.3   Diseases of bone, cartilage, and synovium   1617
         P. J. Maddison

5.17.4 Diseases of bone and cartilage in children   1629
        Barbara M. Ansell

5.18 Disorders of the spine   1639
      5.18.1 Intervertebral disc disease and other
              mechanical disorders of the back   1639
              Malcolm I. V. Jayson
      5.18.2 Cervical pain syndromes   1650
              Allan I. Binder

5.19 Miscellaneous abnormalities of connective tissue 1665
      5.19.1 Rheumatic diseases and neoplasia   1665
              Thomas G. Benedek
      5.19.2 Algodystrophy
              (reflex sympathetic dystrophy syndrome)   1679
              Geoffrey O. Littlejohn
      5.19.3 Rheumatic complications of drugs and toxins 1689
              Robert M. Bernstein

6 Intervention, rehabilitation, and sports medicine

6.1 Surgery in adults   1701
     Justin Cobb and C.B.D. Lavy

6.2 Surgery in children   1713
     Malcolm Swann

6.3. Rehabilitation of adults   1723
      Lynne Turner-Stokes

6.4. Rehabilitation of children   1737
      Renate Häfner and Marianne Spamer

6.5 Corticosteroid injection therapy   1757
     Allan I. Binder

6.6 Sports medicine   1773
     Mark Harries

6.7 Sports injuries   1779
     J. R. Jenner and M. Shirley Emerson

Index   I.1

Contributors list

D. ADU
  Consultant Renal Physician, Queen Elizabeth Hospital, Birmingham, UK
  5.11.3 Classical polyarteritis nodosa, microscopic polyarteritis, and Churg-Strauss syndrome

SANJIV N. AMIN
  Consultant Rheumatologist, Bombay Hospital, India
  5.3.7 Mycobacterial diseases

ANDREW A. AMIS
  Reader in Orthopaedic Biomechanics, Imperial College London, UK
  2.7 Biomechanics of articulations and derangements in disease

BERNARD P. AMOR
  Professor of Rheumatology, Hôpital Cochin, University of Paris V, France
  5.5.5 Reactive arthropathy, Reiter's syndrome, and enteric arthropathy in adults

JANICE R. ANDERSON
  Consultant Neuropathologist, Addenbrooke's Hospital, Cambridge, UK
  4.10 Histopathology

BARBARA M. ANSELL
  Consultant Rheumatologist, Windsor, Berkshire, UK
  5.4.3 Juvenile rheumatoid arthritis (rheumatoid factor positive polyarthritis)
  5.17.4 Diseases of bone and cartilage in children

PAUL A. BACON
  Arthritis and Rheumatism Council Professor of Rheumatology and Head of Department of Rheumatology, University of Birmingham Medical School, UK
  5.11.3 Classical polyarteritis nodosa, microscopic polyarteritis, and Churg-Strauss syndrome

ROSAMONDE E. BANKS
  ICRF Cancer Medicine Research Unit, St James's University Hospital, Leeds, UK
  4.1 Acute phase response
  4.3 Biochemistry

JOHN I. BALL
  Nuffield Professor of Clinical Medicine, Nuffield Department of Clinical Medicine, University of Oxford; Consultant Physician, John Radcliffe Hospital, Oxford, UK
  3.3 Specific immune responses

THOMAS G. BENEDEK
  Professor of Medicine, University of Pittsburgh School of Medicine, Pennsylvania, USA
  5.19.1 Rheumatic diseases and neoplasia

ROBERT M. BERNSTEIN
  Consultant Rheumatologist, Manchester Royal Infirmary, UK
  5.19.3 Rheumatic complications of drugs and toxins

A. K. BHALLA
  Consultant Rheumatologist, Royal National Hospital for Rheumatic Diseases, Bath, Avon, UK
  5.17.1 Osteoporosis and osteomalacia

ALLAN I. BINDER
  Consultant Rheumatologist, Lister Hospital, North Hertfordshire NHS Trust, Stevenage, Hertfordshire, UK
  1.3.9 An anaesthetic perspective
  5.18.2 Cervical pain syndromes
  6.5 Corticosteroid injection therapy

HOWARD A. BIRD
  Reader in Rheumatology, University of Leeds, UK
  4.1 Acute phase response
  4.3 Biochemistry

CAROL M. BLACK
  Professor of Rheumatology, Academic Unit of Rheumatology and Connective Tissue Diseases, Royal Free Hospital Medical School, London, UK
  5.8 Scleroderma and related disorders in adults and children

DAVID R. BLAKE
  Arthritis and Rheumatism Council Professor of Rheumatology and Consultant Physician, St Bartholomew's and Royal London Hospital School of Medicine and Dentistry, Queen Mary and Westfield College, University of London, UK
  2.5 The physiology of the joint and its disturbance in inflammation

TOMÁS S. BOCANEGRA
  Senior Director, Arthritis Clinical Group, Clinical Research, G. D. Searle & Co., Skokie, Illinois, USA
  5.3.9 Parasitic involvement

EMILIO BOUZA
  Professor and Chief of the Division of Clinical Microbiology and Infectious Diseases, Hospital General Universitario 'Gregorio Maranon', Madrid, Spain
  5.3.3 Osteomyelitis and associated conditions

S. J. BOWMAN
  Senior Lecturer in Rheumatology, University of Birmingham, UK
  3.3 Specific immune responses

BARRY BRESNIHAN
Professor of Rheumatology, University College Dublin, and Consultant Rheumatologist, St Vincent's Hospital, Dublin, Ireland
5.13.5 Sarcoidosis

PETER BROOKS
Professor of Medicine, University of New South Wales, St Vincent's Hospital, Sydney, Australia
3.5.1 Non-steroidal anti-inflammatory drugs

CAROLYN P. CACHO
Assistant Professor of Medicine, Case Western Reserve School of Medicine, Cleveland, Ohio, USA
1.3.11 The kidney

ANDREI CALIN
Consultant Rheumatologist, Royal National Hospital for Rheumatic Diseases, Bath, Avon, UK
5.5.1 Spondylarthropathy, undifferentiatated spondylarthritis, and overlap
5.5.3 Ankylosing spondylitis

EVAN CALKINS
Emeritus Professor of Medicine, School of Medicine and Biomedical Sciences, State University of New York at Buffalo; Senior Physician and Coordinator, Geriatric Programs, Health Care Plan, Buffalo, New York, USA
1.1.3 The geriatric age group

JEFFREY P. CALLEN
Professor of Medicine (Dermatology); Chief, Division of Dermatology, University of Louisville School of Medicine, Kentucky, USA
5.13.3 Panniculitis
5.13.4 Neutrophilic dermatoses

T. E. CAWSTON
Professor of Rheumatology, The Medical School, University of Newcastle upon Tyne, UK
5.15 Osteoarthritis

JUSTIN COBB
Consultant Orthopaedic Surgeon, University College Hospital, London, UK
6.1 Surgery in adults

ADRIAN J. CRISP
Consultant Rheumatologist, Addenbrooke's Hospital, Cambridge, UK
5.17.2 Paget's disease of bone

CHAD DEAL
Associate Professor of Medicine, Case Western Reserve University School of Medicine, Cleveland, Ohio, USA
1.3.7 The endocrine system

A. M. DENMAN
Consultant Rheumatologist and Clinical Immunologist, Northwick Park Hospital, Harrow, Middlesex, UK
3.5.2 Antirheumatic drugs
3.5.3 Therapeutic immunomodulation

CHRISTOPHER P. DENTON
Clinical Research Fellow, Academic Unit of Rheumatology, Royal Free Hospital, London, UK
5.8 Scleroderma and related disorders in adults and children

STANLEY C. DERESINSKI
Clinical Professor of Medicine, Stanford University; Director, AIDS Health Services; Associate Chief of Infectious Diseases, Santa Clara Valley Medical Center, San Jose, California, USA
5.3.10 Fungal arthritis

KOMAL B. DESAI
Children's Mercy Hospital, Kansas City, Missouri, USA
5.3.2 Pyogenic arthritis in children

MICHAEL J. DILLON
Consultant Physician and Senior Clinical Nephrologist, The Hospital for Sick Children, London, UK
5.11.8 Primary vasculitis in children

MICHAEL DOHERTY
Professor of Rheumatology, Nottingham University Medical School, UK
5.15 Osteoarthritis

FRANCES DORMON
Consultant in Anaesthetics and Intensive Care, Lister Hospital, Stevenage, Hertfordshire, UK
1.3.9 An anaesthetic perspective

GORDON W. DUFF
Lord Florey Professor of Molecular Medicine, Royal Hallamshire Hospital, Sheffield, UK
3.1 Cells and mediators

ALISON A. EDDY
Associate Professor of Pediatrics, The Hospital for Sick Children, University of Toronto, Ontario, USA
5.7.2 Systemic lupus erythematosus in children

ERKKI EEROLA
Head of Laboratory, Department of Medical Microbiology, Turku University, Finland
1.3.6 The gastrointestinal system

MICHAEL EHRENFELD
Clinical Senior Lecturer, Sackler School of Medicine, Tel Aviv University; Consultant Rheumatologist, Rheumatic Disease Unit, Sheba Medical Center, Tel Hashomer, Israel
1.3.8 Oncology and haematology

M. SHIRLEY EMERSON
Clinical Assistant, Peter Wilson Sports Injury Clinic, Addenbrooke's Hospital, Cambridge, UK
6.7 Sports injuries

PAUL EMERY
ARC Professor of Rheumatology and Rheumatologist, Leeds General Infirmary and St James's University Hospital, Leeds, UK
4.2 Haematology

ADEL G. FAM
Professor of Medicine and Head, Division of Rheumatology, Sunnybrook Health Science Centre, University of Toronto, Ontario, Canada
1.2.2.1 The upper limbs in adults

MARC FELDMANN
Head of Cytokine and Immunology Unit, Kennedy Institute of Rheumatology and Professor of Cellular Immunology, Charing Cross and Westminster Medical School, London, UK
5.4.1 Immunopathogenesis of rheumatoid arthritis

I. T. FERGUSON
Consultant Neurologist, Southmead Hospital, Bristol, UK
1.3.3 Neurological complications

ØYSTEIN FØRRE
Professor and Head, Centre for Rheumatic and Autoimmune Connective Tissue Disease, The National Hospital, Oslo University, Norway
4.7 Gene marker analysis

ANDREW O. FRANK
Consultant Physician in Rheumatology and Rehabilitation, Northwick Park Hospital, Harrow, Middlesex, UK
1.2.1.1 Spinal problems in adults

PATRICIA A. FRASER
Assistant Professor of Medicine, Harvard Medical School; Director of Pediatric Rheumatology, Brigham and Women's Hospital, Boston, Massachusetts, USA
5.1.2 Epidemiology of rheumatic diseases in selected non-European populations

CHARLES S. B. GALASKO
Professor of Orthopaedic Surgery, University of Manchester; Consultant Orthopaedic Surgeon, Manchester Children's Hospitals NHS Trust; Consultant Orthopaedic Surgeon, Salford Royal Hospitals NHS Trust, UK
1.2.1.2 Spinal problems in children

PATRICK J. GALLAGHER
Reader in Pathology, Southampton University Hospitals, UK
4.10 Histopathology

ALLAN GIBOFSKY
Professor, Departments of Medicine and Public Health, Cornell University Medical College, New York, USA
5.3.12 Rheumatic fever

DAFNA D. GLADMAN
Professor of Medicine, University of Toronto, Ontario, Canada
5.5.4 Psoriatic arthritis

DAVID N. GLASS
Professor of Pediatrics and Director, Division of Rheumatology, Children's Hospital Medical Center, Cincinnati, Ohio, USA
5.2 Nosology of the chronic inflammatory rheumatic diseases

ELIZABETH M. GRAHAM
Consultant Medical Ophthalmologist, St Thomas's Hospital and The Hospital for Sick Children, London, UK
1.3.10 The eye

CLIVE E.H. GRATTAN
Consultant Dermatologist, West Norwich Hospital, Norfolk, UK
5.11.4 Small vessel vasculitis

IAN D. GRIFFITHS
Consultant Rheumatologist, Freeman Hospital and Senior Clinical Lecturer, University of Newcastle upon Tyne, UK
1.2.3 Extra-articular features of rheumatic diseases

BRIDGET GRIFFITHS
Lecturer, Department of Rheumatology, University of Leeds, UK
4.2 Haematology

WOLFGANG L. GROSS
Professor of Internal Medicine and Rheumatology; Director, Department of Rheumatology, University of Lubeck and Clinic for Rheumatology in Bad Bramstedt, Germany
5.11.2 Wegener's granulomatosis

RENATE HÄFNER
Paediatric Rheumatologist, Rheuma-Kinderklinik, Garmisch-Partenkirchen, Germany
6.4 Rehabilitation of children

VEDAT HAMURYUDAN
Associate Professor of Medicine, Division of Rheumatology, Cerrahpaşa Medical Faculty, University of Istanbul, Turkey
5.11.7 Behçet's syndrome

TIM HARDINGHAM
Professor of Biochemistry, School of Biological Sciences, University of Manchester, UK
2.3 Articular cartilage

MARK HARRIES
Consultant Physician, Northwick Park and St Mark's NHS Trust; Honorary Clinical Director, British Olympic Medical Centre, Northwick Park Hospital, Harrow, Middlesex, UK
6.6 Sports medicine

DORIAN O. HASKARD
Sir John McMichael Professor of Cardiovascular Medicine, Royal Postgraduate Medical School and Honorary Consultant Physician, Hammersmith Hospital, London, UK
3.2 Lymphocyte traffic in inflammation

BRIAN HAZLEMAN
Consultant Rheumatologist, Addenbrooke's Hospital, Cambridge, UK
5.14 Soft-tissue rheumatism

SIMON HELFGOTT
Assistant Professor of Medicine, Harvard Medical School and Brigham and Women's Hospital, Boston, Massachusetts, USA
1.3.12 Psychiatric issues in rheumatology

PETER HOLLINGWORTH
Consultant Rheumatologist, Southmead Hospital, Bristol, UK
1.3.3 Neurological complications

ANGELA C. HORSFALL
Senior Research Fellow, Charing Cross Medical School and Honorary Senior Scientist, Kennedy Institute, London, UK
5.7.1 Systemic lupus erythematosus in adults

J. LAWRENCE HOUK
Professor of Clinical Medicine, University of Cincinnati Medical Center, Ohio, USA
4.6 Joint fluid

G. R. V. HUGHES
Head of the Lupus Arthritis Research Unit, Rayne Institute, St Thomas's Hospital, London, UK
5.7.3 The antiphospholipid antibody syndrome

GUNNAR HUSBY
Professor, Oslo Sanitetsforening Rheumatism Hospital, The National Hospital, University of Oslo, Norway
5.13.1 Amyloidosis

DAVID A. ISENBERG
Professor of Rheumatology, University College London, UK
1.3.5 The respiratory system
5.7.1 Systemic lupus erythematosus in adults

SILVIU ITESCU
Assistant Professor of Surgical Science; Director, Transplantation Immunology, Department of Surgery, Columbia University College of Physicians and Surgeons, New York, USA
5.3.6 HIV infection

MARY ANNE JACKSON
Professor of Pediatrics, University of Missouri School of Medicine and Pediatrician in Infectious Diseases, Children's Mercy Hospital, Kansas City, Missouri, USA
5.3.2 Pyogenic arthritis in children

MALCOLM I.V. JAYSON
Professor of Rheumatology, Rheumatic Diseases Centre, University of Manchester, UK
5.18.1 Intervertebral disc disease and other mechanical disorders of the back

J. R. JENNER
Consultant in Rheumatology, Addenbrooke's NHS Trust, Cambridge, UK
6.7 Sports injuries

VICTORIA A. JOLLIFFE
Senior Registrar, West Norwich Hospital, Norfolk, UK
5.11.4 Small vessel vasculitis

ADRIAN JONES
Consultant Rheumatologist, Nottingham City Hospital, UK
5.15 Osteoarthritis

D. A. JONES
Professor of Sport and Exercise Sciences, University of Birmingham, UK
2.6 Skeletal muscle damage

GARY M. KAMMER
Professor of Internal Medicine/Rheumatology, The Bowman Gray School of Medicine, Wake Forest University, Winston-Salem, North Carolina, USA
1.3.11 The kidney

WALTER F. KEAN
Clinical Professor of Medicine (Rheumatology) and Head, Service of Rheumatology, McMaster University Medical Centre, Hamilton, Ontario, Canada
1.3.1.1 Pregnancy
1.3.1.2 Antirheumatic drugs in pregnancy and lactation

CAROL A. KEMPER
Clinical Assistant Professor of Medicine, Stanford University; Co-director, AIDS Health Services, Santa Clara Valley Medical Center, San Jose, California, USA
5.3.10 Fungal arthritis

MUNTHER A. KHAMASHTA
Deputy Director, Lupus Arthritis Research Unit, The Rayne Institute; Honorary Senior Lecturer, St Thomas's Hospital, UMDS, London, UK
5.7.3 The antiphospholipid antibody syndrome

PNINA LANGEVITZ
Senior Lecturer in Medicine, Tel Aviv University Medical School; Head of Rheumatic Disease Unit, Sheba Medical Center, Tel Hashomer, Israel
5.13.2 Familial Mediterranean fever

C.B.D. LAVY
Associate Professor, University of Malawi School of Medicine and Honorary Consultant, University College London Hospitals, UK
6.1 Surgery in adults

RONALD M. LAXER
Associate Professor of Pediatrics and Medicine, University of Toronto; Head, Division of Rheumatology, The Hospital for Sick Children, Toronto, Ontario, Canada
5.6.2 Systemic-onset juvenile chronic arthritis

ALISON M. LEAK
Consultant Rheumatologist, Thanet General Hospital, Margate, Kent, UK
1.3.10 The eye

KENG HONG LEONG
Consultant Rheumatologist, Department of Rheumatology and Immunology, Tan Tock Seng Hospital, Singapore
5.13.8 Hyperlipidaemias

MATTHEW H. LIANG
Professor of Medicine, Harvard Medical School, and Professor of Health Policy and Mangement, Harvard School of Public Health, Boston, Massachusetts, USA
1.1.5 Outcomes assessment in rheumatology

GEOFFREY O. LITTLEJOHN
Associate Professor of Medicine and Director of Rheumatology, Monash Medical Centre, Melbourne, Australia
5.19.2 Algodystrophy (reflex sympthetic dystrophy syndrome)

AVI LIVNEH
Senior Physician, Sheba Medical Center and Senior Lecturer, Sackler Faculty of Medicine, Tel Aviv University, Israel
5.13.2 Familial Mediterranean fever

DANIEL J. LOVELL
Associate Professor of Pediatrics, Children's Hospital Medical Center, University of Cincinnati Medical Center, Ohio, USA
1.1.7 Growth and skeletal maturation

C. R. LOVELL
Consultant Dermatologist, Royal United Hospital, Bath, Avon, UK
1.3.2 The skin

MICHAEL E. LUGGEN
Associate Professor of Clinical Medicine, University of Cincinnati Medical Center, Ohio, USA
1.3.4 The cardiovascular system

P.J. MADDISON
Consultant Rheumatologist, Gwynedd Hospitals NHS Trusts, Bangor, UK
1.3.2 The skin
4.5 Autoantibody profile
5.13.7 Multicentric reticulohistiocytosis
5.17.3 Diseases of bone, cartilage, and synovium

RAVINDER N. MAINI
Director, Kennedy Institute of Rheumatology; Head and Professor of Rheumatology, Charing Cross and Westminster Medical School; Consultant Physician, Charing Cross Hospital, London, UK
5.4.1 Immunopathogenesis of rheumatoid arthritis

PAUL MAPP
Research Fellow, Bone and Joint Research Unit, The London Hospital Medical College, UK
2.5 The physiology of the joint and its disturbance in inflammation

NEIL JOHN McHUGH
Consultant Senior Lecturer in Rheumatology, Royal National Hospital for Rheumatic Diseases, Bath, Avon, UK
5.12 Overlap syndromes in adults and children
5.13.8 Hyperlipidaemias

ELIZABETH D. MELLINS
Associate Professor of Pediatrics, Stanford University Medical Center, California, USA
5.6.1 Pauciarticular-onset juvenile chronic arthritis

MARC L. MILLER
Clinical Associate Professor of Medicine, Unversity of Vermont School of Medicine, USA
5.3.1 Pyogenic arthritis in adults

H.M. MOUTSOPOULOS
Professor and Chairman, Department of Pathophysiology, Medical School, University of Athens, Greece
5.10 Sjögren's syndrome

PATRICIA MUÑOZ
Assistant Professor in Clinical Microbiology and Infectious Diseases, Hospital General Maranón, Universidad Complutense, Madrid, Spain
5.3.3 Osteomyelitis and associated conditions

STANLEY J. NAIDES
Associate Professor, Division of Rheumatology, Department of Internal Medicine, University of Iowa College of Medicine, and Clinical Investigator, Veterans Affairs Medical Center, Iowa City, USA
5.3.5 Viral arthritis

BARBARA S. NEPOM
Research Associate Member, Virginia Mason Research Center, and Research Associate Professor, Department of Pediatrics, University of Washington School of Medicine, Washington, USA
5.6.1 Pauciarticular-onset juvenile chronic arthritis

S.P. NEWMAN
Professor of Health Psychology, University College London Medical School, London, UK
1.1.6 Psychological aspects of rheumatic disease

LAUREN M. PACHMAN
Professor of Pediatrics and Head, Division of Pediatric Immunology/Rheumatology, Northwestern University Medical School, Chicago, Illinois, USA
5.9.2 Polymyositis and dermatomyositis in children

ELISABETH PAICE
Consultant Rheumatologist, Whittington Hospital, London, UK
1.1.4 Principles of examination

G. S. PANAYI
Arthritis and Rheumatism Council Professor of Rheumatology, United Medical and Dental Schools of Guy's and St Thomas' Hospitals, London, UK
5.11.5 Polymyalgia rheumatica

E. PASCUAL
Professor of Rheumatology, University of Alicante School of Medicine, Spain
5.3.8 Brucellar arthritis

MURRAY H. PASSO
Associate Professor of Clinical Pediatrics, University of Cincinnati College of Medicine, Children's Hospital Medical Center, Ohio, USA
5.5.2 Spondylarthropathies in childhood

REIJO PELTONEN
Specialist in Infectious Diseases, Department of Medicine, Turku University Central Hospital, Finland
1.3.6 The gastrointestinal system

JOHN S. PERCY
Professor of Medicine, University of Alberta, Edmonton, Canada
1.1.1 The adult patient

ROSS E. PETTY
Professor of Pediatrics, University of British Columbia, Vancouver, Canada
1.1.2 Children and adolescents

RAFAL PLOSKI
Research Fellow, Centre for Rheumatic and Autoimmune Connective Tissue Disease, The National Hospital, Oslo University, Norway
4.7 Gene marker analysis

F. MICHAEL POPE
Head of Medical Research Council Connective Tissue Genetics Group, Addenbrooke's Hospital, Cambridge, UK
2.2 Molecular abnormalities of collagen and connective tissue

MORDECHAI PRAS
Professor of Medicine, Faculty of Medicine, Tel Aviv University, Israel
5.13.2 Familial Mediterranean fever

ANNE-MARIE PRIEUR
Consultant Paediatrician, Unite Fonctionnelle de Rhumatologie Pediatrique, Hôpital Necker-Enfants Malades, Paris, France
5.6.3 Rheumatoid factor- negative polyarthritis in children ('seronegative polyarthritis')
5.13.6 The chronic, infantile, neurological, cutaneous, and articular syndrome (CINCA)

J.-F. QUIGNODON
Paediatric Radiologist, Hôpital des Enfants Malades, Paris, France
4.9.2 Imaging in children

DANIEL W. RAHN
Professor and Vice Chairman, Department of Medicine, Medical College of Georgia, Augusta, USA
5.3.4 Lyme disease

J. RECKLESS
Consultant Physician, Royal United Hospital, Bath, and Honorary Senior Lecturer in Biochemistry and in the Postgraduate Medical School, University of Bath, UK
5.13.8 Hyperlipidaemias

PETER RENTON
Consultant Radiologist, University College Hospital and The Royal National Orthopaedic Hospital, London, UK
4.9.1 Imaging in adults

CHARLES RICHARDSON
Faculty of Medicine and Dentistry, University of Birmingham, UK
4.2 Haematology

MALCOLM P. ROGERS
Associate Professor of Psychiatry, Harvard Medical School and Attending Psychiatrist, Division of Psychiatry, Brigham and Women's Hospital, Boston, Massachusetts, USA
1.3.12 Psychiatric issues in rheumatology

ANN K. ROSENTHAL
Assistant Professor of Medicine, Division of Rheumatology, Medical College of Wisconsin, Milwaukee, USA
5.16 Crystal arthropathies

JOAN M. ROUND
Honorary Research Fellow, School of Sport and Exercise Sciences, University of Birmingham, UK
2.6 Skeletal muscle damage

ANTHONY S. RUSSELL
Professor of Medicine, University of Alberta, Edmonton, Canada
1.1.1 The adult patient

OLIVER SANGHA
Harvard Medical School, Brigham and Women's Hospital, Boston, Massachusetts, USA
1.1.5 Outcomes assessment in rheumatology

HANS-GEORG SCHAIBLE
Professor of Physiology, University of Würzburg, Germany
2.8 The neurophysiology of pain

RAYFEL SCHNEIDER
Assistant Professor of Pediatrics, University of Toronto; Staff Rheumatologist, The Hospital for Sick Children, Toronto, Ontario, Canada
5.6.2 Systemic-onset juvenile chronic arthritis

DAVID G.I. SCOTT
Department of Rheumatology, Norfolk and Norwich Hospital, UK
5.11.1 Classification of vasculitis
5.11.6 Large vessel vasculitis

GEOFFREY SCOTT
Consultant Microbiologist, University College London Hospitals, London, UK
4.4 Microbiology and diagnostic serology

G. H. SEBAG
Paediatric Radiologist, Hôpital Robert Debré, Université Saint Louis, Paris, France
4.9.2 Imaging in children

DAVID D. SHERRY
Director, Pediatric Rheumatology, Children's Hospital and Medical Center, Seattle; Associate Professor of Pediatrics, University of Washington, USA
5.6.1 Pauciarticular-onset juvenile chronic arthritis

YEHUDA SHOENFELD
Professor and Head, Department of Medicine 'B', Chaim Sheba Medical Center, Tel-Hashomer, Israel
1.3.8 Oncology and haematology

ALAN J. SILMAN
ARC Professor of Rheumatic Disease Epidemiology, University of Manchester, UK
5.1.1 Epidemiology and the rheumatic diseases

EARL D. SILVERMAN
Associate Professor of Pediatrics and Immunology, Division of Rheumatology, Hospital for Sick Children, University of Toronto, Canada
5.7.2 Systemic lupus erythematosus in children

ROBERT W. SIMMS
Director, Boston City Hospital Arthritis Clinic; Associate Professor of Medicine, Boston University School of Medicine, Massachusetts, USA
1.2.2.2 The lower limbs in adults

ROGER SMITH
Consultant Physician, Nuffield Orthopaedic Centre, Oxford, UK
2.4 Bone in health and disease

ENRIQUE ROBERTO SORIANO
Consultant Rheumatologist, Hospital Italiano de Buenos Aires, Argentina
5.12 Overlap syndromes in adults and children

TAUNTON R. SOUTHWOOD
Senior Lecturer and Consultant in Paediatric Rheumatology, Department of Rheumatology, University of Birmingham, UK
5.5.2 Spondylarthropathies in childhood

MARIANNE SPAMER
Physiotherapist, Rheuma-Kinderklinik, Garmisch-Partenkirchen, Germany
6.4 Rehabilitation of children

STEPHEN G. SPIRO
Consultant Physician, University College London Hospitals Trust, UK
1.3.5 The respiratory system

CLIFF. R. STEVENS
Head of Vascular Biology, Bone and Joint Research Unit, St Bartholomew's and The Royal London Hospital School of Medicine and Dentistry, London, UK
2.5 The physiology of the joint and its disturbance in inflammation

GEROLD STUCKI
Lecturer, Department of Rheumatology and Physical Medicine, University of Zurich, Switzerland
1.1.5 Outcomes assessment in rheumatology

MALCOLM SWANN
Consultant Orthopaedic Surgeon, Windsor, Berkshire
6.2 Surgery in in children

IRA N. TARGOFF
Associate Professor of Medicine, University of Oklahoma Health Sciences Center; Staff Physician, Department of Veterans Affairs Medical Center and Assistant Member, Oklahoma Medical Research Foundation, Oklahoma City, USA
5.9.1 Polymyositis and dermatomyositis in adults

DOUGLAS THOMPSON
Principal Biochemist, Leeds General Infirmary, UK
4.1 Acute phase response
4.3 Biochemistry

ANTOINE A. TOUBERT
Laboratoire d'Immunogénétique Humaine, INSERM U396, Hôpital Saint-Louis, Paris, France
5.5.5 Reactive arthropathy, Reiter's syndrome, and enteric arthropathy in adults

LYNNE TURNER-STOKES
Director, Regional Rehabilitation Unit, Northwick Park Hospital, London, UK
6.3 Rehabilitation of adults

ATHANASIOS G. TZIOUFAS
Consultant Rheumatologist, Department of Pathophysiology, Medical School, University of Athens, Greece
5.10 Sjögren's syndrome

ANTHONY UNSWORTH
Professor of Engineering and Director of the Centre for Biomedical Engineering, University of Durham, UK
2.7 Biomechanics of articulations and derangements in disease

W.B. VAN DEN BERG
Professor of Experimental Rheumatology and Head, Rheumatology Research Laboratory, University of Nijmegen, The Netherlands
3.4 Animal models of arthritis

MARK J. WALPORT
Professor of Medicine, Royal Postgraduate Medical School, Hammersmith Hospital, London, UK
3.1 Cells and mediators

W. WATSON BUCHANAN
Emeritus Professor of Medicine, McMaster University Faculty of Health Sciences, Sir William Osler Health Institute, Hamilton, Ontario, Canada
1.3.1.1 Pregnancy
1.3.1.2 Antirheumatic drugs in pregnancy and lactation

RICHARD A. WATTS
Consultant Rheumatologist, Ipswich NHS Trust, UK
5.11.1 Classification of vasculitis
5.11.6 Large vessel vasculitis

A. D. B. WEBSTER
Senior Lecturer, MRC Immunodeficiency Research Group, Royal Free Hospital Medical School, London, UK
5.3.11 Immunodeficiency

LAURA F. WEXLER
Professor of Medicine, University of Cincinnati Medical Center, Ohio, USA,
1.3.4 The cardiovascular system

FRANCES B. WHEELER
The Bowman Gray School of Medicine, Wake Forest University, Winston-Salem, North Carolina, USA
1.3.11 The kidney

JOHN T. WHICHER
Professor, Research School of Medicine, University of Leeds, UK
4.1 Acute phase response
4.3 Biochemistry

PATIENCE H. WHITE
Associate Professor of Pediatrics and Medicine, George Washington University; Chairman, Pediatric and Adult Rheumatology, Children's National Medical Center, Washington DC, USA
1.2.2.3 The arm and leg in children

BRYAN D. WILLIAMS
Professor of Rheumatology, University Hospital of Wales, Cardiff, UK
4.8 Immune complex detection

ROBERT WINCHESTER
Professor of Medicine and Pediatrics, College of Physicians and Surgeons, Columbia University, New York City, USA
5.3.6 HIV infection

JAY B. WISH
Professor of Medicine, Case Western Reserve University; Medical Director, Hemodialysis Services, University Hospitals of Cleveland, Ohio, USA
1.3.11 The kidney

FRANK A. WOLLHEIM
Professor of Rheumatology, Lund University, Sweden
5.4.2 Rheumatoid arthritis-the clinical picture

PATRICIA WOO
Professor of Paediatric Rheumatology, University College London, UK
1.1.7 Growth and skeletal maturation
2.1 Molecular genetics and its relevance in rheumatology
5.2 Nosology of the chronic inflammatory rheumatic diseases

B. P. WORDSWORTH
Clinical Reader in Rheumatology, Nuffield Department of Clinical Medicine, Oxford University, UK
3.3 Specific immune responses

HASAN YAZICI
Professor of Medicine and Chief, Division of Rheumatology, Cerrahpaşa Medical Faculty, University of Istanbul, Turkey
5.11.7 Behçet's syndrome

PIERRE YOUINOU
Professor of Immunology, Brest University Medical School, France
5.10 Sjögren's syndrome

ADAM YOUNG
Consultant Rheumatologist, City Hospital, St Albans, Hertfordshire, UK
4.11 Electrophysiology

SEBAHATTIN YURDAKUL
Professor of Medicine, Division of Rheumatology, Cerrahpaşa Medical Faculty, University of Istanbul, Turkey
5.11.7 Behçet's syndrome

JOHN B. ZABRISKIE
Associate Professor and Head, Laboratory of Clinical Microbiology/Immunology, Rockefeller University, New York, USA
5.3.12 Rheumatic fever

DEBORAH ZEMER
Sheba Medical Center, Tel Hashomer, Israel
5.13.2 Familial Mediterranean fever

5

The scope of rheumatic disease

5.1   Epidemiology
    5.1.1   Epidemiology and the rheumatic diseases
    5.1.2   Epidemiology of rheumatic diseases in selected non-
           European populations

5.2   Nosology of the chronic inflammatory rheumatic diseases

5.3   Infections
    5.3.1   Pyogenic arthritis in adults
    5.3.2   Pyogenic arthritis in children
    5.3.3   Osteomyelitis and associated conditions
    5.3.4   Lyme disease
    5.3.5   Viral arthritis
    5.3.6   HIV infection
    5.3.7   Mycobacterial diseases
    5.3.8   Brucellar arthritis
    5.3.9   Parasitic involvement
    5.3.10   Fungal arthritis
    5.3.11   Immunodeficiency
    5.3.12   Rheumatic fever

5.4   Rheumatoid arthritis
    5.4.1   Immunopathogenesis of rheumatoid arthritis
    5.4.2   Rheumatoid arthritis-the clinical picture
    5.4.3   Juvenile rheumatoid arthritis (rheumatoid factor positive
           polyarthritis

5.5   Spondylarthropathies
    5.5.1   Spondylarthropathy, undifferentiatated spondylarthritis,
           and overlap
    5.5.2   Spondylarthropathies in childhood
    5.5.3   Ankylosing spondylitis
    5.5.4   Psoriatic arthritis
    5.5.5   Reactive arthropathy, Reiter's syndrome, and enteric
           arthropathy in adults

5.6   Arthropathies primarily occurring in childhood
    5.6.1   Pauciarticular-onset juvenile chronic arthritis
    5.6.2   Systemic-onset juvenile chronic arthritis
    5.6.3   Rheumatoid factor-negative polyarthritis in children
           ('seronegative polyarthritis')

5.7   Systemic lupus erythematosus
    5.7.1   Systemic lupus erythematosus in adults
    5.7.2   Systemic lupus erythematosus in children
    5.7.3   The antiphospholipid antibody syndrome

5.8   Scleroderma and related disorders in adults and children

5.9   Polymyositis and dermatomyositis
    5.9.1   Polymyositis and dermatomyositis in adults
    5.9.2   Polymyositis and dermatomyositis in children

5.10   Sjögren's syndrome

5.11   Primary vasculitides
    5.11.1   Classification of vasculitis
    5.11.2   Wegener's granulomatosis
    5.11.3   Classical polyarteritis nodosa, microscopic polyarteritis,
           and Churg-Strauss syndrome
    5.11.4   Small vessel vasculitis
    5.11.5   Polymyalgia rheumatica
    5.11.6   Large vessel vasculitis
    5.11.7   Behçet's syndrome
    5.11.8   Primary vasculitis in children

5.12   Overlap syndromes in adults and children

5.13   Miscellaneous inflammatory conditions
    5.13.1   Amyloidosis
    5.13.2   Familial Mediterranean fever
    5.13.3   Panniculitis
    5.13.4   Neutrophilic dermatoses
    5.13.5   Sarcoidosis
    5.13.6   The chronic, infantile, neurological, cutaneous, and articular
           syndrome (CINCA)
    5.13.7   Multicentric reticulohistiocytosis
    5.13.8   Hyperlipidaemias

5.14   Soft-tissue rheumatism

5.15   Osteoarthritis

5.16   Crystal arthropathies

5.17   Diseases of bone and cartilage
    5.17.1   Osteoporosis and osteomalacia
    5.17.2   Paget's disease of bone
    5.17.3   Diseases of bone, cartilage, and synovium
    5.17.4   Diseases of bone and cartilage in children

5.18   Disorders of the spine
    5.18.1   Intervertebral disc disease and other mechanical disorders of the
           back
    5.18.2   Cervical pain syndromes

5.19   Miscellaneous abnormalities of connective tissue
    5.19.1   Rheumatic diseases and neoplasia
    5.19.2   Algodystrophy (reflex sympathetic dystrophy syndrome)
    5.19.3   Rheumatic complications of drugs and toxins

5.1 Epidemiology

5.1.1 Epidemiology and the rheumatic diseases

Alan J. Silman

Introduction

Epidemiology can be defined broadly as the study of the occurrence of diseases in human populations. Occurrence can be considered in terms of the demographic, genetic, and environmental influences and thus, in addition to 'counting', the epidemiological investigation of a disorder aims to uncover risk factors in disease causation. Additionally, and increasingly, epidemiological method is being applied to the study of the natural history of disease and to those factors that influence prognosis.

The term clinical epidemiology refers to a different area of endeavour and describes the application of epidemiology to clinical practice. Areas in this regard of specific relevance to rheumatology are:

(1) the derivation of criteria for diagnostic or classification purposes;

(2) the evaluation of clinical data in terms of their accuracy (validity) and reliability (reproducibility);

(3) the design, conduct, and analysis of intervention studies (clinical trials).

In other areas of medicine (for example, cardiovascular disease), the application of epidemiology to the evaluation of strategies for primary prevention and screening is of much interest. Such activities are, unfortunately, of little relevance in rheumatology, given current knowledge, and will not be considered further. This review will concentrate on the application of epidemiology to understanding the occurrence and causation of disease. Examples are taken, where appropriate, from some of the principal disorders to illustrate the particular points to be made. Detailed epidemiological information of relevance to specific disorders will also be found in the appropriate chapters in this volume.

Criteria for diagnosis

There is no single diagnostic test for most of the major rheumatological disorders. Further, there is considerable overlap, both clinically and pathologically, between the various conditions. As a consequence, sets of criteria covering the main clinical and other facets of each disorder have been formulated with the aim of separating 'cases' from 'non-cases'.

Purpose of criteria

Criteria are useful in so far as they allow like to be compared with like, such that results of clinical and other studies may be compared directly. The American College of Rheumatology has taken an important lead in formulating criteria for most of the principal disorders. It prefers the term 'classification' to 'diagnostic' when applied to the criteria generated for specific disorders, to take account of the atypical case.

Criteria are developed for a number of purposes including population studies of occurrence, aetiological studies, and clinical trials (Fries *et al.* 1994). In trials, there is a need for considerable stringency, i.e. only patients with clearly established disease are eligible for study to prevent dilution of an effect. In that case, the aim of the criteria is maximal specificity (no false positives). By contrast, if the aim is the investigation of familial clustering one would not wish to miss even mild disease in the first-degree relatives of affected probands. Criteria in this situation should opt for maximal sensitivity (few false negatives). In practice, published criteria take no account of the different applications and, as a consequence, they are not always appropriate to the desired task.

Derivation of criteria

Historically, there are three approaches to deriving criteria (Table 1). These are (i) expert consensus, (ii) quasianalytical, and (iii) analytical. The first approach results from the deliberations of a group of 'experts' who reach an agreement between themselves as to what constitutes a case. The second starts as a consensus, but the criteria developed are thereafter tested in patients with and without the disease (determined in an independent manner), and then subjected to subsequent refinement. The third approach is to collect data on the major, potentially diagnostic features and, using a number of statistical approaches (Bloch *et al.* 1990), derive the most discriminatory criteria. The main advantages and disadvantages of these approaches are summarized in Table 1. Diseases for which criteria have been published are listed in Table 2, with their methods of derivation.

The constitution both of cases and the comparison group used for deriving criteria is of fundamental importance for their interpretation. This is best illustrated by example. The 1987 American Rheumatology Association (**ARA**) revised criteria for rheumatoid arthritis (Arnett *et al.* 1988) allow the following subset of signs to satisfy the criteria: either positive rheumatoid factor test or typical radiological erosion, plus swelling in three or more groups of appropriate joints of which at least one should be either a wrist or metacarpophalangeal joint. Such a subset might not be specific

Table 1　Approaches to deriving criteria for rheumatic diseases

Approach	Advantages	Disadvantages
Consensus	Criteria based on clinical good sense and likely to be acceptable	May not maximize discrimination between cases and non-cases
Quasi-analytical	As above but discriminatory power stated	Assumes that appropriate individual items were included in criteria sets; may not maximize discrimination
Analytical	Maximal discrimination between cases and non-cases; excludes bias from preconceived notions	May not reflect clinical sense and thus have difficulty in acceptance

Table 2　Publications of criteria for rheumatic diseases

Disease	Reference	Approach	Common name
Rheumatoid arthritis	Kellgren (1962)	Consensus	The 'Rome' criteria
	Bennett and Wood (1968)	Consensus	The 'New York' criteria
	Arnett et al. (1988)	Analytical	Revised ARA[a]
Ankylosing spondylitis	Bennett and Wood (1968)	Consensus	'New York' revision of 'Rome' criteria
	van der Linden et al. (1984)	Quasi-analytical	'Revised New York'
Systemic lupus erythematosus	Cohen et al. (1971)	Consensus	'Preliminary ARA'
	Tan (1982)	Quasi-analytical	'Revised ARA'
Reiter's syndrome	Wilkins et al. (1982)	Quasi-analytical	
Systemic sclerosis	Masi et al. (1980)	Quasi-analytical	Revised ARA
Osteoarthritis:			
Knee	Altman et al. (1986)	Analytical	ARA
Hand	Altman et al. (1990)	Analytical	ARA
Vasculitis (various types)	Hunder et al. (1990)	Analytical	ARA
Fibromyalgia	Wolfe et al. (1990)	Analytical	ARA

[a]ARA, American Rheumatism Association

enough for routine clinical practice. The sensitivity of the criteria as a whole were, however, very high in the case series studied because they were all current attenders at a specialist hospital facility and had had disease for a mean of 7.7 years. The application of the same criteria to patients attending with early disease to a non-specialist could give a much reduced sensitivity (Silman and Symmons 1995).

The preliminary criteria for the diagnosis of scleroderma (Masi et al 1980) show an extremely high specificity for the major criterion of proximal skin tightness against the comparison group chosen for study from rheumatological practice. Their performance against patients without scleroderma attending a dermatology practice with swollen or tight skin would be substantially different. The purpose of emphasizing this point is not to devalue the criteria themselves, but to argue for caution in their use in circumstances different to those from which they were derived.

Occurrence of disease

The occurrence of diseases is expressed as the number of cases arising in the population 'at risk'. The latter is multiplied by an appropriate power of 10 to yield a sensible number. Thus, it might be appropriate to express the annual incidence of new episodes of back pain as a percentage, whereas the incidence of scleroderma is more conveniently expressed per million population. Frequently there are reports of 'epidemiological' studies that present the relative proportions of diagnoses seen, for example, in a clinical practice, with the interpretation that the proportions represent the relative occurrence of those diseases in the catchment population of the clinic. Such data relying totally on numerator ascertainment, without consideration of the population base, are subject to considerable error. Thus it is difficult to interpret reports from Chinese populations that systemic lupus

Table 3 Measures of disease occurrence

Measure	Description	Appropriate example
Incidence	Rate of occurrence of new cases arising in population conveniently expressed per unit time interval (e.g. per year)	Incidence of rheumatoid arthritis is 0.5 new cases/1000/year
Episode incidence	Rate of occurrence of new episodes of a disease arising in population; usefully applied to conditions where previous episodes may only be weakly related	New episode incidence of painful shoulder is 10/1000/year
Cumulative incidence	Similar to incidence but time interval expressed as fixed period	Cumulative incidence of juvenile chronic arthritis by age 16 is 1/1000
(Point) prevalence	Describes the occurrence of current cases, i.e. those with evidence of disease; implication is based on a particular point in time (notional prevalence day)	Point prevalence of radiographic osteoarthritis of the hip is 15/1000 (on 1 January 1991)
Period prevalence	Similar to episode incidence in so far as it expresses the rate of individuals displaying evidence of disease in a fixed period (e.g. 1 year) but they may not be continually affected during this period; unlike episode incidence does not require development of new episode during that period	One-year period prevalence of low back pain is 50/1000
Cumulative prevalence	Summation of disease occurrence during fixed period; similar to cumulative incidence but would exclude those who had died from cause prior to investigation	Similar to cumulative incidence

erythematosus is more frequent than rheumatoid arthritis, suggesting that either the lupus is more frequent than in the West or that the arthritis is less frequent. There may also be selective differences in attendance at hospital between these two disorders.

Measures of occurrence

A number of measures of occurrence are used in the epidemiology of the rheumatic diseases and these are listed in Table 3. Broadly, prevalence, which describes the proportion of existing cases in a population, is less useful than incidence, which describes the rate of occurrence of new cases. Prevalence is dependent on duration, so the longer a disease persists the greater the likelihood that it will be included in a prevalence estimate.

There are considerable problems in assessing prevalence in rheumatic diseases, because they frequently go into remission without any residual clinical sign of disease. Thus a population prevalence survey can only detect either those with currently active disease (e.g. inflamed joints) or those with evidence of past disease (e.g. joint deformity). Those individuals whose disease resolved without damage will remain undetected. To overcome this investigators may try to assess the existence of past disease, for example by taking a detailed history or reviewing available medical records. This is acceptable, but if such an approach is comprehensive, then it is not point prevalence that is being ascertained (see Table 3) but cumulative prevalence (MacGregor and Silman 1992). Further, the problem with such an approach is that cases who died before being ascertained would obviously be missed. Thus such a cumulative prevalence would underestimate cumulative incidence.

Approaches to estimating disease occurrence in rheumatology

The approach to be used (Table 4) depends both on the frequency of the disease (Safavi et al. 1990) and its severity. Population surveys are prohibitively expensive for rare diseases, but necessary for common ones. Thus it would not be appropriate to ascertain back pain by review of hospital attenders as many cases will not seek medical attention. Conversely it would be reasonable to assume that the majority of cases with scleroderma will seek medical care and thus a population survey is not necessary. The complacency of such an approach, however, was displayed by a population survey from South Carolina suggesting that there is a considerable, unrecognized prevalence in the community of previously unrecognized scleroderma and 'scleroderma spectrum' disorders (Maricq et al. 1989) and that expensive population surveys may be necessary.

It is virtually impossible to derive incidence data from cross-sectional population surveys, as a single survey will miss cases that went into remission or died before the survey. Lawrence (1977) in his classical work in Leigh and Wensleydale in the North of England, undertook a second survey five years after the first and calculated the rate of development of new cases from those that developed the disease in the interval. Again, this approach would miss those that developed the disease and either died or went into remission between the two surveys.

The only realistic options for assessing incidence (see Table 4) are, first, some form of prospective notification system whereby newly developing cases are continuously and prospectively notified to a central source in a similar fashion to cancer registration. Such a

Table 4 Approaches to measuring disease occurrence

Measure	Approach
Incidence	(i) Retrospective review of diagnosed cases from medical facilities
	(ii) Prospective notification or registration scheme
	(iii) Measurement of cases occurring in interval between two population surveys
Episode incidence	(i) Retrospective population survey[a]
	(ii) Prospective notification or registration scheme
Cumulative incidence	(i) Retrospective review of diagnosed cases
	(ii) Retrospective population survey[a]
Point prevalence	(i) Cross-sectional population survey[a]
	(ii) Estimate based on current diagnosed clinic attenders
Period prevalence	(i) Retrospective[a] population survey
	(ii) Prospective population survey

[a]A retrospective population is based on recall for past events whereas a cross-sectional survey aims to investigate current disease status. In practice, both methods can be adopted concurrently, e.g. 'Have you ever had or do you now have painful joints?'

Table 5 Occurrence of major rheumatic diseases: Western populations aged 15+ years

Disease	Annual incidence per 1000	Point prevalence per 1000
Rheumatoid arthritis	0.5	8.0
Psoriatic arthritis	Not available	0.2
Systemic lupus erythematosus	0.05	0.4
Systemic sclerosis	0.01	0.1
Ankylosing spondylitis	0.07	2.0
Knee osteoarthritis	Not applicable	100[a]
Juvenile chronic arthritis[a]	0.1	0.7
Gout	1.0	Not applicable

Rates are based on consensus of most recently available data.
[a]Rates variable and age dependent; this prevalence in age range 35–74 years.
[b]Rates refer to children under 15 years of age.

scheme is logistically difficult and expensive, although a recent example of its use in rheumatoid arthritis is encouraging (Symmons *et al*. 1994). Alternatively, all relevant clinical facilities used by the target population may be reviewed to determine the rate of newly diagnosed cases. The disadvantages of this second approach are, first, its retrospective element relying on sufficient information being recorded in the case records to allow a subsequent diagnostic opinion. Second, such an approach requires an excellent information system with few mistakes in diagnostic coding, entry, or retrieval. Such systems are infrequent, with the Rochester Epidemiology Program being a notable exception.

Rochester Epidemiology Program

The Mayo Clinic in Rochester, Minnesota, together with the Olmsted Medical Practice, provides apparently the only source of medical care to the local population, which was approximately 60 000 in 1980. The record system at the Mayo Clinic is almost unique in being able to extract diagnostic data from the records over at least the past 50 years and as a consequence any diagnosis made on a resident of the County can be retrieved. These data have been used to generate estimates of the incidence of many rheumatic diseases such as rheumatoid arthritis (Linos *et al*. 1980), systemic lupus erythematosus (Michet *et al*. 1985), ankylosing spondylitis (Carbone *et al*. 1992) and temporal arteritis (Chuang *et al*. 1982). There are problems, however,

in interpreting the results. First, the population is really too small for reliably assessing the incidence of some rare disease. Thus there were no male cases of scleroderma recorded in their incidence series (Michet *et al*. 1985), although males with this disorder do exist. Second, the Olmsted population is unusual both in having heavy over-representation of the professional middle classes and also (compared with the rest of the United States) having a relative excess of those of Scandinavian origin.

In most other parts of the world, it is impossible to rely on one clinical facility to ascertain all cases and an obvious alternative approach is to review as many different sources of data as possible. The greater the degree of overlap between the sources, the greater the confidence that ascertainment is complete. Such an approach has been applied to both scleroderma (Silman *et al*. 1988) and systemic lupus erythematosus (Jonsson *et al*. 1990), both studies using many different sources of data. Statistical methods are available which use the amount of overlap to assess the likely range of the true occurrence (McCarty *et al*. 1992).

Overview of the occurrence of the major rheumatic diseases

Table 5 summarizes the typical available estimates of the occurrence of the rheumatic disorders for Western populations. For some diseases, such as rheumatoid arthritis, there have been many studies and the aim has been to produce a 'ball park' figure.

There are a number of points of note. First, in terms of incidence, the inflammatory arthropathies are very rare disorders. Thus less than one new case of rheumatoid arthritis occurs in an adult population of 1000 every two years. Even the prevalence is relatively low at approximately 0.6 to 0.8 per 100, meaning that population surveys of less than 2000 are unlikely to give robust estimates of occurrence. There are, however, considerable differences in the reported prevalence and incidence of many of the rheumatic diseases and it is tempting to ascribe the differences to underlying differences in the populations studied. As an example, the range of incidence rates observed is shown for giant cell arteritis (temporal arteritis) in Table 6. It seems unlikely that these differences represent true biological variation in geographical or temporal occurrence. It is more likely that there is an artefactual explanation for such differences and some of these are:

(1) small sample size leading to random error;

(2) differences in age and sex structure of populations surveyed;

(3) high non-response rate with selective differences in occurrence between responders and non-responders;

(4) differences in completeness of case ascertainment;

(5) differences in case definition;

(6) observer variation in use of case definition.

Small-denominator population size increases the risk of denominator error. Differences in the ascertainment procedure for cases are a principal source of variation. Even when the same apparent source is used (for example, referrals to a specialist rheumatologist), there is likely to be large variation between populations in the threshold for referral. Sources of this variation include the availability of health care services and physician and population perception of disease severity. Lack of standardization in case definition is a major problem. Thus, in the data in Table 6 some studies restricted inclusion to those with a positive biopsy, others relied on a broader clinical diagnosis.

Generally in rheumatology, it is perhaps easy to declare that cases satisfied 'the ARA Criteria' for the relevant disease, but there may be considerable differences in observer interpretation of the various individual constituents of the particular criteria used. The timing of a report is of interest. The effect of time trends on disease is considered below, but differences in diagnostic fashion will obviously have an effect on the reported occurrence rates in different years. Thus reported prevalence rates of up to 20 per cent for rheumatoid arthritis in a survey undertaken 25 years ago (Engel 1968) are more likely to represent a perception of what was then rheumatoid arthritis and what now would be considered unacceptable.

Factors affecting occurrence of the major rheumatic diseases

Age and sex

It is impossible to compare the results from different studies without considering the age and sex structure of the population studied. Differences in crude (i.e. all age and sex combined) estimates of occurrence rates between populations may well be explained by differences in demographic structure. There are very striking effects of age and sex in virtually all the rheumatic diseases, as shown in Table 7. Extreme examples are the very low incidence of ankylosing spondylitis at age 65 and the virtual absence of knee osteoarthritis at age 25. In all disorders considered, a 5-year shift in the mean age or a 10 per cent difference in the proportions of the two sexes in the population studied can have a large effect on the crude estimates. One problem in

Table 6 Variation in reported incidence of polymyalgia rheumatica/giant cell arteritis

Country	Incidence rate per 100 000 (both sexes, age 50+ years)
Israel	0.5
Scotland	4.2
France	9.4
USA	11.7
USA	17.0
Sweden	28.6
England	40.0
USA	54.0
USA	70.0
Denmark	76.6

Source: Silman and Hochberg (1993).

Table 7 Effect of age and sex on incidence of rheumatic disease

Disease	Ratio ages 65:25 years	Sex (F:M)
Rheumatoid arthritis	6:1	2.5:1
Ankylosing spondylitis	0[a]	1:3
Gout	2:1	1:6
Systemic sclerosis	3:1	4:1
Systemic lupus erythematosus	1.5:1	3:1→9:1[b]
Juvenile chronic arthritis (pauciarticular)	N/A	2:1→7:1[b]
Knee osteoarthritis (prevalence)	0[a]	2:1

Data are typical.
[a]No incident cases at this age.
[b]Range given as ratio varies considerably in published studies
Source: Silman and Hochberg (1993).

surveys is that males and those at the two extremes of the age distribution are less likely to participate, resulting in a 'skewed' estimate of occurrence.

There are two approaches to overcoming this problem. First, the data can be presented separately for each age and sex group (e.g. Table 8), although this is frequently not possible or desirable as the numbers in individual age and sex 'strata' may be too small for precise estimates. The data presented on the prevalence of knee

Table 8 Age- and sex-specific prevalence rates for grade 3 osteoarthritis of the right knee

Age (years)	Prevalence			
	Males		Females	
	Number studied	%	Number studied	%
40–44	395	0.0	428	0.0
45–49	362	0.3	386	1.6
50–54	312	2.2	298	2.7
55–59	220	1.4	229	0.4
60–64	178	5.6	186	4.8
65–69	116	6.9	183	9.8
70–74	85	7.1	122	16.4
75–79	59	8.5	117	14.5
80+	27	7.4	77	29.9

Source: Van Saase *et al.* (1989)

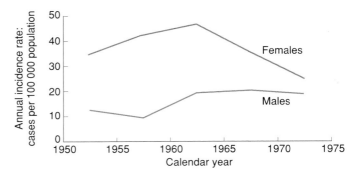

Fig. 1 Published results from 1950 to 1975 in the Rochester studies (reproduced with permission from Linos *et al.* 1980).

osteoarthritis and on the incidence of rheumatoid arthritis are unusual by virtue of having large sample sizes for the disorders considered. Frequently in publications this is not the case. Alternatively, adjustment may be made to some notional standard population to produce a standardized rate. For example, in the Symmons *et al.* study of rheumatoid arthritis incidence (Symmons *et al.* 1994), male and female crude rates of 14.0 and 35.6 per 100 000 were standardized to the United Kingdom 1991 population to produce standardized rates of 12.7 and 34.3 per 100 000 respectively. The only problem is that other reports do not standardize to the same population and readers rarely make the necessary calculations themselves to obtain comparable results.

With the exception of the HLA B27-associated spondylarthropathies and gout, there is a striking female excess (even after age adjustment) in most of the rheumatic diseases for reasons that are mainly unexplained. Such an excess is always a useful starting point for considering aetiological hypotheses and the effect of hormonal and reproductive factors (e.g. Silman and Black 1988; Brennan and Silman 1994). In disorders with an increased occurrence with age then a degenerative aetiology, perhaps as a consequence of a sustained environmental insult, is likely (e.g. osteoarthritis in the presence of obesity). By contrast, disease with a young age at onset may represent a greater genetic contribution or more short-lived environmental influence (e.g. Reiter's syndrome).

Time trends

It is of considerable interest to monitor the trends over time in the occurrence of diseases. From an aetiological view changes in the incidence of disease may represent changing levels of exposure to putative risk factors. From a public health perspective the appropriate health service provision requires knowledge of both current and future

levels of occurrence. Trends in prevalence rates are difficult to interpret because improvement in survival will lead to an increase in prevalence. Thus it is really only appropriate to consider changes in incidence over time, and regrettably, there are few data on incidence at different time periods for most of the major rheumatic diseases, the notable exception being rheumatoid arthritis.

Time trends for rheumatoid arthritis

The earliest reliable data on trends in the incidence of rheumatoid arthritis come from estimates based on cross-sectional surveys of population samples from Leigh and Wensleydale, studied in the 1950s and 1960s. A follow-up survey was undertaken after 5 years in the 620 individuals who had participated in the initial survey in 1954 to 1959. This found that 36 (6 per cent) of the population originally free of rheumatoid arthritis had developed it during the follow-up period (Lawrence 1977). This however, is equivalent to an annual incidence of 12 per 1000, which was six times the rate estimated during the first survey (based on recalled age at onset). It is not likely that the incidence increased sixfold during this period and the data probably seriously overestimate the true occurrence of the disease and probably reflect a case definition of low specificity.

The accurate determination of trends requires the continual monitoring of a population, with access to contemporary medical records; these permitting retrospectively correct diagnostic assignment. Such a system can only work if the monitoring can detect all the cases in a defined population as in the Rochester Epidemiology Program discussed above. Although retrospective examination of medical records will omit those who never seek medical attention for their symptoms and standardization of diagnosis is difficult, the utility of such a system in documenting trends in new cases is clear. Figure 1 shows published results from 1950 to 1975 in the Rochester studies (Linos *et al.* 1980). These show an increasing incidence in the first part of this period, with a marked subsequent decline in females but not in males. Although there have been considerable changes in diagnostic practice over this period, with increasing recognition of the need to separate out the HLA B27-related seronegative arthritides, such an explanation is unlikely, given the patterns observed. Such a diagnostic reassignment would have been expected to alter the trends in both sexes equally. Possible reasons for the difference between the sexes will be considered later in this review. A more recent study from Seattle (Dugowsen *et al.* 1991) aiming to 'capture' all incident cases in women in 1987 in a fixed population, yielded an annual incidence rate of 0.23 per 1000 women aged between 18 and

Table 9 Incidence rate of rheumatoid arthritis in the United Kingdom

	1970–1972		1981–1982	
	Males	**Females**	**Males**	**Females**
Incidence rate per thousand (age adjusted)	1.3	3.2	1.2	2.6

Source: Hochberg (1990).

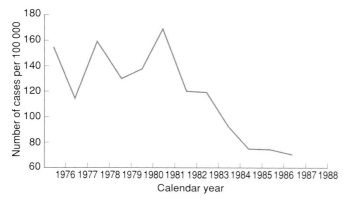

Fig. 2 Time trends in incidence of rheumatoid arthritis (United Kingdom general practice 1967 to 1987). (Reproduced with permission from Silman 1988.)

64 years compared with a rate of 0.46 per 1000 in the same age group in the Rochester population during the period 1950 to 1974, i.e. the rate had halved over the past decade. This decline in the United States is not restricted to white groups. Over the past 25 years there has been a halving in incidence in Pima Indians, a group with one of the world's highest rates (Jacobsson *et al.* 1994).

There are also supporting data from the United Kingdom. The Royal College of General Practitioners conducted morbidity surveys involving a large group of general practitioners who were required to make a diagnosis for every patient consultation. These surveys in 1955, 1970 to 1972, 1981 to 1982, and 1992 all relied on the recorded diagnosis from the general practitioner and were not standardized. The results comparing the two middle surveys show (Hochberg 1990) (Table 9) that there was no significant decline in incidence between these surveys. The other data from this source are from an ongoing survey of all patients attending one of 30 participating general practitioners, who send back to the 'central' unit a 'weekly return' of the numbers attending with a list of specific diagnoses (Royal College of General Practitioners 1976 to 1987). These include rheumatoid arthritis. Analysis of these data (Fig. 2) (Silman 1988) showed a statistically significant decline of approximately 7.5 per 100 000 per year between 1976 and 1987, equivalent to a halving in the incidence rate during this time. Although most of the participating doctors had remained the same during the period of observation the possibility cannot be excluded that there was a decline in completeness of recording during this period.

Whole population data are also available from those countries that have a population morbidity register for specific disorders. Interpretation of trends from such sources is difficult as, in addition to the persistent problem of changes in completeness of registration, there may be selective changes in the severity of cases recorded. Such registers are extensively available in Scandinavia, and data from Finland (Isomaki 1989) have recently been published. This source demonstrated an annual incidence of newly registered patients with seropositive rheumatoid arthritis of 0.46 per 1000 in 1980, which was unchanged from that recorded in the early 1970s.

Time trends for other rheumatic diseases

There are fewer data for the other diseases. There are suggestions that symptomatic osteoarthritis is increasing in incidence, based on an increase in consultations to general practitioners from the Royal College of General Practitioners data (Croft 1990) (Fig. 3). Similar data have shown a 30 per cent increase in the incidence of gout between 1971 and 1981 (Stewart and Silman 1990). There has been a marked increase in the incidence of scleroderma, based on a number of studies covering 35 years of observation of the population of Allegheny County, Pennsylvania (Fig. 4) (reviewed by Williams and Silman 1991). Giant cell arteritis has also doubled in incidence in some countries in the past two decades (Rajala *et al.* 1993). However, there is always a problem with such diseases in that increasing incidence may only represent better case ascertainment as physicians become more confident at making the diagnosis. By contrast, there has been a decline in the incidence of ankylosing spondylitis over six decades in the Olmsted County population (Carbone *et al.* 1992).

Trends in birth cohorts

The onset of many of the rheumatic diseases is difficult to define in time and thus trends in calendar year of presentation or diagnosis may not reflect true temporal patterns of disease. Further, if the presumed environmental exposure which triggers a particular disorder occurs early in life, it might be more appropriate to examine trends in disease in successive generations defined by their cohort of birth. An illustrative example of this in rheumatoid arthritis is that contemporary studies of its incidence demonstrate a marked increase in risk with increasing age (Symmons *et al.* 1994). Although this might represent a true age effect on incidence, an alternative explanation is that the oldest groups in that population were at highest risk based on their year of birth and that follow-up over a long period would confirm that the age-specific incidence rates would fall.

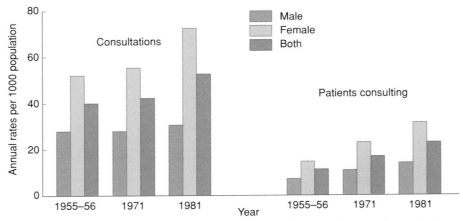

Fig. 3 Incidence of consultations for, and patients consulting with, osteoarthritis and allied conditions in United Kingdom general practice (reproduced with permission from Croft 1990).

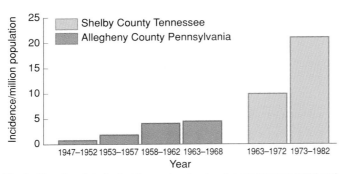

Fig. 4 Time trends in the incidence of systemic sclerosis between 1947 and 1982 in the United States.

Lawrence (1977) was the first to point out the possibility that the risk of rheumatoid arthritis could be related to the period in which an individual was born. In a prospective study in Oberhörlen (West Germany) in the 1960s the maximal incidence was found to be in those aged 65 years and over, whereas the maximal prevalence of existing cases in the cross-sectional survey in the same population was in the decade below that age.

More interesting perhaps, are the data from the Leigh and Wensleydale population surveys (mentioned above) on the prevalence of rheumatoid factor positivity in relation to period of birth (Lawrence 1977). In brief, there were three observations: (i) in urban populations, positivity increases with age in cross-sectional studies; (ii) over a 10-year follow-up period in that urban population there was a tendency for individuals to have a fall in titre; (iii) on analysis by year of birth, the rate of positivity fell in successive cohorts from those born between 1885 and 1894; indicating perhaps that the 1885 to 1894 groups had a peculiarly high risk. Lawrence suggested that the reduction in titre in the older age groups was consistent with an effect of improvement in atmospheric pollution resulting from the Clean Air Acts in 1956.

Clustering in time

A further approach to considering the influence of time on the onset of disease is to look for clustering of disease, i.e. the non-random distribution in time. The most classical example of this was the initial description of the apparent epidemic of juvenile arthritis in Lyme (Steere *et al.* 1977), where both the parents' and the physicians' feelings were that the number of cases seen was greater than would be expected by normal random distribution of sporadic cases. Although there are complex statistical methods available for confirming the non-randomness, it is normally obvious that such a cluster exists, as was the case in Lyme. The ultimate consequence from the follow-up of this cluster was the incrimination of *Borrelia burgdorferi* as the causative organism.

The reporting of apparent clusters of cases in time has occurred in other rheumatic disorders with no well-defined cause. One interesting example is polymyalgia rheumatica/giant cell arteritis, although the role of increased awareness and changes in diagnostic sensitivity in producing such clusters is unknown. A cluster of five cases in Jerusalem was reported in a 7-week period, where their expected annual referral rate was one case. A study in general practice in the United Kingdom was also suggestive of a cluster with six cases of polymyalgia rheumatica and two of giant cell arteritis presenting in 7 months in a population of 4400. Further, one of the most unusual aspects of the epidemiology of polymyalgia rheumatica/giant cell arteritis is the suggestion of seasonality in incidence. The results are confusing, however. Thus, an initial report of clustering in summer (Kinmont and McCullum 1965) was followed by two of a definite winter peak (Coomes *et al.* 1976; Jonasson *et al.* 1979), one with a marked summer peak (Cimmino *et al.* 1990), and one suggesting both a summer and a winter peak (Mowat and Hazleman. 1974). Two more studies showed no such seasonality (Chuang *et al.* 1982; Omland *et al.* 1986) but the results from the positive studies do suggest that clustering in time and indeed in space might be responsible for some of the variable incidence of this disease.

Racial influences

A summary of the principal racial influences in the rheumatic diseases is given in Table 10. The consideration of racial influences is of interest, although any differences that do emerge are inevitably difficult to interpret. The reasons for this are first that there may be racial differences in symptom perception, physician consultation, and physician bias in diagnosis, all of which could lead to apparent

Table 10 Racial differences in the occurrence of rheumatic diseases

	Racial groups with rate:	
	Increased[a]	Decreased
Rheumatoid arthritis	Pima Indians	Black Africans Chinese
Ankylosing spondylitis	Haida Indians	
Systemic lupus erythematosus	American blacks Chinese	
Osteoarthritis	Blackfeet Indians	Caribbean blacks
Juvenile chronic arthritis	Native Americans	Chinese
Gout	Filipinos Tamils Malaysians	Pima Indians

[a]Compared with 'European' group.
Data from numerous sources; groups mentioned are those with the most extreme results.
Source: Silman and Hochberg (1993).

differences in incidence. Second, ethnic groups differ in both genes and environment, the latter both at a macro level—there may be geographical differences due to area of residence—and at a micro level, perhaps due to differences in nutrition or other lifestyle factors. The classical epidemiological method of attempting to distinguish between these explanations is the migrant study. Thus, one aims to compare the incidence of a disease in members of an ethnic group who migrate with that seen in the population who remain in their original environment. One example of this is the study of rheumatoid arthritis in black African populations. Thus a very low prevalence of rheumatoid arthritis was seen in a rural African population in South Africa, but the prevalence approximated to the white persons' rate among those black people who had migrated to an urban environment (Solomon *et al.* 1975). The suggestion is that it is the rural environment rather than the negro race that is protective. However, there has to be caution in interpreting the results of such studies. First the migrants are unlikely to be representative of the 'parent' population in respect of their lifestyle and other factors. Second, the occurrence of disease may lead to migration, thus an individual with rheumatoid arthritis may seek to move nearer to a city for greater access to medical care. One problem in considering comparative studies of racial differences is that one may not be comparing like with like, and different study methods may be involved.

Rheumatoid arthritis is rarer in both developed (Lau *et al.* 1993) and rural (Beasley *et al.* 1983) Chinese groups and in both developed (MacGregor *et al.* 1994a) and rural (Silman *et al.* 1993) black groups than in white populations. Examples of racial differences in a few other selected diseases are considered below.

Osteoarthritis

A single-observer study comparing rural Jamaica with rural England showed a similar overall prevalence of osteoarthritis, although there was a difference in the distribution of affected joints. Jamaicans were more likely to have knee and hand involvement and less likely to have hip and metatarsophalangeal joint involvement (Bremner *et al.* 1968). By contrast, involvement of the distal interphalangeal joint is very common in Pima and Blackfeet Indian groups in North America, with rates of Heberden's nodes as high as 30 per cent in some Blackfeet communities (Bennett and Burch 1968). In North American black populations, radiographic changes in the knee are more common in women but similar in men when compared with a similarly surveyed white population (Felson 1988). Differences in the prevalence of osteoarthritis of the hip are more common, with a relative rarity of disease at this site in Asian Indians, Chinese, and black African populations (Felson 1988).

Juvenile chronic arthritis

The incidence of juvenile chronic arthritis in native Americans in British Columbia, Canada is three times that of a comparable white population (Hochberg 1981). By contrast no cases were found in an extensive survey of 20 000 Chinese children in the same population (Hill 1977). There do not appear to be any differences between black and white children in North America.

Systemic lupus erythematosus

This is up to five times more common in black than in white races, although this excess is more predominant in the United States and West Indian populations than in black African groups (Symmons 1991). South Asians are also at double the risk of white populations (Hopkinson *et al.* 1994). The other at-risk group would appear to be the Chinese, with a number of anecdotal hospital series reporting a relative excess of systemic lupus erythematosus compared with rheumatoid arthritis, in contrast to the normal state in Western Caucasoid populations. There may be environmental factors relevant here however, as the excess is seen in Chinese populations in Malaysia but not in 'Westernized' Chinese for example in San Francisco (Frank 1980). It is likely in this, as in other disorders, that the effect of race is not limited to disease susceptibility but also applies to disease severity.

Geographical influences

The racial distribution of disease can, as was explained above, be interpreted on the basis of geographical differences related to environmental factors. Some of the differences that affect the Third World are considered in Chapter 5.1.2. Geographical, like racial, differences can be useful in framing hypotheses for further testing. Geographical differences may be between countries or even within countries to the level of small, area clusters, in an analogous manner to the clustering in time discussed above for Lyme disease. Clustering without an obvious explanation has been described for connective tissue diseases in general in Georgia, United States (Arnett *et al.* 1990) and for scleroderma in South and West London, where one hypothesis was that this was due to proximity to airports (Silman *et al.* 1990).

Geographical differences between populations for the various diseases have been considered and many of these were well described at a conference nearly 25 years ago (Bennett and Wood 1968), relating particularly to gout and rheumatoid arthritis.

Table 11 Geographical variation in prevalence of rheumatoid arthritis

Population	N	Prevalence of definite rheumatoid arthritis at age 15+ years (%)
Europe		
Leigh and Wensleydale, England	2 234	1.1
Sofia, Bulgaria	4 318	0.9
Rotterdam, Netherlands	19 647	0.9
Sweden (various locations)	39 418	0.9
Samso, Denmark	4 557	0.8
Heinola, Finland	8 000	2.0
Asia		
Shizouko, Japan	3 006	0.8
Kinmet, China	5 629	0.3
Java, Indonesia	4 683	0.2
Africa		
Phokeng, South Africa	801	0.12
Soweto, South Africa	964	0.9
Venda, South Africa	543	Nil
America		
Kingston, Jamaica	530	1.9
Sudbury MA, USA	4 552	0.9
Chippewa Indians, USA	205	6.8
Inuit, Canada	2 055	0.6
Puerto Rico	3 883	0.3
Oceania		
New Zealand	432	1.0
Maori, New Zealand	175	3.9

Source: Silman and Hochberg (1993).

Rheumatoid arthritis

Rheumatoid arthritis has been subject to more population studies than any other rheumatic disease and the breadth of these studies across all five continents is shown in Table 11. The points listed above on methodological explanations for differences in results are relevant in interpreting these studies. Most of the studies are very small and with a disease, such as rheumatoid arthritis, with a less than 1 per cent rate of prevalence, population studies of under 2000 are unlikely to yield useful data. The precision with which the studies were conducted varies, and the published reports do not always allow an accurate appreciation of the methods used,

particularly the diagnostic criteria. Despite these caveats, the most striking feature from these numerous studies is the overall similarity in prevalence between populations, with a standard rate of between 0.5 and 1.0 per cent. This consistency is most unusual in human chronic diseases and may reflect the ubiquity of the causative factors, genetic and/or environmental.

Other rheumatic diseases

Ankylosing spondylitis varies in prevalence according to the underlying population frequency of the HLA-B27 gene. Rates of the disease are substantially higher in Scandinavian than in other European or American Caucasian populations (Rigby 1991). Gout is a disease with a very marked geographical variation in prevalence, probably related to the underlying population levels of serum uric acid. Filipino and Polynesian populations in the Pacific Rim have shown the greatest excess in prevalence compared with that in Caucasoid populations (Decker *et al.* 1968). Interestingly, even within relatively homogeneous populations, there are differences in prevalence. For example, there is a higher rate of gout in England than in either Wales or Scotland (Currie 1979). Juvenile chronic arthritis has also been extensively studied with no major difference found in Western populations or what was the Soviet Union. There have also been a number of prevalence and incidence studies of polymyalgia rheumatica in different populations, although many of the these studies were from populations of the same ethnic origins, mostly either from Scandinavia or from the largely originally Scandinavian population in Olmsted County served by the Mayo Clinic. There are no consistent differences between the populations studied in Scandinavia or the United States. One study from Israel (Friedman *et al.* 1982) had the lowest recorded incidence (0.5 per 100 000), although it is always difficult to be sure as to the role of under-ascertainment. Similarly studies from Southern Europe—France (Barrier *et al.* 1982) and Italy (Salvarani *et al.* 1987)— yielded incidence estimates substantially lower than those from most of the major studies in Northern European and the United States. The one exception is the study from the Southern United States (Smith *et al.* 1983) which, at 2.4 per 100 000 in the white population, had the lowest incidence rate for giant cell arteritis (apart from the Israeli study).

Aetiological models

Most of the rheumatic diseases have a combination of genetic and environmental factors implicated in their aetiology; it is frequently the role of epidemiology to define the nature of these factors and consider their involvement quantitatively. The problem is not a simple one, however, for two reasons: first, there is not a single aetiological model for the majority of the rheumatic diseases. However, knowledge about genetic factors has increased exponentially as data on gene products is replaced by information from DNA sequencing. Thus it is likely that there is an infinite number of point mutations that explain the occurrence of such wholly genetic disorders as the Ehlers–Danlos syndrome, rather than a single genetic cause.

It is, however, useful to consider models for disease causation according to whether a cause is necessary, i.e. the disease for all practical purposes cannot occur in its absence, and/or sufficient, i.e. the disease can occur in the presence of that risk factor alone, as shown in the diagram below.

Table 12 Approaches to studying genetic factors in disease aetiology

Approach	Advantages	Disadvantages
Comparison of occurrence in different ethnic groups	Data may be readily available	Differences between ethnic groups may be more related to environment than genes
Assess whether there is an increased risk in relatives	Families normally willing to participate and provide good data	Environmental factors also cluster within families
		Often difficult to obtain data from control families
		Need to adjust for age and sex as younger members have not had time to develop disease
Comparison of concordance in identical and non-identical twins	Good matching for environmental factors	Twin pairs not available in rare diseases Identical twins may share closer environment than non-identical (especially if of unlike sex)
Comparison of frequency of genetic marker in probands and controls	Data easy to obtain Accurate definition by DNA techniques of markers may enhance specificity	Such population associations do not prove causation Difficult to obtain strength of genetic contribution or type of inheritance
Studies of linkage between marker and disease in multicase families	Strength of genetic contribution and inheritance are possible to determine	Linkage difficult to show and large number of families needed Results from multicase families may not be applicable to sporadic cases

	Cause necessary	
	Yes	**No**
Yes	*Borrelia burgdorferi* and Lyme disease	Organic solvents and scleroderma
Cause sufficient		
No	HLA B27 and ankylosing spondylitis	HLA DRB1*04 and rheumatoid arthritis

Thus Lyme disease follows infection by *Borrelia burgdorferi* and this organism (probably) alone can cause the disease (Steere *et al*. 1983). By contrast, organic solvent exposure is not necessary for the development of scleroderma but is sufficient for some cases (Black *et al*. 1986). It is (almost) true that HLA B27 is necessary for the development of ankylosing spondylitis but it is not sufficient, as the majority of individuals with this antigen will not develop the disease. The most frequent pattern of causation is, however, the last quadrant (bottom right) where a risk factor is neither necessary nor sufficient. Thus the overwhelming majority of individuals with HLA DR4 (HLA DRB1*04) will not develop rheumatoid arthritis and a significant proportion (30 per cent) of individuals with rheumatoid arthritis will not have HLA DR4 (HLA DRB1*04).

It is obvious to most observers that for most of the rheumatic diseases there is not, as in the Lyme model, a single cause, and one is searching for risk factors that may be relevant but are poor discriminators between those who will and will not develop a particular disease. One useful strategy is to describe clinically or pathologically derived subsets within a clinical entity that may allow the better derivation of causes, the so-called splitting approach. This is particularly useful in relation to juvenile chronic arthritis, where such factors as pattern of joint involvement at onset and the production of antinuclear antibodies have been associated with different immunogenetic backgrounds to an increasingly specific level (Fernandez-Vina *et al*. 1990)

Genetic factors

There are a number of epidemiological approaches to assessing the genetic contribution to disease and these are shown, with their advantages and disadvantages, in Table 12.

Family studies

It is obvious from Table 12 that the study of family members of probands with a disease is an important tool in genetic epidemiology, but there are specific problems in relation to the rheumatic diseases which have been summarized for rheumatoid arthritis (Silman 1986); these are listed below.

1. Categorization of relatives into affected and non-affected is frequently difficult as relatives may show some features of the syndrome under investigation but not sufficient to satisfy the relevant criteria. As an example the relatives of probands with ankylosing spondylitis frequently have either clinical or radiographic evidence of sacroiliitis but not both (Burns and Calin 1983) and to categorize them as affected or unaffected would both be wrong. The answer is to use all the available data and analyse subsets, and thus in family studies not to be bound by rigid criteria.

Table 13 Genetic features of the major rheumatic diseases

Disease	Familial clustering (ratio of rate in first-degree relatives to expected population rate)	Monozygotic twin concordance (%)	HLA association (relative risk)
Rheumatoid arthritis	1.7×	12 (population)	DR4 (8×)
Generalized osteoarthritis	3×	43	Inconsistent
Juvenile chronic arthritis	3–4×	40	DR5[a] (2.3–4.8[a])
			DRw8[a] (10–25×)
Ankylosing spondylitis	15–20×	50	B27 (100×)
Systemic lupus erythematosus	9×	≃25	DR2/3 (2–3×)
Systemic sclerosis	6–8×	No data	DR5 (2.5)

Data are based on pooled estimates from many sources. *Source:* Silman and Hochberg (1993).

2. Many of the rheumatic diseases may not become evident until the seventh or subsequent decades and misclassification of those yet to develop the disease may occur. This is different to, for example, the situation with type I diabetes, where development of the disease has normally occurred by the end of the third decade. Some have suggested adjusting for the age of the proband as a suitable method, i.e. if a sibling has not developed the disease by the age at which his or her affected proband developed the disease then he or she can be categorized as non-affected. This is erroneous, as data (for example, in rheumatoid arthritis) have shown that there are considerable differences in the age of onset between affected sibling pairs (Silman *et al.* 1987) and even between concordant monozygotic twins (MacGregor *et al.* 1994b).

3. By contrast for some of the inflammatory joint diseases there is also the problem of misclassification, because the disease has undergone complete remission by the time of the family survey and there is no evidence of past disease either clinically or radiologically. Unless contemporary notes are of high quality, it may be impossible to determine the significance of self-reported past history.

4. It is well recognized that probands derived from hospital series are more likely to have a 'positive' family history than unselected probands chosen from a community survey. This is likely to be due to selection for referral to hospital of an individual with symptoms in the face of a family history, thus explaining the greater familial clustering in hospital series (for example, in rheumatoid arthritis; Wolfe *et al.* 1988). An alternative, but less likely explanation is that hospital cases are more severe, and that the 'genetic contribution' is considered to be one of severity as opposed to susceptibility.

Genetic contribution to specific diseases

In this review it is impossible to provide the detailed data of the genetic contribution to the various rheumatic disorders. A summary of the data from some of the major disorders is shown in Table 13, from which it can be seen that the various strategies outlined above have yielded very different estimates of the role of genetic factors for the different disorders. Recent advances in molecular biology are refining the genetic factors to be considered. An excellent example of this is the 'shared epitope hypothesis' (Gregerson *et al.* 1987), which provides an explanation for the population association between rheumatoid arthritis and different, serologically defined class-II antigens at the DR locus on the basis of the shared possession of a short sequence of amino acids in the third, hypervariable region of the DRB1 gene. Unfortunately for the epidemiologist, although this shared epitope is observed in some 90 per cent of rheumatoid arthritis, it is also found in 50 per cent of the normal population. A quick calculation of the relevant 2 × 2 table gives the results that positive predictive value for the epitope is less than 2 per cent and the specificity is around 50 per cent; in other words, it is a poor discriminator for those destined to develop rheumatoid arthritis.

Non-genetic host factors

This term is a slight misnomer but it is a convenient label for the non-environmental factors present in individuals that are not predominantly genetic in origin. A list of such factors examined in the rheumatic diseases is:

(1) perinatal problems;

(2) family size, position in family;

(3) menstrual/menopausal status;

(4) sex hormonal status;

(5) stature and body form;

(6) reproductive history;

(7) organic comorbidity;

(8) psychiatric comorbidity;

Table 14 Menstrual, hormonal, and reproductive factors in various rheumatic diseases	
Disease	**Menstrual, hormonal, and reproductive risk factors**
Rheumatoid arthritis	Early menarche, nulliparity, early post-partum period, possibly fetal loss in some groups, low testosterone in males
Osteoarthritis	Menopause, previous hysterectomy for menstrual irregularity, possible oestrogen excess
Systemic sclerosis	Infertility, possible fetal loss
Osteoporosis	Early menopause
Systemic lupus erythematosus	Pregnancy

(9) biochemical background;

(10) height and weight.

Data in relation to some of the factors in the list are considered next.

Family size/position in family

In many instances this would be considered as a surrogate for over-crowding or a similar socioeconomic variable. For instance, in a study of rheumatoid arthritis, there was an increased risk of disease in older than younger siblings, suggesting that being first born carries an increased risk (Hazes *et al.* 1990b). This would be unlikely to have a simple socio-economic explanation. By contrast, a study of Behçet's disease suggested that there was a risk connected with large family size (Cooper *et al.* 1986).

Menstrual, hormonal, and reproductive factors

It is appropriate to combine consideration of these variables as suggesting an influence of sex hormones. One of the most interesting aspects of the epidemiology of the major rheumatic diseases (see above) is the marked sex difference in occurrence, which is not easily explained by differences in lifestyle (such as occupation, smoking, or alcohol consumption), as is the case for other chronic disorders. It is thus reasonable to consider whether there are hormonal or reproductive effects that might explain these differences and there has been much recent work on the subject. A summary of some of the findings is shown in Table 14. Many of those factors listed might of course represent the sub- or preclinical effects of the disease rather than the cause, but such factors might be useful in explaining sex differences in occurrence.

Height and weight

There are a number of disorders where anthropometric variables are thought to be of relevance. Tallness may be a risk factor for low back pain. The greatest topic of interest has been the relationship between obesity and, particularly, non-inflammatory joint disease. Although obesity might also be seen as an environmental factor (i.e. excess calorie intake). The mechanical effect of obesity is to increase load on weight-bearing joints, such as the hip and knee, and it is thus of interest to note that obesity is more strongly linked to osteoarthritis of the knee than of the hip (Felson and Radin 1994). Methodologically, it is important to distinguish cause from effect. Thus in the presence of osteoarthritis there may be less physical activity with a greater tendency to obesity. Recent prospective studies have shown conclusively that obesity is a real risk factor not only for osteoarthritis of the knees (Hochberg *et al.* 1995), but also of the hands (Carman *et al.* 1994), suggesting perhaps a 'metabolic' effect.

The effect of comorbidity

Many of the diseases discussed in this volume will be classified as primary or secondary depending on whether there is another under-lying pathology for the joint disease, e.g. polycythaemia and gout. The fact that this is true for a (normally small) proportion of clinical cases does not mean that such comorbidity is of relevance for the disease in general. Of greater relevance is an increased risk of joint disease in the presence of other illness, although the latter does not 'cause' the former. There are some data to support the increased coincidence of some disorders: for example, rheumatoid arthritis and autoimmune thyroid disease (Silman *et al.* 1989), scleroderma and cancer (Abu-Shakra *et al.* 1993), and neurosis and back pain (Leino and Magni 1993) are amongst a large list of such associations.

There are some interesting negative associations, i.e. the presence of one disorder 'protecting' against the development of another. Examples include the mutual exclusivity of schizophrenia and rheumatoid arthritis (Spector and Silman 1987), and osteoporosis and osteoarthritis (Dequeker 1986). The underlying explanation for these negative associations is, however, somewhat obscure.

Environmental factors

Infectious agents

The identification of *Borrelia burgdorferi* as the spirochaete responsible for Lyme disease, has acted as a stimulus to search for viral causes of other inflammatory joint diseases, such as rheumatoid arthritis for which a viral background seemed likely. It is of interest to review the epidemiological data suggesting a viral cause for rheumatoid arthritis as the lessons are applicable more widely.

Seroepidemiological studies

In this approach, antibody frequencies in a diseased and a disease-free population are compared. Numerous studies have confirmed the high titres of antibodies against a variety of Epstein–Barr virus (EBV)-related antigens in patients with rheumatoid arthritis. However, not all studies have been positive and, more importantly, the differences from a control population have not always been either biologically or statistically significant. Given the almost universal exposure to EBV in Western populations, it may be more relevant to look for a quantitative difference in response but this is methodologically more difficult. Epidemiologically, the geographical distribution of infectious mononucleosis and rheumatoid arthritis are similar, and infectious mononucleosis is apparently unknown in countries with a low prevalence of rheumatoid arthritis (Aho and Raunio 1982). One explanation for these observations in the face of the ubiquity of infection with EBV is the effect of age. In countries with a low prevalence of rheumatoid arthritis, infection with EBV is virtually universal by the age of 3 years and the infection is clinically silent; whereas in countries with a high prevalence, infection occurs at a later age and is more likely to be clinically apparent with, for example, infectious mononucleosis. The increased rate of antinuclear antibodies in rheumatoid arthritis is seen, however, in most populations including Mexican and American Indians and Afghans (Vaughan 1979). The evidence for EBV infection as a cause of rheumatoid arthritis is constrained by the lack of clinical evidence that EBV is arthritogenic, unlike, for example, rubella, hepatitis and mumps virus (Depper and Zvaifler 1981).

The other widely studied agent has been human parvovirus (HPV), given that arthritis can follow infection with this agent. A reasonable conclusion is that HPV probably has little relevance (Leading Article 1985) for rheumatoid arthritis, despite two reports from the United Kingdom, the first showing that 19 out of 153 patients with early synovitis had evidence of HPV infection (White et al. 1985) and the second describing joint problems in 17 patients after an HPV outbreak (Reid et al. 1985). Neither study had appropriate control groups and there were no patients with a persistent arthritis.

Retroviruses have also been investigated, owing to the similarity between rheumatoid arthritis and the arthritis produced by lentiviruses in animals, for example caprine arthritis encephalitis. However, attempts in man to show evidence of retrovirus infection in rheumatoid arthritis have been unsuccessful. There are also very good mycoplasma-induced animal models of rheumatoid arthritis and in these chronicity and severity, as in man, are related to genetic factors. Clinical and epidemiological studies in humans have, however, mainly failed to support a mycoplasma source for rheumatoid arthritis.

Lifestyle

In many chronic diseases there is a considerable wealth of epidemiological data linking aspects of lifestyle, such as diet, exercise, and cigarette and alcohol consumption, with the risk of disease. Studies of such variables in the rheumatic diseases have been mostly non-informative, for example, there have been studies supporting (Heliovaara et al. 1993) and refuting (Vessey et al. 1987) an increased risk of rheumatoid arthritis from cigarette smoking. Alcohol is well established to be associated with gout and possibly also osteoporosis. Diet is an aspect of lifestyle that is consistently considered by patients to be the explanation behind their disease, although scientific evidence is hard to find. Problems in studying diet include the accurate recall of diet at the appropriate time before disease onset (which might be many years in a disease with a long latency), and within-individual variation in dietary intake for many nutrients, which results in misclassification if an inappropriate dietary methodology is used, such as a food frequency interview or a 24-h recall.

Occupation

The investigation of occupational exposure as a cause of specific rheumatic syndromes is potentially of importance for those who are exposed, but of relatively minor importance at the population level. It is useful to distinguish the two epidemiological concepts of attributable risk and population attributable risk. Attributable risk, in this setting, estimates the proportion of an exposed individual's risk that is directly due to the exposure, whereas by contrast, the population attributable risk provides an estimate of the proportion of cases that arise in the population as a whole owing to that exposure. Thus there are well-established links between being a footballer (soccer) and the subsequent development of osteoarthrosis of the knee. The attributable risk is high for footballers, i.e. the occupation explained most of their increased risk, whereas in the population as a whole, being a footballer will explain only a small proportion of cases. The consequence of this fairly obvious point is that it is virtually impossible to identify most occupational exposures by undertaking retrospective case–control studies of random series of diagnosed cases, the approach frequently used for testing aetiological hypotheses. It is necessary to undertake prospective studies of occupationally derived cohorts.

Occupational exposure as far as the rheumatic diseases are concerned normally reflects either chemical or toxic exposure, or the outcome of mechanical trauma to joints and associated structures from the physical demands of the job. In practice, occupation is only rarely of interest in the inflammatory rheumatic disorders, although there have been suggestions that some cases of rheumatoid arthritis have an occupational cause (e.g. Klockars et al. 1987). By contrast there have been a number of toxic exposures linked to the development of scleroderma and indeed in this disease, which

Table 15　Mechanical occupational exposures linked to osteoarthritis

Exposure	Site
Sports	
Boxers	Hands
Baseball pitchers	Shoulders
Hurdlers	Hip
Runners	?Knees
Footballers (soccer)	?Knees, ?hips
Footballers (American)	?Knees
Weight lifters	Knees
Other	
Parachutists	Knees
Jack-hammer operators	Wrists, hands
Cotton-mill workers	Hands
Coal miners	Knee
Dockers/shipyard workers	Knee
Farmers	Knee, hip

Source: Felson (1988).

Table 16 Studies investigating possible protective effect of oral contraceptives against the development of rheumatoid arthritis

First author	Study design	Source of cases	Source of controls	Source of data	Odds ratio for ever used
Wingrave (1978)[a]	Prospective cohort[b]	General practice records	n/a	General practice	0.68
Vandenbroucke et al. (1982)	Case-control	Hospital clinic	Soft tissue	Postal questionnaire	
Linos et al. (1983)[a]	Case-control	Diagnostic register	Non-arthritic clinic attenders	Medical record	1.7
Allebeck et al. (1984)	Case-control	Inpatients	Community	Postal questionnaire	0.7
del Junco et al. (1985)[a]	Case-control	Diagnostic register	Non-arthritic clinic attenders	Medical records	1.1
Vandenbroucke et al. (1986)	Case-control	Hospital clinic	Osteoarthritis	Postal questionnaire	0.57
Vessey et al. (1987)	Prospective, cohort[b]	Postal questionnaire	n/a	Family-planning clinic	1.12
Darwish and Arminian (1987)	Case-control	Hospital clinic	Non-arthritic clinic attenders	Interview	1.29
Koepsell et al. (1989)	Incident case-control	Hospital clinic	Community	Interview	0.27
Spector et al. (1990)	Case-control	Hospital clinic	(i) Community (ii) Osteoarthritis	Postal questionnaire	0.56 0.60
Moskowitz et al. (1990)	Case-control	Group health clinic	Pharmacy users	Pharmacy records	2.0
Hannaford et al. (1990a)[a]	Incident case-control	Hospital clinic	Osteoarthritis	Interviews	0.39
Hernandez-Avila et al. (1990)	Prospective cohort[b]	Postal questionnaire	n/a	Postal questionnaire	1.0
Hazes et al. (1990b)[a]	Case-control	Hospital clinic	Sisters	Postal questionnaire	0.37

[a]These are reports from the same population.
[b]These are cohort studies and study population is chosen by their exposure status at basetime. The controls (comparison) group are the non- (or ex-) users.

predominantly affects women, the development in a man might indicate a chemical exposure. Suggested exposures are:

(1) silica dust (coal miners, gold miners, stonemasons);

(2) organic chemicals:

  (a) aromatic hydrocarbons (toluene, benzene, xylene, aromatic mixes — white spirit, dieselene);

  (b) aliphatic hydrocarbons:

    (i) chlorinated (vinyl chloride)
    (ii) non-chlorinated (naphtha-n-hexane);

(3) toxic oil;

(4) epoxy resins;

(5) biogenic amines — metaphenylenediamine;

(6) urea–formaldehyde foam insulations;

(7) drugs

It remains an unanswered (and possibly unanswerable) question as to whether silicone breast implants lead to this disease (Gabriel et al. 1994).

Osteoarthritis provides a useful example of mechanical causes, resulting from occupational exposure, that are linked with the disease; a list of such occupations is shown in Table 15. The scientifically difficult task is to try and combine the study of such occupations so as to achieve some more precise measure of joint stress. From this, overall risk of disease in relation to trauma might be determined, rather than the risk associated with specific occupations. Recent attempts at this exercise for osteoarthritis of the knee, have confirmed the increased risk from jobs with heavy demand and those that involve heavy bending, but the absolute increase in risk is small, less than twofold for the highest compared with the lowest stress group.

Drugs

Pharmaceutical agents are a source of chemical exposure that have been linked to a number of rheumatic diseases. Many of these examples reflect an idiosyncratic response to the drug, or a genetically determined response (e.g. slow or fast acetylators in drug-induced systemic lupus) and are not a clear example of toxicity *per se*. Again, in public health terms, drugs are a relatively weak contributor to overall risk for most rheumatic diseases, systemic lupus being a notable exception. The chief epidemiological interest in relation to the aetiologic effects of drugs has been the hypothesis that the oral contraceptive pill reduces the risk of rheumatoid arthritis, to such an extent that there is a decline in incidence as a result (Vandenbroucke 1983). This has probably been the most investigated area in the epidemiology of rheumatic disease and a clear consensus has now emerged (Silman and Vandenbroucke 1989; Spector and Hochberg 1990). This is that the oral contraceptive pill probably either protects against or postpones the development of severe rheumatoid arthritis, although the mechanism for this is obscure. The studies themselves demonstrate the entire repertoire of investigational methods in epidemiology, and the various problems and biases involved in undertaking this area of research. Table 16 is instructive in so far as it illustrates the variety of approaches used to generate answers to the same question, although no single study is perfect on its own. This list is a fitting description of the current state of epidemiological research into the aetiology of the rheumatic diseases. The conclusions are that there is a lot of interest, that the studies are methodologically difficult but can be completed, that conflicting results can be expected, but that ultimately a useful answer for the basic scientists to follow up may emerge!

References

Abu-Shakra, M., Guillemin, F., and Lee, P. (1993). Cancer in systemic sclerosis. *Arthritis and Rheumatism*, 36, 460–4.

Aho, K. and Raunio, V. (1982). EB-virus and rheumatoid arthritis: new insights into their interrelation. *Medical Biology*, 60, 49–52.

Allebeck, P., Ahlbom, A., Ljungstrom, K., and Allander, E. (1984). Do oral contraceptives reduce the incidence of rheumatoid arthritis? *Scandinavian Journal of Rheumatology*, 13, 140–6.

Altman, R. *et al.*. (1986). Development of criteria for the classification and reporting of osteoarthritis. *Arthritis and Rheumatism*, 29, 1039–49.

Altman, R. *et al.*. (1990). The American College of Rheumatology criteria for the classification and reporting of osteoarthritis of the hand. *Arthritis and Rheumatism*, 33, 1601–10.

Arnett, F.C. *et al.* (1988). The American Rheumatism Association 1987 revised criteria for the classification of rheumatoid arthritis. *Arthritis and Rheumatism*, 31, 315–24.

Arnett, F.C. *et al.* (1990). Connective tissue disease in south east Georgia. A community based study of immunogenetic markers and autoantibodies. *Journal of Rheumatology*, 17, 1029–35.

Barrier, P., Pion, P., and Massari, R. (1982). Epidemiological approach to Horton's disease. *Revue de la Medicine Interne*, 3, 13–20.

Beasley, R.P., Bennett, P.H., and Chun, L.C. (1983). Low prevalence of rheumatoid arthritis in Chinese. Prevalence survey in a rural community. *Journal of Rheumatology*, 10 (Suppl.1), 11–15.

Bennett, P.H. and Burch, T.A. (1968). Osteoarthrosis in the Blackfeet and Pima Indians. In *Population studies of the rheumatic diseases*, (ed. P.H. Bennett and P.H.N. Wood), pp. 407–12. Excerpta Medica, Amsterdam.

Bennett, P.H. and Wood, P.H.N. (ed.) (1968). *Population studies of the rhuematic diseases*, p. 477. Excerpta Medica, Amsterdam.

Black, C., Pereira, S., McWhirter, A., Welsh, K., and Laurent, R. (1986). Genetic susceptibility to scleroderma-like syndrome in symptomatic and asymptomatic workers exposed to vinyl chloride. *Journal of Rheumatology*, 13, 1059–62.

Bloch, D.A., Moses, L.E., and Michel, B.A. (1990). Statistical approaches to classification: methods for developing classification and other criteria rules. *Arthritis and Rheumatism*, 33, 1137–44.

Bremner, J.M., Lawrence, J.S., and Miall, W.E. (1968). Degenerative joint disease in a Jamaican rural population. *Annals of the Rheumatic Diseases*, 27, 326–32.

Brennan, P. and Silman, A.J. (1994). An investigation of gene-environmental interaction in the etiology of rheumatoid arthritis. *American Journal of Epidemiology*, 140, 453–60.

Burns, T. and Calin, A. (1983). The hand radiograph as a diagnostic discriminant between seropositive and seronegative rheumatoid arthritis: a controlled study. *Annals of the Rheumatic Diseases*, 42, 605–12.

Carbone, L.D., Cooper, C., Michet, C.J., Atkinson, E.J., O'Fallon, W.M., and Melton, L.J. (1992). Ankylosing spondylitis in Rochester, Minnesota 1935–1989. Is the epidemiology changing? *Arthritis and Rheumatism*, 35, 1476–82.

Carman, W.J., Sowers, M.F., Hawthorne, V.M., and Weissfeld, L.A. (1994). Obesity as a risk factor for osteoarthritis of the hand and wrist. A prospective study. *American Journal of Epidemiology*, 139, 119–29.

Chuang, T.Y., Hunder, G.G., Ilstrup, D.M., and Kurland, L.T. (1982). Polymyalgia rheumatica. *Annals of Internal Medicine*, 97, 672–80.

Cimmino, M.A., Caporali, R., Montecucco, C.M., Rovida, S., and Baratelli, E. (1990). A seasonal pattern in the onset of polymyalgia rheumatica. *Annals of the Rheumatic Diseases*, 49, 521–3.

Cohen, A.S. *et al.* (1971). Preliminary criteria for the classification of systemic lupus erythematosus. *Bulletin of the Rheumatic Diseases*, 21, 643–8.

Coomes, E.N., Ellis, R.M., and Kay, A.G. (1976). A prospective study of 102 patients with the polymyalgia rheumatica syndrome. *Rheumatic Rehabilitation*, 15, 270–6.

Cooper, C. *et al.* (1986). Is Behçet's disease triggered by childhood infection? *Annals of the Rheumatic Diseases*, 43, 421–3.

Croft, P. (1990). Review of UK data on the rheumatic diseases — osteoarthritis. *British Journal* of Rheumatology, 29, 391–5.

Currie, W.J.C. (1979). Prevalence and incidence of gout in Great Britain. *Annals of the Rheumatic Diseases*, 38, 101–6.

Darwish, M.J. and Armenian, H.K. (1987). A case–control study of rheumatoid arthritis in Lebanon. *International Journal of Epidemiology*, 16, 420–4.

Decker, J.L., Healey, L.A., and Skeith, M.D. (1968). Ethnic variations in serum uric acid: Filipino hyperuricemia, the result of hereditary and environmental factors. In *Population studies of the rheumatic diseases* (ed. P.H. Bennett and P.H.N. Woods), pp. 336–43. Excerpta Medica, Amsterdam.

del Junco, D.J. *et al.* (1985). Do oral contraceptives prevent rheumatoid arthritis? *Journal of the American Medical Association*, 254, 1938–41.

Depper, J.M. and Zvaifler, N.J. (1981). Epstein–Barr-Virus — its relationship to the pathogenesis of rheumatoid arthritis. *Arthritis and Rheumatism*, 24, 755–61.

Dequeker, J. (1986). The relationship between osteoporosis and osteoarthritis. *Clinics in the Rheumatic Diseases*, 11, 261–96.

Dugowson, E.C. *et al.* (1991). Rheumatoid arthritis in women: incidence rates in group Health Cooperative Seattle, Washington, 1987–1989. *Arthritis and Rheumatism*, 34, 1502–7.

Engel, A. (1968). Rheumatoid arthritis in US adults 1960–2. In *Population studies of the rheumatic diseases* (ed. P.H. Bennett and P.H.N. Woods), pp 83–9. Excerpta Medica, Amsterdam.

Felson, D.T. (1988). Epidemiology of osteoarthritis. *Epidemiologic Reviews*, 16, 499–512.

Felson, D.T. and Radin, E.L. (1994). What causes knee osteoarthrosis? Are different compartments susceptibile to different risk factors? *Journal of Rheumatology*, 21, 181–3.

Fernandez-Vina, M.A., Fink, C.W., and Stastny, P. (1990). DQA1 and DQB1 alleles in patients with juvenile arthritis. *Human Immunology Abstracts*, 62.

Frank, A.O. (1980). Apparent predisposition to systemic lupus erythematosus in Chinese patients in West Malaysia. *Annals of the Rheumatic Diseases*, 39, 266–9.

Friedman, G., Friedman, B., and Benbassat, J. (1982). Epidemiology of temporal arteritis in Israel. *Israel Journal of Medical Science*, 18, 241.

Fries, J.F., Hochberg, M.C., Medsger, T.A., Hunder, G.G., and Bombardier, C. (1994). Criteria for rheumatic disease: different types and different functions. *Arthritis and Rheumatism*, 37, 454–62.

Gabriel, S.E., O'Fallon, W.M., Kurland, L.T., Beard, C.M., Woods, J.E., and Melton, L.J. (1994). Risk of connective-tissue diseases and other disorders after breast implantation. *New England Journal of Medicine*, **330**, 1697–702.

Gregersen, P.K., Silver, J., and Winchester, R.J. (1987). The shared epitope hypothesis. An approach to understanding the molecular genetics of susceptibility to rheumatoid arthritis. *Arthritis and Rheumatism*, **30**, 1205–13.

Hannaford, P.C., Kay, C.R., and Hirsch, S. (1990). Oral contraceptives and rheumatoid arthritis: new data from the RCGP oral contraceptives study. *Annals of the Rheumatic Diseases*, **49**, 744–6.

Hazes, J.M.W. *et al.* (1990a). Reduction of the risk of rheumatoid arthritis among women who take oral contraceptives. *Arthritis and Rheumatism*, **33**, 173–9.

Hazes, J.M.W. *et al.* (1990b). Influence of oral contraception on the occurrence of rheumatoid arthritis in female sibs. *Scandinavian Journal of Rheumatology*, **19**, 306–10.

Heliovaara, M., Aho, K., Aromaa, A., Knekt, P., and Reunanen, A. (1993). Smoking and the risk of rheumatoid arthritis. *Journal of Rheumatology*, **20**, 1830–35.

Hernandez-Avila, M. *et al.* (1990) Exogenous sex hormones and the risk of rheumatoid arthritis. *Arthritis and Rheumatism*, **33**, 947–53.

Hill, R. (1977). Juvenile arthritis in various racial groups in British Columbia. *Arthritis and Rheumatism*, **20**, 162.

Hochberg, M.C. (1981). Adult and juvenile rheumatoid arthritis. *Epidemiologic Review*, **3**, 33–44.

Hochberg, M.C. (1990). Changes in the incidence and prevalence of rheumatoid arthritis in England and Wales—1970–1982. *Seminars in Arthritis and Rheumatism*, **19**, 294–302.

Hochberg, M.C., Lethbridge-Cejku, M., Scott, W.W., Reichle, R., Plato, C.C., and Tobin, J.D. (1995). The association of body weight, body fatness, and body fat distribution with osteoarthritis of the knee: data from the Baltimore longitudinal study of aging. *Journal of Rheumatology*, **22**, 488–93.

Hopkinson, N., Doherty, M., and Powell, R.J. (1994). Clinical features and race-specific incidence/prevalence rates of systemic lupus erythematosus in a geographically complete cohort of patients. *Annals of the Rheumatic Diseases*, **53**, 675–80.

Hunder, G.G. *et al.* (1990). The American College of Rheumatology 1990 criteria for the classification of giant cell arteritis. *Arthritis and Rheumatism*, **33**, 1122–8.

Isomaki, H.A. (1989). Rheumatoid arthritis as seen from official data registers: experience in Finland. *Scandinavian Journal of Rheumatology*, **79**, 21–4.

Jacobsson, L.T.H. *et al.* (1994). Decreasing incidence and prevalence of rheumatoid arthritis in Pima Indians over a 25 year period. *Arthritis and Rheumatism*, **37**, 1158–65.

Jonasson, F., Cullen, J.F., and Elton, R.A. (1979). Temporal arteritis. *Scottish Medical Journal*, **24**, 111–17.

Jonsson, H. *et al.* (1990). Estimating the incidence of systemic lupus erythematosus in a defined population using multiple source of retrieval. *British Journal of Rheumatology*, **29**, 185–8.

Kellgren, J.H. (1962). Diagnostic criteria for population studies. *Bulletin of the Rheumatic Diseases*, **13**, 291–2.

Kinmont, P.C. and McCallum, D.I. (1965). The aetiology, pathology and course of giant cell arteritis—the possible role of light sensitivity. *British Journal of Dermatology*, **77**, 193.

Klockars, M., Koskela, R.S., Jarvinen, E., Kolari, P.J., and Rossi, A. (1987). Silica exposure and rheumatoid arthritis: a follow up study of granite workers 1940–81. *British Medical Journal*, **294**, 997–1000

Koepsell, T. *et al.* (1989). Preliminary findings from a case–control study of risk of rheumatoid arthritis in relation to oral contraceptive use. *British Journal of Rheumatology*, **28**, 41.

Lau, E., Symmons, D., Bankhead, C., MacGregor, A., Donnan, S., and Silman, A. (1993). Low prevalence of rheumatoid arthritis in the urbanized Chinese of Hong Kong. *British Journal of Rheumatology*, **20**, 1133–7.

Lawrence, J.S. (1977). *Rheumatism in populations*. Heinemann, London.

Leading Article (1985). Arthritis and parvovirus infection. *Lancet*, i, 436–8.

Leino, P. and Magni, G. (1993). Depressive and distress symptoms as predictors of low back pain, neck-shoulder pain, and other musculoskeletal morbidity: a 10-year follow-up of metal industry employees. *Pain*, **53**, 89–94.

Linos, A. *et al.* (1980). The epidemiology of rheumatoid arthritis in Rochester Minnesota: a study of incidence, prevalence, and mortality. *American Journal of Epidemiology*, **111**, 86–98.

Linos, A., O'Fallon, W.M., Worthington, J.W., and Kurland, L.T. (1983). Case-control study of rheumatoid arthritis and prior use of oral contaceptive. *Lancet*, i, 1299–1300.

MacGregor, A.J. and Silman, A.J. (1992). A reappraisal of the measurement of disease occurrence in rheumatoid arthritis. *British Journal of Rheumatology*, **19**, 1163–5.

MacGregor, A.J., Riste, L.K., Hazes, J.M.W., and Silman, A.J. (1994a). Low prevalene of rheumatoid arthritis in black Caribbeans compared with whites in inner city Manchester. *Annals of the Rheumatic Diseases*, **53**, 293–7.

MacGregor, A.J., Bamber, S., and Silman, A.J. (1994b). A comparison of the performance of different methods of disease classification for rheumatoid arthritis. Results from a nationwide twin study. *Journal of Rheumatology*, **21**, 1420–26.

Maricq, H.R. *et al.* (1989). Prevalence of scleroderma spectrum disorders in the general population of South Carolina. *Arthritis and Rheumatism*, **32**, 998–1006.

Masi, A.T. *et al.* (1980). Preliminary criteria for the classification of systemic sclerosis (scleroderma). *Arthritis and Rheumatism*, **23**, 581–90.

McCarty, D.J., Kwoh, C.K., and LaPorte, R.E. (1992). The importance of incidence registries for connective tissue diseases. *British Journal of Rheumatology*, **19**, 1–7.

Michet, C.J. *et al.* (1985). Epidemiology of systemic lupus erythematosus and other connective tissue diseases in Rochester, Minnesota, 1950 through 1979. *Mayo Clinic Proceedings*, **60**, 105–13.

Moskowitz, M.A. *et al.* (1990). The relationship of oral contraceptive use to rheumatoid arthritis. *Epidemiology*, **1**, 153–6.

Mowat, A.G. and Hazleman, B.L. (1974). Polymyalgia rheumatica. A clinical study with particular reference to arterial disease. *Journal of Rheumatology*, **1**, 190–202.

Omland, O., Sommer, G., and Elling, H. (1986). Incidence of polymyalgia rheumatica/temporal arteritis in a Danish country. *Ugeskrift fur Laeger*, **143**, 981–3.

Rajala, S.A., Ahvenainen, J.E., Mattila, K.J., and Saarni, M.I. (1993). Incidence and survival rate in cases of biopsy-proven temporal arteritis. *Scandinavian Journal of Rheumatology*, **22**, 289–91.

Reid, D.M., Reid, T.M.S., Brown, T., and Rennie, J.A.N. (1985). Human parvovirus-associated arthritis: a clinical and laboratory description. *Lancet*, i, 422–5.

Rigby, A.S. (1991). Review of UK data on the rheumatic diseases—ankylosing spondylitis. *British Journal of Rheumatology*, **30**, 50–3.

Safavi, K.H., Heyse, S.P., and Hochberg, M.C. (1990). Estimating the incidence and prevalence of rare rheumatologic diseases: a review of methodology and available data sources. *Journal of Rheumatology*, **17**, 990–3.

Salvarani, C. *et al.* (1987). Polymyalgia rheumatica and giant cell arteritis: a 5-year epidemiologic and clinical study in Reggio Emilia, Italy. *Clinical and Experimental Rheumatology*, **5**, 205–15.

Silman, A.J. (1986). Epidemiology aspects of family studies in rheumatoid arthritis. *Disease Markers*, **4**, 55–9.

Silman, A.J. (1988). Has the incidence of rheumatoid arthritis declined in the United Kingdom? *British Journal of Rheumatology*, **27**, 77–8.

Silman, A.J. and Black, C. (1988). Increased incidence of spontaneous abortion infertility in women with scleroderma before disease onset. *Annals of the Rheumatic Diseases*, **47**, 441–4.

Silman, A.J. and Hochberg, M.C. (1993). *Epidemiology of the rheumatic diseases*. Oxford University Press, Oxford.

Silman, A.J. and Symmons, D.P.M. (1995). Selection of study population in the development of rheumatic disease criteria: comment on the article by the American College of Rheumatology Diagnostic and Therapeutic Criteria Committee. *Arthritis and Rheumatism*, **38**, 722.

Silman, A.J. and Vandenbroucke, J.P. (1989). Female sex hormones and rheumatoid arthritis. *British Journal of Rheumatology*, **28** (Suppl. 1), 1–73.

Silman, A.J., Ollier, W.E.R., and Currey, H.L.F. (1987). Failure to find disease similarity in sibling pairs with rheumatoid arthritis. *Annals of the Rheumatic Diseases*, **46**, 135–8.

Silman, A.J., Jannini, S., Symmons, D., and Bacon, P. (1988). An epidemiological study of scleroderma in the West Midlands. *British Journal of Rheumatology*, **27**, 286–90.

Silman, A.J., Ollier, W.E.R., and Bubel, M.A. (1989). Auto-immune thyroid disease and thyroid autoantibodies in rheumatoid arthritis patients and their families. *British Journal of Rheumatology*, **23**, 18–21.

Silman, A.J., Hicklin, A.J., and Black, C. (1990). Geographical clustering of scleroderma in South and West London. *British Journal of Rheumatology*, **29**, 92–6.

Silman, A.J. et al. (1993). Absence of rheumatoid arthritis in a rural Nigerian population. *Journal of Rheumatology*, **16**, 618–22.

Smith, C.A., Fidler, W.J., and Pinals, R.S. (1983). The epidemiology of giant cell arteritis. *Arthritis and Rheumatism*, **26**, 1214–19.

Solomon, L., Robin, G., and Valkenburg, H.A. (1975). Rheumatoid arthritis in an urban South African Negro population. *Annals of the Rheumatic Diseases*, **34**, 128–35.

Spector, T.D. and Hochberg, M.C. (1990). The protective effect of the oral contraceptive pill on rheumatoid arthritis. *Journal of Clinical Epidemiology*, **43**, 1221–30.

Spector, T.D. and Silman, A.J. (1987). Does the negative association between rheumatoid arthritis and schizophrenia provide clues to the aetiology of rheumatoid arthritis? *British Journal of Rheumatology*, **26**, 307–10.

Spector, T.D., Roman, E., and Silman, A.J. (1990). The pill, parity, and rheumatoid arthritis. *Arthritis and Rheumatism*, **33**, 782–9.

Steere, A.C. et al. (1977). An epidemic of oligoarticular arthritis in children and adults in three Connecticut communities. *Arthritis and Rheumatism*, **20**, 7–37.

Steere, A.C. et al. (1983). The spirochetal etiology of Lyme disease. *New England Journal of Medicine*, **308**, 733–9.

Stewart, O.J. and Silman, A.J. (1990). Review of UK data on the rheumatic diseases — gout. *British Journal of Rheumatology*, **29**, 485–8.

Symmons, D.P.M. (1991). Review of UK data on the rheumatic diseases — systemic lupus erythematosus. *British Journal of Rheumatology*, **30**, 288–90.

Symmons, D.P.M., Barrett, E.M., Bankhead, C.R., Scott, D.G.I., and Silman, A.J. (1994). The incidence of rheumatoid arthritis in the United Kingdom: results from the Norfolk Arthritis Register. *British Journal of Rheumatology*, **33**, 735–9.

Tan, E.M. (1982). The 1982 revised criteria for the classification of systemic lupus erythematosus. *Arthritis and Rheumatism*, **25**, 1271–7.

van der Linden, S., Valkenburg, H.A., and Catas, A. (1984). Evaluation of diagnostic criteria for ankylosing spondylitis. *Arthritis and Rheumatism*, **27**, 361–8.

Vandenbroucke, J.P. (1983). Oral contaceptives and rheumatoid arthritis. *Lancet*, **ii**, 1282.

Vandenbroucke, J.P. et al. (1982). Oral contraceptives and rheumatoid arthritis: further evidence for a preventive effect. *Lancet*, **ii**, 839–42.

Vandenbroucke, J.P. et al. (1986). Non-contraceptive hormones and rheumatoid arthritis in premenopausal and postmenopausal women. *Journal of the American Medical Association*, **255**, 1299–303.

van Saase, J.L.C.M. et al. (1989). Epidemiology osteoarthritis: Zoetermeer survey. Comparison of radiological osteoarthritis in a Dutch population with that in 10 other populations. *Annals of the Rheumatic Diseases*, **43**, 271–80.

Vaughan, J.H. (1979). Rheumatoid arthritis, rheumatoid factor, and the Epstein–Barr-Virus. *Journal of Rheumatology*, **6**, 381–8.

Vessey, M.P., Villard-Mackintosh, L., and Yeates, D. (1987). Oral contraceptives, cigarette smoking, and other factors in relation to arthritis. *Contraception*, **35**, 457–65.

White, D.G. et al. (1985). Human parvovirus arthropathy. *Lancet*, **i**, 419–21.

Wilkins, R.F. et al. (1981). Reiter's syndrome: evaluation of a preliminary criteria for definite disease. *Arthritis and Rheumatism*, **24**, 844–9.

Williams, G.H. and Silman, A.J. (1991). Review of UK data on the rheumatic diseases — scleroderma. *British Journal of Rheumatology*, **30**, 365–7.

Wingrave, S.J. (1978). Reduction in incidence of rheumatoid arthritis associated with oral contraceptives. *Lancet*, **i**, 569–71.

Wolfe, F., Kleinheksel, S.M., and Khan, M.A. (1988). Prevalence of familial occurrence in patients with rheumatoid arthritis. *British Journal of Rheumatology*, **27**, 150–52.

Wolfe, F. et al. (1990). The American College of Rheumatology 1990 criteria for the classification of fibromyalgia. *Arthritis and Rheumatism*, **33**, 160–72.

5.1.2 Epidemiology of rheumatic diseases in selected non-European populations

Patricia A. Fraser

Epidemiology is the study of the distribution, transmission, and control of disease (Masi 1984). The primary focus of this chapter is the variation in frequencies of rheumatic diseases among several ethnic groups. Ethnicity-specific disease expression also provides clues to aetiological factors for rheumatic diseases. Comparative analysis of the frequencies of specific disease manifestations is a secondary focus of this chapter. The gaps in our knowledge of the causes and the mechanisms of transmission of rheumatic diseases preclude discussion about control and interventions. Observed variations in incidence, prevalence, and clinical and laboratory manifestations of systemic rheumatic diseases between ethnic groups may result from environmental factors. The correlation of exposure to *Mycoplasma pneumoniae* respiratory infections and cyclic variation in incidence of juvenile rheumatoid arthritis in one Canadian province (Oen et al. 1995) emphasizes the importance of region-specific microbial exposure. Inherited factors contribute to susceptibility to rheumatic diseases. These genetic factors may be linked to, or regulated by, multiple loci throughout the human genome. If the genes of interest are polymorphic, their allelic frequencies may vary between ethnic groups. Such genetic variation may be the basis for ethnic differences in susceptibility and disease expression. Survival is one important prognostic feature of disease expression. Ethnic differences in disease mortality may be multifactorial. Studies of the prognosis for systemic lupus erythematosus in African Americans emphasize the importance of socioeconomic factors (Karlson et al. 1995). Future epidemiological studies of the rheumatic diseases should be designed to obtain data on multiple variables such as genetic markers at multiple loci, climate, microbial exposure, cultural or behavioural factors (e.g. dietary habits, tobacco and alcohol use) (Adebajo 1995), and the conundrum of 'socioeconomic status'.

The occurrence and manifestations of juvenile arthritis, rheumatoid arthritis, systemic lupus erythematosus, and the seronegative spondylarthropathies in selected non-European populations are presented in this chapter. Limited data on Caucasians of European descent will be presented for the purpose of comparison. Similarly, features of arthritic disorders will be compared between Native Americans and Eskimos and between Native Americans and Mexicans because of the common origin of Native Americans and Eskimos and because of the significant contribution of Native Americans to the gene pool of Mexicans (Williams et al. 1985).

Interethnic comparisons of the epidemiology of rheumatic diseases are hampered by the lack of uniform sampling and disease definitions, and also by limited or missing data on many ethnic groups. Clinical case series have been included for several ethnic groups when formal epidemiological studies of prevalence or incidence are not available. These data are not equivalent in their scientific rigor to formal epidemiological studies. They are presented for the purpose of completeness of information on rheumatic diseases worldwide.

Juvenile arthritis

Definition

Descriptive terms and definitions of chronic inflammatory arthritis in childhood are numerous. North American diagnostic criteria for juvenile rheumatoid arthritis (Brewer *et al.* 1977) and European criteria for juvenile chronic arthritis (Ansell 1978) provide the foundation for an evolving worldwide nomenclature and classification of juvenile arthritis shown in Table 1 (Ansell 1990) and Table 2 (Fink and Fernandez-Vina 1995).

Occurrence

Juvenile arthritis is the most common, childhood, chronic systemic rheumatic disease in the United States (Cassidy and Nelson 1988). This statistic reflects the frequency of juvenile arthritis in the largest ethnic group, Caucasians, and in Native Americans. Data on the occurrence of juvenile arthritis in Africa, Australia, and Asia are sparse.

Several survey methods have been used to estimate the occurrence of juvenile arthritis and other rheumatic diseases (Gewanter *et al.* 1983). The field population survey is the most accurate method because it includes actual physical examination of the population under study by trained observers. It is also the most costly. Estimates are also based on the number of cases presenting to a central clinic. The size of the source population must be known and it is assumed that all cases from this population base would present to this centre. The review of a medical records database for the diagnoses of interest has been used extensively. This approach also assumes the database captures virtually all of the source population. The practitioner survey interviews practitioners by questionnaire, which may be a preferable method in a population with a decentralized health-care system and has been used effectively to estimate frequencies for childhood rheumatic diseases in the United States (Gewanter *et al.* 1983).

Estimates of prevalence reveal an excess risk of juvenile arthritis among Native Americans when compared to Caucasians in various parts of North America. Juvenile arthritis is twice as common among Native Americans than among Caucasians in western Canada. Susceptibility to juvenile arthritis also varies between Native American tribal groups. In this analysis, data from Eskimo ethnic groups are compared to those from other Naive American tribal groups. The twofold difference in the prevalence of juvenile arthritis between Native Americans in Manitoba and British Columbia (Rosenberg *et al.* 1982) may be due to the high prevalence of juvenile-onset spondylarthropathy among the Native Americans of Manitoba (Hochberg 1984). Similarly designed studies reveal a variable prevalence for juvenile arthritis in several samples of Eskimos and Alaskan Native Americans (Oen *et al.* 1986; Boyer *et al.* 1988; Boyer *et al.* 1990; Boyer *et al.* 1991). The Inuit and Native Americans from the south-east coast of Alaska have the two highest reported prevalence rates for juvenile arthritis (126/100 000 and 83/100 000, respectively) (Oen *et al.* 1986; Boyer *et al.* 1991). Figure 1 includes estimates of the period prevalence of juvenile arthritis in Native Americans, Eskimos (Rosenberg *et al.* 1982; Oen *et al.* 1986; Boyer *et al.* 1988; Boyer *et al.* 1990; Boyer *et al.* 1991), and African Americans in Baltimore (Hochberg *et al.* 1983), and the frequency of juvenile arthritis in Caucasians in the United States (Lawrence *et al.* 1989) and Arabs in Kuwait, another Caucasian population (Khuffash and Majeed 1988).

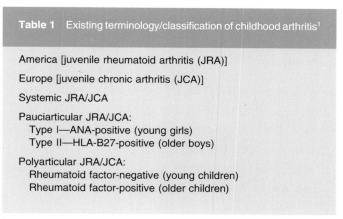

Table 1 Existing terminology/classification of childhood arthritis[1]

America [juvenile rheumatoid arthritis (JRA)]

Europe [juvenile chronic arthritis (JCA)]

Systemic JRA/JCA

Pauciarticular JRA/JCA:
   Type I—ANA-positive (young girls)
   Type II—HLA-B27-positive (older boys)

Polyarticular JRA/JCA:
   Rheumatoid factor-negative (young children)
   Rheumatoid factor-positive (older children)

[1]From Ansell (1990).
ANA, antinuclear antibody.

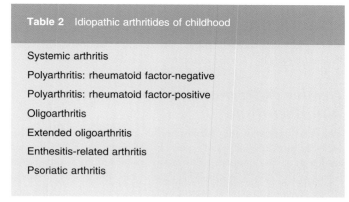

Table 2 Idiopathic arthritides of childhood

Systemic arthritis

Polyarthritis: rheumatoid factor-negative

Polyarthritis: rheumatoid factor-positive

Oligoarthritis

Extended oligoarthritis

Enthesitis-related arthritis

Psoriatic arthritis

Proposed classification from the Task Force of the Pediatric Standing Committee of the International League of Associations for Rheumatology (from Fink and Fernandez-Vina 1995).

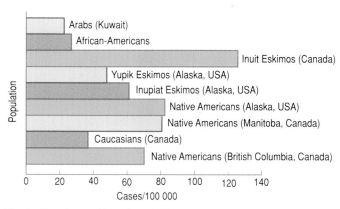

Fig. 1 Prevalence of juvenile arthritis.

Cases of juvenile arthritis have been observed in Chinese in Hawaii (Hicks 1977) and California (Hanson *et al.* 1977), but a formal estimate of the incidence of juvenile arthritis in British Columbia indicates that it is rare in North American Chinese (Hill 1976; Kelsey 1982). The incidence of juvenile arthritis in African Americans approximates that observed in Caucasians in the United States (Lawrence *et*

Table 3   Annual incidence rate per 100 000 of juvenile arthritis

Population	Rate
Chinese (Canada)	0.00
Caucasian (British Columbia, Canada)	2.20
Native American (British Columbia)	7.20
Native Americans (S.E. Alaska, USA)	38.6
Inupiat Eskimo (Alaska, USA)	28.0
Yupik Eskimo (Alaska, USA)	42.5
Inuit Eskimos (Canada)	23.6
African American	6.20
Caucasian (USA)	9.20

al. 1989). Differences in method may account for the disparity in incidence estimates between United States and Canadian Caucasians. Incidence rates by race and ethnicity are listed in Table 3.

Gender differences and laboratory manifestations

The distribution of the different onset types of juvenile arthritis varies by race, ethnicity, and region. For example, onset types varied among three predominantly Caucasian samples in the United States (Hanson et al. 1977; Jacobs 1982; Aaron et al. 1985). In view of the strong genetic component in predisposition to juvenile arthritis and the known variation in the frequency of genetic markers within an ethnic group, the observed difference in the distribution of onset types in United States Caucasians may reflect the particular ethnic composition (e.g. ratio of individuals of northern versus southern

European origin) in these samples. Smaller samples of individuals with juvenile arthritis in other ethnic groups also demonstrate variability in the distribution of onset types. Polyarticular-onset juvenile arthritis was twice as common among Canadian Native Americans as Canadian Caucasians (Rosenberg et al. 1982). Comparison of three samples of patients with juvenile arthritis among black Africans revealed different proportions of onset types and no evidence for a regional trend (Kanyerezi and Mbidde 1980; Gupta et al. 1981; Haffejee et al. 1984). The studies of juvenile arthritis among Kuwaiti Arabs (Khuffash and Majeed 1988), Ugandans (Kanyerezi and Mbidde 1980), Zambians (Gupta et al. 1981), Black and Indian South Africans (Haffejee et al. 1984), and Mexicans (Martinez-Cairo Cueto et al. 1978) are presented in Table 4.

Equal sex ratios among Black and Indian South African (Haffejee et al. 1984) and Mexican individuals with juvenile arthritis (Martinez-Cairo Cueto et al. 1978) contrast with the female predominance in samples of Native American and North American Caucasians with juvenile arthritis (Rosenberg et al. 1982, Aaron et al. 1985) (Table 5). With the exception of two studies on sex ratios (Hanson et al. 1977; Aaron et al. 1985), data were not analysed to demonstrate the age dependence of sex ratios in pauciarticular juvenile arthritis (i.e. girls more often affected than boys in early onset, boys more than girls in late onset).

The frequencies of antinuclear antibodies for individuals with juvenile arthritis in three racial groups in Table 6 are much lower than a recent report from the United States. Szer et al. (1991) noted antinuclear antibody positivity of 83, 42, and 39 per cent for patients with pauciarticular, polyarticular, and systemic juvenile arthritis, respectively. This discrepancy may be due to difficulty in comparing clinical case series and epidemiological studies, or to differences in laboratory methods, or both.

Case series must be utilized when we consider comparisons of rheumatoid factor positivity. With the exception of black Ugandans, rheumatoid factor-positive juvenile arthritis is threefold greater in the non-European populations included, although the proportion of polyarticular-onset juvenile arthritis is not significantly different

Table 4   Juvenile arthritis onset types by author, race, or ethnicity

Race/ethnicity/author and/or locale	Number	Systemic (%)	Polyarticular (%)	Pauciarticular (%)
Caucasians[a] (USA; Jacobs 1982)	260	9.0	16.0	75.0
Caucasians[a] (USA; Hanson et al. 1977)	563	43.0	23.0	34.0
Caucasians[a] (USA; Aaron et al. 1985)	327	15.0	27.0	58.0
Native Americans	34	11.8	58.8	29.4
Arabs (Kuwait)	41	39.0	39.0	22.0
Blacks (Uganda)	41	54.0	37.0	9.0
Blacks (Zambia)	8	37.5	37.5	25.0
Blacks (South Africa)	42	15.0	50.0	35.0
Indians (South Africa)	18	16.6	44.4	39.0
Mexicans	46	28.3	45.6	26.1

[a]Sample composition is >95% US Caucasian.

Table 5 Female:male ratio by onset type or all juvenile arthritis (JA)

Race or ethnicity	Systemic	Polyarticular	Pauciarticular	All JA
Native Americans (British Columbia)				4.1:1
Caucasians (British Columbia)				5.8:1
Blacks/Indians (South Africa)	1.25:1	1.1:1	0.83:1	1:1
Mexicans	0.63:1	2:1	0.7:1	1.1:1
Arabs	2.2:1	33:1	8:1	1.3:1
US Caucasians (Hanson *et al.* 1977)	1.1:1	3.8:1	3.2:1	2:1
US Caucasians (Aaron *et al.* 1985)	1.6:1	5.3:1	2:1	2.4:1
Inuit				1:1

Table 6 Frequency (per cent), of antinuclear antibody by race or ethnicity by onset type or juvenile arthritis (JA) unclassified

Race or ethnic group	Systemic	Polyarticular	Pauciarticular	JA
Native Americans (British Columbia)				53.3
Caucasians (British Columbia)				28.8
Black/Indian (South Africa)				6.8

Table 7 Frequency (per cent) of rheumatoid factor by race or ethnicity by onset subtype or unclassified juvenile arthritis (JA)

Race or ethnicity	Systemic	Polyarticular	Pauciarticular	JA
Native Americans (Alaska)				32.0
Native Americans (British Columbia)				36.0
Caucasians (British Columbia)				9.1
Black (South Africa)				38.0
Indian (South Africa)				33.0
Mexican	30.7	42.8	16.6	33.0
Black (Uganda)				10.0

among these populations. The disparity between the proportions of polyarticular-onset juvenile arthritis and seropositivity may indicate the presence of other stimuli for rheumatoid factor production such as malaria or other recurrent parasitic infections and tuberculosis (Haffejee *et al.* 1984). Estimates of the seroprevalence of rheumatoid factor in juvenile arthritis are presented in Table 7.

Juvenile spondylarthropathies

Juvenile-onset seronegative spondylarthropathies, which include ankylosing spondylitis, Reiter's syndrome, and seronegative enthesopathy and arthropathy syndrome (Rosenberg and Petty 1982), account for at least half of the arthritides of childhood in

Table 8 Juvenile spondylarthropathies (SPA): Prevalence (cases/100 000), incidence (cases/100 000 per year), ratio of SPA:juvenile arthritis (JA), and frequency of HLA-B27 (per cent)

Population	Diagnosis	Number of cases	Prevalence	Incidence	SPA:JA	HLA-B27
Native Americans (British Columbia)	All SPA	14	29.4		0.82:1	70
	SEA	5				
	AS	3				
	RS	4				
Native Americans (Alaska)	All SPA	9			3.75:1	
	SEA	7				
	RS	2				
Yupik Eskimo	All SPA	21			7:1	
	SEA	17				
	RS/AS	4				
Inupiat Eskimo	All SPA	5		47.4	5:1	
	SEA	2				
	RS	2				
	AS	1				
Inuit	All SPA	11	367	105.6	4.5:1	

AS, ankylosing spondylitis; RS, Reiter's syndrome; SEA, seronegative enthesopathy and arthropathy.

native North American populations. Specific criteria for childhood-onset ankylosing spondylitis are necessary since the application of adult criteria have limited value (Singsen 1990) and may result in underestimation of this condition. The demographic, clinical, and laboratory features of juvenile-onset spondylarthropathies (Rosenberg *et al.* 1982; Oen *et al.* 1986; Boyer *et al.* 1988; Boyer *et al.* 1990; Boyer *et al.* 1991) are summarized in Table 8.

Rheumatoid arthritis

Several variables affect comparisons of the prevalence estimates for rheumatoid arthritis.

Definition

The case definition of rheumatoid arthritis varies between studies. This non-uniform disease definition resulted from the evolution of disease criteria for rheumatoid arthritis over time — the Manchester grading system, the 1958 and 1962 American Rheumatism Association criteria, the New York criteria, 1987 revised, for rheumatoid arthritis [(Ropes *et al.* (1958), Lawrence (1961), Kellgren (1962), Lawrence and Wood (1963), and Arnett *et al.* (1988), respectively]. The earliest prevalence estimates to be presented in this section, from New Zealand Maoris (Rose and Prior 1963), rural Japan (Shichikawa *et al.* 1981), Jamaica (Lawrence *et al.* 1966), Puerto Rico (Mendez-Bryan *et al.* 1964), Liberia and Nigeria (Muller 1970), and among the South African Bantu (Solomon *et al.* 1975; Beighton *et al.* 1975), included probable and definite cases of rheumatoid arthritis. In later studies, prevalence rates were based on classical and definite cases of rheumatoid arthritis.

Occurrence

Rheumatoid arthritis does not occur at the same frequency at all ages. Its age distribution may vary between populations. Crude estimates of prevalence in populations with a younger age structure will be lower than age-adjusted prevalence rates since rheumatoid arthritis is a disease of middle age. This potential source of bias is one explanation offered for the very low prevalence of rheumatoid arthritis in several studies from different Asian and African, and African-derived population samples (Mijiyawa 1995).

Population sampling may also affect the comparability of data. Population-based epidemiological studies are preferred, when feasible.

Rheumatoid arthritis occurs in India, Pakistan, Oman, and Iraq at frequencies (0.75–1.98 per cent) similar to that observed in the United Kingdom and the United States (Al-Rawi *et al.* 1978; Pountain 1991; Malaviya *et al.* 1993; Hameed *et al.* 1995). The common methods used to estimate the occurrence of rheumatoid arthritis among samples of Native American facilitate the comparison of prevalence estimates among these groups. It is noteworthy that rheumatoid arthritis was confined to women in an Inuit sample, although records of both sexes were reviewed (Oen *et al.* 1986). In contrast, a field population survey among the Yakima was limited to women (Beasley *et al.* 1973). Variability between ethnic groups was observed between tribal groups and by locale. The majority (76 per cent) of those with rheumatoid arthritis among south-eastern Alaskan Native Americans were of Tlingit ancestry (Boyer *et al.* 1991). The prevalence of rheumatoid arthritis varied among the groups of Native Americans studied (Chippewa, Haida, Nootka and Pima, Yupik, and Inupiat Eskimos) from 0.6 to 7.1 per cent, with the highest rates among the Chippewa and the Pima (7.1 and 5.3 per cent, respectively) (Gofton *et al.* 1964; Harvey *et al.* 1983; Atkins *et al.* 1988; Del Puente *et al.* 1989; Boyer *et al.* 1990; Boyer *et al.* 1991).

Rheumatoid arthritis occurs at a lower frequency in populations of African ancestry when compared to Caucasians. This is best exemplified in a study in Manchester, England, where the age-adjusted prevalence of rheumatoid arthritis was significantly lower in Afro-Caribbeans (Afro-Caribbean: Caucasian 0.36:1) (MacGregor *et al.* 1994), and in a study that failed to detect any cases of rheumatoid arthritis among 2000 rural Nigerians (Silman *et al.* 1993).

Comparison of the prevalence rates of rheumatoid arthritis among populations of black African descent is more problematical and necessitates review of the raw data. This is necessary because several disease definitions were used in the studies of interest. Intercontinental differences in population age structure may also contribute to the observed differences in the prevalence of rheumatoid arthritis. For example, the age distribution in the United States is significantly older than that in most sub-Saharan African nations (Hall 1991). Since rheumatoid arthritis occurs most frequently in young and middle-aged adults, a country such as the United States may have a higher prevalence of rheumatoid arthritis on the basis of the age distribution of its population. The combined prevalence of definite and classical rheumatoid arthritis has been estimated for African Americans (Lawrence *et al.* 1989), while prevalence data for probable and definite rheumatoid arthritis are available from Jamaica and several black African samples. Variability is observed if the prevalence of definite rheumatoid arthritis among samples of black African descent is compared. Although the prevalence of definite rheumatoid arthritis is similar for African Americans, rural Jamaicans, and urban South African Bantu (Lawrence *et al.* 1966; Solomon *et al.* 1975; Lawrence *et al.* 1989), estimates from rural Africa are significantly lower (Beighton *et al.* 1975; Moolenburgh *et al.* 1984; Brighton *et al.* 1988). With the exception of the Jamaican sample, there is a striking difference between urban and rural black populations. This is best illustrated in southern Africa, where rural and urban estimates among the Tswana reveal a more than threefold difference in the prevalence of rheumatoid arthritis (Beighton *et al.* 1975; Solomon *et al.* 1975). It is difficult to draw any conclusions about ethnic differences in predisposition in black African populations. A study of 39 patients with rheumatoid arthritis admitted to a central hospital in Uganda did not show any ethnic predisposition among the Baganda, Banyarwanda, and Banyankole, the major tribal groups in that region (Kanyerezi 1969). A similar investigation in western Nigeria also failed to show heightened susceptibility in any ethnic group (Greenwood 1969).

The hypotheses that rheumatoid arthritis is a relatively new disease in Africa (Adebajo 1991) and that it is due to infection with a slow virus (Buchanan and Murdoch 1979) may explain the difference in urban and rural prevalence estimates for rheumatoid arthritis in Africa in populations of Bantu ancestry. Presumably, urban Bantu dwellers had greater exposure to the putative viral infection than did rural inhabitants. Similarly, the very low prevalence of the disease (0.2–0.5 per cent) among rural and urban Chinese in the People's Republic of China, Taiwan, Hong Kong, three Japanese samples, and Indonesia (Kato *et al.* 1971, Shichikawa *et al.* 1981; Beasley *et al.* 1983; Lau *et al.* 1993; Darmawan *et al.* 1993; Chou *et al.* 1994; Wigley *et al.* 1994) may indicate lack of exposure to the rheumatoid arthritis-associated virus. These hypotheses do not explain the very low prevalence of rheumatoid arthritis (0.1 per cent) in Chile, which is possibly due to the age distribution of the population (Gomez-Carpio *et al.* 1966).

Such theories of differential susceptibility or aetiological agents can neither be confirmed nor refuted until standardized disease definitions are used to estimate the age-adjusted prevalence of rheumatoid arthritis in population-based studies. Table 9 lists 45 prevalence estimates for rheumatoid arthritis.

Comparative analyses of seropositivity in rheumatoid and non-rheumatoid arthritis show rates of seropositivity in non-rheumatoid from 2 to 20 per cent and between 9 to 94 per cent in rheumatoid (Table 10). It is interesting that two studies from Nigeria made more than 20 years apart provide very different estimates of the seroprevalence of rheumatoid factor (Greenwood 1969; Adebajo *et al.* 1993). A longitudinal study of rheumatoid factor and rheumatoid arthritis in the Pima indicated that the titre of rheumatoid factor predicts the risk of developing rheumatoid arthritis in this population (Del Puente *et al.* 1988). This observation may also explain the high prevalence rates of rheumatoid arthritis and of seropositive rheumatoid arthritis (78–94 per cent) among other Native American groups.

Systemic lupus erythematosus

Definition

The analysis of Jamaicans with systemic lupus erythematosus (Wilson and Hughes 1979) utilized 1971 criteria to define the disease (Cohen *et al.* 1971). The remainder of the studies used the 1982 revised criteria (Tan *et al.* 1982).

Occurrence

Although there is little evidence for geographic clustering of systemic lupus erythematosus (Wallace and Quismorio 1995), there are abundant data to support the concept of differential susceptibility to lupus associated with ethnicity. The prevalence of systemic lupus erythematosus among African Americans is more than threefold greater than among Caucasians in the same regions (Siegel and Lee 1973; Fessel 1974). The available rates for systemic lupus in African Americans are stratified by sex and age, with peak prevalence between 15 and 64 years. United States incidence data are two- to threefold greater in African American than Caucasian women (McCarty *et al.* 1995). The same trends are seen in data from Afro-Caribbeans in Birmingham, UK (Johnson *et al.* 1995). The excess risk of systemic lupus erythematosus in populations of African ancestry residing outside continental Africa are unexplained. Genetic admixture of the lupus-prone individuals has been offered as a possible explanation for the excess susceptibility (Symmons 1995). The only study to address admixture in systemic lupus found no difference in its level (approx. 28 per cent) between African Americans patients in Baltimore and local controls (Bias *et al.* 1992). In several samples, age of onset in African-Americans and Afro-Caribbeans is significantly younger than locale-matched Caucasian lupus patients (Johnson *et al.* 1995; McCarty *et al.* 1995). Estimates of systemic lupus erythematosus occurrence in Curacao, a Caribbean island largely populated by descendants of enslaved Africans, differ slightly from other samples of African ancestry. Although the peak incidence occurs among women 45 to 65 years exceeds that for the 15 to 44 age group (186.6 versus 102.9/100 000) (Nossent 1992). The minor discordance between these two rates are not due to differences in mortality rates. Figure 2 summarizes age-specific population, prevalence, incidence, and mortality data for the Curacao sample.

Table 9 Prevalence rates of rheumatoid arthritis

Population	Type of estimate	Criteria for diagnosis	Prevalence (cases/100)	
			Females	Total
Inuit Eskimo	Database	1958		1.82
Yupik Eskimo	Database	1958	1.00	0.60
Inupiat Eskimo	Database	1958	1.10	0.70
Native Americans (Alaska)	Database	1958	3.50	2.40
Haida Native Americans (Canada)	Population	1958, 1962 Manchester[b]	1.50	1.00
Nootka native Americans (Canada)	Population	1958		1.40
Pima Native Americans (USA)	Population	1962[c]	6.95	5.30
Yakima Native Americans (USA)	Population	New York[d]	3.40	
Chippewa Native Americans (USA)	Population	1958		5.30
Wayakama, Japan (rural)	Population	1962		0.50
Hiroshima+Nagasaki, Japan (urban)	Population	1958	0.64	0.47
African Americans	Population	1958		0.9*
Jamaica	Population	1958	6.0/1.6*	4.3/1.1*
Black Caribbean (Manchester, UK)	Population	1987		0.29
Liberia	Population	1962 + Manchester	2.1	2.3
Igbo-Oro (Nigeria)	Population	1962 + Manchester	0.0	1.0
Isheri (Nigeria)	Population	1962 + Manchester	3.7	3.1
Igbo-Oro (Nigeria)	Population	1987	0.0	0.0
Bantu (South Africa—urban)	Population	1962	3.7/1.4*	3.3/0.9*
Tswana (South Africa—rural)	Population	1962	0.4	0.87/0.12*
Basutho (Lesotho—rural)	Central	1962	0.19	0.23/0.20*
Venda (South Africa—rural)	Population	1962		0.0026*
Xhosa (South Africa—rural)	Population	1962		2.2/0.68*
Puerto Rico	Population	1958	1.2	0.93
Maoris, New Zealand	Population	1962		3.3
Kinmen, China (rural)	Population	1962	0.4	0.3*
Hong Kong (urban)	Population	1958, 1962, 1987		0.35
Han (North China, rural)	Population	?		0.34
Han (South China, rural)	Population	?		0.32
Taiwan (rural)	Population	1958		0.26
Taiwan (suburban)	Population	1958		0.78
Taiwan (urban)	Population	1958		0.93
India (rural)	Population	1987		0.75
Pakistan (urban, poor)	Population	1987		0.90
Pakistan (urban, affluent)	Population	1987		1.98
Indonesia (rural)	Population	1958		0.20
Indonesia (urban)	Population	1958		0.30
Oman	Population	1987		0.84
Iraq	Population	1958		1.00

Table 9 Prevalence rates of rheumatoid arthritis (continued)

Population	Type of estimate	Criteria for diagnosis	Prevalence (cases/100)	
			Females	Total
Santiago, Chile	Central	1962		0.10*
Monterrey, Mexico	Central	1987		0.68
El Salvador	Not specified	1987		0.86

*Computed from definite or definite + classical rheumatoid arthritis cases only.
[a]Ropes *et al.* (1958); [b]Lawrence (1961); [c]Kellgren (1962); [d]Lawrence and Wood (1963).

Table 10 Frequency (per cent) rheumatoid factor seropositivity in selected normal and rheumatoid arthritis (RA) samples

Population/locale	Type of sample	Total	Non-RA	RA
USA	Population		2.6	32.0
Uganda	Hospitalized			51.3[a]
Western Nigeria	Hospitalized		11.4	13.0[b]
Ibadan, Nigeria	Central clinic		4.0	47.0[c]
Jamaica	Population	1.6		20.0
Tswana (rural South Africa)	Central clinic			8.90[d]
Tswana (urban South Africa)	Central clinic			12.1[e]
Xhosa (rural South Africa)	Central clinic			17.0[f]
Cape Town, South Africa	Central clinic			85.0[g]
Xhosa (rural South Africa)	Population	17.0	14.7	50.0[h]
Basutho (Lesotho)	Population		12–19	54.8[i]
Chippewa (USA)	Population		10.0	92
Yakima (USA)	Population		3.0	94
Haida (Canada)	Population	3.5	2.0	50
Yupik (Alaska)	Population			78
Inuit (Alaska)	Population			83
Japan (urban)	Population	8.9	7.4	75
China (rural)	Population		1.7	28

[a]Kanyerezi (1969); [b]Greenwood (1969); [c]Adebajo *et al.* (1993); [d]Meyers *et al.* (1983); [e]Meyers *et al.* (1983); [f]Meyers *et al.* (1983); [g]Mody and Meyers (1989); [h]Meyers *et al.* (1977); [i]Moolenburgh *et al.* (1984).

Among Native American women in Alaska aged 15 to 64 years, the prevalence of systemic lupus erythematosus is 280/100 000, which is intermediate between estimates for United States Caucasians and African Americans (140/100 000 and 410/100 000, respectively) (Boyer *et al.* 1991). The Nootka Native Americans in British Colombia have the highest reported prevalence of systemic lupus (500 cases/100 000 population) (Atkins *et al.* 1988), while the Sioux, Crow, and Arapaho exhibited the highest incidence rates of systemic lupus in a survey of 75 Native American peoples (Morton *et al.* 1976). The estimates for the Nootka, Crow, and Arapaho were derived from small populations (2000–3000) and it is likely that the incidence estimate for the Sioux is the most accurate (Hochberg 1990) because they were the most numerous group studied (population = 30 000).

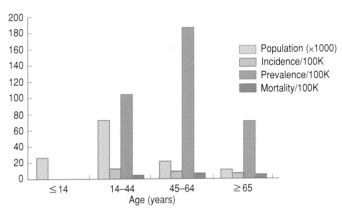

Fig. 2 Age-specific population, prevalence, incidence, and mortality in Curacao.

Black South Africans were over-represented among inpatients with systemic lupus erythematosus in Cape Town (Jessop and Meyers 1973; Fessel 1988). Since admission to hospital with systemic lupus is highly correlated with disease severity, the disproportionate number of Blacks may reflect more severe disease rather than excess risk of lupus. This conclusion in supported by estimates from a central clinic in Johannesburg where the highest prevalence and incidence of systemic lupus was among Asian Indians, with decrements in the frequency among Coloured or mixed-race individuals and Caucasians, and the lowest frequencies in Blacks (Morrison *et al.* 1990).

Higher prevalence rates of systemic lupus erythematosus have been observed among Chinese, Japanese, and Filipinos in Hawaii, and Polynesians in New Zealand, when compared to Caucasians in either locale (Serdula and Rhoads 1979; Hart *et al.* 1983; Catalano and

Table 11 Prevalence (cases/100 000) and incidence (new cases/100 000 per year) of systemic lupus

Population (locale)	Type of sample	Prevalence		Incidence
		All	**15–64 yrs**	
African American female	Not specified	283.0[a]	410.0[b]	8.1[c], 11.4[d]
African American male[e]	Not specified	53.0		
African American female	Population-based registry			9.2[f]
African American male	Population-based registry			0.7[g]
Afro-Caribbean female (UK)	Multisource registry	197.2[h]		
Curacao female	Hospital	83.8		7.9[i]
Curacao male	Hospital	8.5		1.1[j]
Venezuela female	Inpatient	9.27		
Venezuela male	Inpatient	0.8[k]		
Native American-female[l] (Alaska)	Population		280.0	
Eskimo (Alaska)[m]	Population	11.4		
Sioux Native American[n]	Inpatient			16.6
Caucasian female (USA)[o]	Not specified	71.0	140.0	3.90
Caucasian (New Zealand)[p]	Composite[q]	14.6		
Polynesian (New Zealand)	Composite	51	99	
Japanese (Hawaii)[t]	Not specified	27.5		
Chinese (Hawaii)[w]	Not specified	10.3		
Caucasian (South Africa)[x]	Central clinic	23.9		1.95
Black (South Africa)[x]	Central clinic	12.2		1.03
Coloured (South Africa)[x]	Central clinic	20.7		1.60
Indian (South Africa)[x]	Central clinic	69.3		6.33

[a]Fessel (1974), data from Hochberg (1990; Table 4); [b]Fessel (1974), data from Hochberg (1990; Table 4); [c]Siegel and Lee (1973), data from Hochberg (1990); Table 3; [d]data from Hochberg (1990; Table 3); [e]Fessel (1974); [f]McCarty *et al.* (1995); [g]McCarty *et al.* (1995); [h]Johnson *et al.* (1995); [i]Nossent (1992); [j]Nossent (1992); [k]Abadi and Gonzalez (1990); [l]Boyer *et al.* (1991); [m]Boyer *et al.* (1991); [n]Morton *et al.* (1976) [o]Fessel (1974); [p]Hart *et al.* (1983); [q]hospital disk data and practitioner survey; [r]Hart *et al.* (1983); [s]Nakae *et al.* (1987), from Hochberg (1990); Table 2; [t]Catalano and Hoffmeier (1989), from Hochberg (1990; Table 5); [u]Nai-Zheng (1989), from Hochberg (1990); [v]Catalano and Hoffmeier (1989), from Hochberg (1990; Table 5); [w]Catalano and Hoffmeier (1989), from Hochberg (1990; Table 5); [x]Morrison *et al.* (1990).

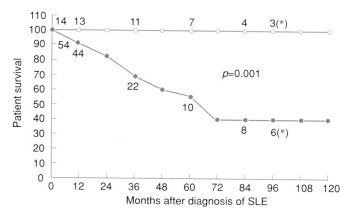

Fig. 3 Survival of lupus patients in Curacao stratified by renal involvement. *Number of patients still in study.

Hoffmeier 1989), but for several reasons we cannot determine whether so-called mongoloid ethnic groups originating in Asia are more susceptible to systemic lupus than are Caucasians. Estimates from China and Japan give rates similar to those computed in Hawaii but there were no local Caucasians available for comparison in those countries. Furthermore, comparisons of international rates among Caucasians also reveal significant variability (Hochberg 1990). The application of similar methods (Hochberg 1990) and an assessment of racial heterogeneity (Fessel 1988) are necessary to determine whether these ethnic groups exhibit a significant predisposition to

systemic lupus. Prevalence and incidence estimates appear in Table 11.

Clinical and laboratory manifestations

The ratio of females to males with systemic lupus erythematosus in the Unites States is 8–10:1 (Siegel and Lee 1973; Fessel 1974) and approaches 12:1 in Venezuela (Abadi and Gonzalez 1990). Case series in Latin America may indicate higher female to male ratios than among United States Caucasians (Alarcon 1986). Populations of black African descent in Jamaica and the United States demonstrate an earlier age of onset than Caucasians (Wilson and Hughes 1979; Ballou *et al.* 1982; Hochberg *et al.* 1985; Ward and Studenski 1990; Smikle *et al.* 1995), more frequent and more severe renal involvement, and greater mortality (Harris *et al.* 1989; Williams *et al.* 1990; Smikle *et al.* 1995) Earlier age of onset is associated with HLA-DR8 in African Americans (Reveille *et al.* 1989). Among African Americans, discoid lupus (Hochberg *et al.* 1985; Ward and Studenski 1990), lupus pneumonitis, serositis, nephritis, hypocomplementaemia, hyperglobulinaemia (Ballou *et al.* 1982; Hochberg *et al.* 1985) and anti-Sm and antiribonucleoprotein (Ward and Studenski 1990) are significantly more common than among United States Caucasians, while photosensitivity is significantly less frequent (Hochberg *et al.* 1985; Ward and Studenski 1990). Photosensitivity occurs with a similar frequency among African Americans residing in a temperate climate and Jamaicans who are exposed to a subtropical climate. Interestingly, photosensitivity is twice as common in black South Africans who also reside in a temperate zone as among African Americans. The propensity for renal involvement in Afro-Caribbeans is best exemplified by the cohort analysis in Curacao. Lupus nephritis

Table 12 Frequency (percentage) of clinical and laboratory manifestations of systemic lupus in selected samples

Feature	USA		Jamaica		Curacao	Southern Africa		
	Ward[a]	Hochberg[b]	Wilson[c]	Smikle[g]	Nossent[h]	Morrison[d] (i/ii/iii)	Taylor[e]	Dessein[f]
Oral/nasal ulcers	21.4			13	19		19	23
Photosensitivity	15.5	11	12	12	25	32/8/27	16	13
Discoid rash	16.0	35					19	27
Renal	51.9	49	40		78	83/66/100	71	60
All CNS			58				13	20
Seizures	14.4				18		6	10
Psychosis	13.4				3		6	
Anti-DNA	63.6	30			97	48/100/86	100	81
Anti-Sm	17.1	24		17	4			
Anti-RNP	26.2	41						
Hypocomplementaemia	61.0	81						

[i]Frequency in South African Blacks; [ii]frequency in Coloureds; [iii]frequency in Indians.
[a]From Ward and Studenski (1990; Tables 2 and 3); [b]from Hochberg *et al.* (1985; Table 3); [c]from Wilson and Hughes (1979; Tables 6 and 8); [d]from Morrison *et al.* (1990); [e]from Taylor and Stein (1986; Table 1); [f]from Dessein *et al.* (1988; Tables 1 and 2); [g]from Smikle *et al.* (1995); [h]from Nossent (1993; Table 1).

Table 13 Prevalence of seronegative spondylarthropathies (SPA)

Population (locale)	Disease	Criteria	Rate (cases/100)
Haida Native Americans (Canada)	AS	New York	6.7
Haida Native Americans (Alaska)	AS	New York	0.8
Other Native Americans (Alaska)	All SPA	Composite[a]	1.1
Yupik Eskimos (Alaska)	AS	Rome	0.2
Yupik Eskimos (Alaska)	RS	ARA (1981)	0.23
Inupiat Eskimos (Alaska)	AS	Rome	0.1
Inupiat Eskimos (Alaska)	RS	ARA (1981)	0.6
Inuit Eskimos (Alaska)	AS	New York	0.34
Inuit Eskimos (Alaska)	RS		0.63
Inuit Eskimos (Greenland)	RS	ARA (1981)	1.08/0.35[b]
Navajo Native Americans (USA)	RS		0.3[c]
Chinese (Kinmen Island)	AS		0.3[d]

AS, ankylosing spondylitis; RS, Reiter's syndrome.
[a]Boyer *et al.* (1991) used New York criteria for AS, American Rheumatism Association 1981 criteria for RS, and working criteria for undifferentiated SPA;
[b]Estimates from Greenland Community's A and B, respectively, from Boyer *et al.* (1990; Table 3);
[c]From Morse *et al.* (1981)
[d]From Beasley *et al.* (1983).

occurred at some time during the follow-up period in 78 per cent of patients (Figure 3) and was associated with greater mortality (Nossent 1993*a*). When multiple prognostic variables were examined, the SLEDAI score which incorporates data on active renal disease was more powerful than the variable for renal involvement alone as a predictor of mortality (Nossent 1993*b*). The frequencies of clinical and laboratory features of systemic lupus erythematosus in African American, Jamaican, and black South African and Zimbabwean samples are listed in Table 12 (Wilson and Hughes 1979; Hochberg *et al.* 1985; Taylor and Stein 1986; Dessein *et al.* 1988; Morrison *et al.* 1990; Ward and Studenski 1990; Nossent 1993*b*; Smikle *et al.* 1995).

Seronegative spondylarthropathies

Definition

The seronegative spondylarthropathies are a group of chronic rheumatic diseases characterized by variable combinations of asymmetrical peripheral arthritis, enthesopathy, involvement of the axial skeleton, mucocutaneous symptoms, higher than expected frequencies of the *HLA-B27* allele, and the absence of rheumatoid factor. Ankylosing spondylitis, Reiter's syndrome/'reactive arthritis', psoriatic arthritis/spondylitis, and inflammatory bowel disease-associated spondylitis are included within the spondylarthropathy category. Also to be included are syndromes that have several features of spondylarthropathies but do not meet the criteria for any one. The term undifferentiated spond(lyo)arthropathy has been designated for these conditions (Boyer *et al.* 1988).

The Rome criteria (Kellgren 1962) and the New York criteria (Bennett and Wood 1968) have been developed to assess the frequency of ankylosing spondylitis in populations. The Rome criteria are more suited to field studies since they do not require radiographs to make the diagnosis of definite ankylosing spondylitis. The criteria for Reiter's syndrome (Willkens *et al.* 1981) and the undifferentiated spondylarthropathies (Boyer *et al.* 1988) have not been used as extensively as those for ankylosing spondylitis. Also problematical is the relation of sacroiliitis to the groups of spondylarthropathy. Is asymptomatic sacroiliitis distinct from clinical spondylarthropathy or does it represent one end of the spectrum of spondylarthropathic disease expression?

Occurrence

Prevalence estimates for spondylarthropathies for several Native American and Eskimo groups and the Chinese (Morse *et al.* 1980; Beasley *et al.* 1983; Oen *et al.* 1986; Boyer *et al.* 1988; Boyer *et al.* 1990; Boyer *et al.* 1991) appear in Table 13. HLA-B27 and spondylarthropathies occur at higher frequencies in several Native American groups than in Caucasians, with the highest recorded rates among the Haida in Canada. The published criteria for Reiter's syndrome were not used in the Navajo (the study preceded the publication of the criteria) nor in one of the Inuit studies, so the accuracy and comparability of these estimates is uncertain.

In sharp contrast to the Native American groups, spondylarthropathy is diagnosed infrequently in African Americans and black Africans (Baum and Ziff 1971). The frequency of spondylarthropa-

Table 14 HLA-B27 frequency in caucasoid, mongoloid, and negroid populations

	Ankylosing spondylitis		Normal controls	
	No. of patients	B27-positive (%)	No. of controls	B27-positive (%)
Caucasian				
Euro-Caucasoids (whites)	2022	79–100	16 162	4–13
Indians and Pakistanis	130	83–100	456	2–8
Iranians	25	92	400	3
Arabs	32	81	355	3
Jews	31	81	456	3
Mongoloid				
Chinese:				
Mainland China	196	69–91	726	2–7
Hong Kong	77	99	102	4
Taiwan	75	95	297	9
Singapore	29	97	238	7
Japanese	72	82	208	<1
Filipino	17	94	529	5–8
Thai	71	86	138	5
North American Indians:				
Haida	17	100	222	50
Navajo	5	80	100	36
Bella Colla	3	100	129	25
Pima	14	100	400	18
Zuni			158	13
Hopi			100	9
Mestizo[a]	239	69–81	1404	3–7
South American Indians[b]			440	0
Negroid				
African blacks[c]			259	0
South African blacks	9	22	798	1
American blacks	67	57	1330	2–4

[a]Mestizo are basically Mongoloid (Asiatic origin) like the rest of the Amerindians, living in Latin American countries, but have had continuous admixture of Caucasian (primarily Spaniard) and to a small extent Negroid genes since the sixteenth century.
[b]Of unmixed ancestry.
[c]From Congo and Zambia; of unmixed ancestry.
From Khan M. A. HLA and ankylosing spondylitis. In Calabro and Dick (ed.) (1987), pp.23–44; with permission.

thies in African Americans is not known. The ratio of Caucasians to African Americans with ankylosing spondylitis (range 20:1–6.5:1) admitted to United States Veterans' hospitals serves as an indirect estimate of the prevalence of ankylosing spondylitis in African Americans (Baum and Ziff 1971). The rarity of spondylarthropathies in West Africans, who are racially heterogeneous and are one of the source populations for African Americans, has been attributed to the low frequency of HLA-B27. For example, the *HLA-B*2703* allele has been found in Gambians but ankylosing spondylitis has not been observed (Hill *et al*. 1991). Because of the low overall frequency of HLA-B27 (2.6 per cent) in Gambians, it is possible that one might not see cases of ankylosing spondylitis since only a proportion of HLA-B27-positive individuals develop ankylosing spondylitis. Alternatively, the absence of ankylosing spondylitis in a population

Table 15 Relative frequencies (per cent) of spondylarthropathy (SPA) subsets and sex ratios in several populations

Population (locale)	SPA	Frequency	Male:female ratio
Native American (Alaska, USA)	AS	32.8	5.3:1
	RS	32.8	0.58:1
	USPA	34.4	0.33:1
Inuit (Alaska, USA)	AS	11.8	
	RS	41.2	
	PSA/S	5.9	
	USPA	41.1	
	All SPA		3.3:1
Yupik Eskimo (Alaska, USA)	AS	22.4	6.5:1
	RS	28.4[a]	
	USPA	32.8[b]	1.6:1
	PSA/S	1.4[s]	
	All SPA		5:1
Navajo Native American (USA)	RS	100.0	
Caucasian (England)	AS	85.0	2.4:1
Shona (Zimbabwe)	AS	47.4	8:1
	RS	52.6	4:1

AS, ankylosing spondylitis; PSA/S, psoriatic arthritis/spondylitis; RS, Reiter's syndrome; USPA, undifferentiated SPA.
[a]No females were observed with this diagnosis; [b]includes cases of USPA and overlap SPA syndromes; [c]no females were observed with this diagnosis.

with HLA-B27 may indicate the absence of environmental factors that interact with HLA-B27 to trigger spondylarthropathies, or that the HLA-B27 molecules in the population do not confer susceptibility to spondylarthropathies (Hill *et al*. 1991). In support of this latter theory, *HLA-B*2703* differs from other *B27* alleles at amino acid position 59 in the α_1-domain. This observation may explain the results of experiments with alloreactive T-cell clones with this allele (Calvo *et al*. 1990) and may indicate that peptide binding for *HLA-B*2703* is different from other B27 subtypes (Woodrow 1991). HLA-B27 frequencies in normal individuals and those with ankylosing spondylitis appear in Table 14.

Distribution of spondylarthropathy subsets and sex ratios

The relative frequencies of the spondylarthropathy subtypes vary within and between racial groups. As shown in Table 15, ankylosing spondylitis is the predominant spondylarthropathy in Caucasians of Northern European descent (Edmunds *et al*. 1991). Equal frequencies of ankylosing spondylitis and Reiter's syndrome are seen in Alaskan Native Americans and Eskimos (Boyer *et al*. 1990, 1991) and the Shona cultural group in Zimbabwe (Stein *et al*. 1990). Cases of ankylosing spondylitis comprise only 11 per cent of spondylarthropathies

among the Alaskan Inuit, where the frequencies of Reiter's syndrome and undifferentiated spondylarthropathy are equal. With the exception of Native Americans in Alaska (Reiter's syndrome and undifferentiated spondylarthropathies are more common in females), males outnumber females with spondylarthropathies (Table 15).

References

Aaron, S. *et al*. (1985). Sex ratio and sibship in juvenile rheumatoid arthritis kindreds. *Arthritis and Rheumatism*, **28**, 753–8.

Abadi, I. and Gonzalez, N. (1990). Epidemiologia de lupus eritematosos sistemico en Venezuela. Sindrome clinico e immunologico. In *Ediciones Anno Acta Medica Colombiana* (ed. M. Sanchez, M. Diaz, F. Rondon, and G. Ucros), pp. 17–22.

Adebajo, A. O. (1991). Rheumatoid arthritis: a twentieth century disease in Africa? *Arthritis and Rheumatism*, **34**, 248–9.

Adebajo, A. O. (1995). Tropical rheumatology. Epidemiology and community studies: Africa. *Baillières Clinical Rheumatology*, **9**, 21–30.

Adebajo, A. O., Charles, P. J., Hazleman, B. L., and Maini, R. N. (1993). Serological profile of rheumatoid arthritis in West Africa. *Rheumatology International*, **12**, 235–8.

Alarcon, G. S. (1986). Epidemiologia de las enfermedades reumaticas en America Latina. *Bol Oficina Sanit Panam*, **101**, 309–27.

Al-Rawi, Z. S., Alazzawi, A. J., Alajili, F. M., and Alwakil, R. (1978). Rheumatoid arthritis in population samples in Iraq. *Annals of the Rheumatic Diseases*, **37**, 73–5.

Ansell, B. M. (1978). Chronic arthritis in childhood. *Annals of the Rheumatic Diseases*, 37,107–20.

Ansell, B. M. (1990). Classification and nomenclature. In *Paediatric rheumatology update* (ed. P. Woo, P. H. White, and B. M. Ansell), pp. 3–5. Oxford University Press.

Arnett, F. C. *et al.* (1988). The American Rheumatism Association 1987 revised criteria for the classification of rheumatoid arthritis. *Arthritis and Rheumatism*, 31, 315–24.

Atkins, C. *et al.* (1988). Rheumatic disease in the Nuu-Chah-Nulth native Indians of the Pacific Northwest. *Journal of Rheumatology*, 15, 684–90.

Ballou, S. P., Khan, M. A., and Kushner, I. (1982). Clinical features of systemic lupus erythematosus. *Arthritis and Rheumatism*, 25, 55–60.

Baum, J. and Ziff, M. (1971). The rarity of ankylosing spondylitis in the black race. *Arthritis and Rheumatism*, 14, 12–18.

Beasley, R. P., Willkens, R. F., and Bennett, P. H. (1973). High prevalence of rheumatoid arthritis in Yakima Indians. *Arthritis and Rheumatism*, 16, 743–8.

Beasley, R. P., Bennett, P. H., and Lin, C. C. (1983). Low prevalence of rheumatoid arthritis in Chinese. *Journal of Rheumatology*, 10 (Suppl.),11–15.

Beighton, P., Solomon, L., and Valkenburg, H. A. (1975).Rheumatoid arthritis in a rural South African Negro population. *Annals of the Rheumatic Diseases*, 34, 136–41.

Bennett, P. H. and Wood, P. H. N. (1968). Report from the subcommittee on diagnostic criteria for ankylosing spondylitis. In *Population studies of the rheumatic diseases* (Proceedings of the Third International Symposium, New York), (ed. P. H. Bennett and P. H. N. Wood), p 314. Excerpta Medica, Amsterdam.

Bias, W. B., Hochberg, M. C., McLean, R. H., and Machan, C. (1992). Systemic lupus erythematosus joint report. In *HLA 1991: Proceedings of the Eleventh International Histocompatibility Workshop and Conference*, Vol. 1, (ed. K. Tsuji, M. Aizawa, and T. Sasazuki), pp. 740–5. Oxford University Press.

Boyer, G. S., Lanier, A. P., and Templin, D. W. (1988). Prevalence rates of spondyloarthropathies, rheumatoid arthritis, and other rheumatic diseases in an Alaskan Inupiat Eskimo population. *Journal of Rheumatology*, 15, 678–83.

Boyer, G. S. *et al.* (1990). Spondyloarthropathy and rheumatoid arthritis in Alaskan Yupik Eskimos. *Journal of Rheumatology*, 17, 489–96.

Boyer, G. S., Templin, D. W., and Lanier, A. P. (1991). Rheumatic diseases in Alaskan Indians of the southeast coast: high prevalence of rheumatoid arthritis and systemic lupus erythematosus. *Journal of Rheumatology*, 18, 1477–84.

Brewer, E. J. *et al.* (1977). Current proposed revision of JRA criteria. *Arthritis and Rheumatism*, 20 (Suppl.), 195–9.

Brighton, S. W. *et al.* (1988). The prevalence of rheumatoid arthritis in a rural African population. *Journal of Rheumatology*, 15, 405–8.

Buchanan, W. W. and Murdoch, R. M. (1979). Hypothesis: that rheumatoid arthritis will disappear. *Journal of Rheumatology*, 6, 324–9.

Calabro, J. J. and Dick, C. (ed.). (1987). *Ankylosing spondylitis. New clinical applications in rheumatology*, Vol. 1. MTP Press, Lancaster.

Calvo, V. *et al.* (1990). Structure and diversity of HLA-B27-specific T cell epitopes: analysis with site-directed mutants mimicking HLA-B27 subtype polymorphism. *Journal of Immunology*, 144, 4038–45.

Cassidy, J. T. and Nelson, A. M. (1988). The frequency of juvenile arthritis. *Journal of Rheumatology*, 15, 535–6.

Catalano, M. A. and Hoffmeier, M. (1989). Frequency of systemic lupus erythematosus (SLE) among ethnic groups of Hawaii. *Arthritis and Rheumatism*, 32 (Suppl. 4), S30.

Chou, C. T., Pei, L., Chang, D. M., Lee, C. F., Schumacher, H. R., and Liang, M. H. (1994). Prevalence of rheumatic diseases in Taiwan: A population study of urban, suburban, rural differences. *Journal of Rheumatology*, 21, 302–6.

Cohen, A. S. *et al.* (1971). Preliminary criteria for the classification of SLE. *Bulletin of the Rheumatic Diseases*, 21, 643–8.

Darmawan, J., Muirden, K. D., Valkenburg, H. A., and Wigley, R. D. (1993). The epidemiology of rheumatoid arthritis in Indonesia. *British Journal of Rheumatology*, 32, 537–40.

Del Puente, A. *et al.* (1988). The incidence of rheumatoid arthritis is predicted by rheumatoid factor titer in a longitudinal population study. *Arthritis and Rheumatism*, 31, 1239–44.

Del Puente, A. *et al.* (1989). High incidence and prevalence of rheumatoid arthritis in Pima Indians. *American Journal of Epidemiology*, 129, 1170–8.

Dessein, P. H. M. C., Gledhill, R. F., and Rossouw, D. S. (1988). Systemic lupus erythematosus in black South Africans. *South Africa Medical Journal*, 74, 387–9.

Edmunds. J. E., Kennedy, L. G., and Calin, A. (1991). Primary ankylosing spondylitis, psoriatic and enteropathic spondyloarthropathy: a controlled analysis. *Journal of Rheumatology*, 18, 696–8.

Fessel, W. J. (1974). Systemic lupus erythematosus in the community incidence, prevalence, outcome and first symptoms: the high prevalence in black women. *Archives of Internal Medicine*, 134, 1027–35.

Fessel, W. J. (1988) Epidemiology of systemic lupus erythematosus. *Rheumatic Disease Clinics of North America*, 14, 15–23.

Fink, C. W. and Fernandez-Vina, M. (1995).Classification of juvenile arthritis. *Bulletin of the Rheumatic Diseases*, 14, 3–5.

Gewanter, H. L., Roghman, K. J., and Baum, J. (1983). The prevalence of juvenile arthritis. *Arthritis and Rheumatism*, 26, 599–601.

Gofton, J. P., Robinson, H. S., and Price, G. E. (1964). A study of rheumatic disease in a Canadian Indian population. II. Rheumatoid arthritis in the Haida Indians. *Annals of the Rheumatic Diseases*, 23, 364–71.

Gomez-Carpio, M. *et al.* (1966). Epidemiologia de la artritis reumatoidea en Chile. *Revista Medica de Chile*, 94, 315–22.

Greenwood, B. M. (1969). Polyarthritis in Western Nigeria. *Annals of the Rheumatic Diseases*, 28, 489–96.

Gupta, K., Chintu, C., and Raghu, M. B. (1981). Juvenile rheumatoid arthritis in Zambian children. *East Africa Medical Journal*, 58, 344–5.

Haffejee, I. E., Raga, J., and Coovadia, H. M. (1984). Juvenile chronic arthritis in Black and Indian South African children. *South Africa Medical Journal*, 65, 510–14.

Hall, P. (1991). Rheumatoid arthritis in sub-Saharan Africa. *Proceedings First AFLAR Congress of Rheumatology* (Abstract 17).

Hameed, K., Gibson, T., Kadir, M., Sultana, S., Fatima, Z., and Syed, A. (1995). The prevalence of rheumatoid arthritis in affluent and poor urban communities of Pakistan. *British Journal of Rheumatology*, 34, 252–6.

Hanson, V. *et al.* (1977). Three subtypes of juvenile rheumatoid arthritis. *Arthritis and Rheumatism*, 20 (Suppl.),184–6.

Harris, E.N., Williams, E., Shah, D.J., and De Ceular, K. (1989). Mortality of Jamaican patients with systemic lupus erythematosus. *British Journal of Rheumatology*, 28, 113–17.

Hart, H. H., Grigor, R. R., and Caughey, D. E. (1983). Ethnic difference in the prevalence of systemic lupus erythematosus. *Annals of the Rheumatic Diseases*, 42, 529–32.

Harvey, J. *et al.* (1983). Rheumatoid arthritis in a Chippewa band. II. Field study with clinical serologic and HLA-D correlations. *Journal of Rheumatology*, 10, 28–32.

Hill, A. S. V. *et al.* (1991). HLA class I typing by PCR: HLA-B27 and an African HLA-B27 subtype. *Lancet*, 337, 640–2.

Hill, R. (1976). Juvenile arthritis in various racial groups in British Columbia. *Arthritis and Rheumatism*, 20 (Suppl.), 162–4.

Hochberg, M. C. (1984). *The epidemiology of juvenile rheumatoid arthritis: review of current status and approaches for future research*. In *Epidemiology of the rheumatic diseases*, (Proceedings of the Fourth International Conference, National Institutes of Health) (ed. R. C. Lawrence and L. E. Shulman), pp. 220–30. Gower Medical, London.

Hochberg, M. C. (1990). Systemic lupus erythematosus. *Rheumatic Disease Clinics of North America*, 16, 617–39.

Hochberg, M. C., Linet, M. S., and Sills, E. M. (1983). The prevalence and incidence of juvenile rheumatoid arthritis in an urban black population. *American Journal of Public Health*, 73, 1202–3.

Hochberg, M. C. *et al.* (1985). Systemic lupus erythematosus: a review of clinico-laboratory features and immunogenetic markers in 150 patients with emphasis on demographic subsets. *Medicine*, 64, 285–95.

Jacobs, J. C. (1982). *Pediatric rheumatology for the practitioner*. Springer-Verlag, New York.

Jessop, S. and Meyers, O. L. (1973). Systemic lupus erythematosus in Cape Town. *South Africa Medical Journal*, 47, 222–5.

Johnson, A. E., Gordon, C., Palmer, R. G., and Bacon, P. A. (1995). The prevalence and incidence of systemic lupus erythematosus in Birmingham, England. *Arthritis and Rheumatism*, 38, 551–8.

Kanyerezi, B. R. (1969). Rheumatoid arthritis in Uganda. *East Africa Medical Journal*, 46, 71–5.

Kanyerezi, B. R. and Mbidde, E. (1980). Juvenile chronic polyarthritis in Ugandan African children. *East Africa Medical Journal*, 57, 484–9.

Karlson, E. W. *et al.* (1995). The independence and stability of socioeconomic predictors of morbidity in systemic lupus erythematosus. *Arthritis and Rheumatism*, 38, 267–73.

Kato, H. *et al.* (1971). Rheumatoid arthritis and gout in Hiroshima and Nagasaki, Japan: a prevalence and incidence study. *Journal of Chronic Diseases*, 23, 659–79.

Kellgren, J. H. (1962). Diagnostic criteria for population studies. *Bulletin of the Rheumatic Diseases*, 13, 291–2.

Kelsey, K. L. (1982). Juvenile rheumatoid arthritis. In *Epidemiology of musculo-skeletal disorders*, pp. 94–7. Oxford University Press.

Khuffash, F. A. and Majeed, H. A. (1988). Juvenile rheumatoid arthritis among Arab children. *Scandinavian Journal of Rheumatology*, 17, 393–5.

Lau, E., Symmons, D., Bankhead, C., MacGregor, A., Donnan, S., and Silman, A. (1993). Low prevalence of rheumatoid arthritis in the urbanized Chinese of Hong Kong. *Journal of Rheumatology*, 20, 1133–7.

Lawrence, J. S. (1961). Prevalence of rheumatoid arthritis. *Annals of the Rheumatic Diseases*, 20, 11–17.

Lawrence, J. S. and Wood, P. H. N. (1963). Criteria for rheumatoid arthritis in populations samples. In *Population studies of the rheumatic diseases* (ed. P. H. Bennett and P. H. N. Wood), pp 164–74. Excerpta Medica, Amsterdam,

Lawrence, J. S. *et al.* (1966). Rheumatoid arthritis in a subtropical population. *Annals of the Rheumatic Diseases*, 25, 59–66.

Lawrence, R. C. *et al.* (1989). Estimates of the prevalence of selected arthritic and musculoskeletal disease in the United States. *Journal of Rheumatology*, 16, 427–41.

McCarty, D. J., Thomas, S. M., Medsger, T. A., Ramsey-Goldman, R., LaPorte, R. E., and Kentworth, C. (1995). Incidence of systemic lupus erythematosus. *Arthritis and Rheumatism*, 38, 1260–70

MacGregor, A. J., Riste, L. K., Hazes, J. M., and Silman, A. J. (1994). Low prevalence of rheumatoid arthritis in black-Caribbeans compared with whites in inner city Manchester. *Annals of the Rheumatic Diseases*, 53, 293–7.

Malaviya, A. N., Kapoor, S. K., Singh, R. R., Kumar, A., and Pande, I. (1993). Prevalence of rheumatoid arthritis in the adult Indian population. *Rheumatology International*, 13, 131–4.

Martinez-Cairo, C. S., Antonio, O. D., and Frati, A. (1978). Arthritis reumatoide juvenil. Estudio de 46 casos. *Boletin Medico del Hospital Infantil de Mexico*, 35, 711–17.

Masi, A. T. (1984) Clinical and epidemiologic perspective of systemic lupus erythematosus. In *Epidemiology of the rheumatic diseases* (Proceedings of the Fourth International Conference, National Institutes of Health) (ed. R. C. Lawrence and L. E. Shulman), pp. 145–63. Gower Medical, London.

Mendez-Bryan, R., Gonzalez-Alcover, R., and Roger, L. (1964). Rheumatoid arthritis: prevalence in a tropical area. *Arthritis and Rheumatism*, 7, 171–6.

Meyers, O. L., Daynes, G., and Beighton, P. (1977). Rheumatoid arthritis in a tribal Xhosa population in the Transkei, Southern Africa. *Annals of the Rheumatic Diseases*, 36, 62–5.

Meyers, O. L. *et al.* (1983). Rheuma — eine Zivilisationskrankheit? *South Africa Medical Journal*, 101, 1224–30.

Mijiyawa, M. (1995). Epidemiology and semiology of rheumatoid arthritis in third world countries. *Expansion Scientifique Francaise*, 62, 121–6.

Mody, G. M. and Meyers, O. L. (1989). Rheumatoid arthritis in blacks in South Africa. *Annals of the Rheumatic Diseases*, 48, 69–72.

Moolenburgh, J. D., Moore, S., Valkenburg, H. A., and Erasmus, M. G. (1984) Rheumatoid arthritis in Lesotho. *Annals of the Rheumatic Diseases*, 43, 40–3.

Morrison, R. C. A. *et al.* (1990). Differences in systemic lupus erythematosus manifestations among racial groups in South Africa. *Arthritis and Rheumatism*, 33 (Suppl. B192), S104.

Morse, H. G. *et al.* (1980). High frequency of HLA-B27 and Reiter's syndrome in Navajo Indians. *Journal of Rheumatology*, 7, 900–2.

Morton, R. O. *et al.* (1976). The incidence of systemic lupus erythematosus in North American Indians. *Journal of Rheumatology*, 3, 186–9.

Muller, A. S. (1970). Population studies on the prevalence of rheumatic diseases in Liberia and Nigeria. Unpublished doctoral thesis, University of Leiden.

Nossent, J. C. (1992). Systemic lupus erythematosus in the Caribbean island of Curacao: an epidemiological investigation. *Annals of the Rheumatic Diseases*, 51, 1197–201.

Nossent, J. C. (1993a). Clinical renal involvement in Afro-Caribbean lupus patients. *Lupus*, 2, 173–6.

Nossent, J. C. (1993b). Course and prognostic value of systemic lupus erythematosus disease activity index in Black Caribbean patients. *Seminars in Arthritis and Rheumatism*, 23, 16–21.

Oen, K. *et al.* (1986). Rheumatic disease in an Inuit population. *Arthritis and Rheumatism*, 29, 65–74.

Oen, K., Fast , M., and Postl, B. (1995). Epidemiology of juvenile rheumatoid arthritis in Manitoba, Canada, 1975–92: cycles in incidence. *Journal of Rheumatology*, 22, 745–50.

Pountain, G. (1991). The prevalence of rheumatoid arthritis in the Sultanate of Oman. *British Journal of Rheumatology*, 30, 24–8.

Reveille, J. D. *et al.* (1989). DNA analysis of HLA-DR and DQ genes in American blacks with systemic lupus erythematosus. *Arthritis and Rheumatism*, 32, 1243–51.

Ropes, M. W. *et al.* (1958). Revision of diagnostic criteria for rheumatoid arthritis. *Bulletin of the Rheumatic Diseases*, 9, 175–6.

Rose, B. S. and Prior, I. A. M. (1963). A survey of rheumatism in a rural New Zealand Maori community. *Annals of the Rheumatic Diseases*, 22, 410–15.

Rosenberg, A. M. and Petty, R. E. (1982). A syndrome of seronegative enthesopathy and arthropathy (SEA syndrome). *Arthritis and Rheumatism*, 25, 1041–7.

Rosenberg, A. M. *et al.* (1982). Rheumatic diseases in Western Canadian Indian children. *Journal of Rheumatology*, 9, 589–92.

Serdula, M. K. and Rhoads, G. G. (1979). Frequency of systemic lupus erythematosus in different ethnic groups in Hawaii. *Arthritis and Rheumatism*, 22, 328–33.

Shichikawa, K. *et al.* (1981). A longitudinal population survey of rheumatoid arthritis in a rural district in Wakayama. *The Ryumachi*, 21 (Suppl.), 35–43.

Siegel, M. and Lee, S. L. (1973). The epidemiology of systemic lupus erythematosus. *Seminars in Arthritis and Rheumatism*, 3, 1–54.

Silman, A. J. *et al.* (1993). Absence of rheumatoid arthritis in a rural Nigerian population. *Journal of Rheumatology*, 20, 618–22

Singsen, B. H. (1990). Rheumatic disease of childhood. *Rheumatic Disease Clinics of North America*, 16, 581–99.

Smikle, M. F., James, O. B., Barton, E. N., and De Ceulaer, K. (1995). Letter to the Editor. *Tropical and Geographical Medicine*, 47, 231.

Solomon, L., Robin, G., and Valkenburg, H. A. (1975).Rheumatoid arthritis in an urban South African Negro population. *Annals of the Rheumatic Diseases*, 34, 128–35.

Stein, M. *et al.* (1990). The spondyloarthropathies in Zimbabwe: a clinical and immunogenetic profile. *Journal of Rheumatology*, 17, 1337–9.

Symmons, D. P. M. (1995). Occasional series: lupus around the world; frequency of lupus in people of African origin. *Lupus*, 4, 176–8.

Szer, W., Sierakowska, H., and Szer, I. S. (1991). Antinuclear antibody profile in juvenile rheumatoid arthritis. *Journal of Rheumatology*, 18, 401–8.

Tan, E. M. *et al.* (1982). The 1982 revised criteria for the classification of systemic lupus erythematosus. *Arthritis and Rheumatism*, 25, 1271–7.

Taylor, H. G. and Stein, C. M. (1986). Systemic lupus erythematosus in Zimbabwe. *Annals of the Rheumatic Diseases*, 45, 645–8.

Wallace, D. G. and Quismorio, F. P. Jr (1995). The elusive search for geographic clusters of systemic lupus erythematosus. *Arthritis and Rheumatism*, 38, 1564–7.

Ward, M. M. and Studenski, S. (1990). Clinical manifestations of systemic lupus erythematosus. *Archives of Internal Medicine*, 150, 849–53.

Wigley, R. D. *et al.* (1994). Rheumatic diseases in China: ILAR–China study comparing the prevalence of rheumatic symptoms in northern and southern rural populations. *Journal of Rheumatology*, 21, 1484–90.

Williams, R. C. *et al.* (1985). GM allotypes in native Americans: evidence for three distinct migrations across the Bering land bridge. *American Journal of Physical Anthropology*, 66, 1–19.

Williams, W. and Shah, D. (1990). Lupus nephritis at the University Hospital of the West Indies, Kingston, Jamaica: A 10-year experience. *Renal Failure*, 12, 25–33.

Willkens, R. F. *et al.* (1981). Reiter's syndrome: evaluation of preliminary criteria for definite disease. *Arthritis and Rheumatism*, 24, 844–9.

Wilson, W. A. and Hughes, G. R. V. (1979). Rheumatic disease in Jamaica. *Annals of the Rheumatic Diseases*, 38, 320–5.

Woodrow, J. (1991). Genetics of the spondyloarthropathies. *Current Science*, 3, 586–91.

5.2 Nosology of the chronic inflammatory rheumatic diseases

Patricia Woo and David N. Glass

Because the causes and pathological mechanisms of the various chronic inflammatory rheumatic diseases are incompletely understood, their classification has traditionally relied on their clinical evolution. Synovitis, a feature of many rheumatic diseases, is not helpful in differentiating between them; it is so common a response to different stimuli that it does not necessarily signal the presence of any given disease. However, features such as the pattern of arthritis (symmetrical or asymmetrical), age at onset, and presence or absence of systemic features, including specific organ involvement, may be used for classification criteria. In juvenile chronic arthritis (juvenile rheumatoid arthritis in North America), for example, the number of joints involved during the first 3 months of illness is an important element in classification (Brewer *et al.* 1977). Aided by the development of a few supportive but generally non-specific laboratory tests, investigators have subdivided the chronic inflammatory rheumatic illnesses in a manner that has proved to be of practical help in patient management. This approach is not so useful in the planning of clinical and laboratory-based investigations, nor in the exchange of information between investigators and clinicians. It necessitates the considerable use of exclusions based on the absence of the development of other diseases. The proper classification of a group of patients can take many years to accomplish as their individual diseases evolve.

Advances in a variety of disciplines, both clinical and experimental, have greatly improved our understanding of the immune response and of relations between infection, inflammation, and autoimmunity (Table 1). This new information can be used to classify the chronic inflammatory rheumatic diseases using a mechanistic/pathological approach (Vaughan 1989).

Relating chronic inflammatory rheumatic diseases to infection, immune responses, and autoimmunity

It has become evident, especially within the last decade, that a few infections may lead directly to chronic rheumatic disease. Prominent examples include Lyme arthritis (an infection with the spirochaete *Borrelia burgdorferi*), rheumatic fever with group A β-haemolytic streptococcal infection, and Reiter's syndrome, which is associated

Table 1 Advances in knowledge on which the hypothesis for infectious–immunological causes is based

Autoimmune phenomena

1. Rheumatic disease sequelae in patients with established infections (e.g. Lyme disease)

2. Autoimmune phenomena in patients with established infections (e.g. tuberculosis)

3. Rheumatic disease and existing self-reactive or autoimmune phenomena (e.g., rheumatoid factors and antinuclear antibodies) with no obvious antecedent infection.

4. Identification of genes with potential roles in broad susceptibility to autoimmunity (e.g. apoptosis-related genes)

5. Disease-modifier genes (e.g., tumour necrosis factor allele in cerebral malaria, and meningococcal meningitis)

A trimolecular complex (MHC gene product, antigen, and T-cell receptor) determines immunological responsiveness

1. Identification of specific trimolecular complexes in animal models of autoimmune disease

2. Identification of components of the trimolecular complex in human chronic inflammatory rheumatic disease confirmed in a transgenic model

Other related immunological advances

3. The superantigen concept, the ability of selected antigens to activate substantial populations of T-cell clones

4. Cytokine profiles Th1 and Th2, with Th1 being associated more with autoimmunity and Th2 being associated with allergic reactions.

5. Transgenic animals allow the exploration of roles for single genes

with a range of gastrointestinal and urogenital infections that are primarily bacterial.

Immunological phenomena, long believed to be involved in most chronic inflammatory rheumatic diseases, are now better documented and understood. Immunologically competent cells such as lymphocytes and plasma cells are universally present in diseased tissues, and immune complexes are often formed locally and within the vascular compartment. The local release of cytokines involved in generating these immune responses is important, as is the profile of cytokines produced (Th1/Th2 from CD4 cells, and Tc1 and Tc2 from CD8 cells). This profile may well reflect the nature of the pathogen and the route of immunization, as well as host factors (Marrack and Kappler 1994; Simon et al. 1994; Mossman and Sad 1996). It is also noteworthy that the selective inhibition of cytokines can alter the manifestations of the disease: for example, treatment with antibody to tumour necrosis factor-α in rheumatoid arthritis (Elliott et al. 1993).

Many of the immunological changes are autoimmune (self-reactive) in nature. At about the same time as rheumatoid factors and antinuclear antibodies with a wide range of specificities were discovered in patients with chronic rheumatic diseases (e.g., rheumatoid arthritis and systemic lupus erythematosus), similar autoimmune phenomena were noted in individuals with established, non-rheumatic, infectious diseases (e.g., chronic forms of bacterial endocarditis and leprosy). This discovery supported the notion that the autoimmune phenomena in patients with chronic rheumatic diseases may have originated from an infectious process.

Meanwhile, understanding of the basic mechanisms of the immune response has greatly improved. Particularly important is the concept of a central role for a trimolecular complex consisting of a T-cell receptor responsive to antigen presentation by proteins of the major histocompatibility complex (**MHC**) genes, which determine the host's response (Davis and Bjorkman 1988). This finding implies that at least two immunological components, HLA and T-cell receptors, underlie susceptibility to many autoimmune rheumatic diseases.

Substantial progress has been made in evaluating this trimolecular complex in animal models of autoimmune disease, most notably the model of allergic encephalomyelitis in which the specific determinants (molecular binding sites) on the antigen (myelin basic protein), the MHC genes, and T-cell receptor have all been identified (Acha-Orbea et al. 1988). The component of the trimolecular complex most extensively studied in human disease is HLA (Todd et al. 1988; see also Chapter 3.3). The direct role of at least one MHC gene (*HLA-B27*) in the spondylarthropathies has been elegantly confirmed in a transgenic model using rats raised in germ-free environments (Hammer et al. 1990; Taurog et al. 1994). Because certain HLA genes are associated with specific rheumatic diseases, HLA typing of patients can be used to aid the classification of their disease.

The study of the T-cell receptor in human autoimmune disease is just beginning, and is likely to prove complex. A limited T-cell repertoire has been documented in rheumatoid arthritis and T-cell receptor genes have been associated with the disease (McDermott et al. 1995). The role of the thymus in regulating the T-cell repertoire (and hence the formation of trimolecular complexes) has also been recognized; further study of this process will clarify the roles that the components of the trimolecular complex have in autoimmune disease. Expansion of certain V_β-chains of the T-cell receptor can be induced peripherally by superantigens. These are thought to make external contacts with the MHC class II molecule and the V_β portion of a T-cell receptor, thereby stimulating entire families of T cells. Bacterial superantigens in man are heat-resistant enterotoxins, such as *Staphylococcus aureus* enterotoxin, causing toxic-shock syndromes and septic arthritis as a result of the production of large quantities of inflammatory cytokines (Bremell and Tarkowski 1995). Murine mycoplasma arthritides superantigen (MAM) can trigger and exacer-

bate murine collagen-induced arthritis, thus providing a model for autoimmunity (Cole and Griffiths 1993).

Another mechanism of 'disturbance' in the T-cell repertoire is the alteration in programmed death (apoptosis) of cells of the immune system. In three strains of lupus-prone mice there are spontaneous mutations of Fas apoptosis antigen, its receptor or its ligand, leading to persistence of autoreactive cells (reviewed in Mountz et al. 1994). Fas mutations have been described in human lymphoproliferative syndrome, which children also have features of autoimmune haemolytic anaemia (Fisher et al. 1995; Rieux-Laucat et al. 1995). In human systemic lupus erythematosus, expression of Fas antigen and Bcl-2 have been studied, but there is no consensus as yet as to their potential roles in immunopathogenesis.

These conceptual advances, discussed more fully in earlier chapters, suggest that many of the chronic rheumatic diseases have infectious causes with complicating immunological responses. In devising a classification that proposes or infers infectious causes complicated by a range of immune responses, several other factors need to be taken into account. While a substantial amount is known about the HLA genes and infectious agents in some arthritides, there is a paucity of knowledge concerning T-cell receptor genes and general autoimmune-predisposing genes. Any classification based on these variables must, therefore, be considered tentative. During the evolution of the disease, the immune response may be directed initially at antigen-recognition sites (epitopes) on the intact infecting organism. Later, antigenic fragments of the organism may persist, providing continuing immunopathological stimulation; the immune response may also become directed against self-antigens. Thus any classification must recognize that clinical stages of the disease may change as a result of changing immune response. Routes of inoculation as well as host genetic factors are responsible for determining whether the immune response will become chronic and the disease progressive. Because the evolution of disease, from a straightforward infection to a complex series of immune responses associated with a range of pathologies, has much to do with genetically defined host variables, genetic studies of patients can help the process of disease classification. The above considerations make it possible to devise classifications based on infectious/immunological causes, even when the likelihood of infectious processes can only be inferred from parallel circumstances in which the presence of infection is well established.

Classification of disease

For the purposes of this discussion, the chronic inflammatory rheumatic diseases can be divided into overlapping categories (see Table 2). The first category comprises the relatively rare diseases in which the products of infection-induced inflammation directly cause tissue damage. The harmful products of inflammation include proteolytic enzymes that are associated with the degradation of synovium and cartilage. Such diseases usually take an acute rather than a chronic course. Pyogenic arthritis, in which the products of the inflammatory process cause the destruction of substantial amounts of synovial and cartilaginous tissue, is an example. Other arthropathies caused by infectious agents include those of rubella and parvovirus, mycobacterial and mycoplasma infections.

Because pyogenic organisms do not normally seed to joints, unusual conditions conducive to rheumatic disease must be present.

Table 2 Categories in the classification of chronic inflammatory rheumatic diseases

Category 1: Localized infection at musculoskeletal sites

1. Basic process	Infection
2. Mechanism	Infection causes tissue inflammation and injury directly; initiating organism can be isolated
3. Examples	Pyogenic arthritis; viral and mycoplasma arthropathies (see Chapters 5.3.1–5.3.10)
4. Susceptibility	Structural changes in joints including arthroplasty; diabetes, complement and immunoglobulin deficiencies (see Chapter 5.3.11)

Category II: Pathogen and pathogen specific immune response

1. Basic process	Infection and organism-specific immune response
2. Mechanism	Immune response to intact organism and/or to injury; persisting antigenic fragments or organisms; probably immune complex-mediated tissue injury
3. Examples	Musculoskeletal syndromes associated with viral hepatitis and streptococcal infections
4. Susceptibility	Not generally established; some complement deficiencies predispose to this type of disease

Category III: Pathogens, immune response, and autoimmunity

(a)

1. Basic process	Infection followed by an organism-specific immune response and cross-reactive immune responses to self-antigens
2. Mechanism	Intact organisms may be isolated but continuing presence is unlikely to be necessary when an autoimmune response is established
3. Examples	Rheumatic fever and other reactive arthropathies (see Chapters 5.3.12, 5.5.1)
4. Susceptibility	Certain MHC class I and class II genes or other, closely linked, receptor genes (see Chapter 3.3)

(b)

1. Basic process	Infection inferred but not established, followed by autoreactivity
2. Mechanism	An autoimmune response which becomes the major phenotype
3. Examples	Rheumatoid arthritis, juvenile chronic arthritis, systemic lupus erythematosus
4. Susceptibility	MHC class I and II genes, T-cell receptor genes and others, e.g., Fas, cytokine, giving general susceptibility to autoimmunity

Local injury or disease may make individual joints especially vulnerable and systemic factors may affect the host's susceptibility to a given pathogen. Some form of mechanical problem in a joint, such as osteoarthritis, is common among these patients. Patients with rheumatoid arthritis, for example, have a greater risk of infection than those with osteoarthritis. Their disease, rheumatoid arthritis, is associated with impaired immune responses, which treatment may aggravate. In addition, arthroplasties carry a particular risk of infection, especially in immunocompromised patients. Therefore, in the patient with rheumatoid arthritis who undergoes an arthroplasty, both local and systemic factors may favour the development of bacterial arthritis (Goldenberg and Reed 1985). Systemic illnesses, for example diabetes mellitus, appear to confer a greater susceptibility (see Chapter 5.3.1). The majority of individuals with septic joints have at least one of these predisposing factors. Less common, but more specific, predisposing factors are host difficulties in handling infectious organisms, as in complement deficiency, hypogammaglobulinaemia, and deficiency of lymphocyte function antigen 1 (Atkinson 1995).

In the second category of rheumatic diseases an immune response directed primarily against a pathogenic organism or fragments of that organism causes inflammation that results in disease. Much of the tissue injury results from immune complexes. Cross-reactivity to self-antigens is not critical. Some rheumatic syndromes associated with streptococcal infection and with hepatitis B virus are typical of this category of illness. The intact infecting organism may sometimes be isolated from the involved joint and provide a source of initial tissue damage, as in category 1, but in other instances the organisms cannot be isolated. In these conditions an immune response directed specifically at antigenic fragments of the organism is likely to be responsible for some components of the pathology of the disease. Such organism-specific responses are well documented. For example, in post-streptococcal syndromes such as glomerulonephritis and vasculitis, immune responses in the form of immune-complex deposition contribute to the inflammatory process. Similarly, in hepatitis syndromes the increased amounts of immune complexes and reduced amounts of complement argue for their inclusion in the second category of diseases, as may the presence of hepatitis antigen in the immune complexes of some patients with vasculitis. Even if persistence of the intact organism is not essential, antigenic fragments may be important in generating a chronic immune response.

Characteristics of the host that affect his or her susceptibility to this category of disease are, at least as presently understood, not organism-specific, and have been identified in a small proportion of individuals at risk. They include some complement, immunoglobulin, and T-cell receptor deficiencies as well as defects of immune-complex clearance.

In a third category of disease, components of the first and second are present, that is, infection causes damage directly and results in an organism-specific immune response. In addition, autoimmunity develops in the form of reactivity with self-antigens including HLA. The best-documented example is probably rheumatic fever, in which the immune response to streptococcal infection becomes directed against host tissue antigens in cardiac muscle (see Chapter 5.3.12). Other diseases likely to be included are the spondylarthropathies, in which it is probable that initial infections with Gram-negative organisms and their plasmids are followed by an immune response directed against the self-antigen HLA-B27 in addition to components of the organisms involved; that is, molecular mimicry (Granfors *et al.* 1989) where the two antigens have common epitopes. We suggest that this theory of the development of HLA-B27-associated rheumatic disease will serve as a model for diseases in which infection is suspected as an initiating event but the organisms are as yet unknown (see below). Explanations other than cross-reactivity or molecular mimicry for the HLA-B27 association with spondylarthropathies are conceivable (Sieper and Braun 1995). Because certain class I or class II HLA genes are associated with each disease in the third category, people who do not carry the implicated gene are not susceptible to the diseases. The particular genes are necessary for the disease to develop but probably do not initiate the disease process.

In an extension of this category are diseases in which infectious agents have not been identified but a strong, autoimmune disease phenotype probably results from the infectious process. The more common chronic inflammatory rheumatic diseases, including rheumatoid arthritis, systemic lupus erythematosus, dermatomyositis and polymyositis, fall into this category. The major laboratory findings in patients in this fourth category are immune responses, and most of the antigenic determinants identified to date are self-antigens. The earliest documented examples of these responses were rheumatoid factors found in rheumatoid arthritis and antinuclear antibodies found in systemic lupus erythematosus. The antibodies may contribute to the pathogenesis, as in congenital complete heart block in the new-born of some patients with systemic lupus erythematosus (Buyon and Winchester 1990). Their presence in these patients, given the overall hypothesis that many of these diseases are infections, has parallels with the presence of the same autoantibodies in patients with various chronic inflammatory infections such as tuberculosis, leprosy, and bacterial endocarditis (in which rheumatoid factors are particularly prominent).

Efforts to identify the infectious agents believed to precipitate these chronic rheumatic diseases have continued to be made. Candidate organisms include Epstein–Barr virus and *Proteus mirabilis* in rheumatoid arthritis, and coxsackie virus in dermatomyositis. It is likely, however, that several agents can precipitate the disease, given the same genetic susceptibility. The host's MHC gene products are important in pathogenesis. Certain HLA class I and class II genes are associated with these diseases, and MHC class III genes may be involved in systemic lupus erythematosus in some populations. Whether the HLA genes are themselves directly involved or serve as markers for MHC non-HLA genes involved in the pathogenesis is unknown. Additional MHC-region genes have been identified: these include those coding for tumour necrosis factors, heat-shock protein, and intracellular transporter genes, any of which may be critical to the disease (see Chapter 4.7).

The concept of a trimolecular complex, discussed above, indicates a role for T-cell receptor genes. T-cell receptors have been implicated in the collagen type-II model of an autoimmune-induced stimulus (Banerjee *et al.* 1988) and in other forms of autoimmunity induced in animals (Acha-Orbea *et al.* 1988). Currently, however, very few T-cell receptor genes have been associated with human disease, their analysis being more complex than that of HLA.

The identification of defects in apoptotic pathways and their association with autoimmunity in both experimental models and in man adds to the importance of the host element in determining the outcome of an infection in terms of subsequent autoimmunity (Watanabe-Fukunaga *et al.* 1992). It is also noteworthy that single

Table 3 New therapeutic strategies
T-cell receptor immunization $V_\beta 17$ in rheumatoid arthritis
Induction of oral tolerance (e.g., to collagen II in rheumatoid arthritis)
Use of antibiotics, sulphasalazine/tetracycline therapy in rheumatoid arthritis and spondylarthropathy

cytokine genes in transgenic animals can create an *in vivo* environment in which arthritis develops (Keffer *et al.* 1991).

Some implications of an infection–immunological classification

Within these broad concepts, an infection would lead to the second and third categories of disease, that is, organism-specific, and then autoimmune responses could develop over time. The occurrence of these diseases in some individuals but not in others needs to be explained. Diseases in categories 2–3 can be regarded as failures of the hosts' initial defence mechanisms. Inherited susceptibility to disease has been suspected for a long time and some of the genetic influences on particular diseases are known, as is clear from the preceding discussion of HLA genes. The multiplicity of genes involved in addition to HLA suggests that autoimmunity is a complex genetic trait, as is the case in insulin-dependent diabetes mellitus (Davies *et al.* 1994). Microsatellite analysis of the human genome and immune models of diabetes mellitus illustrate the complexity of disease-susceptibility genes. It is clear that certain genes are necessary for disease to develop and that others act as 'modifiers,' responsible for the severity of disease, for example the tumour necrosis factor-α_2 allele in cerebral malaria (McGuire *et al.* 1994) and meningococcal meningitis (Girrourdin *et al.* 1992). Other unexplored factors are the virulence of the infecting organisms: for example, adhesive properties of bacteria can be involved in determining the outcome of bacterial infections. Exposure to infectious agents when the immune system is developing may be a cause for polyarthritis. For example, recent evidence suggests that an influenza A_2 epidemic caused an intrauterine infection that predisposed children to the development of a subtype of juvenile chronic arthritis (Pritchard *et al.* 1988). Such host/pathogen relations need to be investigated for their contributions to the chronic inflammatory rheumatic diseases.

The concept of a primary infectious origin for the chronic rheumatic diseases does not include discussion of other antigens known to generate disease (e.g., procainamide-induced systemic lupus erythematosus). Nevertheless, the infectious concept is applicable to many chronic rheumatic diseases, as well as other chronic (autoimmune) inflammatory diseases affecting other organs systems such as the gastrointestinal and renal tracts Further investigation should be promoted because it can be used to develop testable hypotheses aimed at identifying the types of immune responses, the infecting organisms, and genetic predisposing factors causing the disease. In addition, rationales for new therapeutic strategies are also provided (Table 3).

References

Acha-Orbea, H. *et al.* (1988). Limited heterogeneity of T cell receptors from lymphocytes mediating autoimmune encephalitis allows specific immune intervention. *Cell*, 54, 263–73.

Atkinson, J. P. (1995). Some thoughts on autoimmunity. *Arthritis and Rheumatism*, 38, 301–5.

Banerjee, S., Haqqi, T. M., Luthra, H. S., Stuart, J. M., and David, C. S. (1988). Possible role of V T cell receptor genes in susceptibility in collagen-induced arthritis in mice. *Journal of Experimental Medicine*, 167, 832.

Bremell, T. and Tarkowski, A. (1995). Preferential induction of septic arthritis and mortality by superantigen producing staphylococci. *Infection and Immunity*, 63, 4185–7.

Brewer, E. J. *et al.* (1977). Current proposed revision of JRA criteria. *Arthritis and Rheumatism*, 20, 195–9.

Buyon, J. P. and Winchester, R. (1990). Congenital complete heart block. A human model of passively acquired autoimmune injury. *Arthritis and Rheumatism*, 33, 609–14.

Cole, B. C. and Griffiths, M. M. (1993). Triggering and exacerbation of autoimmune arthritis by the mycoplasma arthritides superantigen MAM. *Arthritis and Rheumatism*, 36, 994–1002.

Davis, M. M. and Bjorkman, P. J. (1988). T-cell antigen receptor genes and T-cell recognition. *Nature*, 334, 395–402.

Davies, J. L. *et al.* (1994). A genome-wide search for human type I diabetes susceptibility genes. *Nature*, 371, 130–6.

Elliott, M. J. *et al.* (1993). Treatment of rheumatoid arthritis with chimeric monoclonal antibodies to tumor necrosis factor a. *Arthritis and Rheumatism*, 36, 1681–90.

Fisher, G. H. *et al.* (1995). Dominant interfering *Fas* gene mutations impaired apoptosis in a human autoimmune lymphoproliferative syndrome. *Cell*, 81, 935–46.

Girrourdin, E., Roux-Lombard, P., Grau, G. E., Suter, P., Gallati, H., and Dayer, J. M. (1992). Imbalance between tumour necrosis factor alpha and soluble TNF receptor concentrations in severe meningococcaemia. *Immunology*, 76, 20–3.

Goldenberg, D. L. and Reed, J. I. (1985). Bacterial arthritis. *New England Journal of Medicine*, 312, 764–71.

Granfors, K. *et al.* (1989). Yersinia antigens in synovial fluid cells from patients with reactive arthritis. *New England Journal of Medicine*, 320, 216–21.

Hammer, R. E., Malka, S. D., Richardson, J. A., Tang, J. P., and Taurog, J. D. (1990). Spontaneous inflammatory disease in transgenic rats expressing HLA-B27 and human β_2M: an animal model of HLA-B27-associated human disorders. *Cell*, 63, 1099–112.

Keffer, J. *et al.* (1991). Transgenic mice expressing human tumour necrosis factor: a predictive genetic model of arthritis. *EMBO Journal*, 10, 4025–31.

McDermott, M. *et al.* (1995). The role of T-cell receptor β chain genes in susceptibility to rheumatoid arthritis. *Arthritis and Rheumatism*, 39, 91–5.

McGuire, W., Hill, A. V., Allsopp, R. E., Greenwood, B. M., and Kwiakowski, D. (1994). Variation in the TNF alpha promoter region associated with susceptibility to cerebral malacia. *Nature*, 371, 508–10.

Marrack, P. and Kappler, J. (1994). Subversion of the immune system by pathogens. *Cell*, 76, 323–32.

Mosmann, T. R. and Sad, S. (1996). The expanding universe of T-cell subsets: Th1, Th2 and more. *Immunology Today*, 17, 138–46.

Mountz, J. D., Wu, J., Cheng, J., and Zhou, T. (1994). Autoimmune disease: a problem of defective apoptosis. *Arthritis and Rheumatism*, 37, 1415–20.

Pritchard, M. H., Munro, J., and Matthews, N. (1988). Antibodies to influenza A in a cluster of children with juvenile chronic arthritis. *British Journal of Rheumatology*, 27, 176–80.

Rieux-Laucat, F. *et al.* (1995). Mutations in *fas* associated with human lymphoproliferative syndrome and autoimmunity. *Science*, 268, 1347–9.

Sieper, J. and Braun, J. (1995). Pathogenesis of spondyloarthropathies. Persistent bacterial antigen, autoimmunity or both? *Arthritis and Rheumatism*, 38, 1547–54.

Simon, A. K., Seipelt, E., and Sieper, J. (1994). Divergent T-cell cytokine patterns in inflammatory arthritis. *Proceedings of the National Academy of Sciences (USA)*, 91, 8562–6.

Taurog, J. D. *et al.* (1994). The germ-free state prevents development of gut and joint inflammatory disease in HLA-B27 transgenic rats. *Journal of Experimental Medicine*, 180, 2359–64.

Todd, J. A. *et al.* (1988). A molecular basis for MHC class II-associated autoimmunity. *Science*, 240, 1003–9.

Vaughan, J. H. (1989). Infection and rheumatic diseases: a review. *Bulletin on the Rheumatic Diseases*, 39, 1–7; 1–80.

Watanabe-Fukunaga, R., Brannan, C. I., Copeland, N. G., Jenkins, N. A., and Nagata, S. (1992). Lymphoproliferation disorder in mice explained by defects in Fas antigen that mediates apoptosis. *Nature*, 356, 314–17.

5.3   Infections

5.3.1   Pyogenic arthritis in adults

Marc L. Miller

Septic arthritis caused by pyogenic bacteria is a true medical emergency. Prompt recognition of an infected joint and an immediate start to proper treatment are essential for a good outcome. Despite advances in antimicrobial therapy and in surgical approaches to pyogenic arthritis, the death rate in several large series has ranged up to 10 per cent (Rosenthal *et al*. 1980; Dubost *et al*. 1993), and up to one-third of cases are affected by residual functional impairment, persistent pain, or other complications (Goldenberg and Cohen 1976; Sharp *et al*. 1979; Cooper and Cawley 1986). Therefore, it is important to appreciate the clinical presentations of pyogenic arthritis, underlying risk factors and associated diseases, range of infectious agents, diagnostic techniques, and appropriate medical and surgical treatments.

This chapter will discuss pyogenic bacterial infections in adults only. Paediatric infections will be addressed in Chapter 5.3.2.

Pathophysiology

Bacteria can reach the joint by one of three routes:

(1) by haematogenous spread from a distant infected site;

(2) by direct penetration through the skin to the joint space;

(3) by direct spread from a contiguous infected site.

Haematogenous seeding is by far the most common route for pyogenic joint infection. In the setting of bacteraemia, organisms leave the bloodstream and lodge in the synovium. The synovium is a highly vascular tissue without a limiting basement membrane to block bacterial access to the synovial fluid. However, factors other than the mere presence of bacteria in the bloodstream must be involved as most bacteraemic episodes do not result in septic arthritis and some bacteria that are frequent causes of bacteraemia are rare causes of joint infections. One of these factors is structural changes in the joint. Joints affected by a variety of chronic arthritides (including rheumatoid arthritis, osteoarthritis, Charcot's arthropathy, and gout or pseudogout) and prosthetic joints are at increased risk of pyogenic infections. The presence of synovitis, effusion, granulation tissue, or foreign material increase the likelihood of bacterial colonization (Goldenberg and Reed 1985; Youssef and York 1994).

Characteristics of the infecting organisms are also important. Those organisms that most commonly cause pyogenic arthritis, staphylococci and *Neisseria gonorrhoeae*, have an enhanced ability to adhere to synovial tissue or produce toxins that facilitate colonization (Switalski *et al*. 1993). These organisms are able to infect normal joints in normal hosts. Those organisms with low virulence for joint infection, such as Gram-negative bacilli, typically cause infections in the setting of a structurally abnormal joint or an alteration in host immune defences.

A third contributing factor is alteration in host immunity. This may be due to inherited or congenital immunodeficiency states involving granulocyte function, immunoglobulin production or complement deficiency, or to acquired immunodeficiency due to immunosuppressive therapy or to disease states such as cancer, diabetes, chronic liver disease, or human immunodeficiency virus infection (Rivera *et al*. 1992).

Direct entry of bacteria into the joint space can occur as the result of penetrating trauma, arthrocentesis, arthroscopy, or open surgical procedures such as arthroplasty. The incidence of infection following arthrocentesis is very low, less than 0.06 per cent in two large series (Hollander 1969; Gray *et al*. 1981). The risk of joint infection after arthrocentesis may be increased when an area of cellulitis overlies the joint or in the setting of bacteraemia, in which cases bacteria can be carried by the aspirating needle into the joint space. Persistent drainage from surgical portals should always raise the suspicion of postarthroscopic infection.

Direct spread from an adjacent focus of infection occurs in several clinical settings. Pyogenic arthritis may result from an adjacent osteomyelitis in adults, although this complication is rare, owing to the infrequency of untreated osteomyelitis in the antibiotic era. In adults, but not in children, there is an anastomosis between the metaphyseal and synovial vascular beds allowing direct entry of bacteria from an osseous focus of infection into the joint (Atcheson and Ward 1978). Direct extension of an enteric fistula in inflammatory bowel disease, of a psoas abscess, or of a gluteal abscess in a paraplegic can result in pyogenic arthritis of the hip.

Once infection is established bacteria multiply and spread throughout the synovium and eventually into the synovial fluid. Organisms are phagocytosed by polymorphonuclear leucocytes, resulting in the release of chemotactic factors and activation of complement. Additional phagocytic cells are recruited, resulting in a classic inflammatory reaction. Bacterial products and lysosomal proteolytic enzymes released from leucocytes stimulate the degradation of cartilage. In animal models, the proteoglycan content of cartilage is reduced by 40 per cent within 48 h of the induction of joint infection. Within 2 to 3 weeks, significant loss of collagen develops (Riegels-Nielsen *et al*. 1987). This rapid destruction underscores the importance of prompt detection and initiation of treatment, one aspect of which includes the removal of the products of bacterial and leucocyte degradation by draining the joint. Chronic inflammatory tissue, resembling rheumatoid pannus, that further erodes cartilage and subchondral bone may develop in untreated infections.

Non-gonococcal arthritis

Clinical manifestations

The clinical manifestations, epidemiology, and natural history of gonococcal and non-gonococcal arthritis are sufficiently distinct (Table 1) that infections due to *Neisseria* spp. will be discussed separately.

The typical patient with non-gonococcal bacterial arthritis presents with acute onset of pain, swelling, erythema, warmth, and tenderness of the infected joint (Baker and Schumacher 1993). There may be a tense effusion. The patient usually guards the joint against any movement. The severity of pain, tenderness, and swelling is generally greater than in other causes of joint inflammation and should immediately raise the suspicion of infection. Very rarely, patients present with a subacute or even chronic course and a paucity of inflammatory signs. This presentation is more commonly associated with less virulent organisms.

Localization of pain and tenderness may be difficult, and erythema, warmth, and swelling are not detectable in deep-seated joints. For instance, hip infections produce pain deep in the buttock, in the anterior thigh, or even in the knee, while pain from the sacroiliac joint may be referred to the buttock or posterior thigh and may mimic sciatica.

Systemic signs and symptoms of infection are common but not invariably present. In one large series, 90 per cent of patients with acute bacterial arthritis presented with a temperature of at least 37.8°C (Goldenberg and Cohen 1976); in another, fever was found in only 56 per cent (Rosenthal *et al.* 1980). Marked fever (greater than 39°C) was found in two series in 25 and 39 per cent, respectively (Newman 1976; Cooper and Cawley 1986). Therefore, while the presence of high fever in a patient with an acute arthritis should always raise the suspicion of a pyogenic infection, the absence of fever does not preclude the diagnosis.

The patient may also show signs and symptoms of an infection at a distant site from the joint, such as the skin, respiratory tract, or urinary tract.

While any joint is potentially susceptible to pyogenic infection, the knee is the site in more than half of cases and the hip in another 20 per cent. The remainder of cases is divided largely among the shoulder, wrist, elbow, and ankle (Manshady *et al.* 1980; Rosenthal *et al.* 1980; Cooper and Cawley 1986). Rarely the small joints of the fingers and toes or the axial joints (sacroiliac, sternoclavicular, sternomanubrial, or pubic symphysis) are involved. Typically, pyogenic infections cause monarticular arthritis, but in approximately 20 per cent of cases bacteraemia can lead to polyarticular involvement (Epstein *et al.* 1986; Dubost *et al.* 1993). Certainly a polyarticular presentation should not deter a search for infection in a patient with acute onset of illness, signs of toxicity, or a distant site of infection.

Laboratory studies

Patients with pyogenic arthritis commonly have non-specific laboratory signs of acute infection and inflammation. About half will have a peripheral leucocyte count greater than $10\,000/\text{mm}^3$. The erythrocyte sedimentation rate is generally elevated. In one series, the erythrocyte sedimentation rate was greater than 20 mm/h in 117 of 118 cases of pyogenic arthritis. In 76 of these, the rate was greater than 50 mm/h and in 30 cases greater than 100 mm/h (Newman 1976). Similarly, other acute phase reactants such as C-reactive protein may be elevated. The response of the acute phase reactants parallels the course of the infection and is a good indicator of response to therapy. Blood cultures are positive in about one-third of cases (Rosenthal *et al.* 1980).

The critical test in the evaluation of a patient with suspected pyogenic arthritis is the analysis of synovial fluid. The aspiration of frank pus immediately suggests bacterial infection, although joint fluid in chylous effusions associated with long-standing rheumatoid arthritis or subchondral fractures may have a similar appearance.

Table 1 Distinguishing features of gonococcal and non-gonococcal arthritis

Gonococcal	Non-gonococcal
Most often affects healthy, sexually active, young adults	Most often affects the very young or very old. Underlying joint or other medical conditions
Females more often than males	Males more often than females
Hip uncommonly affected	Hips involved in 20%
Migratory polyarthralgias common	Polyarthralgias uncommon
Rash, tenosynovitis common	Extra-articular manifestations common
Synovial fluid:	Synovial fluid:
Gram's stain positive, 25%	Gram's stain positive, 50–65%
culture positive, 50%	culture positive, 90%
lactate not elevated	lactate elevated
Rapid response to therapy	Response often slow; may require surgical drainage
Full recovery in most cases	10% mortality; one-third with residual joint damage

Effusions due to gout or pseudogout can also at times appear grossly purulent.

The leucocyte count in synovial fluid is greater than $50\,000/\text{mm}^3$ in most cases and often exceeds $100\,000/\text{mm}^3$ (Krey and Bailen 1979). The differential count will show greater than 90 per cent polymorphonuclear leucocytes. When the count is less than $50\,000/\text{mm}^3$, repeat aspiration in the next 24 to 48 h will show an increase to over that figure. Where the infection has been partially treated with antibiotics before aspiration, the count may never exceed $50\,000/\text{mm}^3$. In about half of cases, the glucose in synovial fluid will be decreased to 20 to 40 per cent of that of the simultaneous serum glucose. However, similarly low levels are commonly found in rheumatoid effusions, which diminishes the differential diagnostic value of the synovial fluid glucose in rheumatoid patients (Goldenberg and Reed 1985). A markedly elevated level of lactic acid in the synovial fluid is associated with non-gonococcal pyogenic arthritis but not with non-infectious causes of inflammatory effusions (Riordan et al. 1982). The concentration of lactic acid may be of diagnostic help before cultures of synovial fluid are available or in cases of partially treated infections in which synovial fluid cultures remain negative.

Gram's stain of synovial fluid is positive in 50 to 65 per cent of all cases of non-gonococcal arthritis, approaching 75 per cent in staphylococcal infections but only about 50 per cent in infections caused by Gram-negative bacilli (Goldenberg and Cohen 1976; Newman 1976). Bacteria can be cultured from synovial fluid in nearly all cases of non-gonococcal arthritis. The occasional negative results can be attributed to preceding antibiotic therapy, poor handling of specimens, failure to culture for anaerobic organisms, or theoretically to the localization of organisms to the synovium rather than the fluid during the very early stage of infection. The yield from culture of synovial fluid may be improved by inoculating large volumes of it directly into bottles of blood culture media (Von Essen and Holtta 1986).

Imaging studies

Plain radiographs have limited value in evaluation of the suspected infected joint. Most commonly only periarticular soft-tissue swelling or a joint effusion will be present. The primary value of the radiograph is to demonstrate signs of other causes of acute pain and swelling, such as fracture, chondrocalcinosis, gouty erosions, or avascular necrosis, and to look for underlying chronic joint disease or accompanying osteomyelitis. Plain radiographs can be used to assess the extent of joint damage and cartilage loss in cases in which the diagnosis and treatment of infection have been delayed. The radiographic changes indicative of joint damage may lag behind the clinical signs of infection and may continue to appear even after there has been a response to therapy. Conventional tomography may better demonstrate early bone destruction, particularly in hard-to-visualize joints such as the sternoclavicular.

Except in a few clinical situations, radionuclide scanning also has limited value in the assessment of the suspected infected joint. While pyogenic arthritis of peripheral joints is readily detectable on physical examination, infections of the axial joints are often difficult to localize from the patient's description or by physical examination. In these cases, a technetium-99m bone scan can demonstrate increased activity that suggests involvement of a deep-seated joint (Gordon and Kabins 1980; Vyskocil et al. 1991). For example, in the evaluation of the patient with signs of infection and complaining of diffuse low back or buttock pain, the technetium scan may identify involvement

of the sacroiliac joint. This may help to differentiate joint sepsis from intra-abdominal or retroperitoneal abscess, or from osteomyelitis of the pelvis. The technetium bone scan, however, does not differentiate between infectious and non-infectious inflammatory arthritis and therefore cannot distinguish an infected sacroiliac joint from sacroiliitis due to Reiter's syndrome, or an infected from an uninfected but actively inflamed peripheral joint in rheumatoid arthritis.

The accuracy of detecting joint infections with radionuclide scanning can be improved by scanning with either gallium-67- or indium-111-labelled leucocytes. Gallium scans used in sequence after a positive technetium scan may increase the specificity of technetium scanning. The gallium scan may become positive earlier than the technetium in poorly vascularized joints such as the sacroiliac or sternoclavicular, making it a useful test to consider even when the technetium scan is negative (Lopez-Longo et al. 1987). False-positive gallium scans have been reported in rheumatoid arthritis, thereby limiting the usefulness of this technique in evaluating the possibility of joint sepsis in that condition. Gallium and indium scans are of most value in suspected infection of a prosthetic joint, where they may distinguish an infected from an uninfected, painful, loose prosthesis. Although indium scanning does require the additional steps of removing, labelling, and then reinfusing the patient's leucocytes, it is more sensitive and specific than sequential technetium/gallium scanning and results are available at 24 h rather than 72 h as with gallium scanning (Merkel et al. 1985).

Conventional fluoroscopy or computed tomographic scanning can be of value in guiding diagnostic aspiration of deep-seated joints such as the hip or sacroiliac joint. While computed tomography and magnetic resonance imaging are seldom necessary in the evaluation of septic arthritis, these imaging techniques can be of great value when an infected joint fails to respond as expected to appropriate treatment because of adjacent osteomyelitis or a persistent collection of undrained pus. These techniques can also demonstrate soft tissue masses adjacent to axial joints, so indicating the need for abscess drainage (Wohlgethan et al. 1988).

Bacteriology

A wide variety of organisms has been cultured from infected joints (Table 2). *Staphylococcus aureus* is by far the most common cause of

Table 2 Infecting organisms in non-gonococcal arthritis in adults

Organism	Percentage of cases
Staphylococcus	
aureus	40–50
epidermis	10–15
Streptococcal species	20
Gram-negative bacteria	15
S. pneumoniae	2
H. influenzae	2
Anaerobes	5

non-gonococcal arthritis, accounting for 40 to 50 per cent of cases in adults. *Staph. epidermis* is found in 10 to 15 per cent, various streptococcal species in 20 per cent, and various Gram-negative bacilli in 15 per cent of cases. The incidence of pneumococcal joint infections has been drastically reduced in the antibiotic era, reflecting the more effective treatment of pneumococcal infections of the respiratory tract and the decreased incidence of pneumococcal bacteraemia. *Haemophilus influenzae*, the organism most commonly found in pyogenic infections in children under the age of 2 years, accounts for only about 2 per cent of cases in adults (Goldenberg and Cohen 1976; Newman 1976; Sharp *et al.* 1979; Rosenthal *et al.* 1980; Goldenberg and Reed 1985; Cooper and Cawley 1986; Mikhail and Alarcon 1993; Youssef and York 1994). Anaerobic infections, often polymicrobial, occur in about 5 per cent of cases. Case reports have documented the unusual occurrence of arthritis due to *Listeria monocytogenes*, *Streptobacillus moniliformis*, and *Pasteurella multocida*. While *Staph. aureus* is the most common cause of both monarticular and polyarticular presentations, streptococci and *H. influenzae* are more frequently associated with polyarticular infections than would be expected by the overall incidence of joint infections with these organisms (Epstein *et al.* 1986; Dubost *et al.* 1993).

A variety of streptococcal species, most commonly group A β-haemolytic, but also group B, group C, group G, enterococcus, *Streptococcus milleri* and *Strep. viridans* have been found in infected joints. Group A streptococci are common inhabitants of the skin and respiratory tract and can seed the joints of normal hosts. Group B streptococci, usually associated with neonatal and puerperal sepsis, have been a cause of adult pyogenic arthritis, particularly in patients with prosthetic joints or predisposing medical conditions such as diabetes mellitus. About 40 per cent of reported cases have been diabetics, in whom the death rate was about 15 to 20 per cent. Group B streptococcal joint infections have been associated with significant complications in the form of residual damage and limited range of movement (Small *et al.* 1984; Pischel *et al.* 1985). Similarly, group C and G streptococcal infections appear to affect patients with underlying illnesses, and have been polyarticular in 30 per cent of reported cases (Ike 1990; Burhert and Watanakunakorn 1991). Enterococci are not usually reported as joint pathogens, despite their frequent association with infections of the biliary and urinary tracts, and with bacteraemia. Affected patients generally have either predisposing conditions or pre-existing joint disease.

H. influenzae is an encapsulated organism requiring opsonizing antibody and an effective reticuloendothelial system for optimal clearance. Patients with *H. influenzae* arthritis therefore often have predisposing conditions such as alcoholism, hypogammaglobulinaemia, multiple myeloma, systemic lupus erythematosus, or asplenia. Extra-articular *H. influenzae* infections are frequent, including sinusitis, pneumonia, meningitis, pharyngitis, or cellulitis. Almost half of reported cases have been polyarticular (Borenstein and Simon 1986).

Gram-negative bacilli have emerged as a more frequent cause of septic arthritis in the past two decades. This probably reflects the prolonged survival of patients with serious medical illnesses, the increased use of immunosuppressive drugs, and the increase in intravenous drug abuse. Gram-negative joint infections generally occur in two distinct clinical settings. The first involves elderly patients with underlying systemic illnesses or pre-existing joint disease. Here the presentation is usually abrupt, with frequent fevers and rigors. The most common organism is *Escherichia coli* (Newman *et al.* 1988).

Also reported with some frequency are *Pseudomonas aeruginosa*, *Proteus mirabilis*, *Serratia marcesens*, and *Klebsiella 'pneumoniae'*. Scattered case reports document rare joint infections with a number of Gram-negative organisms including *Aeromonas hydrophila*, *Acinetobacter* spp., *Arizona hinshawii*, *Eikenella corrodens*, *Enterobacter* spp., and *Kingella kingae*; these reports indicate the importance of bacteriological identification by culture in patients with suspected Gram-negative infections.

The second group consists of patients with a history of intravenous drug abuse. These patients tend to be younger and to have no pre-existing joint disease. Their presentation is often more insidious, with a longer duration of illness before diagnosis (Bayer *et al.* 1977; Chandrasekar and Narula 1986). There is a predilection for the axial joints and periarticular soft-tissue abscess or osteomyelitis are frequently encountered. *Ps. aeruginosa* and *Serr. 'marcesens'* have been reported in increased frequency in this group in some but not all series from large urban centres.

Salmonellal arthritis is a rare complication of salmonellosis. *Salmonella typhimurium* is the most common serotype cultured from joints, followed by *Sal. choleraesuis*. Patients with systemic lupus erythematosus or sickle-cell anaemia are at increased risk for salmonella arthritis because the chronic salmonella carrier state is more common in these conditions. This is the result of impaired clearance by the reticuloendothelial system, owing to inhibition of Fc receptors by circulating immune complexes in systemic lupus and to the functional hyposplenism that can accompany either condition. The presentation is usually monarticular but polyarticular cases have been reported. In many cases there is no history of a preceding diarrhoeal illness. The diagnosis of salmonellal arthritis may not be suspected after arthrocentesis because the synovial fluid is often non-purulent, and described as turbid, serosanguinous, or straw-coloured, despite a positive culture from it (Cohen *et al.* 1987; Medina *et al.* 1989).

Rat-bite fever caused by *Streptobacillus moniliformis*, a pleomorphic Gram-negative organism, presents as an acute illness with fever, rash, vomiting, and arthritis that is usually polyarticular. The infection is acquired from bites or close contact with infected rodents or from ingestion of contaminated food or beverages. When articular symptoms are prominent the clinical presentation may be confused with rheumatoid arthritis, adult Still's disease, systemic lupus, or gonococcaemia. Joint effusions can be either sterile and inflammatory or purulent with positive cultures of synovial fluid. Isolation and identification of the organism is difficult, owing to its variable staining characteristics and specific growth requirements (Holroyd *et al.* 1988).

Past. multocida is a small, Gram-negative coccobacillus that causes joint infections after animal bites, most commonly from cats or dogs. In approximately one-third of patients there is no history of a bite. Arthritis with this organism has been reported in both normal hosts and in patients with rheumatoid arthritis, chronic liver disease, or immunosuppression (Weber *et al.* 1984).

L. monocytogenes infections in general have been increasing in recent years, owing to the increased survival of immunocompromised patients. The few case reports of *L. monocytogenes* infections of the joints suggest that these occur in immunocompromised patients or in those with previous joint disease (Kurosh and Perednia 1989).

In recent years there has been increasing recognition of the role of anaerobic organisms in pyogenic arthritis, although the incidence of anaerobic bacterial arthritis is still quite low. Anaerobic joint infections typically occur after joint surgery, after penetrating trauma, or in patients with underlying diseases. In the setting of surgery or trauma, bacteria are introduced directly from the skin or from soil contaminated with faecal organisms. Peptococcal and clostridial species, and *Propionibacterium acnes* predominate. In the setting of underlying disease the anaerobic Gram-negative organisms, particularly *Bacteroides fragilis*, predominate. The route of infection can be haematogenous from a distant site such as the bowel or direct extension from an adjacent site such as a deep sacral decubitus. In about half of cases in all settings a single organism will be cultured, while half will be polymicrobial, usually mixed aerobic and anaerobic organisms (Fitzgerald *et al.* 1982; Brook and Frazier 1993).

Anaerobic joint infections are probably underdiagnosed. There are no specific diagnostic signs and therefore synovial fluid must be cultured for anaerobic organisms whenever the clinical setting suggests the possibility of anaerobic infection. Anaerobic cultures should also be obtained in any patient with suspected joint infection in whom initial aerobic cultures of synovial fluid are negative. Any anaerobic organisms isolated from synovial fluid should not be dismissed merely as contaminants if the clinical setting suggests infection.

Joint infections and rheumatoid arthritis

Patients with rheumatoid arthritis are at increased risk of pyogenic arthritis. While the precise prevalence of joint infections in rheumatoid arthritis is not known, in several large series approximately 10 per cent of all cases of non-gonococcal arthritis occurred in patients with that condition (Goldenberg and Cohen 1976; Rosenthal *et al.* 1980; Cooper and Cawley 1986).

Proliferative synovitis and structural changes in the rheumatoid joint may allow bacteria to become sequestered in the joint more readily and to escape normal host-defence mechanisms. The formation of pannus and damage to cartilage may more readily allow the spread of bacteria from the synovium to subchondral bone. There is some controversy about whether patients with rheumatoid arthritis have an increased risk for infections in general, but they are often treated with immunosuppressive medications, which put them at increased risk of infection. Rheumatoid patients with advanced disease may be significantly debilitated, may be bedridden with greater risk of infections of the respiratory or urinary tracts, and may develop skin ulcerations from vasculitis, all of which increase the risk of infection.

Staph. aureus is the infecting organism in 70 per cent of reported cases, followed by streptococci in 9 per cent, Gram-negative bacilli in 8 per cent, pneumococci in 7 per cent, and anaerobes in 3 per cent. Blood cultures are positive in 20 to 25 per cent of cases. The knee is involved in about half the cases. The hip, shoulder, elbow, wrist, and ankle are each involved in about 10 per cent of cases, while infections in the smaller joints of the hands and feet are unusual. Polyarticular infections are reported in about 30 per cent of cases. The source of infection can be identified in half of these patients. The skin is the most common site of distant infection, followed by the lungs, and the urinary and gastrointestinal tracts (Gardner and Weisman 1990).

Identifying joint infections in the patient with rheumatoid arthritis can be difficult clinically because joint inflammation is part of the underlying disease. Furthermore, fewer than one-half of rheumatoid patients with joint infections present with fever and even fewer develop a leucocytosis (Gardner and Weisman 1990). The erythrocyte sedimentation rate is of limited value in distinguishing infection from disease flare. Both infection and exacerbation of the rheumatoid condition can be monarticular or polyarticular. This difficulty in distinguishing between the two often leads to delay in diagnosis. Joint infection should be suspected in those patients whose disease activity changes abruptly from its normal pattern, particularly if only one or a few joints are involved; in those with systemic signs of toxicity; in those with a remote site of active or recent infection; or in patients on immunosuppressive therapy with long-standing, deforming disease or with accompanying, debilitating illnesses. Whenever one of these clinical states is present, synovial fluid should be obtained, Gram stained, and cultured before considering any treatment (such as an intra-articular steroid injection or systemic anti-inflammatory medication) for a flare-up of rheumatoid disease (Blackburn *et al.* 1986; Goldenberg 1989; Soria *et al.* 1992).

Distinguishing infection from disease exacerbation is further complicated by the occasional patient who develops a 'pseudoseptic' arthritis. In these cases there is an abrupt onset of usually monarticular joint pain and effusion, accompanied by fever. The synovial fluid is purulent, with the leucocyte count usually greater than 100 000/mm³. Gram's stain and culture of the synovial fluid are negative, and the process quickly resolves within a few days without antibiotics (Call *et al.* 1985; Singleton *et al.* 1991). These episodes may be recurrent and identical in presentation in an individual patient, in which case antibiotics may be withheld pending the results of synovial fluid culture. In most instances, however, empirical antibiotic therapy should be started as soon as infection is suspected and cultures obtained. If adequate cultures are negative, then 'pseudoseptic' arthritis should be considered and antibiotics discontinued.

Owing mostly to the delay in establishing the diagnosis, joint infections in rheumatoid patients tend to have a poorer outcome than in other groups with pyogenic arthritis. The death rate in reported series is about 20 per cent, more than doubling in patients with polyarticular involvement (Gardner and Weisman 1990). Only about one-third will recover without any worsening of basic joint function. On occasion osteomyelitis or draining cutaneous fistulas will develop.

Prosthetic joint infections

While the risk of prosthetic joint infection has decreased significantly over the past three decades, infection remains a major cause of failure in arthroplasty. With evaluation and treatment of preoperative infections, improved surgical technique, and perioperative prophylactic antibiotics, infection after hip or knee arthroplasty has been reduced to less than 1 per cent of cases. The incidence of infection for revisions of prosthetic joints is about 5 to 10 times that of primary procedures (Poss *et al.* 1984; Wymenga *et al.* 1992).

A number of factors contribute to the risk of prosthetic joint infection. There is a risk of introducing bacteria whenever the joint space is entered. In addition the presence of foreign material in the joint promotes the growth of bacteria by sequestering organisms from the vascular supply and hence from the host immune-defence mechanisms and antibiotics. Methylmethacrylate cement may inhibit the phagocytic function of polymorphs and promote the production of glycocalyx, a fibrous collection of polysaccharides that enhance bacterial growth (Gristina and Kolkin 1983).

Prosthetic joint infections should be suspected whenever there are systemic or localized signs and symptoms of infection, or in cases of new or increasing prosthetic joint pain, even in the absence of clinical signs of infection. Over 90 per cent of all prosthetic joint infections present with joint pain; fever, and erythema and swelling of the joint occur in less than half of cases. Leucocytosis is unusual while an elevated erythrocyte sedimentation rate is almost always present.

About one-half of infections are detected in the first 12 months after surgery, with one-half of these occurring in the early postoperative period up to 3 months after surgery (Inman *et al.* 1984). Those cases that present in the early postoperative period are usually the result of bacteria introduced at the time of surgery or are due to wound infections. A large proportion of these patients will have or have had wounds complicated by haematoma, stitch abscess, dehiscence, or infection. These patients usually have an acute illness with fever, pain, and local signs of infection, including persistent drainage from the joint. However, infection should still be suspected in the patient with fever, leucocytosis, or elevated erythrocyte sedimentation rate that fails to drop with time, even in the absence of local signs of infection.

Infections occurring between 3 and 12 months postoperatively tend to have a more subacute presentation. Less than half will have local signs of joint infection. Most will present with either joint pain or failure to regain the expected functional level.

The prosthetic joint remains at risk for infection indefinitely. Infections diagnosed more than 1 year after surgery are usually the result of haematogenous seeding from a distant focus such as the urinary tract or skin, from dental work, or from surgical manipulation of the gastrointestinal or urinary tracts. The presentation is usually the insidious onset of pain in the absence of both systemic and local signs and symptoms of infection. There is often a delay of months from onset of pain to diagnosis. Occasionally, late infections present with draining sinus tracts.

Diagnosis of prosthetic joint infection is often difficult. In the early period, infection of the actual joint space must be distinguished from adjacent wound and soft tissue infection. In later infections presenting with only joint pain, the infected prosthesis must be distinguished from the uninfected but painful, loose prosthesis. Plain radiographs are usually normal in early infections. Loosening is defined as greater than 2 mm of lucency at the bone–cement or bone–metal (in cementless prostheses) interface, or any lucency at the metal–cement interface. Other findings in late infections include progressive cortical bone loss around the prosthesis, fractured cement, or a periosteal reaction when the infection has spread through the thickness of cortical bone. Radionuclide scans are useful in the evaluation of prosthetic joint loosening. A negative technetium-99m bone scan is strong evidence against infection and sequential technetium-99m and gallium-67 scanning can help to distinguish infected from non-infected loosening. Similarly, indium-111 uptake favours diagnosis of infection. Joint aspiration is necessary when infection is suspected on a clinical basis or if imaging studies are suggestive of infection or are equivocal. Culturing for anaerobic organisms is imperative. At times, bacteriological diagnosis can only be confirmed by bone biopsy or by culturing material obtained at surgery for removal of the prosthesis.

Staphylococcal species account for 50 to 60 per cent of prosthetic joint infections. *Staph. epidermis* is a more common cause of prosthetic than native joint infections. Various stretococcal species and Gram-negative bacilli each account for 15 to 20 per cent and anae-robes 5 to 10 per cent of cases. Mixed organisms are cultured in 10 to 20 per cent of cases, particularly those occurring in the early postoperative period (Inman *et al.* 1984). Organisms of low virulence that are seldom considered pathogens, such as diphtheroids, propionibac-teria, and lactobacilli, are occasional causes of prosthetic joint infections and must not be dismissed as contaminants if cultured from synovial fluid or biopsy material.

Neisserial arthritis

Gonococcal arthritis

N. gonorrhoeae can cause either localized mucosal infections of the genitourinary tract, rectum, pharynx, or conjunctiva, or disseminated infections of the skin, joints, and less commonly, heart and meninges. Disseminated gonococcal infection complicates approximately 0.1 to 0.3 per cent of localized infections. Seventy-five per cent of cases of disseminated gonococcal infection result from asymptomatic local infections (Eisenstein and Masi 1981). This makes effective preventive measures difficult.

Those strains of *N. gonorrhoeae* associated with disseminated disease differ biologically from those strains associated with sympto-matic, localized disease (O'Brien *et al.* 1983). The strains that disseminate are more likely to be resistant to killing by normal human serum, have specific nutritional requirements when grown in culture, have specific cell-surface proteins, and tend to be more sensi-tive to antibiotics. These characteristics are also shared by those strains that cause asymptomatic localized infections. These strains do not provoke a local inflammatory reaction and thus the organism is not limited to the mucosa, allowing seeding of the bloodstream.

While the incidence of disseminated gonococcal infection has been decreasing in recent years due probably to a decrease in both the prevalence of those strains associated with disseminated disease and to a decline in the overall incidence of gonococcal infections, *N. gonorrhoeae* remains a common cause of bacterial arthritis in young, previously healthy, individuals particularly in urban centres where the largest reservoirs of localized gonococcal infection exist (Rompalo *et al.* 1987). Seventy-five per cent of cases occur between the ages of 15 and 30 years, in parallel with the years of peak incidence for localized gonococcal infections, although any sexually active indi-vidual is potentially at risk (Geelhoed-Duyvestijn *et al.* 1986). Women are affected three to five times more often than men. By contrast, non-gonococcal arthritis more commonly affects the very young or the very old, men, and individuals with underlying diseases or risk factors.

Individuals with inherited deficiencies of the terminal complement components, C5 to C9, have an increased risk of neisserial infection (Ross and Densen 1984). Complement deficiencies should be searched for in individuals with recurrent gonococcal or meningo-coccal infections.

Disseminated gonococcal infection has been classified according to the presence or absence of a purulent effusion (Holmes *et al.* 1971; Masi and Eisenstein 1981; O'Brien *et al.* 1983). About two-thirds of patients present with an acute illness of 3 to 4 days' duration, consisting of fever, rash, tenosynovitis, and migratory polyarthralgias or polyarthritis with non-purulent effusions (group I). The rash, present in 60 to 90 per cent of this group, is a diffuse, maculopapular eruption or a more limited number of vesiculopustular lesions on an erythematous base of approximately 5 mm. in diameter. Less commonly the lesions appear as haemorrhagic pustules or bullas. The rash generally spares the face and scalp but can appear anywhere on the trunk and extremities. The lesions may be painful. Tenosynovitis usually involves multiple sites, particularly at the wrist, fingers, ankles, and toes. It is present in 90 per cent of group I patients. Polyarthralgias and polyarthritis are migratory, with a predilection for upper extremity joints. When effusions are present they are small and cultures of synovial fluid are negative.

Group II patients present with a purulent arthritis that resembles the presentation of non-gonococcal arthritis. Typically, these patients present with an acute illness of 4 to 5 days' duration. Most have a monarticular arthritis, with the knee most commonly involved, followed by the ankle, wrist, and elbow. Involvement of the hip, shoulder, temporomandibular, and axial joints is rare, as is polyarticular involvement. About one-third of patients in this group will also have rash or tenosynovitis and about two-thirds will give a history of polyarthralgia preceding the development of monarthritis.

About 40 per cent of group I patients have positive blood cultures; this rarely if ever occurs in group II patients (O'Brien *et al*. 1983). This strongly negative correlation between positive blood cultures and the presence of purulent joint effusions suggests that group I patients present during the bacteraemic phase of the disseminated infection and group II patients during the phase of joint localization that can follow bacteraemia. Some series have reported progression from group I to II in individual patients (Holmes *et al*. 1971), although others believe that the groups are distinct (O'Brien *et al*. 1983; Koss 1985).

Leucocyte counts in synovial fluid in group II patients range from about 30 000/mm^3 to greater than 200 000/mm^3. This range overlaps with that in non-gonococcal arthritis, although counts tend to be slightly lower in gonococcal infections. The synovial fluid lactate is not increased in gonococcal arthritis. Gram's stain is positive in about one-quarter of cases, and *N. gonorrhoeae* can be successfully cultured from only about half of the purulent effusions (Scopelitis and Martinez-Osuna 1993). There are several explanations for this low rate of recovery of organisms even from purulent effusions. First, *N. gonorrhoeae* is difficult to culture, owing to its fastidious growth requirements. Second, organisms may be sequestered in the synovium and may not have entered the synovial fluid. Third, organisms may exist only transiently in the synovial fluid before they are phagocytosed and can no longer be cultured, but the synovitis persists in response to constituents of the gonococcal cell wall such as lipopolysaccharide. In animal studies, both killed gonococci and purified lipopolysaccharide can induce a purulent synovitis after injection into the joint space (Goldenberg *et al*. 1984). Finally, effusions may be caused or maintained by host immunological reactions to *N. gonorrhoeae*. Immune complexes have been demonstrated in both synovial fluid and the blood of patients with disseminated infection.

As positive cultures of synovial fluid are obtained in only a minority of patients, the diagnosis of disseminated gonococcal infection must often be presumed from a suggestive clinical presentation, together with isolation of *N. gonorrhoeae* from a site other than the joint. In patients with disseminated infection, positive cultures can be obtained from the cervix in 80 to 90 per cent of women, the urethra in 50 to 75 per cent of men, and the blood in 25 per cent. The pharynx and the rectum will be positive in a smaller number of cases (Scopelitis and Martinez-Osuna 1993). To culture *N. gonorrhoeae*

from the joint, synovial fluid should be immediately spread on a prewarmed, chocolate-agar plate and incubated in a atmosphere enriched with carbon dioxide, or sent to the laboratory on transport media. Antibiotic-enriched culture media such as Thayer–Martin are used for isolating *N. gonorrhoeae* from sites that have a native bacterial flora, such as the pharynx, cervix, urethra, and rectum, but are not necessary and in fact may inhibit growth when culturing synovial fluid. Recently, the identification of *N. gonorrhoeae* DNA in culture-negative synovial fluid by the polymerase chain reaction has been reported. This technique potentially can improve diagnostic accuracy and hasten the time to diagnosis but is not yet readily available (Liebling *et al*. 1994)

The differential diagnosis of disseminated gonococcal infection is broad. Reiter's syndrome and disseminated gonococcal infection both commonly affect young, sexually active individuals. Urethritis, rashes, and inflammatory monarthritis or oligoarthritis can occur in both. The onset of illness in Reiter's syndrome tends to be more gradual than in disseminated gonococcal infection. Psoriasiform skin lesions, sacroiliitis, painless oral ulcers, conjunctivitis, and a recent history of a diarrhoeal illness favour the diagnosis of Reiter's syndrome. Analysis of synovial fluid does not distinguish between the two conditions unless a positive culture for *N. gonorrhoeae* is obtained. Not uncommonly the patient with disseminated gonococcal infection presenting with monarthritis must be distinguished from patients with non-gonococcal bacterial arthritis. Table 1 lists the distinguishing features. Other infectious illnesses may present with fever, rash, and polyarthralgias or polyarthritis, such as the prodrome of hepatitis B, subacute bacterial endocarditis, and bacterial arthritis due to *N. meningitidis*, Group A streptococcus, *H. influenzae*, or *Streptobac. moniliformis*. Acute rheumatic fever may present with fever and migratory arthritis distinguishable from disseminated gonococcal infection by evidence of a recent streptococcal infection, accompanying chorea or typical rash, and by rapid response to aspirin. Systemic lupus erythematosus, hypersensitivity vasculitis, and adult Still's disease may all present with fever, rash, and arthritis that at times might be confused with disseminated gonococcal infection, although the nature of the rash and the involvement of other organ systems should help to distinguish most cases.

The course of the disseminated infection is variable. In the pre-antibiotic era, some cases underwent spontaneous remission, while in others there was progression to destructive joint changes. In general the progression to irreversible damage in the cartilage and joint is not as rapid as with organisms such as staphylococci, streptococci, or Gram-negative bacilli. Rash, tenosynovitis, and polyarthralgias respond very promptly to antibiotics, while purulent effusions respond somewhat more slowly.

Meningococcal arthritis

Arthritis due to *N. meningitidis* follows one of several clinical patterns and may be confused with disseminated gonococcal infection (Fam *et al*. 1979; Schaad 1980). Joint manifestations complicate about 2 to 10 per cent of cases of acute meningococcaemia and may follow one of three clinical patterns. In the first, patients develop polyarthralgias, polyarthritis, or tenosynovitis during the acute phase of their meningococcal infection. They are acutely ill with fever, meningitis, and/or a diffuse, erythematous, macular rash or diffuse haemorrhagic skin lesions typical of acute meningococcaemia. When effusions occur in this group they are small and non-purulent. Synovial cultures are negative but *N. meningitidis* can be recovered from blood or cerebrospinal fluid. The articular manifestations respond rapidly to antibiotic therapy. When meningitis is absent, these patients resemble those in group I of disseminated gonococcal infection (see above) (Kidd *et al.* 1985).

The second group of patients, which resembles group II in disseminated gonococcal infection, develops purulent joint effusions that are most commonly monarticular or oligoarticular during the acute phase of meningococcaemia. Cultures of synovial fluid can be positive or negative. In some cases these effusions may be slow to resolve, even after appropriate antibiotics are given and the synovial fluid cultures are sterile.

A small number of patients with acute meningococcaemia will develop articular manifestations only after the acute stage of infection has responded to antibiotics and the patient is clearly improving (Jarrett *et al.* 1980). In these cases, monarticular, oligoarticular, or polyarticular effusions develop 1 to 2 weeks after the onset of the acute illness. Cultures of synovial fluid are negative but immune complexes are detectable in blood and synovial fluid, suggesting an immunological basis for the synovitis, which eventually resolves without further antibiotic therapy.

Patients with purulent arthritis, usually monarticular, but without signs of acute meningococcaemia are classified as primary meningococcal arthritis (Andersson and Krook 1987). The knee and ankle are most commonly involved. Cultures of synovial fluid are positive in 90

per cent of cases. Despite prompt and appropriate therapy these patients are at risk for joint damage and at times may require open drainage. Blood cultures are negative in this group.

Finally, joint manifestations may occur in the setting of chronic meningococcaemia, a condition marked by chronic rash and positive blood cultures. These patients generally present with polyarthralgias rather than frank arthritis. When effusions are present, cultures are negative, suggesting an immune-mediated mechanism.

Management

The three basic principles of management of pyogenic joint infections are: (i) prompt diagnosis and institution of therapy; (ii) appropriate antibiotics; and (iii) adequate drainage of the infected joint.

The most important factors in determining outcome are the length of time before beginning treatment and the length of time to sterilization of synovial fluid cultures (Ho and Su 1982). Therefore, the suspicion of joint infection should arise in any patient with an unexplained, painful or swollen joint, especially those with an acute presentation, with monarticular presentation, with systemic or local signs and symptoms of infection, with risk factors (such as underlying joint disease, recent joint trauma or surgery, diabetes, immunosuppression, or history of intravenous drug abuse), or with active or recent extra-articular infection.

Table 3   Guidelines for initial antibiotic therapy of bacterial arthritis based on Gram's stain

Gram's stain result	Probable pathogen	Antibiotic choice
Gram-positive cocci clusters	*Staph. aureus* (methicillin resistance suspected)	Nafcillin (100–150 mg/kg per day) Vancomycin (1 g every 12 h)
	Staph. epidermis	Vancomycin (1 g every 12 h)
Pairs and chains	Streptococci (enterococcal)	(non-Penicillin G (2.5 million U)
(urinary, biliary, bowel)	Enterococci	Penicillin G (2.5 million U) and gentamycin (1 mg/kg every 8 h)
Gram-negative cocci	*N. gonorrhoeae*	Ceftriaxone (1–2 g every 12 h)
(haemorrhagic rash, meningitis)	*N. meningitidis*	Penicillin G (2.5–5 million U every 6 h)
Gram-negative coccobacilli	*H. influenzae* (ampicillin resistance suspected)	Ampicillin (2 g every 6 h) Cefotaxime (1 g every 8 h)
Gram-negative bacilli	Enterobacteriaceae	Cefotaxime (2 g every 8 h)
	Pseudomonas spp.	Ceftazidime (2 g every 8 h)
No organisms seen		
(healthy young adult)	*N. gonorrhoeae*	Ceftriaxone (1–2 g every 12 h)
(older adult, underlying disease)	Staphylococci Streptococci Enterobacteriaceae	Vancomycin and cefotaxime
(intravenous drug abuser)	Staphylococci *Pseudomonas* (spp. Enterobacteriaceae	Vancomycin and ceftazidime

Reprinted with modification from Parker, R. H. (1988). Acute bacterial arthritis. In *Orthopedic infections*, (ed. D. Schlossberg), p. 74. Springer-Verlag, New York.

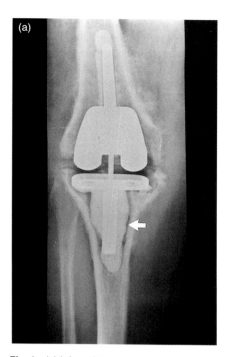
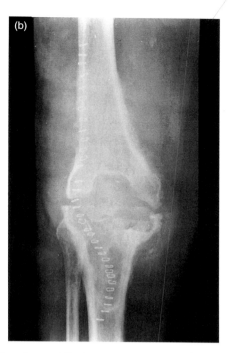
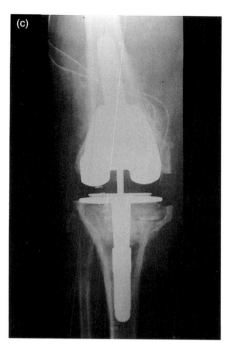

Fig. 1 (a) Infected knee prosthesis. Note the radiolucent zone at the bone–cement interface of the tibial component indicating loosening (arrow); (b) the same knee after complete removal of the infected prosthesis and cement; and (c) the same knee 2 months later after reimplantation of a new prosthesis.

In these settings there should be no delay in aspirating the involved joint or joints. The synovial fluid should be analysed for total and differential cell count, lactate, and crystals, and Gram stained and cultured to differentiate pyogenic infection from other causes of acute joint pain and swelling, including crystal-induced arthritis, exacerbation or presentation of an inflammatory arthritis, haemarthrosis, or trauma. The presence of urate or calcium pyrophosphate crystals, however, does not completely exclude the diagnosis of infection. In rare cases, crystals and infection have occurred in the same joint. The infectious process may 'leach' crystals out of the cartilage or synovium. Blood cultures should be obtained and a search for a distant focus of infection should be undertaken as appropriate for the individual patient.

If Gram's stain is positive or the analysis is otherwise suggestive of pyogenic infection, treatment should begin immediately. The patient should be admitted to hospital and given intravenous antibiotics as soon as all cultures have been obtained. Intra-articular antibiotics should be avoided because adequate concentrations in synovial fluid can be achieved via the parenteral route and because there is a risk of chemical synovitis with the intra-articular route. The concentration of antibiotics in synovial fluid parallels that in serum, and adequate levels can be achieved with standard parenteral doses. Penetration of the drug into the synovial fluid is greatest when the inflammation is most active at the start of therapy and falls off as the infection is controlled. Although they may achieve bactericidal levels in synovial fluid, aminoglycosides are sometimes less effective than other agents, possibly due to inhibition by the reduced pH of infected synovial fluid. Aminoglycosides are therefore inadequate for primary treatment of pyogenic arthritis. Erythromycin does not reach adequate levels in synovial fluid and therefore cannot be used as an alternative to penicillin (Esterhai and Gelb 1991).

Most often the initial choice of antibiotics is empirically guided by the results of Gram's stain, when positive, or by the clinical features when Gram's stain is negative. In choosing antibiotics, one must consider the age of the patient, any underlying disease, and the presence of extra-articular infection. Table 3 provides a guide to the empirical choice of antibiotics. When the results of antibiotic sensitivity testing become known, antibiotic coverage sould then be modified to provide a regimen that has the narrowest spectrum, is the least toxic, and is the least expensive.

In recent years, methicillin-resistant strains of *Staph. aureus* have become more prevalent in both hospital- and community-acquired infections (Ang-Fonte *et al.* 1985). Vancomycin should be the initial drug of choice for suspected *Staph. aureus* infection in those communities and hospitals where resistant strains exist.

Although those strains of *N. gonorrhoeae* that cause disseminated gonococcal infection are more likely to be antibiotic sensitive than those causing localized infections, strains that have chromosomally-mediated resistance to penicillin or are resistant because they produce plasmid-mediated penicillinase have become more common and widespread, and have been reported in disseminated infection (Wise *et al.* 1994). Therefore, in communities with resistant strains, a third-generation cephalosporin should replace penicillin G until antibiotic sensitivities are reported.

The duration of antibiotic therapy must be tailored to the individual presentation and response to therapy and to the infecting organism. In general, intravenous antibiotics should be continued until signs of joint inflammation have resolved, joint effusions have resolved or significantly decreased, and synovial cultures are sterile. Oral antibiotics can then be used to complete the course of treatment, which is usually about 2 weeks in uncomplicated cases but should be extended to 4 weeks or more where there was a significant delay in starting treatment, or a slow response, where infection was with virulent organisms such as *Staph. aureus* or Gram-negative bacilli, and in immunosuppressed patients (Syrogiannopoulos and Nelson 1988). The development of ambulatory intravenous antibiotic delivery systems has allowed earlier hospital discharge in appropriate patients (Williams *et al.* 1989).

The duration of parenteral antibiotic therapy for disseminated gonococcal infection is generally shorter than for non-gonococcal arthritis. In most patients with gonococcal arthritis with a good response to therapy, parenteral antibiotics can be substituted by oral after about 3 days of intravenous therapy to complete a 2-week course. Patients who have dermatitis/tenosynovitis only, without purulent arthritis, can be treated as outpatients, provided they are compliant and closely followed.

Occasional patients with purulent gonococcal effusions will develop a persistent inflammatory effusion, lasting weeks, after a good response to antibiotics and sterilization of synovial fluid. These effusions eventually resolve without further antibiotics. Recovery may be speeded by giving non-steroidal anti-inflammatory drugs.

Infected joints can be drained by closed needle aspiration, tidal irrigation (Ike 1993), arthroscopy, or arthrotomy. Each procedure has its appropriate place in the treatment of septic arthritis depending on the clinical situation. Which modality is chosen is probably not as critical to the ultimate outcome as the duration of time from onset of infection to adequate drainage and sterilization of the joint fluid (Goldenberg *et al.* 1975; Lane *et al.* 1990; Ho 1993).

Initial treatment with serial, closed-needle aspiration avoids the expense and surgical morbidity and mortality of the more invasive procedures and is a satisfactory approach as long as the joint can be completely drained and there is clear evidence of improvement as indicated by resolution of systemic signs of toxicity, serial decrease in synovial fluid white blood-cell count and sterilization of the synovial fluid culture within 48 to 72 h (Broy and Schmid 1986).

The presence of risk factors for a poor outcome include delayed diagnosis, virulent organism, polyarticular involvement, or underlying disease, such as rheumatoid arthritis, and might prompt the early use of a more invasive procedure. Arthroscopy has the advantage of good visualization of the joint space and articular cartilage combined with effective drainage and irrigation, while avoiding the postoperative joint stiffness and slow functional improvement sometimes associated with arthrotomy (Thiery 1989). Arthroscopy is best suited for drainage of the knee joint, although, depending on the skill of the arthroscopist, it can be applied to other smaller joints.

Septic arthritis of the hip should be treated primarily by arthrotomy because of the difficulty and uncertainty of achieving adequate joint drainage by closed aspiration, and the increased risk of osteomyelitis and avascular necrosis in an incompletely drained and decompressed hip. Infection of the deep axial joints complicated by abscess formation requires open drainage.

Regardless of the mode of drainage, early mobilization of the infected joint is important in regaining maximal function. Most often the infected joint will be too painful to allow mobilization during the first few days of therapy. However, passive, range-of-motion exercises should be instituted as soon as pain permits. Both animal and human studies have demonstrated the advantages of a continuous, passive-motion device soon after surgical drainage of the knee. Isometric exercises to restore strength to the limb muscles and progressive ambulation to prevent the complications of prolonged bed rest should also be implemented (Esterhai and Gelb 1991; Mikhail and Alarcon 1993).

Management of the infected prosthetic joint involves the added complication of the presence of foreign material. In general, the prosthesis must be removed to treat the infection effectively. Exceptions include some very early postoperative infections in which the wound and joint can be effectively incised and drained, and where antibiotics are started without significant delay. Another exception is the patient who is not considered a candidate for surgery because of poor medical status and who is infected with an organism of low virulence. In this case, chronic suppression of infection by antibiotics has at times been successful in salvaging the prosthesis and preventing further infectious complications.

In nearly all other instances, the prosthesis, cement, and all necrotic bone and soft tissue should be removed as soon as infection is detected or strongly suspected. Appropriate antibiotics should be started, as outlined in Table 3, keeping in mind the increased frequency of *Staph. epidermis*, Gram-negative bacilli, and anaerobic infections. After 6 weeks of intravenous antibiotics a prosthesis can be reimplanted (Fig. 1) with a greater than 90 per cent chance of success and with a better functional outcome and greater patient satisfaction than with arthrodesis of the knee or excision arthroplasty (Girdlestone procedure) of the hip, which should be reserved for those patients unable or unwilling to tolerate a second surgical procedure (Insall *et al.* 1983). Others have reported success with a one-step procedure in which a new prosthesis is implanted at the time of removal of the infected prosthesis (Goksan and Freeman 1992).

Septic bursitis

The many bursas found throughout the body are lined with a synovial membrane identical to that found in synovial joints. The bursas occupy superficial locations beneath the skin, cushioning the movements of tendons, muscles, and ligaments over bony structures. Bursitis may result from trauma, inflammatory conditions affecting synovial tissues (such as rheumatoid arthritis or gout), or from infection. Most cases of bursal infection are associated with recent trauma to the skin overlying the bursa or with an occupation causing repeated minor trauma to the bursa. Bacteria enter the bursa directly from the skin as a result of trauma, unlike septic arthritis in which the route of infection is most commonly haematogenous seeding. Underlying diseases affecting the bursa, including rheumatoid arthritis and gout, or previous episodes of non-infectious traumatic bursitis, increase the risk of septic bursitis. Immunosuppression, diabetes, and alcoholism may be additional predisposing factors (Canoso and Barza 1993).

Nearly all cases of septic bursitis involve the olecranon or prepatellar bursae. Both of these are closed structures that do not communicate with the adjacent joint. Presentation may be acute, with sudden onset of bursal pain, tenderness, swelling, and erythema leading to diagnosis within a few days of onset. Less commonly, presentation may be subacute or chronic with less dramatic local signs and symptoms present for weeks to months before the diagnosis is established. Involvement of the bursa is readily distinguishable from joint infection by the presence of very superficial, often tense, distension of the bursal sac and preservation of movement in the underlying joint, with little if any pain on motion. Fever is a common but not universal finding. Regional lymphadenopathy and adjacent cellulitis of the forearm or peripatellar skin are frequently present. Desquamation of the skin overlying the infected bursa and spontaneous drainage of the bursa through the skin may occur. Osteomyelitis of the underlying bone may occasionally complicate chronic cases.

The characteristics of synovial fluid from an infected bursa are variable. The gross appearance ranges from clear to frankly purulent. The leucocyte count may range from less than 2000 to several 100 000 cells/mm³, with the proportion of polymorphs ranging from 50 to nearly 100 per cent. In contrast to pyogenic arthritis, the leucocyte count in synovial fluid is often less than 10 000/mm³, so that relatively low counts should not deter one from pursuing the diagnosis of infection in the appropriate clinical setting (Ho *et al.* 1978; Canoso and Barza 1993).

In the absence of previous antibiotic therapy, culture of bursal synovial fluid will be positive in every case. Gram's stain is positive in about two-thirds of cases. *Staph. aureus* is the infecting organism in more than 90 per cent of cases. Sporadic cases are due to *Staph. epidermis* or group A streptococci.

Uncomplicated septic bursitis can be treated effectively with serial, closed-needle aspiration and oral antibiotics. Patients with underlying bursal disease, immunosuppressed patients, or those who fail to respond promptly to treatment as outpatients with oral antibiotics should be admitted to hospital and treated with intravenous antibiotics (Ho and Su 1981; Canoso and Barza 1993). Incision and drainage or excision of the infected bursa may be necessary in those cases with extensive involvement or failure to respond to closed drainage. Empirical antibiotic treatment should be with a semisynthetic, penicillinase-resistant penicillin or vancomycin, if methicillin-resistant *Staph. aureus* is a concern.

References

Andersson, S. and Krook, A. (1987). Primary meningococcal arthritis. *Scandinavian Journal of Infectious Disease*, **19**, 51–4.

Ang-Fonte, G.Z., Rozboril, M.B., and Thompson, G.R. (1985). Changes in non-gonococcal septic arthritis: drug abuse and methicillin-resistant *Staphylococcus aureus*. *Arthritis and Rheumatism*, **28**, 210–3.

Atcheson, S.G. and Ward, J., Jr. (1978). Acute hematogenous osteomyelitis progressing to septic synovitis and eventual pyarthrosis. *Arthritis and Rheumatism*, **21**, 968–71.

Baker, D.G. and Schumacher, H.R., Jr. (1993). Acute monoarthritis. *New England Journal of Medicine*, **329**, 1013–20.

Bayer, A.S., Chow, A.W., Louie, J.S., Nies, K.M., and Guze, L.B. (1977). Gram-negative bacillary septic arthritis: clinical, radiographic, therapeutic, and prognostic features. *Seminars in Arthritis and Rheumatism*, **7**, 123–32.

Blackburn, W.D., Jr., Dunn, T.L., and Alarcon, G.S. (1986). Infection versus disease activity in rheumatoid arthritis: 8 years' experience. *Southern Medical Journal*, **79**, 1238–41.

Borenstein, D.G. and Simon, G.L. (1986). *Hemophilus influenzae* septic arthritis in adults. *Medicine*, **65**, 191–201.

Brook, I. and Frazier, E.H. (1993). Anaerobic osteomyelitis and arthritis in a military hospital: a 10-year experience. *American Journal of Medicine*, **94**, 21–8.

Broy, S.B. and Schmid, F.R. (1986). A comparison of medical drainage (needle aspiration) and surgical drainage (arthrotomy or arthroscopy) in the initial treatment of infected joints. *Clinics in the Rheumatic Diseases*, **12**, 501–22.

Burhert, T. and Watanakunakorn, C. (1991). Group C streptococcus septic arthritis and osteomyelitis: report and literature review. *Journal of Rheumatology*, **18**, 904–7.

Call, R.S., Ward, J.R., and Samuelson, C.O., Jr. (1985). 'Pseudoseptic' arthritis in patients with rheumatoid arthritis. *Western Journal of Medicine*, **143**, 471–3.

Canoso, J.J. and Barza, M. (1993). Soft tissue infections. *Rheumatic Disease Clinics of North America*, **19**, 293–309.

Chandrasekar, P.H. and Narula, A.P. (1986). Bone and joint infections in intravenous drug abusers. *Reviews of Infectious Diseases*, **8**, 904–11.

Cohen, J.I., Bartlett, J.A. and Corey, G.R. (1987). Extra-intestinal manifestations of salmonella infections. *Medicine*, **66**, 349–88.

Cooper, C. and Cawley, M.I.D. (1986). Bacterial arthritis in an English health district: a 10 year review. *Annals of the Rheumatic Diseases*, **45**, 458–63.

Dubost, J. *et al.* (1993). Polyarticular septic arthritis. *Medicine*, **72**, 296–310.

Eisenstein, B.I. and Masi, A.T. (1981). Disseminated gonococcal infection (DGI) and gonococcal arthritis (GCA): I. Bacteriology, epidemiology, host factors, pathologic factors and pathology. *Seminars in Arthritis and Rheumatism*, **10**, 155–72.

Epstein, J.H., Zimmermann III, B., and Ho, G., Jr. (1986). Polyarticular septic arthritis. *Journal of Rheumatology*, **13**, 1105–7.

Esterhai, J.L., Jr. and Gelb, I. (1991). Adult septic arthritis. *Orthopedic Clinics of North America*, **22**, 503–14.

Fam, E.G., Tenenbaum, J., and Stein, J.L. (1979). Clinical forms of meningococcal arthritis. A study of 5 cases. *Journal of Rheumatology*, **6**, 567–73.

Fitzgerald, R.H., Jr., Rosenblatt, J.E., Tenney, J.H., and Bourgault, A. (1982). Anaerobic septic arthritis. *Clinical Orthopaedics and Related Research*, **164**, 141–8.

Gardner, G.C. and Weisman, M.H. (1990). Pyarthrosis in patients with rheumatoid arthritis: a report of 13 cases and a review of the literature from the past 40 years. *American Journal of Medicine*, **88**, 503–11.

Geelhoed-Duyvestijn, P.H.L.M., van der Meer, J.W.M., Lichtendahl-Bernard, A.T., Mulder, L.J., Meyers, K.A.E., and Poolman, J.T. (1986). Disseminated gonococcal infections in elderly patients. *Archives of Internal Medicine*, **146**, 1739–40.

Goksan, S.B. and Freeman, M.A.R. (1992). One-stage reimplantation for infected total knee arthroplasty. *Journal of Bone and Joint Surgery*, **74B**, 78–82.

Goldenberg, D.L. (1989). Infectious arthritis complicating rheumatoid arthritis and other chronic rheumatic diseases. *Arthritis and Rheumatism*, **32**, 496–502.

Goldenberg, D.L. and Cohen, A.S. (1976). Acute infectious arthritis. *American Journal of Medicine*, **60**, 369–77.

Goldenberg, D.L. and Reed, J.I. (1985). Bacterial arthritis. *New England Journal of Medicine*, **312**, 764–71.

Goldenberg, D.L., Brandt, K.D., Cohen, A.S., and Carthcart, E.S. (1975). Treatment of septic arthritis — comparison of needle aspiration and surgery as initial modes of joint drainage. *Arthritis and Rheumatism*, **18**, 83–90.

Goldenberg, D.L., Reed, J.I., and Rice, P.A. (1984). Arthritis in rabbits induced by killed *Neisseria gonorrhoeae* and gonococcal lipopolysccharide. *Journal of Rheumatology*, **11**, 3–8.

Gordon, G. and Kabins, S.A. (1980). Pyogenic sacroiliitis. *American Journal of Medicine*, **69**, 50–6.

Gray, R.G., Tenenbaum, J., and Gottlieb, N.L. (1981). Local corticosteroid injection treatment in rheumatic disorders. *Seminars in Arthritis and Rheumatism*, **10**, 231–54.

Gristina, A.G. and Kolkin, J. (1983). Total joint replacement and sepsis. *Journal of Bone and Joint Surgery*, **65A**, 128–34.

Ho, G., Jr. (1993). How best to drain an infected joint. Will we ever know? *Journal of Rheumatology*, **20**, 2001–3.

Ho, G., Jr. and Su, E.Y. (1981). Antibiotic therapy of septic bursitis: it's implications in the treatment of septic arthritis. *Arthritis and Rheumatism*, **24**, 905–11.

Ho, G., Jr. and Su, E.Y. (1982). Therapy for septic arthritis. *Journal of the American Medical Association*, **247**, 797–800.

Ho, G., Jr., Tice, A.D., and Kaplan, S.R. (1978). Septic bursitis in the prepatellar and olecranon bursae. *Annals of Internal Medicine*, **89**, 21–7.

Hollander, J.L. (1969). Intrasynovial corticosteroid therapy in arthritis. *Maryland State Medical Journal*, **19**, 62–6.

Holmes, K.K., Counts, G.W., and Besty, H.N. (1971). Disseminated gonococcal infection. *Annals of Internal Medicine*, **74**, 979–93.

Holroyd, K.J., Reiner, A.P., and Dick, J.D. (1988). *Streptobacillus moniliformis* polyarthritis mimicking rheumatoid arthritis: an urban case of rat bite fever. *American Journal of Medicine*, **85**, 711–14

Ike, R.W. (1990). Septic arthritis due to group C streptococcus: report and review of literature. *Journal of Rheumatology*, **17**, 1230–6.

Ike, R.W. (1993). Tidal irrigation in septic arthritis of the knee: A potential alternative to surgical drainage. *Journal of Rheumatology*, 20, 2104–11.

Inman, R.D., Gallegos, K.V., Brause, B.D., Redecha, P.B., and Christian, C.L. (1984). Clinical and microbial features of prosthetic joint infection. *American Journal of Medicine*, 77, 47–53.

Insall, J.N., Thompson, F.M., and Brause, B.D. (1983). Two-stage reimplantation for the salvage of infected total knee arthroplasty. *Journal of Bone and Joint Surgery*, 65A, 1087–98.

Jarrett, M.P., Moses, S., Barland, P., and Miller, M.H. (1980). Articular complications of meningococcal meningitis. An immune complex disorder. *Archives of Internal Medicine*, 140, 1656–66.

Kidd, B.L., Hart, H.H., and Grigor, R.R. (1985). Clinical features of meningococcal arthritis: a report of 4 cases. *Annals of the Rheumatic Diseases*, 44, 790–2.

Koss, P.G. (1985). Disseminated gonococcal infection: the tenosynovitis–dermatitis and suppurative arthritis syndromes. *Cleveland Clinic Quarterly*, 52, 161–73.

Krey, P.R. and Bailen, D. (1979). Synovial fluid leukocytosis. *American Journal of Medicine*, 67, 436–42.

Kurosh, N.A. and Perednia, D.A. (1989). *Listeria monocytogenes* septic arthritis. *Archives of Internal Medicine*, 149, 1207–8.

Lane, J.G., Falahee, M.H., Wojtys, E.M., Hankin, F.M., and Kaufer, H. (1990). Pyarthrosis of the knee. Treatment considerations. *Clinical Orthopedics and Related Research*, 252, 198–204.

Liebling, M.R. *et al.* (1994). Identification of *Neisseria gonorrhoeae* in synovial fluid using the polymerase chain reaction. *Arthritis and Rheumatism*, 37, 702–9.

Lopez-Longo, F-J., Menard, H-A., Carreno, L., Cosin, J., Ballesteros, R., and Monteagudo, I. (1987). Primary septic arthritis in heroin users: early diagnosis by radioisotopic imaging and geographic variations in the causative agents. *Journal of Rheumatology*, 14, 991–4.

Manshady, R.M., Thompson, G.R., and Weiss, J.J. (1980). Septic arthritis in a general hospital 1966–1977. *Journal of Rheumatology*, 7, 523–30.

Masi, A.T. and Eisenstein, B.I. (1981). Disseminated gonococcal infection (DGI) and gonococcal arthritis (GA): II. Clinical manifestations, diagnosis, complications, treatment and prevention. *Seminars in Arthritis and Rheumatism*, 10, 173–97.

Medina, F., Fraga, A., and Lavalle, C. (1989). Salmonella septic arthritis in systemic lupus erythematosus. The importance of the chronic carrier state. *Journal of Rheumatology*, 16, 203–8.

Merkel, K.D., Brown, M.L., Dewanjee, M.K., and Fitzgerald, R.H. (1985). Comparison of indium-111 labeled-leukocyte imaging with sequential technitium–gallium scanning in the diagnosis of low-grade musculoskeletal sepsis. *Journal of Bone and Joint Surgery*, 67A, 465–76.

Mikhail, I.S. and Alarcon, G.S. (1993). Nongonococcal bacterial arthritis. *Rheumatic Disease Clinics of North America*, 19, 311–31.

Newman, E.D., Davis, D.E., and Harrington, T.M. (1988). Septic arthritis due to Gram negative bacilli: older patients with good outcome. *Journal of Rheumatology*, 15, 659–62.

Newman, J.H. (1976). Review of septic arthritis throughout the antibiotic era. *Annals of the Rheumatic Diseases*, 35, 198–205.

O'Brien, J.P., Goldenberg, D.L., and Rice, P.A. (1983). Disseminated gonococcal infection: a prospective analysis of 49 patients and a review of pathophysiology and immune mechanisms. *Medicine*, 62, 395–406.

Pischel, K.D., Weisman, M.H., and Cone, R.O. (1985). Unique features of group B streptococcal arthritis in adults. *Archives of Internal Medicine*, 145, 97–102.

Poss, R., Thornhill, T.S., Ewald, F.C., Thomas, W.H., Batte, N.J., and Sledge, C.B. (1984). Factors influencing the incidence and outcome of infections following total joint arthroplasty. *Clinical Orthopedics and Related Research*, 182, 117–26.

Riegels-Nielsen, P., Frimodt-Moller, N., and Jensen, J.S. (1987). Rabbit model of septic arthritis. *Acta Orthopaedica Scandinavia*, 58, 14–9.

Riordan, T., Doyle, D., and Tabaqchali, S. (1982). Synovial fluid lactic acid measurement in the diagnosis and management of septic arthritis. *Journal of Clinical Pathology*, 35, 390–4.

Rivera, J., Monteagudo, I., Lopez-Longo, J., and Sanchezatrio, A. (1992). Septic arthritis in patients with acquired immunodeficiency syndrome with HIV infection. *Journal of Rheumatology*, 19, 1960–2.

Rompalo, A.M., Hook, E.W., III, Roberts, P.L., Ramsey, P.G., Handsfield, H., and Holmes, K.K. (1987). The acute arthritis–dermatitis syndrome: the changing importance of *Neisseria gonorrhoeae* and *Neisseria meningitidis*. *Archives of Internal Medicine*, 147, 281–3.

Rosenthal, J., Boles, G.G., and Robinson, W.D. (1980). Acute non-gonococcal infectious arthritis. *Arthritis and Rheumatism*, 23, 889–92.

Ross, S.C. and Densen, P. (1984). Complement deficiency states and infections: epidemiology, pathogenesis and consequences of neisserial and other infections in an immune deficiency. *Medicine*, 63, 243–73.

Schaad, U.B. (1980). Arthritis in disease due to *Neisseria meningitidis*. *Reviews of Infectious Disease*, 2, 880–8.

Scopelitis, E. and Martinez-Oscina, P. (1993). Gonococcal arthritis. *Rheumatic Disease Clinics of North America*, 19, 363–77.

Sharp, J.T., Lidsky, M.D., Duffy, J., and Duncan, M.W. (1979). Infectious arthritis. *Archives of Internal Medicine*, 139, 1125–30.

Singleton, J.D., West, S.G., and Nordstrom, D.M. (1991). 'Pseudoseptic' arthritis complicating rheumatoid arthritis: a report of six cases. *Journal of Rheumatology*, 18, 1319–22.

Small, C.B., Slater, L.N., Lowy, F.D., Small, R.D., Salvati, E.A., and Casey, J.I. (1984). Group B streptococcal arthritis in adults. *American Journal of Medicine*, 76, 367–75.

Soria, L.M., Sole, J.M.N., Sacanell, A.R., Garcia, J.V., and Escofet, D.R. (1992). Infectious arthritis in patients with rheumatoid arthritis. *Annals of the Rheumatic Diseases*, 51, 402–3.

Switalski, L.M., Patti, J.M., Butcher, W., Gristina, A.G., Speziale, P., and Hook, M. (1993). A collagen receptor on *Staphylococcus aureus* strains isolated from patients with septic arthritis mediates adhesion to cartilage. *Molecular Microbiology*, 7, 99–107.

Syrogiannopoulos, G.A. and Nelson, J.D. (1988). Duration of anti-microbial therapy for acute suppurative osteoarticular infections. *Lancet*, i, 37–40.

Thiery, J.A. (1989). Arthroscopic drainage in septic arthritis of the knee: a multi-center study. *Arthroscopy*, 5, 65–9.

Von Essen, R. and Holtta, A. (1986). Improved method of isolating bacteria from joint fluids by the use of blood culture bottles. *Annals of the Rheumatic Diseases*, 45, 454–7.

Vyskocil, J.J., McIroy, M.A., Brennan, T.A., and Wilson, F.M. (1991). Pyogenic infection of the sacroiliac joint. *Medicine*, 70, 188–97.

Weber, D.J., Wolfson, J.S., Swartz, M.N., and Hooper, D.C. (1984). *Pasteurella multocida* infections. Report of 34 cases and review of the literature. *Medicine*, 63, 133–54.

Williams, D.N., Gibson, J.A., and Bosch, D. (1989). Home intravenous antibiotic therapy using a programmable infusion pump. *Archives of Internal Medicine*, 149, 1157–60.

Wise, C.M., Morris, C.R., Wasilauskas, B.L., and Salzer, W.L. (1994). Gonococcal arthritis in an era of increasing penicillin resistance. *Archives of Internal Medicine*, 154, 2690–5.

Wohlgethan, J.R., Newberg, A.H., and Reed, J.I. (1988). The risk of abscess from sterno-clavicular septic arthritis. *Journal of Rheumatology*, 15, 1302–6.

Wymenga, A.B., van Horne, J.R., Theeuwes, A., Muytjens, H.L., and Slooff, T.J.J.H. (1992). Perioperative factors associated with septic arthritis after arthroplasty. *Acta Orthopaedica Scandinavia*, 63, 665–71.

Youssef, P.P. and York, J.R. (1994). Septic arthritis: a second decade of experience. *Australian and New Zealand Journal of Medicine*, 24, 307–11.

5.3.2 Pyogenic arthritis in children

Mary Anne Jackson and Komal B. Desai

Introduction

A successful outcome to suppurative arthritis in infancy and childhood is contingent upon early recognition and timely antimicrobial and surgical therapy. Despite the advent of newer antimicrobials that penetrate readily into infected joints, complications and permanent changes still arise in some cases of septic arthritis. This chapter reviews the epidemiology and pathogenesis of joint infection, and outlines the approach to diagnosis and management. Changes in the spectrum of childhood skeletal infection in the era of the *Haemophilus influenzae* type b (**Hib**) vaccine are highlighted.

Epidemiology

Acute septic arthritis is a relatively uncommon infection. One estimate suggests that two of every 1000 admissions to general hospitals are for septic arthritis (Smith 1974). Our institution serves a large, urban population in the American midwest where approximately 6000 children are admitted to the hospital each year. In the last fifteen years, an average of 10 admissions each year have been for septic arthritis. In a 30-year study of paediatric skeletal infection reported by Nelson, 682 cases of suppurative arthritis were described with an occurrence of 25 cases among 10 000 annual admissions (Nelson 1991).

Suppurative joint infection is an important disease of childhood. Among 138 cases treated at our institution since 1980, more than half were less than three years of age (Table 1). Although boys are reported to be affected twice as often as girls, in our series this predominance is seen most in the child older than 5 years; in the younger patient, the sex distribution tends to be more equal.

A history of non-penetrating trauma can be elicited in many children with septic arthritis; however, most investigators have questioned its role in the pathogenesis of the infection. In one study (Welkon *et al.* 1986), patients with septic arthritis and sterile cultures more frequently reported a history of trauma than those with culture-confirmed pyarthrosis.

An antecedent infection of the upper respiratory tract or otitis media occurs in 77 per cent of patients with septic arthritis due to *Haemophilus influenzae* type b compared with 18 per cent of those with pyarthrosis due to *Staphylococcus aureus* (Syriopolou and Smith 1987). This observation is consistent with findings in children with meningitis due to *H. influenzae* type b which suggests many have had an antecedent upper respiratory infection or otitis media (Harding *et al.* 1973).

Pathogenesis

In most cases, bacteria enter the joint space haematogenously. Less often, direct inoculation of bacteria into the joint space occurs during an episode of penetrating trauma. Contiguous extension of disease from infected soft tissues is felt to be rare in paediatric practice, and occurs most often in the adult diabetic (Argen *et al.* 1966).

Concomitant osteoarticular infection is a frequent occurrence in the neonate and happens occasionally in the older infant or child.

In neonates, osteoarthritis with destruction of the epiphysis and joint is common because metaphyseal and epiphyseal vessels communicate within the cartilaginous precursor of the ossific nucleus (Trueta 1957). As the ossific nucleus and epiphyseal plate form, separate vessels arise to supply the epiphysis and the communication with metaphyseal vessels disappears at approximately 1 year of age (Ogden 1979).

In children, there are four areas where the bony metaphysis is intracapsular: the proximal femur, proximal humerus, proximal radius, and distal lateral tibia (Morrissy 1989). If bacteria invade the joint from an adjacent osteomyelitis, the clinical presentation is similar to that of isolated joint infection and it is often difficult to differentiate between the two. Data from our institution suggest this type of skeletal infection may occur in up to 20 per cent of cases. In these cases, longer treatment with antibiotics is needed than in primary joint infection. More importantly, these patients have a greater frequency of permanent disability (Jackson *et al.* 1992).

Table 1 Suppurative joint infection, The Children's Mercy Hospital, Kansas City, Missouri 1980 to 1994

Age	Total	%
≤2 months	11	8
3–23 months	58	42
2–5 years	36	26
6–11 years	19	14
>11 years	14	10

Table 2 Distribution of involved joints in suppurative joint infection, The Children's Mercy Hospital, Kansas City, Missouri 1980 to 1994

Joint	Total	%
Knee	46	33
Hip	38	28
Ankle	14	10
Elbow	9	7
Shoulder	8	6
Metatarsal	5	4
Sacroiliac	3	2
Wrist	3	2
Multiple	11	9
Interphalangeal	1	–

Table 3 Aetiology of suppurative joint infection (percentages) by age, The Children's Mercy Hospital, Kansas City, Missouri 1980 to 1994

Age	Sterile	S. aureus	Hib[a]	Cocci[b]	GC[c]	Other[d]
<2 months	9	36	0	36	0	18
2–6 months	40	0	0	60	0	0
7–12 months	26	11	41	15	0	7
13–23 months	36	25	32	0	0	7
24–36 months	29	7	14	36	0	14
3–5 years	35	30	5	20	0	10
6–11 years	35	30	10	10	0	30
>11 years	13	33	0	0	27	20

[a]Haemophilus influenzae type 6.
[b]Streptococci including enterococci, group A and B streptococci, viridans streptococci, pneumococci.
[c]Gonococcal.
[d]P. aeruginosa, acinetobacter, enterobacter, klebsiella, coagulase-negative staphylococci, Eikenella corrodens, salmonella, Brucella spp.

Clinical manifestations

Monoarticular infection of weight-bearing joints is characteristic, with involvement of the knee, hip, or ankle accounting for 70 per cent of cases (Table 2). Usually the child with pyogenic joint infection presents acutely with fever and an exquisitely painful, swollen joint. In some cases, it may be difficult to localize the involved joint, especially in a febrile, irritable infant. A careful examination after giving a short-acting sedative may be needed to locate the affected joint.

Diagnostic evaluation should be pursued promptly, especially in cases of septic arthritis of the hip where compromise of the vascular supply to the femoral head may result in destruction of the capital epiphysis and growth plate. A complete blood count, erythrocyte sedimentation rate (**ESR**), and radiographs of the joint involved should be obtained. In most cases, leucocytosis and elevation of the ESR in the range of 50 to 90 mm/h will be found; however, the diagnosis should not be excluded even if both of these are normal (Nelson and Koontz 1966). Radiographs may reveal periarticular, soft tissue swelling and joint effusion but also may be non-diagnostic (Morrey et al. 1975).

Radioisotope bone scanning is helpful in occasional cases where localization of the diseased joint is difficult. An increase or decrease in uptake on either side of the joint line with limitation to the joint capsule is seen in suppurative arthritis (Tuson et al. 1994). Magnetic resonance imaging has been shown to be a sensitive tool in the diagnosis of septic sacroiliitis (Sandrasegaran et al. 1994). In the child whose hip is painful on examination but plain radiographs are unrevealing, ultrasonography of the hip is useful in identifying fluid and in guiding arthrocentesis (Dorr et al. 1988).

Aspiration of the joint is imperative to confirm the diagnosis. The fluid is usually frankly purulent and low glucose concentrations may be found. In most cases, the white blood cell count in the synovial fluid is greater than 50 000 and a differential count reveals more than 90 per cent polymorphonuclear leucocytes. A Gram-stained smear of the joint fluid will provide a presumptive identification of the causative agent in approximately one-third of cases. Culture of the joint fluid will reveal the precise organism in 50 to 60 per cent of cases. In 10 per cent blood culture will demonstrate the causative agent when cultures of the joint fluid are sterile. Despite careful culture of blood, joint fluid, and other appropriate sites, a microbiological diagnosis will not be obtained in 25 to 30 per cent of cases. If the clinical diagnosis is deemed to be septic arthritis, lack of a defined pathogen should not change the management of the patient.

General aetiology

The most commonly identified, causative bacteria of suppurative arthritis are presented in Table 3. Although *Haemophilus influenzae* type b has historically caused the majority of cases of suppurative arthritis in infants less than two years of age, we have seen no cases due to this pathogen since 1991 (Jackson, in press). Since the implementation of Hib vaccine in the United States in 1985, this organism has virtually disappeared as a cause of invasive disease. Currently, *Staphylococcus aureus* and streptococci account for close to 70 per cent of culture-confirmed cases of suppurative arthritis. Most streptococcal infections are caused by group A and B (neonates) or pneumococci, but, viridans streptococci and enterococci have also been reported (Fink and Nelson 1986). In teenagers with multiple joint involvement, gonococci are the most common pathogens (Keiser et al. 1968). Primary meningococcal arthritis is a rare form of meningococcal disease characterized by polyarticular infection, no involvement of other organs, and excellent prognosis (Schaad et al. 1981). *Pseudomonas aeruginosa* may cause infection in cases of puncture wound to the foot; other Gram-negative organisms cause infection infrequently (Fisher et al. 1985). Occasionally, salmonella arthritis occurs in the setting of salmonellosis or in the sickleaemic patient (Mallouh and Talab 1985). Anaerobes including *Bacteroides* spp., *Fusobacterium* spp. and *Eikenella corrodens* are most commonly involved in joint infection following a human bite (Resnick *et al*. 1985). *Kingella kingae* has been reported to be a possible aetiological agent in some septic arthritis cases and grew only when the initial synovial fluid specimen was inoculated into a blood culture bottle (Dagan 1993).

Specific pathogens in septic arthritis

H. influenzae arthritis

With the advent of conjugate vaccine against *Haemophilus influenzae* type b, the prominence of the pathogen has diminished. Hib vaccine has been used in the United States since 1985, and the more efficacious, conjugate vaccine in infants from 2 months of age since 1990. Between 1986 and 1991, we noted a decline in the incidence of culture-confirmed, septic arthritis from 60 per cent to 20 per cent of infants less than 2 years of age. We have had no cases of Hib arthritis in our institution in the last three years. This changing trend was found in one other study before widespread use of the vaccine; thus the decline in this type of septic arthritis cannot be attributed solely to vaccine-induced immunity, but also to a reduction in nasopharyngeal colonization with this organism (Speiser *et al*. 1985).

Unimmunized infants of less than 2 years or incompletely immunized infants (those infants less than 12 to 15 months of age who have received the appropriate primary vaccine series but no booster) remain susceptible to Hib infection. In such instances, evaluation and management decisions should include Hib as a possible pathogen. As in other cases of disease from invasive *H. influenzae* type b, concomitant meningitis occurs in up to 30 per cent of affected children (Rotbart and Glode 1985). Examination of the cerebrospinal fluid is therefore an essential part of the initial evaluation of the young infant in whom septic arthritis due to *H. influenzae* type b is suspected.

A 1995 report notes the occurrence of the invasive, paediatric disease caused by *H. influenzae* type f, and suggests that reduction in nasopharyngeal Hib carriage may be associated with an increase in carriage of other non-type b strains (Nitta *et al*. 1995). A recent report of skeletal infection due to this organism highlights its ability to cause bone and joint infection (Chusid *et al*. 1992).

Gonococcal arthritis

Suppurative arthritis due to *Neisseria gonorrheae* is one of the manifestations of the disseminated gonococcaemia syndrome (Fig. 1). In more than one-half of cases, polyarticular disease is found, with joints of the arm, especially wrists and fingers, most frequently involved (Bayer 1980). A history of migratory polyarthralgia in a febrile adolescent with arthritis of the wrist is so clinically distinct that a presumptive diagnosis can be made and appropriate therapy begun. Although analysis and culture of joint fluid is mandatory in all patients, the organism is found in joint fluid in less than one-half of cases. It is essential to culture from the pharynx, rectum and vagina/urethra in all patients with a suspected diagnosis of gonococcal arthritis (Angerine and Hall 1976).

Septic arthritis of specific joints

Hip

When the hip is involved in septic arthritis, the child will assume a position of comfort with the hip flexed, externally rotated, and abducted. Asymmetry of the skin folds of the buttocks and thighs may be apparent, and significant limitation of passive hip abduction and extension is typical. Pathological subluxation of the hip may occur, and was found in 8 per cent of children with septic arthritis of the hip at our institution.

There is much potential for permanent disability in cases of septic arthritis of the hip. The femoral capital epiphysis is entirely intra-articular and capsular distension may interfere with the vascular supply to the femoral head. Therefore, in all cases where septic hip is suspected, the diagnosis should be promptly confirmed by aspiration of the joint under fluoroscopy. If purulent material is found, immediate drainage of the hip should be performed.

Sacroiliac joint

Infection of the sacroiliac joint is relatively unusual, accounting for 1 to 2 per cent of cases of septic arthritis. These children tend to be older (mean age, 10 years) and usually do not appear systemically ill. Most have acute onset of fever, with pain in the buttocks, groin, hip or abdomen. Often the patient has an antalgic gait but pain is poorly localized. The duration of symptoms before diagnosis averaged 7 days in one study (Patterson 1970), but chronic symptoms of up to 1 month have been reported (Schaad *et al*. 1980). The most common physical finding in patients with sacroiliac arthritis is a positive Fabere sign (pain with flexion, abduction and external rotation of the hip while stressing the sacroiliac joint by placing pressure on the flexed ipsilateral knee) (Hoppenfeld 1976).

As in many cases of septic arthritis, plain radiographs are often normal. A bone scan may localize the involved sacroiliac joint;

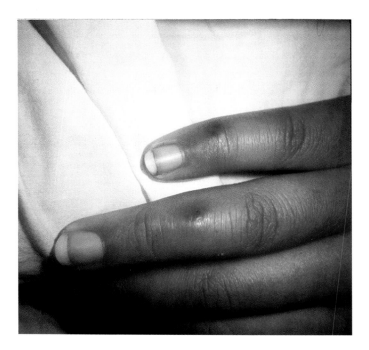

Fig. 1 Typical skin lesions in a teenager with gonococcal arthritis

however, a computed tomographic or magnetic resonance imaging scan is more sensitive and specific (Morgan *et al.* 1981).

Staphyloccocus aureus is the most commonly recognized pathogen and a positive blood culture is often found (Reilly *et al.* 1988). Antistaphylococcal therapy usually results in a prompt clinical response and drainage of the sacroiliac joint is usually unnecessary. *Brucella* spp. have a predilection for sacroiliac involvement and should be considered in individuals who were born or have travelled to endemic areas or have ingested raw milk. Diagnosis of brucella sacroiliitis may be confirmed by culture or serology and therapy should usually include trimethoprim sulphamethoxazole or doxycycline (for patients over 9 years of age) possibly with the addition of rifampicin.

Septic arthritis specific hosts

Neonates (Table 4)

Although suppurative skeletal infection in a newborn infant often reflects systemic infection with *Staphylococcus aureus*, *Candida albicans* or group B streptococci, systemic symptoms and signs are generally not apparent (Pittard *et al.* 1976). Non-specific symptoms such as irritability, lethargy or poor feeding may occur. However, a

Table 4 Characteristics of neonatal skeletal infection

Absence of systemic symptoms and signs

Multiple concomitant osteoarticular sites

Delayed diagnosis

Frequent permanent sequelae

non-toxic appearance and absence of fever is found in more than one-half of cases, and a normal white cell count and ESR are generally found (Fox and Sprunt 1978). Local swelling of an extremity with overlying inflammation and/or flexion contracture are the most common clinical findings. Occasionally, a newborn with hip pyarthrosis may present with abdominal distension secondary to rupture into the abdomen of intra-articular pus (Freiberg and Perlman 1976).

A high index of suspicion is necessary and aspiration of all suspected joints is absolutely essential to confirm the diagnosis. Permanent sequelae are frequent in this age group. Hallel and Salvati (1975) found deformities of the femoral head in 70 per cent of neonates followed up for suppurative arthritis of the hip. Complications from skeletal infection in the neonate can be minimized by a high index of suspicion, detailed evaluation with a careful musculoskeletal examination in any baby with suspected sepsis, and early surgical drainage and antibiotic therapy.

Septic arthritis in chronic joint disease

The diagnosis of suppurative joint infection may be particularly difficult in the patient with underlying chronic disease of the joints, such as those with sickle haemoglobinopathy, haemophilia or systemic juvenile chronic arthritis. Although there is no hallmark for differentiating chronic, active disease from acute suppurative infection of the joint, most infected patients are febrile, have a more toxic appearance, and have marked local manifestations.

In haemophiliacs, septic arthritis has been considered a rare complication of haemarthrosis. Severe joint pain and systemic toxicity that persist despite giving coagulation factors should be considered an indication for needle aspiration of the affected joint. Pneumococci (which have a predilection for diseased joints) and staphylococci are the most common pathogens of septic arthritis in haemophiliacs (Scott *et al.* 1985). Generally, a single joint, usually the

Table 5 Suppurative arthritis following puncture wound

Age (years)	Sex	Joint	Trauma	Pathogen
2	M	Knee	Toothpick	Viridans streptococci
3	M	Knee	Plastic	Group A streptococci
3	M	Knee	Dog bite	Unknown
1	M	Knee	Human bite	*Eikenella corrodens*
4	M	Metatarsal	Nail	*Pseudomonas aeruginosa*
12	M	Knee	Nail	Gram-negative rods
4	M	Metatarsal	Nail	*Pseudomonas aeruginosa*
9	M	Metatarsal	Unknown	*Escherichia coli, Enterobacter cloacae*
7	M	Metatarsal	Nail	*Pseudomonas aeruginosa*
9	M	Metatarsal	Nail	*Pseudomonas aeruginosa*
10	M	Metatarsal	Nail	*Pseudomonas aeruginosa*

knee, is involved and diagnosis may be delayed when a septic joint is superimposed on haemarthrosis. Recently, septic arthritis complicating pneumococcal, staphylococcal or salmonella bacteraemia has been reported in haemophiliacs infected with human immunodeficiency virus. Polyarticular disease with significant destruction occurred despite appropriate therapy (Ragni and Hawley 1989). However, a more favourable outcome has been reported in four recent cases where non-operative management with prompt antimicrobial therapy was advocated (Merchan *et al.* 1992).

Septic arthritis is uncommon in children with sickle haemoglobinopathy. Localized joint pain and fever are usually found, and symptoms and signs tend to persist for 4 days or longer (Syrogiannopoulos *et al.* 1986). Encapsulated bacteria typically cause infection in the patient with sickle haemoglobinopathy. Pneumococci are the most commonly recognized pathogens in such children with septic arthritis, although occasional disease secondary to *H. influenzae* type b is reported (Mallouh and Talab 1986). Salmonella have a predilection for bone in sicklaemic patients and may be found in cases of suppurative arthritis in association with an adjacent osteomyelitis (Seeler and Jacobs 1977).

Joint infection during rheumatoid arthritis is more common in adults than children. Usually, worsening of pain of an isolated joint occurs during a flare-up of the underlying disease; however, there is polyarticular involvement in almost 40 per cent of cases (Kaufman *et al.* 1976). As in other cases where septic arthritis complicates underlying chronic disease of the joint, a high index of suspicion is necessary to avoid a delay in diagnosis and poor subsequent outcome.

Penetrating injuries and arthritis

Suppurative arthritis following a penetrating injury to a joint is well described, although when first reported was most commonly associated with sewing-needle injury to the knee (Samilson *et al.* 1958). The knee is still the joint usually involved, but sewing needles have rarely been implicated as the agent of trauma in the last two decades. The clinical presentation is similar to other cases of pyarthrosis. In our series, 8 per cent of cases of suppurative arthritis followed a penetrating injury (Table 5). All cases were boys, with a mean age of 6 years. A wide variety of pathogens was found; however, *Pseudomonas aeruginosa* arthritis of the metatarsal joint following nail puncture occurred most frequently.

Reactive or so-called traumatic arthritis follows an injury, usually a thorn or splinter puncture, and may be severe and difficult to distinguish from acute suppurative infection. In most cases, symptoms have been present for longer than a week and although there is pain on moving the joint, it is usually not as severe as that associated with a pyarthrosis (Green and Edwards 1987). Exploration of the joint to exclude a foreign body should be considered in cases where traumatic synovitis persists.

Management

The essentials of management of suppurative arthritis in childhood include the combination of an appropriately selected antimicrobial agent and adequate drainage of the pyarthrosis (see Box 1). Simple needle aspiration of the affected joint may be sufficient in some cases. However, emergency surgical

drainage of the joint is mandatory in pyarthrosis of the hip and probably shoulder infection (Patterson 1978). Arthrotomy and drainage should also be considered in cases where the pus is thick, or when significant symptoms and signs persist despite initial needle aspiration of pus from the affected joint (Nade 1983).

When a presumptive diagnosis of septic arthritis is made, parenteral antibiotics should be begun promptly. In older children, an antistaphylococcal penicillin is the drug of choice. For infants who have not received a Hib booster vaccine (those less than 12 to 15 months of age), and for infants who have not received Hib vaccine and are less than 2 years old, I add coverage for *H. influenzae* type b in combination with the antistaphylococcal antibiotic. Cefuroxime is appropriate initial coverage as long as concomitant meningitis is not present. In that case, I prefer to combine an antistaphylococcal penicillin with a third-generation cephalosporin (usually cefotaxime or ceftriaxone) until the results of culture are known. Parenteral antimicrobial agents readily penetrate into infected joints, so intra-articular installation of antibiotics is not necessary.

The efficacy of a sequential intravenous–oral antimicrobial regimen has been demonstrated by numerous prospective studies (for example Feigin *et al.* (1975); Jackson and Nelson (1982)). Usually, intravenous therapy is given for 5 to 7 days. After all surgical procedures and when there is definite clinical improvement, a patient may be considered for an oral regimen if (i) an appropriate oral antimicrobial is available, (ii) the patient is able to take and retain oral medication, and (iii) there is a laboratory at hand to analyse the bactericidal activity of serum samples.

The oral dosage of the selected antibiotic is two to three times that used for otitis media or skin and soft tissue infection. A serum specimen for blood levels should be obtained 1 h after the oral dose is given (after the drug has reached steady-state concentrations) and adequate bactericidal activity should be confirmed. A serum bactericidal activity of at least 1:8 is considered adequate except in cases of streptococcal infection where a titre of 1:32 is needed. Adjustment of the antimicrobial dosage is usually required in 15 per cent of cases. In less than 5 per cent of cases, satisfactory bactericidal activity cannot be achieved and a total parenteral regimen must be used for the duration of therapy (Prober and Yeager 1979). Oral antibiotic regimens should not be used outside the hospital setting in a child unless you feel compliance can be guaranteed.

The optimum duration of antimicrobial therapy for children with suppurative arthritis is dependent upon the duration of symptoms before diagnosis of the pathogen, the response to medical and surgical treatment, and whether or not there is concomitant bone infection. Generally, if the patient's clinical response is good and the ESR returns to normal, 3 weeks of therapy is adequate for staphylococcal and Gram-negative bacillary infection (Syrogiannopoulos and Nelson 1978). Shorter courses have been successful for streptococcal and haemophilus infection, in which a total of 10 to 14 days of therapy may be adequate. In all cases where an oral regimen is used, ESR and serum bactericidal activity should be monitored weekly until therapy is considered complete.

The risk of relapse or recurrent disease is quite small in cases of primary joint infection; however, for the child with pyarthrosis and concomitant bone infection, the potential for relapse or sequelae is significant. Therefore, if compliance cannot be guaranteed, an oral regimen is not appropriate for such patients. Delayed diagnosis, delay in surgical drainage, slow clinical

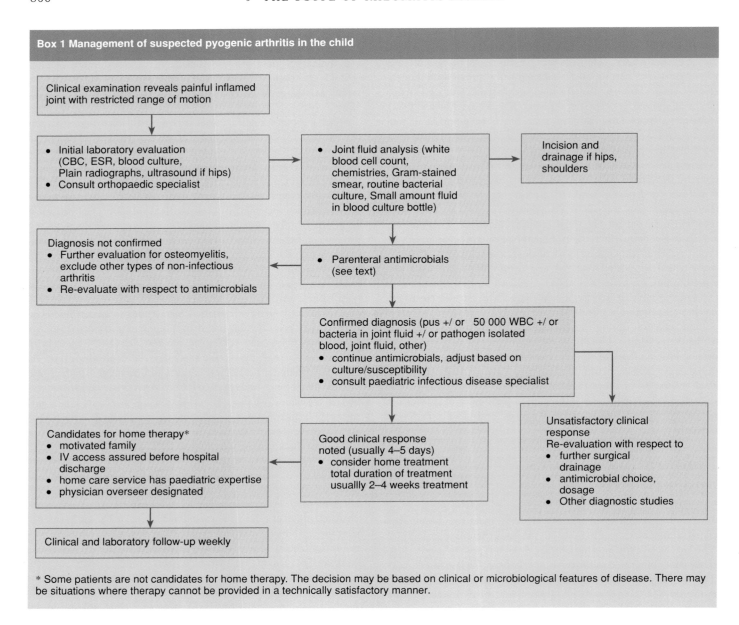

Box 1 Management of suspected pyogenic arthritis in the child

Clinical examination reveals painful inflamed joint with restricted range of motion

- Initial laboratory evaluation (CBC, ESR, blood culture, Plain radiographs, ultrasound if hips)
- Consult orthopaedic specialist

- Joint fluid analysis (white blood cell count, chemistries, Gram-stained smear, routine bacterial culture, Small amount fluid in blood culture bottle)

Incision and drainage if hips, shoulders

Diagnosis not confirmed
- Further evaluation for osteomyelitis, exclude other types of non-infectious arthritis
- Re-evaluate with respect to antimicrobials

- Parenteral antimicrobials (see text)

Confirmed diagnosis (pus +/ or 50 000 WBC +/ or bacteria in joint fluid +/ or pathogen isolated blood, joint fluid, other)
- continue antimicrobials, adjust based on culture/susceptibility
- consult paediatric infectious disease specialist

Candidates for home therapy*
- motivated family
- IV access assured before hospital discharge
- home care service has paediatric expertise
- physician overseer designated

Good clinical response noted (usually 4–5 days)
- consider home treatment total duration of treatment usuallly 2–4 weeks treatment

Unsatisfactory clinical response
Re-evaluation with respect to
- further surgical drainage
- antimicrobial choice, dosage
- Other diagnostic studies

Clinical and laboratory follow-up weekly

* Some patients are not candidates for home therapy. The decision may be based on clinical or microbiological features of disease. There may be situations where therapy cannot be provided in a technically satisfactory manner.

response, and undocumented compliance are all risk factors for chronic disease (Badgley *et al.* 1936; Hallel and Salvati 1975).

Prognosis

In the child over 1 month of age, the prognosis for primary septic arthritis of the knee is good and more than 90 per cent have a satisfactory outcome (Howard *et al.* 1976). However, poor outcome has been estimated to occur in approximately 40 per cent of hip, 20 per cent of ankle and 30 per cent of shoulder infections, particularly if there is an adjacent osteomyelitis (Gillespie 1973; Welkon *et al.* 1986). There should be careful orthopaedic follow-up for at least 6 to 12 months in all children with supporative joint infection.

References

Angerine, C.D. and Hall, C.B. (1976). A case of gonococcal osteomyelitis. A complication of gonococcal arthritis. *American Journal of Diseases of Children*, **130**, 1013–14.

Argen, R.J., Wilson, C.H., and Wood, P. (1966). Suppurative arthritis: clinical features of 42 cases. *Archives of Internal Medicine*, **117**, 661–6.

Badgley, C.E., Yglesias, L., Perham, W.S., and Snyder, C.H. (1936). Study of the end result of 113 cases of septic hips. *Journal of Bone and Joint Surgery*, **18**, 1047–53.

Bayer, A.S. (1980). Gonococcal arthritis syndromes: an update on diagnosis and management. *Postgraduate Medicine*, **67**, 200–8.

Chusid, M.J., Schneider, J.P., Thometz, J.G., and Dunne, W.M. (1992). Osteomyelitis and septic arthritis caused by *Haemophilus influenzae*, type f, in a young girl. *Diagnostic Microbiology and Infectious Diseases*, **15**, 157–9.

Dagan, R. (1993). Management of acute hematogenous osteomyelitis and septic arthritis in the pediatric patient. *Pediatric Infectious Disease Journal*, **12**, 88–93.

Dorr, U., Zieger, M., and Hauke, H. (1988). Ultrasonography of the painful hip. Prospective studies in 204 patients. *Pediatric Radiology*, **19**, 36–40.

Feigin, R.D., Pickering, L.K., Anderson, B., Kooney, R.D., and Shackleford, P.G. (1975). Clindamycin treatment of osteomyelitis and septic arthritis in children. *Pediatrics*, **55**, 213–23.

Fink, C.W. and Nelson, J.D. (1986). Septic arthritis and osteomyelitis in children. *Clinical Rheumatic Disease*, **12**, 423–35.

Fisher, M.C., Goldsmith, J.F., and Gilligan, P.H. (1985). Sneakers as a source of *Pseudomonas aeruginosa* in children with osteomyelitis following puncture wounds. *Journal of Pediatrics*, **106**, 607–9.

Fox, L. and Sprunt, K. (1978). Neonatal osteomyelitis. *Pediatrics*, **62**, 535–42.

Freiberg, J.A. and Perlman, R. (1976). Pelvic abscesses associated with acute purulent infection of the hip joint. *Journal of Bone and Joint Surgery*, **18**, 417–27.

Gillespie, R. (1973). Septic arthritis in childhood. *Clinical Orthopaedics and Related Research*, **96**, 152–9.

Green, N.E. and Edwards, K. (1987). Bone and joint infections in children. *Orthopedic Clinics of North America*, **18**, 555–76.

Hallel, T. and Salvati, E.A. (1975). Septic arthritis of the hip in infancy. End result study. *Clinical Orthopaedics*, **132**, 115–28.

Harding, A.L., Anderson, P., and Howse, V.M. (1973). *Haemophilus influenzae* isolated from children with otitis. In *Haemophilus influenzae* (eds H. Sells and D.T. Karzon), p. 663. University Press, Nashville, TN.

Hoppenfeld, S. (1976). *Physical examination of the spine and extremities*, p. 262. Appleton-Century-Crofts. New York, NY.

Howard, J.B., Highgenboten, C.L., and Nelson, J.D. (1976). Permanent effects of septic arthritis in childhood. *Journal of the American Medical Association*, **236**, 932–5.

Jackson, M.A. and Nelson, J.D. (1982). Etiology and medical management of acute suppurative bone and joint infections in pediatric patients. *Journal of Pediatric Orthopedics*, **2**, 313–23.

Jackson, M.A., Burry, V.F., and Olson, L.C. (1992). Pyogenic arthritis associated with adjacent osteomyelitis: identification of the sequelae-prone child. *Pediatric Infectious Disease Journal*, **11**, 9–13.

Jackson, M.A., Desai, K.B., Burry, V.F., and Olson, L.C. (1995). The changing face of childhood pyogenic arthritis. *Pediatric Infectious Disease Journal*.

Kaufman, C.A., Watanakunakorn, C., and Phair, J.P. (1976). Pneumococcal arthritis. *Journal of Rheumatology*, **3**, 409–19.

Keiser, H., Rubin, F.L., Wolmsky, E., and Kushner, I. (1968). Clinical forms of gonococcal arthritis. *New England Journal of Medicine*, **279**, 234–40.

Mallouh, A. and Talab, Y. (1985). Bone and joint infection in patients with sickle cell disease. *Journal of Pediatric Orthopedics*, **5**, 158–62.

Merchan, E.C.R., Magallon, M., Mauso, F., and Martin-Billar, J. (1992). Septic arthritis in HIV positive haemophiliacs. *International Orthopaedics*, **16**, 302–6.

Morgan, G.J., Schlegelmilch, J.G., and Spiegel, P.K. (1981). Early diagnosis of septic arthritis of the sacroiliac joint by computed tomography. *Journal of Rheumatology*, **8**, 979–82.

Morrey, B.F., Bianco, A.J., and Rhodes, K.H. (1975). Septic arthritis in children. *Orthopedic Clinics of North America*, **6**, 923–34.

Morrissy, R.T. (1989). Bone and joint infection in the neonate. *Pediatric Annals*, **18**, 33–44.

Nade, S. (1983). Acute septic arthritis in infancy and childhood. *Journal of Bone and Joint Surgery*, **65B**, 234–41.

Nelson, J.D. (1991). Skeletal infections in children.. In *Advances in pediatric infecious diseases*, Vol. 6, (eds S.C. Aronoff, W.T. Hughes, S. Kohn, W.T. Speck, and E.R. Wald), pp. 59–76. Mosby Year Book, St. Louis, MO.

Nelson, J.D. and Koontz, W.L. (1966). Septic arthritis in infants and children. *Pediatrics*, **38**, 966–71.

Nitta, D.M., Jackson, M.A., Burry, V.F., and Olson, L.C. (1995). Invasive *Haemophilus Influenzae* type f disease. *The Pediatric Infectious Disease Journal*, **14**, 157–60.

Ogden, J.A. (1979). Pediatric osteomyelitis and septic arthritis: the pathology of neonatal disease. *Yale Journal of Biological Medicine*, **52**, 423–48.

Patterson, D. (1978). Septic arthritis of the hip. *Orthopedic Clinics of North America*, **9**, 135–42.

Patterson, D.C. (1970). Acute suppurative arthritis in infancy and childhood. *Journal of Bone and Joint Surgery*, **52B**, 414–82.

Pittard, W.B., Thullen, J.D., and Fanaroff, A.A. (1976). Neonatal septic arthritis. *Journal of Pediatrics*, **88**, 621–4.

Prober, C.G. and Yeager, A.S. (1979). Use of serum bactericidal titer to assess the adequacy of oral antibiotic therapy in treatment of acute hematogenous osteomyelitis. *Journal of Pediatrics*, **95**, 131–55.

Ragni, M.V. and Hawley, E.N. (1989). Septic arthritis in hemophiliac patients and infection with human immunodeficiency virus. *Annals of Internal Medicine*, **110**, 168–9.

Reilly, J.P., Gross, R.H., Eman, J.B., and Yngve, D.A. (1988). Disorders of the sacroiliac joint in children. *Journal of Bone and Joint Surgery*, **70A**, 31–40.

Resnick, D., Pineda, C.J., Weisman, M.H., and Kerr, R. (1985). Osteomyelitis and septic arthritis of the hand following human bites. *Skeletal Radiology*, **14**, 263–6.

Rotbart, H.A. and Glode, M.P. (1985). *Haemophilus influenzae* type b septic arthritis in children: report of 23 cases. *Pediatrics*, **75**, 254–9.

Samilson, R.L., Bersani, F.A., and Watkins, M.B. (1958). Acute suppurative arthritis in infants and children: the importance of early diagnosis and surgical drainage. *Pediatrics*, **21**, 798–803.

Sandrasegaran, K., Saifuddin, M.B., Coral, A., and Butt, W.P. (1994). Magnetic resonance imaging of septic sacroiliitis. *Skeletal Radiology*, **23**, 289–92.

Schaad, V.B., McCracken, G.H., and Nelson, J.D. (1980). Pyogenic arthritis of the sacroiliac joint in pediatric patients. *Pediatrics*, **66**, 375–9.

Schaad, V.B., Nelson, J.D., and McCracken, G.H. (1981). Primary meningococcal arthritis. *Infection*, **9**, 170–3.

Scott, J.P., Maurer, H.S., and Dias, L. (1985). Septic arthritis in two teenaged hemophiliacs. *Journal of Pediatrics*, **107**, 748–51.

Seeler, R.A. and Jacobs, N.M. (1977). Pyogenic infections in children with sickle hemoglobinopathy. *Journal of Pediatrics*, **90**, 161–2

Smith, T. (1974). On the arthritis of infants. *St. Bartholomew's Hospital Report*, **10**, 189–204.

Speiser, J.C., Moore, T.L., Osborn, T.G., Weiss, T.D., and Zuckner, J. (1985). Changing trends in pediatric septic arthritis. *Seminars in Arthritis and Rheumatism*, **15**, 132–8.

Syriopoulou, V.P. and Smith, A.L. (1987). In septic arthritis. In *Pediatric infectious diseases* (eds R. Feigin and J.Cherry), pp. 773–6. W.B. Saunders, Philadelphia, PA.

Syrogiannopoulos, G.A. and Nelson, J.D. (1978) . Duration of antimicrobial therapy for acute suppurative osteoarticular infections. *Lancet*, i, 37–40.

Syrogiannopoulos, G.A., McCracken, G.H., and Nelson, J.D. (1986). Osteoarticular infections in children with sickle cell disease. *Pediatrics*, **78**, 1090–6.

Trueta, J. (1957). The normal vascular anatomy of the femoral head. *Journal of Bone and Joint Surgery*, **39B**, 358–94.

Tuson, C.E., Hoffman, E.B., and Mann, M.D. (1994). Osotope bone scanning for acute osteomyelitis and septic arthritis in children. *Journal of Bone and Joint Surgery*, **76B**, 306–10.

Welkon, C.J., Long, S.S., Fisher, M.C., and Alburger, P.D. (1986). Pyogenic arthritis in infants and children: a review of 95 cases. *Pediatric Infectious Disease Journal*, **5**, 669–76.

5.3.3 Osteomyelitis and associated conditions

Emilio Bouza and Patricia Muñoz

Introduction

The term osteomyelitis, although specifically applied to medullary infections involving trabecular bone, is used to describe any infection involving bone and marrow (Brause 1990; Laughlin *et al.* 1994; Laughlin *et al.* 1995).

The appearance of new groups of immunosuppressed patients at risk of osteomyelitis, and the emergence of new patterns of antimicrobial resistance in many micro-organisms responsible for bone and joint infections, is a cause of concern (Poiraudeau *et al.* 1993; Rogeaux *et al.* 1993). At the same time, recent and important changes in the field include the application of more precise diagnostic techniques and the use of aggressive surgery with implantation of new prosthetic devices. Finally, the development of non-toxic, highly efficacious, oral antimicrobial agents frequently permits a long-term approach to these difficult-to-treat infections during which the patient remains ambulatory.

First, general aspects of osteomyelitis, with special reference to chronic infections of the long bones, will be discussed. Other forms of osteomyelitis and arthritis will be considered at the end of the chapter.

Classification

The utility of a classification system depends on its ability to predict relevant prognostic, therapeutic, or aetiological data and to provide uniform criteria for comparative studies (Mader *et al.* 1992). A universally applied classification system for stratifying osteomyelitis and prosthetic joint infection would provide a framework to evaluate the efficacy of medical and surgical treatments in different institutions. To date, no attempt at this has been completely successful and there is no single classification system that is satisfactory. Osteomyelitis must, therefore, be classified on the basis of several characteristics. All of them are relevant to planning management and evaluating outcome. The most common criteria are detailed in Table 1.

1. The age of the patient must always be considered, since pathogenesis and aetiology are usually different in neonates, children or adults. Haematogenous osteomyelitis is far more frequent in children. *Staphylococcus aureus*, *Enterobacteriaceae*, and group A and B β-haemolytic streptococci are the most common aetiological agents in neonates. In children under 4 years of age *Haemophilus influenzae* is the most important pathogen, followed by streptococci and *Staph. aureus*. In children older than 4 years *Staph. aureus*, streptococci, and *H. influenzae* predominate.

2. The affected bone is also an important factor. Long bones, particularly those of the lower limbs, are more susceptible to infection because their blood supply is poorer than in short bones. Also, they bear more weight and have worse venous return. Pelvic and cranial bones are infrequently involved (Sexton *et al.* 1993; Bernier *et al.* 1995; Lentz 1995).

3. The host is also very important and special risk groups must be considered. In intravenous drug abusers, atypical locations are more frequently encountered (pubic bones, clavicle or vertebra) and, besides staphylococci and streptococci, Gram-negative rods, mainly *Pseudomonas aeruginosa*, and yeasts must be considered as potential aetiological agents (Chandrasekar and Narula 1986). Patients with haemoglobinopathies, such as sickle-cell disease, have a higher incidence of infections caused by encapsulated bacteria such as *Strep. pneumoniae*, *H. influenzae*, or salmonella (Engh *et al.* 1971). Chronic haemodialysis is also a risk factor for osteomyelitis. The most common sites involved are the ribs and thoracic spine.

4. Most osteomyelitis is caused by Gram-positive bacteria, but practically any other micro-organisms may be responsible for bone infection. Gram-negative bacteria are frequently found in post-traumatic and postsurgical osteomyelitis, and anaerobic and mixed infections should also be considered in osteomyelitis associated with poor vascular supply such as in diabetics (Gerding 1995). Brook and Frazier (1993) isolated anaerobes in 33 per cent of cases of osteomyelitis diagnosed at a military institution. *Mycobacteria*, and particularly *Mycobacterium tuberculosis*, are still an important cause of osteomyelitis, and it is occasionally associated with other micro-organisms (*staphylococci*). Finally, fungal infections of the bone have been described in all agents responsible for systemic mycosis both in the normal and the immunocompromised host.

5. Taking into account the mechanism by which the infecting organisms reach the bone, osteomyelitis can be classified as haematogenous, secondary to a contiguous focus of infection, and caused by direct inoculation. Acute haematogenous osteomyelitis is more common in children and will be discussed later. In adults, haematogenous osteomyelitis frequently involves the spine. This constitutes a diagnostic challenge since clinical and radiological manifestations may be non-specific and rapid evolution may produce significant neurological sequelae (Sapico and Montgomerie 1990; Heary *et al.* 1994). A recent review

Table 1 Classification criteria for osteomyelitis

Criteria	Classification
1. Age	Children — adults
2. Affected bone	Long — short
3. Host	Drug abusers — immunosuppressed — normal
4. Aetiology	Bacterial — non-bacterial
5. Pathogenesis	Haematogenous — contiguous
6. Existence of fracture	Consolidated — non-unions
7. Risk factors	With/without prosthetic material
8. Blood supply	Adequate — inadequate
9. Evolution	Acute — chronic

demonstrates a trend for haematogenous osteomyelitis to have shifted from its known incidence in early age to adulthood, from acute to insidious onset, and from infection by Gram-positive to Gram-negative organisms (Sharma *et al.* 1993).

6. The existence of an underlying fracture, above all with non-union (pseudoarthrosis), is of great importance, since it will influence the surgical approach.

7. The presence of any kind of prosthetic material near the infection site must be carefully sought, since it facilitates persistence of infection, increases the pathogenicity of micro-organisms such as *Staph. epidermidis*, and hinders the efficacy of antimicrobial treatment. Although the withdrawal of prosthetic materials is regularly recommended, it is not always necessary, or possible.

8. Waldvogel *et al.* (1970) classified contiguous osteomyelitis with respect to the integrity of the bone's vascular supply. The most characteristic example of osteomyelitis with poor vascular flow is that associated with infections of the diabetic foot. Neuropathic and vascular changes characteristic of diabetes mellitus put patients at risk for developing chronic foot damage after minor trauma and subsequent bone infection (Gerding 1995).

9. The disease activity in osteomyelitis is classified as acute or chronic. Osteomyelitis is considered acute when the appearance of symptoms is recent, and when there has been no previous therapy. On the other hand, osteomyelitis is chronic when symptoms have been present for 4 to 6 weeks or previous therapy has been given. This classification is important, since therapy and prognosis will be very different. At the present time, less than 6 per cent of haematogenous osteomyelitis becomes chronic but practically all post-traumatic infections are chronic.

Previous classifications have considered these important aspects, the most essential being the presence of vascular compromise, the presence of prosthetic material, and the rate of evolution.

Cierny and Mader (1984) proposed a commendable classification for adult chronic osteomyelitis that takes into account the anatomical status of the bone lesion, the involvement of soft tissues, and the expected host response to infection (Table 2). Accordingly, each case of adult chronic osteomyelitis must be classified with a number and a letter. Nevertheless, the system is imprecise and has not been broadly accepted or generally incorporated into clinical practice. Details of the classification are as follows.

Anatomical classification

Type I Intramedullary infection or infected (but consolidated) fractures with an intramedullary rod. Surgical treatment is simple and will not result in bone instability.

Type II Cortical bone infection (pressure sore). Bone excision is easy, although soft-tissue coverage may be more complicated.

Type III Osteomyelitis affecting cortical bone and marrow, but not including the whole bone circumference (sequestrum). Surgical debridement is complicated, although does not necessarily result in instability.

Type IV Osteomyelitis affecting the whole bone circumference. The surgical approach usually requires ablation of a bone segment and may result in bone instability. Type IV includes infected non-unions and infected articular prostheses.

Physiological classification

Class A Patients and tissues with normal response to infection and surgery.

Class B Patients with local or systemic immune deficiencies, that may predispose to infection (Table 3).

Class C Patients not considered to be suitable surgical candidates, for whom the morbidity of treatment is greater than the risk of disease or exceeds the expected benefit.

Negative aspects of this classification are that it does not consider the aetiology or the bone involved. Surprisingly, the originators obtained relatively uniform results in all the stages, although compromised patients had a statistically inferior prognosis compared with patients who had apparently normal defence mechanisms (Cierny and Mader 1989).

Risk factors for osteomyelitis

Major risk factors for bone infections are contaminated open fractures, previous surgery, insertion of prosthetic material, delayed postoperative wound healing, and previous infections (Gillespie

Table 2 Cierny/Mader classification for adult chronic osteomyelitis

Anatomical	Type I	Medullary
	Type II	Superficial
	Type III	Localized
	Type IV	Diffuse
Physiological	Class A	Normal host
	Class B	Compromised patient
	Class C	Poor-risk candidate

Table 3 Local and systemic factors that affect the immunological, metabolic, and vascular response to osteomyelitis (Cierny/Mader)

Systemic	Local
Malnutrition	Chronic lymphoedema
Renal or hepatic failure	Venous stasis
Immunodeficiency	Large- or small-vessel disease
Neoplasm	Arteritis
Diabetes mellitus	Scars
Extremes of age	Postradiation fibrosis
Smoking (tobacco)	Loss of local sensation
Chronic hypoxia	
Parenteral drug abuse	

1990). In one of the most important series of osteomyelitis, 29 per cent of patients had previous trauma with fracture, 4 per cent trauma without fracture, 42 per cent had recently undergone surgery involving bone, and 11 per cent had a prior open fracture (Guerrero 1989). Pressure sores are closely linked to underlying osteomyelitis, particularly diabetic foot ulcers (Newman et al. 1991). The demonstration of underlying bone involvement frequently requires MRI and indium-111 scintigraphy (Newman et al. 1992).

Aetiology

Gram-positive micro-organisms remain the most common causative agents of osteomyelitis at all ages, although there is a trend towards greater involvement of Gram-negative organisms (Gentry and Rodrguez 1990) (Table 4). Gram-negative organisms should particularly be suspected in patients subject to prolonged stays in hospital or previous surgery, or those admitted to intensive care units or with open fractures (Gentry 1990). In contrast to haematogenous osteomyelitis, which is usually caused by a single pathogen, contiguous chronic osteomyelitis may involve multiple organisms.

Staphylococcus aureus is, undoubtedly, the most common aetiological agent of osteomyelitis of any kind (Guerrero 1987). In recent years, the emergence of methicillin-resistant strains (**MRSA**) (strains resistant to all β-lactam drugs) has been described by many hospitals throughout the world (Ish-Horowicz *et al.* 1992). Nevertheless, osteomyelitis caused by MRSA is less common than might be expected.

Staphylococcus epidermidis is one of the most common agents of bone and joint infection in patients with prosthetic materials, and a high proportion of these infections (more than 50 per cent at our institution) are resistant to methicillin. The aetiological role of *Staph. epidermidis* should only be fully accepted when the isolate is obtained from a usually sterile body fluid or tissue, and skin contamination can be reasonably ruled out. *Staphylococcus epidermidis* infection is extremely rare without the presence of underlying prosthetic material (De Wit *et al.*1993). It is frequently implicated in postsurgical sternal osteomyelitis (Miholic *et al.* 1985).

Although streptococci are of great importance in skin and soft tissue infections, their participation in osteomyelitis is rare (Burkert and Watanakunakorn 1991).

The group B β-haemolytic streptococcus (*Strep. agalactiae*) is exceptional as a cause of osteomyelitis. It is most commonly described in children (Ammari *et al.* 1992; Muñoz *et al.* 1992), or in elderly or immunosuppressed patients (McCarthy and Haber 1987; Elhanan and Raz 1993). Associated bacteraemia may cause high morbidity and mortality (Mateo *et al.* 1993; Farley 1995; Ganapathy and Rissing 1995).

Streptococcus pneumoniae osteomyelitis is also extremely uncommon in adults. It is occasionally described as a single focus of infection in normal children (Jacobs 1991). Cases caused by penicillin-resistant strains have also been reported (Gelfand and Cleveland 1992).

Enterococcus is very rarely implicated in osteomyelitis, and its significance when isolated should be questioned, especially if the biopsy or surgical specimen is not obtained aseptically. The authors have seen two patients with prosthesis-related infections caused by *Enterococcus*, and other cases have been published. In a well-designed study of biopsy confirmed, non-prosthetic osteomyelitis, *Enterococcus* accounted for 3 per cent of the cases (Gentry and Rodrguez-Gomez 1991). Other Gram-positive micro-organisms such as *Listeria* (Housang 1976) or *Bacillus* (Sliman *et al.* 1987; Drobniewski 1993) have only rarely been implicated in osteoarticular infections.

Among the Gram-negative organisms, *Pseudomonas* is one of the most commonly involved in bone infections. It is usually found in osteomyelitis following open fractures or surgical procedures. It is the most frequent cause of calcaneus osteomyelitis following infected puncture wounds of the foot (Dixon and Sydnor 1993; Lavery *et al.* 1994). *Salmonella* osteomyelitis occurs either as a complication of typhoid fever or in patients with various underlying diseases, including immunosuppressed patients and those with sickle-cell disease (Anand and Glatt 1994). Other Enterobacteriaceae have also been described, particularly in infections following open fractures or as a consequence of haematogenous bone involvement in patients with bacteraemia of another origin (Lacour *et al.* 1991; Voss *et al.* 1992).

Conditions predisposing to anaerobic bone infections are vascular disease, bites, a contiguous focus of infection, peripheral neuropathy, haematogenous spread, and trauma. Anaerobes are more frequently detected in osteomyelitis under pressure sores, or in bone infections of the diabetic foot (Hudson 1993). Pigmented *Prevotella* and *Porphyromonas* spp. were mostly isolated in infections of the skull and following bites. Members of the *Bacteroides fragilis* group have been detected in cases of hand and foot infection, and *Fusobacterium* spp. in skull, bite wounds, and haematogenous long-bone infections (Brook and Frazier 1993).

Fungal or nocardial osteomyelitis is found in both normal and immunocompromised hosts (Novak *et al.* 1988; Laurin *et al.* 1991; Pruitt *et al.* 1993; Young 1993; Assaad *et al.* 1994; Straus *et al.* 1994). *Mycobacterium tuberculosis* and, rarely, non-tuberculous mycobacteria, should also be considered as a cause of chronic bone infection (both in normal and immunocompromised hosts) (Cohen and Squires 1992; Jamil *et al.* 1992; Mahan and Jolles 1995; Yao and Sartoris 1995). Viruses are only rarely the cause of bone infections (Berman and Jensen 1990; Kain *et al.* 1990).

Diagnostic procedures

The diagnosis of osteomyelitis and prosthetic joint infections is usually made on the basis of clinical, laboratory, and imaging techniques. Although the problem is usually localized, a complete clinical history and examination must be performed (Levine *et al.* 1993). Information on the presence of any kind of prosthetic material,

Table 4 Changing profile of micro-organisms isolated from osteomyelitis during the last two decades (per cent) (Gentry and Rodriguez 1990)

Micro-organism	1970 (%)	1988 (%)
Staph. aureus	45	27
Other Gram-positive	5	5
Pseudomonas aeruginosa	5	15
Other Gram-negative	8	20
Polymicrobial	37	33

previous surgical and medical therapy, duration of previous antimicrobial courses, and the response must be carefully recorded.

Physical examination should focus on the integrity of involved bone and surrounding tissues, and on evidence of inflammatory signs, pain, bone instability, sinus tracts or neurovascular changes. The nutritional status of the patient should also be considered. The detection of a sinus tract with suppurative drainage will establish the diagnosis in an appropriate clinical setting. Further diagnostic techniques will be required to confirm the diagnosis, if necessary, and to establish the aetiology.

Laboratory investigations

Laboratory data are not essential for the diagnosis of osteoarticular infections. The erythrocyte sedimentation rate is usually high with active infections (92 per cent) and tends to fall after effective therapy. Its accuracy in infected prostheses is variable. In our experience, the erythrocyte sedimentation rate is not useful as an index of either activity or resolution in osteomyelitis.

C-reactive protein is also usually increased, although its measurement is less widely used (Unkila-Kallio *et al.* 1994). Only 35 per cent of patients have leucocytosis at the time of admission.

In summary, no single laboratory measure is reliable enough to be used routinely for the diagnosis of osteomyelitis.

Imaging techniques

Imaging plays an important part in establishing the diagnosis and directing the treatment of osteomyelitis. A variety of imaging methods may be used, including plain radiography, radionuclide imaging, computerized tomography (**CT**), and magnetic resonance imaging (**MRI**). Decisions on the best method can be challenging and should reflect the location of the suspected infection and associated underlying systemic or bone disorder. A brief review of the pathogenesis of osteomyelitis is necessary to help understand when each of imaging techniques is of value (Schauwecker *et al.* 1990; Wegener and Alavi 1991; Crim and Seeger 1994).

Once the micro-organism reaches the bone, a suppurative reaction is produced, followed by a marrow oedema, which can only be readily detected by MRI. The next step consists of vascular congestion, thrombosis, and ischaemia. At this time, soft tissue changes may be detected by CT but not by plain radiology. Finally (after at least 2 to 3 weeks), bone reaction begins, with the production of new periosteal bone, sequestrum, decalcification, and new bone formation, which can be detected even with plain films.

Plain films

The detection of acute osteomyelitis on a plain film requires at least a 35 per cent loss of calcium content in the bone lesion. This usually takes a minimum of 15 days. This is not the issue in chronic osteomyelitis, in which the dilemma is to establish whether radiological changes correspond to active infection, surgical sequelae or just trauma.

The detection of a sequestrum (a clearly defined, isolated necrotic area of bone surrounded by a osteopenic zone) or an involucrum (a hyperdense zone of bone under an elevated periosteum) is considered pathognomonic of osteomyelitis. Other signs that should suggest the presence of active infection are the detection of poorly delineated osteolytic areas, periosteal hyperplasia, or irregular periosteal bone extending into adjacent soft tissue (Gmez 1987).

The presence of periprosthetic bone reabsorption or new periosteal bone formation is highly suggestive of infection in the appropriate clinical setting. Considering their simplicity and low price, conventional radiographs should always be obtained if osteoarticular infection is suspected.

Isotope bone scanning

In most cases of chronic osteomyelitis, clinical and radiological data permit an easy diagnosis (Figs 1, 2, and 3). However, sometimes bone changes from other causes and soft tissue infection make laboratory and radiographic signs unreliable as indicators of osteomyelitis. This happens regularly in acute haematogenous osteomyelitis. In this situation, scintigraphic methods can be helpful. Since it provides physiological data, scintigraphy is also useful in the evaluating therapeutic response. However, anatomical definition is inferior to that of CT or MRI. The following is a description of the widely used techniques, although more sophisticated methods are being developed (Fox and Zeiger 1993).

Technetium-99m methylene diphosphonate
Technetium-99m methylene diphosphonate (**MDP**) is taken up in areas of increased blood flow or osteoblastic activity. A three-phase bone MDP scan (vascular, pool, and late or bone phase) increases specificity, and is the first-line diagnostic imaging technique after a plain radiograph in evaluating suspected osteomyelitis.

Image quality is fairly good, the dose of irradiation is small, the cost is reasonable, and the technique is available in most centres. Preparation is simple, and the technique provides an earlier and more sensitive diagnosis than plain radiography.

However, specificity is poor and the negative predictive value of this technique is more reliable than positive prediction. False positives may be due to neoplasm, fractures, heterotopic ossification, arthritis, neuropathic osteopathy, trauma or arthrosis. It is not very useful in children or following recent surgery to bone.

Gallium-67 citrate
Gallium-67 is taken up in areas where leucocytes or bacteria accumulate and provides quantitative information about inflammatory activity. A comparison with the MDP scan is of great value.

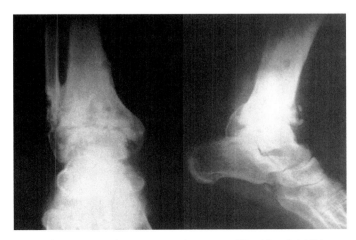

Fig. 1 Plain radiograph: post-traumatic osteomyelitis of the distal tibia.

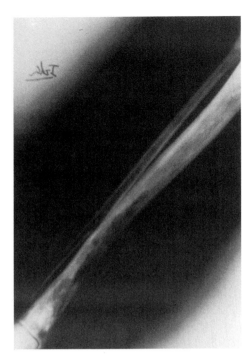

Fig. 2 Haematogenous osteomyelitis of the tibia in an adult with sickle-cell disease.

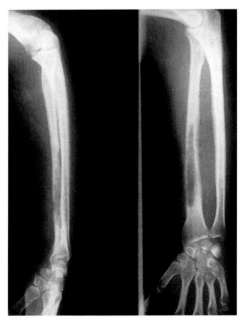

Fig. 3 Haematogenous involvement of bone in a patient with typhoid fever: *Salmonella typhi* osteomyelitis.

Gallium scans become positive earlier than MDP and are sensitive in detecting active bone/joint lesions. A normal gallium scan virtually excludes the presence of an inflammatory process.

False-positive gallium scans in ununited fractures or after recent surgery are common. Images are less precise than MDP scans.

Adult patients with previous bone disorders and possible osteomyelitis or patients with dubious results from MDP scanning should have a gallium scan. Gallium may also be the preferred technique for following response to therapy (Alazraki 1993).

Indium-111 or technetium-99m autologous leucocyte scintigraphy

If the other bone scans are inconclusive, ^{111}In-labelled leucocyte scintigraphy is the next line to take, particularly in adults with other bone disorders.

Patient's leucocytes are obtained and labelled. Afterwards, they are re-infused into the patient and accumulate in the focus of infection where they can be detected.

Indium scans have higher specificity than the previous techniques for the diagnosis of infection, particularly in previously traumatized bone. They provide very good results in osteomyelitis of the diabetic foot, infections associated with delayed or non-union, and prosthetic infections.

Indium scans have higher sensitivity in acute osteomyelitis than in chronic cases (100 per cent vs 60 per cent), probably due to the massive presence of leucocytes in the former (Schauwecker *et al.* 1984). False-positives may occur after trauma, tumours, and other osseous disorders (Nepola *et al.* 1993; Seabold *et al.* 1993). The quality of the image is inferior to that of Tc scintigraphy and it is not very accurate for the axial skeleton. Preparation is complex and long, and the major concerns about this technique are the hazards associated with the handling of blood, and the need to delay imaging for 18 to 24 h, which precludes a rapid result. Potential alternative agents for ^{111}In-labelled leucocytes include labelled immunoglobulin and labelled antigranulocyte antibody reagents.

Indium scans should be reserved for patients with a suspicion of osteomyelitis of the lower extremities not diagnosed with the previous techniques.

None of the types of scintigraphy permits differentiation between septic and non-septic inflammatory processes with sufficient accuracy. For this reason, other techniques are sometimes required.

Computed tomography

This technique accurately detects increased medullary density (typical of the early stages of osteomyelitis), as well as subsequent changes in soft tissues and cortical bone. Its principal advantage is excellent definition of cortical bone, including zones of necrosis, sclerosis, demineralization, periosteal changes, and adjacent soft-tissue swelling. CT does not provide information about the activity of the process and there may be image interference caused by the presence of prosthetic material. Radiation exposure is rather high and it is an expensive technique. CT is especially recommended in chronic osteomyelitis before surgery. It may help to delineate the presence of abscesses, a sinus tract or sequestrum (Maurer *et al.* 1992). It may also be useful for evaluation of infected joint prostheses and osteomyelitis of the spine, pelvis and sternum (Gostishchev *et al.* 1992).

Magnetic resonance tomography (MRI)

Magnetic resonance tomography readily detects the oedema of bone marrow that characterizes the earlier phases of bone infection. Typical features of osteomyelitis on MRI include a low-intensity area in T_1 (less fat) and a hyperintense area in T_2. Bone reaction to fracture or surgery would appear as low marrow intensity in T_1 and normal signal in T_2. Sinus tract and cellulitis would appear as hyperintense areas in T_2.

MRI has proved to be as sensitive as bone scintigraphy in the early detection of osteomyelitis, and, with its superior spatial resolution, it is often more specific than planar scintigraphy in differentiating bone from soft-tissue infection and in separating arthritis, cellulitis, and soft-tissue abscesses from osteomyelitis. In several comparative studies, MRI has been more accurate in detecting the presence and determining the extent of osteomyelitis than scintigraphy, CT scan, and conventional radiography. MRI may facilitate differentiation of acute from chronic osteomyelitis and may help to detect foci of active infection in the presence of chronic inflammation or post-traumatic lesions (Unger *et al.* 1988; Spaeth *et al.* 1991). The patient is not irradiated and newer techniques such as fat-suppressed, contrast-enhanced MRI are significantly more sensitive than scintigraphy, and more specific than non-enhanced MRI or scintigraphy (Morrison *et al.* 1993; Hopkins *et al.* 1995).

MRI also has some drawbacks. It does not provide very precise images of cortical bone and its usefulness decreases in the presence of metallic materials. False-positive results may be obtained in the presence of neoplasm, or intra-/extramedullary inflammation. Experience with MRI is as yet limited and the cost is high. A major indication for MRI is in osteomyelitis of the vertebrae and the foot (Meyers and Wiener 1991), and when diagnosis is still not established after using the previously described techniques.

Microbiological diagnosis

Blood cultures are usually negative in patients with chronic osteomyelitis, and the aetiological diagnosis usually relies on local samples. In acute haematogenous osteomyelitis, blood cultures and/or locally obtained aspirates are the procedures of choice.

It is important to note that only in a small proportion of cases do micro-organisms recovered from sinus tracts reflect the real causative agent present in the bone; *Staph. aureus* is the agent showing the best correlation (Gentry and Rodrguez 1990; Patzakis *et al.* 1994). The overall sensitivity and specificity of sinus-tract cultures for different micro-organisms are summarized in Table 5. Consequently, bone biopsy culture is now the standard method for determining specific antimicrobial therapy (sensitivity and specificity of 87 per cent and 93 per cent, respectively) (Perry *et al.* 1991; Howard *et al.* 1994). Bone biopsy should be taken, using local anaesthesia and imaging control, from the most painful site (Stratton 1989). The specimen must be transported to the laboratory immediately, and stained and cultured for most common pathogens, including aerobes, anaerobes, fungi,

and mycobacteria. Quantitative bone cultures have not been effective in differentiating osteomyelitis from infection or colonization of adjacent soft tissue (Darouiche *et al.* 1994).

The nature of the infection of a joint prosthesis may be particularly difficult to establish. In these cases, joint aspiration with a fine needle is recommended (sensitivity and specificity of 87 per cent and 95, respectively) (Roberts *et al.* 1992).

Finally, mention must be made of the serum bactericidal test, which is considered to be a predictor of therapeutic efficacy in acute and chronic osteomyelitis. This test is based on determining the ability of progressive dilutions of patient's serum to kill the infecting micro-organism. A multicentre study has shown that, in chronic osteomyelitis, peak and trough levels above 1:16 and 1:4, respectively, are desirable (Weinstein *et al.* 1987).

Histological diagnosis

Histological diagnosis of osteomyelitis is useful in all situations but particularly necessary in cases where there is reasonable doubt about the reliability of cultures. It is required in patients already receiving antimicrobial drugs, in osteomyelitis potentially caused by pathogens that are difficult to grow, and in patients where bone samples have to be taken from infected or colonized soft-tissue structures, which may lead to a false-positive result (McGuire 1989).

Bone histopathology also provides more precise information on the anatomical limits of the infected tissue and reassurance that surgical resection has reached healthy, viable bone.

Treatment

The issue of treatment for osteomyelitis has not been completely resolved. Recent research has provided additional insights into the pathogenesis of bone infection. Advances in pharmacology and in surgical techniques have improved our ability to treat such infections. Despite these advances, successful treatment of post-traumatic chronic tibial osteomyelitis depends on adherence to several basic principles: complete debridement of necrotic and infected tissue, obtaining bone stability, the elimination of dead space, and the provision of durable soft-tissue coverage (Dirschl and Almekinders 1993; Meadows *et al.* 1993). Therapy for osteomyelitis requires a multidisciplinary approach, which ideally should include the collaboration of surgeons, infectious disease physicians, rheumatologists, plastic surgeons, radiologists, and many other specialists. The adequate debridement of necrotic tissue is frequently necessary, and the combined orthopaedic and plastic surgical approach has permitted successful salvage of otherwise severely injured lower limbs.

Acute haematogenous osteomyelitis usually responds to antimicrobial therapy. The presence of an abscess, a metaphyseal cavity in haematogenous osteomyelitis, and evidence of spinal-cord compression in vertebral osteomyelitis require surgical treatment.

Chronic osteomyelitis usually implies that dead bone is present, which requires surgical debridement. Because of the chronic nature of the infection and the various presentations and surgical approaches, antibiotic treatment must be individualized. In general, however, at least 4 weeks of therapy is required (Bamberger 1993).

Systemic antimicrobials

The selection of antimicrobial drugs depends on their *in vitro* activity against the responsible pathogens, their penetration into bone tissue,

Table 5 Correlation between cultures from the sinus tract and bone biopsy (Gentry and Rodriguez 1990)

	Sensitivity (%)	Specificity (%)
Bone biopsy	100	100
Sinus tract:	76	86
Staph. aureus	70	90
Other Gram-positive	65	69
Pseudomonas aeruginosa	82	75
Other Gram-negative	88	96

Table 6 Ideal characteristics of antimicrobial agents for the treatment of osteomyelitis

1. Wide spectrum of antimicrobial activity
2. Bactericidal capacity
3. Good oral absorption
4. Long half-life
5. Good penetration in normal and necrotic bone
6. Good activity at low pH and in anaerobic conditions
7. Low toxicity
8. High resistance to bacterial inactivation mechanisms
9. Good clinical efficacy in animal models and humans
10. Low cost

their pharmacological characteristics, toxicity and cost. Table 6 summarizes some of the characteristics of an 'ideal' antimicrobial agent for the treatment of osteomyelitis. The following is a description of some of the antimicrobial agents most frequently used for the therapy of bone and joint infections.

Quinolones

Quinolones are well suited to the treatment of osteomyelitis, since most of them, including ciprofloxacin, ofloxacin and pefloxacin, reach satisfactory levels in bone tissue and their broad spectrum of activity covers most potential pathogens (Overbeck *et al.* 1995; Suh and Lorber 1995). Activity after oral administration is similar to that with parenteral administration. Combined with rifampin they now constitute a frequently used regimen for the treatment of osteomyelitis (Neu 1993). Several trials have shown that the new oral fluoroquinolones are as effective as parenteral cephalosporins and other broad-spectrum agents in treating osteoarticular infections. Tolerance is excellent and permits prolonged courses in ambulatory patients. Ofloxacin has more predictable absorption, although its activity against *Pseudomonas* is less than that of ciprofloxacin. None of them must be used to treat infections caused by MRSA. The widespread overuse of quinolones (1/44 Americans have received ciprofloxacin) has recently raised an alarm (Guay 1992; Greenfield 1993). However, in our opinion, osteoarticular infections can still be considered one of the most clear indications for these drugs.

Co-trimoxazole

Co-trimoxazole is usually active against *Staph. aureus* (including many methicillin-resistant strains) and against some Gram-negative organisms. The authors have treated 17 patients with complicated chronic osteomyelitis, achieving a satisfactory response in 82 per cent after a follow-up of more than two years (Bouza *et al.* 1992). Co-trimoxazole is, on many occasions, the only oral alternative for the therapy of bone and joint infections caused by MRSA.

Vancomycin

Vancomycin is almost uniformly effective against Gram-positive micro-organisms, but has the drawbacks of toxicity and the need for intravenous administration (Ish-Horowicz *et al.* 1992). It may be administered to patients who require parenteral therapy and in osteomyelitis caused by multiresistant Gram-positive micro-organisms (MRSA, *Staph. epidermidis*, etc.) (Refsahl and Andersen 1991). Bone penetration is poor (14 per cent of the serum concentration) and so simultaneous administration of rifampin is recommended.

Teicoplanin

Teicoplanin is a glycopeptide antibiotic with an antimicrobial spectrum of activity similar to that of vancomycin (Wilson and Gruneberg 1994). Nevertheless, it has a longer half-life that permits once-a-day dosing, which is particularly convenient for patients attending day-care hospitals or having antibacterial therapy at home. It can be administered both by intravenous and intramuscular routes, and it is better tolerated than vancomycin. Its efficacy in Gram-positive osteoarticular infections has recently been assessed. Microbiological eradication was achieved in 86 per cent of patients and clinical cure in more than 80 per cent; toxicity precluded termination of therapeutic courses in 12/60 patients. (LeFrock *et al.* 1992; Weinberg 1993).

Rifampin

Rifampin is a bactericidal antimicrobial agent with excellent activity against many Gram-positive micro-organisms. It is considered the most powerful antistaphylococcal agent. It achieves very good bone tissue concentrations (O'Reilly *et al.* 1992), and we feel that, whenever possible, it should be included in the therapeutic regimen of osteoarticular infections. However, it must never be used alone, since resistance develops rapidly if used as a single agent. Patients musts be warned that rifampin may turn body fluids a reddish colour.

Clindamycin

Clindamycin shows good activity against Gram-positive micro-organisms and some anaerobes, and its penetration into bone tissue is satisfactory (98 per cent of the serum concentration). A well-known side-effect of this antibiotic is *Clostridium difficile*-related colitis, especially in elderly patients.

β-Lactam drugs

Among β-lactam drugs, penicillins continue to have an important role. Penicillins are the drugs of choice in osteomyelitis caused by streptococci and staphylococci that are penicillin sensitive. Nevertheless, one should remember that more than 90 per cent of the staphylococci isolated nowadays are resistant to penicillin.

Amoxycillin is the drug of choice in the rare patients with enterococcal osteomyelitis and also in cases due to *Haemophilus* and *Salmonella*. The combination of amoxycillin and clavulanic acid has considerably increased the spectrum of antimicrobial activity of amoxycillin; it can be used in osteomyelitis caused by different *Enterobacteriaceae* and also in cases with anaerobic bacteria present in either mono- or polymicrobial infections.

Piperacillin and piperacillin with tazobactam are suitable agents for the treatment of osteomyelitis caused by *Pseudomonas*, anaerobic bacteria, and mixed infections.

The isoxazolil penicillins and other penicillins resistant to penicillinases are still the preferred drugs (in competition with first-generation cephalosporins) for treatment of most staphylococcal bone and joint infections.

Cephalosporins of all generations have been used in the treatment of osteomyelitis but those of the first generation remain among the drugs of choice for staphylococcal osteomyelitis. Second- and, more particularly, third- and fourth-generation cephalosporins are useful as substitutes for aminoglycosides in the lengthy treatment of Gram-negative osteomyelitis.

Finally, aztreonam is a useful drug for the treatment of Gram-negative osteomyelitis. Imipenem has a very broad spectrum of in vitro activity, including Gram-positive bacteria, *Enterobacteriaceae*, *Ps. aeruginosa* and anaerobes, but should be preserved for cases of osteomyelitis that are particularly difficult to treat or whose aetiology is polymicrobial (Jauregui *et al.* 1993).

Parenteral versus oral antimicrobial agents

Traditionally, parenteral agents were the drugs chosen for the treatment of osteomyelitis. Most still believe that at least the initial treatment of osteomyelitis should be with intravenous antibiotics. Others (us included), however, consider that in clinically stable patients with aetiologically well-documented osteomyelitis, some oral drugs are adequate from the very beginning. For maintenance therapy, intravenous antibiotics have been largely replaced by new, orally active, wide-spectrum agents that permit prolonged treatment in the ambulatory patient (Conrad and Marks 1989; Craig and Andes 1995). The drugs most frequently used for staphylococcal infections are combinations of rifampin with either oral fluoroquinolones or co-trimoxazole. Most Gram-negative infections in adults can be treated with an oral quinolone but for others there are no adequate oral drugs (Tice 1993).

Length of therapy

The use of new, orally active antimicrobials such as quinolones has modified the recommended length of therapy in chronic osteomyelitis. The 6-week benchmark, which was determined largely by experience with childhood haematogenous osteomyelitis, may not be applicable to contiguous-focus osteomyelitis after trauma in adults. At the present time, it is known that 6 weeks may not be sufficient for contiguous chronic osteomyelitis and the availability of oral antibiotics with a low toxicity profile permits a much longer duration of treatment and a higher rate of success. Unfortunately, to our knowledge, no well-designed prospective clinical trials have determined the precise duration of antimicrobial therapy for chronic osteomyelitis. We recommend a minimum of 3 months. This may be extended in certain circumstances, such as poor initial response, unsatisfactory coverage of soft tissues, presence of non-unions, and delayed withdrawal of prosthetic material.

Occasionally, patients not considered to be candidates for surgery require prolonged suppression rather than a curative approach.

Local delivery of antimicrobials

Several devices designed to deliver antimicrobials locally (cement, biodegradable microcapsules) have been developed, although the most widely used are gentamicin-impregnated polymethylmethacrylate beads, which are claimed to allow immediate filling of the bone defect and to provide high antibiotic concentrations. In some centres their use has become standard orthopaedic practice. Chains of beads are packed into the infected bone cavity after debridement, with the end projecting from the scar. During the following 4 to 6 weeks, the chain is progressively pulled out. The procedure is painful and sometimes adhesions prevent complete extraction of the beads.

A recent comparative study, involving 384 patients, suggests that local therapy with gentamicin-impregnated beads is as effective as standard systemic therapy for osteomyelitis. The conclusions may be biased by the fact that most patients received combined surgical and medical treatment (local and systemic antimicrobials). However, the data do suggest that both cost of treatment and toxicity are considerably lower in patients who are treated with local antibiotics alone (Blaha *et al.* 1993). Good results are reported in the treatment of infected non-union (Calhoun *et al.* 1993) and contaminated compound fractures (Ostermann *et al.* 1993). The main drawbacks are the potential danger of leaving foreign material in a septic space with connections to the exterior, and that gentamicin, the most commonly used antimicrobial in these devices, does not seem to be the most potent agent, considering that *Staph. aureus* is the major pathogen. New devices impregnated with more effective antimicrobials such as vancomycin, teicoplanin, or ciprofloxacin are being studied (Dacquet *et al.* 1992; Gerhart *et al.* 1993; DiMaio *et al.* 1994).

Surgical therapy

Antibiotic treatment is not a substitute for surgical debridement of infected, devitalized bone. Absence or inadequacy of surgical treatment is clearly associated with higher rates of initial failures or recurrences. We recommend early surgery whenever possible, before the administration of antimicrobial agents. The purpose of the surgical intervention is not only therapeutic but also may serve to establish the precise aetiological diagnosis.

On some occasions, the need for bone consolidation and stability precludes early surgical therapy and surgery has to be postponed until these occur. In this case, the administration of antimicrobials is 'palliative' until the definitive, and potentially curative, surgical procedure is possible.

The different surgical techniques for bone debridement will not be reviewed in detail in this chapter. However, the principle is that only viable bone should be left in place whenever possible.

Bone viability is of fundamental importance in the surgical management of osteomyelitis. The use of laser Doppler flowmetry as an adjunct to surgery, allowing quantitative evaluation of bone vascularity, has recently proved to be of great value (Duwelius and Schmidt 1992). When axial long bones are involved, aggressive debridement is not easy to perform since adequate wound coverage and mechanical stability may be difficult to achieve or maintain. Treatment of infected non-unions is especially difficult. Prognosis has become more optimistic with the development of new orthopaedic methods, such as the Ilizarov limb reconstruction method. This has proved to be cost-effective when compared with amputation (Cattaneo *et al.* 1992; Williams 1994). Occasionally, osteotomies, bone grafts and transports, or muscular flaps are also necessary (Mahan and Jolles 1995; Yajima *et al.* 1995).

Another situation that requires rapid functional reconstruction is osteomyelitis of the sternum associated with mediastinitis. For this, a wide debridement should be followed (at the same time or soon thereafter) by reconstruction of the chest wall by vascularized pectoral-muscle flaps (Banic *et al.* 1995).

A conservative, non-surgical approach is recommended for asymptomatic or mildly symptomatic osteomyelitis in elderly patients.

Finally, it is important to remember that amputation is sometimes the most functional therapeutic alternative in patients with refractory osteomyelitis of the feet or lower limbs (Lerner *et al.* 1993). We feel that early amputation in chronic and relapsing osteomyelitis of the foot, particularly when associated with poor vascular supply or neuropathic disease, is better for the patient than prolonged disability and antimicrobial therapy condemned to failure.

Administration of hyperbaric oxygen

Hyperbaric oxygen has been used successfully in the treatment of air embolism, in radio-osteonecrosis, in intoxication by carbon monoxide, in clostridial myonecrosis, in severely burned patients, and in other soft-tissue infections. Open, non-randomized studies suggest a potential value of hyperbaric oxygen in the treatment of refractory chronic osteomyelitis (Slack *et al.* 1965; Perrins *et al.* 1966; Depenbusch *et al.* 1972; Davis *et al.* 1986; Mader *et al.* 1990).

In an animal experimental model of chronic *Staph. aureus* osteomyelitis, hyperbaric oxygen was compared to treatment with parenteral cephalothin alone and with a combination of both for 4 weeks. Hyperbaric oxygen was as effective as parenteral cephalothin. At the end of treatment, the original *Staph. aureus* could be recovered from 91 per cent of control animals, 36 per cent of those treated with hyperbaric oxygen only, 47 per cent of those treated with cephalothin alone, and from 40 per cent of those treated with the combination.

Hyperbaric oxygen increases the bactericidal activity of phagocytic cells and the bactericidal effect of drugs as vancomycin and aminoglycosides. Collagen production by fibroblasts occurs more efficiently with oxygen tensions greater than 10 mmHg.

The role of hyperbaric oxygen in the treatment of human osteomyelitis requires definition by well-designed, prospective clinical studies.

Prognosis

Osteomyelitis-associated mortality is usually low, but the tendency for osteomyelitis to recur and become chronic is well known. Patients may experience unpredictable episodes of fistulous discharge. Recurrences are most common within a year of the initial episode, but extremely long intervals have been reported.

Malignant transformation arising from a fistula in patients with chronic osteomyelitis is extremely rare, although isolated cases have been described. This emphasizes the importance of histological examination (Mabit *et al.* 1993; Noonan *et al.* 1993).

Patients and doctors should realize that it is impossible to guarantee whether osteomyelitis can ever be 'cured,' since infections become manifest many years after injury or treatment.

Prophylaxis

Antimicrobial prophylaxis is recommended after open fractures, in which the infection rate is high.

For the implantation of articular prostheses both antimicrobial prophylaxis and environmental air cleaning are recommended. For hip, knee, and other major joint prostheses, the recommended antimicrobial prophylaxis is usually one to three doses of cefazolin starting at the induction of anaesthesia and over the next 24 to 48 h. In addition, antimicrobial prophylaxis is specially important, and widely used, when internal fixation of fractures or joint replacements are performed.

As most osteoarticular infections are proved to be acquired in the operating theatre, highly sophisticated, centrifugal laminar-flow systems have been installed, achieving a 10^4-fold reduction in the concentration of environmental micro-organisms and 10-fold reduction in the incidence of infection. At the present time, the incidence of infection has been reduced to 0.5 per cent in hip prostheses (Lidwell 1986; Schutzer and Harris 1988), while knee and shoulder prostheses are associated with a higher incidence of septic complications (1–4 per cent and 4–7 per cent, respectively) (Bengtsson 1993; Malchau *et al.* 1993).

Some orthopaedic surgeons recommend prophylactic antimicrobial agents for prevention of infection in patients with prosthetic joints undergoing certain invasive procedures. Particular attention should be paid to bacteriuria, the implantation of intravascular devices, drainage, and dental manipulations, for which a prophylactic approach similar to that for endocarditis is recommended.

Chronic post-traumatic osteomyelitis

Most information to date comes from experience with chronic post-traumatic osteomyelitis. The risk of infection after an open fracture varies widely with the site, size, and nature of an open fracture, as shown in Table 7, adapted from Gustilo *et al.* (1990).

Chronic osteomyelitis is usually a local disease that only rarely produces systemic manifestations. The most common symptoms are pain and suppurative discharge. As mentioned previously, the infection is characteristically recurrent and resistant to short courses of therapy. Fever is more common in acute infections or in the presence of soft-tissue abscesses.

The presence of an open draining fistula is always a marker of clinical activity of osteomyelitis.

The main principle of management of infection in non-consolidated bone fractures is to retain fracture fixation whenever possible. When infection becomes apparent, ultrasonography may determine the presence or absence of collections requiring drainage. In the absence of a collection or a wound discharge, only antimicrobial treatment should be provided. If discharge or collections are present, surgical drainage and debridement are necessary, the organisms present must be identified, and antimicrobial treatment prescribed.

Implants should be retained unless fracture has occurred, in which case repeated debridement with removal of all devitalized bone and soft tissue is required. After this, either exchange implants or external fixation are undertaken.

Osteomyelitis in decubitus ulcers

The incidence of osteomyelitis under decubitus ulcers ranges from 28 to 70 per cent (Bohm *et al.* 1988; Bruck *et al.* 1991). Most patients with osteomyelitis have radiological changes but to confirm its activity and aetiology requires needle or surgical bone sampling. Antibiotics are indicated only if osteomyelitis is present. After surgical debridement, soft-tissue coverage is essential. Myocutaneous flaps are superior to skin flaps in securing skin cover.

Table 7 Risk of infection in open fractures (adapted from Gustilo et al. 1990)

Type	Wound	Fracture	Infection
Type I	<1 cm Clean puncture Soft-tissue damage +	Simple, transverse Comminution +	0–2%
Type II	>1 cm Moderate contamination Soft tissue damage ++	Moderate contamination Comminution ++	2–7%
Type III:	Soft tissue damage +++	Instability Comminution +++	
Type III A	Soft-tissue coverage: adequate	Contamination ++	7%
Type III B	Loss of soft tissue Exposure of bone or periosteal stripping	Contamination +++	10–50%
Type III C	Arterial injury		25–50%

Acute haematogenous osteomyelitis in children

Haematogenous osteomyelitis may appear as an acute onset of bone pain or limited motion of an extremity, regardless of the presence or absence of signs of infection such as fever, local tenderness, redness, swelling or heat.

Acute haematogenous osteomyelitis in children is becoming infrequent. Nelson (1990) reports that this diagnosis is made only approx. 15 times per year in a large referral unit for paediatric infectious diseases in the United States. Approximately one-third of the cases occur in children under 2 years of age, another one-third between 2 and 5 years, and the remaining one-third in children more than 5 years old (Nelson 1990).

In most children with acute haematogenous osteomyelitis no predisposing factors are apparent but it is well known that sickle-cell anaemia is associated with a higher risk of haematogenous osteomyelitis, particularly due to *Salmonella* (Adeyokunnu and Hendrickse 1980; Syrogiannopoulos *et al.* 1986). and *Staphylococcus* (Sadat-Ali *et al.* 1985).

Pain, pseudoparalysis (voluntary limitation of movement of one extremity), and fever are the most common clinical manifestations. Initially, local inflammatory signs are rarely present. As mentioned earlier, plain radiographs are frequently negative and isotope bone scanning is required (Herndon *et al.* 1985; Demopulos *et al.* 1988). The disease is almost always monostotic and long-bone metaphyses are the sites most frequently involved. Diagnostic confirmation requires needle aspiration or surgical debridement. Blood cultures are, in contrast to chronic osteomyelitis, frequently positive (in at least one-third of the episodes). Both blood and local samples should be always be obtained because, not uncommonly, only one of the samples is positive. *Staphylococcus aureus* is responsible for at least 50 per cent of the cases. The remaining cases are caused by different micro-organisms, among them *Streptococcus* and *Haemophilus* (Nelson 1990).

When pain is severe, needle or surgical decompression should be undertaken. If the infection opens into the synovial cavity, repeated needle aspiration may be sufficient.

When no pain or large collection of pus is present, antimicrobial treatment alone may be enough. Sequential treatment (intravenous drugs followed by oral antimicrobial agents) has proved adequate (Nelson 1982). A total of 10 to 14 days of intravenous antibiotics is followed by 2 to 6 additional weeks of oral agents. These should have an acceptable flavour, good oral absorption, low toxicity profile and be active against Gram-positives and *Haemophilus*. The indication for measuring serum bactericidal concentrations during follow-up still needs to be defined but trough or peak levels greater than 1/8 or 1/32 have been recommended (Prober and Yeager 1979; Nelson 1990).

Nowadays the prognosis of acute haematogenous osteomyelitis in childhood is much better than in the past. Death from this cause is almost non-existent and evolution to chronicity occurs in less than 5 per cent of cases (Dunkle and Brock 1982; Nelson 1990).

Vertebral osteomyelitis

The spinal column is the most common site of haematogenous osteomyelitis in adults, probably due to vertebrae having abundant red marrow and a slow and tortuous blood flow. Bacteria reach the vertebral bodies preferentially by the arteries but occasionally also through the venous plexus (Wiley and Trueta 1959; Waldvogel *et al.* 1970; Adatepe *et al.* 1986; Sapico and Montgomerie 1990).

More than 50 per cent of the episodes of vertebral osteomyelitis are due to *Staph. aureus*, approx. 30 per cent to *Enterobacteriaceae*, and the remaining 10 to 20 per cent to other micro-organisms such as *Brucella* spp, *M. tuberculosis,* and fungi (Sapico and Montgomerie 1979; Sapico and Montgomerie 1980; Sapico and Montgomerie 1990).

Vertebral osteomyelitis is generally monomicrobial but the association of *M. tuberculosis* with other pathogens, particularly *Staph. aureus,* is more than casual.

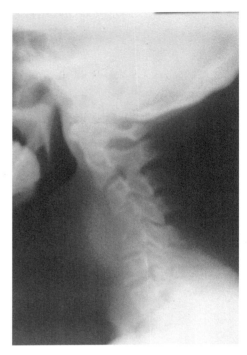

Fig. 4 Cervical vertebral osteomyelitis and prevertebral pyogenic abscess.

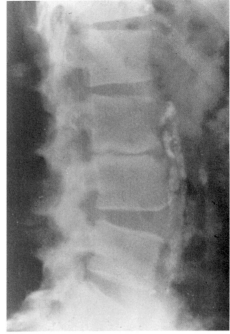

(a)

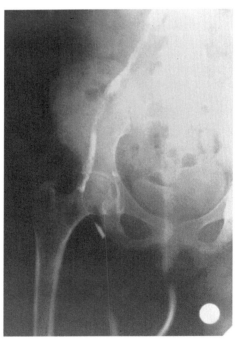

(b)

Fig. 5 Tuberculous vertebral osteomyelitis with a fistulous tract draining to the upper thigh.

Pain that increases with spinal movement is the most common clinical manifestation of vertebral osteomyelitis. Other symptoms depend on the site of involvement. In patients with cervical osteomyelitis and prevertebral abscesses, odinophagia and dysphagia may be present.

Fever and/or an increased white blood-cell count is absent in up to half of the cases. An increased erythrocyte sedimentation rate has traditionally been considered to be a very sensitive marker for the presence of active vertebral infection. In our experience this is not the case and the diagnosis of vertebral osteomyelitis should not be rejected in patients with a normal erythrocyte sedimentation rate.

Overall, the lumbar spine is the most frequent location and is involved in more than 50 per cent of episodes of vertebral osteomyelitis, followed by 35 per cent in the dorsal spine, and the remaining 15 per cent in the cervical spine.

Lumbar osteomyelitis occurs occasionally as a septic metastasis of infections of the pelvis and genitourinary tract (Sapico and Montgomerie 1979); cervical bone infection is frequently a complication of parenteral drug abuse and is seen in patients with other predisposing conditions (Sapico and Montgomerie 1986).

Most cases of vertebral osteomyelitis have abnormalities on plain radiographs when first seen but in very acute presentations, pain may be present but the plain film is normal. Erosive, irregular images in the vertebral bodies and the adjacent intervertebral disc are common. Pre- and paravertebral abscesses and vertebral collapse are common complications (Figs 4 and 5).

Isotope imaging is diagnostically very sensitive in patients with normal or equivocal plain films. Both CT and MRI offer early and well-defined images that are very useful for directing aspiration or surgery (Boddicker *et al.* 1980; Modic *et al.* 1985; Sapico and Montgomerie 1990).

Microbiological confirmation requires either positive blood cultures, vertebral material or both. Only one-quarter of the episodes are documented with blood cultures and consequently bone aspiration should be undertaken whenever possible.

Most cases of vertebral osteomyelitis do not require surgical debridement. Surgery should be reserved for patients with spinal instability, neurological impairment, a large, progressive abscess

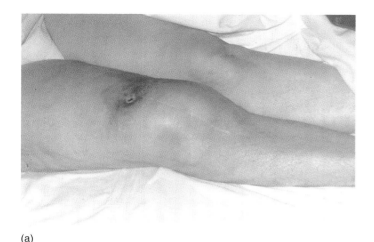

(a)

(b)

Fig. 6 Infected knee prosthesis: (a) fistulous tract; (b) fistulography.

impossible to drain by guided needle aspiration, or cases of unknown aetiology not responding rapidly to antimicrobial therapy.

Considerations governing antimicrobial therapy described previously also apply to vertebral involvement. Immobilization in bed is only required for patients with pain or vertebral instability and casts are not necessary in most cases.

Infected prosthesis (see Chapter 5.3.1)

Infections related to joint prostheses have been divided into those presenting in the first 3 months after surgery (type I), those presenting between 3 months and 1 year postoperatively (type II), and those occurring after 1 year postsurgery (type III) (Coventry 1975). Type I infections are almost exclusively acquired during surgery and may be divided into superficial (involving soft tissues but not the prosthesis), and deep (involving the prosthesis). In group II, most infections are surgically acquired and practically all of them involve the prosthesis. Finally, group III infections are of haematogenous origin and involve the prosthesis. At least 70 per cent of

prosthetic joint infections are monomicrobial and the remaining 20 to 30 per cent are either polymicrobial or not documented (Buchholz *et al.* 1981; Buchholz *et al.* 1984). Among the responsible micro-organisms, *Staph. epidermidis* and *Staph. aureus* are far ahead of other bacteria, followed by Gram-negative rods and anaerobes.

Chronic infection of articular prostheses usually begins as continuous pain, frequently without obvious drainage through a sinus tract, prosthetic dysfunction or complete loosening (Fig. 6). Infections associated with prosthetic material are extremely difficult to treat and often require surgical removal of foreign bodies, which may be very radical when artificial joints are involved. Attempts to implant a new prosthesis are usually made after prolonged courses of antimicrobial therapy, leaving the patient with major incapacity for a long time. Recently, Drancourt *et al.* (1993) reported an acceptable rate of success (74 per cent) on treating osteoarticular prostheses infected with staphylococci with prolonged periods (9–12 months) of ofloxacin and replacing the prosthesis, when necessary, in a one-step procedure.

Type I infections with superficial involvement and no evidence of prosthetic dysfunction should be treated with antimicrobial agents, removal of blood or collections, soft-tissue debridement, and irrigation. A high proportion of these cases (approx. 70 per cent) do not require future prosthetic replacement (Buchholz *et al.* 1984; Fitzgerald 1984; Fitzgerald and Jones 1985). Even in cases with deep infections, antimicrobial therapy and early debridement and irrigation save at least 50 per cent of the prostheses (Drancourt *et al.* 1993).

In patients with type II and III infections the final objective is to preserve a functional, pain-free prosthesis. In patients with no prosthetic dysfunction and with no or minimal pain, a trial of antimicrobial therapy without surgical replacement of the prosthesis can be attempted. We use, whenever possible, oral antimicrobial agents, usually including rifampin in a combination regimen. Treatment is continued for a 6- to 12-month period, provided an adequate response was rapidly obtained. In case of a late relapse, the treatment is individualized depending on many variables such as the age of the patient, functional status, and the risk for surgical replacement.

In patients with pain, prosthetic dysfunction or loosening, surgical replacement is necessary. It may be performed in two stages or in a single step, with a low rate of reinfection (Buchholz *et al.* 1984).

Infectious arthritis

Infectious arthritis must be considered as an emergency, since delays or inadequate treatment may result in great disability. The recognition, diagnosis, and treatment of this condition are therefore very important (Smith 1990).

Infectious arthritis should be suspected in any patient with a swollen joint but especially in children, debilitated patients, immunocompromised persons, those with infection elsewhere (even if on antibiotics), and those with other types of arthritis or a prosthetic joint (Fig. 7). Diagnosis depends on obtaining joint fluid for culture and Gram staining. Initial treatment with appropriate broad-spectrum antibiotics is later best narrowed to suit the individual organism. Treatment requires repeated needle aspiration or surgical drainage plus an antimicrobial course of 2 to 6 weeks (Middleton 1993).

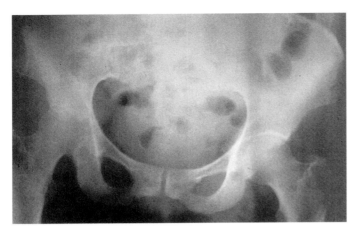

Fig. 7 Right hip infection caused by *Staph. aureus* in an intravenous drug abuser.

Table 8 Epidemiological and clinical characteristics of aetiological agents of infectious arthritis

Risk factor	Micro-organisms
Infants	*Staph. aureus* Enterobacteria Group B streptococci
Children	*Staph. aureus* *H. influenzae* *Streptococcus* spp. Enterobacteria
Adults	*Staph. aureus* Group A streptococci Enterobacteriaceae *N. gonorrhoeae*
Rheumatoid arthritis	*Staph. aureus* *Streptococcus* spp. Enterobacteria
Prosthetic joint, postoperative, intra-articular injection	*Staph. epidermidis* *Staph. aureus* Enterobacteriaceae *Pseudomonas* spp.
Intravenous drug abuse	*Staph. aureus* or *Ps. aeruginosa*
Human bite	*Eikenella corrodens*, oral flora
Cat or dog bite	*Pasteurella multocida*, anaerobes
Rat bite	*Streptobacillus moniliformis*
Tick exposure	*Borrelia burgdorferi*
Unpasteurized dairy products	*Brucella* spp.
Trauma in aquatic environment	*Mycobacterium marinum*
Gardening injury	*Sporothrix schenckii*
Menstruation or pregnancy	*N. gonorrhoeae*

This subject is described in more detail in Chapter 5.3.1. Some clinical and epidemiological features related to aetiological agents of infectious arthritis are shown in Table 8.

Most cases are caused by *Staph. aureus*, although many bacterial and viral pathogens may be involved. Among streptococci, group A β-haemolytic predominates, although group β have been described, mainly in immunosuppressed patients (Barberan *et al.* 1993). *Neisseria gonorrhoeae* is the predominant cause of bacterial arthritis in sexually active adults under 30 years of age with no other risk factor. Transient, disseminated, papular skin lesions precede the appearance of polyarticular symptoms and blood cultures are usually positive. In the rare event of monoarticular infection the micro-organism is only isolated from synovial fluid.

Gram-negative rods usually cause infectious arthritis in patients with underlying conditions, and *Pseudomonas* spp. have been associated sternoclavicular and sacroiliac joint infections in intravenous drug abusers.

Lyme arthritis should be suspected in patients with a history of tick exposure and erythema chronicum migrans. The diagnosis is usually serological.

Chronic monoarticular arthritis is usually caused by mycobacteria or fungus. Infectious arthritis caused by *M. tuberculosis* is infrequent, usually affecting the interphalangeal joints of the hand. *Mycobacterium kansasii* and *M. marinum* arthritis have also been described.

A number of fungi can cause infectious arthritis. *Sporothrix shenckii* infections are usually related to contact with soil and most commonly affect the knee. *Coccidioides immitis* arthritis can occur in endemic areas, in both immunocompetent and immunocompromised patients. Other fungi such as *Candida* (haematogenous spread), *Cryptococcus*, and *Aspergillus* are even rarer agents of infectious arthritis (Christensson *et al.* 1993; Cuende *et al.* 1993).

Many viral infections can produce joint symptoms. Among them, rubella (small joints of the hand), erythema infectiosum (parvovirus B19), and hepatitis B are the most common. Mycoplasmas and urea-plasmas are responsible for about two-fifths of cases of septic arthritis in patients with hypogammaglobulinaemia (Furr *et al.* 1994). Management is dealt with in other chapters.

Prognosis

Bad prognostic factors include: age exceeding 60 years, pre-existing arthritis, infection in hip and shoulder, symptoms for more than 7 days before treatment, involvement of more than four joints, and persistently positive cultures after 7 days of appropriate therapy.

Limitation of motion and persistence of pain are the most common sequel; although a mortality rate between 30 and 100 per cent has been described for polyarticular cases (Bould *et al.* 1993; Pitkin and Eykyn 1993).

References

Adatepe, M. H. *et al.* (1986). Hematogenous pyogenic vertebral osteomyelitis. Diagnostic value of radionuclide bone imaging. *Journal of Nuclear Medicine*, 27, 1680–5.

Adeyokunnu, A. A. and Hendrickse, R. G. (1980). *Salmonella* osteomyelitis in childhood. *Archives of Disease in Childhood*, 55, 175.

Alazraki, N. P. (1993). Radionuclide imaging in the evaluation of infections and inflammatory disease. *Radiologic Clinics of North America*, 31, 783–94.

Ammari, L. K., Offit, P. A., and Campbell, A. B. (1992). Unusual presentation of group B *Streptococcus* osteomyelitis. *Pediatric Infectious Diseases Journal*, 11,1066–7.

Anand, A. J. and Glatt, A. E. (1994). *Salmonella* osteomyelitis and arthritis in sickle cell disease. *Seminars in Arthritis and Rheumatism*, 24, 211–21.

Assaad, W., Nuchikat, P. S., Cohen, L., Esguerra, J. V., and Whittier, F. C. (1994). *Aspergillus* discitis with acute disc abscess. *Spine*, 19, 2226–9.

Bamberger, D. M. (1993). Osteomyelitis. A commonsense approach to antibiotic and surgical treatment. *Postgraduate Medicine*, 94,177–84.

Banic, A., Ris, H. B., Erni, D., and Striffeler, H. (1995). Free latissimus dorsi flap for chest wall repair after complete resection of infected sternum. *Annals of Thoracic Surgery*, 60, 1028–32.

Barberan, J., Rodriguez, R., Gomis, M., Quilez, C., Martin-Gamero, C. P., and Atero, F. (1993). *S. agalactiae*-induced septic arthritis in a patient with vulvar carcinoma. (Letter). *Annales Medicina Interna*, 10, 468–9.

Bengtsson, S. (1993). Prosthetic osteomyelitis with special reference to the knee: risks, treatment and costs. *Annals of Medicine*, 25, 523–9.

Berman, S. and Jensen, J. (1990). Cytomegalovirus-induced osteomyelitis in a patient with the acquired immunodeficiency syndrome. *Southern Medical Journal*, 83, 1231–2.

Bernier, S., Clermont, S., Maranda, G., Turcotte, J. Y. (1995). Osteomyelitis of the jaws. *Journal of the Canadian Dental Association*, 61, 441–2: 445–8.

Blaha, J. D. *et al.* (1993). Comparison of the clinical efficacy and tolerance of genta-micin PMMA beads on surgical wire versus combined and systemic therapy for osteomyelitis. *Clinical Orthopedics*, 295, 8–12.

Boddicker, J. H. *et al.* (1980). Bone and gallium scanning in the evaluation of disse-minated coccidioidomycosis. *American Review of Respiratory Diseases*, 122, 279–87.

Bohm, E., Kuhlmann, I., and Botel, U. (1988). Decubitus ulcer in paraplegic patients: a comparative clinico-pathological study. *Unfallchirurgie*, 14, 335–42.

Bould, M., Edwards, D., and Villar, R. N. (1993). Arthroscopic diagnosis and treat-ment of septic arthritis of the hip joint. *Arthroscopy*, 9, 707–8.

Bouza, E. *et al.* (1992). Eficacia del cotrimoxazol en el tratamiento de infecciones estafiloccicas graves. Abstr. 217 (*Proceedings) V Congreso de la Sociedad Española de Enfermedades Infecciosas y Microbiologa Clnica (SEIMC)*, Barcelona.

Brause, B. D. (1990). Infections with prostheses in bones and joints. In *Principles and practice of infectious diseases*, (3rd edn) (ed. G. L. Mandell, D. R. Gordon, Jr, and J. E. Bennett), pp. 919–30. Churchill Livingstone, New York.

Brook, I. and Frazier, E. H. (1993). Anaerobic osteomyelitis and arthritis in a military hospital: a 10-year experience. *American Journal of Medicine*, 94, 21–8.

Bruck, J. C., Buttemeyer, R., Grabosch, A., and Gruhl, L. (1991). More arguments in favour of myocutaneous flaps for the treatment of pelvic pressure sores. *Annals of Plastic Surgery*, 26, 85–8.

Buchholz, H. W. *et al.* (1981). Management of deep infection of total hip replace-ment. *Journal of Bone and Joint Surgery (B)*, 63, 342.

Buchholz, H. W., von Foerster, G., and Heinert, K. (1984). Management of infected prostheses. *Orthopedics*, 7, 1620.

Burkert, T. and Watanakunakorn, C. (1991). Group G streptococcus septic arthritis and osteomyelitis: report and literature review. *Journal of Rheumatology*, 18, 904–7.

Calhoun, J. H., Henry, S. L., Anger, D. M., Cobos, J. A., and Mader, J. T. (1993). The treatment of infected nonunions with gentamicin polymethylmethacrylate antibiotic beads. *Clinical Orthopedics*, 295, 23–7.

Cattaneo, R., Catagni, M., Johnson, E. E. (1992). The treatment of infected nonunions and segmental defects of the tibia by the methods of Ilizarov. *Clinical Orthopedics*, 280, 143–52.

Chandrasekar, P. H. and Narula, P. (1986). Bone and joint infections in intravenous drug abusers. *Reviews of Infectious Diseases*, 6, 904–11.

Christensson. B., Ryd, L., Dahlberg, L., and Lohmander, S. (1993). *Candida albicans* arthritis in a nonimmunocompromised patient. Complication of placebo intraarticular injections. *Acta Orthopaedica Scandinavica*, 64, 695–8.

Cierny, G. and Mader, J. T. (1984). Adult chronic osteomyelitis. *Orthopedics*, 7, 1557.

Cierny, G. and Mader, J. T. (1989). Adult chronic osteomyelitis: an overview. In *Orthopaedic infections* (ed. R. D. D'Ambrosia and R. L Marier), pp. 31–47. SLACK International, Thorofare, NJ.

Cohen, O. J. and Squires, K. (1992). *Mycobacterium avium* osteomyelitis as the presenting manifestation of AIDS. *Infectious Diseases in Clinical Practice*, 1, 110–13.

Conrad, D. A. and Marks, M. I. (1989). Oral therapy for orthopaedic infections in children and adults. In *Orthopaedic infections* (ed. R. D. D'Ambrosia and R. L Marier), pp. 345–60. SLACK International, Thorofare, NJ..

Coventry, M. B. (1975). Treatment of infections occurring in total hip surgery. *Orthopedic Clinics of North America*, 6, 991.

Craig, W. A. and Andes, D. R. (1995). Parenteral versus oral antibiotic therapy. *Medical Clinics of North America.*, 79, 497–508.

Crim, J. R. and Seeger, L. L. (1994). Imaging evaluation of osteomyelitis. *Critical Reviews of Diagnostic Imaging*, 35, 201–56.

Cuende, E., Barbadillo, C-E., Mazzucchelli, R., Isasi, C., Trujillo, A., and Andreu, J. L. (1993). *Candida* arthritis in adult patients who are not intravenous drug addicts: report of three cases and review of the literature. *Seminars in Arthritis and Rheumatism*, 22, 224–41.

Dacquet, V. *et al.* (1992). Antibiotic impregnated plaster of Paris beads. Trials with teicoplanin. *Clinical Orthopedics*, 282, 241–9.

Darouiche, R. O., Landon, G. C., Klima, M., Musher, D. M., and Markowski, J. (1994). Osteomyelitis associated with pressure sores. *Archives of Internal Medicine*, 154, 753–8.

Davis, J. C. *et al.* (1986). Chronic non-hematogenous osteomyelitis treated with adjuvant hyperbaric oxygen. *Journal of Bone and Joint Surgery (A)*, 68, 1210–17.

Demopulos, G. A., Bleck, E. E., and McDougall, I. R. (1988). Role of radionuclide imaging in the diagnosis of acute osteomyelitis. *Journal of Pediatric Orthopedics*, 8, 558.

Depenbusch, F. I., Thompson, R. E., and Hart, G. B. (1972). Use of hyperbaric oxygen in the treatment of refractory osteomyelitis: a preliminary report. *Journal of Trauma*, 12, 807–12.

De Wit, D., Mulla, R., Cowie, M. R., Mason, J. C., and Davies, K. A. (1993). Vertebral osteomyelitis due to *Staphylococcus epidermidis*. *British Journal of Rheumatology*, 32, 339–41.

DiMaio, F. R., O'Halloran, J. J., and Quale, J. M. (1994). *In vitro* elution of cipro-floxacin from polymethylmethacrylate cement beads. *Journal of Orthopedic Research*, 12, 79–82.

Dirschl, D. R. and Almekinders, L. C. (1993). Osteomyelitis. Common causes and treatment recommendations. *Drugs*, 45, 29–43.

Dixon, R. S. and Sydnor, C. H. (1993). Puncture wound pseudomonal osteomye-litis of the foot. *Journal of Foot and Ankle Surgery*, 32, 434–42.

Drancourt, M., Stein, A., Argenson, J. N., Zannier, A., Curvale, G., and Raoult, D. (1993). Oral rifampin plus ofloxacin for treatment of *Staphylococcus*-infected orthopedic implants. *Antimicrobial Agents and Chemotherapy*, 37, 1214–18.

Drobniewski, F. A. (1993). *Bacillus cereus* and related species. *Clinical Microbiology Reviews*, 6, 324–38.

Dunkle, L. M. and Brock, N. (1982). Long-term follow-up of ambulatory manage-ment of osteomyelitis. *Clinical Pediatrics*, 21, 650.

Duwelius, P. J. and Schmidt, A. H. (1992). Assessment of bone viability in patients with osteomyelitis: preliminary clinical experience with laser Doppler flow-metry. *Journal of Orthopedics and Trauma*, 6, 327–32.

Elhanan, G. and Raz, R. (1993). Group B streptococcal vertebral osteomyelitis in an adult. *Infection*, 21, 397–9.

Engh, C. A., Hughes, J. L., Abrams, R. C., and Bowerman, J. W. (1971). Osteomyelitis in the patient with sickle-cell disease. *Journal of Bone and Joint Surgery*, 53, 1–15.

Farley, M. M. (1995). Group B streptococcal infection in older patients. Spectrum of disease and management strategies. *Drugs and Aging*, 6, 293–300.

Fitzgerald, R. H. (1984). Antibiotic distribution in normal and osteomyelitic bone. *Orthopedic Clinics of North America*, 15, 537.

Fitzgerald, R. H. and Jones, D. R. (1985). Hip implant infection. Treatment with resection arthroplasty and late total hip arthroplasty. *American Journal of Medicine*, 78, S225.

Fox, I. M. and Zeiger, L. (1993). Tc-^{99}m-HMPAO leukocyte scintigraphy for the diagnosis of osteomyelitis in diabetic foot infections. *Journal of Foot and Ankle Surgery*, 32, 591–4.

Furr, P. M., Taylor-Robinson, D., and Webster, A. D. (1994). Mycoplasmas and ureaplasmas in patients with hypogammaglobulinaemia and their role in arthritis: microbiological observations over twenty years. *Annals of the Rheumatic Diseases*, **53**, 183–7.

Ganapathy, M. E. and Rissing, J. P. (1995). Group B streptococcal vertebral osteomyelitis with bacteremia. *Southern Medical Journal*, **88**, 350–1.

Gelfand, M. S. and Cleveland, K. O. (1992). Penicillin-resistant pneumococcal vertebral osteomyelitis. *Clinical Infectious Diseases*, **15**, 746–7.

Gentry, L. O. (1990). Antibiotic therapy for osteomyelitis. *Infectious Disease Clinics of North America*, **4**, 485–99.

Gentry, L. O. and Rodrguez, G. G. (1990). Oral ciprofloxacin compared with parenteral antibiotics in the treatment of osteomyelitis. *Antimicrobial Agents and Chemotherapy*, **34**, 40–3.

Gentry, L. O. and Rodrguez-Gomez, G. (1991). Ofloxacin versus parenteral therapy for chronic osteomyelitis. *Antimicrobial Agents and Chemotherapy*, **35**, 538–41.

Gerding, D. N. (1995). Foot infections in diabetic patients: the role of anaerobes. *Clinical Infectious Diseases*, **20** (Suppl. 2), S283–8.

Gerhart, T. N., Roux, R. D., Hanff, P. A., Horowitz, G. L., Renshaw, A. A., and Hayes, W. C. (1993). Antibiotic-loaded biodegradable bone cement for prophylaxis and treatment of experimental osteomyelitis in rats. *Journal of Orthopedic Research*, **11**, 250–5.

Gillespie, W. J. (1990). Epidemiology in bone and joint infection. *Infectious Disease Clinics of North America*, **4**, 361–76.

Gmez, E. (1987). Radiologa de la infeccin sea. *Enfermedades Infecciosas Microbiologa Clinica*, **5**, 525–30.

Gostishchev, V. K., Karmazanovskii, G. G., Shalykova, L. P., Vasilkova, Z. F., and Vavilova, G. S. (1992). Special methods of examination and their role in the selection of the extent and type of surgical intervention in patients with pelvic osteomyelitis. *Khirurgiia (Moskow)*, **7–8**, 17–21.

Greenfield, R. A. (1993). Symposium on antimicrobial therapy. VII. The fluoroquinolones. *Journal of the Oklahoma State Medical Association*, **86**, 166–74.

Guay, D. R. (1992). The role of the fluoroquinolones. *Pharmacotherapy*, **12**, 71–85S.

Guerrero, A. (1987). Estudio etiolgico de las osteomielitis bacterianas. *Enfermedades Infecciosas Microbiologa Clinica*, **5**, 517–20.

Guerrero, A. (1989). Infecciones del aparato locomotor. In *Monografa en comentarios a la literatura en enfermedades infecciosas*, Vol. 5 (2), (ed. E. Bouza) pp. 9–88. CIMSA, Madrid.

Gustilo, R. B., Merkow, R. L., and Templeman, D. (1990). The management of open fractures. *Journal of Bone and Joint Surgery (A)*, **72**, 299–304.

Heary, R. F., Hunt, C. D., and Wolansky, L. J. (1994). Rapid bony destruction with pyogenic vertebral osteomyelitis. *Surgical Neurology*, **41**, 34–9.

Herndon, W. A. *et al.* (1985). Nuclear imaging for musculo-skeletal infections in children. *Journal of Pediatric Orthopedics*, **5**, 343.

Hopkins, K. L., Li, K. C., and Bergman, G. (1995). Gadolinium-DTPA-enhanced magnetic resonance imaging of musculoskeletal infectious processes. *Skeletal Radiology*, 325–30.

Housang, E. T. (1976). Acute *Listeria monocytogenes* osteomyelitis. *Infection*, **4**, 113.

Howard, C. B., Einhorn, M., Dagan, R., and Yagupski, P. (1994). Fine-needle bone biopsy to diagnose osteomyelitis. *Journal of Bone and Joint Surgery (B)*, **76**, 311.

Hudson, J. W. (1993). Osteomyelitis of the jaws: a 50-year perspective. *Journal of Oral and Maxillofacial Surgery*, **51**, 1294–301.

Ish-Horowicz, M. R., McIntyre, P., and Nade, S. (1992). Bone and joint infections caused by multiply resistant *Staphylococcus aureus* in a neonatal intensive care unit. *Pediatric Infectious Diseases Journal*, **11**, 82–7.

Jacobs, N. M. (1991). Pneumococcal osteomyelitis and arthritis in children. A hospital series and literature review. *American Journal of Diseases of Children*, **145**, 70–4.

Jamil, S., Brennessel, D., Pessah, M., and Hilton, E. (1992). Fluconazole treatment of cryptococcal osteomyelitis. *Infectious Diseases in Clinical Practice*, **1**, 115–17.

Jauregui, L., Matzke, D., Scott, M., Minns, P., and Hageage, G. (1993). Cefepime as treatment for osteomyelitis and other severe bacterial infections. *Journal of Antimicrobials and Chemotherapy*, **32**, 141–9.

Kain, Z., Frogel, M., and Krilov, L. R. (1990). Osteomyelitis associated with varicella infection *Pediatric Infectious Diseases Journal*, **9**, 146–7.

Lacour, M., Duarte, M., Beutler, A., Auckenthaler, R., and Suter, S. (1991). Osteoarticular infections due to *Kingella kingae* in children. *European Journal of Pediatrics*, **150**, 612–18.

Laughlin, R. T., Sinha, A., Calhoun, J. H., and Mader, J. T. (1994). Osteomyelitis. *Current Opinion in Rheumatology*, **6**, 401–7.

Laughlin, R. T., Wright, D. G., Mader, J. T., and Calhoun, J. H. (1995). Osteomyelitis. *Current Opinion in Rheumatology*, **7**, 315–21.

Laurin, J. M., Resnik, C. S., Wheeler, D., and Needleman, B. W. (1991). Vertebral osteomyelitis caused by *Nocardia asteroides*: report and review of the literature. *Journal of Rheumatology*, **18**, 455–8.

Lavery, L. A., Harkless, L. B., Felder-Johnson, K., and Mundine, S. (1994). Bacterial pathogens in infected puncture wounds in adults with diabetes. *Journal of Foot and Ankle Surgery*, **33**, 91–7.

LeFrock, J. L. *et al.* (1992). Teicoplanin in the treatment of bone and joint infections. Teicoplanin Bone and Joint Cooperative Study Group, USA. *European Journal of Surgery*, **567** (Suppl.), 9–13.

Lentz, S. S. (1995). Osteitis pubis: a review. *Obstetrics and Gynecology Survey*, **50**, 310–15.

Lerner, R. K., Esterhai, J. L., Polomano, R. C., and Cheatle, M. D. (1993). Quality of life assessment of patients with posttraumatic fracture nonunion, chronic refractory osteomyelitis, and lower-extremity amputation. *Clinical Orthopedics*, **295**, 28–36.

Levine, S. E., Esterhal, J. L, Heppenstall, R. B, Calhoun, J., and Mader, J. T. (1993). Diagnoses and staging. osteomyelitis and prosthetic joint infections. *Clinical Orthopedics*, **295**, 77–86.

Lidwell, O. M. (1986). The operating environment. *Seminars in Orthopaedics*, **1**, 33.

Mabit, C., Huc, H., Setton, D., Leboutet, M. J,, Arnaud, J. P., and Pecout, C. (1993). Epidermoid carcinoma arising in femoral osteitis. A case. *Revue Chirurgie Orthopédie Reparatrice Apparet Motile*, **79**, 62–5.

McCarthy, J. M. and Haber, J. (1987). Group B streptococcal soft tissue infections beyond the neonatal period. *Western Journal of Medicine*, **147**, 558–60.

McGuire, M. H. (1989). The pathogenesis of adult osteomyelitis. *Orthopedic Reviews*, **18**, 564–70.

Mader, J. T., Adams, K. R., Wallace, W. R., and Calhoun, H. (1990). Hyperbaric oxygen as adjunctive therapy for osteomyelitis. *Infectious Disease Clinics of North America*, **4**, 433–40.

Mader, J. T., Norden, C., Nelson, J. D., and Calandra, G. B. (1992). Evaluation of new anti-infective drugs for the treatment of osteomyelitis in adults. Infectious Diseases Society of America and the Food and Drug Administration. *Clinical Infectious Diseases*, **15**, S155–61.

Mahan, S. and Jolles, P. R. (1995). MAI osteomyelitis. 18-year scintigraphic follow-up. *Clinical Nuclear Medicine*, **20**, 594–8.

Malchau, H., Herberts, P., and Ahnfelt, L. (1993). Prognosis of total hip replacement in Sweden. Follow-up of 92 675 operations performed (1978–1990). *Acta Orthopaedica Scandinavica*, **64**, 497–506.

Mateo, L., Miquel Nolla, J., Rozadilla, A., and del Blanco, J. (1993). Vertebral osteomyelitis caused by *Streptococcus agalactiae*. *Medicina Clinica*, **100**, 398.

Maurer, J., Lehmann-Beckow, D., Vosshenrich, R., Fischer, U., and Grabbe, E. (1992). The place of computed tomography and magnetic resonance tomography in the diagnosis of bone sequestra. *Aktuelle Radiologie*, **2**, 345–9.

Meadows, S. E., Zuckerman, J. D., and Koval, K. J. (1993). Posttraumatic tibial osteomyelitis: diagnosis, classification, and treatment. *Bulletin of the Hospital for Joint Diseases*, **52**, 11–16.

Meyers, S. P. and Wiener, S. N. (1991). Diagnosis of hematogenous pyogenic vertebral osteomyelitis by magnetic resonance imaging. *Archives of Internal Medicine*, **151**, 683–7.

Middleton, D. B. (1993). Infectious arthritis. *Primary Care*, **20**, 943–53.

Miholic, J. *et al.* (1985). Risk factors for severe bacterial infections after valve replacement and aortocoronary bypass operations: analysis of 246 cases by logistic regression. *Annals of Thoracic Surgery*, **40**, 224–8.

Modic, M. T., Feiglin, D. H., and Piraino, D. W. (1985). Vertebral osteomyelitis: assessment using MR. *Radiology*, **157**, 157–66.

Morrison, W. B. *et al.* (1993). Diagnosis of osteomyelitis: utility of fat-suppressed contrast-enhanced MR imaging. *Radiology*, **189**, 251–7.

Muñoz, C., Trujillo, G., Latorre, C., Juncosa, T., and Huget, R. (1992). Osteoarticular infections in children. *Enfermedades Infecciosa Microbiologa Clinica*, **10**, 286–9.

Nelson, J. D. (1982). A critical review of the role of oral antibiotics in the management of hematogenous osteomyelitis. In *Current clinical topics in infectious diseases* (ed. J. S. Remington and M. N. Swartz), p. 64. McGraw-Hill, New York.

Nelson, J. D. (1990). Acute osteomyelitis in children. *Infectious Disease Clinics of North America*, 4, 513–23.

Nepola, J. V., Seabold, J. E., Marsh, J. L., Kirchner, P. T., and el-Khoury, G. Y. (1993). Diagnosis of infection in ununited fractures. Combined imaging with indium-111-labeled leukocytes and technetium-99m methylene diphosphonate. *Journal of Bone and Joint Surgery (A)*, 75, 1816–22.

Neu, H. C. (1993). Synergy and antagonism of fluoroquinolones with other classes of antimicrobial agents. *Drugs*, 45, S54–8.

Newman, L. G. *et al.* (1991). Unsuspected osteomyelitis in diabetic foot ulcers. Diagnosis and monitoring by leukocyte scanning with indium in 111 oxyquinoline. *Journal of the American Medical Association*, 266, 1246–51.

Newman, L. G. *et al.* (1992). Leukocyte scanning with 111In is superior to magnetic resonance imaging in diagnosis of clinically unsuspected osteomyelitis in diabetic foot ulcers. *Diabetes Care*, 15, 1527–30.

Noonan, K. J., Goetz, D. D., Marsh, J. L., and Peterson, K. K. (1993). Rapidly destructive squamous cell carcinoma as a complication of chronic osteomyelitis. *Orthopedics*, 16, 1140.

Novak, R. M., Polisky, E. L., Janda, W. M., and Libertin, C. R. (1988). Osteomyelitis caused by *Rhodococcus equi* in a renal transplant recipient. *Infection*, 16, 186–8.

O'Reilly, T., Kunz, S., Sande, E., Zak, O., Sande, M. A., and Tauber, M. G. (1992). Relationship between antibiotic concentration in bone and efficacy of treatment of staphylococcal osteomyelitis in rats: azithromycin compared with clindamycin and rifampin. *Antimicrobial Agents and Chemotherapy*, 36, 2693–7.

Ostermann, P. A., Henry, S. L., and Seligson, D. (1993). The role of local antibiotic therapy in the management of compound fractures. *Clinical Orthopaedics*, 295, 102–11.

Overbeck, J. P., Winckler, S. T., Meffert, R., Tormala, P., Spiegel, H. U., and Brug, E. (1995). Penetration of ciprofloxacin into bone: a new bioabsorbable implant. *Journal of Investigative Surgery*, 8, 155–62.

Patzakis, M. J., Wilkins, J., Kumar, J., Holtom, P., Greenbaum, B., and Ressler, R. (1994). Comparison of the results of bacterial cultures from multiple sites in chronic osteomyelitis of long bones. *Journal of Bone and Joint Surgery (A)*, 76, 664–6.

Perrins, J. D. *et al.* (1966). OHP in the management of chronic osteomyelitis. In *Proceeding of the Third International Conference on Hyperbaric Medicine* (ed. I. W. Brown and B. G. Cox), pp. 578–84. National Academy of Sciences, National Research Council, Washington DC.

Perry, C. R., Pearson, R. L., and Miller, G. A. (1991). Accuracy of cultures of material from swabbing of the superficial aspect of the wound and needle biopsy in the preoperative assessment of osteomyelitis. *Journal of Bone and Joint Surgery (A)*, 73, 745–9.

Pitkin, A. D. and Eykyn, S. J. (1993). Covert multi-focal infective arthritis. *Journal of Infection*, 27, 297–300.

Poiraudeau, S., Liote, F., Bardin, T., Kuntz, D., and Dryll, A. (1993). Septic arthritis in HIV infection: 5 cases. (Letter). *Annales de Medicine Interne*, 144, 344–5.

Prober, C. G. and Yeager, A. S. (1979). Use of the serum bactericidal titer to assess the adequacy of oral antibiotic therapy in the treatment of acute hematogenous osteomyelitis. *Journal of Pediatrics*, 95, 131.

Pruitt, T. C., Hughes, L. O., Blasier, R. D., McCarthy, R. E., Glasier, C. M., and Roloson, G. J. (1993). Atypical mycobacterial vertebral osteomyelitis in a steroid-dependent adolescent. A case report. *Spine*, 18, 2553–5.

Refsahl, K. and Andersen, B. M. (1991). Coagulase-negative staphylococci-problem bacteria in the hospital. Identification and resistance status. *Nordisk Medicin*, 106, 228–31.

Roberts, P., Walters, A. J., and McMinn, D. J. W. (1992). Diagnosing infection in hip replacements. The use of fine-needle aspiration and radiometric culture. *Journal of Bone and Joint Surgery (B)*, 74, 265–9.

Rogeaux, O., Fassin, D., and Gentilini, M. (1993). Prevalence of rheumatic manifestations in human immunodeficiency virus infection. *Annales de Medicine Interne*, 144, 443–8.

Sadat-Ali, M., Kutty, S., and Kutti, K. (1985). Recent observations on osteomyelitis in sickle-cell disease. *International Orthopedics*, 9, 97.

Sapico, F. L. and Montgomerie, J. Z. (1979). Pyogenic vertebral osteomyelitis. Report of nine cases and review of the literature. *Reviews of Infectious Diseases*, 1, 754–76.

Sapico, F. L. and Montgomerie, J. Z. (1980). Vertebral osteomyelitis in intravenous drug abusers. Report of three cases and review of the literature. *Reviews of Infectious Diseases*, 2, 196–206.

Sapico, F. L. and Montgomerie, J. Z. (1986). Vertebral osteomyelitis. In *Infectious diseases and medical microbiology*, (2nd edn) (ed. A. I. Braude, C. E. Davis, and J. Fierer), pp. 1479–81. Saunders, Philadelphia.

Sapico, F. L. and Montgomerie, J. Z. (1990). Vertebral osteomyelitis. *Infectious Disease Clinics of North America*, 4, 539–50.

Schauwecker, D. S. *et al.* (1984). Evaluation of complicating osteomyelitis with Tc-99m MDP, In-111 granulocytes and Ga-67 citrate. *Journal of Nuclear Medicine*, 25, 849.

Schauwecker, D. S., Braunstein, E. M., and Wheat, L. J. (1990). Diagnostic imaging of osteomyelitis. *Infectious Disease Clinics of North America*, 4, 441–63.

Schutzer, S. F. and Harris, W. H. (1988). Deep wound infection after total hip replacement under contemporary aseptic conditions. *Journal of Bone and Joint Surgery (A)*, 70, 724.

Seabold, J. E., Ferlic, R. J., Marsh, J. L., and Nepola, J. V. (1993). Periarticular bone sites associated with traumatic injury: false-positive findings with In-111-labeled white blood cell and Tc-99m MDP scintigraphy. *Radiology*, 186, 845–9.

Sexton, D. J., Heskestad, L., Lambeth, W. R., McCallum, R., Levin, L. S., and Corey, G. R. (1993). Postoperative pubic osteomyelitis misdiagnosed as osteitis pubis: report of four cases and review. *Clinical Infectious Diseases*, 17, 695–700.

Sharma, S. V., Khare, G. N., Bhalla, N., and Saraf, S. K. (1993). Changing profile of haematogenous osteomyelitis in a teaching hospital. *Indian Journal of Medical Research*, 98, 92–5.

Slack, W. K., Thomas, D. A., and Perrins, D. J. D. (1965). Hyperbaric oxygenation in chronic osteomyelitis. *Lancet*, I, 1093–4.

Sliman, R., Rehm, S., and Shlaes, D. M. (1987). Serious infections caused by *Bacillus* species. *Medicine*, 66, 218–23.

Smith, J. W. (1990). Infectious arthritis. *Infectious Disease Clinics of North America*, 4, 523–38.

Spaeth, H. J. *et al.* (1991). Magnetic resonance imaging detection of early experimental periostitis. Comparison of magnetic resonance imaging, computed tomography, and plain radiography with histopathologic correlation. *Investigative Radiology*, 26, 304–8.

Stratton, C. W. (1989). Microbiologic evaluation of patients with skeletal infections. In *Orthopaedic infections* (ed. R. D. D'Ambrosia and R. L. Marier), pp. 309–20. Slack International Book Distributors, Thorofare, NJ.

Straus, W. L. *et al.* (1994). Clinical and epidemiologic characteristics of *Mycobacterium haemophilum*, an emerging pathogen in immunocompromised patients. *Annals of Internal Medicine*, 120, 118–25.

Suh, B and Lorber, B. (1995). Quinolones. *Medical Clinics of North America*, 79, 869–94.

Syrogiannopoulos, G. A., McCracken, G. H., and Nelson, J. D. (1986). Osteoarticular infections in children with sickle cell disease. *Pediatrics*, 78, 1090.

Tice, A. D. (1993). Osteomyelitis. *Hospital Practice*, 28 (Suppl. 2), 36–9.

Unger, E., Moldofsky, P., Gatenby, R., Hartz, W., and Broder, G. (1988). Diagnosis of osteomyelitis by MR imaging. *American Journal of Radiology*, 150, 605.

Unkila-Kallio, L., Kallio, M. J., Eskola, J., and Peltola, H. (1994). Serum C-reactive protein, erythrocyte sedimentation rate, and white blood cell count in acute hematogenous osteomyelitis of children. *Pediatrics*, 93, 59–62.

Voss, L. M., Rhodes, K. H., and Johnson, K. A. (1992). Musculoskeletal and soft tissue *Aeromonas* infection: an environmental disease. *Mayo Clinic Proceedings*, 67, 422–7.

Waldvogel, F. A., Medoff, G., and Swartz, M. N. (1970). Osteomyelitis: a review of clinical features, therapeutic considerations and unusual aspects. *New England Journal of Medicine*, 198, 260–316.

Wegener, W. A. and Alavi, A. (1991). Diagnostic imaging of musculoskeletal infection. Roentgenography, gallium, indium-labeled white blood cell, gammaglobulin, bone scintigraphy, and MRI. *Orthopedic Clinics of North America*, 22, 401–18.

Weinberg, W. G. (1993). Safety and efficacy of teicoplanin for bone and joint infections: results of a community-based trial. *Southern Medical Journal*, **86**, 891–7.

Weinstein, M. P., Stratton, C. W., Hawley, H. B., and Reller, L. B. (1987). Multicenter collaborative evaluation of a standardized serum bactericidal test as a predictor of therapeutic efficacy in acute and chronic osteomyelitis. *American Journal of Medicine*, **83**, 218–22.

Wiley, A. M. and Trueta, J. (1959). The vascular anatomy of the spine and its relationship to pyogenic vertebral osteomyelitis. *Journal of Bone and Joint Surgery*, **41**, 796–809.

Williams, M. O. (1994). Long-term cost comparison of major limb salvage using the Ilizarov method versus amputation. *Clinical Orthopedics*, **301**, 156–8.

Wilson, A. P. and Gruneberg, R. N. (1994). Use of teicoplanin in community medicine. *European Journal of Clinical Microbiology and Infectious Diseases*, **13**, 701–10.

Yajima, H., Tamai, S., Ishida, H., and Fukui, A. (1995). Partial soleus muscle island flap transfer using minor pedicles from the posterior tibial vessels. *Plastic and Reconstructive Surgery*, **96**, 1162–8.

Yao, D. C. and Sartoris, D. J. (1995). Musculoskeletal tuberculosis. *Radiologic Clinics of North America*, **33**, 679–89.

Young, L. S. (1993). Mycobacterial diseases and the compromised host. *Clinical Infectious Diseases*, **17**, S436–41.

5.3.4 Lyme disease

Daniel W. Rahn

Introduction

Lyme disease is a tick-borne infectious disorder caused by a spirochaete, *Borrelia burgdorferi*. The best clinical marker of disease onset is a characteristic expanding skin lesion, erythema migrans. Weeks to months later the nervous system, heart, and joints may be affected with rare involvement of other organ systems. Lyme disease responds to antibiotics throughout its course, but treatment of early disease is the most successful. Endemic foci of Lyme disease have been described in the United States, Europe, and Asia.

History

'Lyme arthritis' was recognized in November 1975 because of an epidemic of arthritis in children in the region of Lyme, Connecticut (Steere *et al*. 1977*b*). Prospective, community-based study demonstrated the illness to be a multisystem disorder (Lyme disease) (Steere *et al*. 1977*b*; Reik *et al*. 1979; Steere *et al*. 1979; Steere *et al*. 1980; Steere *et al*. 1983*a*), occurring at any age and in both sexes, usually beginning with a characteristic expanding skin lesion, erythema chronicum migrans (Afzelius 1910), now shortened by convention to erythema migrans. Erythema migrans had previously been associated with the bite of the sheep tick, *Ixodes ricinus* (Thone 1968), and with tick-borne meningopolyneuritis (Garin-Bujadoux 1922), but not with arthritis (Bannwarth 1944). Field studies in the Lyme region revealed the presence of a closely related tick, *I. scapularis*, which was subsequently implicated as the principal disease vector (Steere *et al*. 1978; Wallis *et al*. 1978; Steere and Malawista 1979).

In 1982, Burgdorfer and associates (Burgdorfer *et al*. 1982) isolated a spirochaete from *I. scapularis* ticks from Shelter Island, New York.

Patients with Lyme disease were found to have an elevated serological response to this spirochaete and within months this organism had been cultured from blood, skin, and cerebrospinal fluid of patients with various manifestations of Lyme disease (Benach *et al*. 1983; Steere *et al*. 1983*d*).

Much has been learned about Lyme disease but many areas of uncertainty remain. There is no clear consensus among practising physicians regarding the geographic range, clinical spectrum, and optimal treatment of this complex disorder. Why some individuals develop chronic symptoms despite apparent elimination of infecting organisms also remains to be elucidated.

Causative agent: *Borrelia burgdorferi*

Lyme disease is caused by *B. burgdorferi*, a spirochaete 10 to 30 μm long and 0.2 to 0.25 μm wide. It can be grown only in a specialized medium (Barbour–Stoner–Kelly medium) that is not available routinely in clinical laboratories (Weber *et al*. 1993). *Borrelia burgdorferi* replicates slowly *in vitro*, with a generation time of around 12 to 20 h. The organism has an outer membrane that surrounds a periplasmic space, multiple flagella, and a protoplasmic cylinder. Its genetic material is contained on a single linear chromosome and both linear and circular plasmids. Immunodominant, species-specific, outer surface proteins are encoded on plasmids. Other non-species-specific antigens of importance are flagellin (41 kDa) and a high molecular-weight heat-shock protein.

Three different genospecies have been described to date: *B. burgdorferi* sensu stricto, *B. garinii*, and *B. afzelii* (Baranton *et al*. 1992; Canica *et al*. 1993). A serotyping system has been developed based on reactivity to different epitopes of OspA (Wilske *et al*. 1993). North American isolates have shown less variability with regard to OspA, than have European isolates. Genetic differences among isolates appear to explain the different virulence patterns seen in European and North American Lyme disease. *B. afzelii*, isolated predominantly in Europe, has a propensity to persist in the skin causing the chronic skin lesion acrodermatitis chronica atrophicans. The other species appear to have a greater tendency for haematogenous dissemination (van Dam *et al*. 1993; Wienecke *et al*. 1994).

Pathogenesis

Lyme disease develops after an infected tick transmits *B. burgdorferi* to a susceptible host. Following a period of latency, organisms spread outward in skin causing the characteristic skin lesion, erythema migrans. Organisms can be readily cultured from biopsy specimens of the primary skin lesion. Histological staining of lesions of erythema migrans may reveal occasional spirochaetes and there is an inflammatory infiltrate consisting of lymphocytes, histiocytes, and plasma cells. In addition to erythema migrans, *B. burgdorferi* causes another acute skin lesion, benign lymphocytoma (Weber *et al*. 1984), seen primarily in Europe. The infection subsequently disseminates to involve secondary skin sites (secondary annular lesions) and other organs (e.g., central nervous system, heart and joints).

Borrelia burgdorferi has been cultured from involved tissues during all stages of the illness. Positive cultures have been obtained from blood (early) (Benach *et al*. 1983; Steere *et al*. 1983*d*), secondary skin lesions (Åsbrink and Hovmark 1985), cerebrospinal fluid (Steere *et al*. 1983*d*), joint fluid (Snydman *et al*. 1986), iris, ligamentous tissue, and a long-standing lesion of acrodermatitis chronica atrophicans (Åsbrink and Hovmark 1985). As the disease progresses, however, it becomes progressively more difficult to isolate organisms by culture.

Chronic manifestations have primarily involved the nervous system (Reik et al. 1979; Pachner et al. 1985; Halperin et al. 1987; Halperin et al. 1989; Pachner et al. 1989; Logigian et al. 1990), joints (Steere et al. 1987; Steere et al. 1990), and skin (Åsbrink and Olsson 1985). There is mounting evidence to explain how B. burgdorferi might persist in antibiotic-treated patients. In vitro the organism was able to invade and survive within some human cells such as fibroblasts, macrophages and endothelial cells, and thereby evade the action of antibiotics (Comstock and Thomas 1989; Klempner et al.1993; Montgomery et al.1994). Also, B. burgdorferi can cross the blood–brain barrier early in the course of infection where routine oral antibiotic regimens do not produce bactericidal levels. Neurological dysfunction resulting from low-grade infection in the central nervous system may only become apparent clinically months to years later (Garcia-Monco et al. 1990; Pfister et al. 1990; Luft et al. 1992).

Other, parainfectious mechanisms may also contribute to the development of chronic neuropathy and arthritis, at least in some individuals. There is a sharp distinction between the response to antibiotics of individuals with early disease and the inconsistent response of those with chronic neurological involvement (see below). Similarly, the likelihood of Lyme arthritis responding to antibiotics is affected by duration of arthritis and immunogenetic factors, particularly HLA-DR4 (Steere et al. 1979; Steere et al. 1990). Joint inflammation in these individuals may persist after the joint fluid has become negative in the polymerase chain reaction (Nocton et al. 1994). Thus, initial infection may trigger persistent inflammation in immunogenetically susceptible individuals. Clinical heterogeneity and inconsistent antibiotic responsiveness may be explained by differing mechanisms of inflammation at different stages of the illness.

Disabling fatigue has been a particularly troublesome symptom associated with late Lyme disease. Fatigue alone rarely, if ever, responds to antibiotic therapy. Proinflammatory cytokines have been implicated in the pathogenesis of both Lyme arthritis and chronic neurological manifestations, and may account for this pathological fatigue. It is not known whether either live B. burgdorferi or retained bacterial products are necessary to stimulate cytokine release, an issue with obvious implications for therapy.

Immune abnormalities are present in all stages of Lyme disease (Steere et al. 1977; Steere et al. 1979a; Hardin et al. 1979a; Hardin et al. 1979b). At disease onset, immune complexes are often detectable in serum (Hardin et al. 1979a; Hardin et al. 1979b) and the serum IgM is often elevated, both of which are associated with disease dissemination. When arthritis is present, immune complexes are uniformly elevated in joint fluid rather than serum (Hardin et al. 1979a; Hardin et al. 1984). The synovial lesion contains a mixed infiltrate of lymphocytes and plasma cells (Steere et al. 1979). Production of anti-B. burgdorferi antibody in the cerebrospinal fluid is a hallmark of chronic neurological involvement (Halperin et al. 1989; Logigian et al. 1990).

As infection spreads from a local (skin) site to involve other organs, an inflammatory response ensues, which includes immune elements and the release of cytokines. Variation in symptoms and clinical course reflects both direct effects of infection and immunological phenomena triggered by the infection. Systemic symptoms result from disseminated infection, immune-mediated inflammation, and release of cytokines. Organ-specific inflammation occurs when localized infection (e.g. joints and nervous system) stimulates a localized immune response. But in immunogenetically susceptible individuals the immunological response may be prolonged, and perhaps even self-perpetuating. Therapeutic advances will require a clearer understanding of the specific disease mechanisms, particularly regarding the question of persistence of spirochaetes or their antigens throughout the entire course of the illness.

Epidemiology

Cases of Lyme disease have been reported from most states in the United States as well as throughout Europe, the former Soviet Union, China, Japan, and (questionably) Australia (Dekonenko et al. 1988; Burgdorfer 1989). In the United States, endemic foci are clustered in the north-east from Massachusetts to Maryland, the midwest in Wisconsin and Minnesota, and the west along the northern California coast (Steere et al. 1979; Craven and Dennis 1993). Although Lyme disease was first described only 20 years ago, B. burgdorferi has been identified by polymerase chain reaction in preserved mouse tissues collected along the southern New England coast in 1894 (Marshall et al.1994).

A national surveillance case definition was adopted in the United States in 1990 (Table 1). With the use of this case definition, the number of cases reported in the United States has been relatively stable over the past 4 years, with approx. 9000 new cases reported nationally in 1993 (Craven and Dennis 1993). This case count is not an accurate reflection of the true incidence of Lyme disease, however, because most cases are not reported.

The highest incidence of Lyme disease is in children under the age of 15 years and middle-aged adults. Illness generally begins between May 1 and November 30, with the peak in June and July (Steere et al. 1983a). Limited studies have shown a significant prevalence of asymptomatic seropositivity in high-risk populations, the significance of which is unknown at present (Steere et al. 1986).

The primary vectors of Lyme disease are ixodid ticks. Endemic regions correspond to the distribution of I. scapularis (north-east and upper mid-west United States) (Steere et al. 1979), I. pacificus (California) (Steere et al. 1979), I. ricinus (Europe and Russia) (Dekonenko et al. 1988), and I. persulcatus (eastern Russia, China, and Japan) (Burgdorfer 1989). The vector in the north-east United States was previously thought to be a separate species, I. dammini, which has recently been shown to be conspecific with I. scapularis, its current designation (Oliver et al. 1993).

The epidemiology of Lyme disease is explained by the ecology of the tick vectors. The most thoroughly studied, I. scapularis, has a three-stage lifecycle (larva, nymph, and adult) spanning 2 years (Fig. 1). In the north-east United States, both the larval and nymphal stages feed on a variety of small mammals, especially the white-footed mouse (Peromyscus leukopus) (Wallis et al. 1978; Spielman et al. 1985; Mather et al. 1989). Infected nymphs transmit spirochaetes to mice, which in turn pass the infection on to larval ticks. Humans most often acquire infection from nymphs. Adult ticks feed primarily on larger mammals, especially deer. In endemic regions, 20 to 60 per cent of nymphal I. scapularis may be infected with B. burgdorferi (Burgdorfer et al. 1982; Steere et al. 1983d). In contrast the infection rate in I. pacificus in endemic areas of California has been found to be 2 per cent or less (Burgdorfer et al. 1985), where a complex, two-tick enzootic cycle maintains B. burgdorferi in nature (Brown and Lane

Table 1 Lyme disease: US national surveillance case definition

Definition	A systemic, tick-borne disease with protean manifestations: dermatological rheumatological, neurological, and cardiac abnormalities
	The initial skin lesion, erythema migrans, is the best clinical marker (occurs in 60–80% of patients)
Case definition	1. Erythema migrans present or
	2. At least one late manifestation and laboratory confirmation of infection.

General definitions

1. Erythema migrans (EM)
- Skin lesion typically beginning as a red macule/papule and expanding over days or weeks to form a large round lesion, often with partial central clearing
- A solitary lesion must measure at least 5 cm; secondary lesions may also occur
- An annular erythematous lesion developing within several hours of a tick bite represents a hypersensitivity reaction and does not qualify as EM
- The expanding EM lesion is usually accompanied by other acute symptoms, particularly fatigue, fever, headache, mildly stiff neck, arthralgias, and myalgias, which are typically intermittent
- Diagnosis of EM must be made by a physician
- Laboratory confirmation is recommended for patients with no known exposure

2. Late manifestations (these include any of the opposite when an alternative explanation is not found)

Musculoskeletal system:
- Recurrent, brief attacks (lasting weeks or months) of objective joint swelling in one or a few joints, sometimes followed by chronic arthritis in one or a few joints
- Manifestations not considered to be criteria for diagnosis include chronic progressive arthritis not preceded by brief attacks, chronic symmetric polyarthritis, or arthralgias, myalgias or fibromyalgia syndrome alone

Nervous system:
- Lymphocytic meningitis, cranial neuritis, particularly facial palsy (may be bilateral), radiculoneuropathy or, rarely, encephalomyelitis alone or in combination
- Encephalomyelitis must be confirmed by evidence of antibody production against *Borrelia burgdorferi* in cerebrospinal fluid (CSF), shown by a higher titre of antibody in the CSF than in serum
- Headache, fatigue, paraesthesiae, or mildly stiff neck alone are not accepted as criteria for neurological involvement

Cardiovascular system:
- Acute-onset, high-grade (2nd or 3rd degree) atrioventricular conduction defects that resolve in days to weeks and are sometimes associated with myocarditis
- Palpitations, bradycardia, bundle-branch block, or myocarditis alone are not accepted as criteria for cardiovascular involvement

3. Exposure
- Exposure to wooded, brushy or grassy areas (potential tick habitats) in an endemic county no more than 30 days before the onset of EM
- A history of tick bite is not required

4. Endemic county
- A county in which at least two definite cases have been previously acquired or in which a tick vector has been shown to be infected with *B. burgdorferi*

5. Laboratory confirmation
- Isolation of the spirochaete from tissue or body fluid or
- Detection of diagnostic levels of IgM or IgG antibodies to the spirochaete in the serum or the CSF, *or*
- Detection of an important change in antibody levels in paired acute and convalescent serum samples
- States may separately determine the criteria for laboratory confirmation and diagnostic levels of antibody
- Syphilis and other known biological causes of false-positive serological test results should be excluded, when laboratory confirmation is based on serological testing alone

1992). An enzootic cycle involving *Neotoma mexicana* (a wood rat) and *I. spinipalpis* has recently been described in northern Colorado (Maupin *et al.* 1994).

Birds may serve as hosts for larval and nymphal *Ixodes* ticks and provide a natural means of distributing ticks to new areas (Anderson *et al.* 1985; Anderson *et al.* 1986). Birds do not appear to be a reservoir for *B. burgdorferi*, however, and probably do not contribute significantly to the spread of infection.

Various public-health interventions have been designed to reduce the incidence of Lyme disease. Prompt removal of ticks prevents infection in the vast majority of exposed individuals (Shapiro *et al.* 1992). Eliminating deer can reduce the total tick population but is impractical. Distributing permethrine-impregnated (an acaricide) cotton balls in the nesting environment of mice has been shown to reduce the infestation of mice by ticks, which in turn can reduce the tick infection rate, but this too has obvious practical limitations

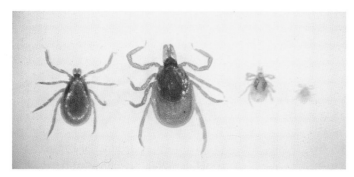

Fig. 1 Larva, nymph, adult female and adult male *Ixodes scapularis* ticks (photo M. Fergione).

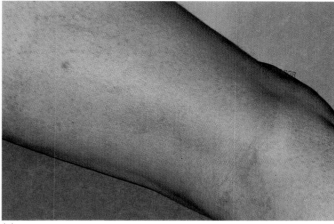

(a)

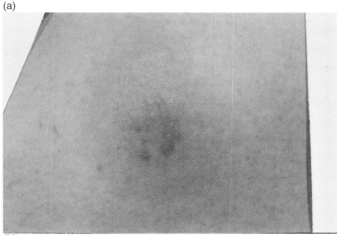

(b)

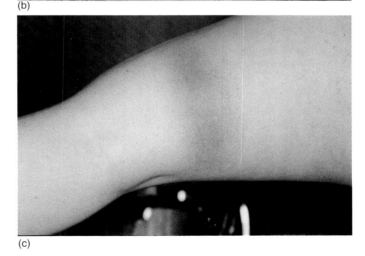

(c)

Fig. 2 (a)–(c) Erythema migrans, various forms.

(Ginsberg 1995). In some regions of the United States the perceived threat of Lyme disease is much greater than objective data can support. The public-health approach in these regions must be focused on education of the public and health professionals rather than disease control. Adequate control of Lyme disease will require close collaboration between ecologists, epidemiologists, public-health officials, physicians, and an informed public.

Clinical features

Most cases of Lyme disease begin with a characteristic skin lesion (erythema migrans) (stage 1). Within days to weeks, the illness disseminates, with the development of secondary skin lesions, headache, and generalized musculoskeletal symptoms. Weeks later, carditis and acute neurological abnormalities may occur (stage 2). Months later, arthritis and chronic neurological abnormalities appear (stage 3). Chronic skin involvement (acrodermatitis chronica atrophicans) also occurs late in disease, predominantly in Europe. As a guide to therapy, it is best to characterize patients as having early localized (erythema migrans), acute disseminated (neurological or non-neurological), or chronic disease. Clinical stages may overlap or be skipped entirely (Hanrahan *et al.* 1984).

Early Lyme disease

Erythema migrans begins as a red macule or papule at the site of a tick bite (Steere *et al.* 1977*c*; Steere *et al.* 1983*a*). After an incubation period of a few days to a month, the lesion expands gradually (0.5–1 cm/day) to a mean diameter of 15 cm (range 3–68 cm). Lesions are flat and non-scaling with a red outer border and partial central clearing (Fig. 2). The centre may be flat, indurated, vesicular or necrotic. The posterior thigh, groin, popliteal fossa, and axilla are particularly common sites. Lesions are warm and minimally tender, and may go unnoticed.

Half of patients in the United States develop multiple secondary lesions within days of onset of infection. Lymphocytoma cutis, a purplish nodule often on the nipple, has been reported as a manifestation of primary infection in Europe (Åsbrink and Olsson 1985). Erythema migrans and secondary lesions fade even without treatment in 3 to 4 weeks but may recur. Spirochaetes can be cultured from the skin of untreated patients even after lesions have resolved (Kuiper *et al.* 1994).

Malaise, fatigue, fever and chills, myalgia, arthralgia, headache, and paraesthesias often accompany erythema migrans (Steere *et al.* 1977*c*; Steere *et al.* 1983*a*). Recent studies have suggested that headache and paraesthesias may reflect early neurological dissemination (Reik *et al.* 1979; Garcia-Monco *et al.* 1990; Luft *et al.* 1992). Systemic signs and symptoms vary from day to day, and may appear before or after erythema migrans (or without it altogether). In untreated patients, symptoms may recur for months (especially fatigue and lethargy) after skin lesions have disappeared. European erythema migrans often has a prolonged, subacute course; secondary skin lesions, prominent systemic symptoms, laboratory abnormalities and subsequent arthritis are uncommon (Åsbrink and Olsson 1985).

Minor laboratory abnormalities associated with early Lyme disease are an increased erythrocyte sedimentation rate, total serum IgM, and serum glutamic oxaloacetic transaminase (Steere *et al.* 1977*b*; Steere *et al.* 1977*c*). Mild anaemia and leucocytosis also are common. Microscopic haematuria and low-grade proteinuria have been reported. Tests for rheumatoid factor or antinuclear antibodies are usually negative.

Disseminated and chronic Lyme disease
Neurological manifestations

Neurological abnormalities develop within several weeks of disease onset in a minority of patients (15 per cent in one series (Reik *et al.* 1979)). Cranial neuropathy (most commonly involving the facial nerve) (Clark *et al.* 1985), meningitis, and radiculoneuropathy alone or in combination (Reik *et al.* 1979; Pachner and Steere 1985; Halperin *et al.* 1987; Halperin *et al.* 1989; Pachner *et al.* 1989). Later in the disease, chorea, demyelinating encephalopathy or myelopathy, chronic encephalopathy, peripheral polyneuropathy, and transverse myelitis may occur (Reik *et al.* 1979; Ackerman *et al.* 1988; Halperin *et al.* 1987; Halperin *et al.* 1989; Logigian *et al.* 1990). Acute and chronic neurological Lyme disease differ in their natural history and response to therapy.

Radiculoneuropathy may affect any dermatome or even several contiguous dermatomes. Symptoms include paraesthesia, pain, sensory deficit and, often, motor weakness. Radiculoneuropathy is often accompanied by meningitis, a complex dubbed Bannwarth's syndrome.

The primary symptom of Lyme meningitis is headache, which may vary in intensity from hour to hour or day to day, and is often accompanied by a mild encephalopathy. Neck stiffness is common but meningismus is not. Spinal fluid contains a lymphocytic pleocytosis and mildly elevated protein, but glucose is normal. Studies with the polymerase chain reaction and rare positive cultures have shown that Lyme meningitis results from direct infection in the cerebrospinal fluid (Keller *et al.* 1992). Both radiculoneuropathy and meningitis eventually remit even without treatment but often only after waxing and waning for months (Reik *et al.* 1979).

Facial palsy, which may be bilateral, is the most common acute neurological manifestation of disseminated, early Lyme disease. Facial paralysis may occur when erythema migrans is present or within a few weeks after its resolution. Even in highly endemic areas, however, facial nerve palsy is usually idiopathic. The course of facial weakness is benign and not distinguishable from that of Bell's palsy; over 95 per cent of individuals experience complete or near complete resolution even without therapy. Fifty per cent of individuals with facial nerve palsy have an associated meningitis, so examination of the cerebrospinal fluid is indicated.

Chronic neurological manifestations emerge months to years after the onset of Lyme disease. Although symptoms vary, memory impairment, and peripheral, sensory polyneuropathy predominate (Reik *et al.* 1985; Halperin *et al.* 1987; Halperin *et al.* 1989; Logigian *et al.* 1990). The cerebrospinal fluid of individuals with chronic encephalopathy usually has a mildly elevated protein but no cells.

Carditis

Carditis develops in less than 5 per cent of cases, generally within several weeks of disease onset (Steere *et al.* 1978). Patients with carditis typically present with palpitations, light-headedness, or syncope due to varying degrees of atrioventricular block. Dilated cardiomyopathy, perhaps reflecting more diffuse myocardial involvement, has also been tentatively linked to Lyme disease (Steere *et al.* 1980; Stanek *et al.* 1990). Carditis remits spontaneously in days to a few weeks and, once resolved, does not recur. Although clinical manifestations are usually limited to the conduction system, subclinical myocardial involvement may be more extensive (McAlister *et al.* 1989). One fatal case involving concurrent *Babesia* infection has been reported (Marcus *et al.* 1985). Carditis should be suspected in individuals in endemic areas who develop heart block without other explanation.

Arthritis

Approximately 60 per cent of untreated individuals develop arthritis from weeks to years after the onset of illness (Steere *et al.* 1977; Steere *et al.* 1979). Frank arthritis may be preceded by months or even years of intermittent migratory myalgias, arthralgias, and periarticular pain. The typical attack begins suddenly with the rapid development of massive swelling of a single large joint, most often the knee. Individual attacks of arthritis usually last a few weeks to a few months and remit spontaneously. Recurrences are common but attacks decrease in frequency by 10 to 20 per cent per year and eventually cease in most patients, even without antibiotic therapy (Steere *et al.* 1987).

Joint-fluid cell counts average about 25 000 cells/mm^3, with a predominance of polymorphonuclear leucocytes (Steere *et al.* 1977*b*). Protein is usually elevated; glucose usually normal. Attempts to culture *B. burgdorferi* from joint fluid have been almost invariably unsuccessful (Snydman *et al.* 1986) but the polymerase chain reaction has revealed *B. burgdorferi* DNA in most untreated patients (Bradley *et al.* 1994; Nocton *et al.* 1994). Arthritis in Lyme disease is almost certainly initiated by direct spirochaetal infection of the joint.

Arthritis becomes chronic in approximately 10 per cent of patients, especially individuals who are HLA-DR4 positive in whom pannus may form and erosions develop despite antibiotic therapy that is curative in other patients (Steere *et al.* 1979; Steere *et al.* 1987; Steere *et al.* 1990). The development of a serological immune response against outer surface proteins A and B has been linked to the development of chronic arthritis (Kalish *et al.* 1993). The synovium in chronic Lyme arthritis looks like that of rheumatoid arthritis (Steere *et al.* 1977*b*; Steere *et al.* 1979). In addition, there may be an obliterative endarteritis and spirochaetes have been seen using a variety of staining techniques. Thus, chronic Lyme arthritis is similar to rheumatoid arthritis, for which it may serve as a model.

Acrodermatitis chronica atrophicans

Acrodermatitis chronica atrophicans (Weber *et al.* 1984; Åsbrink *et al.* 1985) occurs relatively commonly in Europe but is rare in the United States (Kaufman *et al.* 1989). Lesions occur most often on distal extremities and begin as violaceous, infiltrated plaques or nodules that evolve into an atrophic stage. Acrodermatitis chronica atrophicans results from chronic persistence of infection in skin and has been associated with *B. afzelii* (Canica *et al.* 1993; van Dam *et al.*1993; Wienecke *et al.* 1994).

Diagnostic testing

Culture of *B. burgdorferi* from patients is necessary for definitive diagnosis, but has a significant yield only from affected (erythema migrans) skin (Steere *et al.* 1983; Åsbrink and Hovmark 1985; Berger *et al.* 1985). Spirochaetes are rarely visualized by tissue stains (Steere *et al.* 1983; Berger 1984; Johnston *et al.* 1985). Attempts should be made to isolate the organism by culture when erythema migrans is suspected in a patient from a region not previously known to be endemic; in endemic regions, this is not necessary for diagnosis.

Detection of specific anti-*B. burgdorferi* antibody is the most helpful diagnostic test for confirmation of the diagnosis of Lyme disease. Specific IgM antibody appears first after the onset of the disease and reaches a peak within 3 to 6 weeks. IgG antibody develops more slowly, often reaching a peak months later (Steere *et al.* 1983; Craft *et al.* 1984).

In the past, the performance of many commercially available immunofluorescence tests or enzyme-linked immunosorbent assays for *B. burgdorferi* antibodies has been poor, with unacceptably low sensitivity and/or specificity and lack of reproducibility (Schwartz *et al.* 1989; Luger and Krauss 1990; Magnarelli *et al.* 1990). The major problem at present, however, is not performance, which is comparable to that of many other serological tests, but rather that indiscriminate use of serological testing has set the stage for results with very low positive predictive value (Britton *et al.* 1993; Lightfoot *et al.* 1993). As an example, when the likelihood of Lyme disease is estimated to be 5 per cent before testing, a serological test with sensitivity and specificity of 95 per cent will have a positive predictive value of only 50 per cent. Patient selection has a profound effect on the predictive value of serological testing.

Serological tests may be falsely positive or negative for a variety of reasons. *Borrelia burgdorferi* contains epitopes that are cross-reactive with other spirochaetes, including *Treponema pallidum* and oral treponemes. Some patients with rheumatoid arthritis or systemic lupus erythematosus have low-titre, false-positive serological findings. Seronegative Lyme disease also occurs, but rarely, primarily following incomplete antibiotic therapy for early disease.

Western blotting is available as a confirming test (Dressler *et al.* 1993). This technique can distinguish between true seroreactivity against *B. burgdorferi* and false positivity. Both the technique for Western blotting and criteria for positivity must also be standardized, however. A workshop sponsored by the Centers for Disease Control in 1994 produced recommendations that Western blotting be used to confirm all positive enzyme immunoassay results (Table 2). The most cost-effective approach at present may be to reserve Western blotting for equivocal circumstances.

Tests have been developed to measure cell-mediated immunity against *B. burgdorferi* but these have not added clinically useful information because of technical difficulties and the rarity with which the cell-mediated immune response differs from the serological response (Dattwyler *et al.* 1989; Zoschke *et al.* 1991).

Lyme disease of the central nervous system is associated with the production of specific antibody in cerebrospinal fluid. This locally driven immune response leads to a measurable increase in the concentration of specific antibody in the cerebrospinal fluid compared with that in serum. Measurement of antibody in cerebrospinal fluid is a useful adjunct in the diagnosis of neurological involvement in Lyme disease (Halperin *et al.* 1986; Halperin *et al.* 1989; Logigian *et al.* 1990). Positive tests for antibody in cerebrospinal fluid confirm *B. burgdorferi* infection of the central nervous system but negative tests do not rule it out, particularly late in the disease.

The polymerase chain reaction is being applied to the study of Lyme disease as a potential means of elucidating sites of active infection (Nocton *et al.* 1994; Keller *et al.* 1992). It has been validated as a sensitive and specific means of identifying *B. burgdorferi* in ticks (Persing *et al.* 1990). Study of both joint and cerebrospinal fluid of individuals has shown that the polymerase chain reaction has the potential to determine who harbours *B. burgdorferi* DNA. It is not clear whether the presence of DNA from the organism can be considered a surrogate for a positive culture, particularly since polymerase chain reaction-positive fluids are routinely culture-negative. A potential explanation for this observation can be based on the observation that the likelihood of a positive polymerase chain reaction seems to be higher if plasmid rather than genomic DNA targets are used (Persing

---

Table 2 Centers for Disease Control and Prevention Workgroup recommendations on laboratory testing for Lyme disease (draft)

Test performance and interpretation

Recommendation 1.1: Two-test protocol

All serum specimens submitted for Lyme disease testing should be evaluated in a two-step process, in which the first step employs a sensitive screening test, such as an enzyme immunoassay (EIA) or immunofluorescent assay (IFA). All specimens found to be positive or equivocal by a sensitive EIA or IFA should be tested by a standardized Western blot (WB) procedure. Specimens found to be negative by a sensitive EIA or IFA need not be tested further.

Recommendation 1.3: Testing and state of disease

Both IgM and IgG immunoblot procedures should be used for serodiagnosis of suspected cases within the first 4 weeks of disease onset (early Lyme disease). After 4 weeks of disease onset (late Lyme disease), only IgG immunoblot procedures should be used, since IgM band patterns are not reliable for serodiagnosis of late Lyme disease. In the event that a patient with suspected early Lyme disease has a negative serology, testing of a convalescent sample is recommended 2–4 weeks later.

Recommendation 1.5: Reporting of results

An equivocal or positive EIA or IFA result followed by a negative immunoblot result should be reported as negative. An equivocal or positive EIA or IFA result followed by a positive immunoblot result should be reported as positive.

An explanation and interpretation of test results should accompany all reports.

In addition to recommendations presented here, specific recommendations were developed for: WB controls and standardization, criteria for WB positivity, quality assurance practices, test evaluation and clearance, and communication of new developments in testing.

et al. 1994). In culture, spirochaetes shed membrane blebs containing only plasmid DNA into the culture medium (Dorward and Garon 1990). It is plausible that *B. burgdorferi* may shed plasmid-rich DNA blebs into joint or cerebrospinal fluids in the virtual absence of intact organisms, which, in turn, could explain the disparate results for culture and the polymerase chain reaction.

The diagnosis of Lyme disease must be approached clinically. In a setting of risk by epidemiological criteria, an individual with clinical manifestations suggesting Lyme disease should undergo confirming serological testing. If negative, the diagnosis is unlikely. If positive, Lyme disease is likely. Serological status can be confirmed by Western blotting but the diagnosis must still be based on clinical criteria, even in individuals with definite seropositivity (Fig. 3).

Differential diagnosis

Although erythema migrans is the most definitive clinical marker of Lyme disease, a cautionary note is warranted because an expanding erythema cannot be considered diagnostic of early Lyme disease in the absence of the right epidemiological setting. When present in its classical form following exposure in an endemic area, it is virtually diagnostic of Lyme disease, but skin lesions from other causes may mimic erythema migrans. Tick bites alone, without infection, may cause small annular areas of erythema. Efforts should be made to culture *B. burgdorferi* from skin lesions in questionable circumstances, particularly in regions not known to be endemic for Lyme disease.

Secondary lesions superficially resemble erythema multiforme. Several features help to distinguish between these entities: blistering, mucosal lesions, and involvement of the palms and soles are not typical of erythema migrans. Lyme disease has occasionally been associated with an urticarial rash, which must be distinguished from other causes of urticaria. Prominent musculoskeletal symptoms (arthralgias, myalgias and fever) may suggest a viral illness, especially when erythema migrans is absent or missed. Upper respiratory symptoms, which are very common with viral disease, are rare in early disseminated Lyme disease.

The headache, stiff neck, and pleocytosis of cerebrospinal fluid associated with Lyme meningitis are similar to the symptoms and signs associated with viral meningitis. Lyme meningitis has a more protracted course, however, often fluctuating in severity for weeks to months, which helps to distinguish it from viral meningitis. Isolated facial nerve palsy mimics idiopathic Bell's palsy; Lyme disease is one of the very few causes of bilateral facial palsy which is rare with idiopathic Bell's palsy. Generalized lymphadenopathy is occasionally seen in disseminated early Lyme disease. The fever and multiple skin lesions usually present at this stage of illness enable one to determine that the adenopathy is due to Lyme disease. Chronic fatigue may be a major and persistent complaint in Lyme disease but the non-specificity of fatigue is so low that it is not helpful diagnostically..

Disseminated and chronic Lyme disease shares clinical features with many other immune-mediated disorders. The pattern of joint inflammation is similar to that seen with reactive arthritis. The relatively brief duration of individual attacks of joint swelling in Lyme disease and absence of mucosal lesions are useful distinguishing features. In children, the attacks of arthritis, although generally shorter, are similar to those associated with the oligoarticular form of juvenile rheumatoid arthritis, but without iridocyclitis.

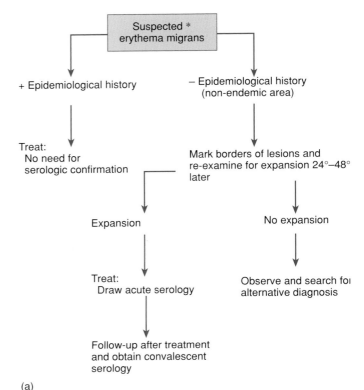

(a)

*If multiple skin lesions are present, institute treatment at time of initial visit regardless of epidemiological history.

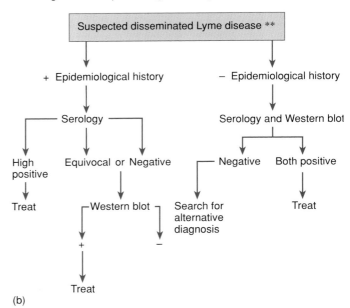

(b)

** Heart block, facial palsy, lymphocytic meningitis, radiculoneuropathy arthritis

Fig. 3 Algorithms for diagnosis of Lyme disease.

Late neurological involvement may mimic multiple sclerosis, Guillain–Barré syndrome, a dementing process, brain tumour, or an affective disorder. A history of previous features of Lyme disease helps, as does a complete neurological evaluation. A unique characteristic of neurological Lyme disease is that it may affect multiple levels of the nervous system: peripheral and cranial nerves, meninges, nerve roots, spinal cord and brain itself. Involvement of many different levels of the nervous system either simultaneously or sequentially is rarely seen in other diseases (Pachner and Steere 1985). In the evaluation of chronic fatigue, it is important to note that chronic fatigue alone is not a manifestation of active Lyme disease.

Diagnostic confusion has resulted from poor understanding of the how to distinguish fibromyalgia from Lyme disease. Fibromyalgia may occur as a sequela to Lyme disease, but there is no evidence that it results from persistent infection (Sigal 1990; Hsu et al. 1993; Steere et al. 1993). Lyme disease appears to be one of many triggers of this common syndrome. Fibromyalgia constitutes up to 25 per cent of presentations in some rheumatology practice and affects up to 3 per cent of the normal population. Misdiagnosis of fibromyalgia as Lyme disease has led to extensive overdiagnosis of Lyme disease (Britton et al. 1993; Hsu et al. 1993; Lightfoot et al. 1993; Steere et al. 1993). The generalized pain, trigger points, debilitating fatigue, and sleep disturbance that characterize fibromyalgia are distinctly different from the joint and nervous system manifestations of Lyme disease. The treatment of fibromyalgia is not affected by a history of preceding Lyme disease.

Treatment

Antibiotic therapy of Lyme disease has advanced considerably over the past decade. Therapy must be tailored to the extent and duration of disease. The leading reason for antibiotic failure is incorrect diagnosis. Early disease responds readily to a variety of agents but the response of certain late manifestations, particularly neurological, is often incomplete. The appropriate endpoint of treatment for late disease may be difficult to determine because resolution may be slow and lag behind the completion of antibiotic therapy. Although the optimal duration of antibiotic therapy for the various stages of Lyme disease is still being determined, no clinical trials have evaluated treatment courses longer than 4 weeks for any stage of Lyme disease. Longer courses should only be administered in the context of a controlled clinical trial. Current recommendations are presented in Table 3.

Early Lyme disease

Early Lyme disease responds promptly to oral antibiotic therapy. Erythema migrans resolves in days and disease progression is halted (Steere et al. 1983b; Dattwyler et al. 1990; Luft et al. 1996). Secondary skin lesions, myalgias, arthralgias, fever, headache, stiff neck, and dysaesthesias indicate more severe infection and have a greater likelihood of incomplete response (Steere et al. 1983b; Dattwyler et al. 1990). Early treatment is important to prevent dissemination and maximize the likelihood of complete response. Because of the potential for early neurological spread, patients should be carefully evaluated for subtle involvement of the central nervous system. If headache or dys-/paraesthesias are present, formal evaluation with lumbar puncture and electrodiagnostic studies is indicated; if abnormal, intravenous antibiotic therapy should be chosen (Garcia-Monco et al. 1990; Pfister et al. 1990; Luft et al. 1992). If treated early, before any systemic immune challenge, patients may be susceptible to reinfection (Shrestha et al. 1985; Aguero-Rosenfeld et al. 1993).

Oral doxycycline, 100 mg twice daily, or amoxicillin, 500 mg three times a day (Dattwyler et al. 1990) (paediatric dose: 30 mg/kg a day), each for 21 days, are the regimens of first choice for early disease. For penicillin-allergic individuals who should not take a tetracycline

Table 3 Treatment recommendations

Early Lyme disease

Amoxicillin, 500 mg 3 times daily for 21 days

Doxycycline, 100 mg twice daily for 21 days

Cefuroxime axetil, 500 mg twice daily for 21 days

Azithromycin, 500 mg daily for 7 days (may be less effective than other regimens)

Neurological manifestations

Bell's palsy (no other neurological abnormalities)

    Oral regimens for early disease suffice

Meningitis (with or without radiculoneuropathy or encephalitis)

    Ceftriaxone, 2 g daily for 14–28 days

    Cefotaxime, 2 g 3 times daily for 14–28 days

    Penicillin G, 20 million units daily for 14–28 days

    Doxycycline, 100 mg twice daily (oral or intravenous) for 14–28 days[e]

    Chloramphenicol, 1 g 4 times daily for 14–28 days

Late neurological disease (peripheral neuropathy or encephalopathy)

    Ceftriaxone, 2 g daily for 28 days

    Cefotaxime, 2 g 3 times daily for 14–28 days

Arthritis[f]

Amoxicillin and probenecid, 500 mg 4 times daily for 30 days

Doxycycline, 100 mg twice daily for 30 days

Ceftriaxone, 2 g daily for 14–28 days

Cefotaxime, 2 g 3 times daily for 14–28 days

Penicillin G, 20 million units daily for 14–28 days

Carditis

Ceftriaxone, 2 g daily for 14 days

Cefotaxime, 2 g 3 times daily for 14 days

Penicillin G, 20 million units daily for 14 days

Doxycycline, 100 mg orally twice daily for 21 days

Amoxicillin, 500 mg 3 times daily for 21 days

Pregnancy

Localized early diseases

    Amoxicillin, 500 mg 3 times daily for 21 days

Disseminated disease

    Penicillin G, 20 million units daily for 14–28 days

Asymptomatic seropositivity

    No treatment necessary

(pregnant or lactating women and children less than 9 years in age), cefuroxime axetil (500 mg twice daily) or erythromycin (250 mg four times a day) may be substituted (Nadelman et al. 1992). For individuals with a history of immediate hypersensitivity reactions to penicillin, cephalosporins should also be avoided. Outcomes with erythromycin or the newer macrolides, azithromycin and clarithromycin, have been less satisfactory than with the other choices (Steere et al. 1983b; Luft et al. 1996).

Maternal–fetal transmission of B. burgdorferi has been associated with stillbirth and neonatal death (Schlesinger et al. 1985; Weber et al. 1988). The direct role of B. burgdorferi in causing these adverse outcomes is unclear. Epidemiological surveys have demonstrated no congenital Lyme disease syndrome, however (Markowitz et al. 1986), and there is no evidence of fetal risk ascribable to maternal seropositivity alone (Strobino et al. 1993). There are no case reports of maternal fetal transmission associated with current recommended treatment. The available data favour aggressive treatment of Lyme disease in pregnancy.

About 10 per cent of patients experience a Jarisch–Herxheimer-like reaction shortly after the institution of therapy (Steere et al. 1983b). Regardless of which drug is selected and the duration of therapy, many patients have persistent symptoms particularly fatigue, for many weeks after its completion (Steere et al. 1983b; Dattwyler et al. 1990). These symptoms do not reflect continuing infection and do not respond to repeated courses of antibiotics, but eventually resolve in most patients. Persistent neurological complaints, however, should raise suspicion of inadequately treated nervous system infection which may progress over time even in seronegative individuals. The importance of careful neurological evaluation of all patients cannot be over-emphasized.

Disseminated and chronic Lyme disease
Neurological disease
Optimal treatment of neurological involvement is still under investigation. Consensus has been slow to emerge because of the differences in the neurological features of European and North American Lyme disease and the slow, often incomplete, resolution of symptoms.

Acute neurological manifestations include meningitis, cranial neuropathy, and radiculoneuritis, and must be distinguished from the chronic manifestations described below. These respond to intravenous penicillin G, 20 million units a day for 10 days (Steere et al. 1983c); longer courses (14–21days) are recommended at present (Rahn and Malawista 1994). Ceftriaxone (Dattwyler et al. 1988) and cefotaxime (Pfister et al. 1989) have both been found effective when given intravenously for 14 days, and are superior to penicillin (Dattwyler et al. 1988). Headache usually begins to subside by the second day of therapy and disappears by 7 to 10 days. Radicular pain also resolves promptly but sensory and motor deficits frequently require 7 to 8 weeks for recovery (Steere et al. 1983c). Most experts currently recommend 4 weeks of therapy for all manifestations of central nervous Lyme disease.

Radiculopathy has been treated successfully in Europe with doxycycline, 100 mg twice daily for 14 days (Dotevall et al. 1988). This regimen has not been studied systematically in the United States. The recently recognized genetic differences between B. burgdorferi isolates (Baranton et al. 1992; Canica et al. 1993) suggest that future treatment should involve attempts to isolate and speciate the offending organism.

Chronic neurological manifestations, including encephalopathy and peripheral neuropathy, usually respond to antibiotic therapy, but response may be delayed or incomplete (Halperin et al. 1987; Halperin et al. 1989; Logigian et al. 1990). Some patients have persistent, nonprogressive deficits after antibiotic therapy. Two to four weeks of treatment are generally recommended, with most authorities recommending 4 weeks.

Many individuals with ill-defined neurological complaints have been diagnosed to have neurological Lyme disease, without a history of exposure, serological confirmation, or even a clearly defined neurological lesion. The costs and risks attributable to misdiagnosis and inappropriate intravenous antibiotic therapy are considerable (Centers for Disease Control 1993; Lightfoot et al. 1993). It is best to withhold therapy until symptoms have been defined as precisely as possible. This may require neuropsychological testing for individuals with cognitive complaints, lumbar puncture for headache, and electrodiagnostic testing to evaluate sensorimotor complaints. Therapeutic trials should not be undertaken for treatment of vague symptoms without an objectively defined endpoint. The American College of Rheumatology has published a guideline recommending against intravenous therapy for seropositive individuals with non-specific symptoms within the spectrum of fibromyalgia (Britton et al. 1993).

Carditis

Carditis responds readily to intravenous antibiotic therapy with one of the above agents (Brown and Lane 1992) but it has also been treated successfully with oral antibiotics, salicylates or glucocorticoids (Steere et al. 1980). Carditis results from myocardial invasion by spirochaetes (de Koning et al. 1989), and should be treated with antibiotics. Prednisone, 40 to 60 mg a day in divided doses, rapidly reverses heart block (Steere et al. 1980) but may interfere with attempts to cure infection. For this reason, glucocorticoids should be given in short courses (fewer than 7 days) or avoided entirely. For patients with allergy to penicillin and cephalosporins, doxycycline (100 mg twice a day for 30 days) is a reasonable alternative choice. Cardiac pacing may be required temporarily (Steere et al. 1980; Clark et al. 1985).

Arthritis

Lyme arthritis responds to oral doxycycline (100 mg twice daily for 4 weeks) or amoxicillin/probenecid (500 mg each, four times daily). Either regimen cures most patients (Steere et al. 1994). Intravenous ceftriaxone is probably as effective when given for at least 2 weeks and offers the advantage of simultaneously treating neurological involvement but this must be balanced against the disadvantages of increased cost and increased risk of toxicity (antibiotic-associated colitis, line sepsis, acute cholecystitis, etc.) (Dattwyler et al. 1988; Steere et al. 1994). Parenteral penicillin is less effective for some patients than oral doxycycline or amoxicillin (Steere et al. 1985).

Treatment failures occur with all regimens, particularly in HLA-DR4 positive individuals (Steere et al. 1990). Longer courses of oral amoxicillin or tetracycline, or longer intravenous therapy with ceftriaxone or penicillin should be considered for those individuals who have not responded to an initial 4-week course, but this requires further study. In one study, there were no polymerase chain reaction-positive joint fluids after either 2 weeks of intravenous ceftriaxone or 8 weeks' oral therapy (Nocton et al. 1994). Antibiotic treatment failures may be treated successfully with synovectomy (Schoen *et al.* 1991). Recurrence after synovectomy has been rare.

Fibromyalgia

Fibromyalgia is the most common primary diagnosis for individuals coming to Lyme disease referral centres for treatment-resistant Lyme disease. In endemic areas in particular, fibromyalgia is often inappropriately treated with repeated, prolonged courses of antibiotics. Regardless of *B. burgdorferi* serological status, fibromyalgia should be treated in conventional ways.

Acrodermatitis chronica atrophicans

The infiltrative lesions of acrodermatitis chronica atrophicans are usually cured by 3 weeks of oral phenoxymethyl penicillin, 2 to 3 g daily in divided doses (Åsbrink *et al.* 1985).

Tick bite management

Ticks should be removed and the site observed for the appearance of erythema migrans. In one randomized, controlled trial in an endemic region in Connecticut, the risk of acquiring Lyme disease following a tick bite approximated the risk of adverse reaction to antibiotics administered prophylactically (Shapiro *et al.* 1992). In this trial, there were no instances of silent seroconversion and no individual developed disseminated disease, so the only risk associated with watchful waiting was a 1 per cent risk of developing erythema migrans. This low risk was much less than the tick infection rate, which was approx. 20 per cent. A cost-effectiveness analysis, based on the assumption that one-third of infected individuals would present with later disease and require intravenous therapy, concluded that prophylactic therapy was only indicated if the risk of acquiring Lyme

---

Box 1 Management of Lyme disease

1. Early Lyme disease with clinical evidence limited to mild to moderate systemic symptoms, and one or multiple lesions of erythema migrans.

Always

    (a) confirm diagnosis by observation of definite erythema migrans lesion(s) in individuals with a positive epidemiological history;
    (b) search for evidence of neurological dissemination with a careful history and neurological examination;
    (c) administer a 21-day course of oral antibiotic selected from the list in Table 3;
    (d) follow up the patient at the end of the antibiotic course to ensure complete resolution of signs and symptoms of Lyme disease;
    (e) counsel the patient about the possibility of relapse, especially neurological.

Often

    (a) confirm the diagnosis serogically with enzyme immunoassay and Western blot, especially if the epidemiological history is questionable or skin lesions are atypical or absent;
    (b) assess at the end of therapy for any persistent symptoms: delayed resolution may occur, especially of systemic symptoms such as fatigue and fibromyalgia-type complaints.

Sometimes

    (a) perform a lumbar puncture if headache, paraesthesiae or facial nerve palsy are present at the time of diagnosis—abnormal spinal fluid should be considered evidence of neurological spread of infection and indicates the need for intravenous antibiotics;
    (b) perform an electrocardiogram if the patient has had complaints possibly indicative of heart block;
    (c) perform post-treatment serological tests if the initial diagnosis was questionable and initial serology was not positive.

2. Disseminated Lyme disease with clinical evidence of dissemination to joints, nervous system heart or other major organs.

Always

    (a) confirm the diagnosis serologically (enzyme immunoassay and Western blot) and rule out alternative diagnoses to explain the clinical presentation;
    (b) characterize the extent of disease before instituting antibiotics—perform a lumbar puncture if neurological signs or symptoms are present and aspirate joint fluid if joint swelling is present;
    (c) administer antibiotic therapy as outlined in Table 3;
    (d) follow up the patient serially until all symptoms are resolved.

Often

    (a) observe the patient for continued resolution of signs and symptoms after completion of a course of antibiotic therapy if all signs of inflammation are not resolved;
    (b) repeat initial studies to monitor for improvement and or progression after therapy (electromyography, nerve conduction studies, joint-fluid analysis, lumbar puncture).

Sometimes

    (a) analyse spinal or joint fluid by polymerase chain reaction if the diagnosis is unclear by clinical and routine serological criteria;
    (b) extend or repeat the course of antibiotic therapy if there is clinical evidence suggesting recurrence of inflammation after an initial response.

disease following a tick bite exceeded 3 per cent (Magid *et al.* 1992). The current evidence favours an expectant, watchful, waiting approach, and not the prophylactic administration of antibiotics.

Vaccine development

Work in progress holds promise for the development of a Lyme vaccine. Vaccination with recombinant polypeptides from outer surface proteins (particularly OspA) have been shown to protect mice from infection and to provide at least limited cross-strain protection (Fikrig *et al.* 1992). Large-scale trials in humans are currently under way. The ability to induce immunity in humans, the range of cross-strain protection provided, and the durability of immunity must be determined (Lovrich *et al.* 1994). The trials currently in progress should define the potential for disease prevention through vaccination.

Summary of practical guidelines for management of Lyme disease

A pragmatic approach to the treatment of Lyme disease requires confirmation of the diagnosis, an assessment of the extent of disease (clinical staging), administration of antibiotic therapy appropriate to the extent of disease, and careful post-treatment follow-up. The choice of specific antibiotic, route of administration, and duration of therapy all are contingent upon an assessment of extent of disease. Generally, early disease (limited to primary and secondary skin sites) is treated with shorter-course antibiotic therapy administered orally, and more extensive disease requires longer oral and intravenous therapy.

My approach to management is summarized in Box 1.

References

Ackerman, R., Rehse-Kupper, B., Gollmer, E., and Schmidt, R.(1988). Chronic neurologic manifestations of erythema migrans borreliosis. *Annals of the New York Academy of Science*, **539**, 16–23.

Afzelius, A. (1910). Verhandlungen der Dermatologischen Gesellschaft zu Stockholm on October 29, 1909. *Archives of Dermatology and Syphilis*, **101**, 404.

Aguero-Rosenfeld, M. E., Nowakowski, J., McKenna, D.F., Carbonato, C.A., and Wormser, G.P. (1993). Serodiagnosis in early Lyme disease. *Journal of Clinical Microbiology*, **31**, 3090–5.

Anderson, J. F., Johnson, R.C., Magnarelli, L.A., and Hyde, F.W. (1985). Identification of endemic foci of Lyme disease: isolation of *Borrelia burgdorferi* from feral rodents and ticks (*Dermacentor variabilis*).

Anderson, J. F., Johnson, R.C., Magnarelli, L.A., and Hyde, F.W. (1986). Involvement of birds in the epidemiology of the Lyme disease agent *Borrelia burgdorferi*. *Infection and Immunity*, **51**, 394–6.

Åsbrink, E. and Hovmark, A. (1985). Successful cultivation of spirochetes from skin lesions of patients with erythema chronicum migrans Afzelius and acrodermatitis chronica atrophicans. *Acta Pathologica Microbiologica et Immunologica Scandinavica* (Sect. B), **93**, 161–3.

Åsbrink, E. and Olsson, I. (1985). Clinical manifestations of erythema chronicum migrans Afzelius in 161 patients. A comparison with Lyme disease. *Acta Dermatologica et Venereologica* (Stockholm), **65**, 43–52.

Åsbrink, E., Hovmark, A., and Hederstedt, B. (1985). Serological studies of erythema chronicum migrans Afzelius and acrodermatitis chronica atrophicans with indirect immunofluorescence and enzyme-linked immunosorbent assays. *Acta Dermatologica et Venereologica* (Stockholm), **65**, 509–14.

Bannwarth, A. (1944). Zur Klinik und Pathogenese der chronischen lymphozytaren Meningitis. *Archiv für Psychiatrie und Nervenkrankheiten*, **117**, 161–85.

Baranton, G., Postic, D., Saint Girons, I., *et al.* (1992). Delineation of *Borrelia burgdorferi* sensu stricto, *Borrelia garinii* sp. nov., and group VS461 associated with Lyme borreliosis. *International Journal of Systematic Bacteriology*, **42**, 378–83.

Barbour, A. G. , Heiland, R.A., and Howe, T.R. (1985). Heterogeneity of major proteins in Lyme disease *Borrelia*: a molecular analysis of North American and European isolates. *Journal of Infectious Diseases*, **152**, 478–84.

Barbour, A. G. (1988). Plasmid analysis of *Borrelia burgdorferi*, the Lyme disease agent. *Journal of Clinical Microbiology*, **26**, 475–8.

Benach, J. L., Bosler, E.M., Hanrahan, J.P., *et al.* (1983). Spirochetes isolated from the blood of two patients with Lyme disease. *New England Journal of Medicine*, **308**, 740–2.

Berger, B. W. (1984). Erythema chronicum migrans of Lyme disease. *Archives of Dermatology*, **120**, 1017–21.

Berger, B.W., Kaplan, M.H., Rothenberg, I.R., and Barbour, A.G. (1985). Isolation and characterization of the Lyme disease spirochete from the skin of patients with erythema chronicum migrans. *Journal of the American Academy of Dermatology*, **3**, 444–9.

Bradley, J. F., Johnson, R.C., and Goodman, J.L. (1994). The persistence of spirochetal nucleic acids in active Lyme arthritis. *Annals of Internal Medicine*, **120**, 487–9.

Britton, M. C., Gardner, P., Kaufman, R.L., *et al.* (1993). Appropriateness of parenteral antibiotic treatment for patients with presumed Lyme disease. A joint statement of the American College of Rheumatology and the Council of the Infectious Diseases Society of America. *Annals of Internal Medicine*, **119**, 518.

Brown, R. N. and Lane, R. S. (1992). Lyme disease in California: a novel enzootic transmission cycle of *Borrelia burgdorferi*. *Science*, **256**, 1439–42.

Burgdorfer, W. (1989). Vector/host relationships of the Lyme disease spirochete, *Borrelia burgdorferi*. *Rheumatic Disease Clinics of North America*, **15**, 775–87.

Burgdorfer, W., Barbour, A.G., Hayes, S.F., *et al.* (1982). Lyme disease—a tick-borne spirochetosis? *Science*, **216**, 1317–19.

Burgdorfer, W., Lane, R.S., Barbour, A.G., Gresbrink, R.A., and Anderson, J.R. (1985). The western black-legged tick, *Ixodes pacificus*: a vector of *Borrelia burgdorferi*. *American Journal of Tropical Medicine and Hygiene*, **34**, 925–30.

Canica, M. M., Nato, F., du Merle, L., *et al.* (1993). Monoclonal antibodies for identification of *Borrelia afzelii* sp. nov. associated with late cutaneous manifestations of Lyme borreliosis. *Scandinavian Journal of Infectious Diseases*, **25**, 441–8.

Centers for Disease Control (1993). Ceftriaxone-associated biliary complications of treatment of suspected disseminated Lyme disease—New Jersey, 1990–1992. *Journal of the American Medical Association*, **269**, 979–80.

Clark, J. R., Carlson, R.D., Casaki, C.T., Pachner, A.R., and Steere, A.C. (1985). Facial paralysis in Lyme disease. *Laryngoscope*, **95**, 1341–5.

Comstock, L. E. and Thomas, D. D. (1989). Penetration of endothelial cell monolayers by *Borrelia burgdorferi*. *Infection and Immunity*, 1626–8.

Craft, J. E., Grodzicki, R.L., and Steere, A.C. (1984). The antibody response in Lyme disease: evaluation of diagnostic tests. *Journal of Infectious Diseases*, **149**, 789–95.

Craven, R. and Dennis, D. (ed.) (1993). *Lyme disease surveillance summary*. U.S. Dept. of Health and Human Services, Fort Collins.

Dattwyler, R. J., Volkman, D.J., Halperin, J.J., and Luft, B.J. (1988). Treatment of late Lyme borreliosis—randomized comparison of ceftriaxone and penicillin. *Lancet*, i, 1191–4.

Dattwyler, R. J., Volkman, D.J., Luft, B.J., *et al.* (1989). Dissociation of specific T- and B-lymphocyte responses to *Borrelia burgdorferi*. *New England Journal of Medicine*, **319**, 1441–6.

Dattwyler, R. J., Volkman, D.J., Conaty, S.M, Platkin, S.P., and Luft, B.J. (1990). Amoxicillin plus probenecid versus doxycycline for treatment of erythema migrans borreliosis. *Lancet*, **336**, 1404–6.

Dekonenko, E. J., Steere, A.C., Berardi, V.P., and Kravchuk, L.N. (1988). Lyme borreliosis in the Soviet Union: a cooperative US–USSR report. *Journal of Infectious Diseases*, **158**, 748–53.

de Koning, J., Hoogkamp-Korstanje, J.A.A., van der Linde, M.R., and Crijns, H.J.G.M.. (1989). Demonstration of spirochetes in cardiac biopsies of patients with Lyme disease. *Journal of Infectious Diseases*, **160**, 150–2.

Dorward, D. W. and Garon, C. F. (1990). DNA is packaged within membrane-derived vesicles of Gram-negative but not Gram-positive bacteria. *Applied Environmental Microbiology*, **56**, 1960–2.

Dotevall, L., Alestig, K., Hanner, P., Norfrans, G., and Hagberg, L. (1988). The use of doxycycline in nervous system *Borrelia burgdorferi* infection. *Scandinavian Journal of Infectious Diseases*, **53**, 74–9.

Dressler, F., Whalen, J.A., Reinhardt, B.N., and Steere, A.C. (1993). Western blotting in the serodiagnosis of Lyme disease. *Journal of Infectious Diseases*, **167**, 392–400.

Fikrig, E., Barthold, S.W., Kantor, F.S., and Flavell, R.A. (1992). Long-term protection of mice from Lyme disease by vaccination with OspA. *Infection and Immunity*, **60**, 773–7.

Garcia-Monco, J. C., Villar, B.F., Alen, J.C., and Benach, J.L. (1990). *Borrelia burgdorferi* in the central nervous system: experimental and clinical evidence for early invasion. *Journal of Infectious Diseases*, **161**, 1187–93.

Garin-Bujadoux, C. (1922). Paralysie par les tiques. *Journal de Medicine*, Lyon, **71**, 765–7.

Ginsberg, H.S. (1995). Vector management to reduce the risk of Lyme disease. In: *Ecology and environmental management of Lyme disease* (ed. M.L. Wilson and R.D. Deblinger), pp. 126–56. Rutgers University Press, Newark, NJ.

Halperin, J. J., Krupp, L.B., Golightly, M.G., and Volkman, D.J. (1986). Lyme borreliosis-associated encephalopathy. *Neurology*, **40**, 1340.

Halperin, J. J., Little, B.W., Coyle, P.K., and Dattwyler, R.J. (1987). Lyme disease: cause of a treatable peripheral neuropathy. *Neurology*, **37**, 1700–6.

Halperin, J. J., Luft, B.J., Anand, A.K., et al. (1989). Lyme neuroborreliosis: central nervous system manifestations. *Neurology*, **39**, 753–9.

Hanrahan, J. P., Benach, J.L., Coleman, J.L., et al. (1984). Incidence and cumulative frequency of endemic Lyme disease in a community. *Journal of Infectious Diseases*, **150**, 489–96.

Hardin, J. A., Steere, A.C., and Malawista, S.E. (1979a). Immune complexes and the evolution of Lyme arthritis: dissemination and localization of abnormal C1q binding activity. *New England Journal of Medicine*, **301**, 1358–63.

Hardin, J. A., Walker, L.C., Steere, A.C., et al. (1979b). Circulating immune complexes in Lyme arthritis: detection of the ^{125}I-C1q binding, C1q solid phase and Raji cell assays. *Journal of Clinical Investigation*, **63**, 468–77.

Hardin, J. A., Steere, A.C., and Malawista, S.E. (1984). The pathogenesis of arthritis in Lyme disease: humoral immune responses and the role of intra-articular immune complexes. *Yale Journal of Biological Medicine*, **57**, 589–93.

Hsu, V. M., Patella, S.J., and Sigal, L.H. (1993). 'Chronic Lyme disease' as the incorrect diagnosis in patients with fibromyalgia. *Arthritis and Rheumatism*, **36**, 1493–500.

Johnston, Y. E., Duray, P.H., Steere, A.C., et al. (1985). Lyme arthritis: spirochetes found in synovial microangiopathic lesions. *American Journal of Pathology*, **118**, 26–34.

Kalish, R. A., Leong, J.M., and Steere, A.C. (1993). Association of treatment-resistant chronic Lyme arthritis with HLA-DR4 and antibody reactivity to OspA and OspB of *Borrelia burgdorferi*. *Infection and Immunity*, **61**, 2774–9.

Kaufman, L. D., Gruber, B.L., Phillips, M.E., and Benach, J.L. (1989). Late cutaneous Lyme disease: acrodermatitis chronica atrophicans. *American Journal of Medicine*, **86**, 828–30.

Keller, T. L., Halperin, J.J., and Whitman, M. (1992). PCR detection of *Borrelia burgdorferi* DNA in cerebrospinal fluid of Lyme neuroborreliosis patients. *Neurology*, **42**, 32–42.

Klempner, M. S., Noring, R., and Rogers, R.A. (1993). Invasion of human skin fibroblasts by the Lyme disease spirochete, *Borrelia burgdorferi*. *Journal of Infectious Diseases*, **167**, 1074–81.

Kuiper, H., van Dam, A.P., Spanjaard, L., et al. (1994). Isolation of *Borrelia burgdorferi* from biopsy specimens taken from healthy-looking skin of patients with Lyme borreliosis. *Journal of Clinical Microbiology*, **32**, 715–20.

Lightfoot, R. W., Benjamin, J.L., Rahn, D.W., et al. (1993). Empiric parenteral antibiotic treatment of patients with fibromyalgia and fatigue and a positive serologic result for Lyme disease. *Annals of Internal Medicine*, **119**, 503–9.

Logigian, E. L., Kaplan, R.F., and Steere, A.C. (1990). 'Chronic neurologic manifestations of Lyme disease. *New England Journal of Medicine*, **323**, 1438–44.

Lovrich, S. D., Callister, S.M., Lim, L.C.L., DuChateau, B.K., and Schell, R.F. (1994). Seroprotective groups of Lyme borreliosis spirochetes from North America and Europe. *Journal of Infectious Diseases*, **170**, 115–21.

Luft, B. J., Steinman, C.R., Neimark, H.C., et al. (1992). Invasion of the central nervous system by *Borrelia burgdorferi* in acute disseminated infection. *Journal of the American Medical Association*, **267**, 1364–7.

Luft, B.J., Dattwyler, R.J., Johnson, R.C., et al. (1996). Azithromycin compared with amoxicillin in the treatment of erythema migrans. *Annals of Internal Medicine*, **124**, 885–91.

Luger, S. W. and Krauss, E. (1990). Serologic tests for Lyme disease: interlaboratory variability. *Archives of Internal Medicine*, **150**, 761–3.

McAlister, H. F., Klementovicz, P., Andrews, C., et al. (1989). Lyme carditis: an important cause of reversible heart block. *Annals of Internal Medicine*, **110**, 339–45.

Magid, D., Schwartz, B., Craft, J., and Schwartz, J.S. (1992). Prevention of Lyme disease after tick bites. *New England Journal of Medicine*, **327**, 534–41.

Magnarelli, L. A. Miller, J.N., Anderson, J.F., and Riviere, G.R. (1990). Cross-reactivity of nonspecific treponemal antibody in serologic tests for Lyme disease. *Journal of Clinical Microbiology*, **28**, 1276–9.

Malawista, S. E., Barthold, S.W., and Persing, D.H. (1994). Fate of *Borrelia burgdorferi* DNA in tissues of infected mice after antibiotic treatment. *Journal of Infectious Diseases*, **170**, 1312–16.

Marcus, L. C., Steere, A.C., Duray, P.H., Anderson, A.E., and Mahoney, E.B. (1985). Fatal pancarditis in a patient with coexistent Lyme disease and babesiosis. Demonstration of spirochetes in the myocardium. *Annals of Internal Medicine*, **103**, 374–6.

Markowitz, L. E., Steere, A.C., Benach, J.L., Slade, J.D., and Broome, C.V. (1986). Lyme disease during pregnancy. *Journal of the American Medical Association*, **255**, 3394–6.

Marshall, W. F., Telford, S.R., Rys, P.N., et al. (1994). Detection of *Borrelia burgdorferi* DNA in museum specimens of *Peromyscus leucopus*. *Journal of Infectious Diseases*, **170**, 1027–32.

Mather, T. N., Wilson, M.L., Moore, S.I., Ribeiro, J.M.C., and Spielman, A. (1989). Comparing the relative potential of rodents as reservoirs of the Lyme disease spirochete (*Borrelia burgdorferi*). *American Journal of Epidemiology*, **130**, 143–50.

Maupin, G. O., Gage, K.L., Piesman, J., et al. (1994). Discovery of an enzootic cycle of *Borrelia burgdorferi* in *Neotoma mexicana* and *Ixodes spinipalpis* from Northern Colorado; an area where Lyme disease is nonendemic. *Journal of Infectious Diseases*, **170**, 636–43.

Montgomery, R. R., Nathanson, M.H., and Malawista, S.E. (1994). Fc and non-Fc mediated phagocytosis of *Borrelia burgdorferi* by macrophages. *Journal of Infectious Diseases*, **170**, 890–3.

Nadelman, R., Luger, S., Frank, E., and Wisniewski, M. (1992). Comparison of cefuroxime axetil and doxycycline in the treatment of early Lyme disease. *Annals of Internal Medicine*, **117**, 273–80.

Nocton, J. J., Dressler, F., Rutledge, B.J., et al. (1994). Detection of *Borrelia burgdorferi* DNA by polymerase chain reaction in synovial fluid from patients with Lyme arthritis. *New England Journal of Medicine*, **330**, 229–34.

Oliver, J. H., Owsley, M.R., Hutcheson, H.J., et al. (1993). Conspecificity of the ticks *Ixodes scapular* and *I. dammini* (Acari: Ixodidae). *Journal of Medical Entomology*, **30**, 54–63.

Pachner, A. R. and Steere, A. C. (1985). The triad of neurologic manifestations of Lyme disease: meningitis, cranial neuritis, and radiculoneuritis. *Neurology*, **35**, 47–53.

Pachner, A. R., Steere, A.C., Sigal, L.H., and Johnson, C.J. (1985). Antigen-specific proliferation of CSF lymphocytes in Lyme disease. *Neurology*, **35**, 1642–4.

Pachner, A. R., Duray, P., and Steere, A.C. (1989). Central nervous system manifestations of Lyme disease. *Archives of Neurology*, **46**, 790–5.

Persing, D. H., Telford, S.R., Spielman, A., and Barthold, S.W. (1990). Detection of *Borrelia burgdorferi* infection in *Ixodes dammini* ticks by using the polymerase chain reaction. *Journal of Clinical Microbiology*, **28**, 566–72.

Persing, D. H., Rutledge, B.J., Rys, P.N., et al. (1994). Target imbalance: disparity of *Borrelia burgdorferi* genetic material in synovial fluid from Lyme arthritis patients. *Journal of Infectious Diseases*, **169**, 664–8.

Pfister, H-W., Preac-Mursic, V., Wilske, B., and Einhaup, K.M. (1989). Cefotazime versus penicillin G for acute neurologic manifestations in Lyme borreliosis: a prospective randomized study. *Archives of Neurology*, **46**, 1190–4.

Pfister, H-W., Preac-Mursic, V., Wilske, B., Einhaupl, K.-M., and Weinberger, K. (1990). Latent Lyme neuroborreliosis: presence of *Borrelia burgdorferi* in the central nervous system: experimental and clinical evidence for early invasion. *Journal of Infectious Diseases*, **161**, 1187–93.

Rahn, D. W. and Malawista, S. E. (1994). *Treatment of Lyme disease*. Mosby–Year Book Inc., St Louis.

Reik, L., Steere, A.C., Bartenhagen, N.H., Shope, R.E., and Malawista, S.E (1979). Neurologic abnormalities of Lyme disease. *Medicine*, **58**, 281–94.

Reik, L. J., Smith, L., Khan, A., and Nelson, W. (1985). Demyelinating encephalopathy in Lyme disease. *Neurology*, 35, 267–9.

Schlesinger, P. A., Duray, P.H., Burke, B.A., and Steere, A.C. (1985). Maternal–fetal transmission of the Lyme disease spirochete, *Borrelia burgdorferi*. *Annals of Internal Medicine*, 103, 67–8.

Schoen, R. T., Aversa, J.M., Rahn, D.W., and Steere, A.C. (1991). Treatment of refractory chronic Lyme arthritis with arthroscopic synovectomy. *Arthritis and Rheumatism*, 34, 1056–9.

Schwartz, B. S., Goldstein, M.D., Ribeiro, J.M.C., Schultz, T.L., and Shahied, S.I. (1989). Antibody testing in Lyme disease. *Journal of the American Medical Association*, 262, 3431–4.

Shapiro, E. D., Gerber, M.A., Holabird, N.B., *et al.* (1992). A controlled trial of antimicrobial prophylaxis for Lyme disease after deer-tick bites. *New England Journal of Medicine*, 327, 1769–73.

Shrestha, M., Grodzicki, R.L., and Steere, A.C. (1985). Diagnosing early Lyme disease. *American Journal of Medicine*, 78, 235–40.

Sigal, L. H. (1990). Summary of the first 100 patients seen at a Lyme disease referral center. *American Journal of Medicine*, 88, 577–81.

Snydman, D. R., Schenkein, D.P., Berardi, V.P., Lastavica, C.C., and Pariser, K.M. (1986). *Borrelia burgdorferi* in joint fluid in chronic Lyme arthritis. *Annals of Internal Medicine*, 104, 798–800.

Spielman, A., Wilson, M.L., Levine, J.F., and Piesman, J. (1985). Ecology of *Ixodes dammini*-borne human babesiosis and Lyme disease. *Annual Reviews of Entomology*, 30, 439–60.

Stanek, G., Klein, J., Bittner, R., and Glogar, D. (1990). Isolation of *Borrelia burgdorferi* from the myocardium of a patient with long-standing cardiomyopathy. *New England Journal of Medicine*, 322, 249–52.

Steere, A. C. and Malawista, S. E. (1979). Cases of Lyme disease in the United States: locations correlated with distribution of *Ixodes dammini*. *Annals of Internal Medicine*, 91, 730–3.

Steere, A. C., Hardin, J.A., and Malawista, S.E., *et al.* (1977*a*). Erythema chronicum migrans and Lyme arthritis. Cryoimmunoglobulins and clinical activity of skin and joints. *Science*, 196, 1121–2.

Steere, A. C., Malawista, S.E., Snydman, D.R., *et al.* (1977*b*). Lyme arthritis: an epidemic of oligoarticular arthritis in children and adults in three Connecticut communities. *Arthritis and Rheumatism*, 20, 7–17.

Steere, A. C., Malawista, S.E., Hardin, J.A, *et al.* (1977*c*). Erythema chronicum migrans and Lyme arthritis: the enlarging clinical spectrum. *Annals of Internal Medicine*, 86, 685–98.

Steere, A. C., Broderick, T.E., and Malawista, S.E. (1978). Erythema chronicum migrans and Lyme arthritis: epidemiologic evidence for a tick vector. *American Journal of Epidemiology*, 108, 312–21.

Steere, A. C., Gibofsky, A., Pattarroyo, M.E., *et al.* (1979). Chronic Lyme arthritis: clinical and immunogenetic differentiation from rheumatoid arthritis. *Annals of Internal Medicine*, 90, 286–9.

Steere, A. C., Batsford, W.P., Weinberg, M., *et al.* (1980). Lyme carditis: cardiac abnormalities of Lyme disease. *Annals of Internal Medicine*, 93, 8–16.

Steere, A. C., Bartenhagen, N.H., Craft, J.E., *et al.* (1983*a*). The early clinical manifestations of Lyme disease. *Annals of Internal Medicine*, 99, 76–82.

Steere, A. C., Hutchinson, G.J., Rahn, D.W., *et al.* (1983*b*). Treatment of the early manifestations of Lyme disease. *Annals of Internal Medicine*, 99, 22–6.

Steere, A. C., Pachner, A.R., and Malawista, S.E. (1983*c*). Neurologic abnormalities of Lyme disease: successful treatment with high-dose intravenous penicillin. *Annals of Internal Medicine*, 99, 767–72.

Steere, A. C., Grodzicki, R.L., Kornblatt, A.N., *et al.* (1983*d*). The spirochetal etiology of Lyme disease. *New England Journal of Medicine*, 308, 733–40.

Steere, A. C., Green, J., Schoen, R.T., *et al.* (1985). Successful parenteral antibiotic therapy of established Lyme arthritis. *New England Journal of Medicine*, 312, 869–74.

Steere, A. C., Taylor, E., Wilson, M.W., Levine, J.R., and Spielman, A.(1986). Longitudinal assessment of the clinical and epidemiological features of Lyme disease in a defined population. *Journal of Infectious Diseases*, 154, 295–300.

Steere, A. C., *et al.* (1987). The clinical evolution of Lyme arthritis. *Annals of Internal Medicine*, 107, 725–31.

Steere, A. C., Dwyer, E., and Winchester, R. (1990). Association of chronic Lyme arthritis with HLA-DR4 and HLA-DR2 alleles. *New England Journal of Medicine*, 323, 219–23.

Steere, A. C., Taylor, E., McHugh, G.L., and Logigian, E.L. (1993). The overdiagnosis of Lyme Disease. *Journal of the American Medical Association*, 269, 1812–16.

Steere, A. C., Levin, R.E., Molloy, P.J., *et al.* (1994). Treatment of Lyme arthritis. *Arthritis and Rheumatism*, 37, 878–88.

Strobino, B. A.Williams, C.L., Abid, S., Chalson, R., and Spierling, P. (1993). 'Lyme disease and pregnancy outcome: a prospective study of two thousand prenatal patients. *American Journal of Obstetrics and Gynecology*, 169, 367–74.

Thone, A. W. (1968). *Ixodes ricinus* and erythema chronicum migrans (Afzelius). *Dermatologica*, 137, 57–60.

van Dam, A. P., Kuiper, H., Vos, K., *et al.* (1993). Different genospecies of *Borrelia burgdorferi* are associated with distinct clinical manifestations of Lyme borreliosis. *Clinical Infectious Diseases*, 17, 708–17.

Wallis, R. C., Brown, S.E., Kloter, K.O., and Main, J. (1978). Erythema chronicum migrans and Lyme arthritis: field study of ticks. *American Journal of Epidemiology*, 108, 322–7.

Weber, K., Schierz, G., Wilske, B., and Preac-Mursic, V. (1984). European erythema migrans disease and related disorders. *Yale Journal of Biological Medicine*, 57, 463–71.

Weber, K., Bratzke, H.J., and Neubert, U. (1988). *Borrelia burgdorferi* in a newborn despite oral penicillin for Lyme borreliosis during pregnancy. *Pediatric Infectious Diseases Journal*, 7, 286–9.

Weber, K., Burgdorfer, W., and Schierz, G. (1993). *Aspects of Lyme disease borreliosis*, Vol. 3, *Ultrastructure of* Borrelia burgdorferi, pp. 20–43. Springer, Berlin.

Wienecke, R., Zochling, N., Neubert, U., *et al.* (1994). Molecular subtyping of *Borrelia burgdorferi* in erythema migrans and acrodermatitis chronica atrophicans. *Journal of Investigative Dermatology*, 103, 19–22.

Wilske, B., Preac-Mursic, V., Gobel, U.B., *et al.* (1993). An OspA serotyping system for *Borrelia burgdorferi* based on reactivity with monoclonal antibodies and OspA sequence analysis. *Journal of Clinical Microbiology*, 340–50.

Zoschke, D. C., Skemp, A.A., and Defosse, D.L. (1991). Lymphoproliferative responses to *Borrelia burgdorferi* in Lyme disease. *Annals of Internal Medicine*, 114, 285–9.

5.3.5 Viral arthritis

Stanley J. Naides

Viruses may affect the joints by a number of mechanisms. The mechanisms employed vary with the infecting virus and are based on mode of tissue entry, tissue tropism, mechanisms of replication, direct viral effects on cellular functions, the ability to establish persistent infection, local immune response, expression of host-like antigens, ability to alter host antigens, host age and genetic makeup, and the infection history of the host. Several viruses directly infect the cells of the synovium. The mechanism of injury may be through lysis of target cells. The target cells may die by one of three mechanisms:

1. Viral infection may result in classic cell necrosis with karyorrhexis.

2. The virus may initiate the cellular machinery for programmed cell death or apoptosis.

3. The virus may express virally encoded antigens on the cell surface which elicit an immune response which targets the killing of virally-infected cells.

Direct infection may also result in non-lytic mechanisms of viral arthritis pathogenesis. Immune activation may occur by transactivation of host genes by viral gene products. The infected cell elicits an immune response with itself as a target or recruits other cytokine-responsive cells. Viral infection may lead to expression of viral antigens on the cell surface. Such antigens may be seen as foreign and elicit an immune response. Alternatively, molecular mimicry of host autoantigens may break immune tolerance resulting in generation of an autoimmune response. Immune complex disease may result when the humoral response generates sufficient antibody to cause deposition of immune complexes either locally, at the site of viral infection, or systemically with deposition of circulating immune complex in synovium.

Parvovirus B19

Human parvovirus B19 was first discovered serendipitously in 1975 (Pattison 1988). It is a member of the family Parvoviridae, consisting of the smallest known DNA viruses, and the genus erythrovirus, autonomously replicating in erythroid precursors. Numerous autonomous parvoviruses are known to infect mammalian animal species. However, these viruses are extremely species specific and are not known to cross species barriers. B19 is a non-enveloped, single-stranded DNA virus measuring approximately 23 nm in diameter. Although infection of other tissue types may occur, reproduction is usually not as brisk in cells other than erythroid progenitors.

Epidemiology

B19 infection is common and geographically widespread. Seroepidemiological studies of community outbreaks of B19 infection demonstrate that a large proportion of B19 infections remain asymptomatic (Mosley 1994) or present as undiagnosed, non-specific viral illnesses. Up to 60 per cent of the general population has serological evidence for past B19 infection (Anderson et al. 1986). Outbreaks of B19 infection occur in late winter and spring, although epidemics have also been reported in summer and autumn. Within a community, B19 outbreaks tend to cycle every 3 to 5 years, representing the period of time for a fresh cohort of susceptible children to enter the school system. Since the seroprevalence of anti-B19 IgG antibodies is only approximately 50 per cent in adults, these periodic outbreaks often involve susceptible adults as well. The risk of infection in adults may be as high as 50 per cent with multiple exposures. Workers in occupations with increased exposure to children, such as school teachers, day-care workers, and hospital personnel, have increased risk of infection (Bell et al. 1989; Gillespie et al. 1990). Sporadic cases occur between outbreaks. Transmission is presumed to be via respiratory tract secretions.

The incubation period between infection and onset of symptoms is 7 to 18 days. In human volunteer studies, introduction of B19 nasally was followed in 7 days by a 'flu-like illness associated with viraemia, viral shedding in nasal secretions, and a reticulocytosis. At approximately 11 days postinfection, an incipient anti-B19 IgM antibody response was associated with clearing of viraemia, cessation of nasal shedding of virus, and a second phase of clinical illness with rash, arthralgia, and arthritis. Onset of the anti-B19 IgG antibody response occurred almost concurrently with the IgM response (Anderson et al. 1985). In natural infections, the temporal distinction between the two phases of clinical illness is often blurred.

Clinical features

Since 1981, well-defined, clinical syndromes have been attributed to B19 infection. B19 is the cause of transient aplastic crisis in the setting of chronic haemolytic anaemia, such as sickle cell disease, hereditary spherocytosis, α- and β-thalassaemias, pyruvate kinase deficiency, glucose-6-phosphate dehydrogenase deficiency, pyrimidine 5'-nucleotidase deficiency, hereditary stomatocytosis, autoimmune haemolytic anaemia, and HEMPAS (hereditary erythrocytic multinuclearity associated with a positive acidified—HAMS—test) (Naides 1992). B19 is the aetiological agent of erythema infectiosum, or fifth disease, a common rash illness of children characterized by bright red 'slapped cheeks' and a macular, maculopapular, and occasionally vesicular or haemorrhagic, eruption on the torso and extremities (Fig. 1). Infection in children may be asymptomatic, and when symptoms do occur they tend to be mild and include sore throat, headache, fever, cough, anorexia, vomiting, diarrhoea, and arthralgia. Erythema infectiosum may also be seen in adults not previously infected. In adults, the rash tends to be more subtle and the bright red 'slapped cheeks' absent. A number of uncommon dermatological manifestations of B19 infection have been reported including a vesiculopustular eruption, purpura with or without thrombocytopenia, Henoch–Schönlein purpura, and a gloves and socks erythema (Mortimer et al. 1985; Feldmann et al. 1994).

B19 infection may be associated with paraesthesias in the fingers. Rarely, progressive arm weakness may occur as may numbness of the toes. In such instances, nerve conduction studies may show mild slowing of nerve conduction velocities and decreased amplitudes of motor and sensory potentials (Faden et al. 1990).

B19 may cross the placenta to infect the fetus. Clinically affected fetuses develop hydrops fetalis on the basis of a B19-induced aplastic crisis, resulting in a high output cardiac failure, or viral cardiomyopathy, both resulting in hydrops fetalis. B19 has been reported to cause less commonly pancytopenia, isolated anaemia, thrombocytopenia, leucopenia, myocarditis, neuropathy, or hepatitis (Naides 1992; Luban 1994). Recent reports have suggested that B19 may be

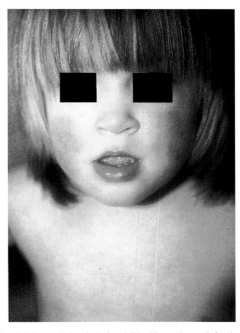

Fig. 1 Classic 'slapped cheeks' of a child with erythema infectiosum, or fifth disease, caused by parvovirus B19. A lacy, macular erythematous eruption is also present on the trunk but is not in focus. (Reproduced from Feder (1994), with permission.)

associated with vasculitis in some cases (Corman and Dolson 1992). Patients with congenital or acquired immune deficiencies, including prior chemotherapy for lymphoproliferative disorders, immunosuppressive therapy for transplantation, or human acquired immune deficiency syndrome (**AIDS**), may fail to clear B19 infection. Such individuals may have chronic or recurrent anaemia, thrombocytopenia, or leucopenia. B19 infection is the leading cause of pure red cell aplasia in patients with AIDS (Frickhofen *et al.* 1990).

Among immune competent children with B19 infection, arthralgia may occur in about 5 per cent and joint swelling in only approximately 3 per cent of children under 10 years of age. In adolescents, joint pain and swelling occurrs in about 12 per cent and 5 per cent, respectively. However, joint pain occurs in about 77 per cent and joint swelling in 60 per cent of adults 20 years of age or older (Ager *et al.* 1966). In adults, B19 infection may be associated with a severe, flu-like illness in which polyarthralgia and joint swelling are prominent. The distribution of involved joints is rheumatoid like with prominent symmetrical involvement of the metacarpophalangeal, proximal interphalangeal, wrist, knee, and ankle joints. Patients usually experience sudden onset polyarthralgia or polyarthritis. Onset of joint symptoms may or may not be preceded by a viral prodrome consisting of fever, malaise, chills, and myalgias. Most present with acute, moderately severe, symmetrical polyarthritis that usually starts in the hands or knees and within 24 to 48 h spreads to include the wrists, ankles, feet, elbows, and shoulders. Spinal involvement is uncommon. Joint symptoms in adults are usually self limited but a minority of adults may have symptoms for prolonged periods of time. Chronic symptoms fall into one of two patterns. Approximately two-thirds of patients have continuous symptoms of morning stiffness and arthralgia with intermittent flares. The remaining one-third of patients will be symptom free between flares. Morning stiffness is prominent. About one-half of the patients meet diagnostic criteria for rheumatoid arthritis. Rheumatoid factor may be present in low to moderate titre during the acute phase of infection but usually resolves. Anti-DNA, antilymphocyte, antinuclear, and antiphospholipid antibodies may also be found acutely. Joint erosions and rheumatoid nodules have not been recorded. Chronic B19 arthropathy may last for up to 8 years, the longest follow-up to date. Several weeks after the initial infection, symptoms of acute synovitis tend to resolve. Pain remains a prominent feature in patients who continue to report morning stiffness. Approximately 12 per cent of patients presenting with 'early synovitis' have B19-induced, rheumatoid-like arthropathy, the majority of whom are women (Naides *et al.* 1990). Adults usually lack the classic 'slapped-cheek' rash seen in children.

The distribution of joint involvement in B19 arthropathy and its symmetry may suggest a diagnosis of a rheumatoid arthritis. About half of all patients with chronic B19 arthropathy meet the criteria of the American Rheumatism Association for a diagnosis of rheumatoid arthritis — morning stiffness which may last for more than an hour, symmetrical involvement, involvement of at least three joints, and involvement of the hand joints. Joint erosions and rheumatoid nodules are absent (Silman 1988). While an initial report suggested that chronic B19 arthropathy may be associated with HLA-DR4, as is seen in classic erosive rheumatoid arthritis, subsequent studies by the same group have demonstrated no increased association with DR4. The absence of rheumatoid nodules or joint destruction aids in the differential diagnosis of B19 arthropathy from classic, erosive rheumatoid arthritis (Naides *et al.* 1990).

Diagnosis

Diagnosis is based on laboratory confirmation in the appropriate clinical setting. A number of approaches and methodologies have been used in the laboratory to confirm B19 infection. Immune electron microscopy, detection of B19 DNA during viraemia, and detection of anti-B19 IgM antibody may be used. However, the most useful modality in the rheumatology clinic is the IgM serology because patients usually have anti-B19 IgM antibodies and have begun to clear viraemia at the time of presentation with polyarthralgia/polyarthritis. Both radioimmunoassays (RIA) and enzyme-linked immunoabsorbent assays (ELISA) have been used to detect B19 antigen and specific antibody to B19 capsid (Cohen *et al.* 1983; Anderson *et al.* 1986; Bell *et al.* 1989; Naides *et al.* 1990). A number of laboratories are developing recombinant B19 antigens for B19 diagnosis in response to the difficulty in obtaining B19 viraemic serum to use as an antigen source.

The anti-B19 IgM antibody response is usually positive for at least 2 months following onset of joint symptoms, but may wane shortly thereafter. However, the IgM antibody may be detectable in occasional patients for 6 months or longer. Because of the high seroprevalence of anti-B19 IgG in the adult population, detection of anti-B19 IgG antibody shortly after presentation of acute-onset joint symptoms in a patient in the absence of anti-B19 IgM suggests past B19 infection and other diagnoses should be pursued. Failure to obtain B19 serological testing at presentation may leave the diagnostic IgM antibody response undetected and result in failure to diagnose B19 arthropathy in those patients in whom joint symptoms persist.

Pathogenesis

Anti-B19 IgM antibody and acute phase IgG antibody (less than 1 week postinoculation) recognize determinants on the major capsid protein, VP2. In convalescent serum, anti-B19 IgG antibody recognizes determinants on the minor capsid protein, VP1 structural protein (Kurtzman *et al.* 1989). B19 VP1 and VP2 are products of alternate transcription of the same open reading frame and VP1 contains an additional 227 N-terminal amino acids not present in VP2. VP1 therefore contains unique determinants not present in the truncated form represented by VP2; these determinants may be in the unique non-overlapping N-terminal region or, alternatively, represent conformational differences in the sequences shared between the two proteins. Western blot analysis of serum from individuals with congenital immune deficiency, prior chemotherapy, or AIDS demonstrated the absence of convalescent anti-B19 IgG antibodies directed against VP1. These sera were unable to neutralize B19 virus in experimental bone marrow culture systems (Kurtzman *et al.* 1989; Sato *et al.* 1991). In the absence of neutralizing antibodies to B19, B19 persists in the bone marrow and may cause chronic or intermittent suppression of one or more haematopoietic lineages.

Management

There is no specific vaccine or treatment for B19 infection at this time. Neutralizing activity to B19 is found in commercially available pooled immunoglobulin since seroprevalence of anti-B19 IgG antibodies in the adult population is approximately 50 per cent (Anderson *et al.* 1986). Intravenous immunoglobulin has been successful in the treatment of bone marrow suppression and B19 persistence in immunocompromised patients. However, this may not be applicable to chronic arthropathy patients. Treatment is symptomatic with non-steroidal anti-inflammatory agents (Naides *et al.* 1990).

Rubella virus

Rubella virus is the sole member of the genus rubivirus in the Togaviridae family of enveloped RNA viruses. The spherical rubella virion measures 50 to 70 nm in diameter with a 30 nm dense core. An envelope is acquired by budding at vesicles or the cell surface. Spike-like projections on the envelope measuring 5 to 6 nm contain haemagglutinin activity that is detected by agglutination of erythrocytes from a variety of animal species (Frey 1994).

Epidemiology

Rubella host range is restricted to humans. Like B19 infection, transmission is by nasopharyngeal secretions with peak incidence in late winter and spring. Widespread rubella vaccination altered the epidemiology of rubella infection, which had occurred in 6 to 9 year cycles prior to vaccination. Most cases were in children. Now the age profile has shifted toward young adults whose risk of infection of 10 to 20 per cent is comparable to that during the prevaccine era. Recent rubella outbreaks in college students and in adults underscores the public health need for maintaining vaccination programmes.

Incubation time from infection to onset of the rash is 14 to 21 days. Viraemia occurs 6 to 7 days before eruption, peaks immediately prior to eruption, and clears within 48 h of the rash. Virus shedding in nasopharyngeal secretions may be detected from 7 days before and until 14 days after eruption, but is maximal just before onset of the rash until 5 to 6 days posteruption (Wolinsky 1990).

Clinical features

The spectrum of clinical disease in children and adults ranges from asymptomatic infection to a classic syndrome of low-grade fever, rash, coryza, malaise, and prominent posterior cervical, postauricular, and occipital lymphadenopathy. Constitutional symptoms may precede the skin eruption by 5 days. The eruption may vary during a brief 2 to 3 day period, starting as a morbilliform facial eruption before spreading to the torso and upper, then lower, extremities. The eruption may coalesce on the face and clear as the extremities become involved. Alternatively, the eruption may be limited to a transient blush.

Joint complaints are common in adult infection, especially in women. Joint symptoms may occur 1 week before or after onset of the rash. Joint involvement is usually symmetrical and may be migratory, resolving over a few days to 2 weeks. Arthralgias are more common than frank arthritis. Stiffness is prominent. The metacarpophalangeal and proximal interphalangeal joints of the hands, the knees, wrists, ankles, and elbows are most frequently involved. Periarthritis, tenosynovitis, and carpal tunnel syndrome may be seen. In some patients, symptoms may persist for several months or years (Smith *et al.* 1987; Ueno 1994).

Live attenuated vaccines have been employed in rubella vaccination with a high frequency of postvaccination arthralgia, myalgia, arthritis, and paraesthesias. The HPV77/DK12 strain is the most arthritogenic of the vaccine strains that have been available. The pattern of joint involvement is similar to natural infection. Arthritis usually occurs 2 weeks postinoculation and lasts less than a week. However, symptoms may persist in some patients for more than a year. The currently used vaccine RA27/3 may cause postvaccination joint symptoms in as many as 15 per cent or more of recipients (Howson and Fineberg 1992; Mitchell *et al.* 1993).

In children, two syndromes of rheumatological interest may occur. In the 'arm syndrome,' a brachial radiculoneuropathy causes arm and hand pain and dysaesthesias that are worse at night. The 'catcher's crouch' syndrome is a lumbar radiculoneuropathy characterized by popliteal fossa pain on arising in the morning. Those affected assume a 'catcher's crouch' position. The pain gradually decreases through the day. Both syndromes occur 1 to 2 months postvaccination. The initial episode may last up to 2 months but recurrences are usually shorter in duration. Episodes of 'arm syndrome' and 'catcher's crouch syndrome' may recur for up to 1 year but there is no permanent damage (Schaffner *et al.* 1974).

Diagnosis

Rubella is readily cultured from tissues and body fluids including throat swabs. Virus is detected in either direct assays of cytopathic effects in tissue culture or in an indirect assay of interference of enterovirus growth in primary African green monkey kidney cell culture. Detection of antirubella IgM antibody or anti-IgG antibody seroconversion is diagnostic of rubella infection. Antirubella IgM and IgG are usually present at the onset of joint symptoms. IgM antibody peaks 8 to 21 days after symptoms then decreases over the next 4 to 5 weeks to undetectable levels in most patients. Therefore, detection of antirubella IgM indicates recent infection, usually in the last 1 to 2 months. Since antirubella IgG rises rapidly over a period of 7 to 21 days after the onset of symptoms, a diagnosis of rubella infection based on IgG serology can only be made with paired acute and convalescent sera. The presence of IgG in a single serum sample only documents immunity (Meurman 1978).

Pathogenesis

Failure to mount an adequate immune response to specific epitopes may allow rubella virus to persist in patients with rubella arthritis. Virus may be detected in synovial fluid during arthritis flares and in lymphocytes years after symptom resolution. Onset of rash and arthritis is coincident with the appearance of antibodies, including neutralizing antibodies to whole virus suggesting a role for antibody or immune complexes in the synovitis (Wolinsky 1990).

Management

Non-steroidal anti-inflammatory agents may be used for symptom control. Low to moderate doses of steroids may be needed to control symptoms and viraemia (Mitchell *et al.* 1993).

Hepatitis B virus

Hepatitis B virus (**HBV**) is a member of the family Hepadnaviridae, genus orthohepadnavirus. HBV is an enveloped, double-stranded DNA, icosahedral virus measuring 42 nm in diameter (Hollinger 1990; Seeger 1994).

Epidemiology

HBV is transmitted by the parenteral and sexual routes. HBV infection occurs worldwide, but prevalence of hepatitis B surface antigen (Australian antigen) is higher in Asia, the Middle East, and sub-Sahara Africa. The prevalence in China may be as high as 10 per cent compared to 0.01 per cent in the United States. There is no known seasonality to primary HBV infections. Most acute infections in endemic regions occur at an early age with many acquired perinatally from infected mothers and it is usually asymptomatic. Incidence of infection in children may be as high as 5 per cent annually, with gradual decline of carriage rates and specific antibody with advanced age. In the west, most infections are acquired during adulthood during sexual or needle exposures. Adult infection is more often associated with acute hepatitis and 5 to 10 per cent of those with hepatitis develop persistent infection. In endemic regions, HBV is a common cause of chronic liver disease and a leading cause of hepatocellular carcinoma (Robinson 1994).

Clinical features

The incubation period from infection to hepatitis is usually 45 to 120 days. A preicteric prodromal period, lasting several days to a month, may be associated with fever, myalgia, malaise, anorexia, nausea, and vomiting. HBV infection may cause an immune-complex-mediated arthritis during this period. Significant viraemia occurs early in infection; soluble immune complexes with circulating hepatitis B virus surface antigen (**HBsAg**) are formed as antihepatitis B surface antigen antibodies (**HBsAb**) are produced. Arthritis onset is usually sudden and often severe. Joint involvement is usually symmetrical with simultaneous involvement of several joints at onset, but arthritis may be migratory or additive. The joints of the hands and knees are most often affected, but wrists, ankles, elbows, shoulders, and other large joints may be involved as well. Fusiform swelling may be seen in the small joints of the hand. Morning stiffness is common. Arthritis and urticaria may precede jaundice by days to weeks and may persist several weeks after jaundice. However, arthritis and rash usually subside soon after the onset of clinical jaundice. While arthritis is usually limited to the preicteric prodrome, those patients who develop chronic active hepatitis or chronic HBV viraemia may have recurrent arthralgias or arthritis. Polyarteritis nodosa is frequently associated with chronic hepatitis B viraemia (Guillevin et al. 1995).

Diagnosis

Urticaria in the presence of polyarthritis should raise the possibility of HBV infection. Acute hepatitis may be asymptomatic but elevated bilirubin and transaminases are usually present when the arthritis appears. Examination of joint fluid is not diagnostic. At the time of arthritis onset, peak levels of serum HBsAg are detectable. Virions, viral DNA, polymerase, and hepatitis Be antigen may be detectable in serum. Antihepatitis B core antigen IgM antibodies are present and indicate acute HBV infection as opposed to past or chronic infection (Hoofnagle 1981).

Pathogenesis

HBV arthritis is thought to be mediated by immune complex deposition in the synovium. Immune complexes containing HBsAg, antibody, and complement components may be detected.

Management

Management is limited to supportive measures including non-steroidal anti-inflammatory agents.

Hepatitis C virus

Hepatitis C virus (**HCV**) is a member of the family Flaviviridae. HCV is an enveloped, single-stranded RNA, spherical virus measuring 38 to 50 nm in diameter (Purcell 1994).

Epidemiology

HCV is distributed worldwide. Using current diagnostic tools, seroprevalence is less than 1 per cent in developed western countries but is higher in Africa and Asia where it may cause a quarter of acute and chronic hepatitis. In Japan, this figure may reach 50 per cent. HCV is transmitted by the parenteral and sexual routes, although the latter is uncommon. HCV is responsible for 95 per cent of post-transfusion hepatitis in countries routinely screening donated blood for HBV. More than half of all cases of non-A, non-B hepatitis are attributable to HCV infection (Bhandari and Wright 1995). HCV genotypic variants have been described and these differ in their pathogenicity, including severity of disease and response to α interferon. To date, 11 HCV subtypes have been delineated (Bhandari and Wright 1995).

Clinical features

Acute HCV infection is usually benign. Up to 80 per cent of post-transfusion infections are anicteric and asymptomatic. Liver enzyme elevations are usually minimal, when present. Community-acquired cases present because of more symptomatic illness in which significant enzyme elevations occur. However, fulminant HCV hepatitis is rare. HCV is strongly associated with HBV-negative hepatocellular carcinoma, especially in Africa and Japan.

Acute onset polyarthritis in a rheumatoid distribution, including the small joints of the hand, wrists, shoulders, knees, and hips, may occur in acute HCV infection (Siegel et al. 1993). Hepatitis C virus is often associated with type II cryoglobulinaemia. It may present as essential mixed cryoglobulinaemia—a triad of arthritis, palpable purpura, and cryoglobulinaemia. Indeed, a majority of patients with essential mixed cryoglobulinaemia have HCV infection. HCV infection is also seen in non-essential secondary cryoglobulinaemia, although less commonly. The presence of anti-HCV antibodies in essential mixed cryoglobulinaemia is associated with more severe cutaneous involvement, for example Raynaud's phenomena, purpura, livedo, distal ulcers, and gangrene. HCV RNA may be found in 75 per cent of cryoprecipitates from patients with essential mixed cryoglobulinaemia and anti-HCV antibodies (Munoz-Fernandez et al. 1994).

Diagnosis

Serological tests utilize an array of antigens in an enzyme immunoassay while a recombinant strip immunoblot assay (**RIBA**) is confirmatory. Second generation RIBA-2 tests for reactivity to four viral antigens; c33c, c22–3, c100–3, and 5–1–1. A positive RIBA-2, especially to c33c and c22–3, is a sensitive assay of HCV infection (Van der Poel 1994). C33c positivity is associated with viraemia. A minority of patients may have HCV RNA detectable by polymerase chain reaction amplification methods in the absence of a positive serology.

Pathogenesis

Chronic HCV infection leads to cirrhosis, end stage liver failure, and hepatocellular carcinoma but the frequency of these sequelae and the mechanisms by which they occur are not known. HCV infection persists despite vigorous antibody response to an array of viral epitopes. A high rate of mutation in the envelope protein is responsible for emergence of neutralization escape mutants and quasispecies (Shimizu *et al.* 1994). Why HCV elicits cryoglobulins remains to be determined.

Management

Interferon α has been shown to be efficacious in the treatment of chronic HCV hepatitis and HCV-associated cryoglobulinaemia. Interferon α2b at a dose of three million units thrice weekly for 6 months suppresses viral titres and ameliorates clinical disease in about half of patients (Jenkins *et al.* 1996). Those with cryoglobulinaemia failing interferon therapy require immunosuppressive therapy. Relapse after completion of the initial course of therapy is common. There is controversy as to whether interferon therapy precipitates autoimmune disease such as autoimmune thyroiditis.

Retroviruses
Human immunodeficiency virus (see Chapter 5.3.6)

Several musculoskeletal syndromes have been described in human immunodeficiency virus (**HIV**) infected patients (Calabrese 1993). Whether reactive arthritis, Reiter's syndrome, and psoriatic arthritis are more prevalent in HIV-infected populations remains somewhat controversial. The incidence and prevalence of these rheumatic diseases may vary between populations studied and may depend on geography, mode of HIV transmission, exposure to different infectious agents, racial and ethnic makeup, risk behaviours, and patient ascertainment (Berman *et al.* 1991). Reiter's syndrome may have a prevalence as high as 11 per cent in some HIV-infected populations. These patients differ from 'idiopathic' Reiter's syndrome patients in that they do not have sacroiliitis or anterior uveitis, nor do they present with the classic triad of arthritis, urethritis, and uveitis. The prevalence of HLA-B27 positivity appears to be lower in the HIV-infected patients as compared to non-HIV associated Reiter's syndrome. In Zimbabwe, where the route of HIV transmission is predominantly heterosexual, approximately 40 per cent of HIV patients with joint symptoms have Reiter's syndrome, and another 40 per cent have a pauciarticular presentation without extra-articular features characteristic of Reiter's syndrome (Davis and Stein 1991). In the United States, psoriatic arthritis limited to a pattern of asymmetric oligoarthritis may be seen in as many as a third of HIV-infected patients with psoriasis, but the overall incidence of psoriasis does not appear to be significantly increased. Whether the different patterns of rheumatic disease expression are attributable to HIV infection itself or coinfection with other agents remains controversial. The caprine arthritis–encephalitis virus, a goat retrovirus, causes an inflammatory destructive arthritis and lends support to the notion that HIV infection alone may have musculoskeletal manifestations.

Initial HIV infection may be associated with a transient 'flu-like illness with arthralgias. Later, three pain syndromes not associated with synovitis may be seen. The concurrence of rheumatoid arthritis and HIV is thought to be very rare. An acute symmetrical polyarthritis involving the small joints of the hands and the wrists has been described in four patients but three had periosteal new bone formation about the involved joints, a feature not seen in rheumatoid arthritis. A subacute oligoarticular arthritis, primarily of the knees and ankles, may cause severe arthralgia and disability but is transient, peaks in intensity within 1 to 6 weeks, and responds to non-steroidal anti-inflammatory agents. The synovial fluid is non-inflammatory. Mononuclear cell infiltrates may be seen in the synovium of the involved joints. As many as 10 per cent of HIV-infected patients may experience 'painful articular syndrome' characterized by intermittent severe joint pain predominantly of the shoulders, elbows, and knees which lasts about a day. The pain may be incapacitating and require short-term narcotic analgesics. Fibromyalgia has been reported in HIV-infected patients with a prevalence as high as 29 per cent in one series. The role of HIV and other potential agents in these pain syndromes remains to be clarified (Calabrese 1993).

Human T lymphocyte leukaemia virus 1

Human T lymphocyte leukaemia virus 1 (**HTLV**) is endemic in Japan where it has been observed to be associated with oligoarthritis and a nodular rash. The patients have positive serology for anti-HTLV antibodies. Type C viral particles are seen in skin lesions. The presence of atypical synovial cells with lobulated nuclei and T-cell synovial infiltrates suggests direct involvement of the synovial tissue by the leukaemic process (Nishioka *et al.* 1993).

Alphaviruses
Chikungunya virus

Chikungunya virus was originally isolated during an epidemic of febrile arthritis in Tanzania in 1952 to 1953. The local tribal word, Chikungunya, 'that which twists or bends up', was applied to the virus and the disease. Retrospectively, it is likely that similar epidemics occurred in Indonesia, Africa, India, Asia, and possibly the southern United States from 1779 to 1828 (Ross 1956; Peters and Dalrymple 1990). Humans are the major reservoir for Chikungunya virus which is transmitted by *Aedes* mosquitoes. The reinfestation of *Aedes aegypti* and the introduction of *Aedes albopictus* into the western hemisphere raises the spectre of an expanded geographic distribution.

Epidemiology

It is transmitted from its reservoir hosts (baboons, monkeys, and, in Senegal, *Scotophilus* bat species) to man by *Aedes* mosquitoes in south and west central Africa, Thailand, Vietnam, and India. *Mansonia africana* and mosquitoes from other genera may also act as a vector (Jupp and McIntosh 1990). In a 1964 epidemic in Bangkok, Thailand, an estimated 40 000 patients out of an urban population of two million were infected (Halstead *et al.* 1969*a*). Thirty-one per cent of the prospectively studied cohort seroconverted to

Chikungunya virus antibody positivity. Communities, particularly urban centres, that have not seen Chikungunya fever, either endemically or epidemically, in a long period of time and that have a number of school age children who have not experienced the virus are at risk for significant outbreaks.

Clinical features

Chikungunya fever has an explosive onset associated with fever and severe arthralgia (Tesh 1982). Constitutional symptoms and rash follow an illness that lasts from 1 to 7 days. The incubation period is usually 2 to 3 days but ranges from 1 to 12 days. Fever elevations occur quickly, reaching 39 to 40°C, and are accompanied by rigors. The acute illness may last 2 to 3 days with a range of 1 to 7 days. Following the acute illness, the fever may resolve for 1 to 2 days before recrudescence. Polyarthralgia is migratory and predominantly affects the small joints of the hands, wrists, feet, and ankles with less prominent involvement of the large joints. Previously injured joints may be more severely affected. Stiffness and swelling may occur but large effusions are uncommon. Severe cases may have persistence of symptoms for months before resolution. Approximately 10 per cent of patients will have joint symptoms at 1 year post infection. Generalized myalgia and back and shoulder pain are common. Skin eruption is characterized by facial and neck flushing followed by macular or maculopapular eruption beginning 1 to 10 days after illness onset. Typically, a rash occurs after 2 to 5 days and is associated with defervescence. The rash may last 1 to 5 days and may recur with fever. It is located on the torso, extremities, and occasionally the face, palms, and soles. It may be pruritic. In some patients, the affected skin desquamates (Halstead *et al*. 1969*d*; Peters and Dalrymple 1990).

Significant haemorrhage usually does not occur but isolated petechiae and mucosal bleeding may occur. Suffusion of the conjunctiva is prominent. Sore throat, pharyngitis, headache, photophobia, retro-orbital pain, anorexia, nausea, vomiting, and abdominal pain may accompany the acute illness. Lymphadenopathy may be tender but is usually not massive. Symptoms in children tend to be milder (Halstead *et al*. 1969*b*; Halstead *et al*. 1969*c*). In symptomatic children, nausea and vomiting, pharyngitis, and facial flushing are prominent features but arthralgia, arthritis, and rash are uncommon. Children may present with a mild dengue-like haemorrhagic fever, headache, pharyngeal injection, vomiting, abdominal pain, constipation, diarrhoea, cough, or lymphadenopathy. Arthralgia and arthritis in children are milder and briefer in duration. A destructive arthropathy may occur in a few adult patients with chronic symptoms (Brighton and Simson 1984). Low titre rheumatoid factor may be found in those with long-standing symptoms.

This infection has not been studied intensively enough to allow conclusions regarding pathogenesis to be made. As noted above, few patients may go on to have chronic symptoms of arthralgia. Case reports would suggest that a few patients go on to have destructive lesions resulting from chronic disease manifestations.

Diagnosis

Chikungunya fever should be considered in any febrile patient resident in or returning from endemic areas. A history of epidemic occurrence should be sought. Mayaro virus, Ross River virus, rubella virus, parvovirus B19, and hepatitis B virus infections may present similarly. Synovial fluid shows decreased viscosity with poor mucin clot and 2000 to 5000 white cells/mm³. Therefore the diagnosis depends on laboratory confirmation.

Virus may be isolated during days two to four. In some patients, viral antigen may be detected in acute sera by haemagglutination assay due to the intensity of the viraemia. Haemagglutination inhibition antibodies develop as viraemia is cleared. Complement fixation antibodies are positive by the third week and slowly decrease over the subsequent year. Neutralizing antibody production parallels haemagglutination inhibition activity. Chikungunya virus-specific IgM antibodies may be found for 6 months or longer (Nakitare *et al*. 1983).

Pathogenesis

Following mosquito bite, intense viraemia occurs within 48 h. Viraemia begins to wane around day three. The appearance of haemagglutination inhibition activity and neutralizing antibody is associated with clearing of the viraemia. Affected skin shows erythrocyte extravasation from superficial capillaries and perivascular cuffing. The virus absorbs to human platelets causing aggregation, suggesting a mechanism for bleeding. Synovitis in Chikungunya fever probably results from direct viral infection of synovium.

Management

Management for the patient is supportive. During the acute attack, range of motion exercises ameliorate stiffness. Non-steroidal anti-inflammatory agents are useful. However, chloroquine phosphate (250 mg/day) has been used when non-steroidal anti-inflammatory agents have failed (Brighton 1984).

O'nyong-nyong virus

O'nyong-nyong fever is closely related to Chikungunya virus. O'nyong-nyong virus was first described in the Acholi province of north-western Uganda in February, 1959. Within 2 years, it had spread through Uganda and the surrounding region, affecting two million people. Serologically determined attack rates ranged from 50 to 60 per cent with 9 to 78 per cent of infected individuals becoming symptomatic (Williams *et al*. 1962; Williams *et al*. 1965*a*; Williams *et al*. 1965*b*). Disease spread at a rate of 2 to 3 km daily. After the epidemic, the virus was not detected again until it was isolated from *Anopheles funestus* mosquitoes in Kenya in 1978. *Anopheles gambiae* also serves as a vector. Serological surveys indicate that O'nyong-nyong virus is endogenous. The non-human vertebrate reservoir for O'nyong-nyong virus is not known.

Clinical features

O'nyong-nyong fever is clinically similar to Chikungunya infections (Shore 1961). The name derives from the Acholi word meaning 'joint breaker'. The incubation period lasts at least 8 days and is followed by sudden-onset polyarthralgia/polyarthritis. Four days later, the appearance of skin eruptions is typically associated with improvement in joint symptoms. The eruption is uniform in nature and lasts 4 to 7 days before fading. The fever is less prominent but postcervical lymphadenopathy may be marked. Although residual joint pain often persists, there appears to be no long-term sequelae.

Diagnosis

Viral isolation by intracerebral injection into suckling mice produces runting, rash, and alopecia (Williams *et al*. 1962). Haemagglutination inhibition or complement fixation tests identify the virus (Williams *et al*. 1962). The differential diagnosis is similar to that of Chikungunya fever. Mouse antisera raised against Chikungunya virus or O'nyong-nyong virus react equally well with O'nyong-nyong virus, but O'nyong-nyong antisera does not react well with Chikungunya virus. The mechanisms of O'nyong-nyong virus pathogenesis are unknown.

Management

Management is symptomatic. Patients recover without sequelae.

Igbo ora virus

Igbo ora virus is serologically similar to Chikungunya and O'nyong-nyong viruses (Moore *et al.* 1975). Infection was first observed in a single patient with fever, sore throat, and arthritis. In 1984, an epidemic of fever, myalgias, arthralgias, and skin eruption occurred in four villages in the Ivory Coast. Igbo ora was coined as 'the disease that breaks your wings'. The virus was isolated from *Anopheles funestus* and *Anopheles gambiae* mosquitoes and from affected individuals.

Ross River virus (epidemic polyarthritis)

Epidemics of fever and rash have been observed in Australia since 1928. Epidemics occurred among soldiers stationed in Australia during World War II. Isolation of Ross River virus from mosquitoes, its serological association with epidemic polyarthritis, and the isolation of the virus from epidemic polyarthritis patients in Australia confirmed Ross River virus is the aetiological agent of epidemic polyarthritis (Aaskov *et al.* 1985). Epidemic polyarthritis from Ross River virus has been seen in New South Wales. Antibodies to Ross River virus have been observed in the sera of endogenous populations in Papua New Guinea, West New Guinea, the Bismarck Archipelago, Rossel Island, and the Solomon Islands (Scrimgeour *et al.* 1987*a*; Scrimgeour *et al.* 1987*b*). From 1979 to 1980, a major epidemic of febrile polyarthritis occurred in the Fiji Islands, affecting over 40 000 individuals (Bennett *et al.* 1980). Serological surveys suggested that a low level of Ross River virus infection was present throughout the Fiji Islands before 1979 but that following the epidemic up to 90 per cent of the residents of some communities had antibody. A similar epidemic occurred in the Cook Islands early in 1980. Weber's line is a hypothetical line separating the Australian geographic zone from the Asiatic zone; west of Weber's line, antibodies to Ross River virus are not found (Peters and Dalrymple 1990).

In Australia, both endemic cases and epidemics occur in tropical and temperate regions. Significant numbers of cases are reported in Queensland and New South Wales, although cases and outbreaks are described in other regions as well. Seroprevalence may reach only 6 to 15 per cent in temperate coastal zones but it is 27 to 39 per cent in the plains of the Murray Valley river system (Boughton *et al.* 1984). High rain fall usually precedes epidemic periods, as this causes increased mosquito populations. Cases occur from the spring to the autumn.

Aedes vigilax is the major vector on the eastern coast of Australia where the mosquito breeds in salt marshes. *Aedes camptorhynchus* similarly breeds in salt marshes of southern Australia. *Culex annulirostris* is a fresh-water breeding vector. Other Australian *Aedes* species and *Mansonia uniformus* may also serve as vectors. Several mammalian species may serve as intermediate hosts, including domestic animals, rodents, and marsupials. In the Pacific islands outbreaks, *Aedes polynesiensis*, *Aedes aegypti*, *Aedes vigilax*, and *Culex annulirostris* may have contributed as well (Peters and Dalrymple 1990).

In Australia, infection rates range from 0.2 to 3.5 per cent per year. During epidemics in Fiji and New South Wales, the majority of those infected were symptomatic (Hawkes *et al.* 1985). While male and female infection rates were similar, there was a predominance of women in presenting cases. Children have a case to infection ratio lower than adults.

A newly described alphavirus in Australia, Barmah forest virus, may present in a fashion similar to epidemic febrile polyarthritis (Lindsay *et al.* 1995).

Clinical features

Arthralgias occur abruptly after a 7 to 11 day incubation period (Fraser 1986). A macular, papular, or maculopapular skin eruption, which may be pruritic, typically follows the onset of arthralgia by 1 to 2 days but in some patients may precede or follow joint symptoms by 11 days or 15 days, respectively. Occasionally, vesicles, papules, or petechias are seen. The trunk and extremities are typically involved although involvement of the palms, soles, and face may occur. The rash resolves by fading to a brownish discoloration or by desquamation. Despite its name, half of patients have no fever, and in those who do, modest fevers may last only 1 to 3 days. Headache, nausea, and myalgia are common. Mild photophobia, respiratory symptoms, and lymphadenopathy may occur.

A majority of patients have severe, incapacitating arthralgia. Joint distribution is often asymmetrical and migratory, with metacarpophalangeal and finger interphalangeal joints, wrists, knees, and ankles commonly involved. Shoulders, elbows, and toes may also be involved. Axial, hip, and temporomandibular involvement occasionally occurs. Arthralgias are worse in the morning and after periods of inactivity. Mild exercise tends to improve joint symptoms. One-third will have frank synovitis. Polyarticular swelling and tenosynovitis are common. As many as one-third have paraesthesias, palm, or sole pain. Some patients have classic carpal tunnel syndrome. Half of all patients are able to resume their activities of daily living within 4 weeks although residual polyarthralgia may be present. Joint symptoms recur but episodes of relapse gradually resolve. A few patients continue to have joint symptoms for up to 3 years (Fraser 1986; Peters and Dalrymple 1990).

Diagnosis

The diagnosis of Ross River virus infection should be considered in anyone with a febrile arthritis in the appropriate geographic setting. Acute rubella arthritis may present in a similar fashion although the signs and symptoms of an upper respiratory infection are more prominent in rubella. Patients may present without a rash. The differential diagnosis then would include early seronegative rheumatoid arthritis, systemic lupus erythematosus, parvovirus B19 infection, hepatitis B virus infection, hepatitis C virus infection, other alphavirus infections, Henoch–Schönlein purpura, and drug hypersensitivities. In those individuals who develop vesicles, differential from varicella or parvovirus B19 infection would need to be considered.

Synovial fluid cell counts range from 1500 to 13 800 cells/mm^3. Monocytes and vacuolated macrophages dominate with few neutrophils. Virus has been isolated only from antibody negative sera. In the Australian epidemics prior to 1979, patients were antibody positive at the time of presentation. However, in the Pacific Island epidemics of 1979 to 1980, patients remained viraemic and serologically negative for up to a week following onset of the symptoms

(Aaskov *et al.* 1981). Ross River virus antigen is detectable by fluorescent antibody staining of C6/36 cells inoculated with acute patient serum. Virus in serum is stable for up to a month at 0 to −10°C (Tesh *et al.* 1981).

Pathogenesis

Ross River viral antigen may be detected by specific immunofluorescence in monocytes and macrophages early but intact virus is not identifiable by electron microscopy or cell culture (Fraser *et al.* 1981). The dermis shows mild perivascular mononuclear cell, mostly T lymphocytic, infiltrate in both erythematous and purpuric eruptions. The purpuric form of eruption also shows extravasation of erythrocytes. Ross River virus antigen may be found in epithelial cells in the erythematous and purpuric lesions, and in the perivascular zone in the erythematous lesion. However, viral antigen was not found in the perivascular zone in the purpuric lesions (Fraser *et al.* 1983).

Management

Management of the acute infection is symptomatic. Aspirin or non-steroidal anti-inflammatory drugs provide relief for joint pain. Occasional patients may develop more persistent joint symptoms but full recovery is usual.

Sindbis virus

Sindbis virus is the prototype alphavirus used for molecular virology studies. It was isolated from *Culex* mosquitoes in the Egyptian village of the same name in 1952.

Epidemiology

Sindbis virus infection occurs in Sweden, Finland, and the neighbouring Karelian isthmus of Russia where it is known locally as Okelbo disease, Pogosta disease, or Karelian fever (Tesh 1982). *Aedes*, *Culex*, and *Culiseta* species transmit the virus to humans. Birds are an intermediate host (Niklasson 1988). Cases are confined to predominately forested areas and individuals involved in outdoor activities or occupations are at risk. Sindbis virus infection has also been reported from Uganda, South Africa, Zimbabwe, central Africa, and Australia, where sporadic cases and small outbreaks occur (Peters and Dalrymple 1990).

Clinical features

Skin eruption and arthralgia are the initial symptoms although one may precede the other by a few days. A fever may be present, although not high. Constitutional symptoms including headache, fatigue, malaise, nausea, vomiting, pharyngitis, and paraesthesias may be present but are usually not severe. The macular skin eruption typically begins on the torso, spreading to the arms and legs, palms, soles, and occasionally head. The eruption evolves to form papules which have a tendency to vesiculate. Vesiculation is particularly prominent on pressure points including the palms and soles. As the eruption fades, a brownish discoloration is left. Vesicles on the palms and soles may become haemorrhagic. The rash may recur during convalescence (Tesh 1982).

Arthralgia and arthritis may involve the small joints of the hands and feet, wrists, elbows, ankles, and knees. Occasionally, the axial skeleton becomes involved. Tendonitis is common, often involving the extensor tendons of the hand and the Achilles tendon. Non-erosive chronic arthropathy is common in both Swedish and Finnish

reports, with up to one-third of patients having arthropathy two or more years after onset. A smaller number had symptoms for as long as 5 to 6 years (Niklasson *et al.* 1988).

Diagnosis

The diagnosis may be established by haemagglutination inhibition and complement fixation tests. Antibodies appear during the first week of illness.

Pathogenesis

Little is known about the pathogenesis of Sindbis virus disease. Virus has been isolated from a skin vesicle in the absence of viraemia. Skin lesions show perivascular oedema, haemorrhage, lymphocytic infiltrates, and areas of necrosis. Antiviral IgM may persist for years, raising the possibility that Sindbis virus arthritis is associated with viral persistence and direct viral effect on the synovium (Niklasson *et al.* 1988).

Management

Management is supportive.

Mayaro virus

Mayaro virus was first recognized in Trinidad in 1954 and has caused epidemics in Bolivia and Brazil. Mayaro virus has a monkey reservoir and is transmitted to man by *Haemogogus* mosquitoes feeding in the south American tropical rain forest. Mayaro virus was responsible for an outbreak in Belterra, Brazil, in 1988, in which 800 out of 4000 exposed latex gatherers were infected with a clinical attack rate of 80 per cent. Illness was characterized by sudden onset of fever, headache, dizziness, chills, and arthralgias in the wrists, fingers, ankles, and toes. About 20 per cent had joint swelling. Unilateral, inguinal lymphadenopathy was seen in some patients. Leucopenia was common. Viraemia was present during the first 1 to 2 days of illness,. After 2 to 5 days, fever resolved but a maculopapular rash on the trunk and extremities appeared. The rash lasted about 3 days. Recovery was complete, although some patients had persistent arthralgias at 2 month follow-up (Hoch *et al.* 1981; LeDuc *et al.* 1981; Pinheiro *et al.* 1981). It is of interest that Mayaro virus has been isolated from a bird in Louisiana (Calisher *et al.* 1974).

Other viruses

Apart from specific viral infections noted above in which arthralgia and/or arthritis is typically a prominent feature, there are a host of commonly encountered viral syndromes in which joint involvement is occasionally seen. Children with varicella have been reported rarely to develop brief monoarticular or pauciatricular arthritis that is thought to be viral in origin. Adults who develop mumps occasionally have small or large joint synovitis lasting up to several weeks. Arthritis may precede or follow parotitis by up to 4 weeks.

Infection with adenovirus and coxsackieviruses A9, B2, B3, B4, and B6 have been associated with recurrent episodes of polyarthritis, pleuritis, myalgia, rash, pharyngitis, myocarditis, and leucocytosis. Epstein–Barr virus associated mononucleosis is frequently accompanied by polyarthralgia but occasional monoarticular knee arthritis occurs. Polyarthritis, fever, and myalgias due to echovirus 9 infection has been reported in a few cases. Arthritis associated with herpes simplex virus or cytomegalovirus infections are likewise rare. Herpes hominis occasionally causes arthritis of the knee known as herpes gladiatorum because it is seen in wrestlers. Vaccinia virus has been associated with postvaccination knee arthritis in only two reported cases.

References

Aaskov, J.G., Mataika, J.U., Lawrence, G.W., Rabukawaqa, V., Tucker, M.M., Miles, J.A., and Dalglish, D.A. (1981). An epidemic of Ross River virus infection in Fiji, 1979. *American Journal of Tropical Medicine and Hygiene*, **30**, 1053–9.

Aaskov, J.G., Ross, P.V., Harper, J.J., and Donaldson, M.D. (1985). Isolation of Ross River virus from epidemic polyarthritis patients in Australia. *Australian Journal of Experimental Biology and Medical Science*, **63**, 587–97.

Ager, E.A., Chin, T.D.Y., and Poland, J.D. (1966). Epidemic erythema infectiosum. *New England Journal of Medicine*, **275**, 1326–31.

Anderson, M.J., Higgins, P.G., Davis, L.R., Willman, J.S., Jones, S.E., Kidd, I.M., Pattison, J.R., and Tyrrell, D.A. (1985). Experimental parvoviral infection in humans. *Journal of Infectious Diseases*, **152**, 257–65.

Anderson, L.J., Tsou, R.A., Chorba, T.L., Wulff, H., Tattersall, P., and Mortimer, P.P. (1986). Detection of antibodies and antigens of human parvovirus B19 by enzyme-linked immunosorbant assay. *Journal of Clinical Microbiology*, **24**, 522–6.

Bell, L.M., Naides, S.J., Stoffman, P., Hodinka, R.L., and Plotkin, S.A. (1989). Human parvovirus B19 infection among hospital staff members after contact with infected patients. *New England Journal of Medicine*, **321**, 485–91.

Bennett, N.M., Cunningham, A.L., Fraser, J.R., and Speed, B.R. (1980). Epidemic polyarthritis acquired in Fiji. *Medical Journal of Australia*, **1**, 316–17.

Berman, A., Reboredo, G., Spindler, A., Lasala, M.E., Lopez, H., and Espinoza, L.R. (1991). Rheumatic manifestations in populations at risk for HIV infection: the added effect of HIV. *Journal of Rheumatology*, **18**, 1564–7.

Bhandari, B.N. and Wright, T.L. (1995). Hepatitis C: An overview. *Annual Review of Medicine*, **46**, 309–17.

Boughton, C.R., Hawkes, R.A., Naim, H.M., Wild, J., and Chapman, B. (1984). Arbovirus infections in humans in New South Wales. Seroepidemiology of the alphavirus group of togaviruses. *Medical Journal of Australia*, **141**, 700–4.

Brighton, S.W. (1984). Chloroquine phosphate treatment of chronic Chikungunya arthritis. An open pilot study. *South African Medical Journal*, **66**, 217–18.

Brighton, S.W. and Simson, I.W. (1984). A destructive arthropathy following Chikungunya virus arthritis—a possible association. *Clinical Rheumatology*, **3**, 253–8.

Calabrese, L.H. (1993). Human immunodeficiency virus (HIV) infection and arthritis. *Infection and Arthritis*, **19**, 477–88.

Calisher, C.H., Gutierrez, E., Maness, K.S., and Lord, R.D. (1974). Isolation of Mayaro virus from a migrating bird captured in Louisiana in 1967. *Bulletin of the Pan American Health Organization*, **8**, 243–8.

Chantler, J.K., Tingle, A.J., and Petty, R.E. (1985). Persistent rubella virus infection associated with chronic arthritis in children. *New England Journal of Medicine*, **313**, 1117–23.

Cohen, B.J., Mortimer, P.P., and Pereira, M.S. (1983). Diagnostic assays with monoclonal antibodies for the human serum parvovirus-like virus (SPLV). *Journal of Hygiene*, **91**, 113–30.

Corman, L.C. and Dolson, D.J. (1992). Polyarteritis nodosa and parvovirus B19 infection. *Lancet*, **339**, 491

Davis, P. and Stein, M. (1991). Human immunodeficiency virus-related connective tissue diseases: a Zimbabwean perspective. (Review). *Rheumatic Disease Clinics of North America*, **17**, 89–97.

Faden, H., Gary, G.W., Jr., and Korman, M. (1990). Numbness and tingling of fingers associated with parvovirus B19 infection. *Journal of Infectious Diseases*, **161**, 354–5.

Feder, H.M.Jr (1994). Fifth disease. *New England Journal of Medicine*, **331**, 1062.

Feldmann, R., Harms, M., and Saurat, J.-H. (1994). Papular-purpuric 'gloves and socks' syndrome: Not only parvovirus B19. *Dermatology*, **188**, 85–7.

Fraser, J.R.E. (1986). Epidemic polyarthritis and Ross River virus disease. *Clinics in Rheumatic Diseases*, **12**, 369–88.

Fraser, J.R., Cunningham, A.L., Clarris, B.J., Aaskov, J.G., and Leach, R. (1981). Cytology of synovial effusions in epidemic polyarthritis. *Australian and New Zealand Journal of Medicine*, **11**, 168–73.

Fraser, J.R., Ratnamohan, V.M., Dowling, J.P., Becker, G.J., and Varigos, G.A. (1983). The exanthem of Ross River virus infection: histology, location of virus antigen and nature of inflammatory infiltrate. *Journal of Clinical Pathology*, **36**, 1256–63.

Frey, T.K. (1994). Molecular biology of rubella virus. *Advances in Virus Research*, **44**, 69–160.

Frickhofen, N., Abkowitz, J.L., Safford, M., *et al.* (1990). Persistent B19 parvovirus infection in patients infected with human immunodeficiency virus type 1 (HIV-1): a treatable cause of anemia in AIDS. *Annals of Internal Medicine*, **113**, 926–33.

Gillespie, S.M., Cartter, M.L., Asch, S., Rokos, J.B., Gary, G.W., Tsou, C.J., Hall, D.B., Anderson, L.J., and Hurwitz, E.S. (1990). Occupational risk of human parvovirus B19 infection for school and day-care personnel during an outbreak of erythema infectiosum. *Journal of the American Medical Association*, **263**, 2061–5.

Guillevin, L., Lhote, F., Cohen, P., Sauvaget, F., Jarrousse, B., Lortholary, O., Nol, L.H., and Trépo, C. (1995). Polyarteritis nodosa related to hepatitis B virus — a prospective study with long-term observation of 41 patients. *Medicine (Baltimore)*, **74**, 238–53.

Halstead, S.B., Nimmannitya, S., and Margiotta, M.R. (1969*a*). Dengue and chikungunya virus infection in man in Thailand, 1962–1964. II. Observations on disease in outpatients. *American Journal of Tropical Medicine and Hygiene* **18**, 972–83.

Halstead, S.B., Scanlon, J.E., Umpaivit, P., and Udomsakdi, S. (1969*b*). Dengue and chikungunya virus infection in man in Thailand, 1962–1964. IV. Epidemiologic studies in the Bangkok metropolitan area. *American Journal of Tropical Medicine and Hygiene* **18**, 997–1021.

Halstead, S.B., Udomsakdi, S., Scanlon, J.E., and Rohitayodhin, S. (1969*c*). Dengue and chikungunya virus infection in man in Thailand, 1962–1964. V. Epidemiologic observations outside Bangkok. *American Journal of Tropical Medicine and Hygiene*, **18**, 1022–33.

Halstead, S.B., Udomsakdi, S., Singharaj, P., and Nisalak, A. (1969*d*). Dengue and chikungunya virus infection in man in Thailand, 1962–1964. III. Clinical, epidemiologic, and virologic observations on disease in non-indigenous white persons. *American Journal of Tropical Medicine and Hygiene*, **18**, 984–96.

Hoch, A.L., Peterson, N.E., LeDuc, J.W., and Pinheiro, F.P. (1981). An outbreak of Mayaro virus disease in Belterra, Brazil. III. Entomological and ecological studies. *American Journal of Tropical Medicine and Hygiene*, **30**, 689–98.

Hollinger, F.B. (1990). Hepatitis B virus. In *Fields virology* (2nd edn) (eds B.N. Fields, D.M. Knipe, R.M. Chanock, M.S. Hirsch, J.L. Melnick, T.P. Monath, and B. Roizman), pp. 2171–236. Raven Press, New York.

Hoofnagle, J.H. (1981). Serologic markers of hepatitis B virus infection. *Annual Review of Medicine*, **32**, 1–11.

Howson, C.P. and Fineberg, H.V. (1992). Adverse events following pertussis and rubella vaccines. Summary of a report to the Institute of Medicine. *Journal of the American Medical Association*, **267**, 392–6.

Jenkins, P.J., Cromie, S.L., Bowden, D.S., Finch, C.F., and Dudley, F.J. (1996). Chronic hepatitis C and interferon alfa therapy: predictors of long term response. *Medical Journal of Australia*, **164**, 150–2.

Jupp, P.G. and McIntosh, B.M. (1990). *Aedes furcifer* and other mosquitoes as vectors of chikungunya virus at Mica, northeastern Transvaal, South Africa. *Journal of the American Mosquito Control Association* **6**, 415–20.

Kurtzman, G.J., Cohen, B.J., Field, A.M., Oseas, R., Blaese, R.M., and Young, N.S. (1989). Immune response to B19 parvovirus and an antibody defect in persistent viral infection. *Journal of Clinical Investigation*, **84**, 1114–23.

LeDuc, J.W., Pinheiro, F.P., and Travassos da Rosa, A.P. (1981). An outbreak of Mayaro virus disease in Belterra, Brazil. II. Epidemiology. *American Journal of Tropical Medicine and Hygiene*, **30**, 682–8.

Lindsay, M.D.A., Johansen, C.A., Broom, A.K., Smith, D.W., and Mackenzie, J.S. (1995). Emergence of Barmah Forest virus in western Australia. *Emerging Infectious Diseases (online)*, **1**, 1–6.

Luban, N.L.C. (1994). Human parvoviruses: implications for transfusion medicine. *Transfusion*, **34**, 821–7.

Meurman, O.H. (1978). Persistence of immunoglobulin G and immunoglobulin M antibodies after postnatal rubella infection determined by solid-phase radioimmunoassay. *Journal of Clinical Microbiology*, **7**, 34–8.

Mitchell, L.A., Tingle, A.J., Shukin, R., Sangeorzan, J.A., McCune, J., and Braun, D.K. (1993). Chronic rubella vaccine-associated arthropathy. *Archives of Internal Medicine*, **153**, 2268–74.

Moore, D.L., Causey, O.R., Carey, D.E., Reddy, S., Cooke, A.R., Akinkugbe, F.M., David-West, T.S., and Kemp, G.E. (1975). Arthropod-borne viral infections of man in Nigeria, 1964–1970. *Annals of Tropical Medicine and Parasitology*, **69**, 49–64.

Mortimer, P.P., Cohen, B.J., Rossiter, M.A., Fairhead, S.M., and Rahman, A.F.M.S. (1985). Human parvovirus and purpura. *Lancet*, **1**, 730–1.

Mosley, J.W. (1994). Should measures be taken to reduce the risk of human parvovirus (B19) infection by transfusion of blood components and clotting factor concentrates? *Transfusion*, **34**, 744–6.

Munoz-Fernandez, S., Barbado, F.J., Martin Mola, E., Gijon-Banos, J., Martinez Zapico, R., Quevedo, E., Arribas, J.R., Gonzalez Anglada, I., and Vazquez, J.J. (1994). Evidence of hepatitis C virus antibodies in the cryoprecipitate of patients with mixed cryoglobulinemia. (Review). *Journal of Rheumatology*, **21**, 229–33.

Naides, S.J. (1992). *Clinical virology manual*, (2nd edn) (eds S. Specter and G. Lancz), pp. 547–69. Elsevier Science Publishers, Essex.

Naides, S.J., Scharosch, L.L., Foto, F., and Howard, E.J. (1990). Rheumatologic manifestations of human parvovirus B19 infection in adults. Initial two-year clinical experience. *Arthritis Rheumatism*, **33**, 1297–309.

Nakitare, G.W., Bundo, K., and Igarashi, A. (1983). Enzyme-linked immunosorbent assay (ELISA) for antibody titers against chikungunya virus of human serum from Kenya. *Tropical Medicine*, **25**, 119–28.

Niklasson, B. (1988). *The arboviruses: epidemiology and ecology* (ed. T.P. Monath), pp. 167–76. CRC Press, Boca Raton.

Niklasson, B., Espmark, A., and Lundstrom, J. (1988). Occurrence of arthralgia and specific IgM antibodies three to four years after Ockelbo disease. *Journal of Infectious Diseases*, **157**, 832–5.

Nishioka, K., Nakajima, T., Hasunuma, T., and Sato, K. (1993). Rheumatic manifestation of human leukemia virus infection. *Rheumatic Disease Clinics of North America*, **19**, 489–503.

Pattison, J.R. (1988). *Parvoviruses and human disease* (ed. J.R. Pattison), pp. 1–4. CRC Press, Boca Raton.

Peters, C.J. and Dalrymple, J.M. (1990). Alphaviruses. In *Fields virology*, (2nd edn) (eds B.N. Fields, D.M. Knipe, R.M. Chanock, M.S. Hirsch, J.L. Melnick, T.P. Monath, and B. Roizman), pp. 713–61. Raven Press, New York.

Pinheiro, F.P., Freitas, R.B., Travassos da Rosa, J.F., Gabbay, Y.B., Mello, W.A., and LeDuc, J.W. (1981). An outbreak of Mayaro virus disease in Belterra, Brazil. I. Clinical and virological findings. *American Journal of Tropical Medicine and Hygiene*, **30**, 674–81.

Purcell, R.H. (1994). Hepatitis C virus. In *Encyclopedia of virology* (eds R.G. Webster and A. Granoff), pp. 569–74. Academic Press, San Diego.

Robinson, W.S. (1994). Hepatitis B viruses. In *Encyclopedia of virology* (eds R.G. Webster and A. Granoff), pp. 554–9. Academic Press, San Diego.

Ross, R.W. (1956). The Newala epidemic. III. The virus: isolation, pathogenic properties and relationship to the epidemic. *Journal of Hygiene*, **54**, 177–191.

Sato, H., Hirata, J., Kuroda, N., Shiraki, H., Maeda, Y., and Okochi, K. (1991). Identification and mapping of neutralizing epitopes of human parvovirus B19 by using human antibodies. *Journal of Virology*, **65**, 5485–90.

Schaffner, W., Fleet, W.F., Kilroy, A.W., Lefkowitz, L.B., Herrmann, K.L., Thompson, J., and Karzon, D.T. (1974). Polyneuropathy following rubella immunization: a follow-up study and review of the problem. *American Journal of Diseases of Children*, **127**, 684–8.

Scrimgeour, E.M., Aaskov, J.G., and Matz, L.R. (1987a). Ross River virus arthritis in Papua New Guinea. *Transactions of the Royal Society for Tropical Medicine and Hygiene*, **81**, 833–4.

Scrimgeour, E.M., Matz, L.R., and Aaskov, J.G. (1987b). A study of arthritis in Papua New Guinea. *Australia and New Zealand Journal of Medicine*, **17**, 51–4.

Seeger, C. (1994). Hepatitis B viruses: molecular biology (human). *Encyclopedia of virology* (eds R.G. Webster and A. Granoff), pp. 560–4. Academic Press, San Diego.

Shimizu, Y.K., Hijikata, M., Iwamoto, A., Alter, H.J., Purcell, R.H., and Yoshikura, H. (1994). Neutralizing antibodies against hepatitis C virus and the emergence of neutralization escape mutant viruses. *Journal of Virology*, **68**, 1494–500.

Shore, H. (1961). O'Nyong-nyong fever: an epidemic virus disease in east Africa. III. Some clinical and epidemiological observations in the northern province. *Transactions of the Royal Society for Tropical Medicine and Hygiene*, **55**, 361–73.

Siegel, L.B., Cohn, L., and Nashel, D. (1993). Rheumatic manifestations of hepatitis C infection. (Review). *Seminars in Arthritis and Rheumatism*, **23**, 149–54.

Silman, A.J. (1988). The 1987 revised American Rheumatism Association criteria for rheumatoid arthritis (editorial). *British Journal of Rheumatology*, **27**, 341–3.

Smith, C.A., Petty, R.E., and Tingle, A.J. (1987). Rubella virus and arthritis. (Review). *Rheumatic Disease Clinics of North America*, **13**, 265–74.

Tesh, R.B. (1982). Arthritides caused by mosquito-borne viruses. *Annual Review of Medicine*, **33**, 31–40.

Tesh, R.B., McLean, R.G., Shroyer, D.A., Calisher, C.H., and Rosen, L. (1981). Ross River virus (Togaviridae: Alphavirus) infection (epidemic polyarthritis) in American Samoa. *Transactions of the Royal Society for Tropical Medicine and Hygiene*, **75**, 426–31.

Ueno, Y. (1994). Rubella arthritis. An outbreak in Kyoto. *Journal of Rheumatology*, **21**, 874–6.

Van der Poel, C.L. (1994). Hepatitis C virus: Into the fourth generation. *Vox Sanguis*, **67** (Suppl. 3), 95–8.

Williams, M.C., Woodall, J.P., and Porterfield, J.S. (1962). O'Nyong-nyong fever: an epidemic virus disease in east Africa. V. Human antibody studies by plaque inhibition and other serological tests. *Transactions of the Royal Society for Tropical Medicine and Hygiene*, **56**, 166–72.

Williams, M.C., Woodall, J.P., Corbet, P.S., and Gillett, J.D. (1965a). O'nyong-nyong fever: an epidemic in east Africa. VIII. Virus isolations from Anopheles mosquitoes. *Transactions of the Royal Society for Tropical Medicine and Hygiene*, **59**, 300–6.

Williams, M.C., Woodall, J.P., and Gillett, J.D. (1965b). O'nyong-nyong fever: an epidemic in East Africa. VII. Virus isolations from man and serological studies up to July 1961. *Transactions of the Royal Society for Tropical Medicine and Hygiene*, **59**, 186–97.

Wolinsky, J.S. (1990). Rubella. In *Fields virology* (2nd edn) (eds B.N. Fields, D.M. Knipe, R.M. Chanock, M.S. Hirsch, J.L. Melnick, T.P. Monath, and B. Roizman), pp. 815–38. Raven Press, New York.

5.3.6 Rheumatological aspects of HIV infection

Robert Winchester and Silviu Itescu

Introduction

The epidemic of human immunodeficiency virus (**HIV**) infection is giving rise to several novel rheumatic conditions, directing renewed attention to the problem of musculoskeletal infection and providing new approaches to the study of the disease mechanisms of certain classic rheumatic illnesses that occur with undiminished intensity and frequency in stages of advanced acquired immune deficiency. The rheumatological aspects of HIV infection vary according to the stage of HIV infection (Table 1). Infection with HIV-1 initiates a complex pattern of injury and host responses that mark distinct stages in the evolution of the disease. For a variable number of years the continuing infection appears to be confined largely to cells of the monocyte lineage. It appears reasonably controlled by a specific immune response, during which time there is a striking degree of viral mutation and consequent diversification. The clinical symptomatology of this phase of the retroviral infection largely reflects the

Table 1 Rheumatological consequences of HIV infection

Events in HIV infection	Consequences on spectrum of rheumatic disease
Chronic immune response to HIV antigens: humoral and cell-mediated	B-cell hyperactivity, autoantibody production and non-specific symptoms of chronic immune stimulation
	Lymphocytic infiltrative syndromes, e.g. DILS and inflammatory myopathy
	Nephropathy
	Vasculitides
	Mikulicz syndrome from B-cell lymphoma
Activation of intact or disregulated residual immune and inflammatory response mechanisms	Highly prevalent Reiter's syndrome and psoriatic arthritis
Selective immune deficiency affecting CD4+'helper' T cells	Opportunistic infections of musculoskeletal system
	Amelioration of CD4-dependent rheumatic diseases, e.g. rheumatoid arthritis

DILS, diffuse infiltrative lymphocytosis syndrome.

ongoing immune response to what have now become endogenous antigens with the potential for cytotoxic cellular and immune complex mechanisms of injury. In some, this phase may be without apparent symptoms. During this phase of clinical — but not viral — latency, the virus evolves toward a form that can more efficiently infect and injure the CD4 T cell. Ultimately, in most individuals and through mechanisms that are poorly understood, progressive deterioration of the immune system develops largely as the result of impairment in the function and numbers of the CD4 lineage of T cells leading to development of an acquired immune deficiency syndrome (**AIDS**).

The rheumatological aspects of HIV infection may be placed in three broad categories (Table 1). The first includes the host response to the HIV infection and specific conditions that appear to arise as a direct result of this response. Because of the endogenous location of the stimulating antigen there is a potential for a sustained immune response characterized by cellular infiltration, the production of certain autoantibodies, and vasculopathic and nephropathic responses that are mediated by immune complexes. The diseases in this group include polymyositis, various vasculitides, and the diffuse infiltrative lymphocytosis syndrome that superficially resembles Sjögren's disease. This mimicking of the features of Sjögren's syndrome by the host response to HIV as well as the rheumatic disorders following infection with HTLV-1 have re-energized interest in the possibility of relationships between autoimmune disorders and retroviruses (Kalden and Gay 1994). The constitutional manifestations associated with chronic viral infection may also simulate non-specific features of conventional inflammatory rheumatic diseases, especially in view of the production of some autoantibodies. The second category of rheumatological diseases comprises joint infections and other musculoskeletal manifestations that arise as a direct consequence of a deficient helper arm of the immune response associated with CD4 T-cell depletion. This group includes infectious arthritis and osteomyelitis resulting from conventional and opportunistic pathogens. The third category of rheumatic illnesses consists of certain conventional rheumatic diseases with an immune pathogenesis, such as Reiter's disease, psoriatic arthritis, and various undifferentiated spondylarthropathy syndromes, which otherwise might not be expected to occur in an immunosuppressed individual, since they are effectively treated by therapeutic immunosuppression. The existence of these diseases in this setting presumably reflects pathogenic mechanisms that operate through residual components of the immune system that have not been impaired significantly by the acquired immune deficiency (Table 2).

Biology of HIV-1 infection
Epidemiology

Approximately 10 million people are infected with HIV-1 (Quinn 1990). HIV is transmitted either sexually or by exchange of blood and other bodily fluids. Accordingly, promiscuity or needle sharing confer a risk for acquisition of HIV. The virus may also be transmitted vertically *in utero*, perinatally at the time of delivery, or postnatally

Table 2 A classification of autoimmune disease according to hypothetical critical immune recognition events

Disease example	Reiter's syndrome	Rheumatoid arthritis
Polymorphic MHC element associated with susceptibility	Class I (e.g. HLA B27)	Class II (e.g. DR4)
Autoantibodies present?	No	Yes
Response to selective immunosuppression of advanced HIV infection	Unchanged to worsened	Ameliorated
T-cell lineage presumably recognizing antigen in context of MHC molecule	CD8 (cytotoxic)	CD4 (help)
Implication for immunopathogenesis	CD8-MHC Class I	CD4-MHC Class II
	T-cell drive	T- and B-cell drive

through breast feeding, with approximately one in four children born to infected mothers becoming persistently infected (Friedland *et al.* 1986; Fischl *et al.* 1987). The predominant mode of transmission differs in various regions of the world and this influences the segment of the population at risk for the infection. In African and Asian countries, heterosexual transmission is the predominant mode of spread and the male:female ratio is approximately 1:1. There is now particularly rapid heterosexual spread of HIV in certain parts of India and South-East Asia. In North America and Europe where the primary modes of transmission have been intravenous drug use and male homosexual relationships, the predominance of cases occur in homosexual or bisexual men, approximately one-third in intravenous drug users, and the rapidly growing balance occurs through heterosexual contact. Although early in the epidemic contaminated blood products represented a major problem that resulted in the infection of a large proportion of haemophiliacs, only 2 per cent of the prevalent cases have resulted from administration of contaminated blood products (Quinn 1990).

Retroviral taxonomy

HIV-1 is a member of the family of retroviridae, defined as RNA viruses replicating via a DNA intermediate that is integrated in the genome of the host cell (Table 3). The family of retroviridae consists of three subfamilies: spumaviridae, oncornaviridae, and lentiviridae. Spumaviruses cause largely inapparent infections. Oncornaviruses, including the human T-cell leukaemia virus type 1 (**HTLV-1**), are transforming viruses that cauRheumatological aspects of se neoplasms in the infected host. HIV is a member of the non-transforming lentivirus subfamily that causes a slowly evolving infection characterized by virus–host interactions that include prolonged periods of clinical stability, weak neutralizing antibody responses, and ongoing, extensive, viral genetic mutation and antigenic drift. In tissue culture the lentiviruses cause cytopathic effects including fusion of selected haematopoietic cell lineages. Lentiviruses also include ovine visna maedi virus and caprine arthritis/encephalomyelitis virus that primarily infect monocyte lineage cells and result in illness in sheep and goats with virus–host interactions similar to those occurring in HIV infection.

Structure and organization

The lentiviruses have a distinctive oblong viral capsid seen on electron microscopy, with a protein core shell consisting of p24 molecules. The HIV virion consists of the retroviral genome, which is a double-stranded 7 to10-kb molecule of RNA associated with lower molecular weight RNA species, nucleoproteins, and several enzymes, including reverse transcriptase, ribonuclease, DNA endonuclease, and a protease (Fig. 1). The virion is encapsulated in an internal protein core shell, which is covered by an outer envelope composed of virally encoded glycoprotein and host cell lipid bilayer membrane containing host-derived proteins such as β_2-microglobulin, HLA molecules, actin, and ubiquitin (Arthur *et al.* 1992).

The genomic RNA of all retroviruses contains three principal genes, *gag*, *pol*, and *env* (Fauci 1988; Greene 1991) that respectively encode structural proteins, reverse transcriptase, and envelope proteins. Each end of the genome contains the long terminal repeat sequence containing the viral promoter for RNA transcription, transcriptional stop signals, and polyadenylation sites (Fig. 2). The *gag*

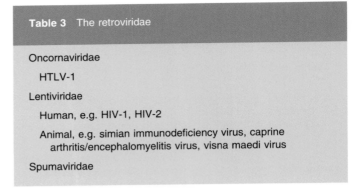

Table 3   The retroviridae
Oncornaviridae
HTLV-1
Lentiviridae
Human, e.g. HIV-1, HIV-2
Animal, e.g. simian immunodeficiency virus, caprine arthritis/encephalomyelitis virus, visna maedi virus
Spumaviridae

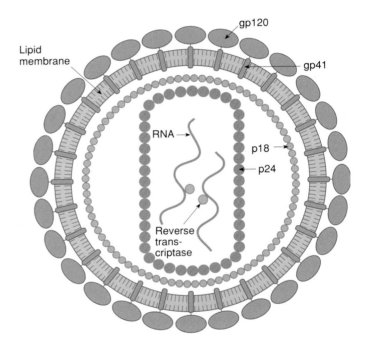

Fig. 1   Schematic representation of HIV-1 structure demonstrating location of various retroviral proteins.

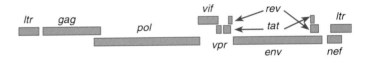

Fig. 2   Genomic organization of HIV-1. The genes encoding *tat* and *rev* exist as two non-contiguous elements, while the structural (*gag*, *pol*, *env*) and accessory genes (*vpr*, *vif*, *nef*) are shown as single elements.

gene (group-associated antigen) encodes the virion structural proteins, including the protein core shell of p24 molecules. The *pol* gene encodes a precursor protein that is sequentially cleaved to produce the RNA-dependent DNA polymerase (reverse transcriptase) of the virus, a protease responsible for the cleavage, and an integrase. The *env* gene codes for two envelope-associated glycoproteins, a smaller transmembrane anchoring protein (gp41 in HIV) and a larger outer membrane protein (gp120 in HIV) which recognizes the target cell viral receptor and against which the host neutralizing antibodies are usually directed. In addition to the *gag*, *pol*, and *env* structural genes, the HIV-1 genome has at least six other accessory genes involved in regulation of viral replication (*tat*, *rev*, and *nef*), virion maturation (*vpr*) and morphogenesis (*vpu* and *vif*) (Fauci 1988; Greene 1991). The rev protein is of interest because it acts rather like the La/SSB molecule and is necessary for transportation of the large pool of unspliced or partially spliced viral mRNAs from the cell nucleus to the cytoplasm, where they are translated (Felber *et al.* 1989).

Lifecycle and replication of HIV

Although the most striking clinical finding of HIV infection, AIDS, results from the infection of the CD4 T-cell lineage, infection of the monocyte plays a particularly central role in the biology of HIV-1 (Meltzer and Gendelman 1992). The monocyte/macrophage is usually the first cell that is infected. While the HIV infection progressively evolves towards a virus that has the ability to infect and injure T cells, this is not apparently a critical feature in the infectious cycle of the virus since the virus is often transmitted to another individual by an HIV-laden monocyte (Meltzer and Gendelman 1992). Macrophages are the major tissue reservoir of the virus at all stages of the infection (Meltzer and Gendelman 1992) with the virus evolving separately in different monocyte lineage compartments (Itescu *et al.* 1994a). As with the visna maedi virus, there is little or no cytopathic effect evident in the HIV-infected monocyte. To gain entry into a host cell (Fig. 3), the viral envelope gp120 molecule binds to the CD4 molecule on the surface of T-helper cells (Klatzmann *et al.* 1984), monocyte lineage cells (Koenig *et al.* 1986; Salahuddin *et al.* 1986), or skin Langerhans cells (Tschachler *et al.* 1987). Subsequently, fusion of cellular and viral membranes occurs, mediated by the HIV-1 gp41 protein. The change in HIV-1 tropism for macrophages or T cells correlates, in part, with structural differences within the HIV-1 gp120 envelope, most notably with the presence of particular residues in a 35-amino acid region within the highly variable principal neutralizing V3 domain (O'Brien *et al.* 1990; Cheng Mayer *et al.* 1991; Hwang *et al.* 1991; Shioda *et al.* 1991; Westervelt *et al.* 1992). Following internalization and uncoating of the virus particle, the viral RNA is reverse transcribed into DNA in the cytoplasm, transported to the nucleus, and integrated as provirus in the host genome.

The central features of HIV replication are depicted in Fig. 3. Regulation of HIV replication involves both host-regulated transcription initiation and virus-regulated post-transcriptional control. In T cells, HIV growth rates are closely linked to the growth state of the host's own T cell, with little or no virus production detected in non-proliferating T cells (Margolick *et al.* 1987). However, activation of these cells, which may occur during certain inflammatory disease states or following stimulation with antigens, mitogens such as phorbol myristate acetate or phytohaemagglutinin, and cytokines such as interleukin 2 (**IL-2**) or tumour necrosis factor-α (TNF-α), dramatically increases viral yields (Siekevitz *et al.* 1987). Coinfection with HTLV-1 also increases HIV-1 replication by a similar action of the transactivating protein of HTLV-1, tax (Siekevitz *et al.* 1987). All of these T-cell activators induce the intracellular production of various nuclear binding factors that mediate the programmes of T-cell activation, such as the NF_KB DNA transcription factor (Nabel *et al.* 1988) (Fig. 4). The presence of NF_KB, EBP-1, and Sp-1 binding sites in the long terminal repeat, promoter region of the virus (Nabel *et al.* 1988), accounts for the observed parallel activation of HIV

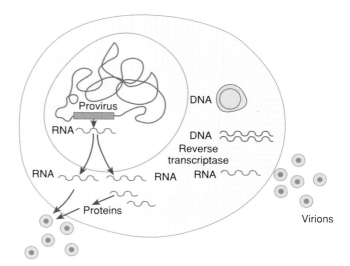

Fig. 3 HIV-1 lifecycle. Events depicted include cellular binding of HIV-1, virion internalization, reverse transcription of RNA genome, integration into host DNA as provirus, proviral transcription, virion transport and assembly, and budding of infectious particles.

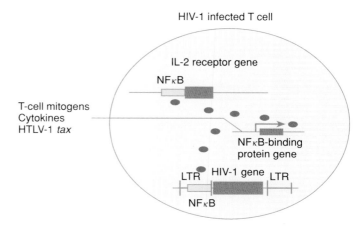

Fig. 4 HIV-1 transactivation. Schematic representation of NFκB-binding protein induction by T-cell mitogens, cytokines, and HTLV-1, and initiation of both viral and host T-cell activation via NFκB elements in the HIV-1 long terminal repeat (LTR) and the interleukin 2R (IL-2R) promoter.

replication and emphasizes how the virus has evolved to exploit normal immunological regulatory circuits of the host. For these reasons, the inflammation of rheumatic diseases arising in the HIV-infected individual may have an adverse impact on the host–viral balance, and it would appear reasonable to consider suppressing the inflammatory aspect of the rheumatic disease in an attempt to diminish the viral transactivation process that might initiate a period of accelerated immune decompensation. Similarly, the initiation of antiretroviral therapy should be considered in all HIV-infected persons developing inflammatory diseases. Indeed, the development of Reiter's syndrome has been rapidly followed by evidence of overt immune deficiency (Winchester *et al.* 1987).

The virus-specific post-transcriptional control of replication involves products of three viral genes: *tat*, *rev*, and *nef*. The tat protein is a powerful transactivator of the HIV genome. It requires specific transactivation responsive (TAR) regions in the viral mRNA transcripts (Muesing *et al.* 1987), leading to as much as a 1000-fold increase in viral mRNA expression. In addition to transactivation of HIV provirus, the tat protein is secreted extracellularly and taken up by uninfected cells (Viscidi *et al.* 1989). The nef protein is associated with cytoplasmic membranes by myristylation, and is a member of the G protein family, both binding GTP and displaying GTPase activity (Guy *et al.* 1987). It is thought to be critical for HIV pathogenesis since HIV strains with defective *nef* genes have been isolated from individuals with non-progressive disease (Kirchhoff *et al.* 1995).

Rheumatological manifestations of the host response to HIV-1 infection

General features

Following infection with HIV-1, specific antibodies develop that are directed against the major structural products of the viral genes *gag*, including p24, *pol* and *env*, including gp120 and gp41. IgM antibodies against gag or env proteins usually appear within 2 weeks of the acute clinical illness associated with primary HIV infection and by 3 months (Tindall *et al.* 1990) are replaced by IgG antibodies. The development of antibodies is occasionally delayed for several months or more. Viral infection can also be directly detected by p24 antigen capture assays, HIV culture, and viral RNA/DNA amplification using the polymerase chain reaction (PCR) (Piatak *et al.* 1993).

B-cell abnormalities

Involvement of the humoral (B-cell) arm of the immune system is reflected by the presence of polyclonal hypergammaglobulinaemia, circulating immune complexes, increased spontaneous B-cell proliferation and development of B-cell lymphomas (Solinger and Hess 1991). These features occur despite an inability to mount antigen-specific B-cell responses (Lane *et al.* 1983) and poor B-cell responsiveness to T-cell factors involved in proliferation and differentiation (Lane and Fauci 1985). Peripheral blood B cells from HIV-infected individuals are polyclonally activated and spontaneously secrete high levels of immunoglobulins (Lane *et al.* 1983). This may be a result of coinfection with known polyclonal B-cell activating viruses such as Epstein–Barr virus or cytomegalovirus (Lane and Fauci 1985), a direct consequence of effects on B cells by HIV-encoded proteins (Pahwa *et al.* 1985), or of B-cell stimulation by IL-6 which is induced in monocytes by HIV infection (Nakajima *et al.* 1989).

As anticipated because of the B-cell hyperreactivity in HIV infection there are a variety of autoantibodies; however, the well-characterized autoantibodies associated with classic rheumatic syndromes are not commonly observed. Rheumatoid factors are rarely detected (Solinger *et al.* 1988; Solinger and Hess 1991). Low titres of antinuclear antibodies are seen in a few patients, without being associated with analogous clinical syndromes in HIV-negative individuals (Solinger *et al.* 1988; Rynes 1990). Circulating immune complexes, measured by the C1q binding assay, are elevated in many HIV-infected individuals at all stages of disease, reflecting at least in part viral–antiviral complexes. However, C3 and C4 levels are not significantly decreased (Mayer-Siuta *et al.* 1988) nor is immune complex disease found in parallel. High titres of IgG anticardiolipin antibodies occur in 20 to 30 per cent of HIV-infected individuals (Bernard *et al.* 1990). While apparently not associated with the

development of thrombotic events, these antibodies have been reported to be associated with thrombocytopenia (Canoso *et al.* 1987) and with cerebral perfusion defects (Rubbert *et al.* 1994). Autoantibodies against circulating lymphocytes have been reported in HIV-positive individuals at all stages of infection (Williams *et al.* 1984; Dorsett *et al.* 1990). These may be lymphocytotoxic, recognizing an extracellular domain of the CD4 molecule that is distinct from the HIV-1 gp120-binding region (Kowalski *et al.* 1989), or directed against the gp41 component of the HIV-1 envelope (Golding *et al.* 1988). In addition to these reactivities, antibodies directed to antineutrophil cytoplasmic antigens (**ANCA**) have been reported in up to 42 per cent of infected individuals (Klaassen *et al.* 1992; Savige *et al.* 1993). In these persons, ANCA antibodies are not associated with cutaneous or systemic vasculitis.

T-cell alterations

The host response to HIV includes an increase in the numbers of CD8+ T cells (Zolla-Pazner *et al.* 1987) that are either HIV-specific MHC class I restricted or unrestricted CD8 cytotoxic cells (Riviere *et al.* 1989). These are particularly prominent early in the course of HIV infection and tend to diminish with disease progression. Shortly after infection, the plasma viral load rises sharply and then decreases within weeks concomitantly with the development of host immune responses including HIV-specific cytotoxic T cells and neutralizing antibodies. At this initial stage the illness may assume a clinical form resembling infectious mononucleosis (De Wolf *et al.* 1988; Connor *et al.* 1993). Both neutralizing antibodies (Looney *et al.* 1988; Rusche *et al.* 1988; Javaherian *et al.* 1989; Koup *et al.* 1994) and cytotoxic T cells (Takahashi *et al.* 1990; Koup *et al.* 1994) elicited by natural infection recognize the immunodominant V3 loop of the envelope gp120 protein, and the high rates of sequence change in this region are thought to confer adaptive value to HIV-1 by allowing it to evade these host immune responses (Zwart *et al.* 1991). In addition, cytotoxic responses to various conserved viral proteins can be detected in most infected individuals throughout the disease course (Walker *et al.* 1987; Koenig *et al.* 1990; Phillips and McMichael 1993).

During this period the HIV envelope evolves to a T-cell tropic form associated with declining numbers of CD4 lymphocytes and increases in viral load. These events are predictive of progression from asymptomatic status to AIDS (Goedert *et al.* 1987; De Wolf *et al.* 1988; Moss *et al.* 1988; Connor *et al.* 1993; Weiss 1993). The median duration from initial infection to the development of frank immune deficiency is 7 to 10 years (Lui *et al.* 1988; Bacchetti and Moss 1989). The HLA genetics of the host appear to influence the course of the infection. Increased rates of progression to CD4 T-cell depletion and opportunistic infections have been reported in individuals with HLA B35 (Scorza-Smeraldi *et al.* 1986; Sheehy *et al.* 1989) and the HLA A1, B8, DR3 haplotype (Steel *et al.* 1988; Kaslow *et al.* 1990). In contrast, slower progression to immune incompetence occurs in infected individuals with the MHC class II alleles DRB1*1102 and DRB1*1301 (Itescu *et al.* 1994). These observations suggest that immunogenetic regulation of the host response to HIV infection may be critical in controlling HIV replication and limiting the progressive increase in viral burden.

Along with the progressive depletion of CD4+ T cells, HIV-infected individuals develop a qualitative helper cell defect, first evident as a deficient T-cell proliferative response to recall soluble antigens, and then to T-cell mitogens (Fahey 1986). These abnormalities are accompanied by diminished production of and response to IL-2 (Prince and John 1987), that results in a predominant T_{H1} pattern of immune deficit. These functional defects are simply demonstrated by cutaneous anergy to routine recall test antigens. They frequently precede the precipitous decline in CD4 cell numbers in late stages of the infection, may occur in the asymptomatic seropositive person with a CD4 count in the range of 400 to 500/mm³, and lead to increased susceptibility to conventional and opportunistic infections. Because of the role of CD4 T cells in inducing CD8 T-cell maturation, the progressive loss of CD4-derived inductive signals ultimately leads to a functional deficiency of CD8 cell cytotoxicity against opportunistic pathogens, such as cytomegalovirus or perhaps HIV itself.

Rheumatic disorders related to T-cell proliferation

In a subset of individuals, the level of CD8 T cells remain high and may reach levels of greater than 2500/mm³. Several distinctive syndromes occur in the setting of these elevated levels of CD8 T cells (Couderc *et al.* 1987; Itescu *et al.* 1989; Malbec *et al.* 1994) including the diffuse infiltrative lymphocytosis syndrome (**DILS**), generalized lymphadenopathy, and pseudotumoural splenomegaly. Each of these syndromes may be seen early in the course of HIV infection, while DILS is also found in long-term survivors.

Diffuse infiltrative lymphocytosis syndrome: a Sjögren's-like disease

The number of entities responsible for keratoconjunctivitis sicca and xerostomia have expanded over the past decade to include chronic graft-versus-host disease following bone marrow transplantation (Fox *et al.* 1986), infection with HTLV-1 (Vernant *et al.* 1988), and HIV-1 infection (Couderc *et al.* 1987; Itescu *et al.* 1989). The sicca syndrome occurring in HIV infection is a part of a syndrome designated 'diffuse infiltrative lymphocytosis', DILS, that differs from classic Sjögren's syndrome in a number of features. It appears to reflect a specific and seemingly beneficial host immune response to HIV (Itescu *et al.* 1994). DILS is encountered in a bimodal age distribution, being seen in children up to age 14 and in adults ranging in age from 22 to 62 years. DILS is not restricted to a particular risk group or ethnicity.

Clinical features

At presentation most patients with DILS meet criteria for AIDS-related complex, or stage 3B (Haverkos *et al.* 1985), with fevers, lymphadenopathy, and weight loss. In part reflecting ascertainment by a rheumatology service, bilateral parotid or submandibular gland enlargement is present in over 90 per cent of patients with DILS, being massive in two-thirds. Xerostomia occurs in 85 per cent, while xerophthalmia and keratoconjunctivitis sicca, diagnosed by Schirmer's test or rose bengal staining of the cornea, occur less frequently, in 40 per cent. Sicca symptoms are less evident in children with DILS. The decreased glandular secretions and associated lymphoid tissue enlargement predisposes to recurrent sinus and middle ear infections. Gallium scanning demonstrates bilateral isotope uptake in the involved tissue (Fig. 5). Computed tomography (CT) scans and magnetic resonance imaging (MRI) techniques show massive symmetrical and often cystic enlargement of major salivary glands (Itescu *et al.* 1993) (Fig. 6). The minor salivary gland tissues have focal lymphocytic infiltration indistinguishable from that of

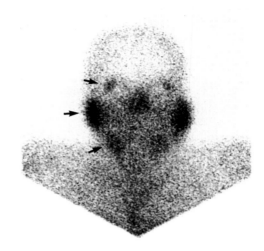

Fig. 5 Gallium scan demonstrating increased uptake bilaterally in the lacrimal, parotid, and submandibular glands (arrows) in an HIV-infected individual with diffuse infiltrative lymphocytosis syndrome.

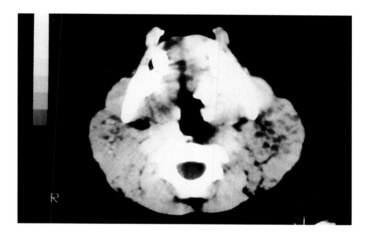

Fig. 6 CT scan of parotid glands in an HIV-infected child with DILS, demonstrating bilateral glandular enlargement with cystic changes.

classic Sjögren's syndrome by conventional microscopy. There is a spectrum from complete preservation of glandular architecture to varying degrees of atrophic duct epithelium, canal dilatation, and interstitial fibrosis. Involved ductules usually express class II MHC molecules, suggesting local effects of cytokine release by infiltrating T cells (Fig. 7).

Extraglandular involvement is particularly prominent. The development and extent of glandular and visceral lymphocytic infiltration in DILS is loosely correlated with the absolute numbers of circulating CD8 T cells, suggesting that lymphocytic infiltration is a direct consequence of the expanded population of circulating CD8 cells in these patients. Pulmonary involvement as a result of lymphocytic interstitial pneumonitis (**LIP**), which occurs in over 50 per cent of patients, appears to be the most serious complication of DILS and may be the initial manifestation of the syndrome. Affected patients may progress to frank respiratory insufficiency and endstage lung disease. Chest radiographs reveal bilateral interstitial infiltrates and gallium scanning often shows diffuse uptake throughout the lung fields. Diagnosis requires histological confirmation, and pulmonary

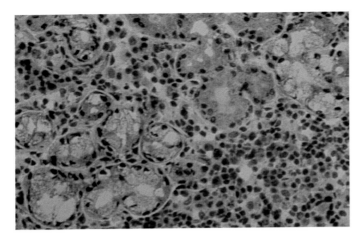

Fig. 7 Immunohistological study of minor salivary gland specimen from a patient with DILS demonstrating staining for HIV gp120 antigens expressed in the cytoplasm of several cells of the monocyte lineage. The positive cells are characterized by abundant cytoplasm and express CD14 lineage markers. They are in a periacinar location and adjacent to a focus of infiltrating lymphocytes.

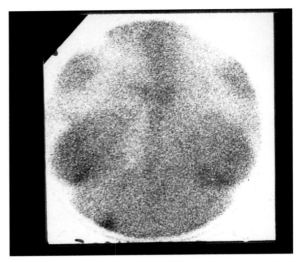

Fig. 8 Gallium scan of a female with DILS illustrating extensive bilateral uptake of the radionuclide in breast tissue. Biopsy of this tissue demonstrated CD8-predominant lymphocytic mastitis with the presence of HIV antigens evident in cells of the monocyte lineage. Analogous findings occur in ovine infection with the visna maedi agent.

infections, particularly *Pneumocystis pneumonia* or *Mycobacterium tuberculosis*, must be excluded. Superimposed bacterial pneumonias can complicate LIP. Enlargement of the tonsils, adenoids, and associated lymphoid tissue may be massive as can be seen in Fig. 6. Gastrointestinal manifestations include lymphocytic hepatitis, causing hepatomegaly and moderate elevations in transaminases and alkaline phosphatase, and gastric lymphocytic infiltration causing disorders in food intake resembling a linitis plastica. Lymphocytic interstitial nephritis, without glomerular involvement, may cause aseptic progressive renal insufficiency and a type IV renal tubular acidosis. Neurological involvement may cause lymphocytic meningitis, unilateral or bilateral palsy of the VIIth cranial nerve, and symmetric sensorimotor neuropathies. Other manifestations have included uveitis, lymphocytic thymoma, and of particular interest, lymphocytic mastitis which is illustrated in Fig. 8. Biopsy of the involved breast tissue revealed a massive CD8 T-cell infiltration, and the presence of HIV viral mRNA and viral proteins p24 and gp120 exclusively in infiltrating monocytes. The appearance of mastitis and LIP are the major features of visna maedi virus disease, suggesting that it may be a model of DILS.

HIV-infected individuals with DILS have a relatively low rate of progression to frank immune deficiency (Itescu *et al.* 1990), for durations of up to 10 years, CD4 T-cell levels decline by less than 10 per cent annually. Opportunistic infections and disseminated fungal or viral infections are rarely seen early in the course of DILS, but there is a considerably increased risk of developing high-grade B-cell salivary gland lymphomas. This complication should be suspected when there is a sudden, generalized increase in the size of the parotid glands, or when there is marked asymmetry. Biopsy is of great importance in making this diagnosis. Circulating cryoglobulins or monoclonal light chains may appear with lymphomatous transformation (Itescu 1991).

Pathogenesis

Immunophenotypic studies have demonstrated that the expanded circulating and infiltrative CD8 lymphocyte population in DILS has a memory phenotype (Itescu *et al.* 1993), expressing CD29 and CD11a/CD18 (LFA-1) molecules involved in effector functions including cell adhesion and cytotoxicity (Martz 1986; Springer *et al.* 1987; Springer 1990). The specific trafficking of CD8 lymphocytes to salivary gland and other tissues in DILS is probably regulated by the interaction between homing receptors on the lymphocytes and their ligands on postcapillary venule endothelial cells, including intercell adhesion molecule 1 (**ICAM-1**), a ligand for CD11a/CD18 (LFA-1) (Springer *et al.* 1987; Springer 1990), perhaps being induced by cytokines such as tumour necrosis factor-α (Springer *et al.* 1987; Springer 1990), produced in high quantities by HIV-infected monocytes (Roux Lombard *et al.* 1989). That the CD8 infiltration occurs in response to local replication of HIV is suggested by the marked diminution in salivary gland size frequently observed following treatment with antiretroviral agents, and by the demonstration of HIV-1 envelope proteins in salivary gland monocyte/macrophage lineage cells located in periacinar and perivascular areas adjacent to lymphoid aggregates and to postcapillary venule endothelial cells that selectively express ICAM-1 (Itescu *et al.* 1993). The T cells infiltrating the minor salivary glands in DILS are relatively oligoclonal, being drawn from a limited number of *V* and *J* gene segment subgroups but exhibiting extensive diversity in VDJ joining (Dwyer *et al.* 1993). The restricted repertoire of both the α- and β-chains of the T-cell receptor exemplified by common structural motifs, both germline and somatically encoded, constitutes compelling evidence that the infiltration of T cells into salivary tissue is the result of a subpopulation of lymphocytes that is responding in a very specific manner to structurally unique antigenic stimuli.

Predisposition to DILS is associated in black subjects with HLA DR5 (Itescu *et al.* 1989) and DR13 (Itescu *et al.* 1994). DNA sequence analysis demonstrates preferential association with the DRB1*1102 (JVM) allele of HLA DR5 (Itescu *et al.* 1994), which is extremely rare in white subjects (Johnson *et al.* 1989; Fernandez-Vina *et al.* 1990), but not with the HLA DR5 allele, DRB1*1101, which is predominant in white subjects. The DRB1*1301 subtype of HLA DRw6, found at the greatest increase in frequency, shares a β_1-chain diversity region motif with DRB1*1102, suggesting that this region may be of importance in predisposing a pattern of response to HIV.

HIV-1 is difficult to isolate and the predominant strains are tropic for monocyte lineage cells. However, viral isolates from individuals with longer disease duration are highly cytopathic and T-cell tropic. Analysis of the HIV-1 V3 domain in the T cells of persons with DILS revealed significantly lower nucleotide evolutionary divergence and amino acid heterogeneity than was observed in controls (Itescu et al. 1994).

Diagnosis

HIV infection should be considered in high-risk individuals presenting with the sicca syndrome, or in all individuals with the sicca syndrome that have atypical features, such as paediatric onset, male gender, prominent extraglandular manifestations, low or absent titres of autoantibodies, and reversed circulating CD4/CD8 T-cell ratio. Tentative criteria for the diagnosis of DILS are: (i) HIV-seropositivity shown by enzyme-linked immunosorbent assay (**ELISA**) and Western blot analysis, (ii) the presence of bilateral salivary gland enlargement or xerostomia persisting for more than 6 months, and (iii) histological confirmation of salivary or lacrimal gland lymphocytic infiltration, in the absence of granulomatous or neoplastic involvement. Typically, two or more foci of at least 50 lymphocytes/ 4 mm^2 of minor salivary gland tissue are seen, or grade 4 according to established criteria (Chisholm and Mason 1968). Rheumatoid factors are found in only 17 per cent of individuals with DILS and antinuclear antibodies with speckled pattern in 13 per cent, all at titres of less than 1:640. Antibodies against SSA/Ro and SSB/La, determined by ELISA using bovine and rabbit substrates as antigen sources (Buyon et al. 1989), are present in only 8 per cent of patients. LIP is an important element of DILS to delineate. After tissue confirmation of lymphocytic interstitial pneumonitis in adults, either by transbronchial or open lung biopsy, gallium scanning and pulmonary function studies are performed to assess the degree of pulmonary involvement. Appropriate biopsies are performed to measure the lymphocytic infiltration of other tissues because of the risk of other complications of HIV infection such as lymphoma or *Mycobacterium avium* infection that could masquerade as a feature of DILS.

Treatment

Treatment with zidovudine or other newer antiretroviral agents should be the first line of therapy. Zidovudine has often, but not uniformly, resulted in diminution of all of the manifestations of DILS including salivary gland enlargement. Discontinuation of zidovudine may result in striking re-enlargement of parotid glands. Circulating T-cell subsets are monitored regularly. Patients responding to zidovudine have demonstrated progressive diminution in CD8 cell numbers and either no change or a concomitant increase in CD4 cells. Symptomatic and progressive visceral involvement, not responsive to zidovudine, is very cautiously treated with 40 to 60 mg of prednisone daily, or other immunosuppressive agents such as chlorambucil, for a period not exceeding 8 to 12 weeks. Prior to commencing this therapy, the degree of circulating HIV antigen load is assessed usually by evaluating for the presence of p24 antigenaemia. Circulating p24 antigen is uncommon in DILS, but if elevated would constitute a relative contraindication to immunosuppressive therapy. More prolonged periods of steroid use and immunosuppression have resulted in the appearance of the development of opportunistic infections. Evidence of enhanced viral replication, ascertained by methods such as p24 antigen assays and cocultivation HIV reverse transcriptase levels, in patients who are being treated with prednisone would be an indication for immediate discontinuation of therapy. Treatment of the salivary gland lymphomas must be aggressive as these are high grade and associated with poor outcome.

Myopathy

Clinical features

HIV-infected individuals may develop a myopathy as a result of polymyositis-like inflammatory muscle disease, zidovudine therapy, or opportunistic infections (e.g. toxoplasmosis) (Snider et al. 1983; Dalakas et al. 1986; Dalakas et al. 1987; Baguley et al. 1988; Dalakas and Pezeshkpour 1988; Till and MacDonell 1990). Most patients with HIV-associated polymyositis present with an insidious onset of proximal muscle weakness and atrophy, as well as muscle pain and tenderness. Systemic features such as fever and weight loss may be present and typical skin lesions of dermatomyositis may be seen, such as heliotrope discoloration, periungual erythema, and erythematous plaques over the wrists and knuckles. In approximately 50 per cent of patients with myopathy, it is the initial manifestation of HIV infection, while in the remainder myopathy develops after the occurrence of opportunistic infections. Differential diagnosis includes vasculitic syndromes, which are usually associated with neuropathies and systemic organ involvement, and pyomyositis, which is usually a discrete unilateral process. Most patients with either inflammatory myopathy associated with HIV-1 or zidovudine-induced myopathy have elevations of muscle enzymes, as well as similar abnormalities on electromyography. Indeed, in one study, 16 per cent of all HIV-infected individuals taking zidovudine for more than 6 months developed abnormally elevated muscle enzymes, though only a few became symptomatic (Till and MacDonell 1990).

Diagnosis and pathogenesis

Muscle biopsy is the procedure of choice for determining the aetiology of HIV-associated myopathy. The entities are heterogeneous. In those with a polymyositis picture, classic myopathic changes are seen, including variation in fibre size, vacuolar change, and fibre destruction. In addition, type II atrophy and nemaline rod myopathy have been described (Dalakas et al. 1986; Dalakas et al. 1987; Panegyres et al. 1988). Most prominent, however, is the inflammatory perivascular and interstitial mononuclear cell infiltrate (Dalakas et al. 1986; Dalakas et al. 1987). In most, the infiltration consists predominantly of CD8+ lymphocytes, although CD4+ T cells and macrophages are also present (Espinoza et al. 1991), raising the possibility that the entity is related to the CD8 T-cell host response. HIV antigens have been demonstrated by immunofluorescence techniques in both muscle tissue and infiltrating mononuclear cells (Dalakas et al. 1986; Espinoza et al. 1991), however HIV-1 has not been cultured from muscle fibres in patients with polymyositis. The possible role of coinfection with HTLV-1, which is tropic for myocytes (Wiley et al. 1989) and may be associated clinically with a myositis (Mora et al. 1988), remains to be determined. In contrast, muscle biopsy in zidovudine-associated myopathy demonstrates similar myopathic changes but much less of an inflammatory infiltrate (Dalakas et al. 1990; Till and MacDonell 1990). In addition, ragged-red fibres suggestive of abnormal mitochondria are consistently observed. Electron microscopic studies confirm mitochondrial damage, with wide variation in size, swelling, degeneration, and laminar bodies present in these organelles (Dalakas *et al.* 1990; Till and MacDonell 1990). These mitochondrial abnormalities may be a result of inhibition by zidovudine of γ-DNA polymerase (Mitsuya and Broder 1986), an enzyme required for mitochondrial DNA replication (Zimmerman *et al.* 1980). High blood lactate:pyruvate ratios, when determined repeatedly, may be a sensitive test for detecting the mitochondrial toxicity of zidovudine (Chariot *et al.* 1994).

Treatment

Therapy of zidovudine-induced myopathy requires discontinuation of the drug. In most cases, clinical improvement and decrease in creatine kinase values occur within 1 to 2 weeks. Careful reinstitution of lower-dose zidovudine may then be attempted. If no improvement occurs after zidovudine withdrawal, or if the affected individual was not taking the drug, muscle biopsy should be performed. Significant inflammatory infiltrates without evidence of mitochondrial changes or opportunistic pathogens indicate an immune-mediated myositis which usually responds to corticosteroid therapy. While these individuals appear to tolerate 40 to 60 mg of prednisone daily, the fact that many patients with polymyositis are at advanced stages of HIV disease, as well as reports of Kaposi's sarcoma developing after treatment with prednisone and methotrexate (Espinoza *et al.* 1991), emphasize the need to taper steroids to the lowest dose effective in symptomatic control and to remain vigilant for possible infectious or malignant complications. Zidovudine therapy should be initiated or continued in polymyositis as it appears to be of benefit in the diminution of myopathic symptoms (Simpson 1988; Dalakas *et al.* 1990).

Vasculitis

Epidemiology

A number of vasculitic syndromes have been reported in HIV-infected individuals (Calabrese 1991; Gherardi *et al.* 1993). This is an area of considerable interest with the strong likelihood that some of these entities will be shown to be directly related to the host response to HIV infection. However, a direct causal relationship between infection with HIV and development of these syndromes remains to be established. Such determinations are complicated by the similarity in clinical manifestations between vasculitides and specific neurological, renal, pulmonary, or cardiac manifestations of HIV infection, and by the coexistence of pathogens such as Epstein–Barr virus, cytomegalovirus, and hepatitis B, which have also been causally related to various vasculitic syndromes (Sergent 1980; Marcellin *et al.* 1991; Louthrenoo 1993; Angulo *et al.* 1994). As with each of the other manifestations in the HIV-infected person, the rheumatologist is challenged by difficult and subtle differential diagnoses. The problems of distinguishing between the host response to hepatitis B and HIV infection has been informatively discussed (Angulo *et al.* 1994).

Clinical features

The reported vasculitic syndromes in HIV infection include involvement of small vessels in the hypersensitivity vasculitis group of either the neutrophilic or mononuclear cell type (Farthing *et al.* 1985; Chren *et al.* 1989; Potashner *et al.* 1990; Gherardi *et al.* 1993), lesions of medium-sized vessels in the polyarteritis nodosa group (Said *et al.* 1988; Gherardi *et al.* 1989; Valeriano *et al.* 1989; Angulo *et al.* 1994; Marks and Kuskov 1995), systemic granulomatous processes (Anders *et al.* 1989; Marks and Kuskov 1995), primary angiitis of the central nervous system (Yanker *et al.* 1986; Scaravalli *et al.* 1989), and involvement of the heart and great vessels (Marks and Kuskov 1995), with a fibroproliferative or aneurysmal process.

The most frequently encountered syndrome, hypersensitivity vasculitis, has been reported to occur either limited to the skin, presenting as palpable purpura, or in association with gut and renal involvement as part of Henoch–Schönlein purpura (Thompson *et al.* 1989; Gherardi *et al.* 1993). In some instances this could be attributed to a drug reaction. Polyarteritis nodosa-like forms of arteritides primarily involve muscles and nerves, and cause symmetric sensorimotor neuropathies, mononeuritis multiplex, muscle pain, and digital ischaemia and gangrene (Calabrese 1991; Jurgensen *et al.* 1995; Libman *et al.* 1995). Skin, gastrointestinal, and renal involvement are less common. Electromyographic studies help differentiate this condition from myopathy, demonstrating a pattern of axonal loss.

Churg–Strauss syndrome, characterized by purpuric skin lesions, bronchospasm, and eosinophilia, has been reported (Cooper and Patterson 1989). Other granulomatous processes, including lymphomatoid granulomatosis, have been reported in HIV-infected individuals, presenting chiefly with pulmonary and central nervous disease (Anders *et al.* 1989). Primary angiitis of the central nervous system may present either as a progressive loss of neurological function or as a fulminating encephalitic illness. Diagnosis is made by angiography or tissue biopsy. Positive serological findings or cultures for HIV in these cases may not be present in the periphery, and may be limited to the cerebrospinal fluid (Yanker *et al.* 1986).

Vasculitis resulting from cytomegalovirus, a major cause of morbidity among all immunocompromised patients because of infection of the endothelial cells by the virus, has been carefully reviewed (Golden *et al.* 1994). Virally induced proliferation and secondary ischaemia and host-mediated immune response to the virus contribute to the consequences of the vasculitis. Cutaneous and gastrointestinal involvement are prominent and must be diagnosed by biopsy.

Pathogenesis

Biopsy of involved skin in hypersensitivity angiitis demonstrates typical small vessel leucocytoclastic vasculitis with IgM and complement deposition within dermal capillaries. In Henoch–Schönlein purpura, the immune deposits in vessel walls contain IgA (Gherardi *et al.* 1993). Hypersensitivity to various drugs, particularly penicillins and sulphonamides, accounts for approximately 20 per cent of small vessel vasculitides (Gherardi *et al.* 1993). Productive infection with cytomegalovirus can be documented by the demonstration of viral inclusions in vascular endothelial cells (Gherardi *et al.* 1993; Golden *et al.* 1994). Polyarteritis nodosa-like disorders are associated with necrotizing vasculitic lesions in medium-sized vessels within muscle or epineurium. ANCA have been detected (Klaassen *et al.* 1992; Savige *et al.* 1993), however these antibodies are found at high prevalence in asymptomatic HIV-infected individuals. Although anticardiolipin antibodies occur in 20 to 30 per cent of HIV-infected individuals (Bernard *et al.* 1990), these antibodies have been reported to be associated with cerebral perfusion defects (Rubbert *et al.* 1994). In contrast, HIV p24 antigen has been reported within the vascular lesions (Bardin *et al.* 1987; Gherardi *et al.* 1993), and HIV RNA has been identified in perivascular cells of monocyte lineage (Gherardi *et al.* 1989; Gherardi *et al.* 1993), suggesting a possible direct role for HIV in the pathogenesis of the polyarteritis nodosa-like syndromes. HIV p24 antigen has also been detected within vascular endothelial cells in the midst of granulomatous inflammation associated with lymphomatoid granulomatosis or with primary central nervous angiitis (Anders *et al.* 1989; Calabrese 1991). The latter is further characterized by multinucleated giant cells within the internal elastic lamina on the surface of the cortex, brainstem, and associated leptomeninges. These findings may also be found in central nervous angiitis associated with herpes zoster infection (Eidelberg *et al.* 1986). The host response to bacterial infections, such as *Neisseria gonorrhoea*, have also been characterized by vasculitis (Ostlere *et al.* 1993).

Treatment

Any drugs possibly contributing to hypersensitivity vasculitis should be withdrawn. Life-threatening vasculitic complications involving the lungs, kidneys, or central nervous system require treatment with corticosteroids or other immunosuppressive agents. Additional treatment required may include antiretroviral agents and prophylactic therapy for herpes zoster and pneumocystis pneumonia. If cytomegalovirus inclusions are demonstrated within involved vascular endothelium, antiviral agents such as ganciclovir or foscarnet should be initiated promptly and immunosuppressive therapy concomitantly reduced (Golden *et al.* 1994).

HIV-associated nephropathy

HIV-associated nephropathy is another entity that is a component of the host response to HIV and which causes differential diagnostic problems for the rheumatologist, especially since, in concert with some of the autoantibodies that characterize the serum of patients with HIV, it may suggest the diagnosis of systemic lupus erythematosus. HIV-associated nephropathy is the most common finding among adult HIV-positive patients who present with nephrotic range proteinuria (D'Agati *et al.* 1989; Bourgoignie 1990). It is a clinicopathological complex characterized by varying degrees of focal segmental and global glomerulosclerosis with collapse of capillary tufts, mesangial cell proliferation, visceral epithelial cell hypertrophy and hyperplasia, microcystic tubular dilatation with tubular atrophy and degeneration, interstitial infiltration with mononuclear cells including a predominance of CD8 T cells, interstitial fibrosis, and endothelial tubuloreticular inclusions. Clinically, HIV-associated nephropathy differs from most idiopathic forms of focal segmental glomerulosclerosis in the greater severity of the renal pathology, the accelerated course to renal failure, and to a lesser degree, tubular damage.

Prevalence

The reported frequency of specific renal involvement in HIV varies to a certain degree according to whether ascertainment is by biopsy of those with symptomatic renal disease or at autopsy of all infected individuals (Bourgoignie 1990). In particular, diffuse mesangial cell hyperplasia and interstitial nephritis appear more frequent at autopsy, 31 and 12.5 per cent, respectively, compared with 5.7 and 1.7 per cent in patients undergoing biopsy, implying they did not

give rise to findings that prompted biopsy (Bourgoignie 1990). In contrast, focal segmental glomerulosclerosis usually results in overt renal disease, accounting for 83 per cent of biopsy diagnoses of renal disease and from 1 to 15 per cent of diagnoses of renal pathology at autopsy according to population and criteria (Bourgoignie 1990). An overall prevalence of at least 7 per cent among HIV-infected adults is a reasonable estimate. The findings in children differ from those of adult series, with diffuse mesangial hyperplasia and focal segmental glomerulosclerosis found in approximately equal frequency (Strauss *et al.* 1989).

Epidemiology

The large majority of HIV-associated nephropathy in adults occurs in the stage of asymptomatic carrier or ARC and only 20 per cent occurs at the time when fully developed AIDS ensues (Haddoum *et al.* 1987; Pardo *et al.* 1987; Bourgoignie *et al.* 1988*a*; Carbone *et al.* 1989). In children, the average age at diagnosis of HIV-associated nephropathy is approximately 3 years (range 6 months to 9 years) (Pardo *et al.* 1987; Connor *et al.* 1988; Strauss *et al.* 1989). Black subjects are far more likely to develop HIV-associated nephropathy than white subjects; this is apparent in all risk groups and in both adults and children, with a ratio of black to white patients approaching 11 to 1 (Bourgoignie *et al.* 1989; Strauss *et al.* 1989; Bourgoignie 1990; Ingulli *et al.* 1991). Because HIV-associated nephropathy develops at a stage of the infection where there is still a reasonably intact immune system which is responding to the virus with a specific immune response, it seems reasonable to hypothesize that this immune response may be the basis of the development of the nephropathy. In this sense HIV-associated nephropathy could be analogous to the development of diffuse infiltrative lymphocytosis syndrome, which is another, and possibly related, host response to HIV infection in which isolated renal tubular acidosis occurs.

Clinical features

Presenting manifestations of HIV-associated nephropathy, other than proteinuria and azotaemia, include nephrotic syndrome in 9 to 60 per cent (Pardo *et al.* 1987; Bourgoignie *et al.* 1988*b*), and hypertension in 39 per cent of individuals in one study (Carbone *et al.* 1989; D'Agati *et al.* 1989), although elsewhere this is less common (Chandler and Treser 1987; Rao *et al.* 1987; Bourgoignie *et al.* 1988*b*; Connor *et al.* 1988; Rao and Friedman 1989). Among adults, endstage renal disease ensues within 4 to 16 weeks (Rao *et al.* 1987; Carbone *et al.* 1989; D'Agati *et al.* 1989). A case of HIV-associated nephropathy with focal segmental membranous glomerulopathy that evolved to central nervous vasculitis and infarction, emphasizes that there may be a spectrum from HIV-associated nephropathy to some of the vasculitides (Bass *et al.* 1994). Cyclosporine and prednisone have been used in small numbers of patients and reported to control HIV-associated nephropathy in some, suggesting a role for participation of the immune response and cytokines in the mechanism of disease (Strauss *et al.* 1989; Ingulli *et al.* 1991; Ifudu *et al.* 1994). Other studies suggest that the progression to renal failure in HIV-associated nephropathy is slowed by zidovudine therapy (Ifudu *et al.* 1994), also directing attention to the importance of HIV replication in the pathogenesis of the syndrome.

Disorders occurring as a direct result of CD4 helper T-cell dysfunction

Musculoskeletal infections, including septic arthritis, osteomyelitis, and pyomyositis

Because of the central role played by the CD4 T cell in regulating both cellular and humoral immunity, the profound cell-mediated and humoral immunodeficiency in the later stages of HIV-1 infection predisposes individuals to a variety of infectious diseases. Infections may primarily develop in the musculoskeletal system as septic arthritis, osteomyelitis, and pyomyositis, or they may be systemic in nature and secondarily involve the musculoskeletal system, with either direct infection of bone joint and muscle or indirectly involving these structures with myalgias and arthralgias. In addition to these diagnostic challenges, the therapeutic approach to treating infection in the immunocompromised host must be altered to reflect the fact that there is an enhanced tendency for the microbial infections to persist after completion of conventional antibiotic therapy regimens, reflecting the failure of effective immune elimination of the residual organisms.

Septic arthritis and osteomyelitis are the two most common secondary infectious complications reported in HIV-infected individuals in case series studied in all parts of the world (Berman et al. 1991; Hughes et al. 1992; Ho 1993; Adebajo and Davis 1994; Goldenberg 1994). Septic arthritis may result from opportunistic or conventional infections that involve various joints, including those commonly affected by septic arthritis such as the hip, knee, wrist, metacarpophalangeal or interphalangeal joints, or those rarely involved such as the sacroiliac and sternomanubrial or sternoclavicular joints. The septic arthritis may be the first manifestation of AIDS, presenting the rheumatologist with the difficult diagnosis of both the septic process and the underlying HIV infection, or the arthritis may occur when an individual with known immune deficiency progresses into an advanced stage.

Organisms cultured from various joints have included, in addition to the anticipated organisms such as *Streptococcus pneumoniae* and *Staphylococcus aureus*, *Sporothrix schenckii* (Lipstein-Kresch et al. 1985), *Cryptococcus neoformans* (Ricciardi et al. 1986), *Histoplasma capsulatum* (Calabrese 1989), and *Mycobacterium avium intracellulare* species (Blumenthal et al. 1990). Other unusual pathogens cultured from septic joints in HIV-infected individuals include *Salmonella* spp. (Winchester et al. 1987; Gutierrez et al. 1993), *Haemophilus influenzae* type B (Lawrence et al. 1991), and *Campylobacter fetus* (Winchester et al. 1987).

Certain patterns of extra-articular involvement are the signatures of particular organisms such as the multifocal cutaneous cellulitis of *Campylobacter (Helicobacter) cinaedi* (Burman et al. 1995) associated with monoarticular or oligoarticular arthritis and an indolent febrile illness. Disseminated sporotrichosis infection may similarly present with diffuse skin lesions and oligo- or polyarthritis (Heller and Fuhrer 1991). Staphylococcal or streptococcal septic arthritis usually presents as an acutely swollen, painful, erythematous process in one or several joints, accompanied by systemic symptoms of bacteraemia. Staphylococcal infections may be widespread, causing septic bursitis (Jacobson et al. 1988; Buskila and Tenenbaum 1989), juxta-articular

osteomyelitis (Masters and Lentino 1984), extensive periarticular soft-tissue involvement, and pyomyositis (Gaut et al. 1988).

Risk factor for HIV acquisition may influence the predominant infectious complications

In addition to the problem attributed to the effect of immune deficiency, the various high-risk behaviour patterns or underlying conditions associated with HIV infection may themselves independently predispose to infection with particular pathogens. *Staph. aureus*, *Pseudomonas aeruginosa*, or *Candida albicans* are usually the most frequently encountered organisms in the arthritis found in intravenous drug users regardless of whether HIV infection is present or absent (Rivera et al. 1992). If these infections, particularly *Pseudomonas*, occur in an individual, they should direct attention to the possibility of parenteral drug abuse (Munoz Fernandez et al. 1991), but some regions experience little Gram-negative disease among addicts (Munoz Fernandez et al. 1991). Among intravenous drug users infected with HIV, *Staph. aureus* infection, most commonly of the hip, accounts for about two-thirds of cases of non-gonococcal septic arthritis (Goldenberg 1991; Munoz Fernandez et al. 1991; Covelli et al. 1993). Pyogenic sacroiliitis or isolated sternoclavicular septic arthritis occurs predominantly among intravenous drug users and is usually caused by infection with *Staph. aureus* or Gram-negative organisms, including *Fusobacterium* as well as *P. aeruginosa* (Guyot et al. 1987).

Conversely, in Africa, where HIV is usually acquired by sexual promiscuity, gonococcal arthritis is the most common musculoskeletal infection and infection by *Staph. aureus*, *P. aeruginosa*, or *C. albicans* is uncommon (Blanche et al. 1993). Among HIV-infected haemophiliacs, the predominant cultured organisms are *Staph. aureus* and *Strep. pneumonia* (Pappo et al. 1989).

There is clear evidence that advanced infection of HIV by itself predisposes to a greatly increased risk of a variety of musculoskeletal infections (Blanche et al. 1993; Adebajo and Davis 1994). Similarly, an increased incidence of septic arthritis among HIV-infected haemophiliacs compared with those uninfected underlines the fact that immune deficiency of HIV infection itself predisposes to septic arthritis (Pappo et al. 1989). It has been argued that infections of the musculoskeletal system complicating HIV infection are rather more prevalent than the literature of reported cases might suggest (Ho 1993).

Osteomyelitis and pyomyositis

In addition to arthritis, osteomyelitis is a common problem. Juxta-articular osteomyelitis may be difficult to distinguish from arthritis, whereas other bony sites may be clinically more distinctive. Organisms reported to have caused osteomyelitis in HIV-infected individuals include *C. albicans* (Boix et al. 1990), *Mycobacterium kansasii* (Crawford and Baird 1987), and *Nocardia asteroides* (Masters and Lentino 1984). Staphylococcal juxta-articular osteomyelitis involving the olecranon process (Masters and Lentino 1984) or distal clavicle (Zimmermann et al. 1989) may present with subacute or chronic joint pain and swelling. Extensive periarticular infections, usually by *Staph. aureus*, can simulate multidigit dactylitis or arthritis.

Pyomyositis is a particular complication of staphylococcal infection and usually occurs in the more advanced stage of AIDS. Acute onset of unilateral thigh pain associated with soft-tissue swelling, erythema and woody induration of the distal thigh is characteristic of pyomyositis (Watts *et al.* 1987; Gaut *et al.* 1988; Goldenberg 1991). In the majority of cases, the cause is a single staphylococcal abscess; however, multiple collections may occur within the quadriceps muscle. Diagnosis is facilitated by imaging techniques, including ultrasound, CT, and MRI scans.

Clinical features and differential diagnosis

Several reviews deal with the changing pattern of musculoskeletal infection during this era and the general principles of diagnosis and therapy (Hughes *et al.* 1992; Ho 1993; Goldenberg 1994). Gram stain and culture of synovial fluid specimens in staphylococcal or streptococcal septic arthritis are diagnostic, and are frequently accompanied by positive blood cultures. Arthritis associated with *M. tuberculosis* may present its usual challenges in diagnosis. Septic arthritis caused by opportunistic organisms tends to be a more indolent and subtle process, often with minimal inflammation. In these patients, the underlying disorder may be suggested by the presence of associated extra-articular manifestations, such as necrotic, crusted skin lesions in sporotrichosis (Lipstein-Kresch *et al.* 1985). Synovial fluid aspirate often reveals low numbers of leucocytes with a relative increase in the proportion of monocytes. Culture of some of these organisms may require special attention from the laboratory and the use of molecular biological methods. The radiological manifestations of musculoskeletal complications of HIV infection have been informatively summarized (Steinbach *et al.* 1993) and emphasize the extensive diagnostic evaluations that may be required to document the extent of structures involved with the infection.

A major problem in the diagnosis of infectious processes of the joints is distinguishing them from the inflammatory non-infectious entities that occur in HIV infection, in particular those of the spondylarthropathy group of illnesses. In addition, other entities that are part of HIV infection but not commonly encountered in rheumatology, such as B-cell lymphoma, Kaposi's sarcoma, and bacillary angiomatosis (an infection by an agent resembling that of trench fever, *Rochalimnaea quintana)* must be considered in the differential diagnosis (Steinbach *et al.* 1993). For example, in pyogenic sacroiliac joint infection, the pronounced pain, exquisite localized tenderness, asymmetry, and lack of involvement of other joints helps differentiate it from inflammatory sacroiliitis associated with the spondylarthropathies. Scintigraphy demonstrating unilateral involvement is also more suggestive of infection, especially when found in the absence of enthesopathy and other arthritis, however, diagnostic aspiration may be required (Guyot *et al.* 1987).

The fact that many patients present with atypical features of the infection because of the attenuated inflammatory response has been emphasized (Hughes *et al.* 1992). Systemic infections such as acute or subacute endocarditis occur with increased frequency in HIV and may present with arthralgias, arthritis, and back pain (Ho 1993). An instructive example of the diagnostic challenges that secondary infections present in the immunologically compromised host is the initial presentation of HIV infection as chronic syphilitic polyarthritis with an efflorescence of autoantibodies that suggested the presence of a rheumatic disease such as rheumatoid arthritis or systemic lupus erythematosus (Burgoyne *et al.* 1992). The rheumatologist has a particular problem in the approach to a patient who is not previously known to be infected with HIV. The general rule that is emerging in endemic areas of HIV infection is that the appearance of acute arthritis should prompt HIV testing (Blanche *et al.* 1993) and, by extension, in Europe and North America where HIV infection is

more stratified, at least a strong suspicion of HIV infection should be entertained. Frequently the atypical manner of presentation directs attention to the probable presence of HIV infection, as for example the presentation of gonococcal arthritis involving a single hip and a sternoclavicular joint (Strongin *et al.* 1991). Atypical, invasive or extensive infection of the musculoskeletal system in a young individual should direct attention to the possibility of an underlying immune deficiency. For example, a report of sternoclavicular arthritis associated with *Strep. pneumoniae* as the presenting manifestation of AIDS illustrates that septic arthritis of a joint that is otherwise seldom involved by infectious processes should prompt a thorough search for predisposing conditions such as HIV infection (Leon *et al.* 1994).

Treatment

Septic arthritis or bursitis is initially treated with broad-spectrum coverage until culture results are available. Some organisms such as streptococcal and staphylococcal joint infections in HIV-positive individuals, or infection with organisms such as *Campylobacter (Helicobacter) cinaedi* (Burman *et al.* 1995), often respond as well to conventional antibiotic treatment as in HIV-negative intravenous drug users (Goldenberg 1991), yet streptococcal and staphylococcal bursitis is difficult to eradicate and requires prolonged therapy (Buskila and Tenenbaum 1989). Opportunistic infections are treated with appropriate antibiotic therapy, including intravenous amphotericin B for fungal infections. Sporotrichosis and allied infections will probably not be eradicated and require chronic maintenance therapy (Heller and Fuhrer 1991).

Some form of joint drainage is initiated soon after the diagnosis is reasonably established, although the precise method is still controversial (Ho 1993; Goldenberg 1994). Surgical drainage is required for appropriate treatment of osteomyelitis and pyomyositis in HIV infection in addition to antibiotics. Several less invasive procedures, such as 'tidal irrigation' or arthroscopic drainage appear to offer the promise of more rapidly controlling the sometimes strikingly rapid destructive consequences of septic arthritis in this group and have the advantage of avoiding the considerable morbidity of an arthrotomy (Ho 1993; Goldenberg 1994). The duration of antibiotic therapy must be given individual consideration in light of an assessment of the integrity of the residual immune function and with the knowledge that most infections in HIV-positive individuals require prolonged therapy and sometimes chronic suppressive therapy. Because most of these individuals are in an advanced stage of HIV infection, they require a comprehensive immunological staging evaluation and most probably appropriate retroviral therapy. Osteomyelitis may require permanent antimicrobial maintenance.

Immune-mediated arthritis occurring with the same or increased intensity and frequency in individuals with selective depletion of CD4 lineage T cells

The epidemiology of rheumatic disease is altered in the setting of HIV infection. The development of certain specific rheumatic disorders, and the absence of others, in individuals infected with HIV is consistent with a classification of immune-mediated rheumatic illnesses according to a hypothetical underlying immune recognition event (Table 2). Classic rheumatic disorders associated with prominent autoantibody and cellular responses, such as rheumatoid arthritis and systemic lupus erythematosus, are rarely found among HIV-infected individuals and, when seen, are often (Bijlsma *et al.* 1988; Amor 1989; Calabrese *et al.* 1989; Molina *et al.* 1995) but not always (Kerr and Spiera 1991), reported to improve with progression of HIV infection. This decrease emphasizes the probable importance of CD4 T cells in their immunopathogenesis.

Reiter's disease, reactive arthritis, psoriatic arthritis, and undifferentiated spondylarthropathy syndromes

Because advancing HIV infection is characterized by progressive immune deficiency, it came as a considerable surprise that certain of the seronegative spondylarthropathies occurred with undiminished, if not increased, frequency in the setting of frank AIDS, despite the fact that these rheumatic diseases respond to iatrogenic immunosuppression (Winchester *et al.* 1987). Both the musculoskeletal system, in the form of the spondylarthropathies (Winchester *et al.* 1987), and the skin, in the form of psoriasiform disease (Duvic 1995), are distinctive clinical markers for advanced HIV infection. The distinctions between the various seronegative spondylarthropathies are blurred in the HIV-infected individual. While HIV-infected patients presenting with classic Reiter's syndrome are at one end of the spectrum and those with classical psoriasis and psoriatic arthritis at the other, many develop features of an undifferentiated spondylarthropathy with or without cutaneous manifestations. Moreover, in the setting of HIV infection, a subset of individuals with Reiter's syndrome have a more distinctively fulminant and extensive disorder simulating psoriatic arthritis with unusually severe enthesopathy, upper limb joint manifestations, and cutaneous involvement which often becomes indistinguishable from pustular psoriasis (Winchester *et al.* 1987). The development of these disorders emphasizes their distinct mechanisms of immunological drive independent from the CD4 lineage as well as the broad spectrum of host–virus relationships that can occur in HIV infection, although psoriasis in isolated form is not associated with decreased survival (Obuch *et al.* 1992). Behçet's disease may fall into this category since its development has been attributed to antecedent HIV infection (Buskila *et al.* 1991). Curiously, ankylosing spondylitis has not been noted to occur at the expected frequency in this group.

Epidemiology

The precise frequency with which Reiter's syndrome, psoriatic arthritis, and the related spondylarthropathies occur in HIV-positive individuals continues to be the subject of inquiry, although there is universal agreement that their prevalence is not decreased and in a number of studies is variably increased (Berman *et al.* 1991; Calabrese *et al.* 1991; Monteagudo *et al.* 1991; Cuellar *et al.* 1994). Prevalence rates of spondylopathic disorders among HIV-infected individuals in the United States ranging up to nearly 5 per cent have been reported when ascertainment was performed by rheumatologists (Berman *et al.* 1988; Winchester *et al.* 1988). Calabrese and colleagues in a longitudinal study found psoriatic arthritis and Reiter's syndrome each at a frequency of 1.7 per cent and undifferentiated forms of oligo- or monoarticular rheumatism at a frequency of

11.1 per cent (Calabrese *et al.* 1991). For some of these patients, the standardized criteria for Reiter's syndrome or psoriatic arthritis are not proving adequate for classification. The uncommon clinical features of the spondylarthropathies that occur in these patients have been pointed out by a number of authors (Winchester *et al.* 1987; Altman *et al.* 1994; Kellner *et al.* 1994). Psoriasiform skin disease, sometimes occurring with spondylarthropathic disease, occurs at increased frequency among those infected with HIV (Cockerell 1991; Duvic 1991; Duvic 1995). It appears that both forms of Reiter's syndrome, the sexually transmitted venereal or endemic form preceded and apparently initiated by urethritis, and the epidemic or postdysenteric form following infection of the gastrointestinal tract, are seen in association with advanced HIV infection. Using strict criteria, the prevalence rates of 'complete' Reiter's syndrome among HIV-infected individuals in the United States were not found to be higher than those for HIV-negative groups matched demographically (Solinger and Hess 1993) and by high-risk behaviour (Clark *et al.* 1989; Hochberg *et al.* 1990). However, in these same studies, the frequency of psoriatic arthritis was over fivefold higher than expected in the HIV-positive cohort when compared with a demographically matched population (Solinger and Hess 1993). Studies from West and sub-Saharan Africa have reported between four- and sixfold higher HIV prevalence rates among patients with various spondylarthropathies than among the local populations (Blanche *et al.* 1993; Mijiyawa 1993). Together, these observations strongly suggest that there is a causal relationship between HIV infection and the development of various spondylarthropathy syndromes; however, their clinical expression may differ in comparison with analogous syndromes in the HIV-negative host.

Psoriasiform lesions, with or without arthritis, may be the first clinical manifestations of HIV infection. Alternatively, in individuals with pre-existent psoriasis, infection with HIV may significantly exacerbate the psoriatic condition, including the joint manifestations. In general, psoriasiform lesions in HIV infection are of greater severity than in HIV-negative individuals and sometimes distinctive in distribution (Duvic *et al.* 1987; Duvic 1995). There is some divergence in studies on the prevalence of the psoriasiform disorders. Certain groups have found an increased prevalence of both psoriasiform lesions and musculoskeletal involvement plus psoriasiform skin lesions in HIV infection (Berman *et al.* 1988; Winchester *et al.* 1988; Solinger and Hess 1990; Calabrese *et al.* 1991). These studies have suggested that the prevalence of arthritis that resembles psoriatic arthritis in HIV infection is 1 to 3 per cent, compared with 0.05 to 0.14 per cent in HIV-negative individuals, and of psoriasiform lesions is 3 to 6 per cent, compared with 1 to 3 per cent in the HIV-negative population. Other studies have found similar prevalence rates of psoriasiform lesions but lower rates of arthritis, approximating those in the general population (Duvic *et al.* 1987; Kaplan *et al.* 1989). Possible explanations for these discrepancies may be differences in categorization of patients between centres, ethnic differences, variable use of diagnostic procedures such as confirmatory skin biopsies, and the high frequency of undifferentiated spondylarthropathy syndromes in HIV infection which do not meet criteria fully for either psoriatic arthritis or Reiter's syndrome.

Clinical features

The predominant finding in HIV-infected individuals with Reiter's syndrome is often relatively severe arthritis and enthesopathy, frequently accompanied by skin and nail disease (Fig. 9)

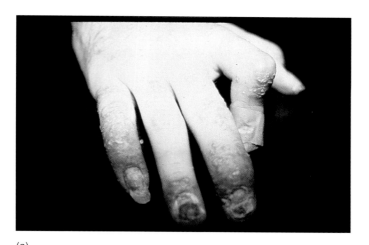

(a)

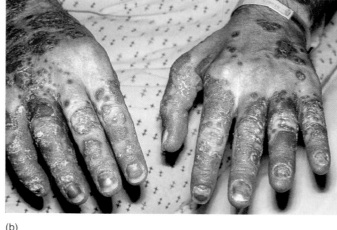

(b)

Fig. 9 Two patterns of HIV-associated spondylarthropathic hand involvement in HLA B27-positive persons; (a) illustrates findings typical of Reiter's syndrome, with onychodystrophy, subungual and acral hyperkeratosis, pseudoparonychia, fusiform swelling, and flexion contracture of the digits; (b) illustrates more extensive psoriasiform involvement of the skin of the hand and other parts of the body. Acral intensification and onychodystrophy are present.

(Winchester *et al.* 1987; Altman *et al.* 1994; Kellner *et al.* 1994). The course of the arthritis in HIV-associated Reiter's syndrome can take two general forms: an accumulative pattern evolving to full intensity over several weeks to months, or, more commonly, a milder intermittent pattern with recrudescences and remissions. The accumulative form is often associated with widespread polyarticular but asymmetric arthritis and is characterized by synovial thickening, erosions, and juxta-articular osteoporosis. The degree of upper extremity involvement and the accumulative pattern suggest features seen in psoriatic arthritis. The intermittent form usually has oligoarticular knee or ankle joint involvement and more closely resembles the clinical evolution of Reiter's syndrome in HIV-negative individuals. Enthesopathy is often unusually severe and profoundly disabling, while ocular involvement may be rather mild or absent. Cutaneous changes are usually striking in both intensity and extent. The distribution of cutaneous lesions is sometimes more like that found in pustular psoriasis.

The foot and ankle are the most commonly involved sites. Severe enthesopathy of the Achilles tendon, plantar fascia, and anterior or posterior tibial tendons may cause some patients to exhibit a characteristic broad-based 'AIDS' gait, walking with the feet in inversion and extension in an attempt to diminish pain by distributing weight on the lateral margins. New bone formation at the insertion of the Achilles tendon and/or plantar fascia may often be seen radiographically as typical fluffy periostitis. Multidigit dactylitis frequently occurs and, in combination with plantar fasciitis and extensor tenosynovitis, may simulate cellulitis or pedal oedema. While synovitis of the knee is prominent, hip disease and shoulder-girdle involvement are uncommon. The prevalence of axial involvement appears to be significantly less common than in the HIV-negative forms of the disease, with sacroiliitis only occasionally being seen, and spinal ankylosis very rarely. Synovitis at the elbow and wrist may result in early flexion contractures and fusion, while asymmetric involvement of the distal interphalangeal joints may cause progressive hand deformities (Fig. 9).

The cutaneous manifestations of HIV-associated Reiter's syndrome vary considerably from individual to individual, but are often very conspicuous and sustained, in contrast to HIV-negative

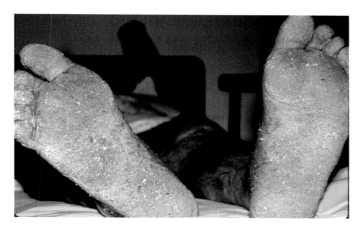

Fig. 10 Severe keratoderma blenorrhagica on the soles of an HIV-infected individual with lower limb arthritis and extensive psoriasiform skin lesions.

Reiter's syndrome. The most prominent is keratoderma blenorrhagicum, a papulosquamous and pustular eruption that usually occurs on the palms and soles. In some instances (Fig. 10), the sole is involved with a uniform dyskeratosis. The rash may spread progressively over the body in a pattern indistinguishable from pustular psoriasis, except that there is a greater tendency for involvement of the groin and intertriginous regions (inverse or sebopsoriasis). A progressive intensification of changes in the distal digits is often very prominent. Acrokeratosis is common, often associated with erythema and periungual pseudoparonychia formation. Severe alterations in the nails of the hands and feet often accompanies involvement of the distal interphalangeal joints, and is manifested clinically as onychodystrophy with or without subungual hyperkeratoses and yellow discoloration of the nails (Fig. 9). Milder degrees of onychodystrophy are present without involvement of the distal interphalangeal joints. Conjunctivitis and iritis appear to be much less prominent than in HIV-negative Reiter's syndrome.

The cutaneous psoriasiform manifestations include lesions of psoriasis vulgaris, guttate psoriasis, keratoderma or pustular psoriasis, sebopsoriasis of the groin and axilla, and erythroderma (Fig.

11). Among the spectrum of psoriasiform skin diseases in HIV-positive patients, atypical features are present that are not seen in classic psoriasis, suggesting the existence of distinct disease mechanisms (Kaplan *et al.* 1987). The spondylarthropathy-like peripheral musculoskeletal involvement is equivalent to that described above in the section on Reiter's disease and oligoarthritis syndromes, but also includes individuals with preponderant distal interphalangeal joint disease including pencil-in-cup deformities. The severity of psoriatic arthritis in HIV-positive individuals has been emphasized (Bulbul *et al.* 1995). Enthesopathy and dactylitis, especially of the foot, are particularly prominent. Onychodystrophy is a common presenting symptom and is highly correlated with arthritis, especially in distal interphalangeal joints of the hands or feet. A significant number of patients with psoriatic skin manifestations or onychodystrophy only have limited musculoskeletal findings, such as dactylitis or enthesopathy, and do not meet the criteria for psoriatic arthritis (Berman *et al.* 1988; Espinoza *et al.* 1988; Winchester *et al.* 1988).

Pathogenesis

The frequency of HLA B27 in HIV-positive Caucasian individuals with Reiter's syndrome approaches 80 per cent (Winchester *et al.* 1987; Berman *et al.* 1988; Forster *et al.* 1988), the same frequency observed in conventional Reiter's syndrome (Tiwari and Terasaki 1985). Over 30 per cent of cases are preceded by gastrointestinal infection with *Shigella flexneri*, *Salmonella* spp., *Yersinia enterocolitica* and *pseudotuberculosis*, and *Campylobacter jejuni* (Winchester *et al.* 1987; Forster *et al.* 1988). Temporal associations of Reiter's syndrome with infection by other organisms, including *Giardia lamblia* and atypical *Mycobacteria* spp., have also been observed but are of unknown significance (Winchester *et al.* 1987). High titres of antichlamydial antibodies have been reported in 33 per cent of HIV-positive individuals not necessarily afflicted with Reiter's syndrome, compared with 1.7 per cent in normal subjects (Gutierrez *et al.* 1990).

Whereas psoriasis vulgaris and psoriatic arthritis in the general population are associated with increased frequencies of HLA class I alleles Cw6, B13, B17, and B38 (White *et al.* 1972; Arnett 1985), no HLA associations have been detected with these disorders in HIV-infected individuals in two independent studies (Duvic *et al.* 1987; Winchester *et al.* 1988), suggesting differences in underlying pathogenesis and further arguing against a necessity for these conditions to occur at similar frequencies. In contrast, the presence of pustular psoriasis, and the arthritis that may accompany it, is associated with an increased frequency of HLA B27 in both HIV-negative and HIV-positive individuals (Arnett 1985; Winchester *et al.* 1988). It is this subgroup that most resembles Reiter's syndrome.

Progressive depletion of CD4 cells in HIV infection may be a permissive factor for greater severity, and possibly increased prevalence, of Reiter's syndrome by allowing the establishment of persistent infection with, or greater invasiveness of, gut micro-organisms such as *C. jejuni* (Perlman *et al.* 1988), or by diminishing help for B-cell dependent bacterial clearance mechanisms, which have been shown to be important in attenuating experimental chlamydial arthritis (Rank *et al.* 1988). In addition to quantitative depletion of CD4 cells, infection with HIV also leads to qualitative defects reflected by diminished interleukin 2 production following antigenic challenge (Antonen and Krohn 1986). Such defects have been observed in HLA B27-positive individuals developing Reiter's syndrome after a salmonella epidemic (Inman *et al.* 1989), and may

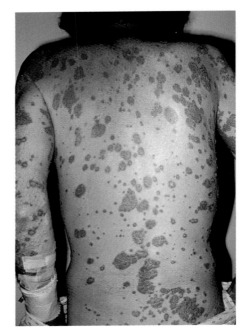

(a)

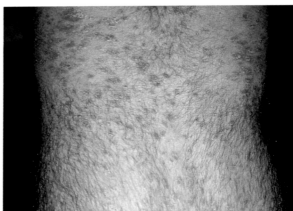

(b)

Fig. 11 Two patterns of psoriasiform skin involvement; (a) shows extensive psoriasiform involvement of the trunk in the HIV-infected patient shown in Fig. 9(a), initially presenting with features of Reiter's syndrome and progressing to severe multijoint arthritis with deformities. Extensive involvement of intertriginous areas (sebopsoriasis) was present; (b) illustrates psoriasis vulgaris in an HIV-positive person without significant arthritis.

contribute to selective microbial persistence and the development of Reiter's syndrome in HIV-infected individuals.

Biopsy of involved tissue in HIV-associated psoriasis is superficially similar to that in the idiopathic variety, demonstrating epidermal proliferation, dermal inflammatory cell infiltrate, tortuous dermal capillaries, and decreased numbers of epidermal Langerhans cells. Similar blood vessel changes, inflammatory cell infiltrate, and proliferative tissue are also present in psoriatic synovium (Espinoza *et al.* 1982). The depletion of epidermal Langerhans cells, which are CD4+ and readily infected by HIV *in vivo* (Belsito *et al.* 1984; Grelen *et al.* 1987), may be a permissive factor for the development of psoriatic lesions. In addition, products of the HIV proviral DNA may directly cause epidermal proliferation (Ensoli *et al.* 1990). In this regard, mice transgenic for the HIV *tat* gene preferentially express the tat protein in the skin and develop epidermal hyperkeratosis and acanthosis (Vogel *et al.* 1988). There is growing evidence for the participation of CD8 T cells in the pathogenesis of psoriasis and in the effect of cytokines (Duvic 1991; Winchester 1994).

The occurrence of these entities in the setting of HIV-induced immunosuppression and CD4 T-cell depletion suggests that the critical cells involved in disease pathogenesis may be residual components of the immune system, such as CD8 T lymphocytes or cells of the monocyte lineage. Indeed, immunopathological studies of synovium from HIV-infected patients with Reiter's syndrome demonstrate a lymphocytic infiltrate that is predominantly CD8+ (Espinoza *et al.* 1990). As the natural ligand for the CD8 structure on the surface of cytotoxic/suppressor cells is an MHC class I molecule such as HLA B27, we have postulated that, in Reiter's syndrome, cells of the CD8 lineage may be critically involved in an immune recognition event interacting with a particular antigen presented by HLA B27 molecules on the surface of cells of the monocyte/macrophage lineage (Meiser *et al.* 1982; Swain 1983) (Table 2). Two mechanistic hypotheses appear likely. In one, the pathogenesis of the spondylarthropathy is the same as when it occurs in a person not infected with HIV, while in the other, HIV-encoded peptides play an aetiological role in the rheumatic disease. HIV has been cultured from synovial fluid (Withington *et al.* 1987), abundant p24 antigen can be demonstrated in synovial tissue (Forster *et al.* 1988; Espinoza *et al.* 1990), and HIV DNA has been detected in synovial dendritic cells (Hughes *et al.* 1990), suggesting that the cellular infiltrate may, at least in part, be reactive to retroviral peptides. Parallel transactivation of HIV in this inflammatory milieu (Siekevitz *et al.* 1987) may act to increase HIV replication within these activated monocytes and T cells and lead to more rapid progression to AIDS. In support of this possibility is the fact that the appearance of Reiter's syndrome is an unfavourable prognostic sign, with many patients developing their first opportunistic infection within several months after the initial manifestations of Reiter's syndrome (Winchester *et al.* 1988).

Infectious agents thought to trigger psoriasis in the general population include streptococci in guttate psoriasis (Whyte and Baughman 1964) and staphylococci in pustular psoriasis (McFayden and Lyell 1971). Both organisms have also been implicated in psoriatic arthropathy (Mustakellio and Lassus 1964; Vasey *et al.* 1982). In HIV infection, the presence of psoriasis or psoriatic arthritis has been reported to be exacerbated by staphylococcal infections in almost 50 per cent of individuals (Duvic *et al.* 1987).

Treatment

The management of these entities is a difficult challenge (Duvic *et al.* 1987; Kaplan *et al.* 1989). Joint erosions, ankylosis, and osteolysis, together with chronic or recurrent enthesopathy, can rapidly lead to fibrosis, deformity, and functional disability. These are frequently compounded by generalized weakness, resulting from progressive muscle loss, and cachexia. Physical and rehabilitative therapy to maintain joint range of motion, prevent contractures, and strengthen muscle function is a central component in the comprehensive care of these patients. Optimal management involves a team-oriented approach including rheumatologists, physical and occupational therapists, and mental health care experts for management of the reactive depression that frequently accompanies the severe physical disability.

While the musculoskeletal pain and inflammation in mild cases may respond to conventional non-steroidal anti-inflammatory agents, severe manifestations of the spondylarthropathy syndromes in HIV infection are more effectively treated with phenylbutazone, given in 100 mg doses twice to three times daily. Monitoring of haematological parameters is recommended during this therapy, although no untoward cytopenias have been observed. Sulphasalazine, at doses of 0.5 to 1.5 g twice daily, may be administered together with phenylbutazone in severe cases. While controlled studies have not been performed, at least one-third of patients respond to this slow-acting drug. Maintenance sulphasalazine therapy is continued while phenylbutazone is gradually withdrawn. Intra-articular corticosteroid injection may sometimes be beneficial, and has not been associated with deleterious effects, in contrast to systemic corticosteroids which may cause extensive candidiasis and opportunistic infections in these patients (Duvic *et al.* 1987; Winchester *et al.* 1987). Prolonged and aggressive antibiotic therapy may, in theory, be of benefit in diminishing microbial persistence. Etretinate has been reported to be particularly efficacious in the treatment of both the joint and cutaneous manifestations of severe Reiter's syndrome previously unresponsive to non-steroidal anti-inflammatory drugs and topical corticosteroids, and in psoriasis (Belz *et al.* 1989; Louthrenoo 1993).

Zidovudine has been reported to improve skin disease (Ruzicka *et al.* 1987; Kaplan *et al.* 1989). In an unblinded study, 90 per cent of HIV-infected persons had either partial or complete improvement of their psoriatic skin disease following zidovudine treatment at a dosage of 1200 mg/day (Duvic *et al.* 1994). The associated arthritis in these individuals, however, did not improve with zidovudine. While zidovudine has no documented beneficial effect on the arthritic symptoms *per se*, therapy with this agent should be considered in all patients with Reiter's syndrome, whether presenting at advanced stages of immunosuppression or as the initial manifestation of HIV infection, in order to prevent the enhanced HIV replication that may secondarily occur as a result of CD4 cell activation. Zidovudine-induced myopathy may become a confounding variable.

Methotrexate and other immunosuppressive agents are capable of strikingly ameliorating the skin and joint disease (Winchester *et al.* 1987; Maurer *et al.* 1994), but they should be used only with great caution because their use has been followed by the development of frank AIDS and death from opportunistic infection (Winchester *et al.* 1987). However, methotrexate administered to three individuals with HIV-associated psoriatic arthritis did not worsen the underlying immune deficiency in two of the three (Maurer *et al.* 1994), suggesting that it may have a limited place when used cautiously. Phototherapy has been asserted to be helpful and without evident problems (Ranki *et al.* 1991; Meola *et al.* 1993), but has also been associated with the appearance or exacerbation of Kaposi's sarcoma (Duvic *et al.* 1987) and the possibility of HIV activation has been emphasized (Duvic 1995). Studies in mice transgenic for HIV have shown that HIV may be activated by ultraviolet radiation, raising concerns for the use of phototherapy in humans (Morrey *et al.* 1991; Vogel *et al.* 1992). These mainstays of therapy in the HIV-negative patient with psoriasis or psoriatic arthritis are probably best reserved for very difficult situations that have failed to respond to all other approaches, because their mode of action parallels the consequences of HIV infection, although continued experimental experience with these therapies may define a risk–benefit balance that is acceptable in certain situations.

References

Adebajo, A. and Davis, P. (1994). Rheumatic diseases in African blacks. *Seminars in Arthritis and. Rheumatism*, 24, 139–53.

Altman, E.M., Centeno, L.V., Mahal, M., and Bielory, L. (1994). AIDS-associated Reiter's syndrome. *Annals of Allergy*, 72, 307–16.

Amor, B. (1989). Rheumatoid arthritis and AIDS. *Journal of Rheumatology*, 16, 845.

Anders, K.H., Latta, H., Chang, B.S., Tomiyasu, U., Quddusi, A.S., and Vinters, H.V. (1989). Lymphoid granulomatosis and malignant lymphoma of the central nervous system in acquired immunodeficiency syndrome. *Human Pathology*, 20,326–34.

Angulo, J.C., Lopez, J.I., Garcia, M.E., Peiro, J., and Flores, N. (1994). HIV infection presenting as renal polyarteritis nodosa. *International Urology and Nephrology*, 26, 637–41.

Antonen, J. and Krohn, K. (1986). Interleukin 2 production in HTLV III/LAV infection. Evidence of defective antigen-induced, but normal mitogen-induced, IL-2 production. *Clinical and Experimental Immunology*, 65, 489–96.

Arnett, F.C. (1985). Psoriatic arthritis: relationship to other spondyloarthropathies. In *Psoriatic arthritis* (ed. L.H. Gerber and L.R. Espinoza), p. 95. Grune and Stratton, Orlando, FL.

Arthur, L.O. *et al.* (1992). Cellular proteins bound to immunodeficiency viruses: implications for pathogenesis and vaccines. *Science*, 258, 1935–8.

Bacchetti, P. and Moss, A.R. (1989). Incubation time of AIDS in San Francisco. *Nature*, 338, 251–3.

Baguley, E., Wolfe, C., and Hughes, G.R. (1988). Dermatomyositis in HIV infection. *British Journal of Rheumatology*, 27, 493–500.

Bardin, T. *et al.* (1987). Necrotizing vasculitis in human immunodeficiency virus (HIV) infection. (Abstract.) *Arthritis and Rheumatism*, 30, S105.

Bass, P.S. *et al.* (1994). AIDS presenting as focal segmental membranous glomerulopathy. *Journal of Clinical Pathology*, 47, 179–81.

Belsito, D.V., Sanchez, M.R., Baer, R.L., Valentine, F., and Thorbecke, G.J. (1984). Reduced Langerhans cell IA antigen and ATPase activity in patients with AIDS. *New England Journal of Medicine*, 310, 1279–82.

Belz, J., Breneman, D.L., Nordlund, J.J., and Solinger, A. (1989). Successful treatment of a patient with Reiter's syndrome and acquired immunodeficiency syndrome using etretinate. *Journal of the American Academy of Dermatology*, 20, 898–903.

Berman, A. *et al.* (1988). Rheumatic manifestations of human immunodeficiency virus infection. *American Journal of Medicine*, 85, 59–64.

Berman, A., Reboredo, G., Spindler, A., Lasala, M.E., Lopez, H., and Espinoza, L.R. (1991). Rheumatic manifestations in populations at risk for HIV infection: the added effect of HIV. *Journal of Rheumatology*, 18, 1564–7.

Bernard, C., Exquis, B., Reber, A., and de Moerloose, P. (1990). Determination of anticardiolipin and other antibodies in HIV-1 infected patients. *Journal of Acquired Immune Deficiency Syndromes*, 3, 536–9.

Bijlsma, J.W., Derksen, R.W., Huber-Bruning, O., and Borleffs, J.C. (1988). Does AIDS 'cure' rheumatoid arthritis? *Annals of the Rheumatic Diseases*, 47, 350–1.

Blanche, P. *et al.* (1993). Acute arthritis and human immunodeficiency virus infection in Rwanda. *Journal of Rheumatology*, 20, 2123–7.

Blumenthal, D.R., Zucker, J.R., and Hawkins, C.C. (1990). *Mycobacterium avium* complex-induced septic arthritis and osteomyelitis in a patient with the acquired immunodeficiency syndrome. *Arthritis and Rheumatism*, 33,757.

Boix, V., Tovar, J., and Martin-Hidalgo, A. (1990). Candida spondylodiscitis, chronic illness due to heroin analgesia in an HIV positive person. *Journal of Rheumatology*, 17, 563.

Bourgoignie, J.J. (1990). Renal complications of human immunodeficiency virus type l. *Kidney International*, 37, 1571–84.

Bourgoignie, J.J., Meneses, R., and Pardo, V. (1988*a*). The nephropathy related to acquired immune deficiency syndrome. *Advances in Nephrology from the Necker Hospital*, 17, 113–26.

Bourgoignie, J.J., Meneses, R., Ortiz, C., Jaffe, D., and Pardo, V. (1988*b*). The clinical spectrum of renal disease associated with human immunodeficiency virus. *American Journal of Kidney Disease*, 12, 131–7.

Bourgoignie, J.J., Ortiz Interian, C., Green, D.F., and Roth, D. (1989). Race, a cofactor in HIV-1-associated nephropathy. *Transplantation Proceedings*, 21, 3899–901.

Bulbul, R., Williams, W.V., and Schumacher, H.R., Jr. (1995). Psoriatic arthritis. Diverse and sometimes highly destructive. *Postgraduate Medicine*, 97, 97–9, 103–6.

Burgoyne, M., Agudelo, C., and Pisko, E. (1992). Chronic syphilitic polyarthritis mimicking systemic lupus erythematosus/rheumatoid arthritis as the initial presentation of human immunodeficiency virus infection. *Journal of Rheumatology*, 19, 313–15.

Burman, W.J., Cohn, D.L., Reves, R.R., and Wilson, M.L. (1995). Multifocal cellulitis and monoarticular arthritis as manifestations of *Helicobacter cinaedi* bacteremia. *Clinical Infectious Diseases*, 20, 564–70.

Buskila, D. and Tenenbaum, J. (1989). Septic bursitis in human immunodeficiency virus infection. *Journal of Rheumatology*, 16, 1374.

Buskila, D., Gladman, D.D., Gilmore, J., and Salit, I.E. (1991). Behçet's disease in a patient with immunodeficiency virus infection. *Annals of the Rheumatic Diseases*, 50, 115–16.

Buyon, J.P. *et al.* (1989). Acquired congenital heart block. *Journal of Clinical Investigation*, 84, 627–34.

Calabrese, L.H. (1989). The rheumatic manifestations of infection with the human immunodeficiency virus. *Seminars in Arthritis and Rheumatism*, 18, 225.

Calabrese, L.H. (1991). Vasculitis and infection with the human immunodeficiency virus. *Rheumatic Diseases Clinics of North America*, 17, 131–47.

Calabrese, L.H., Wilke, W.S., Perkins, A.D., and Tubbs, R.R. (1989). Rheumatoid arthritis complicated by infection with the human immunodeficiency virus and the development of Sjögren's syndrome. *Arthritis and Rheumatism*, 32, 1453–7.

Calabrese, L.H., Kelley, D.M., Myers, A., O'Connell, M., and Easley, K. (1991). Rheumatic symptoms and human immunodeficiency virus infection. The influence of clinical and laboratory variables in a longitudinal cohort study. *Arthritis and Rheumatism*, 34, 257–63.

Canoso, R.T., Zon, L.I., and Groopman, J.E. (1987). Anticardiolipin antibodies associated with HTLV-III infection. *British Journal of Haematology*, 65, 495–8.

Carbone, L., D'Agati, V., Cheng, J.T., and Appel, G.B. (1989). Course and prognosis of human immunodeficiency virus-associated nephropathy. *American Journal of Medicine*, 87, 389–95.

Chander, P. and Treser, G. (1987). Ultrastructural markers of AIDS nephropathy. (Abstract.) *Kidney International*, 31, 335.

Chariot, P. *et al.* (1994). Determination of the blood lactate:pyruvate ratio as a noninvasive test for the diagnosis of zidovudine myopathy. *Arthritis and Rheumatism*, 37, 583–6.

Cheng Mayer, C., Shioda, T., and Levy, J.A. (1991). Host range, replicative, and cytopathic properties of human immunodeficiency virus type l are determined by very few amino acid changes in tat and gp120. *Journal of Virology*, 65, 6931–41.

Chisholm, D.M. and Mason, D.K. (1968). Labial salivary gland biopsy in Sjögren's disease. *Journal of Clinical Pathology*, 21, 656.

Chren, M.M., Silverman, R.A., Sorsensen, R.U., and Elmets, C.A. (1989). Leukocytoclastic vasculitis in a patient infected with human immunodeficiency virus. *Journal of the American Academy of Dermatology*, 21, 1161–4.

Clark, M., Kinsolving, M., and Chernoff, D. (1989). The prevalence of arthritis in two HIV-infected cohorts. (Abstract.) *Arthritis and Rheumatism*, 32, S585.

Cockerell, C.J. (1991). Human immunodeficiency virus infection and the skin. A crucial interface. *Archives of Internal Medicine*, 151, 1295–303.

Connor, E. *et al.* (1988). Acquired immunodeficiency syndrome-associated renal disease in children. *Journal of Pediatrics*, 113, 39–44.

Connor, R.I., Mohri, H., Cao, Y., and Ho, D.D. (1993). Increased viral burden and cytopathicity correlate temporally with CD4+ T-lymphocyte decline and clinical progression in human immunodeficiency virus type 1-infected individuals. *Journal of Virology*, 67, 1772–7.

Cooper, L.M. and Patterson, J.A.K. (1989). Allergic granulomatosis and angiitis of Churg–Strauss: case report in a patient with antibodies to human immunodeficiency virus and hepatitis B virus. *International Journal of Dermatology*, 28, 597.

Couderc, L.J., D'Agay, M.F., Danon, F., Harzic, M., Brocheriou, C., and Clauvel, J.P. (1987). Sicca complex and infection with human immunodeficiency virus. *Archives of Internal Medicine*, 147, 898–901.

Covelli, M., Lapadula, G., Pipitone, N., Numo, R., and Pipitone, V. (1993). Isolated sternoclavicular joint arthritis in heroin addicts and/or HIV positive patients: three cases. *Clinical Rheumatology*, 12, 422–5.

Crawford, E.J.P. and Baird, P.R.E. (1987). An orthopedic presentation of AIDS: brief report. *Journal of Bone and Joint Surgery*, **69B**, 672.

Cuellar, M.L., Silveira, L.H., and Espinoza, L.R. (1994). Recent developments in psoriatic arthritis. *Current Opinion in Rheumatology*, **6**, 378–84.

D'Agati, V., Suh, J.I., Carbone, L., Cheng, J.T., and Appel, G. (1989). Pathology of HIV-associated nephropathy: a detailed morphologic and comparative study. *Kidney International*, **35**, 1358–70.

Dalakas, M.C. and Pezeshkpour, G.H. (1988). Neuromuscular diseases associated with human immunodeficiency virus infection. *Annals of Neurology*, **23**, S38–S48.

Dalakas, M.C., Pezeshkpour, G.H., Gravell, M., and Sever, J.L. (1986). Polymyositis associated with AIDS retrovirus. *Journal of the American Medical Association*, **256**, 2381–3.

Dalakas, M.C., Pezeshkpour, G.H., and Flaherty, M. (1987). Progressive nemaline (rod) myopathy associated with HIV infection. *New England Journal of Medicine*, **317**, 1602–3.

Dalakas, M.C., Illa, I., Pezeshkpour, G.H., Laukaitis, J.P., Cohen, B., and Griffin, J.L. (1990). Mitochondrial myopathy caused by long-term zidovudine therapy. *New England Journal of Medicine*, **322**, 1098–105.

De Wolf, F. *et al.* (1988). Numbers of CD4+ cells and the levels of core antigens of and antibodies to the human immunodeficiency virus as predictors of AIDS among seropositive homosexual men. *Journal of Infectious Diseases*, **158**, 615–22.

Dorsett, B.H., Cronin, W., and Joachim, H.L. (1990). Presence and prognostic significance of antilymphocyte antibodies in symptomatic and asymptomatic human immunodeficiency virus infection. *Archives of Internal Medicine*, **150**, 1025–8.

Duvic, M. (1991). Papulosquamous disorders associated with human immunodeficiency virus infection. *Dermatologic Clinics*, **9**, 523–30.

Duvic, M. (1995). Human immunodeficiency virus and the skin: selected controversies. *Journal of Investigative Dermatology*, **105**, 117S–121S.

Duvic, M., Johnson, T.M., Rapini, R.P., Freeze, T., Brewton, G., and Rios, A. (1987). Acquired immunodeficiency syndrome associated psoriasis and Reiter's syndrome. *Archives of Dermatology*, **123**, 1622–32.

Duvic, M., Crane, M.M., Conant, M., Mahoney, S.E., Reveille, J.D., and Lehrman, S.N. (1994). Zidovudine improves psoriasis in human immunodeficiency virus-positive males. *Archives of Dermatology*, **130**, 447–51.

Dwyer, E., Itescu, S., and Winchester, R. (1993). Characterization of the primary structure of T-cell receptor β-chains in cells infiltrating the salivary gland in the sicca syndrome of HIV-1 infection. Evidence of antigen-driven clonal selection suggested by restricted combinations of VβJβ gene segment usage and shared somatically encoded amino acid residues. *Journal of Clinical Investigation*, **92**, 495–502.

Eidelberg, D., Sotrel, A., Horoupian, D.S., Neumann, P.E., Pumarola-Sune, T., and Price, R.W. (1986). Thrombotic cerebral vasculopathy associated with herpes zoster. *Annals of Neurology*, **19**, 7–14.

Ensoli, B., Barillari, G., Salahuddin, S.Z., Gallo, R.C., and Wong-Staal, F. (1990). Tat protein of HIV-1 stimulates growth of cells derived from Kaposi's sarcoma lesions of AIDS patients. *Nature*, **345**, 84–6.

Espinoza, L.R., Vasey, F.B., Espinoza, T.S., and Germain, B.F. (1982). Vascular changes in psoriatic synovium. A light and electron microscopic study. *Arthritis and Rheumatism*, **25**, 677–84.

Espinoza, L.R., Berman, A., Vasey, F.B., Cahalin, C., Nelson, R., and Germain, B.F. (1988). Psoriatic arthritis and acquired immunodeficiency syndrome. *Arthritis and Rheumatism*, **31**, 1034–40.

Espinoza, L.R. *et al.* (1990). HIV-associated arthropathy: HIV antigen demonstration in the synovial membrane. *Journal of Rheumatology*, **17**, 1195–201.

Espinoza, L.R. *et al.* (1991). Characteristics and pathogenesis of myositis in human immunodeficiency virus infection — distinction from azidothymidine-induced myopathy. *Rheumatic Diseases Clinics of North America*, **17**, 117–29.

Fahey, J.L. (1986). Immunologic aspects of human immunodeficiency virus infection and AIDS. *Clinical Aspects of Autoimmunity*, **1**, 12–33.

Farthing, C.F., Staughton, R.C.D., and Rowland Payne, C.M.E. (1985). Skin disease in homosexual patients with acquired immune deficiency syndrome (AIDS) and lesser forms of human T cell leukaemia virus (HTLV-III) disease. *Clinical and Experimental Dermatology*, **10**, 3.

Fauci, A.S. (1988). The human immunodeficiency virus: infectivity and mechanisms of pathogenesis. *Science*, **239**, 617–22.

Felber, B.K., Hadzopoulou-Cladaras, M., Cladaras, C., Copeland, T., and Pavlakis, G.N. (1989). Rev protein of human immunodeficiency virus type 1 affects the stability and transport of the viral mRNA. *Proceedings of the National Academy of Sciences (USA)*, **86**, 1495–9.

Fernandez-Vina, M., Shumway, J.W., and Stastny, P. (1990). DNA typing for class II HLA antigens with allele-specific or group specific amplification. II. Typing for alleles of the DRw52-associated group. *Human Immunology*, **28**, 51–64.

Fischl, M.A., Dickinson, G.M., Scott, G.B., Klunias, N., Fletcher, M.A., and Parks, W. (1987). Evaluation of heterosexual partners, children and household contacts of adults with AIDS. *Journal of the American Medical Association*, **257**, 640.

Forster, S.M. *et al.* (1988). Inflammatory joint disease and human immunodeficiency virus infection. *British Medical Journal*, **296**, 1625–7.

Fox, R.I., Robinson, C.A., Curd, J.G., Kozin, F., and Howell, F.V. (1986). Sjögren's syndrome: criteria for classification. *Arthritis and Rheumatism*, **29**, 577.

Friedland, G.H. *et al.* (1986). Lack of transmission of HTLV-III/LAV infection to household contacts of patients with AIDS or ARC with oral candidiasis. *New England Journal of Medicine*, **314**, 344.

Gaut, P., Wong, P.K., and Meyer, R.D. (1988). Pyomyositis in a patient with the acquired immunodeficiency syndrome. *Archives of Internal Medicine*, **148**, 1608–10.

Gherardi, R., Lebargy, F., Gaulard, P., Mhiri, C., Bernaudin, J.F., and Gray, F. (1989). Necrotizing vasculitis and HIV replication in peripheral nerves. *New England Journal of Medicine*, **321**, 685–6.

Gherardi, R. *et al.* (1993). The spectrum of vasculitis in human immunodeficiency virus-infected patients. A clinicopathologic evaluation. *Arthritis and Rheumatism*, **36**, 1164–74.

Goedert, J.J. *et al.* (1987). Effect of T4 count and cofactors on the incidence of AIDS in homosexual men infected with human immunodeficiency virus. *Journal of the American Medical Association*, **257**, 331–4.

Golden, M.P., Hammer, S.M., Wanke, C.A., and Albrecht, M.A. (1994). Cytomegalovirus vasculitis. Case reports and review of the literature. *Medicine*, **73**, 246–55.

Goldenberg, D.L. (1991). Septic arthritis and other infections of rheumatologic significance. *Rheumatic Diseases Clinics of North America*, **17**, 149–56.

Goldenberg, D.L. (1994). Bacterial arthritis. *Current Opinion in Rheumatology*, **6**, 394–400.

Golding, H. *et al.* (1988). Identification of homologous regions in HIV-Igp 41 and human MHC class II β1 domain. I. Monoclonal antibodies against the gp41-derived peptide and patients' sera react with native HLA class II antigens, suggesting a role for autoimmunity in the pathogenesis of AIDS. *Journal of Experimental Medicine*, **167**, 914–23.

Greene, W.C. (1991). The molecular biology of HIV type 1 infection. *New England Journal of Medicine*, **324**, 308–17.

Grelen, V., Schnitt, D., Degritter-Dambuyant, C., Nicholas, J.F., and Thivolet, J. (1987). AIDS and Langerhans cells: CD1, CD4 and HLA class II antigen expression. *Journal of Investigative Dermatology*, **89**, 324A.

Gutierrez, F. *et al.* (1990). Serologic evidence for chlamydia infection in human immunodeficiency virus-infected patients. (Abstract.) *Revista Mexicana de Reumatologia*, **5**, 62.

Gutierrez, C., Cruz, L., Olive, A., Tena, X., Romeu, J., and Raventos, A. (1993). Salmonella septic arthritis in HIV patients. *British Journal of Rheumatology*, **32**, 88.

Guy, B. *et al.* (1987). HIV F/3. orf encodes a phosphorylated GTP-binding protein resembling an oncogene product. *Nature*, **330**, 266–9.

Guyot, D.R., Manoli, A.II, and Kling, G.A. (1987). Pyogenic sacroiliitis in IV drug abusers. *American Journal of Roentgenology*, **149**, 1209–11.

Haddoum, F., Dosquet, P., Mougenot, B., Bourrat, E., Viron, B., and Mignon, F. (1987). Nephrotic syndrome disclosing AIDS. *Presse Medicale*, **16**, 1373.

Haverkos, H.W., Gotlieb, M.S., Killen, J.Y., and Edelman, R. (1985). Classification of HTLV-III/LAV-related diseases. *Journal of Infectious Diseases*, **152**, 1095.

Heller, H.M. and Fuhrer, J. (1991). Disseminated sporotrichosis in patients with AIDS: case report and review of the literature. *AIDS*, **5**, 1243–6.

Ho, G., Jr. (1993). Bacterial arthritis. *Current Opinion in Rheumatology*, **5**, 449–53.

Hochberg, M.C., Fox, R., Nelson, K.E., and Saah, A. (1990). HIV infection is not associated with Reiter's syndrome: data from the Johns Hopkins Multicenter AIDS cohort study. *AIDS*, **4**, 1149–51.

Hughes, R.A., Macatonia, S.E., Rowe, I.F., Keat, A.C., and Knight, S.C. (1990). The detection of HIV DNA in dendritic cells from the joints of patients with aseptic arthritis. *British Journal of Rheumatology*, **29**, 166–70.

Hughes, R.A., Rowe, I.F., Shanson, D., and Keat, A.C. (1992). Septic bone, joint and muscle lesions associated with human immunodeficiency virus infection. *British Journal of Rheumatology*, **31**, 381–8.

Hwang, S.S., Boyle, T.J., Lyerly, H.K., and Cullen, B.R. (1991). Identification of the envelope V3 loop as the primary determinant of cell tropism in HIV-1. *Science*, **253**, 71–3.

Ifudu, O., Rao, T.K.S., Tan, C.C., Fleischman, H., Chirgwin, K., and Friedman, E.A. (1994). Zidovudine improves prognosis in HIV-associated nephropathy. *Journal of the American Society of Nephrology*, **4**, 277.

Ingulli, E., Tejani, A., Fikrig, S., Nicastri, A., Chen, C.K., and Pomrantz, A. (1991). Nephrotic syndrome associated with acquired immunodeficiency syndrome in children. *Journal of Pediatrics*, **119**, 710–16.

Inman, R.D., Chiu, B., Johnson, M.E., Vas, S., and Falk, J. (1989). HLA class I-related impairment in IL-2 production and lymphocyte response to microbial antigens in reactive arthritis. *Journal of Immunology*, **142**, 4256–360.

Itescu, S. (1991). Diffuse infiltrative lymphocytosis syndrome in human immuno-deficiency virus infection — a Sjögren's-like disease. In *Rheumatic disease clinics of North America*, Vol. 17, No. 1: *AIDS and rheumatic disease* (ed. R. Winchester), pp. 99–115. W.B. Saunders, Philadelphia.

Itescu, S., Brancato, L.J., and Winchester, R. (1989). A sicca syndrome in HIV infection: association with HLA-DR5 and CD8 lymphocytosis. *Lancet*, **ii**, 466–8.

Itescu, S. *et al.* (1990). A diffuse infiltrative CD8 lymphocytosis syndrome in human immunodeficiency virus (HIV) infection: a host immune response associated with HLA-DR5. *Annals of Internal Medicine*, **112**, 3–10.

Itescu, S., Dalton, J., Zhang, H., and Winchester, R. (1993). Tissue infiltration in a CD8 lymphocytosis syndrome associated with human immunodeficiency virus-1 infection has the phenotypic appearence of an antigenically driven response. *Journal of Clinical Investigation*, **91**, 2216–25.

Itescu, S., Simonelli, P.F., Winchester, R.J., and Ginsberg, H.S. (1994*a*). Human immunodeficiency virus type 1 strains in the lungs of infected individuals evolve independently from those in peripheral blood and are highly conserved in the C-terminal region of the envelope V3 loop. *Proceedings of the National Academy of Sciences* (*USA*), **91**, 11378–82.

Itescu, S., Rose, S., Dwyer, E., and Winchester, R. (1994*b*). Certain HLA-DR5 and -DR6 major histocompatibility complex class II alleles are associated with a CD8 lymphocytic host response to human immunodeficiency virus type 1 characterized by low lymphocyte viral strain heterogeneity and slow disease progression. *Proceedings of the National Academy of Sciences* (*USA*), **91**, 11472–6.

Jacobson, M.A., Geller, H., and Chambers, H. (1988). *Staphylococcus aureus* bacter-emia and recurrent staphylococcal infection in patients with acquired immunodeficiency syndrome and AIDS-related complex. *American Journal of Medicine*, **85**, 172.

Javaherian, K. *et al.* (1989). Principal neutralizing domain of the human immuno-deficiency virus type 1 envelope protein. *Proceedings of the National Academy of Sciences* (*USA*), **86**, 6768–72.

Johnson, A.H., Rosen-Bronson, S., and Hurley, C.K. (1989). Heterogeneity of the HLA-D region in American Blacks. *Transplantation Proceedings*, **21**, 3872–3.

Jurgensen, O., Altermatt, H.J., von Overbeck, J., and Berthold, H. (1995). Necrotizing vasculitis of the tongue. A contribution to the differential diagnosis of ulcerative mucosal changes in HIV-infected patients. *Schweizer Monatsschrift für Zahnmedizin*, **105**, 54–62.

Kalden, J.R. and Gay, S. (1994). Retroviruses and autoimmune rheumatic diseases. *Clinical and.Experimental Immunology*, **98**,1–5.

Kaplan, M.H., Sadick, N., McNutt, S., Meltzer, M., Sarngadharan, M.G., and Pahwa, S. (1987). Dermatologic findings and manifestations of acquired immunodeficiency syndrome (AIDS). *Journal of the American Academy of Dermatology*, **16**, 485–506.

Kaplan, M.H., Sadick, N.S., Weider, J., Farber, B.F., and Neidt, G.W. (1989). Anti-psoriatic effects of zidovudine in HIV-associated psoriasis. *Journal of the American Academy of Dermatology*, **20**, 76–82.

Kaslow, R.A., Duquesnoy, R., VanRaden, M., Kingsley, L., and Mann, D. (1990). A1, Cw7, B8, DR3 HLA antigen combination associated with rapid decline of T-helper lymphocytes in HIV-1 infection. *Lancet*, **335**, 927–30.

Kellner, H., Fuessl, H.S., and Herzer, P. (1994). Seronegative spondylarthropathies in HIV-infected patients: further evidence of uncommon clinical features. *Rheumatology International*, **13**, 211–13.

Kerr, L.D. and Spiera, H. (1991). The coexistence of active classic rheumatoid arthritis and AIDS. *Journal of Rheumatology*, **18**, 1739–40.

Kirchhoff, F., Greenough, T.C., Brettler, D.B., Sullivan, J.L., and Desrosiers, R.C. (1995). Brief report: absence of intact nef sequences in a long-term survivor with nonprogressive HIV-1 infection. *New England Journal of Medicine*, **332**, 228–32.

Klaassen, R.J. *et al.* (1992). Anti-neutrophil cytoplasmic autoantibodies in patients with symptomatic HIV infection. *Clinical and Experimental Immunology*, **87**, 24–30.

Klatzmann, D. *et al.* (1984). Selective tropism of lymphadenopathy-associated virus (LAV) for helper-inducer T lymphocytes. *Science*, **225**, 59–63.

Koenig, S. *et al.* (1986). Detection of AIDS virus in macrophages in brain tissue from AIDS patients with encephalopathy. *Science*, **233**, 1089–93.

Koenig, S. *et al.* (1990). Mapping the fine specificity of a cytolytic T cell response to HIV-1 nef protein. *Journal of Immunology*, **145**, 127–35.

Koup, R.A. *et al.* (1994). Temporal association of cellular immune responses with the initial control of viremia in primary HIV-1 syndrome. *Journal of Virology*, **68**, 4650–5.

Kowalski, M. *et al.* (1989). Antibodies to CD4 in individuals infected with human immunodeficiency virus type 1. *Proceedings of the National Academy of Sciences* (*USA*), **86**, 3346–50.

Lane, H.C. and Fauci, A.S. (1985). Immunologic abnormalities in the acquired immune deficiency syndrome. *Annual Review of Immunology*, **3**, 477.

Lane, H.C. *et al.* (1983). Abnormalities of B cell activation and immunoregulation in patients with the acquired immunodeficiency syndrome. *New England Journal of Medicine*, **309**, 453–8.

Lawrence, J.M., Osborn, T.G., Paro, R., Eaton, C., Hyers, T.M., and Moore, T.L. (1991). Septic arthritis caused by hemophilus influenza type B in a patient with HIV-1 infection. *Journal of Rheumatology*, **18**, 1772–3.

Leon, M., Ramos, M., Saavedra, J., Dominguez, A., Ferrer, T., and Pujol, E. (1994). *S. pneumoniae* sternoclavicular arthritis in a patient with HIV infection. *Anales de Medicina Interna*, **11**, 395–7.

Libman, B.S., Quismorio, F.P., Jr., and Stimmler, M.M. (1995). Polyarteritis nodosa-like vasculitis in human immunodeficiency virus infection. *Journal of Rheumatology*, **22**, 351–5.

Lipstein-Kresch, E., Isenberg, H.D., Singer, C., Cooke, O., and Greenwald, R.A. (1985). Disseminated sporothrix schenkii infection with arthritis in a patient with acquired immunodeficiency syndrome. *Journal of Rheumatology*, **12**, 805–8.

Looney, D.J. *et al.* (1988). Type-restricted neutralization of molecular clones of human immunodeficiency virus. *Science*, **241**, 357–9.

Louthrenoo, W. (1993). Successful treatment of severe Reiter's syndrome asso-ciated with human immunodeficiency virus infection with etretinate. Report of 2 cases. *Journal of Rheumatology*, **20**, 1243–6.

Lui, K.-J., Darrow, W.W., and Rutherford, G.W., III (1988). A model-based estimate of the mean incubation period for AIDS in homosexual men. *Science*, **240**, 1333–5.

Malbec, D., Pines, E., Boudon, P., Lusina, D., and Choudat, L. (1994). CD8 hyper-lymphocytosis syndrome and human immunodeficiency virus infection: 5 cases. *Revue de Medecine Interne*, **15**, 630–3.

Marcellin, P. *et al.* (1991). Latent hepatitis B virus (HBV) infection in systemic necrotizing vasculitis. *Clinical and Experimental Rheumatology*, **9**, 23–8.

Margolick, J.B., Volkman, D.J., Folks, T.M., and Fauci, A.S. (1987). Amplification of HTLV-III/LAV infection by antigen-induced activation of T cells and direct suppression by virus of lymphocyte blastogenic responses. *Journal of Immunology*, **138**, 1719–23.

Marks, C. and Kuskov, S. (1995). Pattern of arterial aneurysms in acquired immunodeficiency disease. *World Journal of Surgery*, **19**, 127–32.

Martz, E. (1986). LFA-1 and other accessory molecules functioning in adhesions of T and B lymphocytes. *Human Immunology*, **18**, 3–37.

Masters, D.L. and Lentino, J.R. (1984). Cervical osteomyelitis related to *Nocardia asteroides*. *Journal of Infectious Diseases*, **149**, 824.

Maurer, T.A., Zackheim, H.S., Tuffanelli, L., and Berger, T.G. (1994). The use of methotrexate for treatment of psoriasis in patients with HIV infection. *Journal of the American Academy of Dermatology*, **31**, 372–5.

Mayer-Siuta, R., Keil, L.B., and De Bari, V.A. (1988). Autoantibodies and circulating immune complexes in subjects infected with human immunodeficiency virus. *Medical Microbiology and Immunology*, **177**, 189–94.

McFayden, T. and Lyell, A. (1971). Coagulase positive staphylococci in pustular psoriasis: evidence for bacteremia and good response to treatment. In *International symposium on psoriasis* (ed. E. Farber and A. Cox), pp. 79–85. Stanford University Press.

Meiser, S.C., Schlossman, S.F., and Reinhertz, E.L. (1982). Clonal analysis of human cytotoxic T lymphocytes: T4+ and T8+ effector cells recognize products of different major histocompatibility complex regions. *Proceedings of the National Academy of Sciences (USA)*, **79**, 4395.

Meltzer, M.S. and Gendelman, H.E. (1992). Mononuclear phagocytes as targets, tissue reservoirs, and immunoregulatory cells in human immunodeficiency virus disease. *Current Topics in Microbiology and Immunology*, **181**, 239–63.

Meola, T., Soter, N.A., Ostreicher, R., Sanchez, M., and Moy, J.A. (1993). The safety of UVB phototherapy in patients with HIV infection. *Journal of the American Academy of Dermatology*, **29**, 216–20.

Mijiyawa, M. (1993). Spondyloarthropathies in patients attending the rheumatology unit of Lomé Hospital. *Journal of Rheumatology*, **20**, 1167–9.

Mitsuya, H. and Broder, S. (1986). Inhibition of the in vitro infectivity and cytopathic effect of human T-lymphotrophic virus type III/lymphadenopathy-associated virus (HTLV-III/LAV) by 2,3-dideoxynucleosides. *Proceedings of the National Academy of Sciences (USA)*, **83**, 1911–15.

Molina, J.F. et al. (1995). Coexistence of human immunodeficiency virus infection and systemic lupus erythematosus. *Journal of Rheumatology*, **22**, 347–50.

Monteagudo, I., Rivera, J., Lopez-Longo, J., Cosin, J., Garcia-Monforte, A., and Carreno, L. (1991). AIDS and rheumatic manifestations in patients addicted to drugs. An analysis of 106 cases. *Journal of Rheumatology*, **18**, 1038–41.

Mora, C.A. et al. (1988). Seroprevalence of antibodies to HTLV-1 in patients with chronic neurological disorders other than tropical spastic paraparesis. *Annals of Neurology*, **23**, S192–S195.

Morrey, J.D. et al. (1991). In vivo activation of human immunodeficiency virus type 1 long terminal repeat by UV type A (UV-A) light plus psoralen and UV-B light in the skin of transgenic mice. *Journal of Virology*, **65**, 5045–51.

Moss, A.R. et al. (1988). Seropositivity for HIV and the development of AIDS or AIDS-related conditions: three year follow-up of the San Francisco General Hospital cohort. *British Medical Journal*, **296**, 745–50.

Muesing, M., Smith, D.H., and Capon, D.J. (1987). Regulation of mRNA accumulation by a human immunodeficiency virus transactivator protein. *Cell*, **48**, 691–701.

Munoz Fernandez, S. et al. (1991). Osteoarticular infection associated with the human immunodeficiency virus. *Clinical and Experimental Rheumatology*, **9**, 489–93.

Mustakellio, K.K. and Lassus, A. (1964). Staphylococcal α-antitoxin in psoriatic arthropathy. *British Journal of Dermatology*, **76**, 544.

Nabel, G.J., Rice, S.A., Knipe, D.M., and Baltimore, D. (1988). Alternative mechanisms for activation of human immunodeficiency virus enhancer in T cells. *Science*, **239**, 1299–302.

Nakajima, K. et al. (1989). Induction of IL-6 (B cell stimulatory factor 2/IFN-β2) production by HIV. *Journal of Immunology*, **142**, 531–6.

O'Brien, W.A. et al. (1990). HIV-1 tropism for mononuclear phagocytes can be determined by regions of gp120 outside the CD4-binding domain. *Nature*, **348**, 69–73.

Obuch, M.L., Maurer, T.A., Becker, B., and Berger, T.G. (1992). Psoriasis and human immunodeficiency virus infection. *Journal of the American Academy of Dermatology*, **27**, 667–73.

Ostlere, L.S., Harris, D., Johnson, M., and Rustin, M.H. (1993). Gastrointestinal and cutaneous vasculitis associated with gonococcal infection in an HIV-seropositive patient. *Journal of the American Academy of Dermatology*, **29**, 276–8.

Pahwa, S. et al. (1985). Influence of the human T-lymphotropic virus/lymphadenopathy-associated virus and functions of human lymphocytes: evidence of immunosuppressive effects and polyclonal B-cell activation by banded viral and lymphocyte preparations. *Proceedings of the National Academy of Sciences (USA)*, **82**, 8198–202.

Panegyres, P.K., Tan, N., Kakulas, B.A., Armstrong, J.A., and Hollingsworth, P. (1988). Necrotising myopathy and zidovudine. *Lancet*, **i**, 1050–1.

Pappo, A.S., Buchanan, G.R., and Johnson, A. (1989). Septic arthritis in children with hemophilia. *American Journal of Diseases of Children*, **143**, 1226.

Pardo, V. et al. (1987). AIDS-related glomerulopathy: occurrence in specific risk groups. *Kidney International*, **31**, 1167–73.

Perlman, D.M. et al. (1988). Persistent *Campylobacter jejuni* infections in patients infected with human immunodeficiency virus (HIV). *Annals of Internal Medicine*, **108**, 540–6.

Phillips, R.E. and McMichael, A.J. (1993). How does the HIV escape cytotoxic T cell immunity? *Chemical Immunology*, **56**, 150–64.

Piatak, M., Jr. et al. (1993). High levels of HIV-1 in plasma during all stages of infection determined by competitive PCR. *Science*, **259**, 1749–54.

Potashner, W., Buskila, D., Patterson, B., Karasik, A., and Keystone, E.C. (1990). Leukocytoclastic vasculitis in association with human immunodeficiency virus infection. *Journal of Rheumatology*, **17**, 1104–7.

Prince, H.E. and John, J.K. (1987). Abnormalities of interleukin 2 receptor expression associated with decreased antigen-induced lymphocyte proliferation in patients with AIDS and related disorders. *Clinical and Experimental Immunology*, **67**, 236–44.

Quinn, T.C. (1990). Global epidemiology of HIV infections. In *The medical management of AIDS* (ed. M.A. Sande and P.A. Volberding), pp. 3–22. W.B. Saunders, Philadelphia.

Rank, R.G., Ramsey, K.H., and Hough, A.J. (1988). Antibody-mediated modulation of arthritis induced by *Chlamydia*. *American Journal of Pathology*, **132**, 372–81.

Ranki, A., Puska, P., Mattinen, S., Lagerstedt, A., and Krohn, K. (1991). Effect of PUVA on immunologic and virologic findings in HIV- infected patients. *Journal of the American Academy of Dermatology*, **24**, 404–10.

Rao, T. and Friedman, E. (1989). AIDS (HIV)-associated nephropathy: does it exist? *American Journal of Nephrology*, **9**, 441–53.

Rao, T.K.S., Friedman, E.A., and Nicastri, A.D. (1987). The types of renal disease in the acquired immunodeficiency syndrome. *New England Journal of Medicine*, **316**, 1062–8.

Ricciardi, D.D., Sepkowitz, D.V., Berkowitz, L.B., Bienenstock, H., and Maslow, M. (1986). Cryptococcal arthritis in AIDS patients. *Journal of Rheumatology*, **13**, 455–9.

Rivera, J., Monteagudo, I., Lopez-Longo, J., and Sanchez-Atrio, A. (1992). Septic arthritis in patients with acquired immunodeficiency syndrome with human immunodeficiency virus infection. *Journal of Rheumatology*, **19**, 1960–2.

Riviere, Y. et al. (1989). HIV-specific cytotoxic responses of seropositive individuals; distinct types of effector cells mediate killing of targets expressing gag and env proteins. *Journal of Virology*, **63**, 2270–7.

Roux Lombard, P., Modoux, C., Cruchaud, A., and Dayer, J.M. (1989). Purified blood monocytes from HIV 1-infected patients produce high levels of TNF-α and IL-1. *Clinical Immunology and Immunopathology*, **50**, 374–84.

Rubbert, A. et al. (1994). Anticardiolipin antibodies in HIV infection: association with cerebral perfusion defects as detected by 99mTc-HMPAO SPECT. *Clinical and Experimental Immunology*, **98**, 361–8.

Rusche, J.R. et al. (1988). Antibodies that inhibit fusion of human immunodeficiency virus-infected cells bind a 24-amino acid sequence of the viral envelope, gp120. *Proceedings of the National Academy of Sciences (USA)*, **85**, 3198–202.

Ruzicka, T. et al. (1987). Treatment of HIV-induced retinoid-resistant psoriasis with zidovudine. *Lancet*, **ii**, 1469.

Rynes, R.I. (1990). HIV and rheumatologic autoimmune phenomena: imitator or illuminator. *Clinical and Experimental Rheumatology*, **8**, 103–6.

Said, G. et al. (1988). The peripheral neuropathy of necrotizing arteritis: a clinicopathological study. *Annals of Neurology*, **23**, 461.

Salahuddin, S.Z., Rose, R.M., Groopman, J.E., Markham, P.D., and Gallo, R.C. (1986). Human T lymphotropic virus type III infection of human alveolar macrophages. *Blood*, **68**, 281–4.

Savige, J.A., Chang, L., and Crowe, S.M. (1993). Anti-neutrophil cytoplasm antibodies in HIV infection. *Advances in Experimental Medicine and Biology*, **336**, 349–52.

Scaravalli, F. *et al.* (1989). Chronic basal meningitis and vasculitis in acquired immunodeficiency syndrome. *Archives of Pathology and Laboratory Medicine*, **113**, 192.

Scorza-Smeraldi, R., Fabio, G., Lazzarin, A., Eisera, N.B., Moroni, M., and Zanussi, C. (1986). HLA-associated susceptibility to acquired immunodeficiency syndrome in Italian patients with human-immunodeficiency-virus infection. *Lancet*, **ii**, 1187–9.

Sergent, J. (1980). Vasculitis associated with viral infection. *Clinics in the Rheumatic Diseases*, **6**, 339.

Sheehy, M.J. *et al.* (1989). A diabetes-susceptible HLA haplotype is best defined by a combination of HLA-DR and -DQ alleles. *Journal of Clinical Investigation*, **83**, 830–5.

Shioda, T., Levy, J.A., and Cheng Mayer, C. (1991). Macrophage and T cell-line tropisms of HIV-1 are determined by specific regions of the envelope gp120 gene. *Nature*, **349**, 167–9.

Siekevitz, M., Josephs, S.F., Dukovich, M., Peffer, N., Wong-Staal, F., and Green, W.C. (1987). Activation of the HIV-1 LTR by T-cell mitogens and the transactivator protein of HTLV-1. *Science*, **238**, 1575–8.

Simpson, D.M. (1988). Myopathy associated with human immunodeficiency virus (HIV) but not with zidovudine. *Annals of Internal Medicine*, **109**, 842.

Snider, W.D., Simpson, D.M., Nielsen, S., Gold, J.W., Metroka, C.E., and Posner, J.B. (1983). Neurological complications of acquired immunodeficiency virus: analysis of 50 patients. *Annals of Neurology*, **14**, 403–18.

Solinger, A.M. and Hess, E.V. (1990). HIV and arthritis. *Arthritis and Rheumatism*, **17**, 562.

Solinger, A.M. and Hess, E.V. (1991). Induction of autoantibodies by HIV infection and their significance. *Rheumatic Diseases Clinics of North America*, **17**, 157–76.

Solinger, A.M. and Hess, E.V. (1993). Rheumatic diseases and AIDS — is the association real? *Journal of Rheumatology*, **20**, 678–83.

Solinger, A.M. *et al.* (1988). Acquired immune deficiency syndrome (AIDS) and autoimmunity — mutually exclusive entities? *Journal of Clinical Immunology*, **8**, 32–42.

Springer, T.A. (1990). Adhesion receptors of the immune system. *Nature*, **346**, 425–34.

Springer, T.A., Dustin, M.L., Kishimoto, T.K., and Marlin, S.D. (1987). The lymphocyte function-associated LFA-1, CD2, and LFA-3 molecules: cell adhesion receptors of the immune system. *Annual Review of Immunology*, **5**, 223–52.

Steel, C.M. *et al.* (1988). HLA haplotype A1, B8, DR3 as a risk factor for HIV-related disease. *Lancet*, **ii**, 1185–8.

Steinbach, L.S., Tehranzadeh, J., Fleckenstein, J.L., Vanarthos, W.J., and Pais, M.J. (1993). Human immunodeficiency virus infection: musculoskeletal manifestations. *Radiology*, **186**, 833–8.

Strauss, J. *et al.* (1989). Renal disease in children with the acquired immunodeficiency syndrome. *New England Journal of Medicine*, **321**, 625–30.

Strongin, I.S., Kale, S.A., Raymond, M.K., Luskin, R.L., Weisberg, G.W., and Jacobs, J.J. (1991). An unusual presentation of gonococcal arthritis in an HIV positive patient. *Annals of the Rheumatic Diseases*, **50**, 572–3.

Swain, S.L. (1983). T cell subsets and the recognition of MHC class. *Immunological Reviews*, **74**, 129.

Takahashi, H., Germain, R.N., Moss, B., and Berzofsky, J.A. (1990). An immunodominant class I-restricted cytotoxic T lymphocyte determinant of human immunodeficiency virus type 1 induces CD4 class II-restricted help for itself. *Journal of Experimental Medicine*, **171**, 571–6.

Thompson, I. *et al.* (1989). Henoch–Schönlein purpura and IgA glomerulonephritis associated with HIV infection. *Abstracts of the Fifth International Conference on AIDS: The Scientific and Social Challenge*, Quebec, MBP278.

Till, M. and MacDonell, K.B. (1990). Myopathy with HIV-1 infection: HIV-1 or zidovudine? *Annals of Internal Medicine*, **113**, 492–3.

Tindall, B., Imre, A., Donovan, B., Penny, R., and Cooper, D.A. (1990). Primary HIV infection: clinical, immunologic and serologic aspects. In *The medical management of AIDS* (ed. M.A. Sande and P.A. Volberding), pp. 68–84. W.B. Saunders, Philadelphia.

Tiwari, J.L. and Terasaki, P.I. (1985). *HLA and disease associations*. Springer Verlag, New York.

Tschachler, E. *et al.* (1987). Epidermal Langerhans cells — a target for HTLVIII/LAV infection. *Journal of Investigative Dermatology*, **88**, 233–7.

Valeriano, J., Lolita, B., and Kerry, L.D. (1989). HIV-associated polyarteritis nodosa (PAN) diagnosed by rectal biopsy; a case report. *Arthritis and Rheumatism*, **32**, S44.

Vasey, F.B. *et al.* (1982). Possible involvement of group A streptococci in the pathogenesis of psoriatic arthritis. *Journal of Rheumatology*, **9**, 719.

Vernant, J.C. *et al.* (1988). T-lymphocyte alveolitis, tropical spastic paresis, and Sjögren syndrome. *Lancet*, **i**, 177.

Viscidi, R.P., Mayur, K., Lederman, H.M., and Frankel, A.D. (1989). Inhibition of antigen-induced lymphocyte proliferation by Tat protein from HIV-1. *Science*, **246**, 1606–8.

Vogel, J. *et al.* (1988). The HIV tat gene induces dermal lesions resembling Kaposi's sarcoma in transgenic mice. *Nature*, **335**, 606.

Vogel, J., Cepeda, M., Tschachler, E., Napolitano, L.A., and Jay, G. (1992). UV activation of human immunodeficiency virus gene expression in transgenic mice. *Journal of Virology*, **66**, 1–5.

Walker, B.D. *et al.* (1987). HIV-specific cytotoxic T lymphocytes in seropositive individuals. *Nature*, **328**, 345–8.

Watts, R.A. *et al.* (1987). Pyomyositis associated with human immunodeficiency virus infection. *British Medical Journal*, **294**, 1524.

Weiss, R.A. (1993). How does HIV cause AIDS? *Science*, **260**, 1273–9.

Westervelt, P. *et al.* (1992). Macrophage tropism determinants of human immunodeficiency virus type 1 in vivo. *Journal of Virology*, **66**, 2577–82.

White, S.H. *et al.*, (1972). Disturbance of HL-A antigen frequency in psoriasis. *New England Journal of Medicine*, **287**, 740.

Whyte, H.J. and Baughman, R.D. (1964). Acute guttate psoriasis and streptococcal infection. *Archives of Dermatology*, **89**, 350–6.

Wiley, C.A., Nerenberg, M., Cros, D., and Soto-Aguilar, M.C. (1989). HTLV-I polymyositis in a patient also infected with the human immunodeficiency virus. *New England Journal of Medicine*, **320**, 992–5.

Williams, R.C., Hasur, H., and Spera, T.J. (1984). Lymphocyte-reactive antibodies in acquired immunodeficiency syndrome. *Journal of Clinical Immunology*, **4**, 118–21.

Winchester, R. (1994). Psoriatic arthritis. In *Dermatology in general medicine* (ed. T.B. Fitzpatrick, A.Z. Eisen, K. Wolff, I.M. Freedberg, and K. Austen). McGraw-Hill, New York.

Winchester, R., Bernstein, D.H., Fischer, H.D., Enlow, R., and Solomon, G. (1987). The co-occurrence of Reiter's syndrome and acquired immunodeficiency. *Annals of Internal Medicine*, **106**, 19–26.

Winchester, R., Brancato, L., Itescu, S., Skovron, M.L., and Solomon, G. (1988). Implications from the occurrence of Reiter's syndrome and related disorders in association with advanced HIV infection. *Scandinavian Journal of Rheumatology*, **74**, 89–93.

Withington, R.H. *et al.* (1987). Isolation of HIV from synovial fluid of a patient with reactive arthritis. *British Medical Journal*, **294**, 484.

Yanker, B.A. *et al.* (1986). Cerebral granulomatous angiitis associated with isolation of human T-lymphotrophic virus III from the central nervous system. *Annals of Neurology*, **20**, 362.

Zimmermann, B., Erickson, A.D., and Mikolich, D.J. (1989). Septic acromioclavicular arthritis and osteomyelitis in a patient with acquired immunodeficiency syndrome. *Arthritis and Rheumatism*, **32**, 1175.

Zimmerman, W., Cher, S.M., Bolden, A., and Weissbach, A. (1980). Mitochondrial DNA replication does not involve DNA polymerase-α. *Journal of Biological Chemistry*, **255**, 11847–52.

Zolla-Pazner, S. *et al.* (1987). Nonrandom development of immunologic abnormalities after infection with human immunodeficiency virus: implications for immunologic classification of the disease. *Proceedings of the National Academy of Sciences (USA)*, **84**, 5404–8.

Zwart, G. *et al.* (1991). Immunodominance and antigenic variation of the principal neutralization domain of HIV-1. *Virology*, **181**, 481–9.

Tuberculosis and leprosy are infectious diseases characterized by chronic inflammation. Tuberculosis is caused chiefly by the organism *Mycobacterium tuberculosis* and much less commonly by *M. bovis* and atypical mycobacteria (*M. avium, intercellulare, scrofulaceum, gordonae, marium*, etc.). Leprosy is caused by *M. leprae*. Most of these infections are readily amenable to modern medical and surgical treatment, which almost always cures the infection.

Tuberculosis

Epidemiology and pathogenesis

Tuberculosis was rapidly declining in the United States, Europe, and Australia until 1985, after which the trend was interrupted by the appearance of acquired immune deficiency disease (Modilevsky *et al.* 1989). Tuberculosis in persons infected by human immunodeficiency virus is characterized by extrapulmonary disease in as many as 70 per cent. At present, one-third of the world's population, estimated at 1.7 billion persons, is infected with *M. tuberculosis*. This reservoir of infection affects around 8 million new patients and results in 19 million deaths annually (Arachi 1991). Fewer than one-tenth of all patients with tuberculosis residing in developed nations suffer from infection of the bones and joints (Davies *et al.* 1994), but the proportion in other populations is much higher.

In the majority of instances, *M. tuberculosis* is transmitted from person to person via the respiratory route. A patient with infectious pulmonary tuberculosis (sputum smear-positive) coughs and produces an aerosol of small droplets, 1 to 5 μm in size, containing bacilli. The small droplets evaporate within a short distance from the mouth, and the desiccated bacilli remain airborne for long periods. Infection of a host occurs when a few bacilli are inhaled. These are sufficiently small to reach the pulmonary alveoli and are phagocytosed by alveolar macrophages.

The *M. tuberculosis* grows slowly, dividing approximately every 10 to 24 h. It has no known endotoxins or exotoxins, and there is no immediate host response to infection. Growth and multiplication of the organism are essentially unimpeded, until a specific cell-mediated immune response develops after 4 to 8 weeks, and only if a threshold number of *M. tuberculosis* organisms is reached. The collection of activated T cells and macrophages forms granulomas that undergo central coagulative necrosis (caseation). Healing then occurs, often with calcification.

Tuberculosis as a clinically manifested disease develops in a minority of the patients who fail to contain the primary infection. In some individuals the disease may appear within a few weeks of primary infection, and in others the bacilli may remain dormant within the macrophages for many years before entering a phase of exponential multiplication to cause the disease. The bacilli reach the bloodstream either by being carried in the lymph to the draining lymph nodes and thence to the thoracic duct, or by erosion of blood vessels in the walls of developing tuberculous lesions in the lungs. The bacilli that enter the bloodstream disseminate throughout the body, and some are deposited in bones or joints.

Immunology

There appears to be variation between individuals in their immune response to mycobacteria, which perhaps is genetically determined. The ability of the host to control infection with *M. tuberculosis* resides in its ability to mount an effective cellular immune response. Cell-mediated immunity develops when T lymphocytes become sensitized after recognizing their specific antigen and then release mediators that modulate macrophage function.

Delayed cellular hypersensitivity is the associated immunological response in the majority of patients with tuberculosis (Stanford 1983; Lucas 1988). Cell-mediated immunity and delayed hypersensitivity are closely related phenomena that occur in the host as a result of T cells becoming specifically activated by *M. tuberculosis*. Both result from the same immunological mechanism and alter the response of the host to subsequent exposure to antigen. Delayed hypersensitivity is responsible for the tuberculin skin-test reaction. There is no single dominant antigen, and the infected (or artificially sensitized) host develops an immune response to an array of mycobacterial proteins. Many of the observed effects of tuberculosis are considered to be due to delayed hypersensitivity (Sifford and Bates 1991) and it has been implicated in caseation and cavitation. Caseation follows the early exudative lesions in the soft tissues and results when blood vessels adjacent to the areas of inflammation thrombose causing tissue necrosis. Delayed hypersensitivity is also involved in the liquefaction of caseous lesions, probably as a result of lymphokine production, which attracts and activates macrophages. Macrophages then release hydrolytic enzymes that digest the necrotic debris.

Mycobacterial infections also stimulate humoral antibody responses, and production of antibodies to polysaccharide and protein antigens has been demonstrated. However, there is no evidence that these antibodies play a part in immunity, hypersensitivity, or the pathogenesis of tuberculosis (Dutt 1989; Ellner *et al.* 1989). Attempts to link HLA phenotype and susceptibility to tuberculous infection have not yielded a significant correlation (Shoemaker 1986).

Clinical manifestations

Primary tuberculous infection is usually asymptomatic and typically occurs in lower or mid zones of the lung as a pneumonitis with enlargement of hilar lymph nodes (primary complex). It may either undergo remission spontaneously or progress at once to clinical disease. After remission, there may be reactivation many months or years later, resulting in a chronic wasting disease. The lungs and respiratory tracts are most frequently affected, followed by lymph nodes, skeleton, pericardium, brain and meninges, abdomen, and skin.

Tuberculosis of a bone or joint is usually a low-grade and slowly progressive infection with a variable degree of local and systemic manifestations (Wolfgang 1978; Butorac *et al.* 1987; Martini *et al.* 1988), depending on the virulence of the organism and the defensive response mounted by the host. The onset of symptoms is insidious; involvement is monoarticular or mono-osseous in the majority of patients. Simultaneous involvement of other viscera (lungs, lymph nodes) is common. There are associated constitutional symptoms (fever, fatigue, weight loss, poor appetite, night sweats). Pre-existing arthritis or old trauma, alcoholism, prolonged use of corticosteroids, and immunodeficiency diseases are significant predisposing factors.

Tuberculosis can affect any part of the spine, although up to about two decades ago the thoracolumbar junction was more commonly affected (Davidson and Horowitz 1970). The infection may begin in and remain confined to a vertebral body, eventually leading to collapse, or it may affect the end-plate of the vertebral body with early involvement of the adjacent disc and the next vertebral end-plate. The formation of a paravertebral abscess is usual, and progressive necrosis of bone and disc with sequestration leads to kyphotic deformity or gibbus at that site. The abscess may remain localized at the same site or track along tissue planes and neurovascular bundles to cause symptoms at a remote site. In the lumbar spine, the abscess may track along the psoas muscle to present as a swelling in groin or thigh; from thoracic vertebrae it may follow the course of a rib and present anteriorly on the chest wall. The local symptoms are pain, muscle spasm, and limited movement. The pain is characteristically worse during sleep, which perhaps is due to relaxation of the protective muscle spasm. In the occasional patient, pain may not be the predominant symptom, and kyphosis or a cold abscess is the first manifestation.

Primary involvement of the posterior elements of vertebrae appears less common. Haematogenous spread of infection to the pedicle is usually the initial event. Destruction of the neural arch and vertebral body posteriorly characterize the disease progression. Later in the course of disease, the medial ends of ribs are eroded, followed by the transverse processes of affected vertebrae. In the majority of cases only a single vertebra is involved (Kumar 1985). Disc spaces remain preserved until late in the disease and paraspinal masses are prominent. Clinical presentation in these patients is often with early paraplegia.

Tuberculosis involving the first and second cervical vertebrae may begin in the retropharyngeal space with secondary involvement of the bone, or more rarely in the bone itself (Lifeso 1987) (Fig. 1). With progression there is increasing ligamentous involvement, with minimal osteolytic erosions, into the odontoid or the arch of the first cervical vertebra. This would allow anterior subluxation of C1 on C2, increasing rotatory subluxation, and proximal translocation of the odontoid. In a final stage of the disease, bone destruction increases, with complete loss of the C1 arch or fracture through the base of the odontoid, leading to a grossly unstable articulation between the occiput and C2. The diagnosis is suspected if an individual with prolonged neck pain has restriction in all ranges of movement. The most serious complication of spinal tuberculosis is involvement of the spinal cord causing a neurological deficit. This may occur incompletely and slowly, with the patient complaining of difficulty in walking, or it can appear more dramatically, with complete spastic paraplegia or quadriplegia and loss of sphincter control. The neurological deficit may be secondary to medullary and radicular inflammation or cord compression by an abscess, tuberculoma, or subluxation of a vertebral body.

Skeletal tuberculosis other than in the spine in adults more commonly occurs in the joints of the lower extremities (Figs 2 and 3). It usually is monoarticular. Weight-bearing joints are more frequently affected, and microtrauma to cartilage is thought to predispose to the infection. The joints commonly involved are the hip, knee, ankle, sacroiliac, wrist, and shoulder in that order (Garrido *et al.* 1988;

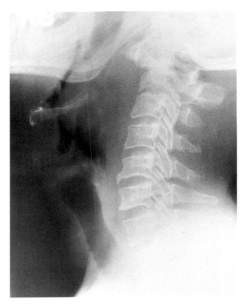

Fig. 1 Tuberculosis of C1 and C2 with a large retropharyngeal abscess.

Pouchot *et al.* 1988). The infected individual usually has a long history of mild or moderate joint or bone pain along with a swelling or large effusion. On examination, there is synovial thickening and mild warmth. There is always significant muscle atrophy around the joint. If a sinus track has formed, there may be signs of superimposed pyogenic infection. Even in the early stages, there is limitation in the range of motion by effusion and synovial thickening. As infection progresses, flexion contractures and joint deformity develop. The end-result may be fibrous or bony ankylosis.

Tuberculous osteomyelitis may affect any long bone (Martini *et al.* 1986). The patient presents with local pain and sometimes a diffuse swelling may be evident, with or without a sinus opening. Involvement of the short bones of the hands or feet is termed tuberculous dactylitis. Soft tissue swelling is usually the first manifestation and the pain appears a few days or weeks thereafter. One or several fingers or toes may be affected.

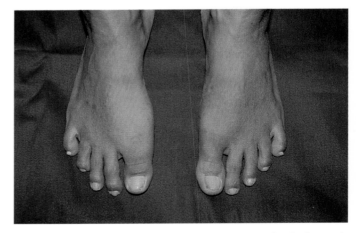

Fig. 2 The base of the right great toe was painful and swollen for 5 years in a 40-year-old premenopausal female; this was an indolent and slowly progressive lesion of tuberculosis.

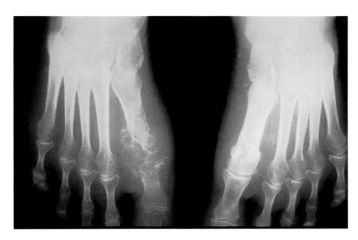

Fig. 3 Radiograph of the feet of the patient in Fig. 2 at 5 years after the onset of pain, revealing remarkable destruction of the bones and joints by tuberculous infection.

Cystic tuberculosis of bone is another type of tuberculous osteomyelitis. Lesions are of variable size and well circumscribed. Multifocal cystic tuberculosis of bone was more common five decades ago, but it seems that solitary lesions are now predominant (Kumar *et al.* 1988). In the adult the common sites are the skull, axial skeleton, and shoulder and pelvic girdles. In children the metaphyses of long bones are often the sites of infection. This predilection is probably due to the vascular structure of the long bones in this region (Edeikin *et al.* 1963). Tubercle bacilli probably lodge in the small terminal branches of the arteries of the metaphyses and grow, caseate, and produce a cystic lesion. A soft tissue swelling is externally visible if the skull bone is affected (LeRoux *et al.* 1990). Most commonly, a circumscribed, punched out lesion, approx. 2 cm in diameter, results. At presentation, most patients are systemically well and manifest a painless swelling, which is firm if the periosteum is intact or soft if not. Headache is uncommon, but if present, it is usually localized to the site of infection. Occasionally, there is a discharging sinus.

Poncet's disease is another pattern of joint involvement (Dall *et al.* 1989). Patients who have active visceral tuberculosis complain of

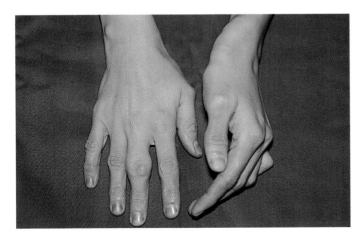

Fig. 4 Tuberculous inflammation of the right middle proximal interphalangeal joint and left abductor pollicis longus tendon sheath in a 36-year-old woman.

polyarthritis or tenosynovitis affecting peripheral joints (Fig. 4), a form of reactive arthropathy. In some patients the symptoms and signs are suggestive of enthesopathy at the ankle, knee, hip, or elbow. There may be mild stiffness after inactivity, and swelling. These symptoms regress within a few weeks after starting treatment. Physicians from the Indian subcontinent do not doubt its existence as a definite entity.

Other, less frequently seen clinical features of tuberculosis include necrotic skin ulcers of erythema nodosum, shoulder-hand syndrome, parotid gland swelling, and red eye caused by uveitis and chorioretinitis. Secondary amyloidosis may appear many years after the tuberculous infection.

Investigations and diagnosis

Tuberculosis is diagnosed if the clinical pattern is suggestive and acid-fast bacilli are demonstrated in the lesions. However, the latter is often not possible and other criteria have to be sought as additional evidence.

To culture tubercle bacilli on the Lowenstein–Jensen medium requires 4 to 8 weeks to detect growth. Nowadays, radiometric techniques using highly selective media allow cultivation in 1 or 2 weeks, but confirmation of the identity of an isolated organism may require more time. Advances in molecular genetics have resulted in impressive DNA hybridization probes that are non-radioactive and easily utilized in a clinical microbiology laboratory. However, these probes require growth of the organism in culture because they are unreliable in detecting the relatively small numbers of organisms in clinical specimens such as tuberculous synovitis.

A smear from the infected site such as a paraspinal abscess usually provides the required evidence because the staining characteristics of *M. tuberculosis* are typical. A slender, curved, often polychromatically beaded rod is seen singly, in pairs, or in clumps of a few organisms, lying side by side. If stained with fluorescent auramine-rhodamine, the bacilli are visualized under the usual high-dry (100 ×) magnification. A more specific stain consists of carbol fuchsin and this requires careful scanning with oil-immersion (1000 ×) microscopy.

A simple smear from clinical specimens such as synovial fluid or infected bone scrapings seldom demonstrates the organism. The technique of polymerase chain reaction holds remarkable promise for this purpose. The key technological element of this procedure is a DNA polymerase that is heat-stable. The function of a DNA polymerase is to generate a complementary strand of DNA using a single strand of DNA as a template. A short segment of complementary DNA annealed to the template (which equates with the a short segment of double-stranded DNA) serves as a primer region. The DNA polymerase can add nucleotides to the primer in a sequential fashion based on the template sequence and result in a longer sequence of double-stranded DNA. The nucleotides are always added in the same direction from any given primer site. If a short primer sequence is added to the double-stranded DNA (chromosomal, plasmid) and the temperature is raised above the melting point of the double strands and then lowered, a number of the primers will anneal to their complementary segments on the chromosome or plasmid. Once annealed, the primer region is elongated by the addition of an appropriate DNA polymerase and deoxyribonucleotide triphosphates. Two primers from opposite ends and strands can anneal and result in a duplication of the target segment. Once the elongation is complete, the temperature is raised so that both the old and newly synthesized strands fall apart. By lowering the temperature, the target region of DNA is logarithmically amplified. Although the reaction mixture goes above 90 °C during each cycle, the heat-stable DNA polymerase is not completely inactivated and can result in millionfold amplifications of the target DNA sequence after 30 to 40 cycles. The temperatures for denaturing, annealing, and elongation steps are easily programmed into automated heat blocks that can reproducibly change temperatures with great precision. Thus, the polymerase chain reaction can amplify minute quantities of DNA to levels that are easily seen on routine agarose gel electrophoresis. However, the major limitation is that minute quantity of contaminating DNA also gets amplified and is seen on the agarose gel as a false-positive result. Present research is seeking to overcome this limitation. Also, the polymerase chain reaction does not differentiate dead from living organisms because it simply amplifies DNA. Thus, identifying a portion of the genome of an organism in a clinical specimen provides the ability to state that the organism was present, and it cannot distinguish between active and treated or inactive tuberculosis (Schluger *et al.* 1994). The correlation of clinical information with the greater sensitivity of the polymerase chain reaction is currently under study.

The typical histological feature is a tuberculous granuloma with partial or complete caseation necrosis. The epithelioid cells are surrounded by a wall of mononuclear cells, which is a lymphocyte mantle comprised mainly of T-suppressor cells. Such typical granulomas are not always seen (particularly in the synovium) and only a tuberculoid infiltrate may be visible. In this infiltrate are seen irregular accumulations of epithelioid cells among mononuclear cells, with or without necrosis and giant cells (Levy *et al.* 1986).

Serological tests for the diagnosis of tuberculosis (Daniel 1989) remain experimental and are not satisfactorily established for routine clinical use. Advances in the definition of species-specific antigenic determinants of *M. tuberculosis* had created a firm basis for the production of standardized serological immunoassays (Brisson-Noel *et al.* 1989). However, in the majority of patients, musculoskeletal tuberculosis is a paucibacillary disease in which the desired sensitivity of these tests is not achievable (Ivanyi 1988). This is attributed to the lack of sufficient antibody formation rather than to limitations in the techniques of detection. A raised erythrocyte sedimentation rate is a non-specific serological measure of inflammation and occasionally is in the normal range though the patient has active tuberculosis.

The likelihood of infection with *M. tuberculosis* can be assessed by intradermal injection of 5 tuberculin units of purified protein derivative (American Thoracic Society 1990). The diameter of any induration is recorded 48 to 72 h later. Reactivity to tuberculin ($\geqslant$ 5 mm induration) is found if the person has been exposed to mycobacteria and has intact cell-mediated immunity. A history of vaccination with bacille Calmette-Guérin is ignored in interpreting the results of tuberculin skin testing in adults, because skin-test reactivity from bacille Calmette-Guérin usually declines by adulthood. If skin testing is done periodically, as in hospital employees, the boosting phenomenon must be considered. In some tuberculin reactors, although the sensitivity to tuberculin declines with time to become a negative skin test, administration of the skin test boosts immunological memory so that a second tuberculin skin test up to 2 years later will be positive. If the person is being tested annually, the positive second response and negative first response are erroneously thought to represent recent infection requiring treatment.

Another shortcoming of the test is cross-reactivity between mycobacterial antigens, and a positive test may result from exposure to environmental non-tuberculous mycobacteria. Tuberculin test sensitivity falls with age, early treatment, and in all conditions that diminish delayed hypersensitivity. In addition, for as yet unknown reasons, about one-tenth of individuals with tuberculosis do not respond to the ordinary intermediate strength of tuberculin (anergy).

Plain radiographs of the skeleton will have features suggestive of tuberculous infection. Osteoporosis is the first sign of active infection. The reactive hyperaemia, which is intense in an exudative lesion, stimulates osteolysis. If long bones are affected (osteomyelitis), small zones of clearly defined radiolucency indicate granular foci. Diffuse demineralization surrounds these osteolytic areas. As caseation takes place, the osteolytic foci become more evident. When the healing process begins, the perifocal bone becomes sclerotic. If the central demineralized area is merely exudative, healing results in reossification with eventual return of the normal trabecular pattern. If central caseation occurs during the active phase of infection, with calcium deposition, then the dense image of a sequestrum is surrounded by an osteolytic ring representing the fibrous wall beyond which the bone is demineralized. In tuberculous dactylitis the soft tissue swelling is obvious and there may be mild or exuberant periostitis of phalanges, metacarpals, or metatarsals (Bush and Schneider 1984). Expansion of the bone accompanied by cystic change is termed spina ventosa. In involvement of a peripheral joint the synovial shadow may be clearly visible in a slightly underexposed radiograph. If the arthritis is destructive, then the joint space narrows due to erosion of cartilage, and the subchondral cortex of bone becomes ragged and osteoporotic. Vague, irregular densities seen in the surrounding soft tissues may signify abscess formation.

The radiographic appearance of spinal tuberculosis depends on the extent of infection (Chang *et al.* 1989). Destructive changes occasionally confined to a vertebral body or part of two posterior elements of the vertebral complex such as the lamina or pars, but these are uncommon and easily confused with malignant disease. More typically seen is reduction of the disc space, with irregularity of adjacent end-plates, surrounded by a soft tissue swelling due to a paravertebral abscess. Later, more extensive destruction and increased abscess formation are evident. Kyphotic or scoliotic deformity develops as vertebral destruction progresses. In children, secondary changes, such as an increase in vertebral height, may develop in uninvolved adjacent vertebrae to produce a compensatory lordosis above and

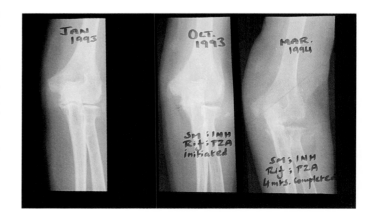

Fig. 5 Progressive radiological destruction in tuberculous infection of the left elbow during the first 5 months of adequate treatment.

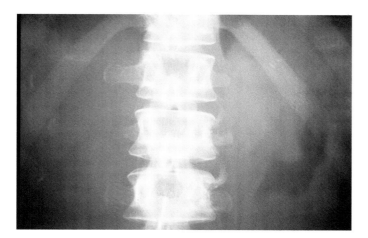

Fig. 6 Erosion of the left transverse process at the L2 vertebra with calcification along the track of caseous fluid to the above and below vertebrae.

below the kyphotic deformity. A severe kyphotic deformity may increase with time, even after healing has occurred, because of the gravitational effect on the deformed spine.

Radiological evidence of healing after successful drug treatment is usually observed late on routine radiographs, both in limb bones or joints (Fig. 5) and the spine. Bone destruction or loss of vertebral height can progress for up to 14 months and recovery of vertebral height is often not seen earlier than 15 months after beginning chemotherapy (Boxer *et al.* 1992). Thus the progression of bone destruction whilst on treatment is not always an adverse feature. Sclerosis is a feature of healing, and appears variably from onset to within 5 months of starting drug treatment. The change from sclerosis to normal bone density takes 5 years or much longer. Paravertebral soft-tissue masses may also take as long as 15 months to resolve. Involvement of adjacent vertebrae is often associated with the reduction in disc space, fusion of the vertebrae, and the formation of syndesmophyte-like bone bridges (Fig. 6).

Computed tomography (**CT**) is provenly superior to conventional radiographs in detecting and monitoring paravertebral abscesses, particularly those situated in the lumbar region (LaBerge and Brant-Zawadski 1984). The CT findings indicative of an abscess include an abnormal mass of low attenuation number, displacement of surrounding structures, obliteration of normal fascial planes, and a 'rind sign' consisting of a rim of increased tissue attenuation. However, none of these features is specific for tuberculosis, with the differential diagnoses being haematoma or neoplasia (Whelan *et al.* 1985), brucellosis, and other pyogenic infections. Tuberculous abscesses are often characterized by macroscopic calcifications. These 'rice bodies', occasionally seen on CT, are diagnostic of tuberculosis infection.

Magnetic resonance imaging (**MRI**) features of vertebral osteomyelitis are characteristic (Smith *et al.* 1989). The T_1-weighted images show a confluent decreased signal intensity at the involved vertebral bodies and intervening disc, whereas the T_2-weighted images demonstrate increased signal intensity. In addition, the normal biconcave configuration of the disc changes and the normal intranuclear cleft is lost. Abscesses can cause an abnormal area of low signal intensity on a T_1-weighted image and a relatively increased signal intensity on T_2-weighted images because of increased fluid content. The MRI can clearly delineate abscesses as distinct from the adjacent spinal cord, psoas muscle, and other surrounding paravertebral soft tissues. To differentiate tuberculous from other pyogenic infections, the clinical features, plain radiographs and CT have to be considered.

Treatment

The cornerstone of the treatment of musculoskeletal tuberculosis is a good regimen of antituberculous drugs, with surgical intervention in selected cases (Cooke 1985; Goldberger 1988; Davidson 1989). Because of increasing drug resistance, drug susceptibility testing is recommended on all *M. tuberculosis* isolates. The available drugs are listed in Table 1. In the treatment of newly diagnosed patients, the regimens should include, whenever possible, the main sterilizing drugs and those most effective in preventing the emergence of resistance. Patients in whom drug resistance is unlikely are prescribed isoniazid, rifampicin, and pyrazinamide. Some of the currently prescribed regimens for adults are:

(1) rifampicin 450–600 mg, isoniazid 300 mg, pyrazinamide 1000–1500 mg, daily for 2 months, followed by rifampicin and isoniazid daily for 6 months;

(2) rifampicin 450–600 mg, streptomycin 0.5–1.0 g, isoniazid 300 mg, pyrazinamide 1000–1500 mg or ethambutol 800 mg for the first 2 months, followed by

    (a) rifampicin 450–600 mg and isoniazid 300 mg daily for 4 months,

    (b) isoniazid 300 mg and ethambutol 800 mg daily for 6 months,

    (c) isoniazid 300 mg, rifampicin 600 mg, and streptomycin 1 g twice weekly for 6 months;

(3) rifampicin 450–600 mg, isoniazid 300 mg daily for 1 month, followed by rifampicin 600 mg and isoniazid 900 mg twice weekly for 8 months;

(4) streptomycin 0.5 g, isoniazid 300 mg, ethambutol 800 mg daily for 3 months, followed by isoniazid and ethambutol for 12 to 18 months.

The duration of treatment is extended if there is no convincing evidence of improvement in clinical features. Surveillance is kept for 12 months after completion of treatment, as most relapses are likely to occur within this period. The introduction of short-course chemotherapy is a major step forward in the treatment of tuberculosis (Hannachi 1988). The twice-weekly drug regimens were developed with the intention to improve patient compliance.

Patients at increased risk for drug resistance should receive isoniazid, rifampicin, pyrazinamide, and ethambutol until susceptibility results are available. Ofloxacin and ciprofloxacin are bactericidal quinolones with low toxicity profiles and penetrate most tissues. They have been used for the treatment of drug-resistant tuberculosis, but reports of prospective controlled trials are not yet available. For adults, ofloxacin 600 mg/day or ciprofloxacin 1000 mg/day may be prescribed in combination with the other drugs.

The surgical treatment of skeletal tuberculosis depends on the tissue involved, whether it is bone, bursa or joint, and the severity of infection. Surgical treatment of bone tuberculosis without joint involvement consists of debridement of the abscess (if it is present)

Table 1 Drugs for tuberculosis

Drug	Daily dose	Bi-weekly dose	Maximum single dose	Adverse reaction	Comment
First-line drugs					
Rifampicin	10–20 mg/kg PO	10–20 mg/kg	600 mg	Nausea, vomiting, hepatitis, febrile reactions, thrombocytopenia	Absorption on empty stomach is complete
Isoniazid	5–10 mg/kg PO	15 mg/kg	300 mg, 900 mg bi-weekly	Hepatitis, peripheral neuropathy, skin rashes	Pyridoxine supplements may be necessary
Pyrazinamide	15–30 mg/kg PO	50 mg/kg	2 g	Hepatitis, skin rashes, arthralgias, hyperuricaemia	Two divided doses daily, active in acidic environment
Ethambutol	15–25 mg/kg PO	50 mg/kg	2.5 g	Optic neuritis	
Streptomycin	15–20 mg/kg IM	25–30 mg/kg	1 g daily, 1.5 g bi-weekly	Auditory neurotoxicity, nephrotoxicity	Total cumulative dose not to exceed 120 g
Second-line drugs					
Ethionamide	15–20 mg/kg PO	1 g		Gastrointestinal intolerance, hepatitis, peripheral neuropathy (rare)	Administer in two or three divided doses
Capreomycin	15–30 mg/kg IM	1 g		Auditory neurotoxicity, nephrotoxicity	
Kanamycin	15–30 mg/kg IM	1 g		Auditory neurotoxicity, nephrotoxicity	
Cycloserine	15 mg/kg PO	1 g		Neuropsychiatric, peripheral neuropathy	Administer in two or three divided doses
p-Amino salicylic acid	150 mg/kg PO	12 g		Gastrointestinal intolerance, hypersensitivity	Administer in four or five divided doses

IM, intramuscular; PO, by mouth (*per os*).

after starting the antituberculous drugs. Suction–irrigation systems are not necessary in tuberculous osteomyelitis. In an occasional patient, if structural instability is anticipated, grafting with cancellous bone chips is done at the time of initial debridement. The treatment of tuberculous arthritis depends on the extent of involvement at the time of detection. Surgery is not indicated if the infection is limited to the synovium (or bursa), with little or no radiographic involvement of the adjacent bone. If the synovium is affected and adjacent bone and cartilage are partially eroded but without gross instability of the joint, there is an argument for synovectomy together with antituberculous drugs to reduce the time needed for convalescence and reduce limitation in the range of joint movement. For advanced joint destruction (complete loss of cartilage and disorganization of the bones), the appropriate surgery is synovectomy, debridement, and fusion of the involved joint. Total arthroplasty is contraindicated in the presence of active tuberculosis. After the infection has been controlled, arthroplasty may be planned for weight-bearing joints (Kim 1988).

All adult patients with spinal tuberculosis are treated with the standardized drug regimen described above (ICMR/BMRC 1989; Medical Research Council 1993). Neurological complications are more frequent when the disease involves the upper and mid-thoracic spine (Omari *et al.* 1989). Surgical intervention is often necessary, especially to obtain adequate specimens for diagnostic purposes. In difficult cases, operative exploration of the lesion is often necessary for the management of complications such as abscesses and sinuses or myelopathy.

Summary of management

The diagnosis of tuberculosis is suspected from the clinical features and appropriate imaging. The final diagnosis is by smear of the aspirate for acid-fast bacilli or from histopathological examination of excised tissue. Appropriate specimens must be obtained before treatment is begun. The material is cultured whenever possible, chiefly to ascertain sensitivity to antituberculous drugs.

The initial drug treatment is with rifampicin, isoniazid, and pyrazinamide for the first 2 months, followed by rifampicin, isoniazid, and ethambutol for 7 or more months. Drug resistance is suspected if there is worsening of clinical signs and symptoms after the first 3 or 4 months of treatment and imaging reveals increased tissue destruction. If reports on culture and antituberculous drug sensitivity are available, then at least four of the appropriate drugs are selected, of which two or three must be bactericidal. In the absence of drug sensitivity reports the treatment must be changed to kanamycin, isoniazid, ethionamide, cycloserine, and ofloxacin or ciprofloxacin. The duration of treatment is then extended by 18 or 24 months.

Surgical intervention is most often necessary to obtain a specimen for diagnosis. In limb bones and vertebrae, necrotic tissue is debrided during the first operation and stabilization, if needed, is done at another operation after 6 or 8 months of drug treatment. Immobilization of the affected region is essential, and for spinal tuberculosis the plaster or acrylic cast must be worn for at least the first 3 months. If spinal instability is demonstrable clinically and on plain radiographs taken in the appropriate postures, then immobilization is prolonged to 6 months or more. Joint infection seldom necessitates synovectomy, except for the occasional patient in whom the diagnosis was delayed and there is a discharging sinus. Most patients not requiring synovectomy can remain ambulatory; if a leg joint is affected, partial weight bearing is recommended for the first 3 or 4 months. This is followed by physiotherapy to build lost muscle mass and tone. Surveillance for 1 year after the end of drug treatment is recommended.

Leprosy

Epidemiology and pathogenesis

The earliest written records describing leprosy come from China and India and date from 600 BC. The true scientific era began when Hensen published his tentative conclusion that the rod-shaped organisms consistently observed in material taken from patients with leprosy were probably responsible for the disease. The World Health Organization estimates that there are over 11 million cases in the world today; that number has not changed much in recent decades, with the majority of patients residing in the poorer nations (Shepard 1982). Leprosy can affect an individual at any age, but cases in infants of less than 1 year old are extremely rare.

Mycobacterium leprae is virtually non-toxic and may infest the human body in large numbers without causing symptoms. Most symptoms of the disease are due to immune reactions against the bacilli. The course after infection in individual patients is variable and determined by the ability of the host to mount an immune response that will limit the bacillary multiplication. There are patients with subclinical infection whose immunological reactivity after exposure to *M. leprae* changes and they do not develop clinical signs. Another group of patients develops skin lesions, which sometimes heal spontaneously, and this is termed the indeterminate form. The third group (estimated as around 10 per cent of all infected) are patients who have the chronic disease, and they chiefly develop dermal and neural involvement. The Ridley and Jopling (1966) classification is accepted widely and provides a good description of variations in clinical course as a basis of accurate clinical diagnosis. It comprises a continuous spectrum with the immunologically stable tuberculoid (TT), in which there are a few lesions containing few

bacilli, at one pole, and the lepromatous (LL) at the other pole, which is a multibacillary disease with fulminant lesions. These poles are bridged by borderline borderline (BB), and borderline lepromatous (BL).

Leprosy is acquired by direct person-to-person transmission (Reich 1987). Spread within family members and others coming into physical contact with patients is facilitated by the indolence of clinical symptoms and the long incubation period, which varies from 6 months to several decades.

Intense bacillaemia is very common in patients with lepromatous leprosy and the organisms can be seen in stained smears of peripheral blood or buffy coats, but signs of toxaemia, including high fever, are absent. Even in the advanced stages of the disease, the lesions are restricted to the skin, peripheral nerves, anterior portion of eyes, upper respiratory tract, and testes. In lepromatous leprosy, collections of bacilli are also found in bone marrow liver, and spleen.

Although the usual course of leprosy is indolent, occasional interruption by the two types of 'reactional states' is observed in patients who are either untreated or already receiving antileprosy drugs. The type 1 lepra reaction can complicate all the three borderline conditions (BT, BB, and BL) and chiefly consists of a change in the course of the disease towards either the lepromatous or tuberculoid pole. The type 2 reaction (or erythema nodosum leprosum) occurs in patients with lepromatous or borderline leprosy, most frequently in the second half of the first year of treatment. Tender subcutaneous nodules develop and the associated features are low-grade fever, lymphadenopathy, and arthritis. Arthritis in this situation is a classical example of an immune-complex deposition disease.

Immunology and histopathology

Although both cell-mediated and humoral immunities occur simultaneously in leprosy, it is the cell-mediated component that assumes significance (Harboe 1985). Individuals capable of developing cell-mediated immunity localize the disease in the form of tuberculoid in the form of tuberculoid leprosy, while those with depleted cell-mediated immunity express it in the lepromatous form.

The ratio of CD4/CD8 lymphocytes is normal in patients with tuberculoid leprosy and it may be decreased or normal in patients with lepromatous leprosy, depending on the bacterial load. At the site of actual inflammation, CD4 cells constitute about 95 per cent of the lymphocyte population in tuberculoid granulomas and CD8 cells dominate to the extent of 85 per cent in lepromatous lesions (Narayanan 1988).

There is speculation that macrophage function is defective in patients with lepromatous leprosy (Birdi *et al.* 1989). T cells from patients with lepromatous leprosy fail to produce interleukin 2 after exposure to *M. leprae*. The nature of the humoral immune response in leprosy is not clearly defined (Sehgal *et al.* 1989). As in other chronic infections, the concentrations of serum gammaglobulins increase in leprosy.

The earliest histopathological events in human leprosy are not known. Perhaps the majority of infections are overcome at the site of entry (possibly the mucosa of the respiratory tract) and the bacilli destroyed. The Schwann cells of the nerves in the upper respiratory tract may be the first to harbour the bacilli and haematogenous spread occurs thereafter. The skin is probably involved via the endothelial cells of small vessels. Bacilli are seen in superficial nerve plexuses and perivascular macrophages in the skin in early lesions,

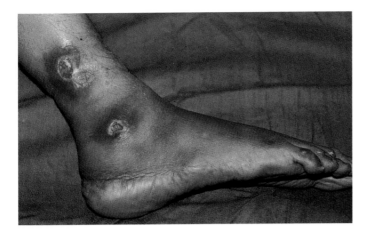

Fig. 7 Trophic ulcers in a patient with tuberculoid leprosy.

with mild local lymphocytic infiltration. In many cases (indeterminate leprosy) these lesions resolve spontaneously with eradication of bacilli. If the bacilli do persist and multiply in skin and/or nerves, the inflammatory reactions are amplified and lesions of leprosy appear. These lesions can be placed along an immunohistopathological spectrum that ranges from organized epithelioid-cell granulomas containing giant cells with few or no bacilli, through intermediate stages with less organized epithelioid cells containing more bacilli, to lepromatous leprosy with mainly macrophages and abundant bacilli. In the reactional state (type 1), there is increased inflammation in the lesions with activation of epithelioid cells and marked oedema. In type 2 states the classical lesions show oedema, polymorphonuclear leucocyte infiltration, and often a necrotizing vasculitis.

The intraosseous lesions of leprosy are characterized by granulomatous tissue reactions that lead to trabecular destruction. The lesions are evident in the epiphysis and metaphyses of tubular bones, and direct involvement of the medullary canal can also occur.

Clinical manifestations

The first signs of leprosy are usually cutaneous. Single or multiple, hypopigmented macules or plaques may appear. Sometimes an anaesthetic patch is first noticed by the patient, but often sensation remains preserved in early lesions, particularly on the face. In tuberculoid leprosy, the fully developed skin lesions are densely anaesthetic and have lost sweat glands and hair follicles. Their distribution is not symmetrical. Nerve involvement occurs early and the superficial nerve leading from lesion is enlarged. The supraorbital, facial, greater auricular, ulnar, median, radial cutaneous, common peroneal, sural, anterior, or posterior tibial nerves may be grossly enlarged and easily palpated. There may be severe paraesthesias initially, followed by muscle atrophy. If the disease progresses and the hands and feet are affected, then contractures develop (Paterson and Rad 1961). Repeated trauma in the absence of protective sensation results in ulcers that get secondarily infected (Fig. 7). In a more advanced stage, osteolysis of the terminal phalanges occurs. In lepromatous leprosy the skin lesions are macules, nodules, papules, or plaques with predilection for the face, wrists, elbows, buttocks, and knees. Involvement of major nerve trunks in common and leads to glove-and-stocking paraesthesias in the extremities.

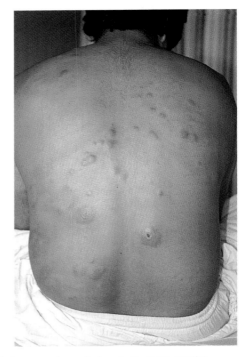

Fig. 8 Erythema nodosum lesions in the lepra reaction.

The incidence of direct involvement of the skeleton in leprosy is probably under-reported. Symmetrical, peripheral, inflammatory polyarthritis of insidious onset with a pattern of exacerbation and remission is observed in some patients (Atkin *et al.* 1989), which is different from the joint involvement of erythema nodosum leprosum or lepra type 1 reaction. Affected joints can include the wrist, knees, and hands and feet. Morning stiffness is variable from 30 min to 1 h. Symptomatic improvement is observed within a few weeks of starting multidrug treatment.

A different pattern of involvement is with changes that are usually confined to the small bones of the face, the hands, and feet (Atkin *et al.* 1987). At the fingers and toes it may appear as a dactylitis. The osseous involvement is probably due to extension of infection from overlying dermal or mucosal areas. The periosteum is contaminated initially (leprous periostitis) and subsequently the cortex and marrow are infected (leprous osteitis and osteomyelitis). In an occasional patient, haematogenous spread of infection can occur, leading to other intramedullary foci in the tubular long bones and the ribs. Overall, the progression of the lesions is very slow.

Neuroarthropathy is a progressive, degenerative joint change due to lesions of peripheral nerves and is observed more frequently in patients admitted to hospital. The skeletal changes may follow the involvement of nerves by two or three decades. The bones of the hands and feet are most susceptible. In the feet the changes usually start in the medial arch and later involve the lateral arch, talus, and calcaneus (Horibe *et al.* 1988). In extreme cases, dissolution of the mid-foot results in separation of the forefoot and the hind foot, and the tibia is driven downwards to become weight-bearing. Infection and bone injury, which can occur separately as sequelae to neuropathy and trophic ulcers, tend to accelerate the skeletal changes, leading to disintegration of the affected bones and joints.

The acute and chronic arthritis associated with the reactional state of erythema nodosum leprosum is common (Karat *et al.* 1966). The development of synovitis and/or dactylitis coincides closely with the appearance of fulminant skin lesions (Fig. 8), and the patient is febrile and toxic.

Investigations and diagnosis

The principal criteria for the diagnosis of leprosy are:

(1) a hypopigmented patch of skin with sensory impairment;

(2) thickening of the peripheral nerves;

(3) the presence of *M. leprae* in slit-skin smears — graded on the Ridley Jopling bacteriological index (**BI**) as 1+ to 6+;

(4) the characteristic histopathological changes in a biopsy specimen of a skin lesion or a peripheral nerve;

(5) positive serological tests.

Patients with lepromatous leprosy frequently have mild anaemia, an elevated erythrocyte sedimentation rate, and hypergammaglobulinaemia; 10 to 20 per cent of patients show a false-positive reaction in serological tests for syphilis, and also antinuclear antibodies.

Myocobacterium leprae is an acid-fast bacillus morphologically and biochemically similar to *M. tuberculosis*. It does not grow in artificial media or tissue cultures but is propagated consistently in the footpads of mice and nine-banded armadillos for the purpose of epidemiological studies and drug evaluation. The bacillus is slow to multiply and the doubling time is around 12 days in optimal conditions in murine footpads. The technique is expensive and time-consuming, and it takes at least 10 months for the organism to grow.

An enzyme-linked immunosorbent assay to detect antibodies to the *M. leprae* specific surface antigen has been developed (Burgess *et al.* 1988). The antigen used in the assay is a phenolic glycolipid 1 and the antibodies detected are predominantly IgM. Titres increase from the tuberculoid to the lepromatous pole of the leprosy spectrum. The early estimates of the sensitivity of this test were 95 per cent for the lepromatous pole and 30 per cent for the tuberculoid pole. This test is not yet available for use in clinical practice. In research laboratories, the polymerase chain-reaction assay is used to detect *M. leprae* DNA in skin biopsy samples (Jamil *et al.* 1993). Owing to its ability to detect small numbers of organisms, the polymerase chain reaction may prove to be a useful tool in paucibacillary disease.

The radiographic features of leprous osteitis are enlarged nutrient foramina, osteoporosis, endosteal thinning, and cyst-like lesions that are best appreciated in the phalanges. Bone sclerosis, which signifies the healing process, may also be seen. In the face, nasal destruction is characteristic. Destruction of the alveolar process and the anterior nasal spine of the maxilla appear to be related to primary involvement of the bone as well as to secondary infection. In patients with neuroarthropathy the typical changes begin with erosion of the terminal tufts of the phalanges and in the more advanced cases the entire length of terminal group of phalanges may be resorbed (MacMoran *et al.* 1987). A rare but specific radiographic finding is calcification of a large peripheral nerve such as the radial or ulnar.

Treatment

Multidrug therapy is the mainstay of treatment for leprosy (Ellard 1988; Hasting *et al.* 1988; Ye 1988). Rifampicin is by far the most potent bactericidal antileprosy drug. Dapsone is well tolerated, and

until two decades ago it was the only drug used (monotherapy) in treatment of all forms of leprosy. Clofazimine is the third drug; it has the additional property of contributing to the control of erythema nodosum leprosum through its anti-inflammatory action. The main drawback of clofazimine is that it causes a deep-brown pigmentation of skin, more evident in light-skinned persons, which is slow to regress after cessation of treatment.

The current multidrug therapy recommended by the World Health Organization for leprosy in adults is, for multibacillary disease (BI > 2+), rifampicin, 600 mg orally once monthly, dapsone 100 mg orally daily, and clofazimine, 300 mg orally once monthly and additionally 50 mg daily. The duration of treatment is at least 2 years and until negative skin tests are obtained, which occasionally extends to beyond 5 years. For paucibacillary disease (BI, 2+) the regimen is rifampicin, 600 mg orally once monthly, and dapsone, 100 mg orally daily. The duration of treatment is 6 months. All drugs are prescribed in full doses from the beginning of treatment and continued without interruption, even during the reactional states.

Evidence of clinical improvement should appear after 8 to 12 weeks from the beginning of treatment. The clinical response to adequate therapy may be confused by reactional states. Mild lepra reactions are controlled by non-steroidal anti-inflammatory drugs such as aspirin or indomethacin. In severe cares, prednisolone (60-100 mg/ daily) may be required. For the reactional state of erythema nodosum leprosum, clofazimine 100 mg orally three times a day for 2 or 3 weeks followed by tapering off to a lower dose may be helpful. An alternative, effective drug is thalidomide, especially for those patients who later take a chronic course with erythema nodosum leprosum. The usual dose of thalidomide is 200 mg orally twice daily, which is then gradually tapered off to a maintenance dose of 50 to 100 mg daily. Thalidomide is absolutely contraindicated in pregnancy.

Non-steroidal anti-inflammatory drugs usually fail to alleviate the symptoms of the polyarthritis, and they regress within a few weeks after starting antibiotic treatment. Those who present with neuroarthropathy are far more difficult to treat, particularly when the feet are involved (Warren 1973). Absolute rest for the affected limbs and control of superimposed infection are mainstays of treatment. Immobilization in plaster until all ulcerative lesions of the skin have healed may be necessary. Regular exercises are required to maintain the flexibility of the other joints until the ulcers heal. Thereafter, graded weight bearing is permitted. Amputation may be indicated if advanced disintegration of bones and joints has occurred, as the patient would be better off with a prosthesis. Advanced deformities of the hands, associated with tendon rupture, can be functionally improved by appropriate tendon-transfer surgery.

Much effort in research is being directed to control of leprosy. Trials with bacille Calmette–Guérin have so far yielded conflicting results, with some revealing only modest efficacy. Two new vaccines (Antia *et al.* 1988), one named the ICRC and the other containing viable bacille Calmette–Guérin with heat-killed *M. leprae*, are currently in field trials.

Summary of management

The diagnosis is usually evident from the clinical examination of the skin, and tender nerves are palpable at the elbows, wrists, and near the head of the fibula. Polyarthritis and enthesitis are sometimes observed in all stages of the disease. Multidrug treatment is the mainstay of therapy, and the duration largely depends on the extent of dermal involvement. Ideally the bacillary count on the slit-skin smear enables one to judge if the patient has pauci- or multibacillary disease. Dapsone and rifampicin are given for 6 or 12 months to patients with paucibacillary disease. Those with multibacillary disease are given dapsone, rifampicin, and clofazimine for 2 years, and if the slit-skin smears remain positive the treatment may be extended to 5 years. The symptoms of arthritis and enthesitis regress within 3 or 4 months of the start of treatment. In late stages, some patients develop a neuropathic foot and subluxation of joints that require surgical rehabilitation. Reactive states are occasionally observed in the first year of treatment and the patient is then given aspirin or low-dose prednisolone for 6 to 8 weeks to alleviate the symptoms, while the multidrug therapy is continued.

References

American Thoracic Society (1990). Diagnostic standards and classification of tuberculosis. *American Review of Respiratory Diseases*, **142**, 725–35.

Antia, N. H. *et al.* (1988). Leprosy vaccine — a reappraisal. *International Journal of Leprosy and Other Mycobacterial Diseases*, **56**, 231–7.

Arachi, A. (1991). The global tuberculosis situation and new control strategy of the World Health Organisation. *Tubercle*, **72**, 1–6.

Atkin, S. L. *et al.* (1987). Clinical and laboratory studies of inflammatory polyarthritis in patients with leprosy in Papua New Guinea. *Annals of the Rheumatic Diseases*, **46**, 688–90.

Atkin, S. L. *et al.* (1989). Clinical and laboratory studies of arthritis in leprosy. *British Medical Journal*, **298**, 1423–5.

Birdi, T. J. *et al.* (1989). The macrophage in leprosy: A review of the current status. *International Journal of Leprosy and Other Mycobacterial Diseases*, **57**, 511–25.

Boxer, D. *et al.* (1992). Radiological features during and following treatment of spinal tuberculosis. *British Journal of Radiology*, **65**, 476–9.

Brisson-Noel, A. *et al.* (1989). Rapid diagnosis of tuberculosis by amplification of mycobacterial DNA in clinical samples. *Lancet*, **ii**, 1069–71.

Burgess, P. J. *et al.* (1988). Serologic tests in leprosy. The sensitivity, specificity and predictive value of ELISA tests based on phenolic glycolipid antigens and the implications of their use in epidemiological studies. *Epidemiology of Infections*, **101**, 159–71.

Bush, D. C. and Schneider, L. H. (1984). Tuberculosis of the hand and wrist. *Journal of Hand Surgery*, **9A**, 391–8.

Butorac, R. *et al.* (1987). Mycobacterial disease in the musculoskeletal system. *Medical Journal of Australia*, **147**, 388–91.

Chang, K. H. *et al.* (1989). Tuberculous arachnoiditis of the spine: findings on myelography, CT and MR imaging. *American Journal of Neuroradiology*, **10**, 1255–62.

Cooke, N. J. (1985). Treatment of tuberculosis. *British Medical Journal*, **291**, 497–8.

Dall, L. *et al.* (1989). Poncet's disease: tuberculous rheumatism. *Review of Infectious Diseases*, **11**, 105–7.

Daniel, T. M. (1989). Rapid diagnosis of tuberculosis: laboratory techniques applicable in developing countries. *Review of Infectious Diseases*, **11** (Suppl. 2), 5471–8.

Davidson, P. T. (1989). The diagnosis and management of disease caused by *M. avium* complex, *M. kansasii* and other mycobacterias. *Clinics in Chest Medicine*, **10**, 431–43.

Davidson, P. T. and Horowitz, I. (1970). Skeletal tuberculosis: a review with patient presentations and discussion. *American Journal of Medicine*, **48**, 77–84.

Davies, P. D. *et al.* (1984). Bone and joint tuberculosis: a survey of notifications in England and Wales. *Journal of Bone and Joint Surgery*, **66B**, 326–30.

Dutt, A. K. (1989). Update in tuberculosis: an overview. *Seminars in Respiratory Infections*, **4**, 155–6.

Edeikin, J. *et al.* (1963). 'Cystic' tuberculosis of bone. *Clinical Orthopedics*, **28**, 163–8.

Ellard, G. A. (1988). Chemotherapy of leprosy. *British Medical Bulletin*, **44**, 775–90.

Ellner, J. J. *et al.* (1989). Immunologic aspects of mycobacterial infections. *Review of Infectious Diseases*, **11** (Suppl. 2), 455–9.

Garrido, G. *et al.* (1988). A review of peripheral tuberculous arthritis. *Seminars in Arthritis and Rheumatism*, **18**, 142–9.

Goldberger, M. J. (1988). Anti tuberculosis agents. *Medical Clinics of North America*, **72**, 661–8.

Hannachi, M. R. (1988). Comparison of 3 chemotherapeutic regimens of short duration (6 months) in osteoarticular tuberculosis — results after 5 years. *Bulletin of the International Union for Tubercular Lung Disease*, **63**, 14–15.

Harboe, M. (1985). Immunology of leprosy. In *Leprosy* (ed. R. C. Hastings), pp. 53–87. Churchill Livingstone, New York.

Hastings, R. C. *et al.* (1988). Chemotherapy of leprosy. *Annual Review of Pharmacology and Toxicology*, **28**, 231–45.

Horibe, S. *et al.* (1988). Neuroarthropathy of the foot in leprosy. *Journal of Bone and Joint Surgery*, **70**, 481–5.

ICMR/BMRC (1989). A controlled trial of short-course regimens of chemotherapy in patients receiving ambulatory treatment or undergoing radical surgery for tuberculosis of spine. *Indian Journal of Tuberculosis*, **36** (Suppl.), 1–21.

Ivanyi, J. (1988). Immunodiagnostic assays for tuberculosis and leprosy. *British Medical Bulletin*, **44**, 635–49.

Jamil, S. *et al.* (1993). Use of polymerase chain reaction to assess efficacy of leprosy chemotherapy. *Lancet*, **342**, 264–8.

Karat, A. B. A. *et al.* (1966). Acute exudative arthritis in leprosy: rheumatoid arthritis like syndrome in association with erythema nodosum leprosum. *British Medical Journal*, **ii**, 770–3.

Kim, Y. H. (1988). Total knee, arthroplasty for tuberculous arthritis. *Journal of Bone and Joint Surgery*, **70A**, 1322–30.

Kumar, K. (1985). A clinical study and classification of posterior spinal tuberculosis. *International Orthopedics*, **9**, 147–52.

Kumar, K. *et al.* (1988). Multifocal osteoarticular tuberculosis. *International Orthopedics*, **12**, 135–8.

LaBerge, J. M. and Brant-Zawadzki, M. (1984). Evaluation of Pott's disease with computed tomography. *Neuroradiology*, **26**, 429–34.

LeRoux, P. *et al.* (1990). Tuberculosis of the skull — a rare condition: case report and review of the literature. *Neurosurgery*, **26**, 851–6.

Levy, A. *et al.* (1986). Early recognition of tuberculous arthritis assisted by CT scan and closed needle synovial biopsy. *Clinical Rheumatology*, **5**, 523–6.

Lifeso, R. M. (1987). Atlanto axial tuberculosis in adults. *Journal of Bone and Joint Surgery*, **69B**, 183–7.

Lucas, S. B. (1988). Histopathology of leprosy and tuberculosis-an overview. *British Medical Bulletin*, **44**, 584–99.

MacMoran, J. W. *et al.* (1987). Bone loss in limbs with decreased or absent sensation: ten year follow up of the hands in leprosy. *Skeletal Radiology*, **16**, 452–9.

Martini, M. *et al.* (1986). Tuberculous osteomyelitis. A review of 125 cases. *International Orthopedics*, **10**, 201–7.

Martini, M. *et al.* (1988). Bone and joint tuberculosis: a review of 652 cases. *Orthopedics*, **11**, 861–6.

Medical Research Council (1993). Controlled trial of short-course regimens of chemotherapy in the ambulatory treatment of spinal tuberculosis. *Journal of Bone and Joint Surgery*, **75B**, 240–8.

Modilevsky, T. *et al.* (1989). Mycobacterial disease in patients with human immunodeficiency virus infection. *Archives of Internal Medicine*, **149**, 2201–5.

Narayanan, R. B. (1988). Immunopathology of leprosy granuloma. Current status: a review. *Leprosy Review*, **59**, 75–82.

Omari, B. *et al.* (1989). Potts' Disease — a resurgent challenge to the thoracic surgeon. *Chest*, **95**, 145–50.

Paterson, D. E. and Rad, M. (1961). Bone changes in leprosy: their incidence, progress and prevention and arrest. *International Journal of Leprosy*, **29**, 393–422.

Pouchot, L. *et al.* (1988). Tuberculosis of the sacroiliac joint: clinical features, outcome, and evaluation of closed needle biopsy in 11 consecutive cases. *American Journal of Medicine*, **84**, 622–8.

Reich, C. V. (1987). Leprosy: cause, transmission and a new theory of pathogenesis. *Review of Infectious Diseases*, **9**, 590–4.

Ridley, D. S. and Jopling, W. H. (1966). Classification of leprosy according to immunity: a five group system. *International Journal of Leprosy*, **34**, 255–73.

Schluger, N. *et al.* (1994). Clinical utility of the polymerase chain reaction in the diagnosis of infections due to *Mycobacterium tuberculosis*. *Chest*, **105**, 1116–21.

Sehgal, V. N. *et al.* (1989). Immunology of leprosy: a comprehensive survey. *International Journal of Dermatology*, **28**, 571–84.

Shepard, C. C. (1982). Leprosy today. *New England Journal of Medicine*, **307**, 1640–1.

Shoemaker, S. A. (1986). Molecular biology and mycobacteriae. *Seminars in Respiratory Infections*, **1**, 265–9.

Sifford, M. and Bates J. H. (1991). Host determinants of susceptibility to mycobacterium tuberculosis. *Seminars in Respiratory Infections*, **6**, 44–50.

Smith, A. S. *et al.* (1989). MR imaging characteristics of tuberculous spondylitis vs. vertebral osteomyelitis, *American Journal of Roentgenology*, **153**, 399–405.

Stanford. J. I. (1983). Immunologically important constituents of mycobacteria. In *Biology of mycobacteria* (ed. C. Ratledge and J. L. Stanford), pp. 85–127. Academic Press, London.

Warren, G. (1973). The management of tarsal disintegration. *Leprosy Review*, **43**, 137–47.

Whelan, M. A. *et al.* (1985). Computed tomography of nontuberculous spinal infection. *Journal of Computer Assisted Tomography*, **9**, 280–7.

Wolfgang, G. I. (1978). Tuberculosis joint infection. *Clinical Orthopedics*, **136**, 257–63.

Ye, G. Y. (1988). Diagnosis of leprosy. *International Journal of Dermatology*, **27**, 263–4.

5.3.8 Brucellar arthritis

E. Pascual

Introduction

Infection of the joints is the most frequent, localized complication of brucellosis, and a common cause of infectious arthritis in the countries where the disease is endemic.

Epidemiology

Brucellosis occurs naturally in domesticated animals. It constitutes an important economic problem and a serious heath hazard in many countries, especially in the Mediterranean region, Arabian peninsula, Indian subcontinent, Mexico, and parts of Central and South America. Of the six recognized species of brucella, only four are known to be human pathogens (Young 1995); *Brucella melitensis*, the most virulent, causes disease in goats, sheep, and camels, *B. abortus* in cattle, *B. suis* in pigs, and *B. canis* in dogs. Multiple viobars have been identified in *B. melitensis*. Localization of brucellae in the male and female reproductive organs accounts for the major clinical manifestation, that is abortion. Human infection is contracted from infected animals and is closely linked to poor methods of animal husbandry, feeding habits, and hygiene standards. The disease is common in some professions due to handling of infected animals or viscera, where the organism is acquired either through breaches in the skin or by infectious aerosol reaching the conjunctiva or the airways. Ingestion of unpasteurized dairy products is the most common cause of infection due to *B. melitensis*. Because of their high infectiveness, brucellae are a common cause of accidental infection in laboratory workers (Miller *et al.* 1987; Young 1995).

Infection acquired during foreign travel, often through consumption of infected, illegally marketed dairy products, is the cause of imported disease (Arnow *et al.* 1984; Revak *et al.* 1989). The possibility of illegal import of such products should be borne in mind (Thapar and Young 1986).

General characteristics of the organism

Brucellae are small, aerobic, non-motile, gram-negative coccobacilli which grow well at $37°C$ in any high quality peptone-based medium enriched with blood or serum. Their growth requires a much longer incubation period than pyogenic organisms and many strains of *B. abortus* and *B. suis* require supplementary CO_2, as described below (Young 1995).

The host defence

Experiments in rats have shown that after entering the blood stream, brucellae are phagocytosed by polymorphonuclear leucocytes. Within hours, phagocytosed organisms can be seen in the mononuclear phagocytic cells of the liver sinusoids, lymph nodes, spleen, and bone marrow — and probably in other organs rich in mononuclear phagocytic cells — where they reproduce (Spink 1964; Smith and Ficht 1990). The frequent isolation of brucellae from bone marrow cultures in diseased humans (Gotuzzo *et al.* 1986) as well as from liver biopsies (Spink 1964) indicates a similar distribution in humans. The permanence and reproduction of the organisms inside the cells may be important in understanding some of the characteristics of the disease.

The tissue response in established disease is a non-specific granulomatous lesion, very similar to sarcoidosis (Hunt and Bothwell 1967). Brucellae cannot be identified in these tissues but can be cultured from them (Spink 1964). Localized areas of suppuration or caseation may occur, most frequently in *B. suis* (Spink 1964) but also in *B. melitensis*.

General characteristics of the disease

The manifestations of brucellosis are non-specific and no combination of signs or symptoms can be considered to be characteristic. *B. melitensis* causes more severe disease than *B. abortus* and *B. suis*, probably because of its greater ability to avoid the host's defences (Smith and Ficht 1990). *B. suis* has a higher tendency to suppurative complications. The large, published series have focused on patients infected by *B. melitensis*, and generalization of this data to disease caused by the other brucellae may be inaccurate. Reference to the other infections will be indicated in the text, as appropriate.

Brucellosis is more common in men than in women both in the Middle East and Mediterranean countries (Colmenero *et al.* 1985; Andonopoulos *et al.* 1986; Mousa *et al.* 1987; Lulu *et al.* 1988; Ariza 1988; Batlle *et al.* 1989). In the same areas, the disease occurs with equal frequency in children of both sexes (Feiz *et al.* 1978; Lubani *et al.* 1986; Gómez -Reino *et al.* 1986; Al-Eissa *et al.* 1990), as happens with adults in Peru (Gotuzzo *et al.* 1987). It may be that where brucellosis is contracted as a professional hazard, more males are affected. Ingestion of milk, which is the usual cause of the disease in children and Peruvian adults (Gotuzzo *et al.* 1987), would result in equal incidence in both sexes.

The incubation period may be as short as 1 week but usually lasts from 2 to 8 weeks (Young 1995). The disease usually presents with fever, often without an undulant pattern, sweats, which may be drenching, and a general feeling of malaise. Weakness, anorexia, myalgia, and arthralgia are common. Patients often recall contact with possibly infected animals or their unpasteurized products but this evidence may be absent. Physical examination may show lymphadenopathies and enlargement of liver or spleen. Localized infections, especially in the skeleton, are common. Other possible causes, such as neurobrucellosis, endocarditis, hepatitis, and epididimo-orchitis, should be considered.

Subclinical disease occurs and may heal spontaneously. Patients may present with relapses following previous subclinical disease or with late, localized complications, simulating a very long incubation period.

The concept of chronic brucellosis was coined before the antibiotic era, to refer to a group of patients who complained of ill health after having suffered from brucellosis, generally due to *B. abortus*. A careful study (Spink 1951) showed that some of these patients had a bacteriologically proven relapse, or localized disease; in others, no explanation was found for the symptoms and it was felt that they were related to an unstable emotional state. It is unclear whether chronic brucellosis in the absence of infection exists and such diagnosis must be handled with care.

Brucellar arthritis

Arthralgia is more common in brucellosis than in other febrile illnesses. It has been recorded in 88 per cent (Thapar and Young 1986), 65 per cent (Colmenero *et al.* 1986), 65 per cent (Ariza 1988), and 58 per cent (Lulu *et al.* 1988) of adult patients studied prospectively, and in 87 per cent (Feiz *et al.* 1978) and 74 per cent (Al-Eissa *et al.* 1990) of the children thus studied; its presence may be a clue to the disease. Bone scans of patients with brucellosis and musculoskeletal symptoms are very frequently abnormal, often in multiple sites (El Desouki 1991). Perhaps some of the minor musculoskeletal symptoms of these patients are due to localized infection. Since the treatment of brucellar arthritis and that of uncomplicated brucellosis is the same, once the diagnosis of brucellosis has been reached, it is not worthwhile conducting a search for arthritis to explain minor or unclear musculoskeletal symptoms.

Infection in the joints is the most common form of localized disease in brucellosis. It appears in 25 per cent (Colmenero *et al.* 1991), 29 per cent (Ariza 1988), 26 per cent (Lulu *et al.* 1988), 24 per cent (Gotuzzo *et al.* 1987), and 22 per cent (Andonopoulos *et al.* 1986) of adult patients studied prospectively, and in 38 per cent (Al-Eissa *et al.* 1990), 28 per cent (Llorens-Terol and Busquets 1980), and 19 per cent (Feiz *et al.* 1978) of children. In areas where brucellosis is endemic, brucellar arthritis may outnumber tuberculous arthritis (Rajapakse 1987). All the above series refer to *B. melitensis*.

The general clinical characteristics of brucellar arthritis are similar to those of infectious arthritis due to other organisms. The disease is generally monoarticular, but in 18 per cent of our patients more than one joint was affected (Batlle *et al.* 1989). The large peripheral joints, sacroiliacs, and the spine are the usual sites of articular involvement. Bursitis and osteomyelitis may occur. Some patients have simultaneous infection in more than one joint. The possibility of reactive arthritis has been considered.

Table 1 Distribution of joint involvement

	Peripheral joints*	Sacroiliacs	Spine
Adults	Frequent	Frequent	Frequent
Children	Frequent	Infrequent (older children)	Exceptional

*In order of frequency; hip, knee, ankle, shoulder, elbow, wrist, and sternoclavicular joint.

Clinical and radiological characteristics

Arthritis of peripheral joints

Large peripheral joints are a common site of localized infection, ranging from 20 to 73 per cent of all arthritides in different adult series (Serre *et al.* 1981; Andonopoulos *et al.* 1986; Gotuzzo *et al.* 1987; Ariza 1988; Al-Rawi *et al.* 1989; Batlle *et al.* 1989) (Table 1). It is of interest that children nearly always show peripheral joint involvement, either with *B. melitensis* (Lubani *et al.* 1986; Gómez-Reino *et al.* 1986; Gotuzzo and Carrillo 1988; Benjamin *et al.* 1992) or *B. abortus* infections (Adam *et al.* 1967). *B. canis* knee arthritis in a child has been reported (Young 1983). In all age groups, the hip followed by the knee are the most common locations. Ankles, shoulders, elbows, wrists, and sternoclavicular joints (Berrocal *et al.* 1993) contribute a small percentage of cases. The smaller hand and feet joints seem to be rarely affected. A 'rheumatoid like' distribution may occur (Gotuzzo *et al.* 1982).

Peripheral joint arthritis often, but not always, predominates over other disease manifestations, and the patient's main complaint is centred on the joint. Usually it occurs during the acute phase of the disease or during a relapse (Gotuzzo *et al.* 1982); fever, or other general symptoms of the disease, frequently accompany the arthritis, which tends to be symptomatic from the start and so patients tend to seek prompt medical attention. The joints are swollen and painful and an effusion is generally seen. Joint inflammation is not as intense as it is in some septic arthritides due to pyogenic organisms, and there is seldom obvious redness or unusual warmth in the skin. Local complications, such as popliteal cyst rupture, may occur (Laajam 1985).

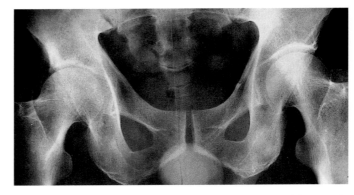

Fig. 1 Radiograph of the hips showing diminished radiological joint space in a patient with brucellar arthritis of his right hip.

If there is delay in the diagnosis or treatment, the structure of the joint is damaged resulting in radiological abnormalities, such as joint space narrowing (Fig. 1) and damage to the joint surfaces, similar to those of other infectious arthritides. The interval between the initiation of the infection and the appearance of structural damage in the joint tends to be longer than in pyogenic arthritides, but probably shorter than in tuberculosis. The sequelae left after appropriate treatment depends on the damage present when treatment was started. If this is started early enough, no sequelae will remain. In children with arthritis of the hip, dislocation and aseptic necrosis have been observed (Benjamin and Khan 1994). Brucellae may infect prosthetic joints (Agarwal *et al.* 1991). Bursitis and tenosynovitis due to *B. melitensis* (Mousa *et al.* 1987), *B. abortus*, and *B. suis* also may occur (Kelly *et al.* 1960).

Sacroiliitis

Involvement of the sacroiliac joint comprises a large percentage of brucellar arthritides. Higher frequencies have been reported in the west Mediterranean countries — 43 per cent in men and 20 per cent in women (Rotés-Querol 1957); 34 per cent (Serre *et al.* 1981); 51 per cent (Ariza 1988); and 36 per cent (Batlle *et al.* 1989) — as compared to countries further east — 11 per cent in Greece (Andonopoulos *et al.* 1986) and 13 per cent and 5 per cent in the Middle East (Mousa *et al.* 1987; Al-Rawi *et al.* 1989). An incidence of 50 per cent was found in Peru (Gotuzzo *et al.* 1982). The reasons for these differences are unclear. Sacroiliitis seems to be an unusual complication of *B. abortus* and *B. suis* (Kelly *et al.* 1960). Sacroiliitis is uncommon in children (Lubani *et al.* 1986; Gómez-Reino *et al.* 1986) but young adults have a clearly increased risk for arthritis in this particular joint (Rotés-Querol 1957; Gotuzzo *et al.* 1982).

Sacroiliitis tends to occur in the acute, febrile phase of the disease, is usually unilateral, and clearly symptomatic from its start. The pain in some of the patients becomes so intense in 2 or 3 days that they can hardly move from the bed (Mousa *et al.* 1987). Radiation of the pain to the buttock, posterior thigh, and even below, is not unusual. In these patients, any movement of the leg is very painful and tests for hip manoeuvres or straight leg elevation may seem positive. In this setting, clinical differentiation of sacroiliitis from hip disease or sciatica may be difficult (Mousa *et al.* 1987; Gotuzzo and Carrillo 1988); gently tapping on the lower surface of the heel while the patient keeps the leg extended, clearly localizes the pain to the sacroiliac area. Other sacroiliac manoeuvres may produce too much pain, and may be difficult to interpret in this group. Standard manoeuvres provide appropriate information in patients with less intense symptoms.

Due to the acute nature of the sacroiliitis, the presenting radiographs do not aid the diagnosis; some blurring of the articular margins and widening of the sacroiliac space (Fig. 2) may occur when the disease is of longer duration (Ariza *et al.* 1993). Computed tomography (CT) scan generally allows earlier demonstration of joint infection. A bone scan provides early evidence of sacroiliitis on most occasions (Mousa *et al.* 1987; Bahar *et al.* 1988; Madkour *et al.* 1988; Cordero Sánchez *et al.* 1990). Brucellar sacroiliitis is a mild disease associated with a good outcome similar to that observed for patients with uncomplicated brucellosis (Ariza *et al.* 1993).

Spondylitis

Infection in the spine is the cause of between 7 and 53 per cent of localized skeletal infection (Rotés-Querol 1957; Serre *et al.* 1981; Gotuzzo *et al.* 1982; Gotuzzo and Carrillo 1988; Ariza 1988; Al-Rawi *et al.* 1989; Batlle *et al.* 1989). Referral patterns to hospitals may account for some of the discrepancies. It is generally seen in older patients (Rotés-Querol 1957; Serre *et al.* 1981; Gotuzzo *et al.* 1982; Lifeso *et al.* 1985; Ariza *et al.* 1985a; Gotuzzo and Carrillo 1988; Colmenero *et al.* 1991) but not in children, neither with *B. melitensis* (Lubani *et al.* 1986; Gómez-Reino *et al.* 1986; Gotuzzo and Carrillo 1988) nor with *B. abortus* (Adam *et al.* 1967). The majority of patients from the United Kingdom or United States described as suffering from skeletal brucellosis are isolated cases or small series and are due to *B. abortus*, or *B. suis* (Kelly *et al.* 1960; Torres-Rojas *et al.* 1979; Manaster 1988); their clinical characteristics are similar to those caused by *B. melitensis*.

The lumbar spine is the most commonly affected segment, followed by the dorsal spine. The cervical spine accounts for a small percentage of the cases. Involvement of more than one disc space is not infrequent (Rotés-Querol 1957; Kelly *et al.* 1960; Serre *et al.* 1981; Ariza *et al.* 1985a; Lifeso *et al.* 1985; Gotuzzo and Carrillo 1988; Sharif *et al.* 1989). In contrast to peripheral arthritis or sacroiliitis, spondylitis is generally a late feature, often occurring in patients with only vague symptoms of a general infectious disorder, and not infrequently afebrile (Serre *et al.* 1981; Lifeso *et al.* 1985; Gotuzzo and Carrillo 1988), although careful register of the temperature may show a low grade fever and patients may complain of some malaise. In other series, 17 out of 20 patients had systemic symptoms, but these patients presented with the spine infection shortly after the start of the disease (Ariza *et al.* 1985a).

Onset of the disease is often insidious, and its hallmark is local pain of variable intensity, often moderate, frequently allowing the patient to maintain a fairly normal life. Pressure or percussion of the spinous processes of the vertebrae corresponding to the affected level often reproduces the pain, and some tenderness may also occur in the paravertebral muscles. Deformities are uncommon (Rotés-Querol 1957). Paravertebral abscesses appear in about 16 per cent of the patients (Ariza *et al.* 1985a) but are generally smaller than those of tuberculosis. In the cervical spine, abscesses may produce retropharyngeal swelling (Lifeso *et al.* 1985). Material obtained from the abscesses is usually sterile (Rotés-Querol 1957; Ariza *et al.* 1985a). Similar abscesses may occur with *B. abortus* (Torres-Rojas *et al.* 1979). Some patients may develop epidural abscesses from the infected disc space and develop a paraplegia. Compression of the medulla or nerve roots is found more frequently in cervical spondylitis, which should be considered a severe manifestation of the disease (Colmenero *et al.*

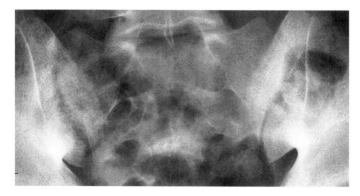

Fig. 2 Radiograph of the sacroiliac joints, showing widening and erosions of the right joint in a patient with long-standing right brucellar sacroiliitis.

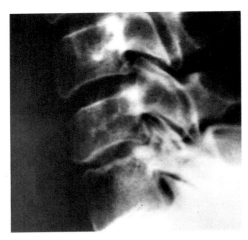

Fig. 3 Lateral radiograph of the lower cervical spine, showing diminished height of the disc space, in a patient with brucellar spondylitis

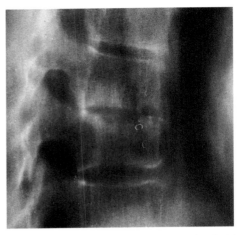

Fig. 5 Lateral tomography of the dorsal spine, showing diminished disc space height and vertebral end-plates erosions in a patient with brucellar spondylitis.

1992). In this case myelography shows extradural compression and these patients may need surgical decompression (Lifeso *et al.* 1985); despite surgery, severe sequelae may occur (Colmenero *et al.* 1991).

In the very early phases, radiographs of the affected segments are normal. After 2 months, nearly all patients show some radiographic alterations (Ariza *et al.* 1985*a*; Lifeso *et al.* 1985). The first sign seen is narrowing of the disc (Fig. 3), without bone abnormalities. Later, two different alterations are seen in the limiting vertebral end-plates: a limited form with an erosion, generally in the anterosuperior vertebral angle, with sclerotic base, which is considered as characteristic of brucellar spondylitis (Pedro Pons' sign) (Fig. 4); and a diffuse form, in which the corresponding vertebral end-plates show erosions, accompanied by disc-space narrowing (Fig. 5). Early signs of repair,

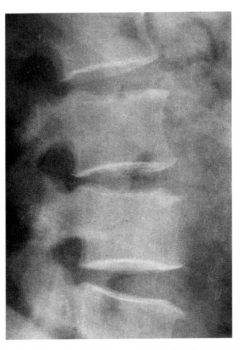

Fig. 4 Lateral radiograph of lumbar vertebrae, showing an upper corner lesion, with sclerotic base (Pedro Pons' sign), considered characteristic of brucellar spondylitis. Diminution in the height of the disc space is also seen.

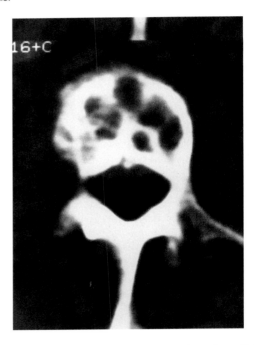

Fig. 6 CT scan through the vertebral end plate of a patient with brucellar spondylitis, showing erosive lesions.

with the appearance of osteophytes, occur (Rotés–Querol 1957; Serre *et al.* 1981; Gotuzzo *et al.* 1982; Ariza *et al.* 1985*a*; Lifeso *et al.* 1985; Gotuzzo and Carrillo 1988; Sharif *et al.* 1989). Both pathological (Rotés–Querol 1957) and radiological (Sharif *et al.* 1989) data suggest that the infection begins in the vertebra and then spreads to the disc. CT scans may show either localized epiphyseal changes (Sharif *et al.* 1989) or diffuse irregularities and erosions in the vertebral end-plates (Fig. 6). Paravertebral abscess formation (Lifeso *et al.* 1985; Manaster *et al.* 1988, Sharif *et al.* 1989) and epidural extension (Manaster *et al.* 1988) are also demonstrated. Experience with magnetic resonance imaging is limited, and has shown lesions of both localized epiphyseal changes and of diffuse disc-space infections; epidural extension was seen in all four patients studied in the absence of neurological damage (Sharif *et al.* 1990).

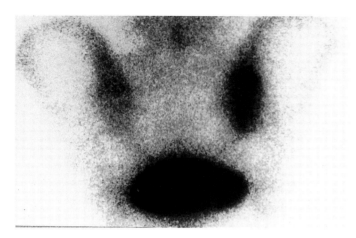

Fig. 7 Bone scan of the posterior pelvis of a patient with left brucellar sacroiliitis of short duration and normal radiograph.

Bone scans frequently show increased uptake at the level of the affected disc space, even when radiologically normal (Bahar *et al.* 1988; Madkour *et al.* 1988; Sharif *et al.* 1989) (Fig. 7). On the other hand, in a prospective study of brucellar spondylitis, bone scans were normal in some patients during the first 3 months of the disease, and later, at times, only slightly abnormal (Ariza *et al.* 1985*a*).

Osteomyelitis

Osteomyelitis is an unusual feature of brucellosis, which may present as local pain and tenderness. *B. melitensis* has a predilection for the ribs and epiphyses of long bones, but may occur in other locations (Rotés-Querol 1957; Serre *et al.* 1981; Mousa *et al.* 1987). *B. suis* seems to prefer the long bones (Kelly *et al.* 1960; Keenan and Guttmann 1982; Bonfiglio *et al.* 1983).

Reactive arthritis

A report (Hodinka *et al.* 1978) of higher frequency of HLA-B27 in patients with brucellar spondylitis raised the possibility of brucellar reactive arthritis. Three HLA-B27-positive patients described as having reactive arthritis after brucellosis were subsequently reported (Dawes and Ghosh 1985). Other studies have failed to find such an association (Alarcón *et al.* 1981; Alarcón *et al.* 1985; Al-Rawi *et al.* 1987). My own experience with 86 prospectively followed patients with brucellar arthritis, is that none of them had any type of chronic arthritis remaining after antimicrobial treatment. As a rule, the symptoms improve clearly after appropriate treatment, both in peripheral and axial arthritides. It is of interest that brucella can be grown from erythema nodosum-like lesions (thought to be a hypersensitivity reaction) occurring in patients with brucellosis (Ariza *et al.* 1989).

The possibility of reactive brucellar arthritis is an open question; such diagnosis should be handled with care and only entertained in those patients in whom unexplained arthritis persists after successful antimicrobial treatment of proven brucellosis.

Other musculoskeletal manifestations

Acute brucellosis may present as a leucocytoclastic vasculitis (Vazquez Doval *et al.* 1991). Patients with brucellosis may also show lesions resembling panniculitis from which brucella can be grown (Ariza *et al.* 1989; Zuckerman *et al.* 1994). Soft tissue abscesses have been reported (Tovar *et al.* 1990)

General laboratory features

With the exception of serological and bacteriological data, the laboratory features of brucellosis are non-specific. The erythrocyte sedimentation rate generally shows some elevation — it was below 44 mm in 70 per cent of the patients with brucellar arthritis (Mousa *et al.* 1987), and normal in 16 per cent in another series (Rotés-Querol 1957). Frequent slight elevations or normal values have been found by others, both in adults (Colmenero *et al.* 1986; Al-Rawi *et al.* 1987; Lulu *et al.* 1988) and children (Gómez-Reino *et al.* 1986; Al-Eissa *et al.* 1990). A similar pattern is seen with *B. abortus* and *B. suis* (Kelly *et al.* 1960). Normal values are not unusual in late, localized forms, as in spondylitis (Serre *et al.* 1981). A normal or low leucocyte count, associated with lymphocytosis is usual (Crosby *et al.* 1984; Colmenero *et al.* 1986; Thapar and Young 1986; Mousa *et al.* 1987). Lymphopenia may be associated with more severe clinical manifestations (Crosby *et al.* 1984). Leucocytosis is unusual but may occur. Thrombocytopenia, anaemia, and pancytopenia may all occur (Crosby *et al.* 1984; Lulu *et al.* 1988).

Abnormality of liver function tests is a common feature of the disease (Colmenero *et al.* 1985; Thapar and Young 1986; Lulu *et al.* 1988), and occurs more frequently in the early phases.

Synovial fluid analysis

Published data of synovial fluid analysis in brucellar arthritis are scarce. Cell counts have been found to be below 50 000/mm³, (Gotuzzo and Carrillo 1988) or even lower — 4460 to 8800/mm³ (Andonopoulos *et al.* 1986); 6000 to 18 000/mm³ (Mousa *et al.* 1987); and 8600 to 11 600/mm³ (Mavridis *et al.* 1987). Glucose levels were within normal limits in the above series. Lactic acid levels have also been found to be normal (Mavridis *et al.* 1984). *B. melitensis* has been isolated from some of the synovial fluids in these studies. Our own unpublished data of the analysis of synovial fluids from 18 prospectively studied brucellar arthritides differ from the above results. The cell counts were 3200 to 90 000/mm³; glucose was low in some of the fluids (0–100 mg/dl, mean 47 ± 33 SD), and lactic acid was also high in some samples (13–138 mg/dl, mean 74 ± 36 SD). *B. melitensis* was recovered from 73 per cent of these fluids, many of them with characteristics suggestive of non-infectious, inflammatory synovial fluid.

Diagnostic investigations

Importance of the clinical features

The clinical features of brucellosis are not specific. The manifestations of brucellar joint disease are similar to those of other infectious peripheral or axial arthritides, and may also resemble some inflammatory arthritides. Nevertheless, in the following circumstances, appropriate testing for brucellosis should always be done:

(1) in all undiagnosed arthritides, with features fitting those of brucellosis, occurring in areas where the disease is endemic or in patients with a history of possible exposure to the disease;

(2) in all cases of undiagnosed acute unilateral sacroiliitis;

Table 2 Percentage of isolation of *Brucella melitensis* in blood cultures

Unselected adults

73 (Thapar and Young 1986)

62 (Colmenero *et al.* 1986)

78 (Ariza 1988)

30 (Lulu *et al.* 1988)

72 (Colmenero *et al.* 1991)

Unselected children

32 (Feiz *et al.* 1978)

75 (Al-Eissa *et al.* 1990)

Brucellar arthritis (adults)

58 (Rotés-Querol 1957)

41 (Batlle *et al.* 1989)

41 (Al-Rawi *et al.* 1989)

Brucellar arthritis (children)

33 (Gómez-Reino *et al.* 1986)

70 (Lubani *et al.* 1986)

(3) in all cases of undiagnosed disc-space infection, especially those with radiological evidence of localized vertebral angle infection or infection of multiple levels.

About one-quarter of the patients do not recall exposure to possibly infected animals or unpasteurized diary products.

Bacteriological diagnosis

Isolation of brucellae from blood, synovial fluid, or other sources should always be attempted when the disease is suspected. It provides a definitive diagnosis and the possibility of differentiating *B. melitensis*, *B. abortus*, and *B. suis*, which cannot be done with the usual serological tests. When brucellosis is suspected, the laboratory should always be warned, since:

1. Brucellae are slow growing organisms and most cultures will be negative if not kept long enough — ideally up to 6 weeks (Rodríguez Torres 1988). In a series of 262 positive blood cultures, the growth was apparent in 8 per cent of the samples during the first week, 36 per cent during the second, 31 per cent during the third, 17 per cent during the fourth, 6 per cent during the fifth, and 2 per cent during the sixth week; the culture was not pursued further (Ariza 1988). More delayed growth was found in a smaller series, with a mean of 37 days (range 20 to 51 days) (Thapar and Young 1986).

2. Brucellae are a common cause of acquired infection in the laboratory and personnel should take special precautions (Miller *et al.* 1987).

Any high quality, peptone-based medium enriched with blood or serum is suitable for growing brucellae (Young 1995); a 10 per cent CO_2 atmosphere increases the yield and is necessary for most strains of *B. abortus*; culture systems with a solid phase are easier and less risky to handle in the laboratory (Rodríguez Torres 1988). Of practical importance, brucellae were isolated from seven blood cultures in a mean time of 2.1 days when processed by the lysis–centrifugation

system; simultaneous standard blood cultures of the same samples were positive in only six cases, and the mean detection time was 20.6 days (Navas *et al.* 1993).

Blood cultures are often positive in disease due to *B. melitensis*. Table 2 shows the isolation rate of the organism from blood cultures obtained in different series of unselected patients and in patients with arthritis. Patients with relapsing disease have the same rate of positive blood cultures as new patients (Ariza 1988).

Although blood cultures should be obtained when patients are febrile, in 30 per cent (Ariza 1988) and 31 per cent (Rodríguez Torres 1988) of afebrile patients the organism grew. Isolation of *B. melitensis* from blood cultures is less frequent in late, localized disease, and in spondylitis (Serre *et al.* 1981; Gotuzzo and Carrillo 1988; Colmenero *et al.* 1991). In these cases, bone marrow culture may be advantageous (Gotuzzo *et al.* 1986). Differences in disease characteristics, or laboratory procedures, probably account for the wide differences found between series; a 7 per cent positive rate was found in a large series in which blood cultures were frequently kept less than 10 days (Mousa *et al.* 1987). The isolation rate of *B. abortus* and *B. suis* is lower than that of *B. melitensis*.

Synovial fluid should always be cultured. *B. melitensis* grew in 73 per cent of the synovial fluids inoculated in blood culture flasks (Carro *et al.* 1988). Other series have obtained a 62 per cent (Gotuzzo and Carrillo 1988), 60 per cent (Andonopoulos *et al.* 1986), and 27 per cent (Gotuzzo *et al.* 1982) growth in the cultured samples. *B. abortus* has been cultured from synovial fluid (Al-Rawi *et al.* 1989) as well as *B. canis* (Young 1983). Material obtained by needle puncture from infected disc spaces (Seignon *et al.* 1980) or surgically from the sacro-iliac joint (Porat and Shapiro 1984) may also grow brucellae. *B. abortus* or *B. suis* may grow in samples obtained from bone, bursa, tendons, and joints (Kelly *et al.* 1960).

Serological diagnosis

The attempts to isolate brucellae from blood or other sources are not always successful; moreover, a long incubation period is required. Under these circumstances, the possibility of serological diagnosis offers great advantages. Serological tests allow the detection of antibodies produced against the lipopolysaccharide of the bacterial cell wall (Diaz *et al.* 1968), which is common to *B. melitensis*, *B. abortus* and *B. suis*, but not *B. canis* which needs a specific antigenic suspension (Polt *et al.* 1982; Devi *et al.* 1987).

The standard tube agglutination test (**STA**) is the most widely used test. The test antigen is generally obtained from *B. abortus*; it reacts against *B. abortus*, *B. melitensis*, and *B. suis* and does not allow differentiation between them (Rodríguez Torres 1988; Young 1995). A positive STA is indicative of contact with brucellae. Although high titres are indicative of current infection, the presence of any positive titre, if the clinical features are compatible, must be investigated further. As in other serological investigations, the individual response, antigen preparations, and laboratory procedures influence the final titre (Rodríguez Torres 1988).

Blocking antibodies may result in a negative STA test at low dilutions, while a positive test is obtained with further serum dilution. This phenomenon occurs mainly in late, localized brucellosis (Rodríguez Torres 1988). The brucellar Coombs' test detects these blocking antibodies and allows the diagnosis to be made (Hall and Manion 1953). The brucellar Coombs' test always gives higher titres than the STA test (Rodríguez Torres 1988). A combination of the STA test and the brucellar Coombs' test allows detection of the large

> **Box 1 Management of brucellar arthritis**
>
> **Antimicrobial therapy:**
> Is the same as that used for uncomplicated brucellosis, i.e. a combination of rifampicin 900 mg/day and doxycycline 200 mg/day over 45 days (relapse rate 5%: relapsing patients : organisms have the same sensitivities as the pre-treatment isolates (relapse is not due to drug resistance). Patients should receive a second course of treatment.
>
> For children under 8:
> Use a combination of trimethoprim–sulphamethoxazole, 10–50 mg/kg/day, given twice daily, for 3 weeks and gentamicin, 5 mg/kg/day twice daily, intramuscularly given the first 5 days
>
> **Local management:**
> • Peripheral joints: no local manoeuvres (e.g. daily drainage) are required.
> • Sacroileitis or spine infection: only bed rest and analgesia until pain eases.
> • Epidural abscesses:
>   Medical treatment may be enough, but the need for surgery is an open question.
>   An antimicrobial regimen including streptomycin and a tetracycline may offer advantages.

majority of infections, and appears adequate for routine clinical practice (Ariza 1988; Rodríguez Torres 1988). If simple agglutination methods (Moyer *et al.* 1987) or the rose bengal slide agglutination test (Altwegg and Bohl 1985; Rodríguez Torres 1988) are used for screening, standard tests must be performed in the positive sera for definite serological diagnosis.

The pattern of the antigenic response may be measured with an enzyme-linked immunosorbent assay. IgM antibodies appear first and may disappear within a mean time of 9 months. IgG peaks at about 2 months but significant titres persist after 18 months or more (Ariza 1988; Gazapo *et al.* 1989). In a large group of serially followed patients, STA and IgM antibodies had a parallel decline, as did the Coombs' test and IgG antibodies (Ariza 1988; Ariza *et al.* 1992*a*). The measurement of specific antibodies allows the detection of occasional patients not discovered by other serological tests (Sippel *et al.* 1982; Gazapo *et al.* 1989; Ariza *et al.* 1992*a*). Detection of an elevation in the IgG antibody during the follow-up is a very useful serological sign for the diagnosis of relapses (Pellicer *et al.* 1988; Gazapo *et al.* 1989; Ariza *et al.* 1992*a*). The definitive diagnosis of a relapse requires either bacteriological or clinical evidence of the disease.

Occupationally exposed workers may have low, abnormal serological test results in the absence of disease. Due to similarities in the cell wall components, serological test for brucellosis may be positive in infections due to *F. tularensis*, *Yersinia enterocolitica* 0 < 9, vibriocholerae, and *Escherichia coli* 0 < 157 (Corbel *et al.* 1983); when a positive result is due to cross-reaction, titres tend to be lower against the cross-reacting antigenic suspension.

Treatment

The treatment of brucellar arthritis is similar to that of uncomplicated brucellosis (Box 1). The regimen recommended at present by the World Health Organization (Joint FAO/WHO expert committee on brucellosis 1986) includes a combination of rifampicin 900 mg combined with doxycycline at 200 mg, both given once a day for 6 weeks. The relapse rate of this regimen (5 per cent), is similar to that of doxycycline 200 mg/day for 45 days, combined with streptomycin 1 g/day for 14 days (4 per cent relapse rate) (Acocella *et al.* 1989). A study conducted after treatment for only 30 days, showed

that the combination of rifampicin 15 mg/kg per day with doxycycline 100 mg every 12 h had a 38 per cent relapse rate, while a combination of tetracycline 0.5 g every 6 h and streptomycin 1 g/day (for only 21 days) had a 7.1 per cent relapse rate (Ariza *et al.* 1985*b*). In another trial, doxycycline 100 mg every 12 h and rifampicin 15 mg/kg per day in a single morning dose, for 45 days, showed a similar efficacy than a combination of doxycycline for 45 days plus streptomycin 1 g/day for 15 days, although the doxycycline–rifampicin combination was less effective in patients with spondylitis (Ariza *et al.* 1992*b*). A recent meta-analysis of six published randomized trials comparing the relative efficacy of rifampicin and doxycycline versus streptomycin and doxycycline, or another tetracycline, concluded that treatment with rifampicin and doxycycline presents a greater number of recurrences and lower number of cures than the classical treatment with streptomycin and tetracycline (Solera *et al.* 1994). Probably a regimen including streptomycin and a tetracycline is to be preferred for patients with severe complications, such as spondylitis of the cervical spine.

Brucellae isolated from patients with relapses show similar drug sensitivities to the pretreatment isolates from the same patients (Ariza *et al.* 1986), indicating that the relapses are not due to drug resistance. A second course of treatment is generally effective in these patients.

A therapeutic study conducted on 1100 children with early disease, showed that very few relapses were seen after oral monotherapy combined with either streptomycin or gentamicin. These combinations fared better than other regimens. It was concluded that children of 8 years or younger should receive trimethoprim–sulphamethoxazole 10 to 50 mg/kg per day, twice daily for 3 weeks, with intramuscular injections of gentamicin 5 mg/kg per day, twice daily for the first 5 days. Children of 9 years or older should receive doxycycline 5 mg/kg per day, twice daily for 3 weeks, combined with intramuscular injections of gentamicin 5 mg/kg per day, twice daily for the first 5 days (Lubani *et al.* 1989). Monotherapy with trimethoprim–sulphamethoxazole (Gómez-Reino *et al.* 1986; Lubani *et al.* 1989) or with rifampicin (Llorens-Terol and Busquets 1980; Lubani *et al.* 1989) results in a higher relapse rate. Treatment of 113 children with 10 to 12 mg/kg trimethoprim, 50 to 60 mg/kg sulphamethoxazole, and rifampicin 15 to 20 mg/kg in two divided doses for 6 weeks resulted in only four relapses and offers a convenient oral therapy for children (Khuri Bulos *et al.* 1993).

Apart from antibiotics, patients with peripheral arthritis do not require repeated evacuation of the joint, as is necessary in pyogenic arthritides. Rarely, large paravertebral abscesses may require drainage. Epidural abscesses with cord compression may need surgery, although it is not clearly established if this more aggressive approach offers advantages over medical treatment alone.

References

Acocella, G., Bertrand, A., Beytout, J., Durrande, J.B., García Rodríguez, J.A., Kosmidis, J., Micoud, M., Rey, M., Rodríguez Zapata, M., Roux, J., and Stahl, J.P. (1989). Comparison of three different regimens in the treatment of acute brucellosis: a multicenter, multinational study. *Journal of Antimicrobial Chemotherapy*, **23**, 433–9.

Adam, A., MacDonald, A., and MacKenzie, I.G. (1967). Monoarticular brucellar arthritis in children. *The Journal of Bone and Joint Surgery*, **49B**, 652–7.

Agarwal, S., Kadhi, S.K., and Rooney, R.J. (1991). Brucellosis complicating bilateral total knee arthroplasty. *Clinical Orthopedics and Related Research*, **267**, 179–81.

Alarcón, G.S., Bocanegra, T.S., Gotuzzo, E., Hinostroza, S., Carrillo, C., Vasey, F.B., Germain, B.F., and Espinoza, L.R. (1981). Reactive arthritis associated with brucellosis: HLA studies. *Journal of Rheumatology*, **8**, 621–5.

Alarcón, G.S., Gotuzzo, E., Hinostroza, S.A., Carrillo, C., Bocanegra, T.S., and Espinoza, L.R. (1985). HLA studies in brucellar spondylitis. *Clinical Rheumatology*, **4**, 312–4.

Al-Eissa, Y.A., Kambal, A.M., al-Nasser, M.N., al-Habib, S.A., Al-Fawaz, I.M., and Al-Zamil, F.A. (1990). Childhood brucellosis: a study of 102 cases. *Pediatric Infectious Diseases Journal*, **9**, 74–9.

Al-Rawi, Z.S., Al-Khateeb, N., and Khalifa, S.J. (1987). Brucella arthritis among Iraqi patients. *British Journal of Rheumatology*, **26**, 24–7.

Al-Rawi, T.I., Thewaini, A.J., Shawket, A.R., and Ahmed, G.M. (1989). Skeletal brucellosis in Iraqi patients. *Annals of the Rheumatic Diseases*, **48**, 77–9.

Altwegg, M. and Bohl, E. (1985). Evaluation of a rapid, reliable, and inexpensive screening test for the serological diagnosis of human brucellosis. *Zentralblatt fur Bakteriologie, Mikrobiologie und Hygiene Series A. Medical Microbiology, Infectious Diseases, Virology and Bacteriology*, **260**, 65–70.

Andonopoulos, A.P., Asimakopoulos, G., Anastasiou, E., and Bassaris, H.P. (1986). Brucella arthritis. *Scandinavian Journal of Rheumatology*, **15**, 377–80.

Ariza, J. (1988). *Brucelosis: perspectiva actual de la enfermedad. Perfil de las inmunoglobulinas específicas en el curso de su evolución*. Doctoral thesis. University of Barcelona.

Ariza, J., Gudiol, F., Valverde, J., Pallarés, R., Fernández Viladrich, P., Rufí, G., Espadaler, L., and Fernández Nogués, F. (1985a). Brucellar spondylitis: a detailed analysis based on current findings. *Reviews of Infectious Diseases*, **7**, 656–64.

Ariza, J., Gudiol, F., Pallarés, G., Rufí, G., and Fernández Viladrich, P. (1985b). Comparative trial of rifampin-doxicicline versus tetracycline-streptomycine in the therapy of human brucellosis. *Antimicrobial Agents and Chemotherapy*, **28**, 548–51.

Ariza, J., Bosch, J., Gudiol, F., Liñares, J., Fernández-Viladrich, P., and Martín, R. (1986). Relavance of in vitro antimicrobial susceptibility of brucella mellitensis to relapse rate in human brucellosis. *Antimicrobial Agents and Chemotherapy*, **30**, 958–60.

Ariza, J., Servitje, O., Pallarés, R., Fernández-Viladrich, P., Rufí, G., Peyrí, J., and Gudiol, F. (1989). Characteristic cutaneous lessions in patients with brucellosis. *Archives of Dermatology*, **125**, 380–3.

Ariza, J., Pellicer, T., Pallares, R., Foz, A., and Gudiol, F. (1992a) Specific antibody profile in human brucellosis. *Clinics in Infectious Diseases*, **14**, 131–40.

Ariza, J., Gudiol, F., Pallares, R., Viladrich, P.F., Rufí, G., Corredoira, J., and Miravitlles, M.R. (1992b) Treatment of human brucellosis with doxycycline plus rifampin or doxycycline plus streptomycin. A randomized, double-blind study. *Annals of Internal Medicine*, **117**, 25–30

Ariza, J., Valverde, J., Nolla, J.M., Rufí, G., Viladrich P.F., Corredoira. J.M., and Gudiol, F. (1993). Brucellar sacroiliitis: findings in 63 episodes and current relevance. *Clincs in Infectious Diseases*, **16**, 761–5.

Arnow, P.M., Smaron, M., and Ormiste, V. (1984). Brucellosis in a group of travelers to Spain. *Journal of the American Medical Association*, **251**, 505–7.

Bahar, R.H., Al-Suhaili, A.R., Mousa, A.M., Nawaz, M.K., Kaddah, N., and Abdel-Dayem, H.M. (1988). Brucellosis: appearance on skeletal imaging. *Clinical Nuclear Medicine*, **13**, 102–6.

Batlle, E., Pascual, E., Salas, E., Plazas, J., Román, J., and Vela, P. (1989). Brucellar arthritis: a study of 86 prospectively collected patients (abstract). *British Journal of Rheumatology*, **28** (suppl. 2), 25.

Benjamin, B. and Khan, M.R. (1994) Hip involvement in childhood brucellosis. *Journal of Bone and Joint Surgery* (British), **76**, 544–7.

Benjamin, B., Annobil, S.H., and Khan, M.R. (1992). Osteoarticular complications of childhood brucellosis: a study of 57 cases in Saudi Arabia. *Journal of Pediatric Orthopedics*, **12**, 801–5.

Berrocal, A., Gotuzzo, E., Calvo, A., Carrillo, C., Castañeda, O., and Alarcon, G.S. (1993). Sternoclavicular brucellar arthritis: a report of 7 cases and a review of the literature. *Journal of Rheumatology*, **20**, 1184–6.

Bonfiglio, M., Mickelson, M.R., and El-Khoury, G.Y. (1983). Case report 221. *Skeletal Radiology*, **9**, 208–11.

Carro, A., Batlle, E., Pascual, E., Castellano, J.A., and Plazas, J. (1988). Blood culture flasks for synovial fluid culture: a more sensitive method for the isolation of bacteria from synovial fluid, particularly brucella mellitensis (abstract). *British Journal of Rheumatology*, **27** (suppl. 2), 33.

Colmenero, D.J., Porras, J.J., Valdivieso, P., Porras, J.A., de Ramón, E., Cause, M., and Juárez, C. (1986). Brucelosis: estudio prospectivo de 100 casos. *Medicina Clínica* (Barcelona), **86**, 43–8.

Colmenero, J.D., Reguera, J.M., Fernandez-Nebro, A., and Cabrera-Franquelo, F. (1991). Osteoarticular complications of brucellosis. *Annals of the Rheumatic Diseases*, **50**, 23–6.

Colmenero, J.D., Cisneros, J.M., Orjuela, D.L., Pachon, J., Garcia-Portales, R., Rodriguez-Sampedro, F., and Juarez, C. (1992). Clinical course and prognosis of Brucella spondylitis. *Infection*, **20**, 38–42.

Corbel, M.J., Stuart, F.A., and Brewer, R.A. (1983). Observations on serological cross-reactions between smooth brucella species and organism of other genera. *Developement Biology Standard*, **56**, 341–8.

Cordero Sánchez, M., Alvarez Ruiz, S., López Ochoa, J., and García Talavera, J.R. (1990). Scintigraphic evaluation of lumbosacral pain in brucellosis. *Arthritis and Rheumatism*, **33**, 1052–5.

Crosby, E., Llosa, L., Miró Quesada, M., Carrillo, P., and Gotuzzo, E. (1984). Hematologic changes in brucellosis. *Journal of Infectious Diseases*, **150**, 419–24.

Dawes, P.T. and Ghosh, S.K. (1985). Tissue typing in brucellosis. *Annals of the Rheumatic Diseases*, **44**, 526–8.

Devi, S.J.N., Polt, S.S., Boctor, F.N., and Peter, J.B. (1987). Serological evaluation of brucellosis: importance of species in antigen preparation. *Journal of Infectious Diseases*, **156**, 658–61.

Diaz, R., Jones, L.M., Leong, D., and Wilson, J.B. (1968). Surface antigens in smooth brucellae. *Journal of Bacteriology*, **96**, 893–901.

El Desouki, M. (1991). Skeletal brucellosis: assessment with bone scintigraphy. *Radiology*, **181**, 415–8.

Feiz, J., Sabbaghian, H., and Miralai, M. (1978). Brucellosis due to *B. mellitensis* in children: clinical and epidemiologic observations on 95 patients studied in central Iran. *Clinical Pediatrics*, **17**, 904–7.

Gazapo, E., Gonzalez Lahoz, J., Subiza, J.L., Baquero, M., Gil, J., and Gómez de la Concha, E.G. (1989). Changes in IgM and IgG antibody concentrations in brucellosis over time: importance for diagnosis and follow-up. *Journal of Infectious Diseases*, **159**, 219–25.

Gómez-Reino, F.J., Mateo, I., Fuertes, A., and Gómez-Reino, J.J. (1986). Brucellar arthritis in children and its successful treatment with trimethoprim-sulphamethoxazole. *Annals of the Rheumatic Diseases*, **45**, 256–8.

Gotuzzo, E and Carrillo, C. (1988). Brucella arthritis. In *Infections in the rheumatic diseases*, (eds L. Espinoza, D. Goldenberg, F. Arnett, and G. Alarcón), pp. 31–41. Grune and Stratton, Orlando.

Gotuzzo, E., Alarcón, G.S., Bocanegra, T.S., Carrillo, C., Guerra J.C., Rolando, I., and Espinoza, L.R. (1982). Articular involvement in human brucellosis: a retrospective analysis of 304 cases. *Seminars in Arthritis and Rheumatism*, **12**, 245–55.

Gotuzzo, E,. Carrillo, C., and Guera, J. (1986). An evaluation of the diagnostic methods for brucellosis—the value of bone marrow culture. *Journal of Infectious Diseases*, **153**, 122–5.

Gotuzzo, E., Seas C., Guerra, J.G., Carrillo, C., Bocanegra, T.S., Calvo, A., Castañeda, O., and Alarcón, G.S. (1987). Brucellar arthritis: a study of 39 Peruvian families. *Annals of the Rheumatic Diseases*, **46**, 506–9.

Hall, W.H. and Manion, R.E. (1953). Comparison of the Coomb's test with other methods for brucella agglutinins in human serum. *Journal of Clinical Investigation*, **32**, 96–106.

Hodinka, L., Gomor, B., Meretey, K., Zahumenszky, Z., Geher, P., Telegdy, L., and Bozsoky, S. (1978). HLA-B27-associated spondylarthritis in chronic brucellosis (letter). *Lancet*, i, 499.

Hunt, A.C. and Bothwell, P.W. (1967). Histological findings in human brucellosis. *Journal of Clinical Pathology*, **20**, 267–72

Joint FAO/WHO expert committee on brucellosis. (1986). World Health Organization, Geneva.

Keenan, M.A. and Guttmann, G.G. (1982). Brucella osteomyelitis of the distal part of the femur. *Journal of Bone and Joint Surgery*, **64A**, 142–4.

Kelly, P.J., Martin, W.J., Shirger, A., and Weed, L.A. (1960). Brucellosis of the bones and joints. *Journal of the American Medical Association*, **174**, 347–53.

Khuri Bulos, N,A., Daoud, A,H., and Azab, S,M. (1993). Treatment of childhood brucellosis: results of a prospective trial on 113 children. *Pediatric Infectious Diseases Journal*, **12**, 377–81.

Laajam, M.A. (1985). Synovial rupture complicating brucella arthritis. *British Journal of Rheumatology*, **24**, 191–3

Lifeso, R.M., Harder, E., and McCorkell, S.J. (1985). Spinal brucellosis. *Journal of Bone and Joint Surgery*, **67B**, 345–51.

Llorens-Terol, J. and Busquets, R.M. (1980). Brucellosis treated with rifampin. *Archives of Diseases of Childhood*, **55**, 486–8.

Lubani, M.M., Sharda, D.C., and Helin, I. (1986). Brucella arthritis in children. *Infection*, **14**, 233–6.

Lubani, M.M, Dudin, K.I., Sharda, D.C., Mana Ndhar, D.S., Araj, G.F., Hafed, H.A., Al-Saleh, Q.A., Helin, I., and Salhi, M.M. (1989). A multicenter therapeutic study of 1100 children with brucellosis. *Pediatric Infectious Diseases Journal*, **8**, 75–8.

Lulu, A.R., Araj, G.F., Khateeb, M.I., Mustafa, M.Y., Yusuf A.R., and Fenech, F.F. (1988). Human brucellosis in Kuwait: a prospective study of 400 cases. *Quarterly Journal of Medicine*, **249**, 39–54.

Madkour, M.M., Sharif, H.S., Abed, M.Y., and Al-Fayez, M.A. (1988). Osteoarticular brucellosis: Results of bone scintigraphy in 140 patients. *American Journal of Radiology*, **150**, 1101–5

Manaster, B.J. (1988). Case report 469. Spondylitis (lumbar spine) due to *Brucella abortus*. *Skeletal Radiology*, **17**, 144–7.

Mavridis, A.K., Drosos, A.A., Tsolas, O., and Moutsopoulos, H.M. (1984). Lactate levels in brucella arthritis. *Rheumatology International*, **4**, 169–71.

Miller, C.D., Songer, J.R., and Sullivan, J.F. (1987). A twenty-five year review of laboratory-acquired human infections at the National Animal Disease Center. *American Industrial Hygiene Association Journal*, **48**, 271–5.

Mousa, A.R., Elhag, K.M., Khogali, M., and Marafie, A.A. (1987). The nature of human brucellosis in Kuwait: study of 379 cases. *Reviews of Infectious Diseases*, **10**, 211–7.

Moyer, N.P., Evins, G.M., Pigott, N.E., Hudson, J.D., Farshy, C.E., Feeley, J.C., and Hausler, W.J. (1987). Comparison of serological screening tests for brucellosis. *Journal of Clinical Microbiology*, **25**, 1969–72.

Navas, E., Guerrero, A., Cobo, J., and Loza, E. (1993). Faster isolation of Brucella spp. from blood by isolator compared with BACTEC NR. *Diagnostic Microbiology and Infectious Disease*, **16**, 79–81.

Pellicer, T., Ariza, J., and Foz, A. (1988). Specific antibodies detected during relapse of human brucellosis. *Journal of Infectious Diseases*, **157**, 918–24.

Polt, S.S., Dismukes, W.E., Flint, A., and Schaefer, J. (1982). Human brucellosis caused by *Brucella canis*: clinical features and immune response. *Annals of Internal Medicine*, **97**, 717–19.

Porat, S. and Shapiro, M. (1984). Brucella arthritis of the sacro-iliac joint. *Infection*, **12**, 205–7.

Rajapakse, C.N.A. (1987). The spectrum of rheumatic diseases in Saudi Arabia. *British Journal of Rheumatology*, **26**, 22–3.

Revak, D.M., Swain, R.A., Guthrie, R.M., and Lubbers, J.R. (1989). Brucellosis contracted during foreign travel. *Postgraduate Medicine*, **85**, 101–4.

Rodríguez Torres, A. (1988). Diagnóstico de la brucelosis humana. *Revista Española de Reumatología*, **15**, 204–14.

Rotés-Querol, J. (1957). Osteo-articular sites of brucellosis. *Annals of the Rheumatic Diseases*, **16**, 63–8.

Seignon, B., Weilbacher, H., Thorel, J.B., Bussières, J.L., Deshayes, P., and Gougeon, J. (1980). La ponction discale dans le diagnostic bactériologique des spondylodiscites bactériennes. *Revue du Rhumatisme et des Maladies Ostéoarticulaires*, **47**, 45–7.

Serre, H., Kalea, G., Brousson, A., Sany, J., Bertrand, A., and Simon, L. (1981) Manifestations ostéo-articulaires de la brucellose. *Revue du Rhumatisme et des Maladies Ostéoarticulaires*, **47**, 143–8.

Sharif, H.S., Aideyan, O.A., Clark, D.C., Madkour, M.M., Aabed, M.Y., Mattsson, T.A., Al-Deeb, S.M., and Moutaery, K.R. (1989). Brucellar and tuberculous spondylitis: comparative imaging features. *Radiology*, **171**, 419–25.

Sippel, J.E., El-Masry, N.A., and Farid, Z. (1982). Diagnosis of human brucellosis with ELISA. *Lancet*, ii, 19–21.

Smith, L.D. and Ficht, T.A. (1990). Pathogenesis of Brucella. *Critical Reviews in Microbiology*, **17**, 209–30.

Solera, J., Martinez-Alfaro, E., and Saez, L. (1994). Metaanalisis sobre la eficacia de la combinacion de rifampicina y doxiciclina en el tratamiento de la brucelosis humana. *Medicina Clinica* (Barcelona), **102**, 731–8.

Spink, W.W. (1951). What is chronic brucellosis? *Annals of Internal Medicine*, **35**, 358–74.

Spink, W.W. (1964). Host-parasite relationship in brucellosis. *Lancet*, ii, 161–4.

Thapar, M.K. and Young, E.J. (1986). Urban outbreak of goat cheese brucellosis. *Pediatric Infectious Diseases*, **5**, 640–3.

Torres-Rojas, J., Taddonio, R.F., and Sanders, C.V. (1979). Spondylitis caused by *Brucella abortus*. *Southern Medical Journal*, **72**, 1166–9.

Tovar, J.V., Moreno, R., Perez, A., Satorres, J., Navarro, F., and Royo, G. (1990). Abscesos gluteos por Brucella melitensis. Probable patogenia yatrogena. *Enfermedades Infecciosas y Microbiología Clínica*, **8**, 588.

Vazquez Doval, F.J., Ruiz de Erenchun Lasa, F., Sola Casas, M.A., Soto de Delas, J., and Quintanilla Gutierrez, E. (1991) Acute brucellosis presenting as leukocytoclastic vasculitis. *Journal of Investigative Allergology and Clinical Immunology*, **1**, 411–3

Young, E.J. (1983). Human brucellosis. *Reviews of Infectious Diseases*, **5**, 821–42.

Young, E.J. (1995). Brucella species. In *Principles and practice of infectious diseases*, (eds G.L. Mandell, J.E. Bennett, and R. Dolin), pp. 2053–60. Churchill Livingstone, New York.

Zuckerman, E., Naschitz, J.E., Yeshurun, D., Wellisch, G., Shajrawi, I., and Boss, J.H. (1994). Fasciitis-panniculitis in acute brucellosis. *International Journal of Dermatology*, **33**, 57–9.

5.3.9 Parasitic involvement

Tomás S. Bocanegra

Improvements in living and sanitary conditions, and aggressive eradication programmes, have reduced the prevalence of most parasitic diseases in Third World countries; however, these conditions continue to be endemic in many areas of the world (Cairncross

1995). In industrialized nations, parasites cause sporadic outbreaks of disease in urban communities (McAmilty *et al.* 1994; MacKenzie *et al.* 1994; Millard *et al.* 1994; Huang *et al.* 1995) and occasionally serious illness in immigrants and travellers (Encarnación *et al.* 1994). More importantly, in the last decade, there are reports of an increasing number of life-threatening infections with parasites in immunosuppressed patients and individuals infected with the human immunodeficiency virus (Pape *et al.* 1994; Ognibene *et al.* 1995; Weiss 1995).

The clinical presentation of parasitic infection varies from localized symptoms to a multisystem disease that may include musculoskeletal manifestations. The incidence of rheumatic manifestations in the different parasitic diseases is not known, but there are reports of a variety of musculoskeletal syndromes. Recently, the importance of considering parasitic disease in the differential diagnosis of patients presenting with rheumatic manifestations was recognized by the description of these syndromes in two major textbooks of rheumatology (Bocanegra 1993; Bocanegra 1994). The diagnosis of parasite-associated musculoskeletal syndrome is established on clinical grounds when manifestations develop in residents or travellers to endemic areas, in patients who have a documented infection with an intestinal or tissue-invasive parasite, and in those whose symptoms do not respond to conventional anti-inflammatory

Table 1 Clinical characteristics of parasite-associated musculoskeletal syndromes

Residence in, or travelling to, endemic areas

Documented parasitic infection

Poor response to conventional treatment

Resolution following eradication of parasite

therapy but resolve after the eradication of the parasite (Bocanegra 1994; Doury 1994) (Table 1).

This chapter will review the rheumatic syndromes that develop in humans as a consequence of parasitic infestation or of the treatment of parasitic diseases.

Protozoal infections

There are reports of rheumatic syndromes with a variety of pathogenic, tissue-invasive, as well as oportunistic protozoa (see Box 1).

Articular syndromes

A symmetrical polyarthritis of the small joints of the hands, wrists, and knees in a rheumatoid pattern may develop in patients infected with *Toxoplasma gondii*. Rheumatoid factor may or may not be present in serum, but all patients have serological evidence of acute toxoplasma infection (IgG toxoplasma antibodies) (Antezana 1979; Gemou *et al.* 1983; Balleari *et al.* 1991).

Arthralgia, back pain, and arthritis occurred in young adults with intestinal amoebiasis (Yonis 1943; Rappaport *et al.* 1951; Doury *et al.* 1977). Patients presented with a polyarthritis of recent onset affecting the small, medium, and large joints of the upper and lower limbs, preceded by mild gastrointestinal symptoms. One patient had concomitant urticaria. Joint symptoms resolved on treatment of the intestinal amoebiasis.

Giardiasis may cause joint symptoms, most commonly in children and young adults. The largest series of patients with articular symptoms associated with *Giardia lamblia* infection was reported by Goobar (1977). The most common pattern was a mild and self-limiting oligoarthritis of the large and medium-sized joints of the upper and lower limbs. The erythrocyte sedimentation rate was elevated but rheumatoid factor was negative with few exceptions. All patients had concomitant gastrointestinal manifestations and most had urticaria. Recently, there have been several other case reports of

Box 1 Musculoskeletal syndrome induced by protozoa

	Articular	Muscular	Vascular	Treatment of choice
Toxoplasma	Polyarthritis	Polymyositis-like	Polyarteritis nodosa-like	Pyrimethamine and sulphadiazine
Amoeba	Arthralgias	None	Focal vasculitis	Metronidazole
Giardia	Oligoarthritis	None	Small vessel vasculitis	Metronidazole or tinidazole
Cryptosporidium	Oligoarthritis	None	None	Paronomycin
Isospora	Oligoarthritis	Focal and generalized myositis	Polyarteritis nodosa-like	Trimethoprim-sulphamethoxazole
Microsporidia	None	Generalized myopathy	None	Albendazole
Trypanosoma	None	Generalized myopathy (*T. rhodesience*), Polymyositis-like (*T. cruzi*)	None	Suranim (*T. rhodesience*) Nifurtimox (*T. cruzi*)
Plasmodium	None	Myalgias	Small vessel vasculitis	Chloroquine

a similar pattern of joint involvement. However, in a few instances the small joints of the hands and feet were affected (Farthing *et al.* 1983; Woo and Panayi 1984; Barton *et al.* 1986; Shaw and Stevens 1987; Brougui and Richard 1990). Articular symptoms did not respond to non-steroidal anti-inflammatory agents but resolved after treatment with metronidazole.

Reactive arthritis may also develop after cryptosporidial gastroenteritis in young adults and children (Hay *et al.* 1987; Sheperd *et al.* 1989). Small, medium, and large joints are affected, but symptoms are usually self-limiting. In addition, there are reports of infectious and reactive arthritis in association with opportunistic infections by *Blastocystis hominis* and *Isospora belli* (Lee *et al.* 1990; Lakhanpal *et al.* 1991; Gonzalez-Dominguez *et al.* 1994; Krüger *et al.* 1994). In one case, *Blastocystis* was recovered from synovial fluid in the knee, supporting the possibility of an infectious cause; in the others, the oligoarthritis was preceded by diarrhoea and resolved after antiparasitic treatment, suggesting a 'reactive' mechanism.

Muscular syndromes

Focal and diffuse myositis may occur in patients infected with protozoa, mostly due to invasion of muscle tissue by the parasite. However, in some cases, an immune-mediated mechanism may play a part.

Isospora hominis (Jeffrey 1974; Bonciou *et al.* 1981) may cause both a localized and a generalized myositis with proximal and distal muscle weakness. Toxoplasmosis may produce an acute and a chronic myositis with clinical manifestations and muscle enzyme abnormalities similar to those seen in idiopathic polymyositis (McNicholl and Underhill 1970; Greenlee *et al.* 1975; Topi *et al.* 1979; Roig-Quilis and Damjanov 1982). Patients usually have a concomitant febrile systemic illness and serological evidence of acute toxoplasma infection. Toxoplasma may or may not be found in the striated muscle. It is possible that toxoplasma is involved in idiopathic polymyositis, based on the higher than expected frequency of antitoxoplasma antibodies in patients with polymyositis and dermatomyositis (Magid and Kagen 1983), the improvement in dermatomyositis on treatment of associated toxoplasmosis (Harland *et al.* 1991), and the expression of major histocompatibility complex class I and II antigens in the inflammatory cells around the muscle fibres (Matsubara *et al.* 1990). However, there is no convincing proof for this hypothesis.

Granulomatous myositis due to microsporidial infection with pleistophora was reported in a patient with severe immunodeficiency (Ledford *et al.* 1985); clusters of parasitic spores were present in the striated muscle fibres. Clinically, the patient presented with muscle wasting, contractures, and cachexia. Muscle wasting is relatively common in American trypanosomiasis (Chagas' disease) caused by *Trypanosoma cruzi* and African trypanosomiasis caused by *T. rhodesiense* and *T. gambiense*, but it is unclear if it is due to direct invasion of the striated muscle by the parasite, denervation, or malnutrition. A symmetrical proximal myositis, similar to idiopathic polymyositis, occurred in a patient with Chagas' disease (Cossermelli *et al.* 1978). Encysted trypanosomes were identified in the muscle biopsy. The muscle weakness improved but did not resolve after treatment of the underlying trypanosomiasis.

Myalgia, muscle necrosis, and elevations of creatine kinase can occur in malaria (DeSilva *et al.* 1988; Swash and Schwartz 1993), and have been attributed to microvascular changes in the striated muscle.

Vascular syndromes

A polyarteritis nodosa-like syndrome is described in patients infected with *Toxoplasma gondii* and *Isospora hominis* (McGill 1957; Carmeni *et al.* 1991). These patients presented with fever, myalgias, weakness, paraesthesias, and weight loss. Muscle biopsy showed necrotizing vasculitis of small and medium arteries.

Localized arteritis due to parasitic invasion of the vessel wall may occur in toxoplasmosis of the central nervous system and in amoebic colitis, and may be the underlying cause of the tissue necrosis frequently observed in these conditions (Huang and Chou 1988; De La Torre and Gorraez 1989; Desphande *et al.* 1992). A systemic, immune complex-mediated vasculitis may occur in infections with *Plasmodium falciparum* and *Giardia lamblia*, resulting in uveitis, urticaria, erythema nodosum, and glomerulonephritis.

Helminthic infections

Musculoskeletal manifestations are more frequently reported in patients infected by helminths than in those with protozoal infections (see Box 2).

Articular syndromes

Arthritis occurs in humans infected with cestodes as definite host (taeniasis) and as intermediate hosts (cysticercosis and hydatid cyst). A symmetrical, 'rheumatoid-like' polyarthritis and an oligoarthritis of the knees have been reported in patients infected with *Taenia saginata* (Bocanegra *et al.* 1981; Bussiere *et al.* 1981). The patient with polyarthritis had elevated amounts of circulating immune complexes and IgE in serum and deposits of IgG and C3 in the synovium. Parasites were not found in the synovial fluid or tissues. Treatment with indomethacin was unsuccessful, but symptoms resolved after treatment of the parasitic infection.

Arthralgias and bone pain may occur in cysticercosis (Surianu *et al.* 1967) and hydatid disease (Fyfe *et al.* 1990). Bone involvement is seen in 1 to 2 per cent of patients with hydatid disease; about half of bone lesions are cysts in the thoracic or lumbar spine (Rao *et al.* 1991). Although the infection is probably acquired in childhood, clinical manifestations do not develop until adulthood, owing to the slow growth of the cyst. Radiographically, bone hydatic cysts present as a lytic lesion without sclerosis and are commonly confused with metastatic malignancy or plasmacytoma. Most commonly, bone hydatid disease affects the body of the vertebra but occasionally may affect the pedicles. Spinal compression with paraplegia may occur and carries a poor prognosis (Argenson *et al.* 1989). The pelvis and femur are affected less frequently, but their involvement may result in pathological fractures (Hooper and McLean 1977; Duran *et al.* 1978). A chronic granulomatous synovitis may occur when a cyst in the para-articular bone or muscle opens into the joint (Vigliani and Campailla 1977; Voutsinas *et al.* 1987). Patients may present with urticaria and eosinophilia in addition to monoarthritis. In one patient (Campoy *et al.* 1995), synovial fluid had increased numbers of eosinophils; synovial biopsy showed granulomas and the remains of hydatid cysts (Fig. 1).

There are reports of a seronegative polyarthritis of the small, medium, and large joints in a few patients with hydatid disease of the liver (Ballina-Garcia *et al.* 1987; Buskila *et al.* 1992). The arthritis did not respond to non-steroidal anti-inflammatory agents but resolved on removal of the hepatic hydatid cysts. The diagnosis of

Box 2 Musculoskeletal syndrome induced by helminthies

	Articular	Muscular	Vascular	Treatment of choice
Taeniasis (intestinal)	Oligoarthritis and polyarthritis	None	None	Praziquantel
Cysticercus	Arthralgias	Myalgias, nodular myopathy	Localized around cysticercus	Albendazole
Hydatid cyst	Bone pain, mono- and polyarthritis	Asymptomatic muscular cysts	Polyarteritis nodosa-like	Albendazole, surgical excision of cyst
Coeneurosis	None	Asymptomatic nodules	None	Surgical excision
Sparganosis	None	Nodular, occasionally migratory	None	Surgical excision
Gnathostoma	None	Nodular myositis, occasionally migratory	None	Albendazole, surgical excision
Strongyloides	Arthralgias, oligo- and polyarthritis	None	Leucocytoclastic vasculitis	Thiabendazole
Ascaris	Oligoarthritis	None	Churg–Strauss syndrome	Mebendazole
Trichuris	Oligoarthritis	None	None	Mebendazole
Ancylostoma	Oligoarthritis	None	None	Mebendazole
Toxocara	Arthralgias, monoarthritis	Localized myositis of the calf	None	Diethylcarbamazine
Dracunculus	Arthralgias, monoarthritis	Myalgias	None	Metronidazole
Filiariae	Arthralgias, mono- and oligoarthritis	Modular myositis (onchocerca)	Leucocytoclastic vasculitis (loa-loa)	Diethylcarbamazine, ivermectin (onchocerca)
Schistosoma	Arthralgias, oligo- and polyarthritis, enthesitis	Diffuse myopathy	None	Praziquantel
Dirofilaria	Oligoarthritis	None	None	Self-limited
Trichina	None	Myalgias, polymyositis-like	Polyarteritis nodosa-like	Mebendazole

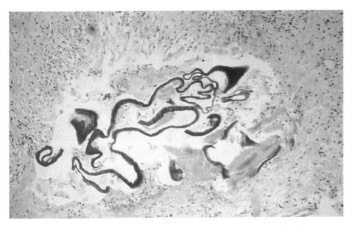

Fig. 1 Hydatid synovitis. Synovial biopsy of the knee showing inflammatory infiltrate, granulomas, and fragments of a hydatid cyst. Sections stained with periodic acid–Schiff. Original magnification × 10. (Reproduced from Campoy *et al.* 1995, with permission).

joint or bone involvement by hydatid disease is difficult and is often established accidentally by the finding of cysts during exploratory surgery. Needle biopsy of the cyst should not be performed, owing to the risk of disseminating the disease. The presence of eosinophilia in peripheral blood or synovial fluid, urticaria, and prior residence in an endemic area for hydatid disease in a patient presenting with arthritis or an unexplained cystic bone lesion should lead the physician to consider hydatid cyst in differential diagnosis. The treatment of bone and joint hydatid disease is of limited success because of the difficulty in removing the cyst and scoleces from the bone. In patients with arthritis associated with hepatic hydatid cysts, the symptoms resolve after the resection of the cyst. However, surgery carries a risk of anaphylactic shock due to the massive release of hydatid antigen in a patient already sensitized to it. Oral treatment with mebendazole may be beneficial in some patients but it has poor penetration of bone.

Joint pain and arthritis may develop in the course of invasive and intestinal infections with *Strongyloides stercoralis* (Bocanegra *et al.*

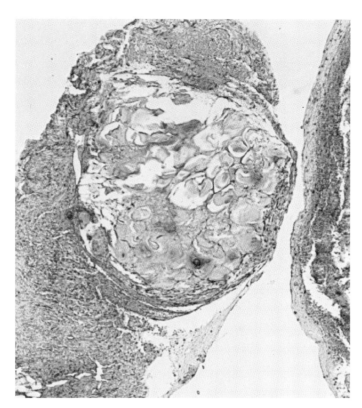

Fig. 2 *Strongyloides* synovitis: synovia from the ankle showing larvae of *Strongyloides stercoralis* surrounded by inflammatory infiltrate (reproduced from Akoglu *et al.* 1984, with permission).

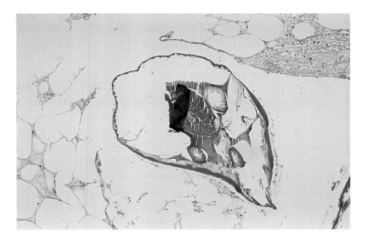

Fig. 3 *Toxocara* panniculitis: skin biopsy showing fragments of *Toxocara* and inflammatory cells in the subcutaneous tissue (reproduced from Kraus *et al.* 1995, with permission).

1981; Patey *et al.* 1990). Two articular syndromes have been reported: one characterized by symmetrical, polyarticular involvement similar to rheumatoid arthritis (Doury *et al.* 1975; Bocanegra *et al.* 1981; Amor *et al.* 1983; Forzy *et al.* 1988) and an oligoarthritis of the knees, ankles, hips, and sacroiliac joints (Amor *et al.* 1983; Akoglu *et al.* 1984; De Jonge-Bok *et al.* 1985; Menkes *et al.* 1987). Patients usually present with eosinophilia in peripheral blood and synovial fluid. Larvae of *Strongyloides* are found in stools and, in some patients, in the synovial fluid or in the synovium (Fig. 2). One patient with polyarthritis had

immune complexes in serum and synovial fluid. HLA-B27 antigen was negative in all patients tested. Articular symptoms resolved in all patients on treatment with thiabendazole.

There are reports of arthralgia and monoarthritis of the knee in infections with *Toxocara canis* (canine ascarids) (William and Roy 1981; Le Luyer *et al.* 1990; Richardson de Corral *et al.* 1990; Van Linthoudt *et al.* 1990; Kraus *et al.* 1995). Some patients presented with panniculitis of the legs due to migration of the parasite through the subcutaneous tissues (Fig. 3). Diagnosis is confirmed by finding the parasite in the affected tissues or by a positive enzyme immunoassay for antitoxocara antibodies. The natural course of the disease is self-limiting, although albendazole has been used in some cases. Isolated cases of seronegative oligoarthritis of leg joints are reported in infections with *Ankylostoma duodenale*, *Ascaris lumbricoides*, and *Trichuris trichiura* (Treusch *et al.* 1981; Bissonnette and Beaudet 1983).

One-third to one-half of patients infected with *Dracunculus medinensis*, a tissue-dwelling nematode, develop arthralgias or myalgias in the legs (Garf 1985). Monoarthritis of the ankle or knee occurred in about 2 per cent of patients (Kothari *et al.* 1968) due to three possible mechanisms: (i) invasion of the joint by the parasite (Reddy and Sivaramappa 1968) with release of microfilariae into the joint — synovial fluid is inflammatory and contains microfilariae of the Guinea worm as well as increased eosinophils; (ii) a reactive arthritis due to the presence of adult worms in the neighbouring soft tissues (McLaughlin *et al.* 1984) — synovial fluid is inflammatory and may show eosinophilia but not microfilariae; (iii) infectious arthritis, most commonly due to staphylococci, which enter the joint through the skin ulcerations and sinus track created by the parasite (Greenwood 1968). Diagnosis is established by the presence of skin ulcerations and calcified parasites near the affected joints. Arthrocentesis and arthroscopy are helpful, particularly in cases of direct joint invasion and infectious arthritis. Non-steroidal anti-inflammatory agents are indicated in reactive arthritis. Antiparasitic treatment rarely results in parasite death and is not recommended. Surgical removal of Guinea worm from the soft tissue is difficult due to the length of the parasite and should not be attempted. However, arthroscopy or arthrotomy are indicated when Guinea worm is located in the joint. Intravenous antibiotics and arthrocentesis are the treatment of choice in infectious arthritis.

Joint pain and arthritis occur in filariasis caused by *Wuchereria bancrofti*, *Loa loa*, and *Onchocerca*. Intermittent polyarthralgias occur during the early phase of *W. bancrofti* filariasis. Arthritis occurs less often and then only in the late, obstructive phase of the infection (Alhadeff 1955). Among patients with arthritis, two-thirds have monoarticular involvement while the other one-third have oligoarthritis (less than four joints affected) (Ismail and Nagaratnam 1973). The joints most frequently affected are the knee, the ankle, and the hip (Salfield 1975). Involvement of the arms is rare, and when present is limited to large joints. The majority of patients do not have other manifestations of filariasis but may show eosinophilia, positive serology for filariasis, or microfilariae in peripheral blood or synovial fluid. Radiographs of the joints are unremarkable except for soft-tissue swelling. Synovial fluid is inflammatory with low cell counts. A few patients have a chylous effusion due to obstruction of the lymphatic vessels (Das and Sen 1968). Synovial biopsy may show mononuclear cell infiltrates and eosinophils or chronic fibrosis. The treatment of choice is ivermectin. Anti-inflammatory drugs alone are ineffective. Arthrocentesis is indicated only for diagnostic purposes but not for treatment. A similar articular syndrome has been noticed in loasis.

Polyarthralgias of large and medium joints of the limbs occurred in up to one-third of patients (Carme *et al.* 1989) and an oligoarthritis affecting the knees and ankles has been seen in a few cases (Bouvet *et al.* 1977). Radiographs of the joints show soft-tissue swelling and occasionally calcified filariae. Synovial fluid is inflammatory, with lymphomononuclear cells, eosinophilia, and occasionally polymorphonuclear cells and microfilariae (Doury *et al.* 1984; Roussel *et al.* 1989). Treatment is similar to that of *W. bancrofti* filariasis.

Infections with *Onchocerca volvulus* may occasionally produce back pain and arthritis of the hip, knee, or metatarsophalangeal joints (De Jou 1941; Commandre *et al.* 1976). Diagnosis is made by identification of microfilariae in skin-punch biopsy (skin-snip examination), in biopsies of subcutaneous nodules (onchocercomas), or in the synovial fluid. The treatment of choice is ivermectin.

Dirofilaria immitis (dog heartworm) rarely infects humans. Most patients are asymptomatic, but a few develop respiratory symptoms including haemoptysis and pulmonary nodules. Arthritis of large leg joints was reported in patients infected with *D. immitis* and *D. tenuis* (Corman 1987; Langer *et al.* 1987). Synovial fluid has a low cell count with a predominance of mononuclear cells. Antiparasitic therapy is unnecessary since dirofilariae do not fully develop in man. Spontaneous death of the parasite leads to resolution of the symptoms.

Schistosomiasis in humans is caused by three species: *Schistosoma mansoni* and *S. japonicum* localized in the veins of the bowel, and *S. haematobium* in the veins of the genitourinary tract. Musculoskeletal manifestations may occur during the acute and chronic phases. Joint and muscle pain occur during the acute, serum sickness-like syndrome known as Katayama fever. Arthritis and enthesitis are seen in chronic schistosomiasis. Atkin *et al.* (1986) reported musculoskeletal manifestations in 80 per cent of patients. In general, these patients were older and had been infected with schistosomes for longer than those without rheumatic symptoms. The three syndromes identified were polyarthritis, in 60 per cent of patients, oligoarthritis in 30 per cent, and enthesitis in 10 per cent. However, enthesitis frequently occurred in patients with oligo- and polyarthritis and, all together, was the most common musculoskeletal syndrome. Polyarthritis affected the small joints of the hands and feet, knees and ankles in a symmetrical pattern, and was accompanied by morning stiffness. Oligoarthritis affected large joints of the legs. Enthesitis was not localized to any particular area. Synovial fluid was inflammatory, with cell counts of 7000 to 30 000/ml and a clear predominance of polymorphonuclear leucocytes. An asymmetrical oligoarthritis of the large leg joints and unilateral sacroiliitis was the most common syndrome in another series of patients with schistosomiasis (Bassiouni and Kamel 1984). Many patients had enthesitis and/or calcaneal spurs. Synovia showed mononuclear cell infiltrates and, in some, ova of schistosomes (Bassiouni and Kamel 1984; Fachartz *et al.* 1993). Low-titre rheumatoid factor, higher levels of IgE and IgM antibodies, and circulating immune complexes were more common in patients with articular symptoms than in those without (Kamel *et al.* 1989; Bebars *et al.* 1992). The treatment of choice is a single oral dose of praziquantel.

Muscular syndromes

Cysticercosis develops in humans infected with *Taenia solium* as intermediate hosts. The most common locations of cysticerci are the central nervous system and the striated muscle. However, occasionally, the cysts may affect the extraocular muscles and the tongue (Stewart *et al.* 1993; Gupta *et al.* 1994). Among those with skeletal muscle involvement, a few develop symptoms consisting of muscle pain and nodules or generalized myopathy (Serre *et al.* 1970; Sawhney *et al.* 1976; Vilhena Lana-Peixoto *et al.* 1985). Deep-seated nodules can be palpated in the muscles of the pelvic and scapular girdles, mostly during muscle contraction. Occasionally, a diffuse, 'pseudohypertrophic' myopathy of the limb muscles is present. Despite an apparently impressive muscle development, many patients are weak. Commonly, patients have seizures or other symptoms indicative of involvement of the central nervous system. Muscle enzymes may be mildly elevated and the electromyogram may show a myopathic pattern. Diagnosis is made by demonstration of multiple muscle cysts by MRI or CT scan (Gupta *et al.* 1994), and muscle biopsy. Cysts contain non-viable larvae and are surrounded by an inflammatory infiltrate with mononuclear cells and eosinophils. Occasionally, cysts are calcified. The treatment of choice is albendazole. A short course of corticosteroids may be needed to prevent exacerbation of symptoms due to inflammation elicited by the dying larvae.

As in cysticercosis, man is an intermediate host of *Echinococcus granulosus* and *E. multilocularis*. Parasite larvae mainly encyst (hydatid cysts) in the liver and lungs. Muscular involvement is infrequent and may affect the chest wall, abdominal wall, pectoralis, sartorius, and proximal limb muscles (Schimrigk and Emser 1978; Menuier *et al.* 1983; Duncan and Tooke 1990; García-Picazo *et al.* 1995). The cysts are usually solitary and asymptomatic, presenting as a soft-tissue mass. CT scans or MRI show a well-defined cyst with a fluid-density signal. Diagnosis and treatment are achieved by complete excision of the cyst. Percutaneous needle biopsy is not recommended, as there is a risk of disseminating the scoleces along the needle tract and of precipitating anaphylactic shock from the release of large quantities of parasitic antigens. Intraoperative cyst aspiration and thorough irrigation of the cavity with hypertonic saline is recommended to inactivate the scoleces and reduce the risk of recurrence. A fibrous and inflammatory reaction with a mononuclear, neutrophilic, and eosinophilic cell infiltrate is seen on histological examination. Muscular manifestations may develop in infections caused by larvae of two other 'flat worms', *Taenia multiceps* (coenurosis) and *Spirometra* spp. (sparganosis). In coenurosis, larvae of *T. multiceps* encyst in the subcutaneous tissues and muscles of the neck, chest or abdomen causing painless nodules (Templeton 1968). In sparganosis acquired by the oral route, larvae of *Spirometra* are released in the intestine and migrate from there to different organs. During this process the larvae burrow through the subcutaneous tissue and muscles causing a slowly growing, occasionally migrating soft-tissue mass (Cho and Patel 1978; Nakamura *et al.* 1990). In both conditions, diagnosis and treatment are achieved by surgical excision of the mass.

Gnathostoma spinigerum (gnathostomiasis) may produce a localized soft-tissue abscess or a nodular, migratory, eosinophilic panniculitis due to migration of the larvae through the skin, subcutaneous tissues, and muscles (Rusnak and Lucey 1993; Stevens and Bryson 1994). Diagnosis is confirmed by positive serology. The treatment of choice is albendazole (Kraivichian *et al.* 1992).

An acute, transient myositis localized to the legs was reported in two children infected with *Toxocara canis* (visceral larva migrans) (Walsh *et al.* 1988). Both cases presented with eosinophilia and diffuse, non-tender swelling of the calf, which resolved spontaneously in 3 days. Diagnosis was established by positive serology (enzyme immunoassay) for *Toxocara*. *Onchocerca volvulus* may produce a nodular, localized, eosinophilic myositis of the abdominal wall (Neumann *et al.* 1985), and schistosomiasis has been associated with a diffuse myopathy of muscles of the shoulder and pelvic girdles (Mansour and Reese 1964).

Muscle involvement occurs during the invasive phase of trichinosis when larvae, released in the intestine by the adult female, migrate through the tissues and reach the striated muscle. The clinical presentation varies from asymptomatic infection to a severe, sometimes fatal, multisystem disease, depending on the immune status of the host and the parasite load; fewer than 10 larvae per gram of muscle rarely cause symptoms. Clinical manifestations characteristic of the invasive phase are: fever, chills, periorbital oedema, subconjunctival, retinal and subungual (splinter) haemorrhages, eosinophilia, myocarditis, and less frequently, encephalitis, nephritis and death. Myalgia and weakness affecting the proximal muscles of the arms and legs develop in two-thirds of patients infected by *T. nelsoni* (Ferraccioli *et al.* 1988). Occasionally, patients may present with manifestations indistinguishable from those of dermato- or polymyositis; that is, proximal muscle weakness, elevated creatine kinase, an electromyogram consistent with myositis, and extensive eosinophilic myositis on muscle biopsy (Herrera *et al.* 1985; MacLean *et al.* 1989; Durán-Ortiz *et al.* 1992; Louthrenoo *et al.* 1993). Larvae of trichinae are present in the muscle fibres (Fig. 4). Larvae of *Trichinella spiralis* are encapsulated while those of *T. pseudospiralis* are unencapsulated and mobile. The treatment of choice is with albendazole or mebendazole. Corticosteroids are indicated only in massive infections with severe myositis, myocarditis or central nervous involvement. Corticosteroids alone may aggravate muscle symptoms (Andrews *et al.* 1994).

Vascular syndromes

Vasculitis was induced in animals experimentally infected with larva migrans (Watzke *et al.* 1984) and is documented in a few patients infected with cestodes and nematodes. Vascular changes have been demonstrated in cysticercosis of the central nervous system and probably contribute to the basal arachnoiditis characteristic of racemous

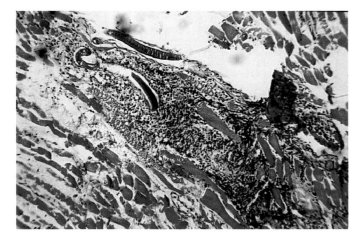

Fig. 4 Trichina myositis. Larvae of *Trichinella spiralis* and inflammatory cell infiltrate in a muscle biopsy of a child with trichinosis. Section stained with haematoxylin and eosin. Original magnification × 100. (Reproduced from Durán-Ortiz *et al.* 1992, with permission.).

cysticercosis (Estañol *et al.* 1986). A case of histologically proven polyarteritis nodosa in a child with hepatic hydatidosis was reported recently (Bakkaloglu *et al.* 1994): treatment with prednisone and cyclophosphamide for 2 months was ineffective, but all symptoms resolved after treatment with mebendazole followed by surgical excision. Leucocytoclastic vasculitis characterized by palpable purpura, arthritis, eosinophilia, and immunoglobulin deposition in the vascular walls has been reported in infections with *Strongyloides stercoralis* (Akoglu *et al.* 1984) and *Loa loa* (Portilla-Sogorb *et al.* 1991). As in other parasite-induced symptoms, all manifestations of vasculitis resolved after antiparasitic treatment. Nematode infections have been associated with more severe forms of necrotizing vasculitis. Reimann *et al.* (1943) and Frayha (1981) described cases of polyarteritis nodosa associated with trichinosis. More recently, Churg–Strauss vasculitis was reported in patients infected with ascarids (Chanham *et al.* 1990) and an *Angiostrongylus*-like nematode (Pirisi *et al.* 1995). In both cases the diagnosis was proven by histology. Grcevska (1993) reported recently a case of renal necrotizing vasculitis associated with glomerulonephritis in a patient infected with ascarids; the renal manifestations resolved completely after eradication of the parasite.

Musculoskeletal symptoms induced by antiparasitic treatment

Arthralgias and arthritis may develop during antiparasitic treatment, especially in patients infected with tissue-invasive parasites. In general, the frequency and severity of the symptoms vary according to the type of parasite, the parasite load, and the drug used. Mild joint and muscle pain occur in 2 to 3 per cent of patients with leishmaniasis treated with stibogluconate (Thakur and Kumar 1990), and in 10 to 15 per cent of patients with opisthochiasis treated with praziquantel (Viravan *et al.* 1986). More severe manifestations (Mazzotti reaction) develop in patients with filariasis treated with diethylcarbamazine or ivermectin (Ottesen 1987; Kumaraswami *et al.* 1988). Mazzotti reactions are seen more commonly in onchocerciasis and in lymphatic filariasis caused by *Bruggia* spp. The clinical manifestations of Mazzotti reaction vary from malaise and minor body aches to a severe, systemic, sometimes fatal reaction. Symptoms develop rapidly in the first few hours after the administration of diethylcarbamazine and consist of pruritus, rash, lymphadenopathy, fever, tachycardia, hypotension, and arthralgias. A second phase of the reaction is characterized by arthritis of the small and large joints, fever, and myalgia, developing in the first 3 to 5 days. Milder and less frequent symptoms have been reported with the use of ivermectin for the treatment of onchocerciasis and lymphatic filariasis.

The use of low initial doses of diethylcarbamazine often diminishes the severity of the early phase of the reaction. The treatment of the Mazzotti reaction is symptomatic; for patients with mild symptoms, analgesics and antipyretics are indicated. Corticosteroids, prednisone 60 mg/day, prevent the development of symptoms and are indicated in patients with heavy infections, although they may decrease the efficacy of diethylcarbamazine.

References

Akoglu, T., Tuncer, I., Erkon, E., Gürcay, A., Ozer, F. L., and Ozcan, K. (1984). Parasitic arthritis induced by *Strongyloides stercoralis*. *Annals of the Rheumatic Diseases*, **43**, 523–5.

Alhadeff, R. (1955). Clinical aspects of filariasis. *Journal of Tropical Medicine and Hygiene*, **58**, 173–9.

Amor, B., Benhamou, C. L., Dougados, M., and Grant, A. (1983). Arthrites a eosinophiles et revue generale de la signification de l'eosinophile articulaire. *Revue Rheumatisme Maladie Osteoarticulaire*, **50**, 659–64.

Andrews, J. R. H., Ainsworth, R., and Abernethy, D. (1994). *Trichinella pseudospiralis* in humans: description of a case and its treatment. *Transactions of the Royal Society of Tropical Medicine and Hygiene*, **88**, 200–3.

Antezana, E. (1979). Polytenosynovitis caused by *Toxoplasma gondii*. *South African Medical Journal*, **56**, 746.

Argenson, C., Griffet, J., Lacour, C., Arcamone, H., Lovet, J., and de Peretti, F. (1989). Hydatid disease of the spine. Report of two cases. *Revue de Chirurgie Orthopedique*, **75**, 267–70.

Atkin, S. L., Kamel, M., El-Hady, A. M,. El- Badawy, S. A., El-Ghobary, A., and Dick, W. C. (1986). Schistosomiasis and inflammatory polyarthritis: a clinical, radiological and laboratory study of 96 patients infected by *S. mansoni* with particular reference to the diarthrodial joint. *Quarterly Journal of Medicine*, **59**, 479–87.

Bakkaloglu, A., Söylemezoğlu, O., Tinaztepe, K., and Saatci, ü. (1994). A possible relationship between polyarteritis nodosa and hydatid disease. *European Journal of Pediatrics*, **153**, 469.

Balleari, E., Cutolo, M., and Accardo, S. (1991). Adult onset Still's disease associated to *Toxoplasma gondii* infection. *Clinical Rheumatology*, **10**, 326–7.

Ballina-Garcia, F. J., Rodriguez-Arboleya, L., Torre-Alonso, J. C., Mori-Garcia, A., and Rodriguez-Perez, A. (1987). Polyarthrite au cours d'une hydatidose hepatique. *Revue du Rheumatisme*, **54**, 779.

Barton, J. J., Burke, J. P., and Casey, E. B. (1986). Reactive arthritis: *Giardia lamblia*, another new pathogen. *Irish Medical Journal*, **79**, 223.

Bassiouni, M. and Kamel, M. (1984). Bilharzial arthropathy. *Annals of the Rheumatic Diseases*, **43**, 806–9.

Bebars, M. A., Soffar, S. A., Abbas, M. M., Ismail, M. S., and Tamara, F. A. (1992). Circulating immune complexes in bilharzial arthropathy. *Journal of the Egyptian Society of Parasitology*, **22**, 51–7.

Bissonnette, B. and Beaudet, F. (1983). Reactive arthritis with eosinophilic synovial infiltrations. *Annals of the Rheumatic Diseases*, **42**, 466–8.

Bocanegra, T. S. (1993). Musculoskeletal manifestations of parasitic diseases. In *Oxford textbook of rheumatology* (1st edn) (ed. P. I. Maddison, D. A. Isenberg, P. Woo, and D. N. Glass), pp. 589–98. Oxford University Press.

Bocanegra, T. S. (1994). Mycobacterial, fungal and parasitic arthritides. In *Rheumatology* (ed. J. H. Klippel and P. A. Dieppe), pp. 4.5.1–4.5.12. Mosby–Year Book Europe, London.

Bocanegra, T. S., Espinoza, L. R., Bridgeford, P. H., Vasey, F. B., and Germain, B. F. (1981). Reactive arthritis induced by parasitic infestation. *Annals of Internal Medicine*, **94**, 207–9.

Bonciou, C., Petronicu, M., and Panateiscu, D. (1981). Observations on a case of chronic myositis due to sarcosporidia. *Archives Romaines do Pathologie Experimentale et Microbiologie*, **40**, 361–3.

Bouvet, J. P., Thérizol, M., and Auquier, L. (1977) Microfilarial polyarthritis in a massive Loa-Loa infestation: a case report. *Acta Tropica*, **34**, 281–4.

Brougui, P. and Richard, P. (1990). Articular manifestations of *Giardia lamblia* infections. *Bulletin de la Societé de Pathologie Exotique et des ses Filiales*, **83**, 688–9.

Buskila, D., Sikenik, S., Klein, M., and Horowitz, J. (1992). Polyarthritis associated with hydatid disease (echinococcosis) of the liver. *Clinical Rheumatology*, **11**, 286–7.

Bussiere, J. L., Ristori, J. M., and Sauvezie, B. (1981). Inflammatory rheumatism associated with intestinal parasitosis. *Nouvelle Presse Médicale*, **10**, 2990.

Cairncross, S. (1995). Victory over guineaworm disease: partial or pyrrhic?, *Lancet*, **346**, 1440.

Campoy, E., Rodriguez-Morena, J., Del Blanco, J., Narvaez, J., Clavaguera, T., and Roig-Escofet, D. (1995). Hydatid disease. An unusual cause of monoarthritis. *Arthritis and Rheumatism*, **38**, 1338–9.

Carme, B., Mamboueni, J. P., Copin, N., and Noireau, F. (1989). Clinical and biological study of Loa-Loa filariasis in Congolese. *American Journal of Tropical Medicine and Hygiene*, **41**, 331–7.

Carmeni, G., Tato, A., Martusciello, S., Valiante, B., Magrino, A., and Meloni, F. (1991). Vascular involvement and toxoplasma infection. *British Journal of Dermatology*, **124**, 14.

Chanham, A., Scott, D. G. I., Neuberger, J., Gaston, J. S. H., and Bacon, P. A. (1990). Churg–Strauss vasculitis and Ascaris infection. *Annals of the Rheumatic Diseases*, **49**, 320–2.

Cho, C. and Patel, S. P. (1978). Human sparganosis in northern United States. *New York State Journal of Medicine*, **78**, 1456–8.

Commandre, F., Lapeyre, L., Viani, J. L., Revelli, G., Lefichoux, Y., and Jozan, S. (1976). Arthritis associated with filarioses. *Rheumatologie*, **18**, 27–33.

Corman, L. C. (1987). Acute arthritis occurring in association with subcutaneous *Dirofilaria tenuis* infection. *Arthritis and Rheumatism*, **30**, 1431–4.

Cossermelli, W. *et al.* (1978). Polymyositis in Chagas' disease. *Annals of the Rheumatic Diseases*, **37**, 277–80.

Das, G. C. and Sen, S. B. (1968). Chylous arthritis. *British Medical Journal*, **2**, 27–9.

De Jonge-Bok, J. M., Overbosch, D., and MacFarlane, J. D. (1985). Parasitic rheumatism presenting as oligoarthritis: a case report. *Tropical and Geographical Medicine*, **37**, 367–8.

De Jou, L. (1941). Surgical localizations of African filarioses: arthritis and suppurations of the soft tissue. *Medicine Tropicale*, **1**, 15–35.

De La Torre, F. E. and Gorraez, M. T. (1989). Toxoplasma-induced occlusive hypertrophic arteritis as the cause of discrete coagulative necrosis in the CNS. *Human Pathology*, **20**, 604.

DeSilva, H. J. *et al.* (1988). Skeletal muscle necrosis in severe falciparum malaria. *British Medical Journal*, **296**, 1039.

Desphande, R. B., Bharucha, M. A., Modhe, J. M., and Bhalerao, R. A. (1992). Necrotizing arteritis in amoebic colitis. *Journal of Postgraduate Medicine*, **38**, 151–2.

Doury, P. (1994). Parasitic arthritis and parasitic rheumatism. *Smaine des Hospitaux Paris*, **7**, 522–8.

Doury, P., Pattin, S., Durosoir, J. L., Voinesson, A., Bienot, B., and Duret, J. C. (1975). Rheumatism and strongyloidiasis. *Nouvelle Presse Médicale*, **4**, 805.

Doury, P., Pattin, S., Dienot, B., Roue, R., and Delayaye, R. P. (1977). Les rheumatismes parasitaires. *Smaine des Hospitaux Paris*, **53**, 1359–63.

Doury, P., Saliou, P., and Charmot, G. (1984). Eosinophilic joint effusions: *propos* of a case. *Revue du Rheumatisme*, **51**, 29–31.

Duncan, G. J. and Tooke, S. M. (1990). Echinococcus infestation of the biceps brachii. A case report. *Clinical Orthopaedics*, **26**, 247–50.

Duran, H. *et al.* (1978). Osseous hydatidosis. *Journal of Bone and Joint Surgery* (A), **60**, 685–90.

Durán-Ortiz, J. S. *et al.* (1992). Trichinosis with severe myopathic involvement mimicking polymyositis. Report of a family outbreak. *Journal of Rheumatology*, **19**, 310–12.

Encarnación, C. F., Giordano, M. F., and Murray, H. W. (1994). Onchocerciasis in New York City. The Moa–Manhattan Connection. *Archives of Internal Medicine*, **154**, 1749–51.

Estañol, B., Corona, T., and Abad, P. (1986). A prognostic classification of cerebral cysticercosis: therapeutic implications. *Journal of Neurology, Neurosurgery and Psychology*, **49**, 1131–4.

Fachartz, O. A., Kumer, V., and Al-Hilou, M. (1993). Synovial schistosomiasis of the hip. *Journal of Bone and Joint Surgery* (B), **75**, 602–3.

Farthing, M. J. G., Chong, S. K. F., and Walter-Smith, J. A. (1983). Acute allergic phenomenon in giardiasis. *Lancet*, **ii**, 1428.

Ferraccioli, G. F., Mercadanti, M., Salaffi, F., Bruschi, F., Melissari, M., and Pozio, E. (1988). Prospective rheumatological study of muscle and joint symptoms during *Trichinella nelsoni* infection. *Quarterly Journal of Medicine*, **69**, 973–84.

Forzy, G., Dhondt, J. L., Leloire, O., Shayeb, J., and Vincent, G. (1988). Reactive arthritis and Strongyloides. *Journal of the American Medical Association*, **259**, 2546–7.

Frayha, R. A. (1981). Trichinosis related polyarteritis nodosa. *American Journal of Medicine*, **71**, 307–82.

Fyfe, B., Amazon, K., Poppiti, R. J., and Razzetti, A. (1990). Intra-osseous echinococcosis: a rare manifestation of echinococcal disease. *Southern Medical Journal*, **83**, 66–8.

García-Picazo, D., Vasquez-Arragón, P., Palomares-Ortiz, G., Cascales-Sánchez, P., and Lopez-Fando de Castro, J. (1995). Multiple hydatid cysts of the liver, bones and muscles. *Revista Española de Enfermedades Digestivas*, **87**, 267–70.

Garf, A. E. (1985). Parasitic rheumatism: rheumatic manifestations associated with calcified Guinea worm: *Journal of Rheumatology*, **12**, 976–9.

Gemou, V., Messaritakis, J., Karpathios, T., and Kingo, A. (1983). Chronic polyarthritis of toxoplasmic etiology. *Helvetia Paediatrica Acta*, **38**, 295–6.

Gonzalez-Dominguez, J., Roldan, R., Vllanueva, J. L., Kindelám, J. M., Jurado, R., and Torre-Cisneros, J. (1994). *Isospora belli* reactive arthritis in a patient with AIDS. *Annals of the Rheumatic Diseases*, **53**, 618–19.

Goobar, J. P. (1977). Joint symptoms in giardiasis. *Lancet*, **i**, 1010–11.

Grcevska, L. and Polenakovic, M. (1993). Renal vasculitis associated with ascaridiasis with good prognosis. *Nephron*, **64**, 327–8.

Greenlee, J. E., Johnson, W. D., Campa, J. F., Adelman, L. S., and Sande, M. A. (1975). Adult toxoplasmosis presenting as polymyositis and cerebellar ataxia. *Annals of Internal Medicine*, **82**, 367–71.

Greenwood, B. M .(1968). Guinea-worm arthritis of knee joint. *British Medical Journal*, **1**, 314.

Gupta, P. K., Jaleel, M. A., Prasad, V. S., Naik, R. T., Sundaram, C., and Dinakar, I. (1994). Unusual clinical manifestations of cysticercosis. *Journal of the Association of Physicians of India*, **42**, 411–12.

Harland, C. C., Marsden, J. R., Vernon, S. A., and Allen, B. R. (1991). Dermatomyositis responding to treatment of associated toxoplasmosis. *British Journal of Dermatology*, **125**, 76–8.

Hay, E. M,. Windfield, J., and McKendrick, M. W. (1987). Reactive arthritis associated with crytosporidium enteritis. *British Medical Journal*, **295**, 248.

Herrera, R., Varela, E., Morales, G., Del Rio, A., and Gallardo, J. M. (1985). Dermatomyositis-like syndrome caused by Trichinae: report of two cases. *Journal of Rheumatology*, **12**, 782–4.

Hooper, J. and McLean, I. (1977). Hydatid disease of the femur. Report of a case. *Journal of Bone and Joint Surgery* (A), **59**, 974–6.

Huang, T. E. and Chou, S. M. (1988). Occlusive hypertrophic arteritis as the cause of discrete necrosis in CNS toxoplasmosis in the acquired immunodeficiency syndrome. *Human Pathology*, **19**, 1210–14.

Huang, P. *et al*. (1995). The first reported outbreak of diarrheal illness associated with *Cyclospora* in the United States. *Annals of Internal Medicine*, **123**, 409–14.

Ismail, M. M. and Nagaratnam, N. (1973). Arthritis possibly due to filariasis. *Transactions of the Royal Society for Tropical Medicine and Hygiene*, **67**, 405–9.

Jeffrey, H. C. (1974). Sarcosporidiosis in man. *Transactions of the Royal Society for Tropical Medicine and Hygiene*, **68**, 17–29.

Kamel, M., Sajwat, E., and El-Tayab, S. (1989). Bilharzial arthropathy. *Scandinavian Journal of Rheumatology*, **18**, 315–19.

Kothari, M. L., Pardnani, D. S., Mehta, L., and Amand, M. P. (1968) Guinea worm arthritis of the knee joint. *British Medical Journal*, **3**, 435–6.

Kraivichian, P., Kulkumthorn, M., Yingyourd, P., Akarabovan, P., and Paireepai, C. C. (1992). Albendazole for the treatment of human gnathostomiasis. *Transactions of the Royal Society of Tropical Medicine and Hygiene*, **86**, 418–21.

Kraus, A., Valencia, X., Cabral, A. R., and De La Vega, G. (1995) Visceral larva migrans mimicking rheumatic diseases. *Journal of Rheumatology*, **22**, 497–500.

Krüger, K., Kamilli, I., and Schattenkirchner, M. (1994). *Blastocystis hominis* infection. A rare cause of arthritis. *Zeitschrift für Rheumatologie*, **53**, 83–5.

Kumaraswami, V. *et al*. (1988). Ivermectin for the treatment of *Wuchereria brancrofti* filariasis: efficacy and adverse reactions. *Journal of the American Medical Association*, **259**, 3150–3.

Lakhanpal, S., Cohen, S. B., and Fleischmann, R. M. (1991). Reactive arthritis from *Blastocystis hominis*. *Arthritis and Rheumatism*, **34**, 251–3.

Langer, H. E., Bialek, R., Mielke, H., and Klose, J. (1987). Human dirofilariasis with reactive arthritis — case report and review of the literature. *Klinische Wochenschrift*, **65**, 746–51.

Ledford, D. K., Overman, M. D,. Gonzalvo, A., Cali, A., Mester, S. W., and Lockey, R. F. (1985). Microsporidiosis myositis in a patient with the acquired immunodeficiency syndrome. *Annals of Internal Medicine*, **102**, 628–30.

Lee, M. G., Rawlins, S. C., Didier, M., and DeCeulaer, K. (1990). Infective arthritis due to *Blastocystis hominis*. *Annals of the Rheumatic Diseases*, **49**, 192–3.

Le Luyer, B., Menager, V., Audebert, C., Le Roux, P., Briquet, M. T., and Boulloche, J. (1990). Arthropathies inflammatoires revelatrices d'une larva migrans a *Toxocara canis*. *Annales Pediatria*, **7**, 445–8.

Louthrenoo, W., Mahanuphab, P., Sanguanmitra, P., and Thamprasert, K. (1993). Trichinosis mimicking polymyositis in a patient with human immunodeficiency virus infection. *British Journal of Rheumatology*, **32**, 1025–30.

McAmilty, J. M., Fleming, D. W., and Gonzalez, A. H. (1994). A community-wide outbreak of cryptosporidiosis associated with swimming at a wave pool. *Journal of the American Medical Association*, **272**, 1597–600.

McGill, R. J. (1957). Sarcosporidiosis in a man with polyarteritis nodosa. *British Medical Journal*, **2**, 333–4.

MacKenzie, W. R. *et al*. (1994). A massive outbreak in Milwaukee of *Cryptosporidium* infection transmitted through the public water supply. *New England Journal of Medicine*, **331**, 161–7.

McLaughlin, G. E., Utsinger, P. D., Trakat, W. F., Resnick, D., and Moidel, R. A. (1984). Rheumatic syndromes secondary to Guinea worm infestation. *Arthritis and Rheumatism*, **27**, 694–7.

MacLean, J. D., Viallet, J., Law, C., and Staudt, M. (1989). Trichinosis in the Canadian Arctic: report of five outbreaks and a new clinical syndrome. *Journal of Infectious Diseases*, **160**, 573–20.

McNicholl, B. and Underhill, D. (1970). Toxoplasmic polymyositis. *Irish Journal of Medical Science*, **3**, 525–7.

Magid, S. K., and Kagen, L. J. (1983). Serologic evidence for acute toxoplasmosis in polymyositis-dermatomyositis: increased frequency of specific anti-toxoplasma IgM antibodies. *American Journal of Medicine*, **75**, 313–20.

Mansour, S. D. and Reese, H. H. (1964). A previously unexpected myopathy in patients with schistosomiasis. *Neurology*, **14**, 355–61.

Matsubara, S., Takamori, M., Adachi, H., and Kida, H. (1990). Acute toxoplasma myositis: an immunohistochemical and ultrastructural study. *Acta Neuropathologica*, **81**, 223–7.

Menkes, C. J., Papo, T., Carter, H., and Renoux, M. (1987). Reactive arthritis caused by strongyloides and ankylosing spondylitis. *Revue du Rheumatisme*, **54**, 504–6.

Menuier, Y., Danis, M., Nozais, J. P., and Gentilini, M. (1983). Muscular hydatid disease: two case reports. *Smaine des Hospitaux Paris*, **59**, 2785–6.

Millard, P. S. *et al*. (1994). An outbreak of cryptosporidiosis from fresh-pressed apple cider. *Journal of the American Medical Association*, **272**, 1592–6.

Nakamura, T., Hara, M., Matsuka, M., Kawabata, M., and Tsuji, M. (1990). Human proliferative sparganosis: a new Japanese case. *American Journal of Clinical Pathology*, **94**, 224–8.

Neumann, H., Herz, R., and Baum, C. (1985). Granulomatous and eosinophilic myositis due to *Onchocerca volvulus*. *Pathology*, **6**, 101–7.

Ognibene, F. P. *et al*. (1995). *Pneumocystis carinii* pneumonia — a major complication of immunosuppressive therapy in patients with Wegener's granulomatosis. *American Journal of Respiratory and Critical Care Medicine*, **151**, 795–9.

Ottesen, E. A. (1987). Description mechanisms and control of reactions to treatment in the human filariases. *Ciba Foundation Symposium*, **127**, 265–83.

Pape, J. W., Verdier, R. I., Boncy, M., Boncy, J., and Johnson, W. D. (1994). Cyclospora infection in adults infected with HIV. Clinical manifestations, treatment and prophylaxis. *Annals of Internal Medicine*, **121**, 654–7.

Patey, O., Bouhali, R., Breuil, J., Chapuis, L., Courillon-Mallet, A., and Lafaix, C. (1990). Arthritis associated with *Strongyloides stercoralis*. *Nouvelle Presse Medicale*, **4**, 805.

Pirisi, M. *et al*. (1995). Fatal human pulmonary infection caused by *Angiostrongylus*-like nematode. *Clinical Infectious Diseases*, **20**, 59–65.

Portilla-Sogorb, J., Sevilla-Linares, A., Carrion, A,. Cordoba, C., and Blesa, M. (1991). Vasculitis Leucocitoclástica por hipersensiblilidad a microfilarias. *Anales de Medicina Interna (Madrid)*, **8**, 30–2.

Rao, S., Parikh, S., and Kerr, R. (1991). Echinococcal Infestation of the spine in North America. *Clinical Orthopedics*, **271**, 164–9.

Rappaport, E. M., Rossien, A., and Roseblum, L. (1951). Arthritis due to intestinal amebiasis. *Annals of Internal Medicine*, **34**, 1224–31.

Reddy, C. R. and Sivaramappa, M. (1968). Guinea-worm arthritis of knee joint. *British Medical Journal*, **1**, 155–6.

Reimann, H. A., Price, A. H., and Herbut, P. A. (1943). Trichinosis and periarteritis nodosa: differential diagnosis, possible relationship. *Journal of the American Medical Association*, **12**, 274–9.

Richardson de Corral, V., Lozano-Garcia, J., and Ramos-Corona, L. E. (1990). Una presentación poco usual de toxocariasis sistémica. *Boletín Médico del Hospital Infantil de México*, **47**, 841–4.

Roig-Quilis, M. and Damjanov, I. (1982). Dermatomyositis as an immunologic complication of toxoplasmosis. *Acta Neuropathologica (Berlin)*, **58**, 183–6.

Roussel, F., Roussel, C., Brasseur, P., Gourmelen, O., and Le Loet, X. (1989). Aseptic knee effusion with Loa-Loa microfilariae in the articular fluid. *Acta Cytologica*, **33**, 281–3.

Rusnak, J. M. and Lucey, D. R. (1993). Clinical gnathostomiasis: a case report and review of the English language literature. *Clinics in Infectious Diseases*, **16**, 33–50.

Salfield, S. (1975). Filarial arthritis in the Sepik district of Papua New Guinea. *Medical Journal of Australia*, **1**, 264–7.

Sawhney, B. B., Chopra, J. S., Banerji, A. K., and Wahi, P. L. (1976). Pseudohypertrophic myopathy in cysticercosis. *Neurology*, **26**, 270–2.

Schimrigk, K. and Emser, W. (1978). Parasitic myositis by *Echinococcus alveolaris*: report of a family with myotonia congenita. *European Neurology*, **17**, 1–7.

Serre, H., Simon, L., Lamboley, C., and Regal, R. (1970). Muscular manifestations of human cysticercosis. *Rheumatologie*, **22**, 537–63.

Shaw, R. A. and Stevens, M. B. (1987). The reactive arthritis of *Giardia lamblia*. A case report. *Journal of the American Medical Association*, **258**, 2734–5.

Sheperd, R. C., Smail, P. J., and Sinha, G. P. (1989). Reactive arthritis complicating cryptosporidial infection. *Archives of Disease in Childhood*, **64**, 743–4.

Stevens, C. O. and Bryson, A. D. (1994). Gnathostomiasis as a cause of soft tissue swellings. *British Journal of Rheumatology*, **33** (Suppl. 65), 36.

Stewart, C. R., Salmon, J. F., Murray, A. D., and Sperryn, C. (1993). Cysticercosis as a cause of severe medial rectus muscle myositis. *American Journal of Ophthalmology*, **116**, 510–11.

Surianu, P., Medrea, B., Popa, M., and Karassi, A. (1967). Rheumatic manifestations of cutaneous cysticercosis. *Presse Médicale*, **65**, 1505.

Swash, M. and Schwartz, M. S. (1993). Malaria myositis. *Journal of Neurology, Neurosurgery and Psychiatry*, **56**, 1238.

Templeton, A. C. (1968). Human coeneurosis: a report of 14 cases from Uganda. *Transactions of the Royal Society for Tropical Medicine and Hygiene*, **62**, 251–5.

Thakur, C. P. and Kumar, K. (1990). Efficacy of prolonged therapy with stibogluconate in post kala-azar dermal leishmaniasis. *Indian Journal of Medical Research*, **91**, 144–8.

Topi, G. C., D'Alessandro, L., Catricala, C., and Zardi, O. (1979). Dermatomyositis-like syndrome due to toxoplasma. *British Journal of Dermatology*, **101**, 589–91.

Treusch, P. J., Swatnam, R. E., and Woelke, B. J. (1981). Eosinophilic joint effusion and intestinal nematodiasis. *Annals of Emergency Medicine*, **10**, 614–15.

Van Linthoudt, D., Mean, A. P., Favre, R., and Ott, H. (1990). Coxarthritis in a child associated with toxocariasis. *Schweizerische Rundschau fur Medizine Praxic (Bern)*, **79**, 1022–4.

Vigliani, F. and Campailla, E. (1977). Meta-echinococcal arthrosynovitis: a clinical, anatomical and pathological entity not previously recognized. *Italian Journal of Orthopaedics and Traumatology*, **3**, 103–10.

Vilhena Lana-Peixoto, M. I., Lana-Peixoto, M. A., and Campos, G. B. (1985). Pseudohypertrophic myopathy due to cysticercosis: a case report. *Arquivos Neuro-psiquiatria (Sao Paolo)*, **43**, 396–402.

Viravan, C., Bunnang, D., Harinasuta, T., Upatham, S., Kurathong, S., and Viyanant, V. (1986). Clinical field trial of praziquantel in opisthorchiasis in Nong Rangya Village, Khon Kaen Province, Thailand. *South East Asian Journal of Tropical Medicine and Public Health*, **17**, 63–6.

Voutsinas, S., Sayakos, J., and Smytnis, P. (1987). Echinococcus infestation complicating total hip replacement. A case report. *Journal of Bone and Joint Surgery* (A), **69**, 1456–8.

Walsh, S. S., Robson, W. J., and Hart, C. A. (1988) Acute transient myositis due to *Toxocara*. *Archives of Disease in Childhood*, **63**, 1087–8.

Watzke, R. C., Oaks, J. A., and Folk, J. C. (1984). *Toxocara canis* infection in the eye: correlation of clinical observations with developing pathology in the primate model. *Archives of Ophthalmology*, **102**, 282–91.

Weiss, L. M. (1995). And now microsporidiosis. *Annals of Internal Medicine*, **123**, 954–6.

William, D. and Roy, S. (1981). Arthritis and arthralgia associated with toxocaral infestation. *British Medical Journal*, **283**, 192.

Woo, P. and Panayi, G. S. (1984). Reactive arthritis due to infestation with *Giardia lamblia*. *Journal of Rheumatology*, **11**, 719.

Yonis, Z. (1943). Amebic arthritis. *Harefuah*, **24**, 135.

5.3.10 Fungal arthritis

Carol A. Kemper and Stanley C. Deresinski

Introduction

Fungal infection of joints is a challenging but uncommon clinical problem whose aetiology is often belatedly recognized. Fungal joint infection most often results from the haematogenous dissemination of the pathogen from a primary portal of infection (usually pulmonary) directly to the synovial tissue or may initially affect para-articular bone with subsequent rupture into a joint space. Less commonly, such infection occurs as the result of direct inoculation of the organism into the joint space or synovial tissue. An inflammatory aseptic arthritis may also occur in association with certain fungal infections (e.g. coccidioidomycosis or histoplasmosis) as a result of the immune response to the organism, rather than a result of infection of the joint itself.

Epidemiology

Only a handful of fungi, perhaps five or six species at most, are responsible for the majority of human mycotic musculoskeletal infections (Schwarz 1984; Bradsher 1988; Fader and McGinnis 1988; Silveira *et al.* 1991; Cuellar *et al.* 1992; Cueller *et al.* 1993) (Table 1), but virtually all of the approximately 100 fungi pathogenic in man have been reported to cause infection of bones and/or joints. The frequency with which arthritis occurs, its clinical presentation, and its outcome varies depending on the specific fungal agent as well as upon host variables. For example, fungal arthritis caused by the endemic dimorphic fungi, such as *Histoplasmosis capsulatum*, *Blastomycosis dermatiditis*, and *Coccidioides immitis*, is often seen in patients without overt immunodeficiency. In contrast, infection resulting from *Candida* spp. is usually found in association with intravascular infection in individuals with readily apparent host factors, such as those with indwelling central venous catheters (often in association with the administration of long-term antibiotic therapy and/ or parenteral nutrition), or those undergoing haemodialysis, or intravenous drug users. Defects in cellular immunity are critical to the dissemination of certain fungi from their initial portal of infection and the secondary infection of joint spaces. Patients with haematological malignancy or the acquired immune deficiency syndrome (AIDS), organ transplants recipients receiving immunosuppressive agents, or those receiving chronic corticosteroids are especially at risk for fungal arthritis. HIV-infected individuals are especially vulnerable to disseminated infection with *Cryptococcus neoformans*, *C. immitis*, and *H. capsulatum*.

Rarely, joint infection occurs secondary to direct inoculation of the organism into the joint during aspiration or injection, trauma, or surgical intervention. Human to human transmission of these mycoses does not, for all practical purposes, occur.

Exposure to *B. dermatitidis*, *C. immitis*, *H. capsulatum*, or *Paracoccidioides brasiliensis* ordinarily occurs within their respective endemic areas (see Table 1). *C. immitis* is limited to endemic zones in North, Central and South America, while *H. capsulatum* is found in areas of both hemispheres, often in association with avian and chiropteran habitats. *B. dermatitidis*, while most often acquired in the United

Table 1 Risk factors for infection and the clinical setting of fungal joint infection

Organism	Endemicity	Host risk factors	Mode of infection	Joint involvement
Candida spp.	Normal human commensal	Haematological malignancy, immunodefficiency, neonates, indwelling catheters, central catheters, long-term antiobiotic use, exogenous steroids	Haematogenous, rarely direct inoculation from trauma or injections	Monoarticular; predominately large joints (knee 70%)
Coccidioides immitis	Arizona, New Mexico, California	Usually immunocompetent host	Haematogenous	Monoarticular >90%; predominately knee and ankle
Blastomyces dermatitidis	Ohio, Missouri, Mississippi river valleys, south-eastern United States, Africa, Middle East	Usually immunocompetent host (>90%)	Haematogenous, rarely direct inoculation	Monoarticular >90%; knee, ankle, elbow, and wrist
Sporothrix schenkii	Worldwide	Alcoholic, diabetic, rarely severely immunocompromised	Haematogenous, may be direct inoculation	50% monoarticular, 50% polyarticular; knee, ankle, wrist, small joints of the hand
Histoplasma capsulatum	Ohio, Missouri, Mississippi river valleys, Central and South America	Both normal and immunodeficient hosts (e.g. AIDS)	Haematogenous	Monoarticular; knee, wrist, small joints of the hand
Cryptococcus neoformans	Worldwide	Organ transplant, AIDS haematological malignancy, diabetes, exogenous steroids	Haematogenous	Monoarticular 65%, polyarticular 35%; knee (60%), ankle, wrist, sterno/acromial-clavicular
Paracoccidioides brasiliensis	Central and South America	Immunocompetent host	Haematogenous	

States, has also been reported from Africa and the Middle East. *P. brasiliensis* is found in Central and South America, although rare cases have been described in North America. For each of these dimorphic fungi, inhalation of conidia or arthroconidia released by the mycelial phase of the organism results in a primary pulmonary infection which is either subacute or acute, and typically self-limited, or which, in some cases, becomes chronic. Secondary dissemination during the acute or chronic phase of pulmonary infection results in a varying incidence of clinical joint infection for each of these diseases. *C. neoformans* and *Sporothrix schenckii* have a worldwide distribution. In contrast to the other fungi, infection with candida is ordinarily the consequence of host invasion by endogenous colonizing organisms.

Clinical picture

The clinical presentation of joint infection is most often indolent, although the onset of some infections, such as those caused by *B. dermatiditis*, *Candida* spp., and, occasionally, other fungi, may be acute, with hot, erythematous and tender joints and accompanying fever. The presentation may thus resemble an acute bacterial septic arthritis. Most cases, however, present with the usual findings of arthritis with decreased range of motion, tenderness and swelling. There is often evidence of joint effusion, but in some cases of chronic infection resulting from *C. immitis*, joint swelling may be because of synovial proliferation rather than the accumulation of fluid. The initial list of differential diagnoses may therefore be quite broad, and includes septic arthritis, rheumatoid arthritis, mycobacterial infection, brucellosis, and pigmented villonodular synovitis. While fungal arthritis may present in the setting of widespread fungal infection, in many instances there is little clinical evidence of extra-articular infection. Large weight-bearing joints, particularly the knee, are the usual targets.

Radiographic examination generally reveals evidence of joint effusion. Other findings which may be seen with varied frequency, depending upon the aetiology, host factors, and the chronicity of the infection, include erosion of juxta-articular cortex, osteoporosis, and associated para-articular osteomyelitis. These radiographic findings are also common to those found in tuberculosis, rheumatoid arthritis, sarcoidosis, metastatic neoplasm, eosinophilic granuloma, and pigmented villonodular synovitis (MacKenzie *et al.* 1988).

Clinically important information about joint integrity and the presence of otherwise unapparent para-articular osteomyelitis may be provided by magnetic resonance imaging which has greater sensitivity and resolution than other conventional techniques (MacKenzie *et al.* 1988; Brown *et al.* 1990). However, the role of this procedure in the clinical evaluation and management of fungal arthritis has not

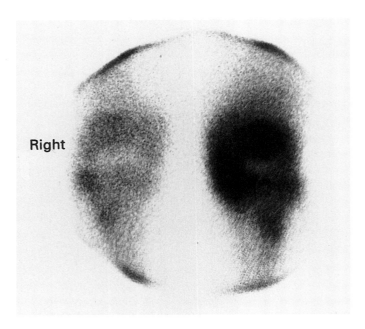

Right

Fig. 1 Bone scintigraphy, using technetium-99m, demonstrating intense uptake of the radionuclide in the left knee of a patient with synovitis caused by *Sporothrix schenckii* (by courtesy of Jesse Hofflin MD).

been critically evaluated. Nuclear medicine techniques, such as scanning after injection of technetium pyrophosphate, may serve to confirm clinical evidence of joint inflammation (Fig. 1).

Synovial fluid examination reveals an elevated white blood cell count. Although candidal and blastomycotic joint infections typically present with frankly purulent synovial fluid with a predominance of polymorphonuclear leucocytes, the other fungi often cause lesser degrees of inflammation with lower cell counts and variable predominance of either polymorphonuclear leucocytes or lymphocytes. The protein concentration is usually in excess of 3.0 g/dl while the glucose concentration is low to normal. Routine direct examination (e.g. Gram stain) usually does not reveal the organism, but cytological preparations are useful in the diagnosis of blastomycosis, cryptococcus, and, to a lesser degree, coccidioidomycosis. Culture of synovial fluid or synovial tissue usually yields the organism.

Synovial tissue histopathology is variable but often non-specific, such as in infection resulting from *S. schenckii* in which the organisms are few and difficult to visualize. Often a granulomatous reaction is observed and the differential diagnosis which must be considered includes fungal infection, brucellosis, mycobacterial infection, syphilis, protothecosis, rheumatoid arthritis, pigmented villonodular synovitis, sarcoidosis, Crohn's disease, foreign body reaction, gout, pseudogout, and oxalosis (Schwarz 1984).

The use of additional diagnostic procedures, such as blood cultures, bone marrow examination and culture, antibody tests, or tests for the detection of fungal antigen in serum or other body fluids, depend upon the clinical setting and the suspected aetiology. Tests of delayed dermal hypersensitivity to fungal antigens are generally not useful for diagnostic purposes.

Some infections may cause tenosynovitis in the absence of osteomyelitis or arthritis. Tenosynovitis may occur as the result of haematogenous dissemination or of direct inoculation, and is most often associated with *S. schenkii* infection, as well as, to lesser degrees, with infections caused by *C. immitis* and *C. neoformans*.

During the primary pulmonary infection with *C. immitis*, an acute self-limited arthritis or periarthritis, commonly referred to as 'desert rheumatism', may be seen in association with erythema nodosum, erythema multiforme, and occasionally hilar adenopathy. Thus the clinical picture may resemble sarcoidosis. An immunological process, probably immune complex deposition, is thought to be aetiologic. Acute aseptic inflammatory arthritis may also be seen in histoplasmosis, as well as in acute blastomycosis.

Management

Amphotericin B remains the therapeutic agent of choice for most serious fungal infections with the exception of those resulting from *Pseudoallescheria boydii* infection in which azole therapy (usually miconazole) is preferred. Several newer oral antifungal agents which may provide similar efficacy with less toxicity are undergoing active investigation.

Amphotericin B, administered intravenously, penetrates into synovial fluid to some extent (Farrell *et al.* 1978). While several authors have advocated directly injecting or irrigating the joint space with amphotericin B, the necessity for this mode of therapy is unproven, and there is concern that a chemical synovitis and articular damage may result. The toxicities of amphotericin are well known and include fever, chills, nausea, vomiting, hypotension, renal dysfunction, hypokalaemia and hypomagnesaemia. The renal toxicity may be dose limiting. Preliminary studies of lipid-associated amphotericin B indicate that higher doses of this drug may be administered with less toxicity than with standard preparations. Whether this is beneficial, however, remains unproven since such preparations also have reduced antifungal activity.

Fluorocytosine (5-FC) enters susceptible fungal cells through a specific permease system and is then converted to 5-fluorouracil. It has a narrow spectrum of activity which includes most *Candida* spp. as well as *C. neoformans*. In most instances, fluorocytosine is not administered as a single agent because of the possibility of the development of drug resistance during therapy. The drug penetrates well into all body fluids, including synovial fluid, and is renally excreted. The major toxicity, bone marrow suppression and resultant cytopenias, is directly related to serum concentrations in excess of 100 μg/ml. Serum concentrations of fluorocytosine should be closely monitored during administration, and dose adjustments must be made in the presence of changing renal function.

The azoles, such as miconazole, ketoconazole, fluconazole and itraconazole, inhibit the C-14 demethylation of lanosterol, thus impairing fungal cell membrane assembly. They have variable pharmacokinetic, toxicity, and antifungal profiles (Fromptling 1988). The intravenous form of miconazole has limited utility because of toxicity and unfavourable pharmacokinetics.

Ketoconazole was the first of the azoles available for oral administration. It has efficacy in a variety of fungal infections including those due to most *Candida* spp. (*Candida* (*Torulopsis*) *glabrata* is resistant), *H. capsulatum*, *B. dermatiditis*, *C. neoformans*, and *C. immitis*. Absorption is impaired in the absence of gastric acid. Ketoconazole penetrates into synovial fluid from the bloodstream. Elimination is non-renal with a terminal half-life of approximately 7.5 h. The most common adverse effect is gastrointestinal. Modest elevations in hepatic transaminases are not uncommon but significant hepatic toxicity rarely occurs. Depressed cortisol and testosterone levels may occur as a result of interference with sterol synthesis, but symptomatic hypocortisolism is very rare. Drug interactions occur with cyclosporin, phenytoin, warfarin, and rifampin (Hawkins Van Tyle 1984), as well as rifabutin; astemizole and terfenadine are contra-indicated in patients receiving ketoconazole.

Fluconazole is a water-soluble bis-triazole with a high degree of bioavailability and the ability to penetrate into body fluids, including synovial fluid, and achieves concentrations similar to those in serum (O'Meeghan *et al.* 1990). Protein binding is low (approximately 10 per cent) and the elimination half-life is approximately 22 h. Clearance is predominantly renal. Drug–drug interactions occur with phenytoin, rifampicin, and rifabutin, as well as with astemizole and terfenadine. Hepatic toxicity is rare; steroid hormone synthesis is not affected. The spectrum of activity is similar to that of ketoconazole (Galgiani 1990).

Another bis-triazole, itraconazole, has a broader spectrum of activity than either ketoconazole or fluconazole. It has now been approved by the United States Food and Drug Administration for use in both blastomycosis and histoplasmosis, and is also very active against *S. schenkii* and most *Aspergillus* species (Tucker *et al.* 1988). Itraconazole is lipophilic, highly protein bound, well absorbed, and has an elimination half-life of approximately 24 h. Elimination is non-renal. Body fluid penetration is less than that of fluconazole. Cortisol synthesis is not impaired by itraconazole. Pharmacokinetic interaction with cyclosporin occurs (Kramer *et al.* 1990); the same precautions regarding drug–drug interactions should be observed with itraconazole as ketoconazole. Gastrointestinal side-effects are common (Tucker *et al.* 1990). Itraconazole, which requires stomach acid for absorption, is not recommended for patients who are receiving antacids, H$_2$ blockers, or those who have achlorhydria, unless adequate serum levels can be demonstrated.

Individual mycoses
Candida *spp.*

Candida albicans is a normal commensal of man and endogenous colonization is the source of most infections by *Candida* spp. Deep tissue infection generally occurs after amplification of colonization during an intervening immunodeficient state or during administration of broad-spectrum antibacterial therapy coupled with breaches in integumentary and mucosal barriers (Crislip and Edwards 1989). Candida infection of joints is typically the consequence of haematogenous dissemination (often from indwelling intravenous catheters in predisposed immunodeficient hosts or in intravenous drug users) (Marina *et al.* 1991). Joints previously afflicted by rheumatoid arthritis appear to be at increased risk of infection with candidal organisms (Campen *et al.* 1990). Less commonly, joint infection occurs secondary to direct inoculation of the organism into the joint during aspiration or injection of corticosteroids (Ginzler *et al.* 1979; Campen *et al.* 1990), trauma, or surgical intervention (including simple arthrotomy) (Arnold *et al.* 1981) (Table 1). Immunocompromise resulting from HIV infection does not appear to predispose to disseminated candidiasis or to candidal arthritis, except in those who use parenteral drugs (Edlestein and McCabe 1991; Munoz-Fernandez *et al.* 1991; Silveira *et al.* 1991). *Candida* spp. which have been implicated in septic arthritis include *C. albicans, Candida tropicalis, Candida parapsilosis, Candida guilliermondi, Candida krusei, Candida zeylanoides,* and *Torulopsis (Candida) glabrata.*

In contrast to many of the other fungal joint infections discussed here, the onset of disease caused by *Candida* spp. is acute in approximately two-thirds of cases (Bayer and Guze 1978). The remaining

Table 2 Clinical and laboratory data helpful in the diagnosis of fungal joint infection

Organism	Serology	Synovial fluid white blood cell count	Synovial glucose	Synovial fluid examination	Cultures
Candida spp.	Not useful	Frankly purulent, <100 000/mm³	Variable, low to normal	20% positive	Blood and/or synovial fluid, >95% positive
Coccidioides immitis	Complement fixation, immunodiffusion diagnostic	<50 000/mm³, mononuclear cells	Low	Rarely positive	Synovial fluid, >95% positive
Blastomyces dermatitidis	Low sensitivity, low specificity	Frankly purulent, <100 000/mm³ polymorphonuclear	Variable, low to normal	By cytological preparation, 88% positive	Synovial fluid, 50% positive
Sporothrix schenkii	Not available	2000–60 000/mm³ lymphocytes and polymorphonuclear	Variable, low to normal	Rarely positive	Synovial tissue more often positive than synovial fluid
Histoplasma capsulatum	Complement fixation, immunodiffusion diagnostic			Not helpful	Blood and/or synovial fluid, 20–25% positive
Cryptococcus neoformans	Cryptococcal antigen diagnostic	200-5000/mm³, no particular cellular predominance	Variable, usually normal	India ink very helpful	Blood and/or synovial fluid, >80% positive
Paracoccidioides brasiliensis	Serum antibody			Not helpful	Usually positive, slow growth (longer than 4 weeks)

patients present with subacute disease. Instances of remarkably indo-lent presentations include those in which the arthritis was present for 9 months prior to diagnosis in a patient with acute myelocytic leukaemia (Gerster *et al.* 1980), and for 12 months in a patient receiving chronic haemodialysis (De Clerk *et al.* 1988). The large joints are most commonly affected.

Synovial fluid examination demonstrates a markedly elevated white blood-cell count (15 000 to 100 000 cells/mm^3) with a predominance of polymorphonuclear leucocytes (Table 2) (Bayer and Guze 1978; Fainstein *et al.* 1982). The protein concentration is elevated while that of glucose is either low or normal. Histological examination of synovium reveals mononuclear cell infiltration but usually an absence of granulomata (Bayer and Guze 1978). The organism is visualized in only 20 per cent of cases on direct examination of syno-vial fluid by Gram stain or other methods. Synovial fluid or tissue consistently yield the organism in culture. Recovery of the organism from blood cultures may provide an important clue to the aetiology of the joint process.

The cornerstone of management consists of systemic antifungal chemotherapy. Intravenously administered amphotericin B, with or without fluorocytosine, remains the standard treatment. However, based on limited data, the azoles (ketoconazole, fluconazole and itraconazole) appear to be as effective as amphotericin in the treat-ment of candidal infection caused by susceptible isolates, at least in non-neutropenic hosts. Several cases of candidal skeletal infection have been successfully managed with either ketoconazole (Gathe *et al.* 1987) or fluconazole alone (Sugar *et al.* 1990; Lafont *et al.* 1994). The potential role of lipopeptides, cilofungin, and lipid-associated amphotericin B is also unknown. Intra-articular ampho-tericin B has been utilized but the necessity or desirability of this method of treatment is questionable. Repeated joint aspiration is usually indicated. Surgical debridement may also be indicated (in addition to antifungal chemotherapy), particularly in cases of hip joint infection.

Candida spp. are causative in almost one-fifth of cases of nosoco-mial septic arthritis in neonates (Dan 1983; Ho *et al.* 1989), occurring exclusively in high-risk infants. Candida arthritis in neonates and in young infants is frequently associated with antibiotic therapy and parenteral administration of nutritional fluids (Yousefzadeh and Jackson 1980). Additional risk factors include prematurity, abdominal surgery, malnutrition, and immunosuppressive disease or therapy (Pope 1982).

In most neonatal cases, candida arthritis presents as just one facet of a systemic disease process and the organism may be recovered from a variety of extra-articular sites including blood, urine and spinal fluid. In the largest reported series (Dan 1983), joint aspirates yielded *C. albicans* in all but one instance. *C. tropicalis* was recovered from the remaining case. One or both knees were involved in 71 per cent of cases; polyarticular infection was seen in one-third of patients. The synovial fluid white blood-cell count was as high as 100 000/mm^3 with a predominance of polymorphonuclear leucocytes. The synovial membrane was hyperemic and purulent with erosion of cartilage. Radiographic evidence of adjacent osteomyelitis was seen in two-thirds of patients and in almost 90 per cent of joints, suggesting that in most cases, infection of the metaphysis was the original site of haematogenous dissemination with subsequent rupture into the articular cavity (Svirsky-Fein *et al.* 1979). Other radiographic findings included periarticular soft tissue swelling and joint effusion and, in the case of hip joint infection, subluxation of the femoral head. The

mortality rate was 14 per cent. Major orthopaedic sequelas were seen in only one-tenth of survivors.

Fungal infection of prosthetic joints is exceedingly rare. In a series of reported cases, ten infections were identified in eight patients; all were caused by *Candida* spp. (Lambertus *et al.* 1988). One case was due each to *C. albicans* and *T. glabrata*, while three each were due to *C. tropicalis* and *C. parapsilosis*. Infection was probably the result of implantation of skin contaminants at the time of the original surgery. The infections were clinically low-grade, indolent, and presented 5 to 36 months after reconstructive arthroplasty. Pain and decreased range of motion were universally present and peri-articular swelling was common. Other signs of inflammation were absent. A sinus tract was seen in one patient. Radiographic examination revealed evidence of loosening and adjacent areas of osteolysis indica-tive of osteomyelitis. Technetium pyrophosphate and gallium nitrate scans are not useful in the setting of a loosened prosthesis (Fitzgerald and Kelly 1979). Synovial fluid white blood-cell counts were less inflammatory than that typically seen in native joint infections (4000 to 15 000/mm^3); polymorphonuclear leucocytes were pre-dominant.

Amphotericin B, with or without fluorocytosine, in combination with removal of the prosthesis and other foreign material, and debridement of affected tissue is the initial treatment of choice. Although no data are yet available, ketoconazole, fluconazole, and itraconazole may have a role in long-term 'maintenance' therapy of such cases. Reimplantation has been successfully reported in one patient 10 months after resection arthroplasty (Younkin *et al.* 1984).

Blastomycosis

Blastomycosis is an uncommonly encountered mycotic infection primarily endemic to parts of the midwestern, south-eastern, and Appalachian areas of the United States, but which is also seen in Africa and the Middle East (see Table 1). *B. dermatiditis* is a thermal dimorph whose mycelial phase is thought to reside in soil. Conversion to the yeast phase occurs after inhalation of spores. Primary pulmonary infection may be subclinical, acute, or subacute, but is usually self-limited; occasional cases may be chronic. Haematogenous dissemination is relatively frequent during the initial phase of the disease, leading to infection at almost any body site. While skin and bones are the most frequent sites of dissemina-tion (25 to 60 per cent) in disseminated blastomycosis, only between 2.5 and 8 per cent of patients develop joint infection (Blastomycosis Cooperative Study of the Veterans Administration 1964; Witorsch and Utz 1968; George *et al.* 1985; McDonald *et al.* 1990). Those patients with particularly severe pulmonary disease, miliary involve-ment, or those who are immunocompromised are at the greatest risk for dissemination (Sarosi and Davies 1981; Recht *et al.* 1982). The risk of endogenous reactivation, which usually occurs during the first 2 to 3 years following the primary pulmonary infection, is small. Very rarely, joint infection is the result of direct inoculation secondary to trauma (Gnann *et al.* 1983).

While many patients with progressive or disseminated disease due to *B. dermatitidis* suffer from potentially predisposing conditions, such as diabetes, alcoholism, renal failure, and malignancy (Klein *et al.* 1986), this organism is not generally considered an opportunistic pathogen. Recht and colleagues described 78 patients with blastomy-cosis, 6 (13 per cent) of whom were immunocompromised, none, however, due to T-lymphocyte dysfunction (Recht *et al.* 1982). Those

6 patients had a similar clinical presentation and therapeutic response as the remaining patients who were not immunocompromised. Nevertheless, rapidly progressive and unusually severe disease has been reported in patients with profoundly impaired immunity, such as patients who have had transplants and those with AIDS (Davies and Sarosi 1991).

Myalgias and arthralgias are common during the acute pulmonary phase of the disease, but erythema nodosum is not (Sarosi *et al.* 1974). A reactive arthritis, similar to that seen with coccidioidomycosis, has been reported (Berger and Kraman 1981).

The arthritis is monoarticular in 95 per cent of cases with the knee most commonly involved, followed by the ankle, elbow and wrist (see Table 2). Joint pain is often acute in onset and patients usually appear toxic. In contrast to coccidioidal arthritis, active pulmonary disease is present in more than 90 per cent of patients with joint involvement, and more than 70 per cent have evidence of additional dissemination to cutaneous or subcutaneous sites (Fountain 1973; Bayer *et al.* 1979*b*). In contrast to those with candidal or sporotrichal arthritis, less than one-third of patients have radiographic evidence of juxta-articular osteomyelitis (Bayer *et al.* 1979*b*).

Synovial fluid findings are similar to those seen in candida arthritis. The fluid is usually cloudy or frankly purulent with white blood-cell counts which may exceed $100 000/\text{mm}^3$ and with a predominance of polymorphonuclear leucocytes. The concentration of protein in the synovial fluid exceeds 3.0 g/dl while the glucose is low to normal (Fountain 1973; Bayer *et al.* 1979*b*; Robert and Kauffman 1988). Cytological examination of synovial fluid may be more sensitive in detecting the organism than is culture. Bayer and colleagues described a series of nine patients who underwent joint fluid examination, eight (88 per cent) of whom had characteristic organisms detected by direct microscopy and seven (78 per cent) of whom had positive cultures of synovial fluid (Bayer *et al.* 1979*b*). In a study of five patients, cultures were positive in three (60 per cent) and KOH preparation were positive in two (40 per cent), but cytological examination of synovial fluid in four of the cases demonstrated the characteristic organisms in all (100 per cent) (George *et al.* 1985). The organism may also be recovered in culture or visualized on histopathology from synovial biopsy specimens. Histopathological examination of infected synovium reveals prominent polymorphonuclear leucocytes, often with microabscesses and occasional granulomata.

While most patients with acute self-limited pulmonary blastomycosis have demonstrable delayed dermal hypersensitivity to blastomycin, this reactivity wanes over time and is not of diagnostic value. Available serological tests have been disappointing with both false-negative and -positive results commonly seen.

Amphotericin B remains the drug of choice for many patients, particularly those who are critically ill, have evidence of progressive disease, or those who are immunosuppressed (Bradsher 1988). The total dose required is usually 1.0 to 2.0 g. In patients with joint infection and otherwise stable disease, itraconazole is very effective (approximate 90 per cent response rate) (Dismukes *et al.* 1992). The usual starting dose is 200 mg once daily, increasing to 400 mg daily as necessary. A loading dose of 200 mg three times daily can be given for the first 3 days. Therapy should be continued for approximately 6 months.

Ketoconazole also has some efficacy in patients without meningeal disease who are not severely immunocompromised (National Institute of Allergy and Infectious Disease Mycoses Study Group

1985; McManus and Jones 1986; Bradsher 1988). Ketoconazole should be initiated at a dose of 400 mg per day and continued for at least 6 months. The dose can be increased to 600 to 800 mg per day in those who are failing to respond to therapy or who develop a new focus of infection.

Fluconazole does not appear to be nearly as effective as itraconazole in the treatment of blastomycosis. There are, however, reported cases of its use in patients with pulmonary and meningeal disease (Pearson *et al.* 1992; Taillan *et al.* 1992).

Sporotrichosis

S. schenckii, a tissue dimorph, is commonly found on decaying vegetation and in soil in many areas of both hemispheres. Infections are both sporadic and epidemic. In contrast to the other soil fungi discussed here, cutaneous disease occurs secondary to inoculation of the organism as a result of trauma to the skin. The lymphocutaneous form, with the development of an ulcer at the site of cutaneous inoculation and proximal nodules in the area of lymphatic drainage, is the most common manifestation of infection (Belknap 1989). Persons at particular risk for this infection include rose cultivators and those who handle soil and spagnum moss (Kedes *et al.* 1964). Primary pulmonary infection may occur presumably as the result of inhalation of spores.

While arthralgias occur in approximately 2 per cent of those with acute cutaneous or lymphocutaneous disease, infection of the joint space with *S. schenkii* is rare, having occurred in only one of 3300 patients (0.03 per cent) in a large outbreak of sporotrichosis (Lurie 1963). Arthritis may occur in the presence of widespread dissemination to other sites, but is much more common as an isolated finding (Bayer *et al.* 1979*a*; Yao *et al.* 1986). Bayer and colleagues described 44 cases of sporotrichal joint infection, 20 per cent of which were associated with systemic and pulmonary disease (Bayer *et al.* 1979*a*). Most cases of sporotrichal arthritis are therefore believed to be caused by haematogenous dissemination of the organism, although some cases may be the result of articular extension of infection from an adjacent site of osteomyelitis or skin infection or, occasionally, from direct inoculation of the organism into the joint. More than 85 per cent of patients with systemic infection have predisposing underlying disease, including myeloproliferative disorders, malignancy, chronic corticosteroid use and alcoholism (Kedes *et al.* 1964; Bayer *et al.* 1979*a*).

Sporotrichal arthritis is an indolent and slowly progressive infectious process which predominantly affects the knee and other large weight-bearing joints, although the small joints of the hand and wrist are also commonly affected (Molstad and Strom 1978; Bayer *et al.* 1979*a*). Calhoun and colleagues described 11 cases of systemic sporotrichosis; 8 involved the skeletal system with a total of 12 joints being affected, including the wrist (63 per cent), knee (38 per cent), ankle (25 per cent), and elbow and phalanx (13 per cent each) (Calhoun *et al.* 1991). Monoarticular and polyarticular involvement occur with equal frequency. Most cases present as a slowly progressive synovitis or tenosynovitis with pain, warmth, swelling and restricted range of motion (Bayer *et al.* 1979*a*; Chang *et al.* 1984).

Radiographic abnormalities are seen in more than 90 per cent of cases, possibly reflecting the chronicity of infection prior to diagnosis. Osteoporosis of contiguous bone is the most common radiographic finding, followed by soft tissue swelling with effusion,

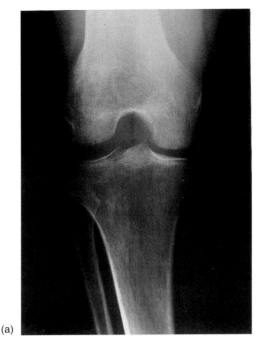

(a)

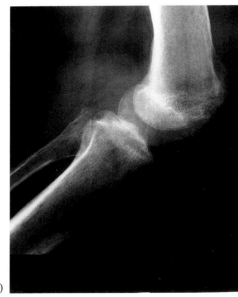

(b)

Fig. 2 (a) and (b). Radiographs of the left knee demonstrating only patchy osteopenia of the distal femur and proximal tibia from a patient with joint infection caused by *S. schenckii*. Bone scintigraphy of the same patient is shown in Fig. 1 (by courtesy of Jesse Hofflin MD).

'punched out' osteolytic lesions, articular cartilage erosion and joint space narrowing (Bayer *et al.* 1979*a*) (see Fig. 2).

Synovial fluid white blood-cell count is reported to range from 2800 to 60 000/mm³. Both lymphocytes and polymorphonuclear leucocytes may be seen (see Table 2). The protein concentration is high while that of glucose is low to normal (Lesperance *et al.* 1988). The diagnosis may be delayed because of the isolated nature of the infection, the rarity of visualizing the organism on smears of synovial fluid, the often non-specific nature of synovial histopathology (which may resemble that of rheumatoid or tuberculous arthritis) (Stratton *et*

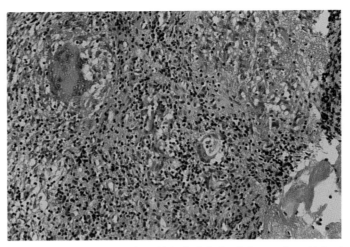

Fig. 3 Granulomatous reaction with typical giant cells in synovium obtained from the same patient described in Fig. 2. Organisms were not visualized with this stain or with Gomori–methanamine silver or periodic acid–Schiff stains, and the diagnosis was made by recovery of the organism in culture from the synovial tissue. Haematoxylin and eosin, original magnification × 200 (by courtesy of Jesse Hofflin MD).

al. 1981), and the paucity of organisms in tissue (Khan *et al.* 1983; Schwartz 1989) (Fig. 3). Asteroid bodies, often said to be pathognomonic of sporotrichosis, may, in fact, be seen in other infections. Isolation of the organism in culture is the cornerstone of diagnosis. Synovial tissue is more likely to yield the organism (usually within five days) than is synovial fluid. Skin tests are only useful for epidemiological surveys. A variety of serological tests have been utilized with varying results (Winn 1988).

While amphotericin B had been recommended for the treatment of skeletal sporotrichosis, newer data indicate that itraconazole is very effective in this infection. In a recent National Institute of Allergies and Infectious Diseases non-comparative clinical treatment trial of 30 patients with both lymphocutaneous and systemic sporotrichosis, one-half of whom had osseous or articular infection, itraconazole (100 to 600 mg daily for 3 to 18 months) was effective in 83 per cent (Sharkey-Mathis *et al.* 1993). However, 6 to 18 months after treatment was discontinued, 7 patients relapsed. Two of these patients have subsequently responded to a second course of therapy. Resolution of infection and normalization of joint mobility and function has been reported in 3 other patients who received itraconazole 200 mg daily (Winn *et al.* 1993).

Despite reasonably effective penetration by the drug into synovial fluid, ketoconazole has effected responses in only approximately two-thirds of patients with systemic sporotrichosis, including patients with joint infection (Dismukes *et al.* 1983; Graybill *et al.* 1983; Horsburgh *et al.* 1983; Pluss and Opal 1986; Calhoun *et al.* 1991). Fluconazole has been similarly disappointing in lymphocutaneous infection (Restrepo *et al.* 1986). Potassium iodide, which is effective in the lymphocutaneous form of the disease, has no role in the treatment of deep tissue infection, such as arthritis. Sporadic cases of skeletal disease have, however, reportedly responded to treatment with potassium iodide (Govender *et al.* 1989).

Intra-articular administration of amphotericin B has also been utilized, but this is unlikely to be necessary (Downs *et al.* 1989). Surgical debridement may also be necessary on occasion, but should be reserved for persistent culture positivity and in cases of tenosynovitis (Winn 1988).

Coccidioidomycosis

C. immitis is endemic to the soils of certain areas of the Lower Sonoran life zone of the Western hemisphere, with most cases resulting from exposure to airborne arthroconidia in Arizona and the the southern central valley of California (see Table 1). Upon reaching the alveoli of the infected host, the organism, a tissue dimorph, converts to the spherule–endospore phase. Approximately one-half of infected patients become symptomatic and, in the vast majority of these, the infection is self-limited with influenza-like symptoms. Transient arthralgias or aseptic inflammatory arthritis, which probably represents an immunologically mediated inflammatory process similar to erythema nodosum (which is also often seen), occur in 3 to 5 per cent of patients with primary pulmonary coccidioidomycosis (Fiese 1958). Treatment consists of giving nonsteroidal anti-inflammatory agents.

Clinically important extrapulmonary dissemination occurs in fewer than 0.5 per cent of cases, although certain groups are at greater risk for dissemination. While many patients with disseminated disease have no impairment in immune function, approximately one-half are immunocompromised by corticosteroids, diabetes, renal failure, or other immunosuppresive therapy. HIV-infection increases both the risk of more frequent and more severe coccidioidomycosis (Galgiani and Ampel 1990).

Joint space infection occurs in up to 25 to 30 per cent of patients with disseminated disease, with occasional extension into adjacent bony areas (Fiese 1958; Deresinski 1980; Deresinski 1994). Monoarticular arthritis occurs in more that 90 per cent of cases, with large weight-bearing joints, particularly the knee and ankle, being most frequently affected (Deresinski 1980; Deresinski 1994). At the time of presentation with joint disease, occult sites of

dissemination are present in up to 25 per cent of cases (Winter *et al.* 1975). Extrapulmonary sites of infection, including meningeal, bone, and joint infection, should therefore be avidly sought for in any patient with disseminated coccidioidomycosis.

While some patients may initially present with an acutely inflamed joint, most infections are indolent with progressive effusion and synovial thickening. The diagnosis of joint infection is often delayed, and chronic infection frequently results in significant articular and bony destruction with resultant loss of joint function (Fig. 4). Occasionally, chronic arthrocutaneous fistulas develop with drainage of synovial fluid (Fig. 5). Baker's cysts may occur as a consequence of knee involvement. Effusion and erosion of articular cortex and adjacent osteoporosis are commonly seen on radiographic examination (Carter 1934; Bayer and Guze 1979). Technetium pyrophosphate radioisotope scans usually localize to the affected joints.

Synovial fluid is inflammatory with total white blood-cell counts as high as $50\,000/mm^3$ (Table 2). Mononuclear cells usually, but not always, predominate. Protein is greater than 3.0 g/dl, glucose is low and mucin clot is poor (Aidem 1968; Deresinski and Stevens 1974). Culture of synovial fluid yields the organism in approximately 50 per cent of cases, usually within 3 to 6 days. Greater yield is seen with culture and histological examination of synovial tissue (Greenman *et al.* 1975). The affected proliferative synovium, which often invades cartilage and articular surfaces, exhibits granulomatous villonodular inflammatory changes with the characteristic endosporulating spherules visible on microscopic examination (Haug and Merrifield 1959). Most importantly, if coccidioidomycosis infection is suspected, the microbiology laboratory must be notified because of the significant biohazard represented by this organism in culture.

Serum complement-fixing antibody to coccidioidin is almost universally present, with the height of the titre reflecting the extent of dissemination, as in other manifestations of disseminated infection with this organism (Deresinski 1980). Delayed dermal hypersensitivity to coccidioidin may be absent.

Patient prognosis depends upon the extent of dissemination to other sites, particularly the central nervous system. Treatment consists of systemic administration of antifungal agents, and

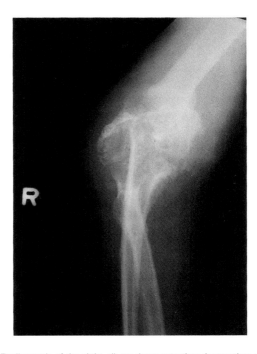

Fig. 4 Radiograph of the right elbow demonstrating destruction of the articular cortex and osteomyelitis of contiguous bone of an elderly women with chronic coccidioidal arthritis of many years duration despite multiple courses of antifungal therapy.

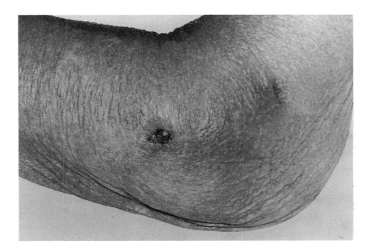

Fig. 5 Chronic coccidioidal arthritis of the same patient as in Fig. 4 demonstrating the right elbow joint fixed in flexion. The sinus tracts intermittently drain material from which *Coccidioides immitis* is recoverable in culture (by courtesy of John S. Hostetler MD).

amphotericin B remains the treatment of choice in many cases. Patients with disseminated disease often receive a total of 1.0 to 2.5 g of amphotericin B. Continued therapy is indicated until remission has been achieved, as defined by objective clinical measures, and improvement in serological and radiographic data. Amphotericin B has also been administered intra-articularly, but the therapeutic necessity or advisability of this is uncertain. Arthrodesis is generally effective, but not desirable.

The need for synovectomy and debridement of infected bone and tissue remain controversial. Despite appropriate medical and surgical intervention, the joint infection often remains progressive and disabling (Lantz et al. 1988). In one study, 7 of 14 patients who received amphotericin alone failed therapy, whereas none of the 14 patients who were treated with a combination of medical and surgical approaches relapsed (Bried and Galgiani 1986). In another similar study, 7 of 9 patients who received amphotericin B and who underwent surgical debridement remained disease-free at least 4 years later (Bisla and Taber 1976). The two remaining patients developed recurrent disease, despite having received more than 3.0 g of amphotericin B each. Patients with complement fixation titres greater than or equal to 1:128 were most likely to fail in response to medical therapy alone (Bried and Galgiani 1986).

Ketoconazole (400 to 800 mg per day) has some efficacy, but the relapse rate is high (approximately 30 per cent) (Galgiani et al. 1988). Although both fluconazole and itraconazole have been used in cases of pulmonary disease and meningitis, relapses are frequent. The optimal dose and duration of therapy remain under study. An unusual case of prosthetic hip joint infection caused by C. immitis responded to long-term therapy with fluconazole (Nomura and Ruskin 1994).

Histoplasmosis

H. capsulatum is endemic to many areas within the temperate zones of the world, but is most heavily concentrated in the Ohio, Mississippi and Missouri River valleys of the United States (Table 1). The organism is a thermal dimorph with the mycelial phase existing in soil, generally in association with bird and bat guano. Large outbreaks occur in urban endemic areas. Speleologists throughout the world may be at risk.

Upon inhalation by the human or animal host, microconidia reach the alveoli where they convert to the yeast phase. While greater than 95 per cent of infections are subclinical, an influenza-like respiratory illness may result from infection. Haematogenous dissemination is rare and occurs most commonly in patients with impaired cellular immunity. Disseminated histoplasmosis is reported in approximately one-third of AIDS patients in Kansas City, Missouri (McKinsey et al. 1989). Persons with HIV infection who travel to or have previously lived in an endemic area are at risk for reactivation disease (Minamoto and Armstrong 1988; Salzman et al. 1988).

Immunologically mediated arthralgias and aseptic inflammatory arthritis, similar to that reported for coccidioidomycosis, are common in primary histoplasmosis (Class and Casio 1972; Rosenthal et al. 1983). Based on previously published reports, one review found that arthralgias occurred in 3 to 21 per cent, and erythema nodosum and erythema multiforme occurred in 1 to 42 per cent of patients with documented histoplasmosis (Schwarz 1984). During a single outbreak of acute histoplasmosis in 381 symptomatic patients, 16 (4.1 per cent) developed arthralgias and 6 (1.6 per cent)

developed aseptic arthritis (Rosenthal et al. 1983). The knees, ankles, wrists, and small joints of the hands were the most common sites of involvement; approximately 50 per cent of the cases were polyarticular. The joint involvement may be additive or migratory, and is often symmetric. Synovial fluid is inflammatory. This clinical problem is self-limited and is treated with non-steroidal anti-inflammatory agents (Sellers et al. 1965).

In contrast to candida and coccidioidomycosis, infection of the synovium or joint space by H. capsulatum is exceedingly rare. It is usually monoarticular and has been reported in both apparently immunologically normal (Key and Large 1942; Omer et al. 1963; Van Der Schee et al. 1990) and compromised hosts (Jones 1985). Juxta-articular osteomyelitis may be present. The diagnosis of histoplasmosis can be made by culture of both blood and infected sites, including synovial fluid, and histological demonstration of the infecting organism. The organism is readily cultivated on a variety of media. The lysis–centrifugation technique hastens recovery from the blood of patients with active dissemination (Paya et al. 1987).

Detection of antigen in serum or urine has been utilized in the diagnosis of disseminated histoplasmosis (Wheat et al. 1986). Although both false-positive and -negative results occur, antibody tests are diagnostically useful. Detection of serum complement-fixing antibody to the yeast phase of the organism of 1:32 or greater should be regarded as presumptive evidence of histoplasmosis. Titres of 1:8 or greater to mycelial-phase antigens or the presence of 'M' or 'H' bands by immunodiffusion are also highly suggestive of histoplasmosis (Kaufmann 1971; Wheat et al. 1982). Histoplasmin skin testing is useful only for epidemiological purposes.

Amphotericin B remains the treatment of choice for severe, life-threatening forms of histoplasmosis. Inadequate information is available concerning the usefulness of the azoles in joint infection caused by H. capsulatum. However, both itraconazole (Sharkey-Mathis et al. 1993) and ketoconazole (National Institute of Allergy and Infectious Disease Mycoses Study Group 1985; Dismukes et al. 1992) have been effective in non-immunocompromised patients with other forms of this disease. In a recent non-comparative treatment trial, itraconazole (200 to 400 mg per day) was effective in 81 per cent of patients with histoplasmosis (Sharkey-Mathis et al. 1993). Patients with chronic pulmonary disease or less than 2 months of therapy were more likely to fail. In patients with AIDS, amphotericin B is often used to suppress the acute infection, but the majority of cases will recur without chronic suppressive therapy. For HIV-infected patients with milder disease, itraconazole alone is effective in approximately 80 per cent (Wheat et al. 1990)).

Cryptococcosis

C. neoformans is worldwide in distribution. Skin test surveys suggest that subclinical infection is quite common in normal hosts. Clinical disease occurs predominantly, but not exclusively, in individuals with defects in cellular immunity (Table 1). The incidence of cryptococcal disease has greatly increased because of the frequency with which patients with HIV are infected with this encapsulated yeast.

The primary pulmonary infection may be subclinical or acute, and haematogenous dissemination may result in diffuse organ involvement. Almost any organ can be involved, but the organism has a particular predilection for the brain and meninges (Perfect et al. 1983). Although osteomyelitis occurs in up to 10 per cent of patients with systemic disease, cryptococcal arthritis, frequently associated with areas of contiguous osteomyelitis, is rare with fewer than 25 cases reported in the literature (Bayer *et al*. 1980; Ricciardi *et al*. 1986; Stead *et al*. 1988). Most patients have severe deficits in cellular immunity, such as those with AIDS, sarcoidosis, diabetes, and renal allograft recipients (Bosch *et al*. 1994). Both gout and calcium pyrophosphate disease appear to increase the risk of cryptococcal infection in affected joints (Sinnott and Holt 1982; Ricciardi *et al*. 1986).

Although soft-tissue swelling, inflammation and frank cellulitis have been reported in cases of cryptococcal joint infection (Bunning and Barth 1984), most cases are indolent in presentation. The knee is involved in approximately 60 per cent of reported cases, followed by an equal number of cases in the sternoclavicular and acromial-clavicular joints, elbow, wrist and ankle (Table 2). Approximately one-third of the cases are polyarticular. Radiographs demonstrate an erosive arthritis and juxta-articular osteomyelitis, and computed tomographic scans often show evidence of parasynovial inflammation. Examination of the synovial fluid reveals a white blood-cell count of 200 to 20 000/mm^3, with a predominance of mononuclear cells. However, the peripheral white blood-cell count and erythrocyte sedimentation rate is often normal (Adams and McDonald 1984; Bunning and Barth 1984; Brand *et al*. 1985).

Amphotericin B should be administered as initial therapy in most cases of disseminated disease. Many experts advocate the concomitant administration of fluorocytosine for approximately 4 weeks. In order to avoid undue toxicity, serum concentrations of fluorocytosine can be monitored weekly and maintained within a range of approximately 50 to 80 μg/ml. Once the systemic disease is under control and the joint disease is improving, consideration can be given to completing treatment with fluconazole (400 mg per day). Itraconazole may also be effective, but the data is limited. Patients with AIDS should remain on life-long suppressive maintenance therapy.

Paracoccidioidomycosis

Paracoccidioidomycosis is endemic only to areas of Central and South America where it is the most commonly encountered respiratory mycosis. *P. brasiliensis* is thermally dimorphic. As is true for the other dimorphic fungi, conidia released by the mycelial phase of the fungus are inhaled and convert to the yeast phase in the alveoli. Acute, self-limited pulmonary infection may occur, although most patients present with chronic pulmonary disease and evidence of chronic haematogenous dissemination, including painful granulomata of the skin, lymphadenopathy, and ulceration of mucous membranes (Sugar 1988). Skeletal disease occurs, but is rare (Table 1); no cases were identified in two reviews describing a total of 66 cases (Londero and Rambos 1972; Murray *et al*. 1974). A case of joint infection, with soft tissue swelling and cartilagenous destruction, has been described (Castaneda *et al*. 1985). Typical budding yeast forms were seen on examination of the synovial fluid and cultures were positive. The diagnosis is usually made on the basis of visualization of the organisms in synovial fluid or tissues, or by culture. Serological tests have been utilized with varying success. Skin tests are useful only for epidemiological surveys.

Although the disease is rarely encountered outside of endemic areas, the diagnosis should be suspected in any individual at epidemiological risk. Paracoccidioidomycosis primarily occurs in persons without evidence of immune dysfunction, but cases of severe disseminated disease have been recently described in immunosuppressed patients (Londero and Rambos 1972; Murray *et al*. 1974; Restrepo *et al*. 1976; Sugar *et al*. 1984; Sugar 1988).

Amphotericin B is effective in the treatment of disseminated paracoccidioidomycosis, although itraconazole and ketoconazole appear as effective in the treatment of milder cases (Stevens and Vo 1982; Sugar 1988; Kwon-Chung and Bennett 1992). Relapses after treatment are common, and chronic suppressive therapy with one of the azoles or a sulphonamide are therefore currently recommended.

Miscellaneous mycoses

A variety of additional fungi have been implicated in joint infections. Various species of *Aspergillus* have resulted in cases of joint infection, often associated with contiguous osteomyelitis (Tack *et al*. 1982; Denning and Stevens 1990; Cosgarea *et al*. 1993). While haematogenous dissemination of the organism was implicated in some cases, introduction of the organism into the joint space has occurred during surgical or arthroscopic procedures, or as a result of trauma.

Skeletal infections caused by *Alternaria* spp. and *Bipolaris hawaiiensis* (Sharkey *et al*. 1990), *Acremonium* spp. (Szombathy *et al*. 1988), *Cunninghamella bertholletiae* (Mostaza *et al*. 1989), *Exiophiala jeanselmei* (Roncoroni and Smayevsky 1988), *Exiophila spinifera* (Sharkey *et al*. 1990), *Fusarium solani* (Jakle *et al*. 1983), *Madurella mycetomi* (Yagi *et al*. 1983; McGinnis and Fader 1988), *Phialophora parasitica* (Kaell and Weitzman 1983), *Saccharomyces* spp. (Feld *et al*. 1982), *P. boydii* (Kemp *et al*. 1982; Ansara *et al*. 1987; Rippon 1988), and *Trichosporon beigelii* (Gardella *et al*. 1985) have also been reported.

References

Adams, R. and McDonald, M. (1984). Cryptococcal arthritis of the acromio-clavicular joint. *North Carolina Medical Journal*, **45**, 23–4.

Aidem, H.P. (1968). Intra-articular amphotericin B in the treatment of coccidioidal synovitis of the knee. Case report. *Journal of Bone and Joint Surgery*, **50A**, 1663–8.

Ansara, R.A., Hindson, D.A., Stevens, D.L., and Kloss, J.G. (1987). *Pseudoallescheria boydii* arthritis and osteomyelitis in a patient with Cushing's disease. *Southern Medical Journal*, **80**, 90–2.

Arnold, H.J., Dini, A., Jonas, G., and Zorn, E.L. (1981). *Candida albicans* arthritis in a healthy adult. *Southern Medical Journal*, **74**, 84–5.

Bayer, A.S. and Guze, L.B. (1978). Fungal arthritis. I. Candida arthritis: diagnostic and prognostic implication and therapeutic considerations. *Seminars in Arthritis and Rheumatism*, **8**, 142–50.

Bayer, A.S. and Guze, L.B. (1979). Fungal arthritis. II. Coccidioidal synovitis: clinical, diagnostic, therapeutic, and prognostic considerations. *Seminars in Arthritis and Rheumatism*, **8**, 200–11.

Bayer, A.S., Scott, V.J., and Guze, L.B. (1979*a*). Fungal arthritis. III. Sporothrichal arthritis. *Seminars in Arthritis and Rheumatism*, **9**, 66–74.

Bayer, A.S., Scott, V.J., and Guze, L.B. (1979*b*). Fungal arthritis. IV. Blastomycotic arthritis. *Seminars in Arthritis and Rheumatism*, **9**, 145–51.

Bayer, A.S., Choi, C., Tilman, D.B., and Guze, L.B. (1980). Fungal arthritis. V. Cryptococcal and histoplasmal arthritis. *Seminars in Arthritis and Rheumatism*, **9**, 218–27.

Belknap, B.S. (1989). Sporotrichosis. *Dermatology Clinic*, **7**, 193–202.

Berger, R. and Kraman, S. (1981). Acute miliary blastomycosis after 'short-course' corticosteroid treatment. *Archives of Internal Medicine*, **141**, 1223–5.

Bisla, R.S. and Taber, T.H. (1976). Coccidioidomycosis of bone and joints. *Journal of Clinical Orthopedics and Related Research*, **121**, 196–204.

Blastomycosis Cooperative Study of the Veterans Administration (1964). Blastomycosis. 1: A review of 198 collected cases in Veteran Administration Hospitals. *American Review of Respiratory Disease*, **89**, 658–72.

Bosch, X., Roman, R., Font, J., Alemany, S., and Coca, A. (1994). Bilateral cryptococcosis of the hip. *Journal of Bone and Joint Surgery*, **76A**, 1234–8.

Bradsher, R.W. (1988). Blastomycosis. *Infectious Disease Clinics of North America*, **1**, 877–98.

Brand, C., Warren, R., Luxton, M., and Barraclough, D. (1985). Cryptococcal sacroiliitis. *Annals of the Rheumatic Diseases*, **44**, 126–7.

Bried, J.M. and Galgiani, J.N. (1986). *Coccidioides immitis* infections of bones and joints. *Clinical Orthopedics*, **211**, 235–43.

Brown, D.G., Edwards, N.L., Greer, J.M., Longley, S., Gillespy, T.I., and Panush, R.S. (1990). Magnetic resonance imaging in patients with inflammatory arthritis of the knee. *Clinical Rheumatology*, **9**, 73–83.

Bunning, R.D. and Barth, W.F. (1984). Cryptococcal arthritis and cellulitis. *Annals of the Rheumatic Diseases*, **43**, 508–10.

Calhoun, D.L. *et al.* (1991). Treatment of systemic sporotrichosis with ketoconazole. *Reviews of Infectious Diseases*, **13**, 47–51.

Campen, D.H., Kaufman, R.L., and Beardmore, T.D. (1990). Candida septic arthritis in rheumatoid arthritis. *Journal of Rheumatology*, **17**, 86–8.

Carter, R.A. (1934). Infectious granulomas of bones and joints with special reference to coccidioidal granuloma. *Radiology*, **23**, 1–16.

Castaneda, O.J., Alarcon, G.S., Garcia, M.T., and Lumbreras, H. (1985). *Paracoccidioides brasiliensis* arthritis. Report of a case and review of the literature. *Journal of Rheumatology*, **12**, 356–8.

Chang, A.C., Destouet, J.M., and Murphy, W.A. (1984). Musculoskeletal sporotrichosis. *Skeletal Radiology*, **12**, 23–8.

Class, R.N. and Casio, F.S. (1972). Histoplasmosis presenting as acute polyarthritis. *New England Journal of Medicine*, **287**, 1133–4.

Cosgarea, A.J., Tejani, N., and Jones, J.A. (1993). Carpal aspergillus osteomyelitis: case report and review of the literature. *Journal of Hand Surgery*, **18A**, 722–6.

Crislip, M.A. and Edwards, J.E. (1989). Candidiasis. *Infectious Disease Clinics of North America*, **3**, 103–33.

Cuellar, M.L., Silveira, L.H., and Espinoza, L.R. (1992). Fungal arthritis. *Annals of the Rheumatic Diseases*, **51**, 690–7.

Cuellar, M.L., Silveira, L.H., Citera, G., Cabrera, G.E., and Valle, R. (1993). Other fungal arthritides. *Rheumatic Disease Clinics of North America*, **19**, 439–55.

Dan, M. (1983). Neonatal septic arthritis. *Israel Journal of Medical Science*, **19**, 967–71.

Davies, S.F. and Sarosi, G.A. (1991). Clinical manifestations and management of blastomycosis in the compromised patient. In *Fungal infection in the compromised patient*, (2nd edn) (ed. D.W. Warnock and M.D. Richardson), pp. 215–29. John Wiley, Chichester.

De Clerk, L., Dequaker, J., Westhovens, R., and Hauglustaine, D. (1988). *Candida parapsilosis* in a patient receiving chronic hemodialysis. *Journal of Rheumatology*, **15**, 372–4.

Denning, D.W. and Stevens, D.A. (1990). Antifungal and surgical treatment of invasive aspergillosis: Review of 2121 published cases. *Reviews of Infectious Diease*, **12**, 1147–201.

Deresinski, S.C. (1980). Coccidioidomycosis of the musculoskeletal system. In *Coccidioidomycosis* (ed. D.A. Stevens), pp. 195–212. Plenum Press, New York.

Deresinski, S.C. (1994). *Coccidioides immitis*. In *Infectious diseases* (ed. J.A. Bartlett, S.L. Gorback, and N.R. Blacklow), pp. 1912–23. W.B. Saunders, Philadelphia.

Deresinski, S.C. and Stevens, D.A. (1974). Coccidioidomycosis in compromised hosts. *Medicine*, **54**, 377–95.

Dismukes, W.E. *et al.* (1992). Itraconazole therapy for blastomycosis and histoplasmosis. National Institute for Allergy and Infectious Disease Mycoses Study Group. *American Journal of Medicine*, **93**, 489–97.

Dismukes, W.E. *et al.* (1983). Treatment of systemic mycoses with ketoconazole: emphasis on toxicity and clinical response in 52 patients. *Annals of Internal Medicine*, **98**, 13–20.

Downs, N.J., Hinthorn, D.R., Mhatre, V.R., and Liu, C. (1989). Intra-articular amphotericin B treatment of *Sporothrix schenkii* arthritis. *Archives of Internal Medicine*, **149**, 954–5.

Edlestein, H. and McCabe, R. (1991). *Candida albicans* septic arthritis and osteomyletitis of the sternoclavicular joint in a patient with human immunodeficiency virus infection. *Journal of Rheumatology*, **18**, 110–11.

Fader, R.C. and McGinnis, M.R. (1988). Infections causes by dermatiaceous fungi: chromoblastomycosis and phaeohyphomycosis. *Infectious Disease Clinics of North America*, **1**, 925–38.

Fainstein, V., Gilmore, C., Hopfer, R.L., Maksymiuk, A., and Bodey, G.P. (1982). Septic arthritis due to *Candida* species in patients with cancer: report of five cases and review of the literature. *Review of Infectious Disease*, **4**, 78–85.

Farrell, J.B., Person, D.A., Lidsky, M.D., Hopfer, R.L., and Musher, D.M. (1978). *Candidal tropicalis* arthritis — assessment of amphotericin B therapy. *Journal of Rheumatology*, **5**, 267–71.

Feld, R., Fornasier, V.L., Bombardier, C., and Hastings, D.E. (1982). Septic arthritis due to *Saccharomyces* species in a patient with chronic rheumatoid arthritis. *Journal of Rheumatology*, **9**, 637–40.

Fiese, M. (1958). *Coccidioidomycosis*. Charles.C. Thomas, Springfield, IL.

Fitzgerald, R.H., Jr. and Kelly, P.J. (1979). Total joint arthroplasty: biologic causes of failure. *Mayo Clinic Proceedings*, **54**, 590–6.

Fountain, F.F., Jr. (1973). Acute blastomycotic arthritis. *Archives of Internal Medicine*, **132**, 684–8.

Fromptling, R.A. (1988). Overview of medically important antifungal azole derivatives. *Clinical Microbiology Review*, **1**, 187–217.

Galgiani, J.N. (1990). Fluconazole, a new antifungal agent. *Annals of Internal Medicine*, **113**, 177–9.

Galgiani, J.N. and Ampel, N.M. (1990). Coccidioidomycosis in human immuno-deficiency virus-infected patients. *Journal of Infectious Disease*, **162**, 1165–9.

Galgiani, J.N., Stevens, D.A., Graybill, J.R., Dismukes, W.E., and Cloud, G.A. (1988). Ketoconazole therapy of progressive coccidioidomycosis. Comparison of 400- and 800-mg doses and observations at higher doses. *American Journal of Medicine*, **84**, 603–10.

Gardella, S. *et al.* (1985). Fatal fungemia with arthritic involvement caused by *Trichosporon beigelii* in a bone marrow transplant recipient. *Journal of Infectious Disease*, **151**, 566.

Gathe, J.C., Harris, R.L., Garland, B., Bradshaw, M.W., and Williams, T.W. (1987). Candida osteomyelitis. Report of 5 cases and review of the literature. *American Journal of Medicine*, **82**, 927–37.

George, A.L., Jr., Hays, J.T., and Graham, B.S. (1985). Blastomycosis presenting as monoarticular arthritis: the role of synovial fluid cytology. *Arthritis and Rheumatism*, **28**, 516–21.

Gerster, J.C., Glauser, M.P., Delacretaz, F., and Nguyen, T. (1980). Erosive candida arthritis in a patient with disseminated candidiasis. *Journal of Rheumatology*, **7**, 911–14.

Ginzler, E., Meisel, A.D., Munters, M., and Kaplan, D. (1979). Candida arthritis secondary to repeated intra-articular corticosteroids. *New York State Journal of Medicine*, **79**, 392–4.

Gnann, J.W., Bressler, G.S., Bodet, C.A., and Avent, C.K. (1983). Human blastomycosis after a dog bite. *Annals of Internal Medicine*, **98**, 48–9.

Govender, S., Rasool, M.N., and Ngcelwane, M. (1989). Osseous sporotrichosis. *Journal of Infection*, **19**, 273–6.

Graybill, J.R., Craven, P.C., Donovan, W., and Matthew, E.B. (1983). Ketoconazole therapy of systemic fungal infections. Inadequacy of standard dosage regimens. *American Review of Respiratory Disease*, **12**, 171–4.

Greenman, R., Becker, J., Campbell, G., and Remington, J. (1975). Coccidioidal synovitis of the knee. *Archives of Internal Medicine*, **135**, 526–30.

Haug, W.A. and Merrifield, R.C. (1959). Coccidioidal villous synovitis. *American Journal of Clinical Pathology*, **31**, 165–71.

Hawkins Van Tyle, J. (1984). Ketoconazole: mechanism of action, spectrum of activity, pharmacokinetics, drug interactions, adverse reactions and therapeutic use. *Pharmacotherapy*, **4**, 343–73.

Ho, N.K., Low, Y.P., and See, H.F. (1989). Septic arthritis in the newborn — a 17 years' experience. *Singapore Medical Journal*, **30**, 356–8.

Horsburgh, C.R., Jr., Cannady, P.B., Jr., and Kirkpatrick, C.H. (1983). Treatment of fungal infections in the bones and joints with ketoconazole. *Journal of Infectious Disease*, **147**, 1064–9.

Jakle, C., Leek, J.C., Olson, D.A., and Robbins, D.L. (1983). Septic arthritis due to *Fusarium solani*. *Journal of Rheumatology*, **10**, 151–3.

Jones, P.G. (1985). Septic arthritis due to *Histoplasmosis capsulatum* in a leukaemic patient. *Annals of the Rheumatic Diseases*, **44**, 128–9.

Kaell, A.T. and Weitzman, I. (1983). Acute monoarticular arthritis due to *Phialophora parasitica*. *American Journal of Medicine*, **74**, 519–22.

Kaufmann, L. (1971). Serological tests for histoplasmosis: their use and interpretation. In *Histoplasmosis: Proceedings of the Second National Conference*, Centers for Disease Controls, Atlanta Georgia, (ed. L. Ajello, E.W. Chick, and M.L. Furcolow), pp. 321–6. Charles C. Thomas, Springfield, IL.

Kedes, L.H., Siemienski, J., and Braude, A.I. (1964). The syndrome of the alcoholic rose gardener. *Annals of Internal Medicine*, **61**, 1139–41.

Kemp, H.B.S., Bedford, A.F., and Fincham, W.J. (1982). *Petriellidium boydii* infection of the knee: a case report. *Skeletal Radiology*, **9**, 114–17.

Key, J.A. and Large, A.M. (1942). Histoplasmosis of the knee. *Journal of Bone and Joint Surgery*, **24**, 281–90.

Khan, M.I., Goss, G., Gotsman, A., and Asvat, M.S. (1983). Sporotrichosis arthritis: a case presentation and review of the literature. *South African Medical Journal*, **64**, 1099–1101.

Klein, B.S. *et al.* (1986). Isolation of *Blastomyces dermatitidis* in soil associated with a large outbreak of blastomycosis in Wisconsin. *New England Journal of Medicine*, **314**, 529–34.

Kramer, M. *et al.* (1990). Cyclosporine and itraconazole interaction in heart and lung transplant recipients. *Annals of Internal Medicine*, **113**, 327–8.

Kwon-Chung, K.J. and Bennett, J.E. (1992). Paracoccidioidomycosis. In *Medical mycology*, (ed. K.J. Kwon-Chung and J.E. Bennett), pp. 594–619. Lea and Febiger, Philadelphia.

Lafont, A. *et al.* (1994). *Candida albicans* spondylodiscitis and vertebral osteomyelitis in patients with intravenous heroin drug addiction. Report of 3 new cases. *Journal of Rheumatology*, **21**, 953–6.

Lambertus, M., Thordarson, D., and Goetz, M.B. (1988). Fungal prosthetic arthritis: presentation of two cases and review of the literature. *Review of Infectious Disease*, **10**, 1038–43.

Lantz, B., Selakovich, W.G., Collins, D.N., and Garvin, K.L. (1988). Coccidioidomycosis of the knee with 26-year follow-up examination. *Clinical Orthopedics*, **234**, 183–7.

Lesperance, M.L., Baumgartner, D., and Kauffman, C.A. (1988). Polyarticular arthritis due to *Sporothrix schenckii*. *Mycoses*, **31**, 599–603.

Londero, A.T. and Rambos, C.D. (1972). Paracoccidioidomycosis. A clinical and mycologic study of forty-one cases observed in Santa Maria, RS, Brazil. *American Journal of Medicine*, **52**, 771–5.

Lurie, H.I. (1963). Five unusual cases of sporotrichosis from South Africa showing lesions in muscles, bone and viscera. *British Journal of Surgery*, **50**, 585–91.

MacKenzie, T.R., Perry, C., Pearson, R., and Gilula, L.A. (1988). Magnetic resonance imaging in patients with inflammatory arthritis of the knee. *Orthopaedics Review*, **17**, 709–19.

Marina, N., Flynn, P., Rivera, G., and Hughes, W. (1991). *Candida tropicalis* and *Candida albicans* fungemia in children with leukemia. *Cancer*, **68**, 594–9.

McDonald, P.B., Black, G.B., and MacKenzie, R. (1990). Orthopaedic manifestations of blastomycosis. *Journal of Bone and Joint Surgery*, **72A**, 860–4.

McGinnis, M.R. and Fader, R.C. (1988). Mycetoma: A contemporary concept. *Infectious Disease Clinics of North America*, **1**, 938–54.

McKinsey, D.S., Gupta, M.R., Riddler, S.A., Driks, M., Smith, D.L., and Kurtin, P.J. (1989). Long-term amphotericin B therapy for disseminated histoplasmosis in patients with the acquired immunodeficiency syndrome (AIDS). *Annals of Internal Medicine*, **111**, 655–9.

McManus, E.J. and Jones, J.M. (1986). The use of ketoconazole in the treatment of blastomycosis. *American Review of Respiratory Disease*, **133**, 141–3.

Minamoto, G. and Armstrong, D. (1988). Fungal infection in AIDS. Histoplasmosis and coccidioidomycosis. *Infectious Disease Clinics of North America*, **2**, 447–56.

Molstad, B. and Strom, R. (1978). Multiarticular sporotrichosis. *Journal of the American Medical Association*, **240**, 556–7.

Mostaza, J.M., Barabao, F.J., Fernandez-Martin, J., Pena-Yandez, J., and Vasquez-Rodriguez, J.J. (1989). Cuneoarticular mucormycosis due to *Cunninghamella bertholletiae* in a patient with AIDS. *Reviews of Infectious Disease*, **11**, 316–18.

Munoz-Fernandez, S. *et al.* (1991). Rheumatic manifestations in 556 patients with human immunodeficiency virus infection. *Seminars in Arthritis and Rheumatism*, **21**, 30–9.

Murray, H.W., Littman, M.L., and Roberts, R.B. (1974). Disseminated paracoccidioidomycosis (South American blastomycosis) in the United States. *American Journal of Medicine*, **56**, 209–20.

National Institute of Allergy and Infectious Disease Mycoses Study Group (1985). Treatment of blastomycosis and histoplasmosis with ketoconazole. *Annals of Internal Medicine*, **103**, 861–72.

Nomura, J. and Ruskin, J. (1994). The prosthetic joint and disseminated coccidioidomycosis [abstract 32]. Centennial Conference on Coccidioidomycosis, Stanford, California,

O'Meeghan, T., Varcoe, R., Thomas, M., and Ellis-Preger, R. (1990). Fluconazole concentration in joint fluid during successful treatment of *Candida albicans* arthritis. *Journal of Antimicrobial Chemotherapy*, **26**, 601–2.

Omer, G.E., Jr., Lockwood, R.S., and Travis, L.O. (1963). Histoplasmosis involving the carpal joint. A case report. *Journal of Bone and Joint Surgery*, **45**, 1699–703.

Paya, C.V., Roberts, G.D., and Cockerill, F.R., III (1987). Laboratory methods for the diagnosis of disseminated histoplasmosis: clinical importance of the lysis-centrifugation blood culture technique. *Mayo Clinic Proceedings*, **62**, 480–5.

Pearson, G.J., Chin, T.W., and Fong, I.W. (1992). Case report: treatment of blastomycosis with fluconazole. *American Journal of Medical Science*, **303**, 313–15.

Perfect, J.R., Durack, D.T., and Gallis, H.A. (1983). Cryptococcemia. *Medicine*, **62**, 98–109.

Pluss, J.L. and Opal, S.M. (1986). Pulmonary sporotrichosis: review of treatment and outcome. *Medicine*, **65**, 143–53.

Pope, T.L., Jr. (1982). Pediatric *Candida albicans* arthritis: case report of hip involvement with a review of the literature. *Progress in Pediatric Surgery*, **15**, 271–83.

Recht, A.D., Davies, S.F., and Eckman, M.R. (1982). Blastomycosis in immunosuppressed patients. *American Review of Respiratory Disease*, **125**, 359–62.

Restrepo, A. *et al.* (1976). The gamut of paracoccidioidomycosis. *American Journal of Medicine*, **61**, 33–42.

Restrepo, A., Robledo, J., Gomez, I., Tabares, A.M., and Gutierrez, R. (1986). Itraconazole therapy in lymphangitic and cutaneous sporotrichosis. *Archives of Dermatology*, **122**, 413–17.

Ricciardi, D.D., Sepkowitz, D.V., Berkowitz, L.B., Bienenstock, H., and Maslow, M. (1986). Cryptococcal arthritis in a patient with acquired immune deficiency syndrome. Case report and review of the literature. *Journal of Rheumatology*, **13**, 455–8.

Rippon, J.W. (1988). In *Pseudoallescheriasis*, (ed. M. Wonsiewicz), pp. 651–80. W.B. Saunders, Philadelphia.

Robert, M.E. and Kauffman, C.A. (1988). Blastomycosis presenting as polyarticular septic arthritis. *Journal of Rheumatology*, **15**, 1138–42.

Roncoroni, A.J. and Smayevsky, J. (1988). Arthritis and endocarditis from *Exiophiala jeanselmei* infection. *Annals of Internal Medicine*, **108**, 773.

Rosenthal, J., Brandt, K.D., Wheat, J.L., and Slama, T.G. (1983). Rheumatologic manifestations of histoplasmosis in the recent Indianapolis epidemic. *Arthritis and Rheumatism*, **26**, 1065–70.

Salzman, S.H., Smith, R.L., and Aranda, C.P. (1988). Histoplasmosis in patients at risk for the acquired immunodeficiency syndrome in a nonendemic setting. *Chest*, **93**, 916–21.

Sarosi, G.A. and Davies, S.F. (1981). The clinical spectrum of blastomycosis. *Internal Medicine*, **2**, 64–70.

Sarosi, G.A, Hammerman, K.J., Tosh, F.E., and Kronenberg, R.S. (1974). Clinical features of acute pulmonary blastomycosis. *New England Journal of Medicine*, **290**, 540–3.

Schwartz, D.A. (1989). Sporothrix tenosynovitis — differential diagnosis of granulomatous inflammatory disease of the joints. *Journal of Rheumatology*, **16**, 550–3.

Schwarz, J. (1984). What's new in mycotic bone and joint diseases. *Pathology Research Practice*, **178**, 617–34.

Sellers, T.F., Price, W.N., and Newberry, W.M., Jr. (1965). An epidemic of erythema multiforme and erythema nodosum caused by histoplasmosis. *Annals of Internal Medicine*, **62**, 1244–62.

Sharkey, P.K. *et al.* (1990). Itraconazole treatment of phaeohyphomycosis. *Journal of the American Academy of Dermatology*, **23**, 577–86.

Sharkey-Mathis, P. *et al.* (1993). Treatment of sporotrichosis with itraconazole. National Institute of Allergy and Infectious Disease Mycosis Study Group. *American Journal of Medicine*, **95**, 279–85.

Silveira, L.H., Seleznick, M.J., Jara, L.J., Martinez-Osuna, P., and Espinoza, L. R. (1991). Musculoskeletal manifestations of human immunodeficiency virus infection. *Journal of Intensive Care Medicine*, **6**, 601–2.

Sinnott, J.T., IV. and Holt, D.A. (1982). Cryptococcal pyarthrosis complicating gouty arthritis. *Southern Medical Journal*, **82**, 1555–6.

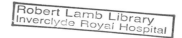

Stead, K.J., Klugman, K.P., Painter, M.L., and Koornhof, H.J. (1988). Septic arthritis due to *Cryptococcus neoformans*. *Journal of Infection*, **17**, 139–45.

Stevens, D.A. and Vo, P.T. (1982). Synergistic interaction of trimethoprim and sulfamethoxazole on *Paracoccidioides brasiliensis*. *Antimicrobial Agents and Chemotherapy*, **21**, 852–4.

Stratton, C.W., Lichtenstein, K.A., Lowenstein, S.R., Phelps, D.B., and Reller, L.B. (1981). Granulomatous tenosynovitis and carpal tunnel syndrome caused by *Sporothrix schenckii. American Journal of Medicine*, **71**, 161–4.

Sugar, A.M. (1988). Paracoccidioidomycosis. *Infectious Disease Clinics of North America*, **1**, 913–24.

Sugar, A.M., Restrepo, A.A., and Stevens, D.A. (1984). Paracoccidioidomycosis in the immunosuppressed host: report of a case and review of the literature. *American Review of Respiratory Disease*, **129**, 340–42.

Sugar, A.M., Saunders, C., and Diamond, R.D. (1990). Successful treatment of *Candida* osteomyelitis with fluconazole. A noncomparative study of two patients. *Microbiology and Infectious Disease*, **13**, 517–20.

Svirsky-Fein, S., Langer, L., Mibauer, B., Khermosh, O., and Rubinstein, E. (1979). Neonatal osteomyelitis caused by *Candida tropicalis*. Report of two cases and review of the literature. *Journal of Bone and Joint Surgery*, **61A**, 455–9.

Szombathy, S.P., Chez, M.G., and Laxer, R.M. (1988). Acute septic arthritis due to *Acremonium. Journal of Rheumatology*, **15**, 714–15.

Tack, K.J., Phame, F.S., Brown, B., and Thompson, R.C., Jr. (1982). *Aspergillus* osteomyelitis: report of four cases and review of the literature. *American Journal of Medicine*, **73**, 295–300.

Taillan, B. *et al.* (1992). Favourable outcome of blastomycosis of the brain stem with fluconazole and flucytosine treatment. *Annals of Medicine*, **24**, 71–2.

Tucker, R., Williams, P., Arathoon, E., and Stevens, D. (1988). Treatment of mycoses with itraconazole. *Annals of the New York Academy of Sciences*, **544**, 451–71.

Tucker, R.M., Denning, D.W., Arathoon, E.G., Rinaldi, M.G., and Stevens, D.A. (1990). Itraconazole therapy for nonmeningeal coccidioidomycosis: clinical and laboratory observations. *Journal of the American Academy of Dermatology*, **23**, 593–601.

Van Der Schee, A.C., Dinkla, B.A., and Festen, J.J.M. (1990). Gonarthritis as only manifestation of chronic disseminated histoplasmosis. *Clinical Rheumatology*, **9**, 92–4.

Wheat, L.J. *et al.* (1982). The diagnostic laboratory tests for histoplasmosis: analysis of experience in a large urban outbreak. *Annals of Internal Medicine*, **97**, 680–5.

Wheat, L.J., Kohler, R.B. and Tewari, R.P. (1986). Diagnosis of disseminated histoplasmosis by detection of *Histoplasmosis capsulatum* antigen in serum and urine specimens. *New England Journal of Medicine*, **314**, 83–8.

Wheat, L.J. *et al.* (1990). Disseminated histoplasmosis in the acquired immune deficiency syndrome: clinical findings, diagnosis and treatment, and review of the literature. *Medicine (Baltimore)*, **69**, 361–74.

Winn, R.E. (1988). Sporotrichosis. *Infectious Disease Clinics of North America*, **1**, 899–911.

Winn, R., Anderson, J., Piper, J., Aronson, N., and Pluss, J. (1993). Systemic sporotrichosis treated with itraconazole. *Clinical Infectious Disease*, **17**, 210–17.

Winter, W.J., Jr., Larson, R.K., Honeggar, M.M., Jacobsen, D.T., Pappagianis, D., and Huntington, R.W. (1975). Coccidioidal arthritis and its treatment. *Journal of Bone and Joint Surgery*, **57A**, 1152–7.

Witorsch, P. and Utz, J.P. (1968). North American blastomycosis: a study of 40 patients. *Medicine*, **47**, 169–200.

Yagi, K.I., Abbas, K., and Prabhu, S.R. (1983). Temporomandibular joint ankylosis due to maduromycetoma caused by *Madurella mycetomi. Journal of Oral Pathology and Medicine*, **38**, 71–3.

Yao, J., Penn, R.G., and Ray, S. (1986). Articular sporotrichosis. *Clinical Orthopedics*, **204**, 207–14.

Younkin, S., Evarts, C.M., and Steigbigel, R.T. (1984). *Candida parapsilosis* infection of a total hip-joint replacement: successful reimplantation after treatment with amphotericin B and 5-fluorocytosine. A case report. *Journal of Bone and Joint Surgery*, **66A**, 142–3.

Yousefzadeh, D.K. and Jackson, J.H. (1980). Neonatal and infantile candidal arthritis with or without osteomyelitis: a clinical and radiographical review of 21 cases. *Skeletal Radiology*, **5**, 77–90.

5.3.11 Immunodeficiency

A. D. B. Webster

Introduction

Joint disease is a relatively common complication of immunodeficiency, and in the majority of cases it can be shown to be due to infection. Immunodeficiency is classified into 'primary' and 'secondary', most cases in the former category being due to inherited single or multiple gene defects, while the common forms of secondary immunodeficiency are associated with lymphoreticular neoplasia, particularly chronic lymphatic leukaemia and myeloma, or infection with the human immunodeficiency virus. It is useful to subclassify patients into those that have a predominantly antibody or cell-mediated immune deficiency, and those with severe combined immunodeficiency (see Table 1).

Antibody deficiency

The principal diseases of the joint that may be associated with primary hypogammaglobulinaemia are shown in Table 2.

Mycoplasma arthritis

Mycoplasmas are prokaryotic organisms which frequently infect mammals but which also occur in fish and reptiles (Taylor-Robinson 1990). There are many different types in humans, the majority colonizing mucosal surfaces and, in general, behaving as commensals. *Mycoplasma pneumoniae* is an exception, being a recognized pathogen that infects the respiratory tract causing pneumonia. Ureaplasmas, so called because they metabolize urea to ammonia, account for about a third of cases of 'non-specific' urethritis in otherwise healthy men, although the infection is usually self-limiting (Taylor-Robinson and McCormack 1980).

Mycoplasmas are normally found on mucosal surfaces and do not penetrate epithelial cells, although they may be taken up by phagocytes and remain viable within such cells (see below). When present in large numbers they do cause inflammation, possibly through direct activation of complement. Different strains have become adapted to different systems within the body: for instance ureaplasmas are mainly found in the urinary tract.

The first descriptions of mycoplasmas in the joints of patients with hypogammaglobulinaemia were published in 1978 (Stuckey *et al.* 1978; Webster *et al.* 1978), but even now there are some sceptics who suggest that the organisms may not cause the arthritis, but are merely 'passengers' in an immunocompromised host. This view stems from the early claim that patients with hypogammaglobulinaemia are prone to rheumatoid arthritis, as well as other autoimmune rheumatic disorders (Good *et al.* 1957). Most of the investigators involved in these early studies now concede that they were probably dealing with an infective arthritis. Surprisingly, mycoplasma arthritis has only been described so far in the primary hypogammaglobulinaemias (e.g. X-linked agammaglobulinaemia and 'common variable' immunodeficiency; see 'rheumatoid arthritis' below), and not in the secondary types associated with chronic lymphatic leukaemia and myeloma. Although cases may have been missed, the severity of the

Table 1 Classification of immunodeficiency

Primary

Selective T-lymphocyte defects

  Thymic aplasia

  Purine nucleoside phosphorylase deficiency

  Class I TAP transporter defect

  T-cell receptor defects

Antibody deficiency

  X-linked agammaglobulinaemia

  X-linked hypertrophy syndrome

  'Common variable' immunodeficiency

  Selective IgA and/or IgG subclass deficiencies

Mixed humoral and cellular immune defects

  Mild

    Ataxia telangiectasia

    Wiskott–Aldrich syndrome

  Severe combined immunodeficiency

    Il-2, -4, -7 γ-chain deficiency

    Janus-associated kinase (JAK)3 deficiency

    Zeta-associated protein kinase (ZAP 70) deficiency

    Recombinase activating gene (RAG 1 or 2) deficiency

    Adenosine deaminase deficiency

    Lymphocyte class-II deficiency

Complement deficiencies

Neutrophil defects

  Neutropenia

  Chronic granulomatous disease

Secondary

Predominant cellular deficiency

  AIDS

  Malignancy

  Cytotoxic chemotherapy

Antibody deficiency

  Drug-induced (gold, sulphasalazine, phenytoin, penicillamine)

  Myeloma

  Chronic lymphatic leukaemia

Neutropenia

  Autoimmune

  Cytotoxic drugs

The above is based on a more comprehensive WHO classification (WHO Scientific Group Report 1995).

Table 2 Joint disease in primary hypogammaglobulinaemia

Disease	Comments
Mycoplasma arthritis	Mainly large joints but any joint can be affected
Monoarthritis of knee	Mainly in children, self-limiting
Tenosynovitis/arthralgia	Usually affects hands and feet; rapid response to immunoglobulin therapy
Echovirus disease	Flexion contractures of elbows and knees
Rheumatoid arthritis	Drugs used to treat rheumatoid arthritis may cause hypogammaglobulinaemia

antibody deficiency may not be enough to predispose to systemic mycoplasma infection in the secondary immunodeficiencies. There are anecdotal reports of mycoplasma septicaemia and/or arthritis in patients on immunosuppressive drugs or following severe trauma, but, surprisingly, most of these patients were not investigated for immunoglobulin deficiency. Although there are claims that mycoplasmas may act as cofactors in the mechanism of the immune deficiency in acquired immune deficiency syndrome (**AIDS**), joint disease has not been described, although chronic mycoplasma infection of the kidneys may contribute to the characteristic nephropathy seen in AIDS (Bauer *et al.* 1991).

The evidence that mycoplasmas are a common cause of arthritis in hypogammaglobulinaemia can be summarized as follows. The organisms can consistently be isolated in high titre from the joint during the active phase; the symptoms usually improve rapidly when antibiotics are given to which the organism is sensitive, and chronic arthritis with joint destruction occurs when antibiotic-resistant organisms are involved. Finally, some patients with severe, generalized infections develop discharging sinuses, often communicating with joints, from which mycoplasmas can be isolated (Taylor-Robinson *et al.* 1985).

Origin of infection

Ureaplasmas are commonly present in the vagina of pregnant women, and it is thought that most neonates become colonized in the respiratory tract shortly after birth, although the organisms then disappear through mechanisms that are not understood (Taylor-Robinson and McCormack 1980). In later life, colonization of the urinary tract may occur from sexual intercourse, and since about a third of healthy women are persistently colonized, most men are exposed to these organisms. Colonization is usually transient and asymptomatic, although a minority of men will develop urethritis. In contrast, there is a high incidence of symptomatic ureaplasma urethritis in both men and women with hypogammaglobulinaemia, which may progress to a chronic cystitis and occasionally pyelonephritis (Webster *et al.* 1981). Fibrosis of the bladder wall with contraction may be the end result of chronic infection. Many patients with hypogammaglobulinaemia who develop ureaplasma arthritis

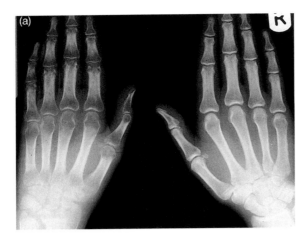
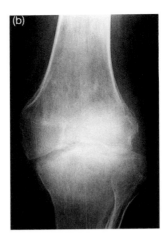

Fig. 1   (a) Chronic infection with *Ureaplasma urealyticum* of the wrist in a 30-year-old man with X-linked agammaglobulinaemia, showing destruction of the left distal ulna, the medial radius, and lunate, with osteoporosis of all joint levels related to disuse. (b) The left knee of the same patient showing destruction of the cartilage, obliteration of the joint space, and disorganization of the joint.

have previously suffered from an episode of urethritis, so it is likely that the origin of the infection is in the urinary tract. Trauma to a joint, which may be minor, often triggers the septic arthritis, suggesting that the organisms are present in small numbers in the circulation and become established at an inflammatory focus within the joint. Once one joint has been infected, there is a tendency for other joints to follow if the infection is not eliminated with appropriate antibiotics. Roifman *et al.* (1986) have suggested that ureaplasmas may cause chronic bronchitis in antibody deficient patients, and although this issue is controversial, the lungs may be a source of systemic infection.

Apart from *M. pneumoniae*, which is acquired by droplet inoculation from an infected person, two other mycoplasmas have been cultured from the inflamed joints of patients with hypogammaglobulinaemia. *M. hominis*, like ureaplasmas, is a commensal in the urinary tract, and is usually acquired through sexual contact. The 10 per cent of 'healthy' women with bacterial vaginosis have particularly heavy colonization of their vaginas with *M. hominis* (Hillier and Holmes 1990); antibody deficient women with this problem may have an increased risk of *M. hominis* arthritis. Women presenting with *M. hominis* arthritis should therefore be tested for bacterial vaginosis and if necessary be given metronidazole to eliminate the bacteria; this should reduce the risk of further systemic spread of the mycoplasma infection. We have seen dual infection in a joint with *M. hominis* and *Ureaplasma urealyticum* in one patient. *M. salivarium* has also been isolated from the joints of a few patients, presumably originating from the upper respiratory tract where it is found in the saliva of about 80 per cent of healthy individuals (So *et al.* 1982). This organism is unequivocally regarded as a commensal and is a good example of commensal overgrowth leading to disease in an immunocompromised host.

Clinical features

Large joints are usually affected, particularly the knees, although the ankles, hips, shoulders, and wrists (including carpal bones) are frequently involved in persistent infections. The fingers and toes are rarely affected, and when this does occur it usually involves a single interphalangeal joint. The initial symptoms are swelling and stiffness

of the affected joint, usually with an obvious effusion when the knee is involved. Nodules may occur on the elbows that have the same histological features as classical rheumatoid nodules. Systemic symptoms are rare and there is usually no fever or blood leucocytosis. Joint pain increases over a few weeks or months, and if the infection persists the synovium will gradually deteriorate through chronic inflammation, leading eventually to fibrosis and fixation of the joint (Fig. 1). This sequence usually takes months, or sometimes years, to reach a conclusion if inappropriate or no treatment is offered.

Some patients may enter a severe phase, presumably reflecting high levels of circulating organisms. Subcutaneous abscesses may then occur, sometimes at sites of minor trauma (e.g. injection sites), but more often adjacent to joints; the skin then breaks down leaving a chronically discharging sinus in communication with the joint space. Even at this relatively late stage, the patient may show no systemic effects of chronic infection, apart from being immobilized and in considerable pain.

Diagnosis

Organisms can be cultured from the synovial fluid, provided that appropriate techniques are used, although cultures may be negative if the patient has recently been treated with antibiotics, particularly erythromycin and tetracyclines. Unfortunately, there are only a few laboratories in the world that are in a position routinely to culture mycoplasmas, despite the fact that the techniques required are relatively straightforward. It should be be remembered that the diagnosis of *M. pneumoniae* infection in immunocompetent patients is usually made retrospectively by positive serology, which is obviously inappropriate in patients with hypogammaglobulinaemia. There are some routine laboratories that will culture for *M. pneumoniae*, although these organisms are slow growing and may take up to 2 weeks to show a positive result. Ureaplasmas, *M. hominis*, and *M. salivarium* need different media, and a positive result can be obtained in 48 h. Organisms can also be isolated from the pus of discharging sinuses, and from synovial tissue removed at biopsy.

Synovial fluid should always be sent for the routine culture of common pathogens, such as staphylococci and *Haemophilus influenzae*, which may rarely cause arthritis in patients with hyogammaglobulinaemia. Microscopic examination of the fluid is not very helpful unless it is clear with a predominant lymphocytosis, in which case mycoplasma arthritis is unlikely. The fluid is usually yellow and/or turbid, and contains many neutrophils. If the routine culture is negative, then the working diagnosis should be mycoplasma arthritis until proved otherwise. Occasionally, there may be confusion between mycoplasma arthritis and other types of arthropathy (see below) that have a raised incidence in patients with hypogammaglobulinaemia. In particular, rheumatoid arthritis in its early stages can be confused with mycoplasma infection, although multiple involvement of finger joints is very much against the latter.

Management

Patients should be given doxycycline as soon as synovial fluid has been aspirated. We use doxycycline intravenously (Pfizer) at a dose of 200 mg at once, followed by 100 mg/day until there is improvement in joint swelling and the level of serum C-reactive protein has become normal, which is a useful marker of disease activity. Treatment should then continue with oral doxycycline at 100 mg/day for at least 3 months. Fortunately, most mycoplasma strains are sensitive to doxycycline and there will be obvious improvement in the joint symptoms within a few days. However, it is useful to arrange sensitivity tests against a range of antibiotics as soon as possible, because occasionally the organism may be resistant. Sensitivity tests should include erythromycin, streptomycin, doxycycline, kanamycin, clindamycin, spectinomycin, netilmicin, ciprofloxacin, and azithromycin, the last being a new macrolide that accumulates in phagocytes, a property which may be of particular advantage in eradicating mycoplasmas. In our experience, patients who are infected with a doxycycline-resistant strain are very difficult to manage and usually progress to multijoint involvement despite various combinations of other antibiotics. However, it is important to test regularly the antibiotic sensitivities of new isolates from joint aspirates in order to keep pace with any changes. Although this can be time consuming for the laboratory, there is a good chance that eventually the infection can be eradicated.

All antibiotics so far tested are static, and consequently long-term therapy is required (Escalante et al. 1985). Surgical interference of the joint should be kept to a minimum; arthroscopy and washing out the joint with saline is unhelpful, although drainage under vacuum of a very tense effusion for 24 h may rarely be necessary. Trauma from surgical interference appears to increase the growth of mycoplasmas, as well as increasing the risk of sinus formation. The joints should be immobilized until there is no longer any swelling, and then if there is damage to the ligaments, the joint must be stabilized by splinting until there is full recovery. Provided the diagnosis is made early and the mycoplasmas are sensitive to tetracyclines, there is usually full recovery.

Patients who steadily deteriorate in spite of treatment with a wide range of antibiotics should be considered for therapy with hyperimmune serum. Unfortunately, regular treatment with intravenous human immunoglobulin has little effect on eradicating mycoplasma infection, because the specific antibody levels are so low in these preparations. However, intravenous human immunoglobulin may have some protective effect against infection. In our series of 18 patients with primary immunodeficiency and mycoplasma arthritis, most presented before treatment with intravenous human immunoglobulin, and in those who developed infection after treatment their trough levels of serum IgG were below 5 g/l (Franz et al. 1997). It is therefore reasonable to treat infected patients with high-dose,

intravenous, human immunoglobulin (i.e. 400 mg/kg per week for 8 weeks), and as a prophylactic measure it is our policy to keep serum IgG levels above 7 g/l.

We have successfully treated two patients with goat serum taken from animals hyperimmunized with the patient's particular strain (Taylor-Robinson et al. 1985). Fortunately, serum sickness does not occur in patients with hypogammaglobulinaemia, who can tolerate repeated infusions of animal serum. The amount of serum given is somewhat arbitrary, and there are no standard immunization schedules for goats. We have raised titres in excess of 1:5000 by first subcutaneously injecting a mycoplasma concentrate in Freund's complete adjuvant, followed by intravenous injections of the concentrate alone at 4-week intervals. It may be better to immunize rabbits using published schedules that are known to produce very high titres of antisera (i.e. $1:10^5$), which might compensate for relatively small amounts of serum obtainable.

Monoclonal antibodies are not yet available, and anyway may have to be raised specifically against the infecting organism because of considerable strain variation in exposed antigenic epitopes. Nevertheless, this is worth considering early in a patient who is difficult to treat, as it will take many months to raise enough antibody.

Role of antibodies in protection against mycoplasmas
The clinical observations on patients with hypogammaglobulinaemia clearly demonstrate that antibodies are important in protection against mycoplasma arthritis. In vitro experiments have shown that the growth of mycoplasmas is readily inhibited by specific antibody, and that, even in the absence of antibody, mycoplasmas will activate the first component of complement. In turn this will activate the complement cascade and split C3, generating opsonic complement, which enables the organisms to be taken up by neutrophils (Webster et al. 1988). However, once within the neutrophil phagolysosome the organisms remain viable, and it is likely that neutrophils transport organisms from mucosae to the joints. The factors that encourage mycoplasma growth within the joints are unknown. It is likely, therefore, that the main function of specific antibodies against mycoplasmas is to control their growth on the mucosal surface. Massive overgrowth of organisms occurs in the absence of antibody. The result is inflammation, with influx of neutrophils and macrophages, followed by phagocytosis of large numbers of mycoplasmas which initiate chronic infection in a susceptible joint.

Bacterial septic arthritis

Patients with hypogammaglobulinaemia are prone to septicaemia and pneumonia due to pneumococci, non-typeable H. influenzae, and staphylococci, any of which can occasionally cause septic arthritis (Asherson and Webster 1980). However, in contrast to mycoplasma arthritis, bacterial arthritis is usually more acute and painful. Bacterial arthritis is extremely rare in patients already established on replacement immunoglobulin therapy, whereas mycoplasma infection still occurs.

Rheumatoid arthritis

Early reports suggested that there was a high incidence of rheumatoid arthritis in patients with hypogammaglobulinaemia, including those with X-linked agammaglobulinaemia (Good et al. 1957). However, it now seems likely that many of these patients suffered from mycoplasma arthritis. Nevertheless, rheumatoid arthritis does occur in

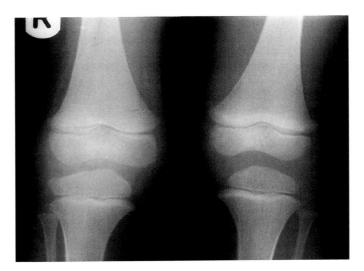

Fig. 2 Epiphyseal hypertrophy in the right knee of a 3-year-old boy with X-linked agammaglobinaemia. There was a sterile effusion; the knee subsequently improved spontaneously.

patients with 'common variable' immunodeficiency, at a frequency of about 2 per cent in our series. It is often difficult to ascertain whether the arthritis precedes or follows the onset of hypogammaglobulinaemia, and there is the added complication that a number of drugs used to treat rheumatoid arthritis (see below) are known to 'cause' or 'trigger' hypogammaglobulinaemia (So *et al.* 1984). Nevertheless, there are patients whose hypogammaglobulinaemia clearly precedes the onset of classical rheumatoid arthritis, with the typical involvement of small joints of the hand, rheumatoid nodules, and gradual destruction of small and large joints. These patients are seronegative for rheumatoid factor and other relevant autoantibodies. This in itself is interesting, because it demonstrates that severe rheumatoid arthritis can occur and progress in the absence of autoantibodies, and supports the view that the disease is driven by cellular interactions.

Drug-associated hypogammaglobulinaemia

Gold, penicillamine, sulphasalazine, and phenytoin have been associated with hypogammaglobulinaemia, and partly explain the apparent raised incidence of rheumatoid arthritis and Still's disease in patients with selective IgA deficiency and other types of hypogammaglobulinaemia (Barclay *et al.* 1979). The immunoglobulin levels usually return to normal after withdrawal of the drug, although this may take many months or even years. The mechanism is unclear, and may be different for the four drugs. In the case of gold, there is evidence that the drug inhibits T-cell proliferation *in vitro* at concentrations likely to be found in tissues (Lipsky and Ziff 1977), but there is no evidence that it affects B-cell differentiation and immunoglobulin synthesis *in vitro*, even when cells are used from patients who have recovered from drug-associated hypogammaglobulinaemia (S. Sukram and A. D. B. Webster, unpublished). One possibility is that the drugs induce 'common variable' immunodeficiency in patients who have genetic predisposing factors for this disease. In this context, it is not yet known whether drug-associated hypogammaglobulinaemia is linked to the same susceptibility genes for common

variable immunodeficiency which are located in the class II and III region on chromosome 6 (Schaffer *et al.* 1989; Howe *et al.* 1991).

Miscellaneous arthritides associated with hypogammaglobulinaemia

Chronic arthritis of the knee

Children with hypogammaglobulinaemia, particularly those with X-linked agammaglobulinaemia, are prone to a chronic insidious arthritis of the knee, which is usually unilateral. There is a chronic and relatively painless effusion, which may persist for many years, sometimes with hypertrophy of the epiphyseal cartilage (Fig. 2). The condition usually recovers spontaneously after a few months or years, leaving very little permanent damage apart from the unsightly appearance of enlarged condyles. Some damage to the cartilage may necessitate meniscectomy in later years.

The synovial fluid is colourless and contains mainly lymphocytes; it is sterile when cultured for bacteria, viruses, and mycoplasmas. Nevertheless, there is still a possibility that this is a low-grade mycoplasma infection, although antimycoplasma drugs such as doxycycline or erythromycin have no effect. Anti-inflammatory drugs are often useful.

Our impression is that this complication is much less common since the introduction of intravenous immunoglobulin therapy in children with hypogammaglobulinaemia, and in one of our cases the arthritis improved after such therapy.

Chronic tenosynovitis/arthritis

This condition was relatively common in British patients with hypogammaglobulinaemia in the 1970s but is now very rare (Webster *et al.* 1976). It usually occurred in adult patients with 'common variable' immunodeficiency as one of the presenting features of the disease. The usual pattern was of a patient suffering from recurrent respiratory infections for many years, who then developed stiffness in the wrists, elbows, and ankles, with swelling of the tendon sheaths on the dorsal aspects of the wrist, hands, and feet. This sometimes led to tendon tethering with cystic swellings that required surgery. The arthritis was usually mild and fluctuating.

The condition was frequently confused with rheumatoid arthritis, but there were no bony erosions. Furthermore, the condition dramatically improved with intramuscular immunoglobulin therapy, suggesting an infectious cause, perhaps by a virus that was neutralized by antibodies in the immunoglobulin therapy. These cases are very rare nowadays in the United Kingdom, although some patients still suffer from mild, fluctuating arthropathy while on intramuscular or intravenous immunoglobulin therapy, which may represent a mild form of the same condition. One of our patients developed tenosynovitis and arthropathy while on intramuscular therapy, but rapidly improved when given intravenous therapy. Finally, it is possible that this condition is caused by low-level mycoplasma infection, as one of our patients initially responded to intravenous immunoglobulin and then relapsed with a confirmed mycoplasma infection which then responded to doxycycline.

Echovirus disease

Patients with severe primary antibody deficiency are prone to chronic echovirus infection of the central nervous system and muscles, and there are reports of arthritis in a few patients (McKinney *et al.* 1987). This is a 'slow' virus disease that mainly affects small vessels in the meninges, subcutaneous tissues, and muscles, leading in the muscles to fibrosis with a 'woody' sensation on palpation. The arms and legs are predominantly affected, and the muscle fibrosis can lead to flexion contractures at the knee and elbows, sometimes producing a characteristic stooped posture (Webster 1984). An erythematous rash may occur transiently, which, together with the subcutaneous oedema, was responsible for the early references to a 'dermatomyositis-like syndrome'. This was thought to provide further evidence that patients with hypogammaglobulinaemia had a predisposition to 'connective tissue disorders'.

The virus can usually be cultured from the cerebrospinal fluid, but occasionally cultures are repeatedly negative and molecular techniques are required to identify viral RNA (Webster *et al.* 1993). The treatment is unsatisfactory, although regular intravenous infusions with high titre, hyperimmune plasma can stabilize the disease, and in a few cases it may have eradicated the infection. Regular injection directly into the cerebrospinal fluid via an Omaya reservoir of pooled immunoglobulin, suitable for intravenous use and preferably with a reasonable titre to the relevant echovirus strain, has been associated with remission in a few patients (McKinney *et al.* 1987). However, most patients gradually deteriorate, sometimes with episodes of partial remission, and ultimately die from involvement of a critical centre in the brain.

Chronic echovirus disease is much less common in the United Kingdom than it was in the 1970s, probably reflecting the increased use of intravenous immunoglobulin during the 1980s. Because each batch of intravenous immunoglobulin is made from a pool of about 20 000 donors, it is likely that significant amounts of antibody to most enteroviral strains are present in these preparations. It is therefore important to maintain serum IgG levels above 7 g/l, particularly in young children with immunodeficiency who may be more susceptible to enteroviruses. This may be difficult to achieve in infants with poor venous access for regular intravenous immunoglobulin therapy. Regular subcutaneous infusions are becoming more popular in this age group but regular monitoring is needed to ensure an adequate serum level.

Defects in cellular immunity

There are a variety of primary defects in cellular immunity, ranging from highly selective T-cell defects to severe combined immunodeficiency. The survival of patients suffering from the latter depends on a successful bone marrow graft (Morgan *et al.* 1987). The best example of a secondary defect in cellular immunity is AIDS, which clinically closely resembles severe combined immunodeficiency. Although patients with selective T-cell defects are not prone to septic or other types of arthritis, those with severe combined immunodeficiency are prone to a wide range of infections, some leading to septic arthritis.

Complement deficiencies

Septic arthritis following pneumococcal, meningococcal, or gonococcal infection may occur in patients with genetically determined homozygous complement deficiencies (Rother 1986). Children with homozygous C2 deficiency, which occurs in about 1 in 10 000 of the population, are prone to pneumococcal and *H. influenzae*

septicaemia, which may be associated with septic arthritis (see Chapter 5.3.2). However, some affected individuals are not prone to infection, presumably because they have other unknown host defence factors against these organisms. Once a patient has developed a septicaemia, it is usually appropriate to recommend regular, prophylactic, oral penicillin therapy, as well as advising the patient to take a broader-spectrum antibiotic (e.g. amoxicillin/clavulanic acid complex) in the event of illness. Patients with defects in other complement components, particularly the late components C7 and C8, are prone to neisserial septicaemia, and occasionally septic arthritis. Prophylactic penicillin may be appropriate for them.

Neutrophil defects

Chronic granulomatous disease (CGD) is one of the primary neutrophil defects described in which joints may be involved, although both primary and secondary neutropenia predisposes to septic arthritis and osteomyelitis, particularly due to staphylococci (White and Gallin 1986). In CGD affected patients are prone to chronic infection with catalase-positive organisms (e.g. salmonella, staphylococci, *Serratia marcescens*), usually causing chronic suppuration of lymph glands with draining sinuses. Staphylococcal and salmonellal osteomyelitis may sometimes occur, although involvement of the joints is very rare.

References

Asherson, G.L. and Webster, A.D.B. (1980). *Diagnosis and treatment of immunodeficiency diseases*. Blackwell, Oxford.

Barclay, D., Ansell, B., Howard, A., Hohermuth, H., and Webster, A.D.B. (1979). IgA deficiency in juvenile chronic polyarthritis. *Journal of Rheumatology*, 6, 219–24.

Bauer, F.A., Wear, D.J., Angritt, P., and Lo, S.C. (1991). *Mycoplasma fermentans* (incognitus strain) infection in the kidneys of patients with acquired immunodeficiency syndrome and associated nephropathy: a light microscopic, immunohistochemical, and ultrastructural study. *Human Pathology*, 22, 63–9.

Escalante, A., Aznar, J., De Miguel, C., and Perea, E.J. (1985). Activity of nine antimicrobial agents against *Mycoplasma hominis* and *Ureaplasma urealyticum*. *European Journal of Sexually Transmitted Diseases*, 2, 85–7.

Franz, A., Webster, A.D.B., Furr, P.M., Taylor-Robinson, D. (1997). Mycoplasmal arthritis in patients with primary immunoglobulin deficiency: clinical features and outcome in 18 patients. *British Journal of Rheumatology* (in press).

Good, R.A., Rotstein, J., and Mazzitello, W.F. (1957). The simultaneous occurrence of rheumatoid arthritis and agammaglobulinaemia. *Journal of Laboratory and Clinical Medicine*, 49, 343–57.

Hillier, S. and Holmes, K.K. (1990). Bacterial vaginosis. In *Sexually transmitted diseases*, (2nd edn) (ed. K.K. Holmes, P.-A. Mardh, P.F. Sparling, and P.J. Wiesner), pp. 547–59. McGraw Hill, New York.

Howe, H.S., So, A.K.L., Farrant, J., and Webster, A.D.B. (1991). Common variable immunodeficiency is associated with polymorphic markers in the human major histocompatibility complex. *Clinical and Experimental Immunology*, 83, 387–90.

Lipsky, P.E. and Ziff, M. (1977). Inhibition of antigen- and mitogen-induced human lymphocyte proliferation by gold compounds. *Journal of Clinical Investigation*, 59, 455–66.

McKinney, R.E., Jr, Katz, S.L., and Wilfert, C.M. (1987). Chronic enteroviral meningoencephalitis in agammaglobulinaemic patients. *Review of Infectious Diseases*, 9, 334–56.

Morgan, G., Levinsky, R.J., Hugh-Jones, K., Fairbanks, L.D., Morris, G.S., and Simmonds, A. (1987). Heterogeneity of biochemical, clinical and immunological parameters in severe combined immunodeficiency due to adenosine deaminase deficiency. *Clinical and Experimental Immunology*, 70, 491–9.

Roifman, C.M., Rao, C.P., Lederman, H.M., Lavi, S., Quinn, P., and Gelfand, E.W. (1986). Increased susceptibility to *Mycoplasma* infection in patients with hypogammaglobulinaemia. *American Journal of Medicine*, 80, 590–4.

Rother, K. (1986). Summary of reported deficiencies. In Hereditary and acquired complement deficiencies in animals and man, (ed. K. and U. Rother), *Progress in Allergy* series, pp. 202–11. Karger, Basle.

Schaffer, F.M., Palermos, J., Zhu, Z.B., Barger, B.O., Cooper, M.D., and Volanakis, J.E. (1989). Individuals with IgA deficiency and common variable immunodeficiency share polymorphisms of major histocompatibility complex class III genes. *Proceedings of the National Academy of Sciences (USA)*, **86**, 8015–19.

So, A.K.L., Furr, P.M., Taylor-Robinson, D., and Webster, A.D.B. (1982). Arthritis caused by *Mycoplasma salivarium* in hypogammaglobulinaemia. *British Medical Journal*, **286**, 762–3.

So, A.K.L., Peskett, S.A., and Webster, A.D.B. (1984). Hypogammaglobulinaemia associated with gold therapy. *Annals of the Rheumatic Diseases*, **43**, 581–2.

Stuckey, M., Quinn, P.A., and Gelfand, E.W. (1978). Identification of *Ureaplasma urealyticum* (T-strain *Mycoplasma*) in patients with polyarthritis. *Lancet*, i, 198–201.

Taylor-Robinson, D. (1990). The mycoplasmatales: mycoplasma, ureaplasma, acholeplasma, spiroplasma and anaeroplasma. In *Topley and Wilson's principles of bacteriology*, (8th edn), Vol. 2, *Systematic bacteriology*, (ed. M.T. Parker and B.I. Duerden), pp. 663–81. Edward Arnold, London.

Taylor-Robinson, D. and McCormack, W.M. (1980). The genital mycoplasmas. *New England Journal of Medicine*, **302**, 1003 and 1063.

Taylor-Robinson, D., Furr, P.M., and Webster, A.D.B. (1985). *Ureaplasma urealyticum* causing persistent urethritis in a patient with hypogammaglobulinaemia. *Genitourinary Medicine*, **61**, 404–8.

Webster, A.D.B. (1984). Echovirus disease in hypogammaglobulinaemic patients. *Clinics in Rheumatology*, **10**, 189–203.

Webster, A.D.B., Loewi, G., Dourmashkin, R.D., Golding, D.N., Ward, D.J., and Asherson, G.L. (1976). Polyarthritis in adults with hypogammaglobulinaemia and its rapid response to immunoglobulin treatment. *British Medical Journal*, **1**, 1314–16.

Webster, A.D.B., Taylor-Robinson, D., Furr, P.M., and Asherson, G.L. (1978). Mycoplasmal (ureaplasma) septic arthritis in hypogammaglobulinaemia. *British Medical Journal*, **1**, 478–9.

Webster, A.D.B., Taylor-Robinson, D., Furr, P.M., and Asherson, G.L. (1981). Chronic cystitis and urethritis associated with ureaplasmal and mycoplasmal infection in primary hypogammaglobulinaemia. *British Journal of Urology*, **54**, 287–91.

Webster, A.D.B., Furr, P.M., Hughes-Jones, N.C., Gorick, B.D., and Taylor-Robinson, D. (1988). Critical dependence on antibody for defence against mycoplasmas. *Clinical and Experimental Immunology*, **71**, 383–7.

Webster, A.D.B., Rotbart, H.A., Warner, T., Rudge, P., and Hyman N. (1993). Diagnosis of enterovirus brain disease in hypogammaglobulinemic patients by polymerase chain reaction. *Clinical Infectious Diseases*, **17**, 657–61.

White, C.J. and Gallin, J.I. (1986). Phagocyte defects. *Clinical Immunology and Immunopatholology*, **40**, 50–61.

WHO Scientific Group Report (1995). Primary immunodeficiency diseases. Report of a WHO Scientific Group. *Clinical and Experimental Immunology*, **99** (Suppl. 1).

5.3.12   Rheumatic fever

Allan Gibofsky and John B. Zabriskie

Introduction

Acute rheumatic fever is a delayed, non-suppurative sequel to a pharyngeal infection with the group A streptococcus. Following the initial streptococcal pharyngitis, there is a latent period of 2 to 3 weeks. The onset of disease is usually characterized by an acute febrile illness, which may show itself in one of three classical ways: (i) the patient may present with migratory arthritis predominantly involving the large joints; (ii) there may be concomitant clinical and laboratory signs of carditis and valvulitis; (iii) there may be involvement of the central nervous system, manifesting itself as Sydenham's chorea. The clinical episodes are self-limiting but damage to the valves may be chronic and progressive, resulting in cardiac decompensation and death.

Although there has been a dramatic decline in both the severity and fatality of the disease since the turn of the century, there are recent reports of its resurgence in the United States (Veasy *et al.* 1987) and in many military installations in the world, reminding us that it remains a public health problem even in developed countries. In addition, the disease continues essentially unabated in many of the developing countries: estimates suggest there will be 10 to 20 million new cases per year in those countries where two-thirds of the world population lives.

Epidemiology

The incidence of rheumatic fever actually began to decline long before the introduction of antibiotics into clinical practice, decreasing, for example, from 250 to 100 patients/100 000 population from 1862 to 1962 in Denmark (Gordis 1985). The introduction of antibiotics in 1950 caused a rapid acceleration of this decline, until in 1980 the incidence ranged from 0.23 to 1.88 patients per 100 000, primarily children and teenagers. A notable exception has been in the Hawaii and Maori populations (both of Polynesian ancestry), where the rate continues to be 13.4/100 000 children admitted to hospital per year (Pope 1989).

As reviewed by Markowitz (1987), only a few M-streptococcal serotypes (types 5, 14, 18, 24) have been implicated in outbreaks of rheumatic fever, suggesting there could be a particular 'rheumatogenic' potential of certain strains of group A streptococci. However,

Table 1   Positive throat cultures—group A β-haemolytic streptococci (Rockefeller University Hospital, rheumatic fever patients; n=78)

M type	RHD	No RHD	Total
Non-typable	1	5	6
1	1	1	2
2	0	1	1
5	1	1	2
6	1	1	2
12	0	2	2
18	2	2	4
19	2	1	3
28	1	0	1
TOTAL	9	11	23

RHD, patients with rheumatic heart disease; no RHD, patients without rheumatic heart disease.

in Trinidad, types 41 and 11 have been the most common strains isolated from rheumatics. In our own series, gathered over 20 years (see Table 1), a large number of different M serotypes were isolated, including six strains that were not typable. Kaplan *et al.* (1989) found that several different M types were isolated from the patients seen during an outbreak of rheumatic fever, and that these strains were both mucoid and non-mucoid in character. Whether or not certain strains are more 'rheumatogenic' than others remains unresolved. What is true, however, is that a streptococcal strain capable of causing a well-documented pharyngitis is almost always potentially capable of causing rheumatic fever, although some notable exceptions have been recorded (reviewed by Whitnack and Bisno 1980).

Pathogenesis

There is little evidence for the direct involvement of group A strepto-cocci in the affected tissues of patients with acute rheumatic fever, but there is a large body of epidemiological and immunological evidence indirectly implicating the group A streptococcus in the initiation of the disease process. For example, (i) it is well known that outbreaks of rheumatic fever closely follow epidemics of either streptococcal sore throats or scarlet fever (Whitnack and Bisno 1980), (ii) adequate treatment of a documented streptococcal pharyngitis markedly reduces the incidence of subsequent rheumatic fever (Denny *et al.* 1950), (iii) approximate antimicrobial prophylaxis prevents recurrences of the disease in patients known to have had acute rheumatic fever (Markowitz and Gordis 1972), and (iv), if one tests the serum of the majority of patients with acute rheumatic fever for three antistreptococcal antibodies (streptolysin O, hyaluronidase, and streptokinase), the vast majority of samples (whether or not the patients recall an antecedent streptococcal sore throat) will have elevated antibody titres to these antigens (Stollerman *et al.* 1956).

A note of caution is necessary concerning the documentation (either clinical or microbiological) of an antecedent streptococcal infection. The rate of isolation of group A streptococci from the oropharynx is extremely low, even in populations who generally do not have access to microbial antibiotics. Further, there appears to be an age-related discrepancy in the clinical documentation of an antecedent sore throat. In older children and young adults, the recollection of a streptococcal sore throat approaches 70 per cent; in younger children, it approaches only 20 per cent (Veasy *et al.* 1987). Thus, it is important to have a high index of suspicion of acute rheumatic fever in children or young adults presenting with signs of arthritis and/or carditis, even in the absence of a clinically documented sore throat.

Another intriguing, and as yet unexplained, observation has been the invariable association of rheumatic fever only with streptococcal pharyngitis rather than other streptococcal lesions. While there have been many outbreaks of impetigo, rheumatic fever almost never follows infection with these impetigo strains. Furthermore, as Potter *et al.* (1978) have pointed out, in Trinidad, where both impetigo and rheumatic fever are concomitant infections, the strains colonizing the skin are different from those associated with rheumatic fever, and did not influence the incidence of acute rheumatic fever.

These observations remain inexplicable. It is clear that group A streptococci fall into two main classes based on differences in the C-repeat regions of the M protein (Bessen *et al.* 1989). One class is clearly associated with streptococcal pharyngeal infection, the other (with some exceptions) belongs to strains commonly associated with impetigo. Thus, the particular strain of streptococcus may be crucial

in initiating the disease process. The pharyngeal site of infection, with its large repository of lymphoid tissue, may also be important in the initiation of the abnormal humoral response by the host to those antigens cross-reactive with target organs (see below). Finally, while impetigo strains do colonize the pharynx, they do not appear to elicit as strong an immunological response to the M-protein moiety as do the pharyngeal strains (Kaplan *et al.* 1970; Bisno and Nelson 1975). This may prove to be an important factor, especially in light of the known cross-reactions between various streptococcal structures and mammalian proteins.

Group A streptococcus

Figure 1 is a schematic cross-section of the group A streptococcus. The capsule is composed of equimolar concentrations of *N*-acetyl glucosamine and glucuronic acid, and is structurally identical to hyaluronic acid of mammalian tissues (Kendall *et al.* 1937).

Numerous past attempts to demonstrate antibodies to this capsule were unsuccessful (Seastone 1939; Quinn and Singh 1957). More recently, Fillit *et al.* (1986) successfully demonstrated high titres to hyaluronic acid, using techniques designed to detect non-precipitating antibodies in the serum of animals. Similar antibodies have been found in man (Faarber *et al.* 1984). Almost no published data implicate this capsule as important in human infections, although Stollerman (1975) commented on the presence of a large mucoid capsule as one of the more important characteristics of certain 'rheumatogenic' strains.

Investigations by Dr Rebecca Lancefield and others, spanning almost 70 years (reviewed by Fischetti 1989), have established that the M-protein molecule (at least 80 distinct serological types) is perhaps the most important virulence factor in human group A streptococcal infections. The protein is a helical, coiled-coil structure; it has striking structural homology with the cardiac cytoskeletal proteins tropomyosin and myosin, as well as with many other coil-coiled structures like keratin, DNA, lamin, and vimentin.

Once the amino acid sequence of a number of M proteins became known, it was possible to localize specifically those cross-reactive areas. The studies of Dale and Beachey (1985) showed that the part of the M protein involved in the opsonic reaction also cross-reacted with human sarcolemmal antigens. Sargent *et al.* (1987) more precisely localized this cross-reaction to the M-protein amino acid residues 164–197.

The evidence implicating these cross-reactions in the pathogenesis of acute rheumatic fever remains scant. Antibodies to myosin have been detected in the serum of patients with acute rheumatic fever, but they are also present in a large percentage of sera obtained from individuals who have had a streptococcal infection but did not subsequently develop acute rheumatic fever (Cunningham *et al.* 1988). The significance of this observation is unclear, since myosin is an internal protein of cardiac muscle cells and therefore not easily exposed to M-protein cross-reacting antibodies.

The group-specific carbohydrate of the streptococcus is a polysaccharide chain consisting of repeating units of rhamnose capped by *N*-acetyl glucosamine molecules. The *N*-acetyl glucosamine is immunodominant and gives rise to the serological group specificity of group A streptococci (McCarty 1970). The cross-reaction between group A carbohydrate and valvular glycoproteins was first described by Goldstein *et al.* (1968), and the reactivity was related to the *N*-acetyl glucosamine moiety present in both structures. Goldstein and

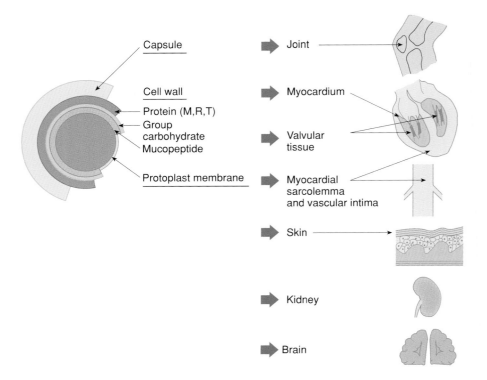

Fig. 1 Schematic representation of the various structures of the group A streptococcus. Note the wide variety of cross-reactions between its antigens and mammalian tissues.

Caravano (1967) noted that serum from patients with rheumatic fever reacted with the heart-valve glycoprotein. More recently, H. M. Fillit (personal communication) has observed strong reactivity of such sera with purified proteoglycan material. Thus, these cross-reactions could involve the sugar moiety present in both the proteoglycan portion of the glycoprotein and the carbohydrate.

It has always been assumed that group A anticarbohydrate antibodies did not play a part in the phagocytosis of group A streptococci. However, the studies of Salvadori *et al.* (1995) have demonstrated that human serum containing high titres of anti-group A carbohydrate antibody were opsonophagocytic for a number of different M-protein-specific strains, and that the opsonophagocytic properties were directed to the *N*-acetyl glucosamine moiety of the group A carbohydrate.

The mucopeptide portion of the cell wall is the 'backbone' of the organism and thus rather rigid in structure. It is composed of repeating units of muramic acid and *N*-acetyl glucosamine, cross-linked by peptide bridges (Chetty and Schwab 1984). It is particularly difficult to degrade and induces a wide variety of lesions when injected into various species, including arthritis in rats (Cromartie *et al.* 1977) and myocardial granulomas in mice that resemble (but are not identical to) lesions in rheumatic fever (Cromartie and Craddock 1966).

The connection between cell-wall mucopeptides and the pathogenesis of rheumatic fever remains obscure. Elevated titres of antimucopeptide antibody have been detected in the serum of patients with acute rheumatic fever, and also in the serum of patients with rheumatoid and juvenile rheumatoid arthritis (Heymer *et al.* 1976), but their pathogenetic relation to the clinical disease has been difficult to establish. There is no evidence that cell-wall antigens are

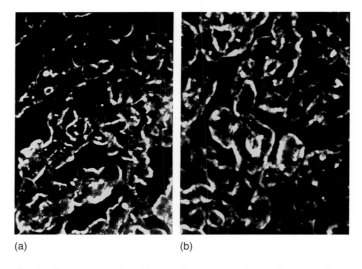

(a)   (b)

Fig. 2 Photomicrographs of immunofluorescent staining of heart sections with (a) rabbit serum immunized with group A streptococcal membranes and (b) serum obtained from a patient with acute rheumatic fever. Note the identical sarcolemmal staining patterns of both sera.

present either in the Aschoff lesion or in the myocardial tissue obtained from patients with rheumatic fever.

Perhaps the most significant cross-reactions lie in the streptococcal membrane structure. We have shown (Zabriskie 1985) that immunization with membrane material elicited antibodies that bound to sections of heart in a pattern similar to that observed with serum from acute rheumatic fever (see Fig. 2).

Kingston and Glynn (1971) were the first to show that animals immunized with streptococcal antigens develop serum antibodies that stain astrocytes. Husby *et al.* (1976) demonstrated that serum from patients with acute rheumatic fever with chorea contains antibodies that were specific for caudate cells. Absorption of the serum with streptococcal membrane antigens eliminated the reactivity with caudate cells.

Numerous other cross-reactions between streptococcal membranes and other organs have also been reported, for example renal basement membranes, basement membrane proteoglycans, and skin, particularly keratin. Here, space does not permit an exhaustive discussion of these cross-reactions, and the reader is referred to our recent review (Froude *et al.* 1989) for more detail. Whether or not these cross-reactions (especially those seen with basement membranes and skin) play a part in the disease awaits further study.

Genetics

The concept that rheumatic fever might be the result of a host genetic predisposition has intrigued investigators for over a century (Cheadle 1889). It has been variously suggested that the disease gene is transmitted in an autosomal-dominant fashion (Wilson *et al.* 1943), an autosomal-recessive fashion with limited penetrance (Taranta *et al.* 1959), or that it is possibly related to the genes conferring blood-group secretor status (Glynn and Holborow 1961).

Renewed interest in the genetics of rheumatic fever came with the recognition that gene products of the human major histocompatibility complex (**MHC**) were associated with certain clinical disease states. Using an alloserum from a multiparous donor, an increased frequency of a B-cell alloantigen was reported in several genetically distinct and ethnically diverse populations of individuals with rheumatic fever, and was not MHC-related (Patarroyo *et al.* 1979).

Most recently, studies were accomplished with a monoclonal antibody (D8/17) prepared by immunizing mice with B cells from a patient with rheumatic fever (Khanna *et al.* 1989). This B-cell antigen was expressed on increased numbers of B cells in 100 per cent of rheumatics of diverse ethnic origin, and only in 10 per cent of normal individuals. The antigen defined by this monoclonal antibody showed no association with, or linkage to, any of the known MHC haplotypes, nor did it appear to be related to B-cell activation antigens.

These findings are in contrast to reports of an increased frequency of HLA-DR4 and HLA-DR2 in white and black patients with rheumatic heart disease (Ayoub *et al.* 1986). Other studies have implicated HLA-DR1 and -DRW6 as susceptibility factors in Black South African patients with rheumatic heart disease (Maharaj *et al.* 1987). Most recently, Guilherme *et al.* (1991) have noted a close association of HLA-DR7 and -DW53 with rheumatic fever in Brazil. These apparently differing results concerning HLA antigens and susceptibility to rheumatic fever prompt speculation that the reported associations might involve genes close to, but not identical with, an unknown gene for that susceptibility. Alternatively, and more likely, susceptibility to acute rheumatic fever is polygenic, and the D8/17 antigen might be associated with only one of the genes (i.e., those of the MHC complex encoding for DR antigens) conferring susceptibility. While the explanation remains to be determined, it is none the less true that the presence of the D8/17 antigen appears to identify a population at special risk for contracting acute rheumatic fever.

Aetiological considerations

While a large body of evidence, both immunological and epidemiological, has implicated the group A streptococcus in the induction of the disease process, the exact pathological mechanisms involved still remain obscure. At least three main theories have been proposed.

The first is concerned with the question of whether persistence of the organism is important. Despite several controversial reports, no investigators have been able consistently to demonstrate live organisms in cardiac tissues or valves in rheumatic fever (Watson *et al.* 1961).

The second theory revolves around the question of whether the deposition of toxic products is required. Although an attractive hypothesis, little or no experimental evidence has been obtained in its support. For example, Halbert *et al.* (1961) suggested that streptolysin O (an extracellular product of group A streptococci) is cardiotoxic and might be carried to the site by circulating complexes containing streptolysin O and antibody. However, in spite of an intensive search for these products (J. B. Zabriskie, unpublished data), no such complexes have been identified *in situ* (Wagner 1960).

Renewed interest in these extracellular toxins has recently emerged with the observation by Schlievert *et al.* (1987) that certain streptococcal pyrogenic toxins (A and C) may act as superantigens. These antigens may stimulate large numbers of T cells through their unique interaction between MHC class II and T-cell receptors of specific V_β types. This interaction does not involve the usual concept of antigen presentation in the context of the MHC complex. Once activated, these cells induce the production of tumour necrosis factor, interferon-γ, and a number of interleukin moieties, thereby contributing to the initiation of pathological damage. Furthermore, it has been suggested (Paliard *et al.* 1991) that in certain disease states such as rheumatoid arthritis, autoreactive cells of specific V_β lineage may 'home' to the target organ. Although an attractive hypothesis, no data on the role of these superantigens in rheumatic fever have as yet emerged.

Perhaps the best evidence to date favours the concept that, in the genetically susceptible individual, there is an abnormal host immune response (both humoral and cellular) to those streptococcal antigens cross-reactive with mammalian tissues. The evidence supporting this concept may be divided into three broad categories as follows.

1. Employing a wide variety of methods, numerous investigators have documented the presence of heart-reactive antibodies in serum from rheumatic fever. The incidence of these antibodies has varied from a low of 33 per cent to a high or 85 per cent in various series. While these antibodies are seen in other individuals (notably those with uncomplicated streptococcal infections and patients with post-streptococcal glomerulonephritis), the titres are always lower than in rheumatic fever and decrease with time during the convalescent period (Zabriskie 1985).

2. Serum in rheumatic fever also contains higher titres of antibodies to both myosin and tropomyosin than serum from patients with uncomplicated streptococcal infections. These myosin affinity-purified antibodies also cross-react with M-protein moieties, suggesting this molecule could be the antigenic stimulus for the production of myosin antibodies in these sera (Cunningham *et al.* 1988).

3. Finally, as indicated above, autoimmune antibodies are a promi-

nent finding in another major clinical manifestation of acute rheumatic fever, chorea, and these antibodies are directed against the cells of the caudate nucleus. The titre of this antibody corresponds with clinical disease activity (Husby *et al.* 1976).

While not necessarily autoimmune in nature, the presence of elevated amounts of immune complexes has been well documented both in serum and joints in acute rheumatic fever (van de Rijn *et al.* 1978). These amounts, which may be as high as those seen in classical post-streptococcal glomerulonephritis, may be responsible for immune-complex vasculitis seen in acute rheumatic fever and may provide the initial impetus for vascular damage, followed by the secondary penetration of autoreactive antibodies. Support for the concept is found in the close clinical similarity of arthritis in rheumatic fever to experimentally induced serum sickness in animals or the arthritis secondary to drug hypersensitivity. Deposition of host immunoglobulin and complement is also seen in the cardiac tissues of patients with acute rheumatic fever, suggesting autoimmune deposition of immunoglobulins in or near the Aschoff lesions.

At a cellular level, there is now ample evidence for the presence of both lymphocytes and macrophages at the site of pathological damage in the heart in patients with acute rheumatic fever (Kemeny *et al.* 1989). The cells are predominantly CD4+ helper lymphocytes during acute stages of the disease (4:1). The ratio of CD4+/CD8+ lymphocytes (2:1) more closely approximates the normal ratio in valvular specimens in chronic rheumatics (see Table 2). A majority of these cells express Ia antigens. A potentially important finding has been the observation that macrophage-like fibroblasts present in the

diseased valves express Ia antigens (Amoils *et al.* 1986) and might be the antigen-presenting cells for the CD4+ lymphocytes.

There was greater reactivity to streptococcal antigens in preparations of mononuclear cells from peripheral blood of patients with acute rheumatic fever than in these cells isolated from patients with nephritis (Read *et al.* 1986). This abnormal reactivity peaked at 6 months after the attack but could persist for as long as 2 years after the initial episode. Once again the reactivity was specific only for those strains associated with acute rheumatic fever, suggesting an abnormal humoral and cellular response to streptococcal antigens unique to rheumatic fever-associated streptococci.

Support for the potential pathological importance of these T cells is further strengthened by the observation that lymphocytes obtained from experimental animals sensitized to cell membranes but not cell walls are specifically cytotoxic for syngeneic embryonic cardiac myofibrils in vitro (Yang *et al.* 1977). In humans, normal mononuclear cells primed in vitro by M-protein molecules from a rheumatic fever-associated strain were also cytotoxic for myofibrils but specificity solely for cardiac cells was lacking (Dale and Beachey 1987). Similar studies have not yet been done with lymphocytes from patients with active acute rheumatic fever.

Clinical features of acute rheumatic fever

The clinical presentation of acute rheumatic fever is rather variable, and the lack of a single pathognomonic feature has resulted in the

Table 2 Composition of mononuclear cellular infiltrates in acute and chronic active rheumatic valvulitis

Patients	Type of valve	Type of valvulitis[a]	HLA-DR+	63D3+[1]	Leu 16+[2]	Leu 4+[3]	Leu 3a+[4]	Leu 2a+[5]	Leu 3a : Leu 2a ratio
Acute valvulitis									
1	Mitral	Acute	58.9	42.6	5.1	49.5	75.6	23.9	3.1
2	Mitral	Acute	49.8	43.1	6.9	43.1	58.7	34.3	1.9
	Aortic	Acute	52.7	51.0	3.9	38.1	65.9	26.5	2.3
3	Mitral	Acute	63.9	42.0	5.5	52.4	75.4	18.9	4.0
4	Aortic	Acute	68.1	56.0	7.4	33.7	71.6	22.0	3.3
Chronic valvulitis									
4	Mitral	Chronic active	49.4	47.4	7.4	44.3	53.7	38.8	1.4
5	Mitral	Chronic active	48.8	39.1	1.4	53.9	45.2	51.5	0.9
	Aortic	Chronic active	67.8	35.0	4.0	36.8	47.5	49.1	1.0
6	Mitral	Chronic active	41.8	23.4	8.0	65.9	57.3	33.3	1.7
	Aortic	Chronic active	69.6	48.7	6.2	30.1	58.2	32.6	1.8
7	Mitral	Chronic active	55.4	24.2	8.1	59.8	64.9	24.7	2.6
8	Mitral	Chronic active	80.4	34.1	13.4	44.4	44.8	50.9	0.9
9	Mitral	Chronic active	46.1	29.6	0.8	65.6	61.6	33.3	1.8

[a]Determined in the frozen valve samples studied.
1, monocytes–macrophages; 2, B cells; 3, pan-T cells; 4, helper cells; 5, suppressor cells.

development of the revised Jones criteria, as illustrated in Table 3 (Jones Criteria Update 1992), which are used to establish a diagnosis. It should be noted that these criteria were established only as guidelines for the diagnosis and were never intended to be 'etched in stone'. Thus, depending on the age, geographical location, and ethnic population, emphasis on one or the other criterion for the diagnosis of acute rheumatic fever may be more or less important. Manifestations of rheumatic fever that are not clearly expressed pose a dilemma because of the importance of clearly identifying a first rheumatic attack in order to establish the need for prophylaxis (see below). Some of the isolated manifestations, particularly polyarthritis, may be difficult or impossible to distinguish from other diseases, especially at their onset. The diagnosis can be made, however, when 'pure' chorea is the sole manifestation, because of the rarity with which this syndrome is due to any other cause.

Arthritis

In the classic, untreated case the arthritis of rheumatic fever affects several joints in quick succession, each for a short time. The legs are usually affected first and later the arms. The terms 'migrating' or 'migratory' are often used to describe the polyarthritis of rheumatic fever, but these designations are not meant to signify that the inflammation necessarily disappears in one joint when it appears in another. Rather, the various localizations usually overlap in time, and the onset, as opposed to the full course of the arthritis, 'migrates' from joint to joint.

Joint involvement is more common, and also more severe, in teenagers and young adults than in children. It occurs early in the rheumatic illness, and is usually the earliest symptomatic manifestation of the disease, although asymptomatic carditis may precede it. Rheumatic polyarthritis may be excruciatingly painful, but is almost always transient. The pain is usually more prominent than the objective signs of inflammation.

When the disease was allowed to express itself fully, unchecked by anti-inflammatory treatment, over half of patients studied show a true polyarthritis, with inflammation in any of from 6 to 16 joints. Classically, each joint is maximally inflamed for only a few days, or a week at the most: the inflammation decreases, perhaps lingering for another week or so, and then disappears completely. Radiographs taken at this point may show a slight effusion but most probably will be unremarkable.

In routine practice, however, many patients with arthritis and/or arthralgias are treated empirically with salicylates or other non-steroidal anti-inflammatory drugs. Accordingly, arthritis subsides quickly in the joint(s) already affected and does not 'migrate' to new joints. Thus, therapy may deprive the diagnostician of a useful sign. In a large series of patients with rheumatic fever and associated arthritis, most of whom had been treated, involvement of only a single large joint was common (25 per cent). One or both knees were affected in 76 per cent, and one or both ankles in 50 per cent. Elbows, wrists, hips, or small joints of the feet were involved in 12 to 15 per cent of patients, and shoulder or small joints of the head were affected in 7 to 8 per cent. Joints rarely affected were the lumbosacral (2 per cent), cervical (1 per cent), sternoclavicular (0.5 per cent), and temporomandibular (0.5 per cent). Involvement of the small joints of the hands or feet alone occurred in only 1 per cent of these patients (Feinstein and Spagnulo 1962).

Analysis of the synovial fluid in well-documented cases of rheumatic fever with arthritis generally reveals a sterile inflammatory fluid. There may be a decrease of the complement components C1q, C3 and C4, indicating their consumption by immune complexes in the joint fluid (Svartman *et al.* 1975).

Post-streptococcal reactive arthritis

A number of investigators (Goldsmith and Long 1982; Arnold and Tyndall 1989; Fink 1991) have raised the question of whether post-streptococcal migratory arthritis, in the absence of carditis both in adults and children, is really acute rheumatic fever, for the following reasons.

(1) The latent period between the antecedent streptococcal infection and the onset of acute rheumatic fever is shorter (1–2 weeks) than the 3 to 4 weeks usually seen in classical acute rheumatic fever.

(2) The response of the arthritis to aspirin and other non-steroidal medications is poor in comparison to the dramatic response seen in classical acute rheumatic fever.

(3) Evidence of carditis is not usually seen in these patients and the arthritis is rather severe.

(4) Extra-articular manifestations such as tenosynovitis and renal abnormalities are often seen in these patients.

While these cases (admittedly rare) do exist, migratory arthritis without evidence of other major Jones criteria, if supported by two minor manifestations (see Table 3), must still be considered acute rheumatic fever, especially in children. Variations in the response to aspirin in these children often are not recorded with serum salicylate

Table 3 Revised Jones criteria for diagnosis of acute rheumatic fever

Major manifestations	Minor manifestations
Carditis	Fever
Polyarthritis	Arthralgia
Chorea	Previous rheumatic fever or rheumatic heart disease
Erythema marginatum	
Subcutaneous nodules	
Laboratory findings	
(1) Elevated acute-phase reactants:	
(a) C-reactive protein	
(b) erythrocyte sedimentation rate	
(2) Prolonged P–R interval rate	
Supporting evidence of proceeding streptococcal infection	
(a) Increased ASO or other streptococcal antibodies	
(b) Positive throat culture for group A haemolytic streptococci	
(c) Recent scarlet fever	

Jones Criteria Update (1992).
ASO, antistreptolysin O.

concentrations, and an unusual clinical course is not sufficient to exclude the diagnosis of acute rheumatic fever; appropriate prophylactic measures should be therefore taken (reviewed by Gibofsky and Zabriskie 1994). Support for this concept may be found in the work of Crea and Mortimer (1959), in which 50 per cent of the children with signs of migratory arthritis alone went on to develop significant valvular damage after a long follow-up.

Rheumatic fever also occurs in adults. Although migratory arthritis is a common presenting symptom, a recent outbreak in San Diego Naval Training Camp (Wallace *et al.* 1989) revealed a 30 per cent incidence of valvular damage in these patients.

The importance of clearly defining this reactive arthritis as a variant of rheumatic fever has obvious implications for secondary prophylactic treatment. As suggested by some investigators, post-streptococcal reactive arthritis is a benign condition without need for prophylaxis. Yet as these patients by and large do fulfil the Jones criteria (one major, two minor), they should be considered as having rheumatic fever and treated as such.

Carditis

Cardiac valvular and muscle damage can manifest in a variety of signs or symptoms, including organic heart murmurs, cardiomegaly, congestive heart failure or pericarditis. Mild to moderate chest discomfort, pleuritic chest pain or a pericardial friction rub are indications of pericarditis. On clinical examination, the patient can have new or changing organic murmurs, most commonly mitral regurgitant murmurs, and occasionally aortic regurgitant murmurs and/or systolic ejection murmurs, caused by acute valvular inflammation and deformity. Rarely, a Carey Coombs mid-diastolic murmur caused by rapid flow over the mitral valve is heard. If the valvular damage is severe enough, together with concurrent cardiac dysfunction, congestive heart failure can ensue, which is the most life-threatening clinical syndrome of acute rheumatic fever. Congestive heart failure needs to be treated intensively and quickly with a combination of anti-inflammatory drugs, diuretics and, occasionally, steroids to acutely decrease the cardiac inflammation. Electrocardiographic abnormalities include all degrees of heart block, including atrioventricular dissociation, but first-degree heart block is not associated with a poor prognosis. Second- or third-degree heart block can occasionally be symptomatic. If heart block is associated with congestive heart failure, a temporary pacemaker can be placed if indicated. The most common manifestation of carditis is cardiomegaly, as seen on radiographs.

In the population of patients recently reviewed from our institution, The Rockefeller University Hospital, who were diagnosed with acute rheumatic fever between 1950 and 1970, with an average of 20 years of follow-up, 90 per cent had evidence of carditis at diagnosis (Table 4). In a classic review of 1000 patients (Bland and Jones 1951), only 65 per cent were diagnosed with carditis. The addition of Doppler sonography to the clinical evaluation of patients during the recent Utah outbreak increased the proportion diagnosed with carditis from 72 to 91 per cent (Veasy *et al.* 1987), indicating that, with more sensitive measurements of cardiac dysfunction, almost all patients with acute rheumatic fever have signs of acute carditis.

Rheumatic heart disease

Rheumatic heart disease is the most severe outcome of acute rheumatic fever. Usually occurring 10 to 20 years after the original attack,

it is the major cause of acquired valvular disease in the world. The mitral valve is mainly involved and the aortic valve less often. Mitral stenosis is a classic finding in rheumatic heart disease and can manifest as a combination of mitral insufficiency and stenosis, secondary to severe calcification of the mitral valve. When symptoms of left atrial enlargement are present, mitral valve replacement may become necessary.

In various studies, the incidence of rheumatic heart disease in patients with a history of acute rheumatic fever has varied. In the classic study of Bland and Jones (1951), after 20 years, one-third of patients had no murmur, another one-third had died, and the remaining one-third was alive with rheumatic heart disease. A majority of the patients who died had rheumatic heart disease. While the dogma is that patients with rheumatic heart disease invariably have had more than one attack of acute rheumatic fever, recent analysis of our patients at the Rockefeller University Hospital disproves this. The population studied was 87 patients who had had only one documented attack of acute rheumatic fever, without any evidence (clinical or laboratory) of a recurrence during a 20-year follow-up under close supervision. Over 80 per cent had carditis at admission and approx. 50 per cent now have organic murmurs (Table 4). Thus, valvular damage manifesting as organic murmurs later in life is still likely to occur in 50 per cent of the patients if they presented with evidence of carditis at initial diagnosis. All of the patients in our population who ended up with rheumatic heart disease had carditis at diagnosis.

Chorea

Sydenham's chorea, chorea minor, or 'St. Vitus dance' is a neurological disorder consisting of abrupt, purposeless, non-rhythmic involuntary movements, muscular weakness, and emotional disturbances. They disappear during sleep, but may occur at rest and may interfere with voluntary activity. Initially, it may be possible to suppress these movements, which may affect all voluntary muscles, with the hands and face usually the most obvious. Grimaces and inappropriate smiles are common. Handwriting usually becomes clumsy and provides a convenient way of following the patient's course. Speech is often slurred. The movements are commonly more marked on one side and are occasionally completely unilateral (hemichorea).

Table 4 Physical signs and symptoms of acute rheumatic fever, Rockefeller University Hospital 1950–1970

	RHD (*n*=40) %	No RHD (*n*=47) %	Total (*n*=87) %	Bland and Jones %
Carditis	100	83.0	90.1	65.3
Arthritis	67.5	68.1	67.8	41.0
Epistaxis	0.0	10.6	5.7	27.4
Chorea	5.0	2.1	3.4	51.8
Pericarditis	2.5	4.3	3.4	13.0
Nodules	7.5	0.0	3.4	8.8
Erythema marginatum	0.0	4.3	2.3	7.1

The muscular weakness is best revealed by asking the patient to squeeze the examiner's hands: the pressure of the patient's grip increases and decreases continuously and capriciously, a phenomenon known as relapsing grip, or milking sign.

The emotional changes manifest themselves in outbursts of inappropriate behaviour, including crying and restlessness. In rare cases, the psychological manifestations may be severe and may result in transient psychosis.

The neurological examination fails to reveal sensory losses or involvement of the pyramidal tract. Diffuse hypotonia may be present.

Chorea may follow streptococcal infections after a latent period, which is longer, on the average, than the latent period of other rheumatic manifestations. Some patients with chorea have no other symptoms, but other patients develop chorea weeks or months after arthritis. In both cases, examination of the heart may reveal murmurs.

Skin lesions

Subcutaneous nodules

The subcutaneous nodules of rheumatic fever are firm and painless. The overlying skin is not inflamed and can usually be moved over the nodules. The diameter of these round lesions varies from a few millimetres to 1 or even 2 cm. They are located over bony surface or prominences, or near tendons; their number varies from a single nodule to a few dozen and averages three or four; when numerous, they are usually symmetrical. These nodules are present for one or more weeks, rarely for more than a month. They are smaller and more short-lived than the nodules of rheumatoid arthritis. Although in both diseases the elbows are most frequently involved, the rheumatic nodules are more common on the olecranon, and the rheumatoid nodules are usually found 3 or 4 cm distal to it. Rheumatic subcutaneous nodules generally appear only after the first few weeks of illness, usually only in patients with carditis.

Erythema marginatum

Erythema marginatum is an evanescent, non-pruritic skin rash, pink or faintly red, usually affecting the trunk, sometimes the proximal parts or the limbs, but not the face. The lesion extends centrifugally while the skin in the centre returns gradually to normal; hence, the name 'erythema marginatum'. The outer edge of the lesion is sharp, whereas the inner edge is diffuse. Because the margin of the lesion is usually continuous, making a ring, it is also known as 'erythema annulare'.

The individual lesions may appear and disappear in a matter of hours, usually to return. A hot bath or shower may make them more evident or may even reveal them for the first time.

Erythema marginatum usually occurs in the early phase of the disease. It often persists or recurs, even when all other manifestations of disease have disappeared. Occasionally, the lesions appear for the first time or, more probably, are noticed for the first time, late in the course of the illness or even during convalescence. This disorder usually occurs only in patients with carditis.

The minor manifestations of rheumatic fever

Temperature is increased in almost all rheumatic attacks and ranges from 38.4 to 40°C. Usually fever decreases in about a week without antipyretic treatment, and may become low grade for another week or two. Fever rarely lasts for more than 3 to 4 weeks.

Abdominal pain

The abdominal pain of rheumatic fever resembles that of other conditions associated with acute microvascular mesenteric inflammation and is non-specific. It usually occurs at or near the onset of the rheumatic attack, so that other manifestations may not yet be present to clarify the diagnosis. In many cases, it may mimic acute appendicitis.

Epistaxis

In the past, epistaxis occurred most prominently and severely in patients with severe and protracted rheumatic carditis. Early clinical studies reported a frequency as high as 48 per cent, but it probably occurs even less frequently now (see Table 3). Although epistaxis has been correlated in the past with the severity of rheumatic inflammation, it is difficult to assess retrospectively the possible thrombasthenic effect of large doses of salicylates administered for prolonged periods in protracted attacks.

Rheumatic pneumonia

Rheumatic pneumonia may appear during the course of severe rheumatic carditis. This inflammatory process is difficult or impossible to distinguish from pulmonary oedema or the alveolitis associated with respiratory distress syndrome due to a variety of pathophysiological states.

Laboratory findings

The diagnosis of rheumatic fever cannot readily be established by laboratory tests. Nevertheless, tests may be helpful in two ways: first in demonstrating that an antecedent streptococcal infection has occurred and second in documenting the presence or persistence of an inflammatory process. Serial chest radiographs may be helpful in following the course of carditis and the electrocardiogram may reflect the inflammatory process on the conduction system.

Throat cultures are usually negative by the time rheumatic fever appears but an attempt should be made to isolate the organism. It is our practice to take three throat cultures during the first 24 h, before giving antibiotics. Streptococcal antibodies are more useful because (i) they reach a peak titre at about the time of onset of rheumatic fever, (ii) they indicate true infection rather than transient carriage, and (ii) by performing several tests for different antibodies, any significant recent streptococcal infection can be detected. To demonstrate a rising titre, it is useful to take a serum specimen when the patient is first seen and another one 2 weeks later for comparison.

The specific antibody tests most frequently used to diagnose streptococcal infections are those directed against extracellular products. They include antistreptolysin O, anti-DNAse B, antihyaluronidase, anti-NADase (anti-DPNase), and antistreptokinase. Antistreptolysin O has been the most widely used test and is generally available in hospitals in the United States.

Titres of antistreptolysin O vary with age, season, and geographical region. They reach peak levels in the young, school-age population. Titres of 200 to 300 Todd units/ml are common, therefore, in healthy children of elementary-school age. After a streptococcal pharyngitis, the antibody response peaks at about 4 to 5 weeks, which is usually during the second or third week of rheumatic fever (depending on how early it is detected). Thereafter, antibody titres fall off rapidly in the next several months, and, after 6 months, they decline more slowly. Since only 80 per cent of documented rheumatics exhibit a rise in the titre of antistreptolysin O, it is recommended that other antistreptococcal antibody tests be performed in the absence of a positive titre. These include anti-DNAse B, hyaluronidase or streptozyme, which is a combination of various streptococcal antigens.

Streptococcal antibodies, when increased, support but do not prove the diagnosis of acute rheumatic fever, nor are they a measure of rheumatic activity. Even in the absence of intercurrent streptococcal infection, titres decline during the rheumatic attack despite the persistence or severity of rheumatic activity.

Acute-phase reactants

Acute-phase reactants are elevated during acute rheumatic fever, just as they are during other inflammatory conditions. Both the C-reactive protein and erythrocyte sedimentation rate are almost invariably abnormal during the active rheumatic process, if it is not suppressed by antirheumatic drugs. Pure chorea and persistent erythema marginatum are exceptions. Particularly when treatment has been discontinued or is being tapered off, the C-reactive protein or erythrocyte sedimentation rate are useful in monitoring 'rebounds' of rheumatic inflammation, which indicate that the rheumatic process is still active. If either remains normal a few weeks after discontinuing antirheumatic therapy, the attack may be considered ended unless chorea appears. Even then, usually, there will be no exacerbation of the systemic inflammation and chorea will be present as an isolated manifestation.

Anaemia

A mild normochromic normocytic anaemia of chronic infection or inflammation may be seen during acute rheumatic fever. Suppressing the inflammation usually improves the anaemia, thus iron therapy is usually not indicated.

Clinical course and treatment of acute rheumatic fever

The mainstay of treatment for acute rheumatic fever has always been anti-inflammatory agents, most commonly aspirin. Dramatic improvement in symptoms is usually seen after the start of therapy. Usually 80 to 100 mg/kg per day in children and 4 to 8 g/day in adults is required for an effect to be seen. Aspirin concentrations can be measured and 20 to 30 mg/dl is the therapeutic range. The duration of anti-inflammatory therapy can vary but the treatment should be maintained until all symptoms are absent and laboratory values are normal. If severe carditis is also present, as indicated by significant cardiomegaly, congestive heart failure or third-degree heart block, steroid therapy can be instituted. The usual dosage is 2 mg/kg per day of oral prednisone during the first 1 to 2 weeks. Depending on clinical and laboratory improvement, the dosage is then tapered over the next 2 weeks and during the last week aspirin may be added in the dosage recommended above sufficient to achieve 20 to 30 mg/dl.

Whether or not signs of pharyngitis are present at the time of diagnosis, antibiotic therapy with penicillin should be started and maintained for at least 10 days, in doses recommended for the eradication of a streptococcal pharyngitis. In addition, all family contacts should be cultured and treated for streptococcal infection, if positive. If compliance is an issue, depot penicillins, such as benzathine penicillin G 600 000 units in children, 1.2 million units in adults, should be given. Recurrences of acute rheumatic fever are most common within 2 years of the original attack but can occur at any time. The risk of recurrence decreases with age. Recurrence rates have been decreasing, from 20 to 2 to 4 per cent in recent outbreaks. This might be due to better surveillance and treatment.

Prophylaxis

Antibiotic prophylaxis with penicillin should be started immediately after the resolution of the acute episode. The optimal regimen consists of oral penicillin VK 250 000 units twice a day, or depot intramuscular injection of 1.2 million units penicillin G every 4 weeks. Recent data suggest, however, that injections every 3 weeks are more effective than every 4 weeks in preventing recurrences of acute rheumatic fever (Lue et al. 1986). If the patient is allergic to penicillin, erythromycin 250 mg/day can be substituted.

The end-point of prophylaxis is unclear; most believe it should continue at least until the patient is a young adult, which is usually 10 years from an acute attack with no recurrence. In our opinion, individuals with documented evidence of rheumatic heart disease should be on continuous prophylaxis indefinitely since our experience has been that rheumatic fever can recur even in the fifth or sixth decades. Another potential problem for recurrences is the presence in the household of young children who could transmit new group A streptococcal infections to rheumatic-susceptible individuals.

Obviously the alternative to long-term prophylaxis in an individual with rheumatic fever will be the introduction of streptococcal vaccines designed not only to prevent recurrent infections in rheumatic-susceptible individuals but also to prevent streptococcal disease in general. While it is not within the scope of this chapter to discuss the prospects for these vaccines (see review by Fischetti 1989), at least a few words are appropriate. Immunization of mice with either C-repeat peptides of M protein or 'cloned' M protein in a vaccinia virus vector protected them against intranasal infection with homologous or heterologous strains of group A streptococci. Whether or not these antigens and/or vectors are protective in man is being investigated. One of the major problems will be to avoid using those parts of the molecule that are cross-reactive with mammalian tissues.

Conclusion

In spite of its disappearance in many areas, rheumatic fever continues to be a serious problem in those geographical areas where two-thirds of the world's population lives. Even in developed countries with full access to medical care, and better nutrition and housing, the recent resurgence of rheumatic fever emphasizes the need for continued vigilance by physicians and other health officials in both diagnosing and treating the disease. The importance of early diagnosis and therapy cannot be overemphasized. Although the joint manifestations are transient and self-limiting, the cardiac sequelae are chronic and life-threatening. Whether the resurgence represents a change in the virulence of the organism or failure to recognize the importance and need for adequate treatment of an antecedent streptococcal infection is an area of intense debate and will therefore require careful and controlled epidemiological surveillance.

Nevertheless, rheumatic fever remains one of the few autoimmune disorders known to occur as a result of infection with a specific organism. The confirmed observation of an increased frequency of a B-cell alloantigen in several populations of rheumatics suggests that it might be possible to identify rheumatic fever-susceptible individuals at birth. If so, then from a public health standpoint, (i) these individuals would be prime candidates for immunization with any streptococcal vaccine that might be developed in the future, (ii) careful monitoring of streptococcal disease in the susceptible population could lead to early and effective antibiotic strategies, resulting in disease prevention, and (iii), in individuals previously infected, who later present with subtle or non-specific manifestations of the disease, the presence or absence of the marker could be of value in arriving at a diagnosis.

The continued study of rheumatic fever as a prime example of microbial–host interactions also has important implications for the study of autoimmune diseases in general and rheumatic diseases in particular. Further insights into this intriguing host–parasite relation may shed additional light on those diseases where infection is assumed to have occurred but has not as yet been identified.

References

Amoils, B. *et al.* (1986). Aberrant expression of HLA-DR antigen on valvular fibroblasts from patients with acute rheumatic carditis. *Clinical and Experimental Immunology*, **66**, 84–94.

Arnold, M. H. and Tyndall, A. (1989). Post-streptococcal reactive arthritis. *Annals of the Rheumatic Diseases*, **48**, 681–8.

Ayoub, E. A., Barrett, D. J., Maclaren, N. K., and Krischer, J. P. (1986). Association of class II human histocompatibility leucocyte antigens with rheumatic fever. *Journal of Clinical Investigation*, **77**, 2019–26.

Bessen, D., Jones, K. F., and Fischetti, V. A. (1989). Evidence for the distinct classes of streptococcal M protein and their relationship to rheumatic fever. *Journal of Experimental Medicine*, **169**, 269–83.

Bisno, A. L. and Nelson, K. E. (1975). Type-specific opsonic antibodies in streptococcal pyoderma. *Infection and Immunity*, **10**, 1356–61.

Bland, E. F. and Jones, T. D. (1951). Rheumatic fever and rheumatic heart disease: a twenty year report on 1,000 patients followed since childhood. *Circulation*, **4**, 836–43.

Cheadle, W. B. (1889). Harvean lectures on the various manifestations of the rheumatic state as exemplified in childhood and early life. *Lancet*, **i**, 821–32.

Chetty, C. and Schwab, J. H. (1984). Chemistry of endotoxins. In *Handbook of endotoxin*, Vol. 1. (ed. E. T. Rietschel Elsenier), pp. 376–410. Elsevier Science Publishers BV, Amsterdam.

Crea, M. A. and Mortimer, E. A. (1959). The nature of scarlatinal arthritis. *Pediatrics*, **23**, 879–84.

Cromartie, W. J. and Craddock, J. B. (1966). Rheumatic-like cardiac lesions in mice. *Science*, **154**, 285–7.

Cromartie, W. J., Craddock, J. B., Schwab, J. H., Anderle, S. K., and Yang, C. H. (1977). Arthritis in rats after systemic injection of streptococcal cells or cell walls. *Journal of Experimental Medicine*, **146**, 1585–602.

Cunningham, M. W. *et al.* (1988). Human monoclonal antibodies reactive with antigens of the group A streptococcus and human heart. *Journal of Immunology*, **141**, 2760–6.

Dale, J. B. and Beachey, E. H. (1985). Multiple cross reactive epitopes of streptococcal M proteins. *Journal of Experimental Medicine*, **161**, 113–22.

Dale, J. B. and Beachey, E. H. (1987). Human cytotoxic T lymphocytes evoked by group A streptococcal M proteins. *Journal of Experimental Medicine*, **166**, 1825–35.

Denny, F. W., Jr, Wannamaker, L. W., Brink, W. R., Rammelcamp, C. H., and Custer, E. A. (1950). Prevention of rheumatic fever: treatment of the preceding streptococcal infection. *Journal of the American Medical Association*, **143**, 151–3.

Faarber, P. *et al.* (1984). Cross reactivity of anti DNA antibodies with proteoglycans. *Clinical and Experimental Immunology*, **55**, 402–12.

Feinstein, A. R. and Spagnulo, M. (1962). The clinical patterns of rheumatic fever: a reappraisal *Medicine*, **41**, 279–305.

Fillit, H. M., McCarty, M., and Blake, M. (1986). Induction of antibodies to hyaluronic acid by immunization of rabbits with encapsulated streptococci. *Journal of Experimental Medicine*, **164**, 762–76.

Fink, C. W. (1991). The role of streptococcus in post streptococcal reactive arthritis and childhood polyarteritis nodosa. *Journal of Rheumatology*, **18**, 14–20.

Fischetti, V. A. (1989). Streptococcal M protein: molecular design and biological behavior. *Clinical and Microbiology Reviews*, **2**, 285–314.

Froude, J., Gibofsky, A., Buskirk, D. R., Khanna, A., and Zabriskie, J. B. (1989). Cross reactivity between streptococcus and human tissue: a model of molecular mimicry and autoimmunity. *Current Topics in Microbiology and Immunology*, **145**, 5–26.

Gibofsky, A. and Zabriskie, J. B. (1994). Rheumatic fever: new insights into an old disease. *Bulletin on the Rheumatic Diseases: Arthritis Foundation*, **42**, 5–7.

Glynn, L. E. and Holborow, E. J. (1961). Relationship between blood groups, secretion status and susceptibility to rheumatic fever. *Arthritis and Rheumatism*, **4**, 203.

Goldsmith, D. P. and Long, S. S. (1982) Poststreptococcal disease of childhood—a changing syndrome. *Arthritis and Rheumatism*, **25**, S18 (Abstr.).

Goldstein, I. and Caravano, R. (1967). Determination of anti group A streptococcal polysaccharide antibodies in human sera by an hemagglutination technique. *Proceedings of the Society of Experimental Biology and Medicine*, **124**, 1209–12.

Goldstein, I., Rebeyrotte, P., Parlebas, J., and Halpern, B., (1968). Isolation from heart valves of glycopeptides which share immunological properties with *Streptococcus haemolyticus* group A polysaccharides. *Nature*, **219**, 866–8.

Gordis, L. (1985). The virtual disappearance of rheumatic fever in the United States: lessons in the rise and fall of disease. *Circulation*, **72**, 1155–62.

Guilherme, L., Weidenbach, W., Kiss, M. H., Snitcowsky, R., and Kalil, J. (1991). Association of human leucocyte class II antigens with rheumatic fever or rheumatic heart disease in a Brazilian population. *Circulation*, **83**, 1995–8.

Halbert, S. P., Bircher, R., and Dahle, E. (1961). The analysis of streptococcal infections. V. Cardiotoxicity of streptolysin O for rabbits *in vivo*. *Journal of Experimental Medicine*, **113**, 759–84.

Heymer, B., Schleifer, K. H., Read, S. E., Zabriskie, J. B., and Krause, R. M. (1976). Detection of antibodies to bacterial cell wall peptidoglycan in human sera. *Journal of Immunology*, **117**, 23–6.

Husby, G., van de Rijn, I., Zabriskie, J. B., Abdin, Z. H., and Williams, R. C., Jr (1976). Antibodies reacting with cytoplasm of subthalmic and caudate nuclei neurons in chorea and acute rheumatic fever. *Journal of Experimental Medicine*, **144**, 1094–110.

Jones Criteria Update (1992). Guidelines for diagnosis of rheumatic fever. *Journal of the American Medical Association*, **268**, 2069–70.

Kaplan, E. L., Anthony, B. F., Chapman, S. S., Ayoub, E. M., and Wannamaker, L. W. (1970). The influence of the site of infection on the immune response to group A streptococci. *Journal of Clinical Investigation*, **49**, 1405–14.

Kaplan, E. L., Johnson, D. R., and Cleary, P. P. (1989). Group A streptococcal serotypes isolated from patients and sibling contacts during the resurgence of rheumatic fever in the United States in the mid 1980's. *Journal of Infectious Diseases*, **159**, 101–3.

Kemeny, E., Grieve, T., Marcus, R., Sareli, P., and Zabriskie, J. B. (1989). Identification of mononuclear cells and T cell subsets in rheumatic valvulitis. *Clinical Immunology and Immunopathology*, **52**, 225–37.

Kendall, F., Heidelberger, M., and Dawson, M. (1937). A serologically inactive polysaccharide elaborated by mucoid strains of group A hemolytic streptococcus. *Journal of Biological Chemistry*, **118**, 61–82.

Khanna, A. K., Buskirk, D. R., Williams, R. C., Jr, Gibofsky, A., Crow, M. K., and Menon, A. (1989). Presence of a non-HLA B cell antigen in rheumatic fever patients and their families as defined by a monoclonal antibody. *Journal of Clinical Investigation*, **83**, 1710–16.

Kingston, D. and Glynn, L. E. (1971). A cross-reaction between *Streptococcus pyogenes* and human fibroblasts, endothelial cells and astrocytes. *Immunology*, **21**, 1003–16.

Lue, H. C., Mil-Wham, W., Hsieh, K. H., Lin, G. J., Hsieh, R. P., and Chou, F. F. (1986). Rheumatic fever recurrences: controlled study of 3 week versus 4 week benzathine penicillin prevention programs. *Journal of Pediatrics*, **108**, 299–304.

McCarty, M. (1970). The streptococcal cell wall. *The Harvey Lectures Series*, **65**, 73–96.

Maharaj, B., Hammond, M. G., Appadoo, B., Leary, W. P., and Pudifin, D. J. (1987). HLA-A, B, DR and DQ antigens in black patients with severe chronic rheumatic heart disease. *Circulation*, **765**, 259–61.

Markowitz, M. (1987). Rheumatic fever: recent outbreaks of an old disease. *Connecticut Medicine*, **51**, 229–33.

Markowitz, M. and Gordis, L. (1972). *Rheumatic fever*, (2nd edn). Saunders, Philadelphia.

Paliard, X. *et al.* (1991). Evidence for the effects of superantigen in rheumatoid arthritis. *Science*, **253**, 325–9.

Patarroyo, M. E. *et al.* (1979). Association of a B cell alloantigen with susceptibility to rheumatic fever. *Nature*, **278**, 173–4.

Pope, R. M. (1989). Rheumatic fever in the 1980s. *Bulletin on the Rheumatic Diseases, Arthritis Foundation*, **38**, 1–8.

Potter, E. V., Svartman, M., Mohammed, I., Cox, R., Poon-King, T., and Earle, D. P. (1978). Tropical acute rheumatic fever and associated streptococcal infections compared with concurrent acute glomerulonephritis., *Journal of Pediatrics*, **92**, 325–33.

Quinn, R. W. and Singh, K. P. (1957). Antigenicity of hyaluronic acid. *Biochemical Journal*, **95**, 290–301.

Read, S. E. *et al.* (1986). Serial studies on the cellular immune response to streptococcal antigens in acute and convalescent rheumatic fever patients in Trinidad. *Journal of Clinical Immunology*, **6**, 433–41.

Salvadori, L. G., Blake, M. S., McCarty, M., Tai, J. Y., and Zabriskie, J. B. (1995). Group A streptococcus-liposome ELISA antibody titers to group A polysaccharide and opsonophagocytic capabilities of the antibodies. *Journal of Infectious Diseases*, **171**, 593–600.

Sargent, S. J., Beachey, E. H., Corbett, C. E., and Dale, J. B. (1987). Sequence of protective epitopes of streptococcal M proteins shared with cardiac sarcolemmal membranes. *Journal of Immunology*, **139**, 1285–90.

Schlievert, P. M., Johnson, L. P., Tomai, M. A., and Handley, J. P. (1987). Characterization and genetics of group A streptococcal pyrogenic exotoxins. In *Streptococcal genetics* (ed. J. Ferretti and R. Curtisis), pp. 136–42. ASM, Washington DC.

Seastone, C. V. (1939). The virulence of group C hemolytic streptococci of animal origin. *Journal of Experimental Medicine*, **70**, 361–78.

Stollerman, G. H. (ed.) (1975). In *Rheumatic fever and streptococcal infection*, p.70. Grune and Stratton, New York.

Stollerman, G. H., Lewis, A. J., Schultz, I., and Taranta, A. (1956). Relationship of the immune response to group A streptococci to the cause of acute, chronic and recurrent rheumatic fever. *American Journal of Medicine*, **20**, 163–9.

Svartman, M., Potter, E. V., and Poon-King, T. (1975). Immunoglobulin components in synovial fluids of patients with acute rheumatic fever. *Journal of Clinical Investigation*, **56**, 111–17.

Taranta, A. *et al.* (1959). Rheumatic fever in monozygotic and dizygotic twins. *Circulation*, **20**, 778–92.

van de Rijn, I. *et al.* (1978). Serial studies on circulating immune complexes in post-streptococcal sequelae. *Clinical and Experimental Immunology*, **34**, 318–25.

Veasy, L. G. *et al.* (1987). Resurgence of acute rheumatic fever in the intermountain area of the United States. *New England Journal of Medicine*, **316**, 421–7.

Wagner, B. M. (1960). Studies in rheumatic fever. III. Histochemical reactivity of the Aschoff body. *Annals of the New York Academy of Sciences*, **86**, 992–1008.

Wallace, M. R., Garst, P. D., Papadimos, T. J., and Oldfield, E. C. (1989). The return of acute rheumatic fever in young adults. *Journal of the American Medical Association*, **262**, 2557–61.

Watson, R. F., Hirst, G. K., and Lancefield, R. C. (1961). Bacteriological studies of cardiac tissues obtained at autopsy from eleven patients dying with rheumatic fever. *Arthritis and Rheumatism*, **4**, 74–85.

Whitnack, E. and Bisno, A. L. (1980). Rheumatic fever and other immunologically mediated cardiac diseases. In *Clinical immunology*, Vol. II. (ed. C. Parker), pp. 894–929. Saunders, Philadelphia.

Wilson, M. G., Schweitzr, M. D., and Lubschez, R. (1943). The familial epidemiology of rheumatic fever. *Journal of Pediatrics*, **22**, 468–82.

Yang, L. C., Soprey, P. R., Wittner, M. K., and Fox, E. N. (1977). Streptococcal induced cell mediated immune destruction of cardiac myofibers in vitro. *Journal of Experimental Medicine*, **146**, 344–60.

Zabriskie, J. B. (1985). Rheumatic fever: The interplay between host genetics and microbe. *Circulation*, **71**, 1077–86.

5.4 Rheumatoid arthritis

5.4.1 Immunopathogenesis of rheumatoid arthritis

Ravinder N. Maini and Marc Feldmann

Historical review

The delineation of rheumatoid arthritis as a disease entity in the contemporary medical literature began to emerge in the eighteenth century. Initially, clinical observations sought to distinguish the disorder from other prevalent joint diseases, such as gout and rheumatic fever, and emphasized distinctive features, for example, its chronicity, joint deformities, female sex distribution, and disability. Thus Sydenham (1676), Landry-Beauvais (1800), Brodie, and others were in all probability describing rheumatoid arthritis in their writings, but it was Alfred Baring Garrod (1859) who first used the term 'rheumatoid' arthritis (Garrod 1859; and for reviews see Short 1974 and Fraser 1982).

The definition of rheumatoid arthritis and its separation from other forms of chronic polyarthritis did not end with Garrod, and has continued to evolve since. A proportion of patients who might previously have been diagnosed as having rheumatoid arthritis would now be readily reclassified as having polyarthritis seen in the context of ankylosing spondylitis, Reiter's syndrome, psoriatic arthritis, or inflammatory bowel disease. The uniform lack of rheumatoid factor (seronegativity), spinal involvement, and HLA-B27 positivity has linked these disorders into the so-called seronegative spondylarthropathies. It is of special historical interest to note that until the late 1950s, despite striking differences in clinical features, ankylosing spondylitis was termed rheumatoid spondylitis by North American physicians in the belief that it was part of the disease spectrum of rheumatoid arthritis. This view was essentially based on the striking histopathological similarity to rheumatoid arthritis of the synovitis and erosive arthropathy of diarthrodial joints in ankylosing spondylitis. However, the inflammatory lesion at the point of tendon and ligamentous attachments to bone (enthesopathy) and the association with HLA B27 proved to be sufficiently distinctive to constitute a basis for differentiation from rheumatoid arthritis.

The possibility that rheumatoid arthritis may result from an infection has had its proponents since the early part of the century. In the early days of modern medicine, rheumatoid arthritis, like other diseases of unknown causes, was thought to result from foci of infection (Hunter 1901; Wilcox 1935). The belief that rheumatoid arthritis may result from infection with *Mycobacterium tuberculosis* is alleged to have motivated Forrestier in France (Forrestier 1935) to use gold salts,

which have some antimicrobial activity, in its therapy. An alternative concept of the aetiology of rheumatoid arthritis arose from microscopical observations of 'fibrinoid' change in rheumatoid joints and nodules. Fibrinoid change in connective tissue in systemic lupus and systemic sclerosis had prompted Klemperer *et al.* (1942) to consider that these diseases might result from diffuse primary degeneration of collagen. This led to the inclusion of rheumatoid arthritis in the group of 'collagen diseases'; however, the development of this new theory was hampered by the observation that the hydroxyproline and collagen content of subcutaneous nodules in rheumatoid arthritis was normal (Ziff *et al.* 1953).

The discovery by Waaler half a century ago (Waaler 1940) of IgM rheumatoid factor in the blood of patients with rheumatoid arthritis was the first immunological marker of rheumatic disease to be recognized and served to distinguish it from other forms of arthritis. However, a proportion of patients with the features of rheumatoid arthritis are persistently seronegative for rheumatoid factor, and this has formed the basis for a subdivision of rheumatoid arthritis, from which the recognized entity of seronegative spondylarthropathies arose. The patients who still remain in the category 'seronegative rheumatoid arthritis' may eventually prove to be a distinct subgroup with a different aetiological basis.

The finding of other autoantibodies circulating in the blood of patients with chronic polyarthritis has provided a continuing impetus for recognition of distinct rheumatic disorders. Notable, and first among these, was the LE cell test described by Hargraves *et al.* (1948), dependent on the presence of antinuclear antibodies, which served to distinguish patients with the polyarthritis of systemic lupus from those with rheumatoid arthritis. The better definition of the antigens with which such autoantibodies react has led to greater confidence in their diagnostic specificity; thus, antibodies to double-stranded-DNA and Sm antigen will distinguish systemic lupus from rheumatoid arthritis with some certainty. Similarly, more contemporary laboratory tests have contributed to the serological basis of disease classification of a patient with polyarthritis superficially resembling rheumatoid arthritis. The presence of anti-La (anti-SS-B) antibodies raises the strong probability of a diagnosis of primary Sjögren's syndrome, the presence of anticentromere or anti-Scl-70 antibodies suggests a diagnosis of systemic sclerosis, of anti-nRNP and anti-Jo-1 a diagnosis of overlap or mixed connective tissue disease, and of antineutrophil cytoplasmic antibody a diagnosis of Wegener's granulomatosis.

The relatively recent historical description of rheumatoid arthritis has prompted the speculation that it is a disease of modern times. A great deal of interest has therefore focused on seeking evidence of the occurrence of rheumatoid arthritis in mediaeval and ancient times. Examination of ancient medical writings and mediaeval paintings has yielded evidence which has satisfied some researchers that rheumatoid arthritis was indeed prevalent in these periods (Short 1974; Dequeker 1987; Dieppe 1988). However, subjectivity of judgement is an obvious problem in assessing such evidence and there appears to be a dearth of convincing descriptions, given that nowadays rheumatoid arthritis is such a common and ubiquitous cause of disability and pain. Another approach in establishing the antiquity of rheumatoid arthritis has been an attempt to gauge its prevalence by using palaeontographic methods. Fossil remains of archaic Indian skeletons found in Alabama and Kentucky in the United States, dated as several thousand years old, have been described as exhibiting changes consistent with an erosive arthritis compatible with rheumatoid arthritis (Rothschild and Woods 1990). However, the basis of ascribing the changes to rheumatoid arthritis has been challenged and the lack of rheumatoid pathology in a study of 800 skeletons excavated in the West Country in England has been used as an argument highlighting the lack of this disorder in ancient times (Rogers and Dieppe 1990).

The implication of the claim that rheumatoid arthritis is a relatively modern disease is the possibility that it might have become widespread as a result of an environmental trigger factor which in itself was new. A report from South Africa purporting to demonstrate an increased prevalence of rheumatoid arthritis in Xhosa tribesmen living in urban surroundings compared with their cousins in rural areas (Solomon et al. 1975) has been interpreted as a recapitulation in a contemporary setting of a global scenario unfolding over the past two centuries. The insight that the epidemiology of acquired immunodeficiency disease (AIDS) has provided into how new diseases of man become established has provided an arena for renewed interest in the possibility that the environmental factor responsible could be an infectious agent.

Aetiology

Rheumatoid arthritis is a disease of unknown cause, but current thinking favours the notion that interplay among genetic factors, sex hormones, and an infectious agent initiates an autoimmune disease mechanism that culminates in a disease with inflammatory and destructive features.

Genetic factors

Genetic factors were implicated by population studies that showed a slight increase in the frequency of rheumatoid arthritis in first-degree relatives of patients with rheumatoid arthritis, especially if seropositive for rheumatoid factor (Lawrence 1970). Concordance rates of disease in identical twins in hospital-based studies were estimated to be of the order of 30 per cent, compared with 5 per cent in non-identical twins (Lawrence 1970), although the figures are lower in community-based studies (Silman et al. 1989), again supporting the concept of a genetic contribution, but arguing against the proposition that rheumatoid arthritis results from a dominant single-gene disorder. The rates of prevalence in the general population, families, and twins have in fact led to the conclusion that rheumatoid arthritis is a polygenic disease, and that non-inherited factors are also of great importance.

Attempts at identifying the genes involved in predisposition to rheumatoid arthritis took a step forward when tissue typing for HLA class II antigen of Caucasian patients showed that 60 to 70 per cent of patients with rheumatoid arthritis were HLA-DR4 positive by

cellular or serological techniques compared with 20 to 25 per cent of control populations (Statsny 1976; Statsny 1978; Panayi et al. 1979). The patients with more severe rheumatoid arthritis, especially those with systemic complications such as vasculitis and Felty's syndrome, were even more likely to have HLA DR4 than patients with less aggressive disease confined to joints (Ollier et al. 1984; Westedt et al. 1986).

The increased frequency of HLA DR4 has also been reported in American black subjects, Japanese, Asian North Indians, and Latin Americans. In Israeli Jews and an Indian immigrant community in the United Kingdom an increased frequency of HLA DR1 has been found. The increase of HLA DR4 or DR1 cannot, however, be found in all races and ethnic groups, and a notable exception was a study of Greek patients in whom no HLA associations could be discovered, irrespective of disease severity or serological status (reviewed by Goldstein and Arnett 1987).

Typing by mixed leucocyte culture has defined several HLA-DR4 subtypes. It is of considerable interest that while the subtypes HLA Dw4 and Dw14 are associated with rheumatoid arthritis in several studies, Dw15 is only associated with rheumatoid arthritis in the Japanese, while Dw10 and Dw13 are not associated with rheumatoid arthritis in any ethnic group. A recent study has shown that in *DR4* homozygotes, *Dw4/Dw14* individuals were at greater risk of developing rheumatoid arthritis than *Dw4/Dw4* (Wordsworth et al. 1992). The significance of this is discussed below.

At the phenotypic level, the importance of HLA class II molecules lies in their participation in a trimolecular reaction involving the HLA antigen-binding cleft formed by the α and β chains of an antigen-presenting cell binding to a processed linear peptide antigen of at least nine amino acids, and the HLA–antigen complex in turn binding to the variable portion of the T-cell receptor. Several research techniques have been used in an attempt to define the similarity of HLA class II molecules common to all patients with rheumatoid arthritis, including patients who are not necessarily HLA-DR4 positive. These include, for example, genotyping of DNA and nucleotide sequencing, using the polymerase chain reaction and enzymatic digestion for restriction fragment length polymorphisms. At the level of expressed surface proteins, HLA epitopes have been sought by using monoclonal antibodies and alloreactive T-cell clones (see Goldstein and Arnett 1987). These studies have lent support to the concept that susceptibility to rheumatoid arthritis is related to a 'shared epitope' on the HLA molecules (Gregersen et al. 1987; Hammer et al. 1995).

Nucleotide sequencing of *HLA-DR* β_1 exons coding amino acid residues 70 to 74 has revealed that HLA DR4 subtypes Dw4, Dw14, and Dw15 share similarities with each other (with a conservative substitution of glutamine with lysine at position 71 in Dw4) and with HLA DR1 (Table 1) (Winchester and Gregersen 1988). The sequence predicts susceptibility to rheumatoid arthritis and, for example, is associated with rheumatoid arthritis in 83 per cent of Caucasians in Britain (Wordsworth et al. 1989). In contrast, negative associations are observed in individuals who are DR4w10, in whom the charged basic amino acids glutamine and arginine in positions 70 and 71 are replaced by the acidic amino acids aspartic and glutamic acid. In Dw13 individuals, in whom a negative association is also observed, arginine is substituted for glutamic acid in position 74. Molecular modelling studies suggest that amino acid residues 70 to 74 are located in the α-helix forming the wall of the peptide-binding groove, and thus likely to be involved in antigen binding and

Table 1 HLA–DR associations with rheumatoid arthritis defined by DR β_1 sequence position 70–74

DR type	Sequence					Association
	70	71	72	73	74	
DR4–W4	Q	K	R	A	A	Positive
–W14	Q	R	R	A	A	Positive
–W15	Q	R	R	A	A	Positive
DR1	Q	R	R	A	A	Positive
DR4–W10	D	E	R	A	A	Negative
–W13	Q	R	R	A	E	Negative

Q, glutamine; K, lysine; R, arginine; A, alanine; D, aspartic acid; E, glutamic acid.

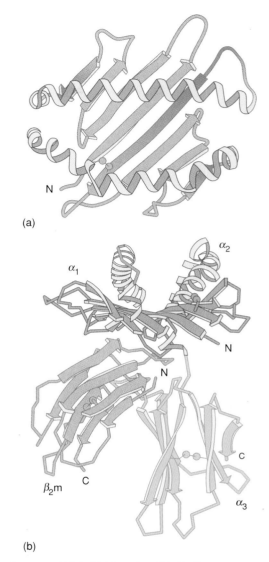

Fig. 1 Structure of HLA. (a) View of peptide-binding groove as seen by T-cell receptor. (b) From side.

subsequent interaction with T-cell receptors (Fig. 1). Acidic substitutions could profoundly alter protein structures and thereby alter affinity for peptide antigens. The predictions that protein structures on the HLA molecule are important in susceptibility to rheumatoid arthritis are supported by serotyping with alloantisera and monoclonal antibodies as well as reactivity with homozygous T cells and T-cell clones (Goronzy *et al.* 1986; Winchester and Gregersen 1988). However, whether the susceptibility to rheumatoid arthritis is due to permissive binding of specific peptides such as those on autoantigens or on environmental antigens, whether superantigens may initiate disease by binding specifically to the HLA molecules (Herman *et al.* 1991), or whether selection or tolerance of the T-cell repertoire are also involved, remains to be elucidated.

The evidence that *Dw4/Dw14* heterozygotes are more likely to develop rheumatoid arthritis than are *Dw4* homozygotes (Wordsworth *et al.* 1992), and the evidence that individuals expressing DR4 (and not DR1) are more likely to have severe disease, challenges the concept that sequences 70 to 74 are the only HLA-D regions that influence disease expression. This is despite the sequence identity of DR1 and DR4w4 in these positions, and a conservative substitution in Dw14 (Table 1). It has been hypothesized that the severity of disease and extra-articular complications are related to homozygosity and the density of disease-associated MHC molecules which critically influence the selection of the T-cell repertoire and tolerance to antigens (Weyand *et al.* 1992; Goronzy and Weyand 1993).

Although HLA genes are of obvious importance in rheumatoid arthritis, it has been calculated from studies of HLA in multicase families that they may only account for 37 per cent of the genetic factors involved (Deighton *et al.* 1989). However, a recent reanalysis has suggested that up to 60 per cent of susceptibility could be determined genetically (Macgregor and Silman 1994). Other susceptibility genes have been sought, and associations with T-cell receptors in gene polymorphisms and deletions of immunoglobulin genes have been observed (Olee *et al.* 1991). The picture is currently incomplete and their relative importance has not been documented.

Infectious agents

Population and twin studies strongly suggest that non-inherited, presumably environmental, factors such as infections may play a

part in the aetiology of rheumatoid arthritis, although rearrangement of the α β genes on T-cell receptors may also contribute to the non-inherited component. As discussed above, although prevalence rates of rheumatoid arthritis from worldwide studies are similar, a population survey designed to seek effects of the environment showed that urbanized tribal South African black subjects suffered from rheumatoid arthritis more than their rural cousins. However, the classical clue of case clustering suggesting an infectious background has not been found for rheumatoid arthritis in any study, unlike Lyme disease. Attempts at demonstrating microbial organisms directly from joints have had a chequered history, since in all instances claims of positive findings — for example, of mycoplasma, diphtheroids, and viruses — have either been attributed to laboratory contamination or have been refuted on grounds of a lack of reproducibility.

Other studies have sought to implicate microbes in the aetiology of rheumatoid arthritis by seeking evidence of immune hyperreactivity to microbial antigens. Increased antibody titres to Epstein–Barr virus (**EBV**) antigens and an induced rheumatoid arthritis nuclear antigen have suggested that this ubiquitous virus, known to infect the majority of people by the late teens, may be of aetiological importance (Venables *et al.* 1981; Venables 1988). Its persistence in B lymphocytes of patients with rheumatoid arthritis in greater than normal amounts because of impaired cellular immunity could lead to the hyperreactivity of B cells, and autoantibody production typical of the disease. Sequence similarity of an EBV capsid antigen to the HLA-DR β$_1$ susceptibility sequence QKRAA (Table 1) (Roudier *et al.* 1988) has suggested a possible explanation for the increased persistence of EBV in rheumatoid arthritis, while immunological cross-reactivity of EBV nuclear antigens to the autoantigens collagen, actin, and cytokeratin and to an antigen in the synovial membrane have suggested mechanisms for the induction of autoimmunity and for localization of immune cells to joints (Baboonian *et al.* 1991). However, these data fail to explain why only a small proportion of individuals infected with EBV might develop rheumatoid arthritis, and conversely, that there are well-documented patients with rheumatoid arthritis who have not been infected with EBV (Venables *et al.* 1981).

At least three bacteria have attracted attention in recent years as candidate agents in the aetiology of rheumatoid arthritis. The first, *M. tuberculosis*, gained current interest following the studies of Cohen *et al.* (1985) on an animal model of rheumatoid arthritis (see adjuvant arthritis in Animal models below). In these studies, mycobacterial protein showed immunological cross-reactivity and sequence similarity to a cartilage link protein, a finding which suggested a possible reason for the localization of the immune response to joints (van Eden *et al.* 1985). The link with human rheumatoid arthritis was suggested by the demonstration of reactivity of synovial T cells to mycobacterial antigens in rheumatoid arthritis (Holoshitz *et al.* 1986). The mycobacterial 65-kDa protein was subsequently shown to belong to the family of heat-shock proteins (**hsp65**) which are expressed in a variety of bacteria and also in the inflamed synovium of rheumatoid arthritis (van Eden *et al.* 1988; de Graeff-Meeder *et al.* 1990). Whether human hsp is a major target of T-cell autoreactivity in rheumatoid arthritis, however, is unproven, as there are significant differences in sequence and epitopes expressed by bacterial and human hsp (Gaston *et al.* 1989). Arguing against a role is the fact that identical responses to hsp65 are found in other inflammatory sites, for example, pleural effusion (Res *et al.* 1990). Attempts to suppress rheumatoid arthritis by vaccination with T cells derived from joints, in a protocol similar to that successfully used in adjuvant arthritis, could have provided support for the importance of mycobacterial immunity, but preliminary attempts have not been impressively successful (Van Laar *et al.* 1991).

In a further study seeking a mechanism dependent on molecular mimicry, antigens homologous to the amino acid sequence QKRAA (see Table 1) present in the hsp DNAj of *Escherichia coli* were reported to elicit T-cell responses only in patients with rheumatoid arthritis (Albani *et al.* 1995). It was suggested by these workers that activated T cells may cross-react with autologous DNAj heat-shock proteins that are expressed in the joints.

The third bacterium proposed as a candidate aetiological agent is *Proteus mirabilis*. Increased levels of IgG antibody to the organism have been detected in patients with rheumatoid arthritis but not ankylosing spondylitis or control subjects (Ebringer *et al.* 1989). It has been claimed that persistence of the organism in the urinary tracts, especially of women, may provide the nidus of infection that

triggers a deleterious immune response culminating in rheumatoid arthritis.

The similarity of retrovirus-induced caprine arthritis to rheumatoid arthritis has attracted interest in the possibility that retroviruses may be of aetiological importance (Trabandt *et al.* 1992). Retroviral GAG proteins have been demonstrated immunohistochemically in the synovium of patients with rheumatoid arthritis (Ziegler *et al.* 1989), and a transgenic mouse carrying the human T-cell leukaemia virus type I that developed chronic arthritis with synovial inflammation and joint erosion similar to rheumatoid arthritis has been described (see Animal models).

Other aetiological factors

Apart from the possible role that infectious agents may play, the predominance of rheumatoid arthritis in females in the premenopausal period compared with males and the protective effect of the contraceptive pill, presumably because of its progesterone content, have suggested that sex hormones may accelerate or retard its onset (Lahita 1990). Other aetiological factors that have been considered include diet (Buchanan *et al.* 1991) and stress (Adler 1985), but their role in initiating disease is debatable, and may be more significant in altering disease expression and outcome.

Autoimmunity

Autoantibodies

The discovery of the autoantibody, IgM rheumatoid factor, in the blood of patients with rheumatoid arthritis was the principal reason for the inclusion in the group of autoimmune diseases. Although high-titre IgM rheumatoid factor is relatively specific for a diagnosis of rheumatoid arthritis in the context of chronic polyarthritis, its occurrence in many autoimmune rheumatic diseases without arthritis and in chronic infections has raised doubts about the role it might play in the pathogenesis of rheumatoid arthritis. However, rheumatoid factor-secreting plasma cells of IgG, IgA, and IgM class can be demonstrated in the rheumatoid synovium (reviewed by Maini *et al.* 1987), thus implicating them at the site of disease. Indeed, cells of the B-lymphocyte lineage constitute 10 to 15 per cent of the population of mononuclear cells in rheumatoid arthritis, produce autoantibodies, are a source of immune complexes that fix complement, and can act as efficient antigen-presenting cells. It seems likely that they contribute to perpetuation of the disease (Andrew *et al.* 1991).

IgG in patients with rheumatoid arthritis shows markedly reduced glycosylation, with a galactose 'pocket' in the Fc region (Parekh *et al.* 1985), in association with low levels of B-cell galactosyl transferase (Axford *et al.* 1987). It has been suggested that this glycosylation defect could result in conformational changes in the Fc region, rheumatoid factors more readily aggregating such molecules. Passive transfer of an acute synovitis in T-cell-primed mice has been shown to be enhanced using IgG containing autoantibodies to type II collagen when the antibodies are present as the agalactosyl glycoform. (Rademacher *et al.* 1994), demonstrating that agalactosyl IgG glycoforms are directly associated with pathogenicity in murine collagen-induced arthritis. However, the role of such glycosylation defects in the aetiology or pathogenesis of rheumatoid arthritis has yet to be established.

Other 'autoantibodies' that occur in rheumatoid arthritis include natural autoantibodies, antinuclear antibodies, anticollagen antibodies, antikeratin antibodies, and an IgG perinuclear factor. Of these, antibodies directed to two distinct epidermal antigens appear to show high diagnostic specificity for rheumatoid arthritis with a sensitivity of about 50 per cent. These are:

1. IgG antikeratin antibodies, which are present in 36 to 60 per cent of patients with rheumatoid arthritis, show a specificity of over 95 per cent in most studies. The antibody activity is directed against an antigen in the keratinized stratified epithelium of the rat oesophagus and is demonstrated by indirect immunofluorescence (Young *et al.* 1979). As a proportion of patients with rheumatoid arthritis without rheumatoid factor were positive in this test, it may be viewed as an additional serological marker of rheumatoid arthritis. Although it has been claimed that the antigen is an epidermal cytokeratin, the supporting data are poorly substantiated, and the identity of the antigen remains unknown.

2. An antibody directed against another epidermal antigen is known as antiperinuclear factor: this is demonstrated by an indirect immunofluorescence technique using buccal mucosal epithelial cells as substrate (Nienhuis and Mandema 1964). These IgG antibodies in rheumatoid arthritis are directed against spherical cytoplasmic granules and, when undiluted serum is used, show a diagnostic specificity of 98 per cent, with a sensitivity of 52 per cent (Westgeest *et al.* 1987). However, antiperinuclear factor has been found by some in a significant proportion of patients with Sjögren's syndrome, systemic lupus, systemic sclerosis, infectious mononucleosis, and metastatic lung cancer. It has been claimed that a positive test for antiperinuclear factor occurs in rheumatoid arthritis in the absence of IgM rheumatoid factor and therefore is of value in diagnosis. The biochemical and molecular properties of the antigen reactive with antibodies to antiperinuclear factor are also poorly characterized. Recent studies have shown colocalization of antiperinuclear factor and profilaggrin in human buccal cells, and evidence has accumulated suggesting that antibodies to antiperinuclear factor and stratified epithelial keratin recognize epitopes on profilaggrin (Berthelot *et al.* 1994; Sebbag *et al.* 1995).

Antinuclear antibodies detected by indirect immunofluorescence occur in up to 40 per cent of sera from patients with rheumatoid arthritis. Antibodies to histones, which also react as rheumatoid factors as a result of an epitope shared with IgG-Fc, have also been described in rheumatoid sera (Hannestad and Stollar 1978). Precipitating antibodies to soluble cellular antigen have been described in rheumatoid vasculitis (Venables *et al.* 1979). An antibody detected by Western blotting to a ribonucleoprotein termed RA33 has been found in 36 per cent of rheumatoid sera, including early in disease, but also occurs in sera from mixed connective tissue disease and systemic lupus. Partial sequencing of RA33 shows it to be identical to the A2 protein of the heterogeneous nuclear ribonucleoprotein (**hnRNP**) complex (Steiner *et al.* 1992; Hassfeld *et al.* 1995).

All the foregoing examples of antibodies appear to be associated specifically with rheumatoid arthritis, but react with antigens that are not restricted to the site of disease in joints. However, another set of antibodies in rheumatoid arthritis is directed against antigens present in cartilage only, such as collagen type II, IX, and XI, and chondrocyte-specific antigens. The published data on the frequency of these antibodies are variable in different series, possibly as a result of the differing derivation of collagen (both homologous and heterologous collagens are used and are not identical), lack of purity of antigens, interference from serum factors, and the wide variety of techniques for detection. In one study, antibodies to collagen II occurred in 29 per cent of patients with rheumatoid arthritis, while antibodies to type IX and XI were present in 40 per cent (Charriere *et al.* 1988). However, antibodies to collagen II and XI were also equally frequent in osteoporosis and Paget's disease, whereas anticollagen IX was relatively restricted to rheumatoid arthritis. Antibodies to collagen I and II are produced locally in rheumatoid joints (Tarkowski *et al.* 1989). Antibodies to chondrocyte membrane antigens occur in rheumatoid arthritis but have been poorly characterized so far (Mollenhauer *et al.* 1988), but a preliminary report suggests that a glycoprotein synthesized by chondrocytes is a specific T-cell autoantigen in rheumatoid arthritis (Rijnders *et al.* 1996).

Induction

In the context of autoimmune diseases in general, as in rheumatoid arthritis, environmental agents are seen as triggers rather than as being directly involved in the disease process. However, how environmental agents induce autoimmunity is not understood. Various hypotheses have been proposed of which the concept of 'antigenic mimicry' is the most popular.

'Antigenic mimicry' implies that an immune response to an extrinsic antigen (usually microbial), closely resembling an autoantigen, induces an immune response that cross-reacts with the autoantigen. If the response is to be long lasting, then the autoantigen must perpetuate it as the extrinsic antigen is eliminated. Despite the popularity of this concept, there are as yet no definite examples in human autoimmunity. Mimicry can occur in autoimmunity, it is the mechanism by which heterogeneous or chemically treated autoantigens can induce experimental autoimmune diseases, for example thyroiditis by using thyroglobulin, or collagen arthritis (see below).

Another concept, proposed by Bottazzo, Feldmann, and colleagues (reviewed Feldmann 1987; Feldmann 1989), was that a local immune response, to any environmental agents, may release enough cytokines into the environment to upregulate local antigen-presenting capacity, so allowing autoantigens, otherwise 'hidden' from the immune system because of lack of HLA class II expression, to be presented to immunocompetent T cells that have escaped elimination or induction of tolerance. This was first proposed for endocrine autoimmune diseases, with the suggestion that the endocrine epithelium becomes the critical source of (atypical) antigen-presenting capacity and of autoantigen. Substantial evidence has since accumulated that this scheme may apply in both experimental models and human disease. Transgenic mice, producing interferon-γ in their islets of Langerhans under the control of the insulin promoter, develop an immune, T-cell-dependent diabetes, with autoreactive T cells lysing islets and rejecting transplanted islets (Sarvetnick *et al.* 1990). In human Graves' thyroiditis, the antigen-presenting capacity of thyrocytes has been documented, as well as the presence of activated autoantigen-reactive T cells, and of local cytokines needed to maintain both antigen-presenting function and T-cell activation (reviewed Feldmann *et al.* 1991). In rheumatoid arthritis, abundant antigen-presenting function resides in macrophages, dendritic cells, B cells, endothelium, and possibly activated T cells, although which of these is most deeply involved in antigen presentation in rheumatoid arthritis is not known. The presence of CD5+ B lymphocytes and their descendants may contribute significantly to local antigen-presenting function by binding to autoantibody containing immune complexes in their immunoglobulin receptor (Andrew *et al.* 1991).

What are the important autoantigens in rheumatoid arthritis? In a local autoimmune disease the autoimmune response is localized by the restricted distribution of critical autoantigens. This can be shown in Graves' disease where antigens synthesized by thyroid epithelial cells—thyroglobulin, thyroid peroxidase, and thyroid-stimulating hormone receptor—are targets of both T- and B-cell recognition (Dayan *et al.* 1991). In rheumatoid arthritis, cartilage autoantigens such as collagen type II, type IX, and type XI recognized by T and B cells would fulfil this role. These antigens as well as other cartilage- or chondrocyte-specific antigens could be of importance in the initial localization to synovial joints. A report of benefit following daily intake of a preparation of purified chicken type II collagen, has excited interest in the possibility of induction of 'by-stander' T-cell tolerance by regulating T cells to joints from the gut lymphoid system (Trentham *et al.* 1993). T cells recognizing hsp65 or the antigen implicated in the autologous mixed lymphocyte reaction, which have been described in rheumatoid arthritis, could not have this role because the antigens are ubiquitous in cell types in most tissues, but may be of importance in maintaining the disease process, and in the extra-articular manifestations.

It is not clear whether rheumatoid arthritis should be considered as a single disease, with all cases having the same aetiology, or whether it should be viewed as a syndrome, with a range of aetiological factors initiating the same pathogenetic mechanism, and so producing a similar constellation of features.

Pathology

Introduction

The most pronounced and invariant pathology is in the synovial joints. There is a typical distribution, the small joints of the hands and feet, knees, and hips being most often implicated, symmetrically. In the different joints there are minor differences in pathology, but there is an overall pattern. There are also extra-articular manifestations, such as nodules and systemic disease.

Involvement of synovial joints

While attempts have been made to study the early events in rheumatoid arthritis, this is difficult, and so the pathology that is well known is from established cases. The involvement of synovial joints in rheumatoid arthritis is both of the synovial fluid and membrane (Zvaifler *et al.* 1994). Synovial fluid volumes are increased, and the cellularity increased; the predominant cell is the polymorph, which is only rarely seen in the lining layer of the synovial membrane. The other major cells in the synovial fluid and membrane are T cells and macrophages, with dendritic cells and cells of the B-lymphocyte lineage in small numbers. Typical numbers in acute cases are about 10^6/ml of polymorphs, and 1 to 3 $\times$ 10^5/ml of mononuclear cells. The exact relationship of the cells in the fluid to those in the membrane is not clear. Those in the fluid originate from the membrane, but how they reach the fluid is not clear. Whether they can re-enter the membrane or directly damage cartilage is also not known.

The involvement of synovial membrane is summarized in Fig. 2. There are several key features:

1. The lining layer, normally two cells thick, is much thickened with increased numbers of both type A (macrophage-like) cells and type B (fibroblast-like) cells, both expressing activation markers.

2. The deeper layers are of increased cellularity, with perivascular accumulations and follicles. These are rich in T cells particularly CD4+ cells. CD8+ T cells are more frequently found in between perivascular accumulations, as are the abundant plasma cells and infrequent B cells. Macrophages are found in the follicles and in between. There are few polymorphs and dendritic cells in the membrane, the majority of which accumulate in fluid.

3. The rheumatoid synovium is particularly vascular. There are markedly increased numbers of vessels, and in some instances high-endothelial venules develop, as in lymph nodes.

4. Many of the cells, of all types, in the rheumatoid joint are activated. Thus HLA class II expression is found on nearly all the cell types, at an increased level, compared with that in normal or osteoarthritic joints. T cells are about 50 per cent class II positive, providing strong evidence of their activation status. B cells are positive, but typically plasma cells are not, as these lose the capacity to express class II. Macrophages express class II, as is often the case when activated, and class II-expressing fibroblasts and endothelial cells can also be seen.

Of interest is the HLA-DQ expression in rheumatoid arthritis, which is significantly greater than in other types of joint inflammation, for example Reiter's syndrome (Barkley *et al.* 1989a). The meaning of this difference is not clearly understood, as the relative roles of the commonest class II antigen, HLA DR, compared with the less common DQ and DP molecules are not known. Certain evidence allies HLA-DQ-restricted T cells to the suppressive immunoregulatory lineage (Sasazuki *et al.* 1986).

Other markers of activation abound. On the macrophage lineage, expression of CD11b (CR3) is increased, as is the related CD11c (p150/95). CD11a (lymphocyte function associated antigen-1) is increased on macrophages and many cell types. On T cells, expression of very late antigen (**VLA**) is increased, as is class II on a major proportion. In contrast interleukin (**IL**)-2 receptor is much less apparent. Endothelial cell expression of the adhesion molecules (**AMs**) ICAM-1 (intercellular), VLA-1, and **ELAM-1** (endothelium–leucocyte) is increased. Tumour necrosis factor (**TNF**) receptors, also markers of activation, are upregulated in rheumatoid joints and are detectable on more than 80 per cent of T cells, on cells of the lining layer, and on cells at the cartilage–pannus junction (Deleuran *et al.* 1992; Brennan *et al.* 1995).

A common feature of activated cells is their increased production of cytokines and expression of cytokine receptors. This is the case in rheumatoid synovium, and the details will be discussed under pathogenesis.

Pannus

The junction between synovial tissue, cartilage, and bone is the site of early erosive damage in rheumatoid arthritis. This site becomes filled and overlaid by vascular tissue termed pannus. The lining layer of pannus is in continuity with the lining layer of hypercellular synovium and has been regarded as being derived from it. The cellular pannus forms a distinct junction with underlying cartilage (see Fig. 3), which shows many characteristics of degradation,

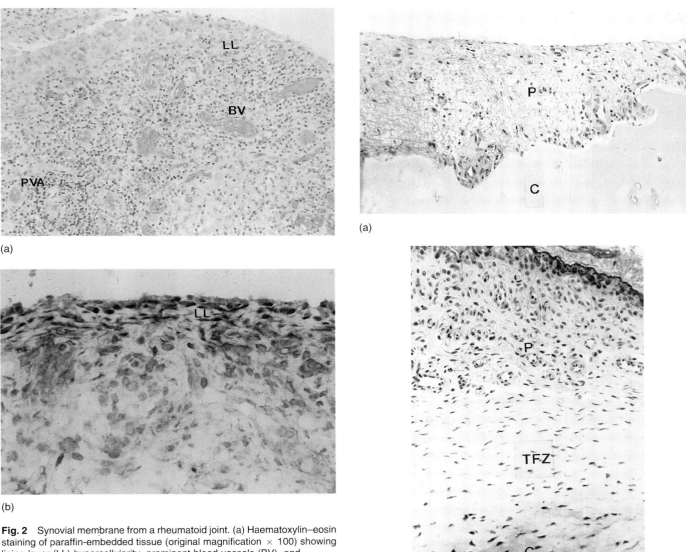

Fig. 2 Synovial membrane from a rheumatoid joint. (a) Haematoxylin–eosin staining of paraffin-embedded tissue (original magnification × 100) showing lining layer (LL) hypercellularity, prominent blood vessels (BV), and perivascular aggregates (PVA) of lymphocytes. The perivascular T lymphocytes are predominantly CD4+, CD45RO+, and CD29+ and a proportion bear activation markers HLA DR and IL-2 receptors. CD8+ T cells are distributed in interaggregate areas, as are plasma cells. (b) Tumour necrosis factor-α (TNF-α), IL-1α, β, and IL-6 are located in LL and in deeper layers: this cryostat section stained with F(ab')$_2$ anti-TNF-α and developed with an immunoperoxidase method shows intracytoplasmic TNF-α.

Fig. 3 Two types of cartilage–pannus junction seen in rheumatoid joints. (a) A distinct, well-defined margin can be seen between pannus (P) and cartilage (C). (b) A transitional fibroblastic zone (TFZ) separates a cellular, vascular pannus (P) from the underlying cartilage (C). Safranin O stain; original magnification × 46. (Reproduced with permission from Allard *et al.* 1987.)

including loss of matrix and water content, and chondrocyte depletion. The conventional view is that pannus has an invasive degradative effect on underlying cartilage, mediated by the secretions of enzymes such as metalloproteinases. This is associated with further loss of cartilage as a result of enzymatic destruction of matrix by chondrocytes themselves, coupled with a lack of synthesis of newly formed matrix. Pannus also appears to erode adjacent bone by a similar process involving degradation of bone matrix, but in addition involving active bone resorption by osteoclasts.

A second type of pannus may also be observed, especially in the marginal cartilage area of weight-bearing joints. This consists of vascular pannus overlying cartilage with an indistinct, intervening, multilayered zone of fibroblast-like cells (Fig. 3). In contrast, the underlying cartilage of this pannus does not show degradative changes with loss of matrix. This type of pannus could represent a fibrotic healing phase, but has alternatively been termed a 'transitional' fibroblastic zone because the cytoplasm of these cells contains cartilage components such as keratan sulphate, chondroitin sulphate, and collagen type II (Allard *et al.* 1987; Allard *et al.* 1991). These cells may be derived from chondrocytes as a result of metaplastic change. However, the possibility has been raised that cells with the same phenotype resident in the subperiosteum, contiguous to synovium in normal joints, may give rise to the transitional fibroblastic zone in rheumatoid arthritis (Allard *et al.* 1990). The finding of proinflammatory cytokines capable of degrading cartilage (such as IL-l and TNF) in pannus cells contiguous with cartilage in the invasive type of erosion contrasts with absence of these cytokines in the transitional fibroblastic zone (Chu *et al.* 1991*a*; Chu *et al.* 1991*b*). Instead, the latter type of pannus shows the presence of only transforming growth factor-β (**TGF-β**), as this factor stimulates collagen and matrix production its presence is compatible with the proposal that the tissue is in an anabolic state of healing or differentiation.

Extra-articular manifestations

Local

These are more common in long-standing and severe cases. Rheumatoid nodules are the most common, and are found in areas susceptible to trauma, such as elbows. They consist of a palisade of macrophages surrounding fibrous tissue.

Systemic

There are disagreements about the extent and frequency of systemic manifestations, and whether rheumatoid arthritis is always manifest systemically. Elevated concentrations of acute-phase proteins such as C-reactive protein, serum amyloid A, or complement components are found in most cases, and these suggest that their production in liver is increased. IL-6 can activate the liver to produce many acute-phase proteins, and it is currently assumed that the increased production of IL-6 (and IL-1) in rheumatoid arthritis (reviewed by Feldmann *et al.* 1996) is responsible.

In more severe cases there may be:

(i) vasculitis;

(ii) fibrosis of the lungs which may progress to significant fibrotic impairment of lung function;

(iii) granuloma formation as characterized by nodule formation;

(iv) serositis as characterized by pericarditis and pleurisy, commonly asymptomatic;

(v) Felty's syndrome: enlargement of the spleen with lymphadenopathy, fever, leg ulcers, and susceptibility to bacterial infections.

Pathogenesis

Introduction

Describing the pathogenesis of a chronic disease, such as rheumatoid arthritis, for which there are no very accurate animal models, is difficult. It is possible to describe, on the basis of human studies, the events occurring when the disease is well established. Accurate description of early events is not possible, only informed speculation can be made. As the pathology — the morphological description of what has happened — has been discussed, consideration of the pathogenesis will be itemized in relation to how these changes may have evolved.

Cell recruitment

The vast majority of the increased number of cells in the rheumatoid joint are of lymphohaemopoietic origin, as shown by immuno-

staining techniques, and their presence in the rheumatoid joint implies that there are mechanisms for increasing cell input, and also for increasing retention. This increase in cellularity is accompanied by angiogenesis in the synovial membrane, thus increasing delivery of cells and molecules to areas of inflammation (Folkman 1995). Neovascularization involves angiogenic cytokines such as **VEGF** (vascular endothelial growth factor), an endothelial-specific mitogen which promotes the growth of new blood vessels (Colville-Nash and Scott 1992) and also renders the vasculature hyperpermeable *in vivo* (Ferrara *et al.* 1991). Much work has focused on the endothelium in rheumatoid arthritis, as blood-borne cells would first have to adhere and migrate through endothelium. Augmented expression of adhesion molecules capable of binding lymphocytes, polymorphs, and monocytes has been noted: ICAM-1, E-selectin, and **VCAM-1** (vascular cell adhesion molecule) are all increased at various pathological sites. Isolated rheumatoid synovial endothelial cells constitutively express ICAM-1 and E-selectin and this expression is upregulated by IL-1 and TNF (Abbot *et al.* 1992). Immunohistochemical techniques have shown that VCAM-1, ICAM-1, and E-selectin are highly expressed by rheumatoid synovial vascular endothelial cells and cells in the lining layer (Koch *et al.* 1992; Morales-Ducret *et al.* 1992; Wilkinson *et al.* 1993).

A local differentiation of T cells in rheumatoid arthritis synovial membrane has been suggested by the predominance of T cells with the phenotype of memory cells (CD45RO+, CD29). Increased expression of VLA-4 on CD45RO+ T cells could indicate selective migration of memory T cells into the inflamed synovial membrane. In fact CD45RO+ T cells have been shown to have a better adherence to endothelial cells than CD45RO-T cells (Pitzalis *et al.* 1987). In addition, synovial T cells in rheumatoid arthritis have a significantly greater capacity to migrate transendothelially compared with those from normal or rheumatoid arthritis peripheral blood (Cush *et al.* 1992).

Equally important in cell recruitment is the action of chemotactic factors, which promote the migration of cells into a site. Some of these mediators have been identified within rheumatoid joints including representatives of the two families of chemokines, the C-X-C(α) chemokines such as IL-8 (Brennan *et al.* 1990*a*), and the C-C(β) chemokines such as **RANTES** (regulated upon activation, T-cell expressed, and secreted) (Rathanaswami *et al.* 1993), **MCP-1** (monocyte chemoattractant protein 1) (Koch *et al.* 1992; Akahoshi *et al.* 1993), **MIP-1α** (macrophage inflammatory protein-α) (Koch *et al.* 1994), and MIP-1β (Villiger *et al.* 1992). As the majority of the cells in the rheumatoid arthritis synovium are macrophages and T lymphocytes, β-chemokines are likely to be important but neutrophil chemoattractants such as IL-8, **GROα** (melanoma growth-stimulating activity), and **ENA-78** (epithelial neutrophil activating peptide) are likely to play a role in neutrophil accumulation within the joint fluid. Split complement components C3a and C5a present in rheumatoid arthritis joints (Jose *et al.* 1990; Abbink *et al.* 1992) are also chemotactic for neutrophils.

T-cell activation in rheumatoid arthritis

The T lymphocyte is one of the most common cells in active rheumatoid arthritis, with an abundance ranging from 20 to 50 per cent of the cells extracted from synovial membrane. CD4+ cells are more abundant than CD8+ in the membrane, but not necessarily in the synovial fluid. The CD4+ cells tend to concentrate in perivascular nodules, whereas the CD8+ are more diffusely scattered. CD4+

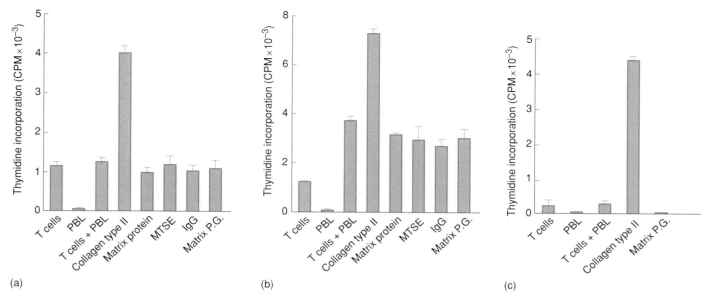

Fig. 4 Proliferative response of collagen type II-specific clones. (a) Clone 4 from the first synovial membrane. (b) Clone 55 with autologous mixed lymphocyte reactivity, from the first synovial membrane. (c) Clone B8 from the second synovial preparation. Results are the arithmetic means ± SEM of a representative experiment from each clone. In other experiments, collagen type I was also used, but there was no response from any of the clones. Cloned T cells (10^4), 2 × 10^4 irradiated, autologous, peripheral blood, mononuclear cells were cultured with or without the antigen indicated. Antigens were used at 100 μg/ml, except MTSE which was at 1 μg/ml. These were the optimal concentrations. PBL, peripheral blood lymphocytes; PG, proteoglycan; MTSE, mycobacterial tuberculosis soluble extract. (Reproduced with permission from Londei *et al.* 1989.)

cells have been subdivided into subsets, depending on their CD45 expression. In normal blood, about one-half are CD45RA+, indicating a 'virgin state'. Essentially all the cells in the rheumatoid joint lack CD45RA and express CD45RO/CD29, indicating a 'primed' or 'memory' state (Pitzalis *et al.* 1987). This is not surprising, as there is evidence for an ongoing immune response, as judged by the expression of T-cell activation markers, such as HLA class II (on 50 per cent), and IL-2 receptors on fewer cells (2 to 12 per cent) (Brennan *et al.* 1988*a*; Londei *et al.* 1989).

T lymphocytes may also be classified according to their T-cell receptor for antigen. In normal blood the great majority (more than 95 per cent) express a heterodimer of α and β chains, whereas a minority use γ and δ chains. Of interest was the observation (Brennan *et al.* 1988*b*) that there was selective enrichment of γδ T cells in active rheumatoid joints, and that some of the γδ T cells recognize mycobacterial antigens (Holoshitz *et al.* 1989). However, elevated γδ cell numbers have not been confirmed in all studies. In patients who have augmented γδ T cells in their blood there is a trend towards increased amounts of CD5+ B cells (Brennan *et al.* 1989*c*).

An important question is whether T cells have a critical role in rheumatoid arthritis. Firestein and Zvaifler (1990), based on low or absent levels of T-cell cytokines in the rheumatoid synovial environment, have proposed that T cells may not be important in the chronic established phase of disease. Indeed, in controlled clinical trials of rheumatoid arthritis with anti-T-cell (for example anti-CD4, anti-CD5) monoclonal antibodies, no beneficial effects were observed (Olsen *et al.* 1994; Van der Lubbe *et al.* 1995). However, our opinion is that in a prolonged, chronic, asynchronous disease with profound immunoregulation, the quantity of cytokines detected need not reflect their importance. Various lines of evidence support this possibility. First is the abundance of T cells in rheumatoid joints.

Virtually none are present in normal joints. Second is their partially activated status and proximity to antigen-presenting cells (see above). Third is the fact that the proportions of different types of T cells present in rheumatoid joints are not the same as in blood (as discussed above), indicating that it is not a reflection of passive trafficking in an inflammatory response. Fourth is the observation that antigen-specific T cells are present, are activated, and persist in rheumatoid joints. For example we found that collagen type II-specific T cells were present, and expressing IL-2 receptors, in three operative specimens in a patient with rheumatoid arthritis, over a period of more than 4 years (Fig. 4) (Londei *et al.* 1989). Finally, **Th1** cells (T-helper 1) appear to predominate in the joint and interferon-γ and IL-2 are expressed, albeit at low levels, but with unexpectedly high IL-10 production (Buchan *et al.* 1988*b*; Simon *et al.* 1994; Cohen *et al.* 1995).

A restricted pattern of V_β chains of the T-cell receptor was observed in rheumatoid joints by one group of workers, suggesting the possibility that activation of lymphocytes was mediated by superantigens (Paliard *et al.* 1991) However, other laboratories have not confirmed this observation. Thus, whereas Paliard *et al.* (1991) reported low $V_\beta 14$ in blood of patients with rheumatoid arthritis compared with the level found in joints, Howell *et al.* (1991) reported that multiple $V\beta$ gene families were transcribed in patients, although sequence similarities were found, in keeping with the hypothesis that superantigen may play a role in rheumatoid arthritis. Clearly much more work is needed in this area, but noting that all known autoimmune diseases and models are T-cell dependent, it is very likely that rheumatoid arthritis is T-cell dependent even in its later stages.

Whilst the function of T cells in rheumatoid arthritis is unresolved, much can be learned from investigations that define the role of T cells in induction and perpetuation of experimental models of arthritis.

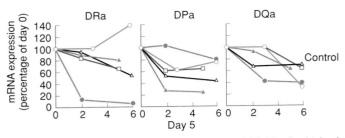

Fig. 5 Fresh isolated synovial membrane and synovial fluid cells obtained from five patients were placed in culture at 1×10^6/ml in the presence or absence of mediators (IFN-γ and IL-2). Cells were harvested at the times indicated for the determination of cytoplasmic RNA. The results are expressed as percentages of the basal level. (●), Patient 1; (△), Patient 2; (▲), Patient 3; (□), Patient 4; (○), Patient 5. (Reproduced with permission from Kissonerghis *et al.* 1989.)

Collagen-induced arthritis is a CD4+ T-cell dependent disease as demonstrated by T-cell depletion (Ranges *et al.* 1985). However, unlike adjuvant arthritis, it is not readily transferred with T cells or T-cell clones. In the case of collagen-induced arthritis, transfer from histoincompatible DBA/1 mice to mice with subacute combined immunodeficiency has demonstrated that T and B cells act in synergy in the full expression of disease (Williams *et al.* 1992*b*; Taylor *et al.* 1995).

B-cell lineage

Plasma cells are abundant in rheumatoid arthritis. Some, but not all are involved in the production of rheumatoid factors. Rheumatoid factor immune complexes have been shown to induce the production of cytokines such as IL-1 and TNF (Fig. 5) (Chantry *et al.* 1989).

The specificity of the antibodies produced in rheumatoid joints has been investigated by the cell fusion technique using the human B-cell fusion partner, SPAZ4. Large numbers of hybridomas producing IgM and IgG were detected (Maini 1989). While a few of these were 'polyreactive', and some produced rheumatoid factors, the majority did not bind to a battery of autoantigens tested. However, it has been claimed that the majority of rheumatoid joints contain B cells producing antibody to collagen type II and IgG Fc (Tarkowski *et al.* 1989).

In examining the B-cell repertoire activated in rheumatoid joints, attempts are being made to ascertain whether there is any evidence of a restricted use of certain genes selected from among the multiple heavy-chain *V* genes available in the genome. In one such study, analysed by northern blotting, an overrepresentation of V_H4 was noted (Brown *et al.* 1992). Such overrepresentation may result from dominance of a B-cell subset in diseased tissues or from selection pressures created by specific antigens or superantigens. Alternatively, regulatory elements in flanking regions active in rheumatoid arthritis may favour recombination of particular individual gene elements and so skew the B-cell repertoire activated (Brown *et al.* 1995). As primed B cells recognizing antigen present antigen to T cells more efficiently than do macrophages (Lanzavecchia *et al.* 1985) and are probably important in the development and maintenance of the immune network in neonatal and adult life (reviewed by Plater-Zyberk *et al.* 1992), a greater understanding of the role of B cells should illuminate the pathogenesis of rheumatoid arthritis.

Antigen-presenting cells

There are abundant cells with antigen-presenting capacity in human rheumatoid joints. Which of these are of major importance in different stages of disease is a controversial question. Macrophages and monocytes represent some 30 to 50 per cent of the cell pool, and there is evidence for their activation, for example increased expression of HLA DQ, and diminished CD14. Dendritic cells are present in increased numbers. Regrettably, due to lack of specific markers for human dendritic cells, their numbers are not easy to quantify. However, cell separation studies by several groups have all demonstrated increased numbers of dendritic cells in rheumatoid synovial fluid, comprising up to 5 to 7 per cent of the mononuclear cells, whereas synovial tissue contained few dendritic cells (March 1987; Tsai *et al.* 1989). Dendritic cells from rheumatoid synovial fluid were potent antigen-presenting cells, but not more so than normal dendritic cells.

CD5+ B cells have Fc receptors and many produce rheumatoid factors. These may permit CD5 B cells to take up immune complexes and present the relevant antigens. The possible importance of CD5+ B cells in antigen presentation in rheumatoid arthritis has been discussed (Maini 1989). Chondrocytes can be activated to express HLA class II and may be critical in the early events of rheumatoid arthritis. ICAM-1 expression in chondrocytes, which facilitates antigen-presenting cell function, has been reported (Davies *et al.* 1992).

Cell interaction

The importance of cell interactions in the rheumatoid joint can be inferred from the immunohistological studies, which show close apposition of T cells and antigen-presenting cells in nodules and in other sites throughout the synovial membrane. However, there are very few T cells in the pannus, suggesting that different interactions may prevail in this specialized site.

Dissociated cells from rheumatoid joints, placed in tissue culture, in the absence of any extrinsic stimulus, rapidly reform into aggregates. This suggests that interactions are of critical importance in the disease process. Experimentally, one can demonstrate that these cell interactions are of importance *in vitro*. We have noted that rheumatoid synovial cells, placed in culture and in the absence of extrinsic stimulation, retain many features of active rheumatoid arthritis. Thus expression of HLA class II persists *in vitro*, at both the protein and mRNA levels, provided that the whole mixture of joint cells is cultured (Fig. 5). If only the adherent cells (chiefly fibroblasts) are cultured, class II expression apparently does not persist in culture (Teyton *et al.* 1987). Below, the persistence of cytokine production in cell cultures from rheumatoid joint not extrinsically stimulated is discussed.

The role of T cells in the persistence of class II expression has been studied by depleting T cells using a combination of lysis with antibody and complement, and antibody-coated magnetic beads. Even with an incomplete depletion of cells, a marked reduction in class II expression was noted after 6 days in culture (C.M. Hawrylowicz *et al.*, unpublished observations). This emphasizes the importance of cell interactions, but does not clarify which T cells are of critical importance, nor which are the critical antigen-presenting cells.

Cytokine expression

As rheumatoid arthritis is mostly manifest in synovial joints, which are the sites of inflammation and destruction, cytokine production in the joints has been investigated by several groups. However, cytokines can also be detected in blood cells by immunostaining, for example IL-1α (Barkley *et al.* 1989*b*). Whether other cytokines can also be detected in the blood cells remains to be established. Elevated serum concentrations of cytokines have been reported, for example, IL-l β (Eastgate *et al.* 1988), but their reproducibility and significance remain to be established in view of the presence of serum cytokine inhibitors.

Rheumatoid joints contain a wide variety of activated cell types, and so it would be expected that many cytokines would be produced locally in the joint. When we began studies on the expression of cytokines in rheumatoid joints in 1985, slot blotting and cDNA hybridization were used to obtain maximum data on cytokine expression from a small number of cells. With these techniques 2×10^6 cells were used, and could provide data on about 6, or sometimes up to 10 cytokines. By densitometry, relative quantification was possible. Further advantages of this technique are its specificity for individual cytokines, ease of performance (same technique for all cytokines), and its resistance to artefacts caused by rheumatoid factors (a problem in binding assays), and to 'toxic' components of synovial fluid in bioassays (Buchan *et al.* 1988*a*; Buchan *et al.* 1988*b*). A disadvantage is that the amounts of cytokine mRNA being measured do not always correlate with the amounts of cytokine protein produced. This is especially a problem with cytokines known to be regulated post-transcriptionally, for example TNF-α. If this type of work was to be begun again, obviously the polymerase chain reaction (**PCR**) would be used, for its much greater sensitivity (Brenner *et al.* 1989). However, the use of PCR is not without problems; for example quantification is very difficult and contamination frequent. Using PCR to explore cytokine expression in rheumatoid arthritis has yielded the same results as slot blotting, that is, predominance of IL-1α and abundance of TNF-α (Brennan *et al.* 1989*a*). *In situ* hybridization has yielded analogous results (Firestein *et al.* 1990), and also provides information about localization, but quantification is difficult.

It is not surprising that virtually all the cytokines sought have been detected because of the wide variety of activated cells. Table 2 summarizes the cytokine expression in the rheumatoid joint. There are some interesting generalizations that can be made. For example, cytokines that are predominantly macrophage products are abundant, at both the mRNA and protein level, for example IL-1, IL-6, TNF, and IL-8. In contrast, cytokines produced by T cells are detectable at the mRNA level, but barely detectable at the protein level, for example interferon-γ, lymphotoxin, and IL-2. The reasons for this discrepancy are not yet known, but TGF-β which inhibits cytokine production post-transcriptionally may be responsible. Local consumption of cytokines by cells with high-affinity receptors may also contribute, as, for example, there are free and cell-bound IL-2 receptors in rheumatoid joint cells (Symons *et al.* 1988).

Cytokines are essential for many processes in rheumatoid arthritis, such as cell growth and expression of HLA class II, reviewed in Feldmann *et al.* (1996). However, it is not clear which cytokines are of major importance in different processes. A critical step in the generation of an immune or inflammatory reaction is activation of macrophages and induction of HLA class II expression. Interferon-γ is potentially the most effective cytokine at inducing such expression in the absence of other factors (Portillo *et al.* 1989). However,

negligible amounts of interferon-γ (or other T-cell lymphokines) are produced by rheumatoid synovial cells (Firestein and Zvaifler 1987; Brennan *et al.* 1989*a*) suggesting that other factors alone or in combination with this interferon-γ are involved. One possible candidate is the haemopoietic growth factor **GM-CSF** (granulocyte–macrophage colony-stimulating factor) which induces HLA-DR expression on human monocytes (Chantry *et al.* 1990) and which could be an important macrophage activator and induce HLA class II expression in the rheumatoid joint (Alvaro-Garcia *et al.* 1989). However, the most significant inhibition of that expression which we observed in the rheumatoid synovial cultures was with anti-TNF antibody (unpublished observation) and was greater than that with antibodies to interferon-γ or GM-CSF. This is unlikely to be a direct effect, as TNF by itself does not induce the expression of HLA class II (for example Pujol-Borell *et al.* 1987). This suggests that many different cytokines may work together to induce this expression (Sadeghi *et al.* 1992*a*; Sadeghi *et al.* 1992*b*) or that other, as yet undefined, molecules may be involved. Alternatively (or in addition) cell–cell interactions through cell adhesion molecules may be necessary to maintain this. Of interest is the observation that TNF-α is a potent inducer of many adhesion molecules including ICAM-1 and VCAM-1 (Pober *et al.* 1986; Rice and Bevilacqua 1989).

The activation and differentiation of B cells is also mediated by cytokines, of which IL-4 and IL-6 are the most important. IL-4 is a potent B-cell growth factor but is detected in negligible amounts in

Table 2 Summary of cytokines produced by rheumatoid synovial cells

Cytokine	mRNA	Protein
IL-1α	+	+
IL-1β	+	+
TNF-α	+	+
LT	+	−
IL-2	+	−
IL-3	−	−
IL-4	?	−
IFN-γ	+	−
GM-CSF	+	+
IL-8	+	+
G-CSF	+	?
M-CSF	−	?
TGF-β	+	+
EGF	+	+
PDGF-A	+	+
PDGF-B	+	+

EGF, epidermal growth factor; G-CSF, granulocyte colony-stimulating factor; GM-CSF, granulocyte–macrophage CSF; IL, interleukin; LT, lymphotoxin; M-CSF, macrophage CSF; PDGF, platelet-derived growth factor; TGF, transforming growth factor; TNF, tumour necrosis factor.
After Brennan *et al.* (1991).

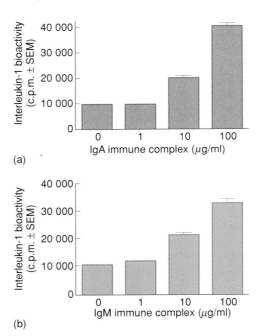

Fig. 6 Both IgA-containing immune complexes (a) and IgM-containing immune complexes (b) induce interleukin 1. Supernatants from monocytes cultured with various concentrations of immune complex for 24 h were assayed for interleukin1 bioactivity using the thymocyte comitogenic assay. Data is shown as [³H]-thymidine incorporation (mean ± SEM of triplicate cultures). Proliferation due to phytohaemagglutinin antigen alone was 3486 ± 450 c.p.m. For both immune complexes significant (p <0.01) interleukin could be detected at concentrations as low as 10 µg/ml. (Reproduced with permission from Chantry et al. 1989.)

rheumatoid synovial cells (unpublished observation) or in synovial fluid. In contrast, high levels of IL-6 have been detected both in rheumatoid synovial fluid and in cells from rheumatoid synovial membrane (Hirano et al. 1988; Field et al. 1991). The presence of high levels of IL-6 in rheumatoid joints may explain the large numbers of plasma cells and few B cells in the synovium and the production of autoantibodies including rheumatoid factors. Lymphotoxin and TNF-α can also act as a B-cell growth factor (Kehrl et al. 1987). The presence of immune complexes containing rheumatoid factor may further contribute to the pathogenesis of rheumatoid arthritis by inducing the production of IL-1 as shown by Chantry et al. (1989) (Fig. 6). The 'cytokine synthesis inhibitor', IL-10, which inhibits T-cell production of interferon-γ, is also a potent B-cell stimulator (Moore et al. 1990).

T-cell growth is controlled by cytokines. For many years, after the discovery of 'T-cell growth factor' and the purification, cloning, and expression of IL-2, it was thought that all T-cell growth was mediated by IL-2. Subsequent work has shown that the position is much more complex. IL-4, initially, described as a B-cell stimulating factor, is also a potent growth factor for many T cells, and IL-7, described as a pre-B growth factor, is also highly active (for example Londei et al. 1990). T-cell activation is found in rheumatoid arthritis, with many cells expressing HLA class II (20 to 50 per cent), and a few (2 to 12 per cent) expressing IL-2 receptors. However, the mechanism of T-cell growth is unclear, as while IL-2 mRNA is found (Buchan et al. 1988b), the protein is not readily detectable. This could be due to absorption by cell-bound receptors, to IL-2 inhibitors such as the soluble IL-2 receptor (Symons et al. 1991), or to post-transcriptional regulation. IL-4 is also not readily detectable, for possibly the same

reasons. Currently it is unknown whether there is IL-7 in rheumatoid joints, but it is clearly an important candidate for T-cell growth regulation in rheumatoid arthritis. A synergy between all these cytokines could permit T-cell growth in the presence of low protein levels of each of these mediators. This possibility requires investigation using cells from rheumatoid joints in culture.

Fibrosis is an important component and complication of rheumatoid arthritis. It participates in deformation of joints, but pulmonary fibrosis can be a damaging systemic complication. Which cytokine drives the fibrosis in the rheumatoid joint (or other tissues) is not currently known. There are abundant candidates present in the rheumatoid joint, for example IL-1α and β, TNF-α, which may act indirectly via induction by platelet-derived growth factor (Raines et al. 1989), and TGF-α and -β. The presence in rheumatoid joints of members of the fibroblast growth family is not known, but is likely.

Cytokine regulation

Initial studies of the expression of IL-1 in rheumatoid joints revealed that all samples contained IL-1 mRNA. After the experimental activation of normal cells in vitro, that of IL-1 mRNA (and the expression of other cytokines) is brief (24 to 48 h), so the fact that all samples from rheumatoid arthritis were positive suggested that cytokine production in the rheumatoid joint may be relatively stable and persistent. In a chronic disease only persistent features can be relevant to the maintenance of the disease process, so the consistence and persistence of cytokine production suggested that it was of importance in the pathogenesis (Buchan et al. 1988a).

Cytokine persistence was directly tested in vitro by culturing dissociated cells from rheumatoid joints in the absence of extrinsic stimulation. The initial results showed that both IL-1α and IL-1β mRNA persisted for up to the 5-day culture period (Fig. 7) (Buchan et al. 1988a). This indicates that the signals necessary to regulate cytokine production are present in the culture, and so can be analysed.

Neutralizing antibodies were chosen as the tool to investigate the signals involved in regulating the production of IL-1. The strongest non-microbial signals for the regulation of this production were the cytokines TNF-α and TNF-β (lymphotoxin), so neutralizing antibodies to these two cytokines were used. The results were clear cut; anti-TNF-α but not anti-TNF-β or control rabbit Ig inhibited IL-1

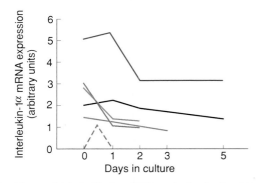

Fig. 7 Persistence of interleukin-1α mRNA production in rheumatoid joint cells in culture. Slot blot analysis of interleukin 1α production by rheumatoid arthritis synovial fluid mononuclear cells cultured in the absence of extrinsic antigen. SF and SM mononuclear cells were cultured for 0 to 5 days, the RNA extracted, blotted on to nitrocellulose, and probed with IL-1α. Integral values were calculated. Different symbols represent different patients. ----- is interleukin-1α mRNA from mitogen-activated peripheral blood mononuclear cells. (Reproduced with modification from Buchan et al. 1988a.)

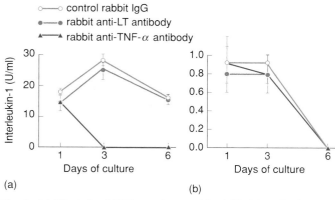

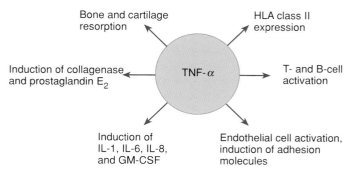

Fig. 9 Effects mediated by TNF-α in rheumatoid arthritis.

Fig. 8 (a) Effect of anti-TNF-α on rheumatoid arthritis joint cell culture. (b) Lack of effect of anti-TNF-α on osteoarthritis joint cell cultures. (Reproduced with modification from Brennan *et al.* 1989*a*.)

production after the first day of culture (Fig. 8(a)) (Brennan *et al.* 1989*b*). Assays at the mRNA level show more rapid kinetics, but the lack of an early effect on the amount of IL-1 protein indicates that already ongoing synthesis of IL-1 was not affected, but that subsequent activation was blocked. As a control, the same antibodies were used on cultures of cells from osteoarthritic joints. Despite the presence of immunoreactive TNF-α there was no effect of anti-TNF-α on the low levels of IL-1 in osteoarthritis (Fig. 8(b)). This is now known to be caused by the TNF in osteoarthritis not being biologically active.

The finding that TNF-α was the single dominant signal regulating the production of IL-1 was surprising. It had been anticipated that multiple signals may be of importance, including immune complexes and perhaps other non-cytokine signals. However, samples from the first seven patients behaved in this way, regardless of their therapy. This led us to investigate what other effects of anti-TNF-α on the disease process may be. It has been postulated that GM-CSF is an important cytokine in rheumatoid arthritis, as it is an inducer of class II on monocytes, and induces cytokine production and macrophage activation (Alvaro-Garcia *et al.* 1989). It was therefore of interest to determine which cytokine regulates the production of GM-CSF in cell cultures from rheumatoid joints. Anti-TNF-α markedly inhibited the production of GM-CSF, but more slowly than inhibition of IL-1, being virtually complete only by day 5 (Haworth *et al.* 1991). We have also found that anti-TNF partially inhibits class II expression and also the aggregation normally found in these cultures. A summary of the effects of TNF in rheumatoid joints is shown in Fig. 9.

The results obtained in rheumatoid arthritis are analogous to those now described in the response of mice to systemic Gram-negative bacteria. Production of TNF-α, IL-1, and IL-6 was monitored; peaks of TNF-α preceded those of IL-1 then IL-6. Anti-TNF-α abrogated the production of IL-1 and IL-6 in this animal model (Fong *et al.* 1989). Thus it seems likely that in rheumatoid arthritis, the dominant position of TNF-α recapitulates the physiological situation.

Following the demonstration that anti-TNF can inhibit the production *in vitro* of IL-1 and other proinflammatory cytokines (IL-6, GM-CSF, IL-8) (Feldmann *et al.* 1996) and the successful amelioration of collagen-induced arthritis in DBA/1 mice by use of anti-TNF (Williams *et al.* 1992*a*), we formulated the hypothesis that TNF-α is at the apex of a cytokine cascade. This gave the rationale to

blockade TNF in 20 patients with active rheumatoid arthritis in an open phase I/II trial lasting 8 weeks (Elliott *et al.* 1993).

The monoclonal antibody used was a chimeric (mouse Fv, human IgG1) neutralizing antibody produced by Centocor, Inc. The benefits of anti-TNF treatment were evident in all patients within a few days and lasted 8 to 26 weeks (median 12 weeks). Improvements in clinical parameters included reduction in pain and morning stiffness, falls in swollen and tender joint counts, increased erythrocyte sedimentation rate and reduced C-reactive protein and serum amyloid A. Following this initial success a randomized, double-blind, placebo-controlled, multicentre trial of anti-TNF in 73 patients was undertaken, the results of which confirmed the open study (Elliott *et al.* 1994) and supported the hypothesis that TNF is of major importance in the pathogenesis of rheumatoid arthritis (Figs 10 and 11).

The mechanism of the anti-inflammatory action of anti-TNF-α antibody is under examination in current studies. A rapid decrease of serum IL-6 following anti-TNF demonstrates the effect of anti-TNF antibody on downregulation of other cytokines (Maini *et al.* 1995). A second, and possibly more important, effect of TNF blockade is in reducing the cellularity of the synovium (Maini *et al.* 1995). This is accompanied by an increase in peripheral blood lymphocyte count and a decrease in expression of adhesion molecules in synovial biopsies taken before and after therapy (Tak *et al.* 1996). There is an associated decrease in circulating levels of E-selectin and ICAM-1 (Paleolog *et al.* 1996). Viewed together, these data suggest that anti-TNF therapy reduces cell traffic into joints by reducing leucocyte–endothelium interactions, thereby reducing the mass of inflammatory tissue and its clinicopathological consequences.

Cytokine antagonists

In 1989, TNF-binding protein, capable of inhibiting the action of TNF, was discovered in the blood and urine of febrile patients (Englemann *et al.* 1989; Seckinger *et al.* 1989). This was subsequently found to be derived from the extracellular domain of the two TNF receptors, probably by proteolytic cleavage. On account of the proposed role of TNF-α in the pathogenesis of rheumatoid arthritis, the role of TNF inhibitor was explored, with the expectation that levels of soluble TNF receptors may be low.

Analysis of serum samples from a variety of arthritic patients has revealed that in rheumatoid arthritis the TNF inhibitor system is enhanced, and there are elevated levels of both soluble TNF receptors (p55 and p75) in serum and in the joint fluids, with an intermediate rise in levels in seronegative arthritis and osteoarthritis (Cope *et al.* 1992). However, these upregulated levels of soluble TNF receptors

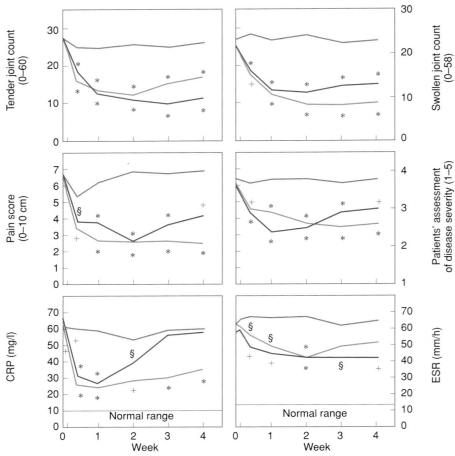

Fig. 10   Changes in clinical assessments in 73 patients treated with placebo (●), 1 mg/kg (▲), or 10 mg/kg (■) anti-TNF monoclonal antibody in a randomized, double-blind trial (p values represent significance versus placebo: + $p < 0.05$; § $p < 0.01$; * $p < 0.001$). (Reproduced by kind permission from an article by Elliott *et al*. 1994, *Lancet*, **344**, 1105–10.)

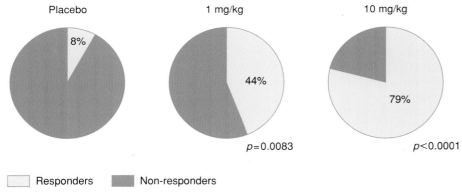

Fig. 11   Overall clinical responses to placebo, 1 mg/kg, or 10 mg/kg anti-TNF monoclonal antibody in 73 patients, 4 weeks after treatment, in a randomized, double-blind trial (p values represent significance versus placebo). (Reproduced by kind permission from articles by Elliott *et al*. 1994, *Lancet*, **344**, 1105–10 and Maini *et al*. 1995, *Immunology Reviews*, **144**, 95–223.)

do not neutralize fully the TNF-α produced by cells from rheumatoid joints in culture, whereas they generally appear to be sufficient to neutralize TNF-α produced by cells from osteoarthritic joints in culture (Brennan *et al*. 1995). Thus, in arthritis there appears to be an attempt at homeostasis, which, however, is inadequate (Cope and Maini 1995). Other soluble cytokine receptors that in the fluid phase

would act as cytokine antagonists have been described, for example, soluble IL-1 (Symons *et al*. 1991), -2 (p55), -4, -6, and -7 receptors and soluble interferon-γ receptor, which may act as regulators of the cytokine network.

There is so far only one cytokine inhibitor described which acts as a receptor antagonist, i.e. the IL-1 receptor antagonist, which is produced in rheumatoid joints (Arend 1991). This is a member of the IL-1 family, with 30 per cent homology to IL-1β. The physiological role of this molecule is unclear, as quantities greatly in excess of those of IL-1 are necessary to exert inhibitory effects, far larger than are physiologically present *in vivo*. Its role may be simply to localize the effects of IL-1 in the environment in which the cytokine is produced. Whatever the exact physiological roles of IL-1 receptor antagonist and soluble TNF receptor, these natural agents with the capacity to interfere with cytokine action are potential therapeutic agents in rheumatoid arthritis (Elliott and Maini 1996).

Immune suppression in rheumatoid arthritis

Despite the evidence for an ongoing autoimmune response at both the T- and B-cell level, there is also considerable evidence that the systemic immune response is suppressed in patients with rheumatoid arthritis. This has been demonstrated as a reduced response to tuberculin (purified protein derivative) testing (Kingsley *et al.* 1987), in IL-2 production, or in T-cell proliferative or cytokine production. Serial studies have shown that the degree of immune suppression is more severe as the patients are clinically more ill. The mechanisms of this suppression are not understood, but could lead eventually to new forms of therapy aimed at reinforcing the endogenous mechanisms of immune suppression.

A number of molecules found in the joints in rheumatoid arthritis may be important contributors to this process. These include prostaglandins and TGF-β. Other potential candidates not yet known to be present include oncostatin M, IL-10, and IL-4. Prostaglandins are produced in the inflammation of rheumatoid arthritis. However, most non-steroidal anti-inflammatory drugs interfere with the production of prostaglandins, and this does not overcome the endogenous suppression, which accordingly is mostly caused by other agents. TGF-β is found in large amounts in supernatants of synovial cell cultures (10 to 20 ng/ml) of which 1 to 2 ng/ml is bioactive (Brennan *et al.* 1990*b*). There is thus sufficient TGF-β to influence immune functions of T and B cells, and cytokine production. However, appropriate neutralizing experiments on synovial cell cultures remain to be done. Oncostatin M is growth inhibitory for a variety of cell types, is produced by activated T cells and macrophages, and so may be expected to be present. IL-10, a product of T cells and B cells, can interfere with antigen-presenting capacity and with the production of interferon-γ. IL-10 has been demonstrated in rheumatoid joints and *in vitro* studies reveal that it is apparently exerting a suppressive effect on endogenous production of TNF-α and IL-1 (Katsikis *et al.* 1993). The beneficial effect of administration of recombinant IL-10 in established collagen-induced arthritis supports its possible therapeutic potential (Walmsley *et al.* 1996)

Animal models (see Chapter 3.4)

Research in unravelling the factors that initiate rheumatoid arthritis, understanding the perpetuation of disease, and devising new strategies for therapy or prevention has to some extent depended on concepts developed and validated in animal models. Recent clinical studies have raised questions that have increased, rather than diminished, the complementary value of the use of animal models.

However, there is as yet no ideal animal model of rheumatoid arthritis that exhibits all key features, namely:

(1) predictable and spontaneous development of an erosive, chronic, symmetrical arthritis punctuated by flares;

(2) female preponderance;

(3) association with the MHC homologue of HLA DR4 or DR1;

(4) high frequency of circulating IgM rheumatoid factor;

(5) synovitis with a cellular response, profile of local production of cytokines, proteases, and inflammatory mediators identical to that observed in rheumatoid arthritis;

(6) cartilage and bone degeneration with pannus formation;

(7) response to disease-modifying antirheumatoid drugs akin to that observed in rheumatoid arthritis.

Despite reservations, the ensuing section gives examples of existing and new models of rheumatoid arthritis, which have contributed to our understanding of this disease.

Collagen-induced arthritis

The distribution of collagen II is essentially restricted to cartilage and the vitreous humour of the eye. Intradermal injection of native collagen II in Freund's adjuvant (but not of collagen types I and III or denatured type II) induces a polyarthritis in rats (Trentham *et al.* 1977), mice (Courtenay *et al.* 1980), and monkeys (Cathcart *et al.* 1986). Heterologous or autologous type II collagens are effective but the former leads to a destructive yet self-limiting disorder, whereas the latter is characterized by a chronic remitting and exacerbating course of disease (Holmdahl *et al.* 1986). T- and B-cell responses to multiple epitopes on collagen II occur, and disease of a milder variety than in the immunized animals has been transferred into syngeneic animals by serum and/or T cells. Rheumatoid factor is detectable and villous synovitis with increased cellularity of the lining layer, infiltration of deeper layers with mononuclear cells (predominantly CD4+ T cells), and pannus formation echo the changes observed in rheumatoid arthritis. The best-documented susceptible mouse, the DBA/1, bears the *H-2q* haplotype; H-2^r mice are also susceptible, but H-2^d mice are resistant to collagen arthritis. Although a polygenic disease, it is of considerable interest that the HLA class II molecules mapping to I-A (the mouse homologue of human HLA DQ) appear to be the element controlling susceptibility and immune responses to type II collagen in DBA/1 (Holmdahl *et al.* 1989). The importance of non-MHC genes, for example, genes regulating complement synthesis and the expression of IgG subclass isotypes, has been deduced from other studies.

The collagen arthritis has significant similarities to rheumatoid arthritis and its importance lies in the ability of an immune response to a constituent of cartilage to induce disease. As B- and T-cell-specific responses to collagen II occur in a proportion of patients with rheumatoid arthritis, especially, and sometimes exclusively, when lymphocytes from the synovial membrane are studied, the model provides evidence that collagen immunity might perpetuate rheumatoid disease. The model has provided useful data on the arthritogenic epitopes on type II collagen and therapeutic manipulations have provided evidence that antibodies directed against CD4+ T cells (Ranges *et al.* 1985), B cells (Helfgott *et al.* 1984), and TNF-α

(Williams *et al.* 1992*a*) are effective in ameliorating established disease.

Adjuvant arthritis

A single intradermal injection of Freund's complete adjuvant (containing *Mycobacterium tuberculosis*) in the footpad or tail of rats induces a severe arthropathy involving the wrists, ankles, paws, and caudal part of the spine and tail (Pearson 1956). The arthropathy in its developed stage consists of synovitis with villous formation, pannus eroding cartilage and bone, marked periostitis with new bone formation, and inflammation and fibrosis of periarticular tissues. After peaking, the inflammatory arthritis declines and is followed by fibrous and bony ankylosis of joints. Extra-articular features can be prominent and include balanitis, conjunctivitis, and cutaneous lesions resembling psoriasis. Although the disease in diarthrodial joints has some similarity to rheumatoid arthritis, the other features are reminiscent of the clinical spectrum of spondylarthropathies, especially Reiter's syndrome. This is further suggested by a consistent lack of IgM rheumatoid factor. Susceptibility is strain dependent; for example, Lewis rats are most susceptible, and Fisher rats are less so. Susceptibility is believed to involve multiple genes with no convincing role for the MHC genes.

The major interest in the model springs from the demonstration that the disease is mediated by T cells that recognize mycobacterial peptides (Cohen *et al.* 1985). Furthermore, there is evidence for molecular mimicry between a mycobacterial antigen and cartilage antigens (van Eden *et al.* 1985), and this is believed to be the key factor in localization of the disease to joints. The relevant antigen has been defined and is a mycobacterial nonapeptide present in a 65-kDa mycobacterial protein that belongs to the family of hsp65 (van Eden *et al.* 1988). The nonapeptide stimulates T-cell clones of the CD4 phenotype, termed A2b and A2c, derived from a parent line, A2, obtained from a rat with adjuvant arthritis. Following *in vivo* inoculation into irradiated syngeneic Lewis rats, A2b causes a severe arthritis, whereas A2c protects from disease induction and causes a rapid remission (Cohen *et al.* 1985). When hsp65 or the nonapeptide are given before Freund's adjuvant, the rats are protected from the disease.

The possibility that T cells equivalent to the suppressive clones isolated from adjuvant arthritis are present in the inflammatory exudate of rheumatoid arthritis has prompted optimism that T-cell vaccination may prove to be a promising therapy. Activated T cells, treated with hydrostatic pressure, or T-cell receptors cross-linked with glutaraldehyde are used as surrogate suppressor–inducers in vaccination protocols. However, preliminary trials have not shown any benefit in rheumatoid arthritis (Van Laar *et al.* 1991).

Streptococcal cell-wall arthritis

A single injection intraperitoneally of an aqueous suspension of group A streptococcal cell-wall fragments into rats induces a polyarthritis (Cromartie *et al.* 1977). The arthritis involves wrists, ankles, and other joints, spares the axial skeleton, and is biphasic with an early phase reaching its maximum at 3 days, followed by the onset of a chronic arthritis 2 to 4 weeks later. Lewis (LEW/N) female rats are the most susceptible to this form of arthritis and exhibit many pathological features of rheumatoid arthritis — a villous synovial thickening with surface fibrin, thickening of the synovial lining layer,

polymorph exudation into joint fluid, mononuclear cell infiltrates with a predominance of CD4+ T cells, angiogenesis, and fibroblast proliferation with pannus formation and associated erosion of underlying cartilage and bone. Low titres of IgM rheumatoid factor are detectable. The active proinflammatory constituent of streptococcal cell-wall is its peptidoglycan component, which has extensive pathophysiological effects involving many cell types; the smallest active subunit of peptidoglycan is muramyl dipeptide, which is itself an activator of macrophages and endothelial cells. Persistence of streptococcal cell-wall owing to its protective carbohydrate side chains, is believed to contribute to the initiation and perpetuation of disease.

The importance of T cells in the pathogenesis of the disease has been demonstrated by transfer of arthritis to nude, T-cell deficient, inbred Lewis rats. Like rheumatoid arthritis, the T-cell abnormalities include depressed responses to mitogen and defective production of IL-2. As hsp65 protects against arthritis induced by streptococcal cell wall (van den Broek *et al.* 1989), it has been suggested that this protein may be the host protein target for the T-cell response. However, the molecular basis of this has not been resolved. Although HLA class II molecules are rapidly induced in endothelial cells in inflamed tissues, the role of MHC antigen-associated susceptibility is ambiguous because a related strain of rats (the Fisher strain) with the same histocompatibility locus is relatively resistant to arthritis.

Of considerable interest are the observations on the hypothalamoadrenal axis in the arthritis induced by streptococcal cell wall. In susceptible female Lewis rats there is an abnormally low gene expression at the mRNA level of the corticotrophin-releasing hormone and encephalin, with a deficient response of adrenal corticotrophic hormone and adrenal corticosteroid (Sternberg *et al.* 1989*a*; Sternberg *et al.* 1989*b*). In contrast, Fisher rats, resistant to arthritis, show relatively rapid and efficient responses from the hypothalamoadrenal axis. That these neuroendocrine responses are important in the pathogenesis of disease is suggested by the observation that giving corticosteroid in small doses simultaneously administered with streptococcal cell wall improves the course of the induced arthritis and, conversely, blockade of the glucocorticoid receptor with RU 486 accelerates disease in resistant Fisher rats (Sternberg *et al.* 1989*a*).

Other models of arthritis

The transient inflammatory arthritis of serum sickness in rabbits induced by antigen and mediated by antigen–antibody complexes (Dixon *et al.* 1958) had antedated the description of chronic arthritis in the rabbit knee induced by intra-articular injection of protein antigens such as fibrin, heterologous gammaglobulin, and ovalbumin into previously sensitized animals that had received antigen in Freund's adjuvant (Dumonde and Glynn 1962). One aspect of interest in the latter model was the demonstration that the arthritis was dependent on antigen–antibody complexes sequestered in cartilaginous tissues (Jasin 1975) which could act as a depot of persistent immunogen and gave rise to a cellular immune response. The induction of arthritis by a similar protocol in neonatally thymectomized or bursectomized chickens demonstrated that arthritis was inducible by both thymus-dependent T and bursa-dependent B cells; however, the fully developed lesion required an intact thymus and bursa (Oates *et al.* 1972).

Infective agents as a cause of arthritis have attracted much interest; and mycoplasmas (Decker and Barden 1975) and erysipelotherix (Drew 1972) are both well-described causes of chronic arthritis in swine. In the former model, a chronic arthritis persisted long after viable organisms could be cultured from joints, blood, or lymph nodes and non-viable antigen persisted for longer periods, and it was suggested thst this might have been responsible for the destructive arthritis. In a model of swine arthritis resembling rheumatoid arthritis studied in Sweden, introduction of fish meal in the diet was causative of arthritis and evidence was obtained that this was associated with population of the gut by *Clostridium perfringens* (Mansson *et al.* 1971). Immune responses to the clostridium were demonstrable, but the organism could not be isolated from the joints and as such represented a form of reactive arthritis.

Caprine arthritis, mainly involving large joints, has generated interest in the arthritogenic potential of the causative lentivirus, which is a lentiform retrovirus, as is the human immunodeficiency virus (Crawford *et al.* 1980). In this disease, possibly acquired by ingestion of milk by goat kids, the virus is harboured by mononuclear phagocytes. Encephalitis also occurs and this feature makes it distinct from rheumatoid arthritis. Chronic destructive joint lesions are described, and these resemble rheumatoid arthritis, as does the mononuclear cell infiltrate in the synovium. However, the lentivirus cannot be isolated from joints. In contrast to rheumatoid arthritis, mononuclear cells rather than polymorphs are dominant in joint fluids and, also unlike rheumatoid arthritis, high levels of interferon activity are demonstrable. Studies of the tropism for joints and the pathogenesis of the inflammatory reaction provide insight into the pathways that might prove important in devising investigations of the possibility that retroviruses may cause rheumatoid arthritis.

The MRL/lpr mouse is generally regarded as a model of systemic lupus and develops a multisystem disease characterized by glomerulonephritis, vasculitis, and antibodies to double-stranded DNA and Sm antigen, associated with marked lymphoproliferation involving a T cell with an $\alpha\beta$ heterodime receptor, but lacking CD4 and CD8 antigens (Andrews *et al.* 1978). This mouse strain, however, also develops an arthritis of the hind limbs with invasion of cartilage by pannus, high levels of rheumatoid factor, and anticollagen type II antibodies; therefore in some respects it shows features of rheumatoid arthritis. Production of rheumatoid factor appears to be under the control of the lymphoproliferation gene. The early destruction of articular tissue is at the marginal junction of the synovium with cartilage and bone, in association with proliferation of fibroblastic cells, and antedates an inflammatory response (O'Sullivan *et al.* 1985). This spontaneous model of arthritis appears to be of importance in delineating the relationship between autoimmunity and nonimmune cellular responses in the synovium and pannus invasion of cartilage and bone, as well as understanding the genetic regulation of rheumatoid factor.

Transgenic mice offer the possibility of assessing *in vivo* the effect of introduced genes on the development of disease. Two models have recently been published which may shed insight into the mechanism of arthritis. The simplest to evaluate is the introduction of a modified human TNF-α gene, under its own promoter, into fertilized ova. The modification of the gene was replacement of the TNF-α 3' untranslated region, which has been shown to confer mRNA instability, with the 3' untranslated region of β-globin, which has a very stable mRNA. With this deregulated TNF-α production, it was found that the mice developed a progressive arthritis by 4 weeks of age. The

arthritis was preventable by the injection of antihuman TNF-α monoclonal antibody from birth onwards. The arthritis is characterized by subchondral erosions and frequent fibrosis, but further analysis is necessary to establish how closely this disease resembles rheumatoid arthritis (Keffer *et al.* 1991). This model, however, confirms the hypothesis that TNF-α is intimately involved in the arthritic process.

Transgenic mice carrying the human T-cell leukaemia virus-1 genome also develop a chronic erosive arthritis (Iwakura *et al.* 1991). In this model, approximately one-third of the mice highly expressing the transgene developed arthritis with synovial inflammation and cartilage erosion, closely resembling a pannus. Low levels of rheumatoid factor were occasionally detected. It was of interest that the mRNA of the *Tax* gene, a transacting transcriptional activator, was highly expressed in the joints. Thus it is likely that the arthritis is the result of increased cytokine expression in the joints. Supporting this is the preliminary observation, cited in Iwakura *et al.* (1991), that IL-1α mRNA is expressed in the joints of these mice, as it is in rheumatoid arthritis.

Conclusions

Our understanding of the pathogenesis of rheumatoid arthritis in molecular terms has progressed rapidly in the past few years. This has provided a number of molecular targets, and therapeutic trials based on these targets have been initiated. The first of these was CD4, and monoclonal anti-CD4 has been used by a number of groups, with beneficial though transient results in a proportion of patients.

Attempts are being made to devise peptide-based therapies which will selectively block the critical HLA peptide-presenting genomes. Neutralization of cytokines such as TNF-α and IL-1 with antibodies or soluble receptors has been successfully applied in clinical trials and has set the stage for an era of promising new therapeutic interventions.

These (and more) therapeutic trials will have an important benefit in helping to evaluate ideas concerning the pathogenesis of rheumatoid arthritis, and even if (as is likely) they are not totally successful, they will contribute to refining our concepts of the pathogenesis of the disease and to more effective therapies.

References

Abbink, J.J., Kamp, A.M., Niujens, J.S., Erenberg, A.J., and Hack, C.E. (1992). Relative contribution of contact and complement activation to inflammatory reactions in arthritic joints. *Annals of the Rheumatic Diseases*, **51**, 1123–8.

Abbot, S.E., Kaul, A., Stevens, C.R., and Blake, D.R. (1992). Isolation and culture of synovial microvascular endothelial cells: characterization and assessment of adhesion molecule expression. *Arthritis and Rheumatism*, **35**, 401–6.

Adler, R. (1985). Psychoneuroimmunologic contributions to the study of rheumatic diseases. In *Immunology of rheumatic diseases* (ed. S. Gupta and N. Talal), pp. 669–96. Plenum Medical Book Company, New York.

Akahoshi, T. *et al.* (1993). Expression of monocyte chemotactic and activating factor in rheumatoid arthritis. *Arthritis and Rheumatism*, **36**, 762–71.

Albani, S. *et al.* (1995). Positive selection in autoimmunity: abnormal immune responses to a bacterial DNAJ antigenic determinant in patients with early rheumatoid arthritis. *Nature New Medicine*, **1**, 448–52.

Allard, S.A., Muirden, K.D., Camplejohn, K.L., and Maini, R.N. (1987). Chondrocyte-derived cells and matrix at the rheumatoid cartilage–pannus junction identified with monoclonal antibodies. *Rheumatology International*, **7**, 153–9.

Allard, S.A., Bayliss, M.T., and Maini, R.N. (1990). The synovial–cartilage junction of the normal human knee: implications for joint destruction and repair. *Arthritis and Rheumatism*, 33, 1170–9.

Allard, S.A., Bayliss, M.T., and Maini, R.N. (1991). Correlation of histopathological features of pannus with patterns of damage in different joints in rheumatoid arthritis. *Annals of the Rheumatic Disease*, 50, 278–83.

Alvaro-Garcia, J.M., Zvaifler, N.J., and Firestein, G.S. (1989). Cytokines in chronic inflammatory arthritis. IV. Granulocyte/macrophage colony stimulating factor-mediated induction of class II MHC antigen on human monocytes: a possible role in rheumatoid arthritis. *Journal of Experimental Medicine*, 170, 865–75.

Andrew, E.M., Plater Zyberk, C., Brown, C.M.S., Williams, D.G., and Maini, R.N. (1991). The potential role of B lymphocytes in the pathogenesis of rheumatoid arthritis. *British Journal of Rheumatology*, 30 (Suppl. 1), 47–52.

Andrews, B.S. *et al.* (1978). Spontaneous murine lupus-like syndrome. *Journal of Experimental Medicine*, 148, 1198–215.

Arend, W.F. (1991). Interleukin-l receptor antagonist — a new member of the IL-l family. *Journal of Clinical Investigation*, 88, 1445–51.

Axford, J.S., Mackenzie L., Lydyard, P.M., Hay, F.C., Isenberg, D.A., and Roitt, I.M. (1987). Reduced B-cell galactosyltransferase activity in rheumatoid arthritis. *Lancet*, ii, 1486–8.

Baboonian, C., Venables, P.J.W., Williams, D.G., Williams, R.O., and Maini, R.N. (1991). Cross-reaction of antibodies to a glycine–alanine repeat sequence of Epstein–Barr virus nuclear antigen-l with collagen, cytokeratin, and actin. *Annals of the Rheumatic Diseases*, 50, 772–5.

Barkley, D., Allard, S.A., Feldmann, M., and Maini, R.N. (1989a). Increased expression of HLA-DQ antigens by interstitial cells and endothelium in the synovial membrane of rheumatoid arthritis patients compared with reactive arthritis patients. *Arthritis and Rheumatism*, 32, 955–63.

Barkley, D., Feldmann, M., and Maini, R.N. (1989b). The detection by immunofluorescence of distinct cell populations producing interleukin-1α and interleukin-1β in activated human peripheral blood. *Journal of Immunological Methods*, 120, 277–83.

Berthelot, J.-M., Vincent, C., Serre, G., and Youinou, P. (1994). APF (antiperinuclear factor). In *Manual of biological markers of disease* (ed. R.N. Maini and W.J. Van Venrooij), B1.2, pp. 1–9. Kluwer, Dordrecht.

Brennan, F.M. *et al.* (1988a). Heterogeneity of T cell receptor idiotypes in rheumatoid arthritis. *Clinical and Experimental Immunology*, 73, 417–23.

Brennan, F.M. *et al.* (1988b). T cells expressing γδ chain receptors in rheumatoid arthritis. *Journal of Autoimmunity*, 1, 319–26.

Brennan, F.M., Chantry, D., Jackson, A.M., Maini, R.N., and Feldmann, M. (1989a). Cytokine production in culture by cells isolated from the synovial membrane. *Journal of Autoimmunity*, 2, (Suppl.), 177–86.

Brennan, F.M., Chantry, D., Jackson, A., Maini, R.N., and Feldmann, M. (1989b). Inhibitory effect of TNFα antibodies on synovial cell interleukin-1 production in rheumatoid arthritis. *Lancet*, ii, 244–7.

Brennan, F.M., Plater Zyberk, C., Maini, R.N., and Feldmann, M. (1989c). Coordinate expansion of 'fetal type' lymphocytes (TCR γδ+T and CD5+β) in rheumatoid arthritis and primary Sjögren's syndrome. *Clinical and Experimental Immunology*, 77, 175–8.

Brennan, F.M. *et al.* (1990a). Detection of interleukin 8 biological activity in synovial fluids from patients with rheumatoid arthritis and production of IL-8 mRNA by isolated synovial cells. *European Journal of Immunology*, 20, 2141.

Brennan, F.M., Chantry, D., Turner, M., Foxwell, B., Maini, R.N., and Feldmann, M. (1990b). Detection of transforming growth factor β in rheumatoid arthritis synovial tissue: lack of effect on spontaneous cytokine production in joint cell cultures. *Clinical and Experimental Immunology*, 81, 278–85.

Brennan, F.M., Gibbons, D.L., Cope, A.P., Katsikis, P., Maini, R.N., and Feldmann, M. (1995). TNF inhibitors are produced spontaneously by rheumatoid and osteoarthritis synovial joint cell cultures: evidence of feedback control of TNF action. *Scandinavian Journal of Immunology*, 42, 158–65.

Brenner, C.A., Tam, A.W., Nelson, D.A., Suzuki, N., Fry, K.E., and Larrick, J.W. (1989). Message amplification phenotyping (MAPPing): a technique to simultaneously measure multiple mRNAs from small number of cells. *BioTechniques*, 7, 1096–2003.

Brown, C.M.S, Longhurst, C., Haynes, G., Plater-Zyberk, C., Malcolm, A., and Maini, R.N. (1992). Immunoglobulin heavy chain variable region gene utilization by B cell hybridomas derived from rheumatoid synovial tissue. *Clinical and Experimental Immunology*, 89, 230–8.

Brown, C.M.S., Fitzgerald, K.J., Moyes, S.P., Mageed, R.A., Williams, D.G., and Maini, R.N. (1995). Sequence analysis of immunoglobulin heavy-chain variable region genes from the synovium of a rheumatoid arthritis patient shows little evidence of mutation but diverse CDR3. *Immunology*, 84, 367–74.

Buchan, G., Barrett, K., Turner, M., Chantry, D., Maini, R.N., and Feldmann, M. (1988a). Interleukin-1 and tumour necrosis factor mRNA expression in rheumatoid arthritis: prolonged production of IL-1α. *Clinical and Experimental Immunology*, 73, 449–55.

Buchan, G., Barrett, K., Fujita, T., Taniguchi, T., Maini, R.N., and Feldmann, M. (1988b). Detection of activated T cell products in the rheumatoid joint using cDNA probes to interleukin 2, IL-2 receptor and interferon γ. *Clinical and Experimental Immunology*, 71, 295–301.

Buchanan, H.M., Preston, S.J., Brooks, P.M., and Buchanan, W.W. (1991). Is diet important in rheumatoid arthritis? *British Journal of Rheumatology*, 30, 125–34.

Cathcart, E.S., Hayes, K.C., Gonnerman, W.A., Lazzari, A.A., and Franzblau, C. (1986). Experimental arthritis in a non-human primate. l. Induction by bovine type II collagen. *Laboratory Investigation*, 54, 26–31.

Chantry, D., Winearls, C.G., Maini, R.N., and Feldmann, M. (1989). Mechanism of immune complex mediated damage: induction of interleukin 1 by immune complexes and synergy with interferon γ and tumour necrosis factor α. *European Journal of Immunology*, 19, 189–92.

Chantry, D., Turner, M., Brennan, F., Kingsbury, A., and Feldmann, M. (1990). Granulocyte–macrophage colony stimulating factor induces both HLA-DR expression and cytokine production by human monocytes. *Cytokine*, 2, 60–7.

Charriere, G., Hartmann, D.J., Vignon, E., Ronziere, M.C., Herbage, D., and Ville, G. (1988). Antibodies to type I, II, IX, XI collagen in the serum of patients with rheumatic diseases. *Arthritis and Rheumatism*, 31, 325–32.

Chu, C.Q., Field, M., Feldmann, M., and Maini, R.N. (1991a). Localization of tumor necrosis factor α in synovial tissues and at the cartilage–pannus junction in patients with rheumatoid arthritis. *Arthritis and Rheumatism*, 34, 1125–32.

Chu, C.Q. *et al.* (1991b). Transforming growth factor β₁ in rheumatoid synovial membrane and cartilage/pannus junction. *Clinical and Experimental Immunology*, 86, 380–6.

Cohen, I.R., Holoshitz, J., van Eden, W., and Frenkel, A. (1985). T lymphocyte clones illuminate pathogenesis and effect therapy of experimental arthritis. *Arthritis and Rheumatism*, 28, 841–5.

Cohen, S.B.A. *et al.* (1995). High level of interleukin-10 production by the activated T cell population within the rheumatoid synovial membrane. *Arthritis and Rheumatism*, 38, 946–52.

Colville-Nash, P.R. and Scott, D.L. (1992). Angiogenesis and rheumatoid arthritis: pathogenic and therapeutic implications. *Annals of the Rheumatic Diseases*, 51, 919–25.

Cope, A.P. and Maini, R.N. (1995). Soluble tumor necrosis factor receptors in arthritis. *Journal of Rheumatology*, 22, 382–4.

Cope, A. *et al.* (1992). Increased levels of soluble tumor necrosis factor receptors in the sera and synovial fluids of patients with rheumatic diseases. *Arthritis and Rheumatism*, 35, 1160–9.

Courtenay, J.S., Dallman, M.J., Dayan, A.D., Martin, A., and Mosedale, B. (1980). Immunisation against heterologous type II collagen induces arthritis in mice. *Nature*, 283, 666–8.

Crawford, T.B., Adams, D.S., Cheevers, W.P., and Cork, L.V. (1980). Chronic arthritis in goats caused by a retrovirus. *Science*, 207, 997–9.

Cromartie, W.J., Craddock, J.C., Schwab, J.H., Anderle, S.K., and Yang, C.H. (1977). Arthritis in rats after systemic injection of streptococcal cells or cell walls. *Journal of Experimental Medicine*, 146, 1585–602.

Cush, J.J., Pietschmann, P., Oppenheimer-Marks, N., and Lipsky, P.E. (1992). The intrinsic migratory capacity of memory T cells contributes to their accumulation in rheumatoid synovium. *Arthritis and Rheumatism*, 35, 1434–44.

Davies, M.E., Sharma, H., and Pigott, R. (1992). ICAM-1 expression on chondrocytes in rheumatoid arthritis: induction by synovial cytokines. *Mediators of Inflammation*, 1, 71–4.

Dayan, C.M. *et al.* (1991). Autoantigen recognition by thyroid-infiltrating T cells in Graves' disease. *Proceedings of the National Academy of Sciences (USA)*, **88**, 7415–19.

de Graeff-Meeder, E.R. *et al.* (1990). Antibodies to the mycobacterium-65 kDa heat-shock protein are reactive with synovial tissue of adjuvant arthritic rats and patients with rheumatoid arthritis and osteoarthritis. *American Journal of Pathology*, **137**, 1013–17.

Decker, J.L. and Barden, J.A. (1975). *Mycoplasma hyortinis* of swine: a model for rheumatoid arthritis? *Rheumatology*, **6**, 338–45.

Deighton, C.M., Walker, D.J., Griffiths, I.D., and Roberts, D.F. (1989). The contribution of HLA to rheumatoid arthritis. *Clinical Genetics*, **36**, 178–82.

Deleuran, B.W. *et al.* (1992). Localization of tumor necrosis factor receptors in the synovial tissue and cartilage–pannus junction in patients with rheumatoid arthritis: implications for local actions of tumor necrosis factor α. *Arthritis and Rheumatism*, **35**, 1170–8.

Dequeker, J. (1987). Rheumatic diseases in visual arts. (General review.) In *Art history and antiquity of rheumatic diseases* (ed. T. Appelboom), p. 84. Elsevier, Brussels.

Dieppe, P.A. (1988). Did Galen describe rheumatoid arthritis? *Annals of the Rheumatic Diseases*, **47**, 84–5.

Dixon, F.J., Vasquez, J.J., Weigle, W.D., and Cochrane, C.G. (1958). Pathogenesis of serum sickness. *Archives of Pathology*, **65**, 18–22.

Drew, R.A. (1972). Erysipelothrix arthritis in pigs as a model of rheumatoid arthritis. *Proceedings of the Royal Society of Medicine*, **65**, 42–6.

Dumonde, D.C. and Glynn, L.E. (1962). The production of arthritis in rabbits by an immunological reaction to fibrin. *British Journal of Experimental Pathology*, **43**, 373–83.

Eastgate, J.A., Symons, J.A., Wood, N.C., Grinlinton, F.M., Di Giovine, F.S., and Duff, G.W. (1988). Correlation of plasma interleukin-1 levels with disease activity in rheumatoid arthritis. *Lancet*, **ii**, 706–9.

Ebringer, A., Khalafpour, S., and Wilson C. (1989). Rheumatoid arthritis and *Proteus*: a possible aetiological association. *Rheumatism International*, **9**, 223–8.

Elliott, M.J. and Maini, R.N. (1996). What are the prospects for therapy based on cytokines and anticytokines in rheumatoid arthritis? In *Cytokines in autoimmunity* (ed. F.M. Brennan and M. Feldmann), pp. 239–56. R.G. Landes, Austin, TX.

Elliott, M.J. *et al.* (1993). Treatment of rheumatoid arthritis with chimeric monoclonal antibodies to tumor necrosis factor α. *Arthritis and Rheumatism*, **36**, 1681–90.

Elliott, M.J. *et al.* (1994). Randomised double-blind comparison of chimeric monoclonal antibody to tumour necrosis factor α (cA2) versus placebo in rheumatoid arthritis. *Lancet*, **344**, 1105–10.

Engelmann, H., Novick, D., and Wallach, D. (1990). Two tumour necrosis factor-binding proteins purified from human urine. *Journal of Biological Chemistry*, **265** (3), 1531–6.

Feldmann, M. (1987). Regulation of HLA class II expression and its role in autoimmune disease. In *Autoimmunity and autoimmune disease*, Ciba Foundation Symposium 129, pp. 88–108. Wiley, Chichester.

Feldmann, M. (1989). Molecular mechanisms involved in human autoimmune diseases: relevance of chronic antigen presentation, class II expression and cytokine production. *Immunology*, Suppl. **2**, 66–71.

Feldmann, M. *et al.* (1991). Cytokine assays: role in evaluation of the pathogenesis of autoimmunity. *Immunological Reviews*, **119**, 105–23.

Feldmann, M., Brennan, F.M., and Maini, R.N. (1996). Role of cytokines in rheumatoid arthritis. *Annual Review of Immunology*, **14**, 397–440.

Ferrara, N., Houck, K.A., Jakeman, L.B., Winer, J., and Leung, D.W. (1991). The vascular endothelial growth factor family of polypeptides. *Journal of Cell Biochemistry*, **47**, 211–8.

Field, M., Chu, C., Feldmann, M., and Maini, R.N. (1991). Interleukin-6 in the synovial membrane in rheumatoid arthritis. *Rheumatism International*, **11**, 45–50.

Firestein, G.S. and Zvaifler, N.J. (1987). Peripheral blood and synovial fluid monocyte activation in inflammatory arthritis. II. Low levels of synovial fluid and synovial tissue interferon suggest that γ-interferon is not the primary macrophage activating factor. *Arthritis and Rheumatism*, **30**, 864–71.

Firestein, G.S. and Zvaifler, N.J. (1990). How important are T cells in chronic rheumatoid synovitis? *Arthritis and Rheumatism*, **33**, 768–73.

Firestein, G.S., Alvaro-Garcia, J.M., and Maki, R. (1990). Quantitative analysis of cytokine gene expression in rheumatoid arthritis. *Journal of Immunology*, **144**, 3347–53.

Folkman, J. (1995). Angiogenesis in cancer, vascular, rheumatoid and other disease. *Nature Medicine*, **1**, 27–30.

Fong, Y. *et al.* (1989). Antibodies to cachectin/tumour necrosis factor reduce interleukin 1β and interleukin 6 appearance during lethal bacteremia. *Journal of Experimental Medicine*, **170**, 1627–33.

Forrestier, J. (1935). Rheumatoid arthritis and its treatment by gold salts. *Journal of Laboratory and Clinical Medicine*, **20**, 827–40.

Fraser, K.J. (1982). Anglo-French contributions to the recognition of rheumatoid arthritis. *Annals of the Rheumatic Diseases*, **41**, 335–43.

Garrod, A.B. (1859). *Nature and treatment of gout and rheumatic gout*. Walton and Maberly, London.

Gaston, J.S., Life, P.F., Bailey, L.C., and Bacon, P.A. (1989). In vitro response to a 65 kDa mycobacterial protein by synovial T cells from inflammatory arthritis patients. *Journal of Immunology*, **143**, 2494–500.

Goldstein, R. and Arnett, F.C. (1987). The genetics of rheumatic disease in man. *Rheumatic Disease Clinics of North America*, **13** (3), 487–510.

Goronzy, J. and Weyand, P.M., (1993). Interplay of T lymphocytes and HLA-DR molecules in rheumatoid arthritis. *Current Opinion in Rheumatology*, **5**, 169–77.

Goronzy, J., Weyand, P.M., and Fathman, C.G. (1986). Shared T cell recognition sites on human histocompatibility leukocyte antigen class II molecules of patients with seropositive rheumatoid arthritis. *Journal of Clinical Investigation*, **77**, 1042–9.

Gregersen, P.K., Silver, J., and Winchester, R.J. (1987). The shared epitope hypothesis. An approach to understanding the molecular genetics of susceptibility to rheumatoid arthritis. *Arthritis and Rheumatism*, **30**, 1205–13.

Hammer, J. *et al.* (1995). Peptide binding specificity of HLA-DR4 molecules: correlation with rheumatoid arthritis association. *Journal of Experimental Medicine*, **181**, 1847–55.

Hannestad, K. and Stollar, B.D. (1978). Certain rheumatoid factors react with nucleosomes. *Nature*, **275**, 671–3.

Hargraves, M.M., Richmond, H., and Morton, R. (1948). Presentation of two bone marrow elements, the 'Tart' cell and 'L-E' cell. *Proceedings of Staff Meetings of the Mayo Clinic*, **23**, 25–8.

Hassfeld, W. *et al.* (1995). Autoimmune response to the spliceosome: an immunologic link between rheumatoid arthritis, mixed connective tissue disease and systemic lupus erythematosus. *Arthritis and Rheumatism*, **38**, 777–85.

Haworth, C., Brennan, F.M., Chantry, D., Turner, M., Maini, R.N., and Feldmann, M. (1991). Expression of granulocyte-macrophage colony-stimulating factor in rheumatoid arthritis: regulation by tumour necrosis factor α. *European Journal of Immunology*, **21**, 2575–9.

Helfgott, S.M., Bazin, H., Dessein, A., and Trentham, D.E. (1984). Suppressive effects of anti-μ serum on the development of collagen arthritis in rats. *Clinical Immunology and Immunopathology*, **31**, 403–11.

Herman, A., Kappler, J.W., Marrack, P., and Pullen, A.M. (1991). Superantigens: mechanism of T-cell stimulation and role in immune responses. *Annual Review of Immunology*, **9**, 745–72.

Hirano, T. *et al.* (1988). Excessive production of interleukin 6/B cell stimulatory factor-2 in rheumatoid arthritis. *European Journal of Immunology*, **18**, 1797–801.

Holmdahl, R., Jansson, L., Larsson, E., Rubin, K., and Klareskog, L. (1986). Homologous type II collagen induces chronic and progressive arthritis in mice. *Arthritis and Rheumatism*, **29**, 106–13.

Holmdahl, R., Karlsson, M., Andersson, M.E., Rask, L., and Andersson, L. (1989). Localisation of a critical restriction site on the 1-A beta chain which determines susceptibility to collagen-induced arthritis. *Proceedings of the National Academy of Sciences (USA)*, **86**, 9475–9.

Holoshitz, J. *et al.* (1986). T lymphocytes of rheumatoid arthritis patients show increased reactivity to a fraction of mycobacteria cross-reactive with cartilage. *Lancet*, **11**, 305–9.

Holoshitz, J., Koning, F., Coligan, J.E., De Bruyn, J., and Strober, S. (1989). Isolation of CD4⁻CD8⁻ mycobacteria-reactive T lymphocyte clones from rheumatoid arthritis synovial fluid. *Nature*, **339**, 226–9.

Howell, M.D. *et al.* (1991). Limited T-cell receptor β chain heterogeneity among interleukin-2 receptor-positive T cells suggests a role for superantigen in rheumatoid arthritis. *Proceedings of the National Academy of Sciences (USA)*, **88**, 10921–5.

Hunter, W. (1901). *Oral sepsis as a cause of septic conditions*. Cassell, London.

Iwakura, Y. *et al.* (1991). Induction of inflammatory arthropathy resembling rheumatoid arthritis in mice transgenic for HTLV. *Science*, **253**, 1026–8.

Jasin, H.E. (1975). Mechanism of trapping of immune complexes into joint collagenous tissues. *Clinical and Experimental Immunology*, **22**, 473–85.

Jose, P.J., Moss, I.K., Maini, R.N., and Williams, T.J. (1990). Measurement of the chemotactic complement fragment C5a in rheumatoid synovial fluids by radio-immunoassay: role of C5a in the acute inflammatory phase. *Annals of the Rheumatic Diseases*, **49**, 747–52.

Katsikis, P., Chu, C.Q., Brennan, F.M., Maini, R.N., and Feldmann, M. (1993). Immunoregulatory role of interleukin 10 (IL-10) in rheumatoid arthritis. *Journal of Experimental Medicine*, **179**, 1517–27.

Keffer, J. *et al.* (1991). Transgenic mice expressing human tumour necrosis factor: a predictive gene model of arthritis. *EMBO Journal*, **10**, 4025–31.

Kehrl, J.H., Alvarez-Mon, M., Delsing, G.A., and Fauci, A.S. (1987). Lymphotoxin is an important T cell derived growth factor for human B cells. *Science*, **238**, 1144–7.

Kingsley, G.M., Pitzalis, C., and Panayi, G.S. (1987). Abnormal lymphocyte reactivity to self—major histocompatibility antigens in rheumatoid arthritis. *Journal of Rheumatology*, **14**, 667–73.

Kissonerghis, A.M., Maini, R.N., and Feldmann, M. (1989). High rate of HLA class II mRNA synthesis in rheumatoid arthritis joints and its persistence in culture: down-regulation by recombinent interleulin 2. *Scandinavian Journal of Immunology*, **29**, 73–82.

Klemperer, P., Pollack, A.D., and Baehr, G. (1942). Diffuse collagen disease: acute disseminated lupus erythematosus and diffuse systemic sclerosis. *Journal of the American Medical Association*, **119**, 331–2.

Koch, A.E. *et al.* (1992). Enhanced production of monocyte chemo-attractant protein-1 in rheumatoid arthritis. *Journal of Clinical Investigation*, **90**, 772–9.

Koch, A.E. *et al.* (1994). Macrophage inflammatory protein-1α. *Journal of Clinical Investigation*, **93**, 921–8.

Lahita, R.G. (1990). Sex hormones and the immune system. Part 1: Human data. *Baillière's Clinical Rheumatology*, **4**, 1–12.

Lanzavecchia, A. *et al.* (1985). Antigen-specific interaction between T and B cells. *Nature*, **314**, 537–9.

Lawrence, J.S. (1970). Rheumatoid arthritis: nature or nurture? *Annals of the Rheumatic Diseases*, **29**, 357–69.

Londei, M. *et al.* (1989). Persistence of collagen type II specific T cell clones in the synovial membrane of a patient with rheumatoid arthritis. *Proceedings of the National Academy of Sciences (USA)*, **86**, 636–40.

Londei, M., Verhoef, A., Hawrylowicz, C., Groves, J., De Berardinis, P., and Feldmann, M. (1990). Interleukin 7 is a growth factor for mature human T cells. *European Journal of Immunology*, **20**, 425–8.

Macgregor, A.J. and Silman, A. (1994). An analysis of the relative contribution of genetic and environmental factors to rheumatoid arthritis susceptibility. *Arthritis and Rheumatism*, **37** (Suppl.), S169.

Maini, R.N. (1989). Exploring immune pathways in rheumatoid arthritis. *British Journal of Rheumatology*, **28**, 466–79.

Maini, R.N., Plater-Zyberk, C., and Andrew, E.M. (1987). Autoimmunity in rheumatoid arthritis: an approach via a study of B lymphocytes. *Rheumatic Diseases Clinics of North America*, **13**, 319–38.

Maini, R.N. *et al.* (1995). Monoclonal anti-TNFα antibody as a probe of pathogenesis and therapy of rheumatoid disease. *Immunology Reviews*, **144**, 195–223.

Mansson, I., Norberg, R., Olhagen, B., and Bjorklund, N.E. (1971). Arthritis in pigs induced by dietary factors: microbiological, clinical, and histologic studies. *Clinical and Experimental Immunology*, **9**, 677–93.

March, L.M. (1987). Dendritic cells in the pathogenesis of rheumatoid arthritis. *Rheumatism International*, **7**, 93–100.

Mollenhauer, J., von der Mark, K., Burmester, G., Gluckert, K., Lütjen-Drecoll, E., and Brune, K. (1988). Serum antibodies against chondrocyte cell surface proteins in osteoarthritis and rheumatoid arthritis. *Journal of Rheumatology*, **15**, 1811–17.

Moore, K.W., Vieira, P., Fiorentino, D.F., Trounstine, M.L., Khan, T.A., and Mosmann, T.R. (1990). Homology of cytokine synthesis inhibitory factor (IL-10) to the Epstein–Barr virus gene BCRF 1. *Science*, **248**, 1230–4.

Morales-Ducret, J., Wayner, E., Elices, M.J., Alvaro-Garcia, J.M., Zvaifler, N.J., and Firestein, G.S. (1992). Alpha 4/beta 1 integrin (VLA-4) ligands in arthritis: I. Vascular cell adhesion molecule 1 expression in synovium and on fibroblast-like synoviocytes. *Journal of Immunology*, **149**, 1424–31.

Nienhuis, R.L.F. and Mandema, E. (1964). A new serum factor in patients with rheumatoid arthritis: the perinuclear factor. *Annals of the Rheumatic Diseases*, **23**, 302–5.

Oates, C.M., Maini, R.N., Payne, L.N., and Dumonde, D.C. (1972). Possible role of lymphokines in the development of ectopic lymphoid foci in the chicken. *Advances in Experimental Medicine and Biology*, **29**, 611–18.

Olee, T. *et al.* (1991). Molecular basis of an autoantibody-associated restriction fragment length polymorphism that confers susceptibility to autoimmune diseases. *Journal of Clinical Investigation*, **88**, 193–203.

Ollier, W. *et al.* (1984). HLA antigen associations with extra-articular rheumatoid arthritis. *Tissue Antigens*, **24**, 279–91.

Olsen, N.J. *et al.* (1994). Multicenter trial of an anti-CD5 immuno-conjugate in rheumatoid arthritis (RA). *Arthritis and Rheumatism*, **37**, S295.

O'Sullivan, F.X., Fassbender, H.G., Gay, S., and Koopman, W.J. (1985). Etiopathogenesis of the rheumatoid arthritis-like disease in MRL/lpr mice. 1. The histomorphologic basis of joint destruction. *Arthritis and Rheumatism*, **28**, 529–36.

Paleolog, E.M., Hunt, M., Elliott, M.J., Woody, J.N., Feldmann, M., and Maini, R.N. (1996). Monoclonal anti-tumour necrosis factor α antibody deactivates vascular endothelium in rheumatoid arthritis. *Arthritis and Rheumatism*, **39**, 1082–91.

Paliard, X. *et al.* (1991). Evidence for the effects of a superantigen in rheumatoid arthritis. *Science*, **253**, 325–9.

Panayi, G.S., Woolley, P.H., and Batchelor, J.H. (1979). HLA-DRW4 and rheumatoid arthritis. *Lancet*, **i**, 730–4.

Parekh, R.B. *et al.* (1985). Association of rheumatoid arthritis and primary osteoarthritis with changes in the glycosylation pattern of total serum IgG. *Nature*, **316**, 452–7.

Pearson, C.M. (1956). Development of arthritis, periarthritis, and periostitis in rats given adjuvants. *Proceedings of the Society of Experimental Biology and Medicine*, **91**, 95–101.

Pitzalis, C., Kingsley, G., Murphy, J., and Panayi, G. (1987). Abnormal distribution of the helper-inducer and suppressor-inducer T lymphocyte subsets in the rheumatoid joint. *Clinical Immunology and Immunopathology*, **45**, 252–8.

Plater-Zyberk, C., Maini, R.N., Brennan, F.M., and Feldmann, M. (1992). CD5+ B and double-negative T cells in rheumatoid arthritis. In *Rheumatoid arthritis* (ed. J. Smolen, J. Kalden, and R.N. Maini), pp. 122–36. Springer, Berlin.

Pober, J.S. *et al.* (1986). Overlapping patterns of activation of human endothelial cells by interleukin 1, tumour necrosis factor, and immune interferon. *Journal of Immunology*, **137**, 1893–6.

Portillo, G., Turner, M., Chantry, D., and Feldmann, M. (1989). Effect of cytokines on HLA-DR and IL-1 production by a monocytic tumour, THP-1. *Immunology*, **66**, 170–5.

Pujol-Borrell, R. *et al.* (1987). HLA class II induction in human islet cells by interferon-γ plus tumour necrosis factor of lymphotoxin. *Nature*, **326**, 304–6.

Rademacher, T.W., Williams, P., and Dwek, R.A. (1994). Agalactosyl glycoforms of IgG autoantibodies are pathogenic. *Proceedings of the National Academy of Sciences (USA)*, **91**, 6123–7.

Raines, E.W., Dower, S.K., and Ross, R. (1989). Interleukin 1 mitogenic activity for fibroblasts and smooth muscle cells is due to PDGK AA. *Science*, **243**, 393–7.

Ranges, G.E., Stiram, S., and Cooper, S.M. (1985). Prevention of type II collagen-induced arthritis by *in vivo* treatment with anti-L₃T₄. *Journal of Experimental Medicine*, **162**, 1105–10.

Rathanaswami, P., Hachicha, M., Sadick, M., Schall, T.J., and McColl, S.R. (1993). Expression of the cytokine RANTES in human rheumatoid synovial fibroblasts. Differential regulation of RANTES and interleukin-8 genes by inflammatory cytokines. *Journal of Biological Chemistry*, **268**, 5834–9.

Res, P.C., Telgt, D., van Laar, J.M., Pool, M.O., Breedveld, F.C., and De Vries, R.R. (1990). High antigen reactivity in mononuclear cells from sites of chronic inflammation. *Lancet*, **336**, 1406–8.

Rice, G.E. and Bevilacqua, M.P. (1989). An inducible endothelial cell surface glycoprotein mediates melanoma adhesion. *Science*, **326**, 1303–6.

Rijnders, A., Boots, A., Verheijden, G., de Keijser, F., and Veijs, E. (1996). Identification of a key autoantigen in rheumatoid arthritis. Sixteenth European Workshop for Rheumatology Research, Stockholm.

Rogers, J. and Dieppe, P.A. (1990). Skeletal paleopathology and the rheumatic diseases. Where are we now? *Annals of the Rheumatic Diseases*, **49**, 885–6.

Rothschild, B.M. and Woods, R.J. (1990). Symmetrical erosive peripheral polyarthritis in arctic Indians: the origin of rheumatoid in the New World. *Seminars in Arthritis and Rheumatism*, **19**, 278–84.

Roudier, J., Rhodes, G., Petersen, J., Vaughan, J., and Carson, D.A. (1988). The Epstein–Barr virus glycoprotein gp110, a molecular link between HLA-DR4, HLA-DR1, and rheumatoid arthritis. *Scandinavian Journal of Immunology*, **27**, 367–71.

Sadeghi, R., Hawrylowicz, C.M., Chernajovsky, Y., and Feldmann, M. (1992*a*). Synergism of glucocorticoids with granulocyte macrophage colony stimulating factor (GM-CSF) but not interferon g (interferon–γ) or interleukin-4 (IL-4) on induction of HLA class II expression on human monocytes. *Cytokine*, **4**, 287–97.

Sadeghi, R., Feldmann, M., and Hawrylowicz, C.M. (1992*b*). Upregulation of HLA class II, but not intercellular adhesion molecule 1 (ICAM-1) by granulocyte-macrophage colony stimulating factor (GM-CSF) or interleukin-3 (IL-3) in synergy with dexamethasone. *European Cytokine Network*, **3**, 373–80.

Sarvetnick, N. *et al.* (1990). Loss of pancreatic islet tolerance induced by B cell expression of interferon-g. *Nature*, **346**, 844–7.

Sasazuki, T. *et al.* (1986). HLA-linked immune suppression maps within HLA-DQ subregion. In *Regulation of immune gene expression* (ed. M. Feldmann and A. McMichael), pp. 197–206. Humana Press, New Jersey.

Sebbag, M. *et al.* (1995). The anti-perinuclear factor and the so-called anti-keratin antibodies are the same rheumatoid arthritis-specific autoantibodies. *Journal of Clinical Investigation*, **95**, 2672–9.

Seckinger, P., Isaaz, S., and Dayer, J.M. (1989). Purification and biologic characterisation of a specific tumour necrosis factor inhibitor. *Journal of Biological Chemistry*, **264**, 11966–73.

Short, C.L. (1974). The antiquity of rheumatoid arthritis. *Arthritis and Rheumatism*, **17**, 193–205.

Silman, A.J., Ollier, W., Hayton, R.M., Holligan, S., and Smith, K. (1989). Twin concordance rates for rheumatoid arthritis: preliminary results from a nationwide study. *British Journal of Rheumatology*, **28** (Suppl. 2), 95.

Simon, A.K., Seipelt, E., and Sieper, J. (1994). Divergent T-cell cytokine patterns in inflammatory arthritis. *Proceedings of the National Academy of Sciences* (*USA*), **91**, 8562–6.

Solomon, L., Robin, G., and Valkenburg, H.A. (1975). Rheumatoid arthritis in an urban South African negro population. *Annals of the Rheumatic Diseases*, **34**, 128–35.

Statsny, P. (1976). Mixed lymphocyte cultures in rheumatoid arthritis. *Journal of Clinical Investigation*, **57**, 1148–57.

Statsny, P. (1978). Association of the B cell alloantigen DRW4 with rheumatoid arthritis. *New England Journal of Medicine*, **97**, 664–761.

Steiner, G. *et al.* (1992). Purification and partial sequencing of the nuclear autoantigen RA33 shows that it is indistinguishable from the A2 protein of the heterogenous nuclear ribonuclearprotein complex. *Journal of Clinical Investigation*, **90**, 1061–6.

Sternberg, E.M. *et al.* (1989*a*). Inflammatory mediator-induced hypothalamic–pituitary–adrenal axis activation is defective in streptococcal cell wall arthritis-susceptible Lewis rats. *Proceedings of the National Academy of Sciences* (*USA*), **86**, 2374–8.

Sternberg, E.M. *et al.* (1989*b*). A central nervous system defect in biosynthesis of corticotropin-releasing hormone is associated with susceptibility to streptococcal cell-wall induced arthritis in Lewis rats. *Proceedings of the National Academy of Sciences* (*USA*), **86**, 4771–5.

Symons, J.A., Wood, N.C., Di Giovine, F.S., and Duff, G.W. (1988). Soluble IL-2 receptor in rheumatoid arthritis. *Journal of Immunology*, **141**, 2612–18.

Symons, J.A., Eastgate, J.A., and Duff, G.W. (1991). Purification and characterization of a novel soluble receptor for interleukin 1. *Journal of Experimental Medicine*, **174**, 1251–4.

Tak, P.P. *et al.* (1996). Reduction in cellularity and expression of adhesion molecules in rheumatoid synovial tissue after anti-TNFα monoclonal antibody treatment. *Arthritis and Rheumatism*, **39**, 1077–81.

Tarkowski, A., Klareskog, L., Carlsten, H., Herberts, P., and Koopman, W.J. (1989). Secretion of antibodies to types I and II collagen by synovial tissue cells in patients with rheumatoid arthritis. *Arthritis and Rheumatism*, **32**, 1087–96.

Taylor, P.C., Maini, R.N., and Plater-Zyberk, C. (1995). The role of the B cells in the adoptive transfer of collagen-induced arthritis from DBA/1 (H-2q) to SCID (H-2d) mice. *European Journal of Immunology*, **25**, 763–9.

Teyton, L. *et al.* (1987). HLA DR, DQ and DP antigen expression in rheumatoid synovial cells: a biochemical and quantitative study. *Journal of Immunology*, **138**, 1730–8.

Trabandt, A., Gay, R.E., and Gay, S. (1992). Oncogene activation in rheumatoid synovium. *Apmis*, **100**, 861–75.

Trentham, D.E., Townes, A.S., and Kang, A.H. (1977). Autoimmunity to type II collagen: an experimental model of arthritis. *Journal of Experimental Medicine*, **146**, 857–68.

Trentham, D.E. *et al.* (1993). Effects of administration of oral type II collagen on rheumatoid arthritis. *Science*, **261**, 1727–30.

Tsai, V., Bergroth, V., and Zvaifler, N.J. (1989). Dendritic cells in health and disease. In *T cell activation in health and disease* (ed. M. Feldmann, R.N. Maini, and J.N. Woody), pp. 33–44. Academic Press, New York.

Van den Broek, M.F., Hogervast, E.J., van Bruggen, M.C., van Eden, W., van der Zee, R., and van den Berg, W.B. (1989). Protection against streptococcal cell-wall-induced arthritis by treatment with the 65 kDa mycobacterial heat shock protein. *Journal of Experimental Medicine*, **170**, 449–66.

Van der Lubbe, P.A., Djikmans, B.A.C., Markusse, H.M., Nassander, U., and Breedveld, F.C. (1995). A randomized, double-blind, placebo-controlled study of CD4 monoclonal antibody therapy in early rheumatoid arthritis. *Arthritis and Rheumatism*, **38**, 1097–106.

van Eden, W., Holoshitz, J., Nevo, Z., Frenkel, A., Klajman, A., and Cohen, I.R. (1985). Arthritis induced by a T lymphocyte clone that responds to mycobacterium tuberculosis and to cartilage proteoglycans. *Proceedings of the National Academy of Sciences* (*USA*), **82**, 5117–20.

van Eden, W. *et al.* (1988). Cloning of the mycobacterial epitope recognised by thymocytes in adjuvant arthritis. *Nature*, **331**, 171–3.

Van Laar, J.M., Miltenburg, A.M., Verdonk, M.J., Daha, M.R., de Vries, R.R., and Breedveld, F.C. (1991). T cell vaccination in rheumatoid arthritis. *British Journal of Rheumatology*, **30** (Suppl. 2), 28–9.

Venables, P.J.W. (1988). Epstein–Barr virus infection and autoimmunity in rheumatoid arthritis. *Annals of the Rheumatic Diseases*, **47**, 265–9.

Venables, P.J.W., Erhardt, C.C., Mumford, P., and Maini, R.N. (1979). The occurrence of antibodies to extractable nuclear antigens (ENA) in extra-articular disease in rheumatoid arthritis (RA). *Annals of the Rheumatic Diseases*, **39**, 146–53.

Venables, P.J.W., Roffe, L.M., Erhardt, C.C., Maini, R.N., Edwards, J.M.B., and Porter, A.D. (1981). Titers of antibodies to RANA in rheumatoid arthritis and normal sera. *Arthritis and Rheumatism*, **24**, 1459–69.

Villiger, P.M., Terkeltaub, R., and Lotz, M. (1992). Production of monocyte chemoattractant protein 1 by inflamed synovial tissue and cultured synoviocytes. *Journal of Immunology*, **149**, 722–7.

Waaler, E. (1940). On the occurrence of a factor in human serum activating the specific agglutination of sheep blood corpuscles. *Acta Pathologica et Microbiologica Scandinavica*, **17**, 172–6.

Walmsley, M. *et al.* (1996). IL-10 inhibits progression of established collagen-induced arthritis. *Arthritis and Rheumatism*, **39**, 495–503.

Westedt, M.L., Breedveld, F.C., Schreuder, G.M.T., d'Amato, J., Cats, A., and de Vries, R.R.P. (1986). Immunogenetic heterogeneity of rheumatoid arthritis. *Annals of the Rheumatic Diseases*, **45**, 534–8.

Westgeest, A.A.A., Boerbooms, A.M.T, Jongmans, M., Vandenbroucke, J.P., Vierwinden, G., and van de Putte, L.B.A. (1987). Anti-perinuclear factor: indicator of more severe disease in seronegative rheumatoid arthritis. *Journal of Rheumatology*, **14**, 893–97.

Weyand, C.M., Xie, C., and Goronzy, J.J. (1992). Homozygosity for the HLA-DRB1 allele selects for extra-articular manifestations in rheumatoid arthritis. *Journal of Clinical Investigation*, **89**, 2033–9.

Wilcox, W.H. (1935). *Reports on chronic rheumatic diseases*, **1**, 72. Lewis, London.

Wilkinson, L.S., Edwards, J.C.W., Poston, R.N., and Haskard, D.O. (1993). Expression of vascular cell adhesion molecule-1 in normal and inflamed synovium. *Laboratory Investigation*, **68**, 82–6.

Williams, R.O., Feldmann, M., and Maini, R.N. (1992*a*). Anti-tumor necrosis factor ameliorates joint disease in murine collagen-induced arthritis. *Proceedings of the National Academy of Sciences (USA)*, **89**, 9784–8.

Williams, R.O., Plater-Zyberk, C., Williams, D.G.. and Maini, R.N. (1992*b*). Successful transfer of collagen-induced arthritis to severe combined immuno-deficiency (SCID) mice. *Clinical and Experimental Immunology*, **88**, 455–60.

Winchester, R.J. and Gregersen, P.K. (1988). The molecular basis of susceptibility to rheumatoid arthritis: the conformational equivalence hypothesis. *Springer Seminars in Immunopathology*, **10**, 119–39.

Wordsworth, B.P., Lanchbury, J.S.S., Sakkas, L.I., Welsh, K.I., Panayi, G.S., and Bell, J.I. (1989). HLA-DR4 subtype frequencies in rheumatoid arthritis indicate that DRbl is the major susceptibility locus within the HLA class II region. *Proceedings of the National Academy of Sciences (USA)*, **86**, 10049–53.

Wordsworth, B.P. *et al.* (1992). HLA heterozygosity contributes to susceptibility to rheumatoid arthritis. *American Journal of Human Genetics*, **51**, 585–91.

Young, B.J.J., Mallya, R.K., Leslie, R.D.G., Clark, C.J.M., and Hamlin, T.J. (1979). Anti-keratin antibodies in rheumatoid arthritis. *British Medical Journal*, ii, 97–9.

Ziegler, B., Gay, R.E., Huang, G., Fassbender, H.G., and Gay, S. (1989). Immunohistochemical localisation of HTLV-l pk and p24-related antigens in synovial joints of patients with rheumatoid arthritis. *American Journal of Pathology*, **135**, 1–5.

Ziff, M., Kantor, T., Bien, E., and Smith, A. (1953). Studies on the composition of fibrinoid material of subcutaneous nodule of rheumatoid arthritis. *Journal of Clinical Investigation*, **32**, 1253–9.

Zvaifler, N.J., Boyle, D., and Firestein, G.S. (1994). Early synovitis, synoviocytes and mononuclear cells. *Seminars in Arthritis and Rheumatism*, **23** (6, Suppl. 2) 11–16.

5.4.2 Rheumatoid arthritis – the clinical picture

Frank A. Wollheim

Introduction

Rheumatoid arthritis is a systemic disease with manifestations in many organs. However, in the majority of cases, involvement of the locomotor system dominates the clinical picture and forms the basis for diagnosis. In a classical textbook from 1957 it was stated that rheumatoid arthritis is 'a chronic systemic inflammatory disorder of unknown etiology characterized by the manner in which it involves the joints' (Short *et al.* 1957). There is no exact definition of rheumatoid arthritis, but several attempts to delineate criteria all are dominated by signs and symptoms from the locomotor system.

Criteria

Criteria are needed both in epidemiological work and for classification in the context of clinical trials. The original American Rheumatism Association (**ARA**) scheme of 1958 lists 11 criteria and no less than 20 exclusions (Ropes *et al.* 1958). With their help one could distinguish classical, definite, probable, and possible rheumatoid arthritis, characterized by decreasing number of criteria (Table 1). The main shortcoming of the ARA criteria is their complexity and low specificity (O'Sullivan and Cathcart 1972). Later, criteria 9, 10, and 11 were dropped to form the scheme of the Rome criteria (Kellgren 1962) (Table 2). The much simpler New York

criteria were proposed in 1966 (Bennett and Burch 1967) (Table 3). These require a history of polyarthritis with clinical signs and either radiological erosions or presence of rheumatoid factor, and do not contain any exclusion criteria. The New York criteria performed better in the Sudbury study (O'Sullivan and Cathcart 1972) but they lack sensitivity for early and atypical cases. More recently the American College of Rheumatology (**ACR**) has developed criteria to replace the 1958 ARA criteria (Arnett *et al.* 1988). Rheumatoid arthritis is diagnosed if at least four of seven criteria are present. Only one category of rheumatoid arthritis is distinguished and exclusions are superfluous, owing to the detailed characterization of the criteria (Table 4). These criteria were developed by observing a number of 'typical' patients considered to be suffering from rheumatoid arthritis by experienced rheumatologists. The mean disease duration was 7.7 years. The performance of these criteria in epidemiological work has only recently been assessed but they may be best used in clinical trials aimed at patients with well-established disease.

Epidemiology

For lack of an obligate pathognomonic test, the diagnosis of rheumatoid arthritis rests on a composite of clinical and laboratory observations. In epidemiological work one has to rely on one of the criteria described above. Their limited precision was demonstrated in the Sudbury study, where only 12 of 40 cases of definite rheumatoid arthritis defined by the ARA criteria still fulfilled the criteria 4 years later. The New York criteria in the same study identified 15 patients with rheumatoid arthritis, and of these 11 were still positive at follow-up (O'Sullivan and Cathcart 1972). This uncertainty, if not evidence for transient disease, should be kept in mind when discussing the epidemiology of rheumatoid arthritis.

Worldwide prevalence

Rheumatoid arthritis has been identified in all populations that have been examined, and prevalence figures ranged between 0.2 and 5.3 per cent (Spector 1990) (Table 5). Nearly all studies indicate point prevalences of between 0.5 and 1 per cent. It is not known whether the high prevalence in Pima Indians is due to environment, genetics, or both and recent figures indicate a decreasing prevalence (Jacobsson *et al.* 1994). The age distribution is a confounding factor in developing countries, perhaps contributing to low figures in Africa.

Incidence

Considering the difficulties involved in establishing early diagnosis of rheumatoid arthritis it is not surprising that only relatively few studies have addressed incidence. The Sudbury population study arrived at the high figure of 29 cases/10 000 per year based on only three observed cases (Table 6), whereas four other studies, using various methods, found annual figures between 9 and 2.9 cases/10 000. The 1987 ACR criteria were used in a prospective population-based registration of all new cases of arthritis in a population of 450 000 people in Norfolk, United Kingdom (Symmons *et al.* 1994), and showed an incidence of 3.4 in women and 1.4/10 000 in men. The incidence increased sharply with age in men from age 45. It increased in women until age 45, then plateaued and fell after age 75. No good longitudinal incidence data are available, although the study of Linos *et al.* (1980) indicated a decline from 9.2 to 4 in women but not men

causing pain on passive pronation or supination, and synovitis of the mid-tarsal joint gives rise to pain on rotating the foot while keeping the heel fixed. These joints may be involved individually. Foot deformities develop with time, e.g. lateral deviation of toes, hammer toes, cock-up toes, and valgus deformity of the ankle. Bursitis, corn formations, and tendinitis are also common.

Knee

The knee joint is the largest human joint. Although not often inflamed at the onset of rheumatoid arthritis, gonarthritis at some stage occurs in 80 per cent or more of all cases. Synovitis is usually easy to identify by tenderness and swelling below the patella. Other signs are exudation, which may be demonstrated by the patella click or the bulge sign. Gonarthritis often leads to quadriceps atrophy and flexion contracture, both of which should initiate prompt and vigilant therapy. The knee joint communicates with bursas in the fossa poplitea, which may become distended and merge into a large Baker's cyst. This may grow and dissect its way down into the calf muscle or rarely into the thigh and sometimes rupture, causing diffuse swelling and pain and may be mistaken for deep-vein thrombosis. Intra-articular pressure may increase to as much as 1100 mmHg in exudative knee joints (Geborek et al. 1989a). This will contribute to decreased muscular function, impede circulation through the synovial membrane, and lead to lactic acidosis and may be a pathogenic factor in the rupture of Baker's cysts. The natural course of long-standing knee involvement is often valgus instability, flexion contracture, and inability to walk. Increased intra-articular pressure may also contribute to bone erosion (Monsees et al. 1985).

Hip

Hip joint involvement is less common and was formerly considered as a late manifestation. However, once started the arthritis often leads to severe disability with pain on weight bearing and limitation of motion, in particular abduction and rotation. Functional limb shortening may sometimes be present secondary to adduction contracture. In a prospective study of recent-onset rheumatoid arthritis, hip involvement was found in 20 per cent. In 7 of 13 patients no symptoms were present despite abnormal swelling found on ultrasonography. Fifteen of 113 patients underwent total hip replacement after a median disease duration of 4 years (Eberhardt et al. 1995). Thus joint failure is more common in the hip than in the knee in early rheumatoid arthritis.

Involvement of the hip must be distinguished from periarticular bursitis or trochanteritis which is characterized by local tenderness, painful motion, and responsiveness to local infiltration with glucocorticoids (Raman and Haslock 1982).

Cervical spine

The cervical spine is involved in approximately 40 to 70 per cent of hospital patients with rheumatoid arthritis (Bland 1974). The dominating symptoms are occipital pain, sometimes worsened by motion, muscle spasm, and crepitation. Synovitis of the faceted joints is commonly present at C1 to C4. The symptoms in most patients improve with immobilization. However, in a small (but important) number of patients severe neurological complications develop secondary to subluxations. This may result in fatal outcome as shown in one study where 11 of 104 patients, dying in a geriatric hospital, had cervical cord compression at autopsy (Mikulowski et al. 1975). This complication will be dealt with below.

Temporomandibular joint

This is affected in one-quarter of patients, usually symmetrically and causing no major disability. In fact patients with unequivocal, palpable, synovial swelling or tenderness often do not report pain on chewing unless specifically asked. In severe destructive cases of rheumatoid arthritis, however, attrition of joint cartilage and bone causes malignment of the teeth with malocclusion (Chalmers and Blair 1973).

Synovitis of the cricoarytenoid joint

This is a well-recognized manifestation in rheumatoid arthritis, occurring in two-thirds of patients in a contemporary hospital-based study (Geterud 1991). The symptoms are sensation of a foreign body, hoarseness, and weak voice, as well as stridor, particularly at night. This may become severe and may eventually cause suffocation. The condition can be detected by palpating local tenderness and finding the vocal cords tender, red, swollen, and immovable on laryngoscopic examination. The laryngeal obstruction can be assessed by computed tomography. This condition is amenable to surgical correction (Geterud 1991).

Rheumatoid nodules

Rheumatoid nodules occur in 30 per cent or less of patients, and when present they are principally in extensor areas of the forearm and pressure areas throughout the skin. Although not specific for rheumatoid arthritis they constitute useful diagnostic and prognostic information, correlating strongly with seropositivity, somewhat with disease activity and progressive disease. Rarely they are the presenting symptom of rheumatoid arthritis, occasionally they are first detected in internal organs, e.g. lungs, heart, and gallbladder.

The histological appearance is that of a central necrotic area surrounded by palisades of fibroblasts, histiocytes, and macrophages. Expression of HLA DR is present among these cells (Hedfors et al. 1983), and collagenase and proteinase production (Palmer et al. 1987) may explain the central necrosis.

Rheumatoid nodules develop in areas over spinal processes and over the neck in patients confined to bed, over the patellae in housewife's knee, and in the inside of the fingers in patients exposed to hand work, demonstrating pressure as an important pathogenetic factor.

It is of particular clinical significance to watch for skin ulcerations over rheumatoid nodules, as this indicates necrotizing vasculitis (Fig. 2).

Disease course

Rheumatoid arthritis is extremely heterogeneous with regard to severity and progression rate. Although early permanent remission may occur in some cases, this is rare once permanent joint damage has started. This does not rule out clinical improvement after initially severely impaired function (Eberhardt et al. 1990b). Long-term follow-up studies (Rasker and Cosh 1989), however, clearly indicate that functional deterioration occurs in most patients surviving 15 years or longer. It is suggested but not well documented that geographical differences may exist in this regard.

Some texts distinguish between cyclic types of disease with remissions and exacerbations and slow but relentless disease progression. In clinical practice, however, features of both types frequently are

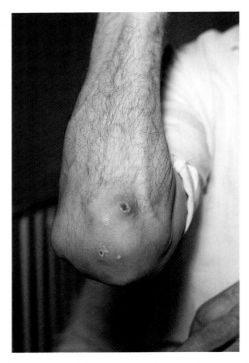

Fig. 2 Subcutaneous nodule over elbow with ulceration in a patient who developed necrotizing vasculitis and gangrene of toes.

Table 8 Some organ manifestations of rheumatoid arthritis		
Organ system	**Manifestation**	**Cumulative frequency (%)**
Lymph nodes	Enlargement, dysfunction	>50
Spleen	Splenomegaly	25
	Felty's syndrome	< 1
Lungs	Pleuritis	>30
	Nodules	5
	Fibrosis	Rare
Heart	Pericarditis	>10
	Myoendocarditis	> 5
	Nodules	5
Muscles	Myositis	Common
	Atrophy	Common
Bone	Osteoporosis	Common
Skin	Nodules	>20
	Vasculitis	> 1
Ophthalmic	Scleritis	1
	Nodules	< 2
	Sjögren's syndrome	10
Neurological	Cord compression	< 1
	Nerve entrapment	Common
	Polyneuropathy	Rare
	Mononeuritis multiplex	< 1

present in a majority of patients. A more useful distinction is that between widespread and more limited chronic joint involvement which can be assessed by careful joint examination (Feigenbaum *et al.* 1979).

Disease activity as manifested by number of swollen joints was low in half of patients with early rheumatoid arthritis followed for 6 years, whereas it was high in 17 per cent and fluctuating in the remainder (van Zeben *et al.* 1994). Disease activity can be monitored by simple measurements, such as joint swelling and tenderness. Erythrocyte sedimentation rate and C-reactive protein measured over time correlate with functional impairment (Hassell *et al.* 1993; Guillemin *et al.* 1994).

Non-articular manifestations

Rheumatoid arthritis is primarily a joint disease, but extra-articular manifestations can be detected in almost any organ system and may occasionally precede the onset of arthritis. Table 8 lists some of these. They are in general more prominent in seropositive and nodular disease.

Lymph nodes

Lymph nodes are enlarged or of abnormal shape in the majority of patients but only rarely palpable. They show up on mammography and give rise to diagnostic concern (Andersson *et al.* 1980). However, in a few cases rheumatoid arthritis may start with widespread palpable lymphadenopathy and a histological picture mimicking Hodgkin's disease. It is of interest that total lymph-node irradiation has a transient suppressive effect on the synovitis in rheumatoid arthritis. Lymphopenia was seen in 15 per cent of cases in one study; it was related to severity but was not influenced by therapy (Symmons *et al.* 1989).

Pulmonary involvement

Pleuritis is most common but frequently asymptomatic. It may be associated with pericarditis and like other pulmonary and cardiac manifestations it is more common in older men. Rheumatoid nodules in the lungs are often asymptomatic and are only seen in seropositive cases. They may be single or multiple and can cause diagnostic problems. Smoking as well as exposure to, for example, silica are pathogenetic factors.

Diffuse interstitial fibrosis and fibrosing alveolitis are rare but serious manifestations, which individuals with HLA DR3 and carriers of the *PiZ* gene are more prone to develop (Geddes *et al.* 1977; Hyland *et al.* 1983). Smoking is also a contributing aetiological factor (Hyland *et al.* 1983).

Cardiac involvement

Pericarditis has been a common finding at autopsy, but causes symptoms in only a few patients. These may range from pain with friction rubs to severe exudative pericarditis with cardiac tamponade requiring surgical intervention (Hara *et al.* 1990). Most cases are, however, benign and self-limiting. Valvular insufficiency, conduction

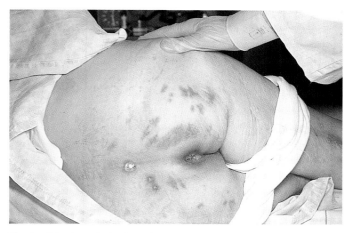

Fig. 3 Skin ulcers in the buttocks in a patient with rheumatoid vasculitis.

Table 9 Secondary Sjögren's syndrome in rheumatoid arthritis compared with primary Sjögren's syndrome

Primary	Secondary
Keratoconjunctivitis sicca	Milder
Xerostomia	Less pronounced
HLA association	HLA DR4; not HLA DR3
Extraglandular manifestations	Not common
Response to therapy	Bromhexin

disturbances, and coronary occlusion may occasionally be due to endocarditis, nodulosis, or vasculitis.

Muscle involvement

Some degree of muscle atrophy is almost invariably present in rheumatoid arthritis, and there is electromyographic evidence of myositis (Moritz 1963). The type II or fast-twitch muscles are most affected (Halla *et al.* 1984). Focal necrosis is also seen. Creatine kinase levels are usually not elevated. Rheumatoid nodules may be seen.

Bone

Generalized axial and appendicular bone loss is seen early in the course of rheumatoid arthritis and has been assessed by dual electron X-ray absorption (DEXA) measurements within 6 months from onset. Bone mineral loss is faster in postmenopausal women and in patients with active disease (Gough *et al.* 1994a). This is a strong argument for early disease suppressive therapy in severe rheumatoid arthritis. This bone loss should be distinguished from the juxta- and periarticular bone loss that probably is a consequence of local cytokine production. Increased bone resorption can also be measured

indirectly by assaying the increased urinary excretion of pyridinoline crosslinks (Gough *et al.* 1994b).

Skin

Cold, clammy hands often accompany flaring rheumatoid arthritis. Palmar erythema is common and may reflect low androgen levels (Spector 1989). Various forms of arteritis manifestations are characteristic signs of systemic disease. Small splinter haemorrhages localize to the nailfolds and may disappear spontaneously. When larger arteries are affected, skin ulcerations develop, often on the lower extremities or where skin is exposed to pressure, e.g. the buttocks (Fig. 3). These ulcerations are very painful, may come in crops, and tend to grow and become chronic. Superinfection is a contributing factor. As mentioned, ulcerations may form over subcutaneous nodules in severe cases.

Leucocytoclastic vasculitis also occurs and is seen as a palpable purpura. This manifestation, as a rule, heals (Fig. 4).

Ocular involvement

Rheumatoid vasculitis gives rise to a severe form of scleritis (Tessler 1985) and rheumatoid arthritis is one of the common causes of scleritis. Scleritis is very painful, gives blurred vision and may last months to years. Episcleritis is a benign condition, resolving within weeks and not highly associated with rheumatoid arthritis. Rheumatoid nodules are not unusual in scleritis, and may cause scleral thinning, secondary glaucoma, and even perforation (scleromalacia). Uveitis and conjunctivitis are not manifestations of rheumatoid arthritis.

Secondary Sjögren's syndrome

Sjögren's syndrome is described in Chapter 5.10. Secondary Sjögren's syndrome in rheumatoid arthritis is not uncommon. It is distinct from primary Sjögren's syndrome (Table 9), and may start many years after onset of the joint disease. Artificial tears, careful oral hygiene to avoid an increase in caries, and bromhexin (*N*-cyclohexyl-*N*-methyl-E-l-2-amino-3,5-dibromobenzylamine, or simpler Bisolvon, Boehringer Ingelheim) in doses of 24 mg thrice daily may help in management.

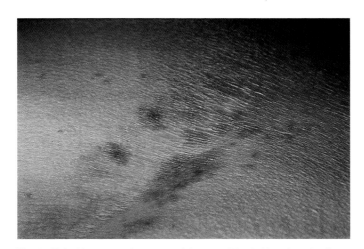

Fig. 4 Palpable purpura in a case of rheumatoid arthritis, where healing occurred without immunosuppressive therapy.

Influence of age, sex, and pregnancy

Age

Several studies have compared the onset of rheumatoid arthritis at older age with that at younger age (Deal *et al.* 1985; Sherrer *et al.* 1986). More recently, van der Heijde (1991) analysed certain features in a prospective 2-year study in patients with recent onset of disease. The only features distinguishing the older patients were a higher biochemical activity, more joint involvement, and persisting marked disease activity after 2 years. Some previous studies have claimed that rheumatoid arthritis with onset in old age is associated with a milder form of the disease, but conversely, Sherrer *et al.* (1986) as well as Sjöblom *et al.* (1984) found age to correlate with a poor prognosis. Van Schaardenburg (1993) compared cases with disease onset over and under 60 years. The only difference was a poorer functional outcome in older seropositive cases, who also had a higher mortality. This is largely due to comorbidity and not to the rheumatoid arthritis as such. However, no population-based data exist and the divergent data may reflect differences in patient selection.

Sex

Female preponderance is present in most series of elderly patients, although to a lesser extent than among younger patients (Silman 1989; Goemaere *et al.* 1990; Jonsson and Larsson 1990). In women, disease onset occurs on average 5 years earlier than in men, and clusters around the menopause. Concomitant health problems, such as osteoporosis and arteriosclerosis, are likely to influence disease course in a negative way. The rate of progression as assessed radiographically in established rheumatoid arthritis did not differ appreciably in relation to gender (Sjöblom *et al.* 1984). Men have a greater risk of developing serious vasculitis complications (Geirson *et al.* 1987).

Pregnancy

The pregnancy-induced amelioration in rheumatoid arthritis, first described by Hench (1938), has been the starting point of both clinical and basic research (Table 10). The relation between sex hormones, the immune system, and autoimmune disease in man and animals is still a much-discussed enigma (Parke 1990). Attempts to ascribe the pregnancy-related remission to a variety of circulating factors, such as α-fetoprotein, adrenal glucocorticoids, or pregnancy-associated immunosuppressive plasma proteins have failed (Klipple and Cecere 1989). The intriguing finding that some 73 per cent of pregnancies induce remission but the remainder do not (Persellin 1977), is elucidated by the recent report (Nelson *et al.* 1993) that improvement correlates with HLA-DQ disparity between mother and fetus. This observation, if confirmed, indicates that an anti-HLA immune response in the mother is implicated. Earlier work in Montpellier (Sany 1994) had used gammaglobulin eluted from human placenta for therapy in rheumatoid arthritis, based on the hypothesis that this contained anti-DR antibodies, which would suppress HLA-DR-expressing cells in the rheumatoid inflammatory tissue. Although such antibodies have indeed been found, this interesting form of therapy has not been pursued.

Sex hormones

Another line of investigation has focused on the role of sex hormones, greatly stimulated by the report on the apparent protective action of oral contraceptives (Wingrave and Kay 1978) and a declining incidence of the disease in women (Linos *et al.* 1980). A number of conflicting results have been published. Whereas most European reports have found relative risks of around 0.5 for developing rheumatoid arthritis in women who currently or have ever used oral contraceptives, the studies from North America have not shown any protective effect. A recent meta-analysis concluded that there was a small but not statistically significant protective effect (Romieu *et al.* 1989).

More detailed analyses indicate that oral contraceptives mainly reduce the risk for developing severe rheumatoid arthritis (van Zeben *et al.* 1990) explaining why, in general, hospital-based studies showed protection, whereas population-based studies did not (Hazes and van Zeben 1991). Postmenopausal use of hormones does not confer protection, according to two recent studies. The reason for this is not known.

In a study from the United States, married women had an increased risk of developing rheumatoid arthritis (Engel 1968), whereas nulliparous women in the United Kingdom had a higher incidence of rheumatoid arthritis in several studies (Spector *et al.* 1990). In women who were both nulliparous and non-users of oral contraceptives, the risk of developing rheumatoid arthritis was even higher. Whereas the correlations are convincing, the mechanisms are unclear.

Attempts to use high-dose oral contraceptives therapeutically in 10 women with rheumatoid arthritis were not successful (Hazes *et al.* 1989). Two controlled trials in postmenopausal women have shown improvements in bone mineral density as well as improved well being and Ritchie index of joint tenderness, although no changes in erthrocyte sedimentation rate were observed (Hall *et al.* 1994; MacDonald *et al.* 1994). Furthermore, the treatment was well tolerated.

Table 10 Some historical developments relating to rheumatoid arthritis (RA) and pregnancy

1938	Hench	Pregnancy-induced improvement of RA
1968	Engel	Marital status as a risk factor for RA
1978	Wingrave and Kay	Reduced incidence of RA in consumers of oral contraceptives
1980	Linos *et al.*	Decreasing incidence of RA in women, 1960–1974
1993	Nelson *et al.*	Maternal–fetal HLA–DQ disparity associated with pregnancy-induced remission

Analysis of androgenic sex hormones in the blood of patients with rheumatoid arthritis has not revealed any abnormalities in women whereas men consistently have low levels, although still within the normal range (Spector 1989). It is possible that this is related to HLA, as the gene for 21-hydroxylase, one of the enzymes involved in the synthesis of sex hormones, is located on the short arm of the sixth chromosome, close to the *HLA-B* locus.

Oestrogen may bind to chondrocytes through oestrogen receptors, or indirectly influence chondrocyte function by inducing cytokine release. In experimental systems, proteoglycan synthesis was inhibited by pharmacological concentrations. T-cell driven models of arthritis are suppressed by oestrogen. It is, however, not known whether these effects are of any relevance in rheumatoid arthritis (Chander and Spector 1991).

Complications

Rheumatoid arthritis is not only a systemic disease with a host of involved organs (see Table 8) but also it is associated with a number of potentially serious complications that contribute to illness and death.

Infections

Patients with rheumatoid arthritis are more afflicted by general infections (Nived *et al.* 1985) and there is anecdotal evidence that respiratory and other infections may trigger flares in rheumatoid arthritis (Wollheim *et al.* 1984). Importantly, rheumatoid arthritis joints are more susceptible to septic arthritis. This may be due to altered T-cell responsiveness and compromised granulocyte function. Local glucocorticoid injections add to the risk for the development of this complication (Östensson and Geborek 1991).

Septic arthritis occurs more often in patients with long-standing disease who are taking oral glucocorticoids. More than one joint may be involved. Usual signs of sepsis, such as fever and leucocytosis, may be absent, and the diagnostic delay may be weeks.

Septic arthritis may easily be overlooked in patients with marked disease activity. The most frequent infecting organism is *Staphylococcus aureus*. The diagnosis may be confirmed by aspiration and positive culture of synovial fluid. However, negative cultures of aspirated fluids are not unusual and cultures of the synovium are a more sensitive and reliable diagnostic method (Kamme and Lindberg 1981). The increased use of immunosuppressive agents probably increases the risk for septic arthritis as well as for other infectious complications. Patients treated with low-dose methotrexate have more respiratory tract and skin infections with relative risks of 1.5 to 2 (van der Veen *et al.* 1994). Furthermore, the introduction of a foreign body in prosthetic joint replacement increases susceptibility to haematogenous septic arthritis.

Neurological involvement

The most common neurological complication in rheumatoid arthritis is entrapment neuropathy secondary to proliferative synovitis. It is most prevalent in the carpal tunnel and in early disease. Rheumatoid arthritis is probably the most common single cause of median-nerve compression (Chamberlain and Bruckner 1970). Carpal tunnel syndrome may be the first symptom that brings the patient to see a doctor. The signs of sensory median-nerve compression are easy to identify as nocturnal paraesthesia of the middle fingers, and may be provoked by forced dorsiflexion of the wrist or percussion over the carpal tunnel. Electromyography shows delayed nerve conduction but is often not more informative than careful clinical examination with testing of motor function. Although median-nerve entrapment in the carpal tunnel is most prevalent, this nerve may also become compressed at the elbow level under the pronator teres muscle. It is important to arrive at a correct diagnosis in these cases, as decompression at the right level will result in prompt restoration of function.

Other entrapments are of the ulnar nerve and rarely the radial nerve at the elbow, as well as the anterior and posterior tibial nerves at the fibular head and in the tarsal tunnel, respectively. The latter gives rise to burning feet and intrinsic foot weakness (Goodgold *et al.* 1965).

An autonomic neuropathy has been defined in rheumatoid arthritis by means of orthostatic electrocardiography (Edmonds *et al.* 1979). It may reflect a microvasculopathy and be related to disturbed skin circulation.

The most alarming form of peripheral neuropathy is called mononeuritis multiplex. It is usually bilateral and most common in the legs. The sudden onset of motor neuropathy signals the presence of aggressive rheumatoid vasculitis and poor prognosis (Geirson *et al.* 1987). The relative incidence of this rare condition is higher in men.

Cervical spine dislocation

Cervical myelopathy associated with rheumatoid arthritis is a well-characterized entity (Marks and Sharp 1981). The symptoms include paraesthesia, numbness, weakness, spastic paralysis, paraplegia, tetraplegia, sensory loss, loss of bladder control, faecal incontinence, and syncope, often in connection with cough or vomiting. Sudden death is also a distinct outcome, particularly if the cervical instability is not recognized (Mikulowski *et al.* 1975).

Cervical subluxation at the atlantoaxial level is present in approximately one-third of patients with rheumatoid arthritis admitted to hospital, and is more prevalent in long-standing disease with pronounced destruction of peripheral joints. The majority of cases are asymptomatic, or suffer from pain without manifest neurological signs. The pain may be mild but is often unbearably intensive. It is usually localized to the neck. Although the atlantoaxial dislocation is augmented by active forward flexion of the head, this manoeuvre rarely precipitates pain.

Some patients suffer from disturbing cracking sensations without pain, when moving the head. Shortening of the neck occurs in extreme cases and an asymmetric posture may be seen.

These patients are particularly vulnerable while under anaesthesia or when involved in accidents and such events may be the starting point of progressive myelopathy.

The diagnosis of unstable subluxation is established by conventional sagittal radiography of the neck in neutral position and anterior flexion, measuring the distance between the anterior odontoid process and atlas (Fig. 5). Subluxation at lower levels between C3 and 4 is another less common complication. However, when present it is much more likely to cause pain and neurological symptoms than atlantoaxial subluxation.

Fractures

Several mechanisms contribute to bone loss in severe rheumatoid arthritis (Woolf 1991). Cytokines, such as interleukin-1 and tumour

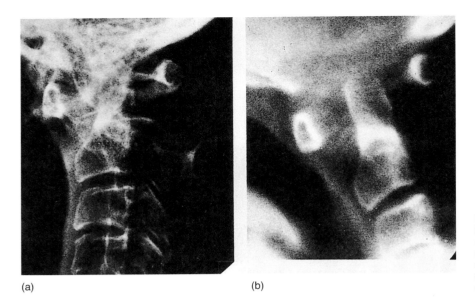

(a)   (b)

Fig. 5 (a) A lateral film of the cervical spine in flexion in a 68-year-old woman with a long history of rheumatoid arthritis shows a marked increase in the distance between the anterior arch of the atlas and odontoid process, measuring 10.2 mm; normally, it should not exceed 3 mm. (b) Trispiral tomogram demonstrates atlantoaxial subluxation in detail.

necrosis factor-α, are generated in the inflammatory process and are known to induce osteoclast activity. Inactivity and nutritional deficiency in combination with frequent administration of glucocorticoids constitute additional risk factors. Postmenopausal women with rheumatoid arthritis are thus at particular risk of developing fragility fractures in connection with minor trauma. Stress fractures, occurring without noticed trauma, are also common (Hooyman *et al.* 1984) and often overlooked, as pain is naturally assumed to be related to rheumatoid inflammation as such (Lakhanpal *et al.* 1986). Whereas bone loss is well documented already in early disease (Gough *et al.* 1994a), the role of glucocorticoids and their proper management are still not settled (Woolf 1991). Although a lower bone-mineral content is found in patients on low doses of glucocorticoids, it is not clear whether this is due to disease activity or drug use (Butler *et al.* 1991). Methotrexate inhibits osteoblast activity and may be yet another risk factor in some patients. Pre-existing osteoporosis is probably a risk factor in patients developing rheumatoid arthritis at a late age. There is no evidence to support the likelihood of impaired healing of fractures, not even in patients with marked disease activity.

Tendon and ligament damage

The destructive process in rheumatoid arthritis involves tendons and ligaments and may cause 'spontaneous' rupture. The most common sites of clinically significant involvement are the hands, wrists, shoulders, neck, knees, and feet.

The flexor tendons of the fingers are affected in more than half of patients by tenosynovitis and rheumatoid nodules, causing stenosis, pain, and occasionally rupture. The extensor tendons are likewise commonly detached and ruptures are frequent, starting with the fifth and spreading to the fourth, third, and second in that order. Reconstructive surgery should be performed at an early stage of this development.

Weakening of ligaments causes joint instability and subluxation of metacarpophalangeal joints, allowing ulnar drift and volar subluxation. Loosening of the distal radioulnar ligament likewise gives instability with piano-key sign and volar luxation of the radius and carpus, and prominence of the ulnar head. Rupture of the rotator cuff and supraspinatus tendon is common, resulting in 'shrugging' of shoulders when abduction is attempted. At the knee, damage to the lateral and cruciate ligaments causes instability and pain, and in the ankles, valgus deformity is common. Atlantoaxial subluxation only occurs in the presence of weakening or rupture of transverse ligaments.

Amyloidosis

Rheumatoid arthritis remains the most common cause of secondary amyloidosis (amyloid A; **AA**) in Europe, occurring in some 2 to 5 per cent of hospital cases (Lender and Wolf 1972). Geographical differences in prevalence may exist. Amyloidosis was found in 17 out of 81 Japanese autopsies performed between 1960 and 1990 (Suzuki *et al.* 1994). No genetic predisposition has been identified in rheumatoid arthritis. Although related to active and widespread disease with prolonged high levels of C-reactive protein and AA in serum, the onset of clinical signs vary between years and decades. The most common type of organ failure in amyloidosis is uraemia, although the skin, liver, and gastrointestinal tract are microscopically involved in a majority of cases. Five-year survival was reduced to 50 per cent in earlier studies (Wegelius *et al.* 1980), but in more recent series, the use of intensive antirheumatic therapy gives a more favourable outlook of 70 to 93 per cent survivors (Ahlmén *et al.* 1987; Berglund *et al.* 1993). It is therefore important to be aware of the occurrence of amyloidosis and perform diagnostic procedures in suspected cases, usually presenting with proteinuria or decreased renal function (see Chapter 5.13.1).

Felty's syndrome

In 1924 Felty observed the occurrence of splenomegaly and neutropenia in five patients with rheumatoid arthritis (Felty 1924). This triad, although shown by Still in juvenile arthritis several decades earlier, has since been called Felty's syndrome. Felty's syndrome is seen in 1 per cent or less of hospital patients with rheumatoid arthritis, and has the same female/male ratio as rheumatoid arthritis itself (Goldberg and Pinals 1980; Campion *et al.* 1990). It has, with few exceptions, only been observed in Caucasians. The rheumatoid arthritis is typically rather destructive, but signs of ongoing synovitis are not prominent despite radiological progression of erosions. Systemic manifestations are common, with subcutaneous nodules, weight loss, and secondary Sjögren's syndrome in over half of the cases. Hepatomegaly and lymphadenopathy are common. Fever, skin pigmentation, and leg ulcers are other characteristics. The diagnosis is established when splenomegaly and a white cell count of less than $2 \times 10^9/mm^3$ are found on three consecutive occasions. Anaemia and thrombocytopenia are usually not pronounced, and in contrast to systemic lupus erythematosus, there is no lymphopenia. The mean disease duration at diagnosis was 20 years on average in one study, but asymptomatic Felty's syndrome may be present and thus undiagnosed for several years.

Skin ulceration and severe systemic infections constitute the main clinical problems in these patients. Repeated upper and lower respiratory infections also contribute to mortality, which is substantial. Eight of 32 patients died in one centre during 5 years' follow-up, and five of these succumbed with fulminant pneumonia. Although neutropenia is related to susceptibility, there is no quantitative correlation to the degree of leucopenia.

Serological abnormalities are present in most cases (Table 11). Of particular interest are antinuclear antibodies that are granulocyte specific (Faber and Elling 1966) and fix complement (Wiik and Munthe 1974). Plasma from patients with Felty's syndrome induced transient granulocytopenia, and failed to stimulate colony formation from bone marrow cells in culture, indicating the pathogenetic importance of circulating factors. A pathogenetic role for granulocyte–macrophage colony-stimulating factor is indicated by a recent observation, where administration of this factor corrected the neutropenia in a patient, but also elicited release of interleukin 6 and flare up of arthritis (Hazenberg et al. 1989).

The occurrence of rheumatoid arthritis in relatives is more common than expected. HLA DR4 is present in close to 100 per cent and homozygosity of HLA DR4 was present in 14 of 28 tested cases in a recent report (Campion et al. 1990). The complement C4B null allele was also associated with Felty's syndrome in 17 of 30 patients. Thus genetic factors clearly distinguish rheumatoid arthritis in Felty's syndrome from other types (Thomson et al. 1988).

The management of Felty's syndrome is still controversial. The effect of splenectomy is not convincing and often transient at best. It confers no protection against sepsis. Anecdotal evidence claims responses to parenteral gold, penicillamine, and methotrexate (Campion et al. 1990). Two cases have apparently responded to cyclosporin in combination with methylprednisolone (Camp et al. 1991). In view of potential risks with all these regimens a conservative approach to the management of Felty's syndrome is warranted in uncomplicated cases.

Laboratory abnormalities

Ideally, laboratory methods, to be clinically useful, should have one or more of the features listed in Table 12. There is presently a proliferation of new tests, many with promising novel features. However, it is not clear which, if any, of these will stand the test of time (di Giovine et al. 1990; Wollheim and Eberhardt 1992).

The rheumatoid factor remains the most important aid in establishing the diagnosis of rheumatoid arthritis. The classical Waaler–Rose test, using sheep cells sensitized with rabbit gammaglobulin, combines relative specificity with reasonable sensitivity. Titres have been replaced by units and the use of World Health Organization standard serum should facilitate comparison between different laboratories.

Another development has been the introduction of enzyme-linked immunosorbent assays (**ELISA**) for the IgG, IgA, and IgM subclasses of rheumatoid factor. These can be made highly sensitive. Thus in one series of patients with early rheumatoid arthritis, 67 per cent were positive in the Waaler–Rose test compared with 85 per cent for IgM rheumatoid factor by ELISA (Eberhardt et al. 1990b). All three classes of rheumatoid factors are present in the majority of seropositive cases. A minority of cases may have only two and occasionally only one immunoglobulin class in the serum. Much attention has been focused on the putative clinical correlations with early selective occurrence of IgA rheumatoid factors, and some investigators find them predictive of erosive disease whereas others do not. It has not been ruled out that technical differences, for instance whether human or rabbit IgG has been used for coating the ELISA plates, may explain the discrepancies. At present, however, ELISAs still should be considered research tools.

A large number of antinuclear antibodies are present in increased amounts in rheumatoid arthritis, but this is of more theoretical than practical interest. Granulocyte-specific antinuclear antibodies are present in two-thirds of patients. Another antibody reacting with a soluble nuclear antigen, called anti-RA 33, was present in one-third and seemed rather specific for this disease (Hassfeld et al. 1989). Other frequently found antibodies that are specific for histones, single-stranded DNA, or Epstein–Barr virus-related antigens are not specific for rheumatoid arthritis.

In the 1960s, reduced amounts of haemolytic complement in synovial fluid were found to distinguish seropositive rheumatoid arthritis from other forms of chronic arthritis (Zvaifler and Pekin 1963; Hedberg et al. 1964). The mechanism behind this characteristic finding is activation and accelerated catabolism of complement products.

Table 11 Serological markers of Felty's syndrome

Antinuclear antibody >80% with HEp-2 cells

Rheumatoid factor >90%, high titre IgG

Cryoglobulins—immune complexes with complement

Complement-fixing granulocyte-specific antinuclear antibodies

Relative hypocomplementaemia

Table 12 Desirable features of laboratory tests in rheumatoid arthritis

1. Diagnostic tool
2. Measure of general disease activity
3. Measure of organ-specific activity
4. Prognostic marker
5. Monitoring of therapeutic effectiveness

Table 13 Acute-phase reactants and rheumatoid arthritis

Analysis	Degree of change	Oestrogen influence	Glucocorticoids	Other comments
ESR	+++	+	−	Best and cheapest screen test
CRP	++++		−	Highest amplitude of change
Orosomucoid	+++	−	+	
α$_1$-Antitrypsin	++	++	−	Liver ++, *PiZ* gene low levels
Haptoglobin	+++	+	−	Liver −, haemolysis − −
Fibrinogen	+++		−	Requires plasma
Caeruloplasmin	+	++	−	
Viscometry	+++			Expensive, not better than ESR
Complement (C3)	+, ±, or −		Variable	
Complement (C4)	+, ±, or −		Variable	C4 null gives low levels

ESR, erythrocyte sedimentation rate; CRP, C-reactive protein.

Surprisingly, assays for complement in synovial fluid have not become widely used. Complement synthesis is high in rheumatoid inflammatory tissue, and plasma concentrations are often raised or normal. However, the relative concentrations of C3 and C4 are low when compared with other acute-phase reactants, and absolute values may be subnormal in the presence of active vasculitis. Detection of cleavage products, e.g. C2a and C3a, is direct evidence of complement activation, and may be useful for investigative purposes.

The acute-phase reaction in rheumatoid arthritis can be measured by a number of methods (Table 13). The erythrocyte sedimentation rate is most widely used and cheapest. Analysis of individual plasma proteins adds little essential information, although C-reactive protein is a more sensitive indicator of activity. It often remains elevated despite clinical remission, and has been found in some studies to correlate with destructive joint changes (Dawes *et al.* 1986; van Leeuwen *et al.* 1993). The erythrocyte sedimentation rate is influenced by anaemia and immunoglobulins, but this does not limit its usefulness in longitudinal monitoring of rheumatoid arthritis.

In recent years an increasing number of more or less tissue-specific markers have been identified and assays constructed for clinical use (Table 14). This field holds promise for better future monitoring of the disease process and response to therapy in rheumatoid arthritis (Wollheim and Eberhardt 1992).

Cytidine deaminase, although not entirely granulocyte specific, has been claimed to be a better marker for inflammation in rheumatoid arthritis than C-reactive protein (Thompson 1987). Calprotectin (L1) may have a similar profile (Berntzen *et al.* 1989). Cytokines and cytokine receptors, although present in trace amounts only, are the subject of numerous studies due to their central position in the pathogenesis of rheumatoid arthritis (di Giovine *et al.* 1996). Increased interleukin 6 levels in synovial fluid but not plasma (Sack *et al.* 1993) and increased amounts of tumour necrosis factor-α and its soluble receptors, and interleukin-2 receptors have been found (Barrera *et al.* 1993).

The concentration of hyaluronate in serum has been correlated with disease activity and morning stiffness in rheumatoid arthritis (Engström-Laurent and Hllgren 1985). Hyaluronate is also a predictor of radiological damage in rheumatoid arthritis (Paimela *et al.* 1991). The type-III collagen *N*-terminal propeptide, P$_{III}$NP, has been used to monitor therapeutic response to disease suppressive therapy and claimed to differ from C-reactive protein (Hørslev-Petersen *et al.* 1988). Cartilage-specific markers have been used and found to vary independently of acute-phase reactants and to correlate with destruction and possibly to stage of disease in rheumatoid arthritis (Wollheim and Saxne 1992; Poole 1994).

Anaemia is common in rheumatoid arthritis and in part related to disease activity as so-called anaemia of chronic disease. This is not responsive to iron therapy, and may be due to hyporesponsiveness to erythropoietin (Means *et al.* 1989). In addition, iron deficiency is present in 30 to 50 per cent of patients with anaemia, as shown by low mean corpuscular volume (Vreugdenhil *et al.* 1990). This may be confirmed by negative iron stains of bone marrow aspirates. Analysis of synovial fluid has traditionally not been much used in evaluation of rheumatoid arthritis. However, it has now been shown that synovial fluid acidosis is related to destruction (Geborek *et al.* 1989b) and that higher concentrations of acid-phosphatase total protein predicted destructive disease (Luukkainen *et al.* 1989). Cytological testing of synovial fluid has been proposed for diagnostic work (Freemont 1991); however, it is not clear whether such observations will become clinically useful in prognostic work.

Lymphopenia was seen in 15 per cent of patients with rheumatoid arthritis. Both CD4 and CD8 cells were equally affected, and changes did not correlate with disease activity or drug therapy (Symmons *et al.* 1989).

Imaging (see also Section 4.9)

As radiography approaches its 100th birthday it remains a cornerstone in the diagnosis and assessment of rheumatoid arthritis. In the last

Table 14 Tissue-specific markers of activity in rheumatoid arthritis

Cell	Marker	Compartment
Granulocytes	Lactoferrin	Synovial fluid
	Cytidine deaminase	Serum, synovial fluid
	L1-calprotectin	Serum, synovial fluid
	Elastase	Synovial fluid, serum
Macrophages	Neopterin	Synovial fluid
	IL-1, TNF, IL-6	Serum, synovial fluid
Lymphocytes	IL-2 receptor	Synovial fluid, serum
	β_2-Microglobulin	Synovial fluid, serum
Synovial membrane (fibroblasts)	$P_{III}NP$	Serum
	Hyaluronan	Serum
	IL-6	Serum, synovial fluid
Endothelial cells	von Willebrand factor	Serum
Cartilage	Proteoglycan fragments	Synovial fluid, serum
	COMP	Synovial fluid, serum
	CMP (148 kDa protein)	Serum
Bone	Deoxypyridinoline	Urine
	Osteocalcin	Serum
	Bone sialoprotein	Serum

CMP, cartilage matrix protein; COMP, cartilage oligomeric protein; IL, interleukin; $P_{III}NP$, type-III collagen N-terminal propeptide; TNF, tumour necrosis factor.

decade, however, scintigraphy, ultrasonography, computed tomo-graphy, and magnetic resonance imaging (**MRI**) have emerged as important complementary techniques. Used in concert, they allow rather comprehensive objective documentation of the anatomic disease progression. However, judicious use, based on well-defined questions, will save patients unnecessary exposure to radiation and society unnecessary costs.

Important issues in early rheumatoid arthritis are concerned with presence or absence of erosive changes and with their quantification in the course of disease. Two methods have emerged to meet the latter need. The Larsen–Dale index (Larsen *et al.* 1977) uses a set of standard radiographs for each joint and distinguishes five stages of involvement, starting with soft tissue swelling and juxta-articular osteoporosis and ending with complete cartilage and advanced bone destruction. This method has the advantage of relative simplicity and has been most used in Europe (Wollheim *et al.* 1988). The Sharp method involves assessing joint space narrowing and counting erosions (Sharp *et al.* 1971). Both are reproducible, but less sensitive to change than the human eye.

Functional impairment correlates with the Larsen index, but is not closely predictable from radiographic changes (Fig. 6). A most impressive example of discrepancy between severe radiographic erosions and preserved function is called 'typus robustus', seen in men, often those employed in heavy manual work.

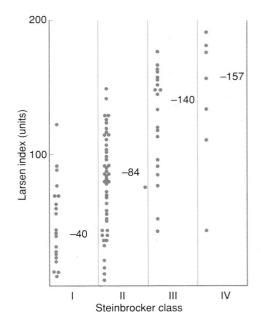

Fig. 6 Larsen index distribution in relation to functional classes according to Steinbrocker. Horizontal bars denote the median.

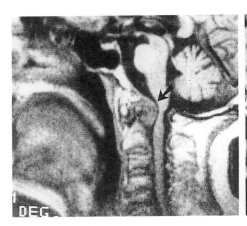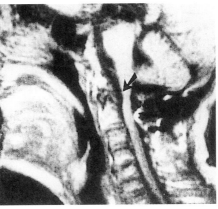

Fig. 7 Preoperative MRI (left) and 4 months postoperative MRI (right) after successful surgical fusion. Arrows indicate periodontoid pannus.

Scintigraphy with technetium pertechnetate is a simple and useful method to visualize synovial activity, and persistent activity predicts occurrence of radiographic erosions (Möttönen 1988). This promising technique needs to be tested as guide for therapy. Scintigraphy with bone-seeking technetium is useful in early detection of avascular necrosis. Other scintigraphic methods involve labelling of granulocytes with a radionuclide, using their localization after reinfusion to diagnose articular or extra-articular inflammation.

Ultrasonography is being used increasingly, as the technique improves. It has replaced arthrography in the diagnosis of Baker's cysts, and is useful for visualizing rotator-cuff lesions in the shoulder and hip joint effusion (Mitchell 1989).

MRI offers superior contrast resolution compared with other imaging techniques (Brahme 1991). It has been possible to visualize joint cartilage and MRI may be the most sensitive tool to detect early joint lesions. In the evaluation of instability of the neck, MRI allows visualization of granulation tissue around the odontoid process and its change after surgical fusion (Fig. 7). MRI also is a sensitive tool to detect effusion and tendon and ligament abnormality. The initial disadvantage of long exposure time has improved with newer, technically more sophisticated equipment.

Treatment

Assessment

Assessment of disease activity, joint damage, and change over time of these variables are essential tools to monitor intervention in rheumatoid arthritis. The traditional methodology of joint examination has been the subject of several evaluations and developments (Preevo et al. 1993). In essence, simple counts are better than weighted ones, swelling is a better indicator than tenderness, and a 28-joint count performs as well as more comprehensive 55- to 66-joint counts (Preevo et al. 1995). In December 1993 the European League Against Rheumatism published a handbook of standard methods for assessing disease activity. Simple self-assessment questionnaires are also available (Kazis et al. 1990). The radiological progression is still considered the gold standard to measure results of treatment. Based on average progression rates from different centres, it has been estimated that regardless of scoring system, due to great variability in progression rate, one would need patient groups of 150 to detect a 50 per cent slowing of radiological progression at a significance level of 0.05 per cent (Sharp et al. 1993). Obviously not many studies of disease suppressive agents meet such standards.

Individual goals

In addition to the physical and radiological assessment it is essential to identify and analyse individual disease-related problems and short-comings, and list them in order of importance to the patient. This is often best accomplished in co-operation with the physiotherapist, occupational therapist, social worker, and metrologist or nurse, also called allied health professionals. Table 15 shows some of the main components of appropriate treatment of rheumatoid arthritis. Some or all of these therapeutic options may be indicated, according to variations in disease severity. It is, however, mandatory that the patient has easy access to a responsible physician with an overview of all the different aspects of management, and it is desirable that the health service provides the necessary organization. Box 1 has a schedule for management of drugs in rheumatoid arthritis.

Pharmacotherapy

The number of drugs used in the treatment of rheumatoid arthritis has increased steadily over the last decades, and there have been remarkable geographic differences in therapeutic traditions, often not scientifically based on proper trials. A new and more aggressive approach to early treatment of rheumatoid arthritis has yet to prove that it will change the long-term outcome. Originating in the feeling that most currently used drugs (Table 16) are only symptom modifying, a new terminology was proposed (Edmonds et al. 1993). It distinguishes between slow acting/disease modifying and 'disease controlling' drugs and requires sustained (2 year!) improvement of function and slowing or prevention of structural joint damage for the

Table 15 Main components of treatment for rheumatoid arthritis
Patient education, adaption, and counselling
Physiotherapy—exercises, joint protection
Occupational therapy—adapt environment, personal aids, orthoses
Medication—pain control, disease suppression
Non-medical pain reduction—transcutaneous nerve stimulation, acupuncture, surgery
Rehabilitation—joint replacement, arthrodesis

Box 1 Management of rheumatoid arthritis (RA)

A. First visit
(a) Diagnosis possible but not certain:
Treatment-symptomatic - NSAID/paracetamol. Consider antimalarials (check colour vision and visual acuity)

(b) Palindromic symptoms and positive rheumatoid factor or ANAs: antimalarials

(c) Unequivocal RA:
(1) Initial information
(2) Symptomatic
   NSAID/paracetamol
   Local glucocorticoids

(3) Assessment including
   Function
   Social
   Radiography of hands and feet
   APPs
   Extra-articular signs ?

(4) Add antimalarials and/or sulphasalazine (1 g twice daily if assessment under (3)) indicates aggressive disease

B. First return visit–usually 3 months later
reassess diagnosis–if change proceed as under A.

If RA (AC): (1) Evaluate response

(a) No remission or progression: add sulphasalazine if not done already (exclude SLE, radiograph lungs, bone marrow, and liver function) Laboratory check every 2 weeks, return visit 3 months
(b) Improvement–continue as A(c), return visit in 6 months

C. Return of B(1)(a)

(1) If stable or improved–continue as above
(2) If progression–try dose escalation to sulphasalazine from 1 g twice daily to 1 g thrice daily
(3) If adverse reaction–shift to methotrexate 7.5 mg once/weekly with folic acid q mg daily. Allow methotrexate dose escalation if needed to 15 mg once weekly.
Return visit 3 months

D. 6 month return of B (1)(b)

Check eyes as under A (a). If improved or stable–continue. If progression– see B (1)(a).

E. 3 month return of C

(1) If stable–continue 3 months
(2) If (a) progression or (b) adverse reactions
   (a) Consider escalation to 25 mg/weekly or shift to parenteral gold or add low dose (<5 mg/kg/day) cyclosporin or add azathioprine

F. If severe extra-articular disease manifestations: prednisolone 15–40 mg and cyclophosphamide or chlorambucil.

G. If proteinuria–consider amyloidosis, which is an indication for immune suppression
If neck involvement–check for instability, consider cervical brace, and/or surgery

H. Low-dose oral glucorticoids only given when needed for symptom control and only with

I. Keep patients on disease suppressive agents unless adverse reactions occur

K. Watch for large joint involvement–especially silent hips–ultrasonography

Table 16 Pharmacotherapy of rheumatoid arthritis

Pain relief

Simple analgesics

Non-steroidal anti-inflammatory drugs

Disease suppression

Chloroquine—hydroxychloroquine

Gold—parenteral

D-Penicillamine

Sulphasalazine

Auranofin

Methotrexate

Azathioprine

Glucocorticoids

Cyclosporin A (now Neoral)

Disease complications

Anaemia: iron, erythropoeitin

Osteoporosis: oestrogens, calcitonin, bisphosphonates

Vasculitis: glucocorticoids, chlorambucil, cyclophosphamide

Amyloidosis: chlorambucil, cyclophosphamide

latter. The distinction obviously can only be made in retrospect and seems to be of little practical use at present.

Non-steroidal anti-inflammatory drugs (NSAIDs) (see also Chapter 3.5.1)

NSAIDs are the dominating group of drugs and are prescribed periodically or continuously for the vast majority of patients. They offer reliable but limited symptomatic relief from pain and stiffness. Their mechanism of action is complex. NSAIDs inhibit constitutional Cox-1 and induced Cox-2 in varying proportions (Mitchell *et al.* 1994), which may have clinical implications. In addition to inhibition of cycloxygenase they also suppress neutrophil function and *in vivo* motility, and according to some investigators cause increase of suppressor lymphocyte function and reduced synthesis of rheumatoid factor (Brooks and Day 1991). They also inhibit platelet aggregation. In experimental systems high doses of NSAIDs have been found to inhibit chondrocyte synthesis of proteoglycans. This has caused speculation of potential harmful effects after long-term use in human disease. However, no convincing documentation of cartilage damage in rheumatoid arthritis has been produced.

It is hard to know with certainty if and how NSAID treatment affects long-term outcome in rheumatoid arthritis. There is, however, no doubt among most observers that they improve quality of life in an important way in most patients with rheumatoid arthritis for long periods.

NSAIDs can be divided into two groups, those with a short and those with a long half-life. The former are often available in slow-release formulation, allowing them to be given once or twice daily, for which improved compliance is claimed. It is not possible to relate serum levels to effect, but a dose–response relationship has been established for some NSAIDs, e.g. naproxen and ibuprofen (Brooks and Day 1991).

NSAIDs contain an asymmetric carbon and inactive (R) and active (S) enantiomers. *In vivo* conversion occurs from (R) to (S) but not from (S) to (R). A variable rate of conversion perhaps contributes to variation in response and adverse effects. A large number of comparative short-term trials have on the whole failed to reveal relevant differences between NSAIDs, although individual patient preference has been suggested (Huskisson *et al.* 1976; Scott *et al.* 1982).

Aspirin was until recently the preferred first line NSAID, based on unsurpassed effectiveness and low price. However, a number of trials have shown it to be less well tolerated than other NSAIDs, and thus it is no longer considered a first choice. This does not apply to non-acetylated salicylates. If optimal dose of one NSAID has no satisfactory effect after 3 to 4 weeks, it is advisable to try another. Combined use of two or more NSAIDs is common practice but its rationale is not well founded; they should be prescribed one at a time. Indomethacin administration at night is popular, due to its combined analgesic and sedative effect.

Adverse effects are very common, and may be life-threatening (Fries *et al.* 1989; Langman 1989). Awareness and careful patient education are essential (Table 17). Gastric ulcer is more common that duodenal and may be asymptomatic. The overall risk factor is 3 to 4, which means that NSAIDs may be associated with one-quarter of all patients admitted to hospital with these conditions. Patients at risk and requiring NSAIDs should receive prophylactic treatment with the prostaglandin E_1-analogue, misoprostol. Risk factors are old age, previous peptic ulcer, and concomitant use of glucocorticoids. There seems to be a hierarchy with regard to upper gastrointestinal toxicity among some NSAIDs (Bateman 1994; Table 18). Small bowel toxicity has also been suggested from biopsy studies, which show membranes and strictures as well as Crohn-like lesions (Bjarnason *et al.* 1988; Banerjee 1989). The practical importance of this is not known. Many patients also become constipated and develop nausea from NSAIDs.

Impaired renal blood flow is likely to occur in patients with pre-existing kidney diseases, and is thought to be related to the reduced presence of procirculatory prostaglandins. All NSAIDs have this effect, although two studies show sulindac to cause less impairment in short-term trials in patients with moderate renal failure (Eriksson *et al.* 1990; Whalton *et al.* 1990). It is important to avoid dehydration, which may precipitate severe renal failure in patients taking NSAIDs.

The effectiveness of thiazides and loop diuretics is reduced by NSAIDs with the possible exception of sulindac, and the same applies to β-blockers and angiotensin-converting enzyme inhibitors. A number of other pharmacokinetic as well as pharmacodynamic drug interactions have been identified (Brooks and Day 1991). Thus it is advisable to treat NSAIDs with respect, and only use them on strict indications of which rheumatoid arthritis, however, is one. Paracetamol (acetaminophen) in adequate dosage of 1 g three times a day is often a useful analgesic when NSAIDs are contraindicated.

Antimalarials

These are highly potent inhibitors of intracellular protein processing, and they accumulate in the cellular acid-vessel system for transport of macromolecules. They also inhibit monocyte production

Table 17 Adverse reactions of non-steroidal anti-inflammatory drugs

Organ	Occurrence	Comment
Gastrointestinal	Common	Upper gastrointestinal bleeding/perforation
		Risk factors: old age, history of ulcer, glucocorticoid
		Drug differences, see Table 18
Renal	Common	Reduced renal blood flow and glomerular filtration
		Fluid retention, renal failure, papillary necrosis
Hypertension	Common	Interference with medications against hypertension and cardiac failure
Hepatic	Not uncommon	Pyrazolones, indole, and proprionic acid derivatives
CNS	Not uncommon	Tinnitus, tiredness, cognitive disturbance in the elderly
Skin	Not uncommon	Rashes, UV sensitivity; rarely erythema multiforme
Variable	Uncommon	Aseptic meningitis (ibuprofen, sulindac, tolmetin), pneumonitis (naproxen), bone marrow dyscrasias

of interleukin1α and interleukin 6 *in vitro* (Sperber *et al.* 1993). They have a well-documented action of moderate disease suppression in rheumatoid arthritis, and cause, at an appropriate dosage, very few adverse reactions (Tett *et al.* 1990; Clark *et al.* 1993). Safety and little need for laboratory surveillance make them an inexpensive first choice among disease suppressing agents. Eye toxicity does not occur in patients without liver disease provided the dose of 4 mg/kg per day for chloroquine or 6 mg for hydroxychloroquine is not exceeded. It is also recommended to stop the drug for 4 to 6 weeks each year to check whether the disease may be in remission. Increased creatinine and 10 per cent lowered creatinine clearance may occur (Landewé *et al.* 1995). Antimalarials may diminish toxicity

of methotrexate to the liver (Fries *et al.* 1991). Given in combination therapy with aureothiomalate, hydroxychloroqine improved efficacy without increasing adverse reactions (Scott *et al.* 1989). Antimalarials in combination with penicillamine, on the other hand, caused more adverse reactions and less therapeutic effect. Thus the antimalarials have a definite place in the management of rheumatoid arthritis of moderate severity, and may become of use in certain combination regimens.

Soluble gold salts

These have been given parenterally since the 1930s and are still considered among the most potent disease-suppressing agents in

Table 18 Odds ratio and 95 per cent CI for bleeding and perforation (Garcia Rodriguez) or acute gastrointestinal bleeding (Langman et al.), and CSM rank order of serious reports of gut toxicity expressed per million prescriptions in the first 5 years of marketing (after Bateman 1994)

Drug	CSM ranking	Garcia Rodriguez		Langman *et al.*	
		Ratio	95%CI	Ratio	95% CI
Overall		4.7	3.8–4.7	4.5	3.6–5.6
Ibuprofen	1	2.9	1.78–5.0	2.0	1.4–2.8
Diclofenac	2	2.9	1.78–5.0	2.0	1.4–2.8
Diclofenac	2	3.9	2.3–6.5	4.2	2.6–6.8
Naproxen	5	3.1	1.7–5.9	9.1	5.5–15.1
Ketoprofen	6	5.4	2.6–11.3	23.7	7.6–74.2
Indomethacin	a	6.3	3.3–12.2	11.3	6.3–20.3
Piroxicam	11	18.0	8.2–39.6	13.7	7.1–26.3
Azapropazone	12	23.4	6.9–79.5	31.5	10.3–96.9

[a]Not ranked by CSM. Marketed before yellow card scheme.
CI, confidence interval

rheumatoid arthritis. The mechanism of action is unknown, but experimental data have shown inhibition of antigen presentation by macrophages, perhaps mediated by enzyme inhibition (Champion *et al.* 1990). This results in diminished lymphocyte function. It is remarkable that all clinically used preparations contain AuI and a sulphydryl ligand in an approximate ratio of 1:1. Aureothiomalate has been most studied, and proven superior to placebo and auranofin, an oral gold preparation, and equal to sulphasalazine in efficacy. Inefficacy, therapeutic escape, and not least, adverse reactions, however, seriously limit its use as a single drug (Sambrook *et al.* 1982). An impressive list of adverse reactions to parenteral gold compounds is shown in Table 19. Transient increase in joint pain, also called nitritoid reaction, rarely causes termination. A most serious, usually fatal complication, aplastic anaemia, may be treated successfully with bone marrow transplantation. Agranulocytosis and thrombocytopenia usually are reversible, but eliminate future use of the drug. Adverse reactions are interestingly not related to dose or circulating levels of gold. Aureothiomalate is administered once weekly in doses between 10 and 50 mg. When clinical remission is achieved, injection frequency is reduced to every 2 to 6 weeks. However, in practice, only half of the patients remain on therapy after 2 years and one-fifth after 4 years.

D-Penicillamine (dimethylcysteine)

In addition to its chelating effects on divalent metals, such as copper, D-penicillamine has a strongly reactive thiol group and forms mixed disulphides through oxidization. Thus free D-penicillamine has a very short half-life *in vivo*. It is excreted mainly in the form of penicillamine–cysteine mixed disulphide, but also forms disulphides with albumin and other proteins possessing reactive sulphydryl compounds. Oxidization and chelation occur readily in the gastrointestinal tract, which is why D-penicillamine should be administered without food or other drugs. Even then only half of the dose is absorbed.

The mechanism of action is not known, but D-penicillamine inhibits T-lymphocyte activation probably through a direct T-cell interaction (Lipsky and Ziff 1980). It also reduces the amount of circulating immune complexes and IgA–α_1-antitrypsin complexes as well as rheumatoid factor (Norberg *et al.* 1980). These effects are synchronous with the therapeutic response. Paradoxically, D-penicillamine causes a number of so-called autoimmune complications. An immune-complex glomerulonephritis, histologically identical with that of systemic lupus erythematosus, is accompanied by proteinuria which may last for a year. Occasionally full-blown systemic lupus develops with hypocomplementaemia and antinative DNA (Joyce 1990). Other autoimmune conditions occasionally induced by D-penicillamine are myasthenia, dermato-/polymyositis and Goodpasture's syndrome. After stopping D-penicillamine, these syndromes slowly remit although polymyositis may be fatal if not detected early.

Other side-effects are bone marrow suppression and various forms of skin lesions, including bullous pemphigoid eruptions. HLA DR3 is a risk factor for development of several of these complications. D-Penicillamine is contraindicated in pregnancy due to its teratogenic effect.

The use of D-penicillamine has diminished but it is still a useful drug in some patients. It is best used in doses from 125 to 750 mg/

Table 19 Adverse reactions to parenteral gold

Post-injection reactions (almost immediate)
   Vasomotor
   Arthralgia, myalgia, malaise

Mucocutaneous
   Chrysiasis
   Dermatitis
   Stomatitis
   Alopecia

Renal
   Proteinuria
   Membranous glomerulonephritis
   Selective haematuria?

Haematological
   Eosinophilia
   Neutropenia
   Thrombocytopenia
   Red cell hypoplasia?
   Pancytopenia
   Aplastic anaemia

Immunological
   Specific IgE antibodies
   Selective IgA deficiency
   Other immunodeficiency syndromes?

Hepatic   Hepatitis with cholestasis
Gastroenterological   Enterocolitis

Pulmonary
   Diffuse pneumonitis
   Bronchiolitis obliterans

Neurological
   Peripheral neuropathy
   Polyneuropathy (Guillain–Barré type)
   Cranial nerve palsies
   Encephalopathy
   Myokymia syndrome

Other
   Corneal, lens chrysiasis
   Metallic taste

From Champion *et al.* (1990).

day, with slowly increasing dosage. Combination with sulphasalazine may be advantageous (Taggart *et al.* 1987).

Sulphasalazine

This was designed as a combined analgesic and antimicrobial agent against a putative intestinal pathogen causing rheumatoid arthritis (Svartz 1942). Although this mechanism of action is still hypothetical, its role as an effective disease-suppressing agent in rheumatoid arthritis is well documented (Porter and Capell 1990). The drug is largely but not completely split into 5-aminosalicylic acid and sulphapyridine by bacteria in the colon, and much of its adverse reactions are sulphapyridine related. However, the effect probably at least in part resides in the intact molecule. The onset of effect is 4 to 12 weeks. There is suggestive evidence for retardation of radiological progression if given in early rheumatoid arthritis (van der Heide *et al.* 1989; Hannonen *et al.* 1993).

The most common adverse reactions are nausea, abdominal pain, dizziness, and irritability, and this is only marginally improved by the use of enteric-coated tablets. An acute pneumonitis develops rarely, usually early. Thrombocytopenia occurs in 1:700 patients in the first 3 months of therapy (Keisu and Ekman 1992) but is rarer later on. Serious bone marrow toxicity is, however, uncommon. Spermiogenesis is affected, causing reversible subfertility (Birnie *et al.* 1981). Although some dose-related adverse reactions are more likely to occur in slow acetylators, fast acetylators are as likely to develop serious idiosyncratic reactions, and acetylator state does not influence response. Sulphasalazine is administered orally in doses starting with 0.5 g and increased to a maintenance dose of 1 g twice or three times daily.

Methotrexate

Methotrexate given once weekly, usually orally in doses of 5 to 15 mg, is widely used as a standard disease-suppressive agent, and placebo-controlled trials as well as follow-up studies of up to 90 months are favourable (Grosflam and Weinblatt 1991; Kremer and Phelps 1992), and superior to azathioprine (Jeurissen *et al.* 1991). Survival on the drug is also better than for parenteral gold, azathioprine, D-penicillamine, sulphasalazine, auranofin, and hydroxychloroquine (Morand *et al.* 1992).

The mechanism of action is not known. In addition to an anti-dihydrofolate reductase effect, methotrexate may have an immunosuppressive effect. Its toxicity may be reduced by administration of folate without loss of therapeutic effect (Morgan *et al.* 1994), indicating at least partly a folate-independent mode of action. The fast onset of clinical response suggests an anti-inflammatory mode of action.

The most common adverse reaction is gastrointestinal intolerance, which usually is not severe. Methotrexate may cause severe septic complications, both fungal and bacterial, and it may be advisable to stop the drug temporarily before arthroplastic surgery. Eosinophilia and pneumonitis arise in some 5 per cent of cases. Renal methotrexate clearance and creatinine clearance decreased by 10 per cent after 6 months (Kremer *et al.* 1995).

The question regarding long-term liver toxicity is still unsettled. Whereas biopsy studies reveal dose-dependent increased liver fibrosis, frank cirrhosis has not occurred with low-dose regimens. Routine liver biopsy is not recommended during initial years of therapy. While NSAIDs increase the toxicity from high-dose methotrexate, this is not reported with low-dose methotrexate, although patients with impaired renal function may be at higher risk.

Combination therapy of methotrexate with gold or azathioprine and hydroxychloroquine, or with hydroxychloroquine and sulphasalazine may be useful (Paulus 1990). A meta-analysis indicates the possibilities of a somewhat lower rate of radiologial progress than for other drugs except parenteral gold (Alarcón *et al.* 1992).

Auranofin

This is a lipophilic gold compound for oral use which is effective in rheumatoid arthritis, although weaker than parenteral gold (Champion *et al.* 1990). A 2-year placebo-controlled prospective study in early rheumatoid arthritis, indicated a retarding effect on radiological progression (Borg *et al.* 1988). The effective dose is 3 mg twice daily. The most common side-effects are diarrhoea and other mild gastrointestinal disturbances. Serious adverse reactions are unusual. The onset of effect is slow, which may be a disadvantage in short-term trials and explain its poor rating in a meta-analysis (Felson *et al.* 1990).

Azathioprine

The purine analogue azathioprine is an effective disease-suppressive drug in rheumatoid arthritis given in doses between 1.5 and 2.5 mg/kg per day, although onset of action is slow (Luqmani *et al.* 1990). Bone marrow toxicity and lymphoma induction are rare complications whereas nausea is common.

Cyclosporin (Neoral)

Cyclosporin is a fungal decapeptide with distinct actions on active T-lymphocytes and possibly antigen-presenting cells, lowering release of interleukin 2. It is an attractive candidate for immune modulation/suppression in rheumatoid arthritis. In doses of 2.5 to 5 mg it was better than placebo in several trials of active rheumatoid arthritis (van Rijthoven *et al.* 1986; Dougados *et al.* 1989; Tugwell *et al.* 1990) and not different from D-penicillamine, azathioprine, and hydroxychloroquine. Evidence for retardation of radiological progression is not convincing (Førre *et al.* 1994), but long-term trials in early rheumatoid arthritis to look into this crucial question are ongoing. A problem with this drug is that it induces hypertension and renal toxicity even in low doses. The long-term consequences of this are not known. Its effect on C-reactive protein is moderate or nil, and the erythrocyte sedimentation rate does not change. Disease activity increases rapidly after the drug is stopped. Cyclosporin must, if used at all, be carefully monitored for adverse reactions, in particular hypertension and nephrotoxicity (Cash and Klippel 1994; Landewé *et al.* 1994).

Glucocorticoids

The introduction of glucocorticoid treatment of rheumatoid arthritis marks the beginning of modern rheumatology, in demonstrating reversibility of what was considered permanent disability (Hench *et al.* 1949). Glucocorticoids have a large number of effects on immune function and regulation, and cell traffic and adhesion. Inhibition of transcription of the interleukin-1β gene is one important effect (Lee *et al.* 1988). It is the most powerful and predictable remedy inducing immediate symptomatic relief in rheumatoid arthritis available to date, but its long-term effects are among the most controversial issues in the treatment of this disease (George and Kirwan 1990; McDougall *et al.* 1994).

High-dose systemic administration may prevent formation of erosions but adverse effects preclude its uninhibited use (Weiss 1989). The list of side-effects is long (George and Kirwan 1990) and diabetes, hypertension, excessive weight gain, cataract, arteriosclerosis, and not least osteoporosis are among them (Lukert and Raisz 1990). New approaches to management of osteoporosis involving bisphosphonate, or oestrogen replacement in postmenopausal women are promising, and long-term trials involving low-dose glucocorticoids may become feasible. Patients with rheumatoid arthritis easily become addicted to oral glucocorticoids and it is therefore a serious decision to start such therapy.

Patients treated with NSAIDs have a low concentration of glucocorticoid receptors (Pelletier *et al.* 1994) as well as autoantibodies to lipocortin-1 with impaired responsiveness to glucocorticoids. Furthermore, the hypothalamic–hypophyseal–adrenal axis is hyporesponsive to, for example, surgical stress (Chikanza et al. 1992). Findings like these will have to be followed-up by formal clinical trials, before increased use of glucocorticoids can be advocated (Saag et al. 1994).

Pulsed intravenous megadoses of 1000 mg methyldprednisolone is no more effective than 100 mg, and this expensive form of administration may be overrated. Intra-articular use of crystalline preparations is, however, both effective and rational, since it delivers the disease-suppressive drug to the involved site. Triamcinolone hexacetonide has the longest lasting effect. If weight-bearing joints are injected a 24-h bed rest should be enforced in order to achieve better effect duration. Iatrogenic septic arthritis is no major problem when using a proper technique, but intra-articular glucocorticoids may predispose to later septic arthritis in the injected joint (Östensson and Geborek 1991).

Alkylating agents

Chlorambucil at 0.1 to 0.2 mg/kg per day and cyclophosphamide at 100 to 150 mg/day, are both active in the suppression of rheumatoid arthritis. No comparative studies have been published, but both drugs induce malignancies after prolonged use (Luqmani et al. 1994), and that limits their use in other than those with severe systemic disease (Table 16). Cyclophosphamide may be given in intravenous pulses of 15 mg/kg, which, however, may be no better than daily oral administration (Luqmani et al. 1994), except for lower risk of bladder toxicity. Both drugs may cause permanent gonadal failure in men and women. Bone marrow suppression is also a prominent feature, although cyclophosphamide may be slightly less toxic for megakaryocytes.

Combination therapy

This has been mentioned in connection with several drugs and is a matter of current interest (Paulus 1990; Brooks and Schwarzer 1991). Theoretically, benefits could be expected both from combining drugs with similar and different mechanisms of action, provided the adverse reactions differed and were dose related. Few controlled trials have been completed, however (Table 20). A promising combination is that of hydroxychloroquine, sulphasalazine, and methotrexate (O'Dell et al. 1994).

Disease-suppressive strategies

Frustrated by lack of evidence for long-term disease modification by employment of established disease-suppressive drugs used according to the conventional 'pyramid', several authors have suggested alternative strategies. These include the early use of potent drug combinations, the inverted pyramid or step-down bridge treatment (Wilske and Healey 1990), the cyclic use of drug combinations (Schwarzer et al. 1990), and the successive use of various suppressive drugs according to monitored disability, the 'sawtooth strategy' (Fries 1990). The common feature is the aim for early, rapid control of disease activity and systemic glucocorticoid administration. Published data supporting these strategies are not available.

Experimental therapy

Limited success with established disease-suppressive agents in conjunction with increased knowledge of the rheumatoid disease process is stimulating active development of new therapies, targeting inflammatory mechanisms (Luqmani et al. 1994). Several lines of progress can be distinguished and an important breakthrough may be close (Table 21). It seems unlikely that one single substance will be able to stop the disease process; rather a multifaceted attack is more likely to be successful in the long term. Different targets depending on the stage and nature of the process may achieve the ultimate 'cure'. Escape mechanisms and redundancy are certainly very prevalent in the pathogenesis of rheumatoid arthritis, so the task is similar to that of Mr Sisyphus.

Monoclonal anti-T-cell antibodies

A number of mouse antibodies which have been either chimeric or more recently humanized have been used in open as well as in a few placebo-controlled trials (Kalden 1994; Luqmani et al. 1994). The results have been equivocal or negative. Antibodies to CD7, although immunologically effective, have been uniformly ineffective did not influence disease symptoms, indicating that established disease is not dependent on CD7+ cells. Some of the anti-CD4 reagents have induced prolonged depletion from circulation of CD4+ helper cells but only transient clinical effects. Campath1H, a humanized antibody to CDw52, a cell surface structure on activated helper T cells, has induced depletion of CD4+ T cells lasting a year or longer, and a few patients died from infections that may have been drug related. In one study, clinical response correlated to diminished concentrations of tumour necrosis factor-α and interleukin 1. At present non-depleting anti-CD4 reagents are in trials with claims of more encouraging results.

Cytokine inhibition

Tissue destruction in rheumatoid arthritis is mediated by interleukin 6, tumour necrosis factor, and interleukin-1, and all three have been targets for immune therapy (Campion 1994). Interleukin-1 antagonism can be achieved by monoclonal antibodies, or by administering recombinant human interleukin-1 receptor. Trials are ongoing, the problem may be administering large enough doses, as the receptor is rapidly used up.

Remarkable short-term clinical remissions have been achieved with large doses of chimeric tumour necrosis factor-α antibody. This was originally developed for use in sepsis, where it, however, did not work. An open study on 20 patients was confirmed in a placebo-controlled trial. Response durations of 14 to 16 weeks were seen after administration of doses of 10 to 60 mg/kg but repeated treatment resulted in shorter periods of response, probably due to immune elimination of the antibody (Elliott et al. 1994a; Elliott et al. 1994b). Similar results are emerging using constructs of human Fc from IgG1 and two 55-kDa receptors for tumour necrosis factor. The striking observation has been made that the patients general well being improves within a day, indicating that this therapy really is affecting essential mechanisms. The effects do not last more than a few weeks, and immunization is a worry.

Diets and oral tolerance

Diets are of considerable interest and after many years of anecdotal accounts of carers, several controlled studies clearly show symptomatic effect of diets rich in unsaturated fish oil or plant-seed oil (Darlington 1994). One plausible mechanism behind the symptomatic effect seems to be reduced synthesis of inflammatory

Table 20 Summary of studies using combination therapy in rheumatoid arthritis

Authors	Year	Combination	No. of patients	Result
Double-blind, randomized				
Bunch *et al.*	1984	D-Penicillamine and hydroxychloroquine	56	Combination not as effective as D-penicillamine alone; more side-effects with D-penicillamine
McKenna *et al.*	1985	Gold and D-penicillamine	45	Combination resulted in earlier response than gold or D-penicillamine alone
Scott *et al.*	1989	Gold and hydroxychloroquine	101	Combination more effective than gold and placebo
Non-blinded, randomized				
Bitter	1984	Gold and D-penicillamine, levamisole or cholambucil; D-penicillamine and levamisole or chlorambucil	71	D-Penicillamine and gold effective Other combinations ineffective
Butler and Tiliakos	1985	Methotrexate, cyclophosphamide, hydroxychloroquine	18	Combination effective; recortication of erosions
Taggart *et al.*	1987	D-Penicillamine and sulphasalazine	30	Combination more effective than sulphasalazine alone
Gibson *et al.*	1987	D-Penicillamine and chloroquine	72	No advantage of combination vs. either drug alone
Non-blinded, non randomized, comparative				
Sievers and Hurri	1963	Gold, hydroxychloroquine/ chloroquine	488	Combination might be of benefit
Martin *et al.*	1982	D-Penicillamine and hydroxychloro-quine	45	Better response from combination than either drug alone at 6 months
McConkey and Sittunayake	1988	Rifampicin and isoniazid	18	Possible beneficial effect from rifampicin
Open, uncontrolled	1974	D-Penicillamine and azathioprine	31	Combination effective Significant toxicity
Berry and Huskisson				
Lewis *et al.*	1977	Gold and azathioprine	70	Good response from combination
McCarty and Carrera	1982	Cyclophosphamide, azathioprine, hydroxychloroquine	17	Combination effective
Singleton and Cervantes	1984	Gold and hydroxychloroquine	18	Combination effective in patients who failed hydroxychloroquine alone
Csuka *et al.*	1986	Cyclophosphamide, azathioprine, hydroxychloroquine	31	Combination effective but significant toxicity
Binder *et al.*	1986	Antilymphocyte globulin, prednisone and cytotoxic	12	Improvement at 3 months not maintained
Dougados *et al.*	1987	Bromocryptine and cyclosporin	6	Combination not effective
Dawes *et al.*	1987	Sulphasalazine and either gold or D-penicillamine	25	Combinations effective
Farr *et al.*	1988	Sulphasalazine and either gold or D-penicillamine	31	Combinations effective
Brawer	1988	Gold and methotrexate	7	Combination effective
Waterworth	1989	Azathioprine and sulphasalazine	13	Combination effective
Shiroky *et al.*	1989	Methotrexate and sulphasalazine	4	Combination effective
Langevitz *et al.*	1989	Methotrexate, azathioprine, hydroxychloroquine	12	Combination effective
Schwarzer *et al.*	1990	Prednisolone, hydroxychloroquine and alternating methotrexate/ sulphasalazine	16	Significant improvement at 3 months but less marked at 6 and 12 months

Reproduced with permission from Schwarzer *et al.* (1990), where references may be found.

Table 21 Experimental therapies in development for rheumatoid arthritis

Target	Principle
The agent	Missing
Activated lymphocytes	Monoclonal antibodies Apharesis/photophoresis Oral tolerance induction/vaccination IL-2 fusion toxin, anti-CD5-ricin conjugate
Macrophage cytokine inhibition	Anti-IL-6 antibodies Anti-IL-1/sIL-1 receptor Anti-TNF/sTNF receptor
Cell adhesion molecules	Anti-ICAM-1
Proinflammation prostanoids	Fish- and plant-seed oil Selective Cox-2-inhibitors
Disease activity	Tetracycline Tenidap Bucillamine Podophyllotoxins Subreum Leflunomide Mycophenolic acid

IL, interleukin; TNF, tumour necrosis factor

arachidonic acid products at the expense of eicosapentaenoic acid products. It has been hard to recruit patients for controlled trials and those entered have usually had relatively mild disease (Kjeldsen-Kragh *et al.* 1991). Elimination diets have also been attempted, usually with unconvincing effects (Darlington 1994).

Animal work has suggested oral tolerance induction in experimental autoimmune disease, such as experimental autoimmune encephalitis and adjuvant and collagen arthritis, by administering the antigen orally (Vischer and van Eden 1994). This principle, although claimed effective in initial open trials has not been confirmed in placebo-controlled trials. The suggested mechanism is that the antigen stimulates bystander suppressive pathways (Miller *et al.* 1992). Similar mechanisms may explain the effectiveness of Subreum (OM 8980), an orally administered *Escherichia coli* preparation (Vischer and van Eden 1994).

Other agents

Several substances are in phase III of clinical development or have actually been licensed in a few countries. Bucillamine is a disulphydryl amino acid similar to D-penicillamine and is much used in Japan. Tenidap is a cyclo-oxygenase inhibitor which also reduces C-reactive protein and is as effective as a NSAID–antimalarial combination (Littman *et al.* 1995). Minocyclin has shown moderate clinical efficacy in a double-blind study, where the interesting observation was a marked reduction in C-reactive protein combined with significant but less impressive clinical effects, indicating that the acute-phase response may not be directly linked to the rheumatoid process (Kloppenburg *et al.* 1994). Podophyllatoxin is a plant extract that in open studies induces prompt reduction in

synovitis, acute-phase proteins, and rheumatoid factor concentration (Berglund *et al.* 1980). Unfortunately, it also causes severe abdominal pain or diarrhoea in most patients. A purified derivative called reumacon has weaker but significant clinical effects (Larsen *et al.* 1989). Intravenous immunoglobulin administration with or without apharesis, photophoresis, lymphapheresis, and infusion of retroplacental immunoglobulins have been tried as immunomodulating therapy. These interesting but extremely expensive procedures have yet to prove their efficacy (Sany 1994).

Surgical therapy

Surgery as a treatment in rheumatoid arthritis was made popular in the early 1960s when orthopaedic surgeons working at the Rheumatism Hospital in Heinola, Finland, showed that synovectomies were well tolerated even in active stages of the disease. Much of rheumatological endeavour since that period has been aimed at reducing the need for surgery. It need not be said that we are still far from this goal.

Synovectomy has become infrequent in most places, although pain relief may last for years. However, no retardation of radiological progression is achieved as was initially hoped (Gschwend *et al.* 1974; Doets *et al.* 1989). Tenosynovectomies have remained popular and the fastest and safest relief for nerve entrapment is still surgical decompression. The main indications for surgery are incapacitating pain and restoration or preservation of function. The state of surgical management was the subject of a recent publication (Kelly and Capell 1990).

The most frequent procedures are reconstructive arthroplasties of the hip. Approximately 10 per cent of a patient cohort with early rheumatoid arthritis were operated on within 5 years from onset in our unit (Eberhardt *et al.* 1995). Also common but much less frequently performed are total knee replacements. Shoulder arthroplasties have only recently become feasible and are still far from ideal (Bennett and Gerber 1994). Elbow reconstruction is also possible although loosening has been a major problem (Wadsworth 1993). Arthroplasty procedures of the wrist, fingers, and ankle joints have been devised but are at an experimental stage. Corrective arthrotomies of the metatarsal toe region are common and successful (Helal and Greiss 1984)

Surgical stabilization of the cervical spine to prevent or relieve compression of the medulla is an important task for highly specialized teams. With improved diagnostic and surgical techniques and results, the indications for this form of therapy can be widened (Zygmunt *et al.* 1988; Milbrink and Wingren 1989).

In order to achieve optimal results the rheumatologists and orthopaedic/hand surgeons must work together, preferably in joint clinics with the help of physiotherapists, occupational therapists, and other allied health professionals. Decisions should result from careful analysis of the problem(s) as seen by the patient and from weighing the possible gains and risks of the procedures. An operation always involves risks and is traumatic and tiresome for the patient. Psychological aspects also confound the issue; sometimes an operation is desired to demonstrate to the family how sick the patient is.

The majority of patients admitted to hospital are subjected to one or more operations with time. Two-thirds of these involve the lower limbs, with the often achieved goal of preserving ambulation. Patients with rheumatoid arthritis are at greater risk for acquiring infections, but less likely to have thromboembolic complications. Disease-suppressing therapy usually can be continued, but methotrexate may be an exception, owing to risk of infection. NSAIDs are given as required in most places, apparently with no important risk of bleeding. They have the added advantage of preventing postoperative calcifying myositis.

Surgical treatment is cost effective, since it reduces costs to society for home service and may preserve productivity and independence (Goldie 1993).

Team rehabilitation

It should be emphasized that rheumatoid arthritis should never be managed without help of a professional team of allied health experts. Patient education is a neglected principle of adapting the individual to cope with a chronic incurable disease and may actually influence pain control and self-esteem favourably (Lindroth *et al*. 1995). Physical therapy may improve self-efficacy, physical capacity, and pain perception (Brighton *et al*. 1993; Stenström 1994). Proper use of technical aids for household and ambulation, adapted environment at home, at work, and in the car are other examples of important therapeutic measures that will reduce helplessness and improve quality of life for the patient. Thus, as mentioned, in most cases a team approach involving doctor(s), physiotherapist, occupational therapist, social worker, and nurse is best suited for the optimal management of rheumatoid arthritis.

Prognosis

There is a growing interest in developing early predictors of long-term outcome in rheumatoid arthritis, which would allow better patient selection for early intervention. Genetic markers and rheumatoid factors have a well-documented relation to disease susceptibility and development of erosions within a year (Gough *et al*. 1994b). The 'shared epitope' in double dose in particular, including DRB1*04 epitopes, also seems to predict a more destructive disease, but the correlation is far too weak to be of use for early therapeutic decisions (Wollheim *et al*. 1995). An *in vitro* test of Ig-synthesis induced by Epstein–Barr virus also can distinguish erosive from non-erosive cases (Jokinen *et al*. 1994). Early functional impairment is a crude but reliable indicator of poor prognosis (Rasker and Cosh 1989). Rheumatoid arthritis is still a severe disease in a large proportion of patients, although as mentioned (Heikkil and Isomki 1994) the proportion of milder cases may be increasing.

References

Ahlmén, M., Ahlmén, J., Svalander, C., and Bucht, H. (1987). Cytotoxic drug treatment of reactive amyloidosis in rheumatoid arthritis with special reference to renal insufficiency. *Clinical Rheumatology*, **6**, 27–38.

Aho, K., Heliövaara, M., Sievers, K., Maatela, J., and Isomki, H. (1989). Clinical arthritis associated with positive radiological and serological findings in Finnish adults. *Rheumatology International*, **9**, 7–11.

Alarcón, G.S. *et al*. (1992). Radiographic evidence of disease progression in methotrexate treated and nonmethotrexate disease modifying antirheumatic drug treated rheumatoid arthritis patients: a meta-analysis. *Journal of Rheumatology*, **19**, 1868–72.

Andersson, I., Marsal, L., Nilsson, B., Sjöblom, K.G., and Wollheim, F.A. (1980). Abnormal axillary lymph nodes in rheumatoid arthritis. *Acta Radiologica Diagnostica*, **21**, 645–9.

Arnett, F.C. *et al*. (1988). The American Rheumatism Associaton 1987 revised criteria for the classification of rheumatoid arthritis. *Arthritis and Rheumatism*, **31**, 315–24.

Banarjee, A.K. (1989). Enteropathy induced by non-steroidal anti-inflammatory drugs. *British Medical Journal*, **298**, 1539–40.

Barrera, P. *et al*. (1993). Circulating soluble tumor necrosis factor receptors, interleukin-2 receptors, tumor necrosis factor α, and interlukin-6 levels in rheumatoid arthritis. Longitudinal evaluation during methotrexate and azathioprine therapy. *Arthritis and Rheumatism*, **36**, 1070–9.

Bateman, D.N. (1994). NSAIDs: time to re-evaluate gut toxicity. *Lancet*, **343**, 1051–2.

Bennett, P.H. and Burch, T.A. (1967). New York symposium on population studies in the rheumatic diseases; new diagnostic criteria. *Bulletin of the Rheumatic Diseases*, **17**, 453–8.

Bennett W.F. and Gerber C. (1994). Operative treatment of the rheumatoid shoulder. *Current Opinion in Rheumatology*, **6**, 177–82.

Berglund, K., Laurell, A.B., Nived, O., Sjöholm, A.G., and Sturfelt, G. (1980). Complement activation, circulating C1q binding substances and inflammatory activity in rheumatoid arthritis: relations and changes on suppression of inflammation. *Journal of Clinical and Laboratory Immunology*, **4**, 7–14.

Berglund, K., Thysell, H., and Keller, C. (1993). Results, principles and pitfalls in the management of renal AA-amyloidosis: a 10–21 year follow-up of 16 patients with rheumatic disease treated with alkylating cytostatics. *Journal of Rheumatology*, **20**, 2051–7.

Berntzen, H.B., Munthe, E., and Fagerhol, M.K. (1989). A longitudinal study of the leukocyte protein L1 as an indicator of disease activity in patients with rheumatoid arthritis. *Journal of Rheumatology*, **16**, 1416–20.

Birnie, G., McLeod, T., and Watkinson, G. (1981). Incidence of sulphasalazine induced male infertility. *Gut*, **22**, 452–5.

Bjarnason, I., Price, A.B., Gumpel, J.M., and Levi, A.J. (1988). Clinicopathological features of nonsteroidal antiinflammatory drug-induced small intestinal strictures. *Gastroenterology*, **94**, 1070–4.

Bland, J.H. (1974). Rheumatoid arthritis of the cervical spine. *Journal of Rheumatology*, **1**, 319–42.

Borg, G. *et al*. (1988). Auranofin improves outcome in early rheumatoid arthritis. Results from a 2 year, double blind, placebo controlled study. *Journal of Rheumatology*, **15**, 1747–54.

Brahme, S.K. (1991). The role of magnetic resonance imaging in rheumatic disorders. *European Journal of Rheumatological Inflammation*, **11**, 100–3.

Brighton S.W., Lubbe, J.E., and van der Merwe C.A. (1993). The effect of a long-term exercise programme on the rheumatoid hand. *British Journal of Rheumatology*, **32**, 392–5.

Brooks, P.M. and Day, R.O. (1991). Nonsteroidal antiinflammatory drugs — differences and similarities. *New England Journal of Medicine*, **324**, 1716–25.

Brooks, P.M. and Schwarzer, A.C. (1991). Combination therapy in rheumatoid arthritis. *Annals of the Rheumatic Diseases*, **50**, 507–9.

Butler, R.C., Davie, M.W.J., Worsfold, M., and Sharp, C.A. (1991). Bone mineral content in patients with rheumatoid arthritis: relationship to low-dose steroid therapy. *British Journal of Rheumatology*, **30**, 86–90.

Camp, J., Sangro, G., Garcia, N., Subira, M.L., and Prieto, J. (1991). Felty's syndrome: response to cyclosporin A with disappaerance of neutrophil autoantibodies. (Letter.) *Arthritis and Rheumatism*, **34**, 353–5.

Campion, E.G. (1994). Leader: The prospect for cytokine based therapeutic strategies in rheumatoid arthritis. *Annals of the Rheumatic Diseases*, **53**, 485–7.

Campion, G. *et al*. (1990). The Felty syndrome: a case-matched study of clinical manifestations and outcome, serologic features, and immunogenetic associations. *Medicine* (Baltimore), **69**, 69–80.

Cash, J.M., and Klippel, J.H. (1994). Second-line drug therapy for rheumatoid arthritis. *New England Journal of Medicine*, **330**, 1368–75.

Chalmers, I.M. and Blair, G.S. (1973). Rheumatoid arthritis of the temporomandibular joint. *Quarterly Journal of Medicine*, **42**, 369–86.

Chamberlain, M.A. and Bruckner, F.E. (1970). Rheumatoid neuropathy: clinical and electrophysiological features. *Annals of the Rheumatic Diseases*, **29**, 609–16.

Champion, G.D., Graham, G.C., and Ziegler, J.B. (1990). The gold complexes. *Baillière's Clinical Rheumatology*, **4**, 491–535.

Chander, C.L. and Spector, T.D. (1991). Oestrogens, joint disease and cartilage. *Annals of the Rheumatic Diseases*, **50**, 139–40.

Chikanza, I.C., Petrou, P., Kingsley, G, Chrousos, G., and Panayi G.S. (1992). Defective hypothalamic response to immune and inflammatory stimuli in patients with rheumatoid arthritis. *Arthritis and Rheumatism*, **35**, 1281–8.

Clark P. *et al.* (1993). Hydroxychloroquine compared with placebo in rheumatoid arthritis. A randomized controlled trial. *Annals of Internal Medicine*, **119**, 1067–71.

Darlington, L.G. (1994). Dietary therapy for rheumatoid arthritis. *Clinical and Experimental Rheumatology*, **12**, 235–9.

Dawes, P.T., Fowler, P.D., Clarke, S., Fisher, J., Lawton, A., and Shadforth, M.F. (1986). Rheumatoid arthritis: treatment which controls the C-reactive protein and erythrocyte sedimentation rate, reduces radiologic progression. *British Journal of Rheumatology*, **25**, 44–9.

Deal, C.L. *et al.* (1985). The clinical features of elderly-onset rheumatoid arthritis. *Arthritis and Rheumatism*, **28**, 987–94.

di Giovine, F.S., Ralston, S.H., and Duff, G.W. (1990). Laboratory and radiologic investigations in the diagnosis and evaluation of rheumatoid arthritis. *Current Opinion in Rheumatology*, **2**, 450–7.

Doets, H.C., Bierman, B.T., and von Soesbergen, R.M. (1989). Synovectomy of the rheumatoid knee does not prevent deterioration. 7-year follow-up of 83 cases. *Acta Orthopaedica Scandinavica*, **60**, 523–5.

Dougados, M., Duchesne, L., Awada, H., and Amor, B. (1989). Assessment of efficacy and acceptability of low dose cyclosporine in patients with rheumatoid arthritis. *Annals of the Rheumatic Diseases*, **48**, 550–6.

Eberhardt, K.B., Rydgren, L.C., Pettersson, H., and Wollheim, F.A. (1990a). Early rheumatoid arthritis — onset, course and prognosis over 2 years. *Rheumatology International*, **10**, 135–42.

Eberhardt, K.B. *et al.* (1990b). Disease activity and joint damage progression in early rheumatoid arthritis: relation to IgG, IgA, and IgM rheumatoid factor. *Annals of the Rheumatic Diseases*, **49**, 906–9.

Eberhardt, K.B., Fex, E., Johnsson, K., and Geborek, P. (1995). Hip involvement in early rheumatoid arthritis. *Annals of the Rheumatic Diseases*, **54**, 45–8.

Edmonds, J.P., Scott, D.L., Furst, D.E., Brooks, P., and Paulus, H.E. (1993). Antirheumatic drugs: a proposed new classification. (Editorial.) *Arthritis and Rheumatism*, **36**, 336–9.

Edmonds, M.E., Jones, T.C., and Saunders, W.A. (1979). Autonomic neuropathy in rheumatoid arthritis. *British Medical Journal*, **3**, 173–5.

Elliot, M.J. *et al.* (1994a). Repeated therapy with monoclonal antibody to tumour necrosis factor α (cA2) in patients with rheumatoid arthritis. *Lancet*, **344**, 1125–7.

Elliot, M.J. *et al.* (1994b). Randomised double-blind comparison of chimeric monoclonal antibody to tumour necrosis factor α (cA2) versus placebo in rheumatoid arthritis. *Lancet*, **344**, 1105–10.

Engel, A. (1968). Rheumatoid arthritis in US adults 1960–62. In *Population studies of the rheumatic diseases* (ed. P.H. Bennet and P.H.N. Wood), pp. 83–8. Excerpta Medica, Amsterdam.

Engström-Laurent, A. and Hllgren, R. (1985). Circulating hyaluronate in rheumatoid arthritis: relationship to inflammatory activity and the effect of corticosteroid therapy. *Annals of the Rheumatic Diseases*, **44**, 83–8.

Eriksson, L.O., Sturfelt, G., Thysell, H., and Wollheim, F.A. (1990). Effects of sulindac and naproxen on prostaglandin excretion in patients with impaired renal function and rheumatoid arthritis. *American Journal of Medicine*, **89**, 313–21.

Faber, E. and Elling, P. (1966). Leucocyte-specific antinuclear factors in patients with Felty's syndrome, rheumatoid arthritis, systemic lupus erythematosus and other diseases. *Acta Medica Scandinavica*, **179**, 257–67.

Feigenbaum, S.L., Masi, A.T., and Kaplan, S.B. (1979). Prognosis in rheumatoid athritis. A longitudinal study of newly diagnosed younger adult patients. *American Journal of Medicine*, **66**, 377–84.

Felson, D.T., Anderson, J.J., and Meenan, R.F. (1990). The comparative efficacy and toxicity of second-line drugs in rheumatoid arthritis. Results of two meta-analyses. *Arthritis and Rheumatism*, **33**, 1449–61.

Felty, A.R. (1924). Chronic arthritis in the adult associated with splenomegaly and leukopenia; a report of five cases of an unusual clinical syndrome. *Bulletin of the Johns Hopkins Hospital*, **35**, 16–20.

Førre, Ø. and the Norwegian Arthritis Study Group (1994). Radiologic evidence of disease modification in rheumatoid arthritis patients treated with cyclosporine. *Arthritis and Rheumatism*, **37**, 1506–12.

Freemont, A.J. (1991). Role of cytological analysis of synovial fluid in diagnosis and research. *Annals of the Rheumatic Diseases*, **50**, 120–3.

Fries, J.F. (1990). Reevaluating the therapeutic approach to rheumatoid arthritis: the 'sawtooth' strategy. *Journal of Rheumatology*, Suppl. **22**, 12–15.

Fries, J.F., Miller, S.R., Spitz, P.W., Williams, C.A., Hubert, H.B., and Block, D.A. (1989). Towards an epidemiology of gastropathy associated with nonsteroidal antiinflammatory drug use. *Gastroenterology*, **96** (Suppl. 2), 647–55.

Fries, J.F., Williams, C.A., and Bloch, D.A. (1991). The relative toxicity of nonsteroidal antiinflammatory drugs. *Arthritis and Rheumatism*, **34**, 1353–60.

Geborek, P., Moritz, U., and Wollheim, F.A. (1989a). Joint capsular stiffness in knee arthritis. Relationship to intraarticular volume, hydrostatic pressures, and extensor muscle function. *Journal of Rheumatology*, **16**, 1351–8.

Geborek, P., Saxne, T., Pettersson, H., and Wollheim, F.A. (1989b). Synovial fluid acidosis correlates with radiological joint destruction in rheumatoid arthritis knee joints. *Journal of Rheumatology*, **16**, 468–72.

Geddes, D.M. *et al.* (1977). α_1-Antitrypsin phenotypes in fibrosing alveolitis and rheumatoid arthritis. *Lancet*, **ii**, 1049–50.

Geirson, A.J., Sturfelt, G., and Truedsson, L. (1987). Clinical and serological features of severe vasculitis in rheumatoid arthritis — prognostic implications. *Annals of the Rheumatic Diseases*, **46**, 727–33.

George, E. and Kirwan, J.R. (1990). Corticosteroid therapy in rheumatoid arthritis. *Baillière's Clinical Rheumatology*, **4**, 621–47.

Geterud, Å. (1991). Rheumatoid arthritis in the larynx. A clinical and methodological study. Ph.D. thesis. University of Gothenburg, Sweden.

Goemaere, S. *et al.* (1990). Onset of symptoms of rheumatoid arthritis in relation to age, sex and menopausal transition. *Journal of Rheumatology*, **17**, 1620–2.

Goldberg, J. and Pinals, R.S. (1980). Felty's syndrome. *Seminars in Arthritis and Rheumatism*, **10**, 52–65.

Goldie, I. (1993). Is there any benefit in the surgery of rheumatoid arthritis? *Current Orthopaedics*, **7**, 120–6.

Goodgold, J., Kopell, H.P., and Speilholz, N.I. (1965). The tarsal tunnel syndrome. *New England Journal of Medicine*, **273**, 742–5.

Gough, A.K, Lilley, J., Eyre S., Holder, R.L, and Emery, P. (1994a). Generalized bone loss in patients with early rheumatoid arthritis. *Lancet*, **344**, 23–7.

Gough, A. *et al.* (1994b). Genetic typing of patients with inflammatory arthritis at presentation can be used to predict outcome. *Arthritis and Rheumatism*, **37**, 1166–70.

Grosflam, J. and Weinblatt, M.E. (1991). Methotrexate: mechanism of action, pharmacokinetics, clinical indications, and toxicity. *Current Opinion in Rheumatology*, **3**, 363–8.

Gschwend, N., Winder, J., and Böni, A. (1974). Indikation und Ergebnisse der Synovektomi. *Therpaeutische Umschau*, **31**, 475.

Guillemin, F. *et al.* (1994). Functional disability in early rheumatoid arthritis: description and risk factors. *Journal of Rheumatology*, **21**, 1051–5.

Hall, G.M., Daniels, M., Huskisson E.C., and Spector, T.D. (1994). A randomised controlled trial of the effect of hormone replacement therapy on disease activity in postmenopausal rheumatoid arthritis. *Annals of the Rheumatic Diseases*, **53**, 112–16.

Halla, J.T. *et al.* (1984). Rheumatoid myositis. *Arthritis and Rheumatism*, **27**, 737–43.

Hannonen, P., Möttönen, T., Hakola, M., and Oka, M. (1993). Sulfasalazine in early rheumatoid arthritis. *Arthritis and Rheumatism*, **36**, 1501–9.

Hara, K.S., Ballard, D.J., Ilstrup, D.M., Connolly, D.C., and Vollertsen, R.S. (1990). Rheumatoid pericarditis: clinical features and survival. *Medicine*, **69**, 81–91.

Hassell, A.B. *et al.* (1993). The relationship between serial measures of disease activity and outcome in rheumatoid arthritis. *Quarterly Journal of Medicine*, **86**, 601–7.

Hassfeld, W. *et al.* (1989). Demonstration of a new antinuclear antibody (anti-rheumatoid arthritis 33) that is highly specific for rheumatoid arthritis. *Arthritis and Rheumatism*, **32**, 1515–20.

Hazenberg, B.P., van Leewen, M.A., van Rijswijk, M.H., Stern, A.C., and Vellenga, E. (1989). Correction of granulocytopenia in Felty's syndrome by granulocyte-macrophage colony-stimulating factor. Simultaneous induction of interleukin-6 release and flare-up of the arthritis. *Blood*, **74**, 2769–70.

Hazes, J.M. and van Zeben, D. (1991). Oral contraception and its possible protection against rheumatoid arthritis. *Annals of the Rheumatic Diseases*, **50**, 72–4.

Hazes, J.M.W., Dijkmans, B.A.C., Vandenbrouke, J.P., and Cauts, A. (1989). Oral contraceptive treatment for rheumatoid arthritis: an open study in 10 female patients. *British Journal of Rheumatology*, **28** (Suppl. I), 28–30.

Hedberg, H., Nordén, Å., Lundquist, A., and Afzelius, B. (1964). Depression of hemolytic complement activity of synovial fluid in adult rheumatoid arthritis. *Acta Medica Scandinavica*, **175**, 347–51.

Hedfors, E. Klareskog, L., Lindblad, S., Forsum, U., and Lindahl, G. (1983). Phenotypic characterization of cells within subcutaneous rheumatoid nodules. *Arthritis and Rheumatism*, **26**, 1333–9.

Heikkil, S. and Isomki, H. (1994). Long-term outcome of rheumatoid arthritis has improved. *Scandinavian Journal of Rheumatology*, **23**, 13–15.

Helal, B. and Greiss, M. (1984). Telescoping osteotomy for pressure metatarsalgia. *Journal of Bone and Joint Surgery*, **22**, 213–7.

Hench, P.S. (1938). The ameliorating effect of pregnancy on chronic atrophic (infectious rheumatoid) arthritis, fibrosis, and intermittent hydrarthrosis. *Proceedings of the Mayo Clinic*, **13**, 161–7.

Hench, P.S., Kendall, E.C., Slocumb, C.H., and Polley, H.F. (1949). The effect of a hormone of the adrenal cortex (17-hydroxy-11-dehydrocorticosterone compound E) and of pituitary adrenocorticotropic hormone on rheumatoid arthritis. *Proceedings of the Staff Meetings of the Mayo Clinic*, **24**, 181–97.

Hooyman, J.R., Melton, L.J., Nelson, A.M., O'Fallon, W.M., and Riggs, B.L. (1984). Fractures after rheumatoid arthritis. *Arthritis and Rheumatism*, **27**, 1353–61.

Hørslev-Petersen, K., Bendtzen, K.D., Engström-Laurent, A., Junker, P., Halberg, P., and Lorenzen, I. (1988). Serum amino terminal type III procollagen peptide and serum hyaluronan in rheumatoid arthritis: relation to clinical and serological parameters of inflammation during 8 and 24 months' treatment with levamisole, penicillamine, or azathioprine. *Annals of the Rheumatic Diseases*, **47**, 116–26.

Huskisson, E.C., Woolf, D.L., Balme, H.W., Scott, J., and Franklyn, S. (1976). Four new anti-inflammatory drugs: responses and variations. *British Medical Journal*, **1**, 1048–9.

Hyland, R.H. *et al.* (1983). A systemic controlled study of pulmonary abnormalities in rheumatoid arthritis. *Journal of Rheumatology*, **10**, 395–405.

Jacobsson, L.T. *et al.* (1994). Decreasing incidence and prevalence of rheumatoid arthritis in Pima Indians over a twenty-five-year period. *Arthritis and Rheumatism*, **37**, 1158–65.

Jeurissen, M.E.C. *et al.* (1991). Methotrexate versus azathioprine in the treatment of rheumatoid arthritis: a forty-eight-week, randomized, double-blind trial. *Arthritis and Rheumatism*, **34**, 961–72.

Jokinen, E.I., Möttönen, T.T., Hannonen, P.J., Mkel, M., and Arvilommi, H.S. (1994). Prediction of severe rheumatoid arthritis using Epstein–Barr virus. *British Journal of Rheumatology*, **33**, 917–22.

Jonsson, B. and Larsson, S.E. (1990). Rheumatoid arthritis evaluated by locomotion score. A population study. *Scandinavian Journal of Rheumatology*, **19**, 223–31.

Joyce, D.A. (1990). D-Penicillamine. *Ballière's Clinical Rheumatology*, **4**, 553–74.

Kalden, J.M. (1994). Biological agents in the therapy of inflammatory rheumatic diseases, including therapeutic antibodies, cytokines and cytokine antagonists. *Current Opinion in Rheumatology*, **6**, 281–6.

Kamme, C. and Lindberg, L. (1981). Aerobic and anaerobic bacteria in deep infections after total hip arthroplasty. Differential diagnosis between infectious and non-infectious loosening. *Clinical Orthopaedics and Related Research*, **154**, 201–7.

Kazis, L.E., Anderson, J.J., and Meenan, R.F. (1990). Health status as a predictor of mortality in rheumatoid arthritis: a five year study. *Journal of Rheumatology*, **17**, 609–13.

Keisu, M. and Ekman, E. (1992). Sulfasalazine associated agranulocytosis in Sweden 1972–1989. Clinical features, and estimation of its incidence. *European Journal of Clinical Pharmacology*, **43**, 215–18.

Kellgren, J.H. (1962). Diagnostic criteria for population studies. *Bulletin of the Rheumatic Diseases*, **12**, 291–2.

Kelly, I.G. and Capell, H.A. (1990). Surgical management of rheumatic diseases. *Annals of the Rheumatic Diseases*, **49** (Suppl 2), 823–82.

Kjeldsen-Kragh, J. *et al.* (1991). Controlled trial of fasting and one-year vegetarian diet in rheumatoid arthritis. *Lancet*, **338**, 899–902.

Klipple, G.L. and Cecere, F.A. (1989). Rheumatoid arthritis and pregnancy. *Rheumatic Disease Clinics of North America*, **15**, 213–39.

Kloppenburg, M., Breedveld, F.C., Terwiel, J.P., Mallee, C., and Dijkmans, B.A.C. (1994). Minocycline in active rheumtoid arthritis. A double-blind, placebo-controlled trial. *Arthritis and Rheumatism*, **37**, 629–36.

Kremer, J.M. and Phelps, C.T. (1992). Long-term prospective study of the use of methotrexate in the treatment of rheumatoid arthritis: update after a mean of 90 months. *Arthritis and Rheumatism*, **35**, 138–45.

Kremer, J.M., Petrillo, G.F., and Hamilton, R.A. (1995). Pharmacokinetics and renal function in patients with rheumatoid arthritis receiving a standard dose of oral weekly methotrexate: association with significant decreases in creatinine clearance and renal clearance of the drug after 6 months of therapy. *Journal of Rheumatology*, **22**, 38–40.

Kurki, P., Aho, K., Palosuo, T., and Heliövaara, M. (1992). Immunopathology of rheumatoid arthritis. Antikeratin antibodies precede the clinical disease. *Arthritis and Rheumatism*, **35**, 914–17.

Lakhanpal, S., McLeod, R.A., and Luthra, H.S. (1986). Insufficiency type stress fractures in rheumatoid arthritis: report of an interesting case and review of the literature. *Clinical and Experimental Rheumatology*, **4**, 151–4.

Landewé, R.B.M., Goei The, H.S., van Rijthoven, W.A.M., Rietveld, J.R., Breedveld, F.C., and Dijkmans, B.A.C. (1994). Cyclosporine in common clinical practice: an estimation of the benefit/risk ratio in patients with rheumatoid arthritis. *Journal of Rheumatology*, **21**, 1631–6.

Landewé, R.B.M. *et al.* (1995). Antimalarial drug induced decrease in creatinine clearance. *Journal of Rheumatology*, **22**, 34–7.

Langman, M.J.S. (1989). Epidemiologic evidence on the association between peptic ulceration and anti-inflammatory drug use. *Gastroenterology*, **96** (Suppl. 2), 640–6.

Larsen, A., Dale, K., and Eek, M. (1977). Radiographic evaluation of rheumatoid arthritis and related conditions by standard reference films. *Acta Radiologica Diagnostica*, **18**, 481–91.

Larsen, A., Petersson, I., and Svensson, B. (1989). Podophyllum derivatives (CPH 82) compared with placebo in the treatment of rheumatoid arthritis. *British Journal of Rheumatology*, **28**, 124–7.

Lee, S.W. *et al.* (1988). Glucocorticoids selectively inhibit the transcription of the interleukin 1β gene and decrease the stability of interleukin 1β mRNA. *Proceedings of the National Academy of Sciences (USA)*, **85**, 1204–8.

Lender, M. and Wolf, E. (1972). Incidence of amyloidosis in rheumatoid arthritis. *Scandinavian Journal of Rheumatology*, **1**, 109–12.

Lindroth, Y., Bauman, A., Brooks, P.M., and Priestley, D. (1995). A five-year follow-up of a controlled trial of an arthritis education programme. *British Journal of Rheumatology*, **34**, 647–52.

Linos, A.D. *et al.* (1980). The epidemiology of rheumatoid arthritis in Rochester Minnesota. A study of its incidence, prevalence and mortality. *American Journal of Epidemiology*, **111**, 87–98.

Lipsky, P.E. and Ziff, M. (1980). Inhibition of human helper T-cell function *in vitro* by D-penicillamine and $CuSO_4$. *Journal of Clinical Investigation*, **65**, 1069–76.

Littman, B.H., Drury, C.E., Zimmerer, R.O., Stack, C.B., amd Law, C.G. (1995). Rheumatoid arthritis treated with tenidap and piroxicam. Clinical association with cytokine modulation by tenidap. *Arthritis and Rheumatism*, **38**, 29–37.

Lukert, B.P. and Raisz, L.G. (1990). Glucocorticoid-induced osteoporosis: pathogenesis and management. *Annals of Internal Medicine*, **112**, 352–64.

Luqmani, R.A., Palmer, R.G., and Bacon, P.A. (1990). Azathioprine, cyclophosphamide and chlorambucil. *Ballière's Clinical Rheumatology*, **4**, 595–619.

Luqmani, R., Gordon, C., and Bacon, P. (1994). Clinical pharmacology and modification of autoimmunity and inflammation in rheumatoid disease. *Drugs*, **47**, 259–85.

Luukkainen, R., Isomki, H., and Kajander, A. (1983). Prognostic value of the type of onset of rheumatoid arthritis. *Annals of the Rheumatic Diseases*, **42**, 274–5.

Luukkainen, R., Kaarela, K., Huhtala, H., Auerma, K., and Merilahti-Palo, R. (1989). Prognostic significance of synovial fluid analysis in rheumatoid arthritis. *Annals of Medicine*, **21**, 269–71.

MacDonald, A.G., Murphy, E.A., Capell, H.A., Bankowska, U.Z., and Ralson, S.H. (1994). Effects of hormone replacement therapy in rheumatoid arthritis. *Annals of the Rheumatic Diseases*, **53**, 54–7.

Marks, J.S. and Sharp, J. (1981). Rheumatoid cervical myelopathy. *Quarterly Journal of Medicine*, **199**, 307–19.

McDougall, R,. Sibley, J., Haga, M., and Russell, A. (1994). Outcome in patients with rheumatoid arthritis receiving prednisone compared to matched controls. *Journal of Rheumatology*, **21**, 1207–13.

Means, R.T., Jr. *et al.* (1989). Treatment of the anemia of rheumatoid arthritis with recombinant human erythropoietin: clinical and *in vitro* studies. *Arthritis and Rheumatism*, **32**, 638–42.

Mikulowski, P., Wollheim, F.A., Rotmil, P., and Olsen, I. (1975). Sudden death in rheumatoid arthritis with atlanto-axial dislocation. *Acta Medica Scandinavica*, **198**, 445–51.

Milbrink, J. and Wingren, A. (1989). Surgical treatment of atlantoaxial subluxation in rheumatoid arthritis. *Journal of Orthopedic Rheumatology*, **2**, 191–9.

Miller, A., Lider, O., and Weiner, H.L. (1992). Antigen-driven bystander suppression after oral administration of antigens. *Journal of Experimental Medicine*, **174**, 791–8.

Mitchell, J.A. *et al.* (1994). Selectivity of nonsteroidal anti-inflammatory drugs as inhibitors of constitutive and inducible cyclooxygenase. *Proceedings of the National Academy of Sciences* (*USA*), **90**, 11693–7.

Mitchell, N. (1989). Imaging techniques in joint disease. *Current Opinion in Rheumatology*, **1**, 29–32.

Monsees, B., Destouet, J.M., Murphy, W.A., and Resnick, D. (1985). Pressure erosions of bone in rheumatoid arthritis: a subject review. *Radiology*, **155**, 53–9.

Morand, E.F., McCloud P.I., and Littlejohn, G.O. (1992). Life table analysis of 879 treatment episodes with slow acting antirheumatic drugs in community rheumatology practice. *Journal of Rheumatology*, **19**, 704–8.

Morgan, S.L. *et al.* (1994). Supplementation with folic acid during methotrexate therapy for rheumatoid arthritis. A double-blind, placebo-controlled trial. *Annals of Internal Medicine*, **121**, 833–41.

Moritz, U. (1963). Electromyograpic studies in adult rheumatoid arthritis. (Thesis.) *Acta Rheumatologica Scandinavica*, Suppl. **5**.

Möttönen, T.T. (1988). Prediction of erosiveness and rate of development of new erosions in early rheumatoid arthritis. *Annals of the Rheumatic Diseases*, **47**, 648–53.

Nelson, J.L., Hughes, K.A., Smith, A.G., Nisperos, B.B., Branchaud, A.M., and Hansen, J.A. (1993). Maternal–fetal disparity in HLA class II alloantigens and the pregnancy-induced amelioration of rheumatoid arthritis. *New England Journal of Medicine*, **329**, 466–71.

Nived, O., Sturfelt, G., and Wollheim, F. (1985). Systemic lupus erythematosus and infection. A controlled and prospective study including an epidemiological group. *Quarterly Journal of Medicine*, **55**, 271–87.

Norberg, R., Wollheim, F.A., and Gedda, P.O. (1980). Circulating protein complexes in D-penicillamine therapy of rheumatoid arthritis. Correlation between IgG and α_1-antitrypsin–IgA complexes and clinical response. *Acta Medica Scandinavica*, **208**, 393–6.

O'Dell, J. *et al.* (1994). Triple DMARD therapy for rheumatoid arthritis: efficacy. *Arthritis and Rheumatism*, **37**, s295.

Östensson, A. and Geborek, P. (1991). Septic arthritis as a nonsurgical complication in rheumatoid arthritis: relation to disease severity and therapy. *British Journal of Rheumatology*, **30**, 35–8.

O'Sullivan, J.B. and Cathcart, E.S. (1972). The prevalence of rheumatoid arthritis: follow-up evaluation of the effect of criteria on rates in Sudbury, Massachusetts. *Annals of Internal Medicine*, **76**, 573–7.

Owsianik, W.D.J. *et al.* (1980). Radiological involvement in the dominating hand in rheumatoid arthritis. *Annals of the Rheumatic Diseases*, **39**, 508–10.

Paimela, L., Heiskanen, A., Kurki, P., Helve, T., and Leirisalo-Repo, M. (1991). Serum hyaluronate level as a predictor of radiologic progression in early rheumatoid arthritis. *Arthritis and Rheumatism*, **34**, 815–21.

Palmer, D.G., Hogg, N., Highton, J., Heissian, P.A., and Denholm, I. (1987). Macrophage migration and maturation within rheumatoid nodules. *Arthritis and Rheumatism*, **30**, 729–36.

Parke, A.L. (1990). Pregnancy and rheumatic diseases. *Ballière's Clinical Rheumatology*, **4**, 1–176.

Paulus, H.E. (1990). The use of combinations of disease-modifying antirheumatic agents in rheumatoid arthritis. *Arthritis and Rheumatism*, **33**, 113–20.

Pelletier, J.-P., Dibattista, J.A., Ranger, P., and Martel-Pelletier, J. (1994). The reduced expression of glucocorticoid receptors in synovial cells induced by nonsteroidal antiinflammatory drugs can be reversed by prostaglandin E_1 analog. *Journal of Rheumatology*, **21**, 1748–52.

Persellin, R.H. (1977). The effect of pregnancy on rheumatoid arthritis. *Bulletin of the Rheumatic Diseases*, **27**, 922–7.

Pincus, T. and Callahan, L.F. (1986). Taking mortality in rheumatoid arthritis seriously — predictive markers, socioeconomic status and comorbidity. (Editorial.) *Journal of Rheumatology*, **13**, 841–5.

Poole, R. (1994). Immunochemical markers of joint inflammation, skeletal damage and repair: where are we now? *Annals of the Rheumatic Diseases*, **53**, 3–5.

Porter, D.R. and Capell, H.A. (1990). The use of sulphasalazine as a disease modifying antirheumatic drug. *Baillière's Clinical Rheumatology*, **4**, 535–51.

Preevo, M.L.L. *et al.* (1993). Validity and reliability of joint counts. A longitudinal study in patients with recent onset rheumatoid arthritis. *British Journal of Rheumatology*, **32**, 589–94.

Preevo, M.L.L., van't Hof, M.A., Kuper, H.H., van Leeuwen, M.A., van de Putte, L.B.A., and van Riel, P.L.C.M. (1995). Modified disease activity scores that include twenty-eight joint counts. Development and validation. A prospective longitudinal study of patients with rheumatoid arthritis. *Arthritis and Rheumatism*, **38**, 44–8.

Raman, D. and Haslock, I. (1982). Trochanteritic bursitis — a frequent cause of 'hip' pain in rheumatoid arthritis. *Annals of the Rheumatic Diseases*, **41**, 602–3.

Rasker, J.J. and Cosh, J.A. (1989). Course and prognosis of early rheumatoid arthritis. *Scandinavian Journal of Rheumatology*, Suppl. **79**, 45–56.

Romieu, I., Hernandez-Avila, M., and Lian, M.H. (1989). Oral contraceptives and the risk of rheumatoid arthritis: a metaanalysis of a conflicting literature. *British Journal of Rheumatology*, **28** (Suppl. I), 13–7.

Ropes, M.W., Bennett, G.A., Cobb, S., Jacox, R., and Jessar, R.A. (1958). 1958 revision of diagnostic criteria for rheumatoid arthritis. *Bulletin of the Rheumatic Diseases*, **9**, 175–6.

Saag, K.G. *et al.* (1994). Low dose long-term corticosteroid therapy in rheumatoid arthritis: an analysis of serious adverse events. *American Journal of Medicine*, **96**, 115–23.

Sack, U., Kinne, R.W., Marx, T., Heppt, P., Bender, S., and Emmrich, F. (1993). Interleukin-6 in synovial fluid is closely associated with chronic synovitis in rheumatoid arthritis. *Rheumatology International*, **13**, 45–51.

Sambrook, P.N., Browne, C.D., Champion, G.D., Day, R.O., Vallance, J.B., and Warwick, N. (1982). Terminations of treatment with gold sodium thiomalate in rheumatoid arthritis. *Journal of Rheumatology*, **9**, 932–4.

Sany, J. (1994). Intravenous immunoglobulin therapy for rheumatic diseases. *Current Opinion in Rheumatology*, **6**, 305–10.

Schwarzer, A.C. *et al.* (1990). The cycling of combination antirheumatic drug therapy in rheumatoid arthritis. *British Journal of Rheumatology*, **29**, 445–50.

Scott, D.L., Roden S., Marshall, T., and Kendall, M.J. (1982). Variations in response to non steroidal anti-inflammatory drugs. *British Journal of Clinical Pharmacology*, **14**, 691–4.

Scott, D.L. *et al.* (1989). Combination therapy with gold and hydroxychloroquine in rheumatoid arthritis: a prospective, placebo-controlled study. *British Journal of Rheumatology*, **28**, 128–33.

Sharp, J.T., Lidsky, M.D., Collins, L,C., and Moreland, J. (1971). Methods of scoring the progression of radiologic changes in rheumatoid arthritis: correlation of radiologic, clinical and laboratory abnormalities. *Arthritis and Rheumatism*, **14**, 706–20.

Sharp, J.T. *et al.* (1993). Radiological progression in rheumatoid arthritis: how many patients are required in a treatment trial to test disease modification? *Annals of the Rheumatic Diseases*, **52**, 332–7.

Sherrer, Y.S., Block D.A., Mitchell, D.M., Young, D.Y., and Fries, J.F. (1986). The development of disability in rheumatoid arthritis. *Arthritis and Rheumatism*, **29**, 494–500.

Short, C.L., Bauer, W., and Reynolds, W.S. (1957). *Rheumatoid arthritis*. Harvard University Press, Cambridge, Massachusetts.

Silman, A.J. (1989). Are there secular trends in the occurrence and severity of rheumatoid arthritis? *Scandinavian Journal of Rheumatology*, Suppl. **79**, 25–30.

Sjöblom, K.G., Saxne, T., Pettersson, H., and Wollheim, F.A. (1984). Factors related to the progression of joint destruction in rheumatoid arthritis. *Scandinavian Journal of Rheumatology*, **13**, 21–7.

Spector, T.D. (1989). Sex hormone measurements in rheumatoid arthritis. *British Journal of Rheumatology*, **28** (Suppl. I), 62–8.

Spector, T.D. (1990). Rheumatoid arthritis. In *Epidemiology of rheumatic diseases* (ed. M.C. Hochberg), pp. 513–37. Saunders, Philadelphia.

Spector, T.D. and Scott, D.L. (1988). What happens to patients with rheumatoid arthritis? The longterm outcome of treatment. *Clinical Rheumatology*, 7, 315–30.

Spector, T.D., Roman, E., and Silman, A.J. (1990). The pill, parity and rheumatoid arthritis. *Arthritis and Rheumatism*, 33, 782–9.

Sperber, K., Quraishi, H., Kalb, T.H., Panja, A., Stecher, V., and Mayer, L. (1993). Selective regulation of cytokine secretion by hydroxychloroquine: inhibition of interleukin 1 alpha (IL-1-α) and IL-6 in human monocytes and T cells. *Journal of Rheumatology*, 20, 803–8.

Stenström, C.H. (1994). Home exercise in rheumatoid arthritis functional class II: goal setting versus pain attention. *Journal of Rheumatology*, 21, 627–34.

Suzuki, A., *et al.* (1994). Cause of death in 81 autopsied patients with rheumatoid arthritis. *Journal of Rheumatology*, 21, 33–6.

Svartz, N. (1942). Salazopyrin, a new sulfanilinamide preparation. *Acta Medica Scandinavica*, 110, 577–98.

Symmons, D.P.M., Farr, M., Salmon, M., and Bacon, P.A. (1989). Lymphopenia in rheumatoid arthritis. *Journal of the Royal Society of Medicine*, 82, 462–3.

Symmons, D.P., Barrett, E.M., Bankhead, C.R., Scott, D.G., and Silman, A.J. (1994). The incidence of rheumatoid arthritis in the United Kingdom: results from the Norfolk Arthritis Register. *British Journal of Rheumatology*, 33, 735–9.

Taggart, A.J., Hill, J., Asbury, C., Dixon, J.S., Bird, H.A., and Wright, V. (1987). Sulphasalazine alone or in combination with D-penicillamine in rheumatoid arthritis. *British Journal of Rheumatology*, 26, 32–6.

Tessler, H.H. (1985). The eye in rheumatic disease. *Bulletin of the Rheumatic Diseases*, 35, 1–8.

Tett, S.E., Cutler, D., and Day, R.O. (1990). Antimalarials in rheumatic diseases. *Baillière's Clinical Rheumatology*, 4, 467–89.

Thompson, M. and Bywaters, E.G.L. (1961). Unilateral rheumatoid arthritis following hemiplegia. *Annals of the Rheumatic Diseases*, 21, 370–7.

Thompson, P.W. (1987). Laboratory markers of joint inflammation and damage. *British Journal of Rheumatology*, 26, 83–5.

Thomson, W., Sanders, P.A., Davis, M., Davidson, J., Dyer, P.A., and Grennan, D.M. (1988). Complement C4B-null alleles in Felty's syndrome. *Arthritis and Rheumatism*, 31, 984–9.

Tugwell, P. *et al.* (1990). Low-dose cyclosporin versus placebo in patients with rheumatoid arthritis. *Lancet*, 335, 1051–5.

Vandenbroucke, J.P., Hazeroet, H.M., and Cats, A. (1984). Survival and cause of death in rheumatoid arthritis: a 25 year prospective follow-up. *Journal of Rheumatology*, 11, 158–61.

van der Heide, D.M.F.M., van Riel, P.L.C.M., Nuver-Zwart, I.H., Gribnau, F.W.J., and van de Putte, L.B.A. (1989). Effects of hydroxychloroquine and sulphasalazine on progression of joint damage in rheumatoid arthritis. *Lancet*, i, 1036–8.

van der Heijde, D.M.F.M. (1991). Disease activity and outcome in rheumatoid arthritis. Thesis, University of Nijmegen, pp. 87–96.

van der Veen, M.J., van der Heide A., Kruize, A.A., and Bijlsma, J.W. (1994). Infection rate and use of antibiotics in patients with rheumatoid arthritis treated with methotrexate. *Annals of the Rheumatic Diseases*, 53, 224–8.

van Leeuwen, M.A. *et al.* (1993). The acute-phase response in relation to radiographic progression in early rheumatoid arthritis: a prospective study during the first three years of the disease. *British Journal of Rheumatology*, 32, 3–13.

van Rijthoven, A.W.A.M. *et al.* (1986). Cyclosporine treatment for rheumatoid arthritis: a placebo-controlled double-blind, multicentre study. *Annals of the Rheumatic Diseases*, 45, 726–31.

van Schaardenburg, D., Hazes, J.M.W., de Boer, A., Zwinderman, A.H., Meijers, K.A.E., and Breedveld, F.C. (1993). Outcome of rheumatoid arthritis in relation to age and rheumatoid factor at diagnosis. *Journal of Rheumatology*, 20, 45–52.

van Zeben, D., Hazes, J.M.W., Vandenbroucke, J.P., Dijkmans, B.A.C., and Cats, A. (1990). Diminished incidence of severe rheumatoid arthritis associated with oral contraceptive use. *Arthritis and Rheumatism*, 33, 1462–5.

van Zeben, D., Hazes, J.M.W., Zwinderman, A.H., Vandenbroucke, J.P., and Breedveld, F.C. (1994). The severity of rheumatoid arthritis: a 6-year followup study of younger women with symptoms of recent onset. *Journal of Rheumatology*, 21, 1620–5.

Vischer, T.L. and van Eden, W. (1994). Oral desensitistaion in rheumatoid arthritis. *Annals of the Rheumatic Diseases*, 53, 708–10.

Vreugdenhil, G., Baltus, C.A.M., van Eijk, H.G, and Swaak, A.J.G. (1990). Anaemia of chronic disease: diagnostic significance of erythrocyte and serological parameters in iron deficient rheumatoid arthritis patients. *British Journal of Rheumatology*, 29, 105–10.

Wadsworth, T.G. (1993). Prosthetic replacement of the arthritic elbow. *Current Opinion in Rheumatology*, 5, 322–8.

Wegelius, O., Wafin, F., Falck, H.M., and Törnroth, T. (1980). Follow-up study of amyloidosis secondary to rheumatic disease. In *Amyloid and amyloidosis* (ed. G.G. Glenner, P.P. de Costa, and A.F. de Freitas), pp. 183–90. Excerpta Medica, Amsterdam.

Weiss, M.M. (1989). Corticosteroids in rheumatoid arthritis. *Seminars in Arthritis and Rheumatism*, 19, 9–21.

Whalton, A., Stout, R.L., Spilman, P.S., and Klassen, D.K. (1990). Renal effects of ibuprofen, piroxicam and sulindac in patients with asymptomatic renal failure. *Annals of Internal Medicine*, 112, 560–76.

Wiik, A. and Munthe, E. (1974). Complement fixing granulocyte-specific antinuclear factors in neutropenic cases of rheumatoid arthritis. *Immunology*, 26, 1127–34.

Wilske, K.R. and Healey, L.A. (1990). Challenging the therapeutic pyramid: a new look at treatment strategies for rheumatoid arthritis. *Journal of Rheumatology*, Suppl. 25, 4–7.

Wingrave, S.J. and Kay, S.R. (1978). Reduction in incidence of rheumatoid arthritis associated with oral contraceptives. *Lancet*, i, 569–71.

Wolfe, F. *et al.* (1994). The mortality of rheumatoid arthritis. *Arthritis and Rheumatism*, 4, 481–94.

Wollheim, F.A. and Eberhardt, K.B. (1992). The search for laboratory measures of outcome in rheumatoid arthritis. *Baillière's Clinical Rheumatology*, 6(1), 69–93.

Wollheim, F.A. and Saxne, T. (1992). Markers of cartilage destruction. In *Rheumatoid arthritis — recent research advances* (ed. J. Smolen). Springer-Verlag, Berlin.

Wollheim, F.A., Carlsson, J., Forsgren, A., and Pettersson, H. (1984). Rapidly progressing rheumatoid arthritis: an example of polycloncal B-cell activation? *Clinical Rheumatology*, 3, 75–9.

Wollheim, F.A., Pettersson, H., Saxne, T., and Sjöblom, K.G. (1988). Radiographic assessment in relation to clinical and biochemical variables in rheumatoid arthritis. *Scandinavian Journal of Rheumatology*, 17, 445–53.

Wollheim, F.A., Saxne, T., Eberhardt, K.B., and Johnson, U. (1995). The shared epitope and COMP as predictors of erosiveness in recent onset RA. (Abstract.) *15th Eruopean Workshop for Rheumatology Research*, Erlangen, 1995.

Woolf, A.D. (1991). Osteoporosis in rheumatoid arthritis. The clinical viewpoint. *British Journal of Rheumatology*, 30, 82–4.

Zvaifler, N.J. and Pekin, T.J., Jr. (1963). Complement components in synovial fluids. *Clinical Research*, 11, 180.

Zygmunt, S., Sveland, H., Brattström, H., Ljunggren, B., Larsson, E.M., and Wollheim, F. (1988). Reduction of rheumatoid periodontoid pannus following posterior occipito-cervical fusion visualised by magnetic resonance imaging. *British Journal of Neurosurgery*, 2, 315–20.

5.4.3 Juvenile rheumatoid arthritis (rheumatoid factor positive polyarthritis)

Barbara M. Ansell

This subset of juvenile chronic arthritis is clinically and genetically indistinguishable from rheumatoid arthritis in adults. The overall incidence is unknown; in a prospective study of 148 patients with juvenile chronic arthritis seen within 3 months of onset, 6 per cent persistently carried IgM rheumatoid factor in the first 3 months and two further patients became seropositive by the 5-year follow-up (Ansell *et al.* 1987). There was a female preponderance of 2:1 and the disease has been seen in patients as young as 3 or 4 years, although more commonly the illness starts in those aged 10 years or more (Ansell 1983). The frequency in this selected referral group may well be an over-estimate as of 1328 patients on the British Paediatric Rheumatology Group register only 2.1 per cent (28) fall into this category. In the British Paediatric Rheumatology Group register the female preponderance was even more marked at 13:1 and the median age of onset was 11.9 years, with the age range 1.9 to 15 years (Symmons *et al.* 1995, personal communication).

As early as 1969 Hanson and his colleagues, in a prospective study of 110 children, recorded the value of the IgM rheumatoid factor as a marker for this variant (Hanson *et al* 1969); patients whose disease started between the ages of 12 and 16 years accounted for more than 80 per cent of those with positive tests for rheumatoid factor; seropositivity also correlated closely with the presence of nodules. Similarly, in a cross-sectional review of 110 patients whose arthritis commenced under 14 years of age, Cassidy and Valkenberg noted a significant correlation between the serological reaction, age of onset, presence of nodules, and bone erosion (Cassidy and Valkenberg 1967).

Mode of presentation

The disease usually presents as a polyarthritis involving the small joints of the hands and feet. A combination of soft tissue swelling of the wrists and carpi with involvement of metacarpophalangeal and proximal interphalangeal and metatarsophalangeal joints was closely associated with the persistent presence of IgM rheumatoid factor (Ansell and Wood 1976). The large joints can also be involved early, particularly knees and ankles, usually in association with small joint involvement. Very occasionally the onset was palindromic (two in 138 patients), while a few had an insidious onset as 'wrist or foot strain' for a few weeks before the polyarthritis became obvious (Ansell 1983). Those with an onset under the age of 10 years tended to have wrists, ankles and hindfeet, and knees affected early with the small joints becoming affected later. Approximately a quarter of our patients ultimately had a family history of seropositive rheumatoid arthritis (parent, grandparent, or sib), which could post-date the child's illness.

Clinical manifestations

Although lassitude, loss of weight, and general malaise were recorded in about half our patients, fever (even low-grade) was rare. Generalized lymphadenopathy was occasionally present, particularly in those with a very acute onset of polyarthritis. Other systemic manifestations were uncommon, although pleural effusion and pericarditis have been seen, and pulmonary fibrosis in a boy and a girl as the presenting feature.

The pattern is one of a progressive arthritis with severe generalized stiffness; shoulders are often badly affected early, while hip involvement can occur at any time from a few months to several years. Neck, elbows, and hindfeet are gradually involved so that by 5 years a deforming arthritis with weight loss is usual.

Dorsal sheath effusions and severe extensor tenosynovitis are not uncommon and can be associated subsequently with rupture of the extensor tendons of the fourth or fifth fingers and the thumb. Flexor tenosynovitis is common and tends to be more nodular than grossly prolific, causing triggering of fingers. As in adults, carpal tunnel syndrome may complicate the picture as can entrapment neuropathy at knee and elbow. Nodules with typical rheumatoid histology have been seen along the forearm in 30 per cent of patients in the first year of disease (Ansell 1983). Cutaneous nodules were not seen until later and vasculitis is very rare early in the course of the disease.

Diagnosis

As low titres of rheumatoid factor can occur in other autoimmune rheumatic disorders (e.g. systemic lupus erythematosus and some types of vasculitis as well as in hypergammaglobulinaemia, as is seen in sarcoidosis), such causes must be excluded. Because transiently positive rheumatoid factor tests can occur in infections (particularly those of viral original but also bacterial infections e.g. subacute bacterial endocarditis), the European League Against Rheumatism (EULAR) criteria suggest that three consecutive positive tests over a 3-month period are required to classify this type of arthritis.

Using standard tests, IgM rheumatoid factor can be present within a few weeks of the first symptoms and in the majority by 3 months; titres tend to rise as the disease becomes established. It is exceptionally rare for the rheumatoid factor test to become positive after more than 1 year of illness (Ansell 1987); once present, unless long-term slow-acting drugs are used early, it tends to remain positive. The importance of positive test results as a hall-mark of a subgroup of children with polyarthritis who generally have a poor outcome has been stressed (Cassidy *et al.* 1989).

Radiological changes tend to be early in all sites and particularly in the hands and feet. Periostitis along the shafts of the metacarpals and metatarsals and at the bases of the proximal phalanges extending on to the epiphyses of the joints have been seen radiologically as early as 6 weeks, although this is more usual between 3 and 6 months (Ansell and Kent 1977) (Fig. 1). Radiological changes tend to progress rapidly with the development of erosions.

Course

In our early studies (Ansell and Wood 1976), the 15-year follow-up showed that a third of the patients had severe limitation of functional

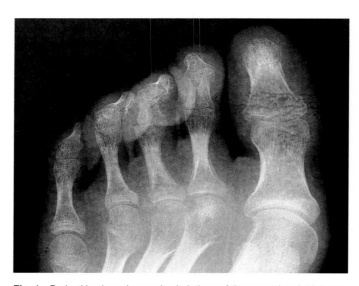

Fig. 1 Periostitis along the proximal phalanx of the second and third toe; note also the severity of the osteoporosis.

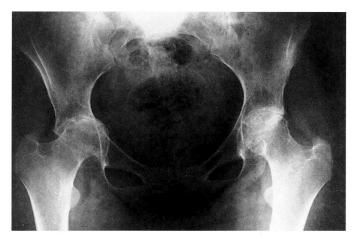

Fig. 2 Both hips were painful and limited in this 14-year-old girl with seropositive disease of 2 years duration. The right shows protrusio with marked narrowing of joint space and erosions; on the left the disease is less advanced.

capacity (i.e. were unable to function independently) and the majority were still active. Slow-acting drugs, usually gold, had been introduced very late in treatment as previously the problems of this subgroup of seropositive juvenile arthritis had not been adequately recognized. Forty per cent had hip involvement, with destructive changes as early as 1 year; radiologically, protrusio, sometimes severe, had occurred within months from the first hip symptoms (Fig. 2).

A review of 138 patients, of whom two-thirds had been followed for at least 10 years, showed that death had occurred from renal failure due to amyloidosis in two, quadriplegia associated with both atlantoaxial and lower cervical subluxation in another, cardiac failure in a further patient, while infections of varying types caused

death in the other three; non-fatal complications included vasculitis and peripheral neuropathy. No specific drug was noted to have been effective in suppressing disease activity, but the frequency of side-effects was a significant factor in preventing the maintenance of treatment schedules for long periods. In the minority where the disease was controlled, healing of erosions could occur (Fig. 3(a), (b)). However, the overall review of 81 serial sets of radiographs (Williams and Ansell 1985), of whom two-thirds had received gold, penicillamine, or chloroquine and 13 per cent had received cytotoxic drugs, while confirming the association between wrist, carpus, and metacarpophalangeal joints in the hands and metatarsophalangeal joints in the feet, showed that lesions in these had progressed radiologically by 5 years (Fig. 4(a),(b),(c)). In addition, a third of the patients showed erosive changes in large joints such as the hips, knees, or shoulders. Between 5 and 10 years from onset of disease, progression radiologically was evident in most patients with additional joints becoming involved in a further third. By this time, 17 per cent had had bilateral total hip replacement and 7 per cent knee replacement; atlantoaxial subluxation was common (Fig. 5). After 15 years or more, the radiological changes tended to stabilize, but various mechanical difficulties, often secondary to poor growth and degenerative change, as well as the primary destructive arthritis, were evident (Fig. 4(c)). The main differences between adults and children appeared to be a tendency to fusion of the carpal bones and distal interphalangeal joint erosion. Another problem in juveniles is alteration in growth in the presence of persistent disease activity.

In addition to joint destruction, lone aortic regurgitation has been a serious complication. Reporting four cases in 1981, Leak et al. commented on the fact that this pursued a particularly aggressive course with sudden deterioration occurring in two patients, one of whom had an urgent aortic valve replacement, at which time

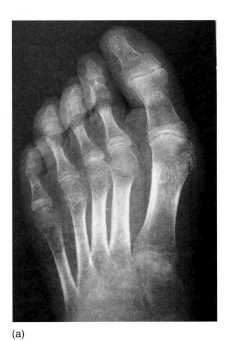
(a)

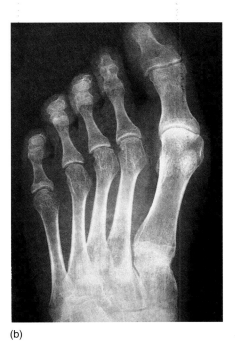
(b)

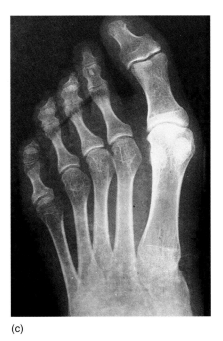
(c)

Fig. 3 (a) Radiograph of feet at presentation with disease duration of 3.5 months; note the erosions in the fifth metatarsals and periostitis along the fourth, third, and second proximal phalanges as well as irregularity in the shape of the first metatarsal head. Penicillamine therapy was commenced at this time and continued. (b) Eighteen months from the first picture there has been healing of the erosions in the fifth metatarsophalangeal joint and improvement in overall porosity with no new erosive changes. (c) This improvement has been maintained during the further 3-year treatment period.

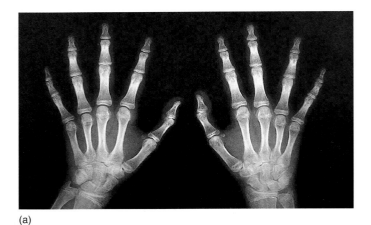

(a)

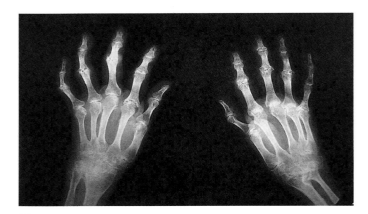

(b)

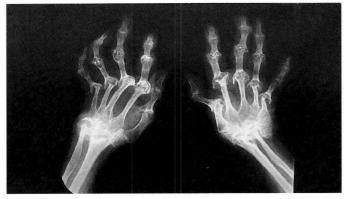

(c)

Fig. 4 (a) At presentation this girl (aged 13.5 years) had crowding of the carpus and changes between the distal row of the carpus; the bases of the metacarpi and particularly the head of the second metacarpals on both sides are thinning. (b) Despite a prolonged course of gold, 5 years from onset there has been gross destructive arthritis affecting the carpus which is fusing, all metacarpophalangeal joints, and proximal and distal interphalangeal joints. (c) Twenty years from onset destruction has occurred, particularly in the metacarpophalangeal joints and at the wrists.

pericarditis was also present, and the other died while awaiting assessment (Leak *et al.* 1981). The patient reported in full developed an aortic diastolic murmur, followed by bouts of chest pain associated with dyspnoea and a rapid deterioration in her clinical state. Histologically, the architecture of the aortic valve had been completely destroyed by multiple necrobiotic foci with the typical features of rheumatoid granulomata. There was active granulomatous tissue growing into the valve. These patients were young at onset (8–11 years) and aortic incompetence was seen to occur as early as 2 years from onset, but it has also been recorded as late as 15 years from onset. All had high titres of IgM rheumatoid factor and a severe destructive arthropathy requiring major joint replacement; three had subcutaneous nodules and one vasculitis. Further cases have been seen since this report; the valvular dysfunction can last only a short time before sudden deterioration (Fig. 6). In view of this, regular cardiac appraisal should be made part of the routine assessment in seropositive juvenile arthritis. Repeated non-invasive assessment can be made by echocardiography; measurement of the left ventricular diastolic dimension and fractional shortening are useful in predicting deterioration in function (O'Rourke *et al.* 1980). Development of the left ventricular dysfunction is an indication for urgent referral for consideration of surgery because the rapid deterioration with the development of angina in a young patient is associated with an increased risk of death (Reicheck *et al.* 1973). In addition to pericarditis and valvular lesions, a single case of endo-myocardial fibrosis has been recorded in seropositive juvenile rheumatoid arthritis (Hughes *et al.* 1988). Whether this is indeed a complication of seropositive juvenile rheumatoid arthritis is not known; the patient had been on treatment with penicillamine at the time of her symptoms.

Pulmonary manifestations have been relatively uncommon in our long-term follow-up, although pleurisy with or without effusion has been seen as well as diffuse interstitial disease. Pulmonary arteritis has also been recorded (Gordon and Snyder 1964). The earliest account of rheumatoid lung disease in a child was that of Brinkman and Shaikoff who reported on a 13-year-old who had had progressive dyspnoea and cyanosis over 3 years (Brinkman and Shaikoff 1959). Nodules in the lungs appear excessively rarely, but pulmonary fibrosis is seen very occasionally (Fig. 7). Bronchiolitis obliterans has been reported in a 12-year-old girl with rheumatoid factor positive juvenile rheumatoid arthritis who was restarted on intramuscular gold about a month after mild side-effects had led to temporary withdrawal; this proved fatal despite intensive therapy (Pegg *et al.* 1994).

Genetic aspects

In a study of 52 Caucasian patients, all of whom had developed widespread erosions by 5 years from onset, 62 per cent were HLA DR4 (Clemens *et al.* 1983). Rheumatoid nodules were more frequent in the DR4 patients. There was no difference with respect to mean age of onset, family history of rheumatoid arthritis, or frequency of toxic reactions to long-acting drugs; the toxic reactions had occurred in 23 per cent and were more common in the DR4-negative patients. Although two patients in our group who were DR4 homozygous had required multiple arthroplasties (one had required replacement of the aortic valve within 5 years), the disease was of similar severity in both the DR4 heterozygotes and DR4-negative patients.

Nepom *et al.* found an association with HLA DW4 and HLA DW14 in seropositive polyarthritis juvenile rheumatoid arthritis subjects from the Pacific north-west United States (Nepom *et al.* 1984). Fraser *et al.* noted that late onset polyarticular juvenile rheumatoid arthritis, irrespective of seropositivity, was associated with one of the three common HLA DR4 extended haplotypes, notably HLA

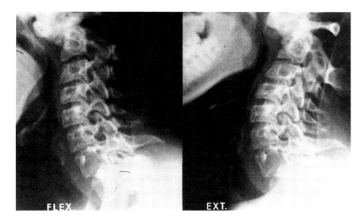

Fig. 5 Atlantoaxial subluxation causing compression on the cord but with relatively little change elsewhere in the cervical spine.

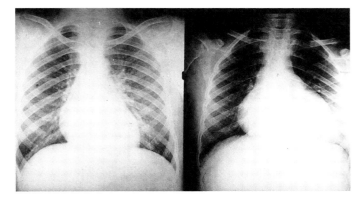

Fig. 6 Rapidly increasing cardiac silhouette over 4 months in a girl who had been noted to have a diastolic murmur 7 months before.

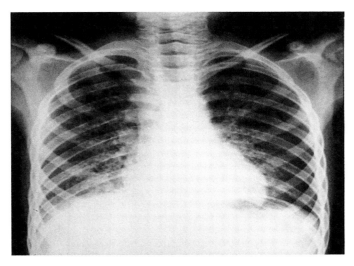

Fig. 7 This 15-year-old patient presented with increasing dyspnoea. Although seropositive, relatively mild juvenile rheumatoid arthritis of some 5-years duration was present affecting the hands and feet only. The duration of the chest symptoms could not be adequately assessed, but he had finger clubbing at presentation.

Box 1 Summary

Seropositive juvenile rheumatoid arthritis is one of the rarer forms of arthritis of childhood. Affecting as it does older children and adolescents, it is important that as soon as the diagnosis is made, they come under a specialist clinic which has information and knowledge and at the same time is able to assess particular drug therapies. To date there has been no good prospective study and from our own personal experience it would seem that patients do better if they are introduced to a slow acting drug within 6 months of the disease, but only through long-term prospective studies, which should be co-ordinated through juvenile rheumatism centres, will this ever be established. In addition to the usual measures of joint protection, maintenance of function, and the use of non-steroidals, the question of local corticosteroid injections into a particularly troublesome joint will also need consideration. As genetically as well as clinically, they are similar to adult rheumatoid arthritis, it would seem that gold or methotrexate are probably the slow acting drugs of choice. There has been no work to date on cyclosporin. Should the onset of disease be under 10 years, it would appear that a proportion of these children will respond to hydrochloroquine; however, if after 6 months the joint count is increasing or the ESR is still very high, it is probably wise to switch to methotrexate or gold.

B44 SC30 DR4 (Fraser *et al.* 1990). The overall results are difficult to interpret, but there may be ethnic differences between the Caucasian subjects in different areas which would strongly influence the frequencies of the alleles and haplotypes under study.

Management

Principles of management are the same as those for adults, namely maintenance of joint position and function and relief of pain by non-steroidal anti-inflammatory drugs. To date, those studied and accepted for children include ibuprofen, tolmetin, naprosyn, piroxicam, and diclofenac. These last three have been particularly valuable in appropriate dosage.

There have been no satisfactory prospective studies on the use of long-acting drugs, both because of the relative rarity of this subgroup of rheumatoid arthritis, and the problem of obtaining an overall picture. Children may attend paediatric clinics while adolescents become diverted to adult clinics; later the majority will attend adult clinics.

It is my impression that the introduction of a long acting drug within 6 months of the first symptoms will cause considerable improvement in some 70 per cent but nearly 30 per cent do not seem to respond satisfactorily to any present medication.

Chloroquine initially, and more recently hydroxychloroquine, in appropriate dosage has been used in some young patients as the sole long-acting drug. In a number, considerable improvement was seen in the first year of therapy (Hasson *et al.* 1993). Such patients were maintained on therapy for a further 2 years. If there was no benefit, another slow-acting drug was introduced.

At present, although there have been no studies of methotrexate in this subgroup, it would seem to be the slow-acting drug most frequently used. Its efficacy appears to be similar to that in adult rheumatoid arthritis and it is well tolerated. However, recurrence of activity has been seen occurring a year or two after control of the disease with no reduction in dosage. The effect on erosions is also not known, in that although no actual healing of erosions has as yet been demonstrated, certainly in some patients after 1 year no further erosions had developed. More work is required on this aspect.

A comparative study of gold and penicillamine early in the onset of disease was undertaken in 1980/81; this involved 24 patients (Ansell *et al.* 1981). At 1 year both gold and penicillamine were found to be effective; gold came into play more quickly. Three patients, two on gold and one on penicillamine, had stopped therapy by 1 year because of side-effects, but of those who were able to continue all had had a reduction in total active joint count and some fall in erythrocyte sedimentation rate. One in each group treated early in the disease became negative for IgM rheumatoid factor and both of these patients were in remission 3 years from commencement of therapy, with healing of erosions. However, even in this state, as in adults, relapses can occur on maintenance therapy. Overall, toxicity with gold and penicillamine is similar to that in adults but in an open study penicillamine appeared to have had the additional complication of myasthenia gravis, which occurred on several occasions, while one of our patients had myositis.

The role of sulphasalazine has not been adequately studied. Combination therapy in the form of gold and an antimalarial has been effective in a small group of patients; all of these had previously failed to respond adequately to gold or an antimalarial alone. In this group of patients with a relatively poor prognosis as regards persistence of disease activity and increasing erosions, multicentre studies are urgently needed.

For some patients, usually when they have become anaemic, have other complications such as weight loss and very severe arthritis, and at times poor growth, corticosteroids may be employed and whenever possible this should be on an alternate-day regimen. In general, cytotoxic therapy has been reserved for those patients whose disease is complicated by amyloidosis, but it has been used with apparent benefit for patients after aortic valve surgery who still had extremely active disease and two who had lung fibrosis and a further two with vasculitis.

In those few patients followed into adult life who have had children, a postpregnancy relapse of their disease has been seen in all but one, even though their disease was in a reasonable state at the commencement of pregnancy.

At the former Medical Research Coucil Rheumatism Unit at Taplow, some 10 per cent of all patients admitted underwent an orthopaedic surgical procedure. Approximately half of these were in patients suffering from seropositive juvenile rheumatoid arthritis, even though such patients accounted for only just over 10 per cent of admissions during that same period. Total replacement hip arthroplasty was one of the more common operations together with stabilization of the thumb and repair of extensor tendon ruptures; other surgery included fusion of the cervical spine and also of the hindfeet. Revision hip surgery has been required in many as the overall loosening rate has been 25 per cent with an average duration from initial surgery of 9.5 years (Witt *et al.* 1991). There has been a steady increase in the number of total replacement knee arthroplasties undertaken; long-term follow-up has not yet been reported. More recently, shoulder and elbow arthroplasty are under consideration in some special centres.

References

Ansell, B.M. (1983). Juvenile chronic arthritis with persistently positive tests for rheumatoid factor seropositive JRA. *Annale de Pediatre*, **30**, 545–50.

Ansell, B.M. (1987). Juvenile chronic arthritis. *Scandinavian Journal of Rheumatology Supplement*, **66**, 47–50.

Ansell, B.M. and Kent, P.A. (1977). Radiological changes in juvenile chronic polyarthritis. *Skeletal Radiology*, **1**, 129–44.

Ansell, B.M. and Wood, P.H.N. (1976). Prognosis in juvenile chronic polyarthritis. *Clinics of Rheumatic Diseases*, **2**, 397–412.

Ansell, B.M., Fink, C., and Wood, P.H.N. (1980). Juvenile arthritis in England: a long term follow-up. *Arthritis and Rheumatism*, **23**, 673.

Ansell, B.M., Hall, M.A., and Ruberio, S.A. (1981). A comparative study of gold and penicillamine in seropositive juvenile chronic arthritis (juvenile rheumatoid arthritis). *Annals of the Rheumatic Diseases*, **40**, 522–3.

Brinkman, E.L. and Shaikoff, L. (1959). Rheumatoid lung disease. Report of a case which developed in childhood. *American Review of Respiratory Disease*, **80**, 732–7.

Cassidy, J.T. and Valkenberg, H.A. (1967). A 5 year prospective study of rheumatoid factor test in juvenile rheumatoid arthritis. *Arthritis and Rheumatism*, **10**, 83–90.

Cassidy, J.T., Levinson, J.E., and Brewer, E.J.Jr. (1989). The development of classification criteria for children with juvenile rheumatoid arthritis. *Bulletin on the Rheumatic Diseases*, **38**, 1–7.

Clemens, L.E., Albert, E., and Ansell, B.M. (1983). HLA studies in IgM rheumatoid factor positive childhood arthritis. *Annals of the Rheumatic Diseases*, **42**, 431–4.

Fraser, P.A. *et al.* (1990). HLA extended haplotypes in childhood and adult onset HLA DR4 associated arthropathies. *Tissue Antigens*, **35**, 56–9.

Gordon, J.D. and Snyder, C.H. (1964). Rheumatoid disease of the lung and cor pulmonale. Observations in a child. *American Journal of Diseases of Children*, **108**, 174–80.

Hanson, V., Drexler, E., and Kornreich, M. (1969). The relationship of rheumatoid factor to age of onset in juvenile rheumatoid arthritis. *Arthritis and Rheumatism*, **12**, 82–6.

Hasson, N., Rooney, M., Ansell, B.M., and Woo, P. (1993). Chloroquine in rheumatoid factor positive polyarticular juvenile chronic arthritis. *Arthritis and Rheumatism*, **36**, Suppl 9, Abstract 123.

Hughes, L.O., Randle, S.M., and Raftery, E.G. (1988). Endomyocardial fibrosis in a white girl with seropositive juvenile chronic arthritis. *International Journal of Cardiology*, **18**, 101–5.

Leak, A.M., Miller-Craig, M.W., and Ansell, B.M. (1981). Aortic regurgitation in seropositive JRA. *Annals of the Rheumatic Diseases*, **40**, 229–34.

Nepom, B.S., Nepom, G.T., Michelson, E., Schaller, J.G., Antonelli, P., and Jansen, J.A. (1984). Specific HLA-DR4 associated histocompatability molecules characterised patients with seropositive juvenile rheumatoid arthritis. *Journal of Clinical Investigation*, **74**, 287–91.

O'Rourke, R.A. and Crawford, M.H. (1980). Editorial. Timing of valve replacement in patients with chronic aortic regurgitation. *Circulation*, **61**, 493–5.

Pegg, S.J., Lang, B.A., Mikhail, E.L., and Hughes, D.M. (1994). Fatal bronchiolitis obliterans in a patient with juvenile rheumatoid arthritis receiving chrysotherapy. *Journal of Rheumatology*, **21**, 549–51.

Reicheck, N., Shelburn, J.C., and Perlock, J.K. (1973). Clinical aspects in rheumatoid valvular disease. Aortic regurgitation. *Progress in Cardiovascular Disease*, **15**, 518–23.

Williams, R.A. and Ansell, B.M. (1985). Radiological findings in seropositive JCA with particular reference to prognosis. *Annals of the Rheumatic Diseases*, **44**, 685–93.

Witt, J.D., Swann, M., and Ansell, B.M. (1991). Total hip replacement in JCA. *Journal of Bone and Joint Surgery*, **73B**, 770–3.

5.5.1 Spondylarthropathy, undifferentiated spondylarthritis, and overlap

Andrei Calin

Historical review

As discussed by Calin, in 1974 Moll and colleagues introduced the term 'spondarthritis'(Moll *et al* 1974; Calin 1984). The concept was further developed in 1976 by Wright and Moll in their text entitled *Seronegative polyarthritis* (Wright and Moll 1976). As pointed out by Wright in a chapter entitled 'Relationships between ankylosing spondylitis and other spondarthritides' in Moll's text on ankylosing spondylitis (Wright 1980), we misquoted their term as 'spondylarthritis' in our 1978 monograph on the subject (Calin and Fries 1978). Since then, common usage has resulted in the widespread acceptance of the terms 'spondylarthritis', 'spondylarthropathy', and 'spondyloarthropathy'. We still favour (Calin 1997) the perhaps best

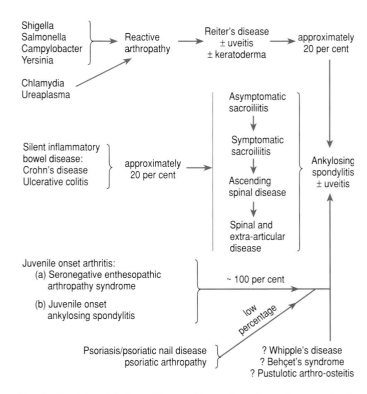

Fig. 1 The inter-related conditions making up the arthropathy group (well differentiated or undifferentiated); * = varying percentage.

known and most commonly applied term 'spondylarthritis', with respect and apologies to Moll, Wright, Khan, and other colleagues who may still prefer one of the other terms (Moll 1980; Wright 1980; Khan 1990). Regardless of preference, all agree that the spondylarthropathies include an exciting and intriguing group of disorders that ranges from asymptomatic sacroiliitis to symptomatic sacroiliitis, widespread multisystem ankylosing spondylitis, enteropathic arthropathies, certain subsets of juvenile onset arthritis, the reactive arthritides, and other entities. These are summarized in Table 1 and Fig. 1. The latter shows how the conditions may overlap with, or develop into, ankylosing spondylitis.

Introduction

The seronegative spondylarthritides are characterized by involvement of the sacroiliac joints, by peripheral inflammatory arthropathy, insertional tendinitis (enthesopathy), and by the absence of rheumatoid factor (Calin 1989).

Table 1 Individual conditions that overlap to form the spondylarthritides

Psoriatic arthropathy

Reiter's syndrome/reactive arthropathy (campylobacter, yersinia, shigella, salmonella)

Enteropathic spondylitis (Crohn's disease and ulcerative colitis)

Uveitis

Ankylosing spondylitis

Juvenile ankylosing spondylitis

Seronegative enthesopathic arthropathy syndrome

Pustulotic arthro-osteitis (considered by the Japanese to be part of spondylarthropathy spectrum (rare in USA and Europe))

Behçet's disease
Whipple's disease } (doubt exists as to whether these should be considered as part of the spectrum)

Undifferentiated spondylitis (i.e. subset of patients who have spondylarthropathic features but who fail to meet criteria for ankylosing spondylitis, Reiter's syndrome, or other condition, e.g. dactylitis, uveitis plus unilateral sacroiliitis)

There are several other important features:

1. Pathological changes are concentrated at the site of insertion of ligaments or tendons into bone rather than the synovium. Further pathological changes may also develop in the eye, the aortic valve, lung parenchyma, and skin.

2. There is clinical evidence of overlap between the various spondylarthritides. Thus, a patient with psoriatic arthropathy may develop uveitis or sacroiliitis and a patient with inflammatory bowel disease may develop ankylosing spondylitis or mouth ulcers.

3. There is a tendency towards familial aggregation, with evidence that these disorders 'breed true' within families (Calin *et al*. 1984).

4. There is an association with HLA-B27, ranging from about 50 per cent (psoriatic and enteropathic spondylitis) to over 95 per cent (primary ankylosing spondylitis). The specific frequency depends on ethnic group and disease type (Table 2).

Table 2 Distribution of HLA-B27 among different healthy and diseased groups

	HLA-B27 (%)
Healthy whites	6–14
(e.g. British)	6
(e.g. Northern Scandinavian)	14
Healthy blacks	<1–4
(e.g. African black)	<1
(e.g. USA black)	4
Indian Asians	2–6
Japanese	1–2
Chinese	5–10
Pakistanis	6–8
Haida Indians	50
Whites:	
Primary ankylosing spondylitis	95
Reactive arthropathy/Reiter's syndrome	80
Enteropathiic spondylarthropathy	50
Uveitis	40–50
Psoriatic spondylitis	50–60
Blacks:	
Primary ankylosing spondylitis	50
Reactive arthropathy	50
Indonesian spondylarthropathy patients	8
Healthy Indonesians	9
Healthy Alaskan Eskimo	25–40

Diagnostic criteria and classification

Classification or diagnostic criteria for several of the disorders belonging to the spondylarthropathy group already exist, for example the Rome (Kellgren *et al*. 1963), the New York (Bennet and Burch 1968), the Van der Linden *et al*. (Van der Linden *et al*. 1984), and other criteria for ankylosing spondylitis. Our group has long favoured the simple approach (i.e. that of symptomatic sacroiliitis) (Calin 1989*a*). Likewise, criteria exist for Reiter's syndrome (Willkens *et al*. 1981) and for psoriatic arthropathy (Vasey and Espinoza 1984).

There is a consensus that these criteria are too restricted, as there is a need to emphasize the existence of a much wider disease spectrum. For example radiographically detected sacroiliitis in the absence of symptoms would not be included in the existing classification. Moreover, patients with asymmetric sacroiliitis in addition to, for example, a dactylitis or uveitis, would be excluded from classification and yet clearly are part of the spondylarthropathy spectrum. Furthermore, patients with such limited or atypical forms of disease would be excluded from the typical clinical or epidemiological study. For this reason the European Spondylarthropathy Study Group (ESSG) has proposed criteria for the entire spondylarthropathy group of patients, which would encompass those with clearly defined entities such as Reiter's syndrome or ankylosing spondylitis on the one hand and those with an undifferentiated spondylarthropathy on the other (Dougados *et al*. 1991). In essence, patients with inflammatory spinal pain or asymmetric synovitis predominantly of the lower limb, together with at least one of the following: positive family history, psoriasis, inflammatory bowel disease, enthesopathic lesions, or asymmetric sacroiliitis, have 'undifferentiated spondylarthropathy', with an acceptable sensitivity and specificity. The proposed classification criteria known as the European Seronegative Study Group (ESSG) criteria for spondylarthropathy, will help broaden our acceptance and understanding of the entire spondylarthropathic disorders (Table 3(a)). Parallel to the ESSG criteria, Amor has developed an excellent point–scale that has good sensitivity and specificity in the assessment of patients with spondylarthritis (Table 3(b)). The two sets are compared in Table 3(c) (Amor *et al*. 1991). Reactive arthritis and enteropathic arthropathy are readily defined with Amor's criteria.

Parallel to the awareness that patients may have a limited or atypical form of spondylarthropathy, there is an appreciation that first degree relatives of HLA-B27-positive probands with classical disease frequently have an inflammatory process that appears to be related in terms of pathology or clinical type to the probands disease and yet would not satisfy any of the above criteria. For this reason several of us have used the term 'undifferentiated spondylarthropathy' (Khan and Van der Linden 1990; Burns and Calin 1984) to describe such individuals. With the proposed new classification (Table 3(a)) all such individuals would be part of the diagnostic group.

Clinical subsets

The interrelated group of conditions constituting the spondylarthropathies have a variety of signs and symptoms (Fig. 2, Table 4). Edmunds *et al*. compared primary ankylosing spondylitis and psoriatic and enteropathic disease in a large controlled study

Table 3 Diagnostic criteria and classification

(a) European Spondylarthropathy Study Group (ESSG) criteria

INFLAMMATORY SPINAL PAIN

SYNOVITIS

or   (asymmetrical* or predominantly in the lower limbs*)

and

one or more of the following
   Positive family history
   Psoriasis
   Inflammatory bowel disease
   Alternate buttock pain
   Enthesopathy
   Sacroiliitis*

*Without sacroiliitis, sensitivity=77 per cent, specificity=89 per cent; with sacroiliitis, sensitivity=86 per cent, specificity=87 per cent.

(b) Criteria for diagnosing spondylarthropathies (Amor 1991)

	Points
A. CLINICAL SYMPTOMS OR PAST HISTORY OF	
1. Lumbar or dorsal pain during the night or morning stiffness of the lumbar or dorsal spine	1
2. Asymmetrical oligoarthritis	2
3. Buttock pain—if affecting alternatively the right or the left buttock	1 or 2
4. Sausage-like toe or digit	2
5. Heel pain or other well-defined enthesopathic pain	2
6. Iritis	2
8. Non-gonococcal urethritis or cervicitis accompanying or within 1 month before onset of arthritis	1
9. Presence or history of psoriasis and/or balanitis and or inflammatory bowel disease (ulcerative colitis, Crohn's disease)	2
B. RADIOLOGICAL FINDING	
10. Sacroiliitis (grade ⩾2 if bilateral grade ⩾3 if unilateral	3
C. GENETIC BACKGROUND	
11. Presence of HLA-B27 and/or familial history of ankylosing spondylitis, Reiter's syndrome, uveitis, psoriasis, or chronic enterocolopathies	2
D. RESPONSE TO TREATMENT	
12. Clear-cut improvement of rheumatic complaints with non-steroidal anti-inflammatory drugs (dramatic improvement or relapse of the pain if NSAIDs discontinued)	2

A patient will be considered as suffering from a spondylarthropathy if the sum of the 12 criteria values is at least 6.

(c) Comparison of the 12 items criteria (Amor 1991) and ESSG criteria

Characteristics	Set of criteria	
	AMOR	ESSG
Sensitivity (%)	91.9	87.1
Specificity (%)	97.9	96.4
Positive predictive value (%)	73.1	60.3
Negative predictive value (%)	99.5	99.2
Likelihood ratio	43.0	24.1
Accuracy	97.5	95.8

Table 4 Comparison of seronegative spondylarthropathies

	Ankylosing spondylitis	Reiter's syndrome	Psoriatic arthropathy	Enteropathic spondylitis	Juvenile arthropathy (juvenile ankylosing spondylitis subset)	Reactive arthropathy	Undifferentiated spondyl-arthropathy
Sex	Male>female	Male=female	Female>male	Female=male	Male>female	Male=female	Male=female
Age at onset (years)	~20	Any age	Any age	Any age	<16	Any age	Any age
Uveitis	++	++	+	+	+	+	±
Conjunctivitis	-	+	-	-	-	+	-
Peripheral joints	Lower>upper	Lower usually	Upper>lower	Lower>upper	Lower>upper	Lower>upper	Upper=lower
Sacroiliitis	Always	Often	Often	Often	Often	Often	±
HLA-B27(%)	95	80	20 (50 with sacroiliitis)	50	90	80	±
Enthesopathy	+	+	+	+	+	+	+
Aortic regurgitation	+	+	?+	?	?	+	±
Familial aggregation	+	+	+	+	+	+	+
Risk for HLA-B27 positive individual (%)	5-20	20	?	?	?	20	?
Onset	Gradual	Sudden	Variable	Gradual	Variable	Sudden	Variable
Urethritis	-	+	-	-	-	±	±
Skin involvement	-	+	++	-	-	-	±
Mucous membrane involvement	-	+	-	+	-	-	±
Symmetry (spinal)	+	-	-	+	+	.	±
Self-limiting	-	±	±	-	±	±	±
Remission, relapses	-	±	±	-	±	±	±

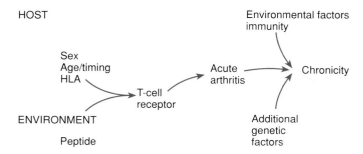

Fig. 2 The relationship between host, environmental, and other factors in determination of phenotypic expression.

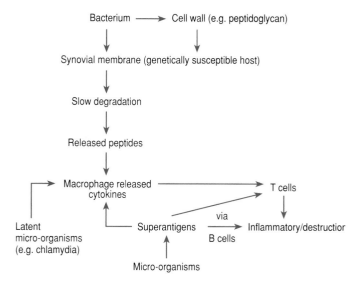

Fig. 3 The putative pathway between the infective trigger and disease pathogenesis.

(Edmunds *et al.* 1991). They are categorized according to the specific articular or extra-articular pattern. Depending on the associated clinical features (i.e. urethritis, eye disease, skin involvement) and the way the disease progresses (i.e. remission, relapse) a specific diagnostic label is given. However, as discussed above, clearly defined criteria are frequently absent and one often meets patients who have a spondylarthropathy but in whom the symptoms and signs are such that one is left with an undifferentiated picture. Family and epidemiological studies confirm this clinical finding. For example a patient may appear with unilateral sacroiliitis and little else, or chest wall symptoms due to intercostal muscle insertional tendinitis, and, for example, uveitis. Clearly, the specific phenotypic expression is the end product of a variety of interrelating genetic and environmental factors. Finally, the link between the skin and arthropathy should be stressed (Rosner *et al.* 1993).

Pathogenesis

Even in the reactive arthropathies where the infective trigger is recognized (e.g. yersinia, shigella, salmonella, campylobacter, chlamydia) and the genetic background (HLA-B27) clearly defined, the precise pathogenesis is not well understood (Schur 1994; Inman and Scofield 1994; De Castro 1994; Khan 1996; Lopez-Larrea *et al.* 1996; Scofield 1996). The various steps may include:

(1) low-grade inflammatory change in the bowel;

(2) the absorption of micro-organisms or parts thereof;

(3) endocytosis of the inciting fragments by antigen-presenting cells;

(4) degrading of the material followed by linking of the putative antigenic peptide with the HLA molecule;

(5) the expression on the cell surface of the combined HLA–peptide complex as a binary product;

(6) finally, this HLA–antigenic peptide composite interacts with the T-cell receptor determinant, the three forming a tertiary product.

An acute arthropathy results and, perhaps, following further unknown environmental factors and poorly defined genetic characteristics (Figs. 2 and 3), the chronic disease state may develop (McClean *et al.* 1993; Scofield *et al.* 1993; Stieglitz and Lipsky 1993; Khan 1993; Rojo *et al.* 1993; Whelan and Archer 1993; De Vries *et al.* 1992; Hermann *et al.* 1993; Taurog *et al.* 1993*a*; Breban *et al.* 1993*a*; Skurnik

et al. 1993; Madden *et al.* 1992). Why the sacroiliac joints are preferentially involved remains unknown (Braun and Sieper 1996).

HLA-B27

The HLA-B27 molecule is a two-chain structure that consists of a polymorphic glycoprotein, termed the heavy or α chain. The α chain is encoded by the HLA complex and is noncovalently linked to a non-HLA-encoded, non-polymorphic protein, β_2-microglobulin. The entire molecule is anchored to the cell membrane by the heavy chain. The extracellular portion of the heavy chain is divided into three domains, termed α_1, α_2, and α_3, each of which contains approximately 90 amino acids. The α_1 and α_2 domains are distal to the cell membrane and it is these that demonstrate the greatest HLA polymorphism. The α_1 and α_2 domains each consist of four β strands and an α helix. The eight β strands of these two domains form a β-pleated sheet or platform, which in turn supports the two α helices. These α helices create a groove which serves as the antigen-binding site for the putative peptide fragment which has been processed from the larger arthritogenic antigen. The two α helices with the bound antigen fragment comprise a ligand which is recognized by the T-cell receptor on a class 1-restricted, CD8-positive T cell.

There are several hypotheses explaining the HLA-B27 association with spondylarthropathy. In contrast to the situation with Reiter's disease, where clearly defined organisms are known to be operative (e.g. chlamydia, shigella, salmonella, campylobacter), the trigger for ankylosing spondylitis remains unclear and could either be one of the above organisms or viruses, or indeed other environmental phenomena (Ebringer 1991).

The first hypothesis suggests that a particular B27 molecule can act as a receptor for the aetiological agent. Support for such an hypothesis comes from observations that other cell surface molecules can act as receptors for viruses, such as CD4 for the human immunodeficiency virus. Individuals with B27 who contact the putative trigger will develop disease.

The second hypothesis suggests that the antigen-binding groove of only certain HLA molecules can accept the processed antigenic fragment that is ultimately responsible for causing disease. Thus, when the ankylosing spondylitis-causing organism enters the cell the antigens are degraded to peptides and only certain HLA molecules accept the antigen. The HLA molecule–antigenic peptide is then presented to the T cell and disease takes place.

The third hypothesis postulates that the T-cell antigen receptor which recognizes the HLA molecule-peptide complex is responsible for disease but because the T-cell recognition is restricted by an HLA molecule there is an association between the disease and B27.

Finally, there is an hypothesis related to the 'molecular mimicry' phenomenon. Here the peptide derived from the organism that causes disease is immunologically identical to HLA-B27. Therefore, the peptide is not recognized as foreign—no immune response is mounted and the disease process develops. Alternatively, the peptide is recognized as foreign and a vigorous immune response is mounted against the organism but the response cross reacts with self tissue causing disease. (For reviews see Khan 1993; Khan 1996; Schur 1994; Inman and Scofield 1994; De Castro 1994).

We still do not know which of these many possibilities—if any— is correct. Interestingly, certain strains of shigella which contain a plasmid (an extrachromosomal piece of DNA) are known to be arthritogenic, causing Reiter's syndrome. Recent data suggest that B27-positive individuals share structural and immunological homology with a sequence of five amino acids present in the plasmid (Stieglitz and Lipsky 1993).

At least 11 variants of the HLA-B27 molecule exist and until recently it was thought that disease predisposition did not appear to be restricted to a particular allele. However, Hill et al. have now described a rapid method of HLA Class 1 typing using the polymerase chain reaction and oligonucleotide hybridization that eliminates requirements for viable lymphocytes and, in addition, allows subtypes to be clearly defined (Hill et al. 1991). The authors studied black subjects in the Gambia, West Africa, and showed that the predominant subtype was HLA-B27.03. This is particularly rare or absent in other racial groups and interestingly the subtype is not recognized by cytotoxic T cells—perhaps explaining why spondylarthritis is rare in black Africa and when it does occur, may not be associated with HLA-B27. HLA-B27.03 differs from the other common HLA-B27 subtypes by a single amino acid substitution of histidine for tyrosine at position 59 of the α_1 domain. This has been predicted by the 'arthritogenic peptide' model of HLA-B27 disease (Benjamin and Parham 1990). This model evokes a central role for cytotoxic T lymphocytes, which react with an HLA-B27-specific peptide carried by a foreign pathogen. It is proposed that HLA-B27-restricted lymphocytes cause disease when they recognize a similar or identical peptide normally expressed in joint tissue. This is in contrast to the 'altered self' and 'molecular mimicry' models where either the cysteine residue at position 67 or neighbouring residues are thought to be of paramount importance. (HLA-B27.03 shares this cysteine residue at position 67 with the other HLA-B27 subtypes.) Using monoclonal anti-HLA-B27 antibodies, several bacterial components have been recognized. The relevance of this cross-reaction remains unclear. Through a computerized search, a klebsiella protein has been identified that carries a stretch of six amino acids identical to residue 72 to 77 of two of the HLA-B27 variants. Moreover, a synthetic peptide carrying the six amino acids of the HLA-B27 protein is reactive with serum antibodies in some patients with disease. Another amino acid residue of interest is that of position 45, which has provided particular interest relating to the '45 pocket'

hypothesis (Benjamin and Parham 1990). The effect of this pocket in peptide presentation is not known but it could have some functional role. The distribution of different HLA-B27 subtypes is given in Table 5.

The immune response to various triggers has been studied at length. For example during yersinia reactive arthropathy, high and persistent IgA anti-yersinia antibodies have been detected (Granfors and Toivanen 1986). This prolonged antibody response to yersinia, as well as the higher chlamydia antibody titres in synovial fluid as compared to that in serum in chlamydial reactive arthropathy (Hughes and Keat 1992), could indicate an antigenic persistence and impaired antigen elimination from the joint. In addition, proliferative responses specific to the organism which causes the infection preceding the arthropathy have been described (Gaston et al. 1989; Hermann et al. 1989). A response to a 65-kDa mycobacterial heat shock protein has been detected in patients with reactive arthropathy but its specificity is only minimal. The persistence of intrasynovial antigenic material is now recognized (Nikkari et al. 1992; Toivanen and Toivanen 1996).

Initial interest was created by Geczy et al. and Ebringer et al. with regard to klebsiella and ankylosing spondylitis (Geczy et al. 1985; Ebringer et al. 1985). The former group reported a specific modification of HLA-B27-positive lymphocytes in patients with ankylosing spondylitis—a phenomenon that has received little support elsewhere. The Ebringer data supported molecular mimicry with cross-reactivity between klebsiella and HLA-B27, a finding supported by other studies with different arthritogenic triggers (van Bohemen et al. 1984; Raybourne et al. 1988). Meanwhile, Schwimmbeck et al. described homology between the 72 to 77 amino acid sequence from HLA-B27.05 subtype and residues 188 to 193 of *Klebsiella pneumoniae* nitrogenase (Schwimmbeck et al. 1987). Likewise, Toivanen et al. have described a similar sequence between HLA-B27 and Yap 1, an outer membrane protein of yersinia (Toivanen et al. 1990). Relevance of the mimicry phenomenon to pathogenesis is complicated by the publication of several studies that fail to agree. Regardless of the putative klebsiella link, there is still no certainty that this organism is arthritogenic in ankylosing spondylitis. It may well be that numerous bacteria (and indeed viruses) can induce disease in genetically susceptible individuals (for review see Kingsley and Sieper 1993; Schoen 1996).

Table 5   Distribution of B27 subtypes in various populations

Population	HLA-B27 subtype
Caucasoids	HLA-B*2704
	HLA-B*2702
Native North Americans	HLA-B*2705
Siberian Chukchis	HLA-B*2704
Chinese	HLA-B*2705
Asian Indians	HLA-B*2705
	HLA-B*2704
	HLA-B*2702
West Africans	HLA-B*2703
	HLA-B*2705

Transgenic rats have now been created that express HLA-B27 and this model will help clarify some of the above issues (Hammer *et al.* 1990). The HLA-B27-carrying rats spontaneously develop a disease characterized by involvement of the gastrointestinal tract, peripheral and axial joints, male genital tract, skin, nails, and heart. In Table 6 this disease is compared with the human spondylarthritides and adjuvant-induced arthritis in the rat (for review see Taurog 1997).

Disease susceptibility relates to the transgene product copy number in lymphoid cells, with the high expressing lines prone to disease. Differences in expression of the HLA-B27 gene product occur by disease onset, but differences in thymic and splenic messenger RNA levels are found *in utero*. HLA-B27 transgenic rats have been studied in cell transfer experiments (Breban *et al.* 1993*b*). The data reveal that disease can be transferred by engraftment of adult bone marrow cells from the diseased animals into irradiated non-transgenic rats. Bone marrow precursor cells are responsible for passage of disease. Moreover, the spondylarthropathy-like illness of rats has been found to be T-cell dependent (Breban *et al.* 1993*b*). These data argue for HLA-B27, itself, being involved in the pathogenesis of disease rather than there being a gene in linkage disequilibrium with HLA- B27 that is operative. When HLA-B27 positive β_2-microglobulin transgenic disease rats are raised in a germ-free environment, disease occurs but in a manner distinct from the regular situation. Specifically, the animals do not develop gut inflammation or arthropathy but they do develop more nail and skin changes as well as genital inflammation. These results suggest that gut flora are involved in some way in the development of spondylarthropathy (Taurog *et al.* 1993*b*).

Reactive arthropathy or intra-articular 'infection'?

Reactive arthropathy (Toivanen and Toivanen 1996) is defined as an inflammatory joint disease that relates to an infective organism that is distant in both time and place from the arthropathy. For example chlamydia induced urethritis may be followed 2 weeks later by uveitis, arthropathy, and other stigmata of Reiter's disease. A similar situation can follow dysenteric infection with campylobacter, yersinia, or other organism. However, there have been studies demonstrating chlamydia, yersinia, and most recently salmonella (Granfors *et al.* 1990) antigenic components within the synovial tissues. Whether the finding of intrasynovial micro-organism-related antigen represents an epiphenomenon or whether the material is central to disease pathogenesis remains unclear but at least at the moment it is not considered that viable organisms are found in the joint space (Highton and Poole 1993; Nikkari *et al.* 1992; Hughes and Keat 1992). Moreover, we have described postsalmonella vaccination arthropathy—a rheumatic condition related to the inoculation of dead organisms (Calin *et al.* 1987).

Interestingly, Lyme disease, which is known to be a multisystem disorder related to *Borrelia burgdorferi*, may produce a 'reactive' phenomenon in addition to the direct infective process (Weyand and Goronzy 1989).

Epidemiology and the spondylarthritides (see van der Linden and van der Heijde 1996)

Epidemiological studies tell us that reactive arthropathy is more common in the epidemic situation than where the organism is endemic. Adults are more at risk than are children in contradistinction to the situation with acute rheumatic fever. In postdysenteric arthropathy, patients frequently suffer only minimal gastrointestinal symptoms. As mentioned, postvaccination (salmonella) Reiter's disease can occur. Ankylosing spondylitis is seen in both the developing and developed world, with an higher age of onset in the latter. Other epidemiological studies demonstrate that ankylosing spondylitis occurs predominantly in the HLA-B27-positive Haida and Pima Indians and the HLA-B27-positive relatives of white patients with ankylosing spondylitis, while Reiter's syndrome occurs among the Navaho Indians and Inupiat Eskimo in addition to white family members of HLA-B27-positive probands with Reiter's disease. Presumably HLA-B27 is not sufficient in itself and, as stated above,

Table 6 Comparison of adjuvant rat model, transgenic (HLA-B27+) rat, ankylosing spondylitis and reactive arthritis (Reiter's syndrome)

	Adjuvant disease	Transgenic rat	Ankylosing spondylitis	Reiter's syndrome/ reactive arthritis
Peripheral joints	+	+ (M > F)	+	+
Axial joints	+	+ (M > F)	++	±
Gastrointestinal tract	?	++ (M=F)	±	±
Male genital tract	+	+	−	±
Skin lesions	+	+	−	±
Nails	?	+	−	±
Heart	?	+	±	±
Eye lesions	+	− (?)	+	±
Enthesitis	+	+	+	+
Synovitis	+	+	+	+

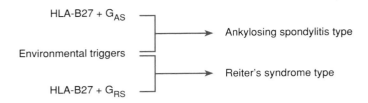

Fig. 4 Epidemiology and the spondylarthritides. G_{AS} = genes determining phenotypic expression of ankylosing spondylitis type. G_{RS} = genes determining phenotypic expression of Reiter's syndrome type.

an additional gene or genes modify the phenotypic expression (i.e. HLA-B27 plus appropriate environmental trigger, plus the ankylosing spondylitis gene results in ankylosing spondylitis while HLA-B27 plus environmental trigger plus the Reiter's gene leads to Reiter's syndrome) (Fig. 4).

The relationship between sex, phenotypic expression, mode of inheritance, and age at onset in the spondylarthropathies has recently been studied by Kennedy and colleagues (Kennedy *et al.* 1993*b*). Epidemiological studies have focused on the presence of spondyl-arthritis in Alaskan Eskimos (Boyer *et al.* 1994), the native population of Chukotka in Russia (Alexeeva *et al.* 1994), the Indonesian Chinese and native Indonesians (Nasution *et al.* 1993), and in Togo (Mijiyawa 1993). The varied prevalence rate is of great interest.

The risk for the HLA-B27-positive individual depends on the nature of that individual. For example if related to an HLA-B27-positive patient with ankylosing spondylitis, the chance of developing that same disease is approximately 1 in 3. HLA-B27-positive relatives of healthy HLA-B27-positive subjects are at much less risk of developing spondylarthropathy. Interplay between different chromosomes almost certainly occurs. Chromosome 6 is clearly important, with HLA-B27, -B60, and -CW6 all relevant. In addition, recent interest focuses on the tumour necrosis factor and class III genes (complement) on the same sixth chromosome. Other possible genetic factors relate to the T-cell receptor β gene (at a locus on the seventh chromosome) and the T-cell receptor α gene, the α_1-antitrypsin gene, and the IgG heavy-chain gene products related to loci on the fourteenth chromosome. Additional gene loci and products thereof include the IgG light λ chain (chromosome 22). Studies using restriction fragment length polymorphisms have failed to confirm the presence of additional genetic material of relevance to disease pathogenesis. For example, no differences have been found between the frequencies of such polymorphisms for tumour necrosis factor between patients and controls (Verjans *et al.* 1991).

Intact antigen is taken up by the cell and partly digested by the so-called large multifunctional protease system, the product from a gene on the short arm of the 6th chromosome. This results in a nonapeptide (i.e. a nine amino acid peptide) reaching the endoplasmic reticulum via the transporter associated with peptide gene product. (The transporter associated with peptide genes are also found in the major histocompatibility complex.) The nonapeptide then becomes associated with the HLA-B27 Class 1 antigen and extrudes on the cell surface as a bimolecular product to face the T-cell receptor gene product. The resulting HLA-B27–antigen–T-cell receptor tri-molecular complex releases cytokines and inflammatory mediators. This has been the focus for study (Maksymowych *et al.* 1994).

Reactive arthropathy appears to be mediated by HLA Class 1-restricted, CD8-positive T cells, given that both psoriatic arthropathy and Reiter's disease thrive in the presence of human immunodeficiency virus infection. This is in contrast to the CD4-positive, T-cell-maintained arthropathy of rheumatoid arthritis, which appears to remit in the presence of human immunodeficiency virus infection. Ankylosing spondylitis, itself, appears unaffected by the virus but few data exist.

The changing epidemiology of rheumatic diseases (Calin *et al.* 1988; Will *et al.* 1990; Will *et al.* 1992)

The spondylarthropathies should perhaps be included in any discussion of changing epidemiological features. There are many reasons why the pattern (perceived or real) of a disease may change. Increased interest and recognition by the medical profession and greater concern and pressure from patients may lead to more emphasis on a particular disease. For example osteoporosis, until recently ignored by rheumatologists, has become a major focus of interest.

Chronic tophaceous gout, once the scourge of medical clinics, is an example of a rheumatic disorder which has all but disappeared, in part due to changing dietary habits and in part because of hypouricaemic agents. By contrast, a recent rise in prevalence of gout in older females relates to the greater use of diuretics.

Rheumatic fever, at least until recently, had become rare in the more affluent communities. The decline in fatal rheumatic carditis accelerated after 1945, perhaps due to an alteration in the pathogenicity of the streptococcal group A M antigen induced by penicillin. Altered streptococcal antigenicity may also be responsible for the recent recognition of a poststreptococcal arthropathy.

Recent studies also suggest that rheumatoid arthritis may be declining in frequency in the developed world, perhaps due to the advent of the contraceptive pill, but it is becoming more severe in the developing world. For example recent published data have demonstrated that as rural black Africans migrate to an urban environment, rheumatoid arthritis increases in frequency and becomes a more destructive disease. Hypothetical explanations for this phenomenon may include either exposure to new antigens present in an urban environment but uncommon in a less crowded rural setting or conversely a reduction in the antigenic load due to fewer parasitic infestations, which in turn could result in less immunosuppression.

There is increasing evidence accumulating from developing countries to suggest that the pattern of ankylosing spondylitis may be changing. This relates to both the age of onset of the disease and the pattern of joint involvement. Ankylosing spondylitis develops at an earlier age in countries with poor living conditions and as these improve the age of onset increases. We have recently suggested that the age of onset of the disease may also be increasing over time in Britain. The influence of potential left and right censoring biases on the United Kingdom data has been emphasized elsewhere, though the importance of this phenomenon is difficult to quantify. Can the conclusion of an increasing age of onset of ankylosing spondylitis in Britain be substantiated by data from other communities? The putative change may be due to a later age of exposure to the presumed 'infective trigger(s)' or altered pathogenicity of the trigger(s), perhaps due to a modifying factor such as the widespread use of antibiotics.

Amor *et al.* in France noted that the age of onset of ankylosing spondylitis was influenced by the geographic background of their patients (Amor *et al.* 1991). They observed that 25 per cent of patients from North Africa develop disease before the age of 15 years whereas only 10 per cent of patients in France did so. Moreover, 47 second generation North Africans with ankylosing spondylitis born and living in France (but whose parents were born in North Africa) were identified from a survey conducted by the French Society of Rheumatology in 1983. None of these 'Beur', as they are known, developed disease before the age of 15. Other studies have also noted a lower frequency of juvenile onset ankylosing spondylitis (at under age 16) in white Caucasian populations as compared to subjects in the developing world. In spite of the inevitable ascertainment biases, there is now a series of studies consistently demonstrating a greater frequency of patients with a lower age of disease onset from developing countries.

An entirely separate epidemiological route has been taken and the changing pattern of new patient referral to the London Hospital has been studied (Will *et al.* 1992). Of interest, patients with non-specific mechanical back pain have become progressively younger over the last three decades whereas new patients with ankylosing spondylitis have become progressively older. These data, together with the French data of Amor, add further support for the changing pattern.

Family studies of sibling pairs with ankylosing spondylitis also suggest that the date of onset in each sib is similar while the age at onset is discordant suggesting exposure to the trigger at about the same time. This emphasises the importance of the environmental trigger determining the time of onset of disease in sibling pairs who have a similar genetic predisposition (Calin and Elswood 1989a).

The age of disease onset also influences the need for total hip replacement. Calin and Elswood have shown that 16 per cent of a juvenile cohort (10-15 years), 10 per cent of an early onset (18-20 years), and 1 per cent of a late onset cohort (30-40 years) had total hip replacements performed (Calin and Elswood 1989b). Amor *et al.* also observed that the frequency of total hip replacement in a spondylitic population correlates well with the mean age of disease onset (Amor *et al.* 1991). A study of total hip replacements performed in patients from four French hospitals between 1977 and 1983 was undertaken. Twenty-two of a total of 71 patients (30 per cent) who had total hip replacements were born in North Africa as compared with only 7.9 per cent of non-surgical patients treated in French hospitals during this same period. The explanation for more severe hip joint involvement in a juvenile cohort is unknown. The developing hip joint may be at greater risk of damage. Conversely, a more marked inflammatory response may result in greater joint destruction in juveniles compared with patients who develop the disease at an older age.

It is of interest that a changing pattern in inflammatory bowel disease is now also recognized and in many studies Crohn's disease, which became progressively more common until the mid-1970s, has now begun to be less prevalent. The intriguing interrelationship between the bowel and ankylosing spondylitis is, of course, well known (Mielants *et al.* 1993; Leirisalo-Repo *et al.* 1994; Mielants *et al.* 1995).

In conclusion, chronic rheumatic diseases should not be considered immutable processes. A changing pattern of disease is to be expected given the interaction of genes and the environment. Ankylosing spondylitis, and perhaps the other spondylarthropathies,

should now be considered as another example of a rheumatic disorder whose characteristics may be altering as a result of a changing environment. We might expect a diminished need for total hip replacement among patients as a consequence of an increasing age of onset of patients in the West and perhaps in developing countries as the environment changes. Physicians will need to be increasingly aware that patients may present with symptoms of disease in their thirties or later. The epidemiological pattern among the other spondylarthropathies is less well defined.

The bowel and spondylarthritis (Mielants *et al.* 1993; Leirisalo-Repo 1994; Mielants *et al.* 1995)

The relationship between the bowel and arthritis is an intimate one. For example an active arthropathy may follow enteropathic infections such as those related to shigella, salmonella, yersinia, campylobacter, and other organisms. Moreover, patients with reactive arthropathy or Reiter's disease related to chlamydia may also develop enteric symptoms as a manifestation of the disease process.

It is well recognized that patients with inflammatory bowel disease (ulcerative colitis and Crohn's disease) may develop both peripheral and axial arthropathy. In general, the peripheral arthritis appears to be a complication of severe bowel involvement with a close relationship between the two components. By contrast, axial disease (sacroiliitis and ascending spinal disease) should be considered a manifestation of the same genetic background, in as much as there is no obvious link between the timing or disease severity of the two entities.

The story has been taken further by Mielants and Veys who performed ileocolonoscopy with biopsies of the gut and described clinical involvement of the terminal ileum as a common finding in the spondylarthropathy patients as a whole (Mielants and Veys 1990; Mielants *et al.* 1993; Mielants *et al.* 1995). Interestingly, the low grade bowel involvement that mimics mild Crohn's disease was often present as a silent phenomenon and appeared unrelated to the HLA-B27 marker. The authors concluded, from multiple studies, that a number of patients with undifferentiated spondylarthropathy could in fact be suffering from a form of subclinical Crohn's disease, of which arthritis is the only clinical manifestation (Leirisalo-Repo *et al.* 1994).

The putative relationship between the bowel, enteric micro-organisms, and arthropathy has been further addressed by way of therapy. Sulphasalazine has been used for years as a treatment for ulcerative colitis, colonic Crohn's disease, and, more recently, for rheumatoid arthropathy. It is metabolized to 5-aminosalicylic acid (active in inflammatory bowel disease) and sulphapyridine (active in rheumatoid disease). Work by Feratz *et al.* suggests efficacy also in ankylosing spondylitis and perhaps the other spondylarthropathies (Feratz *et al.* 1990). Whether this drug works by way of altering the bowel microflora or another mechanism remains unclear.

Titres of serum and secretory IgA (presumed to be of bowel mucosal origin) are raised in patients with ankylosing spondylitis and in patients with yersinia arthropathy, again arguing for a close link between events in the bowel wall and arthritis.

Finally, it is of note that the transgenic rat expressing human HLA-B27 develops a spontaneous arthropathy that mimics

Box 1 Treatment of spondylarthropathy

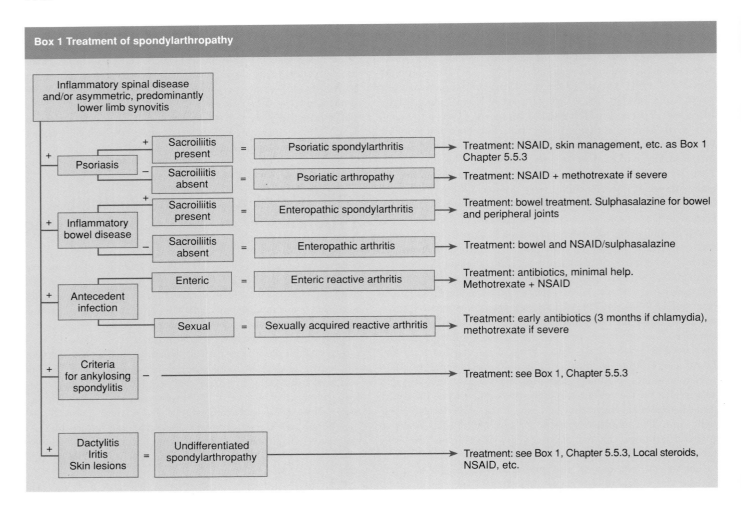

spondylarthritis. Strikingly, the main organ involvement is the bowel with marked diarrhoea (Hammer *et al.* 1990).

Treatment (Box 1)

The management of the various components of spondylarthropathy are discussed in the separate chapters that follow. However, there are some general points that should be stressed. Drug therapy is often disappointing. For example for ankylosing spondylitis, itself, the major thrust of treatment relates to an exercise programme. In contrast to the situation in rheumatoid disease where rest is good for the joints, the patient with ankylosing spondylitis deteriorates with rest and improves with exercise. For those with reactive arthritis, the role of antibiotics has been considered but even the proponents of this approach would agree that outcome is only marginally improved (Leirisalo-Repo 1993; Bardin *et al.* 1992; Lauhio *et al.* 1991; Lauhio *et al.* 1992; Toivanen *et al.* 1993). One difficulty relates to the interpretation of the effect, if any, of an antibiotic. Does this relate to the antimicrobial action or, for example, the anticollagenolytic potential of the drug? There are theoretical reasons why sulphasalazine should be efficacious in the spondylarthropathies given the relationship between bowel inflammation and arthropathy. However, again, improvement is marginal and in large part beneficial only for peripheral joints rather than axial disease (Youssef *et al.* 1992; Kirwan *et al.* 1993; Job-Duslandre *et al.* 1993; Dougados *et al.* 1995).

Natural history and prognosis

Outcome in spondylarthropathy is notoriously difficult to define.

Since our early studies in the 1970s when we showed that Reiter's syndrome is typically not a self-limiting disorder (Calin and Fries 1976), there have been numerous studies showing that for many patients the outcome can be relentlessly progressive. For ankylosing spondylitis, itself, the natural history is varied although most believe that an intensive exercise programme has an excellent effect on disease progression. No longer is it believed that the disease 'burns out' for the majority (Kennedy *et al.* 1993*a*). Amor and colleagues have attempted to define predictive factors for the long-term outcome of spondylarthropathies and have suggested that those individuals with hip involvement, an erythrocyte sedimentation rate over 30, poor response to non-steroidal anti-inflammatory drugs, a decreased Schober's test, dactylitis, oligoarthropathy, and young age at onset have the worse prognosis (Amor *et al.* 1994). Although this study was not a formal prospective investigation, few would disagree that these criteria relate to a less good outcome. Recently, we have defined outcome in terms of metrology, disease activity, function, global status, severity, and radiology (Calin 1995*a*; Calin 1995*b*; Mackay *et al.* 1996).

Finally, the influence of sex in arthritis and its relationship to cartilage damage cannot be ignored (Da Silva and Willoughby 1994).

Conclusion

During the next years we will understand why and how HLA-B27, other genes, the bowel, sex, and environmental triggers interact, resulting in the development of spondylarthropathy in its many guises. Once we understand this intricate, interrelated network we will know how to manage and perhaps cure our patients.

References

Alexeeva, L., Krylov, M., Vturin, V., Mylov, N., Erdesz, S., and Benevolenskaya, L. (1994). Prevalence of spondylarthropathies and HLA-B27 in the native population of Chukotka, Russia. *Journal of Rheumatology*, **22**, 2298–300.

Amor, B. *et al.* (1991). Evaluation des criteres de spondylarthropathies d'Amor et de Liesseg: une etude transversale de 2228 patients. *Annales de Medicine Interne*, **142**, 85–9.

Amor, B., Santos, R.S., Nahal, R., Listrat, V., and Dougados, M. (1994). Predictive factors for the longterm outcome of spondylarthropathies. *Journal of Rheumatology*, **21**, 1883–7.

Bardin T., Enel, C., Comelis, F., Saiski, C., Jorgensen, C., Ward, R., and Lanthrop, M. (1992). Antibiotic treatment of venereal disease and Reiter's syndrome in a Greenland population. *Arthritis and Rheumatism*, **35**, 190–4.

Benjamin, R. and Parham, P. (1990). Guilt by association: HLA-B27 and ankylosing spondylitis. *Immunology Today*, **11**, 137–43.

Bennett, P.H. and Burch, T.A. (1968). *Population studies of the rheumatic diseases*, pp. 456–7. Excerpta Medica Foundation, Amsterdam.

Boyer, G.S. *et al.* (1994). Prevalence of spondylarthropathies in Alaskan Eskimos. *Journal of Rheumatology*, **21**, 2292–7.

Braun, J. and Sieper, J. (1996). The sacroiliac joint in the spondyloarthropathies. *Current Opinion in Rheumatology*, **8**, 275–87.

Breban, M., Hammer, R.E., Richardson, J.A., and Taurog, J.D. (1993a). Transfer of the inflammatory disease of HLA-B27 transgenic rats by bone marrow engraftment. *Journal of Experimental Medicine*, **178**, 1607–16.

Breban, M. *et al.* (1993b). T cells but not thymic exposure to B27 are required for the inflammatory disease of HLA-B27 transgenic rats. *Arthritis and Rheumatism*, **36**, S73.

Burns, T.M. and Calin, A. (1984). Undifferentiated spondylarthopathy. In *Spondylarthropathies* (ed A. Calin), pp. 253–64. Grune and Stratton, Orlando, FL.

Calin, A. (1984). *Spondylarthropathies*. Grune and Stratton, Orlando, FL.

Calin, A. (1989). Ankylosing spondylitis. *Textbook of rheumatology*. WB Saunders, Philadelphia, PA.

Calin, A. (1995a). The Dunlop Dotteridge Lecture. Ankylosing spondylitis: defining disease status and the relationship between radiology, metrology, disease activity, function and outcome. *Journal of Rheumatology*, **22**, 740–44.

Calin, A. (1995b). The Margaret Holroyd Essay. The individual with ankylosing spondylitis: defining disease status and the impact of illness. *British Journal of Rheumatology*, **34**, 663–72.

Calin, A. and Elswood, J. (1989a). Relative role of genetic and environmental factors in disease expression: sib-pair analysis in ankylosing spondylitis. *Arthritis and Rheumatism*, **32**, 77–81.

Calin, A. and Elswood, J. (1989b). The outcome of 138 total hip replacements and 12 revisions in ankylosing spondylitis. *Journal of Rheumatology*, **16**, 955–8.

Calin, A., Elswood, J., Rigg, S., and Skevington, S.M. (1988). Ankylosing spondylitis – an analytical review of 1500 patients: the changing pattern of disease. *Journal of Rheumatology*, **15**, 1234–8.

Calin, A. and Fries J.F. (1976). An 'experimental' epidemic of Reiter's syndrome revisited. *Annals of Internal Medicine*, **84**, 564–6.

Calin, A. and Fries, J.F. (1978). *Ankylosing spondylitis: discussions in patient management*.. Medical Examination Publishing Company, New York.

Calin, A., Goulding, D., and Brewerton, D. (1987). Post salmonella vaccination reactive arthropathy. *Arthritis and Rheumatism*, **30**, 969–70.

Calin, A., Marder, A., Marks, S., and Burns, T. (1984). Familial aggregation of Reiter's syndrome and ankylosing spondylitis: a comparative study. *Journal of Rheumatology*, **11**, 672–77.

Da Silva, J.A.P. and Willoughby, D.A. (1994). The influence of sex in arthritis: is cartilage an overlooked factor? *Journal of Rheumatology*, **21**, 791–6.

De Castro, J.A.L. (1994). Structure, function, and disease association of HLA-B27. *Current Opinion in Rheumatology*, **6**, 371–7.

De Vries, D.D., Dekker-Saeys, A.J., Gyodi, E., Bohn, U., and Ivanyi, P. (1992). Absence of autoantibodies to peptides shared by HLA-B27.5 and klebsiella pneumoniae nitrogenase in serum samples from HLA-B27 positive patients with ankylosing spondylitis and Reiter's syndrome. *Annals of the Rheumatic Diseases*, **51**, 783–9.

Dougados, M. *et al.* (1991). Preliminary criteria for the classification of spondylarthropathy. *Arthritis and Rheumatism*, **34**, 1218–27.

Dougados, M., van der Linden, S., Amor, B., Calin, A., *et al.* (1995). Sulphasalazine in the treatment of spondylarthropathy: a randomized multi-centre double blind placebo controlled study. *Arthritis and Rheumatism*, **38**, 618–27.

Ebringer, A. (1991). Ankylosing spondylitis and klebsiella — the debate continues. Editorial. *Journal of Rheumatology*, **18**, 312–13.

Ebringer, A., Baines, M., Childerstone, M., Ghuloom, M., and Ptaszynska, T. (1985). Etiopathogenesis of ankylosing spondylitis and the cross-tolerance hypothesis. In *Advances in inflammation research. The spondylarthropathies*, Vol. 9 (ed. M. Ziff and S.B. Cohen), pp. 101–28. Raven Press, New York.

Edmunds, L., Elswood, J., Kennedy, L.G., and Calin, A. (1991). Primary ankylosing spondylitis, psoriatic and enteropathic spondylarthropathy: a controlled analysis. *Journal of Rheumatology*, **18**, 696–8.

Ferraz, M.B., Tugwell, P., Goldsmith, C.H., and Atra, E. (1990). Metaanalysis of sulfasalazine in ankylosing spondylitis. *Journal of Rheumatology*, **17**, 11.

Gaston, J.S.H. *et al.* (1989). Synovial T lymphocyte recognition of organisms that trigger reactive arthritis. *Clinical and Experimental Immunology*, **76**, 348–53.

Geczy, A.F., Prendergast, J.K., Sullivan, J.S., Upfold, L.I., Edmonds, J.P., and Bashi, H.V. (1985). Possible role of enteric organisms in the pathogenesis of seronegative arthropathies. In *Advances in inflammation research. The spondylarthropathies*, Vol. 9. (ed. M. Ziff and S.B. Cohen), pp. 129–37. Raven Press, New York.

Granfors, K. and Toivanen, A. (1986). IgA anti-Yersinia antibodies in Yersinia triggering reactive arthritis. *Annals of the Rheumatic Diseases*, **45**, 401–12.

Granfors, K. *et al.* (1990). Salmonella lipopolysaccharide in synovial cells from patients with reactive arthritis. *Lancet*, **335**, 685–8.

Hammer, R.E., Maika, S.D., Richardson, J.A., Tang, J-P., and Taurogi, J.D. (1990). Spontaneous inflammatory disease in transgenic rats expression HLA-B27 and Human bm: an animal model of HLA-B27-associated human disorders. *Cell*, **63**, 1099–112.

Hermann, E., Fleischer, B., Mayet, W.J., Poralla, T., and zum Buschenfelde, K.H.M. (1989). Response of synovial fluid T cell clones to Yersinia enterocolitica antigens in patients with reactive Yersinia arthritis. *Clinical and Experimental Immunology*, **75**, 365–70.

Hermann, E., Yu, D.T.Y., zum Buschenfelde, K.H.M., and Fleischer, B. (1993). HLA-B27-restricted CD8 T cells derived from synovial fluids of patients with reactive arthritis and ankylosing spondylitis. *Lancet*, **342**, 646–50.

Highton, J. and Poole, E. (1993). Sexually acquired reactive arthritis: inflammation or sepsis? *British Journal of Rheumatology*, **32**, 649–52.

Hill, A.V.S, Allsopp, C.E.M., Kwiatkowski, D., Anstey, N.M., Greenwood, B.M., and McMichael, A.J. (1991). HLA class 1 typing by PCR: HLA-B27 and an African B27 subtype. *Lancet*, **337**, 640–2.

Hughes, R.A., Treharne, J.D., and Keat, A.C. (1989). Chlamydial antibody titres in serum and synovial fluid (abstract). *British Journal of Rheumatology*, **28**, 4.

Hughes, R. and Keat, A. (1992). Reactive arthritis: the role of bacterial antigens in inflammatory arthritis. *Baillières Clinical Rheumatology*, **6**, 285–308.

Inman, R.D. and Scofield, R.H. (1994). Etiopathogenesis of ankylosing spondylitis and reactive arthritis. *Current Opinion in Rheumatology*, **6**, 360–70.

Job-Duslandre, C. and Menkes, C.J. (1993). Sulphasalazine treatment for juvenile arthropathy. *Revue du Rheumatisme*, **60**, 489–93.

Kellgren, J.H., Jeffrey, M.R., and Ball, J. (1963). *The epidemiology of chronic rheumatism*, Vol. 1, pp. 326–7. Blackwell Scientific Publications, Oxford.

Kennedy, L.G., Edmunds, L., and Calin, A. (1993a). Does ankylosing spondylitis burn out? A prospective 2-year study. *Journal of Rheumatology*, **20**, 688–92.

Kennedy, L.G., Will, R., and Calin, A. (1993b). Sex ratio in the spondylarthropathies and its relationship to phenotypic expression, mode of inheritance and age at onset. *Journal of Rheumatology*, **20**, 1900–4.

Khan, M.A. (ed) (1990). *Ankylosing spondylitis and related spondyloarthropathies in spine*, Vol. 4, No. 3. Hanley & Belfas, Philadelphia.

Khan, M.A. (1993). Pathogenesis of ankylosing spondylitis: recent advances. *Journal of Rheumatology*, **20**, 1273–7.

Khan, M.A. (1996). Spondylarthropathies (Editorial overview). *Current Opinion in Rheumatology*, **8**, 267–8.

Khan, M.A. and van der Linden, S.M. (1990). Undifferentiated spondyloarthropathies. In *Ankylosing spondylitis and related spondyloarthropathies in spine*, Vol. 3, No. 3 (ed. M.A. Khan), pp. 657–64. Hanley & Belfas, Philadelphia.

Kingsley, G. and Sieper, J. (1993). Current prospectives in reactive arthritis. *Immunology Today*, **14**, 387–91.

Kirwan, J., Edwards, A., Huitfeldt, B., Thompson, P., and Currey, H. (1993). The course of established ankylosing spondylitis and the effects of Sulphasalazine over 3 years. *British Journal of Rheumatology*, **32**, 729–33.

Lauhio, A., Leirisalo-Repo, M., Lahdevirta, J., Saikku, P., and Repo, H. (1991). Double-blind, placebo-controlled study of three-month treatment with lymecycline in reactive arthritis, with special reference to chlamydia arthritis. *Arthritis and Rheumatism*, **34**, 6–14.

Lauhio, A. *et al.* (1992). The anticoliagenolytic potential of lymecycline in the long-term treatment of reactive arthritis. *Arthritis and Rheumatism*, **35**, 195–8.

Leirisalo-Repo, M. (1993). Areantibiotics of any use in reactivearthritis? *Acta Pathologica, Microbiologica, et Immunologica Scandinavica*, **101**, 575–81.

Leirisalo-Repo, M. (1994). Enteropathic arthritis, Whipple's disease, juvenile spondyloarthropathy, and uveitis. *Current Opinion in Rheumatology*, **6**, 385–90.

Leirisalo-Repo, M., Turunen, U., Stenman, S., Helenius, P., and Seppala, K. (1994). High frequency of silent inflammatory bowel disease in spondylarthropathy. *Arthritis and Rheumatism*, **37**, 23–31.

Lopez-Larrea, C. *et al.* (1996). HLA B27. Structure, function, and disease association. *Current Opinion in Rheumatology*, **8**, 296–308.

Mackay, K., Mack, C.S., Pande, I., Rousson, E., and Calin, A. (1996). The Bath Ankylosing Spondylitis Radiology Index (BASRI). *Arthritis and Rheumatism*, **39**, 206.

Madden, D.R., Gorga, J.C., Strominger, J.L., and Wiley, D.C. (1992). The three-dimensional structure of HLA-B27 at 2.1: a resolution suggests a general mechanism for tight peptide binding to MHC. *Cell*, **70**, 1035–48.

Maksymowych, W.P. *et al.* (1994). Polymorphism in an HLA linked proteasome gene influences phenotypic expression of disease in HLA-B27 positive individuals. *Journal of Rheumatology*, **21**, 665–9.

McClean, I.L. *et al.* (1993). HLA-B27 subtypes in the spondyloarthropathies. *Clinical and Experimenal Immunology*, **91**, 214–19.

Mielants, H. *et al.* (1993). Gut inflammation in children with late onset of pauciarticular juvenile chronic arthritis and evolution to adult spondyloarthropathy: a prospective study. *Journal of Rheumatology*, **20**, 1567–72.

Mielants, H. *et al.* (1995). The evolution of spondyloarthropathies in relation to gut histology. *Journal of Rheumatology*, **22**, 2266–72.

Mijiyawa, M. (1993). Spondylarthropathies in patients attending the rheumatology unit of Lome Hospital. *Journal of Rheumatology*, **20**, 1167–9.

Moll, J.M.H. (ed) (1980). *Ankylosing spondylitis*. Churchill Livingstone, Edinburgh.

Moll, J.M.H. *et al.* (1974). Associations between ankylosing spondylitis, psoriatic arthritis, Reiter's disease, the intestinal arthropathies and Behçet's syndrome. *Medicine*, **53**, 343.

Nasution, A.R., Mardjuadi, A., Suryadhana, N.G., Daud, R., and Muslichan, S. (1993). Higher relative risk of spondylarthropathies among B27 positive Indonesian Chinese than native Indonesians. *Journal of Rheumatology*, **20**, 988–90.

Nikkari, S. *et al.* (1992). Yersinia-triggered reactive arthritis: use of polymerase chain reaction and immuno-cytochemical staining in the detection of bacterial components from synovial specimens. *Arthritis and Rheumatism*, **35**, 682–7.

Raybourne, R.B., Bunning, V.K., and Williams, K.M. (1988). Reaction of anti-HLA-B monoclonal antibodies with envelope proteins of Shigella species. Evidence for molecular mimicry in the spondylarthropathies. *Journal of Immunology*, **140**, 3489–95.

Rojo, S., Garcia, F., Villadangos, J.A., and Lopez de Castro, J.A. (1993). Changes in the repertoire of peptides bound to HLA-B27 subtypes and to site specific mutants inside and outside Pocket B. *Journal of Experimental Medicine*, **177**, 613–20.

Rosner, I.A., Burg, C.G., Wisnieski, J.J., Schacter, B.Z., and Richter, D.E. (1993). The clinical spectrum of the arthropathy associated with hidradenitis suppurativa and acne conglobata. *Journal of Rheumatology*, **20**, 4.

Schoen, R.T. (1996). Infectious arthritis and immune dysfunction. *Current Opinion in Rheumatology*, **8**, 317–21.

Schur, P.H. (1994). Arthritis and autoimmunity. *Arthritis and Rheumatism*, **37**, 1818–25.

Schwartz, B.D. (1990). Infectious agents, immunity and rheumatic diseases. *Arthritis and Rheumatism*, **33**, 457–65.

Schwimmbeck, P.L., Yu, D.T.Y., and Oldstone, M.B.A. (1987). Autoantibodies to HLA-B27 in the sera of HLA-B27 patients with ankylosing spondylitis and Reiter's syndrome. Molecular mimicry with Klebsiella pneumonias as potential mechanism of autoimmune disease. *Journal of Experimental Medicine*, **166**, 173–81.

Scofield, R.H. (1996). Etiopathogenesis and biochemical and immunologic evaluation of spondyloarthropathies. *Current Opinion in Rheumatology*, **8**, 309–15.

Scofield, R.H., Warren, W.L., Koelsch, G., and Harley, J.B. (1993). A hypothesis for the immune dysregulation in spondyloarthropathies: contributions from enteric organisms, B27 structure. peptides bound by B27 and convergent evolution. *Proceedings of the National Academy of Science*, **90**, 9330–4.

Skurnik, M., Batsford, S., Mertz, A., and Tolvanen, P. (1993). The putative arthrogenic cationic 19-kilodalton antigen of yersinia enterocolitica is a urease β-subunit. *Infectious Immunology*, **61**, 2498–504.

Stieglitz, H. and Lipsky, P. (1993). Association between reactive arthritis and antecedent infection with shigella flexneri carrying a 2-Md plasmid and encoding an HLA-B27 mimetic epitope. *Arthritis and Rheumatism*, **36**, 1387–91.

Taurog, J.D. (1997). Animal models of the spondylarthropathies. In *Spondylarthropathies* (ed. A. Calin and J. Taurog). Oxford University Press (in press).

Taurog, J.D., Maika, S.D., Simmons, W.A., Breban, M., and Hammer, R.E. (1993a) Susceptibility to inflammatory disease in HLA-B27 transgenic rat lines correlates with level of B27 expression. *Journal of Immunology*, **150**, 4168–72.

Taurog, J.D. *et al.* (1993b) Effect of the germfree state on the inflammatory disease of HLA-B27 transgenic rats: a split result. *Arthritis and Rheumatism*, **36**, S46.

Toivanen, P. *et al.* (1990). Tetrapeptide shared by HLA-B27 and Yersinia outer membrane protein YOP1 is not decisive for antigenicity of YOP1 (abstract). *Clinical Rheumatology*, **9**, 133.

Toivanen, A., Yli-Kerttula, T., Luukkainen, R., Meilahti-Palo, R., Granfors, K., and Seppala, J. (1993). Effect of antimicrobial treatment on chronic reactive arthritis. *Clinical and Experimental Rheumatology*, **11**, 301–7.

Toivanen, A. and Toivanen, P. (1996). Reactive arthritides. *Current Opinion in Rheumatology*, **8**, 334–40.

van Bohemen, C.G., Grumet, F.C., and Zanen, H.C. (1984). Identification of HLA-B27 M1 and M2 cross-reactive antigens in Klebsiella, Shigella and Yersinia. *Immunology*, **52**, 605–9.

van der Linden, S. and van der Heijde, D.M. (1996). Clinical and epidemiologic aspects of ankylosing spondylitis and spondyloarthropathies. *Current Opinion in Rheumatology*, **8**, 269–74.

van der Linden, S., Valkenburg, H.A., and Cats, A. (1984). Evaluation of diagnostic criteria for ankylosing spondylitis. *Arthritis and Rheumatism*, **27**, 361–8.

Vasey, F. and Espinoza, L.R. (1984). Psoriatic arthropathy. In *Spondylarthropathies* (ed. A. Calin), pp. 151–85. Grune and Stratton, Orlando, FL.

Verjans, G.M.G.M., van der Linden, S.M., van Eys, G.J.J.M., de Waal, L.P., and Kijistra, A. (1991). Restriction fragment length polymorphism of the tumor necrosis factor region in patients with ankylosing spondylitis. *Arthritis and Rheumatism*, **34**, 486–9.

Weyand, C.M. and Goronzy, J.J. (1989). Immune responses to borrelia-burgdorferi in patients with reactive arthritis. *Arthritis and Rheumatism*, **32**, 1057–64.

Whelan, M.A. and Archer, J.R. (1993). Chemical reactivity of an HLA-B27 thiol group. *European Journal of Immunology*, **23**, 3278–85.

Will, R., Amor, B., and Calin, A. (1990). The changing epidemiology of rheumatic diseases: should ankylosing spondylitis now be included? *British Journal of Rheumatology*, **29**, 299–300.

Will, R., Calin, A., and Kirwan, J. (1992). Increasing age at presentation with ankylosing spondylitis and rheumatic diseases. *Annals of the Rheumatic Diseases*, **52**, 340–2.

Willkens, R.F. *et al.* (1981). Reiter's syndrome. Evaluation of preliminary criteria for definite disease. *Arthritis and Rheumatism*, **24**, 844–9.

Wright, V. (1980). Relationships between ankylosing spondylitis and other spondarthritides. In *Ankylosing spondylitis* (ed. J.M.H. Moll). Churchill Livingstone, Edinburgh.

Wright, V. and Moll, J.M.H. (1976). *Seronegative polyarthritis*. North Holland, Amsterdam.

Youssef, P.P., Berlouch, J.V., and Jones, P.D. (1992). Successful treatment of human immunodeficiency virus-associated Reiter's syndrome with Sulfasalazine. *Arthritis and Rheumatism*, 35, 723–4.

5.5.2 Spondylarthropathies in childhood

Taunton R. Southwood and Murray H. Passo

Synopsis

Juvenile spondylarthropathy is an umbrella term covering a relatively homogeneous group of diseases in children, usually beginning during the preadolescent or adolescent years. The diagnosis of spondylarthropathy is often more difficult in childhood than during the adult years because symptoms of back pain are uncommon in juvenile spondylarthropathy, particularly at the onset of the illness. Additionally, the radiographic features of spondylitis and sacroiliitis are often absent during childhood. The diagnosis usually rests on a combination of arthritis affecting large joints of the lower limbs and extra-articular inflammatory features including enthesitis, bowel pathology, acute uveitis, and psoriasis. The disease is reported more frequently in boys than girls, and more than 50 per cent of affected children eventually develop ankylosing spondylitis (Burgos-Vargas and Clark 1989; Cabral *et al.* 1992).

Because of the potentially lifelong implications of juvenile spondylarthropathy, every effort should be made to increase patients' and their families' knowledge about the disease and compliance with treatment. However, no published studies confirm that children with spondyarthropathy should be treated any differently from those with other forms of juvenile chronic arthritis. The principles of treatment are summarized as follows, but for further details, reference should be made to the chapters on juvenile chronic arthritis.

Education about the disease for the parents and the patient, presented in an age-appropriate form, is important. Physiotherapy, appropriate limb splinting, and hydrotherapy are aimed at maintaining back posture, flexibility and strength, as well as correcting any reduced range of peripheral joint movement. Orthotics, such as custom-moulded insoles, often alleviate the symptoms of plantar enthesitis. Pharmacotherapy is usually begun with a non-steroidal anti-inflammatory drug. Tolmetin sodium (30 mg/kg per day in three divided doses) and indomethacin (1.5–2.5 mg/kg per day in three divided doses, or as a daily dose if an appropriate slow-release preparation is available) appear to be the most effective. Intra-articular depot corticosteroids (e.g. triamcinolone hexacetonide: 1 mg/kg per joint for large joints, 0.5 mg/kg per joint for smaller joints) are used to control the peripheral arthritis of this condition, and should be considered early in the treatment programme. Sulphasalazine (commencing at a dose of 12.5 mg/kg per day and increasing weekly over a month to 50 mg/kg per day in divided doses) is the slow-acting antirheumatic drug of choice for uncontrolled spondylarthropathy, especially for significant axial involvement, polyarthritis, or severe, persistent oligoarthritis. Regular blood monitoring is required for bone marrow depression and hepatotoxicity, but skin rash and abdominal pain are the most common adverse effects. Methotrexate also may have a role in the long-term control of spondylarthropathy.

It is not uncommon for juvenile spondylarthropathy to run a fluctuating course, and occasionally the doses of non-steroidal anti-inflammatory drugs can be adjusted by the patients or their families to reflect these changes. In those children fortunate enough to experience prolonged remission, pharmacotherapy should be discontinued with caution, as relapse may occur after many symptom-free months or even years.

Aetiology

In considering the aetiology of juvenile spondylarthropathy, both inherited and environmental predisposing factors must be taken into account. Juvenile spondylarthropathy has a strong familial association with ankylosing spondylitis, and other inflammatory diseases such as acute uveitis, psoriasis or inflammatory bowel disease occur with increased frequency in family members (Petty 1990). The genetic predisposition to juvenile spondylarthropathy was first associated with the *HLA-B27* gene over 25 years ago (Ansell *et al.* 1969). Carriage of the gene confers an increased risk of developing ankylosing spondylitis; HLA-B27-positive children of a parent who has both HLA-B27 and ankylosing spondylitis are at least five times more likely to develop the disease than their HLA-B27-negative siblings (Van der Linden *et al.* 1984).

With the advent of molecular techniques, spondylarthropathies have been linked to several of the HLA-B27 subtypes B*2702, 04 and 05 (MacLean 1992), but only B*2705 has been associated with childhood disease. Compelling evidence in support of an aetiological role for HLA-B27 is found in animal models of the disease. Transgenic Lewis rats expressing a high cell-surface density of human B*2705 and β_2-microglobulin develop a spondylarthropathy during the first 6 weeks of life, characterized by peripheral arthritis, spinal inflammation, and inflammatory bowel disease. These features appear to be specific for the *HLA-B27* gene, as they are not seen in the rats expressing the *B*2705* gene in low copy number, or in rats transgenic for *HLA-B7* (Taurog *et al.* 1994). Genetic factors other than HLA-B27 are also likely to play an important part in humans. Jarvinen (1995) has demonstrated a disease concordance rate of 50 per cent for HLA-B27-positive monozygotic twins and only 20 per cent for HLA-B27-positive dizygotic twins.

Environmental factors, including enteric bacteria, are linked to the aetiology of juvenile spondylarthropathy by several intriguing strands of evidence. Enteric infections with salmonella, shigella, campylobacter or yersinia during childhood may be accompanied by peripheral arthritis, and occasionally by typical Reiter's syndrome (arthritis, urethritis, and conjunctivitis). Ninety per cent of children with Reiter's syndrome are HLA-B27 positive, and 80 per cent have had a preceding dysentery. Although the majority of these cases remit spontaneously, at least 1 in 5 develops radiographic evidence of sacroiliac arthritis (Cuttica *et al.* 1992) and there are anecdotal reports of progression to clinical spondyl-arthropathy (Southwood and Gaston 1993). The role of enteric bacteria in the arthritis associated with inflammatory bowel disease is less clear. There is no doubt that many children with inflammatory bowel disease develop arthritis (7–21 per cent). Successful treatment of the bowel inflammation with sulphasala-zine may be accompanied by remission of peripheral arthritis, the benefit of remission appearing to depend on the antibiotic (sulpha-) component, which may alter enteric bacterial colonization. Patients with inflammatory bowel disease who are HLA-B27 positive are more likely to develop ankylosing spondylitis (Lindsley and Schaller 1974; Passo *et al.* 1986).

There are reports that subacute bowel inflammation (histological evidence of acute or chronic ileocolonic inflammation) is found in up to 80 per cent of patients with juvenile spondylarthropathy, and a similar proportion of patients with late-onset pauciarticular juvenile chronic arthritis (Mielants *et al.* 1987; Veys *et al.* 1992; Mielants *et al.* 1993). The finding of chronic mucosal inflammation appeared to predict evolution to ankylosing spondylitis in these patients. There is also evidence that immune responses to enteric bacteria are found in the synovial compartment of children with juvenile spondylarthro-pathy. Approximately 90 per cent of children who have HLA-B27 positive chronic arthritis have lymphocytes in synovial fluid respon-sive to enteric bacteria, compared with only 25 per cent of children with HLA-B27-negative disease (Life *et al.* 1993). However, the stimulus to accumulation of such lymphocytes within the joint space remains unclear. There have been no consistent reports of bacteria or foreign antigenic fragments in the synovial membrane or fluid. Potentially cross-reactive immune responses directed against both bacterial and human heat-shock proteins have been proposed, but there are several arguments against such a directly pathogenetic role. Cells recognizing specific pathogens account for only a tiny minority (1:500) of the synovial cell population (Kingsley, personal communi-cation) and it is possible that the inflammatory milieu of the arthritic joint favours the relatively non-antigen-specific accumulation of memory T lymphocytes.

The importance of enteric colonization has been shown in the *HLA-B27* transgenic rat model. A group of *HLA-B27* transgenic rats maintained in a germ-free environment did not develop the spondylarthropathy or bowel inflammation seen in their littermates. The responsible enteric pathogen or pathogens have yet to be isolated (Taurog 1994). If this model is a true reflection of human disease, the *HLA-B27* gene may predispose an individual to spondylarthropathy by reducing immune resistance to enteric bacteria at the level of the antigen-presenting cell (Feltkamp *et al.* 1996).

Clinical features and outcome

It is frequently difficult to distinguish early or undifferentiated juve-nile spondylarthropathy from juvenile chronic arthritis. The spondylarthropathies are dynamic diseases that may continue to evolve over several years before reaching full expression. A child with arthritis in a peripheral joint(s) may not be suspected of having a spondylarthropathy until classical signs of axial involvement develop during the adult years. This section will deal firstly with the clinical features of the undifferentiated spondylarthropathies, and then with recognizable spondylarthropathies of ankylosing spondylitis, inflam-matory bowel disease, Reiter's syndrome, and psoriasis in childhood (Table 1).

Table 1 Classification of spondylarthropathies in children

Undifferentiated, atypical or prespondylitic syndromes:
  Seronegative enthesopathy and arthropathy (SEA) syndrome
  Late-onset pauciarticular juvenile arthritis
  Ankylosing tarsitis
  HLA-B27 with isolated enthesopathy
  HLA-B27 with isolated dactylitis

Juvenile ankylosing spondylitis

Arthritis associated with inflammatory bowel disease

Reiter's syndrome

Reactive arthritis (? incomplete Reiter's)

Psoriatic arthritis with HLA B-27 and sacroiliitis

Undifferentiated or atypical spondylarthropathy

In a population-based study from Sweden, Andersson Gare *et al.* (1987) reported that 5 per cent of children with chronic arthritis were classified with a spondylarthropathy, but it has been estimated that between 10 and 15 per cent of children diagnosed as having juve-nile chronic arthritis may eventually develop a spondylarthropathy. This poses a diagnostic challenge: to identify characteristic clinical features that predate the onset of back and sacroiliac symptoms, and therefore allow the prediction of outcome with some accuracy in this group of children with arthritis. Several descriptive, retrospective clinical studies of children who eventually developed an identifiable spondylarthropathy have provided useful information for this purpose (Schaller *et al.* 1976; Jacobs *et al.* 1982; Schaller 1983), and can be summarized as follows.

1. A family history of spondylarthropathy (defined as inflammatory low back disease) was described in up to 60 per cent of patients.

2. There was a strong male preponderance in patients; male:female ratios up to 10:1 have been reported.

3. Antecedent insults included febrile illnesses and musculo-skeletal trauma.

4. The arthritis was of 'late onset'; only 40 per cent of the children were symptomatic by their ninth year. The earliest reported onset was at 12 months of age.

5. The arthritis was typically pauciarticular and asymmetrical, predominantly involving the large, weight-bearing joints of the lower limbs.

6. Extra-articular manifestations occurred in 42 per cent of patients, including urethritis, iritis, conjunctivitis, and kerato-derma blennorrhagicum.

7. Enthesopathy was prominent in up to 75 per cent of patients.

Several sets of criteria have been proposed to differentiate childhood spondylarthropathy from other forms of juvenile arthritis. Most re-cently, the term 'late-onset pauci-articular juvenile chronic arthritis' has become fashionable, although there are no studies to indicate the validity of this designation (Table 2).

Table 2 Unclassified or atypical spondylarthropathies in childhood: evidence for progression of disease

Author/series	No. of patients	Period of follow-up (mean years)	SA onset	SEA	JAS at follow-up
1. Rosenberg and Petty (1982)	39	2	13	26	na
2. Cabral et al. (1992) (follow-up to 1 above)	36	11	13	23	12/23
3. Jacobs et al. (1982)	58[b]	5	5[a]		13[a]
4. Sheerin et al. (1988)	36[b]	8.9	5		27[c]
5. Prieur (1987)	65[b]	5[d]	4		7 (JAS) 14 (other SA)
6. Burgos-Vargas and Clark (1989)	20	6.2	0	20	19 (92.3%)
7. Olivieri (1992)	11	5	0	111 (9.1%)	

SA, spondylarthropathy; SEA, seronegative enthesopathy and arthropathy; JAS, juvenile ankylosing spondylitis.
[a]Clinical sacroiliitis—10/43 had radiographic evidence after 5 years.
[b]All HLA-B27 positive.
[c]Included 11/27 with possible JAS (sacroiliac joint tenderness only).
[d]Follow-up at 5 years in 33 patients.

The SEA syndrome

Clinical features

Rosenberg and Petty (1982) described 39 children (35 boys and 4 girls) with a syndrome of seronegative enthesopathy and arthropathy (**SEA syndrome**). The mean age of onset of the first musculoskeletal symptom was 9.8 years (range 1–16 years). This group included 13 patients who fulfilled diagnostic criteria for the diagnosis of juvenile ankylosing spondylitis, inflammatory bowel disease, reactive arthritis, or Reiter's syndrome. The remaining 26 did not have one of these identifiable diseases, but did have the combination of enthesitis and arthritis or arthralgia. Enthesitis was demonstrated by discrete, localized tenderness at the bony insertions of ligaments, tendons or fascias. Principle sites of enthesitis included the calcaneal insertions of the plantar fascia and Achilles tendons, the metatarsal heads and base of the fifth metatarsal, the ischial tuberosities, iliac crests, and patellar tendon insertions. Low back pain and stiffness were present in only nine patients, but many had abnormal flattening of the lumbar curve on forward flexion. HLA typing of 32 children demonstrated that 23 (72 per cent), including the eight patients with juvenile ankylosing spondylitis and one with Reiter's syndrome, were HLA-B27 positive.

Juvenile ankylosing tarsitis has been described in up to 80 per cent of patients with SEA syndrome and 87 per cent of those with juvenile ankylosing spondylitis (Levi et al. 1990; Burgos-Vargas 1991). These patients develop inflammation of synovial sheaths and bursas, tendons, entheses and joints of the feet, leading to radiographic or MRI evidence of ankylosis. Additionally, non-traumatic atlantoaxial subluxation has been reported in two HLA-B27-positive children with SEA syndrome (Foster et al. 1995).

Outcome

There have been several longer-term follow-up studies of patients with SEA syndrome. Cabral et al. (1992) reported on 36 of the original 39 patients described by Rosenberg and Petty (1982), 2.5 to 23.5 years (mean 11 years) after the onset of their symptoms. Assessment of outcome in the patients who did not have ankylosing spondylitis, inflammatory bowel disease, reactive arthritis, or Reiter's syndrome in the original study revealed that the disease had progressed to definite or probable ankylosing spondylitis in half (12 patients). The presence of arthralgia was less specific than definite arthritis for predicting a spondylitic outcome. Burgos-Vargas and Clark (1989) reported 20 Mexican patients with SEA syndrome, and compared their outcome after at least 5 years of follow-up with 25 patients with polyarticular-onset juvenile chronic arthritis and 28 patients with definite ankylosing spondylitis of juvenile onset. Radiographic evidence of sacroiliitis of the ankylosing spondylitis type showed in four patients with SEA syndrome before the third year of follow-up. From the third to the fifth year of follow-up, back complaints and radiographically confirmed sacroiliitis fulfilling the diagnostic criteria for ankylosing spondylitis developed in an increasing proportion of the patients (47.1–75 per cent) and ultimately affected 92.3 per cent. Other than the absence of back problems at the initial presentation, no significant differences in outcome were seen between the group with SEA syndrome and the group with juvenile ankylosing spondylitis.

Olivieri et al. (1992) reported that only 1 of 11 Caucasian HLA-B27-positive children (9.1 per cent) with SEA syndrome developed bilateral sacroiliitis after 5 years of disease. Ethnic and environmental factors were thought to have contributed to the discrepancy between these findings and those of the Mexican population reported by Burgos-Vargas and Clark (1989).

Atypical spondylarthropathy

Clinical features

Hussein et al. (1989) have proposed a set of diagnostic criteria for atypical spondylarthritis in a study of 26 children. Cases were classified according to criteria that were shown to be highly sensitive in differentiating atypical spondylarthropathies from other forms of juvenile chronic arthritis. The major criteria were (i) a family history of spondylarthropathy or oligoarthritis, (ii) enthesopathy, (iii) arthritis of digital joints including big toes, (iv) sacroiliitis, (v) presence of the *HLA-B27* gene, and (vi) recurrent arthralgia or arthritis. Minor criteria were (i) age of onset after 10 years of age, (ii) male sex, (iii) only the lower extremities affected, (iv) acute iritis or conjunctivitis, (v) arthritis of hips, and (vi) onset following an idiopathic enteritis. When four of the six major criteria were present, 96.1 per cent of the patients were correctly classified as having atypical spondylarthropathy, with a sensitivity of 84.6 per cent and a specificity of 100 per cent. The same diagnostic accuracy was achieved when three major and three minor criteria were present. Long-term follow-up studies of patients with atypical spondylarthropathy defined by the above criteria have not been reported.

HLA-B27-positive arthritis

Clinical features
The usefulness of HLA-B27 as a diagnostic marker of the juvenile spondylarthropathies has been discussed by many investigators, but interpretation of a positive HLA-B27 result is complicated by the occurrence of the gene in at least 8 per cent of the normal, non-arthritic childhood population. In addition, HLA-B27 has been associated with a number of different musculoskeletal diseases in children and it is unclear if these all form part of the spondylarthropathic spectrum. For example, there have been reports of children with isolated dactylitis (Siegel and Baum 1988), isolated peripheral enthesitis (Olivieri et al. 1990; Olivieri and Pasero 1992), and isolated hip flexion contractures (Bowyer 1995).

Outcome
A number of investigators have reported the outcome of children with arthritis who are HLA-B27 positive. Jacobs et al. (1982) described 58 such patients who were followed for a mean period of 5 years. The arthritis at the initiation of the illness was often transient and recurrent, pauciarticular and asymmetrical in distribution, and occurred primarily in the knees or ankles. Hip signs were noted in only seven of the patients at onset, but the hips were ultimately affected in 36 per cent. Radiographs of the sacroiliac joints were obtained for 43 of the patients, 10 of whom showed signs of sacroiliitis after a mean symptomatic period of 5 years (range 1–12 years). Other radiographic findings included periostitis, severe osteopenia, calcaneal erosions, or spurs. Rapid destruction of a single joint occurred in 3 of 58 patients.

Prieur (1987) reported a study of 65 children with HLA-B27-associated arthritis. There were 45 boys and 20 girls, with a mean age at onset of symptoms of 10 years (range 2.5–16 years). Just over a quarter of the patients (27 per cent) had arthritis in an upper limb during the first 6 months of disease. Enthesitis was present in 10 patients and 'sausage' digits in one-third. After 5 years' follow- up, 32 per cent had fulfilled criteria for the diagnosis of a defined spondylarthropathy: ankylosing spondylitis (7 patients), Reiter's syndrome (2 patients), psoriatic arthritis (9 patients), and Crohn's disease (3 patients).

Thirty-six HLA-B27-positive children with arthritis who had been followed for a mean period of 8.9 years were described by Sheerin et al. (1988). Five patients had an initial diagnosis of juvenile ankylosing spondylitis (14 per cent), and 24 (67 per cent) initially had peripheral

arthritis without axial involvement. The most frequently involved joint was the knee (15 patients), followed by the ankle (8 patients), and the foot (5 patients). During the follow-up period, 22 patients had symptoms consistent with enthesitis, although it was demonstrable in only 16 patients (44 per cent). Eight patients (22 per cent) had extra-articular manifestations: acute iritis (4 patients), inflammatory bowel disease (1), psoriasis (2), and localized scleroderma (1). One of the patients with psoriasis had recurrent episodes of urethritis suggestive of incomplete Reiter's syndrome. Of the 28 patients in whom radiographs of sacroiliac region had been taken, 13 had normal results. A clinical course consistent with juvenile ankylosing spondylitis ultimately developed in 27 of the 36 patients.

Juvenile ankylosing spondylitis

The Rome and New York criteria for the diagnosis of ankylosing spondylitis (Kellgren et al. 1963; Bennett and Burch 1967) were derived for use in adults, and have not been validated in the paediatric population. However, there is a small proportion of children with arthritis who do fulfil the criteria for the diagnosis of the disease.

Epidemiology
Historical averages in populations of children with arthritis attending paediatric rheumatology clinics have suggested that 5 to 8 per cent have ankylosing spondylitis compared with 75 to 83 per cent with juvenile chronic arthritis (Ladd et al. 1971). The prevalence of juvenile ankylosing spondylitis can also be extrapolated from the numbers of adult patients who report that onset occurred before they were 16 years old. Lawrence et al. (1989) reported an estimated prevalence of ankylosing spondylitis in populations from the United States ranging from 129/100 000 (Carter et al. 1979) to 222/100 000 (Mikkelsen et al. 1967). Generally between 10 and 19 per cent of cases begin before the age of 16 years (Hart and Maclagan 1955). The prevalence depends on the population under study; for example, Burgos-Vargas et al. (1989), describing a Mexican Mestizo population in which ankylosing spondylitis was diagnosed between 1980 and 1987, reported that 54 per cent had onset of symptoms before the age of 16 years. Over 90 per cent of patients in published series of juvenile ankylosing spondylitis were HLA-B27 positive as is true in the adult population (Edmonds et al. 1974; Sturrock et al. 1974; Veys et al. 1976; Hafner 1987; Cassidy and Petty 1995). The sum of these data suggests that the prevalence of juvenile ankylosing spondylitis is approx. 12 to 18/100 000.

Clinical characteristics
Juvenile ankylosing spondylitis in children commonly presents as an arthritis affecting the large joints of the lower limbs, particularly the knees and ankles (Schaller et al. 1969; Ladd et al. 1971; Bywaters 1976; Kleinman et al. 1977; Schaller 1977; Ansell 1980; Garcia-Morteo et al. 1983; Hafner 1987; Burgos-Vargas et al. 1989; Burgos-Vargas and Vazquez-Mellado 1995). Although it is rare for the hips to be involved at presentation, there is a small group of children in whom recurrent, transient hip symptoms eventually develop into ankylosing spondylitis. The early course of the disease is frequently episodic, and other features of an undifferentiated spondylarthropathy may be present. Inflammation of the entheses may be prominent early in the disease course. The most common sites include Achilles tendon insertions, peripatellar insertions including the quadriceps and patellar tendons, and the insertions of the plantar fascia into calcaneum and

Gerster, J. C., Payot, M., and Piccinin, P. (1987) Clinical and echocardiographic assessment in juvenile-onset. *British Journal of Rheumatology*, 26, 155–6.

Gore, J. E., Vizcarrondo, L. E., and Rieffel, C. N. (1981). Juvenile ankylosing spondylitis and aortic regurgitation: a case presentation. *Pediatrics*, 68, 423–6.

Hafner, R. (1987). Die juvenile spondarthritis. Retrospektive untersuchung on 91 patienten. *Monatsschrift Kinderheilkund*, 135, 41–6.

Hamilton, M. L., Gladman, D. D., Shore, A., Laxer, R. M., and Silverman, E. D. (1990). Juvenile psoriatic arthritis and HLA antigens. *Annals of the Rheumatic Diseases*, 49, 694–7.

Hart, F. D. and Maclagan, N. F. (1955). Ankylosing spondylitis. A review of 184 cases. *Annals of the Rheumatic Diseases*, 14, 77.

Hellgren, L. (1969). Association between arthritis and psoriasis in total populations. *Acta Rheumatologica*, 15, 316–26.

Hoppenfeld, S. (1976). Physical examination of the lumbar spine In *Physical examination of the spine and extremities* (ed. S. Hoppenfeld), pp. 261–2. Appleton-Century-Croft, New York.

Hussein, A., Abdul-Khaliq, H., and von der Hardt, H. (1989). Atypical spondyloarthropathies in children: proposed diagnostic criteria. *European Journal of Pediatrics*, 148, 513–17.

Iverson, J. M. I., Nanda, B. S., Hancock, J. A. H., Pownall, P. J., and Wright, V. (1975). Reiter's disease in three boys. *Annals of the Rheumatic Diseases*, 34, 364–8.

Jacobs, J. C., Berdon, W. E., and Johnson, A. D. (1982). HLA-B27-associated spondylarthritis and enthesopathy in childhood: clinical, pathologic, and radiographic observations in 58 patients. *Pediatrics*, 100, 521–8.

Jarvinen, P. (1995). Occurrence of ankylosing spondylitis in a nationwide series of twins. *Arthritis and Rheumatism*, 38, 381–3.

Kean, W. F., Anastassiades, T. P., and Ford, P. M. (1980). Aortic incompetence in HLA B27-positive juvenile arthritis. *Annals of the Rheumatic Diseases*, 39, 294–5.

Kellgren, J. H., Jeffrey, M. R., and Ball, J. (1963). *The epidemiology of chronic rheumatism*, Vol. 1, p. 326. Blackwell Scientific, Oxford.

Kleinman, P., Riverlis, M., Schneider, R., and Kaye, J. J. (1977). Juvenile ankylosing spondylitis. *Pediatric Radiology*, 125, 775–80.

Koo, E., Balogh, Z. S., and Gomor B. (1991). Juvenile psoriatic arthritis. *Clinical Rheumatology*, 10, 245–9.

Kuster, R. M. and Quoss, I. (1983). Juvenile psoriatic arthritis and spondylitis with or without psoriasis: probable and definite courses (Abstr.). *Zeitschrift für Rheumatologie*, 42, 310.

Ladd, J. R., Cassidy, J. T., and Martel, W. (1971). Juvenile ankylosing spondylitis. *Arthritis and Rheumatism*, 14, 579–90.

Lambert, J. R., Ansell, B. M., Stephenson, E., and Wright, V. (1976). Psoriatic arthritis in childhood. *Clinical Rheumatic Diseases*, 2, 339–52.

Levi, S., Ansell, B. M., and Klenerman, L. (1990). Tarsometatarsal involvement in juvenile. *Foot and Ankle Journal*, 11, 90–2.

Life, P., Hassel, A., Williams, K., et al. (1993). Responses to Gram-negative bacterial antigens by synovial T cells from patients with juvenile chronic arthritis: recognition of heat shock protein HSP60. *Journal of Rheumatology*, 20, 1388–96.

Lindsley, C. B. and Schaller, J. G. (1974). Arthritis associated with inflammatory bowel disease in children. *Journal of Pediatrics*, 84, 16–20.

Lockie, G. N. and Hunder, G. G. (1971). Reiter's syndrome in children: a case report and review. *Arthritis and Rheumatism*, 14, 767–72.

MacLean, L. (1992). HLA-B27 subtypes: implications for the spondyloarthropathies. *Annals of the Rheumatic Diseases*, 51, 929–31.

Marks, S. H., Barnett, M., and Calin, A. (1982). A case-control study of juvenile- and adult-onset ankylosing spondylitis. *Journal of Rheumatology*, 9, 739–41.

Mielants, H., Veys, E. M., Joos, R., Covelier, C., De Vos, M., and Proot, F. (1987). Late onset pauciarticular juvenile chronic arthritis: relation to gut inflammation. *Journal of Rheumatology*, 14, 459–65.

Mielants, H. et al. (1993). Gut inflammation in children with late onset pauciarticular juvenile chronic arthritis and evolution to adult — a prospective study. *Journal of Rheumatology*, 20, 1567–72.

Mikkelsen, W. M. et al. (1967). Estimates of the prevalence of rheumatic diseases in the population of Tecumseh, Michigan, 1959–60. *Journal of Chronic Diseases*, 20, 351–69.

Olivieri, I. and Pasero, G. (1992). Long-standing isolated juvenile onset HLA B-27 associated peripheral enthesitis. *Journal of Rheumatology*, 19, 164–5.

Olivieri, I., Barbieri, P., Gemignani, G., and Pasero, G. (1990). Isolated juvenile onset HLA-B27 associated peripheral enthesitis. *Journal of Rheumatology*, 17, 567–8.

Olivieri, I., Foto, M., Ruju, G. P., Gemignani, G., Giustarini, S., and Pasero, G. (1992). Low frequency of axial involvement in Caucasian pediatric patients with seronegative enthesopathy and arthropathy syndrome after 5 years of disease. *Journal of Rheumatology*, 19, 469–75.

Oriente, C. B., Scarpa, R., and Oriente, P. (1994). Prevalence and clinical features of juvenile psoriatic arthritis in 425 psoriatic patients. *Acta Dermatologica Venereologica (Stockholm)*, Suppl. 186, 109–10.

Passo, M. H., Fitzgerald, J. F., and Brandt, K. D. (1986). Arthritis associated with inflammatory bowel disease in children: relationship of joint disease to activity and severity of bowel lesion. *Digestive Disease Science*, 31, 492–7.

Petty, R. E. (1990). HLA-B27 and rheumatic diseases of childhood. *Journal of Rheumatology*, 17, 7–10.

Petty, R. E. (1994). Juvenile psoriatic arthritis, or juvenile arthritis with psoriasis? *Clinical and Experimental Rheumatology*, 12 (Suppl. 10), S55–8.

Prieur, A. M. (1987). HLA B27 associated chronic arthritis in children: review of 65 cases. *Scandinavian Journal of Rheumatology*, 66 (Suppl.), 51–6.

Reid, G. D. and Hill, R. H. (1978). Atlanta-axial subluxation in juvenile ankylosing spondylitis. *Journal of Pediatrics*, 93, 531–2.

Reid, G. D., Patterson, M. W. H., Patterson, A. C., and Cooperberg, P. L. (1979). Aortic insufficiency in association with juvenile ankylosing spondylitis. *Journal of Pediatrics*, 95, 78–80.

Rosenberg, A. M. and Petty, R. E. (1979). Reiter's disease in children. *American Journal of Diseases of Children*, 133, 394–8.

Rosenberg, A. M. and Petty, R. E. (1982). A syndrome of seronegative enthesopathy and arthropathy in children. *Arthritis and Rheumatism*, 25, 1041–7.

Schaller, J. G. (1977). Ankylosing spondylitis of childhood onset. *Arthritis and Rheumatism*, 20, 398–401.

Schaller, J. G. (1983). Pauciarticular arthritis of childhood (pauciarticular juvenile arthritis). *Annales de Pediatrie*, 30, 557–63.

Schaller, J. G. (1985). The spondyloarthropathies (variant diseases) In *Practice of pediatrics*, Vol. 8, (ed. V. E. Kelly), pp. 1–10. Harper and Row, Philadelphia.

Schaller, J. G., Bitnum, S., and Wedgwood, R. J. (1969). Ankylosing spondylitis with childhood onset. *Journal of Pediatrics*, 74, 505–16.

Schaller, J. G., Ochs, H. D., Thomas, E. D., Nisperos, B., Feigl, P., and Wedgewood, R. J. A. (1976). Histocompatibility antigens in childhood onset arthritis. *Journal of Pediatrics*, 88, 926–30.

Sheerin, K. A., Giannini, E. H., Brewer, E. J., Jr, and Barron, K. S. (1988). HLA-B27-associated arthropathy in childhood: long-term clinical and diagnostic outcome. *Arthritis and Rheumatism*, 31, 1165–70.

Shore, A. and Ansell, B. M. (1982). Juvenile psoriatic arthritis — an analysis of 60 cases. *Journal of Pediatrics*, 4, 529–35.

Siegel, D. M. and Baum, J. (1988). HLA-B27 associated dactylitis in children. *Journal of Rheumatology*, 15, 976–7.

Sills, E. M. (1980). Psoriatic arthritis in childhood. *Johns Hopkins Medical Journal*, 146, 49–53.

Singsen, B. H., Bernstein, B. H., Koster-King, K. G., Glovsky, M. M., and Hanson, V. (1977). Reiter's syndrome in childhood. *Arthritis and Rheumatism*, 20 (Suppl.), 402–7.

Southwood, T. R. and Gaston, J.S.H. (1993). Evolution of synovial fluid mononuclear cell responses in a HLA-B27-positive patient with *Yersinia*-associated juvenile arthritis. *British Journal of Rheumatology*, 32, 845–8.

Southwood, T. R. et al. (1989). Psoriatic arthritis in children. *Arthritis and Rheumatism*, 32, 1007–13.

Stamato, T. et al. (1995). Prevalence of cardiac manifestations of juvenile ankylosing spondylitis. *American Journal of Cardiology*, 75, 744–6.

Stewart, S. R., Robbins, D. L., and Castles, J. J. (1978). Acute fulminant aortic and mitral insufficiency in ankylosing spondylitis. *New England Journal of Medicine*, 299, 1448–9.

Sturrock, R. D., Dick, H. M., Henderson, N., Goel, G. K., Lee, W. C., and Buchanan, W. W. (1974). Association of HL-A27 and AJ in juvenile arthritis and ankylosing spondylitis. *Journal of Rheumatology*, 1, 269–73.

Taurog, J.D., Richardson, J.A., Croft, J.T., et al. (1994). The germ free state prevents the development of gut and joint inflammatory disease in HLA-B27 transgenic rats. *Journal of Experimental Medicine*, 180, 2359–64.

Thomas, D. G. and Roberton, D. M. (1994). Reiter's syndrome in an adolescent girl. *Acta Paediatrica*, **83**, 339–40.

Truckenbrodt, H. and Hafner, R. (1990). Die psoriasisarthritis intramuscular kindesalter. *Z Rheumatol*, **49**, 88–94.

Van der Linden, S.M., Valkenburg, H.A., de Jongh, B.M., and Cats, A. (1984). The risk of developing ankylosing spondylitis in HLA-B27 positive individuals. A comparison of relatives of spondylitis patients with the general population. *Arthritis and Rheumatism*, **27**, 241–9.

Veys, E. M., Coigne, E., Mielants, H., and Vergruggen, A. (1976). HLA and juvenile chronic polyarthritis. *Tissue Antigens*, **8**, 61–5.

Veys, E. M., Mielants, H., Joos, R., and Clercq, L. D. (1992) Juvenile spondyloarthropathies in 1992. *Journal of Rheumatology*, **20** (Suppl. 37), 19–25.

5.5.3   Ankylosing spondylitis

Andrei Calin

Historical review

As summarized elsewhere (Calin 1988) Raymond, in 1912, provided convincing illustrations of mummies from Egypt who appeared to have ankylosing spondylitis. The paleopathologist, Sir Mark Ruffer, described a gentleman called Nefermaat who lived some 3000 years before Christ. His mummified remains demonstrated a rigid block of bone from the mid-cervical region to the sacrum. Short described 18 further instances of ankylosing spondylitis from Egyptian sources over the next 3 millennia and other examples exist from the Danish and French neolithic periods. More recent (AD 1200) remains of New Mexican Indians with ankylosing spondylitis have been described. There has, over the last decades, been some debate as to whether these individuals had diffuse idiopathic skeletal hyperostosis or ankylosing spondylitis; although there is no absolute certainty, the fused sacroiliac joints in many instances attest to such patients having ankylosing spondylitis.

In the nineteenth century Bechterew, Strumpell, and Marie promoted the general recognition of ankylosing spondylitis.

Diagnostic criteria

Criteria for the classification and diagnosis of different rheumatic diseases have been developed to help different clinicians in different locations use the same diagnostic labels for similar groups of patients. Originally, criteria were formulated in Rome in 1961 and later revised in New York in 1966 (Bennett and Burch 1968) (Table 1). The most frequent means of satisfying these is a radiographic demonstration of grade 3 or 4 bilateral sacroiliitis (Fig. 1), together with a history of back pain. In fact, few clinicians rely on these criteria and most would consider a patient as having ankylosing spondylitis if symptomatic and with sacroiliitis. Naturally, as discussed in Chapter 5.5.1, there are often exceptions to any list of criteria and, although of major concern to the epidemiologist, the clinician is often satisfied to use 'common sense' rather than rigid criteria. For example, we do recognize ankylosing spondylitis *sine* sacroiliitis on the one hand or atypical forms of disease on the other.

Table 1   Criteria for ankylosing spondylitis

Rome criteria

Clinical criteria

1. Low back pain > 3 months, relieved by rest
2. Thoracic pain and stiffness
3. History of iritis
4. Limited motion of lumbar spine
5. Limited chest expansion

Radiological criteria

1. Bilateral sacroiliitis

Ankylosing spondylitis is diagnosed if bilateral sacroiliitis plus one clinical criterion, or four out of five clinical criteria, are present.

New York criteria

Clinical criteria

1. Limited movement of lumbar spine in three planes
2. Pain in lumbar spine or at dorsolumbar junction
3. Chest expansion < 2.5 cm

Radiological criteria

1. Bilateral sacroiliitis, grade 3–4
2. Unilateral sacroiliitis, grade 3–4, or bilateral sacroiliitis, grade 2

The disease is considered primary if no other rheumatological disorder is present, or secondary if the sacroiliitis is related to psoriatic arthropathy, inflammatory bowel disease or Reiter's syndrome. One great difficulty lies in the prevalence of patients with clinical symptoms and radiological signs of disease but in whom the radiologist has failed to recognize sacroiliitis. Such individuals are often misdiagnosed as having mechanical back pain or other

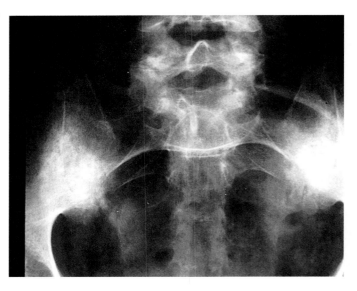

Fig. 1   Pelvic radiograph (anteroposterior view) revealing grade IV sacroiliitis. Note marked juxta-articular sclerosis and destruction of joint with fusion.

inappropriate labels. In essence, a single anteroposterior film of the pelvis is sufficient to define the radiological entity. More sophisticated investigations such as the use of magnetic resonance imaging are always expensive and may be inappropriate and unhelpful (Braun *et al.* 1994).

A review of the Rome Criteria reveals an obvious flaw: the limitation of spinal movement is not defined. The New York Criteria do define limitation of chest expansion as 2.5 cm or less but there is inevitably a major subjective component to chest expansion, and decreased movement typically occurs only late in the course of the disease. Pain, as such, is too sensitive and too non-specific to be used as a criterion and we have developed a simple analysis of the qualitative nature of pain in patients with inflammatory spinal disease (i.e. ankylosing spondylitis). Specifically, (Calin and Fries 1977) (i) patients are typically below 40 years of age at onset; (ii) the onset is insidious; (iii) duration has been at least 3 months at first attendance; (iv) there is an association with morning stiffness; and (v) improvement occurs with exercise. For those with three or more of these features a pelvic radiograph should elucidate whether there is evidence of sacroiliitis. HLA B27 typing has led to immense strides in the understanding of the spondylarthropathy group but should not be considered a diagnostic test or necessary for the diagnosis of ankylosing spondylitis. A patient with symptomatic sacroiliitis lacking HLA B27 still has ankylosing spondylitis and, moreover, the test is frequently negative in secondary forms of ankylosing spondylitis, where only some 50 per cent of those with enteropathic spondylitis or psoriatic spondylitis carry the antigen. Occasionally sacroiliitis is seen as a chance finding in the absence of pain. Presumably the precipitating trigger has been pulled in the susceptible individual, but for reasons not clearly understood, symptoms have never reached a threshold noticed by patient or physician. A review of Bayesian theory reminds us that HLA B27 typing can only be helpful when we are 50 per cent certain of the diagnosis.

By using Bayesian analysis it has been pointed out that if the clinician is 50 per cent certain of the diagnosis, then HLA B27 typing is helpful, whereas at the extremes of a priori probability such testing is of no use. Clearly, the physician is unlikely to know when he or she is 50 per cent confident! The clinician perhaps should simply treat with a non-steroidal anti-inflammatory drug if a diagnosis of ankylosing spondylitis appears possible, rather than relying on further testing such as computed tomography and other investigations (Calin 1980; Calin 1982).

In epidemiological and familial studies patients are sometimes found with unilateral sacroiliitis, dactylitis, syndesmophytes, and other stigmata of 'undifferentiated spondylarthropathy'(see Chapter 5.5.1).

Until the specific environmental trigger(s), gene(s), and biological mechanism(s) leading to disease pathogenesis are fully elucidated, the obsessional use of criteria for classification may be inappropriate.

Epidemiology

During the 1950s it was recognized that ankylosing spondylitis occurred in twins, brothers, fathers, mothers and other relatives of affected individuals. Indeed, Strecher (1957) found the disease to be 30 times more prevalent among relatives of spondylitics than among controls. The author suggested that the disease was inherited as a single autosomal dominant factor with '70 per cent penetrance in men and 10 per cent penetrance in women'. In 1967 Emery and

Lawrence studied 188 available first-degree relatives of 76 probands with ankylosing spondylitis and appropriately matched controls. Sixteen per cent of the first-degree relatives of patients had sacroiliitis, with 20 per cent of the males affected and 8 per cent of the females — a ratio higher than the often quoted 10:1 (male:female) ratio claimed at that time.

The search for an explanation for this increased heritability took a dramatic step forward in 1973 with two reports of the association between ankylosing spondylitis and HLA B27. Indeed, the link between HLA B27 and ankylosing spondylitis could elucidate several observations:

1. The family clustering as discussed above. HLA B27 is inherited as an autosomal codominant characteristic, 50 per cent of first-degree relatives of probands with HLA B27 possessing the antigen.

2. Uveitis is a common accompaniment of ankylosing spondylitis. HLA B27 is found in some 40 per cent of individuals with acute unilateral self-limiting uveitis, even in the absence of underlying rheumatological disease.

3. Many patients with Reiter's disease develop sacroiliitis. Overall, some 80 per cent of patients with reactive arthropathy are HLA B27 positive, those developing sacroiliitis and ascending spinal disease being more closely linked to HLA B27. Whether the sacroiliitis in such patients should be considered a complication of Reiter's syndrome or a further manifestation of the HLA B27 status remains unclear.

4. Juvenile chronic arthropathy, psoriatic arthropathy, and inflammatory bowel disease can all be associated with sacroiliitis and ankylosing spondylitis and it is known that HLA B27 is increased in all three groups who have a spondylarthropathy picture.

For a further discussion of the link between HLA B27 and the spondylarthropathies, the reader is directed to Chapter 5.5.1 and elsewhere. Herein some further clinical aspects may be summarized:

1. Some 5 to 10 per cent of HLA B27 positive individuals develop ankylosing spondylitis after an unknown environmental event and 20 per cent of subjects with HLA B27 develop reactive arthropathy after contact with an arthritogenic agent (chlamydia, salmonella, etc.).

2. Up to 5 per cent of Caucasian patients with ankylosing spondylitis are not HLA B27 positive.

3. Only 50 per cent of those with psoriatic or enteropathic spondylitis are B27 positive.

4. The association between ankylosing spondylitis and HLA B27 in non-Caucasians (around 50 per cent) is much less than that seen in Caucasians.

5. Relatives of probands with both sacroiliitis and HLA B27, even when carrying an identical HLA haplotype, frequently remain disease free.

6. The Pima and Haida Indians, both with a high frequency of HLA B27, develop ankylosing spondylitis frequently but Reiter's syndrome rarely, if ever. By contrast, the Navaho Indians and Alaskan Inupiat Eskimos develop Reiter's syndrome more frequently than ankylosing spondylitis.

7. Ankylosing spondylitis and Reiter's syndrome tend to 'breed true' within families (Calin *et al.* 1984).

8. HLA B27 relatives of HLA B27-positive patients are 20 times more likely to develop ankylosing spondylitis than are HLA B27-positive relatives of healthy HLA B27 subjects. The distribution of HLA B27 among different healthy and disease groups is summarized in Chapter 5.5.2, Table 2, and discussed more fully elsewhere (Calin 1989; Calin and Elswood 1989a; De Castro 1994; Inman and Schfield 1994; Khan 1996; Toivanen and Toivanen 1996; Lopez-Larrea *et al.* 1996; Scofield 1996; Braun and Sieper 1996).

9. Some 11 subtypes of HLA-B27 are now recognized.

Prevalence (see van der Linden and van der Heijde 1996)

With the increased awareness and interest in the disease, many patients who previously were thought to have mechanical back pain, 'seronegative rheumatoid arthritis', and other disorders are now recognized as having ankylosing spondylitis. The true prevalence of ankylosing spondylitis appears to be in the region of 0.25 to 1 per cent with a peak of 2 per cent in northern Norway. The figures contrast sharply with older data reporting a ratio of ankylosing spondylitis to rheumatoid disease of about 1:15.

Several studies of blood donor populations suggest that up to 20 per cent of HLA-B27-positive individuals develop symptomatic ankylosing spondylitis, the majority of whom did not carry a diagnosis. Of interest, some 20 per cent of HLA-B27-positive individuals develop reactive arthropathy/Reiter's syndrome following infection with an arthritogenic trigger. Other studies have suggested that some 10 per cent of individuals with HLA-B27 develop ankylosing spondylitis (Dawkins *et al.* 1981), while up to 20 per cent of Pima and Haida men with HLA-B27 have the condition.

The prevalence and nature of spondylarthropathy varies in different ethnic groups. For example, Boyer *et al.* (1994) identified 104 cases of spondylarthropathy in an Eskimo population, a prevalence of 2.5 per cent in adults aged 20 years and over. They found undifferentiated spondylarthropathy and reactive arthropathy to be more common than ankylosing spondylitis *per se*. Strikingly, they found the prevalence of spondylarthropathy to have an equal sex distribution. Of note, although the prevalence of HLA-B27 is in the range of 20 to 40 per cent, the number of cases of spondylarthropathy was not as high as that found among the Canadian Haida Indians (6 to 10 per cent) (Braun *et al.* 1994). Elsewhere, Alexeeva *et al.* (1994) studied the prevalence of spondylarthritis amongst the native population of Chukotaa in Russia. Among these circumpolar subjects, they found the prevalence of spondylarthropathy to be 2.5 per cent, with 1 per cent having ankylosing spondylitis. HLA-B27 occurred in 34 per cent of the population. Nasution *et al.* (1993) found intriguing data in Indonesia. Specifically, HLA-B27 was found in 62 per cent of the Chinese patients with ankylosing spondylitis compared with under 3 per cent among the healthy controls. In contrast, only 8 per cent of the native Indonesians with disease were HLA-B27 positive compared with 9 per cent of the healthy controls, indicating the lack of association between HLA-B27 and disease in native Indonesians. Finally, Mijiyawa (1993) found spondylarthritis in 31 of 2000 patients

Table 2 Major differences between ankylosing spondylitis in men and in women

	Males	Females
Family history	+	++
Association with psoriasis	++	+
Association with inflammatory bowel disease	++	+++
HLA B27	>90 per cent	>90 per cent
Disease activity	++	+++
Function (severity)	++	+++
Peripheral joint disease:		
Initial	+	++
Subsequent	+	+++
Spinal ankylosis[a]	++	+
Cervical spine symptoms	+	++
Osteitis pubis	+	+++

[a]Skipping thoracic and lumbar spine in females.

in Lomé, Togo. In this population eight patients were HIV carriers. They therefore concluded that spondylarthropathy would appear to be less rare in black Africans than hitherto considered. Moreover, the frequency is likely to rise with the increase in HIV prevalence.

Delay in diagnosis

Until recently delays of between 5 and 10 years were recorded between the onset of symptoms and the diagnosis at last being made. There are now preliminary data suggesting that this delay is decreasing (Calin *et al.* 1988).

Sex distribution

That ankylosing spondylitis may occur much more frequently in females than hitherto suggested has been confirmed by several studies. In our large series in Britain, the sex ratio is in the region of 2.5 to 1 in favour of men, a figure confirmed by other studies. Distinguishing features between men and women with disease are discussed below (and see Table 2) (Will *et al.* 1990a; Kennedy *et al.* 1993).

Racial distribution (see Khan 1990; Khan 1996)

It has long been recognized that ankylosing spondylitis occurs more frequently in Caucasian populations. In fact it appears that ankylosing spondylitis roughly follows the distribution of HLA-B27. For example, in the American Indian where HLA-B27 prevalences have been reported ranging from 18 to 50 per cent, ankylosing spondylitis is particularly frequent, whereas the condition is less common in the black American, where HLA-B27 has a prevalence of 3 to 4 per cent, and correspondingly rarer in black Africans, where HLA-B27 occurs in under 1 per cent. Strikingly, the association with HLA-B27 is less dominant in those races where this phenotype is less frequent (e.g. only 60 to 70 per cent of Japanese patients are HLA-B27 positive; the frequency of which in the general population is correspondingly low (1 to 2 per cent)).

Age distribution (see Kennedy et al. 1994)

Sacroiliac and spinal disease usually develop in the late teenage years or in the early twenties in primary ankylosing spondylitis, whereas in those with secondary forms of disease, older ages at onset are seen. Interestingly, in the developing world, ankylosing spondylitis occurs more frequently at a younger age, teenagers with onset of disease being frequently found. By contrast, in the developed world onset in the mid- to late twenties is relatively more common. As discussed in Chapter 5.5.1, there may well be a changing pattern in disease. Our studies (Will *et al.* 1990*b*; Will *et al.* 1992) have suggested that within France and Britain the age at onset of ankylosing spondylitis is increasing. The fact that different studies using different epidemiological techniques have produced these findings is of particular interest.

Pathological features

The unique pathology of ankylosing spondylitis and the spondylarthritides was clearly defined in 1971 by Ball and developed further by Bywaters (1984). In contrast to the situation in rheumatoid disease the primary pathological site is the enthesis (insertion of ligaments and capsules into bone) rather than the synovium. In addition, the enthesopathic change is characterized by fibrosis and ossification rather than joint destruction and instability. In the spine, enthesopathic changes at the site of insertion of the outer fibres of the anulus fibrosus result in squaring of vertebral bodies (Fig. 2), vertebral end-plate destruction, and syndesmophyte formation (Fig. 3). The enthesis is a metabolically active site, perhaps explaining why early changes in ankylosing spondylitis occur during growth in the teenage years. In spite of our understanding about HLA-B27 and the

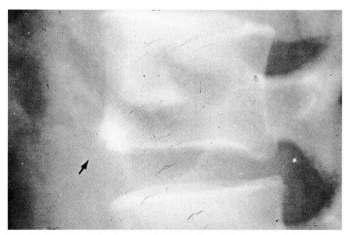

Fig. 2 Squaring of lumbar vertebral body in ankylosing spondylitis. Note sclerosis of bone at site of enthesopathic change at insertion of anterior fibres of the annulus fibrosis.

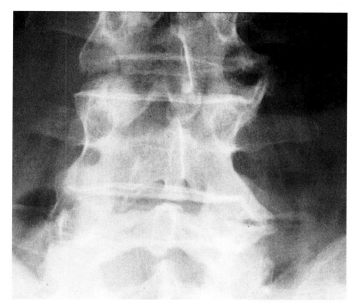

Fig. 3 Note syndesmorphytes between vertebral bodies. These are vertically directed new bone lesions associated with normal joint space.

pathology we still do not understand why the enthesis preferentially becomes affected.

In summary, ossification occurs in the region of the discs, the epiphyseal and sacroiliac joints and extraspinal sites, initiated by lesions at the site of ligamentous insertion. Synovitis itself does occur in peripheral joints and a proliferative synovitis can mimic that seen in rheumatoid disease. For reasons that we do not yet understand, soluble HLA Class II antigens are found in high levels in the synovial fluid in both rheumatoid arthritis and degenerative arthritis but in very low levels in spondylarthritis (Armas *et al.* 1990).

Clinical features

Ankylosing spondylitis will only be diagnosed when there is a high index of suspicion in a patient presenting with back pain of an inflammatory nature. In any such individual the differential diagnosis relates to mechanical dysfunction. The two conditions are contrasted in Table 3.

We have demonstrated a striking loss of bone mineral content in early disease (Will *et al.* 1990*c*). Juxta-articular and generalized osteoporosis are well recognized in rheumatoid disease but the relative role of hormonal factors, immobility, drug therapy, and the disease process is unclear. As discussed, ankylosing spondylitis is characterized by inflammation at the site of the enthesis which can lead to local bone erosion and juxtainsertional osteoporosis, followed by new bone formation. Although it has long been recognized that patients with severe ankylosing spondylitis may develop a dorsal kyphosis with some anterior wedging of the vertebrae, early osteoporosis has not until now been recognized. Whether the pattern of bone loss relates to tumour necrosis factor or other mediators remains unclear. HLA-B27-positive brothers of HLA-B27-positive patients have normal bone density. To what extent this early osteoporosis in patients who have normal spine mobility should be considered an early pathological marker, with changes at the enthesis being secondary in nature, is unknown.

Table 3 Differential findings in mechanical and inflammatory back pain

	Mechanical	Inflammatory
Past history	±	++
Family history	−	+
Onset	Acute	Insidious
Age (years)	15–90	<40
Sleep disturbance	±	++
Morning stiffness	+	+++
Involvement of other systems	−	+
Effect of exercise	Worse	Better
Effect of rest	Better	Worse
Radiation of pain	Anatomic (S1, L5)	Diffuse (thoracic, buttock)
Sensory symptoms	+	−
Motor symptoms	+	−
Scoliosis	+	−
Range of movement decreased	Asymmetrically	Symmetrically
Local tenderness	Local	Diffuse
Muscle spasm	Local	Diffuse
Straight-leg raising	Decreased	Normal
Sciatic nerve stretch	Positive	Absent
Hip involvement	−	+
Neurodeficit	+	−
Other systems	−	+

Spinal symptoms

Late spinal complications

Few patients progress relentlessly to the classical late 'bamboo spine' (Figs. 4 and 5). The fused spine may fracture (Fig. 6) following trivial or even unrecognized injury and microfractures and clinical fractures are relatively common in severe ankylosing spondylitis. The spinal deformity may make it difficult to see a fracture site, particularly in the low neck, and special views may be required. The fracture may be clinically silent or a dramatic event which can be fatal in outcome. A sudden exacerbation of back pain, spontaneously or following mild trauma, may relate to a fracture or a localized defect of the vertebral end plate (destruction of the disc–bone border). Spondylodiscitis is the term given to this lesion and may require rest and analgesia, with pain decreasing over 2 or 3 weeks. This contrasts with the usual exercise programme required for patients. The nature of spondylodiscitis and its prevalence has recently been defined in a cross-sectional study of over 100 patients, some 12 per cent of whom had radiological evidence of discitis, though often asymptomatic in nature (Kabasakal *et al.* 1994).

Extraspinal joint disease

Some 20 to 40 per cent of patients have peripheral joint disease at some stage during their illness. This may be asymmetric and often affects the lower limbs predominantly. Hip (Fig. 7) ankylosis and shoulder disease may provide major disability, with temporomandibular joint dysfunction occurring in up to 10 per cent of patients. HLA-DR4 may be associated with peripheral joint disease.

We have recently shown that there is a striking inverse correlation between the age at onset of disease and hip involvement; the vast majority of individuals requiring a total hip replacement having onset of disease during the teenage years. Hip involvement in those with onset in the twenties or later is vanishingly rare. For those requiring hip replacement, bilateral surgery is frequent. The long-term outcome for those with total hip replacements is excellent, the majority doing well some 10 years after replacement (Calin and Elswood 1989*b*).

Enthesopathic lesions

In view of the pathological disorder it is not surprising that patients have insertional tendinitis at any site typified by involvement of the

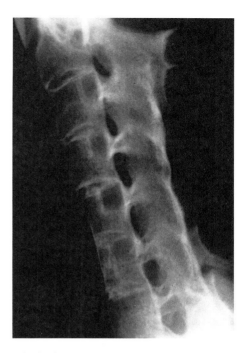

Fig. 4 Cervical spine in severe ankylosing spondylitis. Note fusion of facetal joints and anterior fusion of bodies with squaring of vertebrae.

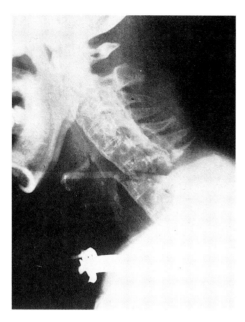

Fig. 6 Fracture of fused cervical spine in ankylosing spondylitis following minimal trauma — note defect in C6.

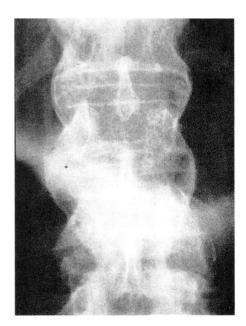

Fig. 5 Fused lumbar spine vertebrae with syndesmorphytes linking vertebrae.

Extra-articular disease

Until recently ankylosing spondylitis was predominantly considered to be a spinal disease with little constitutional systemic involvement. It is now recognized that the disorder may affect all body systems and indeed may not be immunologically silent.

General symptoms

Constitutional features include fatigue, weight loss, low grade fever, hypochromic or normochromic anaemia, and increased erythrocyte sedimentation rate. For many patients, fatigue is the major component. We have shown (Calin *et al.* 1993*a*) that in a comparison of

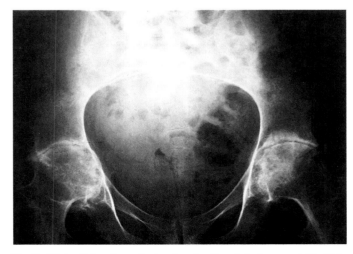

Fig. 7 Bilateral hip arthropathy in a female with ankylosing spondylitis. Note joint space reduction and erosive change in heads of femora.

Achilles tendon, intercostal muscle insertions, plantar fasciitis, and dactylitis.

Apart from low back pain some patients have a 'pleuritic' type of chest pain that may cause sleep disturbance and anxiety. This pain is worse on inspiration and relates to an insertional tendinitis of the small costosternal and costovertebral muscles.

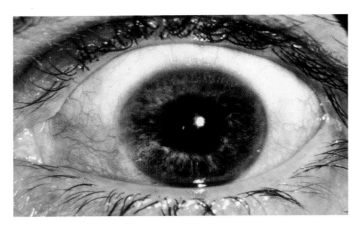

Fig. 8 An example of severe recurrent iritis with both active change and evidence of old damage.

pain, stiffness, and fatigue, the three major features of ankylosing spondylitis, the last of these has been a major component for a large minority. The main difficulty relates to management. Exercise and anti-inflammatory drugs are good for both the pain and stiffness but, to date, fatigue remains a frustrating symptom to treat. Certain features such as an arthropathy and uveitis can occur at any time in the course of the disease; other problems are predominantly associated with severe chronic involvement. Examples of the latter include aortic regurgitation, cord compression, upper lobe pulmonary fibrosis, and amyloid deposition.

Eye disease

Iritis (Fig. 8) occurs in up to 40 per cent of patients with ankylosing spondylitis and, as mentioned, has little correlation with the disease activity in the spine. Although the visual episodes are often self-limiting, local steroid drops or systemic therapy may be required. In a recent study (Edmunds and Calin 1991) we have shown that there is no relationship between the inflammation of the uveal tract and spine. In addition we failed to define any obvious environmental trigger even in those with recurrent disease. For example, there is no seasonal pattern.

Pulmonary involvement

Chronic infiltrative and fibrotic changes in the upper lobe of the lungs may occur. This upper lobe pulmonary fibrosis is now well recognized. Cough, sputum, and dyspnoea may develop with the sputum becoming profuse. Radiographs reveal usually bilateral upper lobe pulmonary fibrosis, sometimes with cyst formation and parenchial destruction. The lesions can be invaded by aspergillus with changes mimicking tuberculosis. Histology reveals patchy pneumonia with round cell and fibroblast infiltration progressing to interalveolar fibrosis. Dense pleural and pulmonary fibrosis can occur. Treatment is of no avail and death may follow massive haemoptysis.

A rigid chest wall may result from fusion of the thoracic joints but pulmonary ventilation is usually well maintained by the diaphragm. In an analysis of deaths in patients with ankylosing spondylitis Court-Brown and Doll (1965) noted deaths from respiratory causes to be some three times higher than in a control population.

Cardiovascular disease

Cardiovascular involvement is well recognized. The stated prevalence of this complication varies from 3.5 per cent of cases within 15 years to 10 per cent with up to 30 years duration. Although heart disease occurs more frequently in those with more severe spondylitis, cardiac conduction defects and other abnormalities may occur in those with minimal disease.

Aortic incompetence, cardiomegaly, and persistent defects in cardiac conduction are the most common findings with complete atrioventricular block occasionally occurring. Pericarditis has been described and cardiac involvement can range from being clinically silent to dominating the picture.

Aortic incompetence is the best studied complication. Up to 20 per cent of patients with ankylosing spondylitis may have anatomic evidence of involvement of the aortic valve but few of these have clinically detectable valvular dysfunction. Scar tissue and intimal fibrous proliferation may affect the aortic valve cusps and aorta behind and above the sinuses of Valsalva. Scar tissue may extend below the base of the aortic valve producing a subaortic fibrous ridge. Occasionally the aortitis is evident before any evidence of ankylosing spondylitis and the condition can thus be considered a *forme fruste*, similar to the occurrence of uveitis in a HLA-B27-positive individual without underlying rheumatological disease.

Amyloidosis

Amyloid is an occasional complication of ankylosing spondylitis. In one study, 3 of 35 patients were found to have amyloid on routine rectal biopsy. Although relatively common the event is rarely of clinical significance.

Renal disease

There appears to be no impairment of renal glomerular function in ankylosing spondylitis, in spite of the recognized pathological changes. In a study of 38 consecutive patients with severe ankylosing spondylitis, investigation of glomerular function failed to show any marked abnormality (Calin 1975). Nevertheless, immunoglobulin A (IgA) nephropathy is well recognized. However this appears to be of relatively little clinical significance.

Neurological syndromes

Involvement of the cauda equina may occur in the later stages of the disease. The syndrome presents with insidious onset of leg and buttock pain with sensory and motor impairment in association with bowel and bladder dysfunction. Lumbar diverticulae are found on myelographic examination. Unfortunately, treatment appears to be of no help, but a single case report suggests the value of a peritoneal shunt in one of our patients in whom the deterioration has been arrested.

Bowel disease (see Mielants et al. 1993a; Mielants et al. 1993b)

As discussed above and in Chapter 5.5.2 there is an intimate relationship between the bowel and ankylosing spondylitis. Low-grade bowel inflammation has been described (on ileocolonoscopy) in the absence of symptoms. The relevance of these findings remains unclear, although we know that the HLA–B27-positive transgenic rat develops a picture typical of spondylarthropathy with a major degree of bowel involvement. There is also a suggestion that there is increased gut permeability in patients and relatives, perhaps relating to disease pathogenesis (Martinez-Gonzalez *et al.* 1994).

Physical examination

Spinal mobility is symmetrically decreased but may still be normal in the earlier stages of disease. A variety of measurements have been described, although the modified Schober is the most useful. The distraction of a line drawn from the midpoint between the posterior iliac spines to an arbitrary site 10 cm above this point is measured and the distraction noted on forward flexion. In a normal individual this 10 cm line increases by some 50 to 100 per cent whereas a patient with active disease may only have a distraction of some 20 per cent or less. Lateral spinal flexion may be measured by noticing the distraction on contralateral flexion of a line drawn in the midaxillary plane. As mentioned above, chest expansion can be reduced, although this may only occur late in the disease. Moreover, in the female—for obvious reasons—chest expansion is difficult to measure precisely. Intermalleolar straddle on abducting the legs is a useful measurement of non-specific pelvic inflammation, and neck mobility can be measured. A formal approach to defining mobility in disease has now been validated (the Bath Ankylosing Spondylitis Radiology Index, BASRI) (Jenkinson *et al.* 1994).

There may be muscle spasm with loss of the normal lumbar lordosis, while some individuals may present with pain but no physical abnormality. Peripheral joints may be normal or grossly involved—particularly in women, who tend to have more peripheral joint disease than men.

Radiological evaluation

The five grades of sacroiliitis introduced by the New York Criteria range from 0 to 4. These are summarized in Table 4. Grade 0 refers to normal joints with clear sacroiliac margins and uniform joint space. There is no juxta-articular sclerosis. Grade 1 signifies suspicious change but no definite abnormality, while grades 2 and 3 relate to an increasing degree of sacroiliitis, as defined by blurring of the joint margin, juxta-articular sclerosis, decreased joint width, and erosive change. Grade 4 describes complete fusion or ankylosis of the joints with or without residual sclerosis.

A single anteroposterior view radiograph of the pelvis is sufficient. Sacroiliitis does not occur as an age-related phenomenon although degenerative change of the sacroiliac joints may occur. Osteitis condensans ilii, a sclerotic condition of unknown cause producing dense bone in one or both iliacs but not the sacrum, may confuse the unwary. However, typically this iliac change allows the joint margin to be defined more clearly and therefore there should be no confusion between the two conditions. It is not unknown for an individual patient to have both sacroiliitis and osteitis condensans ilii.

Patients with bilateral, grade-4 sacroiliitis and no extrapelvic disease are frequently seen. Why some patients do not have progressive disease above the pelvic rim remains unclear.

In view of the enthesopathic nature of the disease it is not surprising that radiological changes occur elsewhere. Thus, vertebral squaring may occur, vertebral-end plate collapse may be seen, and varying degrees of ossification develop. The radiological changes may be contrasted with those seen in diffuse idiopathic hyperostosis (Table 6). Likewise syndesmophytes must be differentiated from

Table 4 Sacroiliac changes in ankylosing spondylitis[a]

Grade
0	Normal	Grade depends on degree
1	Suspicious	of blurring of joint margins,
2	Minimal sacroiliitis	juxta-articular scoliosis,
3	Moderate sacroiliitis	erosive change, and
4	Ankylosis	narrowing

[a]According to New York criteria

Table 5 Radiographic changes in primary and secondary forms of ankylosing spondylitis

	Primary ankylosing spondylitis—and ankylosing spondylitis associated with inflammatory bowel disease	Ankylosing spondylitis associated with Reiter's syndrome and psoriatic arthropathy
Sacroiliac changes	Symmetrical	Asymmetrical
Osteitis pubis	++	+
Facetal joint involvement	+++	+
Squaring of vertebrae	++	+
Syndesmophytes	+++	+
Ossification	++	+
Spread	Ascending	Random

Table 6 Differentiating features of diffuse idiopathic skeletal hyperostosis (DISH) and ankylosing spondylitis

	DISH	Ankylosing spondylitis
Usual age of onset (years)	>50	<40
Thoracolumbar kyphosis	±	++
Limitation of spinal mobility	±	++
Pain	±	++
Limitation of chest expansion	±	++
Radiography:		
Hyperostosis	+	+
SI joint erosion	−	++
SI joint (synovial) obliteration	±	++
SI joint (ligamentous) obliteration	+	++
Apophyseal joint obliteration	−	++
ALL ossification	++	±
PLL ossification	+	?
Syndesmophytes	−	++
Enthesopathies (whiskering) with erosions	−	++
Enthesopathies (whiskering) without erosions	++	+
HLA B27 (white patients) (%)	8	95
HLA B27 (black patients) (%)	2	50

SI, sacroiliac; ALL, anterior longitudinal ligament; PLL, posterior longitudinal ligament.

osteophytes; the latter associated with disc-space narrowing. In essence, syndesmophytes move in a vertical direction whereas osteophytes are typically horizontal. McEwen *et al.* (1971) have defined the radiological differences between primary ankylosing spondylitis and the secondary spondylarthropathies, as summarized in Table 5. The BASRI allows for a simple and rapid assessment of entire spine and hips (Pande *et al.* 1995).

Radionuclide scanning may be more sensitive than radiography but the change is non-specific and is likely to confuse rather than help. Likewise computed tomography and MRI is expensive and usually unnecessary.

Ankylosing spondylitis and diffuse idiopathic skeletal hyperostosis are compared in Table 6. Osteoporosis is now well recognized as is the consequence (i.e. compression fractures) (Donnelly *et al.* 1994; Mullaji *et al.* 1994).

Laboratory abnormalities

Apart from the presence of HLA-B27 in over 95 per cent of white patients, the majority have no evidence of change in laboratory tests. In fact there is little correlation between erythrocyte sedimentation rate and other so-called mediators of inflammatory disease and

disease activity as defined by clinical symptoms and findings. Serum alkaline phosphatase may be elevated and we and others have described elevated serum creatine phosphokinase levels. The explanation for this remains unclear. Circulating immune complexes may be found and one study suggested that psoriasis-associated retrovirus-like particles may be present. Likewise antibodies to proteoglycan occur and antibodies to heat shock protein are described. Interleukin 6 and acute phase reactants have recently been compared (Tutuncu *et al.* 1994). Interleukin 6 is more frequently raised in disease, compared to the situation with erythrocyte sedimentation rate, plasma viscosity or C-reactive protein (approximately 80 per cent compared with 50 per cent).

Ankylosing spondylitis in women

The disease is frequently missed in women unless a high degree of suspicion exists. Moreover certain features of the disease in women make definition of the disease more difficult. The major differences between the disease in men and women are summarized in Table 2. Women tend to have more peripheral joint involvement and the spinal disease progresses less rapidly. However, dramatic spinal involvement in women as in men is sometimes seen. Historically, the delay in diagnosis is greater in women than men but hopefully this difference is now decreasing. Interestingly, the sex distribution of primary ankylosing spondylitis favouring men in the ratio of 2.5 to 1 is even greater in psoriatic spondylitis (4 to 1), but for those with enteropathic disease the ratio is equal. Age is also a factor (Kennedy *et al.* 1993; Kennedy *et al.* 1994).

The sex ratio is said to favour males (about 6:1 in the early teenage years) but this ratio decreases with increasing age. By the late twenties the ratio is down to 2.3 to 1 with intermediate ratios in the ages between. However, our recent data suggest that even in teenagers, the ratio is approximately 3:1 in favour of boys.

Aetiology (see Khan 1993; Khan 1996; Rubin *et al.* 1994; Reveille *et al.* 1994 and further discussion in Chapter 5.5.1)

The cause of ankylosing spondylitis remains unknown. For the last decade interest has focused on a specific klebsiella serotype and the putative relationship between this organism and HLA-B27-positive lymphocytes of patients. However, it appears more likely that many different organisms can precipitate disease in susceptible individuals. The relationship between HLA-B27, other genes (Burney *et al.* 1994), and the environment is under intense scrutiny. As discussed more fully in Chapter 5.5.1 there are several recognized facts that must be taken into consideration:

1. Approximately 5 to 10 per cent of HLA-B27-positive individuals develop ankylosing spondylitis—a similar percentage to those who develop reactive arthropathy following infection with an arthritogenic organism.

2. Relatives of healthy HLA-B27-positive subjects only rarely develop disease while those of HLA-B27-positive patients are more likely to do so.

5.5.4 Psoriatic arthritis

Dafna D. Gladman

Introduction

Psoriatic arthritis is an inflammatory arthritis, associated with psoriasis (Wright and Moll 1976). Its original definition as seronegative for rheumatoid factor, has been replaced by 'usually seronegative' since as many as 15 per cent of the general population, particularly over age 60, may have a positive rheumatoid factor, and rheumatoid factor may be present in more than 10 per cent of patients with psoriasis who do not have arthritis (Gladman *et al.* 1986). The majority of patients with psoriatic arthritis run a benign course. However, in about a fifth of the patients a chronic, progressive, deforming arthritis may develop, resulting in significant joint destruction and limitation of daily activities.

Epidemiology

Psoriasis is a chronic skin condition which affects 1 to 3 per cent of the population (Farber and Scott 1979). The association between psoriasis and arthritis might be fortuitous. Since psoriasis is a common condition, and arthritis, particularly osteoarthritis, is quite prevalent, it is conceivable that psoriasis and some unrelated form of arthritis may occur in the same patient. Indeed, some patients with psoriasis do present with a coincidental rheumatoid arthritis, or osteoarthritis. Cats (1990) has argued that psoriasis is just a measure of disease expression in certain patients with peripheral arthritis and spondylarthropathy. However, epidemiological evidence described below supports the notion that psoriatic arthritis is a distinct form of arthritis associated with psoriasis.

Although the first description of arthritis associated with psoriasis was provided by Aliberti (Eccles and Wright 1985; O'Neill and Silman 1994), psoriatic arthritis was considered to be a variant of rheumatoid arthritis until forty years ago. Epidemiological studies over the past four decades have confirmed the association between psoriasis and arthritis. These studies have shown an increased frequency of arthritis among patients with psoriasis and an increased prevalence of psoriasis among patients with arthritis. Thus, 6 to 42 per cent of patients with psoriasis may have psoriatic arthritis (Table 1), while the prevalence of arthritis in the general population is about 3 per cent. Likewise, the prevalence of psoriasis among patients with seronegative arthritis is reported to be 20 per cent, while arthritis occurs in only 2 to 3 per cent of the general population (Eccles and Wright 1985; O'Neill and Silman 1994). Lawrence *et al.* (1989) recently estimated the prevalence of psoriatic arthritis in the United States to be 0.67 per cent, whereas the overall prevalence for rheumatoid arthritis was estimated at 1.2 per cent.

The discovery of the rheumatoid factor and its association with rheumatoid arthritis helped separate psoriatic arthritis as a distinct entity, since patients with arthritis and psoriasis tended to be seronegative. Radiographical features in psoriatic arthritis were found to be different from those of rheumatoid arthritis (Avila *et al.* 1960). A female preponderance was found in rheumatoid arthritis, whereas the gender ratio among patients with psoriatic arthritis was almost equal (Wright and Moll 1976; Eccles and Wright 1985; O'Neill and Silman 1994). Unlike patients with rheumatoid arthritis, patients with psoriatic arthritis may present with a spondylarthropathy. Psoriatic arthritis is therefore classified with the seronegative spondylarthropathies. The studies by Wright and Moll (1976) are notable for presenting the unique features of psoriatic arthritis, and paving the way for other clinical descriptions.

The frequency of psoriatic arthritis has been reported in 6 to 42 per cent of patients with psoriasis (Leczinsky 1948; Little *et al.* 1975; Leonard *et al.* 1978; Green *et al.* 1981; Scarpa *et al.* 1984; Stern 1985; Zanelli and Wilde 1992; Falk and Vandbakk 1993; Barii-Druko *et al.* 1994). The most quoted prevalence of 6.8 per cent (Leczinsky 1948), is based on a study of the prevalence of rheumatoid-type polyarthritis in a population of inpatients with psoriasis. This frequency does not include other patterns of psoriatic arthritis. More recently, Scarpa *et al.* (1984) and Stern (1985) identified 34 per cent and 20 per cent of their psoriatic patients, respectively, to have psoriatic arthritis, while Green *et al.* (1981) reported arthritis in 42 per cent of their outpatients with psoriasis. A recent study of the prevalence of psoriasis in the Lapp population (Falk and Vandakk 1993) identified 17 per cent of patients with psoriasis who had psoriatic arthritis, while a study from Croatia (Barii-Druko *et al.* 1994) found that 9.8 per cent of patients with psoriasis had psoriatic arthritis. Since psoriasis may affect 1 to 3 per cent of the population, and as many as 30 per cent of psoriatic patients may develop psoriatic arthritis, almost 1 per cent of the population may suffer from psoriatic arthritis, which is the expected prevalence of rheumatoid arthritis. This is indeed close to the estimated prevalence of 0.67 per cent reported for psoriatic arthritis in the United States (Lawrence *et al.* 1989). Little *et al.* (1975) and Leonard *et al.* (1978) suggested that psoriatic arthritis was more common in patients with severe psoriasis. Both groups of investigators reported frequencies of 30 per cent of psoriatic arthritis among patients whose psoriasis required admission to hospital. However, psoriatic arthritis may precede the diagnosis of psoriasis in about 15 per cent of the patients (Wright and Moll 1976; Kammer *et al.* 1979; Gladman *et al.* 1987; Jones *et al.* 1994) (Table 2). Moreover, the highest prevalence of psoriatic arthritis was recorded among patients attending an outpatient dermatology clinic in Cape Town (Green *et al.* 1981).

Clinical features

Psoriatic arthritis affects women and men almost equally, usually in their third or fourth decade (Wright 1956; Kammer *et al.* 1979; Green *et al.* 1981; Scarpa *et al.* 1984; Gladman *et al.* 1987). Nail lesions proved to be the only clinical feature which may identify patients with psoriasis destined to develop arthritis (Gladman *et al.* 1986). These lesions occur in close to 90 per cent of patients with psoriatic arthritis (Little *et al.* 1975; Wright and Moll 1976; Kammer *et al.* 1979; Green *et al.* 1981; Gladman *et al.* 1987) and in 46 per cent of patients with psoriasis uncomplicated by arthritis (Gladman *et al.* 1986).

The arthritis is inflammatory in nature. It may affect any peripheral joint, as well as the axial skeleton and the sacroiliac joints. Patients usually present with pain, associated with stiffness, which is more marked in the morning and improves with activity. More than half the patients complain of morning stiffness of more than 30-min duration (Gladman *et al.* 1987). Evidence of inflammation may be detected clinically by the presence of stress pain or tenderness, as

Table 1 The prevalence of psoriatic arthritis among patients with psoriasis

Authors (year)	Centre	Number of patients studied	Percentage with arthritis
Leczinsky (1948)	Sweden	534	7
Vilanova (1951)	Barcelona	214	25
Little *et al.* (1975)	Toronto	100	32
Leonard *et al.* (1978)	Rochester	77	39
Green *et al.* (1981)	Cape Town	61	42
Scarpa *et al.* (1984)	Naples	180	34
Stern (1985)	Boston	1285	20
Zanelli and Wilde (1992)	Winston-Salem	459	17
Falk and Vandbakk (1993)	Kautokeino	35	17
Barišsić-Druško *et al.* (1994)	Osijek region	553	10

well as effusions (Gladman *et al.* 1990*a*), although these signs may not be as easily detectable as they are in rheumatoid arthritis, since patients with psoriatic arthritis are less tender than patients with rheumatoid arthritis (Buskila *et al.* 1992). The inflamed joints in patients with psoriatic arthritis may have a purplish-red discoloration, a feature which is not often seen in rheumatoid arthritis. The effusions in psoriatic arthritis joints tend to be tense, and are often difficult to detect. There is no predilection to particular joints, with the exception of the distal interphalangeal joints. Roberts *et al.* (1976) suggested that the knees were more commonly involved, as well as the proximal interphalangeal and metacarpophalangeal joints in the three groups they described. Jones *et al.* (1994) found that women tended to have small joints and upper limb involvement, whereas men tended to have axial involvement. Features which appear to differentiate psoriatic arthritis from rheumatoid arthritis clinically are shown in Table 3.

The spondylarthropathy may present with an inflammatory type of back pain, which is associated with stiffness and improves with activity. Clinical evidence of sacroiliitis may be obtained by specific tests, including the Gaenzlen's manoeuvre, the FABER (flexion, abduction, external rotation of the hip) test, and direct pressure over the sacroiliac joints (Gladman *et al.* 1987; Hanly *et al.* 1988). In some patients restricted range of back movements may be documented, by a reduction of flexion–extension as well as lateral flexion and rotation (Gladman *et al.* 1987; Hanly *et al.* 1988). Unlike ankylosing spondylitis, many of the patients with psoriatic spondylarthropathy are asymptomatic, and demonstrate a full range of back movement (Gladman *et al.* 1987; Hanly *et al.* 1988; Gladman *et al.* 1992*b*; Gladman *et al.* 1993). In these patients the diagnosis of the spondylarthropathy is made radiographically.

Clinical spectrum of psoriatic arthritis

Wright and Moll (1976) presented the seminal work on the clinical patterns of psoriatic arthritis. They proposed that these include:

distal arthritis, involving the distal interphalangeal joints (Fig. 1); an asymmetric oligoarthritis involving small or medium-sized joints in an asymmetric distribution (Fig. 2); a symmetric polyarthritis, indistinguishable from rheumatoid arthritis; arthritis mutilans, which is a deforming, destructive, and disabling form of arthritis (Figs 3 and 4); and a spondylarthropathy (Figs 5 and 6). Similar descriptions have been reported by others (Kammer *et al.* 1979; Scarpa *et al.* 1984; Gladman *et al.* 1987; Helliwell *et al.* 1991; Jones *et al.* 1994; Veale *et al.* 1994*b*). The frequency of the various patterns has varied in the literature (Table 2). Although in their initial description of the psoriatic arthritis patterns Wright and Moll (1976) suggested that the most common pattern was asymmetric oligoarthritis, more recent studies confirm that polyarthritis is most commonly seen among patients with psoriatic arthritis. Psoriatic arthritis is asymmetric in distribution in about half the cases, even when polyarticular distribution is noted. Thus, in comparison with rheumatoid arthritis, psoriatic arthritis tends to be characterized as an asymmetric form of arthritis. The exact prevalence of each of the psoriatic arthritis patterns has been difficult to establish, since investigators have not used the exact same definitions, particularly with regards to symmetry. Helliwell *et al.* (1991) suggested a method for defining symmetrical involvement in patients with psoriatic arthritis, such that for each level of joints if the ratio of the number of matched pairs to the total number of joints was more than 0.5 then the distribution was considered symmetrical. Jones *et al.* (1994) showed that using this method more patients were found to have a symmetrical arthritis. Although the distal pattern has been described as typical for psoriatic arthritis, its frequency has varied widely, and some investigators have not been able to identify patients with isolated distal joint involvement. It has also been recognized that the patterns themselves may change with time in individual patients (Gladman 1992). A patient may present initially with an oligoarthritis which later becomes polyarticular, or develop an initial polyarthritis, which persists in only a few joints. Indeed, Jones *et al.* (1994) recently documented these changes in pattern over time in over 60 per cent of their patients with psoriatic arthritis. Moreover,

Table 2 Clinical features of psoriatic arthritis in large series

Features	Roberts et al. (1976)	Kammer et al. (1979)	Scarpa et al. (1984)	Gladman et al. (1987)	Veale (1994)	Jones (1994)
	(N=168)[a]	(N=100)	(N=62)	(N=220)	(N=100)	(N=100)
Male/female ratio	67/101	47/53	29/33	104/116	59/41	43/57
Age of onset (years)	36–45	33–45	40–60	37	34	37.6
Asymmetrical oligoarthritis (%)	53	54[b]	16	11[c]	43	26[f]
Symmetrical polyarthritis (%)	78	25[b]	39.0	19[d]	33	63
Distal (%)	17	?	7.5	12	16	1
Back (%)	5	21	21.0	2[c]	4	6
Mutilans (%)	5	?	2.3	16	2	4
Sacroiliitis (%)	?	?	16.0	27	15	6
Joints before skin (%)	16	30	?	17	?	18

[a]Number of patients in the series.
[b]Includes patients with only distal joints involved.
[c]14 including symmetrical oligoarthritis.
[d]40 including asymmetrical polyarthritis.
[e]33 including peripheral joint plus back involvement
[f]4 were symmetric
?, unspecified.

unless radiographs are performed on all patients, joints which had been previously involved may not be identified, and the spondylarthropathy may be missed (Little *et al.* 1975; Gladman *et al.* 1987; Hanly *et al.* 1988). While the patterns of psoriatic arthritis may facilitate the diagnosis, it is not clear whether they have a prognostic significance.

A typical feature of psoriatic arthritis is the development of dactylitis, which presents as a swelling of a whole digit, with inflammation involving distal and proximal interphalangeal, and occasionally the metacarpophalangeal joints (Fig. 7). Dactylitis occurs in over a third of the patients (Gladman *et al.* 1987). The exact pathogenesis of the dactylitis is unclear. It may be related either to extensive inflammation and effusion in all the joints of a particular digit, with an associated tenosynovitis, or to soft tissue inflammation in the whole digit. The use of more advanced imaging techniques may help delineate the pathogenesis of 'sausage digits'. Indeed, a recent scintigraphy study using human immunoglobulin labelled with technetium-99m demonstrates the inflammation in the digit which is missed by a bone scan (Stoeger *et al.* 1994). Tenosynovitis by itself is also a feature of psoriatic arthritis. Although inflammation of the extensor carpi ulnaris has been considered typical for rheumatoid arthritis, we have seen it quite often among the patients attending the psoriatic arthritis clinic. As in the other spondylarthropathies, such as Reiter's syndrome and ankylosing spondylitis, Achilles tendinitis, heel pain, and plantar fascitis are common among patients with psoriatic arthritis. Enthesitis, or inflammation at sites of tendon insertion, is frequent, particularly at the Achilles tendon, the insertion of the plantar fascia, and ligamentous insertions around the

pelvic bones. These are commonly diagnosed radiographically as spurs (Fig. 8). A recent study from Finland (Lehtinen *et al.* 1994) offers an improved method, using ultrasound, to identify the presence of enthesitis in patients with spondylarthropathy.

The spondylarthropathy of psoriatic arthritis

The frequency of spinal involvement in psoriatic arthritis has varied from 2 per cent, as isolated back disease, to as high as 40 per cent, when associated with peripheral arthritis (Wright and Moll 1976; Lambert and Wright 1977; Kammer *et al.* 1979; Scarpa *et al.* 1984; Gladman *et al.* 1986; Gladman *et al.* 1987; Hanly *et al.* 1988; Moll 1994). Lambert and Wright (1977), found that 40 per cent of 130 patients with psoriatic arthritis had back involvement, based on back pain and reduced spinal mobility. Gladman *et al.* (1987), documented spinal involvement, based on both clinical and radiographical evidence, in 35 per cent of their patients at their first visit to the psoriatic arthritis clinic. This number increased to 51 per cent at follow-up (Gladman *et al.* 1992b). In both studies patients with spinal involvement tended to be male and older than patients without back involvement. Hanly *et al.* (1988) described 52 patients with psoriatic spondylarthropathy who had been followed for a minimum of 30 months, and for a mean of almost 5 years. Despite clinical and radiographical evidence of progression of sacroiliitis and spondylitis, patients' symptoms tended to improve with time, and their spinal mobility was generally good. They suggested that patients with psoriatic arthritis who have spinal involvement are not as symptomatic from their back disease as are patients with

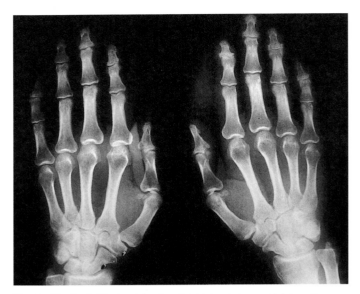

Fig. 1 Distal arthritis, involving the distal interphalangeal joints, with erosions and joint space narrowing.

ankylosing spondylitis, and do not demonstrate the same degree of limitation of back movement that is noted in patients with ankylosing spondylitis (Hanly *et al.* 1988; Scarpa *et al.* 1988). The spondylarthropathy of patients with psoriatic arthritis was indeed found to be less severe than that seen in ankylosing spondylitis. This was evidenced by the lower frequency of symptomatic neck and back disease, as well as less limitation of movement and grade 4 sacroiliitis in patients with psoriatic arthritis compared with those with ankylosing spondylitis (Gladman *et al.* 1993). Moreover, among patients with psoriatic spondylarthropathy, there are

Table 3 Comparison between psoriatic arthritis and rheumatoid arthritis

	Psoriatic arthritis	Rheumatoid arthritis
Female preponderance	Uncommon	Common
Distal interphalangeal involvement	Common	Uncommon
Symmetry	Less common	Common
Erythema over affected joint	Common	Uncommon
Back involvement	Common	Uncommon
Enthesopathy	Common	Uncommon
Skin lesions	Common	Uncommon
Nail lesions	Common	Uncommon
Rhematoid factor	Uncommon	Common
Osteopenia	Uncommon	Common
Osteolysis	Common	Uncommon
Ankylosis	Common	Uncommon

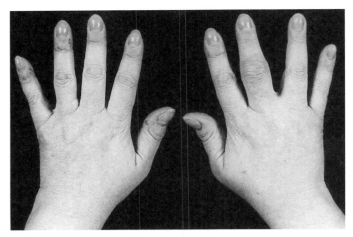

Fig. 2 An asymmetric oligoarthritis involving the third proximal interphalangeal joint on the right. Note the psoriatic lesions in the periungual areas of the left fourth and fifth fingers.

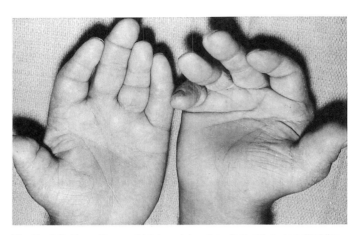

Fig. 3 Arthritis mutilans, which is a deforming, destructive, and disabling form of arthritis, showing the inability to use the hands fully.

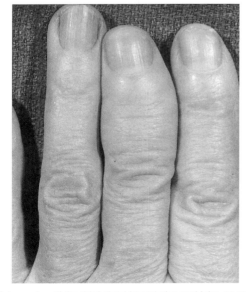

Fig. 4 Telescoping of the third distal interphalangeal joint, seen in patients with psoriatic arthritis, which may be part of arthritis mutilans.

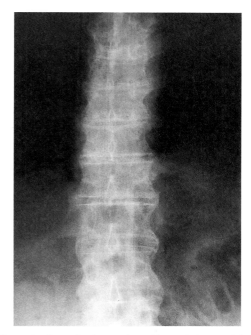

Fig. 5 Thoracolumbar spine in a patient with psoriatic spondylarthropathy, demonstrating syndesmophytes.

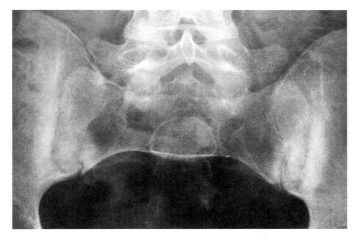

Fig. 6 Bilateral sacroiliitis in a patient with psoriatic spondylarthropathy.

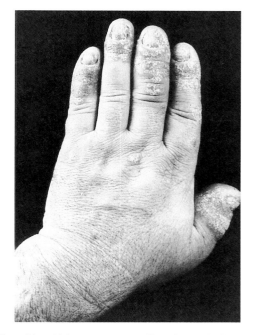

Fig. 7 Dactylitis, which presents as swelling of a whole digit, with inflammation of the distal and proximal interphalangeal, and occasionally the metacarpophalangeal joints, involving the thumb and third finger. Note the psoriatic skin and nail lesions.

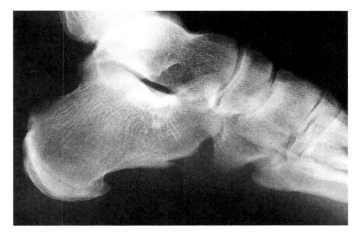

Fig. 8 Spur formation at the insertion of the plantar fascia, representing enthesitis.

gender-related differences in disease expression, with more advanced spondylarthropathy noted among men (Gladman *et al.* 1992*b*). The cervical spine in psoriatic arthritis received special attention in two recent studies. Salvarani *et al.* (1992*a*) studied 57 patients with psoriatic arthritis, of whom 70 per cent had radiographical evidence of cervical spine disease. They identified a high prevalence (23 per cent) of atlantoaxial subluxation. Jenkinson *et al.* (1994) detected cervical spine disease in 57 per cent of their patients with psoriatic arthritis, of whom only 3 had atlantoaxial subluxation. The majority of their patients had spondylitic type changes with apophysial joint narrowing or fusion and syndesmophytes. In both these studies neck involvement was related to prolonged disease duration. At the University of Toronto Psoriatic Arthritis Clinic, only 4 patients with atlantoaxial subluxation have been identified of a total of 450 patients followed over the past 17 years.

Extra-articular features

Skin psoriasis

The skin lesions of psoriasis consist of an erythematous scaly area that varies from a localized plaque on the elbows and knees to an incapacitating, generalized skin involvement with significant effect on the cardiovascular and heat regulating mechanism (Farber and Scott 1979; Goodfield 1994). The skin lesions are classified as: typical psoriasis vulgaris, with major involvement of the extensor surfaces; inverse psoriasis, affecting the flexural areas; pustular psoriasis, which may be localized to the palms and soles, or may be of the more generalized serious form called Von Zambush, and which may pose a threat to life; and the erythrodermic generalized group. The majority of patients with psoriatic arthritis demonstrate the classic psoriasis vulgaris pattern (Wright *et al.* 1979; Gladman *et al.* 1986; Gladman *et al.* 1987). Only 35 per cent of the patients describe a relationship between their skin and joint manifestations (Gladman *et al.* 1987). All areas of the skin may be affected, including the mucosa and the nails. Nail lesions include pitting, ridging, and onycholysis (Wright and Moll 1976). Two or all of these features in the same patient are in favour of a psoriatic origin for the nail dystrophy (Eastmond and Wright 1979). As already mentioned, nail lesions are particularly common among patients with psoriatic arthritis. Occasionally, distal interphalangeal joint disease may follow the development of onycholysis in a particular finger nail, but overall, there has not been a direct correlation between the presence of distal interphalangeal joint disease and nail lesions, since the former occurs in 35 per cent of the patients, whereas the latter occur in almost 90 per cent of the patients with psoriatic arthritis.

Other extra-articular features

The extradermal extra-articular features of psoriatic arthritis are similar to the features described in other seronegative spondylarthropathies and include iritis, which may occur in 7 per cent of the patients (Gladman *et al.* 1987), mouth ulcers, urethritis, colitis, and aortic valve disease (Wright and Moll 1976). A case of a patient with psoriatic arthritis with pyoderma gangrenosum was recently described (Smith and White 1994), and we have seen a case in our psoriatic arthritis clinic. The development of lymphoedema of the upper limb in patients with psoriatic arthritis was recently described in the literature (Mulherin *et al.* 1993). Similar cases have been seen at the University of Toronto Psoriatic Arthritis Clinic. The mechanism of this presentation is not entirely clear, but may represent a similar change to that occurring in dactylitis, with inflammation in both joints and tendons, leading to the clinical picture of 'lymphoedema'. Alternatively, in some of these cases it is possible that a ruptured capsule, as seen in a Baker's cyst in the knee, occurs in the wrist or elbow joint, leading to the soft tissue swelling noted in the distal portion of the upper limb.

Laboratory investigations in psoriatic arthritis

There are no specific laboratory tests which are diagnostic for psoriatic arthritis. Anaemia occurred in 14 per cent of the patients presenting to the psoriatic arthritis clinic (Gladman *et al.* 1987), perhaps reflecting the chronic disease, or an iron deficiency anaemia, secondary to therapy with non-steroidal anti-inflammatory drugs. Indeed, the much higher frequency of anaemia at follow-up (Gladman *et al.* 1990b), was thought to represent the untoward effect of these drugs. Elevated white-cell counts and other acute phase reactants may also be present (Gladman *et al.* 1987). This may reflect the acute phase inflammatory reaction, and may be seen in patients with psoriasis without arthritis. Elevated erythrocyte sedimentation rates may be seen in more than 40 per cent of patients with psoriatic arthritis, and probably reflect both joint and skin inflammation (Gladman *et al.* 1986; Gladman *et al.* 1987). Hyperuricaemia is not uncommon among patients with psoriasis and arthritis (Gladman *et al.* 1986; Gladman *et al.* 1987), and is probably related to the high

turnover of skin cells. However, since both psoriasis and gout may occur in young males, one must rule out the possibility that the arthritis is crystal induced, before making the diagnosis of psoriatic arthritis in a patient with psoriasis. On the other hand, the presence of an acute monoarthritis, even in the first metatarsophalangeal joint in the presence of psoriasis does not mean the patient has gout. In both these situations a careful search for negatively birefringent, uric acid crystals should be carried out on the fluid obtained by joint aspiration.

Patients with psoriatic arthritis are usually seronegative for rheumatoid factor. However, in each series of patients with psoriatic arthritis there are about 10 to 15 per cent of the patients who have a positive rheumatoid factor, albeit in a low titre. It should be noted that patients with psoriasis uncomplicated by arthritis demonstrated the same frequency of a positive rheumatoid factor, despite the fact that they were younger on average than the patients with psoriatic arthritis (Gladman *et al.* 1986). Antinuclear factor has also been demonstrated in the sera of patients with uncomplicated psoriasis and patients with psoriatic arthritis, in the same frequency (Gladman *et al.* 1986). Whether this antinuclear antibody reflects the presence of antibodies to stratum corneum antigens is unclear (Gladman 1985). The demonstration of hypergammaglobulinaemia in patients with psoriatic arthritis provides further evidence for immunological abnormalities in patients with this condition (Gladman 1985).

Radiographical features of psoriatic arthritis

Radiographical abnormalities may be seen in both peripheral joints and the axial skeleton in patients with psoriatic arthritis (Resnick and Niwayama 1981). The features commonly associated with psoriatic arthritis and which help differentiate it from rheumatoid arthritis include: absence of juxta-articular osteoporosis; the predilection for distal interphalangeal joints; 'whittling' (lysis) of terminal phalanges (Fig. 9); lack of symmetry; gross destruction of isolated joint; 'pencil-in-cup' appearance (Fig. 10); ankylosis (Fig. 10); fluffy periostitis (Fig. 11); and both classical and atypical spondylitis (Wright and Moll 1971; Resnick and Niwayama 1981; Figs 5, 6 and 7).

Diagnosis of psoriatic arthritis

There are no available diagnostic criteria for psoriatic arthritis (Gladman 1995). None the less, the diagnosis of psoriatic arthritis is generally based on the definition of the disease: an inflammatory arthritis in the presence of psoriatic skin lesions, usually seronegative for rheumatoid factor. In a patient with psoriasis, the development of an inflammatory arthritis makes the diagnosis easier. The clinical and radiographical features described above help identify the patient with psoriatic arthritis who had not previously demonstrated skin lesions. Thus, a patient who presents with an asymmetric oligoarthritis, or an inflammatory polyarthritis which includes distal interphalangeal joints, or peripheral arthritis with a spondylarthropathy, should be investigated for the presence of psoriasis, and psoriatic arthritis should clearly be considered in the differential diagnosis. The presence of dactylitis is certainly helpful, as is the presence of enthesitis. It should be noted that the skin lesions may be minimal, and indeed 'hidden'. One must therefore search for these lesions, particularly in the umbilical area, the anal cleft, the scalp, and the ears. Nail lesions are not always recognized by the patient, and should be looked for carefully. The common occurrence of distal joint involvement means that psoriatic arthritis needs to be differentiated from osteoarthritis. The distal interphalangeal lesions in patients with psoriatic arthritis are inflammatory in nature, and tend to be swollen, such that for the most part they can be differentiated clinically as softer than the hard bony enlargement of Heberden's nodes. The presence of more proximal joint involvement, particularly the wrist and metacarpophalangeal joints, also helps distinguish psoriatic arthritis from osteoarthritis. However, osteoarthritis is a common condition, particularly with advancing age, and a patient may have Heberden's nodes complicating pre-existing psoriatic arthritis. Reiter's disease occasionally presents a diagnostic difficulty. The skin lesions in pustular psoriasis may be indistinguishable both clinically and pathologically from those of Reiter's syndrome, and the clinical features of the arthritis and the spondylarthropathy are similar. Psoriatic arthritis tends to be polyarticular, which may help. Iritis and mucous membrane lesions may be more common in Reiter's disease.

Pathogenesis of psoriatic arthritis

Understanding the pathogenetic mechanisms of disease is crucial for both the development of appropriate therapeutic approaches and the ultimate cure of a disease. It is likely that similar mechanisms would be operating in the development of both skin and joint disease in psoriatic arthritis. Although the exact pathogenetic mechanisms in psoriatic arthritis remain to be elucidated, factors thought to be important include genetic, immunological, and environmental (Gladman 1992; Abu-Shakra and Gladman 1994).

Genetic factors

More than 40 per cent of patients with psoriasis or psoriatic arthritis have a family history of the skin or joint disease in first-degree family members (Gladman *et al.* 1986; Gladman *et al.* 1987). Further support for genetic factors as possible aetiological mechanisms for psoriatic arthritis has come from the observations of high concordance for psoriasis in monozygotic twins and from clustering of

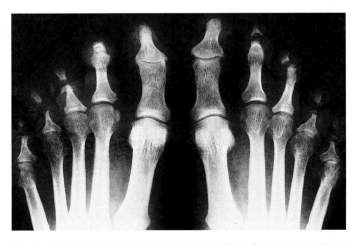

Fig. 9 'Whittling' (lysis) of terminal phalanges of the first and second toes bilaterally.

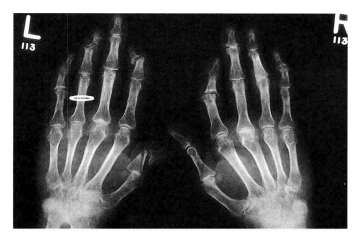

Fig. 10 'Pencil-in-cup' appearance seen in its early phase in the second right proximal, the fifth right distal, and the left fifth distal interphalangeal joints. Fully developed changes are seen in the left index distal and the left thumb interphalangeal joints. In addition, ankylosis is seen in the right distal interphalangeal joint

both psoriasis and psoriatic arthritis within families (Espinoza 1985; Eastmond 1994). The discovery of the HLA system on chromosome 6 of humans, and the ability to detect HLA alloantigens of both class 1 and class 2, has allowed further elaboration of genetic mechanisms in psoriasis and psoriatic arthritis. Population studies in psoriasis revealed an increased frequency of HLA antigens B13, B17, B37, Cw6 and DR7 (Espinoza 1985; Gladman *et al.* 1986; Eastmond 1994). In psoriatic arthritis, increased frequencies of HLA-B13, -B17, -B27, -B38, -B39, -DR4, and -DR7 have been reported (Espinoza 1985; Gladman *et al.* 1986; Sakkas *et al.* 1990). Gladman *et al.* (1986) compared 158 patients with psoriatic arthritis to 101 patients with uncomplicated psoriasis. They found that the HLA-B7 or -B27 antigens were more common among patients with psoriatic arthritis, whereas B17, Cw6, and DR7 were more common among patients with uncomplicated psoriasis. HLA-B27 has clearly been associated with back disease in psoriatic arthritis, thus lending further credence to its grouping with the HLA-B27-associated spondylarthropathy. HLA-DR4 appears to be associated with the peripheral articular pattern of psoriatic arthritis (Gladman *et al.* 1986). A search for other genetic markers in psoriatic arthritis revealed that there were no specific T-cell receptor genes unique to the disease (Sakkas *et al.* 1990). However, Southern blot analysis using DNA probes for the immunoglobulin heavy chain gene (IgH) on chromosome 14q32 suggests that the gene may confer susceptibility to arthritis in patients with psoriasis (Sakkas *et al.* 1991). A recent identification of a gene for familial psoriasis on chromosome 17 is intriguing, but its relationship to psoriatic arthritis is unclear (Tomfohrde *et al.* 1994).

Immunological mechanisms

The clinical and pathological features of both psoriasis and psoriatic arthritis support the role of immunological factors in the pathogenesis of these conditions. The inflammatory nature of the disease, the cellular infiltrates seen both in skin and joint lesions, and the deposition of immunoglobulins in the epidermis as well as the synovial membrane, all support an immune mechanism (Gladman 1985; Panayi 1994). Autoantibodies, such as antinuclear

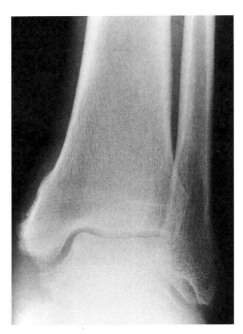

Fig. 11   Fluffy periostitis in the distal end of the tibia.

antibodies, rheumatoid factor, and antibodies against skin antigens, as well as immune complexes, have been found in the sera of patients with psoriasis and psoriatic arthritis, supporting a hyperactive humoral immune mechanism (Gladman 1985). It has recently been hypothesized that antibodies against psoriasis-specific non-histone proteins found in patients with psoriasis, may facilitate displacement of the non-histone complex from DNA which may contain the psoriasis gene (Cormane and Asghar 1987), thus allowing for the development of the disease. This hypothesis is of particular interest since the identification of a psoriasis gene on chromosome 17.

On the cellular side, an imbalance of T-cell activity has been shown, which may result from either lack of T-cell suppression or excess of helper cell activity. Indeed, T-lymphocyte hyporeactivity to mitogens, impaired suppressor cell function, and a decrease in certain T-cell subpopulations have been demonstrated in psoriatic arthritis (Gladman 1985). The presence of activated T cells in psoriatic skin lesions was suggested by the demonstration of T lymphocytes bearing HLA-DR molecules as well as receptors for interleukin 2 in the lesions (Gottlieb 1988). In addition, keratinocytes bearing HLA-DR molecules were found in association with an increased frequency of psoriatic arthritis in patients with psoriasis. This prompted the proposal that these cells serve to present antigen to T cells, leading to mediator release and an inflammatory response (Gottlieb 1988). These T cells have indeed been found to express HLA-DR molecules, receptors for IL-2, and a variety of adhesion molecules, and to secrete proinflammatory cytokines, in particular IL-6 (Abu-Shakra and Gladman 1993). Fibroblasts from the skin and synovium of patients with psoriatic arthritis have an increased proliferative activity and the capability of secretion of increased amounts of IL-1β, IL-6 and platelet-derived growth factors. Activated T cells have been noted in the affected tissues (both skin and joints) in psoriatic arthritis by most investigators (Gladman 1993; Veale *et al.* 1993; Panayi 1994; Veale *et al.* 1994*a*). The results of

several studies suggest that cytokines secreted from activated T cells and other mononuclear proinflammatory cells induce proliferation and activation of synovial and epidermal fibroblasts. It is of interest that both psoriasis and psoriatic arthritis, but not rheumatoid arthritis, have been reported to flare in the presence of the acquired immune deficiency virus (Buskila and Gladman 1990), suggesting that helper T (CD4) cells are not required for the disease process in psoriatic arthritis (Vasey *et al.* 1989). Indeed a decreased helper/ suppressor T-cell ratio has been shown in patients with severe psoriasis (Rubins and Merson 1987). Moreover, deficient helper T-cell function in psoriatic patients was demonstrated using an antibody-specific induction system (Ventura *et al.* 1989). Panayi (1994) recently reviewed the immunological abnormalities seen in psoriatic arthritis. These include the presence of activated T lymphocytes in synovial membranes, an increase in macrophage numbers, and the presence of B cells. Although the presence of activated T cells in the affected tissues (both skin and joints) in psoriatic arthritis has been noted by most investigators (Gladman 1993; Veale *et al.* 1993; Panayi 1994; Veale *et al.* 1994*a*), the presence of an increased number of macrophages has not been uniformly described. This may be related to the stage in the disease at which the observations were made (Gladman 1993). It is still unclear whether the activated T cells are the cause of the arthritis, or the result of as yet unidentified factor.

Over the past 15 years the role of metabolites of arachidonic acid, such as prostaglandins and particularly leukotrienes, in the pathogenesis of both psoriasis and psoriatic arthritis has been evaluated (Voorhees 1983). Levels of leukotriene B4 have been shown to be increased in the psoriatic skin lesions, and injections of this compound has caused intraepidermal microabscesses. Drugs which lower the levels of leukotriene B4 are effective in controlling the skin lesions. However, the evidence is not conclusive. Greaves and Camp (1988) recently proposed an integrated approach to inflammation of human skin, considering the lipoxygenase system, platelet activating factor, and cytokines. This is an attractive proposal which allows for the integration of all the immunological abnormalities described. However, in a recent study, Veale *et al.* (1994*c*) demonstrated that Efamol marine was able to alter prostaglandin metabolism but did not produce a clinical improvement in either skin or joint manifestations in patients with psoriatic arthritis.

Environmental factors

Infection

Some investigators believe that guttate psoriasis is initiated by an infectious agent (Vasey 1985). Support for the role of bacterial antigens in the pathogenesis of psoriasis and psoriatic arthritis comes from indirect observations of enhanced humoral and cellular immunity to Gram-positive bacteria typically found in the psoriatic plaques. However, psoriatic plaques often become secondarily infected, thus the cause–effect relationship of bacteria and psoriasis is complicated. Moreover, Grinlinton *et al.* (1993) demonstrated that the response to streptococcal antigens by γ+ T cells from patients with psoriatic arthritis was also noted by cells from patients with rheumatoid arthritis, suggesting that this reaction may be a feature of inflammatory arthritis.

The exacerbation of psoriasis and psoriatic arthritis seen in the context of acquired immune deficiency virus infection is intriguing (Vasey *et al.* 1989). The possibility that psoriatic arthritis might be virus induced has recently been proposed by Luxembourg *et al.*

(1987). However, an investigation of antigens related to the major internal protein p27 of a psoriasis-associated retrovirus-like particle failed to reveal specificity for psoriatic patients (Rødahl and Iversen 1985). Thus an exact viral aetiology for psoriasis or psoriatic arthritis has yet to be described.

Trauma

In almost all accounts of psoriatic arthritis there are reports of patients whose arthritis developed after trauma. However, the majority of these are anecdotal case reports (Langevitz et al. 1990). Scarpa et al. (1992) reviewed the records of 138 patients with psoriatic arthritis and compared the frequency of a traumatic event prior to the development of the arthritis to that recorded in 138 patients with rheumatoid arthritis. They found that trauma of some type preceded the diagnosis of psoriatic arthritis in 9 per cent of the cases, whereas in rheumatoid arthritis it was found in only 1 per cent of the patients, suggesting a role for trauma in some patients with psoriatic arthritis.

Treatment of psoriatic arthritis

The treatment modalities employed in psoriatic arthritis are in part based on the pathogenetic mechanisms discussed above. They concentrate on control of inflammation, and an attempt to modify the immunological mechanisms thought to be operating in this disease (Gladman 1992).

The treatment of psoriasis

The treatment of psoriatic arthritis includes treatment for the skin condition as well as treatment for the joint disease. The skin lesions are treated by topical medications, aimed at controlling the inflammation and skin proliferation, including tar, anthralin, and corticosteroids (Marks 1980). In refractory cases, systemic medications such as methotrexate (Roenigk et al. 1969), **PUVA** (psoralen and ultraviolet A light) (Parish et al. 1974), retinoic acid derivatives (Klinkhoff et al. 1989), and more recently cyclosporin (Ellis et al. 1991) are used. The possible pathogenetic role of leukotrienes in the development of psoriatic arthritis has resulted in fish oil recently being introduced as a treatment for psoriasis (Gupta et al. 1989a).

The treatment of psoriatic arthritis

Non-steroidal anti-inflammatory therapy

The initial treatment for psoriatic arthritis consists of non-steroidal anti-inflammatory drugs (**NSAIDs**), including enteric-coated acetylsalicylic acid (**ECASA**), ibuprofen, naproxen, indomethacin, tolmetin, piroxicam, diclofenac sodium, and others (Abu-Shakra and Gladman 1993). In patients whose primary problem is that of peripheral arthritis, medications such as ECASA, ibuprofen, naproxen, or diclofenac sodium might be preferred. However, if there is evidence of a spondylarthropathy, it seems that indomethacin or tolmetin would be more appropriate. The latter two drugs would also be appropriate if morning stiffness is prolonged, and may be used in conjunction with other NSAIDs. Several of the NSAIDs have been incriminated in exacerbating the psoriasis (Abel et al. 1986), perhaps through the prostaglandin mechanism. It may therefore be necessary to change medications if an exacerbation of psoriasis occurs.

Disease-modifying drugs for psoriatic arthritis

If the arthritis persists despite the use of non-steroidal anti-inflammatory medications, then the next level of medications is embarked upon, that is, disease-modifying antirheumatic drugs.

Gold

Gold has been studied in a controlled fashion in psoriatic arthritis, using either intramuscular (Dowart et al. 1978) or oral (Carrett and Calin 1989) preparations. It has recently been shown that the intramuscular preparation is superior to the oral gold in patients with this condition (Palit et al. 1990). Moreover, although gold may control the inflammatory process in patients with psoriatic arthritis, it has not prevented progression of erosive disease over a 2-year period (Mader et al. 1995).

Penicillamine

Penicillamine has also been used successfully in psoriatic arthritis (Roux et al. 1979). Both gold and penicillamine are quite slow acting, however, requiring at least 6 months for a therapeutic effect. Therefore, other medications whose onset of action is faster have been tried.

Antimalarials

Although physicians have been reluctant to use antimalarials because of anecdotal reports of flares of psoriasis, and despite the lack of controlled trials, both chloroquine phosphate and hydroxychloroquine have been used (Kammer et al. 1979). Indeed, chloroquine has been shown to reduce disease activity in patients with psoriatic arthritis over a period of 6 months, and the frequency of psoriatic flares was no greater than that observed in the control group (Gladman et al. 1992a).

Methotrexate

Methotrexate, which has been found to be effective in controlling the skin psoriasis, has been used in psoriatic arthritis since 1964, when Black et al. (1964) performed a double-blind study of 21 patients using parenteral methotrexate. There have been two controlled trials of the use of low-dose weekly methotrexate in psoriatic arthritis. Willkens et al. (1984) demonstrated improvement in grip strength, morning stiffness, and joint count in patients with psoriatic arthritis, and physician global assessment was improved in the methotrexate group at 3 months, but only physician global assessment was significantly higher in the methotrexate group compared with the placebo. Zacharia and Zacharia (1987) found significant improvement in pain and functional scores as well as a decrease in the erthrocyte sedimentation rate during treatment with low-dose weekly methotrexate for psoriatic arthritis. Espinoza et al. (1992), in a retrospective uncontrolled study of 40 patients with psoriatic arthritis treated with a mean of dose of 11.2 mg/week of methotrexate during a mean period of 34 months, found that 37 per cent of the patients had an excellent response (no evidence of active synovitis) while 58 per cent had a good response (no more than four active joints and a decrease of at least 50 per cent in the number of those previously involved). Only two patients had discontinued the drug because of toxicity; one with leucopenia and the other stomatitis. Eleven patients developed liver test abnormalities. However, cirrhosis related to methotrexate was not noted. Abu-Shakra et al. (1995) found that while methotrexate reduced the actively inflamed joint count in patients with psoriatic arthritis, it did not prevent disease progression in these patients over a period of 2 years of treatment. None the less, methotrexate is used regularly for the treatment of psoriatic arthritis, particularly in the face of severe psoriasis. Methotrexate has an advantage over gold and penicillamine since it is effective within a few weeks. In addition, because it is given as an intermittent dose, once a week, patients prefer to take it rather than take other medications which are required daily, and often in repeated doses. Concerns about severe liver disease from methotrexate therapy, which resulted from reports in the late 1960s and early 1970s, seem to have been alleviated since more judicious use of intermittent dose has become commonplace.

Sulphasalazine

Sulphasalazine has been shown in two double-blind, placebo-controlled trials to be effective in psoriatic arthritis (Farr *et al.* 1990; Fraser *et al.* 1993). Rahman and Gladman (1995) recently demonstrated that sulphasalazine may not be tolerated by all patients with psoriatic arthritis, but in patients who are able to continue therapy the clinical response is impressive, and there is also improvement in the skin psoriasis.

Azathioprine

Azathioprine has also been used in psoriatic arthritis (Levy *et al.* 1972), but since its effect on psoriasis is not well recognized, it has not been as useful as it is in rheumatoid arthritis. We have recently used azathioprine in patients with psoriatic arthritis who had not responded to or were unable to tolerate methotrexate, with encouraging results.

Retinoids

Retinoids have only been studied in uncontrolled fashion, since it is difficult to blind both patients and observers to their side-effects (Klinkhoff *et al.* 1989). While these drugs may be effective against both skin and joint manifestations, their toxicity appears high. There is a new retinoid being tested at present which may prove less toxic.

Cyclosporin

Cyclosporin has recently been studied as a therapeutic option for both psoriasis and psoriatic arthritis (Gupta *et al.* 1989*b*; Salvarani *et al.* 1992*b*). Although it has been suggested that it is effective and safe, NSAIDs cannot be used concomitantly. Moreover, its adverse effects, particularly on the kidney, preclude its widespread use.

Steroids

Oral steroids are usually avoided in psoriatic arthritis, since on dose reduction they can cause significant flares of the skin psoriasis. However, intra-articular steroids may be used at any time, especially when there is a joint which is particularly inflamed. We tend to avoid injecting joints which are surrounded by psoriatic plaques because of fear of causing infections.

Dietary modification

Based on the pathogenetic mechanisms proposed for both psoriasis and psoriatic arthritis, there may be a role for fish oil preparations or specific immunomodulators in the treatment of both conditions. A pilot study of MaxEpa in psoriatic arthritis was promising (Peloso and Gladman 1992), but a more recent placebo-controlled trial of Efamol marine demonstrated no efficacy in psoriatic arthritis (Veale *et al.* 1994*c*). The use of oral vitamin D_3 for the treatment of psoriatic arthritis has recently been proposed (Huckins *et al.* 1990)

Other medications

Psoralen and ultraviolet A light has been used in psoriatic arthritis with some success (Perlman *et al.* 1979). More recently, the use of extracorporeal photochemotherapy has been proposed (de Misa *et al.* 1994). Buskila *et al.* (1991) described a woman with psoriatic arthritis, who experienced a remarkable improvement of her arthritis while she was taking bromocriptine for primary infertility due to hyperprolactinaemia. Others have also reported similar results (Abu-Shakra and Gladman 1993). Peptide T has also been advocated for the treatment of psoriatic arthritis, but information is currently available only from case reports (Abu-Shakra and Gladman 1993).

Physiotherapy and occupational therapeutic modalities should be used both for symptomatic relief and to avoid development of deformities. Patients may require splints and need to be instructed as to energy conservation and joint protection. In patients with spondylarthropathy, specific back exercises may be necessary.

The approach to the management of a patient with psoriatic arthritis should be to control the inflammatory process, in both the skin and the joints. If conservative measures such as topical medications and NSAIDs are not helpful, disease-suppressive medications should be used. In cases where both skin and joint disease are active, medications such as methotrexate and retinoids should be considered early. Sulphasalazine and azathioprine may also work in these situations. Where the arthritis is a problem, and skin lesions are well controlled with topical medications, then the other medications, including gold, chloroquine, penicillamine, and azathioprine might be used first. Newer modalities, such as cyclosporin, should be reserved for patients with particularly aggressive disease.

Monitoring disease activity during courses of NSAIDs and disease-modifying drugs should be based on the actively inflamed joint count and effusion count, which have been found to be reliable measures of disease activity (Gladman *et al.* 1990*a*) despite the fact that patients with psoriatic arthritis do not demonstrate the same degree of tenderness as do patients with rheumatoid arthritis (Buskila *et al.* 1992). It is important to emphasize that the pain scale has not been shown to correlate with measures of disease severity (Duffy *et al.* 1992; Blackmore *et al.* 1995).

Surgery

Surgery is reserved for patients whose joints have become deformed and damaged. There are no systematic studies of surgery in psoriatic arthritis. There is a concern that the joints do not recover function very well, and that there may be bone formation similar to what has been described in ankylosing spondylitis (Dwosh *et al.* 1976). Our own experience with knee and hip surgery has been good. However, surgical procedures performed on several of our patients in an attempt to correct flexion deformities of the fingers have not been rewarding. Patients developed recurrence or worsening of their deformities, and ended up with a less functional hand than prior to surgery.

Recently an approach to the treatment of temporomandibular joint disease in psoriatic arthritis has been described (Peterson and Shepherd 1992). Hicken *et al.* (1994) recently reviewed their experience with foot and ankle surgery in 17 patients with psoriatic arthritis collected over a 15-year period. There were 27 operations which included forefoot arthroplasty or arthrodesis and toe arthroplasty or arthrodesis. The operations were considered successful in 89 per cent of the cases. Complications occurred in a patient who had a local infection associated with a local flare of psoriasis and required corrective surgery, another patient who required an additional procedure, and a third patient who had delayed union.

The course and prognosis of psoriatic arthritis

The course of psoriatic arthritis is variable. There are patients who have few episodes and who recover completely, but in many the disease is persistent. A third of the patients relate the course of their skin disease and joint disease (Gladman *et al.* 1987). The lack of a systematic approach to disease assessment in psoriatic arthritis has hindered the performance of follow-up studies. Clinical measures of inflammatory activity as well as damage have only recently been validated in psoriatic arthritis (Gladman *et al.* 1990*a*). Roberts *et al.* (1976) concluded in their follow-up study that 'apart from the deforming group the arthritis was not notably progressive'. However, there was time lost from work in at least 60 per cent of all patients, and radiographical progression was recorded in about 15 per cent. Stern (1985) noted that more than 50 per cent of the patients with psoriatic arthritis had some limitation on their daily activities, and they were twice as likely to be unemployed as patients with other joint disease. Hanly *et al.* (1988) and Gladman *et al.* (1990*b*), suggested that the disease is progressive, based on the increased number of deformed and damaged joints observed in their patients, who were followed according to a standard protocol in the University of Toronto Psoriatic Arthritis Clinic. Coulton *et al.* (1989) reported on the outcome of 40 patients admitted to hospital for psoriatic arthritis who were followed for a mean of 8 years. At the end of that period, none of the patients died. However, 35 per cent of their patients were in Steinbrocker's classes III and IV, supporting the notion that a proportion of patients with psoriatic arthritis become disabled. Clear evidence of progression of deformities was demonstrable when patients were compared at presentation and at follow-up, based on duration of follow-up at the psoriatic arthritis clinic (Gladman 1994). None the less, the Health Assessment Questionnaire in patients with psoriatic arthritis does not give the same high scores seen in rheumatoid arthritis (Jones *et al.* 1994; Blackmore *et al.* 1995). This may very well be due to the fact that the questionnaire correlates highly with pain, which is less likely to be an issue for patients with psoriatic arthritis than for those with rheumatoid arthritis (Buskila *et al.* 1992).

It would be of benefit to be able to identify those patients who are destined to develop the more severe disease and treat them appropriately. In an attempt to identify such prognostic factors, Gladman *et al.* (1995) studied 305 patients who entered the psoriatic arthritis clinic with less than ten deformed joints, and identified clinical indicators for progression through four stages: no deformities, one to four deformities, five to nine deformities and ten or more deformities. Patients who had five or more effused joints at presentation to the clinic were more likely to progress, as were patients treated with disease-modifying drugs, while patients who had a low erythrocyte edimentation rate were less likely to develop more deformities during follow-up. There was no correlation with disease duration. Moreover, Gladman *et al.* (1995) recently demonstrated that the HLA antigens B27, B39, and DQw3 were more important than the clinical features in predicting such progression. Thus, prognostic factors for severe disease in psoriatic arthritis are

identifiable and may serve as markers for specific therapeutic modalities.

Approach to the management of psoriatic arthritis

My overall approach to a patient with psoriatic arthritis includes confirming the diagnosis, assessing the extent of disease activity in terms of both joint and skin disease, and assessing the degree of damage that has occurred. This involves a careful history, physical examination, laboratory assessment, and radiographical evaluation. The goal of treatment is control of inflammation which will hopefully lead to control of symptoms, and prevention of deformities and damage, so that the patient may continue to lead an active and productive life.

Once the diagnosis has been made and the patient assessed, my approach to management begins with patient education. I explain to the patient that he/she suffers from an inflammatory arthritis, that the treatment is aimed at controlling inflammation, and therefore medications need to be taken regularly. The role of daily stresses on exacerbations of both skin and joint disease is reviewed. The need to treat both skin and joint manifestations of the disease is also discussed. These topics often need to be repeated during follow-up.

The actual therapeutic approach is then tailored to the individual patient (see Box 1). A patient who has mild disease, with minimal skin lesions and mild arthritis without deformities, is treated with topical ointments for the skin, and non-steroidal anti-inflammatory drugs for the joints. I tend to use enteric-coated acetylsalicylic acid, ibuprofen, naproxen, or diclofenac for polyarticular disease, and those that complain of pain. In patients with oligoarticular disease, and those with spondylarthropathies, I tend to use indomethacin or tolmetin. While there is no scientific proof to support this approach, it seems to be empirically correct. However, since patients vary both in their response to and tolerance of different NSAIDs, this sequence is often changed. More for individuals who clearly express aversion to taking pills, I tend to choose those NSAIDs which can be given once daily.

I also use intra-articular corticosteroid injections for individual joints. I find that in psoriatic arthritis the inflammation is intense and deformity can ensue rapidly. My patients are educated to call immediately when a red, hot joint appears, and to present themselves for joint injections. Although some people feel that intra-articular steroids are not as effective in seronegative disease as they are in rheumatoid arthritis, this has not been my experience. We have been able to control severe inflammation and prevent damage in joints which we injected early (as judged by what happened to other joints in the same individual). This applies to both large and small joints in this disease. I use joint injections as an adjunct to systemic therapy as well, at any point in the disease, provided the joint is not completely destroyed.

In a patient with mild psoriasis but more active and severe arthritis, I tend to use second-line medications early. I use antimalarials, sulphasalazine, methotrexate, gold, and azathioprine, for this type of patient. If the patient demonstrates a spondylarthropathy, I would tend to choose sulphasalazine first, since it seems to control spinal disease as well as peripheral disease, whereas the other medications have not been shown to be as effective for spinal involvement.

In a patient who has severe psoriasis, even if the arthritis is not that severe, I tend to start with methrotrexate, since it has been shown to

Box 1 Therapeutic approach to the management of psoriatic arthritis			
Type of presentation	NSAIDs	Second line	Intra-articular
Mild skin Mild joint	Yes	No	As required
Mild skin Moderate joint	Yes	Sulphasalazine, methotrexate, antimalarials, gold, indomethacin	As required
Severe skin Mild joint	Yes	Methotrexate, sulphasalazine, cyclosporin, PUVA, retinoids	As required
Severe skin Severe joint	Yes	Methotrexate, sulphasalazine, indomethacin, PUVA, cyclosporin, retinoids	As required

be effective for both components of the disease. If the methotrexate is not tolerated, then I switch to either sulphasalazine (unless there is sulpha allergy) or azathioprine. If the methotrexate is tolerated, but not completely effective, I add either an antimalarial or sulphasalazine. In patients with severe psoriasis and mild arthritis I have used PUVA, which works well for the skin and has worked well for the joints.

I reserve the use of cyclosporin and retinoids for patients with severe psoriasis and arthritis who either refuse to take methotrexate, or are unable to tolerate it. These drugs are more toxic than the others and need to be used with caution.

References

Abel, E.A., DiCicco, L.M., Orenberg, E.K., Fraki, J.E., and Farber, E.M. (1986). Drugs in exacerbation of psoriasis. *Journal of the American Academy of Dermatology*, 15, 1007–22.

Abu-Shakra, M. and Gladman, D.D. (1993). Management of refractory psoriatic arthritis. *Rheumatology Reviews*, 2, 201–6.

Abu-Shakra, M. and Gladman, D.D. (1994). Aetiopathogenesis of psoriatic arthritis. *Rheumatology Reviews*, 3, 1–7.

Abu-Shakra, M., Gladman, D.D., Thorne, J.C., Long, J., Gough, J., and Farewell, V.T. (1995). Longterm methotrexate therapy in psoriatic arthritis: clinical and radiologic outcome. *Journal of Rheumatology*, 22, 241–5.

Avila, R., Pugh, D.G., Slocumb, C.H. *et al.* (1960). Psoriatic arthritis. A roentgenologic study. *Radiology*, 75, 691–702.

Barii-Druko, V., Dobri, I., Pai, A, *et al.* (1994). Frequency of psoriatic arthritis in general population and among psoriatics in department of dermatology. *Acta Dermatologica et Venereologica*, 74 (Suppl. 186), 107–8.

Blackmore, M., Gladman D.D., Husted J., Long J., and Farewell V.T. (1995). Measuring health status in psoriatic arthritis. *Journal of Rheumatology*, 22, 886–92.

Black, R.L., O'Brien, W.M., Van Scott, E.J., Auerbach, R., Eisen, A.Z., and Bunim, J.J. (1964). Methotrexate therapy in psoriatic arthritis. Double blind study on 21 patients. *Journal of the American Medical Association*, 189, 743–7.

Buskila, D., Sukenik, S., Holcberg, G., *et al.* (1991). Improvement of psoriatic arthritis in a patient treated with bromocriptine for hyperprolactinemia. *Journal of Rheumatology*, 18, 611–12.

Buskila, D., Langevitz, P., Gladman, D.D., *et al.* (1992). Patients with rheumatoid arthritis are more tender than those with psoriatic arthritis. *Journal of Rheumatology*, 19, 1115–19.

Carrett, S. and Calin, A. (1989). Evaluation of auranofin in psoriatic arthritis: a double blind placebo controlled trial. *Arthritis and Rheumatism*, 32, 158–65.

Cats, A. (1990). Psoriasis and arthritis. *Cutis*, 46, 323–9.

Cormane, R.D. and Asghar, S.S. (1987). Psoriasis specific chromosomal proteins, antibodies against them and disease activity. *Medical Hypotheses*, 22, 369–72.

Coulton, B.L., Thomson, K., Symmons, D.P.M., and Popert, A.J. (1989). Outcome in patients hospitalised for psoriatic arthritis. *Clinical Rheumatology*, 2, 261–5.

de Misa, R.F., Azafia, J.M., Harto, A, *et al.* (1994). Psoriatic arthritis: one year of treatment with extracorporeal photochemotherapy. *Journal of the American Academy of Dermatology*, 30, 1037–8.

Dowart, B.B., Gall, E.P., Schumacher, H.R., and Krauser, R.E. (1978). Chrysotherapy in psoriatic arthritis: efficacy and toxicity compared to rheumatoid arthritis. *Arthritis and Rheumatism*, 21, 513–15.

Duffy, C.M., Watanabe Duffy, K.N., Gladman, D.D., *et al.* (1992). Utilization of the Arthritis Impact Measurement Scales (AIMS) for patients with psoriatic arthritis. *Journal of Rheumatology*, 19, 1727–32.

Dwosh, I.L., Resnick, D., and Becker, M.A. (1976). Hip involvement in ankylosing spondylitis. *Arthritis and Rheumatism*, 19, 683–92.

Eastmond, C.J. (1994). Genetics and HLA antigens. *Baillière's Clinical Rheumatology*, 8, 263–76.

Eastmond, C.J. and Wright, V. (1979). The nail dystrophy of psoriatic arthritis. *Annals of the Rheumatic Diseases*, 38, 226–8.

Eccles, J.T. and Wright, V. (1985). The history and epidemiologic definition of psoriatic arthritis as a distinct entity. In *Psoriatic arthritis*, (ed. L.H. Gerber and L.R. Espinoza), pp. 1–8. Grune & Stratton, Orlando, FL.

Ellis, C.N., Fradin, M.S., Messana, J.M., *et al.*, (1991). Cyclosporin for plaque-type psoriasis. Results of a multidose, double-blind trial. *New England Journal of Medicine*, 324, 277–84.

Espinoza, L.R. (1985). Psoriatic arthritis: further epidemiologic and genetic considerations. In *Psoriatic arthritis*, (ed. L.H. Gerber and L.R. Espinoza), pp. 9–32. Grune & Stratton, Orlando, FL.

Espinoza, L.R., Zakraoni, L., Espinoza, C.G., *et al.* (1992). Psoriatic arthritis: clinical response and side effects of methotrexate therapy. *Journal of Rheumatology*, 19, 872–7.

Falk, E.S. and Vandbakk, ø. (1993). Prevalence of psoriasis in a Norwegian Lapp population. *Acta Dermatological et Venereologica*, 73 (Suppl.), 6–9.

Farber, E.M. and Scott, E.V. (1979). Psoriasis. In *Dermatology in general medicine*, (2nd edn) (ed. T.B. Fitzpatrick *et al.*), pp. 233–47, McGraw-Hill, New York.

Farr, M., Kitas, G.D., Waterhouse, L., Jubb, R., Felix-Davies, D., and Bacon, P.A. (1990). Sulphasalazine in psoriatic arthritis: a double-blind placebo-controlled study. *British Journal of Rheumatology*, **29**, 46–9.

Fraser, S.M., Hopkins, R., Hunter, J.A., *et al.* (1993). Sulphasalazine in the management of psoriatic arthritis. *British Journal of Rheumatology*, **32**, 923–5.

Gladman, D.D. (1985). Immunologic factors in the pathogenesis of psoriatic arthritis. In *Psoriatic arthritis*, (ed. L.H. Gerber and L.R. Espinoza), pp. 33–44. Grune & Stratton, Orlando, FL.

Gladman, D.D. (1992). Psoriatic arthritis: recent advances in pathogenesis and treatment. *Rheumatic Disease Clinics of North America*, **18**, 247–56.

Gladman, D.D. (1993). Toward unravelling the mystery of psoriatic arthritis. *Arthritis and Rheumatism*, **36**, 881–4.

Gladman, D.D. (1994). Natural history of psoriatic arthritis. *Baillière's Clinical Rheumatology*, **8**, 379–94.

Gladman, D.D. (1995) Classification criteria for psoriatic arthritis. *Baillières Clinical Rheumatology* 9, 319–29.

Gladman, D.D. and Farewell, V.T. (1995). The role of HLA antigens as indicators of disease progression in psoriatic arthritis (PSA): multivariate relative risk model. *Arthritis and Rheumatism*, 38, 845–50.

Gladman, D.D., Anhorn, K.A.B., Schachter, R.K., and Mervart, H. (1986). HLA antigens in psoriatic arthritis. *Journal of Rheumatology*, **13**, 586–92.

Gladman, D.D., Shuckett, R., Russell, M.L., Thorne, J.C., and Schachter, R.K. (1987). Psoriatic arthritis (PSA)—an analysis of 220 patients. *Quarterly Journal of Medicine*, **62**, 127–41.

Gladman, D.D., Farewell, V., Buskila, D., *et al.* (1990*a*). Reliability of measurements of active and damaged joints in psoriatic arthritis. *Journal of Rheumatology*, **17**, 62–4.

Gladman, D.D., Stafford-Brady, F., Chang, C.H., Lewandowski, K., and Russell, M.L. (1990*b*). Clinical and radiological progression in psoriatic arthritis. *Journal of Rheumatology*, **17**, 809–12.

Gladman, D.D., Blake, R., Brubacher, B., and Farewell, V.T. (1992*a*). Chloroquine therapy in psoriatic arthritis. *Journal of Rheumatology*, **19**, 1724–6.

Gladman, D.D., Brubacher, B., Buskila, D., Langevitz, P., and Farewell, V.T. (1992*b*). Psoriatic spondyloarthropathy in men and women: a clinical, radiographic, and HLA study. *Clinical And Investigation Medicine*, **15**, 371–5.

Gladman, D.D., Brubacher, B., Buskila, D., Langevitz, P., and Farewell, V.T. (1993). Differences in the expression of spondyloarthropathy: a comparison between ankylosing spondylitis and psoriatic arthritis. Genetic and gender effects. *Clinical And Investigation Medicine*, **16**, 1–7.

Gladman, D.D., Farewell, V.T., and Nadeau, C. (1995). Clinical indicators of progression in psoriatic arthritis (PSA): multivariate relative risk model. *Journal of Rheumatology*, **22**, 675–9.

Goodfield, M. (1994). Skin lesions in psoriasis. *Baillière's Clinical Rheumatology*, **8**, 295–316.

Gottlieb, A.B. (1988). Immunologic mechanisms in psoriasis. *Journal of the American Academy of Dermatology*, **18**, 1276–380.

Greaves, M.W. and Camp, R.D.R. (1988). Prostaglandins, leukotrienes, phospholipase, platelet activating factor, and cytokines: an integrated approach to inflammation of human skin. *Archives of Dermatology*, **280** (Suppl.), S33–S41.

Green, L., Meyers, O.L., Gordon, W., and Briggs, B. (1981). Arthritis in psoriasis. *Annals of the Rheumatic Diseases*, **40**, 366–9.

Grilington, F.M., Skinner, M.A., Birchall, N.M., and Tan, P.L.I. (1993). $\gamma+$ T cells from patients with psoriatic and rheumatoid arthritis respond to streptococcal antigen. *Journal of Rheumatology*, **20**, 983–7.

Gupta, A.K., Ellis, C.N., Telliner, D.C., Anderson, T.F., and Voorhees, J.J. (1989*a*). Double-blind, placebo-controlled study to evaluate the efficacy of fish oil and low-dose UVB in the treatment of psoriasis. *British Journal of Dermatology*, **120**, 801–7.

Gupta, A.K., Matteson, E.I., Ellis, C.N., *et al.* (1989*b*). Cyclosporin in the treatment of psoriatic arthritis. *Archives of Dermatology*, **125**, 507–10.

Hanly, J.G., Russell, M.L., and Gladman, D.D. (1988). Psoriatic spondyloarthropathy: a long term prospective study. *Annals of the Rheumatic Diseases*, **47**, 386–93.

Helliwell, P., Marchesoni, A., Peters, M., Barker, M., and Wright, V. (1991). A re-evaluation of the osteoarticular manifestations of psoriasis. *British Journal of Rheumatology*, **30**, 339–45.

Hicken, G.J., Kitaoka, H.B., and Valente R.M. (1994). Foot and ankle surgery in patients with psoriasis. *Clinical Orthopedics and Related Research*, **300**, 204–6.

Huckins, D., Felson, D.T., and Holick, M. (1990). Treatment of psoriatic arthritis with oral 1,25-dihydroxyvitamin D_3: a pilot study. *Arthritis and Rheumatism*, **33**, 1723–7.

Jenkinson, T., Armas, J., Evison, G., *et al.* (1994). The cervical spine in psoriatic arthritis: a clinical and radiological study. *British Journal of Rheumatology*, **33**, 255–9.

Jones, S.M., Armas, J.B, Cohen, M.G., Lovell, C.R., Evison, G., and McHugh, N.J. (1994). Psoriatic arthritis: outcome of disease subsets and relationship of joint disease to nail and skin disease. *British Journal of Rheumatology*, **33**, 834–9.

Kammer, G.M., Soter, N.A., Gibson, D.J., and Schur, P.H. (1979). Psoriatic arthritis. A clinical, immunologic and HLA study of 100 patients. *Seminars in Arthritis and Rheumatism*, **9**, 75–97.

Klinkhoff, A.V., Gertner, E., Chalmers, A., *et al.* (1989). Pilot study of etretinate in psoriatic arthritis. *Journal of Rheumatology*, **16**, 789–91.

Lambert, J.B. and Wright, V. (1977). Psoriatic spondylitis: a clinical and radiological description of the spine in psoriatic arthritis. *Quarterly Journal of Medicine*, **46**, 411–25.

Langevitz P., Buskila D., and Gladman D. (1990). Psoriatic arthritis precipitated by physical trauma. *Journal of Rheumatology*, **17**, 695–7.

Lawrence, R.C., Hochberg, M.C., Kelsey, J.L., *et al.* (1989). Estimates of the prevalence of selected arthritis and musculoskeletal diseases in the United States. *Journal of Rheumatology*, **16**, 427–41.

Leczinsky, C.G. (1948). The incidence of arthropathy in a ten-year series of psoriasis cases. *Acta Dermatologica et Venereologica*, **28**, 483–7.

Lehtinen, A., Traavisainen, M., and Leirisalo-Repo, M. (1994). Sonographic analysis of enthesopathy in the lower extremities of patients with spondyloarthropathy. *Clinical and Experimental Rheumatology*, **12**, 143–8.

Leonard, D.G., O'Duffy, J.D., and Rogers, R.S. (1978). Prospective analysis of psoriatic arthritis in patients hospitalized for psoriasis. *Mayo Clinic Proceedings*, **53**, 511–18.

Levy, J.J., Paulus, H.E., Barnett, E.V., *et al.* (1972). A double-blind controlled evaluation of azathioprine treatment in rheumatoid arthritis and psoriatic arthritis. *Arthritis and Rheumatism*, **15**, 116–17.

Little, H., Harvie, J.N., and Lester, R.S. (1975). Psoriatic arthritis in severe psoriasis. *Canadian Medical Association Journal*, **112**, 317–19.

Luxembourg, A., Cailla, H., Roux, H., and Roudier, J. (1987). Do viruses play an etiologic role in ankylosing spondylitis and psoriatic arthritis? *Clinical Immunology and Immunopathology*, **45**, 292–5.

Mader, R., Gladman, D.D., Long, J., *et al.* (1995). Injectable gold for the treatment of psoriatic arthritis—long term follow-up. *Clinical And Investigation Medicine*, **18**, 139–43.

Marks, J. (1980). Psoriasis: utilizing the treatment options. *Drugs*, **19**, 429–36.

Moll, J.M. (1994). The place of psoriatic arthritis in the spondarthritides. *Baillière's Clinical Rheumatology*, **8**, 395–417.

Mulherin, D.M., FitzGerald, O., and Bresnihan, B. (1993). Lymphedema of the upper limb in patients with psoriatic arthritis. *Seminars in Arthritis and Rheumatism*, **22**, 350–6.

O'Neill, T. and Silman, A.J. (1994). Historical background and epidemiology. *Baillière's Clinical Rheumatology*, **8**, 245–61.

Palit, J., Hill, J., Capell, H.A., *et al.* (1990). A multicentre double-blind comparison of auranofin, intramuscular gold thiomalate and placebo in patients with psoriatic arthritis. *British Journal of Rheumatology*, **29**, 280–3.

Panayi, G. (1994). Immunology of psoriasis and psoriatic arthritis. *Baillière's Clinical Rheumatology*, **8**, 419–27.

Parish, J.A., Fitzpatrick, T.B., Tanenbaum, L., and Pathak, M.A. (1974). Photochemotherapy of psoriasis with oral methoxsalen and longwave ultraviolet light. *New England Journal of Medicine*, **291**, 1207–11.

Peloso, P. and Gladman, D.D. (1992). Fish oils in the treatment of psoriatic arthritis: an open study. *Arthritis and Rheumatism*, **35** (Suppl. 9), S225 (Abstract).

Perlman, S.G., Gerber, L.H., Roberts, M., *et al.* (1979). Photochemotherapy and psoriatic arthritis. A prospective study. *Annals of Internal Medicine*, **91**, 717–22.

Peterson, A.W. and Shepherd, J.P. (1992). Facia lata interpositional arthroplasty in the treatment of temporomandibular joint ankylosis caused by psoriatic arthritis. *International Journal of Oral and Maxillofacial Surgery*, **21**, 137–9.

Rahman, P.A. and Gladman, D.D. (1995). Sulphasalazine in psoriatic arthritis [Abstract]. *Journal of Rheumatology*, 22, 1601.

Resnick, D. and Niwayama, G. (1981). Psoriatic arthritis. In *Diagnosis of bone and joint disorders*, pp. 1103–29. W.B. Saunders, Philadelphia.

Roberts, M.E.T., Wright, V., Hill, A.G.S., and Mehra, A.C. (1976). Psoriatic arthritis: a follow-up study. *Annals of the Rheumatic Diseases*, 35, 206–19.

Rødahl, E. and Iversen, O.J. (1985). Antigens related to the major internal protein, p27, of a psoriasis associated retrovirus-like particle are expressed in patients with chronic arthritis. *Annals of the Rheumatic Diseases*, 44, 761–5.

Roenigk, H.H., Fowler-Bergfeld, W., and Curtis, G.H. (1969). Methotrexate for psoriasis in weekly oral doses. *Archives of Dermatology*, 99, 86–93.

Roux, H., Schiano, A., Maestracci, D., and Serratrice, G. (1979). Notre experience du traitement du rheumatisme psoriasique par la D-penicillamine. *Revue du Rheumatisme*, 46, 631–3.

Rubins, A.Y. and Merson, A.G. (1987). Subpopulations of T lymphocytes on psoriasis patients and their changes during immunotherapy. *Journal of the American Academy of Dermatology*, 17, 972–7.

Sakkas, L.I., Loqueman, N., Bird, H., Vaughan, R.W., Welsh, K.I., and Panayi, G.S. (1990). HLA class II and T cell receptor gene polymorphisms in psoriatic arthritis and psoriasis. *Journal of Rheumatology*, 17, 1487–90.

Sakkas, L.I., Jachesoni, A., Kerr, L.A., *et al.* (1991). Immunoglobulin heavy chain gene polymorphism in Italian patients with psoriasis and psoriatic arthritis. *British Journal of Rheumatology*, 30, 449–50.

Salvarani, C., Macchioni, P., Cremonesi, T., *et al.* (1992a). The cervical spine in patients with psoriatic arthritis: a clinical, radiological and immunogenetic study. *Annals of the Rheumatic Diseases*, 51, 73–7.

Salvarani, C., Macchioni, P., Boiardi, L., *et al.* (1992b). Low dose cyclosporin A: relation between soluble interleukin-2 receptors and response to therapy. *Journal of Rheumatology*, 19, 74–9.

Scarpa, R., Oriente, P., Pulino, A., *et al.* (1984). Psoriatic arthritis in psoriatic patients. *British Journal of Rheumatology*, 23, 246–50.

Scarpa, R., Oriente, P., Pucino, A., *et al.* (1988). The clinical spectrum of psoriatic spondylitis. *British Journal of Rheumatology*, 27, 123–37.

Scarpa, R., Del Puente, A., di Girolamo, C., *et al.* (1992). Interplay between environmental factors, articular involvement, and HLA B27 in patients with psoriatic arthritis. *Annals of the Rheumatic Diseases*, 51, 78–9.

Stern, R.S. (1985). The epidemiology of joint complaints in patients with psoriasis. *Journal of Rheumatology*, 12, 315–20.

Stoeger, A., Mur, E., Penz-Schneeweiss, D., *et al.* (1994). Technitium-99m human immunoglobulin scintigraphy in psoriatic arthropathy: first results. *European Journal of Nuclear Medicine*, 21, 342–4.

Tomfohrde, J., Silverman, A., Barnes, R., *et al.* (1994). Gene for familial psoriasis susceptibility mapped to the distal end of human chromosome 17q. *Science*, 264, 1141–5.

Torre-Alonso, J.C., Rodriguez-Perez, A., Arribas-Castrillo, J.M., *et al.* (1991). Psoriatic arthritis (PA): a clinical, immunological and radiological study of 180 patients. *British Journal of Rheumatology*, 30, 245–50.

Vasey, F.B. (1985). Etiology and pathogenesis of psoriatic arthritis. In *Psoriatic arthritis*, (ed. L.H. Gerber and L.R. Espinoza), pp. 45–57. Grune & Stratton, Orlando, FL.

Vasey, F.B., Seleznick, M.J., Fenske, N.A., and Espinoza, L.R. (1989). New signposts on the road to understanding psoriatic arthritis. *Journal of Rheumatology*, 16, 1405–7.

Veale, D., Yanni, G., Rogers, S., Barnes L, Bresnihan, B., and Fitzgerald, O. (1993). Reduced synovial membrane macrophage numbers, ELAM-1 expression, and lining layer hyperplasia in psoriatic arthritis as compared with rheumatoid arthritis. *Arthritis and Rheumatism*, 36, 893–900.

Veale, D.J., Barnes, L., Rogers, S., and FitzGerald, O. (1994a). Immunohistochemical markers for arthritis in psoriasis. *Annals of the Rheumatic Diseases*, 53, 450–4.

Veale, D., Rogers, S., and Fitzgerald, O. (1994b). Classification of clinical subsets in psoriatic arthritis. *British Journal of Rheumatology*, 33, 133–8.

Veale, D.J., Torley, H.I., Richards, I.M., *et al.* (1994c). A double-blind placebo controlled trial of efamol marine on skin and joint symptoms of psoriatic arthritis. *British Journal of Rheumatology*, 33, 954–8.

Ventura, M., Colizzi, M., Ottolenghi, A., *et al.* (1989). Cell-mediated immune response in psoriasis and psoriatic arthritis. *Recenti Progressi in Medicina*, 80, 449–54.

Voorhees, J.J. (1983). Leukotrienes and other lipoxygenase products in the pathogenesis and therapy of psoriasis and other dermatoses. *Archives of Dermatology*, 119, 541–7.

Willkens, R.F., Williams, H.J., Ward, J.R., *et al.* (1984). Randomized, double-blind, placebo controlled trial of low-dose pulse methotrexate in psoriatic arthritis. *Arthritis and Rheumatism*, 27, 376–81.

Wright, V. (1956). Psoriasis and arthritis. *Annals of Rheumatic Diseases*, 15, 348–53.

Wright, V. and Moll, J.M.H. (1971). Psoriatic arthritis. *Bulletin of Rheumatic Diseases*, 21, 627–32.

Wright, V. and Moll, J.M.H. (ed.) (1976). Psoriatic arthritis. In *Seronegative polyarthritis*, pp. 169–223. North Holland Publishing Co., Amsterdam.

Wright, V., Roberts, M.C., and Hill, A.G.S. (1979). Dermatological manifestations in psoriatic arthritis: a follow-up study. *Acta Dermatologica et Venereologica*, 59, 235–40.

Zacharias, H. and Zacharias, E. (1987). Methotrexate treatment of psoriatic arthritis. *Acta Dermatologica et Venereologica*, 67, 270–3.

Zanelli, M.D. and Wilde, J.S. (1992). Joint complaints in psoriasis patients. *International Journal of Dermatology*, 31, 488–91.

5.5.5 Reactive arthropathy, Reiter's syndrome, and enteric arthropathy in adults

Bernard P. Amor and Antoine A. Toubert

Historical considerations

A brief historical survey may help in understanding the different names for what is now called reactive arthritis. The occurrence of arthritis following acute diarrhoea or a urethral discharge was intriguing enough to be mentioned occasionally in the ancient medical literature. Hippocrates noted that 'a youth does not suffer from gout until after sexual intercourse', gout at that time meaning acute arthritis. He also mentioned that diarrhoea which stops suddenly may create deposits in the chest and the joints. The observations of Martiniere in 1664, Stoll in 1776, and Brodie in 1818 are also often cited, among many others (see Gounelle and Marche 1941). Clinical descriptions improved when microbiological techniques allowed differentiation of septic from aseptic arthritis. The first description of an identifiable infectious agent triggering aseptic arthritis was made during the First World War by Fiessinger and Leroy (1916), who reported an outbreak of *Shigella dysenteriae* and described four of the dysenteric patients as suffering from what they called an 'oculo-urethro-synovial' syndrome. Hans Reiter (1916) described the same oculo–urethro–synovial triad in a young officer and discussed the role of a treponema called 'treponema arthritidis'. During the Second World War and the period of confusion that followed, epidemics of dysentery (Bauer and Engelman 1942; Marche 1946; Paronen 1948; Masbernard 1959; Noer 1966) were associated with new cases of what was now called 'Reiter's syndrome'. Further observation of these cases showed an unsuspected frequency of relapses and chronic evolution, often unrelated to new infectious episodes (Csonka 1958).

During the same period, the curing of gonococcal infections with penicillin confirmed the identification of non-gonococcal urethritis and disrupted the old and mixed concept of chronic gonococcal arthritis. Among the different aetiological agents of non-gonococcal urethritis, *Chlamydia trachomatis* (Harkness 1950; Ford and Rasmussen 1964; Dunlop *et al.* 1965; Schachter *et al.* 1969; Keat *et al.* 1980; Amor 1985) has progressively become recognized as the one most closely associated with a triad similar to that described by Fiessinger, Leroy, and Reiter after diarrhoea. 'Post-dysenteric or epidemic Reiter' and 'postvenereal or endemic Reiter's syndrome' were defined, and a first set of criteria proposed (Willkens *et al.* 1981). Concurrently, the clinical overlap and genetic links between complete or incomplete Reiter's syndrome, ankylosing spondylitis, and psoriasis appeared more and more impressive as observation periods lengthened (Marche 1954; Khan and Hall 1965; Sairanen 1969).

The association between HLA-B27 antigen, ankylosing spondylitis (Brewerton *et al.* 1973a; Schlosstein *et al.* 1973), and Reiter's syndrome or reactive arthritis (Amor *et al.* 1974; Brewerton *et al.* 1973b) provided strong support to the clinical data.

In 1973 and 1974, Aho and colleagues reported aseptic arthritis following gut infection with *Yersinia enterocolitica*, mostly in HLA-B27-positive individuals, and proposed a new term, 'reactive arthritis', which was so successful that it has progressively replaced all the previous terms (Aho *et al.* 1973; Aho *et al.* 1974).

During the same period, the clinical overlap and genetic links between reactive arthritis, ankylosing spondylitis, and other apparent entities were growing stronger, and the introduction of the concept and the term 'spond(ylo)arthropathies' was welcomed (Moll *et al.* 1974).

Definition

Reactive arthritides are often defined as aseptic arthritis triggered by an infectious agent located outside the joint. This definition is unsatisfactory because in some cases non-viable agents can be identified in the joints, and, moreover, in many patients no triggering agent may be found despite identical clinical features.

Reactive arthritides are now considered as belonging to the spondylarthropathies. Therefore, as a first step, they can be defined as spondylarthropathy according to the criteria shown in Table 1 if the sum of the scores for the 12 items is 6 or more (Amor *et al.* 1990). They can then be defined as reactive arthritis if item 7 (urethritis or cervicitis less than 1 month before an arthritic episode) and/or item 8 (acute diarrhoea less than 1 month before an arthritic episode) are present. The validity of these criteria has been established in a study including 140 spondylarthropathies and 1829 control rheumatic patients (see Table 3(b) of Chapter 5.5.1). The serial recording of the disease pattern of one patient throughout its evolution (Fig. 1) explains this definition.

It may still be useful in clinical practice or for research purposes to subdivide reactive arthritis according to the triggering agent, when it can be identified.

Clinical features

Reactive arthritis, like other spondylarthropathies, combines four syndromes: a peripheral arthritis syndrome, an enthesopathic syndrome, a pelviaxial syndrome, and an extramusculoskeletal syndrome. The combination of these four may vary from one spondylarthropathy to another, in the subgroup of reactive arthritis from one patient to another, and in a given patient during the course of the disease. Nevertheless, the diagnosis of spondylarthropathy will remain unchanged.

General conditions

The onset of reactive arthritis is sometimes acute, with fever as high as 39 °C, severe weight loss, and diffuse, polyarticular involvement. However, in most cases in which synovitis is limited to a few joints, low-grade fever or no fever at all is the rule.

The peripheral arthritis syndrome

The onset is acute and within a few days two to four joints (oligoarthritis), mainly knees and ankles, are painful and swollen with an asymmetrical distribution (item 1). Mono- and polyarthritis may be observed. They are not helpful for diagnosis, but they do not exclude it if the other items of the criteria of spondylarthropathies are present.

Diffuse swelling of an entire finger(s) or toe(s), commonly described as sausage digit or toe, is very specific (item 4).

The enthesopathic syndrome

Localized painful parts of bones at the level of the enthesis, in isolation or associated with arthritis, are described spontaneously or after questioning in 42 per cent of patients. Heel pain is the most frequently recognized enthesopathic pain because it is easier to differentiate from joint pain than enthesopathic pains localized around the knee or the hip.

The pelviaxial syndrome

Highly distinctive features are inflammatory dorsal or low back pain (item 1), or buttock pain (item 3), observed in 50 per cent of patients.

The extramusculoskeletal syndrome

Intestinal and genitourinary symptoms are not only of diagnostic but also of pathophysiological and therapeutic importance; they will be described and discussed in more detail at the end of this chapter.

Mucocutaneous lesions (Montgomery et al. 1959)

Balanitis circinata is a painless, erythematous lesion of the glans penis. The size of the lesion may vary but its boundaries with normal mucosa are always clearly defined (Fig. 2). Similar painless, erythematous, well-defined lesions may be found on the oral mucosa (hard and soft palate, gingiva, tongue, cheeks) (Fig. 3).

Mucosal lesions are not frequent (9–40 per cent) but are very specific. Being painless, they may be ignored by the patient.

Lesions of pustular psoriasis, when localized on the palms and/or the soles of the feet, are called keratoderma blennorrhagica (Fig. 4) and are diagnostically very suggestive, as are hyperkeratosis and parakeratosis of the nails. These lesions are infrequent but are often associated with a severe outcome (Temine *et al.* 1972). Ordinary psoriatic lesions may also be seen.

Visceral involvement, very similar to that observed in other spondylarthropathies, is infrequent (1 per cent), and includes cardiac conduction abnormalities (prolongation of the PR interval, complete heart block) in early disease and aortic insufficiency in late disease. An

Table 1 Criteria for diagnosing spondylarthropathies (Amor 1990)

Criteria	Score
A. *Clinical symptoms or past history of:*	
1. Lumbar or dorsal pain during the night or morning stiffness of the lumbar or dorsal spine	1
2. Asymmetrical oligoarthritis	2
3. Buttock pain—if affecting alternately the right or the left buttock	1 or 2
4. Sausage-like toe or digit	2
5. Heel pain	2
6. Iritis	2
7. Non-gonococcal urethritis or cervicitus accompanying, or within 1 month before, the onset of arthritis	1
8. Acute diarrhoea accompanying, or within 1 month before, the onset of arthritis	1
9. Presence or history of psoriasis and/or balanitis and/or of inflammatory bowel disease (ulcerative colitis. Crohn's disease)	2
B. *Radiological finding*	
10. Sacroiliitis (grade ⩾2 if bilateral; grade ⩾3 if unilateral)	3
C. *Genetic background*	
11. Presence of HLA-B27 and/or familial history of ankylosing spondylitis, Reiter's syndrome, uveitis, psoriasis or chronic enterocolopathies	2
D. *Response to treatment*	
12. Clear-cut improvement of rheumatic complaints with non-steroidal anti-inflammatory drugs (NSAIDs) in less than 48 h or relapse of the pain in less than 48 h if NSAIDs discontinued)	2

A patient will be considered as suffering from a spondylarthropathy if the sum of the 12 criteria scores is at least 6.

association with transient neurological dysfunction such as peripheral or cranial nerve palsy, Parsonage–Turner syndrome, and hemiplegia has been described (Oates and Hancock 1959).

'Pleuritic' chest wall or pseudonephritic pains are probably unrecognized enthesopathic pains of the chest or due to involvement of the costovertebral joints (Benhamou *et al.* 1987).

Ocular lesions

Conjunctivitis is a part of the classical triad and is observed very early, before or at the onset of arthritis; the discharge is sterile and subsides in 1 to 4 weeks. Uveitis is less frequent in early disease but occurs in 15 per cent of patients with recurring disease, often as an incident separate from arthritis.

Intestinal symptoms

Acute diarrhoea may precede the musculoskeletal symptoms by 1 month or less (Table 1; item 8). This diarrhoea, resulting from an outbreak of enterobacterial infection, may affect many individuals, but only some of them will go on to suffer from what has been called epidemic reactive arthritis. Dysenteric symptoms are sometimes very mild in these patients and even milder than in non–arthritic patients. If no medical advice or treatment was required, the symptoms may be ignored if patients are not closely questioned. The provocative agent has commonly disappeared from the gut when the joint symptoms arise, and during an epidemic it is identified in diarrhoeal but not in

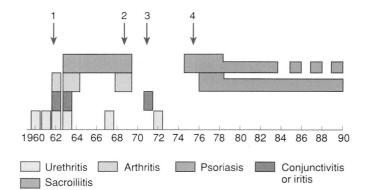

□ Urethritis □ Arthritis □ Psoriasis ■ Conjunctivitis or iritis
■ Sacroiliitis

Fig. 1 Synoptic recording of disease pattern across 30 years of follow-up in a typical patient with Reiter's syndrome. 1. The diagnosis is sexually acquired reactive arthritis. 2. Psoriasis: the diagnosis could be psoriatic arthritis. 3. Isolated iritis. 4. Buttock and back pain/sacroiliitis: the diagnosis could be ankylosing spondylitis. It is clear that this patient does not have four different diseases but only one, a spondylarthropathy, which has taken the clinical aspect of reactive arthritis at onset. He is B27-positive and has enough items (see Table 1) to be defined as spondylarthropathy at all stages of his disease.

arthritic patients. The isolation of a triggering agent from the stool of an arthritic patient is a rare event, except for salmonellae (Hannu and Leirisalo-Repo 1988). An agent is called arthritogenic if, during an outbreak, some cases of reactive arthritis are observed among a number with only dysentery. *Shigella flexneri* type 1 and 2, *Salmonella enteritidis* and *S. typhimurium*, *S. abony*, *S. blocley*, *S. schwarzengrund*, *S. heidelberg*, *S. haifa*, *S. manila*, *S. newport*, *Clostridium difficile* (Puterman and Rubinow 1993), *Vibrio parahaemoliticus* (Tamura *et al.* 1993), *Yersinia pseudotuberculosis*, and *Y. enterocolitica* fall within this definition. *Shigella sonnei*, *S. typhi*, and *Escherichia coli* dysenteric syndrome, in contrast, have so far not been complicated by reactive arthritis. *Yersinia enterocolitica* is often mentioned as the triggering agent in Northern Europe. Infection by *Y. enterocolitica* in Belgium, the country with the highest incidence of this infection, is strongly associated with eating raw pork (Tauxe *et al.* 1987).

Chronic diarrhoea or other gut symptoms are not associated with reactive arthritis; nevertheless, overlap with inflammatory bowel disease-associated arthropathies and the histological finding of silent inflammatory gut lesions in some cases of reactive arthritis make the demarcation blurred and the diagnosis of undifferentiated spondylarthropathies very helpful (see 'Enteric arthropathies in adults' below).

Urogenital symptoms

Non-specific urethritis is generally limited to a mild, painless, and non-purulent urethral discharge. It may be asymptomatic and detected by examination of the first morning urine specimen. Occasionally, however, it is severe and accompanied by prostatitis. In women, cervicitis is usually marked by vaginal discharge but may be asymptomatic.

Urethritis can also be a postdysenteric phenomenon, apparently not sexually acquired, raising the possibility that inflammation may be due to mechanisms other than direct infection.

Non-gonococcal, sexually acquired urethritis was followed by a clinical picture of reactive arthritis in 16 out of 531 men followed prospectively (Keat *et al.* 1987). Agents associated with non-gonococcal urethritis, and particularly *Ch. trachomatis*, which is the most frequently isolated, have therefore been considered as candidates for triggering sexually acquired reactive arthritis. *Chlamydia pneumonia* infection and antibodies against *Ch. pneumoniae* are highly prevalent in the adult population These antibodies make the genus/species tests unhelpful as a means of screening for the serological diagnosis of *Ch. tracomatis* infections (Freidank *et al.* 1993). But is *Ch. pneumoniae* itself able to trigger a reactive arthritis (Braun *et al.* 1994)?

Mycoplasmas and even ureaplasmas that are pathogenic for the human genital tract still require rigorous investigation. It is now clear that sexually acquired reactive arthritis is not attributable to a single micro-organism. Recurrent or repeated infections do not always lead to recurrence of arthritis and may occur in the absence of further sexual intercourse.

In women, reports of reactive arthritis following acute urogenital symptoms are scarce. Of women reviewed 2 to 4 years after the onset of salpingitis, 72 per cent had radiological or scintiscan evidence of sacroiliitis and a substantial proportion of these also had low back pain (Szanto and Hagenfeldt 1979). However, these findings have not, to date, been correlated with any specific microbiological data and raise difficulties of interpretation that remain unresolved.

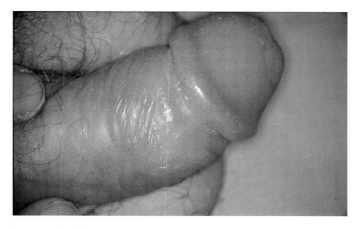

Fig. 2 Balanitis.

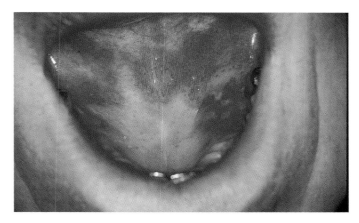

Fig. 3 An erythematous, painless, palatal mucosal lesion.

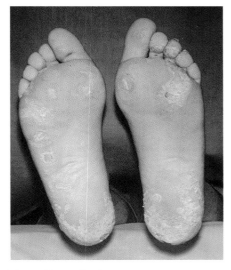

Fig. 4 Keratoderma blennorrhagica.

Genetic background

Family studies of first- and second-degree relatives may be helpful for diagnosis. Questions should not be limited to the history of reactive arthritis, even if multiple cases have been reported in some families

(Wright 1978), but should also concern other rheumatological aspects of spondylarthropathies (ankylosing spondylitis, episodes of oligoarthritis) and their most common extra-articular manifestations or associations (iritis, psoriatic skin lesions, or inflammatory bowel disease). A well-defined family history (Table 1; item 11) may provide a reliable diagnosis in the absence of specific clinical symptoms when testing for HLA-B27 antigen is not desirable for technical or economical reasons, and in HLA-B27-negative individuals (Dougados *et al.* 1991).

Response to treatment

Response to treatment is not a common tool for diagnosis, except when it is dramatic or specific, such as with colchicine in gout, penicillin in gonococcal arthritis, and corticosteroids in polymyalgia rheumatica. Pain at night and morning stiffness in spondylarthropathies are very sensitive to non-steroidal anti-inflammatory drugs. Item 12 in the diagnostic criteria (Table 1) takes advantage of this response and defines its limits (dramatic improvement within 48 h with these drugs or relapse of pain in less than 48 h after their discontinuation).

Laboratory features

The inflammatory nature of the disease is biologically confirmed by an elevated erythrocyte sedimentation rate and an increased concentration of C-reactive protein. Analysis of synovial fluid shows more than 2000 cells/mm^3, with a majority of polymorphonuclear leucocytes; synovial biopsy shows inflammatory changes including vascular congestion and perivascular cell infiltration, mainly of neutrophils. Cultures of synovial tissue or fluid are negative. The synovial complement concentration is normal. HLA-B27 is present in 50 to 80 per cent of cases. In the absence of, or in addition to, a family history, the presence of the HLA-B27 antigen constitutes item 11 in the criteria.

For therapeutic decisions in some cases, but mainly for epidemiological or for research purposes, many biological tests can be performed: these include stool cultures, which might be positive during an outbreak of gastroenteritis but are often negative when arthritic symptoms occur. *Chlamydia trachomatis* may be detected by microimmunofluorescence with specific antisera on urethral or cervical scrapings. Tests for detecting specific antibodies or the stimulation of blood mononuclear cells by bacterial antigen have no significant predictive value for reactive arthritis in the general population or even in the rheumatology clinic (Sieper *et al.* 1993a); the proliferation of mononuclear cells from synovial fluid appears more specific and could give some information on the triggering agent when the preceding infection is asymptomatic (Ford *et al.* 1985; Sieper *et al.* 1993b). The search for the products of triggering agents using specific monoclonal antibodies, or DNA or RNA hybridization, is limited to research purposes (Granfors *et al.* 1989).

In the early stages, no radiographic signs are found except for changes in the sacroiliac joint in 4 per cent of patients, probably present before the onset of reactive arthritis.

Evolution

In the short term

The first oligoarticular episode subsides in 3 to 6 months, during which time symptomatic treatment is generally required. The first episode may be longer in severe polyarticular involvement, or very short and often wrongly attributed to trauma when only one joint is affected. Two sites, the metatarsophalangeal joints and the heels, may remain painful for months and in some cases for 1 to 4 years. Extramusculoskeletal symptoms also subside, but balanitis and psoriatic lesions may persist for longer. When all symptoms are taken into account, 75 per cent of patients are in complete remission at the end of the second year after onset (Fig. 5). One per cent of patients with reactive arthritis, particularly those with keratoderma blennorrhagica, may have a very severe and even fatal outcome (Temine *et al.* 1972).

In the long term and prognosis (Amor 1979; Amor et al. 1994)

Figure 6 is based on synoptic recording of the disease pattern, as shown in Fig. 1, applied to 140 patients with reactive arthritis across 15 years. It shows the percentage of relapses and clinical involvement in these patients over time. Relapses begin 3 to 4 years after the first episode and can consist of recurrence of peripheral arthritis or enthesopathic pain (Fig. 6(a)), of pelviaxial symptoms (Fig. 6(b)), or of iritis or other extra-articular symptoms (Fig. 6(c)); these symptoms can be isolated or associated. Radiographic changes may now be observed. Narrowing of joint spaces and erosions are very uncommon, except when reactive arthritis is associated with psoriatic lesions.

Enthesopathic lesions can be visualized at an early stage by focal uptake of [^{99}Tc^m]methylene diphosphonate (**MDP**) (Fig. 7). Later radiographic changes, such as bone erosions (Fig. 8) and large and fluffy bone spurs, may develop along the metatarsals, the phalanges of the feet, the calcaneum (Fig. 9), and the pelvis.

Sacroiliitis, indistinguishable from that seen in ankylosing spondylitis, is observed in 4 per cent of patients at onset. Its frequency increases with time: it is observed in 37 per cent of patients followed for 15 years or more (see Fig. 6(b)) and is associated with axial lesions of ankylosing spondylitis in 15 per cent of cases. Over 25 per cent of patients were forced to change occupation or were unemployable. The percentage of remissions and the clinical nature of relapses over time are similar in HLA-B27-positive and -negative patients (Table 2). Seven predictive factors of long-term outcome have been selected and weighted (Table 3). If the sum of these factors at entry was 3 or less, a benign outcome could be predicted with a sensitivity of 92 per cent and a specificity of 78 per cent (Amor *et al.* 1994).

Reactive arthritis according to sex, age, and triggering agents

Better knowledge of the disease and more accurate diagnostic criteria have allowed recognition of reactive arthritis in women and children. Nevertheless, the sex ratio (M:F) is still 3:1 and three-quarters of affected patients are young adults under 40 years of age.

As an example, more than 1000 cases of postdysenteric reactive arthritis were observed in Algeria between 1954 and 1960 among young French adults during their military service, whereas the local population, whatever its ethnic origin, remained unaffected. The local population has a frequency of HLA-B27 antigen of 6 per cent and ankylosing spondylitis is as common as in other caucasoid countries but more severe (Will *et al.* 1990). This observation

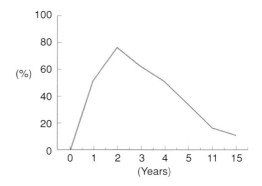

Fig. 5 Complete remission: incidence across 15 years.

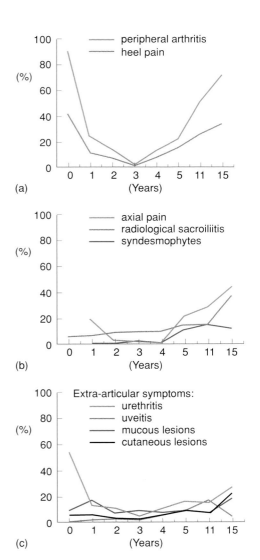

Fig. 6 Synoptic recording, as in Fig. 1, of the disease pattern in 140 patients with reactive arthritis across 15 years. (a) Recurrence of peripheral arthritis or enthesopathic pain; (b) recurrence of pelviaxial symptoms; (c) recurrence of iritis or other extra-articular symptoms.

suggests that some agents, especially those that are water-borne, do not trigger reactive arthritis in very young children.

In patients with yersinial arthritis who were HLA-B27-positive, inflammatory symptoms in the urinary tract, ocular inflammation, and back pain during acute disease were significantly more common than in HLA-B27-negative patients (Leirisalo *et al.* 1982). In contrast, erythema nodosum was more frequent in HLA-B27-negative patients with yersinial arthritis.

Differential diagnosis outside the spondylarthropathy group

Other sexually acquired arthritis

Gonococcal arthritis must be suspected in any cases of acute or subacute arthritis, usually in women. A search for *Neisseria gonorrhoea* in urethral and cervical discharges, and by culture of blood and synovial fluid, must be made concurrently with a search for agents that trigger reactive arthritis. During isolation procedures, if a gonococcal infection is suspected clinically, a therapeutic test using antibiotics exclusively is justified because arthritis will subside dramatically within 3 days and completely within 10 days.

Human immunodeficiency virus (HIV)-associated arthritis

Acute but transitory joint pains are described during the early stage of the disease; they differ from the synovitis of reactive arthritis, but reactive arthritis, like other spondylarthropathies, may be worsened by HIV (Winchester *et al.* 1987; Rowe and Keat 1989). The search for HIV infection is often recommended in even the typical case of reactive arthritis.

Behçet's syndrome

In Behçet's syndrome the painful aphthous ulcerations of oral or genital mucosa are different from the painless mucosal lesions of reactive arthritis. The total or posterior uveitis of Behçet's syndrome may be distinguished from the iritis or anterior uveitis of spondylarthropathies. Strictly oral but recurrent aphthous lesions are sometimes described by spondylarthropathic patients, leading to some confusion in their classification, which may explain some of the discrepancies concerning the frequency of sacroiliitis in Behçet's syndrome.

Parvovirus arthropathies

In parvovirus arthropathies, an acute arthritis associated with lumbar pain may mimic the onset of reactive arthritis. However, the transient erythematous skin lesions and the spontaneous recovery may help in the clinical identification of this disease (White *et al.* 1985).

Lyme disease

Oligoarthritis in Lyme disease (Steere *et al.* 1983) in young people may be confused with reactive arthritis if patients are not asked about a past history of erythema chronicum migrans or a stay in an endemic area. Enthesopathic pains are sometimes described in Lyme disease. When serological indications of Lyme disease are

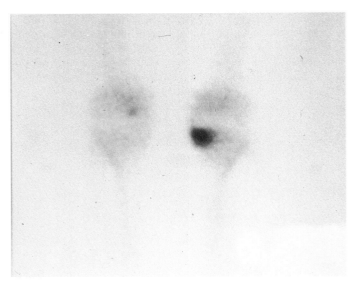

Fig. 7 Enthesopathic lesion visualized by focal uptake of [^{99}Tc^{m}]MDP.

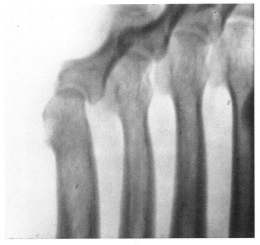

Fig. 9 Enthesopathic erosive lesion of the fifth metatarsal head.

unclear, treatment with high doses of penicillin alone (or other antibiotics), which promptly relieves symptoms in Lyme disease but is ineffective in reactive arthritis, may be helpful.

Differential diagnosis inside the spondylarthropathy group: limits of this concept

Among patients identified as having reactive arthritis in the absence of the typical oculo–urethro–synovial triad, differential diagnosis from the other spondylarthropathies is often disputed because overlaps are numerous. From a practical point of view, these disputes are probably unimportant. However, questions as to the limits of the spondylarthropathy group do arise; they concern psoriatic arthropathies and **SAPHO** (see below).

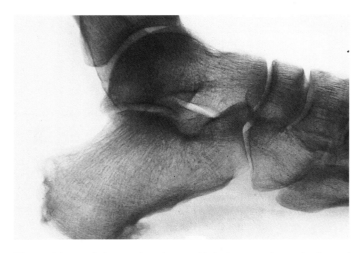

Fig. 8 Advanced changes in enthesopathic lesions: erosion and calcaneal spur.

According to the criteria for spondylarthropathies, patients with psoriatic arthritis are classified into those that meet these criteria and those that do not and in whom psoriasis appears to be associated with other rheumatic disorders such as rheumatoid arthritis.

SAPHO (synovitis, acne, palmoplantar pustulosis, hyperostosis, aseptic osteomyelitis) (Chamot et al. 1987)

The use of this grouping may help to classify patients with different clinical presentations, such as acute pseudoseptic arthritis associated with palmoplantar pustular lesions and multifocal aseptic osteomyelitis whether associated or not with the same skin lesions. The boundaries between palmoplantar pustulosis and psoriasis, the occurrence of bone lesions around the sacroiliac joints, and the presence of HLA-B27 antigen in some patients may make their classification difficult.

Table 2 Percentage of complete remissions according to HLA-B27 antigen status over time

Duration of follow-up (years)	No. of patients	HLA-B27 (percentage remissions)		
		B27	B27+	B27 −
1	123	75	50	55
5–10	69	68	36	38.4
11–15	40	65	17.6	20

Table 3 Seven predictive factors of long-term outcome in spondylarthropathy (Amor et al. 1994)

Factors observed during first 2 years of disease	Mild (n=80)	Severe (n=28)	Risk for severity Ratio	95% CI	Proposed weighting
Hip arthritis	0	7	22.85	4.43–118	4
ESR >30	10	16	7.00	4.84–9.15	3
Poor efficacy of NSAIDs	5	11	8.33	2.56–27.11	3
Limitation of lumbar axis	2	7	7.00	2–25	3
Sausage-like finger or toe	2	5	8.48	1.48–49	2
Oligoarthritis	12	12		1.38–13.1	1
Onset ≤16 years	12	10	3.47	1.058–12.75	1

A sum of 3 or less is predictive of a benign outcome (sensitivity 92.5%; specificity 78%). A sum of 7 or more indicates a risk of severe outcome (sensitivity 50%; specificity 97.5%).
ESR, erythrocyte sedimentation rate; NSAID, non-steroidal anti-inflammatory drug.

The boundaries of reactive arthritis

Postyersinial erythema nodosum may be used to introduce the issue of the boundaries of reactive arthritis. The highly statistical difference in the occurrence of erythema nodosum between HLA-B27-positive and -negative individuals may indicate that postyersinial erythema nodosum is not reactive arthritis but the result of the interaction of the same infectious agent on a different genetic background. Erythema nodosum is not otherwise described among the cutaneous manifestations observed in reactive arthritis triggered by infectious agents other than *Yersinia* spp.

The definition of reactive arthritis given earlier clarifies this issue because postyersinial erythema nodosum does not fit the diagnostic criteria for the spondylarthropathies.

The same can be said for diseases that have sometimes incorrectly been called reactive arthritis, such as rheumatic fever or parasitic arthritis. No relation exists at any level (clinical, pathological, genetic, or therapeutic) between rheumatic fever and reactive arthritis. It is nevertheless suggested that β-haemolytic streptococci may trigger reactive arthritis as well as rheumatic fever in genetically predisposed patients (Valtonen *et al.* 1993). The treatment of carcinoma of the bladder by intravesical injection of bacillus Calmette–Guérin may induce an arthritis which in some cases fits the diagnostic criteria for the spondylarthropathies. Anecdotal reports of arthritis associated with brucellae, *Mycobacterium phlei*, or parasitic infections cannot be classified as reactive arthritis because they are cured by a specific treatment, which is not the case in true reactive arthritis.

Pathogenesis of reactive arthritis

The precise disease mechanism for reactive arthritis is still unknown and research in this field has focused mainly on immunogenetics because of the association between this arthritis and HLA-B27, and on microbiology in view of the clinical data concerning the triggering

of the disease by micro-organisms (Enterobacteriaciae and *Ch. trachomatis*). The interplay between these two areas of research has generated hypotheses that apply not only to reactive arthritis but also to the other forms of spondylarthropathies and even more generally to an HLA–disease association (for a full review of possible pathogenetic mechanisms, see Chapter 5.4.1.). Several controversial aspects of the links between HLA-B27 and reactive arthritis-triggering bacteria have been unravelled by some recent findings. They all point to an important role of the *in situ* antibacterial immune response. Concerning *Ch. trachomatis*, analysis by polymerase chain reaction has shown that the organism could be present in the synovium of reactive arthritis (Rahman *et al.* 1992), albeit in a form lacking the expression of the lipopolysaccharide and major outer-membrane surface antigen (Beutler *et al.* 1994), so reflecting a state of latency and an inability of the host to clear the infection. This phenomenon could be caused by the local production of interferon-γ, consistent with the predominant Th1 phenotype of the T-helper cells in synovial fluid (Simon *et al.* 1993). Another major advance has been the isolation from lymphocytes in the synovial fluid of reactive arthritis of HLA-B27-restricted, CD8 + and bacteria-specific, cytotoxic T lymphocytes (Herman *et al.* 1993). Finally, the absence of arthritis in HLA-B27 transgenic rats (Hammer *et al.* 1990) raised in a germ-free environment (Taurog *et al.* 1994) provides a strong argument for the direct effects of both HLA-B27 and bacterial antigens in the pathogenesis of reactive arthritis and provides a precious tool for future experimental studies.

Management (Box 1)

There is no cure for reactive arthritis, but symptomatic treatments may considerably reduce the discomfort resulting from its musculoskeletal and extra-articular features.

Non-steroidal anti-inflammatory drugs promptly relieve pelviaxial pain but do not always have such clear-cut efficacy for arthritis and enthesopathies. Local injections of corticosteroids are in this instance helpful while awaiting the usual remission, 3 to 6 months later. Arthritic metatarsophalangeal joints should receive local injections very early in the disease course, and should then be passively and actively mobilized to avoid permanent deformity from fibrous retraction. In a double-blind, placebo-controlled study of 3 months, lymecycline significantly decreased the duration of illness in patients with *Ch. trachomatis*-triggered reactive arthritis but not in those with other reactive arthritides (Lauhio *et al.* 1991). A 6-month follow-up of an outbreak of *S. enteritidis* enterocolitis found arthritic symptoms in 17 of 108 patients (15 per cent) that were not prevented by early antibiotic treatment; neither did antibiotics affect the duration of reactive arthritis (Locht *et al.* 1993).

Urethritis following dysentery subsides spontaneously in a few days. Postvenereal or apparently spontaneous urethritis may be aseptic and does not respond to antibiotics. Its chronicity or frequent relapses may disturb the patient and the family. A feeling of guilt and anxiety about sexual misconduct should be allayed and the patient enlightened. Intraurethral instillation of corticosteroid may stop the chronic urethral discharge.

Early conjunctivitis subsides spontaneously. Inflammation of the uveal tract requires steroid eye-drops or subconjunctival injections. However, systemic steroids have no proven, as opposed to anecdotal, role in the management of reactive arthritis. For those patients with relentless progression of the disease, second-line drugs may be given. The efficacy of sulphasalazine (2–3 g/24 h) in ankylosing spondylitis (Dougados *et al.* 1986) has been shown in a 6-month controlled study against placebo. The clinical benefit of this drug is more clearcut in spondylarthropathies with peripheral involvement (Amor *et al.* 1984) such as reactive arthritis. Uncontrolled data suggest that methotrexate (7.5–15 mg/week) and gold salts given in a schedule similar to that used in rheumatoid arthritis may be suitable. In a placebo-controlled study (Calin 1986), azathioprine (1–2 mg/kg body wt daily) was shown to be helpful. However, immunosuppressive therapy should be avoided in young adults, unless other treatment has failed, and must be used as a last resort.

Prevention of reactive arthritis and of relapses

The diversity of agents that may trigger reactive arthritis and the significant number of cases in which no infectious agent at all is identified render preventive treatment, akin to the use of penicillin in rheumatic fever, impracticable.

Nevertheless, the number of patients with sexually acquired reactive arthritis has notably decreased in recent years and this may be due to early treatment of non-gonococcal urethritis. A study in Greenland, where epidemiological conditions are favourable (Bardin *et al.* 1990), seems to indicate that the treatment of non-gonococcal urethritis with tetracycline significantly reduces relapses of the arthritis.

Many workers have observed that in epidemic dysentery, patients with reactive arthritis have not required treatment during the dysenteric episode. This observation may also indicate that the genetic background of reactive arthritis has protects from severe diarrhoea.

Enteric arthropathies in adults

Connections between gut diseases and arthritis have been described for reactive arthritis, where only acute and time-limited dysenteric syndromes occurring within 1 month before the onset of the arthritis are considered as criteria for diagnosis (item 8; Table 1).

However, an association between gut disease and arthritis can be observed in other conditions:

(1) arthritis associated with or complicating chronic inflammatory bowel diseases;

(2) arthritis leading to the discovery of minor and previously not mentioned gut symptoms;

(3) arthritis associated with purely histological gut lesions.

The whole of this puzzle is more or less included within the definition of spondylarthropathies, but a description of each entity, emphasizing the clinical differences, is nevertheless needed. Apparently unrelated to the spondylarthropathies are the arthritis of Whipple's disease, the bypass arthritis–dermatitis syndrome, collagenous colitis, and gluten-sensitive enteropathy.

Issues concerning the bowel flora, diet, and arthritis are mainly speculative and are discussed in Chapter 5.5.1.

Arthritis associated with inflammatory bowel disease

Ulcerative colitis

The association between colitis and arthritis was first described at the end of the nineteenth century (White 1895). It was dismissed as coincident rheumatoid arthritis until 1958, when closer studies showed it to be a seronegative arthritis with distinctive features (Bywaters and Ansell 1958). Different series have shown incidences of arthritis varying from 2.5 to 22 per cent. An incidence of 11.5 per cent in a large unselected series of 269 cases (Wright and Watkinson 1966) is typical. Ulcerative colitis itself occurs in 50/100 000 individuals in England and Scandinavia, but may be less prevalent in other geographical areas.

Crohn's disease

The prevalence of Crohn's disease now exceeds that of ulcerative colitis. The disease has become more frequent in the last 30 years, mainly in northern Europe (Moll 1985), and is making an appearance in southern Europe and in Africa. Arthritis occurs in 10 to 20 per cent in most series.

Arthritis in both ulcerative colitis and Crohn's disease shows many similarities, and both are considered as members of the spondylarthropathy group. Item 9 (present or past history of inflammatory bowel disease) of the criteria shown in Table 1 allows for their classification in this group.

A familial history of inflammatory bowel disease (item 11) associated with any of the other items (sum > 6), in the absence of such disease in the patient, allows only for the diagnosis of spondylarthropathy.

As in other spondylarthropathies, four clinical syndromes, more or less combined, may be described: a peripheral arthritis syndrome, an enthesopathic syndrome, a spinal or axial syndrome, and an extra-articular syndrome.

Peripheral arthritis

Mono- or asymmetrical oligoarthritis is coincident with the onset of inflammatory bowel disease or arises during the course of the disease. There is a close temporal association between exacerbations of the gut and joint disorders. Enteropathic arthritis remits after removal of the diseased bowel segment.

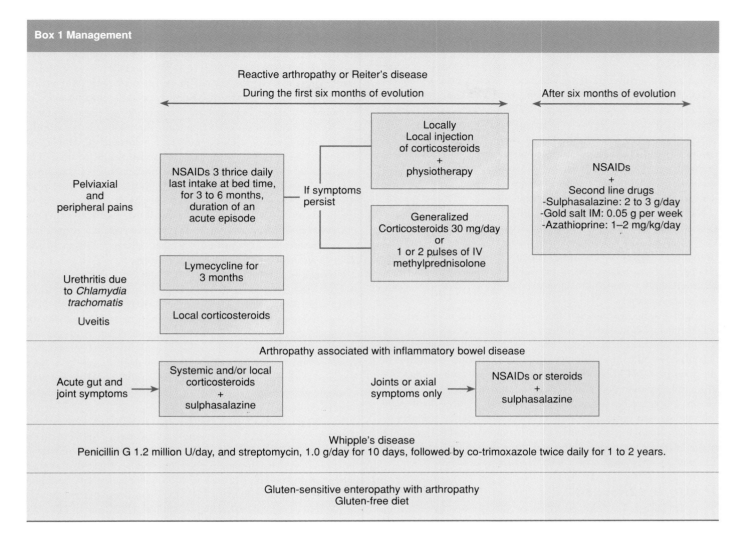

Box 1 Management

Reactive arthropathy or Reiter's disease

During the first six months of evolution — After six months of evolution

Pelviaxial and peripheral pains → NSAIDs 3 thrice daily last intake at bed time, for 3 to 6 months, duration of an acute episode → If symptoms persist → Locally Local injection of corticosteroids + physiotherapy / Generalized Corticosteroids 30 mg/day or 1 or 2 pulses of IV methylprednisolone

NSAIDs + Second line drugs -Sulphasalazine: 2 to 3 g/day -Gold salt IM: 0.05 g per week -Azathioprine: 1–2 mg/kg/day

Urethritis due to *Chlamydia trachomatis* → Lymecycline for 3 months

Uveitis → Local corticosteroids

Arthropathy associated with inflammatory bowel disease

Acute gut and joint symptoms → Systemic and/or local corticosteroids + sulphasalazine

Joints or axial symptoms only → NSAIDs or steroids + sulphasalazine

Whipple's disease
Penicillin G 1.2 million U/day, and streptomycin, 1.0 g/day for 10 days, followed by co-trimoxazole twice daily for 1 to 2 years.

Gluten-sensitive enteropathy with arthropathy
Gluten-free diet

The knees are most commonly involved, closely followed by the ankles. Other joints may be affected, but less frequently. Individual attacks are self-limiting, 50 per cent lasting less than 6 months and only 20 per cent persisting longer than 1 year. Even when recurrent they do not lead to permanent joint damage or deformity (Haslock and Wright 1973). A few cases of erosive large-joint arthritis associated with granulomatous synovitis have been reported in Crohn's disease (Toubert *et al.* 1985). Otherwise the synovial tissue shows non-specific inflammatory changes as in synovial fluid (more than 4000 cells/mm³, the majority polymorphs).

Enthesopathic pain, particularly in the heel, may either be isolated or associated with peripheral arthritis or axial involvement.

Axial involvement

In contrast to peripheral arthritis, sacroiliitis and/or spondylitis are not clearly associated either with the onset of inflammatory bowel disease or with gut exacerbations. Spondylitis is often present years before the onset of colitis or ileitis.

The frequency of ankylosing spondylitis (5 per cent), and asymptomatic sacroiliitis (14 per cent) (Wright and Watkinson 1965) is similar in males and females. HLA-B27 antigen is present in 50 per cent of these patients. HLA-Bw62 is increased in Crohn's disease and in Crohn's arthritis (Mielants and Veys 1990).

Other osteoarticular manifestations

Clubbing of fingers has been reported (Kitis *et al.* 1979) but pulmonary osteoarthropathy may be only coincidental, as are many other more common musculoskeletal disorders.

In Crohn's disease, psoas or retroperitoneal abscess may be complicated by septic arthritis of the hip (Kyle 1971).

Extra-articular syndrome (Greenstein et al. 1976)

Uveitis is observed in 10 per cent of the cases and occurs more frequently in arthritic patients.

Erythema nodosum appears more frequently in Crohn's disease (6.6 per cent) than in ulcerative colitis (4 per cent), while pyoderma gangrenosum is more frequent in ulcerative colitis (5 per cent compared to 1.3 per cent) (Greenstein *et al.* 1976). In the same study, out of 160 patients with Crohn's disease, 17 had both cutaneous and joint lesions, 23 had only arthritis, and 13 only skin lesions. Psoriasis was observed in 1.5 per cent of the patients.

Aphthous stomatitis (4 per cent) is the oral lesion most frequently seen, often associated with erythema nodosum.

Gallstones, kidney stones, and liver disease are not associated with arthritis.

Arthritis with mild, previously unnoticed gut symptoms and asymptomatic gut lesions

When patients suffering from features of spondylarthropathy are asked about gastrointestinal symptoms, some previously unnoticed dysfunctions may be revealed, such as mild but recurrent episodes of diarrhoea, anal fistula, episodes of unexplained weight loss, or a low serum cholesterol. Ileocolonoscopy in those patients often shows Crohn's disease-like lesions (aphthoid ulceration, histiocytic microgranuloma, pyloric metaplasia, and sarcoid-like granuloma). These instances of subclinical inflammatory bowel disease, mainly Crohn's disease, are underestimated (Hogan *et al.* 1980).

Mielants and Veys (1990) have found similar lesions in patients with spondylarthropathies with a negative history for gut symptoms and in patients with ankylosing spondylitis whose next of kin suffered from proven Crohn's disease. In all patients with Crohn's disease-like lesions, the gut inflammation persisted together with the joint inflammation and was more severe in nature, whereas most acute lesions disappeared.

Systematic ileocolonoscopy has been performed in 30 patients suffering from spondylarthropathies without any gut symptoms and in 18 non-arthritic patients who required this examination. Macroscopic and microscopic lesions were classified according to the descriptions of Mielants and Veys (1990). Mild lesions suggestive of gut inflammation were observed in 10 of the 30 patients and in none of the reference group ($p < 0.02$). Microscopically, there were minimal signs of inflammation (lymphocyte and plasma-cell infiltration) at the ileum level in 18 out of 19 patients compared to 11 out of 18 in the reference group ($p < 0.05$), and at the rectum level in 15 out of 19 compared to 8 out of 17 ($p < 0.05$) (Dougados *et al.* 1987).

Whipple's disease

Whipple's disease is a rare, multisystem disorder first described in 1907. Most of 500 documented cases originate from Europe and the United States. Despite its rarity, some reports mention the occurrence of Whipple's disease among individuals living in close proximity to one another (Maizel *et al.* 1970). Three patients in the same village within a 10-year period and two patients who inhabited the same farmhouse, although several years apart, were reported by Capron *et al.* (1973) and Capron *et al.* (1975).

Clinical features

Clinical manifestations (Rubinow 1988) attributable to virtually every organ system may occur in Whipple's disease and frequently may appear years or sometimes decades before the onset of diarrhoea and malabsorption. Polyarthritis, prolonged fever, weight loss, lymphadenopathy, arterial hypotension, hyperpigmentation, polyserositis, and cardiac and pulmonary symptoms are seen with varying frequency. Central nervous abnormalities including personality changes, memory loss, ataxia, presenile dementia, myoclonus, spastic paresis, seizures, ophthalmoplegia, papilloedema, retrobulbar neuritis, and deafness may appear early in the course of the disease. Anaemia and leucopenia are common haematological manifestations. Only on rare occasions have these features been recognized as prodromes of Whipple's disease.

Polyarthritis is the most common prodromal feature: 60 to 90 per cent of patients have articular involvement, which is the sole initial manifestation of the disease in 50 per cent of them.

The attacks of arthritis are characteristically acute in onset, often transient, and intermittent. They last from a few hours only to a few days and usually remit spontaneously. More rarely, the attacks may be of longer duration or even continue relentlessly for several years. Migratory oligoarthritis is more frequent than symmetrical polyarthritis or monoarthritis. Some patients complain only of recurrent arthralgia, whereas in others mild to florid synovitis may be observed. In order of frequency the joints affected are the knees, ankles, wrists, elbows, and small joints of the hands and shoulders. Residual joint deformity is usually absent or mild. The attacks of arthritis do not parallel the occurrence of diarrhoea, and the arthritis appears to subside several months to 2 years before the onset of diarrhoea and weight loss. The arthritis usually resolves within 2 months of instituting antibiotic therapy, and the reappearance of joint symptoms may herald a relapse due to premature discontinuation of that therapy. Subcutaneous nodules and clubbing are infrequent features.

Findings in synovial fluid vary with the clinical severity of the arthritis from more than 20 000 cells/mm³, mainly polymorphs, to lower white counts with a high percentage of mononuclear cells. The histopathological appearances of the synovial membrane parallel the inflammatory response found in the synovial fluid. Large, foamy, vacuolated cells containing periodic acid–Schiff (**PAS**)-positive granules and bacilli in various stages of degradation have been observed during acute episodes of arthritis in two patients, and non-caseating granulomatous lesions with histological features of sarcoidosis (Rouillon *et al.* 1993).

The involvement of axial joints is not as frequent as peripheral arthritis. When strict criteria were applied, only 4 of 95 patients could be classified as either definite ankylosing spondylitis or sacroiliitis. The spondylarthropathy criteria have not been tested on enough patients with Whipple's disease to know how many would be classified in this group of diseases. HLA-B27 antigen is present in over 30 per cent of patients according to Dobbins (1985) and in 1 out of 6 patients described by Khan (1982).

The ability to attribute early arthritic features to Whipple's disease requires a high index of suspicion and astute clinical acumen. Many patients are managed for many years as palindromic rheumatism, atypical rheumatoid arthritis, systemic lupus, or sarcoidosis. With the onset of abdominal pain, diarrhoea, steatorrhea, and weight loss the disease is more readily recognizable.

The diagnosis depends on the presence of PAS-positive macrophages in the jejunum or extraintestinal sites and eventually electron-microscopic demonstration of typical bacilli. Bacterial identification is made possible by applying the polymerase chain reaction to amplify the 16s ribosomal RNA gene sequences in tissue samples (Relman *et al.* 1992).

Pathogenesis

Different organisms easily cultured by routine microbiological methods for the bowel flora have been proposed as Whipple's bacillus. None of them combines the size and the Gram-positive coloration of the intracellular bacilli. By applying the polymerase chain reaction to amplify 16-s ribosomal RNA gene sequences, a previously uncultured new bacterium, *Tropheryma whippelii*, was discovered. It has some homology with the actinomycetes. Other bacteria have also been described (Harmsen *et al.* 1994). A dysfunction of monocytes and macrophages was shown by Bjerknes *et al.* (1985): phagocytosis was normal but no intracellular degradation of *E. coli*, *Streptococcus pyogenes*, or zymogen particles was observed. Degradation was similarly impaired 3 and 9 months after therapy; intracellular binary fission could take place after phagocytosis. Conceivably, impaired degradation of killed or viable bacteria may lead to macrophage overload and impair their antigen-presenting functions.

Treatment

The efficacy of antibiotic therapy in Whipple's disease makes this condition, once universally fatal, totally distinct from arthritis associated with inflammatory bowel disease.

Tetracycline has been the mainstay of most treatment schedules but despite initial resolution in nearly all cases of gastrointestinal and extraintestinal features, within a week to a month after beginning tetracycline (1 g/day), some patients developed late, irreversible lesions of the central nervous system (Knox *et al.* 1976). The present recommendations for the treatment of newly diagnosed patients include parenteral penicillin G, 1.2 million units/day, and streptomycin, 1.0 g/day for 10 days, followed by co-trimoxazole twice daily for 1 to 2 years (Dobbins 1985).

Arthritis–dermatitis syndrome associated with bypass surgery (Utsinger et al. 1988)

Arthritis occurs in 8 to 36 per cent of patients (mostly females) after jejunocolonic bypass. The onset may be at any time in the first 3 years after bypass. The joints commonly affected include the metacarpophalangeal and proximal interphalangeal, wrists, knees, and ankles, sometimes with a symmetrical, rheumatoid-like presentation. The pattern of involvement is most often one of brief remissions. Chronic arthritis, juxta-articular erosions, and spondylitis are very rare. White-cell counts in synovial fluid have ranged from 500 to 39 000 cells/mm^3, of which 10 to 98 per cent are polymorphonuclear leucocytes. Synovial biopsy demonstrates chronic synovitis with lymphocytic predominance but no lymphoid follicles.

Rheumatoid factor and antinuclear antibodies are absent, and the arthritis has no consistent histocompatibility association.

Dermatitis

Skin lesions accompany this arthritis in over 80 per cent of patients. The most common lesions are urticarial or papulovesicular. Lesions progress in 24 to 72 h from initially discrete macules of 2 to 12 mm diameter to pustulovesicles. Lesions are often at different stages of development. Other skin lesions include necrobiosis lipoidica, erythema nodosum, and various forms of cutaneous vasculitis. Jorizzo *et al.* (1983) suggest that the bowel bypass syndrome may occur without actual bypass.

This syndrome is associated with elevated levels of circulating immune complexes and cryoprotein precipitates (Utsinger *et al.* 1988). The antibodies in the complexes are more often to *E. coli* than to *Bacillus fragilis* or to group D streptococci.

Collagenous colitis

This condition was first described by Lindström (1976) and of some 40 patients to date, 10 per cent have had arthritis. Intestinal features consist of intermittent or persistent diarrhoea without bleeding. The majority of the patients are adult women, with a mean age of 56 years. The diagnostic finding is the linear deposition of hyaline material, 1 to 100 μm thick, consisting principally of collagen III, in the subepithelium of the colon. Lymphocytes, plasma cells, and a few eosinophils are also found, and sometimes an inflammatory exudate is present. The histological findings are distinct enough to differentiate the condition from other diseases of the colon (Rams *et al.* 1987). The aetiology is unknown. Treatment is symptomatic. Sulphasalazine and mepacrine have been recommended, with, in some cases, efficacy for both colitis and arthritis (Combe *et al.* 1988).

Gluten-sensitive enteropathy

There are some descriptions of arthropathy in cases of gluten-sensitive enteropathy (Adelizzi *et al.* 1982; Bourne *et al.* 1985; Pinals 1986). Occult coeliac disease in adults (Chakravarty and Scott 1992) and in children (Simoes and Amor 1992) is also associated with arthropathies. Effusive arthritis was present in knees and ankles, and responded promptly to a gluten-free diet. Arthralgia, sclerodactyly, and finger contracture have been described in a 60-year-old man, 10 years after the initial diagnosis of coeliac disease.

References

Adelizzi, R. A., Pecora, A. A., and Chiesa, J. C. (1982). Celiac disease, case report with an associated arthropathy. *American Journal of Gastroenterology*, 77, 481–5.
Aho, K., Ahvonen, P., Lassus, A., Sievers, K. and Tiilikainen, A. (1973). HLA antigen 27 and reactive arthritis. *Lancet*, ii, 157.
Aho, K., Ahvonen, P., Lassus, A., Sievers, K., and Tiilikainen, A. (1974). HLA 27 in reactive arthritis. A study of Yersinia arthritis and Reiter's disease. *Arthritis and Rheumatism*, 17, 521–6.
Amor, B. (1979). Reiter's syndrome: long term follow up data. *Annals of the Rheumatic Diseases*, 38 (Suppl. 1), S32–3.
Amor, B. (1985). Chlamydia and Reiter's syndrome. In *Advances in inflammation research. The spondyloarthropathies*, Vol. 9, (ed. M. Ziff and S. B. Cohen), pp. 203–10. Raven, New York.
Amor, B., Feldmann, J. L., Delbarre, F., Hors, J., Beaujan, M. M., and Dausset, J. (1974). HLA antigen W27. A genetic link between ankylosing spondylitis and Reiter's syndrome ? (Letter). *New England Journal of Medicine*, 290, 572.
Amor, B., Kahan, A., Dougados, M., and Delrieu, F. (1984). Sulfasalazine and ankylosing spondylitis. *Annals of Internal Medicine*, 101, 878.
Amor, B., Dougados, M., and Mijiyawa, M. (1990). Critères de classification des spondylarthropathies. *Revue du Rhumatisme et des Maladies Ostéoarticulaires*, 57, 85–9.
Amor, B., Santos, R. S., Nahal, R., Listrat, V., and Dougados, M. (1994). Predictive factors for the long term outcome of spondyloarthropathies. *Journal of Rheumatology*, 21, 1883–7.
Bardin, T., Enel, C., and Lathrop, M. G. (1990). Treatment by tetracycline or erythromycin of urethritides allows significant prevention of post-venereal arthritic flares in Reiter's syndrome patients. *Arthritis and Rheumatism*, 33, S26 (Abstr. 97).
Bauer, W. and Engelman, E. P. (1942). A syndrome of unknown aetiology characterized by urethritis, conjunctivitis and arthritis (so-called Reiter's syndrome). *Transactions of the Association of American Physicians, Philadelphia*, 57, 307–13.
Benhamou, C. L. *et al.* (1987). Arthrites costo-vertébrales inférieures de la pelvis-pondylite rhumatismale. Révélation pseudo urologique. *Revue du Rhumatisme et des Maladies Ostéoarticulaires*, 54, 203–7.
Beutler, A., Nanagara, R., Schumacher, H. R., and Hudson, A. (1994). Demonstration of *Chlamydia trachomatis* by in situ hybridization in synovial membranes of patients with chronic reactive arthritis. *Arthritis and Rheumatism*, 37, S233 (Abstr. 438).
Bjerknes, R., Laerum, O., and Degaard, S. (1985). Impaired bacterial degradation by monocytes and macrophages from a patient with treated Whipple's disease. *Gastroenterology*, 89, 1139–46.

Bourne, J. T. *et al.* (1985). Arthritis and coeliac disease. *Annals of the Rheumatic Diseases*, **44**, 592–8.

Braun, J., Laitko, S., Treharne, J., Eggens, U., Wu, P., Distler, A., and Sieper, J. (1994). *Chlamydia pneumoniae*, a new causative agent of reactive arthritis and undifferentiated oligoarthritis. *Annals of the Rheumatic Diseases*, **53**, 100–5.

Brewerton, D. A. *et al.* (1973*a*). Ankylosing spondylitis and HLA 27. *Lancet*, **i**, 904–8.

Brewerton, D. A. *et al.* (1973*b*). Reiter's disease and HLA-27. *Lancet*, **ii**, 996–8.

Bywaters, E. G. L. and Ansell, B. M. (1958). Arthritis associated with ulcerative colitis. A clinical and pathological study. *Annals of the Rheumatic Diseases*, **17**, 169–83.

Calin, A. (1986). A placebo controlled, cross-over study of azathioprine in Reiter's syndrome. *Annals of the Rheumatic Diseases*, **45**, 653–5.

Capron, J. P. *et al.* (1973). Maladie de Whipple: deux cas. *La Nouvelle Presse Médicale*, **2**, 2478.

Capron, J. P., Thevenin, A., Delamarre, J., *et al.* (1975). La maladie de Whipple. Etude de 3 cas et remarques épidémiologiques et radiologiques. *Lille Médical*, **20**, 842–5.

Chakravarty, K. and Scott, D. G. I. (1992). Oligoarthritis. A presenting feature of occult coeliac disease. *British Journal of Rheumatology*, **31**, 349–50.

Chamot, A. M., Benhamou, C. L., Kahn, M. F., Beranceck, L., Kaplan, G., and Prost, A. (1987). Le syndrome acné pustulose hyperostose ostéite (SAPHO). Résultats d'une enqute nationale. 85 observations. *Revue du Rhumatisme et des Maladies Ostéoarticulaires*, **54**, 187–96.

Combe, B., Pierrugues, R., Bories, P., Barneon, G., Michel, H., and Sany, J. (1988). Arthrites associées à la colite collagène. A propos de 4 cas traités par la mépacrine. *Revue du Rhumatisme et des Maladies Ostéoarticulaires*, **55**, 929–32.

Csonka, G. W. (1958). The course of Reiter's syndrome. *British Medical Journal*, **1**, 1088–90.

Dobbins, W. O., 3d (1985). Whipple's disease, an historical perspective. *Quarterly Journal of Medicine*, **56**, 523–31.

Dougados, M., Boumier, P., and Amor, B. (1986). Sulphasalazine in ankylosing spondylitis : a double blind controlled study in 60 patients. *British Medical Journal*, **293**, 911–14.

Dougados, M., *et al.* (1987). Iléocolonoscopie systématique au cours des spondyloarthropathies séronégatives. *Revue du Rhumatisme et des Maladies Ostéoarticulaires*, **54**, 279–83.

Dougados, M., *et al.* (1991). The European Spondylarthropathy Study group preliminary criteria for the classification of spondylarthropathy. *Arthritis and Rheumatism*, **34**, 1218–27.

Dunlop, E. M. C., Al-Hussaini, M. K., Garland, J. A., Treharne, J. D., Harper, I. A., and Jones, B. R. (1965). Infection of urethra by TRIC agent in men presenting because of 'non specific' urethritis. *Lancet*, **i**, 1125–8.

Fiessinger, N. and Leroy, E. (1916). Contribution à l'étude d'une épidémie de dysenterie dans la Somme (juillet–octobre 1916). *Bulletins et Mémoires de la Société Médicale des Hopitaux de Paris*, **40**, 2030–69.

Ford, D. K. and Rasmussen, G. (1964). Relationships between genito-urinary infection and complicating arthritis. *Arthritis and Rheumatism*, **7**, 220–7.

Ford, D. K., da Roza D., and Schulzer, M. (1985). Lymphocytes from the site of disease but not blood lymphocytes indicate the cause of arthritis. *Annals of the Rheumatic Diseases*, **44**, 701–10.

Freidank, H. M., Terreri, M. T., Peter, H. H., and Bredt, W. (1993). Comparison of serological tests for the detection of antibodies against *Chlamydia trachomatis* and *Chlamydia pneumoniae* in rheumatological patients. *International Journal of Medical Microbiology, Virology, Parasitology and Infectious Diseases*, **279**, 518–25.

Gounelle, H. and Marche, J. (1941). La maladie rhumatismale post-dysentérique. *Revue du Rhumatisme et des Maladies Ostéoarticulaires*, **8**, 355–401; 415–65.

Granfors, K. *et al.* (1989). Yersinia antigens in synovial-fluid cells from patients with reactive arthritis. *New England Journal of Medicine*, **320**, 216–21.

Greenstein, A. J., Janowitz, H. D., and Sachar, D. B. (1976). The extraintestinal complications of Crohn's disease and ulcerative colitis. A study of 700 patients. *Medicine (Baltimore)*, **55**, 401–12.

Hammer, R. E., Maika, S. D., Richardson, J. A., Tang, J. P., and Taurog, J. D. (1990). Spontaneous inflammatory disease in transgenic rats expressing HLA-B27 and human beta-2 m: an animal model of HLA-B27 associated human disorders. *Cell*, **63**, 1099–112.

Hannu, T. J. and Leirisalo-Repo, M. (1988). Clinical picture of reactive salmonella arthritis. *Journal of Rheumatology*, **15**, 1668–71.

Harkness, A. H. (1950). *Non-gonococcal urethritis*. Churchill Livingstone, Edinburgh.

Harmsen, D., Heeseman, J., Brabletz, T., Kirchner, T., and Muller-Hermelink, H. K. (1994). Heterogeneity among Whipple's-disease-associated bacteria. *Lancet*, **343**, 1288.

Haslock, I. and Wright, V. (1973). The musculo-skeletal complications of Crohn's disease. *Medicine (Baltimore)*, **52**, 217–25.

Hermann, E., Yu, D. T. Y., Meyer zum Büschenfelde, K. H., and Fleischer, B. (1993). HLA-B27-restricted CD8 T cells derived from synovial fluids of patients with reactive arthritis and ankylosing spondylitis. *Lancet*, **342**, 646–50.

Hogan, W. J., Hensley, G. T., and Geenen, J. E. (1980). Endoscopic evaluation of inflammation bowel disease. *Medical Clinics of North America*, **64**, 1083–102.

Jorizzo, J. L. *et al.* (1983). Bowel bypass syndrome without bypass syndrome. Bowel-associated dermatosis syndrome. *Archives of Internal Medicine*, **143**, 457–61.

Keat, A. C., Thomas, B. J., Taylor Robinson, D., Pegrum, G. D., Maini, R. N., and Scott, J. T. (1980). Evidence of *Chlamydia trachomatis* infection in sexually acquired reactive arthritis. *Annals of the Rheumatic Diseases*, **39**, 431–7.

Keat, A., Thomas, B., Dixey, J., Osborn, M., Sonnex, C., and Taylor-Robinson, D. (1987). *Chlamydia trachomatis* and reactive arthritis: the missing link. *Lancet*, **i**, 72–4.

Khan, M. A. (1982). Axial arthropathy in Whipple's disease. *Journal of Rheumatology*, **9**, 928–9.

Khan, M. Y. and Hall, W. H. (1965). Progression of Reiter's syndrome to psoriatic arthritis. *Archives Internal Medicine*, **116**, 911–18.

Kitis, G., Thompson, H., and Allan, R. N. (1979). Finger clubbing in inflammatory bowel disease. Its prevalence and pathogenesis. *British Medical Journal*, **2**, 825–8.

Knox, D. L., Bayless, T. M., and Pittman, F. E. (1976). Neurologic disease in patients with treated Whipple's disease. *Medicine (Baltimore)*, **55**, 467–76.

Kyle, J. (1971). Psoas abscess in Crohn's disease. *Gastroenterology*, **61**, 149–55.

Lauhio, A., Leirisalo-Repo, M., Lahdevirta, J., Saikku, P., and Repo, H. (1991). Double-blind, placebo-controlled study of three-month treatment with lymecycline in reactive arthritis, with special reference to Chlamydia arthritis. *Arthritis and Rheumatism*, **34**, 6–14.

Leirisalo, M. *et al.* (1982). Follow-up study on patients with Reiter's disease and reactive arthritis, with special reference to HLA B27. *Arthritis and Rheumatism*, **25**, 249–59.

Lindström, C. G. (1976). 'Collagenous colitis' with watery diarrhoea — a new entity? *Pathologia Europaea (Bruxelles)*, **11**, 87–9.

Locht, H., Kihlstrom, E., and Lindstrom, F. D. (1993). Reactive arthritis after Salmonella among medical doctors — study of an outbreak. *Journal of Rheumatology*, **20**, 845–8.

Maizel, H., Ruffin, J. M., and Dobbins, W. O., III (1970). Whipple's disease. A review of 19 patients from one hospital and a review of the literature since 1950. *Medicine (Baltimore)*, **49**, 175–205.

Marche, J. (1946). Contribution à l'étude de la maladie rhumatismale post-dysentérique et de certains types de maladies rhumatismales; les syndromes arthro-oculo-uréthro-parotidiens. *Revue du Rhumatisme et des Maladies Ostéoarticulaires*, **13**, 91–5.

Marche, J. (1954). Syndrome de Fiessinger Leroy Reiter et spondylarthrite ankylosante. Parentés et place nosologique. *Revue du Rhumatisme et des Maladies Ostéoarticulaires*, **21**, 320–8.

Masbernard, A. (1959). Le syndrome de Fiessinger–Leroy–Reiter. Enseignements fournis par l'étude de 80 cas observés en Tunisie. *Revue du Rhumatisme et des Maladies Ostéoarticulaires*, **26**, 21–45.

Mielants, H. and Veys, E. M. (1990). The gut in the spondyloarthropathies. *Journal of Rheumatology*, **17**, 7–10.

Moll, J. M. H. (1985). Inflammatory bowel disease. *Clinics in Rheumatic Disease*, **11**, 87–111.

Moll, J. M. H., Haslock, I., Macrae, I. F., and Wright, V. (1974). Associations between ankylosing spondylitis, psoriatic arthritis, Reiter's disease, the intestinal arthropathies and Behçet's syndrome. *Medicine, (Baltimore)*, **53**, 343–64.

Montgomery, M. M., Poske, R. M., Barton, E. M., Foxworthy, D. T., and Baker, L. A. (1959). The mucocutaneous lesions of Reiter's syndrome. *Annals of Internal Medicine*, **51**, 99–109.

Noer, H. R. (1966). An 'experimental' epidemic of Reiter's syndrome. *Journal of the American Medical Association*, **198**, 693–8.

Oates, J. K. and Hancock, J. A. (1959). Neurological symptoms and lesions occurring in the course of Reiter's syndrome disease. *American Journal of the Medical Sciences*, **238**, 79–84.

Paronen, I. (1948). Reiter's disease: a study of 344 cases observed in Finland. *Acta Medica Scandinavica*, **131** (Suppl. 212), 1–114.

Pinals, R. S. (1986). Arthritis associated with gluten-sensitive enteropathy. *Journal of Rheumatology*, **13**, 201–4.

Putterman, C, and Rubinow, A. (1993). Reactive arthritis associated with *Clostridium difficile* colitis. *Seminars in Arthritis and Rheumatism*, **22**, 420–6.

Rahman, M. U., Cheema, M. A., Schumacher, H. R., and Hudson, A. P. (1992). Molecular evidence for the presence of chlamydia in the synovium of patients with Reiter's syndrome. *Arthritis and Rheumatism*, **35**, 521–9.

Rams, H. Roger, A. I., and Ghandur-Mnaymneh, L. (1987). Collagenous colitis. *Annals of Internal Medicine*, **106**, 108–13.

Reiter, H. (1916). Über eine bisher unerkannte Spirochten Infektion (spirochaetosis arthritica). *Deutsche Medizinische Wochenschrift (Leipzig)*, **42**, 1535–6.

Relman, D. A., Schmidt, T. M., MacDermott, R. P., and Falkow, S. (1992). Identification of uncultured bacillus of Whipple's disease. *New England Journal of Medicine*, **327**, 293–301.

Rowe, I. F. and Keat, A. C. S. (1989). Human immunodeficiency virus infection and the rheumatologist. *Annals of the Rheumatic Diseases*, **48**, 89–91.

Rouillon, A., Menkes, C. J., Gester, J. C., Perez-Sawka, I., and Forest, M. (1993). Sarcoid-like forms of Whipple's disease. Report of 2 cases. *Journal of Rheumatology*, **20**, 1070–2.

Rubinow, A. (1988). Whipple's disease. In *Infections in the rheumatic diseases* (ed. L. Espinosa, D. L. Goldenberg, F. Arnett, and G. Alarcon), pp. 361–6. Grune and Stratton, Orlando, FA.

Sairanen, E., Paronen, I., and Mahonen, H. (1969). Reiter's syndrome. *Acta Medica Scandinavica*, **185**, 57–63.

Schachter, J., Barnes, M. G., Jones, J. P., Jnr, Engleman, E. P., and Meyer, K. F. (1966). Isolation of bedsoniae from the joints of patients with Reiter's syndrome. *Proceedings of the Society for Experimental Biology and Medicine*, **122**, 283–5.

Schlosstein, L., Terasaki, P. I., Bluestone, R., and Pearson, C. M. (1973). High association of an HLA antigen, W27, with ankylosing spondylitis. *New England Journal of Medicine*, **288**, 704–6.

Sieper, J., Braun, J., Reichardt, M., and Eggens, U. (1993a). The value of specific antibody detection and culture in the diagnosis of reactive arthritis. *Clinical Rheumatology*, **12**, 245–52.

Sieper, J., Braun, J., Wu, P., Hauer, R., and Laitko, S. (1993b). The possible role of shigella in sporadic enteric reactive arthritis. *British Journal of Rheumatology*, **32**, 582–5.

Simoes, M. and Amor, B. (1992). Juvenile arthritis and coeliac disease. *British Journal of Rheumatology*, **31**, 791.

Simon, A. K., Seipelt, E., Wu, P., Wenzel, B., Braun, J., and Sieper, J. (1993). Analysis of cytokine profiles in synovial T cell clones from chlamydial reactive arthritis patients: predominance of the Th1 subset. *Clinical and Experimental Immunology*, **94**, 122–6.

Steere, A. C. *et al.* (1983). The early clinical manifestations of Lyme disease. *Annals of Internal Medicine*, **99**, 76–82.

Szanto, E. and Hagenfeldt, K. (1979). Sacroiliitis and salpingitis. Quantitative 99m-Tc pertechnetate scanning in the study of sacroiliitis in women. *Scandinavian Journal of Rheumatology*, **8**, 129–35.

Tamura, N., Kobayashi, S., Hashimoto, H., and Hirose, S. (1993). Reactive arthritis induced by *Vibrio parahaemolyticus*. *Journal of Rheumatology*, **20**, 1062–3.

Taurog, J. D. *et al.* (1994). The germfree state prevents development of gut and joint inflammatory disease in HLA-B27 transgenic rats. *Journal of Experimental Medicine*, **180**, 2359–64.

Tauxe, R. V. *et al.* (1987). *Yersinia enterocolitica* infections and pork: the missing link. *Lancet*, 1129–32.

Temine, P., Privat, Y., Marchand, J. P., Chandon, J. P., Follana, J., and Kopp, F. (1972). Les étapes évolutives d'un cas mortel de syndrome de Fiessinger–Leroy–Reiter. *Bulletin de la Société Française de Dermatologie et de Syphiligraphie (Paris)*, **79**, 334–5.

Toubert, A., Dougados, M., and Amor, B. (1985). Erosive granulomatous arthritis in Crohn's disease. (Letter). *Arthritis and Rheumatism*, **28**, 958–9.

Utsinger, P. D., Spalding, D. M., Weiner, S. R., and Clarke, J. (1988). Intestinal immunology and rheumatic disease: inflammatory bowel disease and intestinal bypass arthropathies. In *Infections in the rheumatic diseases* (ed. L. Espinosa, D. Goldenberg, F. Arnett, and G. Alarcon), pp. 317–41. Grune and Stratton, Orlando, FA.

Valtonen, J. M., Koskimies, S., Miettinen, A., and Valtonen, V. V. (1993). Various rheumatic syndromes in adult patients associated with high antistreptolysin O titers and their differential diagnosis with rheumatic fever. *Annals of the Rheumatic Diseases*, **52**, 527–30.

White, M. H. (1895). Colitis. *Lancet*, **i**, 538.

White, D. G., Woolf, A. D., Mortimer, P. P., Cohen, B. J., Blake, D. R., and Bacon, P. A. (1985). Human parvovirus arthropathy. *Lancet*, **i**, 419–21.

Will, R. K., Amor, B., and Calin, A. (1990). The changing epidemiology of rheumatic diseases: should ankylosing spondylitis now be included? *British Journal of Rheumatology*, **29**, 299–300.

Willkens, R. F. *et al.* (1981). Reiter's syndrome: evaluation of preliminary criteria for definitive disease. *Arthritis and Rheumatism*, **24**, 844–9.

Winchester, R. *et al.* (1987). The co-occurrence of Reiter's syndrome and acquired immunodeficiency. *Annals of Internal Medicine*, **106**, 19–26.

Wright, V. (1978). Reiter's disease. In *Copeman's textbook of the rheumatic diseases*, (5th edn.) (ed. J. T. Schott), pp. 549–66. Churchill Livingstone, Edinburgh.

Wright, V. and Watkinson, G. (1965). Sacro-iliitis and ulcerative colitis. *British Medical Journal*, **2**, 675–80.

Wright, V. and Watkinson, G. (1966). Articular complications of ulcerative colitis. *American Journal of Proctology*, **17**, 107–15.

5.6 Arthropathies primarily occurring in childhood

5.6.1 Pauciarticular-onset juvenile chronic arthritis

David D. Sherry, Elizabeth D. Mellins, and Barbara S. Nepom

Pauciarticular-onset juvenile chronic arthritis is the most commonly encountered subset of the chronic childhood arthritides, accounting for 40 to 50 per cent of all patients with juvenile chronic arthritis. By definition its onset occurs before the age of 16 years, active synovitis of at least one joint is present continuously for a minimum of 6 weeks by American Rheumatism Association criteria (Brewer *et al.* 1977) or for 3 months by European League Against Rheumatism criteria (Wood 1978), and a total of four or fewer joints are involved during the first 6 months of disease. Some of the characteristics which make this disease entity quite distinct from other forms of juvenile or adult arthritis include its striking predilection for preschool-age girls, the tendency for involvement of large joints excluding the hip and shoulder, the frequent occurrence of chronic anterior uveitis, the presence of antinuclear antibodies, and unique immunogenetic associations.

In our discussion we do not include a group of patients sometimes called pauciarticular juvenile chronic arthritis type 2. This designation refers to a condition predominantly affecting older boys (over 8 years old), with lower extremity arthritis, in whom HLA B27 is frequently found. These children generally have enthesitis (Rosenberg and Petty 1982) and may have more than four joints involved. The pattern of disease in these children is more consistent with spondylarthropathy than pauciarticular-onset juvenile chronic arthritis (see Chapter 5.5.2).

Epidemiology

Pauciarticular-onset juvenile chronic arthritis is a rheumatic disease distinctly of childhood, and the vast majority of patients are female toddlers. Overall, the disease affects an estimated 20 to 30 per 100 000 children (Gare *et al.* 1987). The female to male ratio is 4:1 (Petty 1979), and may be as high as 7.5:1 among children with iridocyclitis and chronic arthritis (Spalter 1975). The age at onset peaks sharply between 1 and 3 years, but ranges from as young as a few months of age to the teenage years (see Fig. 1 and Cassidy and Petty 1995). Only a limited number of cases in adults have been reported (Chaouat *et al.* 1990; Kenesi-Laurent *et al.* 1991), and the absence of HLA DR5 and of eye involvement in patients in the latter series

raises the possibility that pauciarticular arthritis in adults represents a distinct disease entity. No unique racial or geographic associations have been described for this type of arthritis.

Clinical features

Juvenile chronic arthritis is always a diagnosis of exclusion, as there are no pathognomonic signs, symptoms, or laboratory investigations. Nevertheless, the classic clinical picture is quite recognizable: an otherwise healthy female toddler who has arthritis in only a few joints, such as one knee and one ankle (see Fig. 2(a)). Clinical features are usually mild compared with other forms of juvenile chronic arthritis, reactive arthritis, or joint infections (Morrissy 1990; Sherry 1990; Cassidy and Petty 1995). Non-articular inflammation is rare, except for chronic asymptomatic uveitis (discussed in detail below). Many children complain of little pain and are brought to the physician because joint swelling was noted by a parent. In one study, 26 per cent of patients presented without any pain whatsoever (Sherry *et al.* 1990). Those with symptoms usually complain of morning stiffness, gelling, or pain with use, but typically are not incapacitated and limit their activities only modestly. Constitutional signs and symptoms such as fever, malaise, anorexia, or organomegaly are not a part of pauciarticular-onset juvenile chronic arthritis and, if present, virtually exclude this diagnosis.

In 137 consecutive patients with this condition, we have found that almost half had involvement of the knee, with the ankle joint being the next most frequently affected (Table 1). In general, the joints most frequently involved are reported to be, in order, the knee,

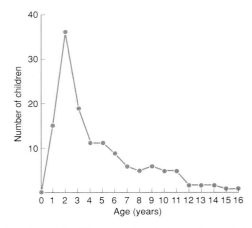

Fig. 1 Age at onset in 137 consecutive children with pauciarticular-onset juvenile chronic arthritis.

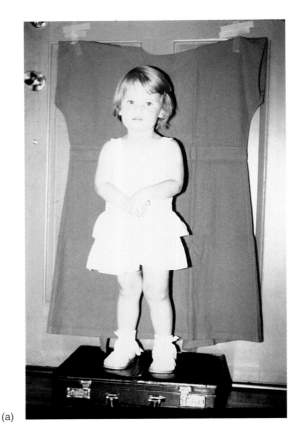

(a)

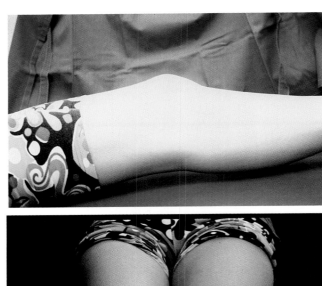

(b)

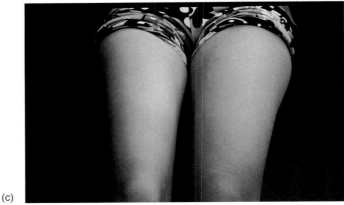

(c)

Fig. 2 Clinical features of pauciarticular-onset juvenile chronic arthritis. (a) Archetypical patient with pauciarticular-onset juvenile chronic arthritis. Note generally healthy young girl with involvement of a single knee. (b) Unilateral flexion contracture as seen frequently in pauciarticular-onset juvenile chronic arthritis. To evaluate for subtle flexion contraction, especially in children with hypermobility, lift both heels equally high and observe for unequal knee height. (c) Thigh atrophy in unilateral disease. This may be a permanent sequela.

ankle, and elbow (Schaller and Wedgwood 1972; Ansell 1977). Involvement of other joints is less frequent, but not uncommon. Children with arthritis in just one or two small joints of the hand do not have the usual pattern of joint involvement, but in our experience, most do not progress to polyarticular changes. Involvement of the shoulder is exceedingly rare. Occasional patients with this pauciarticular-onset arthritis will eventually develop disease of the temporomandibular joint (Strabrun 1991) or cervical spine; the latter can produce torticollis. Arthritis of the hip is so rare in this condition that when that joint is involved at presentation, the diagnosis is suspect and should be made only after extensive evaluation for other causes. There will also be an occasional child who has five or six joints affected over the first 6 months, but whose disease never evolves into the typical polyarticular pattern with symmetrical involvement of many joints including the small joints of the hands. Although meeting criteria for polyarticular-onset juvenile arthritis, these children have a disease more like the pauciarticular-onset disease in terms of their risk for chronic uveitis and long-term prognosis.

Laboratory features

No particular laboratory abnormalities are diagnostic of pauciarticular-onset juvenile chronic arthritis. Acute-phase reactants are usually normal to slightly elevated. Occasionally one will see a child with synovitis of a few joints and a markedly elevated erythrocyte sedimentation rate. This should prompt an extensive search for infection or occult inflammation, such as inflammatory bowel disease or leukaemia. Reactive or viral arthritis may also produce high erythrocyte sedimentation rates. A rare condition, congenital

Table 1 Pattern of joint involvement at presentation in 137 consecutive cases of pauciarticular-onset juvenile chronic arthritis

	%
Single joint	62
Two joints	31
Three joints	4
Four joints	3
Knee	47
Ankle	21
Small hand joint	12
Wrist	5
Elbow	3
Hip	3

hyperfibrinogenaemia, will cause a persistently elevated erythrocyte sedimentation rate without other laboratory features of inflammation.

Antinuclear antibodies (ANA) are present in 40 to 75 per cent of children with pauciarticular-onset chronic arthritis, depending on the analytical technique employed. These are directed to a heterogeneous mixture of nuclear antigens and usually give a homogeneous pattern, although a speckled pattern can also be observed. Antibodies to histones are relatively common; one report identified them in 42 per cent of patients with uveitis-negative, pauciarticular-onset disease (Malleson *et al.* 1992). ANA titres are usually low, less than or equal to three dilutions beyond the threshold of normal. Higher titres, especially in the older patient, should be investigated for specific autoantigens. For example, antibodies to DNA and extractable nuclear antigens would lead to the suspicion of systemic lupus erythematosus or mixed connective tissue disease. Antinuclear antibodies may develop over time; therefore, an initially negative ANA should be repeated within 1 year, owing to its critical importance in determining uveitis risk (see below). Most studies find no connection between the titre of ANA and disease activity. There is no evidence that ANA precede the development of pauciarticular-onset juvenile chronic arthritis; in fact, most healthy children with an isolated positive ANA will not develop any rheumatic disease when followed over several years (Cabral *et al.* 1992).

Rheumatoid factor is distinctly rare, occurring in less than 5 per cent of children with pauciarticular-onset disease. When it is present, it portends a polyarticular, prolonged course with a high risk of erosive arthritis. Non-classical rheumatoid factors (IgG and IgA) have been reported, but the significance of these is unknown.

Synovial fluid or a synovial biopsy are usually obtained only as an aid to excluding other diagnoses. Synovial fluid most often contains less than 25 000 white blood cells/mm³, with most of these being polymorphonuclear. The glucose concentration in synovial fluid is within 10 per cent of the serum glucose concentration; protein concentration is elevated.

A synovial biopsy has features similar to those of adult rheumatoid arthritis, with hyperplasia and hypertrophy of the synovial lining, and vascular endothelial hyperplasia with lymphocytic and plasma cell infiltration. Progression of these inflammatory changes to pannus formation and cartilaginous and eventually bony erosion, although uncommon in pauciarticular- onset arthritis, can occur and is indistinguishable pathologically from other forms of juvenile or adult rheumatoid arthritis (Cassidy and Petty 1995).

Radiographs taken early in the disease process reveal joint effusion or soft tissue swelling. Over time, juxta-articular osteoporosis occurs, followed in more severe cases by joint space narrowing and ultimately erosions. However, many bones are cartilaginous in young children (such as the carpals) or have cartilaginous epiphyses. As these ossify, the articular surface may appear quite irregular or multiple ossification centres may occur, giving the appearance of an erosion. Bilateral views are necessary to assess joint space narrowing or growth abnormalities. The expertise of a paediatric radiologist familiar with the spectrum of normal variants in childhood musculoskeletal imaging should be sought.

Course

In most children with pauciarticular-onset arthritis, the disease remains pauciarticular. Although synovitis may develop in new joints over time, the total number of affected joints remains below five. A relatively short course of active arthritis, usually 2 to 5 years, is typical. Some of these children will have a subsequent episode of chronic arthritis, sometimes many years after the original episode. Each episode seems to mimic the first in terms of joints affected and duration of disease.

An important minority will eventually develop arthritis in many joints, yet only about 20 per cent of all children with disease of pauciarticular onset will later be classified as functional stage III or IV (Stoeber 1981; Cush and Fink 1987). There is a growing impression among paediatric rheumatologists that a larger number of children with pauciarticular-onset chronic arthritis may have long-term, active synovitis than was formerly appreciated (Cush and Fink 1987), and this number may not be reflected in the functional classification data. One North American study showed that patients with three or four arthritic joints at onset, or who had involvement of the ankle, wrist, or smaller joints, were more likely to develop a polyarticular course (Cush and Fink 1987; Wallace and Levinson 1991). However, in a European study, those with monoarticular disease developed polyarticular arthritis slightly more frequently than those with the oligoarticular type (Dequecker and Mardjuadi 1982). It is generally only those converting to a polyarticular course who develop marked joint destruction, similar to those with polyarticular-onset juvenile chronic arthritis. A patient whose disease remains pauciarticular for 5 years is unlikely to progress to polyarticular involvement.

Complications

Articular complications

Children with pauciarticular-onset chronic arthritis are at risk of developing juxta-articular muscle atrophy, bony enlargement of the joint, or leg length inequality (Fig. 2(b and c)). Muscle atrophy may be dramatic. When knee synovitis starts before the age of 3 years, quadriceps muscle atrophy may continue years after disease is past (Vostrejs and Hollister 1988). Bony overgrowth around the affected joint is primarily of cosmetic concern. In those children with unilateral knee involvement, bony overgrowth may lead to a significant leg length discrepancy. When disease begins before 3 years of age, a longer leg develops on the affected side (Vostrejs and Hollister 1988), whereas when disease onset is after the age of 9 years, premature epiphyseal closure can occur, resulting in a shorter leg on the involved side (Simon *et al.* 1981). Mechanically, a longer leg on the involved side may be a problem, since the child will flex the arthritic knee to keep the pelvis level, thus exacerbating a flexion contracture. Rarely, a severe flexion contracture may progress to subluxation. Flexion contracture of the elbow can lead to an apparent foreshortening of the arm, causing a dwarf-like appearance. Effectively controlling joint inflammation can minimize, but not necessarily eliminate, these complications.

Synovial cysts, especially in the popliteal space, are not uncommon (Szer *et al.*1992). Intra-articular triamcinolone hexacetonide (1 mg/ kg) is curative in most, because these cysts communicate with the adjacent joint. Acute onset of intense limb pain and swelling suggests a ruptured cyst.

Ocular complications

In addition to musculoskeletal complications, a chronic, insidious and potentially sight-threatening form of uveitis can occur in

Table 2 Risk factors associated with uveitis in juvenile chronic arthritis

Female gender	
Female–male ratio	4.7–7.5 : 1[a]
Young onset age of arthritis	
Mean onset age (years)	4.0
Oligoarthritis	
Percentage with pauciarticular-onset arthritis	86.6
Percentage with polyarticular-onset arthritis	12.6
Percentage with systemic-onset arthritis	0.8
Antinuclear antibody positivity	
Percentage positive	80–90[b]

[a]Reviewed in Cassidy and Petty (1995).
[b]The percentage of uveitis patients with detectable antinuclear antibodies has risen to 90+ per cent since 1975 when sensitive assays became available (Wolf *et al.* 1987).
Table modified, with permission, from Rosenberg (1987).

Table 3 Uveitis surveillance: recommended frequency of slit-lamp examinations[a]

Systemic onset:	Yearly	
Pauciarticular or polyarticular onset:		
Under 7 years of age at onset:		
ANA positive:	Every 3–4 months for 4 years, then:	
	Every 6 months for 3 years, then:	
	Yearly	
ANA negative:	Every 6 months for 7 years, then:	
	Yearly	
Seven years of age or older at onset:		
	Every 6 months for 4 years, then:	
	Yearly	

These guidelines are for patients who do not develop uveitis during this time. For those patients who develop uveitis, ophthalmological treatment and surveillance will be determined by the ophthalmologist; most patients will require more frequent long-term surveillance.
[a]Taken from the American Academy of Pediatrics Section on Rheumatology and Section of Ophthalmology (1993).

children with pauciarticular-onset chronic arthritis. Described first in a case report in 1910 (Ohm 1910), the association of chronic uveitis and juvenile arthritis is now firmly established and available data suggest it is observed worldwide (for historical review see Rosenberg 1987). The ocular inflammation of juvenile chronic arthritis characteristically affects the anterior uveal tract (the iris and ciliary body); involvement of the posterior uveal tract (the choroid) is infrequent (Key and Kimure 1975).

Prevalence studies of uveitis in patients with pauciarticular-onset juvenile chronic arthritis in the United States and Britain suggest that approximately 20 per cent develop chronic uveitis (reviewed in Sherry *et al.* 1991). Uveitis is also seen in a small fraction of patients with polyarticular onset (5 per cent) and more rarely in those with systemic-onset juvenile chronic arthritis (Key and Kimure 1975; Chylack 1977). The risk of uveitis is associated with the pauciarticular mode of onset of arthritis and not with the later extent of articular disease. In two independent studies, polyarticular disease developed in about 45 per cent of pauciarticular-onset patients with uveitis (Kanski and Shun-shin 1984; Wolf *et al.* 1987). Children with uveitis thus appear to contribute disproportionately to the group with pauciarticular-onset whose disease becomes polyarticular.

In addition to pauciarticular onset of arthritis, other risk factors for the uveitis associated with juvenile chronic arthritis have been identified (Table 2). Young girls who are seropositive for ANA and seronegative for rheumatoid factors are at highest risk. Indeed, the risk of developing uveitis for ANA-positive females whose pauciarticular-onset disease began before the age of 2 years is estimated at greater than 95 per cent (Chylack *et al.* 1979). It is not known why ANA are a serological marker of those at risk. Interestingly, these antibodies are not found in patients with chronic anterior uveitis without juvenile chronic arthritis, although this disease has otherwise

similar characteristics, including a female preponderance (Rosenberg and Romanchuk 1990). In children with uveitis associated with chronic arthritis, the titre of the ANA is usually intermediate (less than 1:640) and does not correlate with the severity of ocular disease (Kanski 1977). No differences in reactivity to defined nuclear antigens are found in the ANA of children with and without uveitis (Malleson *et al.* 1989). One study of children with pauciarticular-onset chronic arthritis reported a correlation between antibodies to a novel 15-kDa nuclear antigen and uveitis, although some individuals with this antibody did not show ANA positivity in other tests (Neuteboom *et al.* 1992).

The uveitis is commonly asymptomatic, even in the face of substantial damage to the eye. In reported series, pain and redness of the eye occur in up to 25 per cent of patients; visual disturbance, photophobia, and headache are less frequent (reviewed in Cassidy and Petty 1995). Detection of disease generally requires slit-lamp ophthalmological examination. Routine surveillance (slit lamp) of at-risk patients is thus essential, at a frequency determined by the presence of risk factors (Table 3). Biomicroscopic signs of active disease include the presence of inflammatory cells and protein flare in the anterior chamber of the eye and fresh keratitic precipitates. On the initial rheumatological evaluation, one should look carefully for evidence of earlier uveitis, such as pupillary irregularities and punctate corneal deposits (Fig. 3). If present, immediate ophthalmic evaluation is appropriate. If not, regular slit-lamp examinations should be arranged.

In most children, uveitis and arthritis develop at different times. Uveitis is documented before onset of arthritis in 10 per cent of affected children (Rosenberg 1987), but asymptomatic (and undetected) uveitis may precede arthritis more often. Among routinely screened children with chronic arthritis, uveitis is usually detected

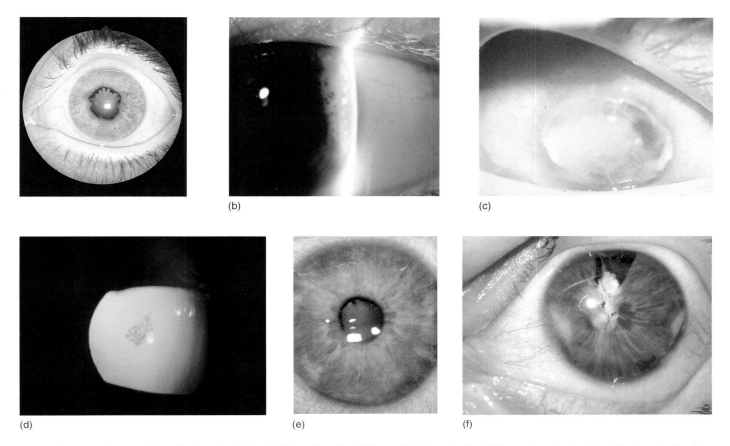

Fig. 3 Ocular involvement in juvenile chronic arthritis. (a) Signs of uveitis visible on clinical examination. This eye has developed pupillary irregularities from synechiae, which adhere the iris to the lens capsule. The dilation of the pupil reveals numerous areas of adhesion. The clouding of the pupillary reflex is caused by keratitic precipitates, which are clumps of inflammatory cells on the posterior surface of the cornea. (b) The white lacy area represents paralimbal band keratopathy, caused by deposition of calcium in Bowman's layer. (c) Extremely severe, untreated band keratopathy. (d) Small posterior subcapsular cataract, seen by retroillumination. Cataract formation may result from either steroid therapy or disease. (e) Chronic iritis with more advanced, complicated cataract. Posterior synechiae are also visible and can induce secondary glaucoma. (f) Ocular findings after surgical intervention for complicated cataract. The pupil has been secondarily scarred down, after removal of cataract membrane. Ocular inflammation predisposes to this degree of scarring, which severely compromises vision. Current surgical techniques attempt to avoid these complications. Note the horseshoe iridectomy, performed for glaucoma, as well as the paralimbal band keratopathy at 3 and 9 o'clock.

within 7 years (median, 2 years) of the onset of arthritis (Kanski and Shun-shin 1984). However, uveitis has developed up to 34 years after joint symptoms (Cassidy *et al.* 1977).

This uveitis is a chronic condition, rarely lasting less than 2 years and often more than 15 years (Smiley 1976). In a study of 20 patients, the course was remitting and relapsing in 60 per cent, persistent in 20 per cent, and limited to a single episode in 20 per cent (Rosenberg 1987). Both eyes are involved in roughly two-thirds of patients (Rosenberg 1987), but both are not necessarily inflamed at the same time. Moreover, children with uveitis of one eye rarely develop involvement of the second eye after more than 1 year of unilateral disease (Kanski 1990). Eye and joint disease evolve independently, and the overall severity of each is likely to differ (Leak and Ansell 1987). In many cases, uveitis persists years after the arthritis has become inactive (Key and Kimure 1975).

A variety of ocular complications can occur in the uveitis associated with juvenile chronic arthritis (Fig. 3). Posterior synechiae, which are fibrous bands adhering the iris to the lens, give the pupil a star-burst or irregular appearance. Band keratopathy, a layer of calcium deposits in Bowman's membrane of the cornea, is another characteristic sequela. The pathogenesis of this condition is unknown and active

iritis may persist for years without the development of keratopathy. Other complications include cataracts, glaucoma, and rarely, phthisis bulbi. Approximately 40 per cent of affected eyes progress to 20/200 visual acuity or below, and approximately 10 per cent of affected eyes will become blind (Rosenberg 1987).

Differential diagnosis

Conditions that may simulate pauciarticular-onset juvenile chronic arthritis can be classified into four major categories: monoarticular conditions, short-lived inflammatory conditions, spondylarthropathies, and complaints of pain without joint inflammation. A list of these conditions, along with some of the features distinguishing them from pauciarticular-onset arthritis, is given in Table 4 (see also related chapters in this text).

Monoarticular conditions

Monoarticular conditions are the most difficult to sort out and include several requiring immediate intervention. However, it is not uncommon for careful examination of a child with monoarticular

Table 4 Differential diagnosis of pauciarticular-onset juvenile chronic arthritis

Condition	Distinguishing features
Monoarticular	
Septic arthritis	Child is ill, high ESR, very painful, joint can be erythematous
	Haemophilus influenza predominates in children under 5 years of age, *Staphylococcus aureus* in those over 5 years
Tuberculosis	Pulmonary disease present
	Lower extremity predominates including hip
	Rapid joint destruction, may be insidious in onset
Trauma	History of direct blow or forced hyperextension
Without intra-articular bleeding	Swelling in 12–24 h, short-lived
With intra-articular bleeding	Swelling in 2 h, very painful, may have adjacent fracture
Pigmented villonodular synovitis	Repeated bleeding into joint causes synovial fluid to be haemorrhagic
Foreign-body synovitis	History of injury; organic material present in synovium
Isolated hip inflammation or pain	Older children usually affected
	Most of these conditions have typical radiographic features
Patellofemoral joint disease	Adolescent females more commonly affected
	Tenderness of undersurface of the patella
Palindromic rheumatism	Episodic and migratory
Thalassaemia	Episodic and migratory; anaemic
Short-lived inflammatory conditions (Usually last 3–6 weeks, occasionally up to 8 weeks)	
Lyme disease	Exposure in an endemic area, rash, fever, other signs of Lyme disease (neurological, cardiac), positive Lyme serology
Viral arthritis	May be associated with rash or immunization
	Rubella, varicella, parvovirus infection have been implicated
Reactive arthritis (including Reiter's)	History of preceding infection (upper respiratory, gastrointestinal, streptococcal, rarely venereal)
	Conjunctivitis, urethritis (dysuria or sterile pyuria)
	Usually older males (over 8 years old)
	May have rash, fever, or enthesitis
Post-streptococcal; acute rheumatic fever	Preceding streptococcal infection
	Migratory arthritis
	May have other signs of rheumatic fever including carditis, erythema migrans, nodules, chorea
Cystic fibrosis	Chronic pulmonary infection, usually with *Pseudomonas* spp.; rash
Spondylarthropathies: (Usually affect older children (over 8 years old); boys more than girls; may have acute iritis, most have enthesitis, frequently HLA-B27 positive, ESR often higher than expected clinically)	
Ankylosing spondylitis	Sacroiliac joint involvement; back pain; back limitation; decreased chest excursion
Psoriatic arthritis	Rash; pitting or other nail changes
Arthritis of inflammatory bowel disease	Bloody diarrhoea, high ESR

(continued on next page)

Table 4 *(continued)*

Condition	Distinguishing features
Pain complaints without joint inflammation (notable for lack of true arthritis)	
Hypermobility	Nocturnal pain in the popliteal space; can occur after specific activities; four of five criteria present: (1) thumb adducts to touch forearm (2) fingers hyperextend to parallel forearm (3 and 4) elbows or knees hyperextend beyond 108° (5) when standing, can bend over and touch palms to floor
Reflex neurovascular dystrophy	Usually pre- to adolescent females with signs of autonomic dysfunction
	More pain and disability than expected or than affect would indicate; incongruent, cheerful affect
	May have abnormal bone scan
Psychogenic musculoskeletal pains	Similar to reflex neurovascular dystrophy but without signs of autonomic dysfunction
	Hyperaesthesia common
Bone pain	Tenderness to palpation of the tibia, ulna, or other assessable bones
	Malignancy can cause some arthritis
	May be episodic
Avulsion fractures	Point-specific pain, such as at tibial tuberosity (Osgood–Schlatter), inferior pole of patella (Sinding–Larson–Johansson), or Achilles tendon insertion (Sever)
Aseptic necrosis	Point-specific pain with radiographic changes, at tarsal navicular (Köhler), carpal lunate (Kienböck), or second or third metatarsal head (Frieberg)
Osteoid osteoma	Site-specific pain, relieved by aspirin
	Abnormal radiograph and bone scan
	50 per cent in tibia
Enthesitis without arthritis	Usually older children (over 8 years old)
	Boys more than girls
	May have acute iritis
	Often HLA-B27 positive

complaints to reveal involvement of other joints. When a single joint is involved, pauciarticular-onset juvenile chronic arthritis is a frequent cause, but the conditions described in Table 4 should also be considered.

Short-lived inflammatory conditions

These conditions cause inflammation in one or several joints which can simulate pauciarticular- onset juvenile chronic arthritis, and include inflammatory reactions to a number of viral and bacterial infections. However, the inflammation is relatively fleeting, usually lasting 1 to 4, but occasionally up to 8 weeks. When evaluating a child within the first weeks of disease, one need not withhold anti-inflammatory treatment in order to establish a diagnosis. Only rarely would juvenile chronic arthritis respond so well as to go into complete remission in such a short time.

Spondylarthropathies

These conditions are discussed at length in Chapter 5.5.2, and are contrasted with pauciarticular-onset juvenile chronic arthritis in Table 4. Briefly, unlike pauciarticular-onset disease, they occur predominantly in adolescents, boys are much more commonly affected than girls, the arthritis is usually limited to the lower extremity and involves both large and small joints, enthesitis is common, and HLA B27 is highly associated (Rosenberg and Petty 1982). Heel pain is often noted in spondylarthropathies but is uncommon in pauciarticular-onset arthritis. Furthermore, the iritis that occurs with the spondylarthropathies, in contrast to that of pauciarticular-onset disease, is typically acute and painful, leading to scleral injection and photophobia.

Pain complaints without joint inflammation

Many children present with musculoskeletal pain that does not emanate from the joint. Younger children in particular may not localize their pain accurately. These conditions can be persistent and underlying arthritis may be suspected, but true arthritis is never seen. The most common examples are listed in Table 4.

Table 5   Non-steroidal anti-inflammatory drug (NSAID) use in children with juvenile chronic arthritis

NSAID	Total daily dose	Maximum daily dose	No. of doses/day	Liquid[a]	Approved[b]
Salicylic acids					
Aspirin	80–100 mg/kg/day	5200 mg	4 or 3		✓
Choline magnesium trilisate	50 mg/kg/day	4500 mg	2	✓	✓
Acetic acids					
Indomethacin	1.5–3 mg/kg/day	200 mg	4 or 3[c]	✓	
Sulindac	300–400 mg/day (adult)	400 mg	2		
Tolmetin	30–50 mg/kg/day	1800 mg	4 or 3		✓
Diclofenac	2.5 mg/kg/day	225 mg	2		
Propionic acids					
Naproxen	10–20 mg/kg/day	100 mg	2	✓	✓
Fenoprofen	40 mg/kg/day	3200 mg	4 or 3		
Ibuprofen	40 mg/kg/day	3200 mg	4 or 3	✓	✓
Fenamic acids					
Meclofenamate	3–7.5 mg/kg/day	400 mg	4 or 3		
Oxicams					
Piroxicam	0.25–0.4 mg/kg/day	20 mg (adult)	4		

[a]✓=Available as liquid preparations.
[b]✓=Approved for use in children by the United States Federal Drug Administration.
[c]Twice daily for slow-release form.

Treatment

As pauciarticular-onset juvenile chronic arthritis often affects the joints and eyes of very young children, a team approach which provides expertise in paediatric rheumatology, ophthalmology, physical therapy, and sometimes psychosocial issues is optimal. The overall guiding principle in treating these children is to keep the joint(s) as normal as possible while the disease is active so that once it becomes quiescent, the child is left with minimal complications. A corollary to this is to treat ocular inflammation early and thoroughly.

Control of intra-articular inflammation is paramount (Emery 1993). Initially non-steroidal anti-inflammatory drugs (**NSAIDs**) are given (see Table 5 and Ansell 1983; Silver 1988; Duffy *et al.* 1989; Hollingworth 1993). While a few studies have demonstrated the effectiveness of particular NSAIDs, such as aspirin, tolmetin, and naproxen (Levinson *et al.* 1977; Moran *et al.* 1979; Kvien *et al.* 1984), there are no consistent findings as to relative efficacy and tolerance. Therefore, the choice of non-steroidal drug is largely empirical, often dictated by the availability of liquid preparations for small

children or by individual response. Twice-daily preparations enhance compliance.

Most NSAIDs are tolerated well by children, with little clinical evidence of gastritis. Chemical hepatitis is their most common untoward effect, with aspirin the leading cause (Bernstein *et al.* 1977). We recommend close monitoring when liver function tests such as aspartate aminotransferase reach a level greater than three times normal, and we generally will stop the medication when the level rises to four times normal.

Pseudoporphyria, a skin disorder characterized by skin fragility, vesiculation, and scarring, has recently been reported as a side-effect of NSAIDs, particularly naproxen, among patients with juvenile chronic arthritis (Levy *et al.* 1990; Lang and Finlayson 1994). Both excessive sun exposure and fair complexion seem to increase risk for this complication. Scarring can also occur in the absence of blistering (Wallace *et al.* 1994).

The association of aspirin with Reye's syndrome, though controversial, is of concern, and it is prudent to interrupt aspirin therapy when influenza or varicella infection is suspected. It is not necessary or practical, however, to stop the drug during every viral syndrome in young children. It has been recommended that children treated with aspirin receive an annual influenza immunization (Committee on Infectious Diseases 1994).

Idiosyncratic reactions to all of the NSAIDs can occur. Neurological complications such as depression or personality changes are uncommon, and can be difficult to detect in very young children. Close attention to parental concerns is warranted.

While children often take NSAIDs for years without side-effects, potentially severe complications can occur, such as blood dyscrasias or renal papillary necrosis. Therefore we recommend careful monitoring during their use, including a complete blood count with platelet count, aspartate aminotransferase, alanine aminotransferase, blood urea nitrogen, creatinine, and urinalysis at least twice a year while on a stable dose.

Often an individual child will not respond, or not respond optimally, to a particular preparation. It can be difficult to determine when to move on to a different NSAID, and especially to a disease-modifying drug. Our guidelines are to try three NSAIDs, preferably from three different biochemical classes, at an optimal dose for 2 months each before moving on to other therapy (Lovell et al. 1984).

Intra-articular steroids are very useful and can be given in a number of different situations (Allen et al. 1986). These injections are warranted in some very young children who have great difficulty taking oral medications, especially those with only a few involved joints. If a single joint is affected, we are more likely to try intra-articular injection early. We will also consider steroid injection when the joint swelling is extreme and unlikely to respond rapidly to NSAID use. Injections can also be very useful if NSAID therapy is not possible owing to severe allergy or toxicity such as renal papillary necrosis.

In addition, we consider synovial cysts an indication for intra-articular injection. Synovial cysts usually completely resolve on injection of the adjacent joint with a steroid preparation (Allen et al. 1986). We will also consider intra-articular steroids if the arthritis is severe (intense symptoms or flexion contracture) or prolonged. Unacceptable duration of arthritis must be determined individually, but in our clinic we will inject a joint if it is markedly swollen over 3 months on optimum NSAID therapy. Finally, medical therapy will sometimes control inflammation successfully except for one recalcitrant joint; in that case, intra-articular injection may be a useful adjunct.

Some joints may not respond to an initial injection but respond well to a second attempt. If successful, joint injection can be repeated to a maximum of three injections per year per joint, or a total maximum of six injections per joint. If the arthritis continues beyond this time, more aggressive treatment is required. Intra-articular steroids may lead to localized cutaneous atrophy, hypopigmentation, or intra-articular calcifications, but these are rarely of clinical significance. We use triamcinalone hexacetonide up to 1 mg/ kg for the larger joints. Triamcinalone acetonide may also be used.

Some children with prolonged or intense arthritis, or with evolution to a more severe polyarticular course, will require more aggressive medical treatment. In these cases, we frequently use sulphasalazine because of its ease of administration, relative safety, and effectiveness in chronic arthritis (Gedalia et al. 1993). Its use is especially attractive in those children whose disease is not erosive, but who have persistent and recalcitrant inflammation. Long-term sequelae such as degenerative joint disease are of concern in patients with persistent inflammation, even in the absence of radiographic changes.

For those children who develop destructive joint changes, more aggressive therapy may be indicated. As in children with polyarticular or systemic-onset chronic arthritis, early recognition and aggressive treatment of destructive disease is critical for optimal outcome. While pauciarticular-onset juvenile chronic arthritis most often carries a favourable prognosis, it is important to monitor patients closely to identify those who will progress to more severe disease. For example, radiographs of affected joints should be obtained yearly in patients with persistent arthritis. Unlike typical adult rheumatoid arthritis, radiographic signs of destructive joint disease may not become evident in juvenile chronic arthritis until many years into the disease course.

For those patients requiring further disease-modifying drugs, there are several options (Rosenberg 1989; Gabriel and Levinson 1990; Giannini et al. 1993), although few studies have been done in pauciarticular-onset juvenile chronic arthritis. There is some controversy as to the effectiveness of hydroxychloroquine, and one study found no difference between it and placebo (Van Kerckhove et al. 1988). Similarly, good data on the use of gold and penicillamine are scant. Methotrexate has been used in some pauciarticular-onset patients with good results (Truckenbrodt and Häfner 1986; Wallace et al. 1989; Giannini et al. 1992); its safety and efficacy make it an increasingly attractive option in this setting. We currently will often use methotrexate if NSAIDs and sulphasalazine have failed. Methotrexate is usually given at a dose between 0.3 and 0.6 mg/kg per week (usually leaning toward the higher dose) as a single oral, subcutaneous, or intramuscular dose. An occasional patient is given as much as 1 mg/kg per week. We monitor blood counts, liver enzymes, and renal function monthly. The role of liver biopsy in ascertaining toxicity is controversial and presently we do not recommend it (Walker et al. 1993).

In those patients whose arthritis completely resolves, the question of when to stop medication arises. The length of treatment depends on the severity and duration of the arthritis; in general, the more difficult it is to achieve remission, the longer the treatment will continue after remission. For example, if the disease lasts 6 to 12 months, we will discontinue medications 3 to 6 months after remission. If the disease lasts longer, medications should be continued for 6 to 12 months past remission. In pauciarticular-onset juvenile arthritis, remission must be a clinical diagnosis, as many children will never have morning stiffness, increased erythrocyte sedimentation rate, or even joint pain. We define remission as the complete clinical absence of active synovitis, in addition to the lack of the conventional signs and symptoms mentioned above. Thus we continue to treat children if they have joint swelling, even if they have no complaints and are fully functional.

Motor activity is so critical to all aspects of childhood, including growth, development, and social interactions, that we are very aggressive in the use of physical therapy to keep the range of motion and muscular strength as normal as possible. However, age-appropriate exercise programmes require experience and creativity. Young children may be particularly difficult to treat because they unconsciously substitute the use of unaffected muscle groups during exercise; for the same reason, normal play activities are not an acceptable alternative to directed physical therapy. Many of these children benefit from seeing a physical therapist experienced in the treatment of these diseases. This can also help decrease parent–child conflicts over exercising.

Although not usually needed, orthotic devices can be very useful in appropriate patients. A few children have tenacious flexion contractures that require serial night splinting or even serial casting to correct. Serial casting is usually carried out three times a week for up to a month. Casting under anaesthesia is done infrequently but can be of great help in difficult situations. Where there is length inequality, shoe lifts on the short side improve gait and encourage full knee extension on the long side; this also helps keep the quadriceps muscle strong, especially the vastus medialis, which contracts only during the last $10°$ of knee extension.

Surgical intervention is rarely necessary. Synovectomy for chronic arthritis is controversial and long-term benefit is limited. In one well-designed study, synovectomy did not prevent progressive joint destruction in adult rheumatoid arthritis (Arthritis Foundation Committee on Evaluation of Synovectomy 1988). Although the complications of arthroscopic synovectomy are much lower than with the open procedure, the effort required in rehabilitation makes this procedure inappropriate for younger children. Chemical and irradiation synovectomies in children have not been adequately studied and we have no experience with these modalities. The rare child with subluxation of the knee may require surgical correction; long-term outcome is uncertain regardless of surgery. Leg length inequality can, rarely, persist into adolescence and is amenable to growth-stopping procedures on the long leg (Simon et al. 1981).

In some patients, eye involvement proves to be more of a therapeutic challenge than the joint disease. Corticosteroid eye drops and mydriatics to prevent synechiae are the typical initial regimen and are generally thought to be effective in preserving vision in eyes with minimal inflammation (Wolf et al. 1987). None the less, in one study, 42 per cent of children had not responded to topical steroids after 6 months, despite early detection and treatment of disease (Chylack 1977). Unresponsive disease is usually treated with subtenon injections of steroid or with oral prednisone; however, these increase the risk of cataract formation and glaucoma. Adjunctive use of NSAIDs may permit a reduction in steroid dose (Olson et al. 1988). Experience with immunosuppressive therapy such as azathioprine or chlorambucil is limited (reviewed in Kanski 1990); cyclosporin A has been used in severe, refractory uveitis. Band keratopathy may require chelation with EDTA or corneal scraping. Surgical intervention may also be necessary for cataracts and glaucoma. In the past, surgical treatment has been only marginally successful in these children, but results with microsurgical techniques and laser therapy are improving (Flynn et al. 1988; Kanski 1990).

The psychosocial aspects of pauciarticular-onset juvenile chronic arthritis bear some mention, especially as they may affect the ability to deliver therapy. The vast majority of patients are young and resilient and do quite well psychologically. They are not particularly limited and are able to carry out developmental tasks without difficulty. However, control issues may become a source of persistent strife between child and parent. This is especially true of the young child who may dislike taking medicine or exercising and the adolescent who is beginning to individuate from the family and deny imperfections. Moreover, even though pauciarticular-onset arthritis may be a mild condition in the spectrum of chronic childhood diseases, it can be a source of substantial distress in individual families. The degree of other stresses in the family, particularly parental dysfunction, may contribute more to the state of psychological health of children with juvenile chronic arthritis than the disease itself (Daltroy et al. 1992). Therefore, appropriate attention to these issues can potentially have a dramatic impact on the well-being of the child.

The child with pauciarticular-onset chronic arthritis is best cared for by an interdisciplinary team consisting of members who are experienced with the complications of this disease and intimately familiar with each other's roles (Brewer et al. 1989). This will enhance both family education and team communication. This team should include physicians (a paediatric rheumatologist, ophthalmologist, and orthopaedist), nurses, physical and occupational therapists, a social worker, and, as needed, other health professionals such as a nutritionist. It is with such a team that a uniform, consistent plan of therapy can be initiated and appropriately altered if complications arise. Preventive measures, especially those dealing with psychological or behaviour factors, can be instituted.

Prognosis

Over 80 per cent of children with pauciarticular-onset chronic arthritis suffer little or no musculoskeletal disability at 15-year follow-up (Ansell and Wood 1976; Stoeber 1981; Dequecker and Mardjuadi 1982). The small percentage of those who do poorly is exclusively made up of those children whose disease follows a polyarticular course (Cush and Fink 1987). The majority of the children who become polyarticular do so within the first 5 years of onset. It has been hoped that certain HLA genes might be associated with the subset of children who progress to a polyarticular course and thus predict those at high risk, but at this time there is no consensus that particular genes are helpful in predicting disease course in an individual child (see below).

The outcome in the associated uveitis varies from remission without residua to significant visual loss. A critical determinant affecting outcome is the extent of disease at initial examination (Wolf et al. 1987). Eyes which are normal or have mild uveitis at first evaluation do significantly better than those with posterior synechiae (Table 6). In addition, early onset of uveitis in relationship to arthritis correlates with poor outcome (Wolf et al. 1987). Ocular prognosis is of greatest concern if uveitis is documented before the onset of arthritis,

Table 6 Frequency of complications of chronic uveitis

Cumulative complications	Initial examination	
	Mild uveitis[a] (% of eyes)	Advanced uveitis[b] (% of eyes)
None	64	
Posterior synechiae	12	100
Cataract	28	81[c]
Band keratopathy	5	77[c]
Glaucoma	17	45[c]
Phthisis bulbi	0	13
Final visual acuity ⩽20/200	3	58[c]

[a]Normal, cells, flare, or keratitic precipitates (n = 58 eyes).
[b]Posterior synechiae (n = 31 eyes).
[c]$p < 0.001$.
Modified from (Wolf et al. 1987).

as progression to symptomatic disease implies significant injury to the eye (Wolf *et al.* 1987). These results strongly suggest that early intervention beneficially influences outcome; indeed, if untreated, uveitis may cause irreversible injury and visual loss in as little as 2 years (Wolf *et al.* 1987). However, there may also be a subgroup of patients with a more benign form of the disease (Smiley 1976). Kanski (1977) reported that 8 out of 26 eyes with continuing active uveitis for more than 10 years remained free of complications or visual loss. Unfortunately, no particular features distinguish such a subset of children at disease onset. The overall prognosis for vision among patients with the uveitis associated with juvenile arthritis has apparently improved in recent years (Sherry *et al.* 1991; Cassidy and Petty 1995). This observed decrease in disease severity is probably due to more comprehensive detection of uveitis, including benign disease, and to more timely treatment.

Aetiology

The aetiology of pauciarticular-onset juvenile chronic arthritis is unknown. Any satisfactory model of pathogenesis must account for the two most striking features of this disease: the preponderance of young female patients and the frequent association of uveitis. The former suggests a possible contribution of an X-linked gene; the latter may reflect tropism of an infectious agent or involvement of an autoantigen common to the eye and the joint.

One attractive hypothesis is that dysregulation of the immune response is important in disease aetiology. This notion is supported by the observation that disease susceptibility is conferred by particular HLA haplotypes (see below). There is also some evidence of aberrant immune reactivity in these patients (reviewed in Miller 1990). Examples include the presence of ANA, elevated levels of circulating immune complexes, and altered *in vitro* immunoglobulin synthesis. Children with pauciarticular-onset chronic arthritis have been found to have an increased C3d/C3 ratio, suggesting activation of the alternate complement pathway. A correlation between C3d/C3 ratios and the titre of IgG antibodies to lipid A was also observed in pauciarticular-onset disease, suggesting these antibodies may play a role in disease pathology (Olds and Miller 1990). In addition, IgA deficiency and pauciarticular-onset disease have been associated. These findings may represent primary immune abnormalities that contribute to pathogenesis or may be secondary to the disease process. Other indices of immune function in these patients, such as lymphocyte subpopulation ratios and responses to mitogens, are usually normal.

The possibility that juvenile chronic arthritis represents a chronic infection or that it is initiated by an environmental trigger has prompted the search for candidate micro-organisms. No single pathogen has been consistently identified with the development of this disease (Phillips 1988). Rubella virus has been isolated from lymphoreticular cells of 7 of 19 children with chronic rheumatic disease, including 2 of 6 with pauciarticular-onset disease (Chantler *et al.* 1985). Persistence of rubella virus in these patients may reflect an aetiological role for the virus or a state of immunodeficiency in the patients. In two small series, antibody to peptidoglycan, a constituent of bacterial cell walls, was elevated in 25 to 50 per cent of pauciarticular patients with chronic uveitis (Burogs-Vargas *et al.* 1986; Moore *et al.* 1989). This finding may be relevant to disease aetiology because humoral immunity to streptococcal cell wall preparations has been implicated in the pathogenesis of chronic synovitis in animal models (Greenblat *et al.* 1980). Alternatively, these antibodies may reflect a state of altered immune reactivity in children with juvenile chronic arthritis. In this regard, it is of interest that defective antibody responses to immunization with bacteriophage were observed in a study of children with each type of juvenile chronic arthritis (Ilowite *et al.* 1987).

The aetiology of the associated uveitis is likewise unknown, but appears to be immune mediated. Histopathological studies show non-granulomatous, inflammatory infiltration, including plasma cells and lymphocytes (Sabetes *et al.* 1979). Ocular fluids from affected eyes contain elevated immunoglobulin levels (Sabetes *et al.* 1979; Rahi *et al.* 1977) and ANA (Rahi *et al.* 1977). The antigenic stimulus that initiates or maintains this process has not been identified. Inflammation of both the joint and eye occur in several diseases (e.g. Kawasaki's disease, seronegative spondylarthropathies, inflammatory bowel disease). The possibility that collagen acts as an autoantigen at both sites has been investigated in patients with juvenile chronic arthritis, but studies have failed to demonstrate a heightened immune response to collagen in children with uveitis (Rosenberg 1987). In one study, 29 per cent of patients with pauciarticular-onset juvenile chronic arthritis and uveitis were found to have serum antibodies to a low- molecular-weight fraction of bovine iris proteins. However, the presence of these antibodies did not correlate with severity of uveal inflammation (Hunt *et al.* 1993). Paradoxically, 30 per cent of children with this chronic arthritis and uveitis manifest a humoral response to a retinal antigen, S (Petty *et al.* 1987). Immunization with this protein induces an acute uveitis in animal models, but its role in chronic uveitis is unclear, as there is at present no animal model of chronic uveitis.

Immunogenetics

Several lines of evidence indicate that genetic factors are involved in disease susceptibility (summarized in Maksymowych and Glass 1988; Cassidy and Petty 1995). Multiple cases of pauciarticular-onset juvenile chronic arthritis within one family are unusual, but some have been reported. In addition, concordance for disease is increased in twins; in many cases, clinical disease manifestations between twins are similar (Clemens *et al.* 1985). Most compelling, a large number of studies indicate that certain genes within the *HLA* complex contribute to disease susceptibility (the *HLA* association studies discussed below are reviewed in Nepom 1991; Nepom and Glass 1992; De Inocencio *et al.* 1993; Fernandez-Vina *et al.* 1994).

These reported *HLA* associations are quite complex, in contrast to those of many other rheumatic diseases where a single allele or family of alleles confers disease risk. In pauciarticular-onset juvenile chronic arthritis, not only are a number of different alleles associated with disease, but products of different loci are involved. The sometimes confusing results of these different studies are further confounded by variations in *HLA* typing methods, inclusion criteria, and ethnic and geographic populations. None the less, the reproducibility of many *HLA* associations by many different investigators substantiates their importance in susceptibility to pauciarticular-onset juvenile chronic arthritis.

Initial studies described *HLA* class I associations with pauciarticular disease, with *HLA A2*, the most consistently identified allele. The consensus of more recent studies using precise DNA-based HLA typing techniques is that alleles of the class II loci are most strongly associated. However, there is some evidence that the *HLA-*

A2 *0201 allele remains significantly associated with disease even after class II associations are taken into account (Fernandez-Vina *et al.* 1994).

Among *HLA* class II genes, several alleles of the *DRB1* locus are the most reproducibly associated with disease. *DR8* (primarily the *DRB1*0801* allele in many studies) shows the strongest correlation, with relative risks of approximately 4 to 12. In a number of different North American and northern and southern European populations, *DR8* accounts for approximately 25 to 50 per cent of patients. The *DR8* association is intriguing, since this allele is infrequent (3 to 10 per cent) in control Caucasian populations, and has not been associated with other autoimmune conditions. Among Caucasians, *DRB1*0801* is strongly linked to the *DQ* genes *DQA1*0401* and *DQB1*0402*, but the association in some studies is stronger with *DR* than *DQ*.

DR5 is also consistently associated with pauciarticular-onset juvenile chronic arthritis, with a relative risk of about 2 to 7 in most studies, slightly lower than that for *DR8*. Several *DR5*+ alleles are present among patients, but *DRB1*1104* alleles are most significantly increased (Melin-Aldana *et al.* 1992; Haas *et al.* 1994).

DR6 has been variably reported to be increased in some populations. The *DRB1*1301* allele appears primarily responsible for this association.

In contrast, *DR4*, which is the *HLA* type most highly associated with both adult and juvenile rheumatoid factor-positive rheumatoid arthritis, is almost never seen in pauciarticular-onset juvenile chronic arthritis. *DR7* also seems to provide protection for this disease.

Interestingly, pauciarticular-onset juvenile chronic arthritis was one of the first diseases shown to be associated with an allele of the *DPB1* locus. Several groups have shown that *DPB1*0201* contributes to disease susceptibility, an effect independent of the *DRB1* contribution and not due to linkage with a particular haplotype. Possessing *DPB1*0201* may not by itself provide enough susceptibility to lead to disease expression; instead, it adds to the risk conferred by the *DRB1* susceptibility alleles.

Gene dosage may play a role in determining the magnitude of risk for this disorder. In addition to the additive contribution of *DPB1* to *DRB1* alleles, some studies have reported increased frequencies of patients heterozygous for two *DRB1* susceptibility alleles. Possessing *A*0201* may also increase risk when added to *DR* and *DQ* susceptibility alleles. Thus, having more than one susceptibility allele may confer additional susceptibility or modulate disease.

Despite quite reproducible *HLA* associations with disease, one cannot rule out the possibility that they are due to involvement of genes linked to these alleles, rather than to the *HLA* genes themselves. Recent studies have examined possible associations with pauciarticular- juvenile chronic arthritis of candidate non-*HLA* genes known to reside near or within the major histocompatibility complex that may contribute to immune processes. So far neither *TAP* nor *LMP* alleles have been reproducibly associated with this disorder (reviewed in Ploski and Førre 1994), although some studies report positive correlations (Donn *et al.* 1994). Other candidate polymorphic genes in the MHC include the genes for tumour necrosis factor, heat-shock protein 70, certain complement components, and other antigen processing genes.

Genes linked to the MHC clearly do not account entirely for disease expression, so, in addition to a hypothesized role for environmental agents, contributing non-*HLA*-linked genes have been sought. The T-cell receptor (**TCR**) for antigen is a leading candidate, but so far no associations with germline TCR polymorphisms have been consistently recognized (Nepom *et al.* 1991). Skewed usage of TCR genes within synovial compartment T cells, however, has been reported (Sioud *et al.* 1992; Bernstein *et al.* 1993). Some groups have found an association of a particular subset of patients with a null allele of the TCR $V\beta6.1$ gene (Maksymowych *et al.* 1992; Charmley *et al.* 1994), while others have not (Ploski *et al.* 1993). Another group has noted an increase of null alleles of several different TCR genes among patients (Barron *et al.* 1993). The relevance of these findings to disease susceptibility awaits further confirmation.

Finally, McDowell *et al.* reported an association of certain disease subsets with an allele of the interleukin-1α gene, a lymphokine encoded on chromosome 2, and not linked to the *HLA* region (McDowell *et al.* 1995). Interestingly, this polymorphism occurs in the promoter region of the gene, suggesting intriguing mechanistic possibilities.

Many investigators have hoped that disease-associated alleles will allow prediction of clinical manifestations of pauciarticular-onset juvenile chronic arthritis, such as which patients are at increased risk for uveitis or progression to polyarticular disease. While an association of iritis, ANA, and *DR5* has been observed by some groups, other studies have not consistently borne this out. *DR8* has also been variably linked to the occurrence of uveitis. Similarly, attempts to link *HLA* alleles to severity of joint disease have been confusing. *DR8*, *DR5*, and a *DR6* haplotype have all been reported to be increased among patients with mild or persistently pauciarticular arthritis. Some reports correlate genes on the *DQA1*0101/DRB1*0101* haplotype with severe arthritis. Another links an interleukin-1α allele with chronic iridocyclitis (McDowell *et al.* 1995). Although at present none of these associations is strong enough for use in predicting specific manifestations in an individual patient, it is hoped that further elucidation of immunogenetic associations with specific aspects of this disorder will ultimately lead to improved understanding of disease pathogenesis as well as clinical utility in the management of patients.

Summary

The typical child with pauciarticular-onset juvenile chronic arthritis is a female toddler with chronic arthritis in a couple of large joints. Up to 70 per cent have antinuclear antibodies present, which select out the 20 per cent who will develop chronic asymptomatic uveitis. Education, physical therapy, and non-steroidal agents are usually required, but complications or severe disease may necessitate further therapy. Ocular disease requires prompt, intensive therapy. Many children have joint disease that is active only a few years and 80 per cent suffer no major functional disability at 15 years after onset. The remaining 20 per cent can have widespread destructive arthritis.

Illustrative cases

Case 1

A 5-year-old girl presents with a 1-month history of a swollen, but not very painful, left knee. She is not stiff in the mornings or after prolonged sitting. There is no history of trauma, piercing injury, tick bite, rash, or travel to an area where Lyme disease is endemic. Family history is negative for arthritis, low back pain, enthesitis, acute iritis, inflammatory bowel disease, and psoriasis.

Physical examination is normal except for increased intra-articular fluid in the left knee. Her leg lengths are closely checked for inequality and they are equal. She does not have a knee flexion contracture. When lying supine with both legs elevated to 45°, the left leg is not as hyperextensible as the right. Her left thigh circumference is 1 cm less than the right when measured at a level 7 cm above the patella. All other joints are normal. Her pupils and corneas are closely observed in a darkened room and reveal no evidence of scarring from chronic uveitis.

At this point we have a young girl who generally feels well, with an isolated swollen left knee. The lack of bony overgrowth indicates that this process has not been prolonged. Because she has no systemic signs, the diagnosis of pauciarticular-onset juvenile chronic arthritis is high on the list. However, a reactive arthritis cannot be ruled out because of the brevity of the episode to date. Lyme disease is unlikely in the absence of travel to an endemic area or a history of exposure.

Laboratory evaluations that would be helpful at this point includes a complete blood count, platelet count, erythrocyte sedimentation rate, urinalysis, ANA, and rheumatoid factor. Had any abnormalities in her eyes been noted, she would have been sent that day to an ophthalmologist; since there were no gross changes, she is instructed to see an ophthalmologist within 2 weeks.

She is begun on an oral anti-inflammatory medication.

Laboratory test results from her first visit show normal blood counts, erythrocyte sedimentation rate, and urinalysis. Rheumatoid factor is absent; ANA are present at 1:80. Report of the slit-lamp examination from the ophthalmologist is normal. Over the next 2 months there is only slight improvement.

At this point the diagnosis of pauciarticular-onset juvenile chronic arthritis is more assured, owing to continuation of symptoms for more than 6 weeks and normal laboratory values except for the positive ANA, which is typical for this condition. In spite of some improvement and minimal functional impairment, however, the arthritis is still active, so other NSAIDs will be tried. Quarterly slit-lamp examinations are scheduled with her ophthalmologist.

After another 2 months on optimal NSAID doses, the patient returns with continued disease.

Persistent swelling in a single joint over this period of time encourages one to think of other diagnoses such as pigmented villonodular synovitis. In addition, if the diagnosis is pauciarticular-onset juvenile chronic arthritis, it would now be reasonable to treat the joint more specifically. Therefore, synovial fluid is removed from her knee and, since infection is not a consideration, intra-articular triamcinolone hexacetonide is given. Her NSAID is continued. Analysis of the fluid shows 12 000 white blood cells (90 per cent polymorphonuclear cells) and 2000 red blood cells.

Her knee becomes much less swollen over the next 2 months, but then fluid reaccumulates.

The relatively large number of red blood cells in the synovial fluid and the recurrent nature of the arthritis makes pigmented villonodular synovitis a concern. Therefore a synovial biopsy is taken. The biopsy shows acute and chronic inflammation, which rules out the diagnosis of pigmented villonodular synovitis. A second injection of intra-articular corticosteroid is given and she subsequently does well. She has no pain or limitation of range of motion. She has a slit-lamp examination of her eyes every 3 months to look for asymptomatic uveitis.

Case 2

At 2 years of age this girl develops arthritis in her knees and one thumb. Laboratory test results show a sedimentation rate of 25 mm/h and normal blood counts. She has a negative rheumatoid factor but does have ANA at a titre of 1:160. She is initially treated with an oral anti-inflammatory medication. An ophthalmologist evaluates her eyes every 3 months for signs of uveitis.

This little girl shows a classic presentation for pauciarticular-onset juvenile chronic arthritis: involvement of fewer than five joints, primarily large joints, with an essentially normal laboratory evaluation except for the typical positive ANA.

After initial improvement arthritis develops in a fourth joint, an elbow. In addition, about 1 year after presentation, evidence of uveitis is noted during routine ophthalmological surveillance; she is treated with local corticosteroids and mydriatics.

Because of ongoing synovitis, she is placed on sulphasalazine. This is a useful choice when arthritis is clearly not under control and a disease-modifying medication is desired, but the situation does not seem to warrant a cytotoxic drug.

This example also points out the critical importance of routine ophthalmological surveillance. Her uveitis is noted early, when simple local measures will usually bring it under control and prevent potentially devastating visual impairment. In this child's case the uveitis and progression of arthritis occurred concurrently, but more often the two do not occur simultaneously.

Her arthritis is well controlled on sulphasalazine and a NSAID, and her uveitis is brought under control. However, at 5 years of age she develops recurrent synovitis. Over a 2-month period, she begins to complain of morning stiffness for the first time, and she develops arthritis in multiple small joints of her hands, feet, wrists, neck, hips, and ankles. Repeat blood samples and radiographs are obtained.

Her laboratory tests remain unchanged, with continued positive ANA and negative rheumatoid factor. Radiographs of multiple joints show juxta-articular osteoporosis but no erosions. Now this child has moved into the category of pauciarticular-onset juvenile chronic arthritis with evolution to a polyarticular course. She is at great risk for progressive, erosive disease because of the widespread nature of her joint involvement, in spite of the lack of radiographically visible erosions. Children, in contrast to most adults, may not show erosions until many years into their disease. Typically, the ANA will remain positive and the rheumatoid factor negative throughout the course. She now requires the addition of methotrexate to her regimen to help control the arthritis, as well as formal physiotherapy two or three times a week to maintain strength, joint range of motion, and functional activities. As her prognosis is now significantly altered, it must be discussed again at length with her parents.

Over the ensuing years, this girl continues to have occasional flares of synovitis, although her arthritis is generally kept under moderate control with methotrexate. She has developed erosions in a number of joints and will probably have permanent sequelae from her arthritis, such as the eventual need for joint replacement. She had two further episodes of uveitis, but both were noted early and treated aggressively and successfully. She continues to have ophthalmological screening every 3 months.

References

Allen, R.C., Gross, K.R., Laxer, R.M., Malleson, P.N., Beauchamp, R.D., and Petty, R.E. (1986). Intraarticular triamcinolone hexacetonide in the management of chronic arthritis in children. *Arthritis and Rheumatism*, **29**, 997–1001.

American Academy of Pediatrics Section on Rheumatology and Section of Ophthalmology (1993). Guidelines for ophthalmologic examinations in children with juvenile rheumatoid arthritis. *Pediatrics*, **92**, 295–6.

Ansell, B.M. (1977). Joint manifestations in children with juvenile chronic polyarthritis. *Arthritis and Rheumatism*, **20**, 204–6.

Ansell, B.M. (1983). The medical management of chronic arthritis in childhood. *Annals of the Academy of Medicine (Singapore)*, **12**, 168–73.

Ansell, B.M. and Wood, P.H.N. (1976). Prognosis in juvenile chronic polyarthritis. *Clinics in the Rheumatic Diseases*, **2**, 397–412.

Arthritis Foundation Committee on Evaluation of Synovectomy (1988). Multicenter evaluation of synovectomy in the treatment of rheumatoid arthritis. Report of the results at the end of five years. *Journal of Rheumatology*, **15**, 764.

Barron, K.S., Deulofeut, J.D., Reveille, J.D., and Robinson, M.A. (1993). T cell receptor (TCR) *V*β null alleles in juvenile rheumatoid arthritis (JRA). *Arthritis and Rheumatism*, **36** (Suppl.), S263.

Bernstein, B.H., Singsen, B.H., King, K.K., and Hanson, V. (1977). Aspirin-induced hepatotoxicity and its effect on juvenile rheumatoid arthritis. *American Journal of Diseases of Children*, **131**, 659–63.

Bernstein, B.H., Miltenberg, A.M.M., van Laar, J.M., Hertzberger, R., and Breedveld, F.C. (1993). T cell receptor rearrangements in juvenile rheumatoid arthritis: a search for oligoclonality. *Clinical and Experimental Rheumatology*, **11**, 209–13.

Brewer, E.J., Jr. *et al*. (1977). Current proposed revision of JRA criteria. *Arthritis and Rheumatism*, **20**, 195–9.

Brewer, E.J., Jr., McPherson, M., Magrab, P.R., and Hutchins, V.L. (1989). Family-centered, community-based, coordinated care for children with special health care needs. *Pediatrics*, **83**, 1055–60.

Burogs-Vargas, R., Howard, A., and Ansell, B.M. (1986). Antibodies to peptidoglycan in juvenile onset ankylosing spondylitis and pauciarticular onset juvenile arthritis associated with chronic iridocyclitis. *Journal of Rheumatology*, **13**, 760–2.

Cabral, D.A., Petty, R.E., Fung, M., and Malleson, P.N. (1992). Persistent antinuclear antibodies in children without identifiable inflammatory rheumatic or autoimmune disease. *Pediatrics*, **98**, 441–4.

Cassidy, J.T. and Petty, R.E. (1995). *Textbook of pediatric rheumatology*, (3rd edn). W.B. Saunders Company, Philadelphia.

Cassidy, J.T., Sullivan, D.B., and Petty, R.E. (1977). Clinical patterns of chronic iridocyclitis in children with JRA. *Arthritis and Rheumatism*, **20**, 224–7.

Chantler, J.K., Tingle, A.J., and Petty, R.E. (1985). Persistent rubella virus infection associated with chronic arthritis in children. *New England Journal of Medicine*, **313**, 1117–23.

Chaouat, D., Chaouat, Y., and Aron-Rosa, D. (1990). Pauciarticular juvenile chronic arthritis with ocular involvement and antinuclear antibody presenting in an adult woman. *British Journal of Rheumatology*, **29**, 236–237.

Charmley, P., Nepom, B.S., and Concannon, P. (1994). HLA and T cell receptor β-chain DNA polymorphisms identify a distinct subset of pauciarticular juvenile rheumatoid arthritis patients. *Arthritis and Rheumatism*, **37**, 695–701.

Chylack, L.T., Jr. (1977). The ocular manifestations of juvenile rheumatoid arthritis. *Arthritis and Rheumatism*, **20**, 217–23.

Chylack, L.T., Dueker, D.K., and Philaja, D.J. (1979). Ocular manifestations of juvenile rheumatoid arthritis: pathology, fluorescein iris angiography and patient care patterns. In *Juvenile rheumatoid arthritis* (ed. J.J. Miller), pp. 149–63. Publishing Sciences Group, Littleton.

Clemens, L.E., Albert, E., and Ansell, B.M. (1985). Sibling pairs affected by chronic arthritis of childhood: evidence for a genetic predisposition. *Journal of Rheumatology*, **12**, 108.

Committee on Infectious Diseases (1994). *1994 Red Book: Report of the Committee on Infectious Diseases* (23rd edn.), p. 280. American Academy of Pediatrics, Elk Grove Village, IL.

Cush, J.J. and Fink, C.W. (1987). Clinical outcome of pauciarticular onset juvenile arthritis. *Arthritis and Rheumatism*, **30** (Suppl.), S34.

Daltroy, L.H. *et al*. (1992). Psychosocial adjustment in juvenile arthritis. *Journal of Pediatic Psychology*, **17**, 277–89.

De Inocencio, J., Giannini, E.H., and Glass, D.N. (1993). Can genetic markers contribute to the classification of juvenile rheumatoid arthritis? *Journal of Rheumatology*, **20** (Suppl. 40), 12–18.

Dequecker, J. and Mardjuadi, A. (1982). Prognostic factors in juvenile chronic arthritis. *Journal of Rheumatology*, **9**, 909–15.

Donn, R.P., Davies, E.J., Holt, P.L., Thomson, W., and Ollier, W. (1994). Increased frequency of TAP2B in early onset pauciarticular juvenile chronic arthritis. *Annals of the Rheumatic Diseases*, **53**, 261–4.

Duffy, C.M., Laxer, R.M., and Silverman, E.D. (1989). Drug therapy for juvenile arthritis. *Comprehensive Therapy*, **15**, 48–59.

Emery, H.M. (1993). Treatment of juvenile rheumatoid arthritis. *Current Opinion in Rheumatology*, **5**, 629–733.

Fernandez-Vina, M., Fink, C.W., and Stastny, P. (1994). HLA associations in juvenile arthritis. *Clinical and Experimental Rheumatology*, **12**, 205–14.

Flynn, H.W., Davis, J.L., and Culbertson, W.W. (1988). Pars plena lensectomy and vitrectomy for complicated cataracts in juvenile rheumatoid arthritis. *Ophthalmology*, **95**, 1114–19.

Gabriel, C.A. and Levinson, J.E. (1990). Advanced drug therapy in juvenile rheumatoid arthritis. *Arthritis and Rheumatism*, **33**, 587–90.

Gare, B.A. *et al*. (1987). Incidence and prevalence of juvenile chronic arthritis: a population survey. *Annals of the Rheumatic Diseases*, **46**, 277–81.

Gedalia, A., Barash, J., Press, J., and Buskila, D. (1993). Sulphasalazine in the treatment of pauciarticular-onset juvenile chronic arthritis. *Clinical Rheumatology*, **12**, 511–14.

Giannini, E.H. *et al*. (1992). Methotrexate in resistant juvenile rheumatoid arthritis. *New England Journal of Medicine*, **326**, 1043–9.

Giannini, E.H. *et al*. (1993). Comparative efficacy and safety of advanced drug therapy in children with juvenile rheumatoid arthritis. *Seminars in Arthritis and Rheumatism*, **23**, 34–46.

Greenblat, J.J., Hunter, N., and Schwab, J.H. (1980). Antibody response to streptococcal cell wall antigens associated with experimental arthritis in rats. *Clinical and Experimental Immunology*, **42**, 450–7.

Haas, J P., Truckenbrodt, H., Paul, C., Hoza, J., Scholz, S., and Albert, E.D. (1994). Subtypes of HLA-DRB1*03, *08, *011, *12, *13 and *14 in early onset pauciarticular juvenile chronic arthritis (EOPA) with and without iridocyclitis. *Clinical and Experimental Rheumatology*, **12** (Suppl. 10), S7–S14.

Hollingworth, P. (1993). The use of non-steroidal anti-inflammatory drugs in paediatric rheumatic diseases. *British Journal of Rheumatology*, **32**, 73–7.

Hunt, D.W., Petty, R.E., and Millar, F. (1993). Iris protein antibodies in serum of patients with juvenile rheumatoid arthritis and uveitis. *International Archives of Allergy and Immunology*, **100**, 314–18.

Ilowite, N.T., Wedgewood, R.J., Rose, L.M., Clark, E.A., Lindgren, C.G., and Owen, M.J. (1987). Impaired in vivo and in vitro antibody responses to bacteriophage OX174 in juvenile rheumatoid arthritis. *Journal of Rheumatology*, **14**, 957.

Kanski, J.J. (1977). Anterior uveitis in juvenile rheumatoid arthritis. *Archives of Ophthalmology*, **95**, 1794–7.

Kanski, J.J. (1990). Uveitis in juvenile chronic arthritis. *Clinical and Experimental Rheumatology*, **8**, 499–503.

Kanski, J.J. and Shun-shin, G.A. (1984). Systemic uveitis syndromes in childhood: analysis of 340 cases. *Ophthalmology*, **91**, 1247–51.

Kenesi-Laurent, M.A., Kaplan, G., and Kahn, M.F. (1991). Oligoarthrites de l'adulte avec facteurs anti-nucleaires. Originalite du syndrome, rapports avec l'oligoarthrite juvenile. *Revue des Rhumatisme et Maladies Osteo-Articulaire*, **58**, 1–6.

Key, S.N. and Kimure, S.J. (1975). Iridocyclitis associated with juvenile rheumatoid arthritis. *American Journal of Ophthalmology*, **80**, 425–9.

Kvien, T.K., Høyeraal, H.M., and Sandstad, B. (1984). Naproxen and acetylsalicylic acid in the treatment of pauciarticular and polyarticular juvenile rheumatoid arthritis. *Scandinavian Journal of Immunology*, **13**, 342–50.

Lang, B.A. and Finlayson, L.A. (1994). Napoxen-induced pseudoporphyria in patients with juvenile rheumatoid arthritis. *Journal of Pediatrics*, **124**, 639–42.

Leak, A.M. and Ansell, B.M. (1987). The relationship between ocular and articular disease activity in juvenile rheumatoid arthritis complicated by chronic anterior uveitis. *Arthritis and Rheumatism*, **30**, 1196–7.

Levinson, J.E. *et al.*, (1977). Comparison of tolmetin sodium and aspirin in the treatment of juvenile rheumatoid arthritis. *Journal of Pediatrics*, **91**, 799–804.

Levy, M.L., Barron, K.S., Eitchenfield, A., and Honig, P.J. (1990). Naproxen-induced pseudoporphyria in juvenile chronic arthritis. *Journal of Pediatrics*, **117**, 660–4.

Lovell, D.J., Giannini, E.H., and Brewer, E.J., Jr. (1984). Time course of response to nonsteroidal anti-inflammatory drugs in juvenile rheumatoid arthritis. *Arthritis and Rheumatism*, **27**, 1433–7.

Maksymowych, W.P. and Glass, D.N. (1988). Population genetics and molecular biology of the childhood chronic arthropathies. *Baillière's Clinical Rheumatology*, **2**, 649–71.

Maksymowych, W.P. *et al.* (1992). Polymorphism in a T-cell receptor viable gene is associated with susceptibility to a juvenile rheumatoid arthritis subset. *Immunogenetic*, **35**, 257–62.

Malleson, P., Petty, R.E., Fung, M., and Candido, E.P.M. (1989). Reactivity of antinuclear antibodies with histones and other antigens in juvenile rheumatoid arthritis. *Arthritis and Rheumatism*, **32**, 919–23.

Malleson, P.N., Fung, M.Y., Petty, R.E., Mackinnon, M.J., and Schroeder, M.-L. (1992). Autoantibodies in chronic arthritis of childhood: relations with each other and with histocompatibility antigens. *Annals of the Rheumatic Diseases*, **51**, 1301–6.

McDowell, T.L., Symons, J.A., Ploski, R., Forre, Ø., and Duff, G.W. (1995). A genetic association between juvenile rheumatoid arthritis and a novel interleukin-1α polymorphism. *Arthritis and Rheumatism*, **38**, 221–8.

Melin-Aldana, H. *et al.* (1992). Human leukocyte antigen-DRB1*1104 in the chronic iridocyclitis of pauciarticular juvenile rheumatoid arthritis. *Journal of Pediatrics*, **121**, 56–60.

Miller, J.J. (1990). Immunologic abnormalities of juvenile arthritis. *Clinical Orthopaedics and Related Research*, **259**, 23–30.

Moore, T.L., El-Najdawi, E., and Dorner, R.W. (1989). Antibody to streptococcal cell wall peptidoglycan-polysaccharide polymers in sera of patients with juvenile rheumatoid arthritis but absent in isolated immune complexes. *Journal of Rheumatology*, **16**, 1069–73.

Moran, H. *et al.*, (1979). Naproxen in juvenile chronic polyarthritis. *Annals of the Rheumatic Diseases*, **38**, 152.

Morrissy, R.T. (ed.) (1990). *Lovell and Winter's pediatric orthopaedics*, (3rd edn). Lippincott, Philadelphia.

Nepom, B. (1991). The immunogenetics of juvenile rheumatoid arthritis. In *Rheumatic disease clinics of North America* (ed. B.H. Athreya). W.B. Saunders, Philadelphia.

Nepom, B.S. and Glass, D.N. (1992). Juvenile rheumatoid arthritis and HLA: Report of the Park City III Workshop. *Journal of Rheumatology*, **19**, 70–4.

Nepom, B.S., Malhotra, U., Schwarz, D.A., Nettles, J.W., Schaller, J.G., and Concannon, P. (1991). HLA and T cell receptor polymorphisms in pauciarticular juvenile rheumatoid arthritis. *Arthritis and Rheumatism*, **34**, 1260–7.

Neuteboom, G.H., Hertzberger-ten Cate, R., de Jong, J., and van den Brink, H.G. (1992). Antibodies to a 15 kDa nuclear antigen in patients with juvenile chronic arthritis and uveitis. *Investigative Ophthalmology and Visual Science*, **33**, 1657–60.

Ohm, J. (1910). Bandformige Hornhauttrubung bei einem neunjahrigen Mädchen und ihre Behandlung mit subkonjunktivalen Jodkaliumeinspritzungen. *Klinische Monatsblätter für Augenheilkunde*, **48**, 243.

Olds, L.C. and Miller, J.J. (1990). C3 activation products correlate with antibodies to lipid A in pauciarticular juvenile arthritis. *Arthritis and Rheumatism*, **33**, 520.

Olson, N.Y., Lindsley, C.B., and Godfrey, W.A. (1988). Nonsteroidal anti-inflammatory drug therapy in chronic childhood iridocyclitis. *American Journal of Diseases of Children*, **142**, 1289–92.

Petty, R.E. (1979). Epidemiology of juvenile rheumatoid arthritis. In *Juvenile rheumatoid arthritis* (ed. J.J. Miller), pp. 11–31. Publishing Sciences Group, Littleton.

Petty, R.E., Hunt, D.W.C., Rollins, D.F., Schroeder, M.L., and Puterman, M.L. (1987). Immunity to soluble retinal antigen in patients with uveitis accompanying juvenile rheumatoid arthritis. *Arthritis and Rheumatism*, **30**, 287–93.

Phillips, P.E. (1988). Evidence implicating infectious agents in rheumatoid arthritis and juvenile rheumatoid arthritis. *Clinical and Experimental Rheumatology*, **6**, 87–94.

Ploski, R. and Førre, Ø. (1994). Non-HLA genes and susceptibility to juvenile chronic arthritis. *Clinical and Experimental Rheumatology*, **12** (Suppl. 10), S15–S17.

Ploski, R., Hansen, T., and Førre, Ø. (1993). Lack of association with T-cell receptor TCRBV6S1*2 allele in HLA-DQA1*0101-positive Norwegian juvenile chronic arthritis patients. *Immunogenetics*, **38**, 444–5.

Rahi, A.S.H., Kanski, J.J., and Fielder, A. (1977). Immunoglobulins and antinuclear antibodies in aqueous humor from patients with juvenile rheumatoid arthritis (Still's disease). *Transactions of the Ophthalmological Society of the United Kingdom*, **97**, 217–22.

Rosenberg, A.M. (1987). Uveitis associated with juvenile rheumatoid arthritis. *Seminars in Arthritis and Rheumatism*, **16**, 158–73.

Rosenberg, A.M. (1989). Advanced drug therapy for juvenile rheumatoid arthritis. *Pediatrics*, **114**, 171–8.

Rosenberg, A.M. and Petty, R.E. (1982). A syndrome of seronegative enthesopathy and arthropathy in children. *Arthritis and Rheumatism*, **25**, 1041–7.

Rosenberg, A.M. and Romanchuk, K.G. (1990). Antinuclear antibodies in arthritis and nonarthritic children with uveitis. *Journal of Rheumatology*, **17**, 60–1.

Sabetes, R., Smith, T., and Apple, D. (1979). Ocular histopathology in juvenile rheumatoid arthritis. *Annals of Ophthalmology*, **11**, 733–7.

Schaller, J. and Wedgwood, R.J. (1972). Juvenile rheumatoid arthritis: a review. *Pediatrics*, **50**, 940–53.

Sherry, D.D. (1990). Limb pain in childhood. *Pediatrics in Review*, **12**, 39–46.

Sherry, D.D., Bohnsack, J., Salmonson, K., Wallace, C.A., and Mellins, E. (1990). Painless juvenile rheumatoid arthritis. *Journal of Pediatrics*, **116**, 921–3.

Sherry, D.D., Mellins, E.D., and Wedgwood, R.J. (1991). Decreasing severity of chronic uveitis in children with pauciarticular arthritis. *American Journal of Diseases of Children*, **145**, 1026–8.

Silver, R.M. (1988). Nonsteroidal anti-inflammatory drugs in the management of juvenile arthritis. *Journal of Clinical Pharmacology*, **28**, 566–70.

Simon, S., Whiffen, J., and Shapiro, F. (1981). Leg-length discrepancies in monarticular and pauciarticular juvenile rheumatoid arthritis. *Journal of Bone and Joint Surgery*, **63A**, 209–15.

Sioud, M., Kjeldsen-Kragh, J., Suleyman, S., Vinje, O., Natvig, J.B., and Førre, Ø. (1992). Limited heterogeneity of T cell receptor variable region gene usage in juvenile rheumatoid arthritis synovial T cells. *European Journal of Immunology*, **22**, 2413–18.

Smiley, W.K. (1976). The eye in juvenile chronic polyarthritis. *Clinical Rheumatology*, **2**, 413.

Spalter, H.F. (1975). The visual prognosis in juvenile rheumatoid arthritis. *Transactions of the American Ophthalmological Society*, **73**, 554.

Stoeber, E. (1981). Prognosis in juvenile chronic arthritis. *European Journal of Pediatrics*, **135**, 225–8.

Strabrun, A.E. (1991). Impaired mandibular growth and micrognathic development in children with juvenile rheumatoid arthritis. A longitudinal study of lateral cephalographs. *European Journal of Orthodontics*, **13**, 423–34.

Szer, I.S., Klein-Gitelman, M., DeNardo, B.A., and McCauley, R.G.K. (1992). Ultrasonography in the study of prevalence and clinical evolution of popliteal cysts in children with knee effusions. *Journal of Rheumatology*, **19**, 458–62.

Truckenbrodt, H. and Häfner, R. (1986). Methotrexate therapy in juvenile rheumatoid arthritis: a retrospective study. *Arthritis and Rheumatism*, **29**, 800–7.

Van Kerckhove, C., Giannini, E.H., and Lovell, D.J. (1988). Temporal patterns of response to D-penicillamine, hydroxychloroquine, and placebo in juvenile rheumatoid arthritis patients. *Arthritis and Rheumatism*, **31**, 1252–8.

Vostrejs, M. and Hollister, J.R. (1988). Muscle atrophy and leg length discrepancies in pauciarticular juvenile rheumatoid arthritis. *American Journal of Diseases of Children*, **142**, 343–5.

Walker, A.M. *et al.* (1993). Determinants of serious liver disease among patients receiving low-dose methotrexate for rheumatoid arthritis. *Arthritis and Rheumatism*, **36**, 329–35.

Wallace, C.A. and Levinson, J.E. (1991). Juvenile rheumatoid arthritis: outcome and treatment for the 1990s. In *Rheumatic disease clinics of North America* (ed. B.H. Athreya), pp. 891–906. W.B. Saunders, Philadelphia.

Wallace, C.A., Bleyer, W.A., Sherry, D.D., Salmonson, K.L., and Wedgwood, R.J. (1989). Toxicity and serum levels of methotrexate in children with juvenile rheumatoid arthritis. *Arthritis and Rheumatism*, **32**, 677–81.

Wallace, C.A., Farrow, D., and Sherry, D.D. (1994). Increased risk of facial scars in children taking non-steroidal antiinflammatory drugs. *Journal of Pediatrics*, **125**, 819–22.

Wolf, M.D., Lichter, P.R., and Ragsdale, C.G. (1987). Prognostic factors in the uveitis of juvenile rheumatoid arthritis. *Ophthalmology*, **94**, 1242–8.

Wood, P.H.N. (1978) Special meeting on: nomenclature and classification of arthritis in children. In *The care of rheumatic children* (ed. E. Munther), p. 47. EULAR, Basel.

5.6.2 Systemic-onset juvenile chronic arthritis

Ronald M. Laxer and Rayfel Schneider

Introduction

While the earliest English language description of systemic-onset juvenile chronic arthritis dates back to 1897 (Still 1897), Espinel has argued eloquently that Caravaggio's 'Il amore dormiente', painted in the early 1600s, is really the first description of this fascinating entity (Espinel 1994). The painting depicts a young boy with jaundice, recessed jaw, distended abdomen, muscle atrophy, and multiple joint deformities. It was, however, Still's classic paper that highlighted the unique features of systemic-onset juvenile chronic arthritis and differentiated it from both rheumatoid arthritis in adults and other forms of chronic arthritis of childhood. Although a great deal has been written about the clinical aspects of systemic-onset juvenile chronic arthritis, there has been little investigation into the aetiology, pathogenesis, and treatment of this severe, and potentially fatal, form of juvenile chronic arthritis.

While arthritis is required to confirm the diagnosis of systemic-onset juvenile chronic arthritis, true joint inflammation may not be present at the onset of the disease. In fact, patients with otherwise classic features of systemic-onset juvenile chronic arthritis have developed arthritis as late as 9 years after the onset (Calabro et al. 1976). In addition to chronic arthritis, the American College of Rheumatology classification criteria require 2 weeks of intermittent fever spikes to at least 103°F (Brewer et al. 1977), while the European League Against Rheumatology criteria (Ansell 1978) require at least one other feature (rash, adenopathy, hepatosplenomegaly, pericarditis) in addition to fever and arthritis.

Epidemiology

Variations in classification criteria for juvenile chronic arthritis and the reports of both population-based studies and specialty clinic or hospital-based studies account for the wide prevalence range (8–220 cases/100 000) and wide incidence range (2.6–13.9 cases/100 000) reported for juvenile chronic arthritis (Hochberg 1981; Gewanter et al. 1983; Towner et al. 1983; Andersson Gare et al. 1987). Although difficult to determine, the prevalence probably approximates to 50 cases/100 000 and systemic-onset disease accounts for approximately 10 to 20 per cent of these patients with a reported range of 7 to 43 per cent (Hanson et al. 1977; Andersson Gare and Fasth 1992).

In contrast to the two- to threefold female predominance for all juvenile chronic arthritis, there is an almost equal sex incidence in systemic-onset disease. However, females may be more commonly affected when the disease begins after age 10 years (Ansell and Wood 1976). Although systemic-onset disease may occur at any age from the neonatal period to adolescence, in two-thirds of patients the onset is under 5 years of age (Ansell 1977) and the mean age at onset is 4 to 6 years (Schaller 1977).

The non-articular features of systemic-onset juvenile chronic arthritis make a viral aetiology an attractive hypothesis, but there is little direct evidence to support this. Seasonal variation in disease onset, with a higher incidence in the late spring, summer, and autumn, has been reported (Lindsley 1987), but is not corroborated by others except for a similar variation in a specific geographic region in a Canadian study (Feldman et al. 1996).

HLA associations

HLA studies have demonstrated genetic heterogeneity in patients with systemic-onset disease (Maksymowych and Glass 1988; Nepom 1991). Inconsistent and weak associations have been reported for a variety of class I antigens. Stronger associations have been reported for class II antigens including DR5 (relative risk 4–7) and DR8 (relative risk 4–5), which have both been associated with pauciarticular juvenile chronic arthritis, and DR4 (relative risk 2–5), which has been associated with rheumatoid factor positive polyarticular disease (De Inocencio et al. 1993). Unlike rheumatoid factor positive arthritis, there has not been a striking association with DR4 homozygosity and there are conflicting reports regarding the prognostic significance of DR4 in systemic disease (Singh et al. 1989; Bedford et al. 1992). As with other HLA associations, the DR4 association with systemic disease does not appear to hold true for all systemic disease populations (Nepom and Glass 1992). An association with Dw7 has also been reported (Stasny and Fink 1979).

Clinical features (Table 1)

Extra-articular manifestations

The hallmark of systemic-onset juvenile chronic arthritis is the systemic toxicity and extra-articular features that occur during 'attacks' or flares of disease.

Fever

Fever is the one extra-articular manifestation that is absolutely essential to make a diagnosis. A typical fever pattern occurs in the majority of cases, and is described as a quotidian, or occasionally double quotidian, fever pattern (Fig. 1). During typical flares, the temperature will spike rapidly in the late afternoon or early evening, to at least 39°C, only to return fairly quickly to normal, or often below normal, even without antipyretics. This fever pattern is very different from the fever of other connective tissue diseases, acute rheumatic fever, malignancy, or infectious fevers, which tend to be more persistent or while spiking do not return to below the baseline. Occasionally, the classic fever pattern is only established when anti-inflammatory treatment is begun. Characteristically, the patient will appear toxic during the spike of fever, may have chills and rigors, and will complain of severe arthralgias and myalgias. The bed sheets are often soaked as the fever resolves. Frequently, rash (see below) is present only during

Table 1 Clinical features during the course of systemic onset juvenile chronic (rheumatoid) arthritis

Very common

    Spiking fever (with chills and sweats)

    Evanescent rash

    Myalgias

    Arthralgias

    Arthritis

Common

    Generalized lymphadenopathy

    Hepatosplenomegaly

    Polyserositis

    Anorexia

    Weight loss

Rare

    Myocarditis

    Coagulopathy

    Ocular involvement

    Central nervous system involvement

    Haemophagocytic syndrome

    Primary pulmonary disease

    Renal involvement

    Amyloidosis

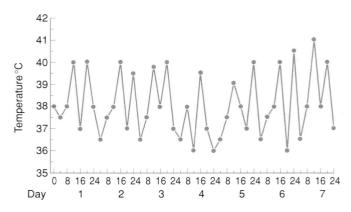

Fig. 1 Temperature chart of a patient demonstrating daily (quotidian) or double-daily fever spikes with rapid return to below the baseline of 37 °C.

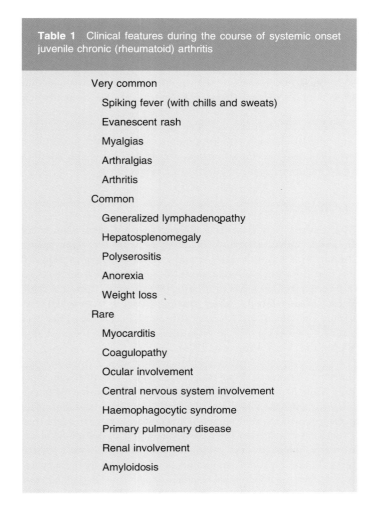

(a)

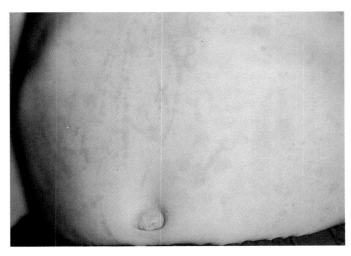

(b)

Fig. 2 (a) Rash of systemic-onset juvenile arthritis showing characteristic salmon-pink macular eruptions with central clearing. (b) Koebner phenomenon (appearance of exaggeration of rash in areas of minor trauma).

the fever spikes. When the fever subsides, the patients are usually much more comfortable and appear less toxic. The fever must be present for at least 2 weeks to satisfy classification criteria, and may persist for months even with treatment. Rarely, fever may follow the development of arthritis (Prieur *et al.* 1984).

Rash

The rash of systemic-onset juvenile chronic arthritis is a salmon-pink colour, and is most prominent over the chest, abdomen, back, and intertriginous areas. Distal involvement of the extremities is uncommon but can occur, as can a facial rash. Individual lesions are 3 to 5 mm in diameter and often demonstrate central clearing within the surrounding pink border (Fig. 2(a)). The rash may coalesce into large lesions. The rash is usually macular but urticarial lesions may occur. While the rash typically comes and goes with the spikes of fever (evanescent), it may sometimes be persistent and even occur without fever or other systemic manifestations. The rash may also demonstrate the Koebner phenomenon — the exaggeration of rash in areas of minor trauma. In systemic-onset juvenile chronic arthritis this may be induced by the bed sheets 'squeezing' the skin with a resultant linear distribution of rash (Fig. 2(b)). If the rash is pruritic (10 per cent of patients), then scratching may also induce the Koebner phenomenon. As the rash does tend to come and go, it is unusual to obtain skin biopsies. Histologically, the lesion typically shows a sparse, perivascular infiltrate with a predominance of polymorpho-nuclear leucocytes (Isdale and Bywaters 1956).

Reticuloendothelial involvement

Reticuloendothelial hyperplasia with hepatomegaly, splenomegaly, and generalized lymphadenopathy is a common feature of systemic-onset juvenile chronic arthritis. Although the organomegaly is usually asymptomatic, rarely patients with active systemic disease may develop massive hepatomegaly accompanied by a severe abdominal pain (Schaller et al. 1970). Mild elevations of serum transaminases occur frequently and are usually not clinically significant. The degree of transaminase elevation does not correlate with the extent of liver enlargement. Aspartate aminotransferase is more frequently elevated than alanine aminotransferase and significant hyperbilirubinaemia is rare. Liver histology in systemic-onset juvenile chronic arthritis is characterized by non-specific periportal inflammatory cell infiltration and Kupfer cell hyperplasia. Fatty change, intrahepatic cholestasis, and fibrosis have been reported less frequently (Tesser et al. 1982; Hadchouel et al. 1985; Agarwal et al. 1994). While transaminase elevations may be seen during active systemic disease, such elevations tend to occur rather sporadically and unpredictably (Rachelefsky et al. 1976). This may make it difficult to determine whether hypertransaminasaemia reflects disease activity or the effect of treatment with potentially hepatotoxic medications including salicylates, non-steroidal anti-inflammatory drugs (NSAIDs), gold, or methotrexate. Chronic liver disease does not occur in systemic-onset juvenile chronic arthritis but has been described in adult-onset Still's disease (Tesser et al. 1982).

Patients with systemic-onset juvenile chronic arthritis may rarely develop hepatomegaly with acute, severe hepatic dysfunction and even fulminant hepatic failure (Hadchouel et al. 1985). This potentially life-threatening syndrome has been associated with neurological involvement (drowsiness and coma) and disseminated intravascular coagulation and bleeding. (For a further description see below under 'Less common features'.)

Serositis

Involvement of serosal surfaces is one of the hallmarks of systemic-onset juvenile chronic arthritis (Yousefzadeh and Fishman 1979). Pericardial involvement is most common and pleuritis is more common than peritonitis. Pericarditis is frequently asymptomatic and is best detected by 2D echocardiography. In one series of children with all forms of juvenile chronic arthritis, pericardial involvement was seen in 45 per cent of autopsy cases, although it was only clinically recognized in 7 per cent, most of whom had systemic-onset juvenile chronic arthritis (Lietman and Bywaters 1963). In another series, 9 out of 57 patients had symptomatic pericardial involvement, which was isolated in five cases but associated with myocarditis in the remaining four (Goldenberg et al. 1992). In the majority, cardiac involvement occurred within the first year but it can occur at any time during the disease course, particularly in association with other systemic manifestations. Most children will have echocardiographic evidence of pericarditis during systemic flares but may not have any clinical signs of pericarditis (Brewer et al. 1977). Occasionally, patients present only with pericarditis and fever before a diagnosis of systemic juvenile chronic arthritis is considered. Therefore, pericardiocentesis may be performed, both for relief of symptoms and diagnosis. Manifestations include tachycardia (out of keeping with the fever), anterior chest pain, and a pericardial friction rub. More severe involvement may lead to dyspnoea, tachypnoea, and even right-sided congestive heart failure. Rarely, cardiac tamponade and constrictive pericarditis may result (Yancey et al. 1981; Pearl 1982; Goldenberg et al. 1990). The electrocardiogram may be normal, show ST wave elevation, or non-specific ST segment changes. The chest radiograph may show enlargement of the cardiothoracic silhouette.

Pleuritis is much less common than pericarditis. Occasionally, large pleural effusions, associated almost invariably with pericarditis, may dominate the clinical picture. Sterile peritonitis may result in severe abdominal pain (Bhettay and Thomson 1985).

Arthritis

Most patients have arthritis at disease onset and those who do not commonly have arthralgias or myalgias with the fever spikes. Patients with only arthralgias or no joint symptoms pose substantial diagnostic challenges. To complicate this, the duration from the onset of fever to the development of arthritis may range from just a few weeks to several years. Most patients, however, develop arthritis within 3 months of disease onset (Ansell 1977). Chronic, persistent arthritis evolves in half to two-thirds of patients (Schaller and Wedgwood 1972; Calabro et al. 1976).

In our series of 38 patients followed for at least 2 years, pauciarthritis was present in 55 per cent at onset and polyarthritis in 35 per cent, while 10 per cent had no objective signs of arthritis. Although more patients had a pauciarticular onset, the majority of those with persistent arthritis evolved to a polyarticular disease. In more than 75 per cent of patients, the wrists, knees, and ankles are involved. Although somewhat less commonly affected, involvement of the cervical spine, hips, and temporomandibular joints is quite characteristic. In fact, hip involvement occurs in about 50 per cent of patients, is almost always bilateral, and is usually associated with polyarthritis. The hip and wrist joints are the most frequent sites of progressive and advanced destructive changes (Figs 3(a, b), and 4), which may occur as early as the first year after onset (Svantesson et al. 1983). Almost one-third of patients who have hip involvement may require total hip arthroplasty (Hayem et al. 1994). Of the small joints, the hands are more commonly affected than the feet. Cricoarytenoid arthritis with resultant laryngeal stridor has been described (Jacobs and Hui 1977). Tenosynovitis of the carpus and tarsus is common.

Less common features

Many organ systems can be involved in addition to those mentioned above. Pulmonary disease (other than pleuritis) is rare, but can involve the pulmonary parenchyma (Calabro et al. 1976; Athreya et al. 1980; Wagener et al. 1981; Zaglul et al. 1982). Primary pulmonary hypertension has been reported (Padeh et al. 1991).

Myocarditis, although rare, can be a serious event with considerable mortality. It has been reported to occur in up to 12 per cent of a series of patients with systemic-onset juvenile chronic arthritis from Brazil, and symptoms include tachycardia, dyspnoea, and congestive heart failure (Goldenberg et al. 1992). Typically, this occurs during systemic flares of disease and usually together with pericarditis. Myocarditis should be suspected in patients who have persistent tachycardia (out of keeping with fever or anaemia), cardiomegaly, and congestive heart failure. The diagnosis can be made by electrocardiography (showing increased PR interval and low voltages) and

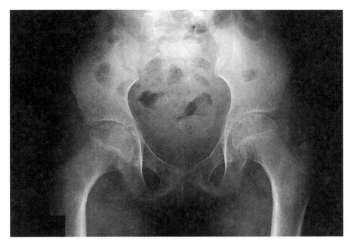

(a)

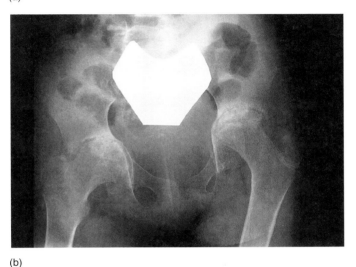

(b)

Fig. 3 Girl with systemic-onset juvenile chronic arthritis since 7 years. Hip radiographs show: (a) At 33 months after disease onset, osteopoenia, joint space narrowing, and erosions. (b) At 4.5 years after disease onset, increased loss of joint space, protrusio acetabulae, subchondral irregularity and erosions, and sclerosis of both sides of the joints. There is also flattening of the left femoral head.

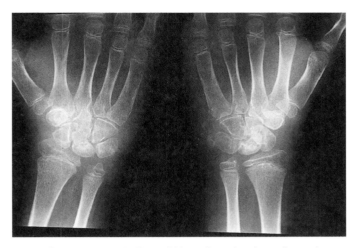

Fig. 4 Same patient as in Fig. 3. Wrist radiographs show advanced changes 2 years after disease onset with moderate narrowing of the carpus, sclerosis, carpal irregularity and erosions, and deformity of the distal radial epiphysis.

echocardiography (showing reduced ventricular function). Because of the high mortality associated with myocarditis, there must always be a high index of suspicion for its development. Although it has been suggested that digitalis may promote arrhythmias (Miller 1977), a recent report did describe using digitalis with good effect (Goldenberg *et al.* 1992). Although cardiac murmurs are common (resulting from anaemia and fever) valvular disease itself is almost never seen, and this helps differentiate systemic-onset juvenile arthritis from acute rheumatic fever with carditis, where valvular inflammation is prominent. However, there are rare reports of valvular abnormalities (Kramer *et al.* 1983; Heyd and Glaser 1990).

Over the last dozen years, several reports have described a syndrome in patients with systemic-onset juvenile chronic arthritis marked by fever, hematocytopenias, hepatic dysfunction, encephalopathy, and disseminated intravascular coagulation with bleeding. This syndrome has been reported under a variety of names. It has occurred

following viral infections as well as following changes in medical therapy, but can also occur spontaneously. Most recently, Stephan *et al.* reported three patients with systemic-onset juvenile chronic arthritis (and one with polyarticular juvenile arthritis) who had 'macrophage activation syndrome' (Stephan *et al.* 1993). This seems to be an appropriate term to include the 'consumptive coagulopathy' described by Silverman *et al.* (Silverman *et al.* 1983), a syndrome of 'acute haemorrhagic, hepatic, and neurological manifestations' described by Hadchouel *et al.* (Hadchouel *et al.* 1985), and the several reports of haemophagocytic syndromes that have followed viral infections (Heaton and Moller 1985; Morris *et al.* 1985) in children with systemic-onset juvenile chronic arthritis. The features of this syndrome include persistent high fever (different from the quotidian fever of systemic-onset juvenile chronic arthritis), lymphadenopathy and hepatosplenomegaly, bruising and mucosal bleeding, hepatic dysfunction, drowsiness, and even coma. The laboratory features include anaemia, neutropenia, thrombocytopenia, and evidence of disseminated intravascular coagulation (low fibrinogen levels, raised levels of fibrin degradation products). Deficiency of clotting factors may result in a raised PT and PTT. In fact, children with systemic-onset juvenile chronic arthritis may have increased levels of factor VIII related antigen, fibrinopeptide A, fibrinogen, and fibrin split products, with normal levels of platelet factor IV, indicative of a vasculopathy (Scott *et al.* 1984), even in the absence of this syndrome. Bone marrow and lymph nodes usually show histiocytic consumption of red cells and platelets (Fig. 5). This syndrome is associated with considerable morbidity and mortality. Early recognition and supportive management is vital in reducing mortality. While some patients do recover with expectant management alone, treatment recommendations have included both corticosteroids and cyclosporin (Hadchouel *et al.* 1985; Stephan *et al.* 1993).

Central nervous system manifestations are dominated by irritability and lethargy during the fever spikes. True organic brain syndrome is rare and no case series has actually examined patients for central nervous system involvement. However, occasional cases of central nervous system vasculitis have been documented and electrocardiographic changes may be seen (Jan *et al.* 1972). Autopsy series have shown perivascular infiltrates of chronic inflammatory cells in

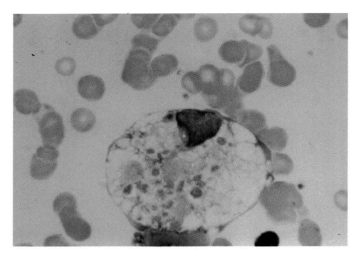

Fig. 5 Bone marrow examination of a patient with macrophage activation syndrome showing histiocytic phagocytosis of red blood cells and platelets (by courtesy of Dr A. Poon).

the brain. Two patients with systemic-onset juvenile chronic arthritis treated with long-standing corticosteroids developed epidural lipomatosis and presented with signs of spinal cord compression requiring emergency laminectomy (Arroyo et al. 1988).

Renal involvement may occur as a complication of treatment or may indicate the onset of amyloidosis. Although mild abnormalities, including proteinuria and mild haematuria (Antilla 1972), may be seen, particularly with fever, significant renal disease is not a component of systemic-onset juvenile chronic arthritis and its presence should raise suspicion about the diagnosis. Significant proteinuria in the presence of long-standing systemic-onset juvenile chronic arthritis is an indication to exclude amyloidosis with appropriate tissue biopsies.

Ocular involvement is distinctly unusual relative to other forms of juvenile chronic arthritis, but asymptomatic uveitis does occur. It is recommended that these patients be screened annually (Anonymous 1993). Several cases of tenosynovitis of the superior oblique muscle (Brown's syndrome) have been reported (Wang et al. 1984; Moore and Morin 1985).

Amyloidosis

Amyloidosis is a serious complication of all subtypes of juvenile chronic arthritis and is associated with significant morbidity and mortality. The clinician should be particularly suspicious of the diagnosis in the systemic subtype in which it occurs most frequently. Although rarely reported in North America, 9 to 10 per cent of patients with systemic-onset disease in European series have developed this complication (Ansell and Wood 1976; Stoeber 1981; Svantesson et al. 1983). The reason for this discrepancy in incidence is unclear. No HLA allele has been associated with amyloidosis; however, a restriction fragment length polymorphism related to the amyloid-P component gene has been associated with the development of amyloidosis in patients with systemic-onset disease (Woo et al. 1987). Serum amyloid-A protein is usually elevated in amyloidosis but is not predictive of its development (Scheinberg and Benson 1980); however, persistent elevation of the C-reactive protein level may predict the development of amyloidosis (Gwyther et al. 1982).

David (David et al. 1993), in the largest series of patients with juvenile chronic arthritis and amyloidosis, reported that 57 per cent of these patients had systemic-onset disease. The interval between the onset of disease and the diagnosis of amyloidosis varied widely from 1.5 to 25 years. Ninety per cent of patients had active synovitis at the time of diagnosis. The presenting clinical features and causes of death in this series are summarized in Table 2. The age at disease onset and the duration of disease activity were not related to the development of amyloidosis (Schnitzer and Ansell 1977). The diagnosis should be suspected in patients with persistent proteinuria. The clinical features are generally accompanied by laboratory evidence of an acute-phase reaction with anaemia, thrombocytosis, elevation of the erythrocyte sedimentation rate and C-reactive protein, hypergammaglobulinaemia, and hypoalbuminaemia. Confirmation of amyloidosis is most reliably achieved by renal, rectal, or even subcutaneous fat biopsy. Scintigraphy using a radio-iodinated serum amyloid-P component has been shown to be a useful, non-invasive technique for detecting amyloid deposits in both suspected and occult sites and may be useful in monitoring the response to therapy (Hawkins et al. 1993).

Treatment is aimed at controlling the underlying inflammatory process since no therapy has been effective in removing amyloid deposits. In the British series (David et al. 1993), chlorambucil was found to have a significant impact on survival. Ten years after amyloidosis was detected, 80 per cent of patients treated with chlorambucil survived compared with less than 25 per cent of patients who did not receive cytotoxic therapy. After 15 years of follow-up, two-thirds of chlorambucil-treated patients were still alive. It should be noted that not all patients with systemic disease are chlorambucil-responsive (Deschenes et al. 1990) and its potential toxicities include malignancy

Table 2	Amyloidosis in juvenile chronic arthritis
	Percentage
Clinical features at diagnosis	
Proteinuria	100
Active juvenile chronic arthritis	90
Oedema	53
Hypertension	25
Abdominal pain	22
Hepatomegaly	22
Splenomegaly	19
Diarrhoea	13
Renal failure	3
Ascites	3
Causes of death	
Renal failure	82
Infection	12
Malignancy	3
Other	3

Modified from David et al. (1993).

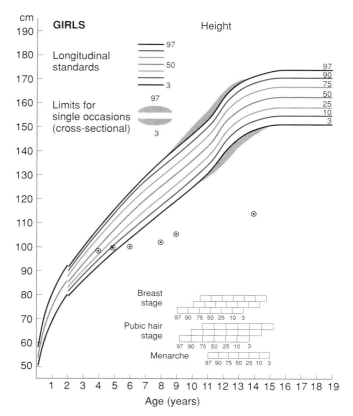

Fig. 6 Growth curve of a 15-year-old girl with severe systemic-onset juvenile arthritis, requiring long-term, high-dose prednisone treatment, showing severe growth delay.

and infertility. There is no conclusive role for other immuno-suppressive agents.

Growth and nutrition

Children with systemic-onset juvenile chronic arthritis frequently have abnormalities of growth, as documented by Still himself (Fig. 6). The systemic features of the disease are associated with hypercatabolism, resulting in breakdown of tissue stores, and also lead to anorexia. Poor energy and nutrient intake has been noted in several studies (Bacon *et al.* 1990; Mortensen *et al.* 1990). In addition, the frequent requirement for corticosteroids will have an effect on growth. Daily intake of corticosteroids equal to or greater than 5 mg/m² will result in growth delay (Blodgett *et al.* 1956). While alternate-day steroid therapy will suppress growth to a lesser degree than daily treatment (Byron *et al.* 1983), this is often difficult to achieve in severely ill systemic-onset juvenile chronic arthritis patients. In addition, Bernstein *et al.* have documented that patients with systemic-onset juvenile chronic arthritis treated with corticosteroids had lower growth velocities than a similar group of systemic lupus erythematosus patients treated with steroids, suggesting that the disease itself has a growth suppressing effect (Bernstein *et al.* 1977).

The role of growth hormone in children with systemic-onset juvenile chronic arthritis is unclear. Levels of growth hormone have been reported as both normal and reduced (Butenandt *et al.* 1974; Allen *et al.* 1991). Low levels of insulin-like growth factors, which mediate the

effects of growth hormone, have been reported (Bennett *et al.* 1988; Aitman *et al.* 1989). Several reports have studied the effects of treatment with growth hormone on children with different forms of juvenile chronic arthritis (Butenandt 1979; Svantesson 1991). Most recently, using doses of 12 and 24 IU/m², given three times per week, increased height velocities were documented. These were more significant in children receiving 24 IU/m² per week, and less marked in systemic-onset versus patients with either pauciarticular or polyarticular-onset disease. It is unclear from this study whether the ultimate height reached will be altered with growth hormone treatment (Davies *et al.* 1994). Most importantly, suppression of disease activity with medications other than corticosteroids and adequate nutrition must be achieved. Currently, treatment with growth hormone should be reserved for patients in prospective studies and for children whose growth is significantly below the third percentile.

Laboratory features

There are no specific laboratory features that are diagnostic of systemic-onset juvenile chronic arthritis. Rather, the common laboratory abnormalities reflect an activation of the acute-phase response, and taken together, are supportive of a diagnosis of systemic-onset juvenile chronic arthritis when other disorders are excluded by appropriate history, physical, and laboratory investigations.

The characteristic haematological abnormalities include anaemia, thrombocytosis, and leucocytosis (Table 3). The anaemia typically is an anaemia of chronic disease. This results in a normochromic normocytic smear, with haemoglobin levels ranging from 9 to 10.5 g/dl. Occasionally, in the face of very active systemic toxicity, haemoglobin values will drop quickly, to values as low as 50 g/l. Frequently, the anaemia of chronic disease is compounded by the effects of medications and nutritional deficiency. For example, occult blood loss secondary to non-steroidal anti-inflammatory drugs and poor iron intake may lead to iron deficiency, thus accentuating the anaemia and resulting in hypochromia and microcytosis (Harvey *et al.* 1987). Despite blood loss and poor iron intake, however, serum ferritin is usually increased and is therefore not helpful in detecting iron deficiency as ferritin is an acute-phase reactant (Craft *et al.* 1977; Pelkonen *et al.* 1986). Bone marrow examination in patients with systemic-onset juvenile chronic arthritis (Fig. 7) usually shows a reactive marrow, with an increased number of plasma cells and with stainable iron. The mechanisms underlying the anaemia of systemic-onset juvenile chronic arthritis are unclear but may reflect an abnormal response to cellular mediators of haematopoiesis (Prouse *et al.* 1987; Silverman *et al.* 1988). Erythroid aplasia, similar to the syndrome of transient erythroblastopenia of childhood, has been reported (Rubin *et al.* 1978). Rarely, acute severe pancytopenia has developed in association with presumed viral haemophagocytic syndromes (Heaton and Moller 1985; Morris *et al.* 1985). Severe reaction to medications have been implicated in cases of consumptive coagulopathy (Silverman *et al.* 1983; Hadchouel *et al.* 1985).

Leucocytosis and thrombocytosis are also hallmarks of systemic-onset juvenile chronic arthritis, so much so that normal counts should always raise suspicion about the diagnosis. Typically, a peripheral blood smear will show a 'left shift' with an increase in the number of immature neutrophils. These neutrophils appear activated, with vacuoles and toxic granules, suggesting infection. White blood cell

Table 3 Haematological abnormalities in systemic onset juvenile chronic arthritis

Common

Anaemia of chronic disease

Iron deficiency anaemia

Neutrophilic leucocytosis

Thrombocytosis

Rare

Acute haemolysis

Haemophagocytic syndrome (disease or drug-induced)

Disseminated intravascular coagulation (disease or drug-induced)

Erythroid aplasia

Other nutritional deficiency anaemias

Leucopenia (disease or drug-induced)

Thrombocytopenia (disease or drug-induced)

Coagulopathy

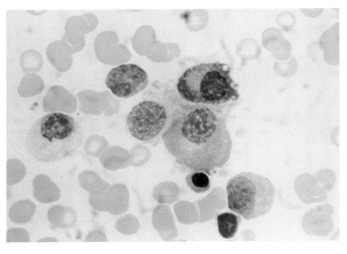

Fig. 7 Bone marrow examination of a patient with newly-diagnosed systemic-onset juvenile arthritis showing reactive plasmacytosis (magnification × 1250, illustration by courtesy of Dr A. Poon).

counts as high as $50 \times 10^9/l$ may be seen. Similarly, thrombocytosis is characteristic of active disease. Rarely, both leucopenia and/or thrombocytopenia can occur, either as isolated events (Sherry and Kredich 1985) or as part of a disseminated intravascular coagulation-like syndrome.

The erythrocyte sedimentation rate is raised, often to greater than 100 mm/h (Westergren). Polyclonal hypergammaglobulinaemia is often observed, although not necessarily at onset (Petty *et al.* 1977); however, both transient and persistent IgA deficiency have been reported (Pelkonen *et al.* 1983). Other indicators of an acute-phase reaction include an elevated C-reactive protein (Gwyther *et al.* 1982) and significant hypoalbuminaemia, which may be multifactorial in

aetiology (poor dietary intake, reduced hepatic synthesis, and intestinal leak). Serum complement levels are often raised, again indicating an acute-phase response (Hoyeraal and Mellbye 1974), and may help differentiate systemic-onset juvenile chronic arthritis from systemic lupus erythematosus. Renal function is normal, although mild proteinuria (which may be fever related) and red and white blood cells in the urine are occasionally observed (Antilla 1972). Elevation of serum transaminases are frequent (see 'Reticuloendothelial involvement' above). Recently, dyslipoproteinaemia has been observed in all juvenile chronic arthritis subtypes, particularly those with systemic-onset juvenile chronic arthritis. This abnormality was felt to reflect active disease and may be mediated by cytokines (Ilowite *et al.* 1989).

While most children with systemic-onset juvenile chronic arthritis are seronegative for antinuclear antibody and rheumatoid factor, up to 37 per cent may be antinuclear antibody positive (Pauls *et al.* 1989; Siamopoulou-Mavridou *et al.* 1991) and 5 per cent rheumatoid factor positive (Cassidy *et al.* 1986; Lang and Shore 1990). No particular antinuclear antibody specificities have been consistently identified. Hidden rheumatoid factor has been reported in upwards of 50 per cent of patients (Moore *et al.* 1984). Immune complexes are found in up to 80 per cent of patients when assessed by a variety of methods (Moore *et al.* 1982). Evidence for complement activation may be found (Miller *et al.* 1986) and levels of complement receptor 1 (CR1) (complement C3b receptors) on erythrocytes were reduced in patients with systemic-onset juvenile chronic arthritis (Thomsen *et al.* 1987).

Abnormalities of immunoregulation, cell number and function, and cytokines have been reported. Unfortunately, most studies include patients with all types of juvenile chronic arthritis and do not specifically address systemic-onset disease alone. Studies of cellular immunity have shown B lymphocyte dysfunction (Tsokos *et al.* 1987; Barron *et al.* 1989), which may result from abnormal T-suppressor-cell function (Alarcon-Riquelme *et al.* 1988; Silverman *et al.* 1990a). In addition, anti-T-cell antibodies have been found in many children with systemic-onset juvenile chronic arthritis (Borel *et al.* 1984).

The clinical and laboratory features of systemic-onset juvenile chronic arthritis are very suggestive of a cytokine mediated process. The fever, skin rash, hypergammaglobulinaemia, hypoalbuminaemia, raised erythrocyte sedimentation rate, and fibrinogen that are characteristic of systemic-onset juvenile chronic arthritis may all be explained by an immune response involving the cytokines interleukin-1 and -6 (**IL-1** and **IL-6**) and tumour necrosis factor-α. In fact, several studies do suggest abnormalities in cytokine production and regulation. Levels of IL-1 are raised and in one study correlated with disease activity (Martini *et al.* 1986). Levels of IL-1β were uniquely raised in systemic-onset juvenile chronic arthritis as opposed to other types of juvenile chronic arthritis (Mangge *et al.* 1995). Prieur *et al.* found a naturally occurring inhibitor to IL-1 during the febrile phase in the urine of patients with systemic-onset juvenile chronic arthritis (Prieur *et al.* 1987). Increased levels of sIL-2R, indicative of immune activation, have been reported by various authors (Silverman *et al.* 1991; Fassbender *et al.* 1992; Lipnick *et al.* 1993). While raised sIL-2R levels are found in all types of juvenile chronic arthritis, levels do appear to be higher in patients with systemic onset, and correlate with active disease. Similarly, raised levels of serum IL-6 have correlated both with disease activity and thrombocytosis in patients with systemic-onset juvenile chronic arthritis (de Bennedetti *et al.* 1991). In addition, reduced levels of sIL-6 receptor but increased levels of IL-6/sIL-6R complexes have been reported (de Bennedetti *et al.* 1994). In preliminary studies, we have found increased levels of soluble tumour necrosis factor receptor P55 and P75, as have others (Mangge *et al.* 1995). Other abnormalities include elevated levels of tumour necrosis factor-α which correlated with disease activity (Mangge *et al.* 1995), elevated soluble CD8 levels (Lipnick *et al.* 1993), and, more recently, increased level of soluble phospholipase A_2 which correlated with active disease (Pruzanski *et al.* 1994). As mentioned, very few of these abnormalities are unique to systemic-onset juvenile chronic arthritis but they are more prominent relative to other subtypes, probably indicating a greater degree of immune activation. Results from studies of the interferon system are conflicting and have not shed light on the pathogenesis of systemic-onset juvenile chronic arthritis (Bacon *et al.* 1983; Arvin and Miller 1984).

Radiological features

The radiological features of juvenile chronic arthritis have been comprehensively reviewed (Reed and Wilmot 1991) but only two studies have detailed the radiological features specific for the systemic-onset subtype (Cassidy and Martel 1977; Lang *et al.* 1995). Table 4 shows the frequency of radiological abnormalities described by Lang *et al.* (Lang *et al.* 1995). The wrists were the most common sites of early and advanced radiological changes followed by the ankles, knees, tarsal joints, hips, and metacarpophalangeal joints. Similar findings were reported by Cassidy *et al.* (Cassidy and Martel 1977) with a significantly greater frequency of early periosteal new bone formation (50 per cent) and epiphyseal and vertebral compression fractures (attributed to the use of corticosteroids). Cervical spondylitis with narrowing, irregularity, and fusion of the apophyseal joints is also common. Ankylosis most commonly affects the C2–C3 level but may include the entire cervical spine (Fig. 8). Cervical spine ankylosis has been reported to be more frequent in systemic-onset disease than other subtypes (Espada *et al.* 1988). Other typical sites of ankylosis are the wrist and tarsus. It is noteworthy that metaphyseal rarefaction, a typical radiological finding of acute leukaemia, has been described in systemic-onset arthritis (Martel *et al.* 1962).

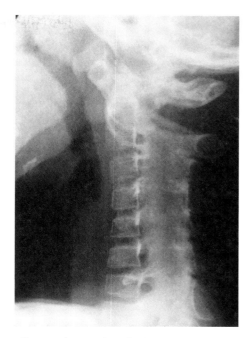

Fig. 8 Boy with systemic-onset juvenile chronic arthritis since 3.5 years. Cervical spine radiograph taken 5 years after disease onset shows ankylosis of the apophyseal joints (C2-C5).

A striking finding in the study by Lang *et al.* (Lang *et al.* 1995) was the early appearance of destructive changes. One-third of patients had erosions and joint space narrowing, 8 per cent had hip subluxation, and one patient developed ankylosis within 2 years of disease onset. These changes were sometimes seen within the first year of disease. Subtle changes of subchondral irregularity and sclerosis seemed to portend the development of erosions. These early destructive changes may be followed by progressive polyarticular disease.

Unusual radiological findings include large humeral cysts, soft tissue calcification unrelated to intra-articular corticosteroid injections (Lang *et al.* 1995), and shoulder synovial cysts (Barbaric and Young 1972). A ring of proliferative osteophytes at the junction of the femoral head and neck, similar to that described in patients with ankylosing spondylitis, has also been described (Mitnick and Mitnick 1980).

Differential diagnosis

When children present with a clinical picture that includes evening fever spikes, evanescent rash in association with the fever, polyarthritis, lymphadenopathy, hepatosplenomegaly, and polyserositis the diagnosis of systemic-onset juvenile arthritis is generally quite straightforward. However, many of these signs and symptoms are often lacking and the clinician must be astute enough to recognize clues that lead to a diagnosis of systemic-onset juvenile arthritis. One of the most important clues is the variation in the clinical signs and symptoms that can occur over a 24-h period. Children may appear very well throughout most of the day, only to look toxic at the time of a fever spike. It is at this time that the rash usually appears. In addition, arthralgias and myalgias can be extremely severe with the fever spikes.

Table 4 Frequency of radiological abnormalities in 42 patients with systemic juvenile chronic arthritis

Radiological feature	Percentage
Soft tissue swelling/osteopenia	81
Joint space narrowing	50
Growth abnormalities	48
Erosions	43
Subluxation	21
Ankylosis	19
Joint destruction	14
Protrusio acetabulae	10
Periosteal new bone formation	10

Modified from Lang *et al.* (1995).

Of utmost importance is that in order to make a diagnosis of juvenile arthritis, a number of exclusions must be made. In the differential diagnosis of systemic-onset juvenile arthritis these include primarily infectious and postinfectious disorders, other inflammatory diseases, and malignancies in addition to some other more rare febrile disorders of childhood.

Infections

Bacterial and viral infections must be searched for diligently. Bacterial infections that may be difficult to diagnose and are associated with prolonged fever include 'hidden' processes such as abscesses and osteomyelitis or diseases associated with intermittent bacteraemia, such as subacute bacterial endocarditis. In the child with localized pain, technecium bone scanning may be indicated to search for osteomyelitis. Abscesses must be searched for by nuclear scanning, ultrasound, or computed tomography (**CT**) scans. Careful examination, assessment of the cardiovascular system for changing murmurs, search for mucocutaneous findings, and frequent blood cultures will lead to a diagnosis of subacute bacterial endocarditis. Mycobacterial and other granulomatous infectious diseases should be excluded with a thorough history of potential exposure to these organisms and appropriate radiographical and serological investigations.

Viral infections may present with fevers, rash, lymphadenopathy, and hepatosplenomegaly, and can therefore closely resemble systemic-onset juvenile arthritis. Important candidates in the differential diagnosis include Epstein–Barr virus, rubella, adenovirus, and hepatitis B in the prehepatitic phase. Serological assays will be helpful in confirming the diagnosis of a viral infection. As with most other diseases, the fever associated with viral illnesses tends to be persistent, rather than quotidian, and patients are not nearly as toxic as patients with systemic-onset juvenile arthritis during the fever spikes. Recently, parvovirus has been implicated as perhaps being of aetiological importance in adult rheumatoid arthritis and juvenile arthritis (Nocton *et al*. 1993). However, it has not been associated with a picture of systemic-onset juvenile arthritis.

Autoimmune rheumatic diseases

'Connective tissue diseases' must be strongly considered in the differential diagnosis. The most important to consider are systemic lupus erythematosus, juvenile dermatomyositis, and systemic vasculitis. Features common to both systemic lupus erythematosus and systemic-onset juvenile arthritis include constitutional symptoms (fever, malaise, anorexia), arthritis/arthralgia, serositis, rashes, lymphadenopathy, and hepatosplenomegaly. However, vasculitic rashes seen in systemic lupus erythematosus are not typically seen in systemic-onset juvenile arthritis, and the rashes of systemic lupus erythematosus are not evanescent. Mucous membrane involvement is common in systemic lupus erythematosus but not in juvenile chronic arthritis. Fever tends to be persistent and not intermittent in systemic lupus erythematosus. Central nervous system and renal disease are almost never seen in juvenile arthritis but are common in systemic lupus erythematosus. Anaemia may be common to both, but leucopenia and thrombocytopenia are seen in systemic lupus erythematosus and almost never in juvenile chronic arthritis, where elevation of the white blood cell and platelet count are the rule. Specific autoantibodies are the hallmark of systemic lupus erythematosus but essentially absent in juvenile chronic arthritis. Reduced C3

and C4 complement levels in systemic lupus erythematosus result from immune complex deposition and consumption. In juvenile chronic arthritis, C3 and C4 tend to be elevated as a reflection of the acute-phase response. For further differences see Chapter 5.7.2.

Juvenile dermatomyositis may present as a systemic illness with arthritis but the heliotrope rash, Gottron's papules, and proximal muscle weakness should differentiate this presentation from systemic-onset juvenile arthritis. While myalgias are very common in patients with systemic-onset juvenile arthritis during fever spikes, true myositis does not occur. Serum levels of muscle enzymes will be helpful in differentiating the two.

Systemic vasculitis may present with fevers, malaise, anorexia, weight loss, arthralgias, and myalgias. The laboratory changes may be similar to those of systemic-onset juvenile arthritis in showing a marked elevation of the acute-phase response. The presence of nodules, vascular bruits, hypertension, mononeuritis multiplex, and cerebral disease help differentiate this from systemic-onset juvenile arthritis. Signs of internal organ involvement (e.g. lung and kidney) will also help in differentiating the two.

Malignancy

Malignancy forms one of the most important differential diagnostic categories—in particular, acute lymphoblastic leukaemia, lymphoma, and neuroblastoma (Schaller 1972). Important differentiating features are that children with malignancy have much more bone pain than patients with juvenile arthritis, and the pain tends to be persistent. Night-time pain is an important symptom in malignant disease (Ostrov *et al*. 1993) but both skin rash and serositis are uncommon. A low to normal white blood cell in the face of what appears to be systemic-onset juvenile arthritis is suggestive of a bone marrow infiltrative process. Lymphoma and neuroblastoma may present with fever and arthritis. Neuroblastoma is more common in young children and may not always be associated with a palpable abdominal mass. Screening of the urine for catecholamines and examining the chest and abdomen by CT scanning is helpful in excluding these. All malignancies may be especially difficult to diagnose in children who may have received even a very short course of corticosteroids for a presumptive diagnosis of juvenile chronic arthritis.

Postinfectious syndromes

Postinfectious syndromes must be considered in the differential diagnosis. The classic postinfectious syndrome is acute rheumatic fever following a group A β-haemolytic streptococcal throat infection. As with systemic-onset juvenile chronic arthritis, acute rheumatic fever may be associated with fever, rash, arthritis, and pericarditis, in association with laboratory markers of acute inflammation. However, the arthritis tends to involve only one or two joints at a time and then 'migrate' to other joints. Painful joints are prominent in acute rheumatic fever but much less so in systemic-onset juvenile arthritis, especially during the afebrile periods. Furthermore, the joints in acute rheumatic fever are often red, but are not in patients with systemic-onset juvenile arthritis. Pericarditis in acute rheumatic fever occurs only in the setting of endocarditis, which is extremely rare in systemic-onset juvenile chronic arthritis. Hepatosplenomegaly and lymphadenopathy are very rare in acute rheumatic fever. The rash, erythema marginatum, is uncommon and not as evanescent as the rash of systemic-onset juvenile arthritis. In acute rheumatic fever, a preceding history of streptococcal infection is necessary. One may have to rely on serology (antistreptolysin-O, antihyaluronidase) as evidence of infection, and a four-fold change in titre is necessary. At least 25 per cent of children with systemic-onset juvenile arthritis will have an increased antistreptolysin-O titre during the febrile phase, which is a reflection of the hypergammaglobulinaemia seen in these patients.

Reactive arthritis following bacterial infections involving the gastrointestinal or genitourinary tracts must be included in the differential diagnosis, and a history of preceding infections must be carefully addressed. Fever may occur in some cases of childhood reactive arthritis. However, the extra-articular features are very different from those of systemic-onset juvenile arthritis and involve the eyes, oral mucosa, and entheses. Inflammatory bowel disease may present with fever and arthritis before the onset of gastrointestinal symptoms. In addition, growth delay may be an early clue to this disorder.

Others

In the child under 1 year of age, chronic infantile neurological, cutaneous, and articular syndrome (**CINCA**) must be entertained in the differential diagnosis. It can be differentiated by its very young age of onset, associated chronic meningitis, uveitis, mental retardation, and epiphyseal changes (see Chapter 5.13.6). Juvenile sarcoidosis may also present with fever and rash; however, the rash is not transient and marked tenosynovial inflammation occurs. A biopsy of the skin or synovium will lead to the diagnosis (Hafner and Vogel 1993). Familial Mediterranean fever, an autosomal recessive disorder, presents with recurrent febrile episodes that generally last 48 to 72 h. These attacks may be associated with polyserositis and arthritis and a marked elevation of the acute-phase response accompanies the attacks. The short-lived, relapsing and remitting nature of the attacks, absence of chronic arthritis, and positive family history (when present) in a person of Mediterranean descent are suggestive of familial Mediterranean fever (Gedalia et al. 1992). The hyper-immunoglobulinaemia D syndrome begins in children below the age of 1 year and is associated with arthritis, lymphadenopathy, and splenomegaly. In contrast to systemic-onset juvenile chronic arthritis, there do not appear to be any residua of the arthritis, and, in contrast to familial Mediterranean fever, amyloidosis has not been reported to occur (Drenth et al. 1994).

The diagnostic workup must be focused to exclude all the entities considered in the American Rheumatism Association classification criteria (Brewer et al. 1977), particularly those mentioned above. It is vitally important to ensure that the child's temperature is recorded and plotted every 4 h to document the intermittent fever pattern of systemic-onset juvenile chronic arthritis. The recommended diagnostic investigations and clues to alternative diagnoses are summarized in Tables 5 and 6.

Disease course and prognosis

Patients with systemic-onset juvenile chronic arthritis may follow a monocyclic course with complete remission within 2 years of disease onset, a polycyclic course characterized by exacerbations of systemic disease activity, or a course of persistent polyarthritis

Table 5 Tests in the initial diagnostic investigation of suspected systemic onset juvenile chronic (rheumatoid) arthritis

Suggested in all patients

    Complete blood count (differential/platelet count), erythrocyte sedimentation rate

    Renal, hepatic function

    Serum immunoglobulins

    Prothrombin time, partial thromboplastin time

    Serum albumin

    Chest radiograph

    Electrocardiograph

    Blood cultures

    Antinuclear antibody

    Abdominal and pelvic ultrasound

    Bone marrow aspiration+biopsy

    Ocular slit lamp examination

    Joint aspirate (if a single joint is involved)

    Plain radiographs of selected affected joints

To be considered in some patients

    Muscle enzymes

    Rheumatoid factor

    Bone and/or gallium scans

    Upper gastrointestinal series/small bowel follow-through

    Tissue biopsies

    Viral serology—parvovirus, adenovirus, others

    Echocardiogram

    Antistreptolysin O/antihyaluronidase titres

    HVA/VMA in urine

    Serum IgD

HVA, homovanillic acid; VMA, vanillylmandelic acid.

Table 6 Manifestations that raise suspicion of another diagnosis

    Leucopenia, thrombocytopenia

    Child looks ill even during afebrile episodes

    Pain out of keeping with degree of synovitis

    Bony tenderness

    'Hard' hepatosplenomegaly/lymphadenopathy

    Recent antibiotic usage

    Monoarthritis

    Persistent diarrhoea

    Significant weight loss

Table 7 Major causes of death in systemic onset juvenile chronic arthritis

Amyloidosis with renal failure

Infection

Hepatic failure

Myopericarditis

Haematological disorders

(Calabro *et al.* 1976). The mean duration of active disease is 5 to 6 years but some patients have persistent disease activity well into their adult years (Schaller and Wedgwood 1972; Svantesson *et al.* 1983). Fifty per cent of patients will have recurrent episodes of fever of variable duration (Schaller 1977) and one-third of patients may have fever for more than 1 year after disease onset (Svantesson *et al.* 1983). Although some North American series report that few patients will have active, systemic disease for more than 5 years (Calabro *et al.* 1976; Baum *et al.* 1980), Prieur *et al.* (Prieur *et al.* 1984) and Häfner and Truckenbrodt (Häfner and Truckenbrodt 1986) report that 25 to 30 per cent of their patients in Europe had persistent systemic symptoms 10 to 15 years after disease onset. Occasionally, patients may have recurrences of active disease following prolonged remissions.

Although the outlook for the extra-articular manifestations is ultimately good, most series report that progressive destructive arthritis occurs in at least one-third of patients (Schaller 1977; Mozziconacci *et al.* 1983; Cabane *et al.* 1990) and accounts for the principal complications of this disease, with most of these patients in functional class III or IV after long-term follow-up. This subgroup of patients would seem to have the worst outcome of all patients with juvenile chronic arthritis. A recent report of 14 patients with systemic-onset disease who were followed for more than 10 years is more optimistic (David *et al.* 1994). These patients had relatively good functional and psychological outcomes, with none in modified Steinbrocker classes III or IV, but total hip replacement surgery was required in 57 per cent.

It has proved difficult to predict reliably the disease course and outcome for the individual patient. Several long-term studies have suggested the following to be possible predictors of poor outcome: disease onset under 5 to 7 years of age, female sex, persistent disease activity for 1 to 5 years (which may be associated with amyloidosis), cardiac disease, thrombocytosis, accelerated radiological changes, and raised IgA levels (Mozziconacci *et al.* 1983; Svantesson *et al.* 1983; Hull 1988). In our own series, prognostic indicators of destructive arthritis were identified within 6 months of disease onset. The two most highly predictive factors found were persistence of systemic symptoms and a platelet count of more than $600 \times 10^9/l$. Three-quarters of our patients with both of these predictors 6 months after disease onset developed joint destruction. In addition, these patients more commonly had pericarditis, hepatosplenomegaly, and hypoalbuminaemia at disease onset than those with a more benign course. They also more commonly developed polyarthritis, leucocytosis ($> 12 \times 10^9/l$) and anaemia ($< 100\,g/l$) at 6 months after the onset of disease (Schneider *et al.* 1992).

Mortality

There are more deaths amongst patients with systemic-onset juvenile chronic arthritis than any other subtype of juvenile chronic arthritis. The reported mortality of 14 per cent in several large European studies (Ansell and Wood 1976; Stoeber 1981; Hafner and Truckenbrodt 1986) is significantly higher than the 2.9 per cent mortality reported for all types of juvenile chronic arthritis (Baum and Gutkowska 1977). The major causes of death associated with systemic-onset arthritis are shown in Table 7. Amyloidosis has been associated with almost half the deaths in European patients with juvenile chronic arthritis and with only 13 per cent of deaths amongst North American patients; this may account for the higher mortality in European series. Infection is the most common cause of death in North American patients and is often associated with corticosteroid therapy. Acute hepatic failure has emerged as a significant cause of death, and in a review of several series accounted for 17 per cent of juvenile chronic arthritis deaths, most in those with systemic-onset disease (Boone 1977). Most deaths occur within the first 10 years of disease onset.

Management (Box 1)

The lack of randomized placebo-controlled trials in patients with systemic-onset juvenile arthritis makes it difficult to evaluate the efficacy of any therapy in this disease. Because of increased medication-related toxicity in these patients, all therapeutic interventions must be carefully monitored. The approach to the management of systemic-onset juvenile chronic arthritis must be a co-ordinated one involving all members of the health-care team. In addition to the articular and extra-articular features of the disease, growth and psychosocial development must be continuously addressed and monitored. The significant financial burdens placed upon families with a chronically ill child must not be overlooked.

Extra-articular features

Initial attempts to control fever should be with NSAIDs. Many paediatric rheumatologists in North America have moved away from salicylates in view of their increased hepatotoxicity relative to other NSAIDs and the potential for Reye's syndrome (Rennebohm *et al.* 1985). Success in controlling fevers has been achieved with both ibuprofen and indomethacin (Brewer 1977). Doses as high as 60 mg/kg in four divided doses of ibuprofen (B.M. Ansell, personal communication) or indomethacin 2 to 3 mg/kg per day seem to be more effective, with less toxicity than acetylsalicylic acid, and should be used prior to treating with corticosteroids for fever alone. Tolmetin sodium in doses up to 40 mg/kg per day may also be effective (Gewanter and Baum 1981). Because NSAIDs are protein bound, it is essential that the serum albumin be measured and the dose adjusted downward if hypoalbuminaemia is present. Failing to do so will result in excessive free drug which can result in toxicity. A minimum of a 1-week trial of an NSAID should be given before it is deemed to have failed; if the patient is not too ill, a second NSAID trial with a different preparation should be attempted.

In our experience, at least 50 per cent of patients will have an inadequate response to NSAIDs. When NSAIDs fail to control systemic toxicity, corticosteroid treatment is indicated. If used in high enough doses, steroids will virtually always result in resolution of fever and systemic toxicity. However, the significant side-effects of daily

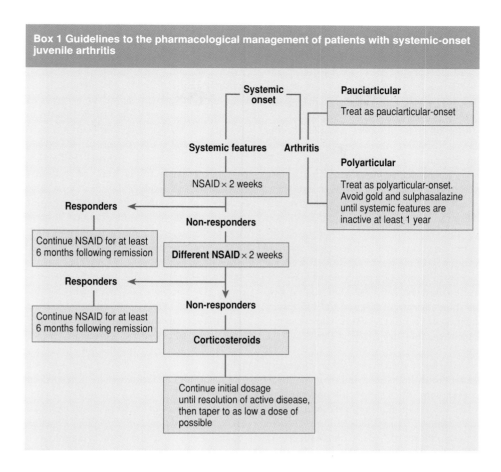

Box 1 Guidelines to the pharmacological management of patients with systemic-onset juvenile arthritis

corticosteroid therapy are well known and as they do not limit the duration of active disease or alter the long-term prognosis, they must be used judiciously. At times, patients, parents, and physicians may have to be willing to settle for some fever provided that the peaks are not too high and not associated with severe systemic toxicity or anaemia. While alternate day dosing is preferable, in our experience, patients who require steroids require at least 1 mg/kg per day, and often in divided doses. Occasionally, symptoms may be so severe that the daily dose may be better administered in three or even four doses over a 24-hour period for a short period of time. High-dose, intravenous pulse methylprednisolone may also be used with severe flares but we have found only very short-term benefits from this treatment.

While the presence of lymphadenopathy, hepatosplenomegaly, and rash usually correlate with more active systemic symptoms and are an indication of active disease, these alone do not justify an increase in treatment.

Anaemia is common in patients with systemic-onset juvenile chronic arthritis and is usually a result of chronic disease. Maintenance doses of iron supplementation may raise the haemoglobin concentration slightly (Koerper *et al.* 1978) but are rarely of great benefit. When the disease is extremely active patients will not respond to oral iron therapy, even if they are iron deficient. Intravenous iron oxide saccharate (Martini *et al.* 1994) at a cumulative dose calculated to reach an ideal haemoglobin of 12.5 g/dl has been recommended as a safe and effective treatment for severe and persistent anaemia in some patients with systemic-onset juvenile

arthritis who are unresponsive to oral iron treatment. In one small study, erythropoietin was also effective in raising the haemoglobin value in systemic-onset juvenile arthritis patients with the anaemia of chronic disease (Fantini *et al.* 1992).

Nutritional deficiencies of folic acid and vitamin B_{12} may need to be addressed. Rarely, during acute systemic flares, the haemoglobin concentration may fall rapidly to as low as 4 to 5 g/dl, necessitating blood transfusion (particularly in the face of cardiac compromise) in addition to corticosteroid therapy.

Attempts to reduce steroid toxicity have led to the use of intravenous immunoglobulin. Three separate studies have now reported on the use of intravenous immunoglobulin in systemic-onset juvenile arthritis. In the first, eight patients with severe juvenile chronic arthritis were treated for at least 6 months, in an open-label study. An impressive improvement in both articular and extra-articular disease and in laboratory abnormalities, as well as in a reduction in the dose of steroids, were noted (Silverman *et al.* 1990*b*). A second study did not seem to show any long-term benefit of intravenous immunoglobulin, although there was an improvement in the laboratory markers of active disease (Prieur *et al.* 1990). The recently completed Pediatric Rheumatology Collaborative Study Group trial did not show a statistically significant improvement in patients treated with intravenous immunoglobulin compared to placebo, although there was a trend towards overall improvement in the intravenous immunoglobulin-treated group (Silverman *et al.* 1994). However, many patients entered the trial so early in the disease course that spontaneous remissions may have occurred. Future studies should be directed at patients who early in their course fall into poor prognostic groups. At the time of writing, intravenous immunoglobulin should still be considered experimental in the treatment of systemic-onset juvenile chronic arthritis and should probably be reserved for patients whose systemic symptoms are not controlled by steroids, or who have significant steroid toxicity.

Serositis, as with the fever of systemic-onset juvenile chronic arthritis, will often respond to NSAIDs. Indomethacin seems to be especially effective for the treatment of pericarditis (Sherry *et al.* 1982). Corticosteroids in low to moderate doses (0.5–1 mg/kg per day) are usually sufficient to control serositis if NSAIDs are not effective. We have found intravenous pulse methylprednisolone 30 mg/kg per day (maximum 1 g) daily for 3 days to be rapidly effective and without toxicity, although of only short-term benefit. If there is significant compromise of cardiac function, pericardiocentesis may be required. Some authors recommend a pleural or pericardial drain for several days. Ventricular tachycardia complicating pericardiocentesis has resulted in a few deaths (Goldenberg *et al.* 1990). There is a report of one patient who, despite these measures, required the emergency placement of a pericardial window (Alukal *et al.* 1984). The efficacy of intrapericardial corticosteroids has not been substantiated and we have not found this necessary.

Myocarditis may occasionally be of such severity that congestive heart failure ensues. Treatment with high-dose oral or intravenous pulse corticosteroids, together with other supportive measures, is indicated. The use of digoxin may result in arrhythmias and sudden death if inflammation is not adequately controlled (Miller 1977), but a recent report did document the efficacy of digoxin (Goldenberg *et al.* 1992).

Articular disease

Many children with systemic-onset juvenile chronic arthritis have arthritis that is only problematic during flares of systemic disease. These children generally have a good outcome and respond well to management of the systemic components of the illness. However, the subset of children with persistent polyarticular disease, even in the absence of systemic manifestations, has progressive erosive disease which is difficult to treat with the standard first and second line agents. Unfortunately, no adequately controlled studies have been conducted in this group of children and our current approach is based largely on anecdotal experience. Currently, it is very difficult to predict at onset the course that patients will follow. It would seem that the earlier definitive treatment is instituted, the more effective treatment will ultimately be. Therefore, prognostic indicators are very important in determining the pharmacotherapeutic approach (Svantesson *et al.* 1983; Schneider *et al.* 1992).

The general approach to the management of the chronic arthritis of systemic-onset juvenile arthritis assumes the same principles as for the management of arthritis in other forms of juvenile arthritis. However, the increased drug-related toxicity is perhaps unique to patients with systemic-onset juvenile arthritis. This may be seen with salicylates, NSAIDs, and disease modifying antirheumatic drugs, including gold (Silverman *et al.* 1983; Hadchouel *et al.* 1985) and sulfasalazine (Cassidy 1990; Hertzberger Ten Cate and Cats 1991; Caspi *et al.* 1992). In fact, many authors consider that both gold and sulfasalazine are contraindicated in patients with systemic-onset juvenile arthritis, particularly if the disease is systemically active.

Currently, methotrexate is the drug of choice for most patients with juvenile arthritis, including systemic-onset juvenile arthritis, needing second-line agents (Giannini *et al.* 1992). To date, it has not been associated with increased toxicity in patients with systemic-onset juvenile arthritis. However, it is also unclear how effective methotrexate actually is for the arthritis of systemic-onset juvenile arthritis, and there is no evidence that it has any effect on systemic symptoms. In fact, there has been a suggestion that systemic-onset patients may be less responsive to methotrexate than patients with other types of juvenile arthritis (Halle and Prieur 1991). In a retrospective review, 63 per cent of patients were deemed to have responded to weekly, low-dose oral methotrexate by 6 months. Analysis showed that early treatment (within 2 years of onset), before the development of radiographical lesions at the time of starting methotrexate, may improve the response (Ravelli *et al.* 1994).

For patients who do not respond to methotrexate, other alternatives must be sought. Chlorambucil has been used in patients with systemic-onset juvenile chronic arthritis who also develop amyloidosis (Deschenes *et al.* 1990), with significantly improved survival (David *et al.* 1993), but systemic features may still not be well controlled (Manners and Ansell 1986). In addition, the risk of leukaemia seems to be particularly increased with this alkylating agent (Palmer and Ansell 1984). Azathioprine may be somewhat effective (Kvien *et al.* 1986). The use of cyclophosphamide has been limited in the literature to case reports (Skoglund *et al.* 1971; Walters *et al.* 1972).

Early studies of cyclosporin in systemic-onset juvenile chronic arthritis (Bjerkhoel and Forre 1988; Ostensen *et al.* 1988) showed only minimal effect on synovitis and systemic symptoms persisted in several patients. The toxicity of cyclosporin seemed to outweigh the benefits. However, a more recent study using somewhat lower doses (unfortunately, uncontrolled) did document efficacy at recommended doses of 5 mg/kg per day in two divided doses (Pistoia *et al.* 1993). Improvement in terms of reduction of arthritis, fever, and prednisone dose was noted as early as 1 month after starting treatment. It is unclear whether cyclosporin is truly remitting, if patients will be able to discontinue cyclosporin, and what the long-term efficacy and toxicity is.

A preliminary study of the use of recombinant γ-interferon in nine patients showed clinical improvement in seven, and an overall marked improvement in laboratory abnormalities (Pernice *et al.* 1989). The immunomodulatory agent thymopentin was effective for the systemic features, but not well-established arthritis, in a small series of children with systemic-onset juvenile chronic arthritis (Bardare *et al.* 1990).

A preliminary, open trial reported the results of repetitive use of pulse treatment with intravenous methylprednisolone (30 mg/kg per day for three consecutive days) with cyclophosphamide (0.4 g/m^2) on the third day, together with methotrexate at a dose of 10 mg/m^2 per week. This 3-day regimen was repeated every 3 months if the disease activity persisted and the patients required oral corticosteroids. Cyclophosphamide was included in subsequent pulses only if the patient had extra-articular disease. While there was an improvement noted in both articular and extra-articular disease, the laboratory features did not show statistically significant improvement. These preliminary results are impressive, and ideally would need to be confirmed in a randomized, placebo-controlled trial. Given the difficulty of conducting these types of trials in juvenile arthritis, the long-term follow-up of these patients must be reported before this approach can be recommended (Shaikov *et al.* 1992).

Adult-onset Still's disease

An entity quite similar in clinical and laboratory manifestations to systemic-onset juvenile chronic arthritis, but occurring in adults, was reported by Bywaters (Bywaters 1971). The so-called 'adult-onset Still's disease' has subsequently been described at all ages and with a worldwide distribution. Females outnumber males slightly. Seventy-five per cent of reported cases range between the ages of 16 and 35 years at the onset, with the overall incidence decreasing with age. Cases have been reported up to age 70. The fever pattern is identical to that of systemic-onset juvenile chronic arthritis (Fig. 1). Approximately 90 per cent have a rash that follows the fever course and may demonstrate a Koebner phenomenon; the rash may be pruritic. One important feature not well appreciated in systemic-onset juvenile chronic arthritis is a complaint of a severe sore throat, during flares of disease (Bujak et al. 1973; Esdaile et al. 1980; Ohta et al. 1987). While arthritis is not necessarily present at the onset, arthralgias are present in virtually all patients with the fever spikes. Although initial series described the arthritis as being quite mild, chronic arthritis with disability may be a sequel in up to 20 per cent of cases (Elkon et al. 1982; Cush et al. 1987; Cabane et al. 1990; Pouchot et al. 1991). As in the childhood form, hepatosplenomegaly and lymphadenopathy are reported in 40 to 75 per cent of cases. Weight loss of at least 10 per cent was recorded in approximately one-third of cases (Ohta et al. 1987). Pericarditis is the most common cardiac manifestation and tamponade may rarely occur. Both myocardial (Sachs et al. 1990) and endocardial (Taillan et al. 1989) involvement are rarely seen. Pulmonary disease appears to be more common than in systemic-onset juvenile chronic arthritis and is usually transient and mild, but severe restrictive lung disease has been observed (Corbett et al. 1983; Cantor et al. 1987). Abdominal pain may relate to hepatitis, adenitis, and sterile peritonitis, although this complaint is usually overshadowed by the other manifestations of adult-onset Still's disease (Bujak et al. 1973; Pollet et al. 1990). Abnormal liver function tests have been reported in up to 76 per cent of patients (Pouchot et al. 1991). Hepatic dysfunction may occur as part of a disseminated intravascular coagulation syndrome, may be related to medications, or as part of the underlying disease (Esdaile et al. 1979). Neurological involvement may rarely occur during systemic flares (Denault et al. 1990) or as a result of infection or complications of therapy (Wouters and van de Putte 1986). A number of ophthalmological manifestations, including inflammatory orbital pseudotumour (Cush et al. 1985), panophthalmitis (Bujak et al. 1973), and Brown's syndrome (Kaufman et al. 1987), have been reported. One case of sensorineural hearing loss, responsive to prednisone, was observed (Markusse et al. 1988). Rarely, renal disease may occur (Wendling et al. 1990).

The disease may follow several courses (Cush et al. 1987; Pouchot et al. 1991). In one series, those with either a mono- or polycyclic systemic course had articular manifestations, primarily during systemic exacerbations, and a good functional outcome. On the other hand, patients with a chronic articular course (either monocyclic systemic or polycyclic systemic) do not fare as well. Those patients with a polyarticular onset, axial arthritis, need for steroids within 2 years of onset, a history suggestive of childhood attacks, and the presence of a juvenile chronic arthritis rash seem to be at a greater overall risk for progressive joint damage and an unfavourable outcome (Cush et al. 1987; Pouchot

et al. 1991). Involvement of the carpus with ankylosis (Medsger and Christy 1975; Pouchot et al. 1991) is particularly common, as is tarsal ankylosis, and involvement of the cervical spine and hips with rapid progression of destructive disease. Distal interphalangeal involvement is also not unusual.

In comparison to same-sex siblings, patients with adult-onset Still's disease had significantly higher levels of pain, psychological disability, and physical disability. Despite these problems, educational achievement, occupational prestige, social functioning, social support, annual family income, and days lost from work did not differ between patients and same-sex siblings (Sampalis et al. 1995).

The treatment of adult-onset Still's disease should follow along the same lines as those of systemic-onset juvenile chronic arthritis. Initial attempts at fever control should be made with either high dose salicylates (100 mg/kg per day) or other NSAIDs, particularly indomethacin. These two agents may be effective together when neither alone gives sufficient therapeutic benefit (Esdaile et al. 1980; Wouters and van de Putte 1986; Cush et al. 1987). The majority of patients will ultimately require moderate to high-dose glucocorticoid therapy at some time during their course. At a median follow-up of 10 years, 50 per cent of patients still required treatment with second-line agents (gold, hydroxychloroquine, or methotrexate) and one-third of these continued to require low-dose prednisone (Sampalis et al. 1995). The effect of slow-acting antirheumatic drugs on the course of the articular disease has not been established and these agents do not have any effect on the systemic features.

The laboratory abnormalities, like those of systemic-onset juvenile chronic arthritis, are non-specific and include leucocytosis with neutrophilia, normochromic, normocytic anaemia, and thrombocytosis. Eosinophilia appears to be common in the Japanese cases (Ohta et al. 1987). Hypoalbuminaemia, hypergammaglobulinaemia, and increased serum complement levels are commonly observed. Raised serum levels of hepatic transaminases, while common, are usually transient and reflect active disease. No consistent HLA associations have been identified (Wouters et al. 1986; Pouchot et al. 1991).

Death may result in a very small number of patients from a wide variety of causes, including liver involvement and systemic amyloidosis (Ohta et al. 1987; Reginato et al. 1987).

References

Agarwal, R.K., O'Neil, K.M., and Bedi, D. (1994). Focal radiolucent hepatic lesions in a patient with juvenile rheumatoid arthritis. *Journal of Rheumatology*, **21**, 580–1.

Aitman, T.J. et al. (1989). Serum IGF-I levels and growth failure in juvenile chronic arthritis. *Clinical and Experimental Rheumatology*, **7**, 557–61.

Alarcon-Riquelme, M.E. et al. (1988). Immunoregulatory defects in juvenile rheumatoid arthritis. Comparison between patients with the systemic or polyarticular forms. *Journal of Rheumatology*, **15**, 1547–50.

Allen, R.C., Jimenez, M., and Cowell, C.T. (1991). Insulin-like growth factor and growth hormone secretion in juvenile chronic arthritis. *Annals of the Rheumatic Diseases*, **50**, 602–6.

Alukal, M.K., Costello, P.B., and Green, F.A. (1984). Cardiac tamponade in systemic juvenile rheumatoid arthritis requiring emergency pericardiectomy. *Journal of Rheumatology*, **11**, 222–5.

Andersson Gare, B. and Fasth, A. (1992). Epidemiology of chronic arthritis in Southwestern Sweden: a 5 year, prospective population study. *Pediatrics*, **90**, 950–8.

Andersson Gare, B. et al. (1987). Incidence and prevalence of juvenile chronic arthritis: a population survey. *Annals of the Rheumatic Diseases*, **46**, 277–81.

Anonymous (1993). American Academy of Pediatrics Section on Rheumatology and Section on Ophthalmology: Guidelines for ophthalmologic examinations in children with juvenile rheumatoid arthritis. *Pediatrics*, **92**, 295–6.

Ansell, B.M. (1977). Juvenile chronic polyarthritis. Series 3. *Arthritis and Rheumatism*, **20** (Suppl), 176–8.

Ansell, B.M. (1978). Heberden oration, 1977. Chronic arthritis in childhood. *Annals of the Rheumatic Diseases*, **37**, 107–20.

Ansell, B., M. and Wood, P.H.N. (1976). Prognosis in juvenile chronic polyarthritis. *Clinics in Rheumatic Diseases*, **2**, 397–412.

Antilla, R. (1972). Renal involvement in juvenile rheumatoid arthritis. *Acta Paediatrica Scandinavica*, **227** (suppl), 1–73.

Arroyo, I.L., Barron, K.S., and Brewer, E.J., Jr (1988). Spinal cord compression by epidural lipomatosis in juvenile rheumatoid arthritis. *Arthritis and Rheumatism*, **31**, 447–51.

Arvin, A.M. and Miller, J.J. (1984). Acid labile alpha-interferon in sera and synovial fluids from patients with juvenile arthritis. *Arthritis and Rheumatism*, **27**, 582–5.

Athreya, B.H. *et al.* (1980). Pulmonary manifestations of juvenile rheumatoid arthritis. A report of eight cases and review. *Clinics in Chest Medicine*, **1**, 361–74.

Bacon, T.H., de Vere-Tyndall, A., Tyrrell, D.A., Denman, A.M., and Ansell, B.M. (1983). Interferon system in patients with systemic juvenile chronic arthritis: *in vivo* and *in vitro* studies. *Clinical and Experimental Immunology*, **54**, 23–30.

Bacon, M.C. *et al.* (1990). Nutritional status and growth in juvenile rheumatoid arthritis. *Seminars in Arthritis and Rheumatism*, **20**, 97–106.

Barbaric, Z.L. and Young, L.W. (1972). Synovial cysts in juvenile rheumatoid arthritis. *American Journal of Roentgenology*, **116**, 655–60.

Bardare, M., Corona, F., Ogliari, M.T., and Cohen, E. (1990). Thymopentin in the treatment of juvenile chronic arthritis. *Clinical and Experimental Rheumatology*, **8**, 89–93.

Barron, K.S., DeCunto, C.L., Montalvo, J.F., Orson, F.M., and Lewis, D.E. (1989). Abnormalities of immunoregulation in juvenile rheumatoid arthritis. *Journal of Rheumatology*, **16**, 940–8.

Baum, J. and Gutkowska, G. (1977). Death in juvenile rheumatoid arthritis. *Arthritis and Rheumatism*, **20**, 253–5.

Baum, J. *et al.* (1980). Juvenile rheumatoid arthritis. A comparison of patients from the USSR and USA. *Arthritis and Rheumatism*, **23**, 977–84.

Bedford, P.A., Ansell, B.M., Hall, P.J., and Woo, P. (1992). Increased frequency of DR4 in systemic onset juvenile chronic arthritis. *Clinical and Experimental Rheumatology*, **10**, 189–93.

Bennett, A.E., Silverman, E.D., Miller, J.J., and Hintz, R.L. (1988). Insulin-like growth factors I and II in children with systemic onset juvenile chronic arthritis. *Journal of Rheumatology*, **15**, 655–8.

Bernstein, B.H. *et al.* (1977). Growth retardation in juvenile rheumatoid arthritis (JRA). *Arthritis and Rheumatism*, **20**, 212–6.

Bhettay, E. and Thomson, A.J.G. (1985). Peritonitis in juvenile chronic arthritis. *South African Medical Journal*, **68**, 605–6.

Bjerkhoel, F. and Forre, O. (1988). Cyclosporin treatment of a child with severe systemic juvenile rheumatoid arthritis. *Scandinavian Journal of Rheumatology*, **17**, 483–6.

Blodgett, F.M., Burgin, L., Iezzoni, D., Sribetz, D., and Talbot, N.B. (1956). Effects of prolonged cortisone therapy on the statural growth, skeletal maturation and metabolic status of children. *New England Journal of Medicine*, **254**, 636–41.

Boone, J.E. (1977). Hepatic disease and mortality in juvenile rheumatoid arthritis. *Arthritis and Rheumatism*, **20**, 257–8.

Borel, Y., Morimoto, C., Cairns, L., Mantzouranis, E.S., Strelkaukas, A.J. and Schlossman, S.F. (1984). Anti-T cell antibody in juvenile rheumatoid arthritis. *Journal of Rheumatology*, **11**, 56–61.

Brewer, E.J. (1977). Nonsteroidal antiinflammatory agents. *Arthritis and Rheumatism*, **20**, 513–25.

Brewer, E.J., Jr *et al.* (1977). Current proposed revision of JRA Criteria. JRA Criteria Subcommittee of the Diagnostic and Therapeutic Criteria Committee of the American Rheumatism Section of The Arthritis Foundation. *Arthritis and Rheumatism*, **20**, 195–9.

Bujak, J.S., Aptekar, R.G., Decker, J.L., and Wolff, S.M. (1973). Juvenile rheumatoid arthritis presenting in the adult as fever of unknown origin. *Medicine*, **52**, 431–44.

Butenandt, O. (1979). Rheumatoid arthritis and growth retardation in children: treatment with human growth hormone. *European Journal of Pediatrics*, **130**, 15–28.

Butenandt, O., Kelch, A., and Rajmann, E. (1974). Growth hormone studies in patients with rheumatoid arthritis with or without glucocorticoid therapy. *Zeitschrift für Kinderheilkunde*, **118**, 53–62.

Byron, M.A., Jackson, J., and Ansell, B.M. (1983). Effect of different corticosteroid regimens on hypothalamic-pituitary-adrenal axis and growth in juvenile chronic arthritis. *Journal of the Royal Society of Medicine*, **76**, 452–7.

Bywaters, E.G. (1971). Still's disease in the adult. *Annals of the Rheumatic Diseases*, **30**, 121–33.

Cabane, J. *et al.* (1990). Comparison of long term evolution of adult onset and juvenile onset Still's disease, both followed up for more than 10 years. *Annals of the Rheumatic Diseases*, **49**, 283–5.

Calabro, J.J., Holgerson, W.B., Sonpal, G.M., and Khoury, M.I. (1976). Juvenile rheumatoid arthritis: A general survey of 100 patients observed for 15 years. *Seminars in Arthritis and Rheumatism*, **5**, 257–98.

Cantor, J.P., Pitcher, W.D., and Hurd, E. (1987). Severe restrictive pulmonary defect in a patient with adult-onset Still's disease. *Chest*, **92**, 939–40.

Caspi, D., Fuchs, D., and Yaron, M. (1992). Sulphasalazine induced hepatitis in juvenile rheumatoid arthritis. *Annals of the Rheumatic Diseases*, **51**, 275–6.

Cassidy, J.T. (1990). Management of JCA: slow-acting anti-rheumatic drugs. In *Pediatric rheumatology update* (eds P. Woo, P.H. White, and B.M. Ansell), pp. 66–80. Oxford University Press, New York.

Cassidy, J.T. and Martel, W. (1977). Juvenile rheumatoid arthritis: clinicoradiologic correlations. *Arthritis and Rheumatism*, **20**, 207–11.

Cassidy, J.T. *et al.* (1986). A study of classification criteria for a diagnosis of juvenile rheumatoid arthritis. *Arthritis and Rheumatism*, **29**, 274–81.

Corbett, A.J., Zizic, T.M., and Stevens, M.B. (1983). Adult-onset Still's disease with an associated severe restrictive pulmonary defect: a case report. *Annals of the Rheumatic Diseases*, **42**, 452–4.

Craft, A.W., Eastham, E.J., Bell, J.I., and Brigham, K. (1977). Serum ferritin in juvenile chronic polyarthritis. *Annals of the Rheumatic Diseases*, **36**, 271–3.

Cush, J.J., Leibowitz, I.H., and Friedman, S.A. (1985). Adult-onset Still's disease and inflammatory orbital pseudotumor. *New York State Journal of Medicine*, **85**, 110–1.

Cush, J.J., Medsger, T.A., Jr, Christy, W.C., Herbert, D.C., and Cooperstein, L.A. (1987). Adult-onset Still's disease. Clinical course and outcome. *Arthritis and Rheumatism*, **30**, 186–94.

David, J., Vouyiouka, O., Ansell, B.M., Hall, A., and Woo, P. (1993). Amyloidosis in juvenile chronic arthritis: a morbidity and mortality study. *Clinical and Experimental Rheumatology*, **11**, 85–90.

David, J. *et al.* (1994). The functional and psychological outcomes of juvenile chronic arthritis in young adulthood. *British Journal of Rheumatology*, **33**, 876–81.

Davies, U.M., Rooney, M., Preece, M.A., Ansell, B.M., and Woo, P. (1994). Treatment of growth retardation in juvenile chronic arthritis with recombinant human growth hormone. *Journal of Rheumatology*, **21**, 153–8.

de Bennedetti, B.F. *et al.* (1991). Correlation of serum interleukin-6 levels with joint involvement and thrombocytosis in systemic juvenile rheumatoid arthritis. *Arthritis and Rheumatism*, **34**, 1158–63.

de Bennedetti, B.F. *et al.* (1994). Serum soluble interleukin 6 (IL-6) receptor and IL-6/soluble IL-6 receptor complex in systemic juvenile rheumatoid arthritis. *Journal of Clinical Investigation*, **93**, 2114–9.

De Inocencio, J., Giannini, E.H., and Glass, D.N. (1993). Can genetic markers contribute to the classification of juvenile rheumatoid arthritis? *Journal of Rheumatology*, **40** (suppl.), 12–18.

Denault, A., Dimopoulos, M.A., and Fitzcharles, M.A. (1990). Meningoencephalitis and peripheral neuropathy complicating adult Still's disease. *Journal of Rheumatology*, **17**, 698–700.

Deschenes, G., Prieur, A.M., Hayem, F., Broyer, M., and Gubler, M.C. (1990). Renal amyloidosis in juvenile chronic arthritis: evolution after chlorambucil treatment. *Pediatric Nephrology*, **4**, 463–9.

Drenth, J.P.H., Haagsma, C.J., and Van der Meer, J.W.M. (1994). Hyperimmunoglobulinemia D and periodic fever syndrome. The clinical spectrum in a series of 50 patients. *Medicine*, **73**, 133–44.

Elkon, K.B. *et al.* (1982). Adult-onset Still's disease. Twenty-year followup and further studies of patients with active disease. *Arthritis and Rheumatism*, **25**, 647–54.

Esdaile, J.M., Tannenbaum, H., Lough, J., and Hawkins, D. (1979). Hepatic abnormalities in adult onset Still's disease. *Journal of Rheumatology*, **6**, 673–9.

Esdaile, J.M., Tannenbaum, H., and Hawkins, D. (1980). Adult Still's disease. *American Journal of Medicine*, **68**, 825–30.

Espada, G., Babini, J.C., Maldonado-Cocco, J.A., and Garcia-Morteo, O. (1988). Radiologic review: the cervical spine in juvenile rheumatoid arthritis. *Seminars in Arthritis and Rheumatism*, **17**, 185–95.

Espinel, C.H. (1994). Caravaggio's 'Il Amore Dormiente': a sleeping cupid with juvenile rheumatoid arthritis. *Lancet*, **344**, 1750–2.

Fantini, F., Gattinara, M., Gerloni, V., Bergomi, P., and Cirla, E. (1992). Severe anemia associated with active systemic-onset juvenile rheumatoid arthritis successfully treated with recombinant human erythropoietin: a pilot study. *Arthritis and Rheumatism*, **35**, 724–6.

Fassbender, K., Michels, H., Vogt, P., Aeschlimann, A., and Muller, W. (1992). Soluble interleukin-2 receptors in children with juvenile chronic arthritis. *Scandinavian Journal of Rheumatology*, **21**, 120–3.

Feldman, B.M. *et al.* (1996). Seasonal onset of systemic-onset juvenile rheumatoid arthritis. *Journal of Pediatrics*, **129**, 513–18.

Gedalia, A., Adara, A., and Gorodischer, R. (1992). Familial mediteranean fever in children. *Journal of Rheumatology*, **19** (Suppl 35), 1–9.

Gewanter, H.L. and Baum, J. (1981). The use of tolmetin sodium in systemic onset juvenile rheumatoid arthritis. *Arthritis and Rheumatism*, **24**, 1316–19.

Gewanter, H.L., Roghmann, K.J., and Baum, J. (1983). The prevalence of juvenile arthritis. *Arthritis and Rheumatism*, **26**, 599–603.

Giannini, E.H. *et al.* (1992). Methotrexate in resistant juvenile rheumatoid arthritis. Results of the U.S.A.-U.S.S.R. double-blind, placebo-controlled trial. *New England Journal of Medicine*, **326**, 1043–9.

Goldenberg, J. *et al.* (1990). Cardiac tamponade in juvenile chronic arthritis: report of two cases and review of publications. *Annals of the Rheumatic Diseases*, **49**, 549–53.

Goldenberg, J. *et al.* (1992). Symptomatic cardiac involvement in juvenile rheumatoid arthritis. *International Journal of Cardiology*, **34**, 57–62.

Gwyther, M., Schwarz, H., Howard, A., and Ansell, B.M. (1982). C-reactive protein in juvenile chronic arthritis: an indicator of disease activity and possibly amyloidosis. *Annals of the Rheumatic Diseases*, **41**, 259–62.

Hadchouel, M., Prieur, A.M., and Griscelli, C. (1985). Acute hemorrhagic, hepatic and neurologic manifestations in juvenile rehumatoid arthritis: possible relationship to drugs or infection. *Journal of Pediatrics*, **106**, 561–6.

Hafner, R. and Truckenbrodt, H. (1986). Course and prognosis of systemic juvenile chronic arthritis—retrospective study of 187 patients. *Klinische Padiatrie*, **198**, 401–7.

Hafner, R. and Vogel, P. (1993). Sarcoidosis of early onset. A challenge for the pediatric rheumatologist. *Clinical and Experimental Rheumatology*, **11**, 685–91.

Halle, F. and Prieur, A.M. (1991). Evaluation of methotrexate in the treatment of juvenile chronic arthritis according to the subtype. *Clinical and Experimental Rheumatology*, **9**, 297–302.

Hanson, V., Kornreich, H., Bernstein, B., King, K.K., and Singsen, B. (1977). Prognosis of juvenile rheumatoid arthritis. *Arthritis and Rheumatism*, **20**, 279–84.

Harvey, A.R., Pippard, M.J., and Ansell, B.M. (1987). Microcytic anaemia in juvenile chronic arthritis. *Scandinavian Journal of Rheumatology*, **16**, 53–9.

Hawkins, P.N. *et al.* (1993). Serum amyloid P component scintigraphy and turnover studies for diagnosis and quantitative monitoring of AA amyloidosis in juvenile rheumatoid arthritis. *Arthritis and Rheumatism*, **36**, 842–51.

Hayem, F., Calede, C., Hayem, G., and Kahn, M.F. (1994). (Involvement of the hip in systemic-onset forms of juvenile chronic arthritis. Retrospective study of 28 cases). *Revue du Rhumatisme, edition Francaise*, **61**, 583–9.

Heaton, D.C. and Moller, P.W. (1985). Still's disease associated with Coxsackie infection and haemophagocytic syndrome. *Annals of the Rheumatic Diseases*, **44**, 341–4.

Hertzberger, Ten Cate R. and Cats, A. (1991). Toxicity of sulfasalazine in systemic juvenile chronic arthritis. *Clinical and Experimental Rheumatology*, **9**, 85–8.

Heyd, J. and Glaser, J. (1990). Early occurrence of aortic valve regurgitation in a youth with systemic-onset juvenile rheumatoid arthritis. *American Journal of Medicine*, **89**, 123–4.

Hochberg, M.C. (1981). Adult and juvenile rheumatoid arthritis: current epidemiologic concepts. *Epidemiologic Reviews*, **3**, 27–44.

Hoyeraal, H.M. and Mellbye, O.J. (1974). High levels of serum complement factors in juvenille rheumatoid arthritis. *Annals of the Rheumatic Diseases*, **33**, 243–7.

Hull, R.G. (1988). Outcome in juvenile arthritis. *British Journal of Rheumatology*, **27**, 66–71.

Ilowite, N.T., Samuel, P., Beseler, L., and Jacobson, M.S. (1989). Dyslipoproteinemia in juvenile rheumatoid arthritis. *Journal of Pediatrics*, **114**, 823–6.

Isdale, I.C. and Bywaters, E.G.L. (1956). The rash of rheumatoid arthritis and Still's disease. *Quarterly Journal of Medicine*, **25**, 377–87.

Jacobs, J.C. and Hui, R.M. (1977). Cricoaretynoid arthritis and airway obstruction in juvenile rheumatoid artyhritis. *Pediatrics*, **59**, 292–4.

Jan, J.E., Hill, R.H., and Low, M.D. (1972). Cerebral complications in juvenile rheumatoid arthritis. *Canadian Medical Association Journal*, **107**, 623–5.

Kaufman, L.D., Sibony, P.A., Anand, A.K., and Gruber, B.L. (1987). Superior oblique tenosynovitis (Brown's syndrome) as a manifestation of adult Still's disease. *Journal of Rheumatology*, **14**, 625–7.

Koerper, M.A., Stempel, D.A., and Dallman, P.R. (1978). Anemia in patients with juvenile rheumatoid arthritis. *Journal of Pediatrics*, **92**, 930–3.

Kramer, P.H., Imboden, J.B., Jr, Waldman, F.M., Turley, K., and Ports, T.A. (1983). Severe aortic insufficiency in juvenile chronic arthritis. *American Journal of Medicine*, **74**, 1088–91.

Kvien, T.K., Hoyeraal, H.M., and Sandstad, B. (1986). Azathioprine versus placebo in patients with juvenile rheumatoid arthritis: a single center double blind comparative study. *Journal of Rheumatology*, **13**, 118–23.

Lang, B.A. and Shore, A. (1990). A review on the current concepts on the pathogenesis of juvenile rheumatoid arthritis. *Journal of Rheumatology*, **17** (Suppl 21), 1–15.

Lang, B.A., Schneider, R., Reilly, B.J., Silverman, E.D., and Laxer, R.M. (1995). Radiologic features of systemic onset juvenile rheumatoid arthritis. *Journal of Rheumatology*, **22**, 168–73.

Lietman, P.S. and Bywaters, E.G.L. (1963). Pericarditis in juvenile rhaumatoid arthritis. *Pediatrics*, **32**, 855–60.

Lindsley, C.B. (1987). Seasonal variation in systemic onset juvenile rheumatoid arthritis. *Arthritis and Rheumatism*, **30**, 838–9.

Lipnick, R.N., Sfikakis, P.P., Klipple, G.L., and Tsokos, G.C. (1993). Elevated soluble CD8 antigen and soluble interleukin-2 receptors in the sera of patients with juvenile rheumatoid arthritis. *Clinical Immunology and Immunopathology*, **68**, 64–7.

Maksymowych, W.P. and Glass, D.N. (1988). Population genetics and molecular biology of the childhood chronic arthropathies. *Baillière's Clinical Rheumatology*, **2**, 649–71.

Mangge, H. *et al.* (1995). Serum cytokines in juvenile rheumatoid arthritis. Correlation with conventional inflammation parameters and clinical subtypes. *Arthritis and Rheumatism*, **38**, 211–20.

Manners, P.J. and Ansell, B.M. (1986). Slow-acting antirheumatic drug use in systemic onset juvenile chronic arthritis. *Pediatrics*, **77**, 99–103.

Markusse, H.M., Stolk, B., van der Mey, A.G., de Jonge-Bok, J.M., and Heering, K.J. (1988). Sensorineural hearing loss in adult onset Still's disease. *Annals of the Rheumatic Diseases*, **47**, 600–2.

Martel, W., Holt, J.F., and Cassidy, J.T. (1962). Roentgenologic manifestations of juvenile rheumatoid arthritis. *American Journal of Roentgenology*, **88**, 400–23.

Martini, A. *et al.* (1986). Enhanced interleukin 1 and depressed interleukin 2 production in juvenile arthritis. *Journal of Rheumatology*, **13**, 598–603.

Martini, A. *et al.* (1994). Intravenous iron therapy for severe anaemia in systemic-onset juvenile chronic arthritis. *Lancet*, **344**, 1052–4.

Medsger, T.A., Jr and Christy, W.C. (1975). Selective carpo-metacarpal arthritis with early ankylosis in adult onset Still's disease. *Arthritis and Rheumatism*, 18, 526–7.

Miller, J.J. (1977). Myocarditis in juvenile rheumatoid artyhritis. *American Journal of Diseases of Childhood*, 131, 205–9.

Miller, J.J., Olds, L.C., Silverman, E.D., Milgrom, H., and Curd, J.G. (1986). Different patterns of C3 and C4 activation in the varied types of juvenile arthritis. *Pediatric Research*, 20, 1332–7.

Mitnick, J. and Mitnick, H. (1980). Kidney enlargement and cervical spine disease in a child. *Journal of the American Medical Association* 243, 465–6.

Moore, A.T. and Morin, J.D. (1985). Bilateral acquired inflammatory Brown's syndrome. *Journal of Pediatric Ophthalmology and Strabismus*, 22, 26–30.

Moore, T.L., Sheridan, P.W., Traycoff, R.B., Zuckner, J., and Dorner, R.W. (1982). Immune complexes in juvenile rheumatoid arthritis: a comparison of four methods. *Journal of Rheumatology*, 9, 395–401.

Moore, T.L. *et al.* (1984). Autoantibodies in juvenile arthritis. *Seminars in Arthritis and Rheumatism*, 13, 329–36.

Morris, J.A., Adamson, A.R., Holt, P.J.L., and Davson, J. (1985). Still's disease and the virus-associated haemophagocutic syndrome. *Annals of the Rheumatic Diseases*, 44, 349–53.

Mortensen, A.L., Allen, J.R., and Allen, R.C. (1990). Nutritional assessment of children with juvenile chronic arthritis. *Journal of Paediatrics and Child Health*, 26, 335–8.

Mozziconacci, P., Prieur, A.M., Hayem, F., and Oury, C. (1983). (Articular prognosis of the systemic form of chronic juvenile arthritis (100 cases)). *Annales de Pediatrie*, 30, 553–6.

Nepom, B. (1991). The immunogenetics of juvenile rheumatoid arthritis. *Rheumatic Disease Clinics of North America*, 17, 825–42.

Nepom, B.S. and Glass, D.N. (1992). Juvenile rheumatoid arthritis and HLA: report of the Park City III workshop. *Journal of Rheumatology Supplement*, 33, 70–4.

Nocton, J.J., Miller, L.C., Tucker, L.B., and Schaller, J.G. (1993). Human parvovirus B19-associated arthritis in children. *Journal of Pediatrics*, 122, 186–90.

Ohta, A., Yamaguchi, M., Kaneoka, H., Nagayoshi, T., and Hiida, M. (1987). Adult Still's disease: review of 228 cases from the literature. *Journal of Rheumatology*, 14, 1139–46.

Ostensen, M., Hoyeraal, H.M., and Kass, E. (1988). Tolerance of cyclosporine A in children with refractory juvenile rheumatoid arthritis. *Journal of Rheumatology*, 15, 1536–8.

Ostrov, B.E., Goldsmith, D.P., and Athreya, B.H. (1993). Differentiation of systemic juvenile rheumatoid arthritis from acute leukemia near the onset of disease. *Journal of Pediatrics*, 122, 595–8.

Padeh, S., Laxer, R.M., Silver, M.M., and Silverman, E.D. (1991). Primary pulmonary hypertension in a patient with systemic-onset juvenile arthritis. *Arthritis and Rheumatism*, 34, 1575–9.

Palmer, R.G. and Ansell, B.M. (1984). Acute leukaemia related to chlorambucil therapy for juvenile chronic arthritis. *Clinical and Experimental Rheumatology*, 2, 81–3.

Pauls, J.D., Silverman, E., Laxer, R.M., and Fritzler, M.J. (1989). Antibodies to histones H1 and H5 in sera of patients with juvenile rheumatoid arthritis. *Arthritis and Rheumatism*, 32, 877–83.

Pearl, W. (1982). Pericarditis in juvenile rheumatoid arthritis. *Pediatrics*, 70, 154–5.

Pelkonen, P., Savilahti, E., and Makela, A.L. (1983). Persistent and transient IgA deficiency in juvenile rheumatoid arthritis. *Scandinavian Journal of Rheumatology*, 12, 273–9.

Pelkonen, P., Swanljung, K., and Siimes, M.A. (1986). Ferritinaemia as an indicator of systemic disease activity in children with systemic juvenile rheumatoid arthritis. *Acta Paediatrica Scandinavica*, 75, 64–8.

Pernice, W., *et al.* (1989). Therapy for systemic juvenile rheumatoid arthritis with γ-interferon. A pilot study of nine patients. *Arthritis and Rheumatism*, 32, 643–6.

Petty, R.E., Cassidy, J.T., and Sullivan, D.B. (1977). Serologic studies in juvenile rheumatoid arthritis: a review. *Arthritis and Rheumatism*, 20, 260–7.

Pistoia, V. *et al.* (1993). Cyclosporin A in the treatment of juvenile chronic arthritis and childhood polymyositis–dermatomyositis. Results of a preliminary study. *Clinical and Experimental Rheumatology*, 11, 203–8.

Pollet, S.M., Vogt, P.J., and Leek, J.C. (1990). Serous peritonitis in adult Still's syndrome. *Journal of Rheumatology*, 17, 98–101.

Pouchot, J. *et al.* (1991). Adult Still's disease: manifestations, disease course, and outcome in 62 patients. *Medicine*, 70, 118–36.

Prieur, A.M., Bremard-Oury, C., Griscelli, C., and Mozziconacci, P. (1984). Pronostic des formes systemiques d'arthrite chronique juvenile. *Archives Francaise de Pediatrie*, 41, 91–7.

Prieur, A.M., Griscelli, C., Kauffman, M.T., and Dayer, J.M. (1987). Specific interleukin-1 inhibitor in serum and urine of children with systemic juvenile chronic arthritis. *Lancet*, 2, 1240–2.

Prieur, A.M., Adleff, A., Debre, M., Boulate, P., and Griscelli, C. (1990). High dose immunoglobulin therapy in severe juvenile chronic arthritis: long-term follow-up in 16 patients. *Clinical and Experimental Rheumatology*, 8, 603–8.

Prouse, P.J. *et al.* (1987). Anaemia in juvenile chronic arthritis: serum inhibition of normal erythropoeisis *in vitro*. *Annals of the Rheumatic Diseases*, 46, 127–34.

Pruzanski, W. *et al.* (1994). Phospholipase A2 in juvenile rheumatoid arthritis: correlation to disease type and activity. *Journal of Rheumatology*, 21, 1951–4.

Rachelefsky, G.S. *et al.* (1976). Serum enzyme abnormalities in juvenile rheumatoid arthritis. *Pediatrics*, 58, 730–6.

Ravelli, A. *et al.* (1994). Factors associated with response to methotrexate in systemic-onset juvenile chronic arthritis. *Acta Paediatrica*, 83, 428–32.

Reed, M.H. and Wilmot, D.M. (1991). The radiology of juvenile rheumatoid arthritis. A review of the English language literature. *Journal of Rheumatology*, 31 (suppl.), 2–22.

Reginato, A.J., Schumacher, H.R., Jr, Baker, D.G., O'Connor, C.R., and Ferreiros, J. (1987). Adult onset Still's disease: experience in 23 patients and literature review with emphasis on organ failure. *Seminars in Arthritis and Rheumatism*, 17, 39–57.

Rennebohm, R.M., Heubi, J.E., Daugherty, C.C., and Daniels, S.R. (1985). Reye syndrome in children receiving salicylate therapy for connective tissue disease. *Journal of Pediatrics*, 107, 877–88.

Rubin, R.N., Walker, B.K., Ballas, S.K., and Travis, S.F. (1978). Erythroid aplasia in juvenile rheumatoid arthritis. *American Journal of Diseases of Children*, 132, 760–2.

Sachs, R.N., Talvard, O., and Lanfranchi, J. (1990). Myocarditis in adult Still's disease. *International Journal of Cardiology*, 27, 377–80.

Sampalis, J.S. *et al.* (1995). A controlled study of the long-term prognosis of adult Still's disease. *American Journal of Medicine*, 98, 384–8.

Schaller, J. (1972). Arthritis as a presenting manifestation of malignancy in children. *Journal of Pediatrics*, 81, 793–7.

Schaller, J.G. (1977). Juvenile rheumatoid arthritis: Series 1. *Arthritis and Rheumatism*, 20, 165–70.

Schaller, J. and Wedgwood, R.J. (1972). Juvenile rheumatoid arthritis: a review. *Pediatrics*, 50, 940–53.

Schaller, J., Beckwith, B., and Wedgwood, R.J. (1970). Hepatic involvement in juvenile rheumatoid arthritis. *Journal of Pediatrics*, 77, 203–10.

Scheinberg, M.A. and Benson, M.D. (1980). SAA amyloid protein levels in amyloid-prone chronic inflammatory disorders. Lack of association with amyloid disease. *Journal of Rheumatology*, 7, 724–6.

Schneider, R. *et al.* (1992). Prognostic indicators of joint destruction in systemic-onset juvenile rheumatoid arthritis. *Journal of Pediatrics*, 120, 200–5.

Schnitzer, T.J. and Ansell, B.M. (1977). Amyloidosis in juvenile chronic polyarthritis. *Arthritis and Rheumatism*, 20, 245–52.

Scott, J.P., Gerber, P., Matyjowski, M.C., and Pachman, L.C. (1984). Evidence for intravasculas coagulation in systemic onset, but not polyarticular, juvenile rheumatoid arthritis. *Arthritis and Rheumatism*, 28, 256–61.

Shaikov, A.V. *et al.* (1992). Repetitive use of pulse therapy with methylprednisolone and cyclophosphamide in addition to oral methotrexate in children with systemic juvenile rheumatoid arthritis–preliminary results of a longterm study. *Journal of Rheumatology*, 19, 612–16.

Sherry, D.D. and Kredich, D.W. (1985). Transient thrombocytopenia in systemic onset juvenile rheumatoid arthritis. *Pediatrics*, 76, 600–3.

Sherry, D.D., Patterson, M.W.H., and Petty, R.E. (1982). The use of indomethacin in the treatment of pericarditis in childhood. *Journal of Pediatrics*, 100, 995–8.

Siamopoulou-Mavridou, A. *et al.* (1991). Autoantibodies in Greek juvenile chronic arthritis patients. *Clinical and Experimental Rheumatology*, 9, 647–52.

Silverman, E.D., Miller, J.J., Bernstein, B., and Shafai, T. (1983). Consumption coagulopathy associated with systemic juvenile rheumatoid arthritis. *Journal of Pediatrics*, 103, 872–6.

Silverman, E.D., Laxer, R.M., Estrov, Z., and Freedman, M.H. (1988). Anemia of systemic onset juvenile arthritis: inhibition of erythropoiesis by interleukin-2 responsive T lymphocytes. *Arthritis and Rheumatism*, **31**, S12.

Silverman, E.D., Somma, C., Khan, M.M., Melmon, K.L., and Engleman, E.G. (1990*a*). Abnormal T suppressor cell function in juvenile rheumatoid arthritis. *Arthritis and Rheumatism*, **33**, 205–11.

Silverman, E.D. *et al.* (1990*b*). Intravenous gammaglobulin therapy in systemic juvenile rheumatoid arthritis. *Arthritis and Rheumatism*, **33**, 1015–22.

Silverman, E.D., Laxer, R.M., Nelson, D.L., and Rubin, L.A. (1991). Soluble inter-leukin-2-receptor in juvenile rheumatoid arthritis. *Journal of Rheumatology*, **18**, 1398–402.

Silverman, E.D. *et al.* (1994). Intravenous immunoglobulin in the treatment of systemic juvenile rheumatoid arthritis: a randomized placebo controlled trial. *Journal of Rheumatology*, **21**, 2353–8.

Singh, G. *et al.* (1989). Histocompatibility antigens in systemic-onset juvenile rheumatoid arthritis. *Arthritis and Rheumatism*, **32**, 1492–3.

Skoglund, R.R., Schanberger, J.E., and Kaplan, J.M. (1971). Cyclophosphamide therapy for severe juvenile rheumatoid arthritis. *American Journal of Diseases of Children*, **121**, 531–3.

Stasny, P. and Fink, C.W. (1979). Different HLA-D associations in adult and juvenile rheumatoid arthritis. *Journal of Clinical Investigation*, **63**, 124–30.

Stephan, J.L. *et al.* (1993). Macrophage activation syndrome and rheumatic disease in childhood: a report of four new cases. *Clinical and Experimental Rheumatology*, **11**, 451–6.

Still, G.F. (1897). On a form of chronic joint disease in children. *Medical-chirurgical Transactions*, **80**, 47–59.

Stoeber, E. (1981). Prognosis in juvenile chronic arthritis. Follow-up of 433 chronic rheumatic children. *European Journal of Pediatrics*, **135**, 225–8.

Svantesson, H. (1991). Treatment of growth failure with human growth hormone in patients with juvenile chronic arthritis. A pilot study. *Clinical and Experimental Rheumatology*, **6**, 47–50.

Svantesson, H., Akesson, A., Eberhardt, K., and Elborgh, R. (1983). Prognosis in juvenile rheumatoid arthritis with systemic onset. A follow-up study. *Scandinavian Journal of Rheumatology*, **12**, 139–44.

Taillan, B. *et al.* (1989). Adult onset still's disease complicated by endocarditis with fatal evolution. *Clinical Rheumatology*, **8**, 541.

Tesser, J.R., Pisko, E.J., Hartz, J.W., and Weinblatt, M.E. (1982). Chronic liver disease and Still's disease. *Arthritis and Rheumatism*, **25**, 579–82.

Thomsen, B.S. *et al.* (1987). Complement C3b receptors on erythrocytes in patients with juvenile rheumatoid arthritis. *Arthritis and Rheumatism*, **30**, 967–71.

Towner, S.R., Michet, C.J., Jr, O'Fallon, W.M., and Nelson, A.M. (1983). The epidemiology of juvenile arthritis in Rochester, Minnesota 1960–1979. *Arthritis and Rheumatism*, **26**, 1208–13.

Tsokos, G.C. *et al.* (1987). Cellular immunity in patients with systemic juvenile rheumatoid arthritis. *Clinical Immunology and Immunopathology*, **42**, 86–92.

Wagener, J.S., Taussig, L.M., DeBenedetti, C., Lemen, R.J., and Loughlin, G.M. (1981). Pulmonary function in juvenile rheumatoid arthritis. *Journal of Pediatrics*, **99**, 108–10.

Walters, D., Robinson, R.G., Dick-Smith, J.B., Corrigan, A.B., and Webb, J. (1972). Poor response in two cases of juvenile rheumatoid arthritis to treatment with cyclophosphamide. *Medical Journal of Australia*, **2**, 1070.

Wang, F.M., Wertenbaker, C., Behrens, M.M., and Jacobs, J.C. (1984). Acquired Brown's syndrome in children with juvenile rheumatoid arthritis. *Ophthalmology*, **91**, 23–6.

Wendling, D., Hory, B., and Blanc, D. (1990). Adult Still's disease and mesangial glomerulonephritis. Report of two cases. *Clinical Rheumatology*, **9**, 95–9.

Woo, P., O'Brien, J., Robson, M., and Ansell, B.M. (1987). A genetic marker for systemic amyloidosis in juvenile arthritis. *Lancet*, **2**, 767–9.

Wouters, J.M. and van de Putte, L.B. (1986). Adult-onset Still's disease; clinical and laboratory features, treatment and progress of 45 cases. *Quarterly Journal of Medicine*, **61**, 1055–65.

Wouters, J.M., Reekers, P., and van de Putte, L.B. (1986). Adult-onset Still's disease. Disease course and HLA associations. *Arthritis and Rheumatism*, **29**, 415–18.

Yancey, C.L., Doughty, R.A., Cohlan, B.A., and Athreya, B.H. (1981). Pericarditis and cardiac tamponade in juvenile rheumatoid arthritis. *Pediatrics*, **68**, 369–73.

Yousefzadeh, D.K. and Fishman, P.A. (1979). The triad of pneumonitis, pleuritis, and pericarditis in juvenile rheumatoid arthritis. *Pediatric Radiology*, **8**, 147–50.

Zaglul, H., Carswell, F., and Simpson, R.M. (1982). A case of persistent pulmonary functional abnormalities in systemic-onset juvenile chronic polyarthritis. *European Journal of Pediatrics*, **138**, 315–16.

5.6.3 Rheumatoid factor-negative polyarthritis in children ('seronegative' polyarthritis)

Anne-Marie Prieur

Polyarticular onset occurs in about 30 per cent of all patients with juvenile chronic arthritis. By definition, it occurs before the age of 16 years with the involvement of a minimum of five joints; the duration varies according to the adopted set of diagnostic criteria. The most accepted diagnostic criteria are either those of the European League Against Rheumatism (**EULAR**) (Wood 1978) or those of the American College of Rheumatology (**ACR**), previously the American Rheumatism Association (**ARA**) (Brewer *et al.* 1977). In the EULAR criteria, polyarthritis with positive rheumatoid factor is excluded, while in the ACR proposal, patients with positive rheumatoid factor are included in the group of polyarticular onset. This helps to explain why this disease is named juvenile chronic arthritis in Europe, but juvenile rheumatoid arthritis in North America. Arthritis must be present for at least 3 months in the EULAR criteria, or for 6 weeks in the ACR criteria. These proposed diagnostic criteria do not take into account the type of course, which obviously is extremely important for the prognosis and outcome. Pauciarticular onset with a polyarticular course will not be considered in this chapter.

The following description will not include the group of so-called 'seropositive' patients. We prefer, for obvious reasons, not to speak of seropositivity or seronegativity, but of rheumatoid factor (**RF**) -positive or -negative. The RF-positive group represents the early onset of adult rheumatoid arthritis and all data available in adults are also true in children (see Chapter 5.4.3). It is uncommon and occurs in less than 10 per cent of the whole polyarticular group in children. Polyarticular onset that is RF negative is the most common and is extremely heterogeneous. Some subgroups are easy to identify, but others need further evaluation to establish convenient and precise criteria for classification. Four subgroups can be identified in the RF-negative group (Table 1). The following discussion is based on the author's experience of more than 15 years in a paediatric rheumatology clinic with an annual referral of more than 1200 patients, one-third of them being first-time referrals.

Frequent manifestations of RF-negative polyarthritis

Extra-articular manifestations

Extra-articular manifestations may be present. Fever can be observed in one-third of patients. It is generally low grade, or a

Table 1 A proposed classification of subgroups of juvenile chronic arthritis with polyarticular onset

	I	II	III	IV	V
M/F ratio	1/9	1/7	1/1	1/1	3/1
Frequency	<10%	40%	15%	15%	20%
Age at onset (years)	8–9	2–3	>8	>6	8–9
Arthritis characteristics	Painful synovitis	Painful synovitis	Boggy synovitis Mild pain	Dry synovitis Marked stiffness	Painful synovitis
Biological inflammation	Marked	Marked	Marked	Mild if any	Marked
Specific features	Positive RF	Positive ANA Negative RF Risk of CAU	None	None	JSA
Genetic markers	HLA DR4	HLA DR5 HLA DR8	?	?	HLA B27
Prognosis	Rapid joint erosions	Severe polyarthritis	Late reduction of joint motion	Progressive stiffness	JAS

ANA, antinuclear antibodies; CAU, chronic anterior uveitis; JSA, juvenile spondylarthropathy according to the ESSG or Amor criteria; JAS, juvenile ankylosing spondylitis; RF, rheumatoid factor.

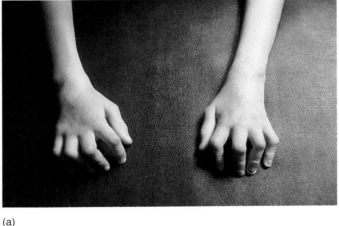
(a)

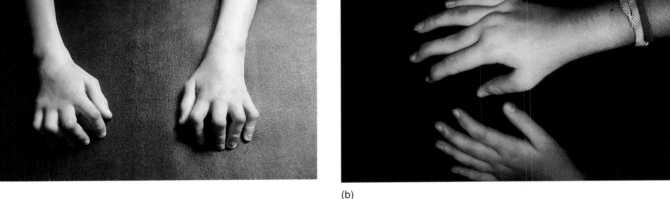
(b)

Fig. 1 Boutonnière deformity (a) and swan-neck deformity (b) of fingers.

high fever often of short duration. By definition, long-lasting swinging fever as described in systemic onset is never observed in the polyarticular type. In very young children, a transient rash lasting 1 or 2 days can occur in the early stages. There is generally no lymphadenopathy, hepatosplenomegaly, or visceral involvement.

Joint manifestations

Joint manifestations dominate the clinical presentation. Generally, the mode of onset is rapidly progressive. The child is referred to the specialist often after several weeks of worsening joint stiffness and/or swelling.

A joint is a complex organ (Chapter 2.5) made up of synovial membrane, articular cartilage, fibrous capsule, ligaments, tendons with their site of attachment on bone (the enthesis), bursas, and tendon sheaths. In children, the joints also have growth cartilage. All these structures may be inflamed during the rheumatic process and chronic inflammation results in joint alterations and deformities. Chronic swelling and limited motion results in local demineralization. Muscular wasting is a consequence of the limitation of motion and it reduces joint motility. Chronic hyperaemia may induce local accelerated growth and growth cartilage fusion. Cartilage and bone erosions are late manifestations. There is potential for cartilage generation in children, which may delay severe functional impairment.

Flexion contracture is the first manifestation of elbow involvement. It may be mild and of little functional significance. Limitation of supination is very common. The shoulders are frequently involved in severe cases, leading to limitation of movment, particularly abduction and external rotation of the glenohumeral joint. In severe cases, growth disturbances and humeral head modifications are observed (Fig. 2).

Lower limb involvement

Lower limb involvement may have significant functional consequences. Individual deformities can affect the performance of other lower limb joints. The foot is a complex joint with many articular

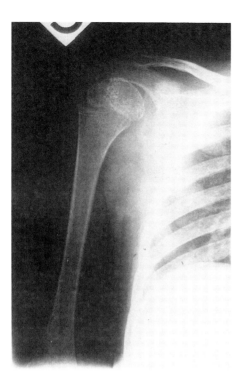

Fig. 2 Shoulder radiograph showing osteoporosis, joint space narrowing, and bony irregularity.

Upper limb involvement

Deformities in the hands and wrists are the consequence of an imbalance between the modified cartilage surfaces, local accelerated growth of bones, and modification of the forces between tendons and ligaments. Reduced carpal length, joint space reduction, and erosions can lead to carpal fusion. A carpal dislocation due to bone lysis is rare but can be observed in severe cases. Radial or ulnar growth reduction induces radial or ulnar deviation. Small joint and associated tendon involvement results in boutonnière or swan-neck deformities of the fingers (Fig. 1).

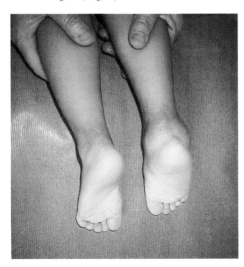

Fig. 3 Retromalleolar tenosynovitis, predominantly on the right side.

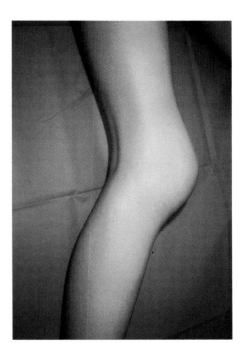

(a)

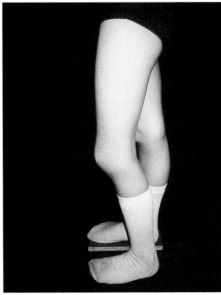

(b)

Fig. 4 Posterior tibial subluxation (a). Increased growth of the left lower limb due to chronic inflammation of the knee (b).

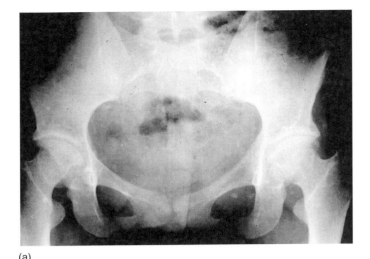

(a)

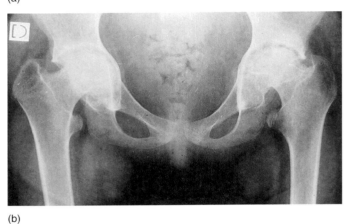

(b)

Fig. 5 Chronic involvement of the hip with shortened femoral neck, irregular head, and joint space narrowing (a); with acetabular protrusion (b).

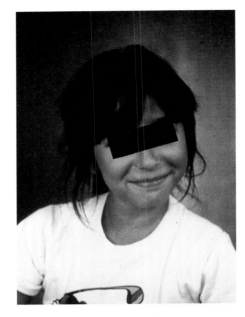

Fig. 6 Torticolis due to cervical spine involvement.

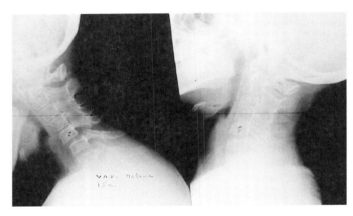

Fig. 7 Cervical spine fusion with underlying hypermobility.

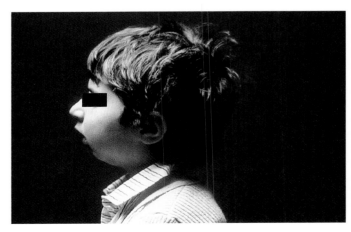

Fig. 8 Microretrognathia.

surfaces in several planes. Foot deformities may also be increased by hip and knee involvement. Tenosynovitis and bursitis are nearly as common as ankle synovitis (Fig. 3). Subtalar joint involvement most often results in valgus deformity or, less commonly, in a varus deformity. As in the carpal area, bony fusion of the tarsus may occur. Mid-tarsal involvement affects the equilibrium of the foot. Metatarsal joint involvement leads to valgus toe deformities.

Flexion contracture of the knee is common, being particularly rapid and severe in the very young child. In the absence of correction, it may rapidly induce a posterior subluxation of the tibia due to capsular retraction (Fig. 4a). The overgrowth of the epiphysis induces a flexion contracture (Fig. 4b). In severe cases, the patella may fuse to the anterior femoral surface.

Hip involvement is characterized by flexion contracture and limitation of motion, particularly of abduction and rotation. This is secondary to the muscle spasm, mainly of the adductors, induced by local synovitis. Chronic inflammation induces anatomic modifications of the bone, with femoral head overgrowth, principally in the external part, and decreased development of the neck, which appears shorter and wider (Fig. 5(a)). Later, aseptic necrosis of the femoral head may occur. Acetabular modifications with erosions or protrusions are possible (Fig. 5(b)). Joint abnormalities at one site in the lower limb may have a reciprocal effect in aggravating deformities at other sites. For example, hip contracture induces a compensatory lumbar lordosis, knee overgrowth increases flexion contractures, and valgus of the knee increases talus deformity.

Spine

Spine involvement is generally clinically expressed at the cervical level. Torticolis and limitation of motion are common (Fig. 6). Radiological changes develop progressively with apophyseal joint fusion most often of the C2–C3 vertebrae, but also of the other cervical spaces. Intervertebral instability below (Fig. 7) and above the fused cervical segment may occur. Subluxation of the atlas on the axis can be observed. A surgical arthrodesis is indicated in case of spinal cord compression. Anaesthetists should be aware of possible difficulties during intubation. Although rarely mentioned, synovitis of the thoracic and lumbar apophyseal joints is possible. A high frequency of spinal scoliosis is described in these children.

Temporomandibular joint

Temporomandibular joint involvement is common. It is often discovered at routine examination. It reduces the normal growth of the mandible and results in micrognathia (Fig. 8). Dental malocclusion is common and may warrant surgical correction when growth is completed.

Laboratory abnormalities

Laboratory features are non-specific in RF-negative polyarthritis. Acute-phase reactants and erythrocyte sedimentation rate can be elevated or normal. The leucocyte count is normal or increased, as is the platelet count. Low blood-cell counts are unusual and suggest an alternative diagnosis.

Specific features of subgroups of RF-negative polyarthritis

Polyarthritis positive for antinuclear antibodies

Although less frequent than the oligoarticular type with positive antinuclear antibodies, this group of patients represents about 40 per cent of the polyarticular onset in our clinic. In a series of 136 children with arthritis positive for antinuclear antibodies, 21 were polyarticular at onset (Peralta and Prieur 1990). As in the oligoarticular-onset group with antinuclear antibodies, there is a female preponderance, although the proportion of boys is higher than in the oligoarticular type. The disease is observed in very young children, two-thirds of the children reviewed in my series (Peralta and Prieur 1990) being less than 3 years old at onset. There is a risk of eye involvement as in the oligoarticular type (21 compared with 42 per cent). To my knowledge, no prognostic study of this particular group of polyarticular onset has been reported. In my experience, very young children with symmetrical involvement of both large and small joints within the first 3 months have a poorer outcome than those with symmetrical polyarticular involvement predominantly of large joints but not necessarily at the same time.

The presence of antinuclear antibodies in the serum characterizes this subgroup of patients. The most frequently used substrate for

diagnosis is the HEp-2 cell. The titres of antinuclear antibodies are usually low and there are no obvious correlations between the titre of the autoantibody and the severity of the disease. The specificity of these antinuclear antibodies is antihistone (Malleson et al. 1989; Østensen et al. 1989; Pauls et al. 1989; Monestier et al. 1990), but there are discrepancies in the frequencies of histone subtypes recognized by the autoantibodies. Anti-H1 and anti-H3 are the most commonly described (Pauls et al. 1989). No correlation has been observed with the presence of uveitis except in one study in which a higher frequency of H3-reacting autoantibodies was found in children with uveitis (Østensen et al. 1989). The autoreactivity to histone fragments is demonstrated either to the C-terminal of H1 (Monestier et al. 1990) or to several fragments within H3 and H4 (Tuaillon et al. 1990; Leak et al. 1993). In a recent study, autoantibodies from sera of 138 children with juvenile chronic arthritis were assessed with 34 histone peptides covering the full length of the four core histones, and two peptides from H1. No correlation was found either with disease subtype or activity, or with the presence of chronic anterior uveitis (Stemmer et al. 1995).

Polyarthritis with boggy synovitis

Some children may present with very thick pannus involving joints in a symmetrical manner. Tenosynovitis is common. Pain remains mild and functional impairment is late. Laboratory tests show a high erythrocyte sedimentation rate (greater than 40 mm/h), marked leucocytosis, and increased levels of acute-phase reactants. There are no autoantibodies. Boys and girls are equally affected.

'Dry' polyarthritis

This group of patients is roughly the counterpart of the previous group. The diagnosis is often delayed as there is no joint swelling but very progressive stiffness. These joint manifestations lead to gait abnormalities including limping. It is not unusual for these children to be referred to a paediatric neurologist, or even to a psychiatrist! However, osteoarticular examination reveals a limited range of motion because of articular stiffness but without obvious synovitis. Joint stiffness seems to be due to capsular and tendon contraction. Muscle wasting occurs. The laboratory profile is normal or mildly inflammatory. There are no autoantibodies.

Polyarthritis with spondylarthropathy features (see Chapter 5.5.2)

Some older patients, particularly boys, can present with polyarthritis (more than four joints), most often in the lower limbs. A careful clinical examination and the presence of relatives with spondylarthropathy suggests the diagnosis of undifferentiated spondylarthropathy. They meet the criteria proposed by the European Spondylarthropathy Study Group or those of Bernard Amor (see Chapter 5.5.5) (Amor et al. 1990; Dougados et al. 1991). Generally in children, the only manifestation is peripheral arthritis with no spinal involvement. Joint pain is often marked. Non-steroidal anti-inflammatory drugs (**NSAIDs**) induce rapid pain relief. Biological evidence of inflammation is more pronounced than in the oligoarticular type of spondylarthropathy. There are no autoantibodies in this group of patients, except for the occasional presence of antinuclear antibodies in the group with psoriatic arthritis. In rare cases, there may be inflammatory bowel disease or reactive arthritis (Reiter's syndrome) with eye and mucosal manifestations. The risk of developing a spondylitis within 5 to 10 years is high. Psoriatic arthritis is considered by many authors to be a spondylarthropathy. However, a higher frequency of girls and a younger age at onset means that its place in the spondylarthropathy group is questionable (Table 2).

Differential diagnosis (Table 3)

Polyarthritis related to an infectious agent

Viruses may induce a joint reaction, particularly in very young children. It may be preceded by an upper respiratory tract infection, with or without fever. Synovial fluid analysis shows a majority of lymphocytes. Joint involvement generally lasts less than 2 weeks. Parvovirus B19, hepatitis, and rubella are among the most common causes of arthritis. Rubella vaccination may be followed by a polyarthritis which can last several weeks. Streptococcal infection or acute rheumatic fever may cause a migratory arthritis (see Chapter 5.3.12). Other signs of rheumatic fever, such as carditis, chorea, and eruption, may be present. Treatment consists of anti-inflammatory drugs, aspirin and/or corticosteroids, and penicillin for at least 5 years. Although this condition now occurs very rarely, we should be aware of its possible resurgence (Kaplan 1990). Lyme borreliosis can be considered when the child has had a tick bite in an endemic area. Typical clinical symptoms are a flu-like illness with erythema chronicum migrans. Some weeks later other symptoms can occur, including neurological, cardiac, ocular, and articular manifestations. Joint involvement is less frequent in Europe than in North America. The diagnosis and treatment is described in Chapter 5.3.4.

Acute infections of the joint or bone are usually easily diagnosed (see Chapter 5.3.2). However, a polyarthritis-like disease can occur in immunodeficiencies (see Chapter 5.3.11). The most frequent immunodeficiency in which this is observed is the X-linked humoral deficiency or Bruton's disease, which occurs in young boys with a history of upper respiratory tract, pulmonary, or gut infection. The diagnosis is made by the absence of serum immunoglobulins. A multifocal, bacterial joint infection should be ruled out first and treated. However, non-bacterial joint swelling is possible, probably resulting from chronic virus infection. Immunoglobulin infusion generally improves chronic joint involvement. Other immunodeficiencies such as acquired humoral deficiencies, or Wiskott–Aldrich and ataxia telangiectasia, can also be complicated by non-bacterial arthritis. In the latter, joint manifestations are rarely the initial symptom.

Autoimmune rheumatic disorders

Autoimmune rheumatic disorders such as systemic lupus erythematosus must also be considered. Polyarthritis is nearly always present in systemic lupus erythematosus and is one of the eleven diagnostic criteria of the ACR (see Chapter 5.7.2). The presence of skin manifestations, serositis, and renal involvement should prompt laboratory investigations to confirm the diagnosis. Cytopenia, anti-DNA antibodies, and decreased complement are the usual findings. Polyarthritis is also prominent in overlap syndromes and mixed connective tissue disease (see Chapter 5.12.1). Polymyositis or dermatomyositis are usually easily diagnosed, but a joint component is possible.

Table 2 Sex ratio and age at onset in the different groups of spondylarthropathies in children[a]

	Sex ratio (% male)	Age at onset (years)
Juvenile ankylosing spondylitis	84	10.7
Reiter's syndrome	75	10.1
Undifferentiated spondylarthropathies	66	11
Inflammatory bowel disease	62	11.4
Juvenile psoriatic arthritis	45	8.8

[a]According to the criteria proposed by the European Spondylarthropathy Study Group and Bernard Amor (Chapter 5.5.5).

Systemic vasculitic syndromes

Systemic vasculitic syndromes (see Chapter 5.11.8) are not exceptional. Kawasaki disease is observed generally in very young children, but the joint symptoms are of secondary importance to the extra-articular manifestations. Polyarteritis nodosa may cause a very severe and painful polyarthritis associated with myalgia. As well as the painful joints, skin involvement includes nodules, with typical changes of medium-sized arteries on biopsy. Cutaneous and articular features without visceral involvement are possible. The differential diagnosis of RF-negative polyarthritis from other other forms of systemic vasculitis such as Wegener's granulomatosis, lymphomatoid granulomatosis, Henoch–Schönlein purpura, and hypocomplementaemic vasculitis is generally easy. Arthritis can occur in relapsing polychondritis. The diagnosis is generally obvious with inflammation of auricular cartilage and nasal chondritis with a saddle-nose deformity.

Behçet's syndrome (see Chapter 5.11.7) can occur in children. These patients may have polyarthritis. The diagnosis is made on the basis of possible familial clustering and ethnic origin, when genital and oral ulcerations are present. Inheritance is autosomal recessive. These children can also develop ocular, intestinal, and neurological manifestations (Koné-Paut et al. 1995). Familial Mediterranean fever (see Chapter 5.13.2) occurs in Sephardic Jews, Armenians, Greeks, Turks, and Arabs. Inheritance is also autosomal recessive and the gene has been mapped on the short arm of chromosome 16. Clinical manifestations include fever, skin rash, serositis, abdominal pain, and possibly arthritis. Colchicine is an effective therapy in preventing attacks and the occurrence of renal amyloidosis.

Sarcoid arthritis produces a distinctive syndrome in children under the age of 4 years, sometimes in the first year of life. The triad of skin rash, uveitis, and huge proliferation of boggy synovium with tenosynovitis is highly suggestive of sarcoid arthritis. Skin or synovial biopsy shows the typical sarcoid granulomata. Joint involvement is relatively painless. Visceral involvement is rare. A familial association has been described (Blau 1985). Vasculopathy has been reported and some authors suggest that this entity should be considered as a 'familial granulomatous

Table 3 Differential diagnosis of RF-negative polyarthritis

Related to an infectious agent	
Reactive arthritis to	
Virus infection: Parvovirus B19, hepatitis, rubella, rubella vaccination	Fever, rash may be present at onset. Upper respiratory tract manifestations
Streptococcus: Post-streptococcal arthritis, rheumatic fever	Streptococcal infection Revised modified Jones criteria
Borreliosis: *Borrelia burgdorferi*	Endemic area. Arthritis rare in Europe
Septic arthritis	
Staphylococcus, *Haemophilus influenzae*	Easy diagnosis Multiple sites in immune deficiencies
Connective tissue disorders	
Systemic lupus erythematosus	ACR criteria. Cytopenia
Mixed connective tissue disease, overlap syndrome	Laboratory characteristics
Poly/dermatomyosistis	Skin lesions, muscle involvement
Systemic vasculitic syndromes	
Kawasaki disease	Young child, high fever, diagnostic criteria
Polyarteritis nodosa	Severe pain, polyarthritis, muscle pain, nodules Biopsy shows vasculitis
Wegener's syndrome, lymphoid granulomatosis	
Henoch–Schönlein purpura	Inflammatory purpura of the lower limbs
Behçet's disease	Genital and oral ulcerations, familial involvement
Familial Mediterranean fever	Sephardic Jews, Armenians, Greeks, Turks Relapsing attacks, abdominal pain
Sarcoid arthritis	In the very young child, association of boggy polyarthritis, rash, uveitis. Also called 'familial granulomatous arteritis'
Haematological disorders	
Sickle cell disease	Ethnic background, abnormal electrophoresis of haemoglobin
Constitutional bleeding disorders	Haemophilia, various deficiency of clotting factors
Acute leukaemia	Bone and joint pain. Abnormal bone marrow
Other causes	
Chronic recurrent multifocal osteomyelitis	Metaphyseal pain, osteolytic lesions of the metaphysis on radiography
Hip involvement	Lamellar coxitis, Legg–Calvé–Perthes disease, transient synovitis
Diabetic arthropathy	Diabetic cheiroarthropathy
Idiopathic osteoporosis	Usually adolescents, no joint involvement, spontaneous fractures, no biological anomalies, spontaneous recovery

arteritis'. Systemic corticosteroids are often necessary to control uveitis and arthritis. Polyarthritis can be observed in the adult type of sarcoidosis in older children.

Haematological disorders

In early childhood, joint involvement in sickle-cell disease may result in hand–foot syndrome. Swelling of the hands and feet is extremely painful. Later, migratory arthritis can be observed. Bone pain can be due either to bone infarction or to osteomyelitis. The diagnosis is based on ethnic origin and haemoglobin electrophoresis. Constitutional bleeding disorders such as haemophilias can be manifested by joint haemorrhage. Generally, the deficiency of clotting factor is identified. Modern therapeutic management aims to prevent haemarthrosis and joint destruction.

Acute leukaemia may induce bone pain and joint swelling due to infiltrates of leukaemic cells. The diagnosis must be confirmed rapidly by examination of a bone marrow smear and specific therapy started without delay. Neuroblastoma with bone metastasis must also be considered in a young child with osteoarticular pain.

Other causes of polyarticular manifestations

Patients with chronic, recurrent, multifocal osteomyelitis can present with bone pain. There is no joint swelling and careful examination localizes the pain to the metaphyseal area. Radiography confirms the diagnosis by the presence of osteolytic lesions in the metaphysis. The lesion is sterile and antibiotics have no effect. The course may be long and relapsing.

Patients with hip pain are sometimes referred as having possible polyarthritis. In an adolescent, the possibility of lamellar coxitis should be ruled out. It is generally unilateral and the laboratory screen is normal, while radiography shows narrowing of the hip space. The cause is unknown and the prognosis is unpredictable. Similarly, Legg–Calvé–Perthes' disease induces osteonecrosis of the femoral head in young boys around the age of 7 years. It is generally unilateral, rarely bilateral. Radiographs are normal at onset, but scintigraphy or MRI may show necrosis at this stage. Orthopaedic management is required. In younger children, transient synovitis of the hip is frequent. It occurs around 6 years of age and may be preceded by upper respiratory tract infection. An increased erythrocyte sedimentation rate is frequent. Bed rest with traction and NSAIDs are necessary. Recovery occurs within a few days. Occasionally hip dysplasia is evident. Some patients develop recurrent episodes of transient synovitis of the hip.

Diabetic arthropathy is observed in uncontrolled diabetes. Exceptionally it may be the first manifestation of diabetes. Diabetic cheiroarthropathy with progressive flexion contractures of the fingers, as a result of increased deposition of collagen in the tissues, is well recognized. Idiopathic juvenile osteoporosis is a painful disease. There are no joint manifestations. Usually, there are no abnormalities of phosphocalcium metabolism. Recovery occurs in adolescence, sometimes with sequelae resulting from spontaneous fractures or vertebral collapse.

Immunogenetics

Most of the immunogenetic studies in polyarticular-onset juvenile arthritis separate the group of 'seropositive' and 'seronegative' forms. RF-positive polyarticular arthritis in children and adults are both associated with HLA DRB1*04 (Ploski et al. 1993). Several authors have observed an association between RF-negative polyarticular arthritis in children and HLA DR8, mainly involving the HLA DRB1*0801 subtype (Morling et al. 1985; Hall et al. 1989; Fernandez-Vina et al. 1990; Barron et al. 1992; Ploski et al. 1993). Ethnic differences may be observed in some populations, such as the studies on Italian (Fantini et al. 1987) and Czech children (Cerna et al. 1994) in which no correlation with HLA DR8 could be found.

HLA DR8, in fact, is associated with several forms of juvenile arthritis including early-onset oligoarticular forms (Malagon et al. 1991) and juvenile spondylarthropathies (Ploski et al. 1995). In contrast, HLA DPB1*0201 is associated with the oligoarticular, but not with the polyarticular forms. The frequency of HLA DPB1*0301 is increased significantly in patients with polyarticular arthritis and juvenile spondylarthropathies. This association between HLA DRB1*0801 and HLA DPB1*0301 in polyarticular-onset disease has been confirmed by several authors. This combination, rarely observed in the normal population or in the oligoarticular types of disease, suggests an interaction between these two alleles, conferring an increased susceptibility to the polyarticular expression of the disease.

However, as seen in Table 4, there are discrepancies between the studies, probably due to various factors including ethnic background, the absence of clinical homogeneity of the patients, the definition of each clinical subgroup, and the number of patients studied. It is evident that uniformly agreed criteria for the improved subgrouping of patients is still required.

Management

The principles of management are those of any childhood chronic disease of the joints, namely to offer pain relief, maintain satisfactory joint function, minimize drug toxicity, and allow the child to grow and be educated as normally as possible. It is sometimes difficult to meet all these requirements and complete trust between the family and the paediatric team must be established.

Non-steroidal anti-inflammatory drugs (NSAIDs)

The use of NSAIDs remains the basis of treatment. In children, only a certain number of drugs have been studied and their licence for use varies in different countries. Acetylsalicylic acid and other NSAIDs such as diclofenac, ibuprofen, and naproxen are available for use in most countries. Recommended doses are indicated in Table 5. In general, all NSAIDs have similar efficacy but tolerance may vary. Aspirin induces the most frequent side-effects, as shown in a comprehensive study (Barron et al. 1982). The mode of administration may be important for compliance. Ideally, aspirin must be administered every 4 h, while other NSAIDs can be given 1 to 3 times over 24 h. The few available pharmacokinetic studies in older children have shown only minor differences to adults. The half-life in synovial fluid is longer than in plasma (Hallé et al. 1991). NSAIDs are usually rapidly effective, but some authors have found that they take several weeks to have full effect (Lovell et al. 1984). The most frequent side-effects are gastrointestinal (mainly abdominal pain), cutaneous (urticaria, rash, and hypersensitivity), and haematological (anaemia). Rare cases of renal damage and disorders of the central nervous system (headache and dizziness) have been reported. Allergic reactions can also occur. Macrophage activation syndrome is exceptional in polyarticular disease, but it must be borne in mind, particularly when aspirin is used (Prieur and Stephan 1994).

Slow-acting antirheumatic drugs

Slow-acting antirheumatic drugs are indicated in the polyarticular forms of juvenile chronic arthritis. The most commonly used agents are gold salts and D-penicillamine. Other thiol derivatives can be used, such as tiopronine and sulphasalazine. Synthetic antimalarials are used, particularly in Scandinavian countries. These treatments all take several weeks to work and carry a risk of side-effects that are now well documented in adults. Their use in children must take account of age and the clinical presentation. An improvement is usually observed during the first 6 months, and there is no point in continuing treatment if no result is obtained after this

Table 4 HLA associations in RF-negative polyarthritis compared with oligoarthritis, with or without a polyarticular course, in three different geographical areas

HLA class II alleles	Relative risk/*P* values			Authors
	Persistent oligoarthritis	Oligoarthritis with polyarticular course	Polyarthritis with negative RF	
DRB1*0101/02	NS	2.5/<0.025	NS	Ploski
	NS	NS	NS	Cerna
DRB1*0401	0.3/<10^{-5}	NS	0.2/<0.01	Ploski
	NS	NS	NS	Cerna
DRB1*07	0.1/<10^{-6}	NS	0.1/<0.05	Ploski
	<0.01	<0.05(E) NS(L)	<0.01	Cerna
DRB1*0801/03	8.4/1076	6.2/<10^{-5}	8.2/<10^{-6}	Ploski
	5.2/<0.001	NS	5.8/<0.001	Fernandez-Vina
	NS	NS(E) <0.0001(L)	NS	Cerna
DRB1*11				Fernandez-Vina
1104	<0.0001	NS(E) <0.0001(L)	NS	Cerna
DRB1*1301	2.0/<0.05	NS	NS	Ploski
	10/<0.0001	NS	NS	Fernandez-Vina
	NS	NS	NS	Cerna
DRB1*1501	NS	<0.01(E) NS(L)	NS	Cerna
DPB1*0201	3.3/10^{-6}	2.6/<0.5	NS	Ploski
	4.3/<0.01	NS	NS	Fernandez-Vina
	<0.001	NS	NS	Cerna
DPB1*0301	NS	NS	2.8/<0.005	Ploski
	NS	NS	NS	Cerna
DPB1*0402	<0.001	<0.001(E) NS(L)	NS	Cerna
DQA1*0101	NS	2.3/<0.05	NS	Ploski
0103	6.2/			Fernandez-Vina
DQA1*0201	0.1/<10^{-3}	NS	NS	Ploski
DQA1*0401	8/<10^{-6}	6.2/10^{-5}	8.2/10^{-6}	Ploski
	NS	NS		Fernandez-Vina
DQB1*0402	8/<10^{-6}	6.2/<10^{-5}	8.2/10^{-6}	Ploski
	NS	NS	NS	Fernandez-Vina
DQB1*0603	8.3/0.0001	NS	NS	Fernandez-Vina
Number of patients in each group				
	170	37	49	Ploski *et al.* (1993)
	42	19	35	Fernandez-Vina *et al.* (1990)
	56	20(E) 22(L)	39	Cerna *et al.* (1994)

E, early; L, late; NS, non-significant.

Table 5 Non-steroidal anti-inflammatory drugs in children

Name	Dose per kg body weight per day (maximum daily dose)
Acetylsalicylic acid	50–100 mg (4 g)
Naproxen	15–20 mg (1.5 g)
Ibuprofen	40–60 mg (2.4 g)
Ketoprofen	3–5 mg (300 mg)
Fenoprofen	40–50 mg (3.2 g)
Flurbiprofen	3–4 mg (300 mg)
Diclofenac	2–3 mg (200 mg)
Sulindac	4–6 mg (400 mg)
Meclofenamate	4–7 g (300 g)
Piroxicam	0.3 mg
Indomethacin	1–3 mg (200 mg)
Tolmetin	20–30 g (1.8 g)

period. Table 6 summarizes the main preparations, their doses, and side-effects.

Several prospective studies have been carried out in the paediatric setting. D-Penicillamine has been the subject of three comparative trials, which yielded somewhat contradictory results. A French study comparing D-penicillamine with placebo showed that the active drug had a degree of efficacy (Prieur *et al*. 1985), while an American–Russian study comparing D-penicillamine, hydroxychloroquine, and placebo showed no difference in efficacy or tolerability among the three groups (Brewer *et al*. 1986). The frequency of side-effects in these two studies was acceptable, whereas a Norwegian team reported side-effects in 25 per cent of patients on D-penicillamine in a comparative study with gold salts (Kvien *et al*. 1985). Certain studies indicate that gold salts given by the oral route were slightly more effective than placebo (Giannini *et al*. 1990), an effect that persisted beyond 5 years (Giannini *et al*. 1991*a*) but did not reach statistical significance. Among the thiol derivatives, tiopronine had similar efficacy and tolerability to D-penicillamine when studied by the author. Several paediatric trials of sulphasalazine have been performed. Sulphasalazine appears to be beneficial in certain conditions, especially spondylarthropathies (Job-Deslandre and Menkes 1991). Published results on slow-acting antirheumatic drugs are only mediocre. A meta-analysis of 6-month efficacy on disease activity confirmed the lack of spectacular improvement (Giannini *et al*. 1991*b*). In addition, most of these studies did not distinguish between the different forms of juvenile chronic arthritis. There is no evidence that combinations of slow-acting antirheumatic drugs are effective in children, although this has not been studied in children in a systematic fashion.

Steroids

Steroids are a very powerful tool but often have unacceptable side-effects in children. They can be given systemically or locally.

Table 6 Slow-acting antirheumatic drugs in children

Name	Dose	Side-effects
Aurothiomalate (Myocrisin®) Aurothiosulphate (Allochrysin) (intramuscular)	Weekly: 0.5 mg, then 1 mg/kg body weight for 3 to 6 months Monthly: 1 mg/kg body weight	Rash Cytopenia Bone marrow aplasia
Auranofin (oral)	0.5 mg/kg body weight per day (max. 9 mg)	Diarrhoea Same as above but less severe
D-Penicillamine (oral)	5, for 1 month then 10 mg/kg body weight per day (if necessary 15 mg/kg per day)	Rash Cytopenia Proteinuria Pneumopathy Autoimmunity: myasthenia, lupus
Tiopronine (oral)	10 for 1 month, then 20 mg/kg body weight per day	Same as D-Penicillamine
Sulphasalazine (oral)	20–30 mg/kg body weight per day	Rash Cytopenia Increased transaminases
Hydroxychloroquine (oral)	5–7 mg/kg body weight per day (max. 200 mg)	Retinopathy Cutaneous symptoms Neuropathies Cytopenia

Systemic steroids generally are not indicated in the polyarticular form of juvenile chronic arthritis. In severe crippling cases, they can be used to improve the functional status. The side-effects of systemic steroids are the main problem in paediatric use. Rapid weight gain can only be avoided by a strict diet, which must be not only sodium-free but also restricted in slow-resorption carbohydrates. The most troublesome cutaneous side-effects are permanent striae, but these are rare if weight gain is controlled by dieting. Arterial hypertension and diabetes can develop. Osteoporosis can lead to very painful vertebral collapse which necessitates immobilization in a corset. The use of deflazacort, available in some countries, apparently lessens the impact of steroids on bone metabolism (Loftus et al. 1993). Aseptic joint necrosis, especially of the hips, is far from rare and complicates underlying diseases that can also involve the joints. The onset of steroid-induced cataracts must be monitored closely. Finally, above all in children, daily steroid therapy arrests growth. This is overcome by alternate-day dosing when possible (Prieur 1993).

Local steroid therapy can be applied to the joints and eyes.

Intra-articular steroid injections have modified totally the prognosis of joint manifestations. They can be used in polyarticular forms when stiffness and flexion contractures cannot be controlled by general therapy. Among the many available products, only triamcinolone hexacetonide gives satisfactory results. It is fairly potent and must therefore be used with care to avoid local complications (mainly cutaneous atrophy at the injection site). Some attempts at multiple joint injection have given encouraging results (Pugh et al. 1995)

This procedure is straightforward for large joints such as the knee, but general anaesthesia may be necessary for small and/or tight joints, especially in the very young child. There is no lower age limit for this type of treatment as long as the precautions for use are respected; this also means that an experienced practitioner must treat the joints of small children. In general, the volume injected must be adapted to the volume of the joint, and the product must not be injected 'under pressure'. The joint must be rested with a splint for 3 days. Complications are rare and mainly consist of cutaneous atrophy at the injection site or asymptomatic intra-articular calcifications. Needless to say, the potency of this preparation contraindicates its use for injecting tendon sheaths, where only water-soluble steroids can be used.

Uveitis, a frequent complication of polyarticular forms of juvenile chronic arthritis with antinuclear antibodies, is treated with steroid-based eye drops and mydriatic agents.

Cytotoxic drugs

Cytotoxic treatments may be of value in severe forms. However, their efficacy is often difficult to determine objectively because of the small number of sound, prospective, multicentre trials. Too many specialists continue to use a given treatment in 'selected cases', meaning that the results are uninterpretable. Ideally, as in oncology, multicentre protocols should be established to accelerate the assessment of the efficacy and tolerability of experimental treatments.

Methotrexate is one of the most widely used immunomodulatory agents. The use of methotrexate in children with rheumatic diseases was proposed when its efficacy and acceptable tolerability were established in adults. The recommended dose, based on a double-blind, placebo-controlled trial, is $10 \, mg/m^2$ per week (Giannini et al. 1992),

but certain authors propose higher doses for particularly resistant forms (Wallace et al. 1991)

The tolerability of methotrexate in children is acceptable (Graham et al. 1992). In combination with NSAIDs, the level of methotrexate in the blood can increase (Dupuis et al. 1990). A few cases of severe liver damage have been reported (Keim et al. 1990). Side-effects, which are generally mild, must be monitored every 1 or 2 months. Many patients (almost 30 per cent) show increased transaminase levels. Values usually return to normal when the dose is reduced or treatment is suspended. After a few months of treatment, nausea is fairly frequent immediately after methotrexate intake, and these patients may benefit from a switch to the intramuscular route. Oral aphthae, cytopenia, and pulmonary manifestations are observed rarely.

Methotrexate seems to have clear efficacy in some cases, especially in pauciarticular juvenile chronic arthritis with the presence of antinuclear antibodies (Hallé and Prieur 1991). A European, multicentre, double-blind trial is underway to confirm this observation.

Azathioprine at a dose of 2 to 2.5 mg/kg body weight per day, is used by certain specialists. It is generally well tolerated. However, the possible long-term risk of cancer must be borne in mind, and this agent should probably only be used in severe cases (Silman et al. 1988). In juvenile chronic arthritis, azathioprine appears to be slightly more effective than placebo (Kvien et al. 1986).

Alkylating agents can be considered in exceptional cases when classical treatments fail to control disease progression. However, chlorambucil (0.2 mg/kg) has a very high mutagenic risk (Prieur et al. 1979). It is thus only recommended for life-threatening complications such as secondary amyloidosis, which hardly ever complicates polyarticular juvenile chronic arthritis. Similarly, the indication for cyclophosphamide in the polyarticular forms is only for exceptional cases.

Cyclosporin is effective in adult rheumatoid arthritis at doses below 5 mg/kg body weight per day (Dougados et al. 1988). Studies involving patients with juvenile chronic arthritis have failed to show marked improvement (Østensen et al. 1988), but further trials are required. The paediatric side-effects of cyclosporin are identical to those observed in adults.

Surgery (see Chapter 6.2)

Surgery plays an increasing role in the management of chronic rheumatic diseases when the medical means are insufficient. The orthopaedic surgeon must participate in the therapeutic discussion. The technical approaches are numerous. Arthroscopy is now efficient for small joints, with adapted equipment. It allows intra-articular examination, biopsies, and synovectomy. Surgery in the form of soft tissue release, osteotomies, surgical realignment, and arthrodesis may be necessary to treat fixed joint deformities. Surgical treatment of growth deformities is mandatory when functional impairment and secondary mechanical problems in adjacent joints develop. Finally, joint arthroplasty must be considered when joint destruction and joint failure lead to major handicap. Anaesthetists must be aware of cervical spine involvement and temporomandibular arthritis, which may make intubation difficult.

Rehabilitation (see Chapter 6.4)

Physical treatments are necessary for any child with chronic arthritis. The techniques involve applied heat (water, paraffin, or hot packs) to

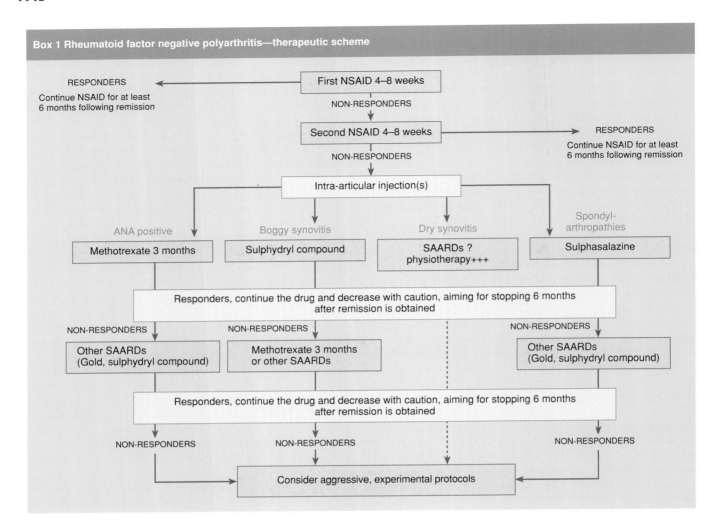

Box 1 Rheumatoid factor negative polyarthritis—therapeutic scheme

induce muscle relaxation. Flexion deformities must be stretched out either actively by the child or passively by the child, parent, or therapist. Correct positioning of the joint must be obtained at rest with appropriate splinting. Prone positions should be recommended for reading or watching television. Each joint requires a specific technique of rehabilitation to prevent deformities. The treatment must be adapted to the severity of the disease, the impact of each joint on total function, and radiological changes. In cases of surgical intervention, both preoperative and postoperative rehabilitation are necessary.

Conclusion

The management of polyarticular juvenile arthritis involves a common approach which is adapted according to the different subtypes of arthritis as shown in the practical guidelines presented in Box 1.

References

Amor, B., Dougados, M., and Mijiyawa, M. (1990). Critères de classification des spondylarthropathies. *Revue du Rhumatisme*, **57**, 85–9.

Barron, K.S., Person, D.A., and Brewer, E.J. (1982). The toxicity of non steroidal antiinflammatory drugs in juvenile rheumatoid arthritis. *Journal of Rheumatology*, **9**, 149–55.

Barron, K. *et al.* (1992). DNA analysis of HLA-DR, DQ, and DP alleles in children with polyarticular juvenile rheumatoid arthritis. *Journal of Rheumatology*, **19**, 1611–16.

Blau, E.B. (1985). Familial granulomatous arthritis, iritis and rash. *Journal of Pediatrics*, **107**, 689–93.

Brewer, E.J., Jr *et al.* (1977). Current proposed revision of JRA criteria. *Arthritis and Rheumatism*, **20**, 195–9.

Brewer, E.J, Giannini, E.H., Kuzmina, N., and Alekseev, L. (1986). Penicillamine and hydroxychloroquine in the treatment of juvenile rheumatoid arthritis. Results of the USA–USSR double blind placebo controlled trial. *New England Journal of Medicine*, **314**, 1269–70.

Cerna, M. *et al.* (1994). Class II alleles in juvenile arthritis in Czech children. *Journal of Rheumatology*, **24**, 159–64.

Dougados, M., Awada, H., and Amor, B. (1988). Cyclosporin A in rheumatoid arthritis, a double blind, placebo controlled study in 52 patients. *Annals of the Rheumatic Diseases*, **47**, 463–9.

Dougados, M. *et al.* (1991). The European spondylarthropathy study group preliminary criteria for the classification of spondylarthropathy. *Arthritis and Rheumatism*, **34**, 1218–27.

Dupuis, L.C. *et al.* (1990). Methotrexate–non steroidal antiinflammatory drug interaction in children with arthritis. *Journal of Rheumatology*, **17**, 1469–73.

Fantini, F. *et al.* (1987). HLA phenotypes in Italian children affected with juvenile chronic arthritis. *Clinical and Experimental Rheumatology*, **5**, 17.

Fernandez-Vina, M.A., Finck, C.W., and Stastny, P. (1990). HLA antigens in juvenile arthritis. Pauciarticular and polyarticular juvenile arthritis are immunogenetically distinct. *Arthritis and Rheumatism*, **33**, 1787–94.

Giannini, E.H. et al. (1990). Auranofin in the treatment of juvenile rheumatoid arthritis — results of the USA–USSR double-blind, placebo controlled cooperative trial.

Giannini, E.H. et al. (1991a). Auranofin therapy in juvenile rheumatoid arthritis: results of the five-year open label extension trial. *Journal of Rheumatology*, 18, 1240–2.

Giannini, E.H. et al. (1991b). Meta-analysis of antirheumatic drug trials in juvenile rheumatoid arthritis. *Arthritis and Rheumatism*, 34, S152.

Giannini, E.H. et al. (1992). Methotrexate in resistant juvenile rheumatoid arthritis. *New England Journal of Medicine*, 326, 1043–9.

Graham, L.D., Myones, B.L., Rivas-Chalon, R.F., and Pachman, L.M. (1992). Morbidity associated with long-term methotrexate therapy in juvenile rheumatoid arthritis. *Journal of Pediatrics*, 120, 468–73.

Hall, P.J. et al. (1989). HLA and complement C4 antigens in polyarticular onset seronegative juvenile chronic arthritis: association of early onset with HLA-DRw8. *Journal of Rheumatology*, 16, 55–9.

Hallé, F. and Prieur, A-M. (1991). Evaluation of methotrexate in the treatment of juvenile chronic arthritis according to the subtype. *Clinical and Experimental Rheumatology*, 9, 297–302.

Hallé, F. et al. (1991). Pharmacokinetics of pirprofen in children with juvenile chronic arthritis. *European Journal of Drug Metabolism and Pharmacokinetics*, 16, 29–34.

Job-Deslandre, C. and Menkes, C.J. (1991). Sulphasalazine in the treatment of juvenile spondylarthropathy. *Arthritis and Rheumatism*, 34, S153.

Kaplan, E.K. (1990). Rheumatic fever. *Current Opinion in Rheumatology*, 2, 836.

Keim, D., Ragadale, C., Heidelberger, K., and Sullivan, D. (1990). Hepatic fibrosis in the use of methotrexate for juvenile arthritis. *Journal of Rheumatology*, 17, 846–8.

Koné-Paut, I., Yurdakul, S., Bahabri, S., Shaefae, N., Ozen, S., and Bernard, J-L. (1995). Epidemiological features of Behçet's disease in children: an international collaborative study of 86 cases. *Arthritis and Rheumatism*, 38, S336.

Kvien, T.K., Hoyeraal, H.M., and Sandstad, B. (1985). Azathioprine versus placebo in patients with juvenile rheumatoid arthritis: a single center double-blind comparative study. *Journal of Rheumatology*, 13, 118–23.

Kvien, T.K., Hoyeraal, H.M., and Sandstad, B. (1986). Gold sodium thiomalate and D-penicillamine. A controlled, comparative study in patients with pauciarticular and polyarticular juvenile rheumatoid arthritis. *Scandinavian Journal of Rheumatology*, 14, 346–54.

Leak, A.M., Tuaillon, N., Muller, S., and Woo, P. (1993). Study of antibodies to histones and histone synthetic peptide in pauciarticular juvenile chronic arthritis. *British Journal of Rheumatism*, 32, 426–31.

Loftus, J.K., Reeve, J., and Hesp, R. (1993). Deflazacort in juvenile chronic arthritis. *Journal of Rheumatology*, 20 (Suppl. 37), 40–2.

Lovell, D.J., Giannini, E.H., and Brewer, E.J., Jr (1984). Time course of response to non steroidal antiinflammatory drugs in juvenile rheumatoid arthritis. *Arthritis and Rheumatism*, 27, 1433–7.

Malagon, C. et al. (1991). The iridocyclitis of early onset pauciarticular juvenile rheumatoid arthritis: outcome in immunogenetically characterized patients. *Journal of Rheumatology*, 19, 160–3.

Malleson, P., Petty, R.E., Fun, M., and Candido, P.M. (1989). Reactivity of anti-nuclear antibodies with histones and other antigens in juvenile rheumatoid arthritis. *Arthritis and Rheumatism*, 32, 919–23.

Monestier, M. et al. (1990). Antihistone antibodies in antinuclear antibody-positive juvenile arthritis. *Arthritis and Rheumatism*, 33, 1836–41.

Morling, N. et al. (1985). HLA antigen frequencies in juvenile chronic arthritis. *Scandinavian Journal of Rheumatology*, 14, 209–16.

Østensen, M., Høyeraal, H.M., and Kåss, E. (1988). Tolerance of cyclosporin A in children with refractory rheumatoid arthritis. *Journal of Rheumatology*, 15, 1536–8.

Østensen, M., Fredriksen, K., Kåss, E., and Rekvig, O.P. (1989). Identification of antihistone antibodies in subsets of juvenile chronic arthritis. *Annals of the Rheumatic Diseases*, 48, 114–17.

Pauls, J.D., Silverman, E., Laxer, R.M., and Fritzler, M.J. (1989). Antibodies to histones H1 and H5 in sera of patients with juvenile rheumatoid arthritis. *Arthritis and Rheumatism*, 32, 877–83.

Peralta, J.L. and Prieur, A.-M. (1990). Arthrite chronique juvénile avec présence d'anyicorps antinucléaires sériques. *Archives de Pediatrie*, 47, 497–502.

Ploski, R. et al. (1993). HLA class II alleles and heterogeneity of juvenile rheumatoid arthritis: DRB1*0101 may define a novel subset of the disease. *Arthritis and Rheumatism*, 36, 465–72.

Ploski, R. et al. (1995). Association to HLA-DRB1*08, HLA-DPB1*0301 and homozygosity for HLA linked proteasome gene in juvenile ankylosing spondylitis. *Human Immunology*, 44, 88–96.

Prieur, A-M. (1993). The place of corticosteroid therapy in juvenile chronic arthritis in 1992. *Journal of Rheumatology*, 30, (Suppl. 37), 32–4.

Prieur, A-M. and Stephan, J-L. (1994). Macrophage activation syndrome in pediatric rheumatic diseases. *Revue du Rhumatism (English Edn)*, 6, 385–8.

Prieur, A-M., Balafrej, M., Griscelli, C., and Mozziconacci, P. (1979). Résultats et risques à long terme des traitements immunosuppresseurs dans l'arthrite chronique juvénile. *Revue du Rhumatism*, 46, 85–90.

Prieur, A-M. et al. (1985). Evaluation of D-penicillamine in juvenile chronic arthritis. A double-blind multicentre study. *Arthritis and Rheumatism*, 28, 376–82.

Pugh, M.T., Grosse, R., and Southwood, T.R. (1995). Multiple joint corticosteroid injections in polyarticular juvenile chronic arthritis: a single-blind one year folloiw-up study. *Arthritis and Rheumatism*, 38, S283.

Silman, A.J. et al. (1988). Lymphoproliferative cancer and other malignancy in patients with azathioprine. A 20 year follow-up study. *Annals of the Rheumatic Diseases*, 47, 988–92.

Stemmer, C., Tuaillon, N., Prieur, A-M., and Muller, S. (1995). Mapping of B-cell epitopes by antibodies to histones in subsets of juvenile chronic arthritis. *Clinical and Experimental Immunopathology*, 76, 82–9.

Tuaillon, N. et al. (1990). Antibodies from patients with rheumatoid arthritis and juvenile chronic arthritis analysed with core histone synthetic peptides. *International Archives of Allergy and Immunology*, 91, 297–305.

Wallace, C., Sherry, D., and Salmonson, K. (1991). Treatment of juvenile rheumatoid arthritis with higher dose methotrexate. *Arthritis and Rheumatism*, 34, S152.

Wood, P.H.N. (1978). Special meeting on nomenclature and classification of arthritis in children. In *The care of rheumatic children* (ed. E. Munthe), p 47. European League Against Rheumatism, Basel.

5.7 Systemic lupus erythematosus

5.7.1 Systemic lupus erythematosus in adults

David A. Isenberg and Angela C. Horsfall

Introduction

Systemic lupus erythematosus has taken the mantle of syphilis as the great mimic of other conditions. It is probably better to think of it as a group of related disorders rather than a single disease entity. By analogy it might also be compared to the Hydra monster of ancient Greek mythology (Fig. 1). This beast, one of the offspring of Echidne and Typhon was notoriously unpleasant and possessed numerous heads. It was said that cutting off one head led to the growth of two or three others. Lupus presents in many unpleasant guises and the successful treatment of, say, joint pain in lupus may be followed by the emergence of skin rash or pleuropericardial involvement. There is another analogy with lupus as no one could agree precisely how many heads the Hydra had or about their appearance—similarly there is disagreement as to how disease activity in lupus should be assessed.

In this chapter we will detail the clinical features of lupus, analyse its serology, appraise the experimental models of the disease, and review studies of its immunopathology and treatment. Drug-induced forms of lupus are considered in Chapter 5.19.1 but the disease in the male and in elderly people is highlighted here, and several controversial areas are discussed. The major historical aspects of lupus, reviewed in detail elsewhere, are indicated in Table 1.

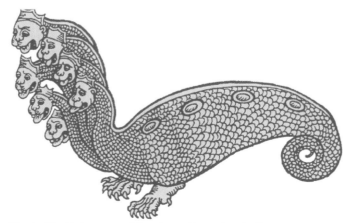

Fig. 1 The Hydra—a useful analogy of lupus (see text).

Definition and classification of lupus

Systemic lupus erythematosus is perhaps best defined as a clinical syndrome with a complex, multifactorial aetiology, characterized by inflammation and the involvement of most of the body's organs or systems. It is subject to many remissions and exacerbations and, although the musculoskeletal system and skin are invariably affected, frequently gives rise to manifestations in the kidney, heart, lungs, and central nervous system. The diversity among its clinical features is matched by an apparent diversity among the autoantibodies detectable in the serum.

The American Rheumatism Association (now the American College of Rheumatology, **ACR**) has published two sets of criteria in 1971 and 1982, which have been widely adopted. Strictly speaking the criteria are for the classification of the disease rather than use as a diagnostic tool, although in practice there is blurring of this distinction. The 1982 revised criteria are set out in Table 2.

The variable clinical and serological expression of lupus makes it easy to obtain a distorted view of the disease. Patients present to a variety of specialists, each of whom will see a different spectrum of the disease. Thus bias amongst the reporting physicians must be borne in mind when assessing reports about lupus. A broad overview of the cumulative percentage incidence of the features of systemic lupus in five large series is shown in Table 3. It must be remembered that the incidence of some clinical features varies between ethnic groups. A recent study of 137 Chinese patients with systemic lupus in Hong Kong reported a relatively low incidence of arthritis (71 per cent) compared with other groups but a high incidence of renal involvement (70 per cent) (Lee *et al.* 1993).

Epidemiology and natural history

Lupus is a worldwide disease. Although it has been estimated that approximately 1 in 250 black women in the United States and the West Indies, about 1 in 1000 Chinese, and 1 in 4300 Caucasians in New Zealand have systemic lupus, there are some curiously conflicting data. In particular, it seems that lupus is rare in most parts of Africa (Fessel 1988). Two recent studies from urban centres in the United Kingdom have highlighted the significant variation in the prevalence of lupus among different ethnic groups sharing much the same environment. The study from Nottingham (Hopkinson *et al.* 1993), while noting a prevalence of 45.4/100 000 per year in women (3.7/100 000 per year in men), implied that the numbers of lupus patients of Afro-Caribbean and Asian origin were overrepresented, but did not quote any figures. In contrast, the study from Birmingham (Johnson *et al.* 1995) reported prevalence rates of 36.2, 90.6 and 206/100 000 among women of Caucasian, Asian, and Afro-Caribbean origin respectively.

Table 1 Historical aspects of lupus

460–370 BC	*Herpes esthiomenos* of Hippocrates; probably a synonym for systemic lupus, according to Lusitanus (AD 1510–1568)
1230–1611	Rogerius (*c.*1230), Paracelsus (1493–1531), Manardi (*c.*1500), Sennert (1611) all credited with mentioning lupus in their writings
1845	Hebra first likened the facial rash to a butterfly shape
1852	Cazenave and Clausit used the term 'lupus érythèmateux'
1875	Hebra and Kaposi differentiated discoid lupus from the systemic or 'aggregated' form
1898	Boeck discussed the possibility that tuberculosis was the cause of many cases of discoid lupus; this was the first of many attempts to link lupus to infectious diseases
1902	Sequira and Baleen found albuminuria to be a common finding in active disseminated lupus
1904	Osler reported many of the clinical features now recognized as symptoms of systemic lupus in at least 2 of 29 cases he described; these features included arthralgia, central nervous system involvement, nephritis, gastrointestinal crisis, endo- and pericarditis
1923	Libman and Sacks described an endocarditis now recognized as a form of systemic lupus
1935	Baehr, Klemperer, and Schifrin reported structural changes in the glomeruli of lupus patients
1941	Klemperer, Pollack, and Baehr coined the term 'diffuse connective tissue disorder'
1948	Discovery of the LE cell test by Hargraves, Richmond, and Marks
1949	Thorn and colleagues used cortisone therapy
1951	Page employed quinacrine (mepacrine), an antimalarial drug, to control lupus with dermal lesions
1954	Dustan, Taylor, Corcoran, and Page observed that hydralazine could induce LE cells; probably the first report of drug-induced lupus
1957–8	Friou and colleagues described antinuclear antibodies in sera from systemic lupus and four laboratories reported the strong association of anti-DNA antibodies and lupus
1959	Bielschowsky, Helyer, and Howie derived the NZB mouse, the first murine model of lupus
1969	Koffler *et al.* correlated immunofluorescent staining pattern of the glomeruli with degree of proteinuria
1971	American Rheumatism Association pubished criteria for the classification of systemic lupus—revised in 1982 and widely accepted
1980–3	Schwartz, and colleagues dissected the spectrum of autoantibody-producing cells in both autoimmune mice and humans with systemic lupus: many of the cloned antibodies were found to have cross-reacting idiotypes
1980–90	Physicians at the National Institutes of Health, including Klippel, Plotz, and Steinberg, demonstrated the use of combinations of prednisolone and intravenous cyclophosphamide given as boluses for the treatment of severe, especially renal, disease
1983–mid-90s	Hughes, Harris, Ascherson, Gharavi, and Khamashta emphasized links between antiphospholipid antibodies and particular clinical features, notably recurrent spontaneous abortion, livedo reticularis, and mutliple thrombotic events
1990s	Widespread acceptance of activity indices (e.g. BILA, SCAM, SLEPAI) and a damage index (SLICC/ALR) for lupus

The important genetic contribution to the aetiology of lupus is emphasized by the study of twin concordance reported by Deapen *et al.* (1992). Of 107 twin pairs studied, concordance among monozygotic pairs was found to be 24 per cent compared with 2 per cent among dizygotic pairs. While the figure for monozygotic twins is lower than previously reported, it is still 12 times that for the dizygotic pairs and may in fact be an underestimate, as not all of the twins were examined personally by the authors and long-term follow-up of the pairs was restricted.

It is widely agreed that lupus is approximately 10 to 20 times more common in women than men. There is also little dispute that the overwhelming majority of patients with lupus will develop their disease between the ages of 15 and 40 years.

Although, in the early part of the century, lupus was considered as a serious and frequently fatal disease, perceptions of it have changed

considerably. This seems to reflect the easier identification of milder cases with the introduction of widely available tests for measuring antinuclear antibodies. The introduction of corticosteroids and immunosuppressive drugs, dialysis, and renal transplantation has improved the chances of survival in the more serious cases. However, as will be discussed, lupus continues to cause considerable morbidity and 10 to 20 per cent of patients succumb from either the disease, a side-effect of its treatment, or both within 10 years of follow-up.

Clinical features

Non-specific features

Lupus, in common with many other chronic diseases, is accompanied by a variety of non-specific or general features. Of these, lethargy is

primary thrombosis. The latter is of particular interest in view of the recognized links with antiphospholipid antibodies. The propensity for corticosteroid therapy to increase the risk factors, such as hypertension, hypercholesterolaemia, and obesity, for coronary artery disease has been emphasized recently (Petri *et al.* 1994). In contrast hydroxychloroquine was associated with a lowered serum cholesterol.

Valves

Conduction defects and rhythm disturbances are recognized as occasional features of lupus, but have rarely been found in more than 10 per cent of patients.

Systolic murmurs have been recorded in up to a third of patients with lupus, but in the majority of cases this probably represents the hypodynamic circulation secondary to the chronic anaemia often found in these individuals. In contrast, diastolic murmurs are rather rare.

The classic endocarditis described by Libman and Sachs (1924), although identified in up to 50 per cent of cases at autopsy, rarely causes clinically significant lesions. Histologically small (1 to 4 cm) vegetations (verrucae) comprising proliferating and degenerating valve tissue with fibrin and thrombi are seen. A recent prospective echocardiographic study of 132 consecutive patients with lupus reported a prevalence of valvular lesions of 22.7 per cent (Khamashta *et al.* 1990). These lesions were most commonly found adjacent to the edges of the mitral and aortic valves and have been shown to contain immunoglobulin and complement components, notably within the walls of the small junctional vessels in the active portions of the verrucous endocardial lesions. These deposits might therefore represent immune complexes deposited via the circulation. In the report referred to above, the valve vegetations were associated with the presence of antiphospholipid antibodies. Leung *et al.* (1990)

also found a correlation between antiphospholipid antibodies and both valvular abnormalities and isolated left ventricular dysfunction in a study using M-mode, 2-D, and Doppler echocardiography.

In Mandell's review (Mandell 1987) of the reports of haemodynamically significant valvular disease in lupus, aortic incompetence and mitral regurgitation were the most frequently found among the paucity of published case reports.

Bacterial endocarditis has been reported on a number of occasions in patients with lupus. It has not been determined whether the most likely cause is a consequence of the underlying immunopathology of the disease or the predisposition to infection. However, reports of bacterial endocarditis in these patients do antedate corticosteroid therapy, suggesting that in some patients at least it is the primary immunopathology which predisposes to secondary bacterial infection. As most of the lesions of Libman–Sachs endocarditis are too small to be assessed accurately by echocardiography, any vegetations which can be identified in a patient with lupus who is febrile should certainly raise the possibility of bacterial endocarditis.

Pulmonary disease

The nature and features of pulmonary disease are indicated in Table 5. By far the commonest feature is pain due to pleurisy, which affects approximately half of lupus patients at some time. This pain may be uni- or bilateral and is usually present at the costophrenic angles anteriorly or posteriorly. Pleural effusions, usually small, also uni- or bilateral, straw-coloured, with a protein level generally greater than 3 g/dl, high mononuclear cell count but normal glucose level, are found in a quarter of the patients. Low levels of pleural fluid complement are quite common compared with effusions in

Table 6 Classification of renal lupus

World Health Organization classification	Deposits			Proliferation			
	Mesangial	Subendothelial	Subepithelial	Mesangial	Endocapillary	Extracapillary	Necrosis
Class I	–	–	–	–	–	–	–
Class IIA	+	–	–	–	–	–	–
Class IIB	+	–	–	+	–	–	–
Class III:	++	+	±	+	+ Focal	+ Focal	+ Focal
Active							
Inactive							
Class IV:	++	++	+	++	++	+	+
Diffuse proliferative							
Membrano- proliferative							
Class V:							
Pure	–	–	+++	–	–	–	–
With II, III, IV	+	±	+++	+'	±	±	±

other conditions, such as heart failure and cancer, but a positive anti-nuclear antibody is recorded very infrequently.

Parenchymal involvement attributable to lupus has been reported in 18 per cent of patients (Haupt *et al.* 1981). These patients had interstitial fibrosis, pulmonary vasculitis, and interstitial pneumonitis. However, these authors argued that many pulmonary lesions such as alveolar haemorrhage, alveolar wall necrosis, and oedema, previously attributed to direct lupus involvement, are probably secondary to factors such as concurrent infection, congestive heart failure, renal failure, and oxygen toxicity. It must be remembered that the immunosuppressive therapy required by many lupus patients does predispose them to concurrent infection. A true lupus pneumonitis is recognized but is rare (less than 2 per cent).

Almost as uncommon is clinically symptomatic diffuse interstitial lung disease. Its manifestations resemble those found in patients with scleroderma and rheumatoid arthritis who may also develop this complication. Thus the slow onset of a chronic non-productive cough with shortness of breath is usually present. Occasionally a more acute presentation occurs after an episode of acute lupus pneumonitis (Weinrib *et al.* 1990).

There is great interest in antiphospholipid antibodies and thrombotic events in systemic lupus. It is accepted that around 10 per cent of patients develop thrombophlebitis and/or a pulmonary embolus. Antiphospholipid antibodies should be sought in patients with these presenting symptoms and also the small number who present with pulmonary hypertension.

Well recognized, but also uncommon, are patients with the so-called 'shrinking lung syndrome' (Hoffbrand and Beck 1965). It is evident that diaphragmatic dysfunction makes a significant contribution to this syndrome.

Abnormal pulmonary function tests (described in detail in Chapter 1.3.5) and notably diminished total lung capacity and flow rates, often show more serious involvement than expected. Haemoptysis is unusual, although commoner than major pulmonary haemorrhage which, while rare, may be life-threatening.

In the relatively few cases studied, immune complex deposition has been correlated with histological evidence of inflammatory lesions in the pleural and pericardial membrane.

Renal involvement

In many published series, renal disease has been the most common cause of death in patients with lupus. However, the clinical symptoms suggesting renal involvement, notably ankle swelling, shortness of breath related to secondary heart failure, and 'frothy' urine, rarely become evident until substantial damage has been done. Thus careful monitoring of the blood pressure for hypertension, the urine for protein, red cells, or casts, and the plasma for raised creatinine and urea levels is most important. Sequira and Balean at The London Hospital appear to have been the first to recognize that nephritis was a component of systemic lupus in 1902, although serious renal disease was thought rare until the 1940s. Histologically, it has been shown that lupus nephritis appears in many guises. The World Health Organization (**WHO**) have subdivided renal lupus into five major categories according to biopsy-derived information. In addition endstage renal disease with sclerosed glomeruli is recognized (see Fig. 5). Kidneys with this appearance are non-functional. These categories are shown in Table 6 and Fig. 5. In brief, the major manifestations are defined as minimal or mesangial change; mild or

focal proliferative; severe or diffuse proliferative, and membranous. The glomerulus appears to bear the brunt of the attack in lupus. The range of glomerular changes include swelling, proliferation of mesangial, endothelial, and parietal epithelial cells, with infiltration by monocytes and polymorphonuclear leucocytes. In addition immune complexes, foci of necrosis, and haemotoxylin bodies can be identified in the glomeruli of lupus patients. While the WHO score has been widely adopted, it has drawbacks. It does not, for example, consider tubulointerstitial disease and makes no allowances for varying degrees of severity within individual categories; neither does it recognize the recently described overlap of lupus nephritis and the multiple small thrombi asssociated with antiphospholipid antibodies (see Fig. 5).

The role of renal biopsy in the management of lupus nephritis

There is a difference of opinion as to precisely when renal biopsy should be undertaken in patients with lupus, and about its value. The ability of lupus nephritis to transform from one variety to another and for the same biopsy to have more than one histological appearance is partly responsible for the conflict. In addition, few studies of the relationships between renal histology and clinical outcome have actually directly addressed the question as to what information the renal histology adds to the clinical data. Goulet *et al.* (1993) used regression tree techniques to show that combinations of serum creatinine, 24-h urine protein levels, nephrotic syndrome, and duration of prior renal disease provide accurate prognostic information about lupus nephritis without recourse to biopsy.

The biopsy itself is not without its problems, including quite heavy haematuria on occasion. It is obviously most important to assess the clotting capability of the patient before undertaking the biopsy. Fries *et al.* (1978) found that renal biopsy contains important prognostic information but that it was less than that of even the simplest clinical classification. Whiting-O'Keefe *et al.* (1982) applied a stepwise regression analysis to data collected over a 12-month period after renal biopsy in 130 patients with lupus to see if biopsy added any useful information to the clinical data. They found the histological classification did not add significantly to the predictive power of the 'before biopsy' model, but that certain features, notably the percentage of glomeruli which had undergone sclerosis in the presence of subendothelial deposits on electron microscopy, did increase the ability to predict the effect of 12 months of treatment of lupus nephritis. These authors felt that renal biopsy did not add important prognostic information over and above the clinical history examination and laboratory tests. A more recent study (Blanco *et al.* 1994) emphasized that chronicity markers, notably hyalinosis, tubular atrophy, and glomerular sclerosis on light microscopy and subepithelial, mesangial, and intramembranous deposits on electron microscopy, are the best indicators of a poor prognosis. More worryingly Schwarz *et al.* (1993) cast doubt upon the ability of pathologists to reproduce activity and chronicity scores accurately.

In contrast, Stamenkovic *et al.* (1986) described treatment based on renal histology of 56 patients with lupus. The mean follow-up period from first biopsy was 8.2 years, by which time 5.3 per cent were dialysis dependent, but nearly 95 per cent had resumed normal renal function. They found that the biopsy provided valuable information about the state of the kidney, independent of the clinical stage of the disease, and have argued that biopsy alone can improve predictions about 'renal survival' in lupus. McLaughlin *et al.* (1994) in a long-term follow-up study of 123 patients with systemic lupus who had a renal biopsy between 1970 and 1984, showed that the biopsy was helpful in assessing prognosis in patients with normal serum creatinine. In those with an elevated serum creatinine, the biopsy did not contribute additional information about the risk of dying.

Although it is not uniformly agreed, it can be recommended that patients with lupus who have haematuria and/or proteinuria and those with diminished glomerular filtration rate should be seriously considered for renal biopsy. However, as the above review of the controversy about the significance (and reproducibility in reporting) of renal biopsies indicates, the information they provide about prognosis should not be overestimated. The opinion of a pathologist with experience in assessing these biopsies is strongly advised.

Nervous system involvement

The first suggestion of involvement of the central nervous system in lupus was altered mental function, described at the end of the last century by Kaposi, and confirmed by Sir William Osler early this century.

Features of neurological disease range from the common, relatively harmless migraine headaches, to major psychotic episodes, and grand mal seizures, recognized in some lupus patients.

Manifestations of lupus affecting the nervous system can be subdivided into central or cerebral effects, peripheral lesions, and psychological aspects. Additional discussion of this topic is found in Chapters 1.2.1.2 and 1.3.4.

Central/cerebral involvement

Up to 40 per cent of lupus patients suffer from migraine, although this may be manifested by teichopsia alone. Of much greater concern are the grand mal seizures which may be an initial manifestation of lupus in perhaps 5 per cent of cases, but are present in up to 20 per cent of patients eventually. As with a number of other features it may be difficult to be certain whether the seizures represent true cerebral disease, or a manifestation of more general problems. They may, for example, be secondary to uraemia and other biochemical disturbances associated with renal involvement. Similarly, hemiplegia (and transverse myelitis) may be consequent upon primary neurological disease or could be secondary to hypertension, or associated with the more recently recognized antiphospholipid antibodies. Cerebellar disease in lupus appears to be uncommon as is aseptic meningitis. A variety of organic brain syndromes with impaired temporal–spatial orientation, poor memory, and intellectual deficit are all well recognized and remain difficult management problems.

There has been a resurgence of interest in a small group of patients with lupus who suffer from the movement disorders, chorea or ballismus. On occasion, chorea due to lupus may be difficult to differentiate from that due to rheumatic fever. However, in the more recently described patients, links with the presence of antiphospholipid antibodies have been stressed. This is discussed in more detail later in the chapter.

Ocular lesions in lupus are well recognized. These include conjunctivitis, episcleritis, and cytoid bodies (white patches seen on retinal examination). In addition, retinal haemorrhage, and occasional papilloedema (usually found in association with malignant hypertension) and macular degeneration have all been described. The potential retinal toxicity of antimalarial drugs is discussed later in the chapter.

Peripheral neuropathy

Approximately 10 per cent of patients with lupus develop a peripheral neuropathy in the course of their disease. These are usually sensory, occasionally sensorimotor. Cranial nerve involvement is rather less common, usually associated with active systemic disease and manifested by visual defects, tinnitus, vertigo, nystagmus, ptosis, and facial palsies. Feinglass *et al.* (1976) reported that the most commonly affected cranial nerves in their study were VII, III, VI, V, and IX in order of decreasing frequency. Optic neuritis was also uncommon, although it may, on rare occasions, be a presenting feature.

Psychological aspects

It has been claimed that up to 70 per cent of patients with lupus suffer a variety of psychiatric abnormalities. However, this label includes depression and anxiety, and most studies have failed to separate the non-specific psychological stresses associated with a debilitating and sometimes painful disease like lupus, from those specifically caused by the disease itself. Whatever the precise cause, a recent report of seven suicides in patients with lupus serves to emphasize that depression must be taken very seriously in systemic lupus (Matsukawa *et al.* 1994).

A lack of significant correlation between indices of general disease activity and psychiatric morbidity has been acknowledged by several authors. However, as with other aspects of lupus, more detailed testing, in this case using psychometric tests and nuclear magnetic resonance imaging, has been claimed to identify subtle degrees of impairment which may not be immediately evident clinically. Thus using a variety of standardized neuropsychological tests Hanley *et al.* (1993) identified cognitive impairment in 21 per cent of their patients with lupus compared with 4 per cent of their rheumatoid and healthy controls. Shortall *et al.* (1995) using a wide ranging set of neurophysiological tests showed that mood and mood disorders in patients with lupus were unrelated to measures of disease activity but were associated with psychological and social factors.

Emotional lability, personality change, impairment of judgement, and difficulty in performing simple tests of cognitive function, such as recall of serial numbers, all suggest organic involvement in lupus. The major psychoses, notably paranoia, schizophrenia, and hypomania, are also well documented. During the 1950s and 1960s, after the introduction of corticosteroids, concern was expressed that large doses of these drugs given for therapeutic purposes might actually be responsible for some of the psychiatric manifestations. Later studies have tended to discount this possibility. For example, Feinglass *et al.* (1976) considered that only 2 of 140 patients had a steroid-induced psychosis.

Investigations of neurological disease

It seems generally agreed that examination of the cerebrospinal fluid in neuropsychiatric disease is not very useful. Patients with lupus may show moderately raised cell counts, some increase in protein and IgG levels, and occasionally low glucose in their cerebrospinal fluid. It has been suggested that C4 levels in the cerebrospinal fluid are low during

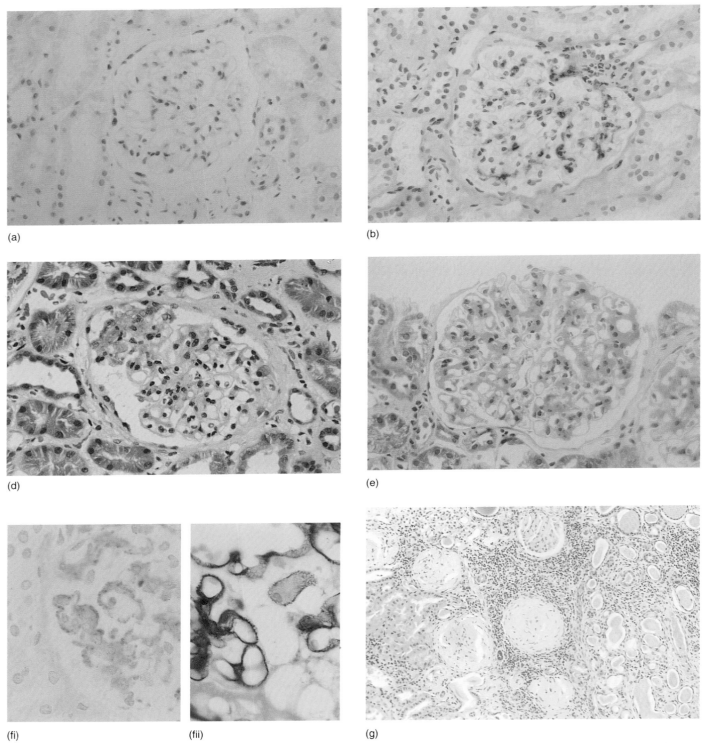

Fig. 5 Renal lupus (by courtesy of Dr M.H. Griffiths). (a) Systemic lupus erythematosus, no renal lesions, WHO class I. In addition to the mesangial immune deposit there is mesangial cell proliferation and the glomerulus appears hypercellular (haematoxylin and eosin). (b) Mesangial lupus nephritis, WHO class IIA. Immune complexes are demonstrable in the mesangium, seen here as granular brown deposits (immunoperoxidase technique for IgG). (c) Mesangial lupus nephritis, WHO class IIB. In addition to mesangial immune deposit there is mesangial cell proliferation and the glomerulus appears hypercellular (haematoxylin and eosin). (d) Focal proliferative lupus nephritis, WHO class III. Segmental proliferation (arrow) is seen in this glomerulus (haematoxylin and eosin). (e) Diffuse proliferative lupus nephritis, WHO class IV. The glomerular capillary walls are irregularly thickened forming, in places, classical 'wire loops' (arrow). There is variable cellular proliferation (haematoxylin and eosin). (f) Membranous lupus nephritis, WHO class V. There is diffuse capillary-wall thickening produced by abundant immune deposits in and on the basement membrane, seen in (i) as granular brown staining (immunoperoxidase technique for IgG). The basement membrane extends out between and around the deposits to produce a series of spikes and circles shown with silver staining in (ii) (hexamine silver technique). (g) Endstage renal disease showing completely sclerosed, non-functional glomeruli. (h) Hyaline thrombus in the glomerulus of a patient with systemic lupus and a high titre of antiphospholipid antibodies.

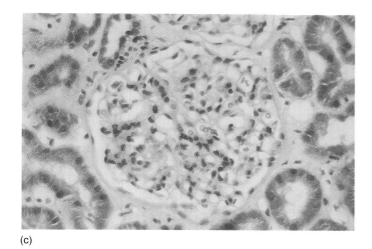

(c)

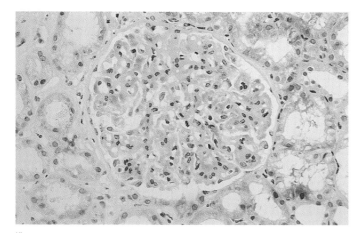

(f)

(h)

Fig. 5 (Continued)

active disease and return to normal as the patient improves. Its potential use, however, is limited by the need for serial determinations. A range of autoantibodies including anti-Sm, antineuronal, antilymphocytotoxic and, most recently, antiribosomal P has been linked to nervous system involvement. Invariably hopes raised in the initial reports have been dashed by later studies (reviewed in Hay and Isenberg 1993). For example, in 1987 in a retrospective study, antiribosomal P antibodies were reported to be highly specific for lupus psychosis (Bonfa *et al.* 1987). Since then there have been at least five other studies (reviewed by Teh and Isenberg 1994) with conflicting findings, and on balance there seems little value in a single measurement of antiribosomal P antibodies to identify patients with lupus psychosis, although serial estimations may be of value in a few individuals.

However, when brain infarction is suspected as a cause for a sudden cerebral event, it is clearly worthwhile testing for antiphospholipid antibodies (see later). The greatest value of cerebrospinal fluid examination is in ruling out concomitant infection, especially as many patients with lupus are treated with major immunosuppressive drugs.

Electroencephalographic studies have been shown by some to be helpful during flares of cerebral disease. The most commonly observed abnormality was diffuse slow-wave activity but focal changes have been found in some 30 per cent of the patients studied. Electroencephalographic changes tend to be associated with seizure activity or focal neurological signs, although on occasion these findings have been reported in patients with purely psychiatric symptoms. Other, more recent, studies have looked at visual, auditory, and somatosensory-evoked potentials. These tests have still to acquire widespread acceptance.

Computed tomography (**CT**) has been used to analyse patients with lupus for approximately 10 years. Unfortunately the results have been conflicting. Thus diffuse cerebral abnormalities have been found in some patients with active disease, but not in others. CT is, however, very helpful in distinguishing between cerebral infarction and cerebral haemorrhage. It has also been claimed that many patients with neuropsychiatric manifestations of lupus have increased cerebral atrophy as evidenced by enlarged sulci, either with or without ventricular enlargement. In fact corticosteroids may promote this atrophy.

The more recent introduction of nuclear magnetic resonance imaging (**MRI**) now offers a further means of investigating cerebral lupus. Figure 6 shows a patient who presented with severe depression, yet who had multiple small infarcts visible on MRI despite normal electroencephalographic and CT scans. High intensity spots are the most common MRI brain abnormality report in systemic lupus, present in at least one-third of patients (Ishikawa *et al.* 1994). However, these spots are neither specific for neuropsychiatric lupus nor do they show good correlation with central nervous involvement.

Haemopoietic involvement

A normochromic, normocytic anaemia, the 'anaemia of chronic disease', is present in up to 70 per cent of patients with lupus. Levels of ferritin in these patients are usually normal. In some individuals other factors contribute to anaemia. Thus some patients have endstage renal disease and many patients are treated with non-steroidal anti-inflammatory drugs, which may cause gastric bleeding. Coombs' positive haemolytic anaemia occurs in approximately 10 per cent of all patients. Much less frequently, a microangiopathic haemolytic anaemia with disseminated intravascular coagulation has been described. It should be noted that a positive Coombs' test is not always associated with haemolysis. An association between pure red cell aplasia and systemic lupus has also now been established.

Leucopenia ($< 4 \times 10^9/l$) and lymphopenia ($< 1.5 \times 10^9/l$) are the most frequent abnormalities of the white blood-cell count in

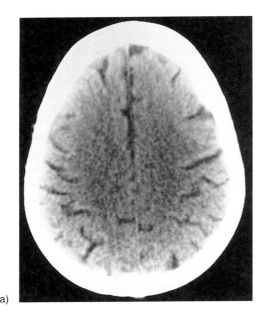

(a)

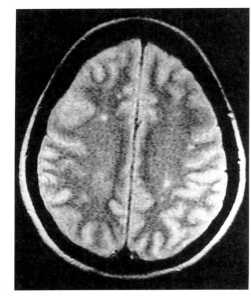

(b)

Fig. 6 Equivalent brain sections seen on CT scaning (a) and MRI scanning (b) in a patient with neuropsychiatric disease. Although some widening of the sulci is seen in (a), several discrete ischaemic areas are present in (b) which are not demonstrated on CT scanning.

patients with lupus. Estimates for the former have ranged from approximately 45 to 65 per cent and for the latter up to 80 per cent. Both T and B lymphocytes are reduced while null cells are increased. Lymphocytotoxic antibodies have been found in over one-third of patients with lupus. In contrast, leucocytosis is rare in lupus in the absence of infection or major corticosteroid therapy.

There are at least three types of clinical presentation of thrombocytopenia associated with lupus. Of these, chronic thrombocytopenia ($< 100 \times 10^9$/l) has been detected in approximately 20 per cent of most series. This is associated rarely with bleeding episodes in patients with lupus, unlike those unusual cases of acute thrombocytopenia where the fall in the platelet count may be both dramatic and life-threatening. Finally, some patients may present with what

initially appears to be an idiopathic thrombocytopenia, usually treated successfully with corticosteroids, which only several years later is followed by other manifestations of the disease. A detailed overview of the haematological manifestations of lupus has been published recently (Keeling and Isenberg 1993).

Other clinical manifestations of lupus

Vascular lesions, notably Raynaud's phenomenon, cutaneous vasculitis, and ulcers and gangrene of the fingers and toes are all well recognized in lupus patients. Approximately one-third of patients have Raynaud's phenomenon, which may antedate the onset of the disease by several years. It is generally relatively easy to control with vasodilating drugs, but on rare occasions it may be associated with gangrene of the extremities (Fig. 7). Unlike the older population which suffers gangrene due to atherosclerosis, the potential for recovery in the patient with lupus is better as the patients are much younger. Active vasculitis in lupus may manifest as necrotic ulcers, small cutaneous infarction, or lupus profundus. Leg ulcers have been recorded in up to 5 per cent of patients with lupus, most commonly around or just above the malleoli.

Although many patients with lupus develop some form of gastrointestinal complaint during the course of their disease, it is often difficult to be certain whether the lupus itself, the drugs used in its treatment, or other unrelated causes are responsible. Certainly anorexia, nausea, vomiting, or diarrhoea will occur at some point during the history of disease in over half of the patients, but frequently the cause will turn out to be iatrogenic. Abdominal pain is found in 10 to 20 per cent of the patients. The causes range from mild non-specific gastroenteritis to life-threatening mesenteric vasculitis. On occasions, an aseptic peritonitis may occur which often requires laparotomy to exclude a perforated ulcer or gangrenous piece of valve.

Pharyngitis and dysphagia are occasional features of lupus as is

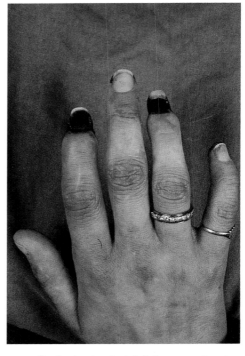

Fig. 7 Gangrene affecting two terminal digits in a young female patient with lupus.

pancreatitis. A problem with treating pancreatitis is that several of the drugs used to manage lupus (corticosteroids, azathioprine, and vasodilators) can precipitate an attack. The subject has been fully reviewed elsewhere (Watts and Isenberg 1989).

Hepatomegaly, which can be detected in approximately a quarter of patients with lupus, is usually a minor enlargement and rarely accompanied by major abnormalities in liver function tests. It is generally agreed that jaundice occurs in less than 5 per cent of patients with lupus. Equally rare is hepatic vasculitis and the Budd–Chiari syndrome, although this latter feature has also been linked to the presence of antiphospholipid antibodies. Splenomegaly is present in approximately 10 per cent of the patients, although the spleen is rarely greatly enlarged.

Apart from the autoantibodies detected in lupus (described later in this chapter) a number of other common blood tests are frequently abnormal in the patients. For example, hypoalbuminaemia has been described in up to 50 per cent of patients, and hypergammaglobulinaemia in up to 60 per cent. IgG and IgM levels, in particular, have been reported to be elevated in patients with lupus; IgA and IgE levels much less frequently so.

The erythrocyte sedimentation rate is increased in the vast majority of these patients, over 90 per cent in some series. Occasionally, however, normal levels are found even in the presence of active disease. In contrast, levels of C-reactive protein are generally, although not always, normal in patients with lupus except for those with a concurrent infection, an erosive arthritis, or possibly serositis. A normal level is thus of some value in helping to rule out infection in these patients although, as levels of C-reactive protein may reflect disease activity in certain individuals, its value is far from absolute.

Lupus and the risk of infection

As indicated in the section on the relationship between lupus and malignancy, the combined effect of the disease itself and its treatment is to render the immune system more prone to infection. It is often impossible to apportion responsibility for such infections to one or the other, but there are major consequences for outcome, discussed later in this chapter. In addition a variety of (generally) non-fatal infectious diseases, such as herpes zoster (Kahl 1994), salmonella (Abramson et al. 1985), and candida (Sieving et al. 1975), are quite common.

Diseases complicating lupus

Sjögren's syndrome is present in approximately 20 per cent of patients. The dryness of the eyes and mouth differs little from those cases of primary disease, although antibodies to Ro and La are present less frequently. Sjögren's syndrome is reviewed fully in Chapter 5.10. Autoimmune thyroid disease (generally hypo- rather than hyperthyroid) has been identified in 5 to 10 per cent of patients with lupus. However, antibodies to thyroglobulin and thyroid microsomes have been found in up to one-third of the patients. The treatment of under- or over-active autoimmune thyroid disease in patients who also have lupus is similar to those without it. Likewise myositis, also detectable in up to 5 per cent of patients with lupus, is treated no differently from patients with the idiopathic disease. A smaller percentage of patients with lupus (perhaps no more than 1 per cent) has myasthenia gravis. This may antedate or postdate the onset of the lupus itself.

Much has been written as to whether systemic lupus and rheumatoid arthritis can coexist. It is certainly very rare to have lupus glomerulonephritis occurring in patients with seropositive erosive rheumatoid arthritis. However, it is generally accepted that up to 5 per cent of patients do have an erosive arthropathy, suggesting that an overlap between these two conditions may exist in some individuals.

Lupus in special situations

Pregnancy and lupus

Even in healthy individuals, pregnancy results in drastic immunological changes. These have been the subject of much interest in the past few years. Oestrogens, for example, are thought to decrease T-suppressor cell function, while androgens have the opposite effect. Oestrogens also tend to increase immune complex clearance thus decreasing their renal deposition. The CD5 + B lymphocytes are also thought to be under oestrogen control. Progesterone is thought to have immunosuppressive properties and its production increases throughout pregnancy. Prolactin, another hormone associated with pregnancy, is a known modulator of lymphocyte responses to antigen in rodents, and human B and T cells are known to have receptors for it. It is thus evident that the effects of pregnancy on the immune system in general are complex and therefore not surprising that patients with lupus with their significantly disordered immune system may suffer deleterious effects during pregnancy.

There are many conflicting data about the effect of pregnancy on the patient with lupus. Despite earlier reports suggesting that sterility might be common among patients, more recent studies have noted that sterility and fertility were little changed by lupus. An exception to this are those patients in renal failure who do have reduced fertility. Similarly, whereas some reports of an increase in maternal mortality in the patients during pregnancy were described in the 1950s and 1960s, the current view is that the majority of pregnancies do not adversely affect the mother with lupus. Thus in a case–control study of 46 patients with 79 pregnancies, lupus flares occurred no more frequently than in non-pregnant controls (Urowitz et al. 1993). The frequency of non-renal complications during pregnancy is relatively low but is a little higher in the period immediately after parturition. Flares of disease, especially renal involvement, may require the introduction of or increase in corticosteroids, and on occasion the baby may have to be induced as early as 30 weeks of gestation.

In contrast to the relatively encouraging outcome for the mother with lupus, fetal outcome is much less certain. A combination of spontaneous abortion and still birth causes a fetal mortality of around 20 per cent. Up to 25 per cent of babies born to mothers with lupus may have to be delivered prematurely, for a combination of reasons relating to fetal distress as well as maternal ill health.

In the past decade the link between recurrent spontaneous abortion and the presence of antiphospholipid antibodies has been established. This is discussed in detail elsewhere in the chapter. The precise mechanism of these fetal deaths remains uncertain.

Mothers with lupus who have antibodies to Ro and/or La also appear to be prone to develop the so-called neonatal lupus syndrome. It appears that approximately 1 in 20 women who have either of these antibodies will have a child with this syndrome, which is notable for

Table 7 Comparison of clinical features and serological abnormalities in six published series of male patients with systemic lupus (%)

Clinical feature	Miller et al. (1983) n=51	Sthoeger et al. (1987) n=49	Kaufman et al. (1989) n=52	Ward et al. (1990) n=62	Cervera et al. (1992) n=76	Koh et al. (1994) n=61
Fever	?	90	50	?	50	?
Malar rash	27	55	40	27	49	56
Discoid rash	6	33	15	10	13	15
Photosensitivity	24	?	33	29	43	30
Oral ulcers	48	21	21	19	19	18
Athritis	94	84	94	71	74	54
Pleuritis	72	41	33	60[b]	74[b]	8
Pericarditis	48	33	33	?[c]	?[c]	7
Renal disease	44	67	65	45	48	72
Neuropsychiatric	18	53	42	26	26	25
Alopecia	26	31	33	?	?	?
Myositis	8	?	?	?	10	?
Lymphadenopathy	26	50	25	?	17	?
Splenomegaly	24	54	?	?	?	?
Hepatic abnormalities	19	50[a]	?	?	?	?
Raynaud's disease	50	14	25	?	30	?
Sicca syndrome	12	?	?	3	16	?
Positive Coombs' test	28	33	?	?	?	?
Haemolytic anaemia	8	?	13	15	?	10
Leucopenia	46	51	44	42	?	36
Lymphopenia	?	?	?	13	?	24
Thrombocytopenia	8	43	40	21	?	36
ANA	100	86	98	?	97	92
Anti-ds DNA	64	69	70	61	86	92
False-negative VDRL	6	30	20	13	?	19
LE cells	82	86	?	?	?	60
Anti-Sm	?	?	23	19	13	10
Anti-RNP	?	?	21	20	9	18
Anti-Ro	?	?	18	?	15	21
Anti-La	?	?	5	22	13	0
Low C3/C4/CH50	84	64	63	52	?	?

Percentages provided here represent cumulative frequencies and have been rounded up to the nearest whole number. ?, data not provided/numbers tested too small to provide meaningful analysis.
[a]Hepatomegaly only.
[b/c]In these studies pleuritis and pericarditis were evidently combined as 'serositis'.
VDRL, Venereal Disease Reference Laboratory.

its congenital conduction defects or skin rashes. This subject is discussed in detail in the next chapter on lupus in children.

Lupus in males

Although lupus in males, especially Caucasian males, is uncommon, many different groups have attempted to identify characteristics of male patients with lupus that distinguish them from women with the disease. A comparison of several reported series (Table 7) shows, however, that no clearly defined criteria have been identified. As discussed by Isenberg and Malik (1994) virtually every claim of a distinctive feature in one series is rebutted in others. In the United States, however, it has been reported that the prognosis is worse for male patients with lupus. Among males with lupus there appears to be no evidence of androgen deficiency, although in one large series 50 per cent had elevated plasma oestrogen levels (Miller *et al*. 1983), but corticosteroid administration might have been expected to decrease these values.

Individuals with Klinefelter's syndrome, who have an unusual XXY karyotype, are more susceptible to systemic lupus. Abnormalities in oestradiol metabolism in these patients may be linked to the persistent oestrogenic stimulation, which might explain the predisposition.

Several families in which systemic lupus predominates in males have been described (Lahita *et al*. 1983) where sons may have inherited the disease from their fathers, analogous with disease in the BXSB mouse, an experimental model of lupus which is described later in this chapter.

Lupus in the elderly

It is clearly a matter of opinion at which point lupus in the young or middle aged becomes lupus in the elderly! Most reports have taken 50 or 55 years as a cut off, although there has been very little attempt to relate chronological age to the menopause, a fact which may well be important in the aetiology of the disease in these patients.

In most large series, lupus commencing in the sixth decade of life represents about 10 per cent of the study population. However, there are conflicting reports on the patterns of presentation, organ involvement, serological findings, and prognosis in this group. It appears that the clinical onset of lupus in the elderly is more insidious, milder, has a lower incidence of severe renal and neurological complications, a lower frequency of antibodies to double-stranded DNA, and hypocomplementaemia, but an increased frequency of serositis, interstitial lung disease, and antibodies to Ro and La. The last of these features suggests that the overlap between lupus and Sjögren's syndrome is frequent in an elderly population.

Among less frequent modes of presentation in the elderly, a polymyalgia rheumatica-like picture has been described, and neuropsychiatric manifestations which might easily be confused with other types of organic disease are important in this group. The time between onset of disease and presentation, and between presentation and diagnosis, are increased compared with younger patients, although this should change with increasing awareness that lupus can occur for the first time well into old age — the oldest case reported so far was diagnosed aged 87.

The antiphospholipid antibody syndrome and lupus

Associations between anticardiolipin antibodies and the lupus anticoagulant with systemic lupus erythematosus have attracted considerable interest in the past 15 years.

Table 8 Clinical features which have been linked to antiphospholipid antibodies in patients with lupus

Venous and arterial thrombosis

Thrombocytopenia

Cerebral disease (including cerebrovascular accident, transient ischaemic attacks, chorea, amaurosis fugax)

Recurrent fetal loss

Pulmonary hypertension

Livedo reticularis

Anticardiolipin antibodies are part of an overlapping spectrum of antiphospholipid antibodies of which the lupus anticoagulant is part. Detailed analysis of anticardiolipin antibodies has distinguished two major varieties. In patients with infectious diseases the antibodies recognize epitopes on cardiolipin itself. However in many patients with lupus, the antibodies are probably binding to a complex or neo-epitope formed by phospholipid and a plasma cofactor β_2-glycoprotein 1 (Galli *et al*. 1990). Thus β_2-glycoprotein 1 dependency was noted for anticardiolipin (40 per cent), antiphosphatidyl serine (20 per cent), and antiphosphatidylinositol (18 per cent) antibodies but not for syphilis or normal sera (Matsuda *et al*. 1994).

A list of the clinical features widely believed to be associated with patients with lupus who have these antiphospholipid antibodies is shown in Table 8. A metanalysis undertaken by Love and Santoro (1990) suggests caution in the interpretation of the published results. In their analysis of 29 published series, they estimated an average frequency of 34 per cent for the lupus anticoagulant and 44 per cent for anticardiolipin antibodies in studies representing over 1000 patients with lupus. However, anticardiolipin antibodies are also prevalent in patients with a wide variety of diseases other than idiopathic lupus, including drug-induced lupus, rheumatoid arthritis, and acute infection. In patients with lupus a statistically significant association has been shown between the presence of either antibody and a history of thrombosis, neurological disorders, and thrombocytopenia (see also Chapter 5.7.3). In a large prospective cohort study of 389 primiparous women assessed at study entry and delivery, 24 per cent were positive for antiphospholipid antibody, 15.8 per cent of whom had fetal loss compared with 6.5 per cent of antibody-negative patients (Lynch *et al*. 1994). Elevated IgG antiphospholipid antibody levels were statistically associated with recurrent fetal loss but not with low birth weight, neonatal distress, or maternal complications.

A small cohort of patients with lupus with anticardiolipin antibodies has been shown to develop impaired renal function due to multiple small thrombi (Leaker *et al*. 1991). These patients have minimal proteinuria and only gradually increasing renal damage. This type of pathology may coincide with the more typical glomerulonephritis.

A number of contentious issues about antiphospholipid antibodies remain. For example, the precise links with other autoantibodies have been the subject of debate. It is widely accepted that anticardiolipin antibodies are associated with the biologically false-positive Venereal Disease Research Laboratory (VDRL) test. However, early studies

Table 9 Deaths from malignancy in patients with systemic lupus erythematosus

Number of patients with lupus studied	Total number of deaths	Number of deaths from malignancy	Reference
365	68	0	Urman and Rothfield (1977)
428	94	0	Karsh *et al.* (1979)
609	128	4	Wallace *et al.* (1979)
1103	272	0	Rosner *et al.* (1982)
150	16	4	Menon *et al.* (1993)

undertaken with monoclonal antibodies which suggested significant overlap between those binding cardiolipin and DNA were not supported by studies in patients with lupus. Although low affinity (generally IgM) antibodies to DNA may bind cardiolipin, higher affinity (generally IgG) antibodies to DNA do not. This would imply separate subpopulations of anti-DNA and antiphospholipid antibodies. This is probably an oversimplification, as a single amino-acid substitution can convert an antiphospholipid antibody into an anti-DNA antibody, supporting the view that these antibodies are very closely related (Diamond and Scharff 1984).

Neither the lupus anticoagulant nor anticardiolipin antibodies appear to correlate with age, duration of disease, or a variety of well-known lupus clinical features, including polyarthritis, vasculitis, or serositis.

Lupus and malignancy

Given that the immune system is so disordered in patients with lupus and that many patients are treated with major immunosuppressive drugs, there has been much recent interest in whether there is an increased risk of malignancy in systemic lupus. Table 9 reviews several published series. A rather low frequency of malignancy change (with no obvious predilection for any particular site) is evident. However, in the most recent series quoted (Menon *et al.* 1993), 7 out of 150 patients developed a malignancy, 5 of whom have died (4 as a direct result of the tumour). An occasional association between systemic lupus and Hodgkin's lymphoma has been described (Bhalla *et al.* 1993).

Assessing lupus disease activity

The assessment of disease activity in lupus is clearly central to patient management, but until recently there has been no consensus on measurement. Liang *et al.* (1988) reviewed, more than 60 different systems (attempting to establish a disease activity index) that have been described in the literature. This, in itself, is good evidence that no one system has won general acceptance. It also reflects the continuing difficulty in determining whether lupus should be thought of

as an individual disease or a group of closely related conditions in the absence of a gold standard, by which to judge disease activity.

In the past 12 years more determined attempts to compare and contrast some of the different activity indices have been undertaken. Thus the **SLAM** (systemic lupus activity measures), **SLEDAI** (systemic lupus erythematosus disease activity index), and **ECLAM** (European Community lupus activity measure) are three global score systems which have been shown to correlate well with each other (Vitali *et al.* 1992). They also correlate well with the **BILAG** system (British Isles Lupus Assessment Group) which was established to provide more detailed information about disease activity in each of eight organs or systems (Hay *et al.* 1993). The BILAG index is based upon the principle of the 'physician's intention to treat.' There has been an encouraging international effort to compare the SLAM, SLEDAI, and BILAG systems in combined studies of both 'paper' and real patients. These systems have repeatedly been shown to correlate with one another and to be reliable in evaluating disease activity in systemic lupus. Most recently they have been shown to be sensitive to change in disease activity over time (Gladman *et al.* 1994). Information about these three indices and a comparison between them, based on an assessment of real, as opposed to 'paper' patients, by seven different physicians is shown in Table 10.

Equally constructive have been attempts by 'lupologists' to agree an index that distinguishes damage (due to lupus or its treatment) from disease activity. The distinction in not simply an academic one. For example, a patient with shortness of breath may have active but reversible vasculitis which could improve with major immunosuppressive therapy. Alternatively the symptom may be due to fibrosis causing irreversible damage for which there would be no requirement for such treatment. Thus a **SLICC** (systemic lupus international collaborating clinics) damage index has been developed (see Table 11) and

Table 10 Correlations (r values) between three indices of activity for systemic lupus erythematosus

	VAS[a]	SLEDAI[c]	SLAM[c]
SLEDAI	0.261	0.732	
SLAM	0.209	0.732	
BILAG[b]	0.162	0.763	0.797

[a]VAS, visual analogue scale completed by the observer. Figures are based on real patient assessments by seven different physicians.
[b]BILAG, British Isles Lupus Assessment Group. This activity index is based on the physician's 'intention to treat' the patient. Lupus activity is divided into eight areas: general features, locomotor system, nervous system, renal involvement, dermatological involvement, pleuropericardial disease, vasculitis, and haematological involvement. Within each system the patients are designated A (action), implying that major immunosuppressive therapy needs to be initiated or increased; B (beware), the patient is known to have active disease but the therapy does not require alteration; C (contentment), remission in symptoms in that organ/system; D (discount), there is no current involvement in this organ/system; or E, there is no (evidence) of activity in the organ/system now or previously (see Hay *et al.* 1993 for further details).
[c]SLAM (systemic lupus activity measures) devised by Dr Liang (Boston) and SLEDAI (systemic lupus erythematosus disease activity index) described by Drs Urowitz, Gladman, and Bombadier are two good global score indices (see Liang *et al.* (1988) for further discussion).

Table 11 SLICC damage index[a]

Item	Score	
Ocular (either eye, by clinical assessment)		
Any cataract ever	1	
Retinal change OR optic atrophy	1	
Neuropsychiatric		
Cognitive impairment (e.g. memory deficit, difficulty with calculation, poor concentration, difficulty in spoken or written language, impaired performance level)		
OR major psychosis	1	
Seizures requiring therapy for 6 months	1	
Cerebral vascular accident ever (score 2 if >once), or resection not for malignancy	1	2
Cranial or peripheral neuropathy (excluding optic)	1	
Transverse myelitis	1	
Renal		
Estimated or measured glomerular filtration rate <50%	1	
Proteinuria 24 h, ⩾3.5 g	1	
OR		
End stage renal disease (regardless of dialysis or transplantation)		3
Pulmonary		
Pulmonary hypertension (right ventricular prominence, or loud P2)	1	
Pulmonary fibrosis (physical and radiograph)	1	
Shrinking lung (radiograph)	1	
Pleural fibrosis (radiograph)	1	
Pulmonary infarction (radiograph) OR resection not for malignancy	1	
Cardiovascular		
Angina OR coronary artery bypass	1	
Mycoardial infarction ever (score 2 if >once)	1	2
Cardiomyopathy (ventricular dysfunction)	1	
Valvular disease (diastolic murmur, or a systolic murmur >3/6)	1	
Pericarditis for 6 months, OR pericardiectomy	1	
Peripheral vascular		
Claudication for 6 months	1	
Minor tissue loss (pulp space)	1	
Significant tissue loss ever (loss of digit or limb, including resection not for malignancy) (score 2 if >one site)	1	2
Venous thrombosis with swelling, ulceration, OR venous stasis	1	
Gastrointestinal		
Infarction or resection of bowel below duodenum, spleen, liver, or gallbladder ever, for whatever cause (score 2 if >one site)	1	2
Mesenteric insufficiency	1	
Chronic peritonitis	1	
Stricture OR upper gastrointestinal tract surgery ever	1	
Pancreatic insufficiency requiring enzyme replacement OR with pseudocyst	1	
Musculoskeletal		
Muscle atrophy or weakness	1	
Deforming or erosive arthritis (including reducible deformities, excluding avascular necrosis)	1	
Osteoporosis with fracture or vertebral collapse (excluding avascular necrosis)	1	
Avascular necrosis (score 2 if >once)	1	2
Osteomyelitis	1	
Ruptured tendon	1	
Skin		
Scarring chronic alopecia	1	
Extensive scarring or panniculum other than scalp and pulp space	1	
Skin ulceration (excluding thrombosis) for more than 6 months	1	
Premature gonadal failure	1	
Diabetes (regardless of treatment)	1	
Malignancy (exclude dysplasia (score 2 if >one site)	1	2

[a]Damage (non-reversible change, not related to active inflammation) occurring since onset of lupus, ascertained by clinical assessment and present for at least 6 months unless otherwise stated. Repeat episodes mean at least 6 months apart to score 2. The same lesion cannot be scored twice.
(The development of this index is described in Gladman *et al.* 1996).

is currently being assessed by many groups in North America and Europe.

Immunopathology of lupus

In this section we review the immunopathology of the disease, both in strains of lupus-prone mice and in humans, by describing the specificity of autoantibodies, dysregulation, and abnormalities at the cellular level, and the genetic background that predisposes to the autoimmune response. Since the first edition of this textbook much interest has focused on apoptosis and the genes or 'autogenes' encoding the proteins important in regulation of apoptosis. Programmed cell death, or apoptosis, is quite distinct from the death of cells by necrosis and is a normal feature of cellular regulation. The current state of knowledge in this area will be addressed in both experimental models and human disease.

Experimental models of lupus

Several strains of mice spontaneously develop clinical and serological symptoms that resemble lupus. The most frequently studied strains are summarized in Table 12 and reviewed by Yoshida *et al.* (1990). Comparison of inbred mouse strains with outbred humans may not be relevant genetically but experimental manipulations in mice have made an important contribution to understanding the immunopathology of lupus.

At the genetic level, three genes have been shown to influence the pattern of disease in susceptible strains. The MRL$^{+/+}$ mice spontaneously develop late-onset lupus with a 50 per cent survival time of 18 months. The MRL-*lpr/lpr* differs by only one gene (*lpr* gene) but this single gene accelerates the disease process to give a 50 per cent survival time of between 2 and 4 months. The introduction of the *gld* gene into non-autoimmune C3H/HeJ mice results in lymphoproliferation and autoimmune disease. In contrast the *xid* gene confers protection against autoimmunity in the NZB/W F$_1$ model by preventing terminal B-cell proliferation and the emergence of autoreactive B-cell clones.

F$_1$ hybrids between an autoimmune strain (NZB) and a non-autoimmune strain (SWR) have an accelerated autoimmune disease with a high incidence of nephritis. All females are dead by 1 year of age. These mice have IgG2b anti-dsDNA antibodies which are cationic and deposit in the glomerular basement membrane. The pathogenic antibodies are derived from the normal SWR parent and carry a nephritogenic idiotypic marker which is not found in the circulation of either parent. The normal parents have deleted 50 per cent of their T-cell receptor Vβ chains and are I-E negative (equivalent to HLA DR in humans), thus they have peripheral T cells with I-E reactive T-cell receptors. The autoimmune parent and the F$_1$ offspring are I-E positive. Autoimmunity arises from the expression of 'forbidden' T-cell receptors by double-negative T-helper cells and suggests an abnormality in thymic selection/deletion.

Additional evidence from lupus mouse models shows that both cellular oncogenes (C-*myc*, N-*ras*, and C-*myb*) and retroviral genes may contribute towards the autoimmune process. Retroviruses have been implicated in murine lupus. A major envelope glycoprotein antigen, gp70, of type C murine retroviruses is present in the sera of all mice. This antigen can thus be regarded as autologous. The antigen may exist free in the circulation, similar to gp120 in HIV-positive patients, or it may exist as part of a xenotropic endogenous retrovirus. It can behave as an acute-phase reactant (stimulated by lipopolysaccharide, etc.). Circulating complexes of gp70 and anti-gp70 antibodies have been identified in the sera of lupus-prone mice, although free anti-gp70 antibodies cannot be detected (Izui *et al.* 1981). Levels of gp70$^+$ immune complexes correlated with nephritis, and gp70 was identified within immune deposits in the kidney (Maruyama *et al.* 1983). A recent report described the preliminary identification of the gp70 receptor as a 100 kDa glycosylated heterodimer on thymic leukaemia cells in mouse and humans.

Table 12 Lupus-prone mouse strains

Strain	Symptoms	Autoantibodies	Defects
(NZB × NZW)F$_1$	F ≫ M Renal defects Hypergammaglobulinaemia	dsDNA ssDNA	TNF deficiency Nephritis delayed by administration of TNF-α
NZB	Autoimmune haemolytic anaeamia	Red blood cells	
MRL$^{+/+}$	F ≫ M, late onset renal disease Lymphadenopathy	Sm, histones, DNA, rheumatoid factor	
MRL-*lpr/lpr*	Early onset similar to +/+ Infection with IL-2/vaccinia recombinant virus gives prolonged survival, decreased antibodies, normal renal function	Sm, histones, DNA, rheumatoid factor	*lpr* gene accelerates, neonatal thymectomy delays disease onset
BXSB	Males only Haemolytic anaemia Glomerulonephritis Lymphadenopathy	DNA, thymocytes, red blood cells	Y chromosome factor Early thymic atrophy
Moth-eaten	M+F Glomerulonephritis Hair loss, infection	DNA, thymocytes, red blood cells	Immunosuppression
(SWR × NZB)F$_1$	F ≫ M early onset lethal glomerulonephritis	IgG$_{2b}$ anti-DNA	Pathogenic antibodies

M, male; F, female; IL-2, interleukin 2; TNF, tumour necrosis factor.

The *Yaa* gene (Y-chromosome-linked autoimmune acceleration) accelerates disease in MRL$^{+/+}$ mice. These mice have increased levels of gp70–anti-gp70 immune complexes but no increase in the levels of circulating antibodies to DNA. Disease expression has been postulated to be controlled by at least four genes, three of which have been mapped to chromosomes 7 and 17.

Mutations in three autosomal recessive autoimmune genes have been identified in autoimmune strains of mice, reviewed by Mountz *et al.* (1994). All of these genes lead to defects in programmed cell death or apoptosis. The Fas protein has been intimately linked with apoptosis and is normally expressed on the cell surface (CD95). MRL-*lpr/lpr* mice have an endogenous retro-viral DNA sequence integrated into the *Fas* gene which results in incorrect membrane expression of the Fas protein and loss of apoptosis. This abnormality would result in failure of self-reactive T cells to undergo apoptosis in the thymus and may account for the accumulation of double-negative T cells (CD4-CD8-) which infiltrate many tissues in these mice. The coining of the expression 'autogene' by Talal encompasses a group of non-MHC, non-immunoglobulin or T-cell receptor genes whose abnormal function contributes to the development of autoimmune disease (Talal 1994). *Fas* may be considered as the first identified autogene. *bcl-2* is an oncogene which inhibits apoptosis, particularly of T cells, and may therefore be considered as a second autogene. Transgenic mice expressing *bcl-2* within B cells show prolonged B-cell survival, production of autoantibodies, prolonged B-cell memory, and inhibition of clonal deletion of self-reactive B lymphocytes, while *bcl-2* transgenic thymocytes display enhanced survival rates in the absence of growth factors and in the presence of lymphotoxic factors (summarized in Aringer *et al.* 1994). The autoimmune consequence of the defect in the *Fas* molecule was highlighted by amelioration of disease in CD2-*Fas* transgenic MRL-*lpr/lpr* mice (Wu *et al.* 1994). The CD2 promoter and enhancer was used to restore *Fas* expression in these mice and resulted in greatly reduced features of autoimmune disease, autoantibody production, and the complete elimination of the development of lymphoproliferative disease. These findings force us to consider that the hyperproliferation and production of abnormal cells in autoimmune disease may be due to defects in the appropriate removal of cells rather than the traditional definition of defects of excessive proliferation and stimulation of certain cells.

Recently a non-autoimmune strain of mice has been used to study human systemic lupus. These mice carry the SCID gene (severe combined immunodeficiency disease) and consequently lack T and B lymphocytes. This deficiency allows human peripheral blood lymphocytes to be grafted into the peritoneum of the mice and survive for up to 7 months. When peripheral blood lymphocytes from patients with lupus were injected into SCID mice over 3 mg/ml of human IgG was found in the circulation. Furthermore, deposits of mouse C3 were found in the renal glomeruli, indicating complement activation by immune complexes. However, no abnormal histology nor deterioration in renal function was associated with these deposits (Duchosal *et al.* 1990). Subsequently, lack of clinical or histological signs of vasculitis associated with lupus in either the skin or kidneys of SCID mice receiving xenografts of lymphocytes from patients with lupus was confirmed by another group (Ashany *et al.* 1992a). Production of autoantibodies by SCID–systemic lupus chimeras requires both T and B cells but is still insufficient to initiate pathological lesions (Geppert and Jasin 1990).

SCID mice have since been used to study aspects of murine lupus. SCID mice were reconstituted with spleen cells from young or old MRL-*lpr/lpr* mice or with *lpr* bone marrow. Seventy per cent of SCID mice receiving mature *lpr* splenocytes produced antibodies to Sm and dsDNA and one-third of these mice had extensive mononuclear and granulocytic infiltrates in lymphoid tissue, liver, and kidneys. However, histology revealed no glomerulonephritis, a marked reduction in the CD4-CD8- T-cells subset compared with the donor spleens, and the absence of massive lymphadenopathy which is associated with infiltration by double-negative T cells in the donor MRL-*lpr/lpr* mice. Nearly all recipients of young donor splenocytes developed acute graft-versus-host disease, dying within 4 weeks of cell transfer, while the majority of the recipients of bone marrow cells developed a wasting disease characterized by lymphoid atrophy and fibrosis in the absence of autoantibody production (Ashany *et al.* 1992b).

The role of self-reactive T cells in renal pathology has been demonstrated by cloning T cells from the interstitium of MRL-*lpr/lpr* mice with lupus nephritis. These T cells are unique and are regulated by the *lpr* gene. They have the phenotype CD4-CD8-αβTCR +, proliferate in response to renal tubular cells, and secrete interferon-γ which induces major histocompatibility (**MHC**) class II antigens and intercellular adhesion molecule 1 (**ICAM-1**) on renal tubular epithelial cells, making these cells capable of triggering T-cell hybridomas to proliferate and secrete interleukin 2 (**IL-2**) (Kelley *et al.* 1993). These double-negative T cells proliferate mostly in the liver and migrate to the periphery. Hepatic mononuclear cells vigorously secrete IL-6 which can be neutralized by antimouse IL-6 antibody and prevent the induction of ICAM-1 on hepatic sinusoidal endothelial cells seen in MRL-*lpr/lpr* mice (Ohteki *et al.* 1993). Upregulation of cell adhesion molecules (ICAM-1, VCAM-1) has also been demonstrated in kidneys of autoimmune mice and may mediate the adherence of pathogenic inflammatory cells in murine lupus nephritis (Wuthrich *et al.* 1990; Wuthrich 1992).

A form of 'experimental lupus' has been induced in normal strains of mice by two 1 μg injections of a human monoclonal anti-DNA antibody bearing the pathogenic 16/6 idiotype. Subsequently mouse IgG carrying the same idiotype was found in mesangial deposits in the kidneys. The mice developed proteinuria, an increased erythrocyte sedimentation rate, and leucopenia and had circulating autoantibodies reactive with a variety of autoantigens (Mendlovic *et al.* 1988). Independent confirmation of this data is awaited as it has not been confirmed by several other laboratories, implicating an environmental factor in the development of this lupus model (Williams and Isenberg 1994). However, transfer of splenocytes from Balb/c mice, in which systemic lupus had been induced by injection of 16/6Id, into SCID mice resulted in transfer of lupus disease, the characteristics of which were more severe if 16/6Id was given at the same time as cell transfer. The SCID recipients had high titres of autoantibodies, multiple immune complex deposits in the kidneys, and glomerular histological changes, including thickening of the glomerular basement membrane, mesangial proliferation, and some fibrotic changes (Segal *et al.* 1992).

Autoantibodies in systemic lupus

The serological hallmark of systemic lupus is the presence of circulating autoantibodies directed against a wide variety of nuclear, cytoplasmic, and plasma membrane antigens which are outlined in

Table 13 Autoantibodies in systemic lupus (SLE)

Antibody	Antigen/epitope	Prevalence (%)	Clinical and other associations
Intracellular			
DNA	dsDNA (ssDNA) (ZDNA)	40–90	IgG, cationic, present in renal eluates. Pathogenic cross-reactions: LAMP/glomerular heparin sulphate
Histone	H1, 2A, 2B, 3, 4	30–80	Drug-induced lupus+anti-ss DNA
Sm	A, B/B′		SLE specific, up to 30% in Afro-Caribbeans, ≃10% in Caucasians
U1RNP	D,N 68 kDa ribonucleoprotein	20–35	Mild disease. Renal involvement, HLA DR4
rRNP	Three subunits: 38, 19, 17, kDa	5–15	Neuropsychiatric lupus?
Ro/SS-A	60,52 kDa protein bound to cytoplasmic RNA (hY1-hY5)	25–40	2°SS, SCLE, CHB. HLA DR2 DQw1(=DQw6) DQw2, DQw3—protective?
La/SS-B	47 kDa protein bound to variety of RNA (Pol III transcripts, viral (EBV, CMV, adeno) U1RNA (Pol II) hY RNA)	10–15	HLA DR3 (2°SS)—SCLE, CHB. κ-chain allotype (Km1)
Heat-shock proteins (hsp)	hsp70 / hsp90	<10 / 25–35	IgM>IgG. Surface expression of hsp90 on monocytes and CD4+T cells and B lymphocytes+↑ cytoplasmic expression in lymphocytes and monocytes
Cell membrane Cardiolipin	Phospholipids / DNA	20–40	Recurrent abortion / Thrombosis
Neuronal antigen	Expressed on neuronal cell line grown *in vitro*	70–90 (+ CNS) / ~10 (− CNS)	In serum and CNS some cross-react with lymphocyte cell surface
Lymphocyte	T cells ≫ B cells / HLA components / CD4+ / CD8+	~75 (IgM) / ~45 (IgG)	Cytotoxic (80%) some cross-react with cell surface antigens of CNS
Red cell	Non-Rh related	<10	Haemolytic anaemia
Platelet		<10	ITP
Extracellular Rheumatoid factor	Fc region of IgG	~25	Usually IgM, cross-react with histones, Ro/SS-A
C1q	Complement component	~56	Rising titres precede renal involvement (prolif. GN)

LAMP, lymphocyte-associated membrane protein; RNP, ribonucleoprotein; CNS central nervous system; 2°SS, secondary Sjögren's syndrome; SCLE, subacute cutaneous lupus erythematosus; CHB, congenital heart block; EBV, Epstein–Barr virus; CMV, cytomegalovirus; ITP, idiopathic thrombocytopenic purpura; Prolif GN, proliferative glomerulonephritis.

Table 13. In a recent study 98 per cent of patients had antinuclear antibodies and 56 per cent had elevated levels of antibodies to dsDNA (Worrall *et al.* 1990).

Antibodies to dsDNA are usually of the IgG isotype. Studies of kidney biopsies from patients with glomerulonephritis show deposition of IgG and complement components indicating a localized immune response and subsequent inflammation. Eluates from affected kidneys show that the IgG has specificity for dsDNA. In addition these antibodies are cationic in charge, clonally restricted, and high affinity (Kalunian *et al.* 1989). Not all circulating anti-DNA antibodies possess these characteristics, suggesting a sub-population of 'pathogenic' antibodies preferentially localized in the kidney. Two mechanisms may account for this deposition. First, circulating immune complexes of DNA–anti-DNA antibodies may

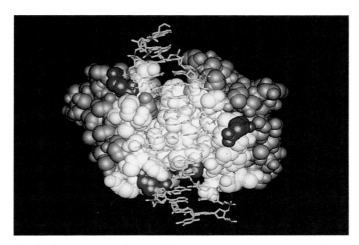

Fig. 8 Computer modelled possible docked complex between an IgG monoclonal anti-dsDNA antibody designated B3 and dsDNA. The light chain is shown on the left-hand side and the heavy chain on the right-hand side. Olive colour=framework residues; white=complementarity determining regions. The arginines (blue) at positions 227A, L54, and H53 all make interactions with the DNA phosphate backbone. (Reproduced from Kalsi *et al.* 1996, with permission from Pergamon Press.)

become trapped in the glomerulus, activate complement, and lead to local inflammation and tissue damage Second, non-complexed anti-DNA antibodies may cross-react with heparan sulphate, the glycosaminoglycan side-chain of heparan sulphate proteoglycan, which is a major constituent of glomerular basement membrane; this anionic side-chain is predominantly responsible for the negative charge of the membrane and may merely reflect antigen non-specific binding of cationic anti-DNA antibodies. Recently this binding was reported to be mediated via bound complexes containing both DNA and histones. Histones have very high affinity for heparan sulphate (Termaat *et al.* 1990) and antihistone antibodies are also a feature of systemic lupus. Evidence of direct pathological consequences of human anti-dsDNA antibodies has been described recently by Ehrenstein *et al.* (1995) using the SCID mouse model.

Heparin has been shown to inhibit the DNA binding of antibodies eluted from kidneys of humans and MRL-*lpr/lpr* mice but did not inhibit DNA binding of serum antibodies. Low, non-anticoagulant doses of heparin administered to MRL-*lpr/lpr* mice prevented the development of severe lupus nephritis and may be useful in treating humans with lupus (Naparstek *et al.* 1990).

Molecular biology techniques have revealed some interesting new data on the nature of the DNA antigen involved in lupus. DNA purified from immune complexes isolated from the sera of patients with lupus was found to be enriched in the deoxynucleotide bases guanosine and cytidine compared with normal genomic DNA. It was highly immunogenic in rabbits, unlike commercial DNA, and bound to anti-DNA antibodies with high avidity. Cloning and sequencing of this DNA revealed 82 per cent homology with the *gag/pol* fragment encoded by the ENV gene of the human immunodeficiency virus, HIV. This finding lends support to a viral aetiology of systemic lupus but a survey of sera from 100 patients with lupus revealed no antibodies to retroviral proteins (p24) (Krapf *et al.* 1989).

Recently a human monoclonal IgG antibody (B3) with specificity for dsDNA has been modelled on the computer, enabling a molecular map of the antigen–antibody interaction to be visualized (Fig. 8). This type of approach will facilitate site-directed mutagenesis

experiments to determine the key amino acids for the recognition of DNA (Kalsi *et al.* 1996).

While antibodies to DNA occur in many patients, antibodies to some of the other nuclear antigens show an association with ethnic origin. Antibodies to Sm are more frequently associated with Afro-Caribbeans than Caucasians. This also relates to the HLA status of the individual (see later) in that many of the Afro-Caribbean patients carry the DR2 haplotype (Olsen *et al.* 1993). Antibodies to U1RNP are usually associated with mild disease, a lower incidence of renal involvement, and the MHC haplotype, DR4.

Antibodies to Ro and La are more frequently associated with Sjögren's syndrome secondary to a diagnosis of lupus. Occasionally these antibodies can be detected in saliva, but not in serum prior to the symptoms associated with salivary gland infiltration (Horsfall *et al.* 1989).

Claims have been made suggesting an association of autoantibodies to ribosomal P protein in patients with lupus with cerebral involvement and psychosis but these findings remain controversial.

Autoantibodies to C1q may be elevated in systemic lupus and are indicative of proliferative glomerulonephritis (Siegert *et al.* 1993).

Abnormalities and dysregulation at the cellular level

Systemic lupus is characterized by multiple functional defects among cells of the immune system — T and B lymphocytes, natural killer cells, and accessory cells (antigen presenting cells) (Table 14). Numbers of circulating lymphocytes may be altered profoundly. Hyperactive B cells may be increased in number with coexistent T lymphocytopenia. Numbers of both lymphocyte populations are extremely variable and fluctuate between normal and abnormal levels with respect to disease activity and duration.

The increase in activated B cells contributes to the hypergammaglobulinaemia associated with reactivity to self antigens outlined in Table 13. On circulating B cells, receptors for the cytokine, IL-2, are increased while CR1 (the receptor for C3b) expression is decreased. There is increased cytoplasmic expression of the heat shock protein, **hsp**90, in B cells and CD4 + T cells (but not CD8 + T cells) compared with normal cells. Some of the excess hsp90 in patients with elevated levels is localized on the lymphocyte cell surface and therefore accessible to the immune system (Erkeller-Yuksel *et al.* 1992).

Among the two major T-cell populations, CD4 + (helper/inducer) and CD8 + (suppressor/cytotoxic), there is a marked reduction of a subset of T cells bearing the CD4 + and CD45R + phenotype. This population of cells helps to induce suppression by providing a signal to the CD8 + population. The reduction in this subset may explain the failure of T cells to suppress the hyperactive B cells. Anti-T-cell autoantibodies may be responsible for the depletion of this particular subset. A study has reported that the titre of anti-T-cell antibodies is directly proportional to the ratio of CD4/CD8 killing and that flares of disease are associated with an increase in CD4/CD8 killing and disease remission is accompanied by a corresponding decrease in the ratio. Parallel changes in anti-T-cell titres reflect the disease activity (Yamada *et al.* 1993). Many of the T cells with the classical αβ T-cell receptor (**TCR**) chains lack the CD4 or CD8 phenotypes normally associated with these cells. As 'double negatives' they have probably escaped thymic deletion. A recent report described that of all activated T cells cloned *in vitro* from patients with lupus only 15 per

Table 14 Cellular abnormalities and cytokine dysregulation

Cell type/cytomine	Dysregulation
Monocyte/macrophages	↓ TNF-α production — genetic defect
Lymphocytes	
B cells	↑ Numbers activated B cells→hypergammaglobulinaemia→IgG autoantibodies reactive with self antigens (cell membrane, cytoplasmic proteins, nuclear antigens, extracellular proteins) and non-self (polyclonal) ↑ IL-2R, ↓ CR1 expression, ↑ surface expression of hsp90 but not hsp70 compared with normal cells
T cells:	↓ CD4+CD45R+ (subset Th, suppressor/inducer) ↑↑ CD48-8-TCRαβ+Th (escape thymic deletion since double negative?)
In vivo	IFN-γActivated T cells are class II+ (DP,DR) Defective suppression Impaired cytotoxicity Activated peripheral T cells (only 15%→anti-DNA help), cloned→Tγ∂ cells reactive with hsp60
In vitro	and→help to anti-DNA+ B cells (not class II restricted) (blocked by antibody to hsp65 but not hsp70)
Cytokines	
IL-1	↓ Does not activate T cells? Insufficient production by accessory cells or defective T-cell IL-1 receptor. Not corrected by addition of IL-1 in vitro.
IL-2	Normal or ↓ IL-2 production by CD4+ and CD8+T cells. Impariment not reversed by addition of IL-2. IFN-γ+IL-2 restores T-cell proliferation in vitro? Functional activity vs. level of IL-2. Low affinity IL-2r expressed on CD4+T cells.
IL-4	↑ IL-4 (antigen-primed T cells→IL-4→all B cells)
IL-6	No response to inflammation/acute-phase reactants
IL-10	↑ in patients. Administration accelerates disease in NZB/W mice. Antibodies against IL-10 delay disease onset and ↑ TNF-α.
TNF-α	MHC linked production, probably protective therefore levels may be critical
IFN-γ	Normal levels produced. NK cells refractory. Administration of rIL-2 exacerbates disease.

TNF-α, tumour necrosis factor-α; IL-2r, interleukin-2 receptor; hsp, heat-shock protein; Th, T-helper cell; TCR, T-cell receptor; IFN-γ, interferon-8; MHC, major histocompatibility complex; NK, natural killer cells; rIL-2, recombinant interleukin 2.

cent actually provided 'help' for B cells to make pathogenic anti-DNA antibodies, i.e. antibodies of IgG isotype, cationic charge, specific for native DNA, and clonally restricted in spectrotype. The majority (83 per cent) of these T cells were CD4 + and expressed the classical αβ TCR, responded to endogenous antigen presented by autologous B cells, and were class II restricted. The remaining 17 per cent were CD4-CD8- (double negative) and were not class II restricted. Of these, 70 per cent expressed the alternative γ TCR and proliferated in response to endogenous heat shock or stress proteins of the hsp60 family expressed by lupus B cells (Rajagopalan et al. 1990). Sequencing of the T-cell receptors showed V and Vγ gene usage not found in normal healthy adults and resembled that of fetal thymocytes early in ontogeny (Rajagopalan et al. 1992).

Increased DNA mutations have been observed in T cells in patients with lupus, which may result in T-cell death and increased release of non-degraded DNA by necrosis rather than apoptosis, in turn contributing to the production of anti-DNA antibodies (Gemelig-Meyling et al. 1992).

Several authors have suggested that a biochemical defect of T cells underlies the impairment of T-cell responses in systemic lupus. There are two possible defects in the T-cell cAMP pathway; one at the level of adenylate cyclase and another at the level of cAMP-dependent protein kinase. Cross-linking of cell surface receptors and lymphocyte movement to sites of inflammation (homing) have effects on the cAMP pathway. These events enhance the intracellular turnover of cAMP, promote occupancy of cAMP receptors, activate cAMP-dependent phosphorylation, and induce directed mobility of surface molecules to a pole of the cell (capping). The cAMP pathway thus mediates the mobility of certain transmembrane and glycolipid-anchored cell surface molecules resulting in ligands bound to T-cell membrane molecules to be selectively internalized or cleared from the cell surface by capping and endocytosis or by shedding.

In comparison with normal T cells, lupus T cells showed markedly abnormal capping of cell surface proteins (CD4 and 8) during active and inactive disease and showed decreased cAMP production in response to adenosine, associated with an inability to switch phenotype and express suppressor activity. Cell permeable cAMP did not bypass potential adenylate cyclase defects nor restore suppressor activity (reviewed by Kammer and Stein 1990).

The appearance of class II molecules, usually HLA DR, on T cells is taken as a marker of activation. Peripheral T cells with increased expression of HLA DP at the cell surface and as mRNA transcripts have been found in patients with lupus. The frequency of HLA DP expression exceeded that of HLA DR and correlated well with disease activity. The ratio of HLA DP + T cells is inversely proportional to the extent of IL-2 production during *in vitro* response to mitogen (Hishikawa *et al.* 1990; Kanai *et al.* 1993).

Some patients with lupus show decreased responses to immunization *in vivo* (primary immune response) and decreased responses to B-cell challenge *in vitro*. Other patients show normal or even increased responses to immunization. Disease activity and immunosuppressive therapy obviously influence the response in individual patients (reviewed by Turner-Stokes and Isenberg 1988).

Antigen-specific T cells have now been cloned from patients with lupus. Patients who have circulating antibodies to the ribosomal P2 protein have T cells which can proliferate *in vitro* to recombinant P2 and are inhibited in the presence of antibodies to MHC class II antigens. These T cells are CD4 + and thus may help B cells to produce antigen-specific antibodies (Crow *et al.* 1994). HLA DR restricted T cells have also been cloned from a patient with lupus and shown to induce IgG anti-DNA antibodies *in vitro* from high density (activated) B cells from DR-matched patients with lupus, and IgM anti-DNA antibodies from B cells from DR-matched normal individuals (Murakami *et al.* 1992). An HLA DR4-restricted T-cell clone has been derived from a healthy individual and recognized the protein but not the RNA moiety of UsnRNP. The T-cell clone had a cytokine profile characteristic of Th1 cells (see the following section) and did not provide helper activity for autoantibody synthesis *in vitro* (Wolff-Vorbeck *et al.* 1994).

Cytokines

In the first edition of this textbook we wrote that 'the role of cytokines in the immunopathology of lupus is uncertain although likely to be of importance'. This prudent statement is underlined by the explosion of literature in this area and the demonstration of effective anticytokine antibody therapy of autoimmune disease. The characterization of different subsets of T-helper (**Th**) cells is directly related to their cytokine profiles and several autoimmune diseases may now be classified according to the predominance of a particular T-helper cell subset. We present a simplified summary of the major findings in this area and refer the reader to a recent excellent review by Horwitz and Jacob (1994).

Table 15 summarizes the major differences between Th1 and Th2 cells in terms of cytokine profiles and function, and outlines the cytokines found in serum or produced spontaneously after stimulation of peripheral blood mononuclear cells. Th1 cells support cell-mediated immunity while Th2 cells provide B-cell help and also suppress cell-mediated immunity. The balance between cytokines from Th1 and those from Th2 cells is thus critical in determining the outcome of the immune response and any imbalance could have profound pathological effects.

At the most simplistic level systemic lupus could be expected to be a disease where Th2 cells predominate resulting in too much help for B cells and overproduction of antibodies. In support of this concept, increased levels of IL-10 have been found in patients with lupus; this cytokine suppresses Th1 cells and thus impairs cell-mediated immunity, a characteristic feature of the disease. In

Table 15 T-cell subsets and cytokines

	Subsets of CD4+T cells	
	T-helper 1 cell	**T-helper 2 cell**
Function	Cell-mediated immunity	B-cell help
Cytokines:	IFN-γ	IL-4
	IL-10 (humans only)	IL-10
	IL-12	
	TNF-α	

Cytokine profiles in patients with active systemic lupus

Cytokine	Serum level[a]	Spontaneous	Stimulation *in vitro*
IFN-γ	↑	low	↓
TNF-α	↑ (or normal)	↓(DR2 DQw1; ↑ nephritis) ↑(DR3,4; ↓nephritis)	↓
IL-1	n.d.	↑ PBM production	↓ monocyte production
IL-2	↑	low	↓
IL-4	n.d.	low	low
IL-6	↑	↑	–
IL-10	↑ (or normal)	↑ (or normal)	normal

[a]Serum levels of cytokines are difficult to interpret since these may be affected by soluble cytokine receptors which are shed from cells. Among the known shed receptors are those for IL-1, IL-2, IL-6, TNF-α, and IFN-γ. Soluble TNF-αR and IL-2R levels are increased in systemic lupus and correlate with disease activity and lupus nephritis. n.d., not detected.

mice continuous administration of anti-IL-10 delays the onset of disease.

Tumour necrosis factor (**TNF-α**) is produced by T (Th1) and B lymphocytes, natural killer cells, and mononuclear phagocytic cells. Another cytokine (TNF-β), originally called lymphotoxin, is produced by activated lymphocytes. The genes for both TNF-α and -β are closely linked and located within the major histocompatibility complex (MHC). *In vitro* TNF-α production by mitogen-activated peripheral blood lymphocytes varies according to the HLA class II haplotype of the donor. Elevated production is found in DR3 and DR4 subjects, whereas low production is found in DR2 and DQw1 positive donors. The DR2, DQw1 genotype in patients with lupus is associated with lupus nephritis. DR3 + patients with lupus are not predisposed to lupus nephritis and have elevated levels of TNF-α production. The DR4 haplotype is associated with high TNF-α inducibility and negatively correlated with lupus nephritis (Jacob *et al.* 1990a).

Paradoxically high levels of TNF-α are more frequently associated with rheumatoid arthritis and, as such, therapeutic benefit has been reported using monoclonal antibodies to TNF-α. Two of 20 patients treated with anti-TNF-α antibody developed anti-dsDNA antibodies and other serological abnormalities characteristic of lupus, although neither developed clinical symptoms of the disease. All antibodies disappeared when therapy was stopped (Maini *et al*. 1994).

Both macrophage and natural killer cell-mediated cytotoxicity are frequently impaired in patients with lupus. γ-Interferon-induced enhancement of both types of cytotoxicity is also impaired despite normal levels of γ-interferon production by lupus Th1 cells. Lupus natural killer cells fail to release soluble factors necessary for killing. Recombinant γ-interferon has been used to induce remission in patients with rheumatoid arthritis, but it exacerbated disease in both patients with lupus (Machold and Smolen 1990) and lupus-prone strains of mice (Jacob *et al*. 1990b).

Accessory cells in lupus seem to produce insufficient amounts of IL-1 to provide the necessary activation signal for T cells. This effect cannot be overcome *in vitro* by the addition of exogenous IL-1, suggesting that a defect may exist at the level of the IL-1 receptor on T cells. Alternatively the defect could exist at a distal point in some biochemical pathway.

Both CD4 + and CD8 + T cells have been described to produce either normal or decreased amounts of IL-2 in response to exogenous antigens, mitogens, allo- and autoantigens. Reduced IL-2 generation would have a profound effect on T-cell responses. This impairment is not reversed by the addition of exogenous IL-2. However, *in vitro* treatment of lupus accessory cells with γ-interferon plus the addition of IL-2 has been shown to restore T-cell proliferation and the expression of T-suppressor activity. The variability of experimental data in this context raises the question of whether IL-2 functional activity varies between patients rather than merely reflecting levels of IL-2.

Studies *in vitro* on the response to IL-2 of the CD4 + T-cell subset (helper/inducer) indicate that there is altered expression of IL-2 receptors. The CD8 + T-cell subset (suppressor/cytotoxic) has IL-2 receptors but fails to respond as there is no IL-2 signal from CD4 + T cells. This is a secondary defect. The primary disorder relates to the CD4 + subset which expresses IL-2 receptors of low affinity. Functional IL-2 receptors are of high affinity. Variable synthesis of both types of receptors may be governed by altered intracellular synthesis and/or transport.

Apoptosis

The study of programmed cell death in human lupus is now an active area of research. As with experimental models of lupus, an underlying defect of apoptosis prevails in human disease. Decreased apoptosis in systemic lupus has been described in association with an increased production of the soluble form of the *Fas* molecule, which is capable of inhibiting apoptosis after a stimulus to proliferate (Cheng *et al*. 1994).

bcl-2 is a proto-oncogene located at the inner membrane of mitochondria, the endoplasmic reticulum, and the nuclear membrane and exerts a regulatory function during development and maintenance of adult tissue by preventing apoptosis in specific cell types. It is involved in T-cell development and thymic selection and is found in long-lived B lymphocytes within the follicular mantle zone. Over-expression of *bcl-2* in circulating lymphocytes from patients with lupus has been described in both CD4 + and CD8 + T cells but not B cells, and levels of *bcl-2* expression have been shown to correlate

with disease activity (Aringer *et al*. 1994). A more recent study of a larger group of patients with lupus has described enhanced *bcl-2* expression in a subpopulation of CD3 + T cells lacking CD4 and CD8 (double-negative T cells). The percentage of these cells expressing *bcl-2* correlated strongly with disease activity (Rose *et al*., unpublished observations). Defects in apoptosis in systemic lupus may therefore involve two genes—either abnormal transcription of the *Fas* gene resulting in a soluble rather than cell membrane-associated product, or increased transcription and expression of the *bcl-2* gene product, both of which are capable of inhibiting apoptosis.

Cell adhesion molecules

Interest in the adhesive mechanisms which facilitate cell–cell and cell–matrix interactions has expanded considerably over the past few years. Adhesion is mediated by several molecules which vary in affinity and structure on the surface of the cells which express them. Adhesion molecules belong to one of three main families: selectins, integrins, or the immunoglobulin superfamily; the important members and their cell distribution, function, and ligands are summarized in Table 16. The mechanism of leucocyte emigration through the vascular endothelium into tissue is simplistically summarized in Fig. 9. As leucocytes roll in the direction of blood flow, random contact is made with the endothelium. Transient adhesion of leucocytes to the endothelium occurs through low affinity binding to E-selectins. The cells become activated and then bind with higher affinity to vascular integrins. Once cells are firmly attached transendothelial migration occurs and, under the influence of extravascular chemoattractants, subendothelial migration into the extracellular matrix occurs.

Up-regulation of the surface expression of three distinct adhesion molecules, E-selectin, VCAM-1, and ICAM-1, has been shown in biopsies of skin, which is non-lesional and has not been exposed to the sun, from 16 patients with lupus. Levels of adhesion molecules were directly correlated with disease activity and in serial biopsy specimens they decreased with clinical improvement (Belmont *et al*. 1994). These findings suggest that excessive complement activation in association with primed endothelial cells induces leucocyte–endothelial cell adhesion and leuco-occlusive vasculopathy. Furthermore, UV irradiation of keratinocytes *in vitro* induces release of epidermal and dermal cytokines and increases ICAM-1 expression, which *in vivo* may lead to vascular activation culminating in the photosensitive lupus syndromes (Norris 1993).

Soluble forms of adhesion molecules are elevated in the circulation of patients with lupus compared with healthy controls. Elevated levels of soluble ICAM-1 (sICAM-1) have been reported to show significant association with skin involvement and disease activity (Sfikakis *et al*. 1994). Lupus patients also have elevated levels of a soluble form of VCAM-1 (Wellicome *et al*. 1993). The importance of these observations may become apparent from studies in murine lupus which have demonstrated up-regulation of ICAM-1 in nephritic MRL-*lpr/ lpr* and NZB/W kidneys, particularly in the brush borders of proximal tubules, glomerular mesangium, and endothelium of larger vessels (Wuthrich *et al*. 1990). Similarly VCAM-1 is also up-regulated in MRL-*lpr/lpr* kidneys, not only in the endothelium but also in cortical tubules and glomeruli. Kidney tissue sections from nephritic MRL-*lpr/lpr* mice also display increased adhesiveness for T-cell and macrophage cell lines which can be blocked by monoclonal antibodies to ICAM-1 and VCAM-1 (Wuthrich 1992).

Table 16 Adhesion molecules

Family	Member	Cell	Ligand	Function
Selectins	ELAM-1	Endothelial	Leucocyte Surface Carbohydrate	Inflammation, leucocyte extravasation
	CD62	Platelets	?	T-cell recruitment to inflammatory sites
	LECAM-1	T and B cells	?	PMN, lys, monos binding to endothelium
Integrins	LFA-1 (CD11a/CD18)	Lys, PMN, monos Macrophages	ICAM-1,2,3	Tc/target cells, MLR, antigen-specific T-cell proliferation, leucocyte adhesion to endothelium
Immunoglobulin supergene	ICAM-1 (CD54)	Monocytes Endothelial cells CD43	LFA-1 (CD11a/18) MAC-1 (CD11b/18)	T–T, T–B, T–APC interactions. Induced by IFN-γ, IL1β, TNF-α
	VCAM-1	Endothelial cells (act), tissue Mφ	VLA-4	Leucocyte recruitment

ELAM, endothelial leucocyte adhesion molecule; CD, cluster differentiation, LECAM, leucocyte adhesion molecule; LFA, leucocyte function associated molecule; ICAM, intercellular adhesion molecule; PMN, Lys, Monos: polymorphonuclear cells, lymphocytes, monocytes; Tc, T-cytotoxic cells; MLR, mixed lymphocyte reaction; APC, antigen-presenting cell; VCAM-1, vascular cell adhesion molecule; Mφ, macrophages; VLA-4, very late antigen.

Genetic components

The idea that genetic factors may play a role in susceptibility to lupus stems from the high rate of concordance for disease in monozygotic twins, increased frequency of lupus and immunological abnormalities in relatives of patients with lupus, and the prevalence of lupus among certain ethnic groups. The genes which may influence or predispose to lupus include those which determine sex, colour, complement haplotype, tissue type (HLA), antibody variable regions, and T-cell receptors (Table 17).

Sex and ethnic background

At the most basic genetic level systemic lupus affects females more than males and shows an ethnic bias in that Afro-Caribbeans are more affected than Orientals, in turn more affected than Caucasians. These basic differences are reflected in other ways. Sex hormones are known to influence disease in both mice and humans with autoimmune disease. Androgens are immunosuppressive and oestrogens are immunoenhancing. This explains the susceptibility of women to autoimmune diseases compared with men (Ansar Ahmed *et al.* 1985).

For example, androgens reduce while oestrogens enhance the spontaneous antibody production in mixed strains of mice (NZB × CBA and NZB × C3H). In MRL-*lpr/lpr* mice, testosterone treatment reduces lupus-like symptoms without affecting lymphoproliferation. In humans where pregnancy occurs during active disease, exacerbations often occur as oestrogen levels rise.

Complement

Lupus is associated with deficiencies of the early classical pathway of complement components C1, C4, and C2. Two alleles are inherited for each complement component thus deficiencies may be partial or complete (homozygous). Congenital deficiencies of C2 and C4 are frequently in linkage disequilibrium with HLA DR3 and DR2, HLA haplotypes associated with lupus. C4 is composed of two distinct but homologous proteins, C4A and C4B. These bind to immune complexes and prevent precipitation. C4A deficiency is rare in the general population but complete (homozygous) deficiency has been found in 10 to 15 per cent of white patients with lupus. Partial C4A deficiency occurs in 10 to 20 per cent of controls but in 50 to 80 per cent of patients with lupus (Kemp *et al.* 1987). A single null C4A allele increases the relative risk for lupus by 3 and two null alleles by 17. Deficiencies of C4A can arise by two mechanisms; one is a 30 kilobase deletion of the DNA encoding all C4A along with a small portion of C4B and occurs in DR3 + patients (Kemp *et al.* 1987), and the other does not involve a deletion but may be the result of a regulatory gene linked to the MHC causing reduced synthesis of C4A (Fronek *et al.* 1988). The consequence of C4A deficiency in lupus is that immune complex clearance and solubilization is seriously impaired, leading to deposition in lungs and kidneys and subsequent inflammation. C4 is important in drug-induced lupus as the drugs bind to the active site of C4 and prevent covalent binding to immune complexes. C4A is inhibited more than C4B, resulting in a relative deficiency of C4A with consequent defective clearance of immune complexes (Gatenby 1991).

Complement receptors, CR1 and CR2, have been studied in lupus. The CR1 ligands are C3b and C4b bound to immune complexes. The receptor is present on peripheral B lymphocytes, erythrocytes, monocytes, and tissue macrophages and binds, internalizes, processes, and transports immune complexes which have activated complement. Low expression of CR1 on erythrocytes and peripheral blood leucocytes was described in patients with lupus and their healthy family members (Walport and Lachmann 1988).

Table 17 Genetic components associated with systemic lupus erythematosus (SLE)

	Genetic factors		
Complement	C1, C4 deficiencies (>75% prevalence, severe disease) C2 deficiency (~35% prevalence, severity similar to non-C deficient lupus patients) C4 50–80% of patients partially deficient CR1 deficiencies (acquired rather than genetic)		
MHC associations	HLA: A1, B8, DR3—English/Irish patients DR3 and DQw2—anti-Ro/La antibodies DQw1—anti-Ro antibodies DQw6,7,8—lupus anticoagulant DR2—Afro-Caribbean patients with anti-Sm DR2, DQw1 (DQw6), DQ2—susceptibility to nephritis DR4, DQw3—protective? DRw8—early onset SLE (<20 years) Decreased expression of class II on APC Susceptibility may depend upon a single amino acid substitution (histidine→tyrosine at position 30 in sequence of DQw1.19b β gene from single SLE patient compared with healthy control)		
T-cell receptor			
Human	Little data on human TCR family usage Anti-Ro response related to TCR-β gene product in SLE Genomic DNA restriction fragment length polymorphism in humans no deletions, insertions in TCRα,β,γ chain genes.		
Mouse	Cβ deletion in TCR of NZW and NZB × NZW F_1 mice: (a) normal TCR (90 kDa); (b) 'light' TCR (70–85 kDa); latter increases as animals age and as disease and lymphadenopathy develop		
Antibody V genes			
Germ-line encoded	Human monoclonal anti-DNA/Sm germline encoded but use same V gene families as Ab to non-self; thus may not need somatic mutation; genetic predisposition to develop anti-Sm Ab in SLE patients and first degree healthy relatives		
Somatic mutation	↑ somatic mutation (e.g. low concordance between homozygous twins) Autoantibody response generally IgG; somatic mutation increases with immunoglobulin class switch		
Idiotypic analysis	Preferential use of V gene family with or without autoantibody activity (proband vs. family members). Specific deposition of anti-DNA pathogenic/nephritogenic idiotypes in kidney:		
		16/6	*IdGN*	*9G4*
	Percentage SLE	42	75	27
	Percentage disease controls	0	6	0
Ethnic origin	Blacks≫whites; most probably linked to MHC		
Sex and endocrine factors?	Females≫males; oestrogen enhances the immune response; testosterone is immunosuppressive		

MHC, major histocompatibility complex; APC, antigen-presenting cell; TCR, T-cell receptor.

This was originally interpreted as an inherited defect which could predispose to the disease. More recently this defect is thought to be acquired, as normal erythrocytes infused into patients with lupus also showed a decrease in CR1 receptors. Levels of CR1 deficiency in patients with lupus correlate with disease activity. Controversy still abounds in this area as to the precise nature of this defect and is confounded further by the possibility of a functional defect of CR1 receptors on polymorphonuclear neutrophils.

Complement receptor 2, **CR2** (CD21), has recently been described on peripheral T cells in healthy individuals. The ligands for CR2 are C3d, C3g, and Epstein–Barr virus (EBV). The receptor is present on mature, circulating, and lymph node cells, follicular dendritic cells and on 10 to 40 per cent of peripheral blood CD4 + or CD8 + T cells. In patients with active or inactive lupus, B-cell CR2 expression is significantly diminished. This may be a consequence of the activated state of lupus B cells reflecting the loss of CR2 as cells differentiate into immunoglobulin-secreting cells and then plasma cells, or the levels may be modulated by high levels of circulating immune complexes or cytokines. Expression of CR2 on T cells from patients with inactive lupus is similar to that found in healthy individuals, but is increased in some patients with active lupus (90 per cent of CD4 + and CD8 + peripheral T cells expressing increased levels of CR2). In this context CR2 is important in signalling and its increased expression on T cells may play a role in cell adhesion or cytotoxicity (Levy *et al.* 1992).

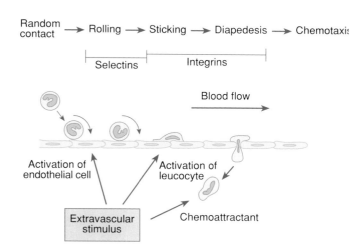

Fig. 9 Adhesive interactions during leucocyte emigration

Major histocompatibility complex

The associations between the MHC and systemic lupus must take into account the ethnic origin of the patient. A recent report highlights this aspect by demonstrating that only in Caucasian patients of English/Irish descent is lupus associated with an MHC extended haplotype (HLA B8, SCO1, DR3) (Schur *et al.* 1990). In black American people DRw52b is positively associated with renal disease and negatively associated with antinuclear RNP antibodies. DR3 (DRw17) and DQw2 are highly associated with the ability to produce anti-Ro/anti-La antibodies. These antibodies are associated with subacute cutaneous lupus, lymphopenia, neonatal lupus and complete congenital heart block. DR4 is associated with the ability to make anti-RNP and with a reduced risk for lupus nephritis. In contrast to the protection conferred by DR4, DR2 confers susceptibility to nephritis. Associations with DQw1 and with DQβ1.AZH and DQβ2 are more recent findings. Early-onset systemic lupus (before 20 years of age) is associated with DRw8 and the frequency of neuropsychiatric involvement correlates negatively with a DQα fragment (Reveille *et al.* 1989). Compared with the normal ethnic population, Afro-Caribbean patients with antibodies to Sm have an increased frequency of DR2 and a reduced frequency of DR3, regardless of anti-DNA antibody status (Olsen *et al.* 1993).

DQw7 correlates significantly with lupus anticoagulant, although there are patients who have lupus anticoagulant but lack the DQw7 haplotype. However these patients all have DQw8. Amino acids in position 71 to 77 of the third hypervariable region of DQB1 chains were identical in DQw7, DQw6, and DQw8 individuals, leading to the proposal that this region might constitute the 'epitope' for mediation of this autoimmune response (Arnett *et al.* 1991). For a more complete description of the known associations between MHC class II genes and autoantibody subsets the reader is referred to an excellent review by Arnett and Reveille (1992).

T-cell receptors (TCR)

Patients with anti-Ro antibodies show association with TCR-β gene products compared with patients with lupus lacking this antibody specificity (Frank *et al.* 1990). The association with this particular gene segment is with the specificity of the autoantibody produced rather than risk factors for the disease. The anti-Ro antibody response

is also associated with HLA-DQw1 (Harley *et al.* 1986) which may be important for recognition by the Ro-specific TCR (Scofield *et al.* 1994). In the lupus-prone mouse strains no evidence of unusual or abnormal TCR gene usage has been demonstrated compared with non-autoimmune mice of the same genetic background (Theofilopoulos *et al.* 1989).

The p70 (Ku) autoantigen has been described as a non-histone nuclear protein recognized by antibodies from patients with lupus. It has been shown that the p70 antigen is a DNA-binding protein and specifically binds to the TCR-β-chain gene enhancer thus playing a role in regulation of TCR-β gene expression (Messier *et al.* 1993).

A human non-specific suppressor factor has been isolated and characterized from lupus ascitic fluid and can inhibit proliferation of T and B cells and suppress IgG production *in vitro*. Suppression was inhibited by anti-TCR-α antibodies but not by those directed against the β chain (Xavier *et al.* 1994).

B-cell immunoglobulin receptors and antibody V genes

The most frequently studied antibodies are those directed against DNA, particularly since anti-idiotypic antibodies raised against the variable regions of murine anti-DNA antibodies have been shown to cross-react with V regions on human anti-DNA antibodies. Many idiotypic markers have been defined on antibodies to DNA and the interpretation of the data has led to much confusion. Only the major findings and their significance with respect to lupus will be discussed.

Several groups have described anti-DNA associated idiotypes defined by anti-idiotype antibodies raised either as monoclonal antibodies in mice or as polyclonal antibodies by immunization of rabbits. In most cases, the immunogen, or anti-DNA antibody-bearing idiotypes, is a human monoclonal antibody made by fusing human B lymphocytes with an immortalized human myeloma/lymphoblastoid cell line to form stable hybridomas which secrete the human antibody of interest. The 16/6 idiotype is located on the heavy chain of a human IgM monoclonal anti-DNA antibody derived from a human lupus spleen hybridoma. The anti-idiotype to the monoclonal antibody bound not only to the parent molecule but to anti-DNA antibodies from different patients with lupus and to IgG lacking anti-DNA activity from healthy relatives, spouses, and family members of patients. Serum levels of the 16/6 idiotype correlated with disease activity and deposits of 16/6 positive immunoglobulin were found in skin and kidney biopsies from patients with lupus(reviewed by Watts and Isenberg 1990).

Among the other DNA antibody idiotypes which have been described are two idiotypic markers which distinguish between nephritogenic antibodies and non-nephritogenic antibodies (Hahn *et al.* 1990). Neither of these idiotypes correlated with HLA class II haplotypes known to be associated with lupus nephritis. High serum levels of idiotypes associated with lupus nephritis are thought to arise from polyclonal B cell activation rather than from idiotype-specific up-regulation associated with one or more of the class II genes that predispose to nephritis. On the contrary, two lupus-associated idiotypes on a somatically mutated anti-DNA antibody have been described, providing evidence that such an antibody reflects the selection pressure of antigen (Davidson *et al.* 1990). However, new data on hybridomas from non-autoimmune strains of mice (Balb/c) shows that pathogenic IgG antibodies with specificity for DNA can be produced by these mice. These antibodies were derived from germ-line genes and were not the products of somatic mutation normally found on antibodies of the same specificity from autoimmune strains of mice. This suggests that such germ-line encoded antibodies are under extremely strict regulation in normal animals. The defect in autoimmunity appears to lie in the products of somatic mutation, possibly at the level of anti-idiotypic regulation (Shefner and Diamond 1990).

The immunoglobulin receptors on B cells are also able to 'present' antigen to T cells. This occurs by binding to antigen-specific immunoglobulin receptors which are then able to internalize antigen and express processed antigen on the cell surface in the context of MHC class II. This process has been demonstrated in mice using snRNP autoantigens which are presented to autoreactive T cells (Mamula *et al.* 1994).

Summary of immunopathological events in systemic lupus

Systemic lupus erythematosus is a multifactorial disease in which the relative contribution of each factor increases the relative risk of disease susceptibility. A significant contribution arises from genetic components, such as those encoding tissue type (MHC), complement components, cell receptors, cytokines, and their respective receptors, together with environmental elements, such as drugs, toxins, diet, and infectious agents. The acquisition of each gene will increase the relative risk of disease development. Genetic predisposition may be so strong that a relatively minor environmental insult may be sufficient to trigger disease, whereas a modest genetic predisposition together with a strong environmental stimulus would be sufficient to lead to manifestations of disease. The latter would encompass idiopathic lupus and drug-induced lupus.

Systemic lupus is characterized by abnormal immune function. Increased numbers of hyperactive B cells, together with impaired cell-mediated immunity, suggest the dominance of Th2 cells and their cytokines in mediating hypergammaglobulinaemia and the appearance of IgG antibodies with specificity for both self and non-self antigens. There is evidence that B cells expand both in response to specific antigen and in a polyclonal fashion.

Molecular mimicry may also contribute to the autoantibody response seen in lupus. Do autoantibodies arise by molecular mimicry (e.g. with viral or bacterial proteins such as anti-U1RNP antibodies and influenza B virus (Guldner *et al.* 1990)) or do they become anti-self and/or pathogenic through somatic mutation of evolutionary 'useful' antibodies and thus bind to host structures/determinants (Diamond and Scharff 1984)?

The transfer of peripheral blood lymphocytes from patients with lupus into SCID mice, described above, which showed deposition of mouse complement and human IgG in the kidneys, suggests that all the information required to cause the histological change associated with lupus resides in the peripheral blood lymphocytes (Duchosal *et al.* 1990). The exact nature of this information remains to be elucidated.

The treatment of lupus

It is evident that the diverse effects of lupus require a variety of treatments. These will be divided into pharmacological and other

Table 18   Treatment of lupus—general measures

1. Rest as appropriate; try to avoid stress.
2. Avoid over-exposure to heat and sunlight. Use sun protection factor 15+ (30+ in USA) if in a sunny country; avoid exposing an arm on an open car window.
3. Try to adhere to a low fat diet and consider adding fish oil derivatives.
4. Vaccination, for foreign travel etc., apart from 'live' vaccines in patients on immunosuppressives, is not contraindicated though the precise nature of the immune response differs from that in healthy individuals.
5. Medium or high oestrogen contraceptive pills should be avoided—progesterone only or the lowest possible oestrogen pill (or other methods of contraception) are advised.
6. The use of hormone replacement in the menopause remains controversial. Many patients do tolerate it without flaring, but not all.

approaches. However, it must be stressed that a number of general measures may be most useful (see Table 18).

Pharmacological

Patients with lupus are treated with four main groups of drugs, often in combination. Recommendations about precisely when to commence therapy, the initial dose of a given drug, the likely response of a given symptom, and the duration of treatment vary widely. In Table 19 the broad indications for use of these four types of drugs are shown. In Table 20 suggestions are provided as to the initial doses and duration of treatment with the antimalarials, corticosteroids, and cytotoxic drugs. These are intended purely as guidelines and there will undoubtedly be patients who require larger doses for longer periods of time.

In general the patient with mildly active lupus can be managed with combinations of non-steroidal anti-inflammatory drugs and antimalarials. Patients with lupus are at no lesser risk of gastrointestinal and renal complications of the non-steroidal anti-inflammatory drugs than other patients and thus the usual type of monitoring (clinical history, blood tests) is required. Hydroxychloroquine (Plaquenil) is the antimalarial drug of choice. It is still recommended by some authorities that ophthalmological examinations are undertaken approximately every 9 months to ensure that no retinal damage is occurring.

Corticosteroids in the main are required when non-steroidal anti-inflammatory drugs and antimalarials are insufficient to relieve the patients symptoms. Thus severe arthritis, pleuritis, pericarditis, autoimmune haemolytic anaemia, thrombocytopenia, nephritis, and a wide range of neuropsychiatric problems frequently require treatment with corticosteroids.

Corticosteroids are usually prescribed and taken by mouth but they may also be given intramuscularly and intravenously. Intravenous or pulse therapy has been widely used in the past 15 years. If given over a

Table 19 Drug therapy in systemic lupus

	NSAID	Antimalarial	Corticosteroids	Cytoxic agents
Malaise	−	+	+	−
Fever	+	−	+	−
Serositis	+	−	+	−
Arthralgia	+	+	+	−
Arthritis	+	+	+	+
Myalgia	+	+	+	−
Myositis	−	−	+	+
Malar/discoid rash	−	+	+	−
Pneumonitis	−	−	+	+
Carditis	−	−	+	+
Vasculitis	−	−	+	+
CNS disease	−	−	?[a]	?
Renal	−	−	+	+
Haemolytic anaemia	−	−	+	+
Thrombocytopenia	−	−	+	+
Raynaud's	−	−	?	?
Alopecia	−	−	?	?

+=usually beneficial; −=not beneficial; ?=dubious/controversial.
[a]widely prescribed but doubts remain that steroids are beneficial in many cases.

Table 20 Recommendations for drug usage in lupus

Symptom	Drugs to try	Dose and duration
Arthralgia	Non-steroidal anti-inflammatory drugs	No special recommendations
Myalgia Lethargy Arthralgia	Hydroxychloroquine	Start 400 mg/day for 3–4 months then reduce to 200 mg/day for 3–4 months, then to 200 mg five times week for 3 to 4 months; repeat courses may be necessary and retinal checks every 6–9 months are generally recommended
Arthritis Pleuritis Pericarditis	Prednisolone	20–40 mg per day initially for 2–4 weeks, reducing in 5–10 mg increments per week, if patient is responding; treatment is likely to be required for several months
Autoimmune haemolytic anaemia/thrombocytopenia	Prednisolone often accompanied by azathioprine	60–80 mg prednisolone for 1–2 weeks reducing in 10 mg increments in response to the blood test results; aim for 2.5–3 mg/kg azathioprine; treatment will last for several months
Renal	Prednisolone plus azathioprine or cyclophosphamide	Depending upon the severity of the renal lesion, anything from 30–80 mg/day is required; cyclophosphamide can be given by intravenous boluses (750 mg–1 g) monthly for 6 months, then every 3 months for 2 years; some groups prefer prednisolone and azathioprine at 2–3 mg/kg in the first instance; treatment is likely to be required for several years
Central nervous system	Prednisolone plus an appropriate drug, e.g. an antidepressant, anticonvulsant, etc.	Controversial — but 20–100 mg prednisolone have been prescribed (sometimes accompanied by azathioprine or intravenous cyclophosphamide pulses); treatment is likely to be required for months

Box 1 Flow diagram of the management of systemic lupus that forms the basis of our practice

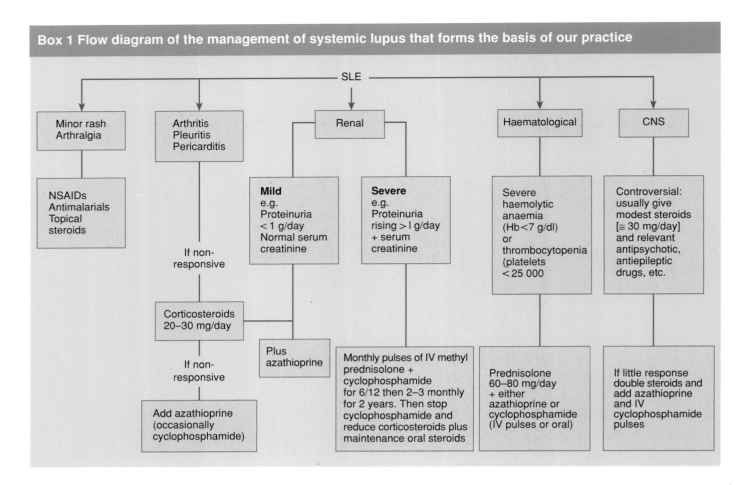

15 to 20-min period there is a danger of reactive arthropathy, and in our experience intravenous pulses are best given slowly over a 3 to 4-h period. We use pulse therapy: for example, 1 g on 3 successive days for patients with severe disease which does not seem to be responding to oral corticosteroids. Although some claims have been made about the advantages of this type of approach, the evidence that anything more than a temporary benefit is obtained is controversial.

Some centres have attempted to use alternate-day oral steroid regimes, although the evidence that there is a reduction in the number or the severity of side-effects compared with daily use is lacking. The major side-effects, however corticosteroids are prescribed, are increased risk of infection, osteoporosis, diabetes, hypertension, cushingoid facies, abdominal striae, and insomnia. Corticosteroids are thus no panacea.

Various control trials of cytotoxic drugs in lupus have been reported. The group from the National Institutes of Health at Bethesda has argued strongly that intravenous boluses of cyclophosphamide, monthly for 6 months, subsequently once every 3 months for 2 years, are the treatment of choice in patients with severe renal involvement (Boumpas *et al.* 1991; Boumpas *et al.* 1992; Boumpas *et al.* 1993). The problems of side-effects with this drug (profound nausea, alopecia, infertility especially in patients over 30, and bone marrow suppression) have made others more wary about its routine use. In common with many European groups we prefer to use steroids and maintenance azathioprine in the first instance for patients with mild/moderately active renal disease. Occasionally however, we have seen patients being treated with steroids and

azathioprine for other manifestations who develop severe renal disease and require cyclophosphamide urgently. For patients with endstage renal disease, kidney dialysis and kidney transplantation are available. Interestingly, it is rare for a patient with lupus with a transplanted kidney to develop lupus nephritis in the new organ. A flow diagram of the way we use drugs to treat the various aspects of lupus is shown in Box 1.

Other treatments

In the late 1970s and early 1980s there was a great vogue for using plasma exchange. The concept was that the removal of circulating, presumptively pathogenic, immune complexes offered a therapeutic advantage. In practice, it became evident that in some patients a 'rebound' phenomenon occurred in which patients' symptoms and signs dramatically improved but returned within a few days or weeks. This form of treatment requires good venous access, much patience on the part of both physician and patient, and is extremely expensive. A double-blind study using a sham exchange procedure has been performed in mild lupus. The frequency and degree of clinical improvement was the same in both groups (Wei *et al.* 1983). In common with most units we now reserve plasma exchange for those patients seemingly resistant to conventional drug therapy. Attempts are currently being made to achieve a more synchronized deletion of immunoglobulins followed by cyto-toxic therapy. Autologous stem cell transplants are also now being considered for lupus.

Lymphoid radiation

Fractionated total lymphoid irradiation, a radiotherapy technique adapted from the method used to treat Hodgkin's disease was shown to improve the survival of NZB/W mice. There have been conflicting opinions as to its value in human patients with lupus. This treatment had not found widespread acceptance. Another form of radiation using ultraviolet A1, has been shown to reduce disease activity in patients in a provisional study (McGrath 1994).

Diet therapy

Many patients with lupus are anxious to know if some form of dietary modification might be of help. It is now well established that diet content can affect the course of disease in NZB/W and MRL-*lpr/lpr* mice. Although some benefits have been demonstrated from total calorie restriction, a restricted amino acid diet, and one in which dietary zinc is reduced, the influence of dietary fat on autoimmunity, certainly in the mouse, appears to be particularly important. In addition, supplementation of the diet by fish oils has been shown to be beneficial. In a recent double-blind, cross-over study in which patients with lupus were put on to low fat diets, those who were concurrently taking 10 g of fish oil per day were shown to have done significantly better over a 3-month period (Walton *et al.* 1991).

Intravenous high-dose gammaglobulins

Intravenous high-dose gammaglobulins may be effective in the treatment of immune thrombocytopenic purpura, immune neutropenia, and myasthenia gravis. It has also been used with moderate success in patients with lupus with low platelet counts. A claim that it was of value in patients with severe renal lupus has not been substantiated. When this approach does not work for patients with thrombocytopenia, splenectomy is beneficial in four or five out of six cases, provided the problem has not been left to become long-term and chronic (Silvestris *et al.* 1994).

Sex hormone therapy

Given the marked predilection of lupus for females, it is not surprising that attempts have been made to treat the condition by manipulating the level of sex hormones.

However, the clinical use of sex hormones in lupus and other autoimmune diseases has neither been extensive nor particularly successful. One drug, danazol, an androgen with reduced virilizing capacity has been used by several groups; as is so often the case with new drugs, the initial optimism has given way to the view that it adds little to the treatment of lupus.

Treatment of experimental lupus

The occurrence of spontaneous lupus in mice has the advantage that manipulation of the disease *in vivo* may be studied. Early studies in the MRL-*lpr/lpr* strain showed that neonatal removal of the thymus delayed the onset of disease to resemble that of the congenic MRL[+/+] strain. This implicated T cells in the pathogenesis of the disease. Attempts to down-regulate autoantibody production by treatment with anti-idiotype were initially successful in suppressing idiotype-positive anti-DNA antibodies in MRL-*lpr/lpr* mice. Subsequently new clones of idiotype-negative anti-DNA-positive antibodies emerged (Hahn and Ebling 1984). Treatment of both NZB/W F1 and MRL-*lpr/lpr* mice with a monoclonal antibody directed against

the CD4 receptor on T helper/inducer cells also improved the clinical status of these animals (Wofsy and Seaman 1985; Santoro *et al.* 1988).

Infection of lupus-prone NZB/W F$_1$ mice with the parasite *Plasmodium chabaudi* retards the development of their autoimmune disease. Survival was prolonged and high-grade proteinuria and IgG anti-DNA antibodies were delayed for 6 months when parasite inoculation was given either before (3 months) or after (7 months) the onset of the clinical symptoms. Similar beneficial effects, although less pronounced, were obtained when mice were treated with IgG or IgM or cryoglobulin preparations isolated from *P. chabaudi*-infected BALB/c mice, while similarly prepared fractions from uninfected mice had little effect. In surviving mice, levels of anti-DNA antibodies, particularly the IgG1 isotype, were significantly decreased. Flow cytometric analysis of various T-cell subsets showed that the number of T cells expressing Vβ 8.1,2, Vβ 10 and Vβ 14 TCR antigens, which increased with age, were significantly reduced. The mode of therapeutic action is thought to arise from the malarial induction of high levels of natural antibodies bearing the D23 idiotype characteristic of polyreactive natural autoantibodies with enhanced activity against Fab and Fc fragments of IgG. These antibodies have immunoregulatory properties and attempt, at least transitorily, to rescue a natural autoantibody network that is deficient in B/W mice (Hentati *et al.* 1994). These experiments may parallel the findings of human disease treated with intravenous gammaglobulin.

As with human disease, experimental models of lupus have become the focus of much research into cytokine-directed therapeutic intervention. In NZB/W F$_1$ mice, administration of interferon-γ aggravated the autoimmune response, whereas monoclonal antibodies to interferon-γ (Jacob *et al.* 1990b) and replacement therapy with recombinant tumour necrosis factor-α (TNF-α) delayed disease development (Jacob and McDevitt 1988). Significantly serum TNF-α levels increased in anti-IL-10 treated NZB/W mice while disease onset was delayed. Simultaneous treatment with a neutralizing antibody to TNF-α at the same time as anti-IL-10 treatment resulted in the rapid onset of lupus and increased mortality supporting the concept that TNF-α is protective in this model. Similarly the role of IL-10 was confirmed to accelerate disease by direct administration of recombinant IL-10 (Ishida *et al.* 1994).

In the same strain of mice, chronic treatment with rat monoclonal antibodies to IL-6 prevented anti-dsDNA antibody production, decreased proteinuria, and prolonged life, provided that mice attained tolerance to rat immunoglobulin by a single injection of anti-CD4 antibodies at the start of therapy (Finck *et al.* 1994). Treatment of MRL-*lpr/lpr* mice for 5 weeks at 15 weeks of age with neutralizing antibodies to the IL-6 receptor showed improvements in glomerular structure and function and a decrease in anti-dsDNA antibodies after 2 weeks of treatment but a gradual increase by week 4 (Kiberd 1993).

A novel 'T-cell vaccination' in MRL-*lpr/lpr* mice has shown a highly significant amelioration of disease parameters. Intravenous administration of irradiated *lpr* cells recovered from hyperplastic lymph nodes of adult diseased animals to young MRL-*lpr/lpr* mice resulted in selective depletion of Vβ 8.2 T cells in lymph nodes, in addition to eliciting a surge in peripheral T cells capable of conferring disease protection in adoptive transfer experiments (De Alboran *et al.* 1992).

The major reversal of disease in MRL-*lpr/lpr* mice has been described in the section on experimental models of lupus and refers

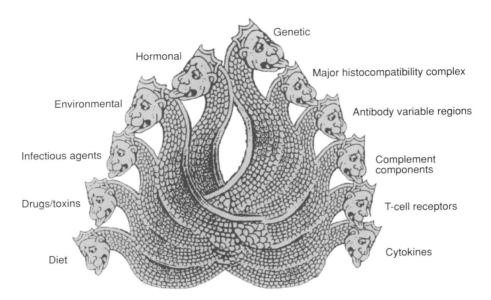

Hormonal

Genetic

Environmental

Major histocompatibility complex

Infectious agents

Antibody variable regions

Drugs/toxins

Complement components

Diet

T-cell receptors

Cytokines

Fig. 10 The Hydra—an analogy of the multiple factors involved in lupus.

to the introduction of the *Fas* gene under the control of the CD2 promoter and enhancer (Wu *et al.* 1994).

Treatment of autoimmune mice with drugs used for humans allows not only efficacy but also the mode of action to be tested. For example, dexamethasone given to MRL-*lpr/lpr* mice from 4 weeks of age, prevents lymphadenopathy and renal injury (proteinuria), suppresses a fourfold increase in MHC class II antigen expression (22 weeks), but has no effect on the costimulatory molecules ICAM-1 and TNF-α (Jevnikar *et al.* 1992). Similarly, methylprednisolone down-regulates renal expression of endothelin-1 and its receptors, TGF-β and TNF-α mRNA in NZB/W mice and suppresses development of renal histological lesions (Nakamura *et al.* 1993).

A low fat diet has been reported to delay disease symptoms in MRL-*lpr/lpr* mice (Morrow *et al.* 1986). Since then the nature of marine long-chain fatty acids in the diet has been investigated in female NZB/W mice fed diets containing 10 per cent fish oil, with control mice fed diets containing 10 per cent corn oil. Compared with control mice those maintained on a diet rich in marine oils had an extended life span, later onset of proteinuria, increased proliferative responses to T-cell mitogens, and decreased circulating anti-dsDNA antibodies. Splenocyte analysis compared with controls showed decreased Ig+, higher lymphocyte ECAM-1 expression, elevated mRNA for IL-2, IL-4, and TGF-β, and higher TGF-β, lower c-Myc and c-Ha-Ras proteins. Changes in membrane fatty acid composition may contribute to the altered immune function and gene expression during the development of murine lupus (Fernandes *et al.* 1994).

Prognosis and survival

Studies on duration of disease and overall survival rates have frequently been confounded by the numbers of patients lost to follow-up and inadequate attention paid to the ethnic group, age of onset, and socio-economic status of individual patients. With these possible confounding factors in mind, and the division of patients with lupus into those with overt nephritis and those without, it is reasonable to state that the 5-year survival in lupus is presently 90 per cent or greater, but at 15 years only 60 per cent of those with nephritis will still be alive compared with around 85 per cent of those without nephritis. In the United States, it has been claimed that black patients with lupus, males, those from poorer socio-economic groups, and possibly children, have poorer survival, especially if nephritis is present. It has also been suggested that there exists a bimodal mortality curve. Patients who die within 5 years usually have very active disease, with a requirement for substantial doses of steroids and other immunosuppressives. Those patients dying much later tend to do so from cardiovascular disease and possibly infection. Overall most patients with lupus die from active generalized disease, nephritis, sepsis, and cardiovascular disease. Evidence that patients are more predisposed to malignancy has been discussed earlier in the chapter but this seems to be a relatively minor cause of death in lupus.

Summary

In the introduction to this chapter an analogy was drawn between systemic lupus erythematosus and the Hydra monster of Greek legend. In Fig. 10 this analogy is reiterated to confirm the multiple factors involved in the aetiology and pathogenesis of lupus. It is evident that this remarkable disease presents a wide spectrum of clinical features and is characterized by multiple autoantibodies, although clearly not due to random polyclonal B-cell activation. The treatment and general management of lupus continues to present a challenge. While lupus may for some patients represent a relatively mild set of problems, many others require large doses of immunosuppressive drugs which carry long-term concerns about side-effects.

References

Abramson, S., Kramer, S.B., Radin, A., and Holzman, R. (1985). Salmonella bacteremia in systemic lupus erythematosus. Eight year experience at a municipal hospital. *Arthritis and Rheumatism*, **28**, 75–9.

Ansar Ahmed, S., Penhale, W.J., and Talal, N. (1985). Sex hormones, immune responses and autoimmune diseases: mechanisms of sex hormone action. *American Journal of Pathology*, **121**, 531–51.

Aringer, M. *et al.* (1994). High levels of bcl-2 protein in circulating T lymphocytes, but not B lymphocytes, of patients with systemic lupus erythematosus. *Arthritis and Rheumatism*, **37**, 1423–30.

Arnett, F.C. and Reveille, J.D. (1992). Genetics of systemic lupus erythematosus. [Review.] *Rheumatic Disease Clinics of North America*, **18**, 865–92.

Arnett, F.C., Olsen, M., Anderson, K., and Reveille, J.D. (1991). Molecular analysis of major histocompatibility complex alleles associated with the lupus anticoagulant. *Journal of Clinical Investigation*, **87**, 1490–5.

Ashany, D., Hines, J., Gharavi, A., Mouradian, J., and Elkon, K.B. (1992*a*). Analysis of autoantibody production in SCID-systemic lupus erythematosus (SLE) chimeras. *Clinical and Experimental Immunology*, **88**, 84–90.

Ashany, D., Hines, J.J., Gharavi, A.E., Mouradian, J., Drappa, J., and Elkon, K.B. (1992*b*). MRL/lpr — severe combined immunodeficiency mouse allografts produce autoantibodies, acute graft-versus-host disease or a wasting syndrome depending on the source of cells. *Clinical and Experimental Immunology*, **90**, 466–75.

Belmont, H.M., Buyon, J., Giorno, R., and Abramson, S. (1994). Up-regulation of endothelial cell adhesion molecules characterizes disease activity in systemic lupus erythematosus. The Shwartzman phenomenon revisited. *Arthritis and Rheumatism*, **37**, 376–83.

Bhalla, R. *et al.* (1993). Systemic lupus erythematosus and Hodgkin's lymphoma. *Journal of Rheumatology*, **20**, 1316–20.

Blanco, F.J., De La Mata, J., Lopez-Fernandez, J.I., and Gomez-Reino, J.J. (1994). Light, immunofluorescence and electron microscopy renal biopsy findings as predictors of mortality in 85 Spanish patients with systemic lupus erythematosus. *British Journal of Rheumatology*, **33**, 260–6.

Bonfa, E. *et al.* (1987). Association between lupus psychosis and anti-ribosomal P protein antibodies. *New England Journal of Medicine*, **317**, 265–71.

Boumpas, D.T. *et al.* (1991). Pulse cyclophosphamide for severe neuropsychiatric lupus. *Quarterly Journal of Medicine*, **81**, 975–84.

Boumpas, D.T. *et al.* (1992). Controlled trial of methyl prednisolone versus two regimens of pulse cyclophosphamide in severe lupus nephritis. *Lancet*, **340**, 741–5.

Boumpas, D.T. *et al.* (1993). Risk for sustained amenorrhea in patients with systemic lupus erythematosus receiving intermittent pulse cyclophosphamide therapy. *Annals of Internal Medicine*, **119**, 366–9.

Callen, J.P. and Klein, J. (1988). Subacute cutaneous lupus erythematosus. *Arthritis and Rheumatism*, **31**, 1007–13.

Cervera, R. *et al.* (1992). Systemic lupus erythematosus: clinical and immunologic patterns of disease expression in a cohort of 1000 patients. *Medicine (Baltimore)*, **72**, 113–24.

Cheng, J. *et al.* (1994). Identification of a soluble form of the fas molecule that protects cells from fas-mediated apoptosis. *Science*, **263**, 1759–61.

Crow, M.K. *et al.* (1994). Autoantigen-specific T cell proliferation induced by the ribosomal P2 protein in patients with systemic lupus erythematosus. *Journal of Clinical Investigation*, **94**, 345–52.

Davidson, A., Manheimer-Lory, A., Aranow, C., Peterson, R., Hannigan, N., and Diamond, B. (1990). Molecular characterisation of a somatically mutated anti-DNA antibody bearing two systemic lupus erythematosus-related idiotypes. *Journal of Clinical Investigation*, **85**, 1401–9.

Deapen, D. *et al.* (1992). A revised estimate of twin concordance in systemic lupus erythematosus. *Arthritis and Rheumatism*, **35**, 311–8.

De Alboran, I.M. *et al.* (1992). lpr T cells vaccinate against lupus in MRL/lpr mice. *European Journal of Immunology*, **22**, 1089–93.

Diamond, B. and Scharff, M. (1984). Somatic mutation of the T15 heavy chain gives rise to an antibody with autoantibody specificity. *Proceedings of the National Academy of Sciences (USA)*, **81**, 841–4.

Dubois, W.L. and Tuffenelli, D.L. (1964). Clinical manifestations of systemic lupus erythematosus. *Journal of the American Medical Association*, **190**, 104–11.

Duchosal, M.A., McConahey, P.J., Robinson, C.A., and Dixon, F.J. (1990). Transfer of human systemic lupus erythematosus in severe combined immunodeficient (SCID) mice. *Journal of Experimental Medicine*, **172**, 985–8.

Ehrenstein, M.R., Katz, D.R., Griffiths, M.H., Papadeki, L., Winkler, T.H., Kalden, J.R., and Isenberg, D.A. (1995). Human IgG anti-DNA antibodies deposit in kidneys and induce proteinurea in SCID mice. *Kidney International*, **48**, 705–11.

Erkeller-Yuksel, F., Isenberg, D.A., Dhillon, V.B., Latchman, D.S., and Lydyard, P.M. (1992). Surface expression of heat shock protein 90 by blood mononuclear cells from patients with systemic lupus erythematosus. *Journal of Autoimmunity*, **5**, 803–14.

Estes, D. and Christian, C. (1971). The natural history of systemic lupus erythematosus. *Medicine*, **50**, 85–95.

Feinglass, E.J., Arnett, F.C., Dorsch, D.A., Zizic, T.M., and Stevens, M.B. (1976). Neuropsychiatric manifestations of systemic lupus erythematosus: diagnosis, clinical spectrum and relationship to other features of the disease. *Medicine*, **55**, 323–37.

Fernandes, G., Bysani, C., Venkatraman, J.T., Tomar, V., and Zhao, W. (1994). Increased TGF-beta and decreased oncogene expression by omega-3 fatty acids in the spleen delays onset of autoimmune disease in B/W mice. *Journal of Immunology*, **152**, 5979–87.

Fessel, W.J. (1988). Epidemiology of systemic lupus erythematosus. *Rheumatic Disease Clinics of North America*, **14**, 15–23.

Finck, B.K., Chan, B., and Wofsy, D. (1994). Interleukin 6 promotes murine lupus in NZB/NZW F1 mice. *Journal of Clinical Investigation*, **94**, 585–91.

Frank, M.B., McArthur, R., Harley, J.B., and Fujisaku, A. (1990). Anti-Ro (SS-A) autoantibodies are associated with T cell receptor β genes in systemic lupus erythematosus patients. *Journal of Clinical Investigation*, **85**, 33–9.

Fries, J., Porta, J., and Liang, M.H. (1978). Marginal benefit of renal biopsy in systemic lupus erythematosus. *Archives of Internal Medicine*, **138**, 1386–9.

Fronek, Z. *et al.* (1988). Major histocompatibility complex associations with systemic lupus erythematosus. *American Journal of Medicine*, **85**, 42–4.

Furie, R.A. and Chartash, E.K. (1988). Tendon rupture in systemic lupus erythematosus. *Seminars in Arthritis and Rheumatism*, **18**, 127–33.

Galli, M. *et al.* (1990). Anticardiolipin antibodies (ACA) directed not to cardiolipin but to a plasma protein cofactor. *Lancet*, **335**, 1544–7.

Gatenby, P.A. (1991). The role of complement in the aetiopathogenesis of systemic lupus erythematosus. [Review.] *Autoimmunity*, **11**, 61–6.

Gemelig-Meyling, F., Dawisha, S., and Steinberg, A. (1992). Assessment of in vivo frequency of mutated T cells in patients with systemic lupus erythematosus. *Journal of Experimental Medicine*, **175**, 297–300.

Geppert, T.D. and Jasin, H.E. (1990). Immunoglobulin (Ig) and autoantibody production in mice with severe combined immunodeficiency (SCID) injected with lymphocytes from patients with systemic lupus erythematosus (SLE). *Arthritis and Rheumatism*, **33** (Suppl.), 599.

Gladman, D.D. *et al.* (1994). Sensitivity to change of 3 systemic lupus erythematosus disease activity indices: international validation. *Journal of Rheumatology*, **21**, 1468–71.

Gladman, D.D. *et al.* (1996). The development and initial validation of the Systemic Lupus International Collaborating Clinics/American College of Rheumatology damage index for systemic lupus erythematosus. *Arthritis and Rheumatism*, **39**, 363–9.

Goulet, J.R., Mackenzie, T., Lewinton, C., Hayslett, J.P., Campi, A., and Esdaile, J.M. (1993). The long term prognosis of lupus nephritis: the impact of disease activity. *Journal of Rheumatology*, **20**, 59–65.

Grigor, R., Edmonds, J., Lewkonia, R., Bresnihan, B., and Hughes, G.R.V. (1978). Systemic lupus erythematosus. A prospective analysis. *Annals of the Rheumatic Diseases*, **37**, 121–8.

Guldner, H.H., Netter, H.J., Szostecki, C., Jaeger, E., and Will, H. (1990). Human anti-p68 autoantibodies recognise a common epitope of nuclear ribonucleoprotein and influenza B virus. *Journal of Experimental Medicine*, **171**, 819–29.

Hahn, B.H. and Ebling, F.M. (1984). Suppression of murine lupus nephritis by administration of anti-idiotypic antibody to anti-DNA. *Journal of Immunology*, **132**, 187–90.

Hahn, B.H. *et al.* (1990). Idiotypic characteristics of immunoglobulins associated with human systemic lupus erythematosus. *Arthritis and Rheumatism*, **33**, 978–84.

Hanley, J.G. *et al.* (1993). Cognitive impairment and autoantibodies in systemic lupus erythematosus. *British Journal of Rheumatology*, **32**, 291–6.

Harley, J.B., Reichlin, M., Arnett, F.C., Alexander, E.L., Bias, W.B., and Provost, T.T. (1986). Gene interaction at HLA-DQ enhances autoantibody production in primary Sjögren's syndrome. *Science*, 232, 1145–7.

Haupt, P.M., Moore, W.G., and Hutchins, G.M. (1981). The lung in systemic lupus erythematosus. Analysis of the pathologic changes in 120 patients. *American Journal of Medicine*, 71, 791–7.

Hay, E.M. and Isenberg, D.A. (1993). Autoantibodies in central nervous system lupus. *British Journal of Rheumatology*, 32, 329–32.

Hay, E.M. *et al.* (1993). The BILAG index: a reliable and valid instrument for measuring clinical disease activity in systemic lupus erythematosus. *Quarterly Journal of Medicine*, 86, 447–58.

Hentati, B., Sato, M.N., Payelle-Brogard, B., Avrameas, S., and Ternynck, T. (1994). Beneficial effect of polyclonal immunoglobulins from malaria-infected BALB/c mice on the lupus-like syndrome of (NZB × NZW)F1 mice. *European Journal of Immunology*, 24, 8–15.

Hishikawa, T. *et al.* (1990). HLA-DP + T cells and deficient interleukin-2 production in patients with systemic lupus erythematosus. *Clinical Immunology and Immunopathology*, 55, 285–96.

Hoffbrand, B.I. and Beck, E.R. (1965). 'Unexplained' dyspnoea and shrinking lungs in systemic lupus erythematosus. *British Medical Journal*, 1, 1273–7.

Hopkinson, N.D., Doherty, M., and Powell, R.J. (1993). The prevalence and incidence of systemic lupus erythematosus in Nottingham, UK, 1989–1990. *British Journal of Rheumatology*, 32, 110–15.

Horsfall, A.C., Rose, L.M., and Maini, R.N. (1989). Autoantibody synthesis in salivary glands of Sjögren's patients. *Journal of Autoimmunity*, 2, 559–68.

Horwitz, D.A. and Jacob, C.O. (1994). The cytokine network in the pathogenesis of systemic lupus erythematosus and possible therapeutic implications. *Springer Seminars in Immunopathology*, 16, 181–200.

Isenberg, D.A. (1983). Immunoglobulin deposition in skeletal muscle in primary muscle disease. *Quarterly Journal of Medicine*, 52, 297–310.

Isenberg, D.A. and Malick, J. (1994). Male lupus — the Loch Ness syndrome revisited. *British Journal of Rheumatology*, 33, 307–8.

Isenberg, D.A. and Snaith, M.L. (1981). Muscle disease in SLE: a study of its nature, frequency and cause. *Journal of Rheumatology*, 8, 917–24.

Ishida, H., Muchamuel, T., Sakaguchi, S., Andrade, S., Menon, S., and Howard, M. (1994). Continuous administration of anti-interleukin 10 antibodies delays onset of autoimmunity in NZB/W F1 mice. *Journal of Experimental Medicine*, 179, 301–10.

Ishikawa, O., Ohnishi, K., Miyachi, Y., and Ishizaka, H. (1994). Cerebral lesions in systemic lupus erythematosus detected by magnetic resonance imaging. Relationship to anti-cardiolipin antibody. *Journal of Rheumatology*, 21, 87–90.

Izui, S., Elder, J.H., McConahey, P.J., and Dixon, F.J. (1981). Identification of retroviral gp70-anti-gp70 antibodies involved in circulating immune complexes in NZB × NZW mice. *Journal of Experimental Medicine*, 153, 1151–60.

Jacob, C.O. and McDevitt, H.O. (1988). Tumour necrosis factor-α in murine autoimmune 'lupus' nephritis. *Nature*, 331, 356–8.

Jacob, C.O., Fronek, Z., Lewis, G.D., Koo, M., Hansen, J.A., and McDevitt, H.O. (1990a). Heritable major histocompatibility complex class II-associated differences in relevance to genetic predisposition to systemic lupus erythematosus. *Proceedings of the National Academy of Sciences (USA)*, 87, 1233–37.

Jacob, C.O., van der Meide, P.H., and McDevitt, H.O. (1990b). *In vivo* treatment of (NZB × NZW) F1 lupus-like nephritis with monoclonal antibody to γ interferon. *Journal of Experimental Medicine*, 166, 798–803.

Jevnikar, A.M., Singer, G.G., Brennan, D.C., Xu, H.W., and Kelley, V.R. (1992). Dexamethasone prevents autoimmune nephritis and reduces renal expression of Ia but not costimulatory signals. *American Journal of Pathology*, 141, 743–51.

Johnson, A.E., Gordon, C., Palmer, R.G., and Bacon, P.A. (1995). The prevalence and incidence of systemic lupus erythematosus (SLE) in Birmingham, UK, related to ethnicity and country of birth. *Arthritis and Rheumatism*, 38, 551–8.

Kahl, L.E. (1994). Herpes zoster infections in systemic lupus erythematosus: risk factors and outcome. *Journal of Rheumatology*, 21, 84–6.

Kalsi, J. *et al.* (1996). Functional and structural analysis of the binding of four human monoclonal anti-DNA antibodies. *Molecular Immunology*, 33, 471–83.

Kalunian, K.C. *et al.* (1989). Idiotypic characteristics of immunoglobulins associated with systemic lupus erythematosus. *Arthritis and Rheumatism*, 32, 513–22.

Kammer, G.M. and Stein, R.L. (1990). T lymphocyte dysfunctions in systemic lupus erythematosus. *Journal of Laboratory and Clinical Medicine*, 115, 273–82.

Kanai, Y., Tokano, Y., Tsuda, H., Hashimoto, H., Okumura, K., and Hirose, S. (1993). HLA-DP positive T cells in patients with polymyositis/dermatomyositis. *Journal of Rheumatology*, 20, 77–9.

Karsh, J., Klippel, J., Balow, J.E., and Decker, J.L. (1979). Mortality in lupus nephritis. *Arthritis and Rheumatism*, 22, 764–9.

Kaufman, L.D., Heinicke, M.H., Hamberger, M., and Corevic, P.D. (1989). Male lupus: retrospective analysis of the clinical and laboratory features of 52 patients, with a review of the literature. *Seminars in Arthritis and Rheumatism*, 18, 189–97.

Keeling, D.M. and Isenberg, D.A. (1993). Haematological manifestations of systemic lupus erythematosus. *Blood Reviews*, 7, 199–207.

Kelley, V.R., Diaz-Gallo, C., Jevnikar, A.M., and Singer, G.G. (1993). Renal tubular epithelial and T cell interactions in autoimmune renal disease. [Review.] *Kidney International*, 39 (Suppl.), S108–15.

Kemp, M.E., Atkinson, J.P., Skanes, V.M., Levine, R.P., and Chaplin, D.D. (1987). Deletion of C4A genes in patients with systemic lupus erythematosus. *Arthritis and Rheumatism*, 30, 1015–22.

Khamashta, M.A. *et al.* (1990). Association of antibodies against phospholipids with heart valve disease in systemic lupus erythematosus. *Lancet*, 335, 1541–4.

Kiberd, B.A. (1993). Interleukin-6 receptor blockage ameliorates murine lupus nephritis. *Journal of the American Society of Nephrology*, 4, 58–61.

Koh, W.H., Fong, K.R., Boeg, N.L., Feng, P.H. (1994). Systemic lupus erythematosus in 61 oriental males. A study of clinical and laboratory manifestations. *British Journal of Rheumatology*, 33, 339–42.

Krapf, F.E., Herrmann, M., Leitman, W., and Kalden, J.R. (1989). Are retroviruses involved in the pathogenesis of SLE? Evidence demonstrated by molecular analysis of nucleic acids from SLE patients' plasma. *Rheumatology International*, 9, 115–21.

Lahita, R.G., Chiorazzi, N., Gibofsky, A., Winchester, R.J., and Kunkel, H.G. (1983). Familial systemic lupus erythematosus in males. *Arthritis and Rheumatism*, 26, 39–44.

Leaker, M., McGregor, A., Griffiths, M., Snaith, M., Neild, G., and Isenberg, D.A. (1991). Insidious loss of renal function in patients with anti-cardiolipin antibodies and absence of overt nephritis. *Annals of the Rheumatic Diseases*, 30, 422–5.

Lee, S.S., Li, C.S., and Li, P.C.H. (1993). Clinical profile of Chinese patients with systemic lupus erythematosus. *Lupus*, 2, 105–9.

Leung, W.H., Wong, K.L., Lau, C.P., Wong, C.K., and Liu, H.W. (1990). Association between antiphospholipid antibodies and cardiac abnormalities in patients with systemic lupus erythematosus. *American Journal of Medicine*, 89, 411–9.

Levy, E., Ambrus, J., Kahl, L., Molina, H., Tung, K., and Holers, V.M. (1992). T lymphocyte expression of complement receptor 2 (CR2/CD21): a role in adhesive cell–cell interactions and dysregulation in a patient with systemic lupus erythematosus (SLE). *Clinical and Experimental Immunology*, 90, 235–44.

Liang, M.H., Sacher, S.A., Neal Roberts, W., and Esdaile, J.M. (1988). Measurement of systemic lupus erythematosus activity in clinical research. *Arthritis and Rheumatism*, 31, 817–25.

Libman, E. and Sachs, B. (1924). A hitherto undescribed form of valvular and mural endocarditis. *Archives of Internal Medicine (Chicago)*, 33, 701–9.

Love, P.E. and Santoro, S.A. (1990). Anti-phospholipid antibodies: anticardiolipin and the lupus anticoagulant in systemic lupus erythematosus (SLE) and in non-SLE disorders. *Annals of Internal Medicine*, 112, 682–98.

Lynch, A. *et al.* (1994). Anti-phospholipid antibodies in predicting adverse pregnancy outcome — a prospective study. *Annals of Internal Medicine*, 15, 470–5.

Machold, K.P. and Smolen, J.S. (1990). Interferon-γ induced exacerbation of systemic lupus erythematosus. *Journal of Rheumatology*, 17, 831–2.

Maini, R.N., Elliott, M.J., Charles, P.J., and Feldmann, M. (1994). Immunological intervention reveals reciprocal roles for tumour necrosis factor-α and interleukin-10 in rheumatoid arthritis and systemic lupus erythematosus. *Springer Seminars in Immunopathology*, 16, 327–36.

Mamula, M.J., Fatenejad, S., and Craft, J. (1994). B cells process and present lupus autoantigens that initiate autoimmune T cell responses. *Journal of Immunology*, 152, 1453–61.

Mandell, B. (1987). Cardiovascular involvement in systemic lupus erythematosus. *Seminars in Arthritis and Rheumatism*, 17, 120–141.

Maruyama, N. *et al.* (1983). Genetic studies of autoimmunity in New Zealand mice. IV. Contribution of NZB and NZW genes to the spontaneous occurrence of retroviral gp70 immune complexes in (NZB xNZW)F1 hybrid and the correlation to renal disease. *Journal of Immunology*, **130**, 740–6.

Matsuda, J., Saitoh, N., Gohchi, I., Gotoh, M., and Tsukamoto, M. (1994). Detection of β2-glycoprotein 1- dependent antiphospholipid antibodies and anti-β2-glycoprotein 1 antibody in patients with systemic lupus erythematosus and in patients with syphilis. *International Archives of Allergy and Immunology*, **103**, 239–44.

Matsukawa, Y., Sawada, S., Hayama, T., Usui H., and Horie, T. (1994). Suicide in patients with systemic lupus erythematosus: a clinical analysis of seven suicidal patients. *Lupus*, **3**, 31–5.

McGrath, H., Jr. (1994). Ultraviolet-A1 irradiation decreases clinical disease activity and autoantibodies in patients with systemic lupus erythematosus. *Clinical and Experimental Rheumatology*, **12**, 129–135.

McLaughlin, J.R., Bombardier, C., Farewell, V.T., Gladman, D.A., and Urowitz, M.B. (1994). Kidney biopsy in systemic lupus erythematosus. III. Survival analysis, controlling for clinical and laboratory variables. *Arthritis and Rheumatism*, **4**, 559–67.

Mendlovic, S. *et al.* (1988). Induction of a systemic lupus erythematosus-like disease in mice by a common human anti-DNA idiotype. *Proceedings of the National Academy of Sciences* (*USA*), **85**, 2260–4.

Menon, S., Snaith, M.L., and Isenberg, D.A. (1993). The asociation of malignancy with SLE: an analysis of 150 patients under long term review. *Lupus*, **2**, 177–81.

Messier, H. *et al.* (1993). p70 lupus autoantigen binds the enhancer of the T-cell receptor β-chain gene. *Proceedings of the National Academy of Sciences* (*USA*), **90**, 2685–9.

Miller, M.H., Urowitz, M.B., Gladman, D.D., and Killinger, D.W. (1983). Systemic lupus erythematosus in males. *Medicine*, **G2**, 327–34.

Morrow, W.J., Homsy, J., Swanson, C.A., Ohashi, Y., Estes, J., and Levy, J.A. (1986). Dietary fat influences the expression of autoimmune disease in MRL/lpr/lpr mice. *Immunology*, **59**, 439–43.

Mountz, J., Wu, J., Cheng, W., and Zhou, T. (1994). Autoimmune disease. A problem of defective apoptosis. *Arthritis and Rheumatism*, **37**, 1415–20.

Murakami, M., Kumagai, S., Sugita, M., Iwai, K., and Imura, H. (1992). *In vitro* induction of IgG anti-DNA antibody from high density B cells of systemic lupus erythematosus patients by an HLA DR-restricted T cell clone. *Clinical and Experimental Immunology*, **90**, 245–50.

Nakamura, T. *et al.* (1993). Renal expression of mRNAs for endothelin-1, endothelin-3 and endothelin receptors in NZB/W F1 mice. *Renal Physiology and Biochemistry*, **16**, 233–43.

Naparstek, Y. *et al.* (1990). Binding of anti-DNA antibodies and inhibition of glomerulonephritis in MRL-lpr/lpr mice by heparin. *Arthritis and Rheumatism*, **33**, 1554–9.

Norris, D.A. (1993). Pathomechanisms of photosensitive lupus erythematosus. [Review.] *Journal of Investigative Dermatology*, **100**, 58S–68S.

Ohteki, T., Okamoto, S., Nakamura, M., Nemoto, E., and Kumagai, K. (1993). Elevated production of interleukin 6 by hepatic MNC correlates with ICAM-1 expression on the hepatic sinusoidal endothelial cells in autoimmune MRL/lpr mice. *Immunology Letters*, **36**, 145–52.

Olsen, M.L., Arnett, F.C., and Reveille, J.D. (1993). Contrasting molecule patterns of MHC class II alleles associated with the anti-Sm and anti-RNP precipitin autoantibodies in systemic lupus erythematosus. *Arthritis and Rheumatism*, **36**, 94–104.

Petri, M., Lakatta, C., Magder, L., and Goldman, D. (1944). Effect of prednisone and hydroxychloroquine on coronary artery disease risk factors in systemic luypus erythematosus: a longitudinal data analysis. *American Journal of Medicine*, **96**, 254–9.

Pistiner, M., Wallace, D.J. Nessim, S., Metzger, A.L., and Klinenberg, J.R. (1991). Lupus erythematosus in the 1980s: A survey of 570 patients. *Seminars in Arthritis and Rheumatism*, **21**, 358–63.

Rajagopalan, S., Zordan, T., Tsokos, G.C., and Datta, S.K. (1990). Pathogenic anti-DNA antibody-inducing T helper cell lines from patients with active lupus nephritis: isolation of CD4-8-T helper cell lines that express the γ T-cell antigen receptor. *Proceedings of the National Academy of Sciences* (*USA*), **87**, 7020–4.

Rajagopalan, S., Mao, C., and Datta, S.K. (1992). Pathogenic autoantibody-inducing γ/ T helper cells from patients with lupus nephritis express unusual T cell receptors. *Clinical Immunology and Immunopathology*, **62**, 344–50.

Reveille, J.D., Schrohenloher, R.E., Acton, R.T., and Barger, B.O. (1989). DNA analysis of HLA-DR and DQ genes in American blacks with systemic lupus erythematosus. *Arthritis and Rheumatism*, **32**, 1243–51.

Rosner, S. *et al.* (1982). A multicenter study of outcome in systemic lupus erythematosus. II. Causes of death. *Arthritis and Rheumatism*, **256**, 612–7.

Santoro, T.J., Portanova, J.P., and Kotzin, B.L. (1988). The contribution of L3T4 + T cells to lymphoproliferation and autoantibody production in MRL-lpr/lpr mice. *Journal of Experimental Medicine*, **167**, 1713–8.

Schur, P.H., Marcus-Bagley, D., Awdeh, Z., Yunis, E.J., and Alper, C.A. (1990). The effect of ethnicity on major histocompatibility complex complement allotypes and extended haplotypes in patients with systemic lupus erythematosus. *Arthritis and Rheumatism*, **33**, 985–92.

Schwartz, M.M., Lan, S., Bernstein, J., Hill, G.S., Holley, K., and Lewis, E.J. (1993). Irreproducibility of the activity and chronicity indices limits their utility in the management of lupus nephritis. *American Journal of Kidney Disease*, **21**, 374–7.

Scofield, R.H. *et al.* (1994). Cooperative association of T cell β receptor and HLA-DQ alleles in the production of anti-Ro in systemic lupus erythematosus. *Clinical Immunology and Immunopathology*, **72**, 335–41.

Segal, R., Globerson, A., Zinger, H., and Mozes, E. (1992). Induction of experimental systemic lupus erythematosus (SLE) in mice with severe combined immunodeficiency (SCID). *Clinical and Experimental Immunology*, **89**, 239–43.

Sfikakis, P.P., Charalambopoulos, D., Vayiopoulos, G., Oglesby, R., Sfikakis, P., and Tsokos, G.C. (1994). Increased levels of intercellular adhesion molecule-1 in the serum of patients with systemic lupus erythematosus. *Clinical and Experimental Rheumatology*, **12**, 5–9.

Shefner, R. and Diamond, B. (1990). A novel class of autoantibody. *Arthritis and Rheumatism*, **33**, S27.

Shortall, E., Isenberg, D., and Newman, S.P. (1995). Factors associated with mood and mood disorders in SLE. *Lupus*, **4**, 272–9.

Siegert, C.E., Daha, M.R., Tseng, C.M., Coremans, I.E., van Es, L.A., and Breedveld, F.C. (1993). Predictive value of IgG autoantibodies against Clq for nephritis in systemic lupus erythematosus. *Annals of the Rheumatic Diseases*, **52**, 851–6.

Sieving, R.R., Kauffman, C.A., and Watanakunakorn, C. (1975). Deep fungal infection in systemic lupus erythematosus — three cases reported, literature reviewed. *Journal of Rheumatology*, **2**, 61–72.

Silvestris, F., Cafforio, P., and Dammacco, F. (1994). Pathogenic anti-DNA idiotype-reactive IgG in intravenous immunoglobulin preparations. *Clinical and Experimental Immunology*, **97**, 19–25.

Spronk, P.E., ter Borg, E.J., and Kallenberg, C.G.M. (1992). Patients with systemic lupus erythematosus and Jaccoud's arthropathy: a clinical subset with an increased C reactive protein response. *Annals of Rheumatic Diseases*, **51**, 358–61.

Stamenkovic, I., Favre, H., Doneth, A., Assimacopoulos, A., and Chatelanet, F. (1986). Renal biopsy in systemic lupus erythematosus irrespective of clinical findings. Long term follow up. *Clinical Nephrology*, **26**, 109–15.

Sthoeger, Z.M., Geltner, D., Rider, A., and Bentwich, Z. (1987). Systemic lupus erythematosus in 49 Israeli males—a retrospective study. *Clinical and Experimental Rheumatology*, **5**, 233–40.

Talal, N. (1994). Oncogenes, autogenes and rheumatic diseases. *Arthritis and Rheumatiem*, **37**, 1421–2.

Tan, E.M. *et al.* (1982). The 1982 revised criteria for the classification of systemic lupus erythematosus (SLE). *Arthritis and Rheumatism*, **25**, 1271–7.

Teh, L. and Isenberg, D.A. (1994). Antiribosomal P protein antibodies in systemic lupus erythematosus—a reappraisal. *Arthritis and Rheumatism*, **37**, 307–15.

Termaat, R.-M. *et al.* (1990). Cross-reactivity of monoclonal anti-DNA sulphate is mediated via bound DNA/histone complexes. *Journal of Autoimmunity*, **3**, 531–45.

Theofilopoulos, A.N., Singer, P.A., Kofler, R., Kono, D.H., Duchosal, M.A., and Balderas, R.S. (1989). B and T cell antigen receptor repertoires in lupus/arthritis murine models. *Springer Seminars in Immunopathology*, **11**, 335–68.

Turner-Stokes, L. and Isenberg, D.A. (1988). Immunisation of patients with rheumatoid arthritis and systemic lupus erythematosus. *Annals of the Rheumatic Diseases*, **47**, 529–31.

Urman, J.D. and Rothfield N.F. (1977). Corticosteroid treatment in systemic lupus erythematosus: survival studies. *Journal of the American Medical Association*, **238**, 2272–6.

Urowitz, M.B., Gladman, D.D., Farewell, V.T., Stewart, J., and McDonald, J. (1993). Lupus and pregnancy studies. *Arthritis and Rheumatism*, **36**, 1392–7.

Valeri, A. *et al.* (1994). Intravenous pulse cyclophosphamide treatment of severe lupus nephritis: a prospective five year study. *Clinical Nephrology*, **42**, 71–8.

Vitali, C. *et al.* (1992). Disease activity in SLE: report of the consensus study group of the European Workshop for Rheumatology Research III: development of a computerized clinical chart and its application to the comparison of different indices of disease activity. *Clinical and Experimental Rheumatology*, **10**, 549–54.

Wallace, D.J., Podell, T., Weiner, J., Klinenberg, J.R., Forouzesh, S., and Dubois, E.L. (1981). Systemic lupus erythematosus: survival pattern. Experience with 609 patients. *Journal of the American Medical Association*, **245**, 934–8.

Walport, M.J. and Lachmann, P.J. (1988). Erythrocyte complement receptor type I, immune complexes and the rheumatic diseases. *Arthritis and Rheumatism*, **31**, 153–8.

Walton, A.J.E., Snaith, M.L., Locniskar, M., Cumberland, A.G., Morrow, W.J.W., and Isenberg, D.A. (1991). Dietary fish oil reduces the severity of symptoms in patients with SLE. *Annals of the Rheumatic Diseases*, **33**, 463–6.

Ward, M.M. and Studensky, S. (1990). Systemic lupus erythematosus in men — a multivariate analysis of gender differences in clinical manifestations. *Journal of Rheumatology*, **17**, 220–4.

Watts, R. and Isenberg, D.A. (1989). Pancreatic complications of the autoimmune rheumatic diseases. *Seminars in Arthritis and Rheumatism*, **19**, 158–65.

Watts, R. and Isenberg, D.A. (1990). DNA antibody idiotypes: an analysis of their clinical connections and origins. *International Review of Immunology*, **5**, 279–93.

Wei, N., Klippel, J.H., and Husto, D.P. (1983). Randomised trial of plasma exchange in mild SLE. *Lancet*, **i**, 17–22.

Weinrib, L., Sharma, O.P., and Quismario, F.P. (1990). A long term study of interstitial lung disease in systemic lupus erythematosus. *Seminars in Arthritis and Rheumatism*, **16**, 479–81.

Wellicome, S.M., Kapahi, P., Mason, J.C., Lebranchu, Y., Yarwood, H., and Haskard, D.O. (1993). Detection of a circulating form of vascular cell adhesion molecule-1: raised levels in rheumatoid arthritis and systemic lupus erythematosus. *Clinical and Experimental Immunology*, **92**, 412–18.

Whiting-O'Keefe, Q., Henke, J.E., Sheard, M.A., Hopper J., Jr., Biava, C.G., and Epstein, W.V. (1982). The information content from renal biopsy in systemic lupus erythematosus. Stepwise linear regression analysis. *Annals of Internal Medicine*, **96**, 718–27.

Williams, W. and Isenberg, D.A. (1994). Idiotypes and autologous anti-idiotypes in human autoimmune disease — some theoretical and practical observations. *Autoimmunity*, **17**, 343–52.

Wofsy, D. and Seaman, W.E. (1985). Successful treatment of autoimmunity in NZB/NZW F1 mice with monoclonal antibody to L3T4. *Journal of Experimental Medicine*, **161**, 378–91.

Wolff-Vorbeck, G. *et al.* (1994). Characterization of an HLA-DR4-restricted T cell clone recognizing a protein moiety of small ribonucleoprotein (UsnRNP). *Clinical and Experimental Immunology*, **95**, 378–84.

Worrall, J.G., Snaith, M.L., Batchelor, J.R., and Isenberg, D.A. (1990). SLE: a rheumatological view. Analysis of the clinical features, serology, and immunogenetics of 100 SLE patients during long term follow up. *Quarterly Journal of Medicine*, **74**, 319–30.

Wu, J., Zhou, T., Zhang, J., and Mountz, J. (1994). Correction of autoimmune disease in CD2-fas transgenic mice. *Proceedings of the National Academy of Sciences (USA)*, **91**, 2344–8.

Wuthrich, R.P. (1992). Vascular cell adhesion molecule-1 (VCAM-1) expression in murine lupus nephritis. *Kidney International*, **42**, 903–14.

Wuthrich, R.P., Jevnikar, A.M., Takei, F., Glimcher, L.H., and Kelley, V.E. (1990). Intercellular adhesion molecule-1 (ICAM-1) expression is upregulated in autoimmune murine lupus nephritis. *American Journal of Pathology*, **136**, 441–50.

Wysenbeek, A.J., Leibovici, L., Weinberger, A., and Guadj, D. (1993). Fatigue in systemic lupus erythematosus: prevalence and relation to disease expression. *British Journal of Rheumatology*, **32**, 633–5.

Xavier, R.M., Nakamura, M., and Tsunematsu, T. (1994). Isolation and characterization of a human nonspecific suppressor factor from ascitic fluid of systemic lupus erythematosus. Evidence for a human counterpart of the monoclonal nonspecific suppressor factor and relationship to the T cell receptor α-chain. *Journal of Immunology*, **152**, 2624–32.

Yamada, A., Minota, S., Nojima, Y., and Yazaki, Y. (1993). Changes in subset specificity of anti-T cell autoantibodies in systemic lupus erythematosus. *Autoimmunity*, **14**, 269–73.

Yoshida, S., Castles, J.J., and Gershwin, M.E. (1990). The pathogenesis of autoimmunity in New Zealand mice. *Seminars in Arthritis and Rheumatism*, **19**, 224–42.

5.7.2 Systemic lupus erythematosus in children

Earl D. Silverman and Alison A. Eddy

Systemic lupus erythematosus (SLE) in children and adolescents has many features in common with adult-onset SLE. This chapter, rather than fully reviewing all the possible presentations and manifestations of SLE will highlight the differences between paediatric SLE and adult-onset lupus. This chapter will not cover many topics such as immunopathogenesis, cytokines, and animal models which are outlined in Chapter 5.7.1, nor will it cover antiphospholipid antibodies in depth. Rather, it should serve as a complementary chapter and will place its emphasis on unique features and provide an overview of general features of paediatric SLE. We suggest reading both chapters on SLE. A separate section of this chapter will cover neonatal lupus erythematosus, a disease caused by maternally-transmitted autoantibodies.

Incidence

Although SLE has been recognized for many decades, most physicians rarely consider it in the paediatric age group. Currently there has been no good epidemiological study focusing on paediatric SLE and very few large population studies give details of its incidence prior to the age of 20. A large population study from New York showed an incidence of 6 cases per 100 000 white females of less than 15 years of age as compared with an overall incidence of 25 cases per 100 000 white females of all ages. The incidence rate rapidly rose to 18.9 cases per 100 000 white females aged between 15 and 25 years. Therefore, the true incidence of SLE beginning prior to age 19 was between 6 and 18.9 cases per 100 000 in white females, and was higher in black (20 to 30 per 100 000) and Puerto Rican females (16 to 36.7 per 100 000) (Siegel and Lee 1973).

Most other series of SLE patients with a large number of paediatric cases state that 20 per cent of all cases of SLE have onset prior to age 18 (Kaufman *et al.* 1986; Reeves and Lahita 1987). Therefore, using the best available data, the incidence of SLE beginning prior to age 18 is 10 to 20 cases per 100 000 children and adolescents, with an overall prevalence of 10 to 20 cases per 10 000 people less than 18 years old. These rates are higher in Hispanic, black and oriental people.

Early reports had suggested that there was a high percentage of male cases prior to puberty, while after puberty the percentage of cases occurring in females rose to make up 85 to 90 per cent of cases (as seen in most adult studies). In our series we had an overall male: female ratio of 1:4.3. When further divided by age, we found a male: female ratio of 1:5.5 between 6 and 10 years (prepubertal); 1:3.4 in the age 11 to 13 group (peripubertal); and 1:4.5 between the ages of 14 and 18 (postpubertal). Our data are consistent with more recent larger reviews (King *et al.* 1977; Lehman *et al.* 1989b). These data may reflect both an increased awareness of the possibility of SLE in males and the larger series size would eliminate any potential false bias of previous small studies. Whatever the reasons, the overall ratio of male:female cases of approximately 1:4.5 suggests that there is a higher percentage of male cases in paediatric SLE than in adult cases of SLE.

In the paediatric series, the average age at diagnosis varied from 11 to 14 years (median 12.2 years). The time from onset of symptoms to diagnosis varied from 8 months to 3.3 years (median 1.2 years). This median time of 1.2 years from symptoms to diagnosis emphasizes the difficulty in diagnosis or the lack of awareness of SLE in this age group. The features of SLE at presentation are shown in Table 1; while features at any time during the course of the disease are shown in Table 2 (Zetterstrom and Berglund 1956; Gribetz and Henley 1959; Cook *et al.* 1960; Jacobs 1963; Robinson and Williams 1967; Walravens and Chase 1976; Fish *et al.* 1977; King *et al.* 1977; Abeles *et al.* 1980; Caeiro *et al.* 1981; Yancey *et al.* 1981; Schaller 1982; Glidden *et al.* 1983; Emery 1986; Kaufman *et al.* 1986; Lehman *et al.* 1989a; El-Garf and Salah 1990; Lacks and White 1990). These are shown as the range of each feature in: (i) previously published paediatric series; and (ii) our series of 86 patients. Details are given in the organ-specific sections. However, general systemic symptoms such as fever, malaise and weight loss are common, as is evidence of systemic inflammation shown by lymphadenopathy and/or hepatosplenomegaly — this is both at diagnosis and throughout the course of the disease.

Table 1 Clinical features: at diagnosis

	Other series (%)	Our series (%)
Fever	60–90	55
Arthritis	60–88	78
Skin rash (any)	60–78	79
Malar rash	22–60	36
Renal	20–80	61
Cardiovascular	5–30	14
Pulmonary	18–40	18
Central nervous system	5–30	25
Gastrointestinal	14–30	19
Hepatosplenomegaly	16–42	30
Lymphadenopathy	13–45	34

Table 2 Clinical features: anytime during the course

	Other series (%)	Our series (%)
Fever	80–100	86
Arthritis	60–90	80
Any skin rash	60–90	86
Malar rash	30–80	38
Renal	48–100	69
Cardiovascular	25–60	17
Pulmonary	18–81	18
Central nervous system	26–44	34
Gastrointestinal*	24–40	24
Hepatosplenomegaly	19–43	30
Lymphadenopathy*	13–45	34

*Not included in follow-up data in many paediatric series

Musculoskeletal disease

Arthritis and arthralgia are among the most common symptoms in paediatric SLE occurring in more than 90 per cent of cases. Most patients with arthritis have a symmetric polyarthritis affecting both large and small joints. The arthritis usually responds to the treatment of other major organ involvement or to treatment of the general systemic symptoms. Unlike juvenile chronic arthritis, the arthritis is usually episodic and is easy to treat. Severely painful joints are common and usually the pain is out of proportion to the physical findings. The peripheral joints including the fingers, hands, wrists and knees are the commonest joints involved, with involvement of hips and ankles more unusual. In most cases there is no radiographic evidence of joint destruction. However, in 1 to 2 per cent of cases of lupus arthritis there is a deforming erosive arthritis as seen in seropositive juvenile chronic arthritis. This type of arthritis is usually associated with a positive rheumatoid factor, and at least in adults, has been referred to as 'Rhupus'. A more common cause of joint deformities is secondary to ligamentous laxity and periarticular fibrosis, the so-called Jaccoud's arthritis. This can result in deformity of the hand with multiple joint subluxations but with good preservation of function. Radiographs show only osteoporosis without evidence of erosions or joint space loss. Jaccoud's arthritis is more of a periarticular rather than an articular disease (Martini *et al.* 1987). However, in most patients with arthritis of SLE, the arthritis does not result in deformity. Both 'Rhupus' and Jaccoud's arthritis combined occur in less than 5 per cent of paediatric SLE patients with arthritis. Tenosynovitis is common and patients with knee effusions can develop Baker's cysts. Of particular interest have been the reports of patients with American College of Rheumatology (ACR) criteria for juvenile chronic arthritis who develop SLE years later. We have seen a patient with 'classic' systemic-onset juvenile chronic arthritis, including evanescent rash and spiking fever, who after 2 years in remission for her juvenile chronic arthritis developed

SLE, including a photosensitive rash and positive antinuclear antibodies (which previously had been negative). Initial reports had shown a transformation from polyarticular rather than systemic juvenile chronic arthritis to SLE (Ragsdale *et al.* 1980; Saulsbury *et al.* 1982), however a more recent report has also demonstrated transformation from systemic juvenile-onset chronic arthritis to SLE (Citera *et al.* 1993).

Analysis of synovial fluid usually shows only mild inflammation with a total white blood-cell count of generally less than 2000 cells/ml. Synovial biopsies show a mild vasculitis or perivasculitis and the diagnostic histological lesion is the hematoxylin body. This may be the equivalent of the LE cell in the joint. However, synovial biopsies are indicated rarely.

Myalgia, as part of the generalized disease process, occurs in approximately 50 to 60 per cent of paediatric cases, while true myositis with proximal muscle weakness or tenderness occurs in less than 10 per cent of cases. When present there is usually a slow progression of weakness and rarely is there involvement of the intercostal or cricopharyngeal muscles. It is seen more commonly in patients with so-called 'overlap syndromes' or with mixed connective tissue disease. Primary muscle involvement must be differentiated from muscle weakness secondary to steroid treatment. This complication is a much talked about steroid side-effect but in our experience it is uncommon. The treatment of steroid-induced myopathy would be to decrease rather than increase the steroid dose and would result in an improvement in muscle strength.

The other steroid-induced musculoskeletal side-effects include avascular necrosis, osteoporosis with fracture or vertebral body collapse, and even growth failure if prolonged high-dose steroids are required. Growth failure may be alleviated partially by alternate-day dose regimens but even using these it still remains a problem. One hope may be through the use of recombinant growth hormone to promote growth, but no studies have been undertaken yet in this group of patients.

Avascular necrosis occurs in approximately 10 to 15 per cent of paediatric cases and appears to be more common in children than adults (Smith *et al.* 1976). In our experience, avascular necrosis occurs more commonly in SLE than other paediatric autoimmune diseases where prolonged high-dose steroids are used. The reason for this is not readily apparent. Unlike adults, in our experience, paediatric patients with Raynaud's phenomenon and vasculitis do not appear to be at a greater risk of this complication. Usually avascular necrosis is related to the dose and duration of therapy but there have been case reports of it developing prior to or without steroid usage (Abeles *et al.* 1978; Kalla *et al.* 1986). In contrast to avascular necrosis, vertebral collapse is rarer in SLE than in other autoimmune rheumatic diseases and in particular juvenile dermatomyositis. The incidence of vertebral collapse is probably related not only to steroid dose and duration but also to the amount of weight gain and physical activity. The most common lesion involves the thoracolumbar spine with cervical spine lesions occurring more rarely.

The last musculoskeletal side-effect of steroid therapy is increased incidence of fractures secondary to steroid-induced osteoporosis. This appears to be less common in children than adults and may reflect relative differences in bone mineral content between the groups. Treatment or prevention of steroid-induced side-effects is controversial in adults and there has not been a good study in children. The best hope lies with the new generation of 'bone-sparing' steroids and keeping patients active while minimizing weight gain.

Treatment of musculoskeletal involvement

The arthritis of SLE frequently occurs with disease flares elsewhere and usually responds to the treatment for the more serious complication. However, if isolated, the use of a non-steroidal anti-inflammatory drug with an antimalarial drug has a high success rate. The only word of caution is that SLE patients seem to be more susceptible to hepatotoxicity induced by non-steroidal anti-inflammatory drugs, particularly aspirin. We commonly use naproxen (10 to 20mg/kg per day), tolmetin (20 to 30 mg/kg per day) and avoid ibuprofen because of the reports of aseptic meningitis occurring in SLE patients. When the arthritis is more severe or unresponsive we commonly add hydroxychloroquine at a dose of 5 mg/kg per day, although others have advocated the use of chloroquine. Antimalarial therapy appears to be of benefit not only for the arthritis but also for rash and overall disease control. The major side-effects are retinal macular deposition of the drug and gastrointestinal distress. Therefore, we recommend ophthalmological examination every 6 months and taking the drug immediately before bed to lessen gastrointestinal upset. Prednisone at low to moderate dose may be required. For suggested therapy of arthritis see Box 1.

Mucocutaneous involvement

Cutaneous involvement has been reported in 50 to 80 per cent of paediatric SLE patients at the time of diagnosis and in up to 85 per cent of patients during the course of the disease. A malar rash, in the classic 'butterfly distribution', is the most common rash occurring in 30 to 60 per cent of cases at diagnosis and in up to 80 per cent of patients during the course of the disease. The rash may be mild, requiring no treatment, but can be severe and cosmetically unacceptable requiring treatment with steroids, either topically or systemic, and/or antimalarial drugs. The appearance of a malar rash often heralds a disease flare and while usually non-scarring it can be present as a crusted or scaling rash. A truly photosensitive rash only occurs in approximately one-third of paediatric patients. The photosensitive rash can occur not only on the face but in any sun-exposed area, especially the arms and legs (Fig. 1). This photosensitive rash may be maculopapular or papulosquamous and may be associated with anti-Ro and anti-La antibodies. The other anti-Ro/La antibody-associated rash is annular erythema. This rash is commonly

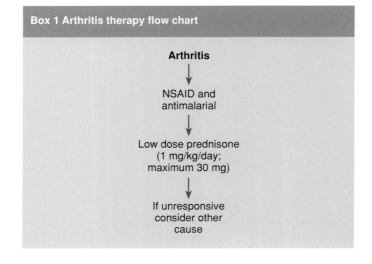

Box 1 Arthritis therapy flow chart

Arthritis
↓
NSAID and
antimalarial
↓
Low dose prednisone
(1 mg/kg/day;
maximum 30 mg)
↓
If unresponsive
consider other
cause

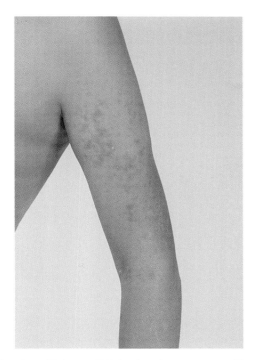

Fig. 1 A patient with known SLE developed a severe, vasculitic rash on arms and legs following sun exposure.

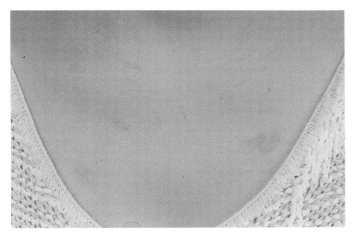

Fig. 2 Annular erythema on the neck of an SLE patient with anti-Ro and anti-La antibodies.

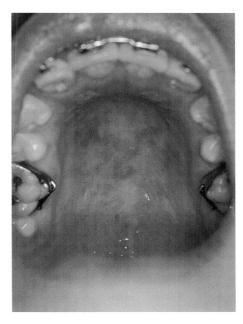

Fig. 3 Hyperaemia and petechiae on hard palate secondary to vasculitis.

photosensitive and occurs on the face or neck (Deng *et al.* 1984) (Fig. 2). True discoid lupus lesions are seen rarely in patients under the age of 18 years. In patients with a photosensitive rash, sun exposure may not only exacerbate the skin disease but may cause a systemic flare. Therefore, we recommend avoidance of sunbathing along with the use of sun-blocking agents, with high SPF (sun protecting factor) blocking both ultraviolet A and B wavelengths, and protective clothing including long-sleeved shirts and hats. It must also be remembered that unshielded fluorescent lamps may emit ultraviolet B radiation.

A true vasculitic skin rash has been reported in 10 to 20 per cent of patients. It occurs commonly in fingers or toes and can result in splinter haemorrhages and digital infarcts. Oral or nasal ulcers are caused by the same vasculitic process and they are probably a reflection of alterations seen in other vascular beds. Even when isolated, they may signify active disease. Painless ulcers are more common on the hard palate but may occur on the soft palate. A petechial rash on the hard palate may precede true ulceration while a chronic sore throat may represent mildly active vasculitis. Similarly, hyperaemia of the nasal mucosa usually precedes ulceration or perforation (Fig. 3). Most paediatric series do not comment on the incidence of these lesions but they probably occur in 10 to 20 per cent of patients. For suggested therapy of mucocutaneous disease see Box 2.

Alopecia, no longer part of the revised ACR criteria for SLE, is common and occurs in up to 50 per cent of paediatric patients. Diffuse hair loss during washing or brushing is more common than patchy hair loss. In some patients there is a delay in the hair loss, which may follow a disease flare or increase after the introduction of steroids. Rarely is the hair loss significant enough to cause a cosmetic problem. Scarring is unusual.

Raynaud's phenomenon appears to be less common in paediatric lupus, occurring in only 10 to 20 per cent of patients. In some patients local therapy including avoidance of cold, use of insulated mittens rather than gloves and hand/feet warmers will suffice. However, many patients will have more severe disease requiring the use of calcium-channel blocking agents or other vasodilating medication, including topical therapy with prostaglandins or nitroglycerin paste. Paediatric patients appear to tolerate calcium-channel blocking agents better than adults do. Patients with Raynaud's phenomenon rarely have normal vascular tone and will often have vasodilation at rest or severe vasoconstriction after only slight provocation. Raynaud's phenomenon may precede overt clinical SLE by months and may initially involve only a few digits and later involve all fingers and toes. Although usually easy to control, Raynaud's may result in distal digital infarction or gangrene.

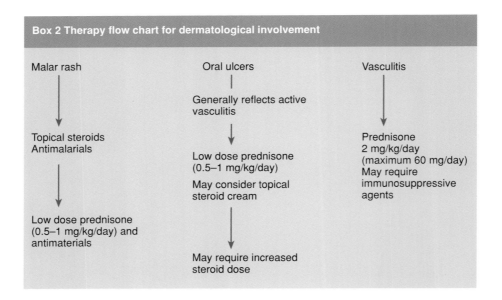

Box 2 Therapy flow chart for dermatological involvement

Malar rash → Topical steroids Antimalarials → Low dose prednisone (0.5–1 mg/kg/day) and antimaterials

Oral ulcers → Generally reflects active vasculitis → Low dose prednisone (0.5–1 mg/kg/day) May consider topical steroid cream → May require increased steroid dose

Vasculitis → Prednisone 2 mg/kg/day (maximum 60 mg/day) May require immunosuppressive agents

Central nervous system

Involvement of the central nervous system, which occurs in 20 to 50 per cent of paediatric patients, can be the most interesting yet frustrating target in SLE. The interest stems from the protean manifestations but the frustration stems from the difficulty in diagnosis and assessment of patients with neuropsychiatric SLE (NP-SLE). Central nervous involvement can occur in isolation or it may be associated with disease flares in other organs. The only correlation between central nervous disease and disease elsewhere appears to be the association with vasculitis and thrombocytopenia. Table 3 lists the different manifestations of nervous system involvement seen.

Neuropsychiatric SLE

The most difficult SLE patients to diagnose and treat are the patients with psychiatric disorders. As a group psychiatric disorders are seen in 10 to 20 per cent of paediatric SLE cases. When a known lupus patient presents with florid psychosis or organic brain syndrome, the diagnosis is easy. However, many patients present with affective or mood disorders. The difficulty is determining whether the abnormalities detected are a direct result of the disease, secondary to steroid treatment, or 'reactive' to the disease or changes in body image. Several different investigations have been proposed to differentiate active disease from other causes of central nervous abnormalities (see below).

It can be very difficult to differentiate neuropsychiatric SLE-induced cognitive impairment and concentration difficulties from other causes of poor school performance. Studies in adults have suggested that cognitive impairment may occur in up to 80 per cent of all SLE patients (Carbotte *et al.* 1986). Defects in cognitive function may reflect active disease or residual defects from previous central nervous involvement (Fisk *et al.* 1993). This is emphasized by a longitudinal study which demonstrated that cognitive functional abnormalities may resolve and therefore they do not necessarily reflect irreversible damage (Hanly *et al.* 1994). To date there has been only one study in paediatric SLE that suggests that cognitive function defects are common (Papero *et al.* 1990). This has also been our

experience. Although affective disorders occur less frequently than cognitive impairment, it must be recognized that patients can present with a major affective disorder with very few other signs of lupus.

Seizures occur in approximately 10 to 20 per cent of paediatric SLE cases and may be the presenting sign. Focal seizures are more common than *grand mal* seizures. Seizures are generally easily treated with anticonvulsant medication and usually do not require high-dose steroids for control. Seizures may not be primary but rather secondary to metabolic disturbances caused by uraemia, hypertension, cerebral infarction or central nervous infection. Structural abnormalities should be ruled-out in all patients with new onset or increasing frequency of seizures.

Movement disorders including chorea, cerebellar ataxia, hemiballismus, tremor and Parkinsonian-like movements, occur in 5 to10 per cent of cases. Interestingly chorea appears to be over-represented in the paediatric age group. In one review of 52 cases of SLE-associated chorea, 34 had chorea that developed before the age of 18 years, with the chorea preceding other manifestations of SLE by more than 1 year in 20 per cent of all cases (Bruyn and Padberg 1984). Recently we have had cases of chorea that preceded the development of overt SLE by many years and chorea that developed in patients with long-standing SLE. It has been demonstrated that there is an association between chorea and antiphospholipid antibodies. The exact mechanism which leads to chorea is unknown, although it rarely appears to be the result of an infarction that can be demonstrated on neuroimaging studies. The decline in the incidence of rheumatic fever means that the diagnosis of SLE or antiphospholipid antibody syndrome should be considered in all patients presenting with chorea.

Neuropathies

Both cranial and peripheral neuropathies can occur, with cranial nerve involvement being the more common. Cranial nerve involvement usually affects cranial nerves II, III, IV, and VI resulting in abnormalities of vision, pupils, or extraocular movements. Less frequently facial palsy (VII), trigeminal neuropathy (V) or nystagmus and vertigo (VIII) occur. When peripheral neuropathies occur, a sensory or mixed sensorimotor involvement is more common than

Table 3 Neuropsychiatric lupus

Psychiatric

  Psychosis

  Depression

Central nervous system

  Organic brain syndrome

  Cognitive function deficits

  Seizures

  Cranial nerve palsy

  Optic atrophy

  Papilloedema

  Parkinson-like syndrome

  Coma

  Headache—unremitting or migrainous

  Transverse myelitis

  Aseptic meningitis

  Cerebrovascular accident—infarction

  Pseudotumour cerebri

Movement disorders

  Chorea

  Hemiballismus

  Cerebellar ataxia

  Tremor

  Hemiparesis

Peripheral nervous system

  Peripheral neuropathy

  Guillain–Barré syndrome

  Paraparesis

  Myasthenia-like syndrome

Infection

  Bacterial

  Viral

  Fungal

  Opportunistic

phospholipid antibodies, or thrombocytopenia. Transverse myelitis may present with acute paraplegia or quadriplegia; in this latter syndrome antiphospholipid antibodies must be sought.

Headache

Headache requires a separate category as this is a common symptom occurring in approximately 20 per cent of cases. The differentiation of the type of headache is important. The severe, unremitting lupus headache is the most serious and reflects active disease or may represent cerebral vein thrombosis (see below). A special problem occurs with migraine headache secondary to SLE, which must be differentiated from non-lupus associated vascular instability, particularly in patients with a family history of migraine headaches (Isenberg *et al.* 1982). A headache may be the presentation of pseudotumour cerebri, which has been described as the presenting diagnosis in paediatric SLE. Migraine headaches may reflect active central nervous SLE (Miguel *et al.* 1994).

Most worrying is the association of severe headache with cerebral vein thrombosis. Although cerebral vein thrombosis has been felt to be rare, we have recently recognized this complication in patients with headache. The headache associated with cerebral vein thrombosis may occur without any other neurological manifestation (Uziel 1995). We recommend neuroimaging studies for patients with persistent or severe headaches (see below).

Investigation

As the differential diagnosis neuropsychiatric SLE is large, so is the list of investigations. Abnormalities of cerebrospinal fluid cell count, protein and complement levels have been described. However, the findings are inconsistent and complement levels cannot be routinely obtained. It has been suggested that measurements of the integrity of the blood–brain barrier and of immunoglobulin synthesis in the cerebrospinal fluid may correlate with neuropsychiatric SLE, but the demonstration of these abnormalities is not specific for SLE (Hirohata *et al.* 1985; McLean *et al.* 1995). Furthermore, large controlled, prospective studies are not available in SLE to test the utility of measuring these parameters. However, the simplest test, examination and culture of cerebrospinal fluid, remains important when the possibility of infection or haemorrhage exists. An elevated cerebrospinal fluid protein and/or white blood-cell count, in the absence of infection, is suggestive of cerebritis.

The correlation of antineuronal antibodies and cognitive function has sparked much interest recently. One prospective adult study suggested that a combination of the measurement of antineuronal antibodies with a large battery of sophisticated neurophysiological cognitive function tests correlated well with fluctuations of disease (Long *et al.* 1989). Our limited experience has suggested that this combination of testing may be of benefit in diagnosis and disease monitoring. Despite its promise, cognitive function testing requires more time and expertise than is routinely available. Furthermore, longitudinal studies of cognitive function may be required to determine whether a defect is old, permanent or temporary (Hanly *et al.* 1994).

Serial measurement of more routine autoantibodies and routine blood tests may not correlate with neuropsychiatric SLE (Miguel *et al.* 1994). Patients may have normal serology and complement levels despite active SLE of the central nervous system. One exception may be the association of antiribosomal P antibody and depression. Initial studies had suggested that although antiribosomal P antibodies are

an isolated motor neuropathy. However, mononeuritis or mononeuritis multiplex can occur and isolated cases of Guillain–Barré-like syndrome have been seen.

Paresis, while seen in approximately 5 per cent of adult cases, is less common in children. Hemiparesis in association with other major neurological findings, rarely seen in children, is usually secondary to cerebral vascular accident. Hemiparesis and/or cerebral vascular accidents may occur as the result of active SLE but also may occur when the SLE is complicated by the presence of hypertension, anti-

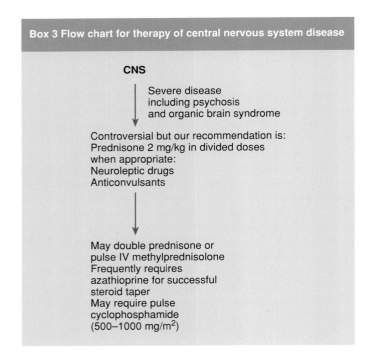

Box 3 Flow chart for therapy of central nervous system disease

CNS

↓

Severe disease
including psychosis
and organic brain syndrome

↓

Controversial but our recommendation is:
Prednisone 2 mg/kg in divided doses
when appropriate:
Neuroleptic drugs
Anticonvulsants

↓

May double prednisone or
pulse IV methylprednisolone
Frequently requires
azathioprine for successful
steroid taper
May require pulse
cyclophosphamide
(500–1000 mg/m^2)

present in approximately 15 per cent of all lupus patients, these auto-antibodies occur in most lupus patients with depression (Bonfa et al. 1987). However, other studies have failed to demonstrate this high degree of association with psychosis or depression (Teh et al. 1993). Importantly, preliminary studies suggest that the presence of the antiribosomal P antibodies may distinguish depression secondary to SLE from other causes including reactive, steroid-induced or other non-SLE causes of depression (Schneebaum et al. 1991). We have recently examined antiribosomal P antibodies in paediatric SLE and found that the antibodies were present only in patients with psychosis secondary to SLE and not in patients with other causes of psychosis. However, many patients with psychosis did not have these antibodies, and many SLE patients with the antibodies did not have psychosis. Therefore, although anti-ribosomal P antibodies were specific for psychosis secondary to SLE, they had a low sensitivity in SLE patients with psychosis and a low specificity for psychosis in our SLE population (Press et al. 1996).

Radiological investigation of the central nervous system may be helpful in demonstrating specific structural lesions such as infarction, embolus and subdural or intracranial haemorrhage. However, neither computed tomography (CT) nor magnetic resonance imaging (MRI) have been shown to be consistently helpful in measuring overall disease activity in the central nervous system (O'Connor 1988). The use of MRI to determine the presence of diffuse disease activity in the central nervous system remains controversial (Isshi et al. 1994; Jarek et al. 1994). Although abnormalities have been described, these findings may not correlate with clinical disease.

An SLE patient with persistent or severe headache should be investigated for the presence of intracranial thrombosis and in particular cerebral vein thrombosis. The best investigation is by a combination of CT and MRI scans. A CT scan, with 'wide-windows' should be performed in all patients when this diagnosis is considered (Uziel 1993). This examination will detect the presence of infarction and thrombosis. The use of 'wide-windows' will allow for the appropriate

visualization of the cerebral veins. The neuroradiologist should be advised of the possibility of this diagnosis as the use of 'wide-windows' is not part of the routine CT scan. The diagnosis of cerebral vein thrombosis may be confirmed by the absence of flow on an MR venogram. An MR venogram is a very sensitive examination but it may not be readily available and may require sedation, while a CT scan is easier to perform and more readily available.

In most series, the use of nuclear medicine brain scans has not been shown to be of any diagnostic use. However, the use of single-photon-emission computed tomography nuclear brain scans (SPECT) holds promise. These scans may be a functional assessment of brain activity (Holman 1991). SPECT scans appear to be a sensitive test, both in adults and children, to measure active disease in the central nervous system (Rubbert et al. 1993; Szer et al. 1993; Kodama et al. 1995). However, the ability of this test to differentiate active SLE from other causes of abnormalities in the central nervous system remains to be determined. In addition patients without overt central nervous disease may have an abnormal SPECT scan. Whether the perfusion abnormalities in this latter group of SLE patients reflects subclinical dysfunction of the central nervous system or the generalized disease process, remains to be determined. Positron-emission tomography (PET) scans are not universally available and are considered generally as a research tool.

Treatment of central nervous system disease

The therapy of central nervous system disease varies with the manifestation. Currently the treatment of isolated cognitive disorders is controversial, although one adult study has suggested that these defects may be steroid-responsive. Obviously when infection is present the therapy is dictated by the microbiological identification of the organism. However, it must be remembered that these patients are susceptible to encapsulated organisms, Gram-negative organisms and opportunistic infections.

Active psychosis and/or organic brain syndrome are potentially life-threatening complications of central nervous system disease and should be treated aggressively with high-dose corticosteroids. In our experience these patients frequently require immunosuppressive therapy with azathioprine, to allow for the successive tapering of the steroid dose. For resistant central nervous disease, treatment with cyclophosphamide may be required. In addition, the use of psychotropic drugs may be needed for the control of the psychosis. We do not recommend the isolated use of psychotropic medication without the use of steroids. Although reported by others, we have not seen a case of steroid-induced psychosis. For suggested therapy of severe central nervous system disease see Box 3.

Treatment of seizures should be directed at finding their cause, whether they are secondary to infarction, active central nervous system disease or metabolic disturbance. Anti-convulsant medication may be required to control the seizures, but in many cases it is needed only for a short-term if the underlying cause of the seizure can be corrected.

As previously described, headaches can occur for a variety of reasons in these patients. The treatment is therefore dictated by the cause. If the headache is mild and it resolves with the use of routine analgesia then no further investigation or therapy is required. However, persistent headache resistant to analgesia may reflect active SLE or may be secondary to an intracranial thrombosis (in particular cerebral vein thrombosis). The management of 'lupus' headache secondary to active SLE requires better control of the SLE, which may include the use of steroids. We suggest that cerebral vein thrombosis requires anticoagulation, initially at high dose for 3 to 6 months followed by long-term low-dose anticoagulation (Uziel 1995). However, the need for and duration of long-term anticoagulation is controversial.

Renal disease

Renal involvement occurs in a significant number of children with SLE. In a literature review of 540 children followed at centres other than our own, 72 per cent developed nephritis during the course of their disease, similar to our overall incidence of 61 per cent in 138 children with SLE. The high susceptibility of the kidneys to injury in this disease is not entirely understood but it is due in part to haemodynamic factors; to the unique architecture of the glomerular capillary wall that permits direct exposure of blood-borne molecules to the glomerular basement membrane; and to the expression of renal antigens that may react with the autoantibodies present in these patients. The pathogenesis of SLE is reviewed in Chapter 5.7.1.

In most published series of childhood SLE, prognosis is most closely related to the severity of the renal disease. The World Health Organization (WHO) developed a morphological classification of

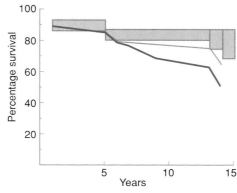

Fig. 4 Long-term survival of 70 children with SLE followed at The University of Minnesota. The patient survival rates for the subset of 21 children with diffuse proliferative lupus nephritis (DPLN) begins to deviate from the entire group (shaded area) at 7 years. Survival of the DPLN group without dialysis or renal transplantation is illustrated by the bolder line (Platt 1982).

lupus nephritis that was modified by the Pathology Advisory Group for the International Study of Kidney Disease in Children in 1980 (Table 4). Although the latter classification is more complex, it is our impression that it provides more useful information when making patient management decisions. Unfortunately, neither classification accurately evaluates extraglomerular (tubular, interstitial and vascular) disease. It has been our practice to biopsy any child with clinical or laboratory evidence of renal involvement, because a diagnosis of diffuse proliferative lupus nephritis (DPLN) adversely affects long-term outcome and thus influences our initial patient management; an approach that is supported by the experience of others (Esdaile *et al.* 1994). In the report by Platt *et al.* (Platt *et al.* 1982), 59 per cent (21) of the children with biopsy-proven DPLN were alive without endstage renal failure 10 years after diagnosis compared with an 85 per cent 10-year survival rate for all 70 children with SLE (Fig. 4). It is important to note that the outcome of patients with DPLN did not deviate from that of the entire group for 7 years, emphasizing the need for long-term clinical trials to validate the efficacy of treatment protocols. A more recent paediatric series (McCurdy *et al.* 1992) reported a 62 per cent incidence of renal

---

Table 4 International Study of Kidney Disease in Children: classification of lupus nephritis

I. *Normal*

A. Nil

B. Normal by light microscopy, but deposits present

II. *Pure mesangiopathy*

A. Mild (+)

B. Moderate (++)

III. *Segmental and focal proliferative glomerulonephritis*

A. Active necrotizing

B. Active and sclerosing

C. Sclerosing

IV. *Diffuse proliferative glomerulonephritis*

A. Without segmental necrotizing lesions

B. With segmental necrotizing lesions

C. With segmental active and sclerotic lesions

D. Inactive, sclerotic

V. *Diffuse membranous glomerulonephritis*

A. Pure membranous

B. Associated with lesions II (A or B)

C. Associated with lesions III (A, B, or C)

D. Associated with lesions IV (A, B, C, or D)

IV. *Advanced sclerosing glomerulonephritis*

From Kunkel (1980).

Table 5 Histological patterns of SLE nephritis

	General (%)[a] (n=368)	Seven paediatric series (%)[b] (n=424)	HSC 1979–1995 (%) (n=79)
Mesangial	27	24	19
Focal proliferative	18	24	20
Diffuse proliferative	39	44	39
Membranous	16	8	22

[a]Data obtained from Pollak and Pirani (1993)
[b]Data obtained from Cassidy *et al.* (1977), King *et al.* (1977), Abeles *et al.* (1980), Platt *et al.* (1982), Glidden *et al.* (1983), Yang *et al.* (1994), Cameron (1994).

Table 6 Clinical manifestations at the time of biopsy of children with diffuse proliferative lupus nephritis[a]

	Mean ± 1SD	Median	Range	Percentage
Age (y)	13 ± 4	14	4–17	
Female				67
Microhaematuria				100
Proteinuria (mg/kg per day)	46 ± 36	35	3–129	
≥50				50
25–49				10
≤24				40
Serum albumin (g/l)	30 ± 7	30	16–47	
≥35				30
26–34				50
≤25				20
GFR[b] ml/min per 1.73 m^2	95 ± 33	102	17–151	
≥100				52
60–99				33
≤59				14
Hypertension				33
C3[c] (g/l)	0.47 ± 0.15	0.49	0.09–0.70	

[a]Diffuse proliferative lupus nephritis diagnosed at our institution since 1979; clinical data available on 29/33 children.
[b]GFR, glomerular filtration rate determined by ^{99}Tc-DPTA or Schwartz equation.
[c]C3, third component of complement; normal value is 0.8–1.8 g/l in our laboratory.

insufficiency in 24 children who developed DPLN between 1970 and 1983. Hopefully, earlier diagnosis of, and newer therapeutic approaches to, DPLN will improve the long-term outcome.

Unfortunately, approximately 40 per cent of patients with SLE nephritis have the most severe subtype, DPLN. Since 1979, when electron microscopy was introduced as a routine part of the evaluation of renal biopsies performed at our institution, 39 per cent of 79 children with biopsy-confirmed lupus nephritis had DPLN (Table 5). Three additional patients underwent histological transformation to DPLN from focal proliferative and mesangial lupus nephritis within 9, 14, and 17 months respectively. Although it is relatively easy for the clinician to predict that a patient presenting with SLE and severe clinical manifestations of nephritis will have DPLN confirmed on renal biopsy, we have been impressed that this lesion may be present even in children with mild clinical manifestations. The profile of 29 children at the time of biopsy-confirmed DPLN illustrates this point (Table 6).

Severe proteinuria, even in the nephrotic range, does not always predict the presence of DPLN. Two children in our series with an unequivocal diagnosis of SLE had nephrotic syndrome at presentation and minimal glomerular histological changes consistent with the diagnosis of mesangial lupus nephritis (Fig. 5). Electron microscopy revealed that the foot processes of the glomerular epithelial cells were fused. The nephrotic syndrome responded quickly to

high-dose prednisone therapy and both girls were in complete remission within 10 days. We believe that their nephrotic syndrome was more typical of a 'minimal lesion-type disease' similar to previously reported cases (Abuelo 1984; Bakir et al. 1989). Since 1979, our incidence of membranous lupus nephritis has been 22 per cent, a frequency that is higher than most published paediatric series (8 per cent of 424 published cases). Whether this is because of an increase in the appreciation of this lesion by ultrastructural studies or due to a changing incidence of epimembranous disease in the past decade is unclear. A previous report of 70 children, who had biopsies taken at this institution between 1970 and 1985, revealed an 8 per cent incidence of membranous lupus nephritis (Baumal et al. 1987). Nephrotic-range proteinuria was present at the time of renal biopsy in 56 per cent of the current series of children with membranous nephropathy, and nephrotic syndrome subsequently developed in another 13 per cent; microscopic haematuria was present in 63 per cent of patients. Importantly, a diagnosis of SLE should be considered in any child with membranous nephropathy, a form of nephropathy that is rare in children and usually not of the idiopathic type.

In our experience the presence of focal necrotizing lesions, even in patients with focal proliferative lupus nephritis, is a bad prognostic sign. These lesions were present in 50 per cent of our patients with biopsy-proven focal proliferative disease, all of whom required treatment with a cytotoxic drug (azathioprine, cyclophosphamide or

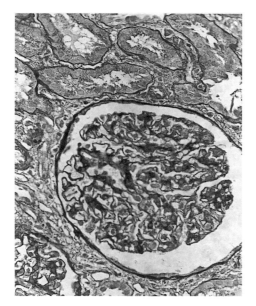

(a)

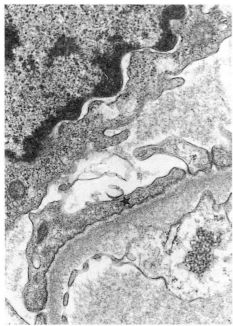

(b)

Fig. 5 Renal biopsy of a 14-year-old girl with SLE associated with nephrotic syndrome. (a) A few glomeruli showed a mild increase in mesangial matrix without mesangial cell proliferation. Several immune deposits were demonstrated in mesangial regions by immunofluorescence and electron microscopy. (b) Marked fusion of the foot processes of glomerular epithelial cells (star) was present. The nephrotic syndrome was in complete remission after 10 days of prednisone therapy. These clinical and histological features are typical of a 'minimal lesion-type disease'.

methotrexate) before their disease could be controlled adequately. In a long-term follow-up study of childhood lupus nephritis of all classes, renal insufficiency was reported in 53 per cent of patients who had focal necrotizing glomerular lesions on the initial biopsy (McCurdy *et al.* 1992). Although rare, focal necrotizing glomerulonephritis in the absence of significant glomerular immune deposits (pauci-immune) has been reported in patients with SLE (Akhtar *et al.* 1994).

In addition to providing a histological classification, renal biopsies can be used to evaluate the degree of active and chronic renal damage.

Semiquantitative scoring indices have been developed and although some controversy regarding the utility of these scores exists, they are particularly valuable in predicting the long-term outcome in patients with DPLN. A high score for the chronicity index is a bad prognostic sign. Austin and his colleagues from the National Institute of Health (NIH) (Austen *et al.* 1984) reported that patients with DPLN and any evidence of chronic damage on the initial renal biopsy had a much higher incidence of renal failure (Fig. 6). This group has recently reanalysed their experience, following the introduction of intensive treatment regimes that include intravenous pulse cyclophosphamide or methylprednisolone for patients with severe lupus nephritis (Austin *et al.* 1994). By multivariant survival analysis the combination of cellular crescents and interstitial fibrosis was shown to be the strongest histological predictor of a poor long-term prognosis at 80 months ($p = 0.0003$). In our series of patients followed since 1979, the three patients who have developed endstage renal disease all had advanced chronic disease on the renal biopsy done at the initial presentation and they developed irreversible renal failure within 3 years of diagnosis.

The evaluation of acute tubulointerstitial injury in lupus nephritis has been neglected until recently. Acute interstitial inflammation is commonly observed in patients with DPLN (75 per cent in our series) where it may or may not be associated with tubulointerstitial immune deposits. In our patient population, four patients without DPLN also had significant interstitial inflammation: three with membranous lupus nephritis (Fig. 7) and in one with atypical mesangial lupus nephritis associated with the nephrotic syndrome. Two of the later four patients had foci of immune deposits along tubular basement membranes. A study by Alexopoulos *et al.* (Alexopoulos *et al.* 1990) reported a positive correlation between the number of interstitial mononuclear cells and both renal function and the degree of chronic renal damage. Magil *et al.* reported a poorer outcome in patients, with tubulointerstitial immune deposits present in more than 20 per cent of the renal biopsy specimen (Magil *et al.* 1984).

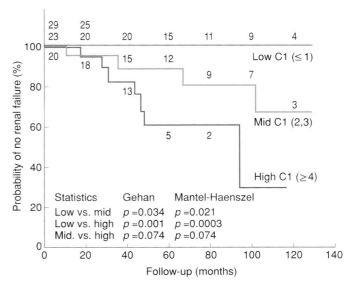

Fig. 6 Cumulative survival curves of 72 lupus patients with diffuse proliferative lupus nephritis (DPLN) demonstrating the negative impact of histological evidence of chronic renal damage on the long-term outcome of renal function. The chronicity index (CI; maximum score of 12 points) adversely affects renal survival rates (reproduced from Austin *et al.* (1984) with permission).

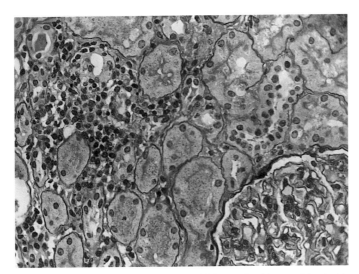

Fig. 7 Light photomicrograph of the renal biopsy of a 14-year-old girl with lupus nephritis illustrating the presence of interstitial inflammation. In this patient immunofluorescence and electron microscopy demonstrated the presence of immune deposits along tubular basement membranes. Interstitial inflammation is a common finding in lupus nephritis and often occurs in the absence of extraglomerular immune complex deposition.

Lupus interstitial nephritis should be considered in the differential diagnosis of older children presenting with renal tubular disorders (Bagga *et al.* 1993). We hope soon to gain a better understanding of the pathogenesis and treatment of the tubulointerstitial disease in lupus nephritis since chronic tubulointerstitial damage predicts a poor long-term prognosis.

As recently reviewed by Appel *et al.*, a variety of renal vascular lesions may be observed in SLE patients, including those associated with vascular immune complex deposits, non-inflammatory necrotizing vasculopathy, thrombotic microangiopathy and true renal vasculitis (Appel *et al.* 1994). Studies of renal vascular lesions in childhood SLE have not been published. Experience in adults suggests a worse prognosis than in patients without vascular lesions.

Regular evaluation of the urine is important in all SLE patients. Many patients with renal involvement develop urinary abnormalities within 3 years of diagnosis, but a longer lag period can occur (Tucker *et al.* 1995). One of our patients recently developed focal proliferative lupus nephritis 5 years after the initial diagnosis of SLE which was made at 11 years of age. The importance of follow-up is illustrated by the fact that there is now a 72 per cent incidence of renal disease in our patients that were reported in the 1993 edition of this chapter, while only 42 per cent of patients referred to our clinic since 1991 have so far had clinical evidence of nephritis.

Hypertension is a common manifestation in patients with SLE. An elevated blood pressure prior to steroid therapy suggests that the patient has DPLN or renovascular disease. The latter is unusual but has been observed in patients with the antiphospholipid antibodies who have a hypercoaguable state. One patient followed at our institution presented with an infarct to the lower pole of one kidney as the result of a segmental occlusion of the renal vein, in the absence of evidence of glomerulonephritis.

It is rare that patients present with haematuria due to a bleeding diathesis. We treated an 11-year-old girl who had gross haematuria resulting from factor-II deficiency. The bleeding reversed with plasma therapy and factor-II levels were normalized by treatment with steroids (Eberhard *et al.* 1994).

Urological manifestations of SLE are not widely recognized but are clearly documented in the literature. Urinary frequency may occur as a result of autoimmune cystitis. However, it is always important to rule out an infectious cause, particularly in immunosuppressed patients.

Treatment of nephritis

There is probably no topic in medicine more disputed than the management of patients with SLE. Once renal involvement is documented, immunosuppression is indicated and steroids remain the mainstay of therapy. The majority of patients with mesangial and focal proliferative disease are successfully managed with steroids alone, although those with associated focal segmental necrotizing lesions have a poorer prognosis and are likely to require additional treatment including the use of cytotoxic agents. Evaluation of newer treatment protocols for patients with DPLN is impeded by the need to follow adequate numbers of patients for 10 to 15 years in order to observe meaningful differences. Although our patients with DPLN are not managed by a rigid protocol, several principles of therapy have evolved.

1. Initial treatment always includes high-dose steroids (prednisone 2 mg/kg per day; maximum 60 mg/day), divided three times daily for 4 to 8 weeks, consolidated to once daily and then tapered slowly over several months. Most patients are maintained on low-dose prednisone for years in an attempt to minimize the risk of subsequent relapses.

2. Azathioprine (2 to 3 mg/kg per day) is initiated within the first month of diagnosis because we believe that the best information available today suggests that patients given cytotoxic drugs in addition to prednisone have a better long-term outcome. Although preliminary data suggests that cyclophosphamide might be a better cytotoxic drug for these patients (Austin *et al.* 1986), the majority of our patients do well without it. Since the long-term toxicities of cyclophosphamide (especially malignancy and infertility) are correlated with the lifetime accumulated dose, we are reluctant to use this drug initially in these children facing a lifetime of chronic illness. Concern about accelerated atherosclerosis by prolonged steroid use (Rubin *et al.* 1985) further rationalizes our use of azathioprine as a steroid-sparing agent. An interesting alternative that we have not used (Cameron 1994) is a protocol that includes an initial 8- to 12-week course of oral cyclophosphamide (3 mg/kg ideal body weight for height, reduced if renal insufficiency is present) followed by maintenance therapy with azathioprine.

3. Intravenous pulse cyclophosphamide given in a slightly modified version of the NIH protocol is used primarily to treat patients whose renal disease is controlled inadequately by steroids plus azathioprine. To date we have treated seven DPLN patients with intravenous cyclophosphamide. Although cyclophosphamide is an important addition to the therapeutic armamentarium, renal relapses following cessation of therapy clearly occur and cyclophosphamide is not universally effective. We have only seen a sustained remission in one in seven patients treated at our institution. Two patients experienced significant disease reactivation (carotid artery thrombosis and renal failure; recurrence of nephrotic syndrome and deterioration of renal function) after completion of

the 6 monthly doses during the 3-month period before the seventh dose was administered. One patient who was also maintained on high-dose prednisone appeared resistant to intravenous cyclophosphamide. After 8 monthly doses she remained hypo-complementaemic, serologically active and had a deterioration in her protein excretion from 0.7 to 2.4 g/24 h. Two additional patients were treated with cyclophosphamide for non-compliance with prednisone and azathioprine. One of these patients had normal renal function after a 2-year course of treatment but in follow-up remained non-compliant. He now has chronic renal failure after 9 years of the disease. The second patient refused to take prednisone during cyclophosphamide therapy. The protocol was discontinued after 7 doses due to non-responsive disease. One year ago this patient consented to treatment with prednisone and azathioprine and is currently in remission. The final patient that we treated had significant chronic renal disease at presentation. Her therapy was discontinued after 4 doses. Although she required dialysis during her initial admission and eventually came off dialysis for 2.5 years, we would no longer recommend cyclophosphamide therapy in this kind of patient (see next point).

4. The chronicity index should be taken into consideration when making decisions about the use of cytotoxic drugs. If advanced chronic disease is present indicating that endstage renal disease is inevitable and severe extrarenal manifestations of SLE are not present, then cytotoxic drugs are not justified. The survival of SLE patients on dialysis and following renal transplantation is very good (Bumgardner 1988; Nossent et al. 1991). The risk of recurrent lupus nephritis in renal allografts is very low. Unfortunately the overall incidence of malignancy following solid organ transplantation is approximately 4 per cent (Penn 1988) and we are concerned about increasing this risk, particularly by treating such a patient with cyclophosphamide.

5. High-dose pulse steroids and plasmapheresis may have a role in the management of patients presenting with acute fulminating renal disease. Methotrexate therapy may be useful in selected patients with long-term disease that is difficult to control (Abud-Mendoza et al. 1993), but its role has not been established. Methotrexate should be restricted to patients with good renal function to avoid serious drug toxicities.

6. Over the past couple of years we have treated an increasing number of renal flares with intravenous methylprednisolone at a dose of 30 mg/kg (maximum 1000 mg) daily for 3 consecutive days each month for 6 months. Two of the five children recently treated were patients with DPLN unresponsive to intravenous cyclophosphamide. Short-term results have been encouraging but whether a sustained long-term benefit will be achieved is not yet clear.

Close follow-up of these patients is essential in order to monitor disease activity, complications of therapy, the patient's understanding of their disease and compliance with treatment. In the evaluation of the renal response to therapy, follow-up urinalysis and quantification of urinary protein excretion rates are obvious. The presence of either red cell or white cell casts may precede a renal relapse. Persistent proteinuria one year after the initiation of treatment predicts a worse long-term prognosis (Fraenkel et al. 1994). We feel that two additional parameters are useful markers of renal disease activity. The first is the serum complement profile, particularly levels for the third component of complement (C3). As demonstrated by Laitman et al., patient outcome is improved if CH50 levels are normalized during the initial phase of therapy and if they remain normal during the maintenance phase (Laitman et al. 1989). Since SLE relapses tend to be mimetic, nephritis is likely to recur during this period. Although we do not consider serological abnormalities alone (i.e., hypocomplementaemia, increasing anti-DNA antibody levels) an indication to retreat a patient, clinically active disease frequently ensues and these patients need to be followed closely (Fig. 8).

Preservation of renal function is an obvious goal in patients with lupus nephritis. Unfortunately, obtaining an accurate measurement of the glomerular filtration rate is not easy. Taking inulin clearance as the 'gold standard', Meyers and his colleagues (Shemesh et al. 1985) have demonstrated that creatinine clearance determinations overestimate the glomerular filtration rate during the acute phase of lupus nephritis, probably as a result of tubular secretion of creatinine (Table 7). Isotopic tests (e.g. 99Tc-DTPA) appear to provide a more accurate measure of glomerular filtration rate in these patients.

The optimal treatment of patients with lupus membranous nephropathy is unknown. We agree with Appel et al. that the long-term outcome of these patients is less favourable than was suggested originally (Appel et al. 1987). A subset of these patients appears

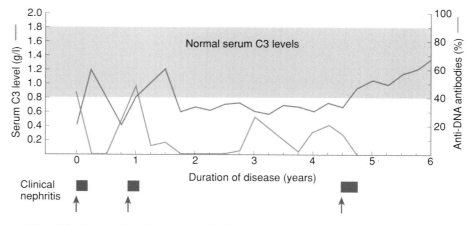

Fig. 8 Schematic summary of the clinical course of a girl with congenital C4 deficiency who developed SLE at 4 years of age associated with diffuse proliferative lupus nephritis. The value of monitoring serum C3 levels (solid line) is highlighted by her clinical course. Initial prednisone therapy (arrow) failed to maintain the C3 level in the normal range. She developed a clinical relapse of nephritis 10 months after the initial presentation, that was treated with prednisone and azathioprine (arrow). One year later the C3 level fell below the normal range. However, she remained clinically well for 3.5 years before findings of recurrent nephritis were documented and high-dose immunosuppression was reinitiated (arrow).

Table 7 Creatinine clearance is an unreliable measure of glomerular filtration rate in lupus nephritis[a]

Inulin clearance (ml/min per 1.73m^2)	n	Creatinine /inulin clearance
>80	13	1.20±0.08
40–80	10	1.57±0.11
<40	21	2.21±0.16

[a]As illustrated by the study of Shemesh *et al.* (1985) the creatinine clearance does not provide an accurate measure of the true glomerular filtration rate (assessed by inulin clearance rates) in patients with lupus nephritis. The more severe the reduction in renal function, the greater is this discrepancy.
c = clearance.

Haematological involvement

Anaemia, thrombocytopenia, and leucopenia are very common laboratory abnormalities seen in 50 to 75 per cent of patients with SLE. The most common anaemia is normochromic normocytic, which when persistent usually becomes a microcytic and hypochromic anaemia. There is both a decrease in the serum iron level and in the iron-binding capacity, with increased iron in macrophages. The serum ferritin is normal or elevated, as ferritin production is increased as part of the acute-phase response. In our experience, in the absence of an immune-mediated haemolytic anaemia (see below), the anaemia is rarely severe.

The Coombs' test is positive in approximately 30 to 40 per cent of our patients but less than 10 per cent of patients have overt haemolysis. Haemolysis is seen generally only in the presence of immunoglobulin on the surface of erythrocytes. The likely explanation for the lack of haemolysis when only complement is present is that red blood cells bind immune complexes through their C3b receptor (Wilson *et al.* 1989). Therefore, the presence of complement components (C3b) on the red blood cell probably represents the presence of immune complexes rather than of autoantibodies directed against erythrocytes. Furthermore, complement activation products, C4d and C3b, may non-specifically coat red blood cells and therefore, can be detected in a Coombs' test. When present, the autoimmune haemolytic anaemia may be a warm or cold. Although rarer than the warm, cold autoimmune haemolytic anaemia is usually associated with Raynaud's phenomenon or cold intolerance and patients more commonly present with haemolysis. Drug-induced haemolytic anaemia in our patients is not a common problem. Haemolysis secondary to autoimmune haemolytic anaemia is usually mild but occasionally it may be severe enough to require treatment with high-dose steroids for prolonged periods of time or even azathioprine or cyclophosphamide. Occasionally transfusions are required, but if the anaemia is secondary to an indirect Coombs' test then the cross-match will be incompatible and type O

destined to develop chronic renal failure and we believe that they should be treated with high-dose steroids. Less clear is the indication for alkylating agents. There is some encouraging preliminary evidence that alkylating agents are beneficial in the treatment of patients with the severe idiopathic form of membranous nephropathy (Imperiale *et al.* 1995) and it is tempting to speculate that alkylating agents may also be useful in patients with membranous nephropathy due to SLE. Unfortunately appropriate clinical trials have not yet addressed these important issues. A recent review by Sloan *et al.* (1996) reported that long-term prognosis in patients with SLE membranous nephritis was determined by the degree of associated glomerular inflammation seen on biopsy. The only patient at our institution with membranous SLE and diffuse endocapillary proliferation developed endstage renal disease.

For an overview of suggested therapy for renal disease see Box 4.

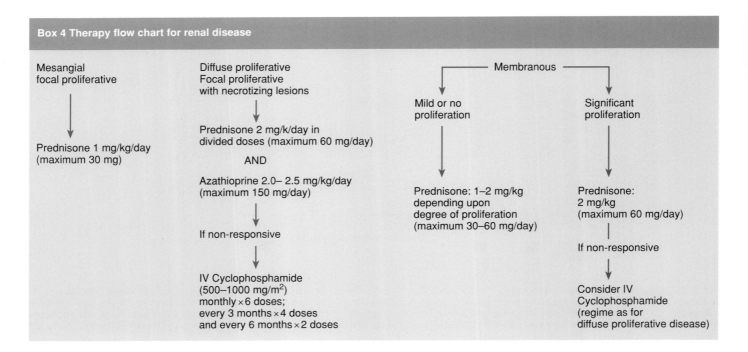

Box 4 Therapy flow chart for renal disease

Mesangial focal proliferative
↓
Prednisone 1 mg/kg/day (maximum 30 mg)

Diffuse proliferative Focal proliferative with necrotizing lesions
↓
Prednisone 2 mg/k/day in divided doses (maximum 60 mg/day)
AND
Azathioprine 2.0– 2.5 mg/kg/day (maximum 150 mg/day)
↓
If non-responsive
↓
IV Cyclophosphamide (500–1000 mg/m^2) monthly × 6 doses; every 3 months × 4 doses and every 6 months × 2 doses

Membranous

Mild or no proliferation
↓
Prednisone: 1–2 mg/kg depending upon degree of proliferation (maximum 30–60 mg/day)

Significant proliferation
↓
Prednisone: 2 mg/kg (maximum 60 mg/day)
↓
If non-responsive
↓
Consider IV Cyclophosphamide (regime as for diffuse proliferative disease)

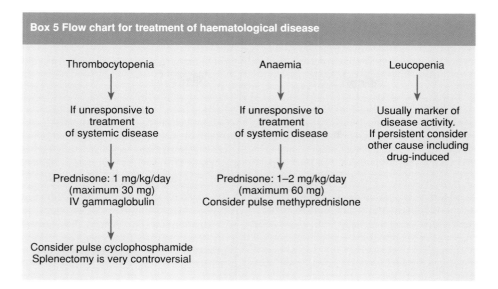

Box 5 Flow chart for treatment of haematological disease

Rh-negative blood is recommended. For an overview of suggested therapy for anaemia see Box 5.

Thrombocytopenia is present in 15 to 45 per cent and in our experience, it may be the initial presentation in up to 15 per cent of paediatric cases. The thrombocytopenia is secondary to peripheral destruction rather than bone marrow suppression. It can occur early in the disease course and may present as classic idiopathic thrombocytopenic purpura, which would be better referred to as autoimmune thrombocytopenic purpura. We have found that these patients have a positive antinuclear antibody and most patients will have decreased complement levels (uncommon in isolated idiopathic thrombocytopenic purpura). Patients with autoimmune thrombocytopenic purpura may have a transient response to intravenous immunoglobulin treatment. The presentation of isolated idiopathic thrombocytopenic purpura progressing to SLE is more common in children than adults. The development of SLE may take 20 years or more. Most patients with idiopathic thrombocytopenic purpura and autoimmune haemolytic anaemia, so-called Evans syndrome, will probably develop SLE. Interestingly, many patients with thrombocytopenia secondary to SLE will respond to therapy with intravenous immunoglobulin.

Despite the high incidence of thrombocytopenia in paediatric SLE, bleeding is unusual and usually occurs only when the platelet count is less than 10 000. Most patients with thrombocytopenia will respond to steroid therapy. If the patient becomes either steroid-resistant or steroid-dependent then pulse steroid therapy or intravenous immunoglobulin therapy should be tried, with cyclophosphamide reserved for resistant cases (Lipnick et al. 1990). Splenectomy is very controversial as some reports have suggested not only a lack of effect but also an unacceptably high increase in infections of these patients postsplenectomy. These findings are not universal and splenectomy may have a role in resistant, persistent life-threatening thrombocytopenia. For an overview of suggested therapy for thrombocytopenia see Box 5.

In addition to thrombocytopenia, acquired abnormalities of platelet function have been described. These include serum inhibitors that decrease aggregation and block uptake and storage of adenosine diphosphate and serotonin. Collagen-induced aggregation may be absent and adenosine diphosphate and adrenaline-induced aggregation impaired (Decker et al. 1979). These defects generally present as purpura while overt bleeding is rare.

Leucopenia is seen in 20 to 40 per cent of cases of paediatric SLE. Both lymphopenia and granulocytopenia can be seen. The lymphopenia may be secondary to the presence of circulating lymphocytotoxic antibodies which may be cold- or warm-reacting; IgM or IgG; and directed against resting or activated cells (Peake et al. 1988). In many patients lymphopenia is a sensitive marker of general disease activity and will rarely if ever require specific therapy. A lymphopenia may also be secondary to therapy with azathioprine or cyclophosphamide. Granulocytopenia is usually secondary to a central depression of granulopoiesis or splenic sequestration and more rarely antigranulocyte antibodies. Drugs including prednisone, azathioprine, and cyclophosphamide decrease granulocyte function and/or numbers. All of these problems probably contribute to the increased susceptibility to infection seen in SLE patients.

Other unusual haematological problems in SLE include myelofibrosis, and thrombotic thrombocytopenic purpura. Myelofibrosis, although rarely seen, is more common in the paediatric age group while there have been reports of thrombotic thrombocytopenic purpura progressing to SLE. Thrombotic thrombocytopenic purpura, as opposed to haemolytic-uraemic syndrome, is rarely seen in childhood. When it does occur, the diagnosis of SLE should be considered. An interesting association is the development of SLE in adolescents with sickle-cell anaemia; the SLE usually develops prior to the age of 18 (Katsanis et al. 1987).

Following thrombocytopenia, the presence of the lupus anticoagulant is the most common coagulation defect. This abnormality presents with an elevated partial thromboplastin time and occurs in 20 to 30 per cent of paediatric cases. The prothrombin time is usually normal or minimally elevated and if markedly prolonged a second defect is probably present (see below). The lupus anticoagulant reacts with the phospholipid portion of the prothrombin activator complex. This antibody cross-reacts with anticardiolipin antibodies, which are seen commonly in paediatric SLE (Shergy et al. 1988), and may be responsible for the false-positive VDRL (Veneral Disease Research Laboratory). Patients with the lupus anticoagulant do not bleed but rather have an increased incidence of deep vein thrombosis, thromboemboli, and less commonly arterial thrombosis. The increased partial thromboplastin time will usually resolve with steroids; however, treatment should not be directed to this laboratory finding alone, but reserved for patients who have clotting problems. When a venous or arterial thrombosis occurs, then patients should be subjected to anticoagulation with heparin followed by warfarin. We recommend that these patients receive full anticoagulant treatment for 3 to 6 months followed by long-term low-dose anticoagulation. We suggest that the INR should be maintained between 1.5 and 2.0. A recent adult study supports the view of long-term anticoagulation although the suggested INR range is higher (Khamashta et al. 1995). In many patients the presence of the anticoagulant correlates with disease activity, especially with vasculitis. The anticoagulant may be IgG, IgM or both. The full spectrum of diseases associated with antiphospholipid antibodies and the lupus anticoagulant is fully discussed in Chapters 5.7.1 and 5.7.3. However it must be remembered that patients with antiphospholipid antibodies may not only present with venous or arterial events, but chorea may be the only manifestation of these autoantibodies. These patients with chorea are at risk for thrombosis or other manifestations of the antiphospholipid antibody syndrome.

Specific inhibitors of other factors of the coagulation cascade have been described. The most common of these is prothrombin deficiency which is associated usually with the lupus anticoagulant. These patients, unlike those with the anticoagulant only, present with bleeding and a prolonged prothrombin and partial thromboblastin time. This defect is reported in approximately 5 per cent of adult patients with the lupus anticoagulant or in less than 1 per cent of all adult SLE patients. Prothrombin deficiency appears to be more common in paediatric SLE and a review of our patients demonstrated this abnormality in approximately 4 per cent of our SLE patients (Eberhard et al. 1994). As expected these patients presented with bleeding rather than clotting. Many patients with prothrombin deficiency have an associated mild thrombocytopenia, but the platelet counts are generally greater than 50 000. The aetiology is unknown and it may result from an acquired production defect or secondary to the presence of an antiprothrombin antibody. We have found that the prothrombin deficiency will rapidly respond to steroid therapy. More rarely a steroid-responsive acquired von Willebrand's defect has been described.

Splenomegaly is quite common occurring in 20 to 30 per cent of paediatric cases. In our series of patients splenomegaly was seen commonly in patients less than 10 years of age and may be the result of the generalized inflammatory state. Functional asplenia has been described and this abnormality of splenic function may increase the incidence of sepsis (Malleson 1989).

The final haematological complication we will discuss is the association of SLE and cancer. Despite the frequent use of immunosuppressive therapy and abnormal immunoregulation, malignancy as a cause of death is rare. There may be a higher incidence of neoplasia than in the general population, but most tumours are of epithelial origin and are easily treated. There have been case reports of lymphoma, including Burkitt's lymphoma, in patients with SLE; from the other perspective, patients with lymphoma may have many features suggestive of SLE, including the presence of a high titre of antinuclear antibodies (Posner et al. 1990). We have seen cases of lymphomas presenting as 'SLE' including a positive, high-titre, speckled antinuclear antibody. Therefore, the presence of a high-titred antinuclear antibody does not help in differentiating these two disorders.

Cardiac involvement

Symptomatic pericarditis is the most common cardiac manifestation occurring in approximately 5 to 25 per cent of patients with SLE and is commonly associated with pleurisy (De Inocencio and Lovell 1994). The diagnosis is made by physical examination, chest radiography, electrocardiogram and confirmed by echocardiogram. Cardiac tamponade rarely occurs. Studies in adults have suggested that echocardiographic evidence of pericarditis may occur in up to 75 per cent of patients (Doherty and Siegel 1985). Similar studies have not been performed in children. Most cases of pericarditis will rapidly respond to either nonsteroidal anti-inflammatory drugs alone, or low to moderate dose of corticosteroids. We suggest the initial use of indomethacin at a dose of 3 mg/kg per day divided into three doses. Indomethacin appears to work well in patients with SLE and is well tolerated in the paediatric patient. Rarely pulse intravenous methylprednisolone is required and on occasion pericardiocentesis is necessary if tamponade is impending. Antimalarials may be of benefit in the long-term management of pericarditis.

The diagnosis of myocarditis or endocarditis is uncommon, with clinically detectable or significant myocarditis in less than 10 per cent of patients (Badui et al. 1985). However, autopsy studies in adults have shown evidence of myocarditis in 25 to 50 per cent of patients. There is no similar autopsy data available in children. Occasionally, patients with myocarditis may present with first degree atrioventricular block or arrhythmia. A study from 1985 showed that Libman–Sacks endocarditis as present in 30 to 50 per cent of all hearts from patients with SLE at autopsy, while echocardiographic evidence of small vegetations may occur in 2 to 5 per cent of cases (Doherty and Siegel 1985). These vegetations commonly occur at valvular rings and commissures. However, clinically significant lesions causing aortic or mitral stenosis or regurgitation are very rare.

Unlike Libman–Sacks endocarditis which appears to be declining with steroid usage, atherosclerotic heart disease and myocardial infarction are increasing with greater steroid usage and longevity of patients (Rubin et al. 1985). Other risk factors, especially hypertension and hyperlipidaemia further increase the risk of myocardial infarction. The presence of either the lupus anticoagulant or antiphospholipid antibodies may further predispose to thrombosis and myocardial infarction. Hyperlipidaemia can either be the result of a primary hyperlipidaemia of SLE or secondary to treatment with steroids, which alters lipid profiles including cholesterol, triglycerides and both high-density and low-density lipoprotein levels (Ilowite et al. 1988). Although myocardial infarction during childhood or adolescence is rare, the incidence of myocardial infarction in young adults (under 25 years of age) with initial onset of SLE in the paediatric age is increasing. When myocardial infarction or chest pain occurs in young patients or shortly following the diagnosis of SLE, the presence of coronary arteritis must be suspected (Friedman et al. 1990). Although it occurs in less than 1 per cent of cases, aggressive treatment of this potentially life-threatening complication with high-dose steroids and immunosuppressive agents is required. We have found recently that many paediatric patients may have asymptomatic abnormalities of cardiac perfusion, which can be demonstrated by nuclear cardiac imaging. The clinical significance of these abnormalities is unknown but they may predispose these patients to early ischaemic heart disease.

Congenital heart block and neonatal lupus erythematosus will be dealt with in another section.

Pulmonary involvement

Pulmonary involvement is common in paediatric SLE occurring in 25 to 75 per cent of cases. The manifestations range from severe life-threatening pulmonary haemorrhage or infection to asymptomatic abnormalities of pulmonary function tests (see Table 8 for a complete list of pulmonary complications). Decreased carbon monoxide diffusing capacity is the most common abnormality in both paediatric and adults patients; in one paediatric series it was seen in 100 per cent of unselected patients (Delgado *et al.* 1990). The next most common abnormality in the pulmonary function test is a restrictive pattern in 35 to 60 per cent of cases, while an obstructive defect is uncommon. The functional defects are probably secondary to chronic fibrotic changes that in turn are secondary to mild subclinical lupus pneumonitis, as suggested by the diffusing capacity abnormalities and restrictive rather than obstructive defects. These abnormalities rarely require specific therapy.

Pleural involvement occurs in up to 50 per cent of cases at some time during the disease course and is seen commonly in association with pericarditis. However, isolated pleuritis, presenting as chest pain, can occur during a systemic flare and may be unilateral. Pleural fluid examination reveals decreased levels of C3 and C4, an increased white blood-cell count, normal glucose and can show a positive antinuclear antibody. There have been reports of a positive antinuclear antibody only in the pleural fluid but not the peripheral blood. When the pleuritis is mild, treatment can consist of anti-inflammatory doses of non-steroidals, but usually prednisone, at a low to moderate dose, is required for complete resolution of symptoms. Similar to patients with pericarditis, antimalarials may be of benefit in the long-term management of pleuritis.

Dyspnoea, a common symptom, can be secondary to acute or chronic pneumonitis, pulmonary infection, pulmonary haemorrhage or shrinking lung syndrome. The dramatic presentation of acute pneumonitis with fever, cough, dyspnoea, hypoxia and chest pain occurs in only 3 to 10 per cent of patients (Carette *et al.* 1984). Pulmonary haemorrhage has a reported death rate of up to 50 per cent and in many paediatric studies this complication accounts for

10 to 20 per cent of deaths despite its occurrence in less than 5 per cent of patients (Nadorra and Landing 1987). Pulmonary haemorrhage or acute pneumonitis must be differentiated from congestive heart failure, pulmonary infection, and non-cardiogenic pulmonary oedema that are the side-effects of drugs and secondary to uraemia, pancreatitis, or sepsis. The clinical differentiation of acute SLE pneumonitis from pulmonary haemorrhage may be aided by a fall in haemoglobin, the presence of haemoptysis and an increased carbon monoxide diffusing capacity on pulmonary function tests seen in pulmonary haemorrhage. The treatment for both is similar and the acute management may require intubation and ventilation in addition to aggressive immunosuppressive therapy, which may include high-dose prednisone and cyclophosphamide. Pulmonary haemorrhage may be the initial and sole manifestation of paediatric SLE and this disease should be considered in young patients presenting with pulmonary haemorrhage even in the absence of other disease manifestations.

In the acutely ill patient the possibility of pulmonary infection must be considered. There is an increased incidence of infection even prior to steroid or immunosuppressive treatment. In addition to the more common bacterial and viral causes of pneumonia, these patients are at risk for opportunistic infection including fungal, parasitic and protozoan infection. We have seen a patient on prednisone and azathioprine who developed *Pneumocystis carinii* pneumonia and others have described patients with this complication while on methotrexate and prednisone. When patients present with acute respiratory failure and fever, we recommend treatment with broad-spectrum antibiotics and high-dose steroids including pulse therapy. If the above-mentioned opportunistic relevant infections are suspected clinically, then antifungal, antiprotozoan, antilegionella, antipneumocystis and even antinocardia therapy should be considered. If the patient does not improve quickly then a diagnostic open lung biopsy is necessary. The use of bronchial washings obtained via bronchoscopy should be considered early, especially if intubation is required.

In contrast to acute pneumonitis, chronic or interstitial pneumonitis has an insidious onset. Clinically significant disease is uncommon and usually follows long-standing SLE. When severe, most patients have clinically evident pulmonary involvement and present with cough and chest pain leading to dyspnoea and a decreased diffusing capacity. An autopsy study of 26 paediatric patients with SLE showed a mild chronic interstitial pneumonitis in all patients, with additional pulmonary lesions in 18 patients (Nadorra and Landing 1987). Most of the chronic lesions were asymptomatic prior to death.

A more unusual cause of dyspnoea is the shrinking lung syndrome. This disorder is diagnosed by chest radiography that demonstrates an elevated diaphragm in the clinical setting of dyspnoea, which might be mild. A paediatric review demonstrated radiographic evidence of an elevated diaphragm in 12 per cent of patients (Delgado *et al.* 1990). They hypothesized that this syndrome was caused by a combination of inspiratory muscle dysfunction, recurrent pleuritis and atelectasis. The long-time outcome is generally good despite the lack of effective therapy, as it is usually a slowly progressive disease. Pulmonary function tests show abnormal diaphragm function and restrictive airway disease.

One of the most fascinating pulmonary manifestations of SLE is pulmonary hypertension (Asherson and Oakley 1986). Difficult to treat, pulmonary hypertension fortunately is rare and is seen usually

---

Table 8 Pulmonary involvement in childhood SLE

Pleuritis

Diaphragm involvement including shrinking lungs

Pneumonitis (acute or chronic)

Vasculitis

Pulmonary haemorrhage

Pulmonary emboli

Isolated pulmonary function test abnormalities

Drug-induced changes

Pulmonary hypertension

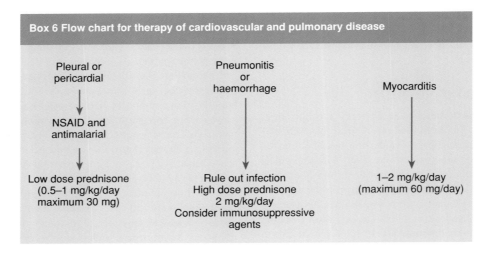

only with long-standing disease. These patients present with classic signs and symptoms of primary pulmonary hypertension but it may evolve from one of five processes. The first is best regarded as primary pulmonary hypertension of SLE. There is no known cause or predisposing clinical setting. The second cause is secondary to pulmonary artery thrombosis or emboli and is seen in patients with antiphospholipid antibodies and/or with severe Raynaud's phenomenon. The third cause is secondary to chronic left ventricular failure. The fourth is secondary to chronic hypoxic from diffuse interstitial lung disease, with the hypertension usually out of proportion to the parenchymal disease. The final cause is obstruction of peripheral pulmonary vasculature secondary to vasculitis. Overall, the outcome of pulmonary hypertension is poor but luckily it is a rare manifestation, especially in children. An overview of suggested therapy for cardiovascular and pulmonary disease is given in Box 6.

Gastrointestinal disease

Gastrointestinal involvement occurs in 20 to 40 per cent of paediatric patients. The most common complaint is abdominal pain that can be the result of peritoneal inflammation (serositis), vasculitis, pancreatitis and/or direct bowel wall involvement (enteritis). In many patients, the abdominal pain heralds a disease flare in another system. The presentation of serositis may vary from mild crampy or colicky pain to severe pain with a rigid abdomen. It can be difficult to differentiate peritoneal inflammation as a manifestation of the underlying SLE from infective peritonitis.

Bowel wall inflammation presenting as crampy, abdominal pain and diarrhoea can be caused by a primary enteritis or be secondary to a mesenteric vasculitis or thrombosis (Hoffman and Katz 1980). The latter two are generally more acute and may be accompanied by bloody diarrhoea and nausea or vomiting. These disorders must be differentiated because vasculitis with thrombosis may require urgent surgery owing to the risk of bowel ischaemia, while most cases of non-thrombotic enteritis will respond to steroids. Involvement of other organ systems may aid in the diagnosis as there is an association of severe enteritis with central nervous system disease and lupus cystitis (Orth *et al.* 1983). This disorder requires aggressive immunosuppressive therapy and although this is an unusual association, paediatric cases have been described. We have seen a patient present with cystitis who rapidly developed severe enteritis with bowel perforation,

disease of the central nervous system and nephritis. Despite aggressive immunosuppressive therapy, the patient died (Eberhard *et al.* 1991a).

An autopsy study of 26 young patients demonstrated that abdominal pain occurred in 65 per cent of all paediatric patients and gastrointestinal bleeding in 46 per cent. Dysphagia and symptoms of reflux were unusual. In 15 out of 25 autopsies a gastrointestinal 'vasculopathy' was found with ischaemic lesions, and a non-specific infiltrate was found in 96 per cent. In 20 per cent of the cases, autopsy findings of ischaemic bowel were clinically asymptomatic (Nadorra *et al.* 1987). These authors suggested that chronic lupus enteritis, as defined by the presence of a non-specific infiltrate, was common at autopsy. However, these patients probably had severe SLE, as they died before reaching adulthood.

Pancreatitis, although it must always be considered, is a rare cause of abdominal pain in paediatric patients. There are very few reports in the literature, with an overall incidence of less than 2 per cent. In order to determine the true incidence of pancreatic dysfunction in SLE, we prospectively evaluated pancreatic function and performed pancreatic ultrasonography in 36 patients. We did not find any significant pancreatic pathology over the 2 year study period and could not find any association of pancreatic function abnormalities with steroid or azathioprine use (Eberhard *et al.* 1992). However, others have reported pancreatitis associated with disease flares, some of which responded to increased steroid dose (Nadorra *et al.* 1987). Rarely a pancreatic pseudocyst may be present at diagnosis.

Liver disease

Hepatomegaly occurs in 40 to 50 per cent of paediatric patients, while abnormalities of liver function tests may occur in up to 25 per cent. However, the elevation of liver enzymes is usually mild and transient. When there is marked elevation of liver function tests another cause must be sought (Miller 1977). The clinical features of autoimmune chronic active hepatitis, so-called 'lupoid hepatitis', may mimic SLE. Both these diseases preferentially occur in adolescent females. Many patients with the autoimmune form of chronic active hepatitis have a malar rash, arthritis and autoantibodies including anti-DNA antibodies, but they rarely have renal involvement (Hall *et al.* 1985; Hall *et al.* 1986). The differentiation between SLE and autoimmune hepatitis may require a liver biopsy. When jaundice is a prominent feature in a known SLE patient then a second disease such as obstruction, haemolysis or viral hepatitis is probably the cause.

Liver involvement may be part of the generalized vasculitis and may explain the increased salicylate sensitivity seen in 10 to 20 per cent of SLE patients. However, salicylate toxicity rarely results in significant, permanent pathological changes. A similar percentage of patients with systemic juvenile arthritis, another disease with systemic vasculitis, develop salicylate sensitivity. An increased incidence of hepatotoxicity to other drugs including azathioprine, and even cyclophosphamide, has been reported. Rarely systemic vasculitis has resulted in hepatic rupture secondary to liver infarction. These patients present with an acute abdomen and usually have evidence of active vasculitis and Raynaud's phenomenon elsewhere.

Endocrine involvement

Thyroid involvement is the most common endocrine organ involved in SLE. In a prospective study we found that antithyroid antibodies are present in 45 per cent of paediatric patients and clinical hypothyroidism was present in 15 per cent (Eberhard *et al.* 1991b). The development of hypothyroidism usually preceded or was coincidental with the development of SLE. The association of these two diseases may reflect similar genetic susceptibility or a common inciting agent. Hyperthyroidism, although less common than hypothyroidism, occurs with an increased incidence in SLE patients than the general paediatric population. Steroid-induced diabetes mellitus occurs in up to 10 per cent of patients but a lower percentage require insulin treatment. There does not appear to be an increased incidence of diabetes mellitus in the absence of steroid therapy. Delayed puberty and menstrual abnormalities are seen commonly. However, these abnormalities are probably secondary to chronic illness and active disease, rather than as a direct result of the disease process. Rarely hypoparathyroidism has been reported in association with SLE. This diagnosis should be considered in the presence of unexplained hypocalcaemia.

Autoantibodies

The hallmark of SLE is the production of autoantibodies. There is a long list of antibodies directed against histone, non-histone, RNA-binding, cytoplasmic and nuclear proteins. Many articles have reviewed the structure and function of the autoantigens and their role in autoimmune disease. A good review of autoantibodies is found in Chapter 5.7.3 and therefore, in this section we will focus on the limited literature regarding specific autoantibodies and disease manifestation in paediatric SLE.

The most common autoantibody is antinuclear. Depending on the series and method of detection, a positive antinuclear antibody is seen in 85 to 100 per cent of paediatric patients. As in adults, adolescent patients negative for this antibody have been described. The incidence of true antinuclear antibody-negative SLE has decreased with the use of human cell line substrates and procedures that eliminate the loss of some of the extractable nuclear antigens. Historically, anti-DNA antibodies were present in 78 to 87 per cent of cases depending on the series. The older series tend to have a higher incidence than the more recent series. This probably reflects the increase in awareness of paediatric SLE without anti-DNA antibodies and we have found anti-DNA antibodies in approximately 70 per cent of our cases. Studies in adults

have suggested that patients with renal disease have higher avidity antibodies than patients with central nervous system disease, in whom anti-DNA antibodies are less common. Similar studies have not been undertaken in children. A paediatric study demonstrated that a lower percentage of paediatric SLE patients had a lower percentage of patients with IgG anti-DNA antibodies than adults, while conversely IgM anti-DNA antibodies were present in a higher percentage of paediatric patients. The anti-DNA antibodies measured were directed against single-stranded DNA (Shergy *et al.* 1989). Similarly there was an increased percentage of paediatric patients with IgM anti-Sm, anticardiolipin and anti-70 kDa ribonucleoprotein antibodies when compared with adult SLE patients (Ward *et al.* 1990). The authors suggested that this was the result of a time-related maturation of the immune response. Therefore, evidence for not only IgG antibodies but also IgM antibodies should be sought in paediatric patients. In enzyme-linked immunosorbent assays (ELISA), the overall incidence of anti-Sm antibodies was 58 per cent, anticardiolipin antibodies were present in 50 per cent of patients, and anti-70 kDa ribonucleoprotein antibodies were present in more than 90 per cent of patients.

Rheumatoid factor has been seen in 12 to 29 per cent of patients by conventional methods. To date there has been no study of the incidence of rheumatoid factor as detected by ELISA. Anticardiolipin antibodies may be present in up to 30 per cent of patients and the lupus anticoagulant is present in approximately 20 per cent of cases. No studies have examined the incidence of anti-Ro and/or anti-La antibodies in paediatric patients, but similar to adults, the presence of anti-Ro and anti-La antibodies defines a population which is at risk of a photosensitive rash and subacute cutaneous lupus.

As previously stated in the haematology section, the presence of anticardiolipin antibodies, the lupus anticoagulant and antiphospholipid antibodies is associated with an increased risk of thrombosis. These autoantibodies are common in paediatric patients and these patients are at increased risk for thrombosis (Shergy *et al.* 1988; Molta *et al.* 1993; Ravelli *et al.* 1994). In our experience, thrombosis may occur in up to 50 per cent of patients with detectable antiphospholipid antibodies. The thrombosis may be arterial or venous. Furthermore, these patients are at risk for the development of other manifestations of the antiphospholipid antibody syndrome including chorea, avascular necrosis, epilepsy, migraine headache, and livedo reticularis (Ravelli *et al.* 1994). There have been recent reports of neonatal thrombosis as the result of the transplacental passage of maternal antiphospholipid antibodies (see section on neonatal lupus erythematosus).

Antiribosomal P antibodies have been addressed in more detail in the section on central nervous system disease. These antibodies appear to be present in approximately 15 per cent of all patients with SLE and there is an increased incidence of antiribosomal P antibodies in patients with psychosis. In patients with psychosis titres of antiribosomal P antibodies may vary with disease activity in the central nervous system. These autoantibodies may be either IgM or IgG.

Similar to the findings seen in spouses of adults with SLE, autoantibodies have been found to be increased in the sera of relatives of paediatric SLE patients. More recently, the presence and titre of anti-Ro antibodies in the asymptomatic mothers of children with SLE correlated with the onset of SLE prior to age 10 and with the male sex (Lehman *et al.* 1989a). The reasons for these observations are not clear.

Neonatal lupus erythematosus

The neonatal lupus erythematosus syndrome (NLE) is a disease of the newborn defined by the demonstration of maternal autoantibodies and characteristic clinical features in the neonatal period. NLE is assumed to be the result of fetal and/or neonatal damage caused by the transplacental passage of maternal IgG autoantibodies. The major clinical manifestations are cardiac and dermatological, with complete congenital heart block being the most significant lesion (Reed *et al.* 1983; Watson *et al.* 1984; Lee *et al.* 1986). More rarely haemolytic anaemia, thrombocytopenia, urinary abnormalities and liver dysfunction are seen (Watson *et al.* 1984; McCune *et al.* 1987). Most early reports suggested that children with NLE are born to mothers with anti-Ro antibodies (Reed *et al.* 1983; Watson *et al.* 1984; Lee *et al.* 1986). However, in larger studies, we and others have demonstrated that the presence of anti-La antibodies in association with anti-Ro antibodies is a more specific disease maker, especially in patients with congenital heart block, and that the presence of anti-La antibodies was a greater risk factor for the development of congenital heart block than the presence of anti-Ro antibodies alone (Buyon and Winchester 1990; Silverman *et al.* 1991). In addition, antibodies directed against 52 kDa Ro were more specific than antibodies directed against the 60 kDa form in determining the risk of development of NLE, although other studies have suggested the importance of antinative 60 kDa Ro antibodies (Buyon *et al.* 1993; Lee *et al.* 1994; Reichlin *et al.* 1994).

The clinical spectrum

Cardiac lesions

The characteristic cardiac lesion of NLE is isolated congenital heart block although there have been case reports of congenital heart block in association with endomyocardial fibroelastosis, valvular insufficiency and patent ductus arteriosus. Ho *et al.* described the histopathology of eight hearts with complete congenital heart block, seven of which were associated with maternal anti-Ro antibodies (Ho *et al.* 1986). There was no mention of the maternal anti-La antibody status. These seven hearts all showed identical abnormalities in the conducting system, namely, a lack of contact between atrial myocardial tissue and the more distal part of the atrioventricular conduction (Lev *et al.* 1971).

In some cases of congenital heart block, in addition to the above mentioned changes, ventricular endomyocardial fibrosis and small inflammatory infiltrates have been described (Hogg 1957). The histopathology of the lesion suggests either early interference with normal organogenesis, or intrauterine inflammatory lesions resulting in subsequent scarring (Carter *et al.* 1974). We believe the latter hypothesis to be true for the following reasons: (i) bradycardia is usually a later intrauterine event corresponding to the time when maternal autoantibodies begin to cross the placenta; (ii) immunofluorescent studies have shown deposition of IgG, complement components and fibrin indicating at least an initial inflammatory event; and (iii) case reports of mothers with SLE which describe the sudden onset of fetal bradycardia and congestive heart failure at 23 to 24 weeks and the reversal of intrauterine congestive heart failure and myocarditis but not the heart block with treatment of the mother with dexamethasone, with or without plasmapheresis. Taken together these data suggest there is initially an inflammatory lesion in the fetal heart. The inflammatory lesion hypothesis is supported by the pathological

demonstration of fibrosis at the chordae tendinae and the ventricular septum (Smith and Ho 1994; Weber and Myers 1994).

Investigators have attempted to use animal models to determine the cause of congenital heart block. Anti-Ro and/or anti-La antibodies may alter membrane action potential of rabbit conduction tissue and these abnormalities may resemble the cardiac conduction disorders seen in NLE (Alexander *et al.* 1992; Garcia *et al.* 1994). However, these conduction changes were not specific for anti-Ro/La sera derived from mothers of children with NLE, and sera obtained from mothers who had delivered unaffected children had similar effects on the rabbit conducting tissue (Garcia *et al.* 1994).

Congenital heart block was described originally as a relatively benign condition. However, studies of large series of patients with this condition are not as optimistic. Of our 60 patients with congenital heart block, approximately 50 per cent have required pacemaker therapy. The pacemaker may not be necessary neonatally but rather in later life. We have had neonatal deaths and later deaths as a result of pacemaker failure. A follow-up report of 14 children with congenital heart block showed that 3 of the children (21 per cent) died neonatally of congestive heart failure secondary to the block and a further 5 required pacemakers (McCune *et al.* 1987). Therefore, although congenital heart block has been felt to be rather benign, most series have demonstrated both intrauterine and neonatal deaths with the potential for further deaths to occur secondary to pacemaker failure.

Skin lesions

The skin lesions of NLE are very similar to those of subacute cutaneous lupus erythematosus in which at least 80 per cent of patients have anti-Ro antibodies (Deng *et al.* 1984). Both Ro and La antigens have been documented in human skin (Harmon *et al.* 1984; Lee *et al.* 1985), and exposure to ultraviolet light increases the expression of Ro on the surface of keratinocytes (LeFeber *et al.* 1984). This feature may explain the photosensitive nature of the skin rash in both NLE and subacute cutaneous lupus erythematosus (Fig. 9). Maternally transmitted factors other than anti-Ro and anti-La antibodies may play a role in the development of cutaneous NLE. Although cutaneous NLE is almost universally associated with anti-Ro and/or anti-La

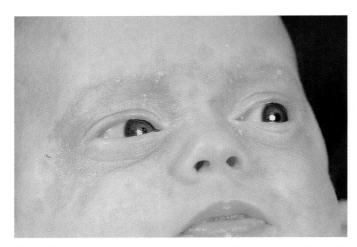

Fig. 9 The face of a 3-month-old baby delivered to a healthy mother with anti-Ro and anti-La antibodies. Note the scaly erythematosus areas around the eyes. This rash healed without scarring following the use of topical steroid cream.

antibodies, there have been reports of the condition with anti-U1 ribonucleoprotein antibodies, instead of anti-Ro or anti-La antibodies. In our prospective study, we demonstrated maternal anti-Ro antibodies in 100 per cent of cutaneous NLE patients, while anti-La antibodies were present in 75 per cent of sera.

Liver disease

Enlargement of the liver, spleen or both occurs in approximately 30 per cent of cases of NLE. The enlargement of these organs may be secondary to congestive heart failure, but there may also be primary hepatic enlargement. In most cases, the liver disease is associated with other clinical manifestations of NLE. These patients presented with liver enlargement, elevated levels of hepatic enzymes and evidence of cholestasis (Laxer *et al.* 1990). The histological changes seen on biopsy include giant cell transformation, ductal obstruction and extramedullary haematopoiesis. The liver changes generally are not severe and recovery from the liver disease usually occurs despite the presence of residual fibrosis on repeat biopsy. However, we and others have seen cases of severe intrahepatic cholestasis secondary to NLE (Lee *et al.* 1993; Rosh *et al.* 1993).

Haematological problems occasionally occur including thrombocytopenia, rarely leading to bleeding, and a mild haemolytic anaemia. Urinary abnormalities include transient pyuria or urethritis, but to date there have been no cases of nephritis.

Treatment

Cutaneous NLE rarely requires treatment as usually it is self-limited and usually heals without scarring. In the unusual case with more severe or scarring lesions, topical steroids may be required. The liver disease of NLE will usually spontaneously resolve by the age of six months and does not require steroid treatment. However, if the cholestasis is severe, these infants may require a formula high in medium-chain triglycerides.

The treatment or prevention of congenital heart block is much more complex than the treatment of cutaneous NLE. Previously, it had been suggested that all mothers at risk for delivering a child with congenital heart block should be treated with plasmapheresis and dexamethasone throughout the pregnancy (Buyon *et al.* 1988). However, this form of treatment will subject both the mother and the fetus to significant risks during the pregnancy, and up to 90 per cent of mothers will deliver a normal child without congenital heart block, despite having previously delivered a child with this condition (McCune *et al.* 1987; Buyon *et al.* 1988). Therefore, the current recommendation is to monitor the fetus using fetal echocardiography to assess the developing heart, prior to the initiation of potentially toxic treatment. When congenital heart block and fetal hydrops is discovered during gestation, treatment of the mother with dexamethasone and plasmapheresis may reverse the fetal congestive heart failure but not the heart block. However, the efficacy of this therapy in altering the natural history of congenital heart block is controversial and unproven. Children diagnosed with this condition should be delivered in a high-risk neonatal centre which can provide cardiac pacing. If the fetal bradycardia is recognized as congenital heart block rather than fetal distress, then unnecessary early, emergency delivery may be prevented. However, further prospective collaborative studies are required to determine the population at risk for this block and how to prevent it.

References

Abeles, M., Urman, J.D., and Rothfield, N.F. (1978). Aseptic necrosis of bone in systemic lupus erythematosus. *Archives of Internal Medicine*, **138**, 750–54.

Abeles, M., Urman, J.D., Weinstein, A., Lowenstein, M., and Rothfield, N.F. (1980). Systemic lupus erythematosus in the younger patient: survival studies. *Journal of Rheumatology*, **7**, 515–22.

Abud-Mendoza, C., Sturbaum, A.K., Vazquez-Compean, R., and Gonzalez-Amaro, R. (1993). Methotrexate therapy in childhood systemic lupus erythematosus. *Journal of Rheumatology*, **20**, 731–3.

Abuelo, J.G., Esparza, A.R., and Garella, S. (1984). Steroid-dependent nephrotic syndrome in lupus nephritis. *Archives of Internal Medicine*, **144**, 2411–12.

Akhtar, M., Al-Dalaan, A., and El-Ramahi, K.M. (1994). Pauci-immune necrotizing lupus nephritis: report of two cases. *American Journal of Kidney Diseases*, **23**, 320–25.

Alexander, E., Buyon, J.P., Provost, T.T., and Guarnieri, T. (1992). Anti-Ro/SS-A antibodies in the pathophysiology of congenital hearth block in neonatal lupus syndrome, an experimental model. *Arthritis and Rheumatism*, **35**, 176–89.

Alexopoulos, E., Seron, D., Hartley, R.B., and Cameron, J.S. (1990). Lupus nephritis: correlation of interstitial cells with glomerular function. *Kidney International*, **37**, 100–109.

Appel, G.B., Cohen, D.J., Pirani, C.L., Meltzer, J.I., and Estes D. (1987). Long-term follow-up of patients with lupus nephritis. A study based on the classification of the World Health Organization. *American Journal of Medicine*, **83**, 877–85.

Appel, G.B., Pirani, C.L., and D'Agati, V. (1994). Renal vascular complications of systemic lupus erythematosus. *Journal of the American Society of Nephrology*, **4**, 1499–515.

Asherson, R.A. and Oakley, C.M. (1986). Pulmonary hypertension and systemic lupus erythematosus. *Journal of Rheumatology*, **13**, 1–5.

Austin III, H.A., Muenz, L.R., Joyce, K.M., Antonovych, T.T., and Balow, J.E. (1984). Diffuse proliferative lupus nephritis: identification of specific pathologic features affecting renal outcome. *Kidney International*, **25**, 689–95.

Austin III, H.A. *et al.* (1986). Therapy of lupus nephritis. Controlled trial of prednisone and cytotoxic drugs. *New England Journal of Medicine*, **314**, 614–19.

Austin III, H.A., Boumpas, D.T., Vaughan, E.M., and Balow, J.E. (1994). Predicting renal outcomes in severe lupus nephritis: contributions of clinical and histologic data. *Kidney International*, **45**, 544–50.

Badui, E. *et al.* (1985). Cardiovascular manifestations in systemic lupus erythematosus. prospective study of 100 patients. *Angiology — Journal of Vascular Diseases*, **36**, 431–41.

Bagga, A., Jain, Y., Srivastava, R.N., and Bhuyan, U.N. (1993). Renal tubular acidosis preceding systemic lupus erythematosus. *Pediatric Nephrology*, **7**, 735–6.

Bakir, A.A., Rhee, H.L., Ainis, H., and Dunea, G. (1989). Nephrotic syndrome, hematuria, and hypocomplementemia in a case of mesangial lupus nephritis evolving later to a membranous lesion. *American Journal of Medicine*, **86**, 609–11.

Baumal, R., Farine, M., and Poucell, S. (1987). Clinical significance of renal biopsies showing mixed mesangial and global proliferative lupus nephritis. *American Journal of Kidney Disease*, **10**, 236–40.

Bonfa, E. *et al.* (1987). Association between lupus psychosis and anti-ribosomal P protein antibodies. *New England Journal of Medicine*, **317**, 265–71.

Bruyn, G.W. and Padberg, G. (1984). Chorea and systemic lupus erythematosus. *European Neurology*, **23**, 435–48.

Bumgardner, G.L. *et al.* (1988). Single-center 1–15-year results of renal transplantation with systemic lupus erythematosus. *Transplantation*, **46**, 703–9.

Buyon, J.P., and Winchester, R. (1990). Congenital complete heart block. *Arthritis and Rheumatism*, **33**, 609–14.

Buyon, J.P. *et al.* (1988). Complete congenital heart block: risk of occurrence and therapeutic approach to prevention. *Journal of Rheumatology*, **15**, 1104–8.

Buyon, J.P. *et al.* (1993). Identification of mothers at risk for congenital heart block and other neonatal lupus syndromes in their children. *Arthritis and Rheumatism*, **36**, 1263–73.

Caeiro, E., Michielson, F.M.C., Bernstein, R., Hughes, G.R., and Ansell, B.M. (1981). Systemic lupus erythematosus in childhood. *Annals of the Rheumatic Diseases*, **40**, 325–31.

Cameron, J.S. (1994). Lupus nephritis in childhood and adolescence. *Pediatic Nephrology*, **8**, 230–49.

Carbotte, R.M., Denburg, S.D., and Denburg, J.A. (1986). Prevalence of cognitive impairment in systemic lupus erythematosus. *Journal of Nervous and Mental Disease*, **174**, 357–64.

Carette, S., Macher, A.M., Nussbaum, A., and Plotz, P.H. (1984). Severe, acute pulmonary disease in patients with systemic lupus erythematosus: ten years of experience at the National Institutes of Health. *Seminars in Arthritis and Rheumatism*, **14**, 52–9.

Carter, J.B., Blieden, L.C., and Edwards, J.E. (1974). Congenital Heart Block. *Archives of Pathology*, **97**, 51–7.

Cassidy, J.T., Sullivan, D.B., Petty, R.E., and Ragsdale, C. (1977). Lupus nephritis and encephalopathy. Prognosis in 58 children. *Arthritis and Rheumatism*, **20**, 315–22.

Citera, G., Espada, G., and Maldonado Cocco, J.A. (1993). Sequential development of 2 connective tissue diseases in juvenile patients. *Journal of Rheumatology*, **20**, 2149–52.

Cook, C.D., Wedgwood, J.P., Craig, J.M., Hartmann, J.R., and Janeway, C.A. (1960). Systemic lupus erythematosus: description of 37 cases in children and a discussion of endocrine therapy in 32 of the cases. *Pediatrics*, **26**, 570–85.

Decker, J.L., Steinberg, A.D., Reinertsen, J.L., Plotz, P.H., Balow, J.E., and Klippel, J.H. (1979). Systemic lupus erythematosus: evolving concepts. *Annals of Internal Medicine*, **91**, 587–604.

De Inocencio, J. and Lovell, D.J. (1994). Cardiac function in systemic lupus erythematosus. *Journal of Rheumatology*, **21**, 2147–56.

Delgado, E.A., Malleson, P.N., Pirie, G.E., and Petty, R.E. (1990). The pulmonary manifestations of childhood onset systemic lupus erythematosus. *Seminars in Arthritis and Rheumatism*, **19**, 285–93.

Deng, J-S., Sontheimer, R.D., and Gilliam, J.N. (1984). Relationships between antinuclear antibodies and anti-Ro/SSA antibodies in subacute cutaneous lupus erythematosus. *Journal of the America Academy of Dermatology*, **11**, 494–9.

Doherty, N.E. and Siegel, R.J. (1985). Cardiovascular manifestations of systemic lupus erythematosus. *American Heart Journal*, **110**, 1257–65.

Eberhard, A., Shore, A., Silverman, E., and Laxer R. (1991*a*). Bowel perforation and interstitial cystitis in childhood systemic lupus erythematosus: a case report. *Journal of Rheumatology*, **18**, 746–7.

Eberhard, A., Laxer, R., Eddy, A., and Silverman, E. (1991*b*). Presence of thyroid abnormalities in children with systemic lupus erythematosus. *Journal of Pediatrics*, **119**, 277–9.

Eberhard, A., Couper, R., Durie, P., and Silverman, E. (1992). Exocrine pancreatic function in children with systemic lupus erythematosus. *Journal of Rheumatology*, **19**, 964–7.

Eberhard, A., Sparling, C., Sudbury, S., Ford, P., Laxer, R., and Silverman, E. (1994). Hypoprothrombinemia in childhood systemic lupus erythematosus. *Seminars in Arthritis and Rheumatism*, **24**, 12–18.

El-Garf, A. and Salah, S. (1990). Juvenile systemic lupus erythematosus among Egyptian children. *Journal of Rheumatology*, **17**, 1168–70.

Emery, H. (1986). Clinical aspects of systemic lupus erythematosus in childhood. *Pediatric Clinics of North America*, **33**, 1177–90.

Esdaile, J.M., Joseph, L., Mackenzie, T., Kashgarian, M., and Hayslett, J.P. (1994). The benefit of early treatment with immunosuppressive agents in lupus nephritis. *Journal of Rheumatology*, **21**, 2046–51.

Fish, A.J., Blau, E.B., Westberg, N.G., Burke, B.A., Vernier, R.L., and Michael, A.F. (1977). Systemic lupus erythematosus within the first two decades of life. *American Journal of Medicine*, **62**, 99–117.

Fisk, J.D., Eastwood, B., Sherwood, G., and Hanly, J.G. (1993). Patterns of cognitive impairment in patients with systemic lupus erythematosus. *British Journal of Rheumatology*, **32**, 458–62.

Fraenkel, L., Mackenzie, T., Joseph, L. Kashgarian, M., Hayslett, J.P., and Esdaile, J.M. (1994). Response to treatment as a predictor of longterm outcome in patients with lupus nephritis. *Journal of Rheumatology*, **21**, 2052–7.

Friedman, D.M., Lazarus, H.M., and Fierman, A.H. (1990). Acute myocardial infarction in pediatric systemic lupus erythematosus. *Journal of Pediatrics*, **117**, 263–6.

Garcia, S. *et al.* (1994) Cellular mechanism of the conduction abnormalities induced by serum from anti-Ro/SSA-positive patients in rabbit hearts. *Journal of Clinical Investigation*, **93**, 718–24.

Glidden, R.S., Mantzouranis, E.C., and Borel, Y. (1983). Systemic lupus erythematosus in childhood: clinical manifestations and improved survival in fifty-five patients. *Clinical Immunology and Immunopathology*, **29**, 196–210.

Gribetz, D. and Henley, W.L. (1959). Systemic lupus erythematosus in childhood. *Mount Sinai Journal of Medicine*, **26**, 289–96.

Hall, S., McCormick, Jr., J.L., Greipp, P.R., Michet, Jr., C.J., and McKenna, C.H. (1985). Splenectomy does not cure the thrombocytopenia of systemic lupus erythematosus. *Annals of Internal Medicine*, **102**, 325–8.

Hall, S., Czaja, A.J., Kaufman, D.K., Markowitz, H., and Ginsburg, W.W. (1986). How lupoid is lupoid hepatitis? *Journal of Rheumatology*, **13**, 95–8.

Hanly, J.G., Fisk, J.D., Sherwood, G., and Eastwood, B. (1994). Clinical course of cognitive dysfunction in systemic lupus erythematosus. *Journal of Rheumatology*, **21**, 1825–31.

Harmon, C.E., Deng, J-S., Peebles, C.L., and Tan, E.M. (1984). The importance of tissue substrate in the SS-A/Ro antigen-antibody system. *Arthritis and Rheumatism*, **27**, 166–73.

Hirohata, S., Hirose, S., and Miyamoto, T. (1985). Cerebrospinal fluid IgM, IgA, and IgG indexes in systemic lupus erythematosus. *Archives of Internal Medicine*, **145**, 1843–6.

Ho, Y.S., Esscher, E., Anderson, R.H., and Michaelsson M. (1986). Anatomy of congenital complete heart block and relation to maternal anti-Ro antibodies. *American Journal of Cardiology*, **58**, 291–4.

Hoffman, B.I. and Katz, W.A. (1980). The gastrointestinal manifestations of systemic lupus erythematosus: a review of the literature. *Seminars in Arthritis and Rheumatism*, **9**, 237–47.

Hogg, G.R. (1957). Congenital acute lupus erythematosus associated with subendocardial fibroelastosis. *American Journal of Clinical Pathology*, **28**, 648–53.

Holman, B.L. (1993). Functional imaging in systemic lupus erythematosus: an accurate indicator of central nervous system involvement? *Arthritis and Rheumatism*, **36**, 1193–95.

Ilowite, N.T., Samuel, P., Ginzler, E., and Jacobson, M.S. (1988). Dyslipoproteinemia in pediatric systemic lupus erythematosus. *Arthritis and Rheumatism*, **31**, 859–63.

Imperiale, T.F., Goldfarb, S., and Berns, J.S. (1995). Are cytotoxic agents beneficial in idiopathic membranous nephropathy? A meta-analysis of the controlled trials. *Journal of the American Society of Nephrology*, **5**, 1553–8.

Isenberg, D.A., Meyrick-Thomas, D., Snaith, M.L., McKeran, R.O., and Royston, J.P. (1982). A study of migraine in systemic lupus erythematosus. *Annals of the Rheumatic Diseases*, **41**, 30–32.

Isshi, K., Hirohata, S., Hashimoto, T., and Miyashita, H. (1994). Systemic lupus erythematosus presenting with diffuse low density lesions in the cerebral white matter on computed axial tomography scans: its implication in the pathogenesis of diffuse central nervous system lupus. *Journal of Rheumatology*, **21**, 1758–62.

Jacobs, J.C. (1963). Systemic lupus erythematosus in childhood: report of thirty-five cases, with discussion of seven apparently induced by anticonlvulsant medication, and of prognosis and treatment. *Pediatrics*, **32**, 257–64.

Jarek, M.J., West, S., Baker, M.R., and Rak, K.M. (1994). Magnetic resonance imaging in systemic lupus erythematosus patients without a history of neuropsychiatric lupus erythematosus. *Arthritis and Rheumatism*, **37**, 1609–13.

Kalla, A.A., Learmonth, I.D., and Klemp, P. (1986). Early treatment of avascular necrosis in systemic lupus erythematosus. *Annals of the Rheumatic Diseases*, **45**, 649–52.

Katsanis, E., Hsu, E., Luke, K.-H., and McKee, J.A. (1987). Systemic lupus erythematosus and sickle hemoglobinopathies: a report of two cases and review of the literature. *American Journal of Hematology*, **25**, 211–14.

Kaufman, D.B., Laxer, R.M., Silverman, E.D., and Stein, L. (1986). Systemic lupus erythematosus in childhood and adolescence — the problem, epidemiology, incidence, susceptibility, genetics, and prognosis. *Current Problems in Pediatrics*, **16**, 555–624.

Khamashta, M.A., Cuadrado, M.J., Mujic, F., Taub, N.A., Hunt, B.J., and Hughes, G.R.V. (1995). The management of thrombosis in the antiphospholipid-antibody syndrome. *New England Journral of Medicine*, **332**, 993–7.

King, K.K., Kornreich, H.K., Bernstein, B.H., Singsen, B.H., and Hanson, V. (1977). The clinical spectrum of systemic lupus erythematosus in childhood. *Arthritis and Rheumatism*, **20** (Suppl.), 287–94.

Kodama, K. *et al.* (1995). Single photon emission computed tomography in systemic lupus erythematosus with psychiatric symptoms. *Journal of Neurology, Neurosurgery, and Psychiatry*, **58**, 307–11.

Kunkel, H.G. (1980). The immunopathy of systemic lupus erythematosus. *Hospital Practice*, **15**, 47.

Lacks, S. and White, P. (1990). Morbidity associated with childhood systemic lupus erythematosus. *Journal of Rheumatology*, **17**, 941–5.

Laitman, R.S., Glicklich, D., Sablay, L.B., Grayzel, A.I., Barland, P., and Bank, N. (1989). Effect of long-term normalization of serum complement levels on the course of lupus nephritis. *American Journal of Medicine*, **87**, 132–8.

Laxer, R.M. *et al.* (1990). Liver disease in neonatal lupus. *Journal of Pediatrics*, **116**, 238–42.

Lee, L.A., Harmon, C.E., Huff, J.C., Norris, D.A., and Weston, W.L. (1985). The demonstration of SS-A/Ro antigen in human fetal tissues and in neonatal and adult skin. *Journal of Investigative Dermatology*, **85**, 143–6.

Lee, L.A., Norris, D.A., and Weston, W.L. (1986). Neonatal lupus and the pathogenesis of cutaneous lupus. *Pediatric Dermatology*, **3**, 491–7.

Lee, L.A., Reichlin, M., Ruyle, S.Z., and Weston, W.L. (1993). Neonatal lupus liver disease. *Lupus*, **2**, 333–8.

Lee, L.A., Frank, M.B., McCubbin, V.R., and Reichlin, M. (1994). Autoantibodies of neonatal lupus erythematosus. *Journal of Investigative Dermatology*, **102**, 963–6.

LeFeber, W.P. *et al.* (1984). Ultraviolet light induces binding of antibodies to selected nuclear antigens on cultured keratinocytes. *Journal of Clinical Investigation*, **74**, 1545–51.

Lehman, T.J.A. (1989*a*). Intermittent intravenous cyclophosphamide therapy for lupus nephritis. *Journal of Pediatrics*, **144**, 1055–60.

Lehman, T.J.A., McCurdy, D.K., Bernstein, B.H., King, K.K., and Hanson, V. (1989*b*). Systemic lupus erythematosus in the first decade of life. *Pediatrics*, **83**, 235–9.

Lev, M., Silverman, J., Fitzmaurice, F.M., Paul, M.H., Cassels, D.E., and Miller, R.A. (1971). Lack of connection between the atria and the more peripheral conduction system in congenital atrioventricular block. *American Journal of Cardiology*, **27**, 481–90.

Lipnick, R.N., Tsokos, G.C., Bray, G.L., and White, P.H. (1990). Autoimmune thrombocytopenia in pediatric systemic lupus erythematosus: alternative therapeutic modalities. *Clinical and Experimental Rheumatology*, **8**, 315–19.

Long, A.A., Denburg, S.D., Carbotte, R.M., Singal, D.P., and Denburg, J.A. (1989). Serum lymphocytotoxic antibodies and neurocognitive function in systemic lupus erythematosus. *Annals of the Rheumatic Diseases*, **49**, 249–53.

Magil, A.B., Ballon, H.S., Chan, V., Lirenman, D.S., and Rae, A. (1984). Diffuse proliferative lupus glomerulonephritis. Determination of prognostic significance of clinical, laboratory, and pathologic factors. *Medicine*, **63**, 210–20.

Malleson, P.N. (1989). The role of the renal biopsy in childhood onset systemic lupus erythematosus: a viewpoint. *Clinical and Experimental Rheumatology*, **7**, 563–6.

Martini, A., Ravelli, A., Viola, S., and Burgio, R.G. (1987). Systemic lupus erythematosus with Jaccoud's arthropathy mimicking juvenile rheumatoid arthritis. *Arthritis and Rheumatism*, **30**, 1062–4.

McCune, A.B., Weston, W.L., and Lee, L.A. (1987). Maternal and fetal outcome in neonatal lupus erythematosus. *Annals of Internal Medicine*, **106**, 518–23.

McCurdy, D.K. *et al.* (1992). Lupus nephritis: prognostic factors in children. *Pediatrics*, **89**, 240–46.

McLean, B.N., Miller, D., and Thompson, E.J. (1995). Oligoclonal banding of IgG in CSF, blood–brain barrier function, and MRI findings in patients with sarcoidosis, systemic lupus erythematosus, and Behçet's disease involving the nervous system. *Journal of Neurology, Neurosurgery, and Psychiatry*, **58**, 548–54.

Miguel, E.C. *et al.* (1994). Psychiatric manifestations of systemic lupus erythematosus: clinical features, symptoms, and signs of central nervous system activity in 43 patients. *Medicine*, **73**, 224–32.

Miller, J.J.I. (1977). Drug-induced lupus-like syndrome in children. *Arthritis and Rheumatism*, **20** (Suppl.), 308–11.

Molta, C. *et al.* (1993). Childhood-onset systemic lupus erythematosus: antiphospholipid antibodies in 37 patients and their first-degree relatives. *Pediatrics*, **92**, 849–53.

Nadorra, R.L. and Landing, B.H. (1987). Pulmonary lesions in childhood onset systemic lupus erythematosus: analysis of 26 cases, and summary of literature. *Pediatric Pathology*, **7**, 1–18.

Nadorra, R.L., Nakazato, Y., and Landing, B.H. (1987). Pathologic features of gastrointestinal tract lesions in childhood-onset systemic lupus erythematosus: study of 26 patients, with review of the literature. *Pediatric Pathology*, **7**, 245–59.

Nossent, H.C., Swaak, T.J.G., and Berden, J.H.M. (1991). Systemic lupus erythematosus after renal transplantation: patient and graft survival and disease activity. *Annals of Internal Medicine*, **114**, 183–8.

O'Connor, P. (1988). Diagnosis of central nervous system lupus. *Canadian Journal of Neurological Sciences*, **15**, 257–60.

Orth, R.W., Weisman, M.H., Cohen, A.H., Talner, L.B., Nachtsheim, D., and Zvaifler, N.J. (1983). Lupus cystitis: primary bladder manifestations of systemic lupus erythematosus. *Annals of Internal Medicine*, **98**, 323–6.

Papero, P.H., Bluestein, H.G., White, P., and Lipnick, R.N. (1990). Neuropsychologic deficits and antineuronal antibodies in pediatric systemic lupus erythematosus. *Clinical and Experimental Rheumatology*, **8**, 417–24.

Peake, P.W., Greenstein, J.D., Timmermans, V., Gavrilovic, L., and Charlesworth, J.A. (1988). Lymphocytotoxic antibodies in systemic lupus erythematosus: studies of their temperature dependence, binding characteristics, and specificty in vitro. *Annals of the Rheumatic Diseases*, **47**, 725–32.

Penn, I. (1988). *Development of new tumors after transplantation*. J.B. Lippincott Co., Philadelphia.

Platt, J.L., Burke, B.A., Fish, A.J., Kim, Y., and Michael, A.F. (1982). Systemic lupus erythematosus in the first two decades of life. *American Journal of Kidney Diseases*, **11**, 212–22.

Pollak, V.E. and Pirani, C.L. (1993). In *Dubois' lupus erythematosus*, (4th edn) (ed. D.J. Wallace and B.H. Hahn), pp. 525–41. Lea and Febiger, Philadelphia.

Posner, M.A., Gloster, E.S., Bonagura, V.R., Valacer, D.J., and Ilowite, N.T. (1990). Burkitt's lymphoma in a patient with systemic lupus erythematosus. *Journal of Rheumatology*, **17**, 380–82.

Press, J. *et al.* (1996). Antiribosomal P antibodies in pediatric patients with systemic lupus erythematosus and psychosis. *Arthritis and Rheumatism*, **39**, 671–6.

Ragsdale, C.G., Petty, R.E., Cassidy, J.T., and Sullivan, D.B. (1980). The clinical progression of apparent juvenile rheumatoid arthritis to systemic lupus erythematosus. *Journal of Rheumatology*, **7**, 50–55.

Ravelli, A., Martini, A., and Burgio, G.R. (1994). Antiphospholipid antibodies in paediatrics. *European Journal of Pediatrics*, **153**, 472–9.

Reed, B. *et al.* (1983). Autoantibodies to SS-A/Ro in infants with congenital heart block. *Journal of Pediatrics*, **103**, 889–92.

Reeves, W.H. and Lahita, R.G. (1987). Clinical presentation of systemic lupus erythematosus in the adult. In *Systemic lupus erythematosus*, pp.355–75. John Wiley, New York..

Reichlin, M. *et al.* (1994). Concentration of autoantibodies to native 60-kd Ro/SS-A and denatured 52-kd Ro/Ss-A in eluates from the heart of a child who died with congenital complete heart block. *Arthritis and Rheumatism*, **37**, 1698–703.

Robinson, M.J., and Williams, A.L. (1967). Systemic lupus erythematosus in childhood. *Australian Paediatric Journal*, **3**, 36–47.

Rosh, J.R., Silverman, E.D., Groisman, G., Dolgin, S., and LeLeiko, N.S. (1993). Intrahepatic cholestasis in neonatal lupus erythematosus. *Journal of Pediatric Gastroenterology and Nutrition*, **17**, 310–12.

Rubbert, A. *et al.* (1993). Single-photon-emission computed tomography analysis of cerebral blood flow in the evaluation of central nervous system involvement in patients with systemic lupus erythematosus. *Arthritis and Rheumatism*, **36**, 1253–62.

Rubin, L.A., Urowitz, M.B., and Gladman, D.D. (1985). Mortality in systemic lupus erythematosus: the bimodal pattern revisited. *Quarterly Journal of Medicine*, **55**, 87–98.

Saulsbury, F.T., Kesler, R.W., Kennaugh, J.M., Barber, J.C., and Chevalier, R.L. (1982). Overlap syndrome of juvenile rheumatoid arthritis and systemic lupus erythematosus. *Journal of Rheumatology*, **9**, 610–12.

Schaller, J. (1982). Lupus in childhood. *Clinics in the Rheumatic Diseases*, 8, 219–28.

Schneebaum, A.B. *et al.* (1991). Association of psychiatric manifestations with antibodies to ribosomal P proteins in systemic lupus erythematosus. *American Journal of Medicine*, 90, 54–62.

Shemesh, O., Golbetz, H., Kriss, J.P., and Myers, B.D. (1985). Limitations of creatinine as a filtration marker in glomerulopathic patients. *Kidney International*, 28, 830–38.

Shergy, W.J., Kredich, D.W., and Pisetsky, D.S. (1988). The relationship of anticardiolipin antibodies to disease manifestations in pediatric systemic lupus erythematosus. *Journal of Rheumatology*, 15, 1389–94.

Shergy, W.J., Kredich, D.W., and Pisetsky, D.S. (1989). Patterns of autoantibody expression in pediatric and adult systemic lupus erythematosus. *Journal of Rheumatology*, 16, 1329–34.

Siegel, M. and Lee, S.L. (1973). The epidemiology of systemic lupus erythematosus. *Seminars in Arthritis and Rheumatism*, 3, 1–54.

Silverman, E.D., Mamula, M., Hardin, J.A., and Laxer R.M. (1991). Importance of the immune response to the Ro/La particle in the development of congenital heart block and neonatal lupus erythematosus. *Journal of Rheumatology*, 18, 120–24.

Sloan, R.P., Schwartz, M.M., Korbet, S.M., Borok, R.Z., and the Lupus Nephritis Collaborative Study Group (1996). Long-term outcome in systemic lupus erythematosus membranous glomerulonephritis. *Journal of the American Society of Nephrology*, 7, 299–305.

Smith, F.E., Sweet, D.E., Brunner, C.M., and Davis IV, J.S. (1976). Avascular necrosis in SLE. An apparent predilection for young patients. *Annals of the Rheumatic Diseases*, 35, 227–32.

Smith, N.M. and Ho, S.Y. (1994). Heart block and sudden death associated with fibrosis of the conduction system at the margin of a ventricular septal defect. *Pediatric Cardiology*, 15, 139–42.

Szer, I.S., Miller, J.H., Rawlings, D., Shaham, B., and Bernstein, B. (1993). Cerebral perfusion abnormalities in children with central nervous system manifestations of lupus detected by single photon emission computed tomography. *Journal of Rheumatology*, 20, 2143–8.

Teh, L.S. *et al.* (1993). Anti-P antibodies are associated with psychiatric and focal cerebral disorders in patients with systemic lupus erythematosus. *British Journal of Rheumatology*, 32, 287–90.

Tucker, L.B., Menon, S., Schaller, J.G., and Isenberg, D.A. (1995). Adult- and childhood-onset systemic lupus erythematosus: a comparison os sonet, clinical features, serology and outcome. *British Journal of Rheumatology*, 34, 866–72.

Uziel, Y., Laxer, R.M., Blaser, S., Andrew, M., Scneider, R., and Silverman, E.D. (1995). Cerebral vein thrombosis in childhood systemic lupus erythematosus. *Journal of Pediatrics*, 126, 722–7.

Walravens, P. A. and Chase, H.P. (1976). The prognosis of childhood systemic lupus erythematosus. *American Journal of Diseases of Children*, 130, 929–33.

Ward, M.M., Dawson, D.V., Kredich, D.W., and Pisetsky, D.S. (1990). Expression of IgM and IgG autoantibodies in pediatric and adult systemic lupus erythematosus. *Clinical Immunology and Immunopathology*, 55, 273–84.

Watson, R.M., Lane, A.T., Barnett, N.K., Bias, W.B., Arnett, F.C., and Provost, T.T. (1984). Neonatal lupus erythematosus. A clinical, serological and immunologenic study with review of the literature. *Medicine Baltimore*, 63,362–78.

Weber, H.S. and Myers, J.L. (1994). Maternal collagen vascular disease associated with fetal heart block and degenerative changes of the atrioventricular valves. *Pediatric Cardiology*, 15, 204–6.

Wilson, W.A., Armatis, P.E., and Perez, M.C. (1989). C4 concentrations and C4 deficiency alleles in systemic lupus erythematosus. *Annals of Rheumatic Diseases*, 48, 600–604.

Yancey, C.L., Doughty, R.A., and Athreya, B.H. (1981). Central nervous system involvement in childhood systemic lupus erythematosus. *Arthritis and Rheumatism*, 24, 1389–95.

Yang, L-Y, Chen, W-P., and Lin, C-Y. (1994). Lupus nephritis in children—a review of 167 patients. *Pediatrics*, 94, 335–40.

Zetterstrom, R. and Berglund, G. (1956). Systemic lupus erythematosus in childhood a clinical study. *Acta Paediatrica Hungarica*, 45, 189–204.

5.7.3 The antiphospholipid antibody syndrome

Munther A. Khamashta and G. R. V. Hughes

Introduction

In 1983, few rheumatologists would have predicted the interest that the introduction of the anticardiolipin test would generate in subsequent years (Harris *et al.* 1983). New autoantibodies turn up frequently in patients with systemic lupus erythematosus and there may have seemed little reason why anticardiolipin antibodies should have merited any more than passing interest. However, these particular autoantibodies had unusual characteristics that attracted the attention of investigators from a variety of disciplines (Fig. 1). One reason may have been the novelty of phospholipid molecules as antigens, given that most attention up to that time had focused on protein, DNA, and even polysaccharide antigens (Harris *et al.* 1994). In addition, these antibodies exhibited an easily detectable biological effect, as evidenced by their ability to prolong clotting times of

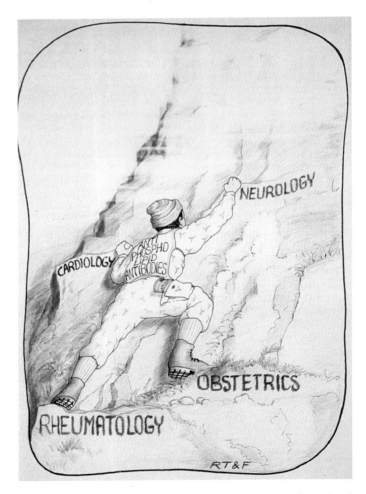

Fig. 1 Antiphospholipid antibodies—linking many specialties (reproduced with permission of the Editor of *Clinical and Experimental Rheumatology*).

plasma. More intriguing was their association with an unusual combination of clinical complications that included venous and arterial thrombosis, pregnancy loss, and thrombocytopenia (Hughes 1983; Hughes 1993).

During the last decade, considerable progress has been made in understanding antiphospholipid antibodies and the disorder with which they are associated, but many questions remain unanswered, particularly those of pathogenesis and optimal treatment (Khamashta and Asherson 1995). A chronology of the major developments in the unfolding of the antiphospholipid syndrome story is listed in Table 1.

Detection of antiphospholipid antibodies

Antiphospholipid antibodies are detected by a variety of laboratory tests, the most useful for identifying patients with the antiphospholipid syndrome being the lupus anticoagulant and the anticardiolipin

Table 1 Antiphospholipid antibodies and the antiphospholipid syndrome—history

1906	Wasserman reaction (reagin)
1941	Reagin binds cardiolipin
1952	False-positive test for syphilis
1959	Cofactor requirements for lupus anticoagulant activity
1960s	Lupus anticoagulant: association with thrombosis
1970s	Lupus anticoagulant is due to immunoglobulin
1975	Lupus anticoagulant: association with recurrent abortions
1983	Anticardiolipin antibodies: detection by radioimmunoassay
1985	Anticardiolipin antibodies: detection by ELISA
1980s	Clinical description of the antiphospholipid syndrome
1987	Diagnostic criteria for the antiphospholipid syndrome
1989	Lupus anticoagulant and anticardiolipin: separate antibody subgroups
1990	Cofactor requirements for anticardiolipin antibody binding
1990	Anticardiolipin cofactor: β_2-glycoprotein I
1991	Lupus anticoagulant cofactor: prothrombin
1991	Animal models: passive immunization
1992	Animal models: active immunization
1992	Lupus anticoagulant cofactor: β_2-glycoprotein I
1992	Anti-β_2-glycoprotein I: association with thrombosis
1994	Phospholipid binding site: fifth domain of β_2-glycoprotein I

ELISA, enzyme-linked immunosorbent assay.

antibody tests. These antibodies are distinct and separable immunoglobulins present alone or in combination in the plasma of people with the antiphospholipid syndrome. The autoantibodies sometimes bind phospholipids utilized in the Venereal Disease Research Laboratories (**VDRL**) test; hence, some patients may have a false-positive test for syphilis. However, the VDRL test is not positive frequently enough to make it valuable in diagnosing the antiphospholipid syndrome.

The lupus anticoagulant is a functional assay measuring the ability of antiphospholipid antibodies to prolong clotting via their inhibition of the conversion of prothrombin to thrombin or the activation of factor X (both reactions are catalysed by phospholipids). Tests for the lupus anticoagulant have been difficult to standardize, and no single test appears to be adequate (Permpikul et al. 1994; Triplett 1994). The test begins with an attempt to demonstrate an abnormal coagulation screening test, such as a prolonged activated partial thromboplastin time, dilute Russell viper venom time, or kaolin clotting time. If any of these is positive, the test is repeated, using a sample in which the patient's plasma has been mixed with normal plasma. If the patient's disorder is a clotting deficiency, the test should become normal. If, on the other hand, lupus anticoagulant or some other clotting inhibitor is present, the clotting time will remain prolonged. The presence of lupus anticoagulant is confirmed by the return to normal of the clotting test after addition of freeze–thawed platelets or excess phospholipids, either of which bind the antibodies. The lupus anticoagulant test must be performed on platelet-poor plasma. The test cannot be performed reliably if the patient is receiving heparin or oral anticoagulants.

The most sensitive test for antiphospholipid antibodies is the anticardiolipin antibody test, introduced in 1983 and extensively improved since that time (Gharavi et al. 1987; Harris et al. 1987; Harris et al. 1990; Khamashta and Hughes 1993). This test uses enzyme-linked immunosorbent assay to determine antibody binding to solid plates coated either with cardiolipin or other phospholipids. Serum or plasma samples may be used for the anticardiolipin assay. The availability of reference sera which are isotype specific (IgG and IgM) has greatly improved interlaboratory testing and quantification of anticardiolipin antibodies (Harris et al. 1990). IgG and IgM isotype concentrations are expressed as GPL and MPL units, respectively. One unit represents the binding activity of $1\,\mu g/ml$ of affinity purified anticardiolipin antibody. Results are expressed as low, medium, and high positive according to levels below 20 units, between 20 and 80 units, and above 80 units, respectively. IgA anticardiolipin reference sera are now also available. Many laboratories currently measure all three isotypes and sensitive kits are commercially available. Flow cytometry has also been used to test for anticardiolipin antibodies (Stewart et al. 1993). This sytem allows the simultaneous measurement of antiphospholipid antibody isotypes with different phospholipid specificity. The routine detection of other phospholipids, such as phosphatidylserine, phosphatidylinositol, and phosphatidic acid, gives little additional information.

In our experience, although a strong association between the anticardiolipin and the lupus anticoagulant results was found, these tests were discordant in 40 per cent of cases. The majority of patients with positive anticardiolipin antibodies were found to be positive for the IgG isotype (93 per cent). IgM anticardiolipin antibodies were demonstrated in only a quarter of the patients (Khamashta et al. 1995). The unrelated behaviour of lupus anticoagulant and anticardiolipin antibodies in the course of disease and in individual

Table 2 Clinical features of the antiphospholipid syndrome

Major features

    Venous thrombosis: deep venous thrombosis, Budd–Chiari syndrome, and pulmonary thromboembolism

    Arterial thrombosis: strokes, transient ischaemic attacks, and multi-infarct dementia

    Recurrent pregnancy loss

    Thrombocytopenia

Associated clinical features

    Leg ulcers, livedo reticularis, thrombophlebitis, and Sneddon's syndrome

    Heart valve lesions and myocardial infarctions

    Transverse myelitis, chorea, and epilepsy

    Haemolytic anaemia, Coombs' positivity, and Evans' syndrome

    Pulmonary hypertension

Others (less common)

    Migraine headache

    Splinter haemorrhages

    Labile hypertension and accelerated atherosclerosis

    Ischaemic necrosis of bone

    Addison's disease

    Guillain–Barré syndrome and pseudo-multiple sclerosis

    Amaurosis fugax

    Renal artery and vein thrombosis and microangiopathy

    Retinal artery and vein thrombosis

    Digital gangrene

patients indicates that both assays are required if most cases with the antiphospholipid syndrome are to be identified.

Clinical features

The antiphospholipid syndrome is a thrombophilic disorder in which patients may develop both venous and arterial occlusion. The clinical ramifications are extensive (Table 2). Table 3 illustrates the frequency of the major manifestations of the antiphospholipid syndrome in our patients.

Thrombosis

Although some antiphospholipid antibodies prolong *in vitro* clotting tests, haemorrhage is rare in patients with these antibodies. When haemorrhage does occur, other causes such as severe thrombocytopenia or clotting factor inhibitors should be excluded (Harris *et al.* 1993).

Instead of being associated with haemorrhage, antiphospholipid antibodies are paradoxically associated with thrombosis. Thrombosis can occur anywhere in the venous or arterial circulation. Vessels of all sizes may be affected, and the vascular pathological appearance has consistently been of bland occlusion without inflammatory infiltrate (Fig. 2) (Lie 1994). Thus, it is unlikely that thrombotic occlusion of blood vessels in patients with the antiphospholipid syndrome is caused by vasculitis, which may be seen in other patients with autoimmune rheumatic disorders. The distinction is important not only for discovering the pathogenesis of the vascular lesions, but also for the choice of treatment.

In the venous circulation, thrombosis of the deep and superficial veins of the lower extremities has been reported most frequently (occasionally after the use of oral contraceptive pills containing oestrogen). It is often recurrent and may be accompanied by pulmonary embolism. It has been estimated that up to 19 per cent of patients with deep vein thrombosis and/or pulmonary thromboembolism are suffering from antiphospholipid coagulopathy and may demonstrate a positive lupus anticoagulant test, antibodies to cardiolipin, or both. Some patients with antiphospholipid antibodies also have pulmonary hypertension, perhaps caused by recurrent pulmonary emboli or intravascular thromboses (Asherson *et al.* 1990). Other reported venous sites of thrombosis include the axillary, ocular, renal, and hepatic veins and the inferior vena cava.

Table 3 Clinical manifestations of 171 patients with antiphospholipid syndrome[a]		
Clinical features	**No. of patients**	**Percentage**
Thrombosis	147/171	86
Venous:	80/147	54
Lower limbs DVT	54/80	67
Pulmonary embolism	19/80	24
Other	7/80	9
Arterial:	67/147	46
Stroke	32/67	48
TIA	24/67	36
Other	11/67	16
Thrombocytopenia	40/171	23
Pregnancy loss	48/147 (female)	33
First trimester	61/169 (pregnancies)	36
Second trimester	78/169 (pregnancies)	46
Third trimester	30/169 (pregnancies)	18

[a]St Thomas' Hospital Lupus Clinic database (1985–1994)
DVT, deep venous thrombosis; TIA, transient ischaemic attack

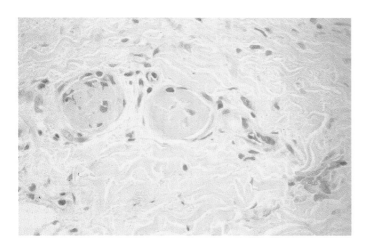

Fig. 2 Typical bland thrombus without inflammatory infiltrate in the vessel of a patient with primary antiphospholipid syndrome.

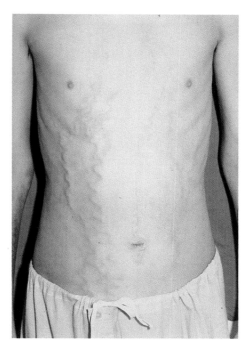

Fig. 3 Budd–Chiari syndrome in a 20-year-old patient with primary antiphospholipid syndrome (by courtesy of Dr L. Pallares, Servicio de Medicina Internal, Hospital Son Dureta, Palma de Mallorca, Spain).

The antiphospholipid syndrome is now considered one of the most frequent causes of the Budd–Chiari syndrome (Fig. 3) (Pelletier *et al.* 1994). Antiphospholipid antibodies have recently been implicated in the development of adrenal vein thrombosis leading to Addison's disease (Asherson and Hughes 1991). Interestingly, most documented cases with adrenal insufficiency associated with antiphospholipid antibodies were in patients with history of previous venous thromboses.

Unlike other known clotting disorders, arterial thromboses are a major feature of the antiphospholipid syndrome. Occlusion of the intracranial arteries has been reported most frequently, with the majority of patients presenting with stroke and transient ischaemic attacks. Magnetic resonance imaging scans show changes that vary from single lesions to multiple widely-scattered infarcts (Fig. 4) (Asherson *et al.* 1989a; Stimmler *et al.* 1993). In some patients, untreated recurrent cerebral thrombosis has led to multi-infarct dementia and psychiatric features have been prominent in the

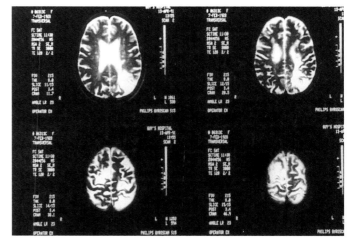

Fig. 4 Cerebral magnetic resonance imaging scan showing multiple widely-scattered infarcts in a patient with primary antiphospholipid syndrome.

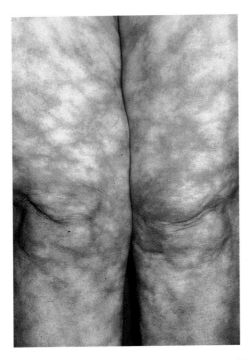

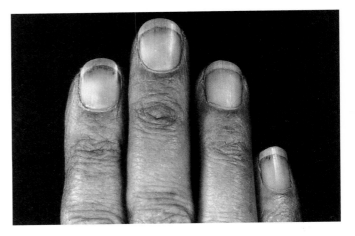

Fig. 6 Subungual splinter haemorrhages in a patient with primary antiphospholipid syndrome.

Fig. 5 Extensive livedo reticularis in a patient with primary antiphospholipid syndrome.

presentation of some of our patients with the antiphospholipid syndrome. Antiphospholipid antibodies are now internationally recognized as an important aetiological factor and may be present in 7 per cent of all patients who have suffered a stroke (Montalban *et al.* 1991). They should be sought especially in young patients with strokes, where they may account for up to 18 per cent (Nencini *et al.* 1992). The prevalence of myocardial infarction in patients with antiphospholipid antibodies has yet to be established. A figure of 4 per cent was derived from our studies assessing patients with lupus and related disorders (Asherson *et al.* 1989b). Another study, found that one-fifth of all young patients with myocardial infarction had antiphospholipid antibodies (Hamsten *et al.* 1986). Other arterial thromboses have involved the retina, mesenteric and peripheral arteries. Malignant hypertension with renal insufficiency secondary to thrombosis of the renal glomeruli and renal thrombotic microangiopathy (without classical lupus nephritis) has also been associated with the presence of antiphospholipid antibodies (Fig. 5) (Amigo *et al.* 1992; Asherson *et al.* 1993a; Piette *et al.* 1994).

Occasionally, patients positive for antiphospholipid antibody develop acute medical collapse with severe thrombocytopenia, adult respiratory distress syndrome, and multiple organ (notably cerebral and renal) failures. The aetiology of this usually fatal condition is unknown, though the limited reports available suggest widespread thrombosis as the pathogenesis. The syndrome often appears to have had a trigger, such as preceding viral infection. We have chosen to call this rare but life-threatening presentation the 'catastrophic antiphospholipid syndrome' (Asherson 1992a).

Fetal loss

Recurrent spontaneous pregnancy losses are one of the most consistent complications of the antiphospholipid syndrome. Losses can

occur at any stage of pregnancy, although miscarriages associated with antiphospholipid antibody are strikingly frequent (about 50 per cent of cases) during the second and third trimester. This differs from the pattern of pregnancy loss in the normal population, which usually occurs during the first trimester and is most often due to non-immunological factors, i.e. morphological or chromosomal abnormalities (Branch 1994). The rate of miscarriage in patients positive for antiphospholipid antibody is still uncertain, although the epidemiology is being studied and, increasingly, testing for this antibody is becoming a routine investigation in women with recurrent miscarriages. Fewer than 2 per cent of apparently normal pregnant women have either anticardiolipin antibody or lupus anticoagulant in any titre and less than 0.2 per cent have high titre antibody (Lockwood *et al.* 1989; Harris and Spinnato 1991). Hence, screening normal pregnant women has little value. Previous pregnancy history is of importance in determining the significance of a positive laboratory test for antiphospholipid antibodies. It has been estimated that if a patient with lupus has a positive lupus anticoagulant, or at least moderate levels of IgG anticardiolipin antibodies, the risk of spontaneous abortion during the first pregnancy is 30 per cent and if she has a history of at least two spontaneous abortions, the risk is 70 per cent during the following pregnancy (Lockshin *et al.* 1987). In our series, the presence of antiphospholipid antibodies was an important predictor of poor fetal outcome, as was a poor obstetric history (Buchanan *et al.* 1992; Lima *et al.* 1995). These findings are in keeping with the results of other authors (Branch *et al.* 1992).

The mechanism of pregnancy loss associated with antiphospholipid antibody remains uncertain. Progressive thrombosis of the microvasculature of the placenta and subsequent infarction resulting in placental insufficiency, fetal growth retardation and, ultimately, fetal loss, is a plausible explanation. Not all placentas examined, however, have shown areas of thrombosis or infarction and other mechanisms may be operative in these patients (Out *et al.* 1991). The aborted fetus is often normal except for evidence of growth retardation. It seems, therefore, that placental disease rather than fetal abnormality is responsible for fetal deaths related to antiphospholipid antibody. Pre-eclampsia is common in pregnant patients with the antiphospholipid syndrome and may provide clues to the pathogenesis of pregnancy loss related to this antibody (Branch *et al.* 1992).

Thrombocytopenia

Thrombocytopenia is common in patients with antiphospholipid antibodies, though not severe enough to cause haemorrhage (Khamashta and Machin 1991). The platelet count often remains stable for many years; then, for reasons that are often obscure, the count drops, sometimes catastrophically. A survey of sera from patients presenting with idiopathic thrombocytopenic purpura, found anticardiolipin antibodies in 30 per cent of the cases (Harris *et al.* 1985). This finding raises the possibility that patients with the antiphospholipid syndrome may present only with severe thrombocytopenia and will later develop pregnancy loss or thrombosis. This form of presentation was observed in a very small number of our patients with the syndrome. Some patients with antiphospholopid antibodies and thrombocytopenia also develop haemolytic anaemia with positive direct Coombs' test. This is widely known as Evans' syndrome. In a study of 12 patients with Evans' syndrome and systemic lupus, 10 patients had evidence of antiphospholipid antibodies (Deleze *et al.* 1989). Similarly, in 70 patients with the primary antiphospholipid syndrome, 10 per cent were described as having Evans' syndrome (Asherson *et al.* 1989c).

Other manifestations

Epilepsy and chorea are less frequent manifestations of the antiphospholipid syndrome and have, intriguingly, been seen to improve in some patients treated with anticoagulants (Asherson *et al.* 1987; Herranz *et al.* 1994). Transverse myelopathy, though rare, is strongly associated with the presence of antiphospholipid antibodies (Alarcon-Segovia *et al.* 1989). Occasionally, in some patients with bizarre, transient/recurrent neurologial signs (resembling multiple sclerosis), antiphospholipid antibodies have been detected in the absence of other immunological abnormalities. Its recognition is important as anticoagulation therapy may be effective in these patients. Migraine is a common finding in patients with the antiphospholipid syndrome, and often pre-dates the diagnosis by many years. However, recent prospective studies have not demonstrated a significant statistical association between migraine headaches and the presence of antiphospholipid antibodies (Montalban *et al.* 1992; Tsakiris *et al.* 1993).

Heart valve disease, particularly mitral valve involvement, is strikingly associated with antiphospholipid antibodies (Khamashta *et al.* 1990; Cervera *et al.* 1991; Galve *et al.* 1992). In some cases this is due to a combination of valvular thrombosis and degeneration. In our prospective echocardiographic studies, the valves were involved in more than one-third of the patients with lupus or primary antiphospholipid syndrome. Most patients with heart valve disease associated with antiphospholipid antibodies are asymptomatic, though heart insufficiency requiring surgical valve replacement has been reported. Emboli from sterile valvular vegetations can cause multiple cerebral lesions. Large intracardiac thrombosis associated with antiphospholipid antibodies can mimic atrial myxoma.

One of the most striking physical signs in patients positive for antiphospholipid antibody is livedo reticularis (Fig. 5), sometimes widespread, sometimes subtle, e.g. confined to a small area on the back of the wrist. In one prospective study of patients with livedo reticularis, 43 per cent had anticardiolipin antibodies (Asherson *et al.* 1989d). We found that surprisingly few patients with Sneddon's syndrome (a triad of livedo reticularis, ischaemic cerebrovascular

disease, and hypertension) were positive for antiphospholipid antibody, suggesting either that this syndrome results from many coagulopathies or that antiphospholipid antibodies are indeed important but that in our study the antibodies had long since disappeared. More dramatic skin manifestations associated with vascular thrombosis include widespread skin ulceration, notably in the lower extremities. Clinically, some patients with antiphospholipid antibodies may develop nail splinter haemorrhages (Fig. 6) and clubbing, posing major diagnostic difficulties, in those with heart valve disease, in differentiating from bacterial endocarditis (Mujic *et al.* 1995a).

Avascular necrosis of bone is an uncommon complication in lupus patients and clearly associated with high steroid dosage. We have noted an increased risk of avascular necrosis in individuals positive for antiphospholipid antibody, possibly as a result of small arterial occlusions, notably of the head of the femur (Asherson *et al.* 1993b).

Many patients with the antiphospholipid syndrome seem to develop widespread arteriopathy. The systemic narrowing of major arteries is similar in many respects to the widespread endarterial disease seen in some patients after heart–lung transplantation. Thus, antiphospholipid antibodies might be associated with accelerated vascular disease, including atherosclerosis (Lahita *et al.* 1993; Vaarala *et al.* 1993; Vaarala *et al.* 1996).

Epidemiology

The epidemiology of antiphospholipid antibodies is still being investigated worldwide. Efforts are being made in clinics throughout the world to assess the importance of this factor in recurrent abortion, stroke, myocardial infarction, epilepsy, and so on. In cardiovascular disease, Hamsten *et al.* (1986) found that 21 per cent of young patients in Sweden with myocardial infarction were antiphospholipid positive—this figure has not been reached in other studies. A collaborative United Kingdom/Spanish study found a prevalence of antiphospholipid positivity of 6.8 per cent in a large cohort of patients with stroke (Montalban *et al.* 1991). More recently, Nencini *et al.* (1992) in a study of 'young' stroke patients found that 18–per cent were positive for antiphospholipid antibody. In many of the other specialties, there is not enough data for adequate analysis. In obstetrics, the associations are now more clearly defined, though still with wide disparity between series, due possibly more to variations in test standardization than to clinical selection. Lynch *et al.* (1994) in a recent, large, prospective cohort study of 389 nulliparous mothers assessed at study entry and delivery, showed that 95 (24 per cent) were positive for antiphospholipid antibody of which 15.8 per cent had pregnancy loss, compared with 6.5 per cent of the women who were negative for antiphospholipid antibody.

Antiphospholipid antibodies are detected in patients with a variety of autoimmune, infectious, malignant, and drug-induced disorders, as well as in some apparently healthy individuals. Other than patients with the antiphospholipid syndrome, the single disorder in which these antibodies have been reported most frequently is systemic lupus erythematosus, in which lupus anticoagulants are reported in 10 to 20 per cent of cases, and anticardiolipin antibodies in 20 to 40 per cent of cases (Love and Santoro 1990; Cervera *et al.* 1993).

The specificities of antiphospholipid antibodies probably differ in various disorders. Large retrospective studies of patients with thrombotic complications suggest that those with high concentrations of IgG anticardiolipin antibodies appear to be at greatest risk for

Table 4 Criteria for the classification of the antiphospholipid syndrome[a]

Clinical	Laboratory
Venous thrombosis	IgG anticardiolipin antibodies (moderate/high titres)
Arterial thrombosis	
Recurrent fetal loss	IgM anticardiolipin antibodies (moderate/high titres)
Thrombocytopenia	
	Positive lupus anticoagulant test

[a]Patients with the syndrome should have at least one clinical plus one laboratory finding during their disease. Antiphospholipid antibody test must be positive on at least two occasions more than 3 months apart.

thrombosis, whereas the risk of clotting appears to be much lower in patients with infection-related or drug-induced antiphospholipid antibodies. Families positive for antiphospholipid antibody exist, and HLA studies have suggested associations with DR7, DR4, DRw53, DQw7, and C4 null alleles (Wilson *et al.* 1988; Arnett *et al.* 1991; Asherson *et al.* 1992; Wilson *et al.* 1995).

Diagnosis

Tests for anticardiolipin and lupus anticoagulant are essential to a diagnosis of the antiphospholipid syndrome. This syndrome is best defined as the occurrence of venous or arterial thrombosis, pregnancy losses, or thrombocytopenia associated with persistently positive tests for anticardiolipin or lupus anticoagulant. Patients may have one, two, or all three clinical features present, but they must also be positive for at least one of the two laboratory tests (Table 4). Many of the patients reported to have the syndrome have lupus and can be regarded as having secondary antiphospholipid syndrome. Some patients do not have any underlying systemic disease. These patients may be regarded as having primary antiphospholipid syndrome (Alarcon-Segovia and Sanchez-Guerrero 1989a; Asherson *et al.* 1989c; Mackworth-Young *et al.* 1989). For research and classification purposes, the term primary is useful, although there appear to be few differences in complications related to antiphospholipid antibody or in antibody specificity in the presence or absence of systemic lupus erythematosus (Vianna *et al.* 1994). Although some patients with primary antiphospholipid syndrome progress to systemic lupus, most do not show such progression (Mujic *et al.* 1995b).

Apart from lupus and primary antiphospholipid syndrome, antiphospholipid antibodies can occur in a wide variety of rheumatic, inflammatory, drug-induced, malignant, or infectious disorders. Usually, they are of low titre, of the IgM isotype, and unassociated with thrombotic events (Asherson 1992b). Antiphospholipid antibodies, using standardized techniques, are detected in less than 1 per cent of apparently normal persons and in up to 3 per cent of the elderly population without clinical manifestations of the antiphospholipid syndrome.

Differential diagnosis

Careful family and personal history and physical examination of patients with unexplained thromboses are of the utmost importance as thrombotic events and, notably, venous thromboses, often have explanations other than the antiphospholipid syndrome. It is advisable that thrombophilia testing, as suggested in Table 5, be performed in all patients, before initiating anticoagulant treatment.

Deficiencies in protein C, protein S, or antithrombin III are usually associated with recurrent venous thromboses. Echocardiographic studies should be performed in patients with cerebral infarcts as arterial emboli originating from cardiac valvular lesions are particularly common.

The most striking feature of the antiphospholipid syndrome is the frequent observation of life-threatening thrombosis in the setting of thrombocytopenia. A number of other conditions can result in thrombocytopenia and thrombosis, including heparin-induced thrombocytopenia and thrombotic thrombocytopenic purpura.

Heparin-induced thrombocytopenia develops in 1 to 5 per cent of patients receiving standard heparin and somewhat less frequently in

Table 5 Laboratory investigation of unexplained thromboses

Full blood count including platelets and blood microscopy (e.g. schistocytes)

Protein C

Activated protein C resistance (ratio)

Protein S (free and total)

Antithrombin III

Activated partial thromboplastin time

Prothrombin time

Reptilase time

Fibrinogen concentration

Fibrin split products

Plasminogen concentration

Serum and urine homocysteine

Antinuclear antibodies

Complement profile (C3, C4 and CH50)

Lupus anticoagulant

Anticardiolipin antibodies (IgG and IgM)

Syphilis serology

Others[a]:   Anticardiolipin antibody (IgA)

Anti-β_2-glycoprotein I antibody

Antibodies against other phospholipids: antiphosphatidylserine, antiphosphatidic acid, antiphosphatidylinositol, antiphosphatidylethanolamine, antiphosphatidylcholine

[a]For patients with a clinical picture highly suggestive of the antiphospholipid syndrome but negative for standard tests for anticardiolipin antibodies and lupus anticoagulant.

those who receive preparations of low molecular weight. Approximately 10 to 20 per cent of patients with substantial heparin-induced thrombocytopenia have venous or arterial thrombosis, including pulmonary, cardiac, and cerebral thrombosis. Thrombocytopenia typically develops approximately a week after exposure in persons not previously treated with heparin and sooner in those with previous exposure.

Thrombotic thrombocytopenic purpura is associated with neurological syndromes, but it is chiefly a microvascular disorder and confusion, seizures, or changes in the level of consciousness are more frequent than isolated, cerebral, large vessel thrombosis. Microangiopathic haemolysis with evidence of schistocytes in peripheral blood is usually a prominent finding. Elevation in the serum level of lactate dehydrogenase is found in nearly all cases and is a sensitive marker of the severity of the disorder.

We suggest that the tests for IgA anticardiolipin, anti-β_2-glycoprotein I, and antibodies against other phospholipids be ordered only for patients strongly suspected of having the antiphospholipid syndrome despite negative assays for IgG and IgM anticardiolipin and for lupus anticoagulant (Viard et al. 1992; Amengual et al. 1996).

Pathogenesis

Precisely how antiphospholipid antibodies relate to thrombosis is unknown. Several mechanisms have been proposed to explain the prothrombotic nature of the antiphospholipid syndrome. The range of possible mechanisms include effects of antiphospholipid antibodies on platelet membranes, on endothelial cells, and on clotting components such as antithrombin III, protein C, and protein S (Table 6) (Khamashta et al. 1989; Roubey 1994).

In 1990, three groups independently reported that the anticardiolipin antibodies detected by enzyme-linked immunosorbent assay are not directed against cardiolipin alone, because purified IgG from anticardiolipin-positive patients did not bind to cardiolipin unless a

Table 6 Proposed mechanisms of thrombosis mediated by antiphospholipid antibody

Decreased prostacyclin production and/or release by endothelial cells

Inhibition of factor XII/prekallikrein-mediated fibrinolytic activity

Decreased protein C activation

Decreased free protein S levels

Interference with thrombomodulin function on endothelial cells

Decreased antithrombin III activation

Increased platelet activation and aggregation

Interference with the function of plasma β_2-glycoprotein I

Increased tissue factor expression

Decreased function of annexin V (placental anticoagulant protein I)

Direct vascular damage

Complement activation

Vascular activation and release of von Willebrand factor multimer

plasma protein cofactor was present (Galli et al. 1990; Matsuura et al. 1990; McNeil et al. 1990). This protein was β_2-glycoprotein I. It has since become clear that anticardiolipin antibody in patients with the syndrome is dependent on both cardiolipin and β_2-glycoprotein I for optimum binding, though the relative importance of the two molecules, or their combination, is uncertain. Recent data indicate that certain lupus anticoagulants also require a plasma protein cofactor. This cofactor has been identified as prothrombin or β_2-glycoprotein I (Bevers et al. 1991; Oosting et al. 1992).

β_2-Glycoprotein I (apolipoprotein H) is a 50-kDa protein present at approximately 200 μg/ml in normal plasma. Although its physiological role is not known, in vitro data suggest that β_2-glycoprotein I may play a role in coagulation. β_2-Glycoprotein I binds to anionic phospholipids and inhibits the contact phase of intrinsic blood coagulation, platelet aggregation dependent on adenosine diphospate, and the prothrombinase activity of platelets. Although these data suggest an anticoagulant role for β_2-glycoprotein I, deficiency of this protein is not a clear risk factor for thrombosis. Patients with antiphospholipid antibodies have normal or somewhat elevated levels of β_2-glycoprotein I (Roubey 1994).

β_2-Glycoprotein I has its critical role in the recognition of cardiolipin by anticardiolipin antibodies in patients with autoimmune disease, but not from patients with infection (Hunt et al. 1992; Hunt et al. 1994). Anticardiolipin antibodies associated with syphilis bind to cardiolipin in the absence of β_2-glycoprotein I but this binding is inhibited by its presence, presumably because the antibodies and β_2-glycoprotein I bind to similar phospholipid structures. This difference in antigenic specificity may explain why the autoimmune type of anticardiolipin antibody is associated with the lupus anticoagulant and clinical complications such as thrombosis and recurrent fetal loss, whereas anticardiolipin antibodies associated with infection are not (Roubey 1994).

One hypothetical model for the mechanism of thrombosis proposes persistent endothelial cell damage and/or platelet activation, resulting in increased exposure of anionic phospholipid surfaces. Plasma proteins such as β_2-glycoprotein I and prothrombin are relatively abundant and may bind to the lipid surface, exposing novel epitopes. The immune response is directed to modified plasma proteins, therefore, rather than to lipids (Fig. 7) (Comfurius et al. 1995).

We have recently established five, monoclonal, IgM anticardiolipin antibodies from three patients with the antiphospholipid syndrome and showed that binding to anionic phospholipids was absolutely dependent on the presence of β_2-glycoprotein I (Ichikawa et al. 1994). Furthermore, a mixture of β_2-glycoprotein I and cardiolipin inhibited the binding of monoclonal anticardiolipin antibodies to β_2-glycoprotein I, but cardiolipin or β_2-glycoprotein I alone did not. These results suggest that anticardiolipin antibodies may recognize a cryptic epitope, which appears as a result of β_2-glycoprotein I binding to anionic phospholipids. Recent studies by Matsuura et al. (1994) confirmed that anticardiolipin antibodies bind to an epitope on β_2-glycoprotein I that is expressed when β_2-glycoprotein I binds to γ-irradiated microtitre plates. Interestingly, immunization of healthy mice and rabbits with β_2-glycoprotein I resulted in high titres of anti-β_2-glycoprotein I and anticardilipin antibodies, whereas cardiolipin alone was not immunogenic (Gharavi et al. 1992).

It has recently been demonstrated that the fifth C-terminal domain of β_2-glycoprotein I contains the major phospholipid binding site, a region critical for binding anticardiolipin antibodies (Hunt et al.

1993). Using synthetic peptides spanning the fifth domain, it has been shown that the major phospholipid binding site is restricted to the sequence Cys[281]–Lys–Asn–Lys–Glu–Lys–Lys–Cys[288] (Hunt and Krilis 1994). A preparation of β_2-glycoprotein I clipped in the C-terminus between Lys[317] and Thr[318] completely loses both its ability to bind negatively-charged phospholipid and to act as a cofactor. In addition, anticardiolipin antibodies purified from patients with autoimmune disease could bind directly to β_2-glycoprotein I but not to wells coated with the preparation of β_2-glycoprotein I cleaved between Lys[317] and Thr[318]. These results were confirmed recently using monoclonal, anticardiolipin antibodies derived from patients with the antiphospholipid syndrome (Wang et al. 1995).

Animal models are providing useful clues to the pathogenesis of the antiphospholipid syndrome (Blank et al. 1991; Bakimer et al. 1992). Passive transfer and active immunization of BALB/c mice with human or mouse anticardiolipin monoclonal antibodies induced features of the antiphospholipid syndrome. The experimental antiphospholipid syndrome was characterized by serological markers (a panel of antiphospholipid antibodies, prolonged activated partial thromboplastin time, indicating the presence of the lupus anticoagulant), haematological findings (thrombocytopenia),and clinical manifestations (recurrent fetal resorption, the equivalent of human fetal loss). A role for antiphospholipid antibodies in causing thrombosis has been more difficult to demonstrate. Pierangeli and Harris (1994) provided recently the most persuasive evidence yet for a cause-and-effect role for antiphospholipid antibodies in thrombosis. In an in vivo mouse model, the femoral vein was exposed and damaged by a standardized 'pinch' injury. A fibreoptic transilluminator was placed underneath the vessel and the clotting process observed through a stereoscopic operating microscope. Infusion of anticardiolipin antibodies dramatically enhanced both the size of the thrombus formed locally as well as the time of persistence of the clot.

The basis of the heterogeneity of the clinical features of the antiphospholipid syndrome is not well understood. If one hypothesizes that these antibodies are pathogenic on the basis of their antigenic specificity, it is not clear why certain patients have venous thrombosis as opposed to arterial thrombosis or thrombocytopenia or recurrent fetal loss, or some combination of these manifestations (Roubey 1994). It is also not clear why only about 30 per cent of individuals with antiphospholipid antibodies will develop the clinical syndrome, although greater risk is associated with higher antibody titres (Harris et al. 1986; Ginsburg et al. 1992).

Treatment

One of the reasons for the widespread interest in the antiphospholipid syndrome has been its effect on approaches to therapy. Before its recognition, most features of systemic lupus erythematosus were attributed to inflammatory phenomena, requiring anti-inflammatory measures such as corticosteroids. Now it is recognized that features as diverse as fits, miscarriage, endocardial disease, and hypertension may all be the result of a thrombotic process. This concept has spread beyond the confines of systemic lupus, and pinpointing antiphospholipid-associated thrombosis and taking appropriate anticoagulation measures have become important considerations in specialties as diverse as neurology and obstetrics (Hughes and Khamashta 1994). Table 7 shows our preferred treatment for the different clinical features associated with antiphospholipid antibodies.

Identification and treatment of additional risk factors for thrombosis

In treating patients with the antiphospholipid syndrome, attention should first be given to removal or reduction of other risk factors that might predispose to thrombosis. Treatment of hypertension and hypercholesterolaemia is required, along with advice to stop smoking and, for female patients, counselling against use of oral contraceptives containing oestrogen (Levine et al. 1992; Vianna et al. 1994). Prophylaxis with heparin administered subcutaneously at the time of surgery should be considered for all patients.

Prophylactic treatment of asymptomatic patients with antiphospholipid antibodies

Antiphospholipid antibodies persist for many years, possibly a lifetime. Thus, one of the unresolved key clinical questions is what additional factors lead to the sudden development of thrombosis, which occurs only in a minority of these patients (Hughes 1993).

The controversy concerning whether or not prophylactic treatment is indicated for patients with antiphospholipid antibodies who have no history of thrombosis remains unresolved. Most clinicians do not consider this sufficient reason for prophylactic anticoagulation, though prophylaxis should certainly be given to cover high-risk situations such as surgery. In our daily practice, we recommend that patients with a persistently positive test for lupus anticoagulant and/or with moderate to high levels of IgG anticardiolipin antibody and no history of thrombosis, be treated with low-dose aspirin (75 mg/day). These patients should be monitored carefully because they have the greatest risk of thrombosis (Khamashta and Wallington 1991; Hunt and Khamashta 1996).

In pregnancy, inappropriate treatment of women who do not have the antiphospholipid syndrome must be avoided. Anticardiolipin tests are positive at low titres in up to 2 per cent of the normal obstetric population, and such findings do not appear to be associated with an adverse outcome (Lockwood et al. 1989; Harris and Spinnato 1991). The risk is relatively low for primiparas, even if they have high titres of antiphospholipid antibody, and therefore their recommended prophylactic treatment is either close observation only or observation plus low-dose aspirin (Lockshin 1993).

Prevention of recurrent thrombosis

Optimal management of patients with thrombotic features associated with antiphospholipid antibodies remains a problem. Controlled treatment trials have proved difficult to perform in these patients because of the limited number of eligible patients with antiphospholipid syndrome available for study at a single centre and the necessity of long-term follow-up. There is now good evidence that those with thrombosis will be subject to recurrences, but there is still no consensus regarding the duration and extent of prophylactic antithrombotic treatments in these patients (Khamashta 1996). Many patients with the antiphospholipid syndrome in whom anticoagulation has been stopped have had major recurrent thromboses (Asherson et al. 1985; Rosove and Brewer 1992; Derksen et al. 1993).

Table 7 Preferred treatment for the different clinical manifestations associated with antiphospholipid antibodies

Clinical situation	Suggested treatment
1. Asymptomatic individuals	Observations ± low-dose aspirin
2. Thrombotic events:	
Deep vein thrombosis ± pulmonary embolism	Life-long oral anticoagulants (INR ⩾ 3)
Large vessel arterial occlusion (i.e. stroke)	Life-long oral anticoagulants (INR ⩾ 3) ± low-dose aspirin
Transient ischaemic attack	Low-dose aspirin
Catastrophic antiphospholipid syndrome	Oral anticoagulants (INR ⩾ 3)+plasmapheresis ± corticosteroids or immunosuppressives
3. Pregnancy:	
No previous history of thrombosis or abortions	Observation ± low-dose aspirin
History of 1st trimester abortions	Low-dose aspirin
History of 2nd or 3rd trimester fetal loss	Low-dose aspirin ± subcutaneous heparin
Previous history of thrombosis ± pregnancy loss	Low-dose aspirin+subcutaneous heparin
4. Thrombocytopenia:	
Mild (100 000–150 000)	Observation
Moderate (50 000–100 000)	Observation ± low-dose aspirin
Severe (< 50 000)	Corticosteroids ± intravenous gammaglobulin

INR, international normalized ratio.

We have recently assessed our experience of the management of anti-phospholipid-associated thrombosis in 147 patients over a 10-year period (Khamashta *et al.* 1995). Our study showed that long-term and intensive oral anticoagulation (international normalized ratio 3) was the most effective therapeutic option in the secondary prevention of venous and arterial thrombosis in these patients. Moreover, our study has shown that the first 6 months after stopping warfarin therapy were associated with the highest rate of recurrences (1.30 thrombotic events per year). This high probability of recurrent thromboses in patients with antiphospholipid antibodies and previous thromboembolic disease without oral anticoagulation, suggests that these patients require indefinite warfarin therapy. The benefits of long-term anticoagulation should, however, be balanced by the risks of bleeding. In our series, bleeding complications occurred in 29 patients (0.071 occasions per patient–year) and in 7 (0.017 occasions per patient–year) they were severe, suggesting that the benefits of warfarin in the antiphospholipid syndrome are greater than the risks. There was no evidence that low–dose aspirin (75 mg/day) alone prevented further thrombotic events in our patients. A similar finding was observed in the study of Rosove and Brewer (1992). It should be emphasized, however, that some patients with transient ischaemic attacks may respond to low–dose aspirin or dipyridamole therapy.

A significant number of patients require high doses of warfarin (up to 20 mg/day) to maintain the international normalized ratio in therapeutic range (3.0 to 4.0). In our experience, most of these patients were receiving other drugs and, notably, azathioprine at the same time as warfarin therapy. An important drug interaction has been pointed out recently between azathioprine and warfarin (Singleton and Conyers 1992; Rivier *et al.* 1993). When azathioprine is reduced or discontinued, anticoagulation may increase with the potential for bleeding if the international normalized ratio is not carefully monitored in these patients.

The role of steroids and immunosuppressive drugs in treatment of patients with antiphospholipid antibodies and thrombosis is uncertain. Such drugs have severe side-effects when given for prolonged periods and we, and others, have found that antiphospholipid antibodies are not always suppressed by these agents (Out *et al.* 1989; Harris *et al.* 1993). Furthermore, in our series of patients with the antiphospholipid syndrome, corticosteroids and immunosuppressive therapy, prescribed in some patients to control lupus activity, did not prevent further thrombotic events (Asherson *et al.* 1991; Khamashta *et al.* 1995). The use of these drugs is probably justified only in patients with repeated episodes of thrombosis despite adequate anticoagulant therapy, i.e. catastrophic antiphospholipid syndrome. In this rare but life-threatening condition, plasmapheresis has also been used (Asherson 1992; Asherson and Piette 1996).

It is of interest to note that our studies have shown that there were no broad significant differences in the levels of anticardiolipin antibodies between those patients who developed recurrent

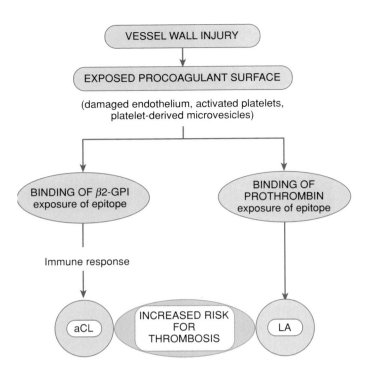

Fig. 7 Hypothesis explaining the generation of antiphospholipid antibodies as a normal response of the body to a potentially dangerous situation. This hypothesis predicts the possible existence of antibodies directed against all lipid-binding plasma proteins. As a consequence, it also explains the coexistence of anticardiolipin antibodies and lupus anticoagulant that is frequently observed in patients with the antiphospholipid syndrome. (Reproduced with the permission of the Editor of *Lupus* and from Dr P. Comfurius.)

thromboembolic events and those who did not (Asherson *et al.* 1991; Khamashta *et al.* 1995). These findings further support the recommendation that treatment aimed at suppressing antibody formation is not warranted in patients with thrombosis associated with antiphospholipid antibodies.

The use of intra-arterial fibrinolysis has been described to be of benefit in patients with acute myocardial infarction associated with antiphospholipid antibodies. Prostacyclin analogues (iloprost) were also successfully used in patients with severe ischaemic necrotic toes associated with antiphospholipid syndrome (Zahavi *et al.* 1993). Elective pulmonary thromboendarterectomy can be very effective and lifesaving in selected patients with chronic large-vessel thrombo-embolic pulmonary hypertension (Sandoval *et al.* 1996).

Prevention of fetal losses

The treatment of patients with recurrent pregnany loss associated with antiphospholipid antibodies remains controversial and there are no clear guidelines for management. However, consensus is being reached on some aspects. An appropriate approach would be to assemble a multidisciplinary team (rheumatologist, obstetrician, and clinical haematologist), exclude causes of pregnancy loss other than the antiphospholipid syndrome, and select a drug regimen which has some reported efficacy and which will cause the least harm for the mother and fetus. Most importantly, the woman should be followed carefully throughout her pregnancy with

frequent ultrasound evaluation for early detection of intrauterine growth retardation, and Doppler studies to monitor the flow-velocity waveforms of umbilical and uterine arteries (Harris 1990; Kerslake *et al.* 1992; Buchanan *et al.* 1993; Kamashta and Hughes 1996).

Over the past 7–years there has been a re-evaluation of the significance of antiphospholipid antibodies in pregnancy and, whilst an increased rate of fetal loss is seen in this group, experience suggests that with close monitoring this can be significantly reduced (Trudinger *et al.* 1988; McHugh *et al.* 1989). Recent data from our pregnancy clinic show that the greatest impact on fetal outcome in our series of patients with systemic lupus erythematous and antiphospholipid syndrome has been the regularity and quality of obstetric care, judicious monitoring, and timely intervention (Buchanan *et al.* 1992; Lima *et al.* 1995). In view of these findings, many of the high-dose (40 to 60 mg/day) prednisolone strategies, which were the treatments of choice in the early 1980s for patients with recurrent abortions associated with antiphospholipid antibodies, are being abandoned. These doses regularly produce severe cushingoid effects, hypertension, and diabetic manifestations. Furthermore, controlled clinical trials now favour low-dose aspirin (75 mg/day) and subcutaneous heparin (10 000 to 15 000 IU/day) in those with a history of thrombosis, over corticosteroid therapy (Lockshin *et al.* 1989; Cowchock *et al.* 1992). In our recently reported study of pregnant women with the antiphospholipid syndrome, pregnancy outcome improved from 19 to 70 per cent using low-dose aspirin in all patients and subcutaneous heparin in those with previous thrombosis (Lima *et al.* 1996).

The presence of antiphospholipid antibodies in pregnant women in the absence of a previous history of thrombosis or fetal loss is not an indication for treatment. If, however, the patient does have a history of previous thrombosis and is being given warfarin, careful management is needed. Warfarin may be teratogenic, even early in the first trimester. The risks of continuing warfarin and also the problems with using heparin should be carefully explained to the patient. For the benefit of the fetus, warfarin should ideally be converted to subcutaneous heparin prior to conception, as heparin does not cross the placenta. Some women prefer to continue with warfarin until the first missed period, and then convert at this time.

Standard heparin or heparins of low molecular weight can be used during pregnancy, although the latter are not licensed for this purpose. There is no theoretical advantage of either. However, as one can monitor the levels of heparin with a low molecular weight very accurately with anti-Xa activity, we prefer to use them (Hunt *et al.* 1997). Their other practical advantage is that the patient can be started on one injection daily, in contrast to the necessary two or even three injections a day with standard subcutaneous heparin. Heparin doses need to be increased during pregnancy as the plasma volume expands. The patients can be converted back to warfarin after delivery.

Despite widespread use of heparin in pregnancy, there are relatively few reports of obstetric complications. The risks associated with heparin treatment include dose-related problems such as bleeding or osteopenia and idiosyncratic reactions such as immune thrombocytopenia, alopecia, and local reactions. The possibility of maternal osteoporosis is a limiting factor in the use of heparin. Heparin of low molecular weight, which has a long half-life and can be given once daily, may have less effect on bone. The combined use of corticosteroids and heparin may result in severe osteopenia.

Aspirin has been an integral part of treatment for women with the antiphospholipid syndrome. It was used on the basis of several reports suggesting that prostacyclin synthesis or release by endothelial cells was decreased *in vitro* by antiphospholipid antibodies. This would lead to an imbalance in the thromboxane/prostacyclin ratio and to platelet aggregation and vasospasm. Aspirin given in doses of under 150 mg/day preferentially blocks arterial thromboxane synthesis. Such dosages are associated with few (if any) maternal or fetal risks.

For patients who continue to have pregnancy loss despite a heparin and low-dose aspirin regimen, high-dose intravenous gamma-globulin (0.4 g/kg on 4 days each month) might be considered. The treatment should be initiated as soon as pregnancy is ascertained and continued throughout the pregnancy; it has proved very effective but is expensive. Fluid overload and hypertension are the major complications.

Clearly, optimal management of patients with recurrent pregnancy loss associated with antiphospholipid antibodies remains a problem, but the recent establishment of animal models for the antiphospholipid syndrome provides an excellent opportunity to develop rational and more-targeted therapies. A recent example is the demonstration by Fishman *et al.* (1993) that mice with experimental antiphospholipid syndrome are deficient in interleukin-3 and that fetal losses in these mice could be prevented by administration of recombinant interleukin-3. This novel approach has not yet been used in patients with antiphospholipid syndrome.

Treatment of thrombocytopenia

Mild thrombocytopenia with platelet counts between 100 000 and 150 000/mm³ are common in patients with antiphospholipid antibody and usually does not require intervention (Khamashta and Machin 1991). In a minority of cases it can be severe. In these cases, corticosteroid therapy should always be the treatment of choice. However, it should be noted that there have been several case reports of peripheral thrombocytopenia unresponsive to steroid therapy, with platelet counts returning to normal following low-dose aspirin therapy (Alarcon-Segovia and Sanchez-Guerrero 1989b). Aspirin, by reducing the degree of spontaneous platelet activation, also presumably reduces binding of antiphospholipid antibody and immune-type platelet destruction (Khamashta *et al.* 1988). Intravenous gammaglobulin infusion, danazol, and dapsone have been given successfully to some patients with severe thrombocytopenia associated with antiphospholipid antibody. There is no published experience reported with splenectomy in these patients, though we have one patient (a 33-year-old male) with severe thrombocytopenia and antiphospholipid antibodies in whom splenectomy failed to improve the platelet count. This procedure should be considered with caution in view of an increased thromboembolic risk related to post-splenectomy thrombocytosis.

Antiphospholipid syndrome in childhood

There have been relatively few reports of clinical associations of antiphospholipid antibodies in children and the spectrum of clinical findings remains at present unknown. Antiphospholipid antibodies in childhood-onset systemic lupus erythematosus have been described in several small clinical reports, occurring in one-third of the patients. The clinical manifestations are similar to those encountered in adults, particularly recurrent deep-vein thrombosis, strokes, and chorea. Devastating thrombotic complications of the antiphospholipid syndrome in children have been reported including digital ischaemia and myocardial infarction (Tucker 1994). The risk of maternal transmission of antiphospholipid antibodies to infants during pregnancy is unknown, though there have been several case reports of thrombotic events in neonates of mothers with the antiphospholipid syndrome (Silver *et al.* 1992).

Prognosis

Although there are a number of studies of prognostic factors in systemic lupus erythematosus, only a few have addressed the possible role of the antiphospholipid syndrome in the mortality rates of these patients. Drenkard *et al.* (1994) have recently analysed the influence of the antiphospholipid syndrome in the survival of their series of 667 patients with systemic lupus erythematosus. Thrombocytopenia and arterial occlusions were the manifestations related to antiphospholipid antibody that were associated with decreased survival. The syndrome itself was also associated with increased mortality rate, independently of other variables. A negative impact of positivity for IgM anticardiolipin antibody on the probability of survival of lupus patients also was found in another study (Gulko *et al.* 1993).

References

Alarcon-Segovia, D. and Sanchez-Guerrero, J. (1989*a*). Primary antiphospholipid syndrome. *Journal of Rheumatology*, **16**, 482–8.

Alarcon-Segovia, D. and Sanchez-Guerrero, J. (1989*b*). Correction of thrombocytopenia with small dose aspirin in the primary antiphospholipid syndrome. *Journal of Rheumatology*, **16**, 1421–3.

Alarcon-Segovia, D., Deleze, M., Oria, C.V., Sanchez-Guerrero, J., and Gomez-Pacheco, L. (1989). Antiphospholipid antibodies and the antiphospholipid syndrome in systemic lupus erythematosus: a prospective analysis of 500 consecutive patients. *Medicine (Baltimore)*, **68**, 353–65.

Amengual, O., Atsumi, T., Khamashta, M.A., Koike, T., and Hughes, G.R.V. (1996). Specificity of ELISA for antibody to β2-glycoprotein I in patients with antiphospholipid syndrome. *British Journal of Rheumatology*, **35**, 1239–43.

Amigo, M.C. *et al.* (1992). Renal involvement in the primary antiphospholipid syndrome. *Journal of Rheumatology*, **18**, 1181–5.

Arnett, F.C., Olsen, M.L., Anderson, K.L., and Reveille, J.D. (1991). Molecular analysis of major histocompatibility complex alleles associated with the lupus anticoagulant. *Journal of Clinical Investigation*, **87**, 1490–5.

Asherson, R.A. (1992*a*). The catastrophic antiphospholipid syndrome. *Journal of Rheumatology*, **19**, 508–12.

Asherson, R.A. (1992*b*). Antiphospholipid antibodies and syndromes. In *Systemic lupus erythematosus* (2nd edn) (ed. R.G. Lahita), pp. 587–635. Churchill Livingstone Inc., New York.

Asherson, R.A. and Hughes, G.R.V. (1991). Hypoadrenalism, Addison's disease and antiphospholipid antibodies. *Journal of Rheumatology*, **18**, 1–3.

Asherson, R.A. and Piette, J.C. (1996). The catastrophic antiphospholipid syndrome: acute multi-organ failure associated with antiphospholipid antibodies: a review of 31 patients. *Lupus*, **5**, 414–17.

Asherson, R.A., Chan, J.K.H., Harris, E.N., Gharavi, A.E., and Hughes, G.R.V. (1985). Anticardiolipin antibody, recurrent thrombosis and warfarin withdrawal. *Annals of the Rheumatic Diseases*, **44**, 823–5.

Asherson, R.A., Derksen, R.W.H.M., Harris, E.N., and Hughes, G.R.V. (1987). Chorea in systemic lupus and lupus-like disease: association with antiphospholipid antibodies. *Seminars in Arthritis and Rheumatism*, **16**, 253–9.

Asherson, R.A. *et al.* (1989*a*). Cerebrovascular disease and antiphospholipid anti-bodies in systemic lupus erythematosus, lupus-like disease and the primary antiphospholipid syndrome. *American Journal of Medicine*, **86**, 391–9.

Asherson, R.A., Khamashta, M.A., Baguley, E., Oakley, C., Rowell, N.R., and Hughes, G.R.V. (1989*b*). Myocardial infarction and antiphospholipid antibo-dies. *Quarterly Journal of Medicine*, **73**, 1103–15.

Asherson, R.A. *et al.* (1989*c*). The primary antiphospholipid syndrome: major clinical and serological features. *Medicine (Baltimore)*, **68**, 366–74.

Asherson, R.A., Mayou, S.C., Merry, P., Black, M.M., and Hughes, G.R.V. (1989*d*). The spectrum of livedo reticularis and anticardiolipin antibodies. *British Journal of Dermatology*, **120**, 215–21.

Asherson, R.A., Higenbottam, T.W., Dinh Xuan, A.T., Khamashta, M.A., and Hughes, G.R.V. (1990). Pulmonary hypertension in a lupus clinic: experience with twenty-four patients. *Journal of Rheumatology*, **17**, 1292–8.

Asherson, R.A., Baguley, E., Pal, C., and Hughes, G.R.V. (1991). Antiphospholipid syndrome: five year follow up. *Annals of the Rheumatic Diseases*, **50**, 805–10.

Asherson, R.A., Doherty, D.G., Vergani, D., Khamashta, M.A., and Hughes, G.R.V. (1992). Major histocompatibility complex associations with primary antipho-spholipid syndrome. *Arthritis and Rheumatism*, **35**, 124–5.

Asherson, R.A., Khamashta, M.A., and Hughes, G.R.V. (1993*a*). Hypertension and the antiphospholipid antibodies. *Clinical and Experimental Rheumatology*, **11**, 465–7.

Asherson, R.A. *et al.* (1993*b*). Avascular necrosis of bone and antiphospholipid antibodies in systemic lupus erythematosus. *Journal of Rheumatology*, **20**, 284–8.

Bakimer, R., Fishman, P., Blank, M., Sredni, B., Djaldetti, M., and Shoenfeld, Y. (1992). Induction of experimental antiphospholipid syndrome in mice by immunization with human monoclonal anticardiolipin antibody (H-3). *Journal of Clinial Investigation*, **89**, 1558–63.

Bevers, E.M., Galli, M., Barbui, T., Comfurius, P., and Zwaal, R.F.A. (1991). Lupus anticoagulant IgG's (LA) are not directed to phospholipids only, but to a complex of lipid-bound human prothrombin. *Thrombosis and Haemostasis*, **66**, 623–32.

Blank, M., Cohen, J., Toder, V., and Shoenfeld, Y. (1991). Induction of anti-phospholipid syndrome in naive mice with mouse lupus monoclonal and human polyclonal anticardiolipin antibodies. *Proceedings of the National Academy of Science (USA)*, **88**, 3069–73.

Branch, D.W. (1994). Thoughts on the mechanism of pregnancy loss associated with the antiphospholipid syndrome. *Lupus*, **3**, 275–80.

Branch, D.W., Silver, R.M., Blackwell, J.L., Reading, J.C., and Scott, J.R. (1992). Outcome of treated pregnancies in women with antiphospholipid syndrome: an update of the Utah experience. *Obstetrics and Gynecology*, **80**, 614–20.

Buchanan, N.M.M., Khamashta, M.A., Morton, K.E., Kerslake, S., Baguley, E.A., and Hughes, G.R.V. (1992). A study of 100 high risk lupus pregnancies. *American Journal of Reproductive Immunology*, **28**, 192–4.

Buchanan, N.M.M., Khamashta, M., Kerslake, S., Hunt, B.J., and Hughes, G.R.V. (1993). Practical management of pregnancy in systemic lupus erythematosus. *Fetal and Maternal Medicine Review*, **5**, 223–30.

Cervera, R. *et al.* (1991). High prevalence of significant heart valve lesions in patients with the primary antiphospholipid syndrome. *Lupus*, **1**, 43–7.

Cervera, R. *et al.* (1993). Systemic lupus erythematosus: clinical and immunologic patterns of disease expression in a cohort of 1000 patients. *Medicine (Baltimore)*, **72**, 113–24.

Comfurius, P., Bevers, E.M., Galli, M., and Zwaal, R.F.A. (1995). Regulation of phospholipid asymmetry and induction of antiphospholipid antibodies. *Lupus*, **4** (Suppl. 1), 19–22.

Cowchock, F.S., Reece, E.A., Balaban, D., Branch, D.W., and Plouffe, L. (1992). Repeated fetal losses associated with antiphospholipid antibodies. A collaborative randomized trial comparing prednisolone with low-dose heparin treatment. *American Journal of Obstetrics and Gynecology*, **166**, 1318–23.

Deleze, M. *et al.* (1989). Hemocytopenia in systemic lupus erythematosus. Relationship to antiphospholipid antibodies. *Journal of Rheumatology*, **16**, 926–30.

Derksen, R.H.W.M., de Groot, P.H.G., Kater, L., and Nieuwenhuis, H.K. (1993). Patients with antiphospholipid antibodies and venous thrombosis should receive long term anticoagulant treatment. *Annals of the Rheumatic Diseases*, **52**, 689–92.

Drenkard, C., Villa, A.R., Alarcon-Segovia, D., and Perez-Vazquez, M.E. (1994). Influence of the antiphospholipid syndrome in the survival of patients with systemic lupus erythematosus. *Journal of Rheumatology*, **21**, 1067–72.

Fishman, P. *et al.* (1993). Prevention of fetal loss in experimental antiphospholipid syndrome by *in vivo* administration of recombinant interleukin-3. *Journal of Clinical Investigation*, **91**, 1834–7.

Galli, M. *et al.* (1990). Anticardiolipin antibodies (ACA) directed not to cardiolipin but to a plasma protein cofactor. *Lancet*, **336**, 1544–7.

Galve, E. *et al.* (1992). Valvular heart disease in primary antiphospholipid syndrome. *Annals of Internal Medicine*, **116**, 293–8.

Gharavi, A.E., Harris, E.N., Asherson, R.A., and Hughes, G.R.V. (1987). Anticardiolipin antibodies: isotype distribution and phospholipid specificity. *Annals of the Rheumatic Diseases*, **46**, 1–6.

Gharavi, A.E., Sammaritano, L.R., Wen, J., and Elkon, K.B. (1992). Induction of antiphospholipid autoantibodies by immunization with β_2-glycoprotein I. *Journal of Clinical Investigation*, **90**, 1105–9.

Ginsburg, K.S. *et al.* (1992). Anticardiolipin antibodies and the risk for ischemic stroke and venous thrombosis. *Annals of Internal Medicine*, **117**, 997–1002.

Gulko, P.S., Reveille, J.D., Koopman, W.J., Burgard, S.L., Bartolucci, A.A., and Alarcon, G.S. (1993). Anticardiolipin antibodies in systemic lupus erythema-tosus: clinical correlates, HLA associations and impact on survival. *Journal of Rheumatology*, **20**, 1684–93.

Hamsten, A., Norberg, R., Bjorkholm, M., de Faire, U., and Holm, G. (1986). Antibodies to cardiolipin in young survivors of myocardial infarction: an asso-ciation with recurrent cardiovascular events. *Lancet*, **i**, 113–16.

Harris, E.N. (1990). Maternal antibodies and pregnancy: the antiphospholipid antibody syndrome. *Baillière's Clinical Rheumatology*, **4**, 53–68.

Harris, E.N. and Spinnato, J.A. (1991). Should anticardiolipin tests be performed in otherwise healthy pregnant women? *American Journal of Obstetrics and Gynecology*, **165**, 1272–7.

Harris, E.N. *et al.* (1983). Anticardiolipin antibodies: detection by radioimmu-nossay and association with thrombosis in systemic lupus erythematosus. *Lancet*, **ii**, 1211–14.

Harris, E.N. *et al.* (1985). Anticardiolipin antibodies in autoimmune thrombocyto-penic purpura. *British Journal of Haematology*, **59**, 231–4.

Harris, E.N., Chan, J.K.H., Asherson, R.A., Aber, V.R., Gharavi, A.E., and Hughes, G.R.V. (1986). Thrombosis, recurrent fetal loss and thrombocytopenia. Predictive value of the anticardiolipin test. *Archives of Internal Medicine*, **146**, 2153–6.

Harris, E.N., Gharavi, A.E., Patel, S.P., and Hughes, G.R.V. (1987). Evaluation of the anticardiolipin antibody test: report of an international workshop held 4th April 1986. *Clinical and Experimental Immunology*, **68**, 215–22.

Harris, E.N. and the Kingston Anti-phospholipid Groups (KAPS) (1990). The second international anticardiolipin standardisation workshop/The Kingston Anti-phospholipid Antibody Study (KAPS) Group. *American Journal of Clinical Pathology*, **94**, 476–84.

Harris, E.N., Khamashta, M.A., and Hughes, G.R.V. (1993). Antiphospholipid antibody syndrome. In *Arthritis and allied conditions* (12th edn) (ed. D.J. McCarty and W.J. Koopman), pp. 1201–12. Lea and Febiger, Philadelphia.

Harris, E.N., Gharavi, A.E., Asherson, R.A., Khamashta, M.A., and Hughes, G.R.V. (1994). Antiphospholipid antibodies — middle aged but robust. *Journal of Rheumatology*, **21**, 978–81.

Herranz, M.T., Rivier, G., Khamashta, M.A., Blaser, K.U., and Hughes, G.R.V. (1994). Association between antiphospholipid antibodies and epilepsy in patients with systemic lupus erythematosus. *Arthritis and Rheumatism*, **37**, 568–71.

Hughes, G.R.V. (1983). Thrombosis, abortion, cerebral disease and lupus anticoa-gulant. *British Medical Journal*, **287**, 1088–9.

Hughes, G.R.V. (1993). The antiphospholipid syndrome: ten years on. *Lancet*, **342**, 341–4.

Hughes, G.R.V. and Khamashta, M.A. (1994). The antiphospholipid syndrome. *Journal of the Royal College of Phyicians of London*, **28**, 301–4.

Hughes, G.R.V. and Khamashta, M.A. (1996). *Management of the Hughes syndrome. Clinical and Experimental Rheumatology*, **14**, 115–17.

Hunt, B.J. *et al.* (1997). Thromboprophylaxis with low molecular weight heparin (Fragmin) in high risk pregnancies. *Thrombosis and Haemostasis*, **77**, 39–43.

Hunt, J. and Krilis, S. (1994). The fifth domain of β_2-glycoprotein I contains a phospholipid binding site (Cys^{281}–Cys^{288}), and a region recognized by anticardiolipin antibodies. *Journal of Immunology*, **152**, 653–9

Hunt, J.E., McNeil, H.P., Morgan, G.J., Crameri, R.M., and Krilis, S.A. (1992). A phospholipid-β_2-glycoprotein I complex is an antigen for anticardiolipin antibodies occurring in autoimmune disease but not with infection. *Lupus*, **1**, 83–90.

Hunt, J.E., Simpson, R.J., and Krilis, S.A. (1993). Identification of a region of β_2-glycoprotein I critical for lipid binding and anticardiolipin cofactor activity. *Proceedings of the National Academy of Sciences (USA)*, **90**, 2141–5.

Hunt, J.E., Adelstein, S., and Krilis, S.A. (1994). New basic aspects of the antiphospholipid syndrome. *Clinical and Experimental Rheumatology*, **12**, 661–8.

Ichikawa, K., Khamashta, M.A., Koike, T., Matsuura, E., and Hughes, G.R.V. (1994). β_2-Glycoprotein I reactivity of monoclonal anticardiolipin antibodies from patients with the antiphospholipid syndrome. *Arthritis and Rheumatism*, **37**, 1453–61.

Kerslake, S. *et al.* (1992). Early Doppler studies in lupus pregnancy. *American Journal of Reproductive Immunology*, **28**, 172–5.

Khamashta, M.A. (1996). Management of thrombosis in the antiphospholipid syndrome. *Lupus*, **5**, 463–6.

Khamashta, M.A. and Asherson, R.A. (1995). Hughes syndrome — antiphospholipid antibodies move closer to thrombosis in 1994. *British Journal of Rheumatology*, **34**, 493–4.

Khamashta, M.A. and Hughes, G.R.V. (1993). Detection and importance of anticardiolipin antibodies. *Journal of Clinical Pathology*, **46**, 104–7.

Khamashta, M.A. and Hughes, G.R.V. (1996). Pregnancy in systemic lupus erythematosus. *Current Opinion in Rheumatology*, **8**, 424–9.

Khamashta, M.A. and Machin, S.J. (1991). Hematological immune cytopenias and antiphospholipid antibodies. In *Phospholipid binding antibodies* (ed. E.N. Harris, T. Exner, G.R.V. Hughes, and R.A. Asherson), pp. 247–54. CRC Press, Boca Raton, Florida.

Khamashta, M.A. and Wallington, T. (1991). Management of the antiphospholipid syndrome. *Annals of the Rheumatic Diseases*, **50**, 959–62.

Khamashta, M.A. *et al.* (1988). Immune mediated mechanism for thrombosis: antiphospholipid antibody binding to platelet membranes. *Annals of the Rheumatic Diseases*, **47**, 849–54.

Khamashta, M.A., Asherson, R.A., and Hughes, G.R.V. (1989). Possible mechanisms of action of the antiphospholipid binding antibodies. *Clinical and Experimental Rheumatology*, **7** (Suppl. 3), 85–9.

Khamashta, M.A. *et al.* (1990). Association of antiphospholipid antibodies with heart valve disease in systemic lupus erythematosus. *Lancet*, **335**, 1541–4.

Khamashta, M.A., Cuadrado, M.J., Mujic, F., Taub, N.A., Hunt, B.J., and Hughes, G.R.V. (1995). The Management of thrombosis in the antiphospholipid-antibody syndrome. *New England Journal of Medicine*, **332**, 993–7.

Lahita, R.G., Rivkin, E., Cavanagh, I., and Romano, P. (1993). Low levels of total cholesterol, high density lipoprotein, and apolipoprotein A1 in association with anticardiolipin antibodies in patients with systemic lupus erythematosus. *Arthritis and Rheumatism*, **36**, 1566–74.

Levine, S.R., Brey, R.L., Joseph, C.L.M., and Havstad, S. (1992). Risk of recurrent thromboembolic events in patients with focal cerebral ischemia and antiphospholipid antibodies. *Stroke*, **23** (Suppl. 1), 29–32.

Lie, J.T. (1994). Vasculitis in the antiphospholipid syndrome: culprit or consort? *Journal of Rheumatology*, **21**, 397–9.

Lima, F., Buchanan, N.M.M., Khamashta, M.A., Kerslake, S., and Hughes, G.R.V (1995). Obstetric outcome in systemic lupus erythematosus. *Seminars in Arthritis and Rheumatism*, **25**, 184–92.

Lima, F., Khamashta, M.A., Buchanan, N.M.M., Kerslake, S., Hunt, B.J., and Hughes, G.R.V (1996). A study of sixty pregnancies in patients with the antiphospholipid syndrome. *Clinical and Experimental Rheumatology*, **14**, 131–6.

Lockshin, M.D. (1993). Which patients with antiphospholipid antibody should be treated and how? *Rheumatic Disease Clinics of North America*, **19**, 235–47.

Lockshin, M.D., Qamar, T., Druzin, M.L., and Goei, S. (1987). Antibody to cardiolipin, lupus anticoagulant, and fetal death. *Journal of Rheumatology*, **14**, 259–62.

Lockshin, M.D., Druzin, M.L., and Qamar, T. (1989). Prednisolone does not prevent recurrent fetal death in women with antiphospholipid antibody. *American Journal of Obstetrics and Gynecology*, **160**, 439–43.

Lockwood, C.J. *et al.* (1989). The prevalence and biologic significance of lupus anticoagulant and anticardiolipin antibodies in a general obstetric population. *American Journal of Obstetrics and Gynecology*, **161**, 369–73.

Love, P.E. and Santoro, S.A. (1990). Antiphospholipid antibodies: anticardiolipin and the lupus anticoagulant in systemic lupus erythematosus (SLE) and non-SLE disorders: prevalence and clinical significance. *Annals of Internal Medicine*, **112**, 682–98.

Lynch, A. *et al.* (1994). Antiphospholipid antibodies in predicting adverse pregnancy outcome. *Annals of Internal Medicine*, **120**, 470–5.

Mackworth-Young, C.G., Loizou, S., and Walport, M.J. (1989). Primary antiphospholipid syndrome: features of patients with raised anticardiolipin antibodies and no other disorder. *Annals of the Rheumatic Diseases*, **48**, 362–7.

Matsuura, E., Igarashi, Y., Fujimoto, M., Ichikawa, K., and Koike, T. (1990). Anticardiolipin co-factor(s) and differential diagnosis of autoimmune disease. *Lancet*, **336**, 177–8.

Matsuura, E., Igarashi, Y., Yasuda, T., Triplett, D.A., and Koike, T. (1994). Anticardiolipin antibodies recognize β_2-glycoprotein I structure altered by interacting with an oxygen modified solid phase surface. *Journal of Experimental Medicine*, **179**, 457–62.

McHugh, N., Reilly, P.A., and McHugh, L.A. (1989). Pregnancy outcome and autoantibodies in connective tissue disease. *Journal of Rheumatology*, **16**, 42–6.

McNeil, H.P., Simpson, R.J., Chesterman, C.N., and Krilis, S. (1990). Antiphospholipid antibodies are directed against a complex antigen that includes a lipid-binding inhibitor of coagulation: β_2-glycoprotein I (apolipoprotein H). *Proceedings of the National Academy of Sciences (USA)*, **87**, 4120–4.

Montalban, J., Codina, A., Ordi, J., Vilardell, M., Khamashta, M.A., and Hughes, G.R.V. (1991). Antiphospholipid antibodies in cerebral ischemia. *Stroke*, **22**, 750–3.

Montalban, J. *et al.* (1992). Lack of association between anticardiolipin antibodies and migraine in systemic lupus erythematosus. *Neurology*, **42**, 681–2.

Mujic, F., Lloyd, M., Cuadrado, M.J., Khamashta, M.A., and Hughes, G.R.V. (1995*a*). Prevalence and clinical significance of subungual splinter haemorrhages in patients with the antiphospholipid syndrome. *Clinical and Experimental Rheumatology*, **13**, 327–31.

Mujic, F., Cuadrado, M.J., Lloyd, M., Khamashta, M.A., Page, G., and Hughes, G.R.V. (1995*b*). Primary antiphospholipid syndrome evolving into systemic lupus erythematosus. *Journal of Rheumatology*, **22**, 1589–92

Nencini, P., Baruffi, M.C., Abbati, R., Massai, G., Amaducci, L., and Inzitari, P. (1992). Lupus anticoagulant and anticardiolipin antibodies in young adults with cerebral ischemia. *Stroke*, **23**, 189–93.

Oosting, J.D., Derksen, R.H.W.M., Entjes, H.T.I., Bouma, B.N., and DeGroot, P.G. (1992). Lupus anticoagulan activity is frequently dependent on the presence of β_2-glycoprotein I. *Thrombosis and Haemostasis*, **67**, 499–502.

Out, H.J., DeGroot, P.G., Hasselaar, P., van Vliet, M., and Derksen, R.H.W.M. (1989). Fluctuations of anticardiolipin antibody levels in patients with systemic lupus erythematosus: a prospective study. *Annals of the Rheumatic Diseases*, **48**, 1023–8.

Out, H.J., Kooijman, C.D., Bruinse, H.W., and Derksen, R.H.W.M. (1991). Histopathological findings in placentae from patients with intra-uterine fetal death and antiphospholipid antibodies. *European Journal of Obstetrics and Gynaecology and Reproductive Biology*, **341**, 179–86.

Pelletier, S. *et al.* (1994). Antiphospholipid syndrome as the second cause of nontumorous Budd–Chiari syndrome. *Journal of Hepatology*, **21**, 76–80.

Permpikul, P., Mohan Rao, V., and Rapaport, S.I. (1994). Functional and binding studies of the roles of prothrombin and β_2-glycoprotein I in the expression of lupus anticoagulant activity. *Blood*, **83**, 2878–92.

Pierangeli, S.S. and Harris, E.N. (1994). Antiphospholipid antibodies in an *in vivo* thrombosis model in mice. *Lupus*, **3**, 247–51.

Piette, J.C., Cacoub, P., and Wechsler, B. (1994). Renal manifestations of the antiphospholipid syndrome. *Seminars in Arthritis and Rheumatism*, **23**, 357–66.

Rivier, G., Khamashta, M.A., and Hughes, G.R.V. (1993). Warfarin and azathioprine: a drug interaction does exist. *American Journal of Medicine*, **95**, 342.

Rosove, M.H. and Brewer, P.M.C. (1992). Antiphospholipid thrombosis: clinical course after the first thrombotic event in 70 patients. *Annals of Internal Medicine*, **117**, 303–8.

Roubey, R.A.S. (1994). Autoantibodies to phospholipid-binding plasma proteins: a new view of lupus anticoagulants and other 'antiphospholipid' antibodies. *Blood*, **84**, 2854–67.

Sandoval, J., *et al.* (1996). Primary antiphospholipid syndrome presenting as thromboembolic pulmonary hypertension. Treatment with thromboendartectomy. *Journal of Rheumatology*, **23**, 772–5.

Silver, R.K., MacGregor, S.N., Pasternak, J.F., and Neely, S.E. (1992). Fetal stroke asociated with elevated maternal anticardiolipin antibodies. *Obstetrics and Gynecology*, **80**, 497–9.

Singleton, J.D. and Conyers, L. (1992). Warfarin and azathioprine: an important drug interaction. *American Journal of Medicine*, **92**, 217.

Stewart, M.W. *et al.* (1993). Detection of antiphospholipid antibodies by flow cytometry: rapid detection of antibody isotype and phospholpid specificity. *Thrombosis and Haemostasis*, **70**, 603–7.

Stimmler, M.M., Coletti, P.M., and Quismorio, F.P. (1993). Magnetic resonance imaging of the brain in neuropsychiatric systemic lupus erythematosus. *Seminars in Arthritis and Rheumatism*, **22**, 335–49.

Triplett, D.A. (1994). Assays for detection of antiphospholipid antibodies. *Lupus*, **3**, 281–7.

Trudinger, B.J., Stewart, G.J., Cook, C.M., Connelly, A., and Exner, T. (1988). Monitoring lupus anticoagulant-positive pregnancies with umbilical artery flow velocity waveforms. *Obstetrics and Gynecology*, **72**, 215–8.

Tsakiris, D.A. *et al.* (1993). Lack of association between antiphospholipid antibodies and migraine. *Thombosis and Haemostasis*, **69**, 415–7.

Tucker, L.B. (1994). Antiphospholipid syndrome in childhood: the great unknown. *Lupus*, **3**, 367–9.

Vaarala, O. (1996). Antiphospholipid antibodies and atherosclerosis. *Lupus*, **5**, 442–7.

Vaarala, O., Alfthan, G., Jauhiainen, M., Leirisalo-Repo, M., Aho, K., and Palosuo, T. (1993). Cross-reaction between antibodies to oxidised low-density lipoprotein and to cardiolipin in systemic lupus erythematosus. *Lancet*, **341**, 923–5.

Vianna, J.L. *et al.* (1994). Comparison of the primary and secondary antiphospholipid syndrome: a European multicenter study of 114 patients. *American Journal of Medicine*, **96**, 3–9.

Viard, J.P., Amoura, Z., and Bach, J.P. (1992). Association of anti-β_2 glycoprotein I antibodies with lupus-type circulating anticoagulant and thrombosis in systemic lupus erythematosus. *American Journal of Medicine*, **93**, 181–6.

Wang, M.X. *et al.* (1995). Epitope specificity of monoclonal anti-β_2 glycoprotein I antibodies derived from patients with the antiphospholipid syndrome. *Journal of Immunology*, **155**, 1629–36.

Wilson, W.A., Perez, M.C., Michalski, J.P., and Armatis, P.E. (1988). Cardiolipin antibodies and null alleles of C4 in black Americans with systemic lupus erythematosus. *Journal of Rheumatology*, **15**, 1768–72.

Wilson, W.A. *et al.* (1995). Familial anticardiolipin antibodies and C4 deficiency genotypes that co-exist with MHC DQB1 risk factors. *Journal of Rheumatology*, **22**, 227–35.

Zahavi, J., Charach, G., Schafer, R., Toeg, A., and Zahavi, M. (1993). Ischaemic necrotic toes associated with antiphospholipid syndrome and treated with iloprost. *Lancet*, **342**, 862.

5.8 Scleroderma and related disorders in adults and children

Carol M. Black and Christopher P. Denton

'Scleroderma', a word meaning hard skin, is a part of many syndromes including localized, limited, and generalized scleroderma. Related to these are environmentally induced 'scleroderma-like' diseases, overlap syndromes, undifferentiated autoimmune rheumatic disease, and localized fibroses (Table 1). Most of these disorders in the scleroderma spectrum can occur at any stage of life, although the pattern of scleroderma occurring in childhood is different from that in the adult (see below). The disease we call scleroderma or systemic sclerosis has been confused with other diseases that have cutaneous features resembling it, for example scleromyxoedema, scleroedema, and primary amyloidosis (Table 2).

The milestones in the history of scleroderma (see Table 3) bear testimony to the gradual realization of the heterogeneity of the disorder. The last 50 years have seen an explosion of interest in the disease and its mechanisms, which has fostered collaboration between many branches of basic science and clinical medicine. For a more detailed discussion of the fascinating history of this disease the reader is referred to the excellent historical review by Rodnan, the 'father' of modern-day clinical scleroderma (Rodnan and Benedek 1962).

The group of syndromes called localized scleroderma includes morphoea (limited and guttate), linear scleroderma with the *en coup de sabre* variety, and generalized morphoea. These syndromes are almost never associated with systemic involvement but may demonstrate abnormal autoimmune serology and inflammatory histological changes in skin (Falanga 1989). These forms of scleroderma predominate in childhood.

Raynaud's phenomenon now best classified as either primary or secondary (the terms Raynaud's disease and Raynaud's syndrome should be abandoned and replaced by these more accurate, simple descriptive terms) and can be a forerunner one of the autoimmune rheumatic diseases such as generalized scleroderma (see below).

When generalized scleroderma is called systemic sclerosis the term is preferable to progressive systemic sclerosis because not all systemic sclerosis is progressive.

Systemic sclerosis is a multisystem disease, predominantly affecting females and of unknown cause. It is characterized pathologically by the overproduction of several elements of the connective tissue, notably collagen (Mauch *et al.* 1993), widespread vascular damage with the development of microvascular obliteration, and tissue infiltration of mononuclear inflammatory cells often in a perivascular distribution (Prescott *et al.* 1992). It embraces a clinical spectrum ranging from widespread skin thickening (diffuse scleroderma) to skin thickening either limited to the face and distal extremities (limited scleroderma) or absent (systemic sclerosis *sine* scleroderma).

There is no single diagnostic test for systemic sclerosis and, for the purposes of separating it from other autoimmune rheumatic diseases and identifying cases to permit comparison of reported series, preliminary criteria were developed and published in 1980 (Subcommittee for Scleroderma Criteria of the American Rheumatism Association Diagnostic and Therapeutic Criteria Committee 1980; Pope and Bellamy 1993). These criteria had a 97 per cent sensitivity and 98 per cent specificity for definite systemic sclerosis, but they are less sensitive for limited cutaneous disease, which is the largest subset, and they fail to identify at least 10 per cent of such patients. In the future, criteria taking full account of the limited-disease subset, and

Table 1 Spectrum of scleroderma and scleroderma-like syndromes	
Raynaud's phenomenon	Primary Raynaud's
	Secondary Raynaud's
Scleroderma — localized	Morphoea (plaque, guttate, generalized)
	Linear
	En coup de sabre
Scleroderma — systemic	Limited cutaneous systemic sclerosis
	Diffuse cutaneous systemic sclerosis
	Scleroderma *sine* scleroderma
Chemically induced[a]	Environmental/occupations
	Drugs
Scleroderma-like diseases	Metabolic
	Immunological/inflammatory
	Localized systemic sclerosis and visceral diseases

[a]See Table 8.

Table 2 Scleroderma-like syndromes

Metabolic/inherited	Scleroedema of Buschke ⎱ with or without paraproteinaemia
	Scleromyxoedema ⎰
	Insulin-dependent diabetes mellitus (digital sclerosis)
	Carcinoid syndrome
	Acromegaly
	Phenylketonuria
	Porphyrias (congenital and porphyria cutanea tarda)
	Lichen sclerosis et atrophicus
	Acrodermatitis chronica atrophicans
	Amyloidosis
	Inherited premature ageing syndromes — progeria, Rothmund's, Werner's
Immunological/inflammatory	Chronic graft-versus-host disease
	Eosinophilic fasciitis
	Overlap syndromes (systemic sclerosis with rheumatoid arthritis, systemic lupus, Sjögren's, polymyositis/dermatomyositis)
	Undifferentiated autoimmune rheumatic disease
Localized systemic sclerosis and visceral diseases	Idiopathic pulmonary fibrosis
	Amyloidosis
	Sarcoidosis
	Infiltrating carcinomas
	Infiltrating cardiomyopathy
	Oesophageal and intestinal hypomotility syndromes

also including clinical, pathological, and immunological data (such as recent-onset Raynaud's phenomenon, capillary abnormalities, and circulating antibodies) should be developed. There is a readily identifiable group of presclerotic patients who should be included in diagnostic criteria, classification, and subsetting.

Classification of systemic sclerosis is difficult (Masi 1988), and a number of different systems have been proposed (LeRoy *et al.* 1988). Central to all of them is the extent of skin involvement, and whether a two-subset or three-subset model is superior is still debated. Currently the most widely used classification defines two subsets, based on the extent of skin involvement together with a number of reliable clinical laboratory and natural history associations. The two-subset model divides the disease into limited cutaneous systemic sclerosis and diffuse cutaneous systemic sclerosis (Table 4) (LeRoy *et al.* 1988). Over 60 per cent of patients with systemic sclerosis fall into the limited cutaneous subset, where visceral involvement is a late event and tends to occur 10 to 30 years after the onset of Raynaud's. The term limited cutaneous systemic sclerosis is preferable to CREST (**C**alcinosis, **R**aynaud's, (O)**E**sophageal dysphagia, **S**clerodactyly, **T**elangiectasia syndrome), because cutaneous manifestations often extend beyond sclerodactyly and calcinosis may be present only late or radiologically. Diffuse cutaneous systemic sclerosis, the more serious form of the disease, is much more rapid in onset, with organ failure often present within 5 years of the first symptoms.

This model will almost certainly be changed and developed as knowledge of the pathogenesis of the disorder advances, and the ever-increasing numbers of autoantibodies are matched to clinical subsets. Within each subset, there is great variability in the pace of the disease: for example, some patients with diffuse cutaneous systemic sclerosis develop extensive internal-organ complications within 2 to 4 years; others have widespread skin disease but only grumbling interstitial lung disease. Some patients with limited cutaneous systemic sclerosis may never develop clinically apparent pulmonary hypertension or mid-gut disease whereas other individuals develop this complication, usually late on, but occasionally as early as 5 to 7 years after diagnosis. Thus, not only is there disease heterogeneity, but differential progression within a subset. Notwithstanding these problems a useful and practical scheme is to divide the disease into early and late stages (see Table 5). This is a useful concept because it permits the doctor, patient, and patient's family to anticipate certain developments, which will concentrate attention on early detection and correct management of complications.

Epidemiological considerations

Scleroderma is an uncommon disorder and virtually all of the descriptive epidemiology is derived from retrospective or prospective reviews of patients attending hospitals or institutions serving a

Table 3 History of scleroderma

1753	Curzio	Description of young woman of Naples with 'excessive hardness of skin'—possibly scleroderma, but probably scleroedema of Buschke
1847	Gintrac	First use of name 'Sclerodermie'
1847	Forget	First description of joint involvement in scleroderma
1854	Addison	First description of linear scleroderma
1862	Raynaud	Description of 'local asphyxia and symmetrical gangrene of the extremities'
1878	Weber	Coexistence of scleroderma and calcinosis noted
1892	Osler	Tendency for scleroderma patients to die of pulmonary or renal disease noted
1893	Hutchinson	Association of scleroderma and Raynaud's phenomenon noted
1903	Ehrmann	Association of scleroderma and dysphagia recorded
1910	Thibierge and Weissenbach	'Rediscovery' of coexistence of scleroderma and calcinosis
1924	Matsui	First clear description of visceral involvement, with sclerosis of lungs, gastrointestinal tract and kidneys
1943	Weiss	Clear description of myocardial involvement in scleroderma
1945	Goetz	Coined the term 'progressive systemic sclerosis'
1964	Winterbauer	Described the CREST subset (calcinosis, Raynaud's, oesophagitis, sclerodactyly, and telangiectasia)

defined denominator population: there is only one true population-based study (Maricq *et al.* 1989). A summary of salient epidemiological data is given in Table 6 (Silman 1995). The demographic conclusions that may be drawn from these data are that the disease is rare in childhood, and that its incidence increases steadily with age amongst adults. Its rarity suggests that the genetic and/or environmental exposures necessary for disease susceptibility occur infrequently in the population. Scleroderma is a disorder with a female excess (4F:1M overall, and in the child-bearing years 15F:1M). The disease occurs most frequently and severely in young black women, but overall there are no prominent racial, seasonal, or socioeconomic differences. Of great interest is the possibility that the disease clusters in certain areas. A clustering has been described close to international airports in the United Kingdom (Silman 1995), a cluster of patients with a variety of autoimmune rheumatic diseases is reported from The Republic of Georgia (Freni-Titulaer *et al.* 1989), and a clearer cluster of systemic sclerosis in a region of Italy close to Rome (Valesini *et al.* 1993). Unlike some other autoimmune rheumatic diseases, the genetic contribution to the disease would appear to be relatively weak, although it is stronger for individual organ involvement (e.g. the lung). Finally, again in contrast to other autoimmune rheumatic diseases, a growing number of environmental agents have been implicated in systemic sclerosis (see Table 7).

Aetiology and pathogenesis

Although the basic aetiology of systemic sclerosis is unknown, it is almost certainly multifactorial with genetic and environmental factors playing a part (Briggs *et al.* 1990). As mentioned earlier,

systemic sclerosis occurs mostly in females and sex may be the strongest genetic marker. There are, however, several lines of evidence that indicate familial or genetic predisposition to systemic sclerosis. First, although rare, there are familial clusters of systemic sclerosis and related diseases, particularly Raynaud's phenomenon. Autoantibodies associated with systemic sclerosis are found in high frequency in blood relatives of patients with systemic sclerosis, although the incidence of antinuclear antibodies in spouses suggests an environmental component. Thirty-six per cent of relatives with antinuclear antibodies had clinical features of autoimmune rheumatic disease not observed in spouses (Briggs *et al.* 1993). The presence of autoantibodies in the blood of patients' spouses in the United Kingdom study was not confirmed in an Australian study. Thirdly, many centres worldwide have observed abnormal frequencies of the major histocompatibility complex (MHC) antigens associated with systemic sclerosis. The association is complex (see Table 8) and the strongest link is between HLA-DRw52a and patients with systemic sclerosis who have lung fibrosis (relative risk 16.7).

As one of the primary roles of MHC class II molecules is the presentation of processed antigen to the T-cell receptor on helper T lymphocytes resulting in an antigen-specific immune response, autoantibody subsets in scleroderma might be expected to show correlations with class II MHC polymorphism and indeed they do, although again, they appear to be complex. In the initial reports, anticentromere antibody was found to be associated with HLA-DR5 (-DR11), -DR4 (-D13 subtypes), -DR1, and -DR8. These findings appear to reflect linkage disequilibrium of *HLA-DR5* (*-DR11*) and many *HLA-DR4* (*-D13* subtypes) with *HLA-DQ7*, and *-DR1* with *-DQ5*. These HLA-DR specificities share no unique amino-acid

Table 4 Classification of the subsets of systemic sclerosis (SSc)

1. *'Pre-scleroderma'*

   Raynaud's phenomenon plus nailfold capillary changes, disease-specific circulating antinuclear autoantibodies, (antitopoisomerase-I, anticentromere (ACA), or nucleolar), and digital ischaemic changes

2. *Diffuse cutaneous SSc (dcSSc)*

   Onset of skin changes (puffy or hidebound) within 1 year of onset of Raynaud's

   Truncal and acral skin involvement

   Presence of tendon friction rubs

   Early and significant incidence of interstitial lung disease, oliguric renal failure, diffuse gastrointestinal disease, and myocardial involvement

   Nailfold capillary dilatation and drop out

   Antitopoisomerase-I (Scl-70) antibodies (30% of patients)

3. *Limited cutaneous SSc (lcSSc)*

   Raynaud's for years (occasionally decades)

   Skin involvement limited to hands, face, feet, and forearms (acral)

   A significant (10–15%) late incidence of pulmonary hypertension, with or without interstitial lung disease, skin calcification, telangiectasiae and gastrointestinal involvement

   A high incidence of ACA (70–80%)

   Dilated nailfold capillary loops, usually without capillary drop out

4. *Scleroderma* sine *scleroderma*

   Raynaud's +/−

   No skin involvement

   Presentation with pulmonary fibrosis, scleroderma renal crisis, cardiac or gastrointestinal disease

   Antinuclear antibodies may be present (Scl70, ACA, nucleolar)

sequences, which raised the possibility that another linked gene might be more highly correlated with this antibody response. More recently, in a study by Reveille *et al.* (1992*a*), oligotyping showed that the anticentromere antibody response was most closely associated with *HLA-DQB1* alleles in linkage disequilibrium with *HLA-DR1*, -DR4, -DR5 (DR11), and -DR8. These *HLA-DQB1* alleles had in common a polar tyrosine or a glycine at position 26 of the outermost domain of the HLA-DQB molecule, as opposed to a hydrophobic leucine residue. In a British study (Briggs *et al.* 1993) implication of the *HLA-DQB1* locus was inferred, as virtually all of the anticentromere antibody-positive patients had either HLA-DR1 or -DR4. However, McHugh *et al.* (1994) have indicated that, although at least one *HLA-DQB1* allele not coding at position 26 of the first domain appears necessary, it may not be sufficient for the generation of

anticentromere antibody. Reveille and colleagues have also extended the known associations of antitopoisomerase antibodies with HLA-DR5, -DR2, and -DR52a to include four *HLA-DQB1* alleles (Reveille *et al.*1993*b*). Japanese workers have found a similar allele association (Kuwana *et al.* 1993). Localization of 'susceptible epitopes', however, has been less definitive. Suggestions include an American population in which a tyrosine at position 30 or the TRAELDT sequence spanning positions 71 to 77 of the *HLA-DQB1* outermost domain is seen (Reveille *et al.* 1992), and a Japanese population with systemic sclerosis in which a tyrosine at position 26 of the *HLA-DQB1* outermost domain is present (Kuwana *et al.* 1993). In a British study an HLA-DPB1 association was suggested, with the presence of an acidic amino-acid residue at position 69 in the third hypervariable region of the outermost domain. Autoantibodies to the anti-Pm/Scl antigen (see below) are nearly 100 per cent correlated with the presence of the *HLA DR3-DQw2* haplotype (Reveille *et al.* 1992).

Important racial and ethnic differences in the frequencies of these autoantibodies have been described, with Western Europeans and North American whites having a significantly higher frequency of anticentromere autoantibodies and a lower frequency of antitopoisomerase-1 than American blacks, Choctaw native Americans, Thai, and Italians (Kallenberg 1994). Particular forms of the disease may not be so strongly influenced by sex. For example, certain chemically induced systemic sclerosis-like disorders tend to be associated with males, partly due to an occupational bias. The range of known agents that can induce a systemic sclerosis-like disease is large and growing (Table 7), although it must be noted that in formal epidemiological studies, no excess was found. It is almost certain that sporadic cases can follow certain occupational exposures, but that both the absolute and attributable risks are low. There are some MHC associations with the environmentally induced cases, for example toxic oil syndrome is characterized by a raised incidence of HLA-DR4, while vinyl chloride disease is primarily associated with HLA-DR5, HLA-DR3 being a marker of severity. There is (see Table 8) inconsistency in the frequencies for genetic markers of susceptibility between patients from different study centres. This may reflect at least in part different agents present at these various geographical locations. The newest arrivals to the group of environmentally induced, systemic sclerosis-like syndromes are the eosinophilic–myalgic syndrome associated with the oral ingestion of the essential amino acid l-tryptophan (discussed elsewhere) and a renewed interest in the possible association between disease development and silicone breast implants. Much of the work in this area has been generated by the need to obtain accurate data because of considerable litigation, particularly in the United States. Hochberg (1994) has carefully reviewed the epidemiological aspects of the literature and has reasonably concluded that none of the available studies has demonstrated a statistical association between augmentation mammoplasty with silicone gel-filled prostheses and scleroderma or other autoimmune rheumatic disorders.

Autoimmune considerations

An increasing number of immune abnormalities are being reported in systemic sclerosis and the designation of systemic sclerosis as an autoimmune disease now has widespread support. Some of the clinical features of scleroderma bear similarities to other autoimmune disorders such as systemic lupus erythematosus, dermatomyositis,

Table 5 Characteristic findings in the early and late stages of systemic sclerosis subsets

Diffuse cutaneous	Early (<3 years after onset)	Late (>3 years after onset)
Constitutional	Fatigue and weight loss	Minimal, weight gain typical
Vascular	Raynaud's often relatively mild	Raynaud's more severe, more telangiectasia
Cutaneous	Rapid progression involving arms, trunk, face	Stable or regression
Musculoskeletal	Prominent arthralgia, stiffness, myalgia, muscle weakness, tendon friction rubs	Flexion contractures and deformities, joint/muscle symptoms less prominent
Gastrointestinal	Dysphagia, heartburn	More pronounced symptoms, midgut and anorectal complications more common
Cardiorespiratory	Maximum risk for myocarditis, pericardial effusion, interstitial pulmonary fibrosis	Reduced risk of new involvement but progression of existing established visceral fibrosis
Renal	Maximum risk period for scleroderma renal crisis	Renal crisis less frequent, uncommon after 5 years

Limited cutaneous	Early (<10 years after onset)	Late (>10 years after onset)
Constitutional	None	Only secondary to visceral complications
Vascular	Raynaud's typically severe and long-standing Telangiectasia	Raynaud's persists, often causing digital ulceration or gangrene
Cutaneous	Mild sclerosis with little progression; trunk, face	Stable, calcinosis more prominent
Musculoskeletal	Occasional joint stiffness	Mild flexion contractures
Gastrointestinal	Dysphagia, heartburn	More pronounced symptoms, midgut and anorectal complications more common
Cardiorespiratory	Usually no involvement	Lung fibrosis may develop but progresses slowly
		Maximum risk for developing isolated pulmonary hypertension and secondary right ventricular failure
Renal	No involvement	Rarely involved

and rheumatoid arthritis, and there are also patients who have overlap syndromes or who have sequential development of more than one autoimmune rheumatic disease. Cases of familial systemic sclerosis and familial associations of systemic sclerosis with other autoimmune diseases such as rheumatoid arthritis and systemic lupus erythematosus occur and have already been mentioned.

There is considerable evidence that abnormalities in both humoral and cell-mediated immunity occur in systemic sclerosis, although the precise importance of these immunological events in the pathogenesis remains uncertain. Some of this evidence is summarized in Table 9, and discussed below. The lack of a generalized immune dysfunction in systemic sclerosis suggests that the derangement of immune-cell dysfunction may be *specific* to certain antigens or cell types (Padula *et al.* 1986; Lupoli *et al.* 1990).

The association of systemic sclerosis with particular major HLA antigens and the close association of certain HLA alleles with scleroderma-specific antibodies (see Table 8) is indirect evidence for T-cell involvement in systemic sclerosis. There is considerable evidence for

T-cell activation in systemic sclerosis, including an increased ratio of circulating CD4+:CD8+ cells (Degiannis *et al.* 1990; White 1994), reflecting an increased number of CD4+ and/or a reduced number of CD8+ lymphocytes. A particular role for γ T-cells has been suggested (White 1994) and others have reported increased numbers of lymphokine-activated killer and natural killer cells (Kantor *et al.* 1992) in blood samples from patients with systemic sclerosis. Furthermore, several studies have found increased soluble interleukin-2 receptor in scleroderma, sometimes appearing to correlate with disease activity (Kahaleh 1991). Support for the possibility that activated T-cells are important in pathogenesis is provided by the presence of infiltrates of CD3+, CD4+, CD450+, interleukin 2-producing, HLA-DR-positive+, leucocyte function-associated antigen-1-positive, a/β+ T cells in lesional tissues (Prescott *et al.* 1992). Also, chronic graft-versus-host disease in humans shows several histological and clinical similarities with systemic sclerosis, and is known to be a T-cell-mediated process (Chosidow *et al.* 1992). Humoral abnormalities in systemic sclerosis are most clearly reflected

Table 6 Epidemiological facts in systemic sclerosis

Mortality	USA 1969–77	1.5 males and 3.5 females per million population
	UK 1974–85	1.0 males and 4.0 females per million population
Incidence (new cases detected/ population at risk/time period)	Rates variable Before 1980 report	2–10 per million population per year
	Pittsburgh study (1963–82)	19.1 per million population per year
	UK 1980–85	3.7 per million population per year
Prevalence (number of cases living at particular time or during time interval)	Estimates: 1947–52	4 per million (hospital studies)
	1977–79	126 per million (hospital studies)
	1985	253 per million (community studies)
	1986	290 per million (point prevalence)
	1986	30.8 per million (hospital and community)
	1988	19 per million (hospital study)
Survival		
Cumulative survival rates using life-table methods	Overall	60–70% @ 5 years 40–50% @ 10 years
	By subset: localized cutaneous	80% @ 6 years 50% @ 12 years
	diffuse cutaneous	30% @ 6 years 15% @ 12 years
	Older patients reduced survival	
Factors associated with decreased survival — increasing skin involvement, organ involvement etc.		

by the presence of autoantibodies with well-defined target epitopes; mapping of the precise binding sites for some of these is currently being undertaken in several centres (Bona and Rothfield 1994). Although circulating immune complexes have been reported in systemic sclerosis, most studies have not found functional complement abnormalities (Seibold *et al.* 1982), probably because most systemic sclerosis-associated autoantibodies do not activate the complement cascade (White 1994).

Nevertheless, autoantibody production is an early and almost universal feature of systemic sclerosis. The number of autoantibody targets identified in systemic sclerosis continues to grow (see Table 10) but the major ones are topoisomerase-1, centromeric proteins, and RNA polymerases I, II, and III. About 97 per cent of patients have detectable antinuclear antibodies when HEp-2 lines are used as the detection tissue. Characteristic staining patterns for antinuclear antibodies within the nuclear and subnuclear structures are relatively specific (Tan 1989) and can be confirmed by more sophisticated tests. A diffusely grainy pattern of staining is associated with the presence of antibodies to topoisomerase-1 (Scl-70), a nuclear enzyme important in the unwinding of DNA for replication and RNA transcription. Antibodies to Scl-70 occur in up to 40 per cent of patients with diffuse systemic sclerosis and 15 per cent of those with limited disease. The occurrence of this antibody varies considerably between laboratories and studies have shown that the immunoblot technique is more sensitive than indirect immunofluorescence and should be the 'gold standard' for this test. An anticentromere staining pattern occurs in up to 80 per cent of patients with the limited form of systemic sclerosis. Antigens recognized by positive sera have been

identified as CENP-A, CENP-B, and CENP-C, with molecular weights of 19, 80, and 140 kDa, respectively (Earnshaw *et al.* 1986). A correlation has been shown (Jabs *et al.* 1993) between anticentromere antibodies and aneuploidy in patients with systemic sclerosis, and it is possible that anticentromere antibodies could disrupt centromere function and allow chromosomes to segregate inappropriately during mitosis, leading to a high rate of chromosomal breakage and sister chromatid exchange, although to date no correlation has been found between the presence of anticentromere antibody and chromosomal changes. Anti-RNA polymerase (**RNAP**) antibodies are the latest systemic sclerosis-specific antibodies to be described. They occur mainly in patients with diffuse disease, and antibodies against RNAPI, -II, and -III have been described (Bona and Rothfield 1994). The RNAPs are multiprotein complexes and are components of the transcription complex (Reeves *et al.* 1994). Each RNAP is composed of collections of smaller proteins shared by other RNAPs and two large distinct proteins. RNAPI synthesizes ribosomal RNA precursors in the nucleoli, whereas RNAPs II and III are found in the nuclei. RNAPII synthesises most of the small nuclear RNAs found in ribonucleoprotein particles that mediate pre-mRNA splicing and synthesize precursors of mRNA, and RNAPIII synthesizes small RNAs including single-strand ribosomal RNA and transfer RNA. Anti-RNAP antibodies target both the smaller shared subunits and the larger distinct proteins, which explains antibody reactivity against several RNAPs in one serum sample.

The relation between HLA status and autoantibody production is also of increasing interest in scleroderma. It would appear that certain

Table 7 Environmental agents implicated in the development of scleroderma

Silica

Stone masons

Coal miners

Gold miners

Foundry workers

Organic chemicals

Aliphatic hydrocarbons

Chlorinated:
vinyl chloride
trichlorethylene
perchlorethylene

Non-chlorinated:
naphtha-n-hexane

Aromatic hydrocarbons

Benzene

Toluene

Xylene

Mixtures, e.g. diesel fuel, white spirit

Epoxy resins

Foam insulin (urea-formaldehyde)

Metaphenylene diamine (biogenic amine)

Toxic oil (aniline-treated rapeseed oil)

Augmentation mammoplasty (silicone, paraffin)

Drugs

L-5-Hydroxytryptophan

Pentazocine

Carbidopa

Appetite suppressans

Diethylpropion hydrochloride

Mazindol

Fenfluramine

Bleomycin

Cocaine

Amide-type local anaesthetics

the various autoantibodies (see Table 8). These antibodies not only mark out certain subsets of patients with systemic sclerosis but are of increasing importance in defining a subgroup of Raynaud's patients likely to develop scleroderma.

The antinuclear antibody profile is not as clear-cut in juveniles as in the adult form, although some trends are emerging. Serum antinuclear antibodies have been reported in 25 to 55 per cent of juveniles with localized scleroderma, the association being most marked in the linear group and in patients with extensive cutaneous lesions. Antibodies to single-stranded DNA also appear to be correlated with the extent of localized disease, whereas antibodies to double-stranded DNA are rarely found. It is interesting that in the generalized form of childhood scleroderma no anticentromere antibodies have been reported, even in those children with disease identical to that found in the adult.

A pathogenetic role for autoantibodies in systemic sclerosis has long been sought. Defined epitopes seem to be targets for the autoantibodies and there has been recent work showing homology between target autoantigens in systemic sclerosis and retroviral proteins, suggesting molecular mimicry, which may have significance in disease pathogenesis. There are reports that some of these antibodies are also able to enter intracellular compartments (Levine *et al.* 1991; Ma *et al.* 1991) and thereby to mediate intracellular events, such as the reported ability of anticentromeric antibodies to disrupt the centromere. In addition, autoantibodies might be able to activate cells that bear the target autoantigens; for example, patients with systemic sclerosis produce antibodies that bind *Fc*γRI (CD64), II (CD32), and III (CD16) (Boros *et al.* 1993). It has been suggested that some of the autoantibodies in serum from systemic sclerosis may mediate antibody-dependent cytotoxicity, and potential effector cells have been found in the skin of some patients (White 1994). Another speculation is that these antibodies might contribute to the pathology if they mediated complement-dependent cellular lysis or phagocytosis. However, these ideas must be kept in perspective balanced against the lack of correlation of antibody titre with disease duration or activity. Circulating antibodies to the extracellular matrix proteins, collagens I, III, IV and VI, and laminin have also been found in systemic sclerosis, but their role is undetermined (Mackel *et al.* 1982).

Macrophages, mast cells, eosinophils, and basophils are found in increased numbers and in an activated state in tissues of patients with systemic sclerosis. These cells are capable of producing soluble mediators and can thereby modify endothelial and fibroblast function; for example, mast cells produce histamine, which stimulates both proliferation and matrix synthesis by fibroblasts and causes retraction of endothelial cells.

The initiating stimulus in idiopathic scleroderma is unknown, although the identification of chemical precipitants for environmentally induced systemic sclerosis as discussed above (e.g. vinyl chloride and epoxy resin) may provide some clues to the processes involved, particularly in view of the similar immunogenetic associations for both idiopathic and chemically induced disease (Black *et al.* 1983).

The most obvious major targets for the immune response in systemic sclerosis are endothelial cells and the fibroblasts. Stimulation of collagen synthesis could involve an increasing number of cytokines known to modulate the properties of fibroblasts. It is possible that cascades of such cytokines or autocrine/paracrine loops stimulate or maintain the disease process. It is now appreciated that the repertoire of mediators and cytokines produced by immune

of these antibodies are closely related to particular HLA alleles, for example it has recently been shown that class II MHC haplotype is an important factor determining *in vitro* responsiveness to topoisomerase antigen, both in patients with systemic sclerosis and in healthy control individuals (Kuwana *et al.* 1995). It is important to consider that there may be racial differences in HLA associations for

Table 8 Immunogenetic associations of scleroderma

Allele	First author	Year	Size of population	Geo[a]	Disease association	Autoantibody association
DR1	Lynch	1982	237	USA	dcSSc	
	Whiteside	1983	125	USA	Weak dcSSc	ACA
	Alarcon	1985	44	USA	SSc	
	Livingstone	1987	35	USA	Weak dcSSc	
	Steen	1988	191	USA	lcSSc	ACA
	Black	1984	54	Eur	lcSSc	ACA
	Luderschmidt	1987	136	Eur	CREST	ACA
	Genth	1990	118	Eur	SSc	ACA
DR1 & 4	Briggs	1993	115	Eur	SSc	ACA
DR2	Kondo	1985		Jap	Ssc	—
DRw6	Sasaki	1991	Families	Jap	Ssc familial	ACA
DR3	Germain	1981	14	USA	CREST	
	Livingstone	1987	35	USA	lcSSC	
	Kallenberg	1981	28	Eur	SSc	
	Ercilla	1981	21	Eur	Ssc	
	Black	1983	21	Eur	Severe VCD	
	Black	1984	54	Eur	Weak dcSSc	
	Myers	1989	21	Eur	IPF	
	Luderschmidt	1987	136	Eur	Male SSc	
DRw52a	Briggs	1992	75	Eur	IPF	
	Langevitz	1992	126	Can	PHT	
DR5	Gladman	1981	34	Can	Severe SSc	
	Alarcon	1985	44	USA	SSc	
	Livingstone	1987	35	USA	Weak SSc	
	Steen	1988	206	USA	dcSSc	SCl-70
	Harvey	1983	44	Eur	VCD	
	Black	1984	54	Eur	lcSSc	ACA
	Luderschmidt	1987	136	Eur	SSc	ACA & Scl-70
	Genth	1990	118	Eur	SSc	ACA
	Barnett	1989	46	Aus	dcSSc	
DR11	Dunckley	1989	41	Aus	SSc	
DRw15	Jazwinska	1990	18	Jap	SSc	
DQA2	Briggs	1993	115	UK	SSc	
DQ57	Reveille	1992a	116	USA	SSc	ACA
DQB1, DQw3	Reveille	1992b	161	USA	SSc	Scl-70
DQB1	Kuwana	1993	62	Jap	SSc	Scl-70
DPB1	Briggs	1993	115	UK	SSc	SCl-70

[a]Geo, geographic location of study: Aus, Australia; Can, Canada; Eur, Europe; Jap, Japan.
Other abbreviations: ACA, anticentromere antibody; dc-, lcSSc, diffuse cutaneous, localized cutaneous systemic sclerosis; IPF, interstitial pulmonary fibrosis; PHT, pulmonary hypertension; VCD, vinyl chloride disease (remainder as in text).

Table 9 Summary of evidence for immune-system involvement in systemic sclerosis

Immunogenetic associations (see Table 8)

Autoantibody associations (see Table 10)

Increased circulating levels of soluble CD4, soluble IL2 receptor and lymphocyte-derived cytokines (IL2, IL4, IL6, IL8) in *some* patients

Circulating T cells that are reactive to laminin, collagen (type I), and show increased adhesion to endothelial cells and fibroblasts

Elevated levels of IL5 and IL8 in bronchoalveolar lavage fluid

Perivascular T-cell infiltrates (DR+, 1, 2 integrin expression) in lesional skin

Increased tissue expression of lymphocyte-binding cell-surface adhesion molecules in lesional and prelesional skin and lung tissue

Clinical and pathological similarities with chronic graft-versus-host disease

IL, interleukin.

cells, fibroblasts, and endothelial cells is large. It is possible that the aberrant properties of connective tissue cells (e.g. excess synthesis of collagen, fibronectin, and glycosaminoglycans) and the endothelial-cell damage and vasculopathy, are consequences of the immunological events in systemic sclerosis.

To date, the only well-established animal model of an immune, scleroderma-like disorder is that of the chronic graft-versus-host disease in mice (Bocchieri and Jimenez 1990). There is also a human counterpart following bone marrow transplantation in which patients develop Raynaud's, dermal sclerosis, and vasculopathy (Roumm *et al.* 1984; Chosidow *et al.* 1992). Although these models are interesting, they should be viewed with caution. Graft-versus-host disease is certainly induced by T cells but the final lesion is damage to endothelium, epithelium, or both, related to the actions of natural killer cells, lymphokines (e.g. interleukin 1) and tumour necrosis factor. This damage can occur in many organs, for example lung, gut and skin, and can therefore mimic the end-point of many damaging processes. Such mimicry may be totally irrelevant to the initiating process or even the damaging events.

Pathogenesis

Although the pathogenesis of systemic sclerosis is still uncertain, it is likely that the development of both the *fibrous* and the *vascular* lesion is complicated and involves events that may occur simultaneously or in sequence (Fig. 1).

Fibrosis is a hallmark of a number of diseases that includes scleroderma, pulmonary fibrosis, atherosclerosis, liver cirrhosis, and keloids. It is important to remember that the formation of fibrous tissue can be a normal physiological response, for example in wound healing. However, in fibrotic disorders the regulation of this normal response is altered, and in systemic sclerosis it is a widespread, non-organ-specific phenomenon. Excess deposition of collagen and extracellular matrix protein in the skin and internal organs of patients with

Table 10 Autoantibodies in scleroderma

Antigen	Molecular identity	Immunofluorescence pattern	Disease subtype and frequency
Scl 70 (topoisomerase I)	100-kDa protein degrades to 70 kDa	Nuclear (diffuse fine speckles)	Up to 40% with diffuse cutaneous SSc[a] 10–15% limited
Kinetochore centromere	17-, 80-, 140-kDa proteins at inner and outer kinetochore plates	Centromere	70–80% in limited cutaneous SSc 9–29% with primary biliary cirrhosis
RNA polymerase I, II, III	Complex of 13 proteins 12.5–210 kDa	Nucleolar (punctate)	23%—especially diffuse; high prevalence of internal organ involvement
Fibrillarin	34-kDa protein—component of U3RNP[c]	Nucleolar (clumpy)	6% (immunofluorescence) 60% by fibrillarin fusion protein assay Clinical association uncertain ? less articular disease
PM-Scl	Complex of 11 proteins 20–110 kDa	Nucleolar (homogeneous)	3%—high prevalence of myositis; more renal involvement
To or Th	40-kDa protein associated with 7-2 & 8-2-kDa RNAs	Nucleolar (homogeneous)	Rare—localized cutaneous SSc
Mitochondrial M2	70-kDa protein—dihydrolipo-amide acyltransferase	Cytoplasmic (rod like)	25% of CREST[b] (95% primary biliary cirrhosis)

[a]SSc, systemic sclerosis; [b]CREST, see Table 3; [c]RNP, ribonucleoprotein.

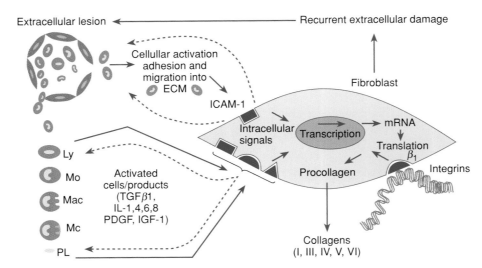

Fig. 1 Hypothesis for pathogenesis of the scleroderma lesion. Complex interactions between cells of the immune system, vasculature, and connective tissue matrix lead to the development of an activated fibrogenic fibroblast phenotype.

systemic sclerosis was first demonstrated histopathologically many years ago, and this was confirmed by physical and biochemical means. Subsequently, techniques for culturing fibroblasts have provided valuable insight into the mechanisms involved in the synthesis of extracellular matrix components. Skin fibroblasts from scleroderma, or at least a subset of them, synthesize increased quantities of fibronectin, proteoglycan core proteins, and particularly collagens types I and III and to a lesser degree IV and VI.

Fibroblasts grown from areas of dermal sclerosis continue to synthesize increased amounts of collagen for several passages *in vitro* (LeRoy 1974; Uitto *et al.* 1979). It has also been demonstrated that the amounts of mRNA for these matrix proteins are increased and have been localized predominantly to areas surrounding dermal blood vessels. Nucleic-acid hybridization techniques have since confirmed that not all fibroblasts are activated to produce more normal collagen but rather a group of high-collagen producers is responsible. The increase in collagen RNA could arise through increased an transcription rate or by a reduction in the breakdown of the mRNA, and there is evidence that both mechanisms may operate. The transcriptional rate of genes encoding pro-α2(I) collagen (*COL1A2*) is increased in fibroblasts from systemic sclerosis, suggesting a change in regulatory transcription factors in these cells.

The mechanism for transcriptional regulation of collagen synthesis is still unproven but De Crombrugghe *et al.* (1990) have demonstrated a pathway that could have a direct bearing on the transcriptional defect in scleroderma. Following stimulation by transforming growth factor-β, fibroblasts containing the promoter–enhancer regions of the α2(I) collagen gene linked to a chloramphenicol acetyl transferase reporter show a marked enhancement of collagen gene expression. This appears to be through the interaction of a transacting DNA-binding protein, nuclear factor 1, and the specific promoter of the collagen gene. Such elegant experiments provide a prototype for the study of the activation of a pleomorphic genetic response such as fibrosis, which is not, of course, restricted to systemic sclerosis. Neither is the cytokine stimulus likely to be transforming growth factor-β alone. The activation and perpetuation of systemic sclerosis is a complex affair and other mediators such as platelet-derived growth factor, interleukins 1 and 4, and fibroblast growth factors may

be involved. The cytokines possibly act in a cascade, and the timing and site of a biopsy might be critical for its correct interpretation.

One aspect of control that seems to be normal in fibroblasts from systemic sclerosis is that provided by negative feedback from propeptides. In addition, it should be noted that fibroblasts in scleroderma have changes in their proliferative properties. Scleroderma fibroblasts, unlike those from normal skin, display persistent proliferation in serum-free medium, but they are not transformed or immortalized cells, and they have similar doubling times, life-span and monolayer culture patterns to those of normal fibroblasts. What is, however, without doubt is that they are dysregulated with respect to the synthesis of extracellular matrix; whether this abnormality is wholly acquired or whether it is partially inherited and then activated by an inciting event is unknown.

Vascular lesions

Vascular injury is critical to the pathogenesis of systemic sclerosis and may be the primary event (Campbell and LeRoy 1975). The damage in systemic sclerosis is widespread and can be recognized as:

1. Vasomotor instability or Raynaud's phenomenon with repeated 'transient' interruption of tissue perfusion in the digits and internal organs (systemic Raynaud's), which is often an early event in disease development.

2. Microvascular abnormalities with structural changes characterized by proliferative intimal arterial lesions and obliteration of the vessels, leading to chronic ischaemia. Vascular damage can be visualized in the nailfold capillaries but it is also present in the small blood vessels of virtually all the viscera, muscle, subcutaneous tissues, and skin.

3. Intravascular pathology that is manifest by decreased red-cell deformability, increased platelet activity, and enhanced thrombus formation.

Many factors may be important in the vascular damage but it is the endothelial cell that is thought to have a pivotal role. The endothelium is now known to produce numerous molecules (see Table 11) and to

Table 11 Molecules synthesized by the vascular endothelium

1. *Growth factors and cytokines*

   Platelet-derived growth factors (PDGF)

   Transforming growth factor-β (TGF-β)

   Insulin-like growth factor (s)

   Basic fibroblast growth factor

   Interleukin 1α and β

   Interleukin 6

   Colony-stimulating factor(s)

   Platelet-activating factor

2. *Extracellular matrix and adhesion proteins*

   Collagens: types III, IV and V

   Sulphated proteoglycans

   Fibronectin

   Thrombospondin

   von Willebrand factor

   E-selectin

   Intercellular adhesion molecule 1 (ICAM-1)

   Vascular cell adhesion molecule 1 (VCAM-1)

3. *Anticoagulation factors*

   Antithrombin III

   Thrombomodulin

   Protein S

4. *Vasoactive proteins*

   Nitric oxide (endothelial-dependent relaxation factor)

   Endothelin (endothelial-dependent vasoconstriction factor)

   Prostacyclin (prostaglandin PGI$_2$)

   Prostaglandin E$_2$

regulate many aspects of vascular stability including control of vascular tone, permeability, thrombotic potential, and leucocyte trafficking (Pearson 1990; Kahaleh and Mattuci-Cerinic 1995).

Evidence for endothelial-cell dysfunction

The considerable evidence for endothelial-cell dysfunction in scleroderma is summarized below:

(1) direct observation of abnormal nailfold capillaries;

(2) increased capillary permeability to tracer molecules, with a slowing of flow and increased periods of stasis;

(3) changes in circulating levels of endothelial-cell products such as von Willebrand factor, endothelin 1, plasminogen activator, angiotensin-converting enzyme, and prostacyclin/thromboxane metabolites;

(4) the presence of a circulating cytotoxic factor identified as granzyme 1, a serine protease present in granules of activated T cells;

(5) the presence of autoantibodies that bind to endothelial cells—these autoantibodies are distinct from other circulating antibodies characteristic of scleroderma.

(6) increased endothelial cell-surface expression *in vivo* and elevated circulating levels of the adhesion molecules, intracellular adhesion molecule 1 (**ICAM-1**), vascular cell adhesion molecule 1 (**VCAM-1**), and E-selectin.

The mechanism for vasospasm in systemic sclerosis is likely to be complex. Interactions between extracellular matrix products such as nitric oxide, endothelin 1 and prostacyclins, platelet-released products (serotonin and β-thromboglobulin) and neuropeptides (calcitonin gene-related peptide and vasoactive intestinal polypeptide) may all contribute to the abnormal vascular tone (Kahaleh and Mattuci-Cerinic 1995).

The mechanism for the development of injury in the extracellular matrix is unknown but both immune (cell-mediated and humoral) and non-immune cytotoxicity have been implicated, and recently, several reports have shown that extracellular matrix can be damaged before there is an obvious inflammatory infiltrate. Prescott *et al.* (1992) studied sequentially the pathological changes in the perivascular spaces in the skin of patients with scleroderma and normal controls. Functional and structural endothelial change with subendothelial oedema was recognized as the first defect, followed by platelet aggregation and lymphocyte migration of both CD+ and CD8+ T cells. Tissue fibrosis occurred after the inflammation had subsided. Supporting evidence for this finding comes from the work of Harrison *et al.* (1991) in which damage to endothelial/epithelial surfaces is shown to be the first ultrastructural change to occur in lung biopsies from patients with systemic sclerosis. Lung sections appearing normal under light microscopy, with no evidence of infiltrating inflammatory cells, were, on electron microscopy, shown to contain widespread endothelial/epithelial damage. The nature of the primary vascular trigger to immune stimulation is critical to our understanding of the disease: environmental agents or an endothelium-seeking virus are possible candidates. In addition, intense vasospasm, which occurs both in the extremities and in internal organs in patients with systemic sclerosis, could lead by reperfusion injury and free-radical damage to structural and functional change in the endothelium and subsequent immune activation (Blann *et al.* 1993).

Following injury to, and activation of, the vascular endothelium adhesion molecules such as E-selectin, VCAM-1 and ICAM-1 are up-regulated in response to cytokines and other factors. These endothelial adhesion molecules bind to specific ligands on T and B lymphocytes, platelets, neutrophils, monocytes and natural killer cells, facilitating their adhesion to vascular endothelium and subsequent migration through what have now become 'leaky vessels' into the extracellular matrix, ultimately with the potential for fibroblast activation. Therefore if endothelial change could be detected, and stabilized at an early stage, it would almost certainly influence the clinical expression and progression of the disease.

The clinical picture

Scleroderma, as discussed earlier, is not one condition but a spectrum of heterogeneous conditions occurring at any age and including localized and systemic forms. Within each subtype the rate of progression and extent of damage varies. Occasionally, localized scleroderma may become systemic and sometimes localized scleroderma and eosinophilic fasciitis merge or overlap, either appearing together or sequentially. In addition, there are sclerotic conditions induced by a variety of occupational, environmental, and metabolic stimuli.

Juveniles may develop any form of scleroderma, but fortunately, there is a predilection for the localized forms in which the skin, subcutaneous fascia, muscle, and bone are the main organs to be attacked. In the localized form the skin at first shows a marked inflammatory reaction, followed by matrix deposition, fibrosis, and ultimately atrophy. The linear lesions are most associated with subcutaneous involvement and growth defects, but in general there are no systemic features (Hanson 1976).

Childhood-onset scleroderma is rare in comparison to the adult disease and to juvenile chronic arthritis. Fewer than 3 per cent of all cases of scleroderma are childhood-onset (Dabich *et al.* 1974), and such children comprised fewer than 3 per cent of all patients seen in a paediatric rheumatology clinic (Hanson 1976). Ascertainment of childhood scleroderma may be biased by referral patterns and subspecialty orientation. In a paediatric rheumatology centre, systemic sclerosis is seen much less frequently than localized scleroderma, approximately one case to every 15 of localized disease. In a busy dermatology clinic, morphoea is more commonly seen and scleroderma *en coup de sabre* may be misdiagnosed as alopecia areata: consequentially, the real prevalence of these conditions is unknown. Like its adult counterpart, childhood-onset scleroderma occurs in all races, with a female predominance. There appears to be no significant familial incidence. HLA studies with sufficient numbers of children in each group are only now being undertaken, and preliminary information presented would suggest that the HLA associations in the childhood disease are quite different from those found in adult scleroderma.

Localized scleroderma

This is separated from systemic sclerosis not only by the absence of vasospasm, structural vascular damage and involvement of internal organs, but also by the distribution of the dermal lesions, which may, depending on the subtype, follow a dermatomal pattern. The varied clinical features have led to the separation of three main varieties of localize scleroderma, morphea, linear, and *en coup de sabre*.

Morphoea

This may be circumscribed or generalized. In circumscribed morphoea (Fig. 2) there may be just one or two lesions with no generalized spread. The changes often begin with small, violaceous or erythematous skin lesions, which enlarge and progress to firm 'hidebound' skin with variable degrees of hypo- or hyperpigmentation. These lesions eventually settle into a waxy, white appearance with subsequent atrophy. Pruritis is often a problem with the early lesion. Lesions vary in diameter between 1 and 10 cm. The condition generally resolves within 3 to 5 years, although sometimes a patch may persist for over 25 years. In generalized morphoea there are many patches covering a large surface area. The acral parts are

Fig. 2 Localized morphoea showing discrete lesions with central depigmentation and circumferential inflammation.

usually spared, but the trunk and legs are often involved. Generalized morphoea can be disfiguring and may continue to extend, resulting in contractures, disability, and troublesome ulceration that may occasionally become malignant. In guttate morphoea there are multiple small, hypopigmented and pigmented papules 2 to 10 mm in diameter, with minimal sclerosis, and the lesions closely resemble those of lichen sclerosus et atrophicus. These lesions usually localize to the neck, shoulders, and anterior chest wall.

Linear scleroderma

The sclerotic areas occur in a linear, band-like pattern, often in a dermatomal distribution (Fig. 3). They often cross joint lines, and are associated with atrophy of the soft tissue, muscle, periosteum, bone, and occasionally synovium; they can lead to extensive growth defects in a limb or a part thereof, which can be extremely disfiguring.

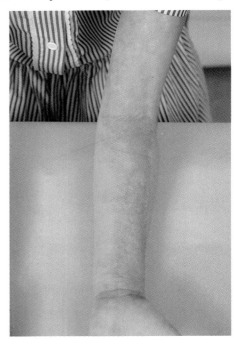

Fig. 3 Linear scleroderma occurring in childhood. Defective growth of the involved limb is a major clinical problem in childhood-onset disease.

Fixed valgus or various deformities also occur, and scoliotic changes in the spine can develop as a result of inequalities in limb length. If the toes or fingers are involved, 'hammer toes' or 'claw hand' may develop. All of these changes are much more noticeable in a growing child and most cases of linear systemic sclerosis tend to occur in childhood, as do most cases of *en coup de sabre*, a specialized form of linear disease.

En coup de sabre

Linear scleroderma occurring on the face or scalp may assume a depressed, ivory appearance. The lesion was considered originally reminiscent of the scar from a sabre wound so it was termed '*coup de sabre*'. The linear lesion is often associated with hemiatrophy of the face on the same side. It may also be associated with vascular abnormalities of the brain (David *et al.* 1991), and also with morphoea lesions elsewhere. It is also not uncommon for patients to present with morphoea and then later develop linear lesions (Falanga *et al.* 1986). This evolution should be anticipated extremely carefully, as the linear lesions tend to have much greater morbidity than the circumscribed patches of morphoea. The linear lesions may be quietly progressive for a long period, and lengthy follow-up is important.

In addition, in children there has been described a small group with morphoea and/or linear lesions who also have a synovitis, which can be demonstrated by infrared thermography (Allen *et al.* 1987). These patients have a raised erythrocyte sedimentation rate, rheumatoid factor, and circulating autoantibodies. Such cases are unusual, but they have an accelerated course with rapid development of contractures. An additional intermediate and interesting group of juveniles was described by Ansell *et al.* (1976). These children's disease is often mistaken for polyarticular juvenile chronic arthritis, since they may present with extensor and/or flexor tendon nodules in the hands, nodules at the elbows, knees or ankle joints, stiffness and a limitation of joint movement, but with little evidence of synovitis. At the time of presentation, there may only be a small area of localized or linear scleroderma, distant from the joint symptoms. The erythrocyte sedimentation rate and rheumatoid factor are usually normal, but autoantibodies are often present. There is both a clinical and a biochemical association, the nature of which is unclear, between localized scleroderma and eosinophilic fasciitis, in which large sclerotic patches may also occur.

Evaluation of all forms of scleroderma is difficult. In the localized forms, charting of the involved areas is often cumbersome and imprecise. However, the size of the lesion can be recorded, leg length, limb circumferences, and posture can be monitored, and muscle function and neurological status assessed. Charting of new lesions is also essential. In addition, thermography can be used to assess the activity of localized disease (Birdi *et al.* 1992).

Raynaud's phenomenon and the presclerotic state

It is fortunate that almost all cases of generalized systemic sclerosis arise in patients with Raynaud's phenomenon. The overall prevalence of this phenomenon has been variably assessed as between 3 and 10 per cent of adults worldwide, although it may affect as many as 20 per cent of young women. The prevalence varies somewhat depending on climate, skin colour, ethnic background, and occupational exposure to vibrating machines (Belch 1989).

The clinical syndrome was first described by Maurice Raynaud in 1862 as episodic digital ischaemia provoked by cold and emotion. It is classically manifest by episodic pallor of the digits followed by cyanosis, suffusion, and/or pain and tingling. The blanching reflects vasospasm in the digital vessels, the cyanosis the deoxygenation of static venous blood, and the redness reactive hyperaemia following the return of blood flow. Continuous blanching, blueness or pain is not Raynaud's phenomenon and to have implications for autoimmune rheumatic disease the phenomenon must be biphasic and episodic.

The episodic vasospasm can also be observed in the tip of the nose, the nipples, the mouth, and the ear lobes. More recently, and of great interest, there are reports of a systemic 'vasospasm', which may affect the cerebral, coronary, pulmonary, renal or upper gastrointestinal blood supply. With the published evidence of vasospasm in many organs, it is interesting to speculate that abnormalities of the vasculature may exist throughout the whole Raynaud's patient (Belch 1990). A careful history is still the best way to diagnose the phenomenon, although this can be supported in the laboratory with measurements of digital and organ blood flow.

Important clues to secondary Raynaud's on clinical evaluation are: the development of Raynaud's either in very young children or after the age of 45 years; severe symptoms occurring all year round; digital ulcerations, which rarely, if ever occur in primary Raynaud's; asymmetry of symptoms; and the reoccurrence of chilblains in an adult (Lally 1992). Two simple, inexpensive, non-invasive procedures have high predictive power for detecting patients in the Raynaud's group who will have systemic sclerosis in the future; serum autoantibody determination and nailfold capillary microscopy. These tests should be performed in all Raynaud's patients. The antinuclear antibodies were discussed earlier in the chapter and the presence of disease-specific autoantibodies plus abnormal nailfold capillaries is a powerful predictive tool.

Autoantibodies

The number of autoantibodies present in the serum of patients with scleroderma is varied (Table 9) (Pollard *et al.* 1989; Bona and Rothfield 1994). However, three of these antibodies have particular importance: anticentromere, antitopoisomerase-1 (Scl-70), and antinucleolar antibodies. Anticentromere antibodies react with the centromere portion of chromosomes and particularly with the kinetochore plates that attach the centromere to the spindle during mitosis; they appear to be a constant finding over time, appear early in the disease, and have a predilection for the subset of limited cutaneous systemic sclerosis. In contrast, antitopoisomerase 1 is an antibody found in up to 60 per cent of patients with diffuse cutaneous systemic sclerosis. This proportion tends to vary considerably between laboratories, and retrospective analysis and patient selection may have influenced results. The specificity of antinuclear antibodies as determined by immunoblots was also found to be predictive of the subtypes of systemic sclerosis. A prospective study of primary Raynaud's and undifferentiated autoimmune rheumatic disease (Kallenberg *et al.* 1988), using the immunoblot method, found that the presence of antinuclear antibodies at the time of entry into the study was associated with the evolution of an autoimmune rheumatic disease, usually scleroderma. Furthermore, in those who initially presented with Raynaud's disease alone, anticentromere antibody had a predictive value for the development of limited cutaneous systemic sclerosis (sensitivity 60 per cent, specificity 98 per cent) and Scl-70 for diffuse cutaneous systemic sclerosis (sensitivity 38 per cent, specificity 100 per cent). Antinucleolar antibodies now being characterized biochemically are present in many patients with scleroderma and further definition may improve their diagnostic specificity. Thus it seems that the presence of antinuclear antibodies, particularly anticentromere antibody and Scl-70, in a patient with apparent Raynaud's disease may mark the probability of later progression to one of the subsets of systemic sclerosis (Wollersheim *et al.* 1989).

Nailfold capillaroscopy

The most distal parts of the skin and its appendages receive their nutrient blood supply from capillary loops that arise from and return to a vascular plexus deeper in the skin. These capillary loops can be seen in the skinfold of the finger nail, where the capillary is visible over its long axis (Fig. 4). Direct observation of the nailfold capillary bed dates back almost 70 years and was introduced by German investigators. Recent refinements have permitted permanent photographic recording of a row of horizontal capillary loops at the nailfold, just proximal to the cuticle (Carpentier and Maricq 1990). The characteristic patterns seen in patients destined to develop autoimmune rheumatic disease are:

(1) the enlargement of all three portions of the capillary loop — arterial, apical and venular;

(2) the loss of capillaries either diffusely or in localized areas often adjacent to enlarged capillaries.

Dilatation without avascular areas is reported to be characteristic of limited cutaneous systemic sclerosis and dilatation with avascular areas characteristic of diffuse cutaneous systemic sclerosis. The capillary patterns are present early in the disease and are remarkably constant over time.

Comment

Tests for autoantibodies and nailfold capillaroscopy together detect more than 90 per cent of patients destined to have generalized systemic sclerosis. Of the 3 to 10 per cent of the population with Raynaud's up to 15 per cent are positive for one or both procedures. These recent observations are now leading to a shrinkage in the number of patients with true Raynaud's disease and an expansion in the number of patients who potentially have autoimmune rheumatic disease.

There is no evidence that symptomatic treatment of Raynaud's phenomenon in any way influences the evolution of scleroderma. However, once the mechanisms of fibrosis and vascular damage are better understood, the predictive power of these two tests, possibly coupled with other serological or genetic markers, ought to allow for a more preventive approach.

Scleroderma once established is a multisystem, multistage disease and each target organ progresses through stages of inflammation, fibrosis, atrophy, not necessarily at the same time or with the same speed. The eventual effect of these pathological processes is to impair organ function. In the following sections some organs, particularly those whose involvement may be fatal, will be discussed in detail; others will be summarized and/or tabulated.

Cutaneous involvement (Figs 5 and 6)

The changes in the skin usually proceed through three phases: early, classic, late. The early stage can be difficult to diagnose and a high

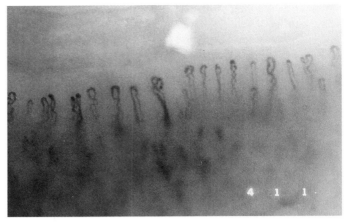

(a)

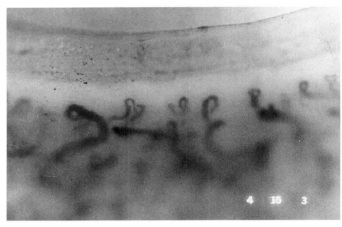

(b)

Fig. 4 (a) Photographs of normal nailfold capillaries showing normal spacing, orientation, and indentations. (b) Photograph of nailfold capillaries of a patient with scleroderma showing avascular areas and capillaries that are dilated and irregular in shape and distribution with disturbed orientation. Original magnification × 65. (By courtesy of Dr Frances Lefford, Department of Anatomy and Developmental Biology, University College London.)

level of suspicion is needed in the oedematous phase when the only feature may be puffiness of the hands and feet, most marked in the mornings. The face may feel slightly taut at this stage and Raynaud's may be present. On examination there is a non-pitting oedema with intact epidermal and dermal appendages. The subsequent, often sudden, development of firm, taut, hidebound skin proximal to the metacarpophalangeal joints, adherent to deeper structures such as tendons and joints, causing limitation of their movement and subsequent contractures, permits a definitive diagnosis in over 90 per cent of patients. The skin may be coarse, pigmented, and dry at this stage. The epidermis thins, hair growth ceases, sweating is impaired, and skin creases disappear.

Changes limited to the fingers alone (sclerodactyly) do not carry the same implication. The classical changes, once fully developed, can remain static for many years. Careful mapping of the degree and extent of skin involvement is the single best clinical technique for detecting the patient at risk for life-threatening involvement of internal organs. A number of scoring systems to quantify skin sclerosis have been developed. Most are two-dimensional instruments

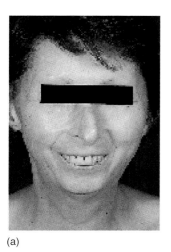
(a)

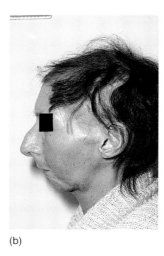
(b)

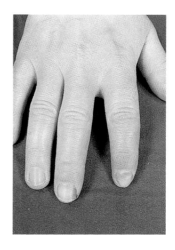
(a)

Fig. 5 (a, b)Typical facial appearance of diffuse cutaneous systemic sclerosis, with tight shiny skin, contrasting with the widespread facial telangiectasis often present in advanced, limited cutaneous systemic sclerosis.

that attempt to summate the severity of skin involvement at a number of different sites in the body. A modified version of the original Rodnan skin score, consisting of a 0 to 3 grading at 17 skin sites (maximum score 51), has been shown to be better in terms of greater observer agreement and lower bias than a method in which the observer attempts to shade on a mannequin the full extent of skin involvement. The interobserver variability in the use of the modified Rodnan skin score in studies from both the United Kingdom and United States is similar (Clements *et al.* 1990). An overall within-patient variability in scoring (derived from multiple examinations) is about five skin-thickness units, which is similar to the variability found in scoring joint tenderness in rheumatoid arthritis (Ritchie score), justifying its use in clinical trials to follow-up the outcome of skin involvement.

Taut hypo- or hyperpigmented skin proximal to the elbows, knees or clavicles qualifies a patient as having diffuse cutaneous systemic sclerosis and such patients require more frequent multi-system evaluation. Patients with diffuse cutaneous systemic sclerosis have a preponderance of visceral involvement in the first 5 years of symptoms. The exact beginning of the late phase is usually impossible to define, but at some point, and this may be 2 to 15 years after the appearance of the classical changes, the pattern moves into a final phase. The taut truncal arm and leg skin softens, and in some patients, but for the pigmentation, it would be difficult to know that they had ever had systemic sclerosis. Nevertheless, the hands in diffuse cutaneous systemic sclerosis nearly always show the ravages of the early, actively fibrotic period, and tautness and contractures usually remain even after resolution elsewhere. Other skin manifestations include digital pitting scars, loss of fingerpad tissue, ulcers, telangiectasias, and calcinosis. Skin biopsy is usually no more sensitive than the experienced touch in diagnosing the full-blown disease, but may provide useful sugges-tive information in the early oedematous phase.

In the early phase there are collections of mononuclear cells in the dermis, particularly around blood vessels. The soluble products of these monocytes and lymphocytes may have pathogenetic signifi-cance in the disease process. In the classic phase, fibrosis replaces

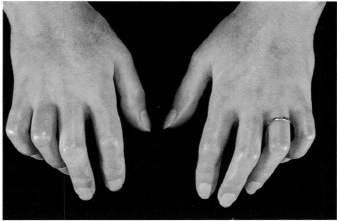
(b)

(c)

Fig. 6 The three phases of skin involvement in the hands of a patient with systemic sclerosis: (a) initial puffiness of the skin; (b) tight shiny skin with induration, loss of finger pulp, and contractures; (c) late changes of contractures with atrophic skin and ulceration.

the cellular infiltrate and may extend deep into the connective tissue to surround tendons, nerves, muscle bundles, and joint capsules. In the final stage, the fibrosis may be less evident, with epidermal thinning and loss of appendages the major findings.

Systemic features of disease

General manifestations

The patient with systemic sclerosis must cope with a complex set of symptoms that range from features common to chronic diseases through to complaints attributable to specific visceral involvement; fatigue and lethargy are common throughout the illness, although usually more pronounced in its early phases. Weight loss is almost universal in the diffuse cutaneous form and is less common in the limited variety. Fever is uncommon and if present, other causes such as infection or underlying malignancy should be excluded. Reactive depression is a frequent accompaniment to this often relentless and disfiguring disorder. Patients often feel isolated and support groups provide an invaluable service.

Gastrointestinal tract

The gastrointestinal tract is probably the most commonly involved internal organ system in systemic sclerosis (Shorrock and Rees 1988; Silver 1990). Over 90 per cent of patients with limited cutaneous and diffuse cutaneous systemic sclerosis have oesophageal hypomotility and serious gastrointestinal disease has been estimated to occur in 50 per cent of patients with limited cutaneous systemic sclerosis. It is probable that when systemic sclerosis affects an area of the gastrointestinal tract it does so in a sequential manner with progressive dysfunction (Cohen *et al.* 1980; Greydanus and Camilleri 1989). This concept is important when designing therapeutic regimens. The earliest lesion is neural dysfunction. The basis for this lesion is uncertain, although in the oesophagus there is both physiological and anatomical evidence that it is due to arteriolar changes in the vasa nervorum (D'Angelo *et al.* 1969; Russell *et al.* 1982; Greydanus and Camilleri 1989). An alternative explanation would be compression of nerve fibres by fibrous tissue (Dessein *et al.* 1992). This produces functional change before the next step, which is impairment of muscle contractility. These functional changes may remain asymptomatic for a long period but, if looked for, they usually respond well to prokinetic drugs. Once smooth-muscle atrophy is established, symptoms usually appear. The muscle can respond partially to prokinetic drugs but the response is weak. The final lesion, as with all other organs in systemic sclerosis, is muscle fibrosis superimposed on neural dysfunction and atrophy. At this stage, restoration of function is not possible.

The earliest clinical symptoms may be quite subtle. Patients can, often recall a specific event when there was difficulty in swallowing a pill or bolus of hard food. They may also experience retrosternal discomfort or even overt pain, which can be nocturnal. There are patients (forming part of the continuum of systemic sclerosis and who should be included in the group with limited cutaneous systemic sclerosis) who demonstrate Raynaud's phenomenon, abnormal nail-fold capillaries, anticentromere antibodies, and decreased motility or at least decreased lower oesophageal-sphincter pressure, but no skin sclerosis. Measurement of lower oesophageal pressure is frequently unacceptable to the patient and therefore in clinical practice the oesophageal transit time (quantitative oesophageal scintigraphy) is usually the preferred screening test. It is non-invasive, cost-effective, and is highly acceptable to patients. In those who have an abnormal scan and those who have frank dysphagia or heartburn, barium studies and/or direct oesophagoscopy may be required to

identify structural divisions such as hiatus hernia and oesophageal strictures. Fortunately, Barrett's metaplasia and oesophageal stricture are rare. All patients with systemic sclerosis should be recommended to raise their bed ends with blocks, take small frequent meals, and not eat late at night. The therapies available for oesophageal disease are numerous and their place in management is summarized in Table 12.

Recent studies have also emphasized that oesophageal disease is not predicted by disease subset or duration and may be relatively asymptomatic. Often investigations are not undertaken in the non-complaining patient, but perhaps we should pursue studies early in the disease so that distal hypomotility can be detected and treated aggressively. Such action may delay or prevent irreversible, pathological change.

Small-bowel disease with hypomotility is a major problem in scleroderma and can lead to weight loss, cachexia, malabsorption, and death. The classical symptoms are of a change in bowel pattern, with loose, frequent, floating, foul-smelling stools, and abdominal distension, but a patient may also present with weight loss (otherwise unexplained) or a nutritional anaemia. There are numerous possible ways of investigating the small bowel (some as yet research tools), and each test has its exponent. Details are given in Table 12.

Once the disease is established, bacterial overgrowth with its associated malabsorption is a recurring problem, often punctuated by abrupt episodes of distension and adynamic ileus or pseudo-obstruction as it is now called. The management of such patients is difficult and includes the rotational use of antibiotics, attempts to stimulate the bowel directly with cisapride, and ultimately total parenteral nutrition administered by the patient at home. There are greater than 50 per cent 5- and 10-year survival rates for patients on total parenteral nutrition, which is a distinct improvement over survival rates before total parenteral nutrition was available.

Atony and hypomotility of the rectum and sigmoid colon is frequent and occurs early. It is often missed clinically because patients are reluctant to discuss symptoms such as anal incontinence, a problem for which there is no relief. Constipation is usually manageable with the use of dietary manipulation and stool volume expanders. Codeine can cause constipation and should be avoided.

Surgery to the large bowel or any other part of the gastrointestinal tract must be viewed with great caution. Careful manometry and radiographic localization of affected segments of stomach, small intestine, and colon may allow judicious surgical resection or venting procedures, but these are not without risk and are not always successful.

Pancreatic exocrine function is frequently reduced, but rarely to an extent that is clinically important. Primary biliary cirrhosis may occur and it is associated with the subgroup of limited cutaneous systemic sclerosis. As the gastrointestinal manifestations of systemic sclerosis are frequent, and debilitating if not life-threatening, the goal in this area must be early detection, support, and control, thus permitting as active a life as possible.

Cardiac disease

Vascular, microvascular, and a vasospastic phenomena are, as in all other organs, a feature of cardiac scleroderma (Follansbee 1986). The clinical symptoms are diverse and sometimes difficult to separate from pulmonary or renal disease. They are largely non-specific, including dyspnoea, orthopnoea, paroxysmal nocturnal dyspnoea, oedema, palpitations, and atypical chest pain. Angina pectoris is uncommon and such a history should be regarded as a potential

Table 12 Gastrointestinal-tract pathology in systemic sclerosis

Site	Disorder	Symptom	Investigation	Treatment
Mouth	Tight skin	Cosmetic	None	Facial exercises
	Dental caries	Toothache	Dental radiograph	Dental treatment
	Sicca syndrome	Dry mouth	Salivary gland biopsy	Artificial saliva
Oesophagus	Hypomotility	Dysphagia	Barium swallow	Cisapride Avoid NSAIDs and nifedipine
	Reflux oesophagitis	Heartburn	Oesophageal scintiscan	Omeprazole Bed elevation No late meals Metoclopramide
	Stricture	Dysphagia	Manometry Endoscopy	Dilatation Omeprazole
Stomach	Gastric paresis	Anorexia Nausea Early satiety	Scintigram	Cisapride Metoclopramide
	NSAID-related ulcer	Dyspepsia	Barium meal	H_2-blockers, then misoprostol
Small bowel	Hypomotility Stasis Bacterial overgrowth	Weight loss Postprandial bloating Malabsorption Steatorrhoea	Barium follow-through ^{14}C glycocholate or hydrogen breath test Jejunal aspiration Faecal microscopy	Rotational antibiotics* Cisapride** Metoclopramide** Pancreatic supplements Octreotide (low dose) Enteral and parenteral Nutritional support
	Pseudo-obstruction NSAID ulceration	Abdominal pain Distension	Plain abdominal radiograph	Conservative management: 'drip and suck'
	Pneumatosis intestinalis	Diarrhoea with blood; benign pneumoperitoneum	Plain abdominal radiograph	
Large bowel	Hypomotility	Alternating constipation and diarrhoea	Barium enema	Dietary manipulation Cisapride may help Stool expanders (e.g. ispaghula)
	Colonic pseudodiverticula	Rare perforation	Barium enema	(Resection)
	Pseudo-obstruction	Abdominal pain Distension	Plain abdominal radiograph	Conservative management: 'drip and suck'
Anus	Sphincter involvement	Faecal incontinence	Rectal manometry	?? stimulation ? surgery

*Useful antibiotics: ciprofloxacin, amoxycillin, metronidazole, oral vancomycin, trimethoprim changing every 4 weeks with occasional 'antibiotic holiday' may reduce development of resistant strains.
**Prokinetic drugs only useful in early neuropathic disease, not later, when smooth muscle is destroyed.
NSAID, non-steroidal anti-inflammatory drug.

indicator of an underlying complicating factor such as coronary atherosclerosis. No definite predisposition to coronary atherosclerosis has been demonstrated in this disease, although recently the occurrence of large-vessel disease in association with systemic sclerosis has been emphasized. Youssef *et al.* (1993) found a threefold increase in evidence of large-vessel disease among patients with systemic sclerosis compared with the predicted population prevalence of 2.3 per cent for symptomatic vascular disease. Large-vessel disease seems to be associated with limited cutaneous systemic sclerosis and anticentromere antibody-positive patients. Cardiovascular manifestations of systemic sclerosis include myocardial fibrosis, pericarditis, a variety of arrhythmias, conduction abnormalities and pulmonary

Table 13 Cardiopulmonary manifestations of systemic sclerosis

Lung disease	Pathology	Frequency	Clinical features	Investigation	Treatment
Pulmonary fibrosis	Alveolitis with mixed cellular infiltrate, predeliction for bases, progresses to lung fibrosis	More frequent and severe in dcSSc D3/DR52a/anti-topoisomerase predictive in caucasoid population	Dry cough, dyspnoea, reduced expansion, bibasal crepitations, clubbing (late sign)	CXR (may be normal FVC, TLC, DLCO and KCO (reduced) HRCT definitive test DTPA clearance (fast)	No good trials; prednisolone (alternate-day regimen preferred) and cyclophosphamide (oral/intravenous) most widely used agents
Pleural disease	Pleurisy, effusion rare	Uncommon	Pleuritic chest pain, dyspnoea, pleural rub	CXR	NSAIDs or low-dose oral prednisolone
Bronchiectasis	Suppurative inflammation of airways	Rare	Chronic productive cough, focal coarse crepitations	CT scan	Appropriate antibiotics, postural drainage
Spontaneous pneumothorax	Rupture of cyst into pleural cavity	Rare	Chest pain, severe acute dyspnoea	CXR	Intercostal drainage, (? pleuradesis)
Lung carcinoma	Scar type (especially alveolar-cell carcinoma)	Rare	Variable	CT/bronchoscopy	Supportive if unresectable
Pulmonary hypertension (PHT)	Can be isolated PHT in lcSSc or secondary to interstitial fibrosis in dcSSc	10–15% overall	Dyspnoea, loud P2, left parasternal heave Right ventricular failure implies advanced disease	ECG, KCO and DLCO reduced Doppler-echo or right heart catheter can determine PA pressure	Dismal prognosis overall Prostacyclin infusion, oral anticoagulation and long-term oxygen may help
Cardiac disease					
Arrhythmias	Extrasystoles Rhythm disturbance		Palpitation, syncope	ECG (may need 24-h tape)	Treat if haemodynamically significant
Conduction defects	Due to fibrosis of conduction tissue		Syncope	ECG	Assess individual risk Permanent pacemaker may be needed
Pericardial involvement	Pericarditis Pericardial effusion	10–15% clinically 35% at autopsy	Chest pain, dyspnoea	ECG, echocardiogram	NSAIDs or low-dose prednisolone
Myocardial involvement	Myocarditis	Rare	Congestive cardiac failure	ECG, MUGA scan, echocardiogram	Prednisolone Diuretics, ACEIs
	Myocardial fibrosis	30–50% dcSSc	Congestive cardiac failure	MRI may be discriminatory	

ACEI, angiotensin-converting enzyme inhibitor; CT, computed tomography; CXR, chest radiograph; *DL*CO, carbon monoxide diffusing capacity; DTPA, see text; ECG, electrocardiogram; FVC, forced vital capacity; HRCT, high-resolution CT; *K*CO, carbon monoxide transfer coefficient; MRI, magnetic resonance imaging; MUGA, multiple-gated acquisition; NSAID, non-steroidal anti-inflammatory drug; PA, pulmonary arterial; dc/lcSCc, diffuse cutaneous/localized cutaneous systemic sclerosis.

hypertension, and rarely myocarditis. Cardiac involvement has a poor prognosis, which is probably most directly related to the extent of myocardial fibrosis present. There are many diagnostic techniques useful in evaluating cardiac scleroderma, but the investigation must be carefully matched to the clinical feature (see Table 13).

Two features have been singled out for discussion, myocardial fibrosis because it is the hallmark of cardiac scleroderma, and

pulmonary hypertension, with its sequelae including right heart failure, which often presents abruptly and which has such a devastating course. The nature and distribution of the myocardial fibrosis has a number of distinctive features. It is distributed randomly throughout both ventricles and develops throughout the entire thickness of the ventricular wall. It bears no relation to the extramural vascular supply and in some areas is so confluent that it gives the appearance of a circumscribed myocardial infarction. An additional distinctive histological feature of the myocardial fibrosis is the coexistence of contraction-band necrosis. This is typically seen in circumstances of myocardial ischaemia followed by reperfusion. In patients with scleroderma this suggests that vasoconstriction of the small, intramyocardial coronary arteries (a myocardial Raynaud's phenomenon) might be contributing to the pathogenesis of myocardial scleroderma. It would appear from work by Follansbee et al. (1990) that patients who develop left ventricular dysfunction in the absence of other apparent underlying causes commonly have advanced myocardial fibrosis associated with contraction-band necrosis, whilst patients who develop ventricular dysfunction in the clinical context of altered myocardial loading conditions (that is, systemic hypertension, pulmonary fibrosis, pulmonary hypertension) tend to have less myocarditis.

Pulmonary hypertension occurs in systemic sclerosis, usually in patients with the limited cutaneous type. It is attributable directly to pulmonary vascular disease, which can be suspected if on testing pulmonary function there is an isolated marked decrease in diffusing capacity for carbon monoxide (< 50 per cent of predicted normal) in the absence of significant restrictive ventilatory abnormalities. Pathologically, pulmonary arteries of all sizes show marked intimal and medial hyperplasia; of great interest is the finding by Follansbee et al. (1990) that, although the clinical syndrome seems confined to the group with limited cutaneous systemic sclerosis, intimal thickening and narrowing, albeit to a lesser degree, occurred in patients with diffuse cutaneous systemic sclerosis. In addition to the obstructive vascular lesions, the pulmonary vasculature appears to be abnormally reactive, with significant pulmonary vasoconstriction occurring on exposure to cold, again analogous to a peripheral Raynaud's phenomenon. That systemic sclerosis can be an overwhelmingly vascular disease is perhaps nowhere more convincingly demonstrated than in the subset of patients with severe pulmonary hypertension. It has an extraordinarily poor prognosis; death is usually due to rapidly progressive respiratory insufficiency accompanied by severe right-ventricular hypertrophy and failure.

The treatment of the cardiac manifestations of systemic sclerosis is primarily supportive, empirical, and of moderate value (see Table 13). Caution is necessary when treating patients with large pericardial effusions in diffuse scleroderma to avoid intravascular volume depletion, because of their predisposition to develop renal failure. Patients with systemic sclerosis and coexisting coronary arterial disease are often not good candidates for bypass surgery because of the distal vascular and interstitial disease that will reduce flow despite the presence of a satisfactory graft.

Pulmonary involvement

Pulmonary involvement ranks only second to oesophageal in frequency of visceral disease, and with considerable improvements in the management of renal disease it is now the major cause of death in scleroderma.

A study (Altmann et al. 1990) on patients with diffuse skin disease, pulmonary involvement but no cardiac or renal disease found a median survival of 78 months with 60 per cent dead at 5 years. Early diagnosis enabling the institution of effective therapy to halt disease progression is therefore a critical aim in the management of the patient with systemic sclerosis. Fortunately, this is becoming possible with the aid of modern techniques such as high-resolution computed tomography (Wells et al. 1993b; Wells et al. 1994), [^{99}Tc^{m}]diethylene triamine

pentacetate (**DTPA**) scanning and analysis of bronchoalveolar lavage fluid (Wells et al. 1993a). There is also evidence that the genetic markers HLA-DR3/DR52a (Briggs et al. 1990; Langevitz et al. 1992) and specific autoantibodies Scl-70, anti-U3 ribonucleoprotein, and antihistone antibodies may help separate this group at presentation.

The two major clinical manifestations of lung involvement are fibrosing alveolitis and pulmonary vascular disease. Other potential complications include aspiration pneumonia, pleural disease, spontaneous pneumothorax, drug-induced pneumonitis, associated pneumoconiosis, and neoplasm. Pulmonary fibrosis occurs in more than three-quarters of the patients with systemic sclerosis and pulmonary vascular disease in approx. 50 per cent. Autopsy studies have always yielded higher percentages than clinical studies.

In contrast to pulmonary hypertension, as discussed above, with other cardiac manifestations, interstitial lung disease often develops insidiously but established fibrosis is irreversible with present-day therapy. Early diagnosis is therefore vital and in the future genetic markers may help to identify this group at presentation. Pulmonary manifestations of systemic sclerosis are listed in Table 13.

The most common symptoms of respiratory involvement are breathlessness, especially on exertion, and a dry cough. Chest pain is infrequent and haemoptysis rare, and if either are present then the presence of additional pathology should be sought. On physical examination the most frequent finding is of bilateral basal crepitations (Alton and Turner-Warwick 1988).

The classical radiographic features consist of reticulonodular shadowing, usually symmetrical and most marked at the lung bases. However, the chest radiograph is an insensitive indicator of fibrosing alveolitis, and should be used only as an initial screen or to exclude infection or aspiration secondary to oesophageal abnormalities. There are many symptomatic patients (often mildly so) with normal chest radiographs despite interstitial lung disease, and lung function tests can be discriminatory. The single-breath diffusion test (DLco) is abnormal in over 70 per cent of patients with diffuse cutaneous systemic sclerosis (including asymptomatic patients with no complaints and an unremarkable chest radiograph). A reduction in DLco is the earliest proven abnormality in patients with systemic sclerosis who develop interstitial lung disease; lung function tests that show normal volumes but reduced transfer of gases in the face of normal imaging are suggestive of pure pulmonary vascular disease (see above). Measurement of the alveolar–arterial oxygen difference during exercise also appears to be a sensitive indicator of lung disease in systemic sclerosis.

Over the past 5 years the application of thin (3 mm)-section, high-resolution CT scanning of the lungs has revolutionized the approach to diffuse lung diseases and has revealed the character and distribution of fine structural abnormalities not visible on chest radiographs (Harrison et al. 1989) (Fig. 7). Using this technique, the earliest detectable abnormality is usually a narrow, often ill-defined, subpleural crescent of increased density in the posterior segments of the lower lobes. When more extensive, the shadowing often takes on a more characteristic reticulonodular appearance yet frequently retaining a subpleural distribution. It also becomes associated with fine, honeycomb air spaces and ultimately larger, cystic air spaces— an appearance that mirrors the macroscopic appearance. In a semi-quantitative comparison of the predictive value of these CT appearances to mirror the biopsy evidence of an inflammatory alveolitis, a 'ground glass' pattern of opacification on CT was associated with a predominantly cellular biopsy whereas a reticular pattern of

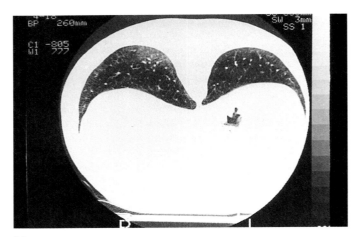

(a)

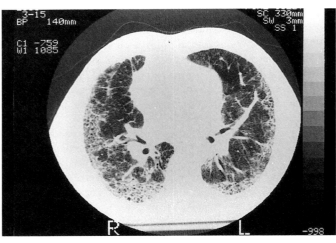

(b)

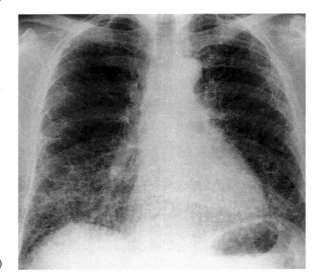

(c)

Fig. 7 Thin-section CT scan images illustrating: (a) ground-glass appearance of early pulmonary involvement posteriorly, associated with a normal chest radiograph; (b) extensive honeycomb shadowing and cystic air spaces involving both lower lobes, with corresponding chest radiographic appearances of advanced interstitial lung disease (bibasilar reticulonodular shadowing) (c). (With grateful acknowledgement to Drs A. Wells, R. du Bois and B. Strickland, Departments of Respiratory Medicine and Radiology, Royal Brompton Hospital, London.)

abnormality was found in patients whose subsequent lung biopsy confirmed a particularly fibrotic disease process (Muller and Miller 1990; Wells *et al.* 1992). CT scans also confirm the presence of pleural disease or mediastinal lymphadenopathy, which is commonly present. It is important to perform prone as well as supine scans, particularly in more subtle cases, to exclude the contribution of gravity to the radiographic appearances from vascular and interstitial pooling in the dependent areas. In addition to identifying early disease, high-resolution CT scanning can identify a pattern of disease that predicts a better response to therapy and a better prognosis (Wells *et al.* 1993). Furthermore, the extent of disease present, as defined by CT within the lavaged lobe, correlates with the predominant type of inflammatory cell obtained by bronchoalveolar lavage of that same lobe: lymphocytes are present in excess before CT identifies disease; eosinophils appear as the lung becomes abnormal; neutrophils are found in most abundance when at least 50 per cent of the lavaged lobe is involved in the disease process. In other words, the predominant type of inflammatory-cell traffic into the lungs depends upon extent of disease, and this would suggest that different inflammatory cells are involved in different stages of the pathogenesis.

In predicting the histological pattern CT, although useful, has not replaced lung biopsy as the 'gold standard' investigation (Fig. 8). As yet, patients who appear to have early changes on CT should still be considered for a thorascopic biopsy for staging of the disease. In the evaluation of diffuse lung disease, bronchoalveolar lavage has now been used for almost 20 years to sample cells and non-cellular material from the lower respiratory tract. The presence of abnormal numbers of granulocytes, particularly neutrophils and eosinophils (Harrison *et al.* 1989; Miller *et al.* 1990), is typical for a patient with fibrosing alveolitis occurring alone or in the context of systemic sclerosis. Excess lymphocytes are found in some individuals. In a typical patient with fibrosing alveolitis, bronchoalveolar lavage would produce an increase in total cell returns of three- to sixfold (up to 6×10^5/ml of fluid return); of these, up to 20 per cent may be neutrophils or eosinophils. Excess lymphocytes may be found (up to 20 per cent of the total cells) and an increase in mast cells may be observed in a small percentage of patients.

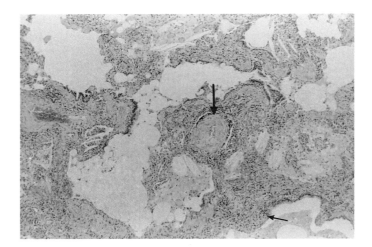

Fig. 8 Open lung biopsy of patient with systemic sclerosis showing interstitial chronic inflammation and fibrosis (small arrow) and thick-walled arteriole showing intimal fibrosis (large arrow). Haematoxylin and eosin, ×300. (Courtesy of Dr Mary N. Sheppard, Department of Lung Pathology, Royal Brompton Hospital London.)

The prognostic value of bronchoalveolar lavage has been demonstrated in several studies (Harrison *et al.* 1989; Silver *et al.* 1990). Silver *et al.* (1990) reported that patients with scleroderma with persistent alveolitis have greater deterioration in their pulmonary function than alveolitis-negative patients with systemic sclerosis.

The use of DTPA clearance in the management of systemic sclerosis has been the subject of extensive study and has been shown to be of value. It identifies early disease and also identifies a group of patients whose disease will run a more stable, non-progressive course; that is, those with normal clearance (Wells *et al.* 1993). The speed of clearance of the isotope is dependent upon the integrity of the epithelial barrier and therefore anything that disrupts this, either inflammation or fibrosis, will increase the rate of clearance (Barrowcliffe and Jones 1987). DTPA clearance is highly sensitive: cigarette smoking will produce increased clearance rates and the test is, therefore, only of value in non-smokers or those who have given up smoking for at least 1 month before the assessment (Mason *et al.* 1983).

In systemic sclerosis, clearance of DTPA may be abnormal even when chest radiography and pulmonary function tests are normal (Harrison *et al.* 1989). In established disease, clearance is enhanced in comparison with normal individuals. Furthermore, the speed of, and change in, clearance can predict subsequent changes in pulmonary function tests. Patients whose clearance is persistently abnormal are more likely to have a deterioration in pulmonary function tests at follow-up subsequent to the DTPA measurements. In contrast, persistently normal DTPA clearance predicts stable disease and therefore provides a good prognostic index; a study showed significant improvement in pulmonary function tests in 75 per cent of patients whose clearance returned to the normal range whereas similar improvements were not seen in those whose clearance remained normal or abnormally fast (Wells *et al.* 1993).

Considerable space has been devoted here to the lung because it is the organ that represents a major challenge in systemic sclerosis for the next decade, and because the available diagnostic tests have improved. The frequency of reassessments depends on the subset and length of disease. Those with diffuse cutaneous disease should be studied yearly or more frequently if necessary, whilst those with limited cutaneous disease have less need for frequent follow-up in the first 5 years of their illness and could be assessed at 2 years, but with increasing time must be watched on an annual basis for the development of pulmonary complications, either fibrosis or vascular disease.

Renal disease

Although renal disease has now been superseded by lung involvement as the major cause of systemic sclerosis-related death, it remains one of the most important complications of scleroderma and, despite its life-threatening nature, it is amenable to treatment, although the prognosis is much better if appropriate management is instituted early. Both post- and ante-mortem studies suggest that epithelial and endothelial renal lesions occur before there is clinical evidence of renal disease in systemic sclerosis (Kovalchik *et al.* 1978), and certainly precede any histological evidence of fibrosis. This supports the view that epithelial, and particularly endothelial, damage are important early events in the pathogenesis of scleroderma (Prescott *et al.* 1992). The best characterized pattern of renal involvement in systemic sclerosis is an acute or subacute renal hypertensive crisis.

This generally occurs in patients with diffuse systemic sclerosis within 5 years of disease onset. The overall incidence of scleroderma renal crisis is uncertain, with differences in the reported frequency even in series from the same unit. This variation probably reflects differences in incidence in the various subsets of systemic sclerosis. In high-risk patients the incidence may be as great as 20 per cent but overall is probably less than 10 per cent (Steen 1984). Traub (1994) proposed the following criteria to diagnose scleroderma renal crisis: abrupt onset of arterial hypertension greater than 160/90 mmHg; hypertensive retinopathy of at least grade III severity; rapid deterioration of renal function and elevated plasma renin activity. Other typical features include the presence of a microangiopathic haemolytic blood film and hypertensive encephalopathy, often complicated by generalized convulsions. It is generally considered important to perform a renal biopsy, once hypertension has been adequately controlled, especially if renal replacement therapy is being contemplated. This allows histological confirmation of the diagnosis and the exclusion of other causes for renal failure of abrupt onset, such as glomerulonephritis or the haemolytic–uraemic syndrome. Histologically, systemic sclerosis renal crisis typically shows fibrinoid necrosis, mucoid or fibromucoid proliferative intimal lesions (when extensive, termed onion skinning) in renal arteries, particularly the arcuate and interlobular vessels; glomerular thrombi occur and ultimately glomerulosclerosis (Fig. 9). The extent of the glomerular lesion can be useful in predicting the eventual degree of functional recovery. Patients usually present with the clinical features of severe hypertension, including headaches, visual disturbances, hypertensive encephalopathy (especially seizures), and pulmonary oedema. Occasionally a similar pattern of renal dysfunction occurs without hypertension (normotensive renal crisis), suggesting that the pathological features are not simply the end-organ consequences of raised arterial pressure (Helfrich *et al.* 1989). A more insidious pattern of renal involvement in systemic sclerosis is also reported in which there is a slow reduction in glomerular filtration rate accompanied by proteinuria. This is

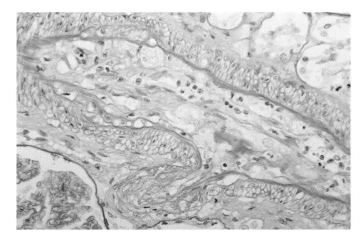

Fig. 9 An artery in the corticomedullary region. This section has been stained by the Alcian-blue/diastase-periodic acid–Schiff method. The lumen of the blood vessel has been entirely effaced by proliferation and swelling of the intima. Intimal cells can be seen to have developed an unusual bubbly, blue (mucoid) cytoplasm that is characteristic of scleroderma-related acute renal arteriopathy. There is a scattered small-lymphocytic infiltrate as well. (By courtesy of Dr A. P. Dhillon, Department of Histopathology, Royal Free Hospital Medical School, London.)

believed to reflect a more benign vascular and fibrotic process than scleroderma renal crisis.

Management of renal systemic sclerosis requires a high index of suspicion to enable early diagnosis and treatment of the renal crisis. Creatinine clearance or isotope glomerular filtration rate should be checked twice yearly in diffuse cutaneous systemic sclerosis for the first 5 years and annually thereafter. In limited cutaneous systemic sclerosis there is much less risk and a less frequent measurement of the glomerular filtration rate is sufficient. Blood pressure should be well controlled (often antihypertensive treatments also help Raynaud's symptoms) and in diffuse cutaneous systemic sclerosis the use of angiotensin-converting enzyme inhibitors is particularly appropriate since there is some anecdotal evidence that they protect from hypertensive crisis (Steen *et al.* 1990). High-dose corticosteroids have now been formally demonstrated in a case–control study to increase the risk of renal crisis in diffuse cutaneous systemic sclerosis and doses above 20 mg prednisolone equivalent daily should be avoided (Steen *et al.* 1994).

Once diagnosed, an acute renal crisis in systemic sclerosis must be treated as a medical emergency. The patient should be admitted immediately and reasonable control of the blood pressure is a priority. Extreme caution must be taken, however; to avoid a precipitous or excessive drop in arterial pressure and also to prevent relative or actual hypovolaemia associated with vasodilatation of constricted vascular beds, both of which can further diminish renal perfusion and compound the renal lesion of systemic sclerosis with acute tubular necrosis. For this reason, powerful parenteral antihypertensives (e.g. intravenous nitroprusside or labetolol) should be avoided; an internal jugular or subclavian venous cannula should be inserted to monitor central venous filling pressure; and an indwelling arterial cannula for pressure monitoring should be considered. Hypertension should be treated with angiotensin-converting enzyme inhibitors (captopril or enalapril up to maximum dose) and calcium-channel blockers (starting with long-acting nifedipine initially), aiming to reduce both diastolic and systolic pressure by 20 mmHg in the first 48 h and ultimately maintaining diastolic pressure at 80 to 90 mmHg. Intravenous prostacyclin, which is believed to help the microvascular lesion without precipitating hypotension, is often administered from diagnosis. Fish-oil capsules are sometimes prescribed in view of their unproven but theoretically beneficial properties (McCarthy and Kenny 1992). Renal function should be closely monitored by twice-weekly creatinine clearance and daily serum creatinine estimations. Regular full blood counts, clotting screening, and estimations of fibrin degradation product are important to monitor the degree of microangiopathic haemolytic anaemia, which often reflects the activity of the disease process. Short-term haemodialysis should be given if necessary and peritoneal dialysis often works well if long-term renal replacement therapy is needed. Interestingly, it has been observed that after a renal crisis, skin sclerosis and other features of systemic sclerosis improve (Denton *et al.* 1994), particularly if a patient is undergoing maintenance dialysis. The reason for this is unknown; it may result from the removal or inactivation of circulating mediators or simply reflect the natural history of the disease. It should be remembered that there is also often considerable recovery in renal function after an acute crisis, sometimes allowing dialysis to be discontinued, and improvement can continue for up to 2 years. Therefore any decisions regarding renal transplantation should not be made before this time.

Musculoskeletal system

Muscle
Skeletal muscle is often involved in scleroderma (Russell 1988). In many instances the weakness and atrophy results from disuse secondary to joint contractures or chronic disease. However, about 20 per cent have a primary myopathy (Medsger 1979), which is a subtle process distinctive for the disease. This chronic myopathy is characterized by mild weakness and atrophy of muscles, minimal elevation of creatine phosphokinase, few or no changes on electromyography, and subtle histological features showing focal replacement of myofibrils with collagen and perimysial and epimysial fibrosis without inflammatory change. This form of myopathy, which can last for many years, is non-progressive, does not warrant intervention, and is often unresponsive to anti-inflammatory mediation. A minority of patients exhibit an inflammatory myositis, indistinguishable from polymyositis; caution must be observed if this occurs in the context of early diffuse disease, when treatment with high-dose steroids might precipitate renal failure, and an alternative treatment should be considered. An atypical inflammatory myositis that requires special histochemical stains to demonstrate the differences in fibre size and composition has been reported in association with myocarditis in a few cases of systemic sclerosis. This form of myopathy, which can last for many years, is often unresponsive to non-steroidal or glucocorticoid anti-inflammatory medications.

Joints
A symmetrical polyarthritis, usually seronegative, anodular and non-erosive, is the presenting feature in a small number of patients destined ultimately to develop systemic sclerosis. By 2 years, frequently much earlier, the synovitis has subsided and classic cutaneous systemic sclerosis is present, often developing abruptly over 1 to 3 months.

The fibrosis characteristic of the classical disease affects the tendons (causing tendon friction rubs), the ligaments, and joint capsules, restricting movement; fibrosis is also found in the synovium. The synovium in systemic sclerosis is often covered by an excessive amount of fibrin; the reason for this is unknown.

Joint destruction is unusual. Management of soft tissue and joint problems is closely linked to skin care and to overall skeletal mobility. True bone changes in the form of distal tufts are usually a late change occurring in the second and third decade of the disease, and are thought to be due to a lack of a vascular supply adequate enough to preserve viable bone. This can occur in patients with long-standing Raynaud's phenomenon without connective tissue disease. Other sites of bone reabsorption, for example the mandible and ribs, have been recorded late in the disease.

Other organ involvement
Other organs involved in systemic sclerosis are listed in Table 14.

Systemic sclerosis and pregnancy
The greater incidence of scleroderma in women has focused interest on the potential interrelations between scleroderma, hormones, and pregnancy. It is of interest that women with Raynaud's phenomenon have an increased likelihood of low birthweight babies and fertility problems both before and after the onset of disease. It is unknown

Table 14 Other organ involvement in scleroderma

Organ	Effect	Pathological process	Frequency
Thyroid	Spectrum of autoimmune thyroid disorders — especially hypothyroid	Thyroid antibodies present in >50%	20–40%
Liver	Primary biliary cirrhosis (PBC)	Antimitochondrial antibodies in 25% patients with systemic sclerosis Anticentromere antibodies in 9–25% patients with PBC	3% CREST
	Abdominal pain, bile peritonitis	Vasculitis of gallbladder	Rare
	Calcification of liver		Very rare
	Extrahepatic obstructive jaundice	Mucosal ulceration	Very rare
	Nodular regenerative hyperplasia of the liver		Very rare
Nervous system	Trigeminal neuralgia	Collagen deposition in epineurium	Most common neurological change
	Carpal tunnel syndrome		3%
	Sensorimotor peripheral neuropathy	Vascular damage of vasa nervorum	
	Autonomic neuropathy		Possibly up to 80% — under-recognized
	Prolonged action of local anaesthetics		
	Subacute combined degeneration of the cord	Malabsorption of vitamin B_{12} Secondary to small-bowel involvement	Rare
Impotence	Erectile failure (libido intact)	Vascular fibrosis of cavernosal arteries	26–60% males

whether these findings are a reflection of the vasospasm affecting pregnancy or whether they reflect a common aetiological link.

The question of pregnancy in systemic sclerosis can be approached from two angles: the effect of scleroderma on pregnancy and its outcome, and the effect of pregnancy on the development and course of systemic sclerosis (Black 1990b).

Case-controlled studies have provided conflicting evidence on the outcome of pregnancy. British and Italian studies have shown an increase in the spontaneous abortion rate in women destined to develop systemic sclerosis. The British workers also found a higher rate of infertility, habitual abortion, and a higher probability that the pregnancy would end in stillbirth or neonatal death. An American study, however, showed only an increase in intrauterine growth retardation and prematurity, but not in miscarriage or fetal death.

The outcome of the pregnancy for the mother is also a subject of discussion. The American workers found no increase in maternal morbidity or mortality. However, the 23 case reports since 1932 (which may well select more interesting and thus severe cases) gave nine deaths, eight in patients with diffuse cutaneous systemic sclerosis, and at least five due to renal failure. Disease progressed in twelve of these patients, regressed in two, regressed during pregnancy but progressed afterwards in two, and developed during the pregnancy in one. In reports of larger series, totalling 103 pregnancies (mainly in women with limited disease), the disease developed during pregnancy in 9, progressed in 32, remitted in 11, and was stable in 35. There were 24 spontaneous abortions, 5 perinatal

deaths, 6 cases of toxaemia, and 2 maternal deaths. These reports reinforce the worse prognosis in diffuse disease. Of some encouragement are three more recent case reports. One describes a successful pregnancy in a patient with renal involvement, controlled with angiotensin-converting enzyme inhibitors throughout. The second patient, who had a renal crisis 6 years before treated with angiotensin-converting enzyme inhibitors for 5 years, managed without therapy to reach 38 weeks' gestation before becoming hypertensive and needing caesarean section for delivery of a healthy baby. The third case described a patient with limited cutaneous systemic sclerosis, livedoid vasculitis with foot ulceration, and a positive ribonucleoprotein autoantibody, and three previous spontaneous abortions, one neonatal death (28 weeks' gestation) and a 4-year period of secondary infertility. She was delivered of a healthy baby at 33 weeks, taking nifedipine before and throughout pregnancy for the foot ulceration.

The most feared complication in pregnancy is renal disease, which usually presents with hypertension especially in the third trimester, and is thus difficult to distinguish from toxaemia. Renal scleroderma should be considered in all but the most typical cases of pre-eclamptic toxaemia. In contrast to ordinary pre-eclamptic toxaemia, patients with systemic sclerosis can be vulnerable in the postpartum period, and must be watched very carefully.

Advice to patients with systemic sclerosis at pregnancy is difficult, since studies are limited and retrospective. Patients with diffuse skin involvement, especially with lung, renal or cardiac involvement, tend to have a worse prognosis, and should be offered therapeutic abortion. The patient with limited disease should be told of the possible development of complications, and the variable and unpredictable outcome, and may then request abortion. Very close monitoring of any patient with systemic sclerosis is then necessary throughout pregnancy.

Drug therapy

Although there is currently no treatment that can induce complete remission of the disease there are therapies available that can offer partial relief, control end-organ damage, and improve quality of life for the patient with scleroderma. The choice and evaluation of any treatment regimen are not easy. This is because (a) the disease is complex and the relation between immune dysfunction, vascular damage, and fibrosis speculative; (b) the disorder is heterogeneous and its extent, severity, and rate of progression are highly variable — therapy must therefore be closely tailored to the individual patient systems involved; (c) there is a tendency towards spontaneous stabilization and/or regression after a few years, particularly within the more benign and numerically larger subset of limited cutaneous systemic sclerosis; and (d) there is a paucity of both clinical and laboratory features for ascertaining improvement (or deterioration) in the disease, especially with respect to visceral change. Therapeutic trials of disease-modifying drugs are essential but their design is critical in this disease. There is growing acceptance that any trial of disease-modifying drugs must be controlled (preferably placebo-controlled), that patients should have early diffuse disease (less than 3 years' duration), and that studies must be of sufficient duration (1 year minimum).

Such is the frustration of the condition that numerous vitamins, hormones, 'alternative' medicines, acupuncture, and surgical procedures have been used. Most have been heralded with great enthusiasm, only to be abandoned once critically assessed.

There are no truly effective antifibrotic therapies. Some of the newer, putative antifibrotic agents that have been used in scleroderma are summarized in Table 15. D-Penicillamine and colchicine have been used in the treatment of scleroderma for many years. Neither drug stops the fibrotic process, but consensus opinion is that D-penicillamine is the more useful. To derive maximum benefit the drug must be used correctly. The most suitable subjects for treatment are those with diffuse active skin disease. Long-term treatment in a dose between 500 and 750 mg is needed. D-Penicillamine should be used throughout the active phase into the stable period and the dose maintained until there is no further improvement in skin thickening. The drug may then be reduced, but low-dose treatment should be maintained for many years — some recommend 10 years.

The ideal group to target and treat would be the 'at risk' patients, those in the presclerotic state. Many such patients can now be identified by circulating antibodies, cytokine production, and nailfold changes. Unfortunately, adequate preventative therapy is still wanting. An extension of this idea and one that can, for example, be applied to the lung is the earliest possible diagnosis of internal organ involvement so that containment therapy may be attempted.

As the immune system may be involved early in the disease, immunomodulatory and immunosuppressive agents have been employed, particularly for early diffuse systemic sclerosis. Table 16 summarizes their use and evaluation. Both antimetabolites and alkylating agents have been used. Chlorambucil, a hopeful therapy in

1985, failed in a placebo-controlled trial. The same fate befell 5-fluorouracil. Cyclophosphamide still has an undetermined place; as a single agent its efficacy is unproven. In combination with steroids or plasma exchange it may also have a role — unfortunately as yet there are no controlled data. The use of the antimetabolites 6-thioguanine and azathioprine has been reported but again all the data are anecdotal. Methotrexate is now being approached in a more rational manner. Pilot studies have been hopeful and controlled trials are being undertaken. Attempts to target the immune system by lymphoplasmapheresis and total lymphoid irradiation again failed and currently under investigation are the use of rabbit antithymocyte globulin, and photophoresis. Monoclonal antibody therapy may hold hope for the future.

Cyclosporin has been used in a few patients with positive results but high doses of the drug were followed by reports of hypertension and renal failure, both of which might be attributed to either the drug or systemic sclerosis (Denton *et al.* 1994). Physicians must be mindful of the fact that trough blood levels are multiplied two- to fourfold in patients taking calcium-channel blockers. Therefore a lower dose (5 mg/kg body wt per day) has been tried with encouraging results, but awaits confirmation in a controlled study.

The interferons α and γ are currently being investigated in controlled trials after initial pilot studies. Recombinant interferon-γ has immunoregulatory activities and is a potent inhibitor of collagen production by normal and scleroderma fibroblasts *in vitro*. Interferon-α, although theoretically less potent than interferon-γ as an inhibitor of collagen synthesis, does not activate the class II cell-surface antigens — this may be a distinct advantage in a disease that is HLA-linked. None of these drugs should be used for late-stage, stable, diffuse or limited cutaneous disease.

Long-term high-dose steroids have no place in the management of systemic sclerosis; indeed they are potentially toxic (Steen *et al.* 1994) and may be implicated in 'normotensive renal crisis'. Steroid usage has been restricted to patients with myositis, symptomatic serositis, the early oedematous phase of the skin disease, and refractory arthritis and tenosynovitis. The lowest possible but therapeutically effective dose should be sought.

Raynaud's, as described above, is a prominent feature of systemic sclerosis and occurs in over 97 per cent of cases. It is an aspect of the disease that can be relieved, though the response is variable. This idiosyncratic response may reflect the stage of the disease. If structural damage is present and severe, the patient will respond rather poorly to vasodilators alone. In uncomplicated cases, simple measures may suffice. As the attacks become more frequent, prolonged oral drug therapy, possibly on an intermittent basis, may be needed. Intravenous therapy and limited surgery are restricted to the most severe cases (see Table 17).

Because of the widespread vascular damage there has been a search to find drugs to protect injured endothelial cells and to prevent platelet aggregation and subsequent release of platelet-derived mediators. This search has been disappointing to date. Ketanserin, a serotonin antagonist, although useful in Raynaud's phenomenon, does not improve structural vascular disease. Dipyridamole and aspirin, although reducing the circulating plasma concentrations of β-thromboglobulin or circulating platelet aggregates, were not clinically effective in a randomized double-blind trial. Captopril, the angiotensin-converting enzyme inhibitor that has been so successful in the treatment of renal crisis, has been considered for the primary and possibly prophylactic treatment of vascular disease.

Table 15 Novel potential antifibrotic therapies for systemic sclerosis

Therapy	Mechanism	Comments
Anticytokine antibodies	Block mediators of fibroblast activation (e.g. TGFβ)	Toxicity likely to be problematic
Enzyme antagonists	Lysyl and prolyl hydroxylase inhibitors to block post-translational modification of collagen	No data yet
Pretranslational inhibition	Block collagen gene transcription or mRNA translation using antisense nucleotides or gene therapy	Hypothetical and dependent upon progress in understanding of collagen gene regulation

Table 16 Immunology therapies for systemic sclerosis

Treatment	Mechanism of action	Comments	Efficacy in clinical trials
1. *Selective immunosuppression*			
Cyclosporin	Inhibits T-helper-cell actions by reducing IL-2 release	Reported beneficial effects on skin sclerosis may be confounded increased incidence of renal crisis	Yes (open study; Zachariae *et al.* 1990) Yes (open study; Clements *et al.* 1994)
Antithymocyte globulin Antilymphocyte globulin	Temporary suppression of cell-mediated immunity	Possible benefit; confirmation of pilot work is essential, especially because of considerable therapy-associated morbidity	Yes (open study; Tarkowski *et al.* 1993) Possible benefit in placebo-controlled pilot study (Sinclair *et al.* 1993, unpublished communication)
Photopheresis	Extracorporeal photoactivated 8-methoxypsoralen inhibits activated T cells	Benefit has been reported but good placebo-controlled clinical trial is needed	No (open study; Zachariae *et al.* 1993) Yes (controlled trial comparing with D-penicillamine therapy; Williams *et al.* 1995) Multicentre placebo-controlled trial currently in progress
Plasmapheresis	Removes circulating immune mediators	Equivocal results but anecdotal benefit	Possible benefit
Pooled human gammaglobulin	Possible inhibition of lymphocyte function via regulatory idiotype cross-reactivity		Not formally evaluated
2. *Non-selective immunosuppression*			
Methotrexate	Folic acid antagonist	Currently under formal evaluation in dcSSc	Controlled trial in progress
Cyclophosphamide Chlorambucil Azathioprine	Alkylating agents suppressing production of immunocompetent leucocytes	Anecdotal benefit reported in open studies but controlled trial of chlorambucil failed to show superiority over placebo Cyclophosphamide often combined with corticosteroids	Yes (cyclophosphamide in SSc lung fibrosis—open study; Akesson *et al.* 1994) No (chlorambucil, controlled trial; Clements *et al.* 1994)

IL-2, interleukin 2; dc/SSc, diffuse cutaneous/systemic sclerosis.

Table 17 Treatment options for Raynaud's phenomenon

Treatment	Examples	Comments
1. *Simple measures*		
Non-drug	Hand warmers Protective clothing	Universally helpful; also useful to minimize cold exposure and ambient temperature changes in work environment
Pharmacological	Evening primrose oil	Evening primrose oil has been shown effective in controlled clinical trial
	Fish-oil capsules	
2. *Oral vasodilators*		
Calcium-channel blockers	Nifedipine Nicardipine Felodipine Amlodipine	Retard responses, often idiosyncratic; therefore best to try several drugs in rotation to find most effective
5-Hydroxytryptamine antagonist	Ketanserin	Only available on named-patient basis but shown effective in clinical trials
ACE inhibitors	Captopril Enalapril	In Raynaud's secondary to dcSSc may protect from hypertensive renal crisis
3. *Topical vasodilators*	GTN patches	Shown effective in short-term use but often cause headaches
4. *Parenteral vasodilators*	Carboprostacyclin (iloprost) prostaglandin E$_1$	Effective and reasonably tolerated Given for severe frequent attacks of Raynaud's, digital ulceration or gangrene, and before digital surgery
5. *Antibiotics*	Flucloxacillin Erythromycin	Important in secondary infection in Raynaud's; prolonged oral administration may be necessary
6. *Surgical procedures*		
Lumbar sympathectomy	Chemical or operative	For severe Raynaud's of lower limbs
Digital sympathectomy (radical microarteriolysis)		Useful treatment for isolated ischaemic of 1 or 2 digits
Debridement amputation	Surgical or auto-	Such surgery should be conservative to allow maximum possibility of spontaneous healing

ACE, angiotensin-converting enzyme; GTN, glycerol trinitrate; dcSSc, diffuse cutaneous sytemic sclerosis.

Our own approach to the management for some of the important subgroups of patients within the scleroderma spectrum of disorders is summarized below, and in Box 1. The management of localized scleroderma in adults and children is summarized in Table 18.

Our approach to management of Raynaud's and scleroderma

1. Raynaud's phenomenon without other features of autoimmune rheumatic disease

At presentation

Detailed history and examination to look for evidence of asymptomatic autoimmune rheumatic disease. Thoracic-inlet radiographic imaging to exclude simple structural lesion (e.g. cervical rib).

Baseline nailfold capillaroscopy and autoantibody profile (antinuclear antibodies, extractable nuclear antigen, anticentromere antibody) are important to determine whether the patient has primary Raynaud's phenomenon or is likely to develop features of an autoimmune rheumatic disease in the future. Infrared thermography with a standard cold challenge can be used to confirm diagnosis in equivocal cases and assess severity of vasospasm.

Follow-up

If capillaroscopy and autoantibodies are normal/negative, then simple approaches with advice on non-pharmacological relief (hand-warmers, thermal gloves), supplemented as necessary by vasodilator drugs. If the Raynaud's is of short duration (i.e., less than 2 years) the patient is followed annually until the fourth year after onset of symptoms. If capillaroscopy or autoantibody studies are positive, then give the same advice and treatment but follow up at 6 months, and then yearly for 5 years, with repeat capillaroscopy and autoimmune profile. Discharge from regular follow-up at 5 years if no

Table 18 Management of localized scleroderma in adults and children

Pattern of disease	Clinical features	Treatment	Prognosis
Localized morphoea	One or a few circumscribed sclerotic plaques with hypo- or hyperpigmentation and an inflamed violaceous border	Often unnecessary Serial measurement to assess progress	Good prognosis; lesions less active within 3 years but pigmentary changes often persist
Generalized morphoea	Widespread pruritic lesions, often symmetrical and following the distribution of superficial veins	Suppress inflammatory component using corticosteroids: in children oral doses up to 15 mg/day have been recommended; infusion i.v. may be better D-Penicillamine is often used: in children 3 mg/kg/day initially (maximum) 15 mg/kg/day); adult daily maintenance dose at least 500 mg Methotrexate and systemic or intralesional interferon may be effective, and cyclosporin has been used in refractory cases	Internal organ pathology very rare; Raynaud's seldom associated Generally improves within 5 years of onset, although textural and pigmentary changes can remain
Linear scleroderma	Sclerotic areas occurring in linear distribution often on limbs and asymmetrical; in childhood can lead to serious growth defect of affected limbs; careful, serial measurement of muscle bulk and limb length essential	Suppression of inflammation with oral or i.v. steroids (as above) Maintenance treatment with D-penicillamine or methotrexate Physiotherapy and appropriate regular exercise to minimize growth defect in childhood-onset form	Long-term effects of childhood-onset form minimized by effective suppression of inflammatory process, and by good physiotherapy Ultimately the disease tends to resolve, but it can remain active for many years
En coup de sabre	Linear scleroderma affecting the face of scalp, involving underlying subcutaneous tissues, muscles periosteum and bone; underlying cerebral abnormalities have been reported	Therapeutic options as for linear, sclerodermas; systemic treatment only for active inflammatory lesions	Scarring, growth defects, and alopecia persist but inflammatory component usually resolves

other disease features have developed, and Raynaud's has not required parenteral vasodilator drugs.

2. *Diffuse cutaneous systemic sclerosis*

At presentation

History and physical examination generally establish the diagnosis. Assess the extent of visceral disease by baseline hand and chest radiography, lung function tests, oesophageal motility study (scintigraphy or barium swallow), creatinine kinase, creatinine clearance and urinary protein excretion, Doppler echocardiography (with estimation of pulmonary arterial systolic pressure), and electrocardiogram. High-resolution CT lung scan, DTPA clearance, and bronchoscopy with studies of bronchoalveolar lavage fluid are usually performed in highly specialized units. Right-heart catheter studies and open lung biopsies are occasionally necessary to supplement the information obtained from other less invasive investigations. Once diagnosis is confirmed, tissue typing and autoantibody profiles may be useful to identify groups with poor prognosis. Raynaud's symptoms, if prominent, can respond well to intravenous prostacyclin infusions.

Immunosuppressive therapy (e.g. antithymocyte globulin) may be considered for the most severe cases within 3 years of onset. Antifibrotic therapy is clearly the most appropriate approach for established diffuse cutaneous systemic sclerosis but unfortunately agents of proven efficacy are lacking. In our unit, for patients with progressive and extensive diffuse cutaneous systemic sclerosis, interferon-α is the first-line agent, monitored by serial skin sclerosis score. The results of formal controlled trials in diffuse cutaneous systemic sclerosis are keenly awaited. Lung fibrosis is treated by combination therapy with prednisolone and cyclophosphamide, as outlined in detail above.

Follow-up

This is especially important during the first 5 years from disease onset. Vigilant monitoring for renal involvement should include regular checks of blood pressure, 6-monthly 24-h urine collection for protein excretion and creatinine clearance. Six-monthly lung function tests and electrocardiograms, with yearly oesophageal motility and echocardiographic studies are generally performed in our own unit.

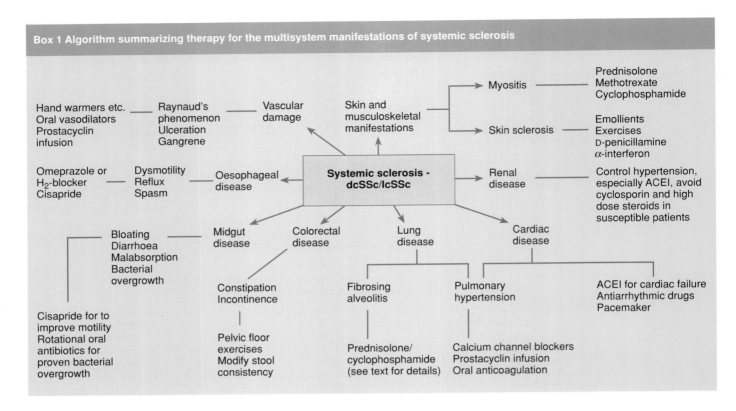

Box 1 Algorithm summarizing therapy for the multisystem manifestations of systemic sclerosis

3. Limited cutaneous systemic sclerosis

At presentation

By the time of presentation the history is usually of some years duration and the physical signs, even if minimal, are generally diagnostic. Diligent attention to the assessment of internal organs is necessary, especially as the disease duration lengthens. The main risks in this scleroderma subset are of pulmonary hypertension, often in the absence of significant interstitial fibrosis, and involvement of the small and large bowel.

Treatment in this group is largely symptomatic and as yet no satisfactory drugs to halt the underlying processes are available. It may, however, be important to treat these patients at an asymptomatic stage in the hope of preventing or slowing down the chronic vascular damage. Current treatment in this group is directed mainly towards the vascular features (Raynaud's and pulmonary vascular disease, when present) and gastrointestinal complications. Reflux oesophagitis is almost universal but fortunately responds well to proton-pump inhibitors such as omeprazole, which we prefer to use rather than H₂-blockers, although the latter also often give good symptomatic relief. Oesophageal spasm may respond to cisapride. In contrast, although midgut disease and anorectal complications are less frequent, they are far more difficult to manage.

Follow-up

Annual follow-up is generally undertaken, with assessment of visceral disease, including renal function by creatinine clearance. These patients often require long-term vasodilator therapy, usually intensified during the winter months. Later in the disease (especially after

10 years of established limited cutaneous systemic sclerosis), pulmonary hypertension more likely. Patients carrying antitopoisomerase 1 (Scl-70) antibody are particularly susceptible to lung fibrosis and their lung function should be carefully monitored.

Education and support forms a particularly important component of the management of patients with systemic sclerosis, who should be made aware of the various support groups and the importance of non-pharmacological aspects of care including appropriate exercises, skin care, and the importance of being in a stable, warm ambient temperature.

Conclusion

Currently therefore, although there is no curative treatment for scleroderma, a careful consideration of the subset and stage of disease of the individual patient can maximize the use of the drugs currently available. It is hoped, more importantly, that the level and degree of activity of research into the cause and pathogenesis of the condition may eventually result in early rational effective treatment.

Acknowledgement

The authors are grateful to Dr Aine Burns, Consultant Nephrologist at the Royal Free Hospital, London, for her help with the section on renal disease in scleroderma.

References

Alarcon, G. S., Philips, R. M., and Wasner, C. K. (1985). DR antigens in systemic sclerosis: lack of clinical correlations. *Tissue Antigens*, **26**, 156–8.

Allen, R. G., Ansell, B. M., Clark, R. P., Goff, M. R., Waller, R., and Williamson, S. (1987). Localised scleroderma: treatment response measured by infrared thermography. *Thermology*, **2**, 550–3.

Altmann, R. D., Medsger, T. A., Jr, Bloch, D. A., and Michel, B. A (1990). Predictors of survival in systemic sclerosis (scleroderma). *Arthritis and Rheumatism*, **34**, 403–13.

Alton, E. and Turner-Warwick, M. (1988). Lung involvement in scleroderma. In *Systemic sclerosis (scleroderma)* (ed. C. M. Black and M. I. V. Jayson). Wiley, Chichester.

Ansell, B. M., Nasseh, G. A., and Bywaters, E. G. L. (1976). Scleroderma in childhood. *Annals of the Rheumatic Diseases*, **35**, 189–97.

Barnett, A.J., Tait, B.D., Barnett, M.A., and Toh, B.H. (1989). T lymphocyte subset abnormalities and HLA antigens in scleroderma. *Clinical and Experimental Immunology*, **76**, 24–9.

Barrowcliffe, M. P. and Jones, L. G. (1987). Solute permeability of the alveolar capillary barrier. *Thorax*, **42**, 1–10.

Belch, J. J. F. (1989). Raynaud's phenomenon. *Current Opinions in Rheumatology*, **1**, 490–8.

Belch, J. J. F. (1990). Raynaud's phenomenon. *Current Opinions in Rheumatology*, **2**, 937–41.

Birdi, N. *et al.* (1992). Childhood linear scleroderma: a possible role of thermography for evaluation. *Journal of Rheumatology*, **19**, 968–72.

Black, C. M. (1990a). Scleroderma — systemic sclerosis. In *Oxford textbook of clinical nephrology* (ed. J. S. Cameron, A. M. Davidson, J. P. Grunfeld, D. N. S. Kerr, and E. Ritz). Oxford University Press.

Black, C. M. (1990b). Systemic sclerosis and pregnancy. *Baillière's Clinical Rheumatology*, **4**, 105–24.

Black, C. M. (1990c). Systemic sclerosis: is there a treatment yet? *Annals of the Rheumatic Diseases*, **49**, 735–7.

Black, C. M. and Denton, C. P. (1995). The management of systemic sclerosis. *British Journal of Rheumatology*, **34**, 3–7.

Black, C. M. *et al.* (1983). Genetic susceptibility to scleroderma-like syndrome induced by vinyl chloride. *Lancet*, **i**, 53–5.

Black, C. M. *et al.* (1984). HLA antigens, autoantibodies and clinical subsets of scleroderma. *British Journal of Rheumatology*, **23**, 267–71.

Blann, A. D., Illingworth, K., and Jayson, M. I. V. (1993). Mechanisms of endothelial cell damage in systemic sclerosis and Raynaud's phenomenon. *Journal of Rheumatology*, **20**, 1325–30.

Bocchieri, M. H. and Jimenez, S. A. (1990). Animal models of fibrosis. *Rheumatic Disease Clinics of North America*, **16**, 153–67.

Bona, C. and Rothfield, N. (1994). Autoantibodies in scleroderma and tightskin mice. *Current Opinions in Immunology*, **6**, 931–7.

Boros, P., Muryoi, T., Spiera, H., Bona, C., and Unkeless, J. C. (1993). Auto-antibodies directed against different classes of FcR are found in sera of autoimmune patients. *Journal of Immunology*, **50**, 2018–24.

Briggs, D., Black, C. M., and Welsh, K. I. (1990). Genetic factors in scleroderma. *Rheumatic Disease Clinics of North America*, **16**, 31–51.

Briggs, D., Stephens, C., Vaughan, R., Welsh, K. I., and Black, C. M. (1993). A molecular and serologic analysis of the major histocompatibility complex and complement component C4 in systemic sclerosis. *Arthritis and Rheumatism*, **36**, 943–54.

Campbell, P. M. and LeRoy, E. C. (1975). Pathogenesis of systemic sclerosis: a vascular hypothesis. *Seminars in Arthritis and Rheumatism*, **4**, 351–68.

Carpentier, P. H. and Maricq, H. R. (1990). Microvasculature in systemic sclerosis. *Rheumatic Disease Clinics of North America*, **16**, 75–91.

Chosidow, O. *et al.* (1992). Sclerodermatous chronic graft-versus-host disease. Analysis of seven cases. *Journal of the American Academy of Dermatology*, **26**, 49–55.

Clements. P. J., Lachenbruch, P. A., Ng, S. C., Simmons, M., Sterz, M., and Furst, D. E. (1990). Skinscore: a semi-quantitative measure of cutaneous involvement that improves prediction of prognosis in systemic sclerosis. *Arthritis and Rheumatism*, **33**, 1256–63.

Clements, P.J., Lachenbruch, P.A., Sterz, M.A., *et al.* (1994). Cyclosporine in systemic sclerosis. Results of a forty-eight week open safety study in ten patients. *Arthritis and Rheumatism*, **36**, 75–83.

Cohen, S., Laufer, I., Snape, W. J., Shiau, Y-F., Levine, G. M., and Jimenez, S. A. (1980). The gastrointestinal manifestations of scleroderma: pathogenesis and management. *Gastroenterology*, **79**, 155–66.

Dabich, L., Sullivan, D. B., and Cassidy, J. T. (1974). Scleroderma in the child. *Journal of Paediatrics*, **85**, 770–5.

D'Angelo, W. A., Fries, J. F., Masi, A. T., and Shulman, L. E. (1969). Pathologic observations in systemic sclerosis (scleroderma). *American Journal of Medicine*, **46**, 428–40.

David, J., Wilson, J., and Woo, P. (1991). Scleroderma *en coup de sabre*. *Annals of the Rheumatic Diseases*, **50**, 260–2.

De Crombrugghe, B., Vuorio, T., and Karsenty, G. (1990). Control of type I collagen genes in scleroderma and normal fibroblasts. *Rheumatic Disease Clinics of North America*, **16**, 109–23.

Degiannis, D., Seibold, J., Czarnecki, M., Raskova. J., and Raska, K. (1990). Soluble and cellular markers of immune activation in patients with systemic sclerosis. *Clinical Immunology and Immunopathology*, **56**, 259–70.

Denton, C. P., Abdullah, A., Sweny, P., and Black, C. M. (1994). Acute renal failure occurring in scleroderma treated with cyclosporin A — a report of three cases. *British Journal of Rheumatology*, **33**, 90–2.

Dessein, P. H., Joffe, B. I., Metz, R. M., Millar, D. L., Lawson, M., and Stanwix, A. E. (1992). Autonomic dysfunction in systemic sclerosis: sympathetic overactivity and instability. *American Journal of Medicine*, **93**, 143–50.

Dunckley, H., Jazwinska, E. C., Gatenby, P. A., and Serjeatson, S. W. (1989). DNA DR-typing shows HL-DRw11 RFLPs are increased in frequency in both progressive systemic sclerosis and CREST variants of scleroderma. *Tissue Antigens*, **33**, 418–20.

Earnshaw, W. C., Bordwell, B., Marino, C., and Rothfield, N. (1986). Three human chromosomal autoantigens are recognised by sera from patients with anticentromere antibodies. *Journal of Clinical Investigation*, **77**, 426–30.

Ercilla, M. G. *et al.* (1981). HLA-antigens and scleroderma. *Archives of Dermatological Research*, **271**, 381–5.

Falanga, V. (1989). Localised scleroderma. *Medical Clinics of North America*, **73**, 1143–56.

Falanga, V., Medsger, T. A., Jr, Reichlin, M., and Rodnan, G. P. (1986). Linear scleroderma. Clinical spectrum and laboratory abnormalities. *Annals of Internal Medicine*, **104**, 849–57.

Follansbee, W. P. (1986). The cardiovascular manifestations of systemic sclerosis (scleroderma). *Current Problems in Cardiology*, **11**, 242–98.

Follansbee, W. P. *et al.* (1990). Myocardial fibrosis in systemic sclerosis (scleroderma): a case controlled clinicopathologic study. *Journal of Rheumatology*, **17**, 656–62.

Freni-Titulaer, L. J. W. *et al.* (1989). Connective tissue disease in south eastern Georgia: a case-control study. *American Journal of Epidemiology*, **129**, 404–9.

Genth, E. *et al.* (1990). Immunogenetic associations of scleroderma associated autoantibodies. *Arthritis and Rheumatism*, **33**, 657–65.

Germain, B. F. *et al.* (1981). Increased prevalence of DRw3 in the CREST syndrome. *Arthritis and Rheumatism*, **24**, 857–9.

Gladman, D. D. *et al.* (1981). Increased frequency of DR5 in scleroderma. *Arthritis and Rheumatism*, **24**, 854–6.

Greydanus, M. P. and Camilleri, M. (1989). Abnormal post-cibal gastric and small bowel motility due to neuropathy or myopathy in systemic sclerosis. *Gastroenterology*, **96**, 110–15.

Hanson, V. (1976). Dermatomyositis, scleroderma and polyarteritis nodosa. *Clinical Rheumatic Diseases*, **2**, 445–67.

Harrison, N. K. *et al.* (1989). Pulmonary involvement in systemic sclerosis: the detection of early changes by thin section CT scan, bronchoalveolar lavage and ^{99m}Tc-DTPA clearance. *Respiratory Medicine*, **83**, 403–14.

Harrison, N. K. *et al.* (1991). Structural features of interstitial lung disease in systemic sclerosis. *American Review of Respiratory Diseases*, **144**, 706–13.

Harvey, W. (1983). Submucous fibrosis. In *Proceedings of the scleroderma symposium*. Smith Kline and French Laboratories Ltd, Welwyn Garden City.

Helfrich, D. J., Banner, B., Steen, V. D., and Medsger, T. A., Jr (1989). Renal failure in normotensive patients with systemic sclerosis. *Arthritis and Rheumatism*, **32**, 1128–34.

Hochberg, M. C. (1994). Silicone breast implants and rheumatic disease. *British Journal of Rheumatology*, **33**, 601–2.

Jabs, E. W., Tuck-Muller, I. C. M., Anhalt, G. J., Earnshaw, W. C, Wise, R. W., and Wigley, F. (1993). Cytogenetic survey in systemic sclerosis and association with autoantibodies to RNA polymerases I and III. *Journal of Clinical Investigation*, **91**, 1399–404.

Jazwinska, E. C. *et al.* (1990). HLA-DRw15 is increased in frequency in Japanese scleroderma patients. *Disease Markers*, **8**, 323–6.

Kahaleh, M. B. (1991). Soluble immunologic products in scleroderma sera. *Clinical Immunology and Immunopathology*, **58**, 139–44.

Kahaleh, M. B. and Mattuci-Cerinic, M. (1995). Raynaud's phenomenon and scleroderma: dysregulated neuroendothelial control of vascular tone. *Arthritis and Rheumatism*, **38**, 1–4.

Kallenberg, C. G. (1994). Antitopoisomerase and anticentromere antibodies in the sclerodermatous complex. *Clinical Reviews in Allergy*, **12**, 221–35.

Kallenberg, C. G. M., Wonda. A. A., Hoet, M. H., and Van Venrooij, W. J. (1988). Development of connective tissue disease in patients presenting with Raynaud's phenomenon: a six-year follow-up with emphasis on the predictive value of antinuclear antibodies as detected by immunoblotting. *Annals of the Rheumatic Diseases*, **47**, 634–41.

Kantor, T. V., Whiteside, T. L., Friberg, D., Buckingham, R. B., and Medsger T. A., Jr (1992). Lymphokine activated killer cells and natural killer cell activities in patients with systemic sclerosis. *Arthritis and Rheumatism*, **35**, 694–9.

Kondo, H. *et al.* (1985). Histocompatibility antigens in progressive systemic sclerosis. In *Systemic sclerosis (scleroderma)* (ed. D. M. Black and A. R. Myers). Gower Medical, New York.

Kovalchik, M. T., Guggenheim, S. J., Robertson, J. S., and Steigerwald, J. C. (1978). The kidney in progressive systemic sclerosis: a prospective study. *Annals of Internal Medicine*, **89**, 881–7.

Kuwana, M., Kaburaki, J., Okano, Y., Inoko, H., and Tsuji, K. (1993). The *HLA-DR* and *DQ* genes control the autoimmune response to DNA topoisomerase 1 in systemic sclerosis (scleroderma). *Journal of Clinical Investigation*, **92**, 1296–301.

Kuwana, M., Medsger, T.A., and Wright, T.M. (1995). T cell proliferative response induced by DNA topoisomerase 1 in patients with systemic sclerosis and healthy donors. *Journal of Clinical Investigation*, **96**, 586–96.

Lally, E. V. (1992). Raynaud's phenomenon. *Current Opinions in Rheumatology*, **4**, 825–36.

Langevitz, P., Buskila, D., Gladman, D. D., Darlington, G. A., Farewell, V. T., and Lee, P. (1992). HLA alleles in systemic sclerosis: associations with pulmonary hypertension and outcome. *British Journal of Rheumatology*, **31**, 609–13.

LeRoy, E. C. (1974). Increased collagen synthesis by scleroderma skin fibroblasts *in vitro*. A possible defect in regulation or activation of scleroderma fibroblasts. *Journal of Clinical Investigation*, **54**, 880–9.

LeRoy, E. C. *et al.* (1988). Scleroderma (systemic sclerosis): classification, subsets, and pathogenesis. *Journal of Rheumatology*, **15**, 202–5.

Levine, B., Hardwick, J. M., Trapp, B. D., Crawford, T. O., Bollinger, R. C., and Griffin, D. E. (1991). Antibody mediated clearance of alpha virus infection in neurones. *Science*, **254**, 865–70.

Livingstone, J. Z. *et al.* (1987). Systemic sclerosis (scleroderma): clinical, genetic and serological subsets. *Journal of Rheumatology*, **14**, 512–18.

Luderschmidt, C. *et al.* (1987). Associations of progressive systemic scleroderma to several HLA-B and HLA-DR alleles. *Archives of Dermatology*, **123**, 1188–91.

Lupoli, S., Amlot, P., and Black, C. M. (1990). Normal immune responses in systemic sclerosis. *Journal of Rheumatology*, **17**, 323–37.

Lynch, C. J. *et al.* (1982). Histocompatibility antigens in progressive systemic sclerosis (scleroderma). *Journal of Clinical Immunology*, **2**, 314–18.

Ma, J., Chapman, G. V., Chen, S. L., Melick, G., Penny, R., and Briet, S. N. (1991). Antibody penetration of viable human cells: I. Increased penetration of human lymphocytes by anti-RNP IgG. *Clinical and Experimental Immunology*, **84**, 83–91.

McCarthy, G. M. and Kenny, D. (1992). Dietary fish oil in rheumatic diseases. *Seminars in Arthritis and Rheumatism*, **21**, 318–75.

McHugh, N. J. *et al.* (1994). Anti-centromere antibodies (ACA) in systemic sclerosis patients and their relatives: a serological and HLA study. *Clinical and Experimental Immunology*, **96**, 267–74.

Mackel, A. M., De Lustro, F., Harper, F. E., and LeRoy, E. C. (1982) Antibodies to collagen in scleroderma. *Arthritis and Rheumatism*, **25**, 522–31.

Maricq, H. R. *et al.* (1989). Prevalence of scleroderma spectrum disorders in the general population of South Carolina. *Arthritis and Rheumatism*, **32**, 998–1006.

Masi, A. T. (1988). Classification of systemic sclerosis (scleroderma): relationship of cutaneous subgroups in early disease to outcome and serologic reactivity. *Journal of Rheumatology*, **15**, 894–8.

Mason, G. R., Uzzler, J. M., Effros, R. M., and Reid, E. (1983). Rapidly reversible alterations of pulmonary epithelial permeability induced by smoking. *Chest*, **83**, 6–11.

Mauch, C., Eckes, B., Hunzelman, N., Oono, T., Kozlowska, E., and Krieg, T. (1993). Control of fibrosis in systemic scleroderma. *Journal of Investigative Dermatology*, **100**, 92–6S.

Medsger, T. A., Jr (1979). Progressive systemic sclerosis — skeletal muscle involvement. *Clinical Rheumatic Diseases*, **5**, 103–13.

Miller, K. S., Smith, E. A., Kinsella, M., Schabel, S. I., and Silver, R. M. (1990). Lung disease associated with progressive systemic sclerosis. Assessment of interlobar variation by bronchoalveolar lavage and comparison with non-invasive evaluation of disease activity. *American Review of Respiratory Disease*, **141**, 301–6.

Muller, N. L. and Miller, R. R. (1990). Computed tomography of chronic diffuse infiltrative lung disease. *American Review of Respiratory Disease*, **142**, 1206–15; 1440–8.

Myers, A. R. *et al.* (1989). Class II major histocompatibility complex antigens and pulmonary fibrosis in systemic sclerosis. (Abstract). *Arthritis and Rheumatism*, **32** (Suppl.), S77.

Padula, S. J., Clark, R. B., and Korn, J. H. (1986). Cell mediated immunity in rheumatic diseases. *Human Pathology*, **17**, 254–63.

Pearson, J. D. (1990). The endothelium: its role in systemic sclerosis. *Annals of the Rheumatic Diseases*, **50**, 866–71.

Pollard, K. M., Reimer, G., and Tan, E. M. (1989). Autoantibodies in scleroderma. *Clinical and Experimental Rheumatology*, **7** (Suppl. 3), 57–62.

Pope, J. E. and Bellamy, N. (1993). Outcome measurements in scleroderma clinical trials. *Seminars in Arthritis and Rheumatism*, **23**, 22–33.

Prescott, R. J., Freemont, A. J., Jones, C. J., Hoyland, J., and Fielding, P. (1992). Sequential dermal microvascular and perivascular changes in the development of scleroderma. *Journal of Pathology*, **166**, 255–63.

Reeves, W. H., Satih, M., Wang, J., Chou, C-H, and Ajmani, A. K. (1994). Antibodies to DNA, DNA binding proteins, and histones. *Rheumatic Disease Clinics of North America*, **20**, 1–28.

Reveille, J. D., Owerbach, D., Goldstein, R., Moreda, R., Isern, R. A., and Arnett, F. C. (1992*a*). Association of polar amino acids at position 26 of the *HLA-DQB1* first domain with the anticentromere autoantibody response in systemic sclerosis (scleroderma). *Journal of Clinical Investigation*, **89**, 1208–13.

Reveille, J. D., Durban, E., Macleod, St Clair, *et al.* (1992*b*). Association of amino acid sequences in the *HLA-DQB1* first domain with the anti-topoisomerase 1 autoantibody response in scleroderma. *Journal of Clinical Investigation*, **90**, 973–80.

Rodnan, G. P. and Benedek, T. G. (1962). An historical account of the study of progressive systemic sclerosis (diffuse scleroderma). *Annals of Internal Medicine*, **57**, 305–19.

Roumm, A. D., Whiteside, T. L., Medsger, T. A., Jr, and Rodnan, G. P. (1984). Lymphocytes in the skin of patients with progressive systemic sclerosis. *Arthritis and Rheumatism*, **29**, 645–53.

Russell, M. L. (1988). Muscle and nerve in systemic sclerosis (scleroderma). In *Systemic sclerosis: scleroderma* (ed. C. M. Black and M. I. V. Jayson). Wiley, Chichester.

Russell, M. L., Friesen, D., Henderson, R. D., and Hanna, W. M. (1982). Ultrastructure of the oesophagus in scleroderma. *Arthritis and Rheumatism*, **25**, 1117–23.

Sasaki, T., Denpo, K., Ono, H., and Nakjima, J. (1991). HLA in systemic sclerosis (PSS) and familial scleroderma. *Journal of Dermatology*, **18**, 18–24.

Seibold, J. R., Medsger, T. A., Jr, Winkelstein, A., Kelly, R. H., and Rodnan, G. P. (1982). Immune complexes an progressive systemic sclerosis (scleroderma). *Arthritis and Rheumatism*, **25**, 1167–73.

Shorrock, C. J. and Rees, W. D. W. (1988). Gastrointestinal manifestations of systemic sclerosis. In *Systemic sclerosis: scleroderma* (ed. C. M. Black and M. I. V. Jayson). Wiley, Chichester.

Silman, A. J. (1995). Scleroderma. *Ballière's Clinical Rheumatology*, **9**, 471–8.

Silver, R. M. (1990). Clinical aspects of systemic sclerosis (scleroderma). *Annals of the Rheumatic Diseases*, **50** (Suppl. 4), 854–61.

Silver, R. M., Miller, K. S., Kinsella, M. B., Smith E. A., and Schabel, S. I. (1990). Evaluation and management of scleroderma lung disease using bronchoalveolar lavage. *American Journal of Medicine*, **88**, 470–6

Steen, V. D. (1984). Factors predicting the development of renal involvement in progressive systemic sclerosis. *American Journal of Medicine*, **76**, 799–86.

Steen, V. D., Powell, D. L., and Medsger, T. A., Jr (1988). Clinical correlations and prognosis based on serum autoantibodies in patients with systemic sclerosis. *Arthritis and Rheumatism*, **31**, 196–203.

Steen, V. D., Constantino, J. P., Shapiro, A. P., and Medsger, T. A., Jr (1990). Outcome of renal crisis in systemic sclerosis: relation to the availability of converting enzyme inhibitors (ACE). *Annals of Internal Medicine*, **113**, 352–7.

Steen, V. D., Conte, C., and Medsger, T. A., Jr (1994). Case-control study of corticosteroid use prior to scleroderma renal crisis. (Abstract). *Arthritis and Rheumatism*, **37** (Suppl.), S360.

Subcommittee for Scleroderma Criteria of the American Rheumatism Association Diagnostic and Therapeutic Criteria Committee (1980). Preliminary criteria for the classification of systemic sclerosis (scleroderma). *Arthritis and Rheumatism*, **23**, 581–90.

Tan, E. M. (1989). Antinuclear antibodies: diagnostic markers for autoimmune diseases and probes for cell biology. *Advances in Immunology*, **44**, 93–151.

Tarkowski, A. and Lindgren, I. (1994). Beneficial effects of anti-thymocyte globulin in severe cases of progressive systemic sclerosis. *Transplantation Proceedings*, **26**, 3197–9.

Traub, Y. M. *et al.* (1984). Hypertension and renal failure (scleroderma renal crisis) in progressive systemic sclerosis. Report of a 25 year experience with 68 cases. *Medicine*, **62**, 335–52.

Uitto, J., Bauer, E., and Eisen, A. Z. (1979). Scleroderma: increased biosynthesis of triple-helical type I and type III procollagens associated with unaltered collagenase by skin fibroblasts in culture. *Journal of Clinical Investigation*, **64**, 921–30.

Valesini, G. *et al.* (1993). Geographical clustering of scleroderma in a rural area in the province of Rome. *Clinical and Experimental Rheumatology*, **11**, 41–7.

Warrick, J. H., Bhalla, M., Schabel, S. I., and Silver, R. M. (1991). High resolution computed tomography in early scleroderma lung disease. *Journal of Rheumatology*, **18**, 1520–8.

Wells, A. U., Hansell, D. M., Harrison, N. K., Lawrence, R., Black, C. M., and du Bois, R. M. (1993a). Clearance of inhaled 99m-Tc DTPA predicts the clinical course of fibrosing alveolitis. *European Respiratory Journal*, **6**, 797–802.

Wells, A. U., Hansell, D. M., Rubens, M. B., Cullinan, P., Black, C. M., and du Bois, R. M. (1993b). The predictive value of appearances on thin section computed tomography in fibrosing alveolitis, *American Review of Respiratory Disease*, **148**, 1076–82.

Wells, A. U., Hansell, D.M., Rubens, M.B., *et al.* (1994). Fibrosing alveolitis associated with progressive systemic sclerosis: the relationship between bronchoalveolar lavage cellularity and computed tomographic appearances. *American Journal of Respiratory and Critical Care Medicine*, **150**, 462–8.

White, B. (1994). Immunologic aspects of scleroderma. *Current Opinion in Rheumatology*, **6**, 612–15.

Whiteside, T.L., Medsger, T.A. Jr., and Rodnan, G.P. (1983). HLA-DR antigens in progressive systemic sclerosis. *Journal of Rheumatology*, **10**, 128–31.

Williams, W.V., Rook, A.H., Freundlich, B.F., *et al.* (1995). T-cell receptors in scleroderma skin. The effect of photopheresis. *Annals of the New York Academy of Sciences*, **756**, 424–7.

Wollersheim, H., Thien, T., Hoet, M. H., and Van Venrooy, W. J. (1989). The diagnostic value of several immunological tests for antinuclear antibody in predicting the development of connective tissue disease in patients presenting with Raynaud's phenomenon. *European Journal of Clinical Investigation*, **19**, 535–41.

Youssef, P., Englert, H., and Bertouch, J. (1993). Large vessel occlusive disease associated with CREST syndrome and scleroderma. *Annals of the Rheumatic Diseases*, **52**, 564–9.

Zacheriae, H., Halkier-Sorensen, L., Heickendorff, L., Zacheriae, E., and Hansen, H.E. (1990). Cyclosporin A treatment of systemic sclerosis. *British Journal of Dermatology*, **122**, 677–81.

Polymyositis and dermatomyositis

5.9.1 Polymyositis and dermatomyositis in adults

Ira N. Targoff

Introduction

Polymyositis and dermatomyositis are the most common forms of 'idiopathic inflammatory myopathy', a category that also encompasses inclusion body myositis, and several rare forms. Inflammatory myopathy may also be induced by drugs or infections. Dermatomyositis is distinguished from polymyositis by the presence of a characteristic rash. Weakness affecting skeletal muscle is the major clinical manifestation of most patients, although the skin rash or other extramuscular features may predominate in some.

Wagner first described a case as polymyositis in 1863, while Unverricht first used the term dermatomyositis in 1887. Early studies often included cases that would not fit our present concept. The wide acceptance of the diagnostic criteria of Bohan and Peter (1975) has served to standardize subsequent studies and promote recognition.

Epidemiology

Incidence and prevalence

Estimates of the annual incidence of polymyositis/dermatomyositis have ranged from 1 to 9 cases per million per year, and prevalence from 2.4 to 10.7 cases per 100 000 (Cronin and Plotz 1990; Sigurgeirsson *et al.* 1992; Ahlstrom *et al.* 1993). For example, Oddis *et al.* (1990a) in Pittsburgh, Pennsylvania, found 5.5 per million per year, with an increased incidence over time (2.5 cases per million per year in the first decade, 8.9 per million per year in the second) that could reflect better detection and recognition, or a true increase.

Polymyositis is more common than dermatomyositis in most studies of adults (Bohan *et al.* 1977; Tymms and Webb 1985), but the ratio (less than 2:1) is low and may vary with the population, referral patterns, or criteria for dermatomyositis. Some studies found dermatomyositis to be more common (Ramirez *et al.* 1990; Love *et al.* 1991; Koh *et al.* 1993). Overlap syndromes with other autoimmune rheumatic diseases occur in 15 to 20 per cent.

Risk factors

Polymyositis/dermatomyositis is fourfold more common in the United States in black patients than white patients (Cronin and Plotz 1990). The female:male ratio is 2:1 overall, but lower in myositis with malignancy, and higher during the childbearing years (5:1) and in patients with associated autoimmune rheumatic diseases (Bohan *et al.* 1977). Polymyositis and dermatomyositis may begin at almost any age, but the peak in adults is usually from 40 to 60 years; it tends to develop later in white than in black women (Oddis *et al.* 1990a), and later with cancer (Love *et al.* 1991).

Cases of adult polymyositis and dermatomyositis among family members are very rare, but have been observed (Gurley *et al.* 1992; Garlepp 1993). A family history of myopathy should make one question the diagnosis of polymyositis/dermatomyositis. Other autoimmune disease in relatives of polymyositis and dermatomyositis patients is not unusual (Mbauya *et al.* 1993).

Temporal and geographic factors

Most studies have not found variation in the incidence of adult-onset polymyositis /dermatomyositis with time of year, although one study found a higher rate from March to May (Manta *et al.* 1989). However, certain autoantibody-defined subgroups show significant seasonal differences in the onset of myositis: anti-Jo-1-associated myositis begins more often in the spring, and anti-**SRP**-(signal recognition particle)-myositis more often in the autumn (Leff *et al.* 1991).

Polymyositis and dermatomyositis occur in all parts of the world, but in developing countries infectious myositis is more common. Occasional local clusters of myositis have been reported, which may have atypical features (Nagaraja *et al.* 1992). Certain autoantibodies appeared to differ in prevalence in different regions (Love *et al.* 1992).

Clinical picture

Classification

Several classification systems have been proposed to define subgroups of patients with idiopathic inflammatory myopathies that are more clinically homogeneous (Dalakas 1988a; Miller 1994; Medsger and Oddis 1995), and able to predict course and responsiveness. Disagreement remains, however, due to our lack of knowledge of aetiology.

Most recent studies have used the Bohan and Peter (1975) classification (Table 1), or modifications. Pure polymyositis is separated from dermatomyositis, but not in the presence of malignancy, juvenile onset, or an associated autoimmune rheumatic disease. Patients are usually considered to have dermatomyositis rather than polymyositis only when the rash is observed, but some also include patients without overt skin lesions who have characteristic muscle pathology (Byrne and Dennett 1993). Inclusion-body myositis is a clinically and histologically distinct entity, and should probably be classified separately even when associated with malignancy or autoimmune

Table 1 Classification of idiopathic inflammatory myopathies[a]

   I. Primary idiopathic polymyositis

   II. Primary idiopathic dermatomyositis

   III. Polymyositis or dermatomyositis with malignancy

   IV. Juvenile dermatomyositis (or polymyositis)

   V. Overlap syndrome of polymyositis or dermatomyositis with
      another autoimmune rheumatic disease

   VI. Inclusion-body myositis[a]

   VII. Rare forms of idiopathic myositis
      (a) Granulomatous myositis
      (b) Eosinophilic myositis
      (c) Focal myositis
      (d) Orbital myositis

[a]Classes I to V correspond to Bohan and Peter's original classification (Bohan and Peter (1975).
[a]Patients with inclusion body myositis in association with malignancy or other autoimmune rheumatic diseases should be considered to be class VI.

rheumatic diseases (see later section). Several rare but distinctive forms of idiopathic myositis have also been defined (Table 1).

Certain specific autoantibodies can define subgroups of patients that differ from the overall myositis population with regard to clinical features, response to therapy, prognosis, and HLA type (Love et al. 1991). These autoantibodies can be used to classify patients in a way that is complementary to clinical classification.

Clinical features

Myositis

Weakness

Muscle weakness is the main clinical feature of both polymyositis and dermatomyositis, occurring in almost all patients. It usually develops insidiously over weeks to months, generally more slowly in polymyositis than dermatomyositis (Casademont et al. 1993). More indolent cases may be seen, progressing over years (more in polymyositis than dermatomyositis), that must be distinguished from inclusion-body myositis. More rapid onset occurs occasionally.

The weakness is typically symmetrical, affecting the large proximal muscles around the shoulders, hips, thighs, trunk and neck. The lower extremities are often involved first, but in most patients both upper and lower extremity involvement occurs (Plotz et al. 1989; Henriksson and Lindvall 1990). Patients often have impairment in performance of daily activities such as standing from a chair, getting out of a car, climbing stairs, reaching (e.g. into cabinets), working overhead (hanging clothes, etc.), or combing their hair. The gait may be affected. Getting out of bed, sitting from a supine position, or raising the head off the pillow may become difficult. Weakness of distal muscles is uncommon in polymyositis/dermatomyositis, but may occur late in the course (in about 10 per cent of caes, Love et al. 1991). Patients may note impairment of chewing or dysphagia (see below). Involvement of the face is unusual, and involvement of extraocular muscles is rare, and should suggest other diagnoses (Dalakas 1991). Within regions of weakness, there is usually diffuse involvement, unlike some myopathies in which weakness and atrophy may be highly selective for specific muscles.

Other muscle manifestations

Myalgia and muscle tenderness occur in about half of patients, usually as mild aching or soreness. They are usually not predominant, but may be more severe when myositis develops acutely, and occasionally can lead to confusion with polymyalgia rheumatica (Hopkinson et al. 1991). There may be atrophy in chronic disease, seen in 9 per cent by Love et al. (1991), more commonly in polymyositis than dermatomyositis. Contractures may occur with disease of long duration.

Examination

Muscle strength can be assessed as part of initial evaluation and later monitoring of progress by observing activities and by direct muscle testing. Walking, standing from a squatting position or low chair without using the arms, sitting up or raising the head from a supine position, and raising the arms overhead, should be tested, or multiple repetitions timed (Csuka and McCarty 1985; Moxley 1994). Deltoids, biceps, iliopsoas, quadriceps, and other proximal muscles should be manually tested directly, and graded by systems such as the Medical Research Council scale. In order to overcome insensitivity and subjectivity, and standardize and quantify such testing, there is continuing interest in the use of biomechanical measures of muscle strength with machines that can measure applied force (Moxley 1994). Fafalak et al. (1994) found that improved strength by a mechanical measure correlated well with a functional assessment scale. All types of muscle strength testing depend on effort, and may be complicated by fatigue or pain of arthritis or myalgia.

Cutaneous manifestations

Rash

The dermatomyositis rash, found in about 30 to 40 per cent of adults with myositis, most commonly precedes the weakness by weeks to several months, or even longer (Hochberg et al. 1986; Rockerbie et al. 1989). At presentation, 93 per cent of adult dermatomyositis patients of Bohan et al. (1977) had a rash but only 53 per cent weakness. The activity of the rash may parallel that of the weakness or may be independent, and can persist after the myositis resolves.

Gottron's lesions

Erythematous or violaceous, sometimes scaly, papules or plaques (Gottron's papules) or macular patches (Gottron's sign) may occur over the metacarpophalangeal and proximal (and less often distal) interphalangeal joints (Fig. 1) (Franks 1988), and also over the extensor surfaces of the knees, wrists, elbows or medial malleoli (Fig. 2). These lesions may be found in 70 to 80 per cent of dermatomyositis patients, and are considered pathognomonic (Euwer and Sontheimer 1994). Telangiectasia and atrophy can occur. The erythematous finger rash of systemic lupus erythematosus differs in that it usually occurs between the knuckles.

Erythematous and/or poikilodermatous rash

A macular erythematous or violaceous eruption may involve the upper chest, neck, shoulders, extremities, hands, scalp and face. It may develop into poikiloderma, varied hyper- and hypopigmentation

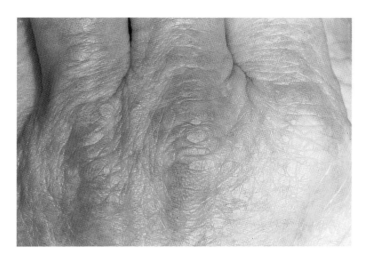

Fig. 1 Skin over the metacarpcphalangeal joints of a patient with dermatomyosis shows the characteristic erythematous lesions of Gottron's sign. (By courtesy of the Department of Dermatology, University of Oklahoma Health Sciences Center.)

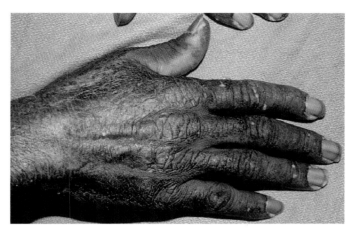

Fig. 3 Hand of a patient with dermatomyositis shows Gottron's papules over the proximal interphalangeal and metacarpophalangeal joints, with marked linear extensor erythema extending from the joints along the tendons. In black patients, the lesions may appear hyperpigmented. (By courtesy of Dr Frank C. Arnett, University of Texas at Houston Health Sciences Center.)

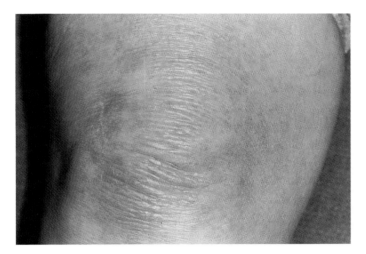

Fig. 2 Skin over the knee of a patient with dermatomyositis shows a characteristic erythematous, violaceous lesion. (By courtesy of the Department of Dermatology, University of Oklahoma Health Sciences Center.)

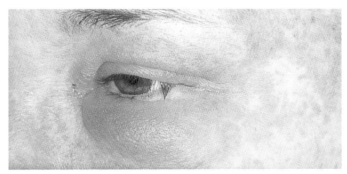

Fig. 4 A severe heliotrope rash of dermatomyositis, with the characteristic lilac colour and accompanying periorbital oedema. (By courtesy of the Department of Dermatology, University of Oklahoma Health Sciences Center.)

with atrophy and fine telangiectasias. Typical of dermatomyositis are the 'V' sign (involvement at the anterior base, 'V', of the neck; 36 per cent of cases), and the 'shawl' sign (back of neck, upper torso, and shoulders in a shawl-like pattern; 22 per cent) (Love *et al.* 1991). Erythema may extend from the joints along the course of the extensor tendons (linear extensor erythema, Franks 1988; Fig. 3). Kasteler and Callen (1994) noted a high frequency of scalp involvement (82 per cent), marked by erythema, atrophy, scale, and sometimes alopecia that can be misdiagnosed as psoriasis or seborrheic dermatitis. Rash on the malar areas, forehead and chin may lead to confusion with systemic lupus erythematosus, although involvement of the naso-labial folds may be a clue (Plotz *et al.* 1989).

Patients often report exacerbation or development of new lesions after sun exposure (Callen 1987), and this has also been documented after therapeutic ultraviolet or experimental solar-simulated light (Cheong *et al.* 1994; Euwer and Sontheimer 1994). The distribution also suggests photosensitivity, but can occur without sun exposure (Franks 1988).

Heliotrope

The heliotrope rash, found in about 30 to 60 per cent of dermato-myositis, is a purplish, lilac-coloured suffusion (resembling a heliotrope flower) around the eyes, particularly the upper eyelids and surrounding area (Fig. 4), often associated with periorbital oedema. It is characteristic but not pathognomonic of dermatomyositis, since a similar appearance may occasionally be seen in allergy, trichinosis, lupus, or other conditions (Euwer and Sontheimer 1994). It may be difficult to see in black patients.

Other cutaneous features

Periungual telangiectasia and/or haemorrhages are also seen in dermatomyositis (Franks 1988). Nailfold capillaries may show marked changes similar to those in scleroderma, including throm-bosis and haemorrhage, giant capillary loops, and capillary loss, that may parallel disease activity (Fig. 5). The cuticles may be thickened, roughened, and irregular (Fig. 6) (Caro 1988).

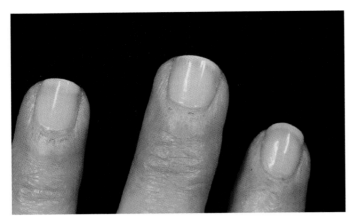

Fig. 5 Nailfold vascular changes in a patient with amyopathic dermatomyosistis for 4 years. Capillary dilatation, dropout, and haemorrhage are evident without microscopy. Gottron's papules were present over the proximal interphalangeal joints of the index and middle fingers, with suggestive lesions visible over the distal interphalangeal joints. (By courtesy of Dr Lela Lee, Department of Dermatology, University of Oklahoma Health Sciences Center.)

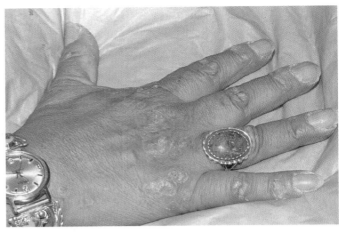

(a)

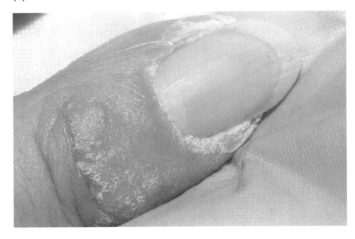

(b)

Fig. 6 (a) Hand of a patient with anti-Mi-2-positive dermatomyosistis with severe weakness of 2 months duration. Typical Gottron's papules are seen over the metacarpophalangeal, and proximal and distal interphalangeal joints, with more scale than in Fig. 7. There is cuticular hyperkeratosis around many nails, and mechanic's hand change on the thumb. (By courtesy of Dr E. Taylor-Albert, University of Oklahoma Health Sciences Center). (b) Thumb of the patient in (a). Cuticular changes are evident. A Gottron's papule is over the interphalangeal joint.

Hyperkeratosis and scaling with fissuring and hyperpigmentation may appear as dirty horizontal lines along the lateral and palmar aspects of the fingers ('mechanic's hands') (Fig. 7). This lesion was associated strongly with antisynthetase autoantibodies (Love *et al.* 1991) (see below). Although often seen without other signs of dermatomyosistis, the histology resembles dermatomyosistis (Mitra *et al.* 1994).

Calcinosis can occur in adults but is more common in juvenile dermatomyosistis. It can be extensive, and usually occurs late. Cutaneous vasculitis, especially of the fingers, is not infrequent in adult dermatomyosistis (Ramirez *et al.* 1990); cutaneous ulcers associated with severe vasculopathy of juvenile dermatomyosistis (Roberts and Fink 1988) may rarely be seen in adults (Fig. 8). Other rare manifestations include panniculitis (Fusade *et al.* 1993), and erythroderma (Ramirez *et al.* 1990).

Amyopathic dermatomyosistis

There is increasing recognition of patients with typical cutaneous dermatomyosistis who do not develop myositis (Fig. 9). Some of the patients have subclinical myositis demonstrable by testing (see below), and some later develop overt myositis, but some have no sign of myositis for as long as 12 years (Rockerbie *et al.* 1989; Stonecipher *et al.* 1993). 'Amyopathic dermatomyosistis' (or 'dermatomyosistis sine myositis') is applied to those with rash alone for at least 2 years without treatment. Such patients cannot satisfy criteria for dermatomyosistis, which are based on the myositis, and alternative criteria and a separate classification category have been proposed (Euwer and Sontheimer 1993). The risk of malignancy and systemic complications appears similar to usual dermatomyosistis (Euwer and Sontheimer 1993; Euwer and Sontheimer 1994).

Manifestations in other systems

Systemic signs

Fatigue and malaise are common and must be distinguished from muscle weakness. Weight loss may be impressive in some patients (Tymms and Webb 1985). Fevers are seen in about 40 per cent

overall, but are associated strongly with antisynthetases (87 per cent, versus 23 per cent without antibody, Love *et al.* 1991).

Pulmonary disease

Pulmonary involvement resulting from muscle weakness, treatment, or the underlying disease (Table 2), occurs in 40 to 50 per cent of patients (Dickey and Myers 1984), contributing to morbidity and mortality (Arsura and Greenberg 1988).

Respiratory muscle weakness

Clinical respiratory muscle weakness develops in 4 to 7 per cent of patients (Dickey and Myers 1984), but a measurable decrease in respiratory muscle strength may be more common (Braun *et al.* 1983). Both inspiratory and expiratory muscles may be affected, including the diaphragm. Total lung capacity and vital capacity are decreased, while residual volume may be increased. Respiratory

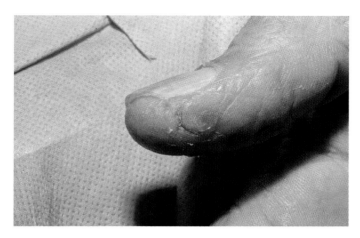

Fig. 7 Thumb of a patient with anti-Jo-1-positive polymyositis. The edge of the thumb shows fissuring and some hyperkeratosis as in mechanic's hands. (By courtesy of Dr Frank C. Arnett, University of Texas at Houston Health Sciences Center.)

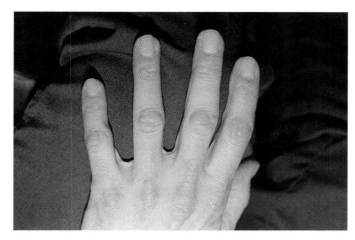

Fig. 9 Skin over the finger joints of a patient with cutaneous dermatomyositis for less than 6 months, but without evident muscle disease, showing characteristic lesions. The metacarpophalangeal region shows Gottron's papules (raised erythematous lesions with fine scale) with additional erythema extending along the tendons, most evident on the middle finger, consistent with linear extensor erythema. Classic Gottron's papules have formed over the proximal interphalangeal and, to a lesser extent, the distal interphalangeal joints. (By courtesy of Dr Lela Lee, Dept. of Dermatology, University of Oklahoma Health Sciences Center.)

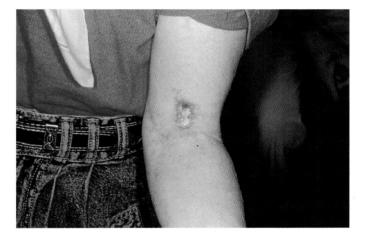

Fig. 8 Cutaneous ulcer in a 32-year-old woman with dermatomyositis. Endothelial cell swelling and change (vasculopathy) without inflammatory invasion of the vessel wall (vasculitis) was seen by biopsy. (By courtesy of the Department of Dermatology, University of Oklahoma Health Sciences Center.)

Table 2 Features of polymyositis/dermatomyositis in addition to muscle and skin involvement
Pulmonary
Due to weakness:
Ventilatory failure
Aspiration pneumonia
Due to treatment:
Hypersensitivity pneumonitis
Opportunistic infection
Due to disease:
Interstitial lung disease
Pulmonary hypertension
Pulmonary vasculitis
Cardiac
Heart block
Arrhythmias
Cardiomyopathy
Gastrointestinal
Oesophagus (dysphagia)
Striated muscle dysfunction
Cricopharyngeal dysfunction
Lower oesophageal dysfunction
Stomach, intestines
Decreased motility
Arthritis
Mild, responsive
Deforming, minimally erosive

failure requiring assisted ventilation may result, and may develop rapidly. It is usually responsive to or prevented by treatment. Most of these patients have had involvement of the pharyngeal and tongue muscles with dysphagia and impaired speech. Patients at risk should be monitored closely, commonly in hospital, using serial pulmonary function testing to judge respiratory muscle strength (expiratory pressure, peak flow, etc.). Rarely, weakness may involve respiratory muscles selectively or disproportionately, and be the presenting feature (Sano *et al.* 1994). Pharyngeal and tongue involvement also increase risk of aspiration, as does impaired cough and difficulty turning or sitting up in bed. Most patients with aspiration have had dysphagia (Lakhanpal *et al.* 1987).

Pulmonary complications of treatment

New interstitial infiltrates in patients with polymyositis/dermato-myositis on immunosuppressive agents may cause diagnostic confusion between the disease itself (see below) and effects of treatment, including opportunistic infections and drug reactions. Methotrexate hypersensitivity pneumonitis can occur in polymyositis/dermatomyositis, which can present acutely with fever, cough, dyspnoea, bilateral interstitial infiltrates, and with lymphocytic infiltrates on biopsy. It usually improves after withdrawal of the drug, but corticosteroids may be required. Pulmonary reactions may rarely occur with azathioprine.

Interstitial lung disease

Interstitial lung disease is found in 10 to 30 per cent of polymyositis and dermatomyositis overall (Hochberg *et al.* 1986; Love *et al.* 1991), and may be more easily diagnosed by pulmonary function testing than by chest radiography. It is much more frequent in patients with antisynthetases. Interstitial lung disease in polymyositis/dermatomyositis is similar to idiopathic interstitial lung disease (Targoff 1990). A small proportion have a fulminant course with fever and rapidly progressive dyspnoea that may be fatal within weeks. A second group has a more chronic course, and a third group may have asymptomatic test abnormalities. Chest radiography shows a reticulonodular pattern, often more prominent in the lower lobes (Fig. 10), and pulmonary function tests show a restrictive defect with decreased diffusing capacity and hypoxaemia with exercise, early signs that can be used to assess progress.

Interstitial lung disease may occur in polymyositis/dermatomyositis of any type (including cancer-associated). The severity of the interstitial lung disease is unrelated to that of the myositis, even occurring in amyopathic dermatomyositis (Euwer and Sontheimer 1994). It may precede myositis in up to 40 per cent of cases (Schwarz *et al.* 1976), and limitations from interstitial lung disease may mask muscle weakness in others. Elevated creatine kinase, myositis-specific autoantibodies, or the dermatomyositis rash may be clues to underlying polymyositis/dermatomyositis.

Lung histology shows interstitial mononuclear cell infiltrates (Fig. 11) with a variable amount of fibrosis. Often there is a loss of type I cells, proliferation of type II cells, and increased numbers of free alveolar macrophages. Tazelaar *et al.* (1990) identified four histological patterns among 15 patients: bronchiolitis obliterans with organizing pneumonia (6 patients), usual interstitial pneumonitis, diffuse alveolar damage, and cellular interstitial pneumonia. Those with bronchiolitis obliterans had the best prognosis, as in other studies (Hsue *et al.* 1993), while all three with diffuse alveolar damage died. Direct immunofluorescence has been negative for immunoglobulin or complement deposition in most studies.

There may be medial and/or intimal thickening of small pulmonary arteries or arterioles as in pulmonary hypertension, which may occur in association with interstitial fibrosis (Schwarz *et al.* 1976). Pulmonary vasculitis may also occur (Lakhanpal *et al.* 1987). Hebert *et al.* (1990) found pulmonary hypertension in 7 of 11 patients using echocardiography, but the clinical significance is unclear.

There have been at least 21 case reports of spontaneous pneumomediastinum in dermatomyositis (adult and juvenile, not polymyositis), usually associated with interstitial lung disease, often with normal creatine kinase (Matsuda *et al.* 1993). The mechanism for this potentially fatal complication is unclear.

Cardiac disease

The potential for cardiac involvement in polymyositis/dermatomyositis was recognized early, but was considered unusual. More

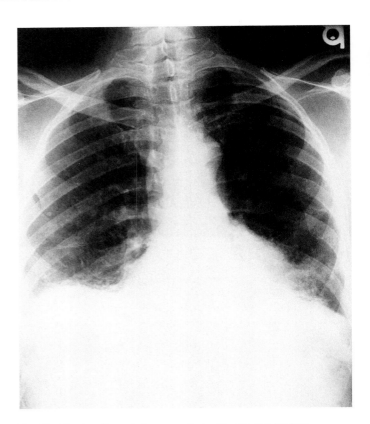

Fig. 10 Chest radiograph from a patient with anti-Jo-1-positive polymyositis that shows severe interstitial fibrosis affecting predominantly the lower lobes.

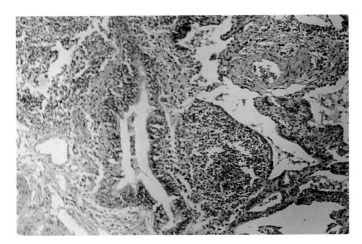

Fig. 11 Lung pathology from a patient with anti-Jo-1-positive polymyositis, showing severe mononuclear cell infiltration and thickening of the interstitium.

recent studies have found signs of cardiac involvement in excess of 70 per cent of cases (Taylor *et al.* 1993). It is commonly asymptomatic, but may contribute to mortality (Hochberg *et al.* 1986). The activity of the cardiac disease may be independent of the myositis (Rechavia *et al.* 1985). The major manifestations include conduction disturbances, arrhythmias, and myocarditis.

The frequency of conduction block varies, but only occasionally does advanced heart block occur requiring a pacemaker. Taylor *et al.* (1993) found ECG abnormalities in 81 per cent, but 58 per cent were non-specific ST and T-wave changes, and significant conduction block was uncommon. Fibrosis of the conducting system was correlated with conduction disturbance in some cases (Haupt and Hutchins 1982), and inflammation has also been seen.

The most common arrhythmias seen are extrasystoles and tachyarrhythmias, and are usually mild (Taylor *et al.* 1993). Love *et al.* (1991) found palpitations in 26 per cent, more in polymyositis (57 per cent) than dermatomyositis (19 per cent) or other subgroups. A Holter monitor should be considered in patients with palpitations or ECG abnormalities.

Congestive heart failure resulting from myocarditis is uncommon in polymyositis and dermatomyositis, and is found in about 3 per cent (Bohan *et al.* 1977). Myocarditis was seen in a quarter of patients in an autopsy study (Haupt and Hutchins 1982), where severe cardiac disease would be overrepresented. A diffuse interstitial and perivascular mononuclear cell infiltrate may be seen, similar to that in skeletal muscle, with replacement fibrosis and sometimes small vessel disease with medial smooth muscle hyperplasia (Denbow *et al.* 1979).

A reported increase in mild mitral valve prolapse, possibly from myocarditis, was not seen in other studies (Taylor *et al.* 1993). Pericardial effusions are seen in 5 to 25 per cent of polymyositis/dermatomyositis by echocardiogram, but are usually asymptomatic (Tami and Bhasin 1993). Significant pericarditis without systemic lupus erythematosus overlap is rare.

Gastrointestinal disease

Dysphagia may occur in up to 30 per cent (Tymms and Webb 1985), particularly with more severe disease. It predisposes to aspiration and has been associated with a poor prognosis. Dysphagia can result from weakness of the muscles of swallowing (pharyngeal muscles or striated muscles of the upper oesophagus), correlating with disease activity and responding to treatment (Dietz *et al.* 1980). It may be worse while recumbent, and can cause regurgitation of liquids into the nose with attempted swallowing. Changes in the voice (nasal speech or hoarseness) may be associated. Histology is similar to that of other striated muscle, dysphagia but may occasionally be the presenting or sole complaint.

Abnormalities of oesophageal motility have been reported to be common, involving both upper and lower oesophagus (DeMerieux *et al.* 1983). Involvement is similar to scleroderma, but can occur without other evidence of overlap. It is not associated with inflammation, and does not respond to treatment. Decreased motility and lower oesophageal sphincter pressure may lead to dysphagia, heartburn, reflux, and stricture. Gastric emptying may also be delayed (Horowitz *et al.* 1986).

Cricopharyngeal muscle dysfunction from inflammation and/or fibrosis may lead to a distinctive dysphagia marked by a sensation of food sticking in the back of the throat, or coughing with swallowing. It can be distinguished from weakness by cine-oesophagoscopy and oesophageal manometry, and is important to identify since it may require surgical myotomy (Kagen *et al.* 1985).

Intestinal vasculitis with perforation, as well as pneumatosis cystoides intestinalis, well recognized in juvenile dermatomyositis, are extremely rare in adults, but reported (Ramirez *et al.* 1990).

Malignancy

Association

The link with malignancy was noted in 1916, and was at one point thought to be frequent. Later studies found a much lower frequency, and some questioned the reality of an association (Lakhanpal *et al.* 1986). Most recent studies, however, find a modest increase in malignancies within 1 to 2 years of onset in dermatomyositis, and possibly also polymyositis. Malignancy may be antecedent, concurrent, or subsequent to myositis onset.

The frequency of malignancy in dermatomyositis has ranged from 6 to 43 per cent (Bernard and Bonnetblanc 1993). A large population-based study in Sweden (Sigurgeirsson *et al.* 1992) found increased malignancy in dermatomyositis and polymyositis: 15 per cent of 392 dermatomyositis patients (relative risk, **RR**= 2.4 for men, 3.4 for women) and 9 per cent of 396 polymyositis patients (RR=1.8 for men, 1.7 for women). Cancer deaths were increased in dermatomyositis but not polymyositis, supporting a true association in dermatomyositis, rather than intensive searching. The case–control study of Manchul *et al.* (1985) found that 71 adult polymyositis/dermatomyositis patients had significantly more total antecedent plus concurrent malignancies (21.1 per cent) than matched controls (5.6 per cent with inflammatory disease, 1.4 per cent others), with no difference beyond 6 months after myositis. A meta-analysis that included these studies found a significant overall association with cancer (odds ratio = 4.4 for dermatomyositis, 2.1 for polymyositis), with risk before and after onset for dermatomyositis (Zantos *et al.* 1994).

The activity of the myositis may appear linked to that of the malignancy ('paraneoplastic', 22 per cent of dermatomyositis cancers, Bonnetblanc *et al.* 1990), supporting the validity of an association. The myositis may resolve with treatment of the cancer, be resistant until it is resected, or flare with its recurrence. In the majority, cancer and myositis have an independent course (Callen 1993).

Tumours

A wide variety of tumours have been reported in polymyositis/dermatomyositis patients. Tumours that are frequent in the general population (lung, breast, etc.) are frequent in polymyositis/dermatomyositis. However, a number of studies have indicated an increase in ovarian cancer out of proportion to that of other tumours (Cox *et al.* 1990; Cherin *et al.* 1993b; and others). Sigurgeirsson *et al.* (1992) found a relative risk of 8.2 for ovarian cancer in women with dermatomyositis, and 16.7 during the 5 years after dermatomyositis diagnosis. Three of five patients of Whitmore *et al.* (1994) had amyopathic dermatomyositis; the skin disease was resistant until treatment of the cancer. Tumours were typically stage III or IV serous carcinoma. In Asia, an increase in nasopharyngeal carcinomas has been suggested (Koh *et al.* 1993), which may reflect an increase in such tumours in the population of the region.

Evaluation

The extent of testing that should be performed to uncover an occult malignancy in recent-onset polymyositis/dermatomyositis is controversial. Most of the associated malignancies show abnormalities detectable by a thorough initial evaluation, and all agree with the importance of this step (Callen 1994; Bernard and

Bonnetblanc 1993). It should include careful history and physical examination, rectal examination and stool occult blood testing, breast examination and screening mammography and pelvic examination with Pap smear in women, complete blood counts, chemistries, urinalysis, and chest radiograph, and a prostate-specific antigen test in men. Any abnormalities should be pursued, and the evaluation should be repeated yearly, at least during the 2 to 3 year theoretical risk period.

In addition, most would give special attention to excluding ovarian cancer in women. Ovarian cancer is often missed in dermatomyositis patients, even sometimes by pelvic CT or ultrasound (Sigurgeirsson et al. 1992). Whitmore et al. (1994) recommend routine serial gynaecological examinations, transvaginal ultrasound, and CA-125 levels (even after oophorectomy).

There is disagreement as to the extent of further searching recommended in the absence of abnormalities. Schulman et al. (1991), citing examples of occult cancers, recommend routine upper and lower gastrointestinal barium studies and abdominal and chest CT, with repeat evaluation for myositis flares. Others limit additional testing to those with higher risk, resistant disease, or weight loss. The highest risk is in those aged over 45 with dermatomyositis rather than polymyositis, with no autoimmune rheumatic diseases overlap syndromes or myositis-specific auto-antibodies (**MSAs**) (Love et al. 1991) (although cases with MSAs have occurred). Malignancy may be higher with cutaneous vasculitis, or with capillary damage even without a dermatomyositis rash (Casademont et al. 1993).

Other features, overlap syndromes, and associated conditions

Raynaud's phenomenon and arthralgia/arthritis, common features of autoimmune rheumatic diseases, may occur as part of polymyositis/dermatomyositis. They are more common in polymyositis/dermatomyositis when antisynthetases are present. Patients with polymyositis/dermatomyositis may have overlap syndromes in which diagnostic criteria for other conditions are also fulfilled. Conditions commonly overlapping with polymyositis/dermatomyositis include systemic lupus erythematosus (found in almost half of overlap patients by Love et al. 1991), scleroderma, Sjögren's syndrome (about 20 per cent), and rheumatoid arthritis (6 per cent). The distinction between an autoimmune rheumatic disease overlapping with polymyositis/dermatomyositis versus an autoimmune rheumatic disease with myositis as a manifestation, is not well defined. The relative severity of clinical features, and the serological picture may be helpful.

Renal disease is very rare in pure polymyositis/dermatomyositis without overlap, but focal mesangial proliferative glomerulonephritis has been seen (Frost et al. 1993), including cases with antisynthetases. Renal injury may occur from myoglobinuria.

A variety of other autoimmune conditions have been reported in association with polymyositis and dermatomyositis, including Graves' or Hashimoto's disease, inflammatory bowel disease, cryoglobulinaemia, primary biliary cirrhosis, dermatitis herpetiformis, coeliac disease, Behçet's disease, thrombotic thrombocytopenic purpura, myasthenia gravis, and others. Whether these conditions have a true association with polymyositis/dermatomyositis is unclear.

Pregnancy and polymyositis/dermatomyositis

Active polymyositis/dermatomyositis appears to confer increased risk to both the mother and the fetus, with potential for exacerbations, fetal loss and premature births. However, in established polymyositis/dermatomyositis, controlled at the time of pregnancy, most patients do not have flares, and many pregnancies are successful (Ishii et al. 1991; Oddis and Hill 1993). Those with myositis onset during pregnancy (and those with relapse) often have severe myositis requiring high-dose steroids, and have a high rate of adverse fetal outcome (Rosenzweig et al. 1989; Satoh et al. 1994). Thus, patients should optimally be in remission before becoming pregnant. If treatment is needed during pregnancy, prednisone is often used. Immunosuppressive medications should be avoided if possible, particularly methotrexate. Intensive evaluation for malignancy in pregnant patients who develop polymyositis/dermatomyositis without other indications would be inadvisable. No effect of polymyositis/dermatomyositis on fertility has been identified.

Laboratory investigations

Muscle factors

Enzyme

Creatine kinase
Serum levels of enzymes released from damaged muscle can be helpful for diagnosis and disease monitoring (Targoff 1988; Rider and Miller 1995). Creatine kinase is the most widely used due to its sensitivity, relative specificity for muscle, ready availability, and correlation with disease activity.

Elevations
Elevated creatine kinase levels are present in most patients (80 to 90 per cent) when first seen, and in more than 95 per cent at some time during their course (Bohan et al. 1977; Hochberg et al. 1986). The mean increase of creatine kinase (about 10-fold), and the potential to rise 100-fold or more, is greater than that of other enzymes measured. The creatine kinase usually rises with exacerbations, and can precede them by 5 to 6 weeks or more. A fall in the enzyme usually indicates improvement, and can precede recovery of strength by 3 to 4 weeks. There is a general correlation of creatine kinase level and disease activity for most individual patients over time (Kroll et al. 1986).

Normal creatine kinase
The creatine kinase may be normal in some patients despite active myositis. This is more common in dermatomyositis (Rider and Miller 1995) than polymyositis, possibly due to easier diagnosis of dermatomyositis when the creatine kinase is normal. Some dermatomyositis patients have normal creatine kinase because myositis has not yet developed. Lesser elevations may be seen in advanced or chronic disease, especially with severe atrophy, but elevations may still occur. Creatine kinase levels are lower in patients with autoimmune rheumatic diseases in general (Wei et al. 1981), possibly leading to lower levels in overlap patients. Creatine kinase has been correlated inversely with measures of inflammation in rheumatoid arthritis (Sanmarti et al. 1994). The enzymatic measurement of creatine kinase (generation of ATP from creatine phosphate and

ADP) may be reduced falsely by an inhibitor found in some myositis sera (Kagen and Aram 1987). Steroids may lower the creatine kinase level even if they do not suppress disease activity. Levels that are within the normal range in patients with active disease may still be higher than the baseline for that individual.

One study of seven polymyositis/dermatomyositis patients with a normal creatine kinase found that the prognosis was worse than expected, with more interstitial lung disease and malignancy (Fudman and Schnitzer 1986); others have also found more interstitial lung disease (Koh *et al.* 1993; Matsuda *et al.* 1993), but many see no relation (Rider and Miller 1995).

Other causes of creatine kinase elevation

Creatine kinase may be elevated in a wide variety of conditions other than myositis (Table 3). It is released in conditions leading to muscle necrosis, but not usually simple atrophy (as in disuse, denervation, steroid myopathy, hyperthyroidism). Strenuous, prolonged exercise, particularly when unaccustomed, may raise the creatine kinase level in normal people for 2 days (Rider and Miller 1995). Physical injury to muscle can raise the creatine kinase, including intramuscular injections, electromyography, or muscle biopsy. Drugs can raise the creatine kinase level through a variety of mechanisms, including toxic effects, induction of myositis or myopathy, or decreasing excretion of the enzyme (see below). Various myopathies, as well as carrier states, may increase creatine kinase, including dystrophies, metabolic myopathies, and others. Some disease states other than myopathies may lead to increased creatine kinase, such as diabetic nephrotic syndrome associated with oedema (Taniyama *et al.* 1987). Others may raise total creatine kinase through effects on the creatine kinase-BB isoenzyme, such as gastrointestinal or lung tumours.

The normal range for creatine kinase may differ between patient groups. It is higher for men than for women, higher for black than for white people, and higher with increased muscle mass (Black *et al.* 1986). The composition of the group used to determine the normal range is therefore important in interpretation of the result.

Isoenzymes

Serum creatine kinase-MB isoenzyme can be elevated in polymyositis and dermatomyositis, but this has not correlated with cardiac involvement (Hochberg *et al.* 1986). High levels of creatine kinase-MB may occur without evidence of cardiac involvement, and severe cardiac involvement may occur despite a normal level of this isoenzyme (Targoff 1988). Regenerating or chronically stressed skeletal muscle fibres may contain significant creatine kinase-MB (Wolf 1991), and are the likely source in polymyositis/dermatomyositis.

Macro-creatine kinase type 1, a complex of antibody with creatine kinase, was found in 36 of 8322 patients tested for isoenzymes, and half had myositis (Lee *et al.* 1994). Modification of creatine kinase-MM after release leads to formation of subisoenzymes. A high MM3:MM1 subisoenzyme ratio suggests deteriorating disease (Annesley *et al.* 1985).

Other enzymes

Several other enzymes are released during muscle damage that may occasionally be helpful for disease monitoring. More than 98 per cent of patients will have an elevation of at least one serum enzyme at some time during their course (Hochberg *et al.* 1986). Aldolase is elevated usually in polymyositis and dermatomyositis, in some cases when creatine kinase is not, but is not as specific for muscle and does not correlate as well with disease activity (Bohlmeyer *et al.* 1994).

Table 3 Factors affecting creatine kinase (CK) levels

Causes of elevated CK levels

1. Strenuous prolonged exercise

2. Muscle trauma:
   (a) Injury
   (b) Needlestick
   (c) Electromyography
   (d) surgery

3. Diseases affecting muscle[1]:
   (a) Myositis
       Infectious
       Idiopathic
   (b) Metabolic
   (c) Dystrophy
   (d) Myocardial infarction[a]
   (e) Rhabdomyolysis
   (f) Amyotrophic lateral sclerosis (effect on muscle indirect)

4. Drugs[2]:
   (a) Toxic myopathy
   (b) Induction of myositis (D-penicillamine)
   (c) Direct elevation of CK (inhibition of excretion)
       barbiturates, morphine, diazepam

5. Endocrine and metabolic abnormalities:
   (a) Hypothyroidism
   (b) Hypokalaemia
   (c) Hyperosmolar state or ketoacidosis
   (d) Diabetic nephrotic syndrome
   (e) Renal failure

6. Others:
   (a) CNS disease[b]
       cerebral ischaemia
       head injury
       psychosis
       delirium tremens
   (b) Tumours (gastrointestinal, bronchial, others[b])
   (c) Pneumococcal sepsis

7. Normal:
   (a) Ethnic group
   (b) Increased muscle mass
   (c) Technical artefact

Causes of low CK levels in active polymyositis/dermatomyositis

1. Circulating inhibitor

2. Additional autoimmune rheumatic disease

3. Steroid treatment without disease suppression

4. Advanced disease with atrophy

5. Unexplained

[1]See Table 5
[2]See Table 6
[a]Elevated proportion of CK-MB
[b]Predominantly or elevated proportion of CK-BB

Lactate dehydrogenase (LDH) is also elevated, predominantly LDH-5, although LDH-1 may increase without necessarily correlating with cardiac involvement (Targoff 1988). Aspartate transferase correlates very well with biopsy-proven muscle inflammation, and was found useful in combination with creatine kinase and aldolase in assessing enzyme elevations (Hood *et al.* 1991). Carbonic anhydrase III, an isoenzyme found exclusively in skeletal and not cardiac muscle, rises with skeletal muscle damage, including polymyositis/dermatomyositis (Osterman *et al.* 1985).

Myoglobin

Myoglobin is unique to skeletal and cardiac muscle. Very little is present normally in serum or urine, but it is detectable in the serum of most patients with active polymyositis/dermatomyositis (Targoff 1988). It can serve as a disease activity marker, rising with exacerbation and falling with remission, and can predict exacerbation in some cases. It may occasionally be elevated when the creatine kinase is not. It has the advantages of tissue specificity, rapid clearance, and sensitive, non-enzymatic detection. A new immunoturbidimetric assay may make testing more available, but is slightly less sensitive than radioimmunoassay (Lovece and Kagen 1993). It should be measured in samples taken at a standard time during the day because of diurnal variation.

Other muscle factors

Creatine is produced in the liver, pancreas, and kidney, and taken up by the muscle. Creatine excretion rises with muscle disease due to defects in uptake and retention. The creatine or the creatine/ [creatinine+creatine] ratio in a 24 h urine sample (normal less than 6 per cent) is elevated in most polymyositis/dermatomyositis patients, and can vary with disease activity. Its clinical utility is limited by many disadvantages. Elevation, found whenever muscle mass is reduced, is less specific than creatine kinase, and may persist in inactive polymyositis/dermatomyositis as a result of atrophy. It is cumbersome to collect and difficult to obtain clinically.

Measures of muscle mass correlate with strength, but not necessarily inflammation; they can be used to provide a longer-term view. Tests that measure muscle mass, including 24 h urinary creatinine, 3-methyl histidine excretion (reflecting skeletal muscle protein turnover), and total body potassium (measuring total body mass), have been used in studies but are not currently practical for clinical use (Moxley 1994). Dual radiography/absorptiometry may be used in the future (Kanda *et al.* 1994).

Autoantibodies

Indirect immunofluorescence is positive in 50 to 80 per cent of patients with polymyositis or dermatomyositis (Reichlin and Arnett 1984; Love *et al.* 1991). Nuclear or speckled patterns are most common, nucleolar may be seen, and cytoplasmic patterns provide clues to an antisynthetase or anti-SRP (Fig. 12). A high antinuclear antibody (**ANA**) titre favours polymyositis or dermatomyositis over other myopathies or neuropathies, and a MSA strongly supports polymyositis/dermatomyositis when present (see below). Antisynthetases may alert the physician to an increased risk for interstitial lung disease, or identify underlying polymyositis/dermatomyositis in patients who present with prominent extra-muscle features.

A general correlation of anti-Jo-1 titre with disease activity has been observed (Miller *et al.* 1990b), and in some cases a rise in anti-Jo-1 predicted exacerbation. Occasional disappearance of anti-Jo-1 correlates with disease remission. The usefulness of titres as an index of disease activity is not established, but they may provide support if serial measurements are available.

Other tests

The erythrocyte sedimentation rate is elevated in about half of active cases, but is correlated poorly with disease activity or response to treatment. Similarly, the C-reactive protein may be normal or slightly high despite active disease (Gabay *et al.* 1994). Rheumatoid factor is positive in about 10 to 20 per cent of patients, most commonly in the overlap group. Circulating immune complexes and cryoglobulins have been reported in some patients, but their significance is unclear. Elevated gammaglobulins may be seen; hypogammaglobulinaemia should raise the suspicion of echovirus or other infection. Patients with polymyositis with monoclonal gammopathies have been described, including some in which sarcolemmal deposition of paraprotein was found (Kiprov and Miller 1984). Complement is usually normal, but myositis has occurred in C2 deficiency (Targoff 1988). Proteinuria is usually the result of myoglobinuria, with rare exceptions (see below).

Diagnosis

The criteria of Bohan and Peter (1975) (Table 4), often with modifications such as that of Dalakas (1991), have been used widely for diagnosis and clinical studies. Muscle enzymes, electromyography and muscle biopsy remain essential in evaluation of patients and establishing the diagnosis of polymyositis and dermatomyositis. Autoantibody testing and magnetic resonance imaging (MRI) can also greatly aid in diagnosis. Recent attempts have been made to devise new criteria that take advantage of newer tests and other features (Medsger and Oddis 1995; Tanimoto *et al.* 1995). Even when the criteria are satisfied, other causes of muscle disease must be excluded.

Electromyography

Electromyography and nerve conduction studies cannot establish the diagnosis of polymyositis/dermatomyositis with certainty, but can demonstrate that the process is myopathic and consistent with these diseases, and can help to exclude many other neuropathies and certain myopathies. Electromyography may reveal muscle involvement in patients presenting with rash or extra-muscle features, and can identify areas of involvement to help direct biopsies (on the contralateral side) and provides some information regarding activity. Ninety per cent of patients with active polymyositis/dermatomyositis have an abnormal electomyograph (Bohan *et al.* 1977; Henriksson and Lindvall 1990). Testing of multiple muscles is important, since involvement may be limited, and to demonstrate the distribution of involvement. Paraspinal muscle involvement is common, and may be the only abnormal area.

Motor unit action potentials in polymyositis/dermatomyositis typically are myopathic (low amplitude, short duration). Polyphasic potentials (complex potentials with increased turns) are increased, and may be attributed to asynchronous firing of fibres (Bertorini 1988a). Over time, long-duration, high amplitude polyphasic potentials may be seen (attributed to reinnervation of regenerating or denervated fibres) (Uncini *et al.* 1990). Patients with myositis have early recruitment and full interference patterns (more fibres required to achieve a given force), in contrast to the decreased recruitment and interference seen in neuropathies (Greenlee 1988).

Spontaneous activity at rest is seen in three-quarters of patients (Henriksson and Lindvall 1990). Increased insertional activity gener-

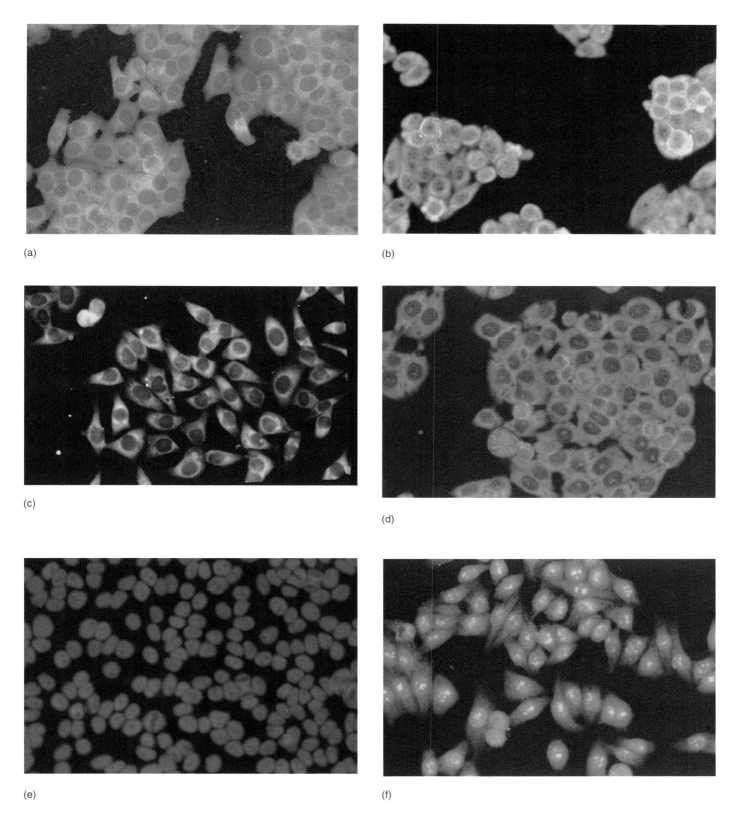

Fig. 12 Indirect immunofluorescence on HEp-2 cells using sera with myositis-associated autoantibodies. (a) Anti-Jo-1 autoantibodies (reacting with histidyl-tRNA synthetase): finely speckled cytoplasmic pattern of fluorescence. (b) Anti-PL-7 autoantibodies (antithreonyl-tRNA synthetase): cytoplasmic pattern (more homogeneous at higher concentration). (c) Anti-SRP autoantibodies (antisignal recognition particle): cytoplasmic pattern. (d) Anti-KJ autoantibodies (reacting with a translation factor): cytoplasmic pattern with slight nucleolar staining. (e) Anti-Mi-2 autoantibodies (reacting with an unidentified nuclear protein): nuclear pattern, sparing nucleoli, without cytoplasmic staining. (f) Anti-PM-Scl autoantibodies (reacting with a complex of 11 proteins): intense nucleolar staining with significant nuclear staining.

Table 4 The diagnosis of polymyositis and dermatomyositis
(a) Criteria for the diagnosis of polymyositis (PM) and dermatomyositis (DM)[a]

1. Compatible weakness
   symmetrical proximal muscle weakness, developing over
   weeks to months

2. Elevated serum muscle enzymes
   creatine kinase, aldolase

3. Electromyographic findings typical of PM or DM
   Most common: myopathic potentials (low amplitude, short
      duration, polyphasic potentials)
   Most characteristic: triad of
   (a) myopathic potentials
   (b) fibrillations, positive sharp waves, increased insertional
      activity
   Hepatitis B or C(c) complex repetitive discharges

4. Muscle biopsy findings typical of PM or DM
   Necrosis, phagocytosis, regeneration, inflammation.

5. Dermatological features of DM
   (a) Gottron's papules or sign, involving finger joints, knees,
      elbows, and/or medial malleoli
   (b) Heliotrope sign
   (c) Erythematous and/or poikilodermatous rash

[a]Reference: Bohan and Peter (1975)

(b) Other useful diagnostic findings

1. Autoantibodies:
   (a) myositis-specific autoantibodies: low sensitivity, high
      specificity (Table 8);
   (b) positive ANA: sensitivity 60%.

2. Imaging
   (a) MRI: increased signal on T_2 images
   (b) MRS: elevated inorganic phosphate/phosphocreatine

3. Other dermatological findings:
   Nailfold capillary changes, calcinosis, mechanic's hands.

ated by needle trauma to the muscle fibre is very common, as are fibrillations and positive sharp waves, sometimes more evident in the paraspinal muscles. Often associated with denervation, fibrillations in polymyositis/dermatomyositis have been attributed to damage to intramuscular nerves, nerve endings or motor end plates, or to segmental muscle fibre necrosis that denervates the distal fibre (Greenlee 1988). Complex repetitive discharges (bizarre high-frequency discharges) may also be seen in a third to a half of patients. In contrast to myotonic discharges, these start and stop abruptly, and usually have constant amplitude. They have been attributed to inflammatory damage to the sarcolemma. Spontaneous activity has been associated with active inflammation; it is less common with chronic disease, and may subside with treatment.

Single-fibre electromyography in myositis shows increased jitter and blocking, although less prominent than in myasthenia gravis.

Computerized quantitative analysis may reveal increased fibre density (more potentials per motor unit) (Bertorini 1988a). A myopathic interference pattern was the most common abnormality (83 per cent) on quantitative electromyography (Barkhaus *et al.* 1990).

Imaging

Magnetic resonance imaging (MRI)

Numerous studies in recent years have demonstrated the value of MRI in polymyositis/dermatomyositis for diagnosis and assessment of disease activity. MRI can identify sensitively areas of muscle inflammation, atrophy, or fatty replacement (Reimers *et al.* 1994). It is non-invasive and can be repeated sequentially. Use is often limited by cost or availability, but in certain situations it can provide critical information that may not be available by other methods, affecting treatment decisions (Park *et al.* 1994).

T_2-weighted images are best for showing areas of active muscle inflammation, where increased water content is seen as increased intensity; this is not seen with T_1-weighted images (Park *et al.* 1990). Increased fat is seen on both images. Some studies have used fat suppression techniques to improve image contrast (Fraser *et al.* 1991; Hernandez *et al.* 1992). Gadolinium was not helpful (Reimers *et al.* 1994). The thighs are most often studied.

Involvement seen using MRI is often focal and patchy, with differences in intensity between and within muscles, and the technique can therefore be more sensitive than biopsy for detecting clinical activity (Fraser *et al.* 1991). Park *et al.* (1990) found that the vastus lateralis was the most involved muscle in their dermatomyositis patients, with a predominance of anterior over posterior thigh muscle involvement. Fraser *et al.* (1991) did not find anterior predominance in dermatomyositis or polymyositis patients, but found a correlation of atrophy and disease duration. Fatty infiltration is more common in polymyositis than dermatomyositis, and in chronic disease.

Fraser *et al.* (1991) also noted a correlation between MR images or quantitative signal intensity scores with disease activity, although Reimers *et al.* (1994) did not. By correlating with clinical activity, MRI can help assess therapeutic response; abnormalities can return to normal within months on treatment (Fujino *et al.* 1991; Park *et al.* 1994). Persistent abnormalities can indicate activity. MRI may show high intensity in active disease, even when enzymes, electromyography, and/or biopsy are normal (Park *et al.* 1994; Stonecipher *et al.* 1994), although exceptions with negative MRI in active disease may occur (Stiglbauer *et al.* 1993).

Magnetic resonance spectroscopy (MRS)

P-31 MRS has been used in the study of various myopathies to assess energy utilization and reserve by measuring phosphate metabolites in muscle. The inorganic phosphate/phosphocreatine ratio rises in myopathies indicating a decrease in energy reserve, and is correlated with disease activity (Park *et al.* 1994). Phosphocreatine and ATP are decreased at rest, decrease further with exercise, and show delayed recovery to baseline (Park *et al.* 1990). Phosphocreatine changed more than ATP, and was thus better for assessing disease activity. However, the decline of ATP with exercise was felt to relate to the severe fatigue that may occur. The impaired energy utilization and muscle metabolism may contribute to muscle weakness in polymyositis/dermatomyositis.

While not specific, MRS may help monitor disease activity and response to therapy. It can be abnormal in some patients with normal creatine kinase (Park *et al.* 1994), but can continue to be abnormal in some patients whose inflammation has resolved (reflecting persistent muscle abnormalities). When MRI and MRS were discordant, MRS was felt to be more useful for assessing disease status. Park *et al.* (1995) also found that patients with amyopathic dermatomyositis, who have normal MRI and MRS at rest, often have subtle MRS abnormalities with exercise (reduced total oxidative capacity, V_{max}), which may explain their fatigue.

Other methods

Ultrasound of muscle was abnormal, most often with hyperechogenicity as a result of fat and atrophy, in 83 per cent of 70 patients with myositis, including some with normal creatine kinase or electromyographs (Reimers *et al.* 1993). It is less expensive and more readily available than MRI, but is less sensitive and specific (Stonecipher *et al.* 1994), and does not provide as much information. It may help direct the biopsy.

Technetium-99m and thallium uptake may be increased in muscles affected by active polymyositis. Although non-specific, this also might be useful for directing a biopsy. Gallium-67 scanning has been used to identify myositis in Lyme disease and other infections. Scanning with indium-labelled antimyosin can reveal areas of muscle necrosis in dermatomyositis (DeGeeter *et al.* 1989). With a monoclonal antibody specific for cardiac myosin, the scan can detect myocarditis in polymyositis (Le Guludec *et al.* 1993).

Biopsy

Indications

Most patients in whom polymyositis or dermatomyositis is suspected should have a muscle biopsy. It can provide the most convincing evidence supporting the diagnosis, and can definitively exclude certain relevant conditions. There are cases in which the diagnosis can be established for clinical purposes without the biopsy. With proximal weakness, elevated enzymes, and a typical electromyograph, those with a classic dermatomyositis rash, confirmed myositis-specific autoantibodies, or autoimmune rheumatic diseases overlap syndromes with specific antibodies (anti-U1RNP, anti-PM-Scl) do not usually require a biopsy, although others feel that all adults should have a biopsy (Urbano-Marquez *et al.* 1991).

Methods

Open muscle biopsy gives the best picture of the muscle architecture. A large specimen may decrease sampling error, allows proper orientation, and provides enough muscle for all studies. Complications from the procedure (bleeding, infection, nerve damage, etc.) are very low (Pamphlett 1988), but the 4 to 8 cm incision commonly used creates a significant scar, especially in obese patients. Needle biopsy, with a 0.5 cm incision, causes substantially less morbidity, is often more easily and rapidly arranged, and is adequate for diagnosis of polymyositis/dermatomyositis in most cases (O'Rourke *et al.* 1994). Multiple specimens may be taken through the same incision site for enzyme histochemistry and electron microscopy (**EM**), and to reduce sampling error (Haddad *et al.* 1994). The low morbidity allows repeat biopsy or later open biopsy if needed. However, processing of samples is more difficult,

more artefact is encountered (particularly in EM), and open biopsy is required for certain functional enzyme studies.

The best information is obtained from muscle with active disease but not endstage fibrosis or atrophy. Muscles used for electromyography or intramuscular injection should not be used for biopsy. The quadriceps or deltoid are most often used due to accessibility, but focal disease may result in non-diagnostic samples. As noted, certain diagnostic procedures have been used to localize disease activity to direct the biopsy (electromyography, MRI, ultrasound). MRI is most promising since it can show focal involvement, but is not always successful (Pitt *et al.* 1993; Reimers *et al.* 1994).

EM should be performed when inclusion-body myositis or mitochondrial myopathies are considerations, or to exclude certain other conditions. Enzyme histochemistry may be helpful to exclude myophosphorylase deficiency and other metabolic myopathies which may masquerade as polymyositis. Co-ordination with the pathologist can help to optimize processing and evaluation of specimens.

Muscle pathology

Inflammation is a hallmark of myositis. The infiltrates are predominantly lymphocytes, but include macrophages, plasma cells, and sometimes eosinophils, basophils, and neutrophils. The amount of inflammation is variable, and up to 25 per cent may show no inflammation, usually attributed to a focal process.

In polymyositis, inflammatory infiltrates more often predominate in the endomysial area around the muscle fibres, usually without perifascicular atrophy (Fig. 13). Necrosis of individual muscle fibres may be observed. The fibres appear swollen with homogeneous contents, losing the normal striations of the contractile proteins. There is invasion of mononuclear cells, phagocytosis, and regeneration (Fig. 14), the latter marked by sarcoplasmic basophilia, large vesicular, internalized nuclei, and prominent nucleoli. In later stages, there is atrophy, fibrosis, and fatty replacement. Steroid treatment may enhance type II fibre atrophy. Non-caseating granulomas were recently observed in muscle from anti-Jo-1-associated polymyositis (Moder *et al.* 1993).

In typical dermatomyositis, infiltration predominates in the perimysial area (around the fascicles) and around small blood vessels,

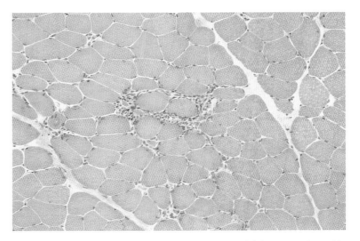

Fig. 13 Muscle biopsy (haematoxylin and eosin stain) from a patient with polymyositis. Endomysial inflammation (infiltration with mononuclear cells between fibres within the fascicle) is seen; a pattern characteristic of biopsies from patients with polymyositis.

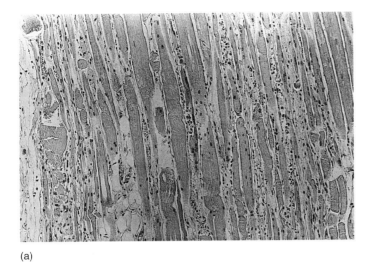

(a)

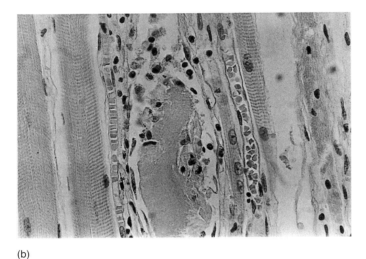

(b)

Fig. 14   Muscle biopsy from a patient with anti-Jo-1-positive polymyositis. (a) Inflammation with necrosis and degeneration of muscle fibres. (b) Necrosis with loss of characteristic striations and integrity of fibre. (By courtesy of M. Reichlin, MD.)

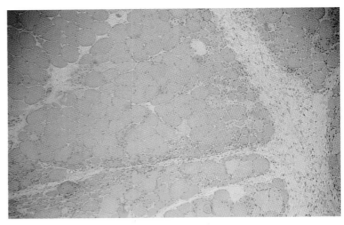

Fig. 15   Muscle biopsy (haematoxylin and eosin stain) from a patient with anti-Jo-1- positive myositis. The histological appearance is characteristic of dermatomyositis, but the patient had no cutaneous manifestations. The most intense infiltration is perimysial, with some extension into the endomysial area in a perifascicular distribution. Perifascicular atrophy (atrophy of the fibres at the periphery of the fascicle) is marked. Involvement of the vessel in the interstitial area is seen.

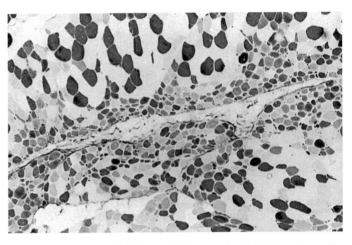

Fig. 16   Muscle biopsy (ATPase stain) from a patient with dermatomyositis. The pattern of perifascicular atrophy is evident.

sometimes extending into the endomysial area (Fig. 15). Microvascular changes are often seen, with perifascicular atrophy (decreased fibre size at the periphery of the fascicle), a characteristic (although not specific) feature of dermatomyositis (Figs 15 and 16). This may result from capillary loss, which is greater in the perifascicular region, or to a direct effect of perifascicular inflammation (Kalovidouris 1994). It is most common in juvenile dermatomyositis (90 per cent), and also occurs in adult dermatomyositis (50 per cent) (Bertorini 1988b). Circumscribed areas of myofibrillar loss are also typical, attributed to ischaemic damage. There is some overlap of the polymyositis and dermatomyositis patterns (Ringel *et al.* 1986). Despite prominent vascular damage, frank necrotizing vasculitis is unusual (Fig. 17).

EM shows endothelial cell injury, with swelling, hyperplasia, vacuolization, degeneration, and regeneration. There is endothelial cell necrosis and capillary thrombosis, and loss of capillaries resulting in decreased capillary density (Emslie-Smith and Engel

1990). The endothelial cells contain characteristic tubuloreticular inclusions ('undulating tubules'), that resemble viral structures but are believed to result from endothelial cell damage (Fidzianska and Goebel 1989). They may be seen in endothelial cells in other tissues (skin, lungs, joints, and lymphocytes). They can be induced by interferon-α, and may occur in other diseases, although usually not polymyositis.

Other EM findings are non-specific (Carpenter 1988). In dermatomyositis, Z disc streaming may be found. In polymyositis, aggregates of dense, membrane-bound material may be seen in some cases, and reduplication of the basal lamina.

Skin pathology

Skin biopsy can support the diagnosis of dermatomyositis, but generally cannot establish it. The biopsy should be taken from lesional

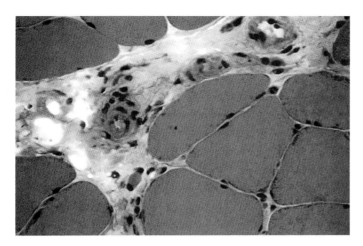

Fig. 17 Muscle biopsy from a patient with severe myositis associated with Sjögren's syndrome, showing inflammation surrounding small vessels.

skin (rather than as part of the muscle biopsy), usually from the chest or extremities. Liquefaction degeneration of the basal cell layer with prominent vacuolar changes is seen (Janis and Winkelman 1968). There is often a mild mononuclear cell infiltrate in the upper dermis and dermal–epidermal junction. There may be basement membrane thickening. Oedema and increased mucin can be seen in the dermis. The mucin (mostly hyaluronic acid) may be severe enough to be clinically evident (Igarashi *et al.* 1985). With poikiloderma, there is telangiectasia and epidermal atrophy. In Gottron's papules, typical dermatomyositis changes may be seen, with less atrophy, but with the addition of epidermal changes, including acanthosis and mild papillomatosis (Hanno and Callen 1985).

These findings may resemble systemic lupus erythematosus, but the dermal–epidermal infiltrate is milder in dermatomyositis, and there is more dermal mucin. Immunoglobulin deposition is much less prominent in dermatomyositis. Occasionally, mild deposition is seen at the dermal–epidermal junction in dermatomyositis lesional (but not non-lesional) skin (Kasper *et al.* 1988).

Differential diagnosis

The diagnosis of dermatomyositis is easier than that of polymyositis when the rash is florid. In polymyositis and less typical dermatomyositis, other conditions that can cause muscle weakness, myalgias, or elevated creatine kinase levels must be excluded. In all patients, tests for thyroid disease should be performed, and the role of medications should be considered. Most patients, particularly those with risk factors, should be tested for retroviral infection, and those at risk for other specific infections should be tested, such as specific exclusion of parasitic infection in those with eosinophilia or who are from endemic areas.

In patients with weakness without systemic features, other myopathies (inclusion-body myositis, metabolic or mitochondrial myopathies, drug-induced myopathies) or neuropathies (myasthenia gravis, amyotrophic lateral sclerosis) should be considered. In patients with weakness and signs of acute illness or autoimmune rheumatic disease, such as fever, arthritis, etc., the major conditions to be distinguished may be infectious or rheumatic. In a small number of cases, the patient will present with extra-muscle features

only, either cutaneous lesions or autoimmune rheumatic features, resembling other autoimmune rheumatic diseases, or undifferentiated autoimmune rheumatic disease syndromes. Conditions that may be confused with polymyositis/dermatomyositis are listed in Table 5; special considerations are discussed below.

Human immunodeficiency virus (HIV)

Patients with HIV infection may develop myositis indistinguishable from polymyositis. Weakness, myalgia and elevated creatine kinase are seen, but rarely a rash. Electromyography shows myopathy, and biopsy shows inflammation with lymphocytic infiltration and necrosis (Dalakas 1993).

The pathogenesis of HIV-myositis appears similar to idiopathic polymyositis. CD8+ cytotoxic T cells and macrophages predominate, with very few CD4+ cells (Illa *et al.* 1991). As in polymyositis, there is endomysial infiltration, surrounded and invaded fibres, and expression of MHC-1 on most muscle fibres, all consistent with cell-mediated attack (Dalakas 1993). Numerous studies had failed to find HIV inside intact muscle fibres (Leon-Monzon *et al.* 1993), and it did not infect muscle cells *in vitro*, but HIV was found in cells infiltrating muscle or in degenerating fibres. However, a recent study using the more sensitive *in situ* polymerase chain reaction (**PCR**) found HIV in myocyte nuclei in four of seven cases (Seidman *et al.* 1994), plus HIV RNA indicating transcriptional activity. It remains to be shown whether myositis results from primary infection, secondary infection with a myositis-inducing virus, induction of autoimmune responses, or dysregulation.

HIV-myositis must be distinguished from the myopathy that can occur with zidovudine (Dalakas *et al.* 1990), which can cause weakness, myalgias, wasting, elevated creatine kinase, and myopathic electromyographs (Dalakas 1993). It is more frequent with longer therapy and higher doses. Zidovudine inhibits mitochondrial DNA synthesis, resulting in muscle mitochondrial toxicity *in vitro* and in experimental animals. Muscle shows ragged red fibres and abnormal mitochondrial structure and function (Mhiri *et al.* 1991). Inflammation is sometimes seen, but may relate to coexistent HIV-myositis; this combination may be required for symptomatic myopathy (Dalakas *et al.* 1990; Lane *et al.* 1993).

HIV has also been associated with a nemaline rod myopathy (Simpson and Bender 1988) and other non-inflammatory myopathy and muscle wasting. Patients with AIDS are also at risk for myositis from other infections, such as tuberculosis or microsporidia (Preston 1993), and for pyomyositis. Symptoms related to a myopathy may occur in up to 30 per cent of patients with AIDS, although a recognized inflammatory myopathy requiring treatment is much less common. Since polymyositis may be the first manifestation of disease, testing for HIV infection is recommended in most patients with myositis.

Human T-cell lymphotropic virus type I (HTLV-1)

HTLV-1 has also been associated with myositis, with or without HTLV-1-associated myelopathy, and may be a major cause of polymyositis in endemic areas. In Jamaica, Morgan *et al.* (1989) found HTLV-1 antibodies in 11 of 13 polymyositis patients, but only in 7 of 93 others. The polymyositis was clinically similar to idiopathic polymyositis, with weakness, elevated creatine kinase, and compatible histology, and none of the patients had other HTLV-1-associated conditions. HTLV-1 was also increased in polymyositis patients in an endemic area in Japan, although not as dramatically (Higuchi *et*

Table 5 Differential diagnosis of polymyositis/dermatomyositis

Other forms of inflammatory myopathy (myositis)

Infectious myositis

1. Viruses:
    (a) Retroviruses:
        HIV: PM-like myositis, other infections
        HTLV-1

    (b) Picornaviruses (enteroviruses):
        Echovirus (In Ig deficiency)
        Coxsackievirus

    (c) Other viruses:
        Influenza
        Hepatitis B or C
        Others (Epstein–Barr virus, cytomegalovirus, adenovirus, etc.)

2. Bacteria:
    Pyomyositis
    Lyme myositis
    Other (tuberculosis, mycoplasma, leprosy, streptococci, etc.)

3. Protozoa: toxoplasmosis, American trypanosomiasis

4. Parasites: trichinosis, cysticerosis

5. Fungi: candida

Idiopathic

1. Inclusion-body myositis

2. Autoimmune rheumatic diseases
    (a) Scleroderma
    (b) Systemic lupus erythematosus
    (c) Sjögren's syndrome
    (d) Rheumatoid arthritis
    (e) Vasculitis (polyarteritis nodosa, Wegener's granulomatosis, rheumatoid arthritis)
    (f) Polymyalgia rheumatica

3. Other idiopathic myositis
    (a) Granulomatous myositis (giant cell, sarcoid, etc.)
    (b) Eosinophilic myositis
    (c) Eosinophilia–myalgia and toxic oil syndromes
    (d) Focal myositis
    (e) Orbital myositis

Other myopathies

Dystrophies

1. Limb girdle

2. Fascioscapulohumeral

Congenital myopathies

1. Nemaline rod, central core, etc.

2. Mitochrondrial myopathies

Metabolic

1. Myophosphorylase deficiency (McArdle's)

2. Phosphofructokinase deficiency

3. Myoadenylate deaminase deficiency

4. Acid maltase deficiency

5. Lipis storage diseases
    (a) Carnitine deficiency
    (b) Carnitine palmitoyl transferase deficiency

6. Carcinomatous myopathy

7. Acute rhabdomyolysis

Other neurological disorders

1. Motor neurone diseases

2. Myasthenia gravis or Eaton–Lambert

3. Guillain-Barré syndrome

Endocrine/metabolic disorders

Thyroid:

1. Hypothyroidism

2. Hyperthyroidism

Hypercortisolism

1. Endogenous

2. Steroid myopathy

Parathyroid:

1. Hyperparathyroidism

2. Hypoparathyroidism

Metabolic:

1. Hypocalcaemia

2. Hypokalaemia

Diabetes and neurological complications

Malnutrition

Drugs See Table 6

al. 1992). HTLV-1 is infrequent in polymyositis in non-endemic areas (Nishikai and Sato 1991; Nelson *et al.* 1994), but it may occur. HTLV-1 testing should be performed in patients at risk.

As with HIV, studies of infiltrating lymphocytes and MHC-1 expression in HTLV-1-myositis suggest T-cell mediated cytotoxicity (Leon-Monzon *et al.* 1994). One study found evidence of HTLV-1-associated proteins in muscle fibres (Wiley *et al.* 1989), but this was not confirmed (Higuchi *et al.* 1992; Leon-Monzon *et al.* 1994), and HTLV-1 did not infect muscle cells *in vitro*. The reason myositis develops in HTLV-1 infection is not known.

Bacterial pyomyositis

Pyomyositis has been well known in tropical areas for many years (Chiedozi 1979), most commonly affecting young males, with one or more spontaneous muscle abscesses, usually from *Staphylococcus aureus*. Pyomyositis in non-tropical areas is now increasingly reported, affecting older patients, often non-staphylococcal, with AIDS, diabetes, and chronic illness as predisposing factors (Rodgers *et al.* 1993; Gomez-Reino *et al.* 1994). Other muscle disease may be a factor in some cases. Although usually localized, a syndrome that could be confused with polymyositis has been seen (Wolf *et al.* 1990). Diagnosis can be made with ultrasound, CT, or MRI.

Other neurological conditions

Sensory abnormalities are against polymyositis/dermatomyositis, but diseases with exclusively diffuse motor involvement, such as amyotrophic lateral sclerosis or myasthenia gravis, can resemble polymyositis. Fasciculations and prominent atrophy may be clues in the former, and extraocular or eyelid muscle involvement in the latter.

Many myopathies are inherited and a family history of myopathy is an important point against polymyositis/dermatomyositis. Adult onset narrows the myopathies to consider, although a few associated with early onset occasionally present later (Table 5). In favour of dystrophy would be lack of inflammation on biopsy; myotonia; involvement of selective muscles (such as pectorals, biceps, triceps, etc.); and lack of response to therapy.

Mitochondrial myopathy may sometimes present in adults with pure limb myopathy without extraocular muscle involvement or encephalopathy. 'Ragged red fibres' on biopsy, due to subsarcolemmal accumulation of abnormal mitochondria, should prompt further testing with EM. Varga *et al.* (1993) described two cases of asymptomatic primary biliary cirrhosis associated with a severe, new onset mitochondrial myopathy with fatal outcome resembling polymyositis, raising the possibility of antimitochondrial antibody-induced mitochondrial myopathy.

Genetic defects in glycogen or glucose metabolism usually present with episodic fatigue, cramping, or pain related to exercise (Martin *et al.* 1994). Some, however, such as deficiencies of myophosphorylase (McArdle's disease), phosphofructokinase, myoadenylate deaminase, or acid maltase, may have an atypical presentation with late-onset progressive weakness that can be misdiagnosed as polymyositis (Higgs *et al.* 1989; Plotz 1992). The forearm ischaemic exercise test (Martin *et al.* 1994) is often used to screen for such disorders; several cause impaired rise in lactate but not ammonia, while myoadenylate deaminase causes impaired rise in ammonia but not lactate. There may also be clues on muscle biopsy (such as increased glycogen deposition). When metabolic myopathies are suspected, enzyme histochemistry and other tests for specific enzyme defects should be performed.

Drug-induced myopathies

Numerous drugs can induce myopathy (Table 6). Most have a toxic effect rather than inducing autoimmunity, and some have associated neuropathy, but the picture of weakness, myalgia, and elevated creatine kinase, often with electromyographic changes characteristic of myopathy, can look like polymyositis/dermatomyositis (Le Quintrec and Le Quintrec 1991; Zuckner 1994). D-Penicillamine is discussed later.

Table 6 Drugs causing myopathy

Implicated in autoimmune myopathy	
1. D-Penicillamine	0.2–1.4% of rheumatoid arthritis patients taking drug
2. Cimetidine	Case report of inflammatory myopathy
3. L-Tryptophan	Eosinophilia–myalgia syndrome
4. Zidovudine	Mitochondrial changes and myositis; role in myositis unclear
Myopathy with weakness, myalgia, elevated creatine kinase	
1. Colchicine	Neuromyopathy, elevated creatine kinase; when normal doses used with renal insufficiency
2. Chloroquine, hydroxychloroquine	Vacuolar myopathy, curvilinear bodies
3. Lipid-lowering agents	
(a) lovastatin	Higher frequency with lovastatin; increases when used in combination with cyclosporin (30%), and some increase with clofibrate, gemfibrozil (5%), or niacin
(b) clofibrate	
(c) gemfibrozil	
(d) niacin	
4. Cyclosporin	
5. Alcohol	
6. Ipecac, emetine	
7. Vincristine	
8. Aminocaproic acid	
9. Carbimizole, propyl-thiouracil	
10. NSAIDs	Rare; aspirin, phenylbutazone
Rhabdomyolysis picture	
1. Alcohol	
2. Drugs of abuse	Trauma, muscle crush, and direct drug effect
(a) cocaine	
(b) amphetamines	
(c) heroin	
(d) phencyclidine	
(e) barbiturates	
3. Lovastatin	
4. Anaesthetics	Malignant hyperthermia
5. Psychotropics	Neuroleptic–malignant syndrome
Muscle effects, normal CK	
1. Diuretics etc.	Drug-induced hypokalaemia
2. Corticosteroids	Creatine kinase usually normal

Colchicine may cause a non-inflammatory, vacuolar neuromyopathy (Kuncl *et al.* 1987), most often occurring with maintenance therapy at usual doses with renal insufficiency. A rise in creatine kinase is a sensitive indicator. A vacuolar myopathy may also be caused by chloroquine or less severely hydroxychloroquine, with characteristic myeloid and curvilinear bodies (Estes *et al.* 1987; Plotz 1992). Cardiomyopathy and neuropathy with loss of reflexes may be seen. Case reports of vacuolar myopathy with other drugs have appeared.

Muscle toxicity is a common side-effect with various cholesterol-lowering agents, possibly related to effects on sarcolemma (Dalakas 1992a). It can occur with HMG-CoA-reductase inhibitors (especially lovastatin) or fibrates or nicotinic acid alone, but is more severe with higher creatine kinases when combined (Pierce *et al.* 1990). Renal insufficiency may predispose to fibrate myopathy. Lovastatin myopathy is also more frequent in combination with cyclosporine, as after heart transplants.

Alcohol abuse may lead to either an acute necrotizing myopathy with prominent pain and high creatine kinase, or a chronic myopathy with proximal-muscle weakness, atrophy, and milder creatine kinase elevation (Charness *et al.* 1989). Several drugs of abuse, including cocaine, may lead to myopathy, creatine kinase elevation, or rhabdomyolysis, either due to pressure injury during unconsciousness, or without trauma (Rubin and Neugarten 1989). Abuse of ipecac in bulimia can induce a proximal, polymyositis-like myopathy, and as with other drug abuse, may be hidden (Plotz 1992).

In the eosinophilia–myalgia syndrome associated with L-tryptophan ingestion (Kaufman 1994), proximal myopathy was seen in two-thirds of cases. Aldolase was sometimes elevated, but not creatine kinase. Mononuclear and eosinophilic interstitial infiltrate (perimyositis) was seen, but fibre necrosis was rare. Similar findings occurred in the Spanish toxic oil syndrome.

Endocrine and steroid myopathies

Hypothyroidism is a common cause for elevated creatine kinase level with or without weakness, and can resemble polymyositis (Plotz 1992). Thyroid function should be tested in all patients when myositis is considered. Hypokalaemia from any cause can lead to myopathy, with creatine kinase elevation; severe hypokalaemic myopathy has been associated with chronic licorice ingestion (Sintani *et al.* 1992). Other endocrine or metabolic problems can also cause myopathy (Table 5).

Use of corticosteroids for treatment of any condition may lead to proximal muscle weakness, associated with accentuated type II fibre atrophy (Khaleeli *et al.* 1983). Its onset is usually insidious, with lower extremity predominance. It tends to occur with higher doses for extended periods, and is more likely with multiple daily doses or longer acting, fluorinated preparations. In 10.6 per cent of patients taking dexamethasone steroid myopathy developed, with peak onset between the 9th and 12th weeks (Dropcho and Soong 1991). It usually improves if the dose is lowered. An acute form can occur associated with high-dose intravenous therapy and neuromuscular blocking agents in patients on respirators (Zuckner 1994).

In polymyositis/dermatomyositis, steroid myopathy can be confused with recurrent myositis. Elevated creatine kinase, increased spontaneous activity on electromyography, and inflammation detected by MRI or biopsy should all be absent in pure steroid myopathy. It may develop while the myositis is still active,

indicating the likely need for a steroid-sparing drug. Often, if the situation is not life-threatening and remains unclear, dosage reduction is tried.

Aetiology and pathogenesis

Aetiology

Abundant evidence supports an autoimmune pathogenesis for polymyositis and dermatomyositis, but the reason they develop is unknown. It is generally felt that an inciting factor, exogenous or endogenous, acts in a genetically susceptible host, and that different inciting agents can lead to similar pictures. For example, D-penicillamine, HIV infection, various malignancies, and autoimmune rheumatic diseases, have been associated with autoimmune inflammatory myopathies that may be clinically indistinguishable from each other or from cases without recognized associations. Despite the paucity of familial cases, genetic predisposition is undoubtedly important, evident in the HLA associations, and suggested by animal models.

Potential aetiological factors

Infectious
A variety of infections can induce a syndrome resembling polymyositis/dermatomyositis in humans or animals, and unrecognized infections could be responsible for at least some idiopathic cases. Studies noting temporal variation in onset overall or for MSA-defined subgroups support this (Plotz *et al.* 1995). Mechanisms that might explain how infections such as viruses could induce autoimmune inflammatory myopathy include: persistent infection, molecular mimicry with cross-reaction of infectious agent and muscle protein, presentation or alteration of muscle antigens, production of immune complexes, effects on the immune system, or others (Targoff 1991; Behan and Behan 1993).

Picornaviruses
A variety of viruses (influenza, hepatitis, etc.) can cause myositis that resembles polymyositis, but repeated efforts to culture viruses from muscle in typical polymyositis and dermatomyositis have been unsuccessful. Picornaviruses, small RNA viruses that include enteroviruses (coxsackie, polio, echo), animal viruses such as encephalomyocarditis, and others, have been suspected as possible aetiologic factors in polymyositis/dermatomyositis (as well as myocarditis and other autoimmune conditions). One reason is their tendency to infect muscle, evident in animal models (see below) and human infection (e.g. myocarditis, rhabdomyolysis, chronic coxsackievirus A9 myopathy; Kuroda *et al.* 1986). Although self-limited in normal patients, enteroviral infection, particularly echovirus, can cause a dermatomyositis-like syndrome, usually accompanied by meningoencephalitis and sometimes by arthritis, in patients with agammaglobulinaemia (McKinney *et al.* 1987).

There is some evidence to support a viral role in polymyositis/dermatomyositis. More frequent antibodies to coxsackievirus-B, but not other viruses, were found in recent-onset juvenile dermatomyositis (83 per cent versus 25 per cent in matched controls; Christensen *et al.* 1986). Similarly, antibodies to coxsackievirus-A or B were more frequent in adult dermatomyositis, polymyositis, or myositis/malignancy (but not overlap, anti-Jo-1, or polymyositis/interstitial lung disease) compared with normal or rheumatoid arthritis controls (Nishikai 1994). Picornaviruses cannot be demonstrated by culture or immunofluorescence in typical polymyositis/dermatomyositis (Ytterberg 1994), and the picornavirus-like structures reported in early studies of diseased muscle by EM were probably not of viral origin. Data using molecular probes has been conflicting. Some studies have found evidence of coxsackievirus by hybridization (Yousef et al. 1990; Bowles et al. 1993), but others found no evidence of any enterovirus by in situ methods (Rosenberg et al. 1989; Hilton et al. 1994). Rosenberg et al. (1989) did find 60 per cent of adult dermatomyositis biopsies (but not polymyositis or controls) to be positive in muscle macrophages with a mouse picornavirus probe (Theiler's). Reactive material in the positive studies has not been characterized further, and Hilton et al. (1994) suggested they were detecting non-specific effects. Most studies using the PCR have been negative for enterovirus and other viruses (Leff et al. 1992; Leon-Monzon and Dalakas 1992; Jongen et al. 1993). In contrast, Behan and Behan (1993), using large samples, found polymerase chain reaction evidence of enterovirus in 56 per cent, with positives in all polymyositis/dermatomyositis groups, and in 4 per cent of controls; hybridization was seen in macrophages, endothelial cells, and occasional muscle fibres.

Thus, evidence is not consistent or convincing, and a role for ongoing picornavirus infection in polymyositis/dermatomyositis seems unlikely for most cases, although a potential role for subgroups of patients or isolated cases remains. Persistent infection is not necessarily required for an initiating role.

Retroviruses

HIV and HTLV-1 myositis discussed above suggest that polymyositis/dermatomyositis may be induced by as yet unidentified retroviruses, and understanding the mechanisms of these conditions may provide insight into the aetiology and pathogenesis of idiopathic polymyositis. No evidence of retrovirus by PCR was found (Leff et al. 1992; Nelson et al. 1994). Retroviruses are also under study in other autoimmune conditions, such as rheumatoid arthritis, Sjögren's syndrome and systemic lupus erythematosus (Kalden and Gay 1994).

Toxoplasmosis

Cases have been reported of Toxoplasma gondii infection causing a picture resembling polymyositis/dermatomyositis (reviewed in Ytterberg 1994), with some responding at least partially to treatment of the Toxoplasma. Antibodies to Toxoplasma were more frequent in polymyositis patients than controls, and IgM antibodies, suggesting recent or active infection, were also more frequent in polymyositis/dermatomyositis patients (24 per cent versus 3 per cent of systemic lupus erythematosus) (Magid and Kagen 1983). The significance of the tests is unclear, and a role for Toxoplasma in the polymyositis/dermatomyositis of these patients has not been established. Active Toxoplasma infection is not found in the muscle in most typical cases of these diseases by culture or biopsy. Bretagne et al. (1994) failed to find Toxoplasma DNA by a PCR method in the muscle of three patients with polymyositis/dermatomyositis with elevated titres. Reactivation of Toxoplasma by disease or treatment has been suggested as a cause for the positive titres (Behan et al. 1983). It remains possible that some cases of apparently idiopathic polymyositis/dermatomyositis result from unrecognized Toxoplasma or related infection.

Non-infectious causes

Drug, chemical, and environmental factors

Unlike most other drugs that cause myopathy, D-penicillamine induces a polymyositis-like inflammatory myopathy (Takahashi et al. 1986). The mechanism is unknown, and there is no clear relation to dose or duration. It usually responds when the drug is stopped, but steroids are often needed and deaths have occurred. Cardiac involvement can occur (Wright et al. 1994), as well as the dermatomyositis rash and even anti-Jo-1 (Jenkins et al. 1993). This emphasizes that ingested environmental agents could induce idiopathic polymyositis/dermatomyositis. A small number of other drugs, such as cimetidine and propylthiouracil, have been associated with an inflammatory myopathy.

An important lesson from D-penicillamine polymyositis/dermatomyositis is that genetic factors may affect the risk for disease among patients with equal exposure to the aetiological agent (Garlepp 1993). It was more frequent among Japanese patients (1.2 per cent) and Asian Indian patients (1.4 per cent) than Caucasian patients (0.2 to 0.4 per cent). It was associated with HLA DR4 in Caucasians, in contrast with idiopathic polymyositis/dermatomyositis. This may relate to the use of the drug in rheumatoid arthritis, but a link with DR4 was not seen in Asian Indians with rheumatoid arthritis, who did show an association with DR2 (80 versus 47 per cent) (Taneja et al. 1990). Thus, immunogenetic background may affect susceptibility.

Environmental toxins are also of potential significance in the induction of autoimmune disease (Love and Miller 1993). Possible examples include cases of polymyositis developing after poisoning by the natural fish toxin ciguatera (Stommel et al. 1991), or with silica exposure. There has been recent focus on polymyositis/dermatomyositis after cosmetic procedures. Cukier et al. (1993) identified eight patients with dermatomyositis (and one with polymyositis) developing an average of 6.4 months after bovine collagen dermal implant or test exposure. However, an analysis by Rosenberg and Reichlin (1994), including review of individual cases, found the observed frequency to be lower than the estimated expected frequency. A link between polymyositis/dermatomyositis and silicone breast implants has also been postulated. Love et al. found that 13 women with polymyositis/dermatomyositis after implants differed in the frequency of clinical features, autoantibodies, and HLA types from 76 without implants (Love et al. 1992). However, its significance as an aetiological or adjuvant factor remains to be demonstrated (Houpt and Sontheimer 1994).

Malignancy

The mechanism for the association of dermatomyositis and malignancy (noted above) is unknown. The tumour might lead to polymyositis/dermatomyositis by causing immune dysregulation, producing immune complexes, or inducing specific antimuscle reactions, but a common factor might lead to both conditions (persistent viral infections, toxins, genetic predispositions, immunological abnormalities).

Other factors

A large survey to determine risk factors for developing polymyositis/dermatomyositis found an increased frequency of recent heavy muscular exertion and emotional stress in patients (Lyon et al. 1989), but immunization was not correlated, and recent upper respiratory infections were negatively associated.

Immunogenetics

Associations with MHC genes indicate the importance of genetic susceptibility in polymyositis/dermatomyositis (Garlepp 1993). HLA DR3 has been associated with polymyositis in several studies, such as those of Love et al. (1991) (DR3 in 45 per cent in polymyositis/dermatomyositis versus 23 per cent in controls), and Ehrenstein et al. (1992) (DR3 in 75 per cent polymyositis versus 27 per cent in controls). The association is clearer in white than in black patients. C4A null, associated with B8/DR3, showed no independent association with polymyositis/dermatomyositis (Moulds et al. 1990). MHC associations do not differ between clinically defined subgroups, but are stronger with myositis-specific autoantibodies than with polymyositis/dermatomyositis overall. Compared with other patients, HLA DR3 is more frequent in patients with anti-Jo-1 (Goldstein et al. 1990; Love et al. 1991), but not other antisynthetases. Both anti-Jo-1 and other antisynthetases were associated with HLA DRw52, with or without DR3. This suggested that a short sequence on the DRβ1 chain may be crucial in antisynthetase production (Goldstein et al. 1990). DQα associations have also been reported, including an association of anti-Jo-1 with DQα4 (Gurley et al. 1991). Reveille et al. (1992) found that most black or white antisynthetase patients showed DQA1*0501 or DQA1*0401 (associated with DR52-bearing DR types), and Japanese antisynthetase patients showed DQA1*0101, *0102, or *0103. Immunoglobulin allotypes may also predispose to development of antisynthetases; patients with anti-Jo-1 had higher Gm 3;5, and the combination of Gm 3;5 and DR3 was markedly increased (92 versus 15 per cent) (Enz et al. 1992).

Anti-PM-Scl is most common among Caucasians, and was not found in a large study of Japanese patients (Hirakata et al. 1992). It is strongly associated with DR3, as first noted by Genth et al. (1990) (DR3 in all 12 patients with anti-PM-Scl versus 23.5 per cent of controls, $p < 0.001$), and later Marguerie et al. (1992) (DR3 in all 22 patients with anti-PM-Scl and 50 per cent homozygous), and Oddis et al. (1992) (DR3 in 15 out of 20 patients with anti-PM-Scl versus 22 per cent of controls). DR7 was associated with anti-Mi-2 (75 per cent versus 16 per cent without MSA), and DR5 with anti-SRP (57 per cent versus 20 per cent) (Love et al. 1991).

Pathogenetic mechanisms

Autoimmunity in polymyositis/dermatomyositis is suggested by the inflammatory picture, the response to steroids, and the association with other autoimmune diseases. Studies of both the cellular and humoral immune abnormalities have supported this impression, and have provided important insight into the mechanisms involved (Kalovidouris 1994; Plotz et al. 1995).

Cellular immunity

Infiltrating lymphocytes

Lymphocytes in muscle inflammatory infiltrates have been characterized using monoclonal antibodies to cell surface markers (Engel et al. 1990). T cells, many of which are activated (expressing DR antigens), are prominent in areas of severe inflammation (Rowe et al. 1983). CD4+ T cells are most abundant in untreated adults with acute disease, and decrease with treatment. In moving from the perivascular to the endomysial area, the proportion of CD8+ suppressor/cytotoxic T cells increases, and that of CD4+ T cells and B cells decreases (Arahata and Engel 1984; Mantegazza et al. 1993).

Dermatomyositis biopsies show a higher proportion of B cells and a lower proportion of CD8+ T cells than polymyositis.

In polymyositis, many non-necrotic muscle fibres are surrounded and invaded by mononuclear cells; such fibres are very rare in dermatomyositis. A majority of surrounding and most of the invading cells are CD8+ T lymphocytes (Engel and Arahata 1984), indicating direct involvement of CD8+ T cells in fibre injury. A high proportion of invading cells are activated, and most are cytotoxic rather than suppressor (Arahata and Engel 1988a). Killer and natural killer cells do not seem to contribute to muscle damage (Arahata and Engel 1988b). Necrotic fibres become infiltrated predominantly by macrophages. By EM, cytotoxic T cells and macrophages become apposed against the fibre and send 'spike-like processes' into it, which then proliferate, but the membrane remains intact (Arahata and Engel 1986). Many endomysial (not perimysial) cells may show perforin and granzyme A, granule proteins of cytotoxic T cells that may participate in fibre damage, as well as TIA-1 protein related to apoptosis (Cherin et al. 1993a; Orimo et al. 1994).

The T-cell receptors of the infiltrating lymphocytes also suggest an antigen-directed T-cell attack in polymyositis. T-cell receptor rearrangements and marked restriction in V gene usage are seen, although the V genes used differed between studies. Using PCR techniques, Mantegazza et al. (1993) found preferential usage of Vα1, Vα5, Vβ1, and Vβ15, while O'Hanlon et al. (1994a) showed predominance of Vα1 and Vβ6, with Jβ gene conservation, among anti-Jo-1 patients with polymyositis, but not dermatomyositis. By histochemistry, V-gene usage differed between cells in the perimysial areas and those in the endomysial areas that are attacking the muscle fibres (Lindberg et al. 1994a). Bender et al. (1995), confirming this, found that sequences of T-cell receptor V genes from different invading T cells of an individual were often identical, suggesting local clonal expansion, evidently in response to a muscle antigen. One patient had a unique form of polymyositis, in which the infiltrating T cells had almost exclusively γ/-T-cell receptors (Hohlfeld et al. 1991b). It was hypothesized that the antigens may be heat-shock proteins, a common target of such T cells. The T cells may have been derived from a single T-cell clone (Pluschke et al. 1992).

Thus, the predominant mechanism for immunologically mediated muscle injury in polymyositis, but not dermatomyositis, appears to be T-cell cytotoxicity, directed at an unidentified antigen, presumably on the muscle fibre surface. The fibre is surrounded and invaded by activated, clonally expanded, cytotoxic T cells. Additional mechanisms, such as cytokines, may come into play in the final destruction of the fibre.

T-cell attack on muscle fibres does not appear to occur in dermatomyositis, but cellular immunity may still play a role, possibly contributing to the vessel injury. Saito et al. (1989) found that mononuclear cells (mostly CD8+ T cells) from patients with dermatomyositis, but not polymyositis, showed cytotoxicity against cultured fibroblasts in a non-MHC restricted manner.

Muscle fibres

While expression of MHC-1 antigens on muscle fibres is normally low or absent, in polymyositis and inclusion-body myositis muscle many fibres strongly express MHC-1, making them vulnerable to antigen-directed T-cell mediated cytotoxicity (Karpati et al. 1988). MHC-1 was seen on all fibres that were invaded by CD8+ lymphocytes (Emslie-Smith et al. 1989). However, it can also be seen in dermatomyositis, where surrounded and invaded fibres are rare.

MHC-2 antigens have been found on muscle fibres in most active polymyositis and dermatomyositis biopsies (Kalovidouris 1994), but not in normal muscle or that of other myopathies. ICAM-1 (intercellular adhesion molecule 1) is induced on muscle fibres under attack, in the area of invasion, and may be important in adhesion of invading cells (De Bleecker and Engel 1994).

Since strength often returns with treatment of polymyositis and dermatomyositis sooner than would be expected if regeneration were required, much of the weakness may relate to muscle cell dysfunction. This may result from cytokines or other factors released by infiltrating mononuclear cells, that can interfere with calcium binding to the sarcoplasmic reticulum and suppress muscle contractility (Kalovidouris 1986). A possible additional mechanism may be relative acquired enzyme deficiencies such as myoadenylate deaminase (Sabina *et al.* 1990).

Peripheral blood lymphocytes

Early studies of peripheral blood lymphocytes in polymyositis/dermatomyositis showed increased proliferation in response to muscle extract in some studies (Targoff 1991), greater in active untreated cases, but generally of a low level, and not myositis-specific. Kalovidouris *et al.* (1989) later found significant lymphocyte stimulation in response to autologous or allogeneic muscle much more frequently in active (76 per cent) than treated myositis (12.5 per cent) or controls, consistent with sensitization of lymphocytes to muscle.

Peripheral lymphocytes from patients with polymyositis/dermatomyositis showed toxicity for muscle cells in culture in some studies (Targoff 1991), but this was not specific for polymyositis/dermatomyositis and did not require MHC compatibility, suggesting a non-antigen-specific mechanism such as natural killer cells. Recently, Hohlfeld and Engel (1991a) tested cultured muscle-infiltrating cytotoxic T cells against cultured autologous muscle, and some lines did show some evidence of cytotoxicity by chromium-51 release, but further study is needed to demonstrate clearly antigen-directed T-cell cytotoxicity in polymyositis/dermatomyositis.

In active polymyositis/dermatomyositis, a high proportion of peripheral blood T cells show activation markers (Miller *et al.* 1990a), decreasing with treatment. As expected, those with dermatomyositis show fewer activated T cells, but more B-cells than those with polymyositis. There is increased trafficking of lymphocytes to muscle. Peripheral lymphocytes show decreased mitogen responsiveness in polymyositis, and decreased autologous mixed lymphocyte responses (Plotz *et al.* 1989).

Cytokines

Cytokines could be important in the development, enhancement, or perpetuation of the autoimmune response, or in tissue injury and cytotoxicity. Lymphocytes cultured with autologous muscle elaborate cytotoxic factors (Johnson *et al.* 1972). Interferon-γ, present in polymyositis/dermatomyositis muscle (Isenberg *et al.* 1986), can enhance MHC-1 and induce MHC-2 expression on cultured muscle fibres *in vitro* (Kalovidouris 1992) and enhance T-cell adhesion to muscle by increasing ICAM-1 expression (Kalovidouris *et al.* 1994). Interferon-γ can inhibit proliferation and differentiation, an effect enhanced by tumour necrosis factor-α (TNF-α), thus possibly directly injuring or preventing repair of muscle fibres (Kalovidouris *et al.* 1993). Polymyositis has occurred after interferon therapy.

The serum levels of IL-2 receptor and IL-1α are elevated in active polymyositis and dermatomyositis (Wolf and Baethge 1990) and fall with treatment, possibly reflecting activated lymphocytes. IL-1 receptor antagonist was markedly elevated in some patients with active disease, and fell with treatment (Gabay *et al.* 1994), while spondylarthropathies and rheumatoid arthritis show instead higher IL-6 and C-reactive protein, possibly reflecting the relative prominence of activated T cells in polymyositis/dermatomyositis.

Humoral immunity

Microvascular injury

Direct T-cell mediated attack against muscle fibres does not seem to be important in dermatomyositis, with little endomysial infiltrate, and few surrounded and invaded non-necrotic fibres. However, the intense B-cell and CD4+ T-cell infiltrate in the perivascular area suggests a local humoral response (Arahata and Engel 1984) (Table 7).

Vasculopathy involving the small vessels and capillaries, with resultant ischaemic damage and perifascicular atrophy, is an important mechanism of muscle injury in dermatomyositis (Emslie-Smith and Engel 1990; Heffner 1993). Long associated with juvenile dermatomyositis, it is often found in typical adult dermatomyositis, but generally not polymyositis. Casademont *et al.* (1993) found that

Table 7 Differences between polymyositis and dermatomyositis

	Dermatomyositis	Polymyositis
Skin rash	Yes	No
Microvascular injury	Yes	No
Perifascicular atrophy	Common	Uncommon
Endomysial infiltration	Less common	Common
Surrounded and invaded fibres	Rare	Frequent
Deposition of membrane attack complex	Yes	No
Anti-Mi-2	15–20%	<1%
Anti-SRP	<1%	5%

87 per cent of patients with muscle capillary damage had a dermatomyositis rash.

Emslie-Smith and Engel (1990), studying muscle biopsies from adults with clinical dermatomyositis that showed little or no structural change by routine examination ('early dermatomyositis'), found definite microvascular abnormalities by EM in all cases, including endothelial cell injury, microtubular inclusions, and decreased capillary density (confirmed quantitatively), not seen in polymyositis or inclusion-body myositis. Biopsies showing overt dermatomyositis had even lower capillary density and more advanced vascular changes, including capillary necrosis.

Microvascular damage in muscle is felt to be mediated by complement. Kissel *et al.* (1986) found deposition of complement membrane attack complex (**MAC**) in the walls of muscle microvasculature, indicating local activation of complement, in most cases of juvenile dermatomyositis and some cases of adult dermatomyositis, but not polymyositis. It is greater in areas where ischaemic damage is recent (fibres with 'punched-out' central myofibrillar loss) than in those with perifascicular atrophy (a later change), and is less evident in long-standing disease (Kissel *et al.* 1991). Emslie-Smith and Engel (1990) found membrane attack complex deposition in 9 of 10 'early dermatomyositis' biopsies. Since injury to the microvasculature can occur before inflammatory infiltrates and muscle fibre damage are evident, it may be the primary target in the pathogenesis of dermatomyositis.

The factors leading to complement activation are not known. Deposition of immunoglobulin in muscle blood vessels, not seen in normal people, has been found in dermatomyositis in some studies, especially juvenile dermatomyositis and autoimmune rheumatic disease overlap, and less commonly polymyositis, but is not specific (Isenberg 1983). Its relation to the membrane attack complex deposition is unknown. Deposition has also been seen in the periphery of the fibre (sarcolemma and basement membrane), and in the fibre itself.

Autoantibodies

The clearest evidence of abnormality of humoral immunity in polymyositis/dermatomyositis is the presence of autoantibodies to nuclear and cytoplasmic antigens in up to 89 per cent of patients (Reichlin and Arnett 1984) (Fig. 12). A positive ANA is found in 40 to 80 per cent, more commonly in overlap and less in myositis with malignancy. The specificities of these antibodies have been studied in detail (Targoff 1994), and are heterogeneous, possibly reflecting heterogeneity of the disease (Table 8). About half of patients have autoantibodies of recognized specificity, some of which are found primarily in polymyositis/dermatomyositis, referred to as MSAs (Miller 1993). Others have an association with myositis, but may be found in other conditions. Most MSAs are associated with a characteristic clinical picture, and an individual generally has only a single MSA, so that MSAs can define clinical subgroups (Love *et al.* 1991).

Myositis-specific antibodies (MSAs)

Antisynthetases

About 30 per cent of patients with polymyositis/dermatomyositis have antibodies to an aminoacyl-tRNA synthetase, an enzyme that attaches one specific amino acid to its cognate tRNAs. Five antisynthetases occur in polymyositis/dermatomyositis sera (Table 8). These enzymes are antigenically distinct, and an individual patient has antibodies to only one. By far the most common is antibody to

histidyl-tRNA synthetase (anti-Jo-1) (Mathews and Bernstein 1983), found in 20 per cent of patients with polymyositis/dermatomyositis.

A group of clinical features have been associated with anti-Jo-1 in several studies (Table 9; Marguerie *et al.* 1990; Love *et al.* 1991). The limited number of patients with non-Jo-1 antisynthetases studied have had a similar clinical picture (Targoff and Arnett 1990; Targoff *et al.* 1992; Targoff *et al.* 1993). Apart from myositis, the most striking feature is interstitial lung disease, found in 50 to 90 per cent with the antibodies, but less than 10 per cent of other patients with polymyositis/dermatomyositis. The interstitial lung disease can dominate the picture, and some patients have this without overt myositis (more common with anti-PL-12). Two-thirds of patients with anti-Jo-1 have inflammatory polyarthritis (Oddis *et al.* 1990b), usually mild and responsive to treatment, but a third of these may have finger deformity, usually non-erosive, occasionally with calcinosis (rare erosive disease may represent rheumatoid arthritis overlap; O'Neill and Maddison 1993). Raynaud's phenomenon (62 per cent), fever (87 per cent), and mechanic's hands (71 per cent) are other important features (Love *et al.* 1991). Marguerie *et al.* (1990) found that sclerodactyly (72 per cent) and sicca (59 per cent) were also frequent. Their response to therapy may be less complete, with more relapses. A third to a half of the patients have dermatomyositis (some find a lower proportion among anti-Jo-1 patients). Malignancy is uncommon but has occurred. Patients with these antibodies are also immunogenetically distinctive (see above).

The set of clinical features associated with antisynthetases has been referred to as the 'anti-synthetase syndrome' (Targoff 1994). It may resemble other autoimmune rheumatic diseases syndromes, including mixed connective tissue disease (with joint disease, scleroderma and Raynaud's phenomenon; Marguerie *et al.* 1990) or systemic lupus erythematosus (fever, pneumonitis, polyarthritis, and positive ANA). However, myositis is usually more prominent and less responsive to treatment, significant interstitial lung disease is more frequent, and features of systemic lupus erythematosus are rare in the absence of other autoantibodies.

Other anticytoplasmic myositis-specific antibodies

Antibodies to other cytoplasmic antigens are found in a small proportion of patients with polymyositis/dermatomyositis (Table 8), the most important of which is antibody to the signal recognition particle (anti-SRP), a ribonucleoprotein involved in protein translocation into the endoplasmic reticulum. Anti-SRP is found almost exclusively in adult polymyositis (Targoff *et al.* 1990), with no increase in interstitial lung disease, arthritis, or Raynaud's phenomenon. Some patients with anti-SRP have an acute, fulminant course, resistant to treatment (Love *et al.* 1991). Antibodies to translation factors have been identified rarely in patients with polymyositis/dermatomyositis, including anti-KJ, which was associated with a picture similar to the antisynthetase syndrome (Targoff *et al.* 1989). Anti-Mas, directed at a tRNA-related antigen, was identified in rare patients with inflammatory myopathy and alcoholism (Love *et al.* 1991), but is not myositis-specific. Several MSAs are directed at cytoplasmic antigens related to tRNA or protein synthesis, but more patients with polymyositis/dermatomyositis have antinuclear than anticytoplasmic antibodies.

Antinuclear myositis-specific antibody

Anti-Mi-2, which reacts with a nuclear antigen of unknown function, is strongly associated with dermatomyositis (Targoff 1994). Ninety-five per cent of patients with anti-Mi-2 have dermatomyositis, and 15 to 20 per cent with dermatomyositis have the antibody. The rash

Table 8 Autoantibodies in polymyositis/dermatomyositis (PM/DM)

Antibody	Antigen	Percentage of all PM/DM	Myositis subgroup
Myositis-specific antibodies		30–40	
Anticytoplasmic			
Antisynthetase: Aminoacyl-tRNA synthetases:		25–30	
Anti-Jo-1	Histidyl-tRNA synthetase	18–20	Antisynthetase syndrome
Anti-PL-7	Threonyl-tRNA synthetase	<3	Antisynthetase syndrome
Anti-PL-12	Alanyl-tRNA synthetase/tRNAala3	<3	Antisynthetase syndrome
Anti-OJ	Isoleucyl-tRNA synthetase	<2	Antisynthetase syndrome
Anti-EJ	Glycyl-tRNA synthetase	<2	Antisynthetase syndrome
Anti-SRP	Signal recognition particle	4	PM
Antinuclear			
Anti-Mi-2	Nuclear protein complex	8	DM
Anti-56-kDa	56 kDa nuclear protein	85–90	All
Myositis-associated antibodies			
Antitranslation			
Anti-KJ	Unidentified translation factor	<1	PM, Raynaud/s interstitial lung disease
Anti-Fer	Elongation factor-1α	<1	ND
Myositis overlap antibodies			
Anti-PM-Scl	Nucleolar/nucleolar protein complex	8	PM/DM–scleroderma overlap
Anti-U1RNP	U1 small nuclear ribonucleoprotein	12	PM/DM–overlap syndromes
Anti-U2RNP	U2 small nuclear ribonucleoprotein	<2	PM
Anti-U5RNP	U5 small nuclear ribonucleoprotein	<2	PM
Anti-KU	DNA binding protein dimer	<2	PM–scleroderma or systemic lupus erythematosus
Anti-Ro/SSA	RNA–protein particle	10	Systemic lupus erythematosus; Sjögren's overlap
Anti-La/SSB	RNA–protein	5–7	Systemic lupus erythematosus; Sjögren's overlap

Most characteristic subgroup is shown, but most may occur in others.
ND=Not determined
Antisynthetase syndrome: See Table 9.

is often florid (Fig. 6), with a higher frequency of the 'V' and 'shawl' signs than others with dermatomyositis (Love *et al*. 1991). Patients with anti-Mi-2 tend to do better than those with antisynthetases. No increase in interstitial lung disease or Raynaud's phenomenon is seen.

Myositis–overlap antibodies
Several autoantibodies are seen in patients with myositis–scleroderma or other overlap syndromes. Although not MSAs, since some patients do not have myositis, these antibodies can be very helpful in evaluating a patient with suspected myositis.

Anti-PM-Scl
Anti-PM-Scl reacts with a nucleolar protein complex of unknown function containing at least 11 polypeptides. Patients with anti-PM-Scl have myositis (5 to 10 per cent of patients with polymyositis/dermatomyositis), scleroderma, or, most commonly, a myositis–scleroderma overlap syndrome, often with arthritis (Marguerie *et al*. 1992; Oddis *et al*. 1992). Cutaneous scleroderma is usually limited when present. The myositis is often mild and tends to be responsive to treatment. Raynaud's phenomenon and interstitial lung disease are common and calcinosis may be increased. Jablonska *et al*. (1993) describe 'scleromyositis', a syndrome with features of polymyositis/dermatomyositis and scleroderma with anti-PM-Scl that may resemble mixed autoimmune rheumatic disease. In Japan, anti-PM-Scl is rare, but anti-Ku is commonly found in polymyositis–scleroderma overlap (Hirakata *et al*. 1992). Anti-Ku is rare in polymyositis/dermatomyositis in the United States, but found more often in systemic lupus erythematosus and scleroderma.

Table 9 Features of antisynthetase syndrome

	Love *et al.* (n=47) (%)	Marguerie *et al.* (n=29) (%)
Myositis	100	83
Arthritis/arthralgia	94	90
Interstitial lung disease	89	79
Raynaud's phenomenon	62	93
Fever	87	NR
Flares during taper	60	NR
Mechanic's hands	71	NR
Sclerodactyly	NR	72
Sicca	NR	59
Myalgia	84	NR
Calcinosis	NR	24
DM rash	54	38
Anti-Ro/SSA	25	24
HLA DR3	73	NR
Mortality	21	17
Female:male ratio	2.7	1.4
Percentage anti-PL-12	2	21

References: Lover *et al.* (1991); Marguerie *et al.* (1990). NR=not recorded.

Anti-snRNPs

Anti-U1RNP is found in 10 to 15 per cent of polymyositis/dermatomyositis, often with autoimmune rheumatic disease overlap features such as Raynaud's phenomenon, arthritis or dactylitis. Myositis is often found in patients with overlap syndromes or systemic lupus erythematosus who have U1RNP. The myositis tends to be more responsive to treatment (Lundberg *et al.* 1992; Jablonska *et al.* 1993). Three per cent of patients with polymyositis/dermatomyositis have anti-Sm, usually with systemic lupus erythematosus overlap. Antibodies specific for the U2 snRNP (usually with anti-U1RNP) occur in a small number of patients with polymyositis–scleroderma (Craft *et al.* 1988), and anti-U5RNP (without anti-U1RNP/Sm) appears to be myositis-specific (Rider *et al.* 1994).

Patients with anti-U3RNP, a scleroderma-specific antibody, have a higher frequency of inflammatory myositis than others with diffuse scleroderma (Okano *et al.* 1992). Anti-Ro/SSA, often with anti-La/SSB, is found in 10 per cent of polymyositis/dermatomyositis, more commonly with antisynthetases; Sjögren's syndrome or systemic lupus erythematosus overlap may be present, but is not always evident. Antibodies associated with other autoimmune rheumatic diseases, such as anticentromere, occur in occasional patients with polymyositis/dermatomyositis, usually as part of overlap syndromes.

Other myositis-associated autoantibodies

The sera of 87 per cent of patients with polymyositis/dermatomyositis reacts with a 56-kDa protein of nuclear ribonucleoprotein particles (Arad-Dann *et al.* 1989). Anti-56 kDa is common in all subgroups, but more in dermatomyositis than polymyositis. It is not completely specific, being found in 10 per cent of other autoimmune rheumatic diseases (usually in lower titre), but was not found in serum of normal subjects or patients with other muscle diseases. The titre varied with disease activity. It may be a more general marker for myositis, and have a different significance than other MSAs.

Antiendothelial cell antibodies, of interest in view of the endothelial injury in dermatomyositis, and antibodies to heat shock proteins, occur in some patients with polymyositis and dermatomyositis, but they are common in other conditions, and their significance in polymyositis/dermatomyositis is unknown (Cervera *et al.* 1991). Antibodies to muscle proteins such as myosin occur in up to 90 per cent of polymyositis/dermatomyositis (Wada *et al.* 1983; Koga *et al.* 1987), and may vary with disease activity. Although more frequent in polymyositis/dermatomyositis than other muscle diseases, they are not specific, and could be secondary to muscle damage. The possibility that they contribute to muscle injury is of interest, but their role is unknown.

Possible relation to pathogenesis

The reason for production of these antibodies is unknown, and may relate to aetiological factors (Targoff 1994). HLA and other genetic factors seem to be important (see above). There is increasing evidence that production is driven and perpetuated by the recognized antigens (Miller *et al.* 1990c), but they may not initiate the responses. It is often speculated that myositis-inducing viruses lead to the antibodies through such mechanisms as molecular mimicry, formation of immunogenic complexes between host and viral factors, etc. (Targoff 1991). Hypotheses must explain how patients with antibodies to different members of the same enzyme family, present in every cell, have a similar clinical syndrome manifested in specific organs.

It is not known if the antibodies play a direct role in pathogenesis (Naparstek and Plotz 1993). Antisynthetases consistently inhibit antigen function, but they have not been shown to enter intact cells. They could injure muscle through immune complexes, reaction with cell surface antigens, etc., but there is as yet no evidence of this. A correlation of anti-Jo-1 titre with myositis activity (Miller *et al.* 1990b), including the development of anti-Jo-1 shortly before the onset of weakness (Miller *et al.* 1990a), suggests a pathogenetic role, but against such a role is their common occurrence in polymyositis, where cell-mediated fibre damage is most important, and low frequency in juvenile dermatomyositis, where humoral injury occurs.

The epitopes of the myositis-associated autoantibodies are under study; predominant epitopes are often found (Raben *et al.* 1994). They generally differ from those of animal antisera, and tend to be conformational (Targoff 1994). Specific immunological features of the antibodies may provide clues to their origin.

Animal models

Experimental autoimmune myositis

Certain strains of guinea pig, rat, or mouse develop myositis (but not weakness or rash) as a result of immunizations with homologous or heterologous muscle homogenates in adjuvant (Rosenberg 1993). Inflammation and necrosis occur, but no vascular changes or perifascicular atrophy. Muscle damage is mediated by cellular immune mechanisms, and lymphoid cells can transfer disease. Humoral reaction to muscle is seen, and serum could transfer disease in one

(Matsubara *et al.* 1993) but not other studies. The histology resembles human polymyositis, but with more macrophages in the inflammatory infiltrate (80 to 90 per cent). Experimental autoimmune myositis demonstrates that cell-mediated immunity can mediate muscle injury, but is limited by differences from human polymyositis/dermatomyositis.

SJL/J mice are uniquely susceptible to experimental autoimmune myositis, and with aging, develop a similar and more severe myositis spontaneously. Immunological defects and neoplasms occur in these mice, which may contribute. This spontaneous model may provide insight into aetiological factors (Rosenberg 1993).

Viral models

Picornaviruses

Coxsackie and several other picornaviruses can produce a polymyositis-like myositis in mice. Neonatal Swiss mice infected with coxsackie-B1 Tuscon strain develop an acute illness followed by a chronic inflammatory myositis resembling polymyositis, with proximal muscle weakness, myopathic electromyographs, and mononuclear cell infiltration, with degenerating and regenerating muscle fibres (Strongwater *et al.* 1984). Myositis progresses beyond the period in which the virus can be cultured (6 months versus 2 weeks), but viral nucleic acid persists longer than culturable virus (Tam *et al.* 1994). Production of the myositis depends on the strain of virus and of mouse used, and requires cell-mediated immunity (Ytterberg *et al.* 1987).

Infection of adult mice with a myotropic strain of encephalomyocarditis virus produces an inflammatory myositis and myocarditis in some mouse strains (Miller *et al.* 1987). As with coxsackievirus, development of the myositis requires specific strains of virus and genetic background (susceptibility was H2 restricted). Further, viral nucleic acid could be detected at 4 weeks, when virus could no longer be cultured but muscle inflammation persisted (Cronin *et al.* 1988); thus viral persistence may be important in chronicity. The mice do not develop myositis-associated autoantibodies. Thus, picornaviruses can produce an immune-mediated myositis, supporting their potential as aetiological agents in some cases of idiopathic polymyositis/dermatomyositis.

Retroviruses

Macaque monkeys develop a syndrome resembling AIDS after infection with the D-type simian retrovirus SRV-1. Up to half of infected monkeys develop a myositis that closely resembles polymyositis as part of their disease (Dalakas *et al.* 1987), with weakness, elevated enzymes, and a biopsy showing inflammation, necrosis, phagocytosis, and fibrosis. The mechanism is unclear, although the virus could infect cultured muscle cells. The model may be useful in the study of retrovirus-associated myositis, as well as idiopathic polymyositis/dermatomyositis.

Canine dermatomyositis

A condition resembling dermatomyositis occurs spontaneously in collies and Shetland sheep dogs (Hargis and Prieur 1988), with autosomal dominant inheritance. Juvenile dogs develop muscle weakness and atrophy, difficulty eating, and an erythematous, scaly rash over the periorbital areas, face, and distal extremities. Muscle histology shows inflammation, fibre necrosis, regeneration, and atrophy, and vasculitis may occur. Serological tests are usually negative. The model has significant differences from human myositis, but

is most similar to juvenile dermatomyositis. Dogs may spontaneously develop an eosinophilic myositis of the muscles of mastication. Occasionally, polymyositis is seen.

Management

Treatment should be started promptly, since significant delay has been associated with poorer outcome (see below). Treatment is most urgent, and sometimes initiated pending completion of the evaluation, in patients with rapid onset of severe weakness, dysphagia, respiratory insufficiency, myocardial involvement, or systemic signs. Most cases can be managed outside the hospital, but admission may be required for patients with respiratory insufficiency or severe dysphagia, those requiring intravenous medications, or clarification of diagnosis.

A general approach to treatment is outlined in Table 10. Guidelines for initial treatment, dosage reduction, and choice of agents should be adapted to the situation of the patient. Most patients are first given a trial of corticosteroids alone. Initial therapy with a combination of steroids and immunosuppressives also has some support (Bunch 1981). Some have recently suggested other agents for first-line treatment, such as cyclosporine (Grau *et al.* 1994) or for certain patients, intravenous gammaglobulin (Dalakas 1994a). Immunosuppressives and recently intravenous gammaglobulin are used when additional therapy is required.

Corticosteroids

While not demonstrated by prospective randomized controlled trials, the effectiveness of steroids in improving muscle strength is accepted generally, and readily apparent from observation of treated patients. It is further suggested by studies demonstrating improved outcome with earlier treatment.

Initial treatment

Treatment is usually begun at high doses (prednisone 1 mg/kg per day, usually 60 to 80 mg/d, or equivalent), often in divided doses that are considered to increase effectiveness. Dalakas (1994a; Dalakas 1994b) recommends 80 to 100 mg/d as a single morning dose, feeling that this increases its benefits.

The high initial dose (prednisone more than 60 mg/d) is continued until the creatine kinase has returned to normal and the strength has substantially improved, usually 1 to 2 months (Oddis 1991). Adequate initial treatment is important, and is associated with better responses (Oddis and Medsger 1988). When begun as divided doses, the daily amount is usually consolidated to a single morning dose after the acute period or before beginning dosage taper.

Very high-dose intravenous 'pulse' methylprednisolone, in regimens such as 1 g/day for 3 days, is sometimes used initially to achieve a more immediate effect in severely ill patients, or later when disease is unresponsive to oral steroids, or for exacerbations during steroid taper (Oddis 1993). Matsubara *et al.* (1994) found that pulse therapy (0.5 g/day for 3 days per week for 1 to 9 weeks) added to oral therapy increased the rate of and shortened the time to remission. Although some have used alternate-day steroids in milder cases from the outset to reduce side-effects (Hoffman *et al.* 1983), it is less reliable, and not recommended in most cases (Dalakas 1994b).

Table 10 A strategy for treatment of newly diagnosed active idiopathic polymyositis or dermatomyositis

1. *Significant but not severe weakness*
   A. Begin:
      Prednisone, 1 mg/kg/day ($\geqslant$ 60 mg/day), divided dose
   B. After initial response:
      (i) Consolidate to single daily dose
      (ii) Continue for at least 1 month until creatine kinase normal
   C. Continues to do well:
      Decrease dose such that maintenance level (5 to 10 mg/day) achieved by 6 months ($\approx$ 10 to 25% per month)
   D. Maintenance:
      (i) Prednisone 5 to 10 mg/day for at least 1 year
      (ii) Then taper by approximately 1 mg per 3 months until stopped.

2. *Severe (but not life threatening) weakness*
   A. Begin:
      (i) High-dose pulse methyl-prednisolone (1 g/day for 3 days)
      (ii) Then prednisone, 1 mg/kg.day ($\geqslant$ 60 mg/day), divided dose
   B. Then follow 1 above.

3. *Rapidly progressive, severe weakness and/or concerning features (severe dysphagia, respiratory muscle weakness)*
   A. Begin:
      (i) intravenous gammaglobulin 1 g/kg.day $\times$ 2 days
      (ii) Then follow 2 above

4. *Inadequate response of creatine kinase and strength by 4 to 8 weeks or significant steroid side-effects*
   A. Add second line agent.
      (i) If no contraindications methotrexate 10 mg/week, then gradual increase to response, or 20 mg/week oral or if needed, higher parenterally.
      (ii) If contraindication to or failure of methotrexate:
         Less severe (can wait for response):
            Switch to azathioprine 100 mg/week, then gradual increase to 2 to 3 mg/kg.day.
         Clinically severe unfavourable MSA:
            Add azathioprine or switch to cyclosporin

5. *Side-effects with immunosuppressive agents or failure to respond to two second-line agents*
   Add intravenous gammaglobulin 2 g/kg.month

6. *Creatine kinase responds but strength not recovering as expected*
   A. Further evaluation needed.
      (i) Consider factors in section on response to corticosteroids
      (ii) MRI
   B. If disease active, add second-line agent
   C. If disease not active, taper steroids (possible steroid myopathy)

7. *Steroid side-effects during taper*
   A. Convert to alternate day
   B. If flare or not tolerated, see 4 above.

8. *Other considerations*
   (a) Rehabilitation: consider for all patients. Begin with passive range of motion. Cautiously add resistive exercises when creatinine kinase normalizes. Slowly advance.
   (b) Interstitial lung disease: if progressive and requiring treatment and high-dose prednisone unsuccessful, consider cyclophosphamide intravenous pulse (0.5 to 1.0 g/m^2/month); if very severe or intravenous failure, oral cyclophosphamide, 1 to 2 mg/kg/day.
   (c) Myositis in systemic lupus erythematosus or scleroderma: in patients with mild myositis and favourable antibody but require treatment for myositis, consider lower initial dose (prednisone $\approx$ 30 mg/day).
   (d) Cutaneous dermatomyositis without myositis: watch for myositis, especially in first 2 years, with prompt treatment as above if seen. Topical steroids and sunscreens initially. Hydroxychloroquine 200 to 400 mg/day for non-responders who require additional treatment. If no
      myositis, moderate-dose steroids or methotrexate are used only when indicated for the cutaneous lesions.
   (e) Respiratory failure due to weakness: intravenous gammaglobulin and/or high-dose pulse methylprednisolone used at any point, plus supportive care.

Response

It is important to monitor patients closely during treatment for degree of improvement, new complications, or side-effects. Both muscle strength (assessed as above) and creatine kinase levels are used to judge improvement. The response to steroids in polymyositis/dermatomyositis tends to be slower than that in systemic lupus erythematosus or rheumatoid arthritis, and it may take months to achieve the full effect (Plotz *et al.* 1989), with a mean time to recovery of normal strength of more than 3 months (Tymms and Webb 1985).

The creatine kinase usually normalizes weeks to months earlier than the strength, generally indicating adequate suppression of disease activity. Creatine kinase levels in the high normal range may indicate disease activity and may decrease with treatment.

Oddis and Medsger (1989) found that treatment using the following guidelines was more likely to result in prolonged suppression of disease: (i) start with 60 mg/day or more of prednisone for at least 1 month; (ii) continue initial treatment until or after the creatine kinase becomes normal; and (iii) taper steroids slowly, with average reduction from first reduction to maintenance dosage of 10 mg/month or less.

Most patients respond at least partially to treatment with steroids. If there is no improvement or if significant weakness persists, possibilities include: (i) incorrect diagnosis: the basis for the diagnosis should be reviewed, and further evaluation considered, such as repeat biopsy looking in particular for inclusion-body myositis or metabolic myopathy; (ii) malignancy: although myositis with malignancy may be quite responsive (Joffe et al. 1993), failure to respond or weight loss on steroids should suggest a more extensive search (Plotz 1992); (iii) steroid myopathy: when creatine kinase falls but weakness persists, not explained by the expected lag of strength behind creatine kinase, steroid myopathy should be considered; (iv) permanent loss of strength: some patients cannot recover full strength despite complete suppression of disease activity, often those with prolonged delay before treatment, atrophy, or prominent fibrosis on biopsy; (v) resistance: disease activity may be unresponsive to steroid therapy. Persistent elevation of the creatine kinase usually means that the disease has not been controlled. Occasional patients have resolution or stabilization of weakness while creatine kinase remains elevated, often at low levels. Such elevations may not reflect ongoing disease activity (Oddis 1994); MRI may help to assess activity in these situations.

Dosage reduction

When the initial goals are reached, the dosage is gradually reduced over 6 to 8 months, usually at 15 to 25 per cent per month (Table 10). Some recommend routine conversion to an alternate-day regimen after the initial high-dose daily regimen (Dalakas 1988b), usually accomplished gradually, as by reduction of the low-day dosage by about 10 mg per week. This may be advantageous in patients who have developed or are at high risk for significant steroid side-effects. Steroids are usually continued for 1 to 2 years or longer at a low, maintenance dose (Oddis 1994) that is high enough to successfully prevent recurrence but low enough to keep the risk of side-effects low (prednisone 5 to 10 mg/day or 10 to 20 mg every other day).

Less aggressive or less prolonged therapy may be adequate in some patients. In a primary care setting, Hoffman et al. (1983) could successfully discontinue treatment in 41 per cent of patients without recurrence. The myositis in the autoimmune rheumatic diseases overlap syndromes associated with anti-U1RNP and anti-PM-Scl may be more responsive and require less therapy than other myositis (Jablonska et al. 1993). However, the standard regimens should be considered more reliable for most patients with polymyositis/dermatomyositis.

Exacerbations of disease may occur during taper, and are more likely if dosage is reduced rapidly. A rise in the creatine kinase level, sometimes within the normal range, frequently precedes exacerbation (Oddis and Medsger 1989). If creatine kinase elevation occurs after initial response, causes other than disease flare should be considered, particularly when no other signs are present. Exacerbation without creatine kinase elevation may occur, even if the enzyme was elevated originally, but if weakness increases without creatine kinase elevation, steroid myopathy should be considered. Other tests, such as MRI, electromyography, or repeat needle biopsy, can help assess disease activity in these cases. Exacerbation is treated usually with an increase in steroid dosage above those which last maintained control of the disease, although full-dose is usually not necessary, and/or addition of an immunosuppressive agent (Oddis 1991).

The side-effects of corticosteroids in polymyositis/dermatomyositis are similar to those in other situations. Steroid myopathy poses a special problem, as noted above. Steroid-induced hypokalaemia may also lead to further weakness and should be avoided. Due to the prolonged high-dose steroids used in polymyositis/dermatomyositis, osteoporosis and aseptic necrosis are significant problems, contributing to disability. Adequate calcium and vitamin D intake should be maintained. Tymms and Webb (1985) found aseptic necrosis in 8.6 per cent of patients with polymyositis/dermatomyositis receiving high-dose steroids. Gastric protection is commonly used. Diabetes, hypertension, cataracts, and opportunistic infections (including tuberculosis) may be seen.

Immunosuppressives

Immunosuppressive agents are required in about a quarter to a half of patients. Indications include: (i) steroid resistance, with failure to respond to high-dose steroids after 6 to 12 weeks, (excluding considerations mentioned above); (ii) persistent disease activity after prolonged therapy despite initial improvement; (iii) inability to taper the prednisone without recurrence; or (iv) severe steroid side-effects. Immunosuppressives would be considered earlier in those with very severe or acute disease, or factors suggesting poorer response, such as certain autoantibodies (anti-synthetases or anti-SRP) (Plotz et al. 1995). Generally, the trend is toward earlier and more frequent use of immunosuppressive agents because of steroid side-effects and possibly improved response (Steinberg 1993).

Methotrexate and azathioprine are the immunosuppressives used most extensively. Retrospective analysis (Joffe et al. 1993) suggests a higher response rate and more rapid onset of effect with methotrexate, and some (Oddis 1994) use it first if an immunosuppressive is required and there are no contraindications. However, azathioprine may have less toxicity and has demonstrated efficacy in a controlled study (Bunch 1981), and some prefer it as first choice (Ramirez et al. 1990; Urbano-Marquez et al. 1991; Dalakas 1992b).

Joffe et al. (1993) found that patients with antisynthetases were more likely to respond to methotrexate than to azathioprine. Methotrexate should be used with caution in this setting because of the frequent interstitial lung disease in antisynthetase patients, which can lead to diagnostic confusion with hypersensitivity pneumonitis, or difficulty tolerating it. They also found that men were more likely to respond to methotrexate than azathioprine.

Methotrexate

Methotrexate has been used over a broad dosage range in polymyositis/dermatomyositis. Early studies frequently employed a high-dose regimen administered intravenously (intramuscular injec-tions may interfere with creatine kinase monitoring in polymyositis/dermatomyositis), begun at 10 to 15 mg/week, and gradually increased to 0.5 to 0.8 mg/kg per week (30 to 50 mg/week). After an adequate response, methotrexate was tapered by extending the dosing interval to 2, 3, and 4 weeks, or by decreasing the weekly dose. Metzger *et al.* (1974) found good to excellent responses in 15 of 22 patients (68 per cent), at an average of 13 weeks.

Weekly low-dose oral regimens are now more often used (Plotz *et al.* 1989; Oddis 1994), starting at 7.5 to 10 mg/week and increasing gradually as required to a maximum of 20 to 25 mg/week. Parenteral therapy should be considered for the higher dose ranges, or if gastro-intestinal intolerance develops. Response times may range from 3 to 44 weeks. The prednisone dose can usually be reduced ('steroid-sparing'). Exacerbations may occur with methotrexate taper in responsive patients.

Although methotrexate toxicity in polymyositis/dermatomyositis is usually mild, severe toxicity (hepatotoxicity, fatal hypersensitivity pneumonitis) has occurred. As in rheumatoid arthritis, patient selec-tion is important (avoid in renal insufficiency, hepatic damage, alcoholism). The monitoring guidelines for rheumatoid arthritis should be considered a minimum; the higher doses often used in polymyositis/dermatomyositis may require closer observation, and elevated transaminases from muscle injury may interefere with their use in monitoring. Zieglschmid-Adams *et al.* (1995) observed hepatic fibrosis (grade IIIA) with methotrexate in 2 of 10 patients with derma-tomyositis on usual doses; diabetes was a risk factor. Euwer and Sontheimer (1994) feel that toxicity in dermatomyositis may resemble that of psoriasis more than rheumatoid arthritis. Other side-effects include stomatitis, infections, teratogenicity, bone marrow suppres-sion, and gastrointestinal bleeding. A methotrexate-associated reversible lymphoma was reported in dermatomyositis (Kamel *et al.* 1993).

Azathioprine

Bohan *et al.* (1977) noted improvement with azathioprine in about 35 per cent of polymyositis/dermatomyositis, and a steroid-sparing effect in 50 per cent. Ramirez *et al.* (1990) noted benefit in 75 per cent of those with an adequate course. In a controlled trial (Bunch 1981), patients beginning therapy with azathioprine plus prednisone had better long-term outcome with less disability and less prednisone requirement than those receiving prednisone alone, although there was no difference in short-term outcome after 3 months. It is used orally at 1.5 to 3.0 mg/kg per day, with doses of 100 to 150 mg/d being most common. Dalakas (1992b) recommends 3 mg/kg per day, with an adequate trial requiring 3 to 6 months. Steroids may be gradually reduced as response occurs. Cytopenias or bone marrow suppression may occur, and complete blood counts including platelets must be monitored. The possibility of malignancy is a concern, but the risk appears low in polymyositis/dermatomyositis. Other side-effects are similar to those in other situations.

Alkylating agents

Cyclophosphamide and chlorambucil are generally reserved for those who have failed to respond to other agents (Steinberg 1993), or have other manifestations such as severe interstitial lung disease. They generally have a higher risk of serious side-effects, particularly increased malignancy but also bone marrow suppression, infertility, and, for cyclophosphamide, haemorrhagic cystitis.

Reports regarding the value of oral cyclophosphamide in poly-myositis/dermatomyositis have been conflicting (Plotz *et al.* 1989); some found it lacked efficacy, but others had success. It is usually used at a dose of 1 to 2 mg/kg per day, with close monitoring of the white blood count. Monthly intravenous pulse cyclophos-phamide has been used in an effort to limit side-effects. Cronin *et al.* (1989), used this in patients with long-standing, refractory disease, and found poor efficacy and high toxicity (fever, nausea, infections, etc.). Bombardieri *et al.* (1989), however, had a high success rate in patients without previous cytotoxic therapy using short courses (2 to 3 weeks) of 0.5 g intravenous pulses at 1 to 2 week intervals, with a repeat course for flares. De Vita and Fossaluzza (1992) had good results with a similar regimen, begin-ning with 3 weeks of low pulses, then 0.5 to 1 g/m² per month for non-responders, with individual regimens as needed.

Chlorambucil has also been successful in a small number of reported patients. Of five patients treated with chlorambucil at 4 mg/day by Sinoway and Callen (1993), all had some improvement by 4 to 6 weeks, and normal strength by 13.5 months, but with minimal effect on the skin disease. Little toxicity was seen (two with leucopenia), and the drug could be stopped in four patients.

Cyclosporin (Neoral)

Several case reports or small series have described beneficial effects of cyclosporin in polymyositis/dermatomyositis, more in children but some in adults, including in severe, resistant disease (Oddis 1994). Grau *et al.* (1994) compared their experience in 10 consecu-tive patients with dermatomyositis treated initially with cyclosporin (usually 5 mg/kg per day), with their previous 45 patients treated initially with prednisone. Cyclosporin-treated patients responded earlier and achieved complete remission in less than half the time (mean 8.6 weeks), with a comparable failure rate and less frequent serious toxicity. Nephrotoxicity is the greatest concern. Although many reports used doses of greater than 5 mg/kg per day, following the recent guidelines of Feutren and Mihatsch (1992) would be prudent (doses of 5 mg/kg or less per day, and creatinine kept less than 30 per cent over baseline). Tacrolimus (FK506) was also effective in a preliminary report (Oddis *et al.* 1994).

Combination therapy

Combinations of immunosuppressives, such as methotrexate and azathioprine or chlorambucil and methotrexate, often with predni-sone, have been used in patients with refractory disease, or to limit toxicity by using smaller doses. The methotrexate/azathioprine combination and high-dose methotrexate with leukovorin rescue are under study (Steinberg 1993).

Intravenous gammaglobulin

There is increasing evidence of the efficacy of high-dose intra-venous gammaglobulin in polymyositis and dermatomyositis, and increasing experience with its use. Dalakas *et al.* (1993) showed that intravenous gammaglobulin was significantly better than placebo in a double-blind, cross-over trial in 15 adults with dermatomyositis. There was major improvement in 9 of 12 with intravenous gammaglobulin (0 of 11 with placebo) and none worsened (versus 5 of 11 with placebo). The rash improved in

Basta, M. and Dalakas, M.C. (1994). High-dose intravenous immunoglobulin exerts its beneficial effect in patients with dermatomyositis by blocking endomysial deposition of activated complement fragments. *Journal of Clinical Investigation*, **94**, 1729–35.

Behan, W.M. and Behan, P.O. (1993). The role of viral infection in polymyositis, dermatomyositis and chronic fatigue syndrome. *Baillière's Clinical Neurology*, **2**, 637–57.

Behan, W.M.H., Behan, P.O., Draper, I.T., and Williams, H. (1983). Does *Toxoplasma* cause polymyositis. *Acta Neuropathologica*, **61**, 246–52.

Bender, A., Ernst, N., Iglesias, A., Dornmair, K., Wekerle, H., and Hohlfeld, R. (1995). T cell receptor repertoire in polymyositis: clonal expansion of autoaggressive CD8+ T cells. *Journal of Experimental Medicine*, **181**, 1863–8.

Bernard, P. and Bonnetblanc, J.M. (1993). Dermatomyositis and malignancy. *Journal of Investigative Dermatology*, **100**, 128S–132S.

Bertorini, T.E. (1988*a*). Electromyography in polymyositis and dermatomyositis (PM/DM). In *Polymyositis and dermatomyositis* (ed. M.C. Dalakas), pp. 217–34. Butterworths, Boston.

Bertorini, T.E. (1988*b*). Histopathology of the inflammatory myopathies. In *Polymyositis and dermatomyositis* (ed. M.C. Dalakas), pp. 157–94. Butterworths, Boston.

Black, H.R., Quallich, H., and Gareleck, C.B. (1986). Racial differences in serum creatine kinase levels. *American Journal of Medicine*, **81**, 479–87.

Bohan, A. and Peter, J.B. (1975). Polymyositis and dermatomyositis. Parts 1 and 2. *New England Journal of Medicine*, **292**, 344–7, 403–7.

Bohan, A., Peter, J.B., Bowman, R.L., and Pearson, C.M. (1977). A computer-assisted analysis of 153 patients with polymyositis and dermatomyositis. *Medicine*, **56**, 255–86.

Bohlmeyer, T.J., Wu, A.H.B., and Perryman, M.B. (1994). Evaluation of laboratory tests as a guide to diagnosis and therapy of myositis. *Rheumatic Disease Clinics of North America*, **20**, 845–56.

Bombardieri, S., Hughes, G.R., Neri, R., Del Bravo, P., and Del Bono, L. (1989). Cyclophosphamide in severe polymyositis [letter]. *Lancet*, **i**, 1138–9.

Bonnetblanc, J.M., Bernard, P., and Fayol, J. (1990). Dermatomyositis and malignancy: a multicenter cooperative study. *Dermatologica*, **180**, 212–16.

Bowles, N.E. *et al.* (1993). Persistence of enterovirus RNA in muscle biopsy samples suggests that some cases of chronic fatigue syndrome result from a previous, inflammatory viral myopathy. *Journal of Medicine*, **24**, 145–60.

Boyd, A.S. and Neldner, K.H. (1994). Therapeutic options in dermatomyositis/polymyositis. *International Journal of Dermatology*, **33**, 240–50.

Braun, N.M., Arora, N.S., and Rochester, D.F. (1983). Respiratory muscle and pulmonary function in polymyositis and other proximal myopathies. *Thorax*, **38**, 616–23.

Bretagne, S., Costa, J.M., Cosnes, A., Authier, F.J., Vidaud, M., and Gherardi, R.K. (1994). Lack of *Toxoplasma gondii* DNA in muscles of patients with inflammatory myopathy and increased anti-*Toxoplasma* antibodies. *Muscle and Nerve*, **17**, 822–4.

Bunch, T.W. (1981). Prednisone and azathioprine for polymyositis: Long-term followup. *Arthritis and Rheumatism*, **24**, 45–48.

Byrne, E. and Dennett, X. (1993). Idiopathic inflammatory myopathies: clinical aspects. *Baillière's Clinical Neurology*, **2**, 499–526.

Calabrese, L.H., and Chou, S.M. (1994). Inclusion body myositis. *Rheumatic Disease Clinics of North America*, **20**, 955–72.

Calabrese, L.H., Mitsumoto, H., and Chou, S.M. (1987). Inclusion body myositis presenting as treatment-resistant polymyositis. *Arthritis and Rheumatism*, **30**, 397–403.

Callen, J.P. (1987). Dermatomyositis. *Disease-a-Month*, **33**, 237–305.

Callen, J.P. (1993). Dermatomyositis and malignancy. *Clinics in Dermatology*, **11**, 61–5.

Callen, J.P. (1994). Myositis and malignancy. *Current Opinion in Rheumatology*, **6**, 590–94.

Caro, I. (1988). A dermatologist's view of polymyositis/dermatomyositis. *Clinics in Dermatology*, **6**, 9–14.

Carpenter, S. (1988). Resin histology and electron microscopy in inflammatory myopathies. In *Polymyositis and dermatomyositis* (ed. M.C. Dalakas), pp. 195–215. Butterworths, Boston.

Casademont, J., Grau, J.M., Masanes, F., Herrero, C., and Urbano-Marquez, A. (1993). Analysis of the outcome of idiopathic inflammatory myopathies with particular emphasis on muscle capillary damage. *Scandanavian Journal of Rheumatology*, **22**, 292–8.

Cervera, R. *et al.* (1991). Antibodies to endothelial cells in dermatomyositis: Association with interstitial lung disease. *British Medical Journal*, **302**, 880–81.

Charness, M.E., Simon, R.P., and Greenberg, D.A. (1989). Ethanol and the nervous system. *New England Journal of Medicine*, **321**, 442–54.

Cheong, W.-K., Hughes, G.R.V., Norris, P.G., and Hawk, J.L.M. (1994). Cutaneous photosensitivity in dermatomyositis. *British Journal of Dermatology*, **131**, 205–8.

Cherin, P. *et al.* (1991). Efficacy of intravenous gammaglobulin therapy in chronic refractory polymyositis and dermatomyositis: an open study with 20 adult patients. *American Journal of Medicine*, **91**, 162–8.

Cherin, P., Herson, S., Coutellier, A., Bletry, O., and Piette, J.C. (1992). Failure of total body irradiation in polymyositis: report of three cases. *British Journal of Rheumatology*, **31**, 282–3.

Cherin, P., Crevon, M.C., Hauw, J.J., Galanaud, P., Herson, S., and Emilie, D. (1993*a*). Mechanisms of lysis by cytotoxic cells in inflammatory myopathies: study of perforin and serine esterase gene expression by in situ hybridization and protein TIA-1 expression by immunohistochemistry, from muscular biopsies. *Arthritis and Rheumatism*, **36**, S84 (Abstract).

Cherin, P. *et al.* (1993*b*). Dermatomyositis and ovarian cancer: A report of 7 cases and literature review. *Journal of Rheumatology*, **20**, 1897–9.

Cherin, P. *et al.* (1994). Intravenous gamma globulin as first line therapy in polymyositis and dermatomyositis: an open study in 11 adult patients. *Journal of Rheumatology*, **21**, 1092–7.

Chiedozi, L.C. (1979). Pyomyositis: review of 205 cases in 112 patients. *American Journal of Surgery*, **137**, 255–9.

Chou, S.M. (1986). Inclusion body myositis: a chronic persistent mumps myositis? *Human Pathology*, **17**, 765–77.

Chou, S.M. (1993). Inclusion body myositis. *Baillière's Clinical Neurology*, **2**, 557–77.

Christensen, M.L., Pachman, L.M., Schneiderman, R., Patel, D.C., and Friedman, J.M. (1986). Prevalence of coxsackie B virus antibodies in patients with juvenile dermatomyositis. *Arthritis and Rheumatism*, **29**, 1365–70.

Cole, A.J., Kuzniecky, R., Karpati, G., Carpenter, S., Andermann, E., and Andermann, F. (1988). Familial myopathy with changes resembling inclusion body myositis and periventricular leucoencephalopathy. A new syndrome. *Brain*, **111**, 1025–37.

Cox, N.H., Lawrence, C.M., Langtry, J.A.A., and Ive, F.A. (1990). Dermatomyositis: disease associations and an evaluation of screening investigations for malignancy. *Archives of Dermatology*, **126**, 61–5.

Craft, J., Mimori, T., Olsen, T.L., and Hardin, J.A. (1988). The U2 small nuclear ribonucleoprotein particle as an autoantigen. Analysis with sera from patients with overlap syndromes. *Journal of Clinical Investigation*, **81** 1716–24.

Cronin, M.E. and Plotz, P.H. (1990). Idiopathic inflammatory myopathies. *Rheumatic Disease Clinics of North America*, **16**, 655–65.

Cronin, M.E., Love, L.A., Miller, F.W., McClintock, P.R., and Plotz, P.H. (1988). The natural history of encephalomyocarditis virus-induced myositis and myocarditis in mice. Viral persistence demonstrated by in situ hybridization. *Journal of Experimental Medicine*, **168**, 1639–48.

Cronin, M.E., Miller, F.W., Hicks, J.E., Dalakas, M.C., and Plotz, P.H. (1989). The failure of intravenous cyclophosphamide therapy in refractory idiopathic inflammatory myopathy. *Journal of Rheumatology*, **16**, 1225–8.

Csuka, M.E. and McCarty, D.J. (1985). Simple method for measurement of lower extremity muscle strength. *American Journal of Medicine*, **78**, 77–81.

Cukier, J., Beauchamp, R.A., Spindler, J.S., Spindler, S., Lorenzo, C., and Trentham, D.E. (1993). Association between bovine collagen dermal implants and a dermatomyositis or a polymyositis-like syndrome. *Annals of Internal Medicine*, **118**, 920–28.

Cumming, W.J.K. (1989). Thymectomy in refractory dermatomyositis. *Muscle and Nerve*, **12**, 424.

Dalakas, M., Gravell, M., London, W.T., Cunningham, G., and Sever, J.L. (1987). Morphological changes of an inflammatory myopathy in Rhesus monkeys with simian acquired immunodeficiency syndrome (42556). *Proceedings of the Society of Experimental Biology and Medicine*, **185**, 368–76.

Dalakas, M.C. (1988a). A classification of polymyositis and dermatomyositis. In *Polymyositis and dermatomyositis* (ed. M.C. Dalakas), pp. 1–16. Butterworths, Boston.

Dalakas, M.C. (1988b). Treatment of polymyositis and dermatomyositis with corticosteroids: a first therapeutic approach. In *Polymyositis and dermatomyositis* (ed. M.C. Dalakas), pp. 235–53. Butterworths, Boston.

Dalakas, M.C. (1991). Polymyositis, dermatomyositis, and inclusion-body myositis. *New England Journal of Medicine*, 325, 1487–98.

Dalakas, M.C. (1992a). Inflammatory and toxic myopathies. *Current Opinion in Neurology and Neurosurgery*, 5, 645–54.

Dalakas, M.C. (1992b). Clinical, immunopathologic, and therapeutic considerations of inflammatory myopathies. *Clinics in Neuropharmacology*, 15, 327–51.

Dalakas, M.C. (1993). Retroviruses and inflammatory myopathies in humans and primates. *Baillière's Clinical Neurology*, 2, 659–691.

Dalakas, M.C. (1994a). Current treatment of the inflammatory myopathies. *Current Opinions in Rheumatology*, 6, 595–601.

Dalakas, M.C. (1994b). How to diagnose and treat the inflammatory myopathies. *Seminars in Neurology*, 14, 137–45.

Dalakas, M.C. and Engel, W.K. (1988). Total body irradiation in the treatment of intractable polymyositis and dermatomyositis. In *Polymyositis and dermatomyositis* (ed. M.C. Dalakas), pp. 281–91. Butterworths, Boston.

Dalakas, M.C., Illa, I., Pezeshkpour, G.H., Laukaitis, J.P., Cohen, B., and Griffin, J.L. (1990). Mitochondrial myopathy caused by long-term zidovudine therapy. *New England Journal of Medicine*, 322, 1098–105.

Dalakas, M.C. *et al.* (1993). A controlled trial of high-dose intravenous immune globulin infusions as treatment for dermatomyositis. *New England Journal of Medicine*, 329, 1993–2000.

Dau, P.C. (1981). Plasmapheresis in idiopathic inflammatory myopathy: experience with 35 patients. *Archives of Neurology*, 38, 544–52.

De Bleecker, J.L. and Engel, A.G. (1994). Expression of cell adhesion molecules in inflammatory myopathies and Duchenne dystrophy. *Journal of Neuropathology and Experimental Neurology*, 53, 369–76.

De Vita, S. and Fossaluzza, V. (1992). Treatment of idiopathic inflammatory myopathies with cyclophosphamide pulses: clinical experience and a review of the literature. *Acta Neurologica Belgica*, 92, 215–27.

DeGeeter, F., Deleu, D., Debeuckelaere, S., DeConinck, A., Somers, G., and Bossuyt, A. (1989). Detection of muscle necrosis in dermatomyositis by ^{111}In-labelled antimyosin Fab fragments. *Nuclear Medicine Communications*, 10, 603–7.

DeMerieux, P., Verity, M.A., Clements, P.J., and Paulus, H.E. (1983). Esophageal abnormalities and dysphagia in polymyositis and dermatomyositis. *Arthritis and Rheumatism*, 26, 961–8.

Denbow, C.E., Lie, J.T., Tancredi, R.G., and Bunch, T.W. (1979). Cardiac involvement in polymyositis: a clinicopathologic study of 20 autopsied patients. *Arthritis and Rheumatism*, 22, 1088–92.

Dickey, B.F. and Myers, A.R. (1984). Pulmonary disease in polymyositis/dermatomyositis. *Seminars in Arthritis and Rheumatism*, 14, 60–76.

Dietz, F., Logeman, J., Sahgal, V., and Schmid, F.R. (1980). Cricopharyngeal muscle dysfunction in the differential diagnosis of dysphagia in polymyositis. *Arthritis and Rheumatism*, 23, 491–5.

Dropcho, E.J. and Soong, S. (1991). Steroid-induced weakness in patients with primary brain tumors. *Neurology*, 41, 1235–9.

Dwyer, J.M. (1992). Manipulating the immune system with immune globulin. *New England Journal of Medicine*, 326, 107–16.

Ehrenstein, M.R., Snaith, M.L., and Isenberg, D.A. (1992). Idiopathic myositis: a rheumatological view. *Annals of the Rheumatic Diseases*, 51, 41–4.

Emslie-Smith, A.M., and Engel, A.G. (1990). Microvascular changes in early and advanced dermatomyositis: a quantitative study. *Annals of Neurology*, 27, 343–56.

Emslie-Smith, A.M., Arahata, K., and Engel, A.G. (1989). Major histocompatibility complex class I antigen expression, immunolocalization of interferon subtypes, and T cell-mediated cytotoxicity in myopathies. *Human Pathology*, 20, 224–31.

Engel, A.G., and Arahata, K. (1984). Monoclonal antibody analysis of mononuclear cells in myopathies. II: phenotypes of autoinvasive cells in polymyositis and inclusion body myositis. *Annals of Neurology*, 16, 209–15.

Engel, A.G., Arahata, K., and Emslie-Smith, A.M. (1990). Immune effector mechanisms in inflammatory myopathies. *Research Publications — Association for Research in Nervous and Mental Diseases*, 68, 141–57.

Enz, L.A., Love, L.A., Targoff, I.N., Pandey, J.P., and Miller, F.W. (1992). Associations among Gm phenotypes, HLA alleles, and myositis-specific autoantibodies (MSA) in idiopathic inflammatory myopathy (IIM). *Arthritis and Rheumatism*, 35, S52 (Abstract).

Escalante, A., Miller, L., and Beardmore, T.D. (1993). Resistive exercise in the rehabilitation of polymyositis/dermatomyositis. *Journal of Rheumatology*, 20, 1340–44.

Estes, M.L. *et al.* (1987). Chloroquine neuromyotoxicity: clinical and pathologic perspective. *American Journal of Medicine*, 82, 447–55.

Euwer, R.L. and Sontheimer, R.D. (1993). Amyopathic dermatomyositis: a review. *Journal of Investigative Dermatology*, 100, 124–7S.

Euwer, R.L. and Sontheimer, R.D. (1994). Dermatologic aspects of myositis. *Current Opinion in Rheumatology*, 6, 583–9.

Fafalak, R.G., Peterson, M.G., and Kagen, L.J. (1994). Strength in polymyositis and dermatomyositis: best outcome in patients treated early. *Journal of Rheumatology*, 21, 643–8.

Feutren, G. and Mihatsch, M.J. (1992). Risk factors for cyclosporine-induced nephropathy in patients with autoimmune diseases. *New England Journal of Medicine*, 326, 1654–60.

Fidzianska, A. and Goebel, H.H. (1989). Tubuloreticular structures (TRS) and cylindric confronting cisternae (CCC) in childhood dermatomyositis. *Acta Neuropathologica*, 79, 310–16.

Figarella-Branger, D., Pellissier, J.F., Bianco, N., Devictor, B., and Toga, M. (1990). Inflammatory and non-inflammatory inclusion body myositis: Characterization of the mononuclear cells and expression of the immunoreactive class I Major histocompatibility complex product. *Acta Neuropathologica*, 79, 528–36.

Franks, A.G., Jr. (1988). Important cutaneous markers of dermatomyositis. *Journal of Musculoskeletal Medicine*, 5, 39–63.

Fraser, D.D., Frank, J.A., Dalakas, M.C., Miller, F.W., Hicks, J.E., and Plotz, P.H. (1991). Magnetic resonance imaging in the idiopathic inflammatory myopathies. *Journal of Rheumatology*, 18, 1693–700.

Frost, N.A., Morand, E.F., Hall, C.L., Maddison, P.J., and Bhalla, A.K. (1993). Idiopathic polymyositis complicated by arthritis and mesangial proliferative glomerulonephritis: case report and review of the literature. *British Journal of Rheumatology*, 32, 929–31.

Fudman, E.J. and Schnitzer, T.J. (1986). Dermatomyositis without creatine kinase elevation: a poor prognostic sign. *American Journal of Medicine*, 80, 329–32.

Fujino, H., Kobayashi, T., Goto, I., and Onitsuka, H. (1991). Magnetic resonance imaging of the muscles in patients with polymyositis and dermatomyositis. *Muscle and Nerve*, 14, 716–20.

Fusade, T., Belanyi, P., Joly, P., Thomine, E., Mihout, M.F., and Lauret, P. (1993). Subcutaneous changes in dermatomyositis. *British Journal of Dermatology*, 128, 451–3.

Gabay, C. *et al.* (1994). Elevated serum levels of interleukin-1 receptor antagonist in polymyositis/dermatomyositis. A biologic marker of disease activity with a possible role in the lack of acute-phase protein response. *Arthritis and Rheumatism*, 37, 1744–51.

Garlepp, M.J. (1993). Immunogenetics of inflammatory myopathies. *Baillière's Clinical Neurology*, 2, 579–97.

Garlepp, M.J., Baing, B., Zilko, P.J., Ollier, W., and Mastaglia, F.L. (1994). HLA associations with inclusion body myositis. *Clinical and Experimental Immunology*, 98, 40–45.

Genth, E. *et al.* (1990). Immunogenetic associations of scleroderma-related antinuclear antibodies. *Arthritis and Rheumatism*, 33, 657–65.

Goldstein, R. *et al.* (1990). HLA-D region genes associated with autoantibody responses to Jo-1 (histidyl-tRNA synthetase) and other translation-related factors in myositis. *Arthritis and Rheumatism*, 33 1240–48.

Gomez-Reino, J.J., Aznar, J.J., Pablos, J.L., Diaz-Gonzalez, F., and Laffon, A. (1994). Nontropical pyomyositis in adults. *Seminars in Arthritis and Rheumatism*, 23, 396–405.

Grau, J.M., Herrero, C., Casademont, J., Fernandez-Sola, J., and Urbano-Marquez, A. (1994). Cyclosporine A as first choice therapy for dermatomyositis. *Journal of Rheumatology*, 21, 381–2.

Greenlee, R. (1988). The neurologist's approach to polymyositis. *Clinics in Dermatology*, **6**, 23–35.

Gurley, R.C., Love, L.A., Targoff, I.N., Leff, R.L., Plotz, P.H., and Miller, F.W. (1991). Associations among myositis-specific autoantibodies (MSA) and HLA-DQA1 alleles. *Arthritis and Rheumatism*, **34**, S137 (Abstract).

Gurley, R.C. *et al.* (1992). Familial myositis cases emphasize the roles of genetic and environmental factors in the pathogenesis of idiopathic inflammatory myopathy (IIM). *Arthritis and Rheumatism*, **35**, S89 (Abstract).

Haddad, M.G., West, R.L., Treadwell, E.L., and Fraser, D.D. (1994). Diagnosis of inflammatory myopathy by percutaneous needle biopsy with demonstration of the focal nature of myositis. *American Journal of Clinical Pathology*, **101**, 661–4.

Hanno, R. and Callen, J.P. (1985). Histopathology of Gottron's papules. *Journal of Cutaneous Pathology*, **12**, 389–94.

Hargis, A.M. and Prieur, D.J. (1988). Animal models of polymyositis/dermatomyositis. *Clinics in Dermatology*, **6**, 120–29.

Haupt, H.M. and Hutchins, G.M. (1982). The heart and cardiac conduction system in polymyositis-dermatomyositis: a clinicopathologic study of 16 autopsied patients. *American Journal of Cardiology*, **50**, 998–1006.

Hebert, C.A., Byrnes, T.J., Baethge, B.A., Wolf, R.E., and Kinasewitz, G.T. (1990). Exercise limitation in patients with polymyositis. *Chest*, **98**, 352–7.

Heffner, R.R., Jr. (1993). Inflammatory myopathies. A review. *Journal of Neuropathology and Experimental Neurology*, **52**, 339–50.

Henriksson, K.G. and Lindvall, B. (1990). Polymyositis and dermatomyositis 1990 — diagnosis, treatment and prognosis. *Progress in Neurobiology*, **35**, 181–93.

Hernandez, R.J., Keim, D.R., Chenevert, T.L., Sullivan, D.B., and Aisen, A.M. (1992). Fat-suppressed MR imaging of myositis. *Radiology*, **182**, 217–19.

Hicks, J.E. (1988). Comprehensive rehabilitative management of patients with polymyositis and dermatomyositis. In *Polymyositis and dermatomyositis* (ed. M.C. Dalakas), pp. 293–317. Butterworths, Boston.

Higgs, J.B., Blaivas, M., and Albers, J.W. (1989). McArdle's disease presenting as treatment resistant polymyositis. *Journal of Rheumatology*, **16**, 1588–91.

Higuchi, I. *et al.* (1992). Failure to detect HTLV-1 by in situ hybridization in the biopsied muscles of viral carriers with polymyositis. *Muscle and Nerve*, **15**, 43–7.

Hilton, D.A., Fletcher, A., and Pringle, J.H. (1994). Absence of coxsackie viruses in idiopathic inflammatory muscle disease by *in situ* hybridization. *Neuropathology and Applied Neurobiology*, **20**, 238–42.

Hirakata, M., Mimori, T., Akizuki, M., Craft, J., Hardin, J.A., and Homma, M. (1992). Autoantibodies to small nuclear and cytoplasmic ribonucleoproteins in Japanese patients with inflammatory muscle disease. *Arthritis and Rheumatism*, **35**, 449–56.

Hochberg, M.C., Feldman, D., and Stevens, M.B. (1986). Adult onset polymyositis/dermatomyositis: an analysis of clinical and laboratory features and survival in 76 patients with a review of the literature. *Seminars in Arthritis and Rheumatism*, **15**, 168–78.

Hoffman, G.S., Franck, W.A., Raddatz, D.A., and Stallones, L. (1983). Presentation, treatment, and prognosis of idiopathic inflammatory muscle disease in a rural hospital. *American Journal of Medicine*, **75**, 433–8.

Hohlfeld, R. and Engel, A.G. (1991*a*). Coculture with autologous myotubes of cytotoxic T cells isolated from muscle in inflammatory myopathies. *Annals of Neurology*, **29**, 498–507.

Hohlfeld, R., Engel, A.G., Ii, K., and Harper, M.C. (1991*b*). Polymyositis mediated by T lymphocytes that express the gamma/delta receptor. *New England Journal of Medicine*, **324**, 877–81.

Hood, D., Van Lente, F., and Estes, M. (1991). Serum enzyme alterations in chronic muscle disease. *American Journal of Clinical Pathology*, **95**, 402–7.

Hopkinson, N.D., Shawe, D.J., and Gumpel, J.M. (1991). Polymyositis, not polymyalgia rheumatica. *Annals of the Rheumatic Diseases*, **50**, 321–2.

Horowitz, M., McNeil, J.D., Maddern, G.J., Collins, P.J., and Shearman, D.J.C. (1986). Abnormalities of gastric and esophageal emptying in polymyositis and dermatomyositis. *Gastroenterology*, **90**, 434–9.

Houpt, K.R. and Sontheimer, R.D. (1994). Autoimmune connective tissue disease and connective tissue disease-like illnesses after silicone gel augmentation mammoplasty. [Review]. *Journal of the American Academy of Dermatology*, **31**, 626–42.

Hsue, Y.T., Paulus, H.E., and Coulson, W.F. (1993). Bronchiolitis obliterans organizing pneumonia in polymyositis. A case report with longterm survival. *Journal of Rheumatology*, **20**, 877–9.

Igarashi, M., Aizawa, H., Tokudome, Y., and Tagami, H. (1985). Dermatomyositis with prominent mucinous skin change. Histochemical and biochemical aspects of glycosaminoglycans. *Dermatologica*, **170**, 6–11.

Illa, I., Nath, A., and Dalakas, M.C. (1991). Immunocytochemical and virological characteristics of HIV-associated inflammatory myopathies: similarities with seronegative polymyositis. *Annals of Neurology*, **29**, 474–81.

Isenberg, D.A. (1983). Immunoglobulin deposition in skeletal muscle in primary muscle disease. *Quarterly Journal of Medicine*, **207**, 297–310.

Isenberg, D.A., Rowe, D., Shearer, M., Novick, D., and Beverley, P.C.L. (1986). Localization of interferons and interleukin 2 in polymyositis and muscular dystrophy. *Clinical and Experimental Immunology*, **63**, 450–58.

Ishii, N., Ono, H., Kawaguchi, T., and Nakajima, H. (1991). Dermatomyositis and pregnancy: case report and review of the literature. *Dermatologica*, **183**, 146–9.

Jablonska, S., Chorzelski, T.P., Blaszczyk, M., Jarzabek-Chorzelska, M., Kumar, V., and Beutner, E.H. (1993). Scleroderma/polymyositis overlap syndromes and their immunologic markers. *Clinics in Dermatology*, **10**, 457–72.

Janis, J.F. and Winkelman, R.K. (1968). Histopathology of the skin in dermatomyositis: a histopathologic study of 55 cases. *Archives of Dermatology*, **97**, 640–50.

Jenkins, E.A., Hull, R.G., and Thomas, A.L. (1993). D-Penicillamine and polymyositis: the significance of the anti-Jo-1 antibody. *British Journal of Rheumatology*, **32**, 1109–10.

Joffe, M.M. *et al.* (1993). Drug therapy of the idiopathic inflammatory myopathies: predictors of response to prednisone, azathioprine, and methotrexate and a comparison of their efficacy. *American Journal of Medicine*, **94**, 379–87.

Johnson, R.L., Fink, C.W., and Ziff, M. (1972). Lymphotoxin formation by lymphocytes and muscle in polymyositis. *Journal of Clinical Investigation*, **51**, 2435–49.

Jongen, P.J., Zoll, G.J., Beaumont, M., Melchers, W.J., van de Putte, L.B., and Galama, J.M. (1993). Polymyositis and dermatomyositis: no persistence of enterovirus or encephalomyocarditis virus RNA in muscle. *Annals of the Rheumatic Diseases*, **52**, 575–8.

Kagen, L.J. and Aram, S. (1987). Creatine kinase activity inhibitor in sera from patients with muscle disease. *Arthritis and Rheumatism*, **30**, 213–17.

Kagen, L.J., Hochman, R.B., and Strong, E.W. (1985). Cricopharyngeal obstruction in inflammatory myopathy (polymyositis/dermatomyositis): report of three cases and review of the literature. *Arthritis and Rheumatism*, **28**, 630–36.

Kalden, J.R. and Gay, S. (1994). Retroviruses and autoimmune rheumatic diseases. *Clinical and Experimental Immunology*, **98**, 1–5.

Kalovidouris, A.E. (1986). Mononuclear cells from patients with polymyositis inhibit calcium binding by sarcoplasmic reticulum. *Journal of Laboratory and Clinical Medicine*, **107**, 23–8.

Kalovidouris, A.E. (1992). The role of cytokines in polymyositis: interferon-gamma induces class II and enhances class I major histocompatibility complex antigen expression on cultured human muscle cells. *Journal of Laboratory and Clinical Medicine*, **120**, 244–51.

Kalovidouris, A.E. (1994). Mechanisms of inflammation and histopathology in inflammatory myopathy. *Rheumatic Disease Clinics of North America*, **20**, 881–98.

Kalovidouris, A.E., Pourmand, R., Passo, M.H., and Plotkin, Z. (1989). Proliferative response of peripheral blood mononuclear cells to autologous and allogeneic muscle in patients with polymyositis/dermatomyositis. *Arthritis and Rheumatism*, **32**, 446–53.

Kalovidouris, A.E., Plotkin, Z., and Graesser, D. (1993). Interferon-gamma inhibits proliferation, differentiation, and creatine kinase activity of cultured human muscle cells. II. A possible role in myositis. *Journal of Rheumatology*, **20**, 1718–23.

Kalovidouris, A.E., Horn, C.A., and Plotkin, Z. (1994). The role of cytokines in polymyositis. III. Recombinant human interferon-gamma enhances T cell adhesion to cultured human muscle cells. *Arthritis and Rheumatism*, **37**, 907–14.

Kamel, O.W. *et al.* (1993). Brief report: reversible lymphomas associated with Epstein–Barr virus occurring during methotrexate therapy for rheumatoid arthritis and dermatomyositis. *New England Journal of Medicine*, **328**, 1317–21.

Kanda, F., Fujii, Y., Takahashi, K., and Fujita, T. (1994). Dual-energy X-ray absorptiometry in neuromuscular diseases. *Muscle and Nerve*, **17**, 431–5.

Karpati, G., Pouliot, Y., and Carpenter, S. (1988). Expression of immunoreactive major histocompatibility complex products in human skeletal muscles. *Annals of Neurology*, **23**, 64–72.

Kasper, C.S., White, C.L., III, and Freeman, R.G. (1988). Pathology and immunopathology of polymyositis/dermatomyositis. *Clinics in Dermatology*, **6**, 64–75.

Kasteler, J.S. and Callen, J.P. (1994). Scalp involvement in dermatomyositis: often overlooked or misdiagnosed. *Journal of the American Medical Association*, **272**, 1939–41.

Kaufman, L.D. (1994). The evolving spectrum of eosinophilia myalgia syndrome. *Rheumatic Disease Clinics of North America*, **20**, 973–94.

Khaleeli, A.A. *et al.* (1983). Corticosteroid myopathy: a clinical and pathological study. *Clinics in Endocrinology*, **18**, 155–66.

Kiprov, D.D. and Miller, R.G. (1984). Polymyositis associated with monoclonal gammopathy. *Lancet*, ii, 1183–6.

Kissel, J.T., Mendell, J.R., and Rammohan, K.W. (1986). Microvascular deposition of complement membrane attack complex in dermatomyositis. *New England Journal of Medicine*, **314**, 329–34.

Kissel, J.T., Halterman, R.K., Rammohan, K.W., and Mendel, J.R. (1991). The relationship of complement-mediated microvasculopathy to the histologic features and clinical duration of disease in dermatomyositis. *Archives of Neurology*, **48**, 26–30.

Koga, K., Abe, S., Hashimoto, H., and Yamaguchi, M. (1987). Western-blotting method for detecting antibodies against human muscle contractile proteins in myositis. *Journal of Immunological Methods*, **105**, 15–21.

Koh, E.T., Seow, A., Ong, B., Ratnagopal, P., Tjia, H., and Chng, H.H. (1993). Adult onset polymyositis/dermatomyositis: clinical and laboratory features and treatment response in 75 patients. *Annals of the Rheumatic Diseases*, **52**, 857–61.

Kroll, M., Otis, J., and Kagen, L.J. (1986). Serum enzyme, myoglobin and muscle strength relationships in polymyositis and dermatomyositis. *Journal of Rheumatology*, **13**, 349–55.

Kuncl, R.W., Duncan, G., Watson, D., Alderson, K., Rogawski, M.A., and Peper, M. (1987). Colchicine myopathy and neuropathy. *New England Journal of Medicine*, **316**, 1562–8.

Kuroda, Y., Neshige, R., Oda, K., and Shibasaki, H. (1986). Chronic polymyositis: presence of coxsackievirus A9 antigen in muscle. *Japanese Journal of Medicine*, **25**, 191–4.

Lakhanpal, S., Bunch, T.W., Ilstrup, D.M., and Melton, L.J. (1986). Polymyositis-dermatomyositis and malignant lesions: does an association exist? *Mayo Clinic Proceedings*, **61**, 645–53.

Lakhanpal, S., Lie, J.T., Conn, D.L., and Martin, W.J. (1987). Pulmonary disease in polymyositis/dermatomyositis: a clinicopathological analysis of 65 autopsy cases. *Annals of the Rheumatic Diseases*, **46**, 23–9.

Lane, R.J., McLean, K.A., Moss, J., and Woodrow, D.F. (1993). Myopathy in HIV infection: the role of zidovudine and the significance of tubuloreticular inclusions. *Neuropathology and Applied Neurobiology*, **19**, 406–13.

Le Guludec, D. *et al.* (1993). New application of myocardial antimyosin scintigraphy: diagnosis of myocardial disease in polymyositis. *Annals of the Rheumatic Diseases*, **52**, 235–8.

Le Quintrec, J.-S. and Le Quintrec, J.-L. (1991). Drug-induced myopathies. *Baillière's Clinical Rheumatology*, **5**, 21–38.

Lee, K.N., Csako, G., Bernhardt, P., and Elin, R.J. (1994). Relevance of macro creatine kinase type 1 and type 2 isoenzymes to laboratory and clinical data. *Clinical Chemistry*, **40**, 1278–83.

Leff, R.L. *et al.* (1991). Distinct seasonal patterns in the onset of adult idiopathic inflammatory myopathy in patients with anti-Jo-1 and anti-signal recognition particle autoantibodies. *Arthritis and Rheumatism*, **34**, 1391–6.

Leff, R.L. *et al.* (1992). Viruses in idiopathic inflammatory myopathies: absence of candidate viral genomes in muscle. *Lancet*, **339**, 1192–5.

Leff, R.L., Miller, F.W., Hicks, J.E., Fraser, D.D., and Plotz, P.H. (1993). The treatment of inclusion body myositis: a retrospective review and a randomized, prospective trial of immunosuppressive therapy. *Medicine*, **72**, 225–35.

Leon-Monzon, M. and Dalakas, M.C. (1992). Absence of persistent infection with enteroviruses in muscles of patients with inflammatory myopathies. *Annals of Neurology*, **32**, 219–22.

Leon-Monzon, M., Lamperth, L., and Dalakas, M.C. (1993). Search for HIV proviral DNA and amplified sequences in the muscle biopsies of patients with HIV polymyositis. *Muscle and Nerve*, **16**, 408–13.

Leon-Monzon, M., Illa, I., and Dalakas, M.C. (1994). Polymyositis in patients infected with human T-cell leukemia virus type I: the role of the virus in the cause of the disease. *Annals of Neurology*, **36**, 643–9.

Lilley, H., Dennett, X., and Byrne, E. (1994). Biopsy proven polymyositis in Victoria 1982–1987: analysis of prognostic factors. *Journal of the Royal Society of Medicine*, **87**, 323–6.

Lindberg, C., Oldfors, A., and Tarkowski, A. (1994a). Restricted use of T cell receptor V genes in endomysial infiltrates of patients with inflammatory myopathies. *European Journal of Immunology*, **24**, 2659–63.

Lindberg, C., Persson, L.I., Bjorkander, J., and Oldfors, A. (1994b). Inclusion body myositis: clinical, morphological, physiological and laboratory findings in 18 cases. *Acta Neurologica Scandinavia*, **89** 123–31.

Lotz, B.P., Engel, A.G., Nishino, H., Stevens, J.C., and Litchy, W.J. (1989). Inclusion body myositis: observations in 40 patients. *Brain*, **112**, 727–47.

Love, L.A. and Miller, F.W. (1993). Noninfectious environmental agents associated with myopathies. *Current Opinions in Rheumatology*, **5**, 712–18.

Love, L.A. *et al.* (1991). A new approach to the classification of idiopathic inflammatory myopathy: myositis-specific autoantibodies define useful homogeneous patient groups. *Medicine*, **70**, 360–74.

Love, L.A. *et al.* (1992). Geographical and seasonal clustering in the onset of idiopathic inflammatory myopathy (IIM) in groups defined by myositis-specific autoantibodies (MSA). *Arthritis and Rheumatism*, **35**, S40 (Abstract).

Love, L.A. *et al.* (1992). Clinical and immunogenetic features of women who develop myositis after silicone implants (MASI). *Arthritis and Rheumatism*, **35**, S46 (Abstract).

Lovece, S. and Kagen, L.J. (1993). Sensitive rapid detection of myoglobin in serum of patients with myopathy by immunoturbidimetric assay. *Journal of Rheumatology*, **20**, 1331–4.

Lundberg, I., Nennesmo, I., and Hedfors, E. (1992). A clinical, serological, and histopathological study of myositis patients with and without anti-RNP antibodies. *Seminars in Arthritis and Rheumatism*, **22**, 127–38.

Lyon, M.G., Bloch, D.A., Hollak, B., and Fries, J.F. (1989). Predisposing factors in polymyositis-dermatomyositis: results of a nationwide survey. *Journal of Rheumatology*, **16**, 1218–24.

Magid, S.K. and Kagen, L.J. (1983). Serologic evidence for acute toxoplasmosis in polymyositis-dermatomyositis. *American Journal of Medicine*, **75**, 313–20.

Manchul, L.A. *et al.* (1985). The frequency of malignant neoplasms in patients with polymyositis-dermatomyositis: a controlled study. *Archives of Internal Medicine*, **145**, 1835–9.

Manta, P., Kalfakis, N., and Vassilopoulos, D. (1989). Evidence for seasonal variation in polymyositis. *Neuroepidemiology*, **8**, 262–5.

Mantegazza, R. *et al.* (1993). Analysis of T cell receptor repertoire of muscle-infiltrating T lymphocytes in polymyositis. Restricted V alpha/beta rearrangements may indicate antigen-driven selection. *Journal of Clinical Investigation*, **91**, 2880–86.

Marguerie, C. *et al.* (1990). Polymyositis, pulmonary fibrosis and autoantibodies to aminoacyl-tRNA synthetase enzymes. *Quarterly Journal of Medicine*, **77**, 1019–38.

Marguerie, C. *et al.* (1992). The clinical and immunogenetic features of patients with autoantibodies to the nucleolar antigen polymyositis-Scl. *Medicine*, **71**, 327–36.

Martin, A., Haller, R.G., and Barohn, R. (1994). Metabolic myopathies. *Current Opinion in Rheumatology*, **6**, 552–8.

Mathews, M.B. and Bernstein, R.M. (1983). Myositis autoantibody inhibits histidyl-tRNA synthetase: a model for autoimmunity. *Nature*, **304**, 177–9.

Matsubara, S., Shima, T., and Takamori, M. (1993). Experimental allergic myositis in SJL/J mice immunized with rabbit myosin B fraction: immunohistochemical analysis and transfer. *Acta Neuropathologica*, **85**, 138–44.

Matsubara, S., Sawa, Y., Takamori, M., Yokoyama, H., and Kida, H. (1994). Pulsed intravenous methylprednisolone combined with oral steroids as the initial treatment of inflammatory myopathies. *Journal of Neurology, Neurosurgery and Psychiatry*, **57**, 1008–16.

Matsuda, Y., Tomii, M., and Kashiwazaki, S. (1993). Fatal pneumomediastinum in dermatomyositis without creatine kinase elevation. *Internal Medicine*, **32**, 643–7.

Mbauya, A.L., Plotz, P.H., Wilder, R.L., and Miller, F.W. (1993). Increased prevalence of autoimmune disease in first degree relatives of patients with idiopathic inflammatory myopathy (IIM). *Arthritis and Rheumatism*, 36, S255 (Abstract).

McKendry, R.J.R. (1987). Influence of age at onset on the duration of treatment in idiopathic adult polymyositis and dermatomyositis. *Archives of Internal Medicine*, 147, 1989–91.

McKinney, R.E., Katz, S.L., and Wilfert, C.M. (1987). Chronic enteroviral meningoencephalitis in agammaglobulinemic patients. *Review of Infectious Diseases*, 9, 334–56.

Medsger, T.A., Jr. and Oddis, C.V. (1995). Classification and diagnostic criteria for polymyositis and dermatomyositis. *Journal of Rheumatology*, 22, 581–5.

Medsger, T.A., Jr., Robinson, H., and Masi, A.T. (1971). Factors affecting survivorship in polymyositis: a life-table study of 124 patients. *Arthritis and Rheumatism*, 14, 249–58.

Mendell, J.R., Sahenk, Z., Gales, T., and Paul, L. (1991). Amyloid filaments in inclusion body myositis: novel findings provide insight into nature of filaments. *Archives of Neurology*, 48, 1229–34.

Metzger, A.L., Bohan, A., Goldberg, L.S., Bluestone, R., and Pearson, C.M. (1974). Polymyositis and dermatomyositis: combined methotrexate and corticosteroid therapy. *Annals of Internal Medicine*, 81, 182–9.

Mhiri, C. *et al.* (1991). Zidovudine myopathy: a distinctive disorder associated with mitochondrial dysfunction. *Annals of Neurology*, 29, 606–14.

Miller, F.W. (1993). Myositis-specific autoantibodies: touchstones for understanding the inflammatory myopathies. *Journal of the American Medical Association*, 270, 1846–9.

Miller, F.W. (1994). Classification and prognosis of inflammatory muscle disease. *Rheumatic Disease Clinics of North America*, 20, 811–26.

Miller, F.W., Love, L.A., Biswas, T., McClintock, P.R., Notkins, A.L., and Plotz, P.H. (1987). Viral and host genetic factors influence encephalomyocarditis virus-induced polymyositis in adult mice. *Arthritis and Rheumatism*, 30, 549–56.

Miller, F.W., Love, L.A., Barbieri, S.A., Balow, J.E., and Plotz, P.H. (1990a). Lymphocyte activation markers in idiopathic myositis: changes with disease activity and differences among clinical and autoantibody subgroups. *Clinical and Experimental Immunology*, 81, 373–9.

Miller, F.W., Twitty, S.A., Biswas, T., and Plotz, P.H. (1990b). Origin and regulation of a disease-specific autoantibody response: antigenic epitopes, spectrotype stability, and isotype restriction of anti-Jo-1 antibodies. *Journal of Clinical Investigation*, 85, 468–75.

Miller, F.W., Waite, K.A., Biswas, T., and Plotz, P.H. (1990c). The role of an autoantigen, histidyl-tRNA synthetase, in the induction and maintenance of autoimmunity. *Proceedings of the National Academy of Sciences USA*, 87, 9933–7.

Miller, F.W. *et al.* (1992). Controlled trial of plasma exchange and leukapheresis in polymyositis and dermatomyositis. *New England Journal of Medicine*, 326, 1380–84.

Mitra, D., Lovell, C.L., Macleod, T.I., Tan, R.S., and Maddison, P.J. (1994). Clinical and histological features of 'mechanic's hands' in a patient with antibodies to Jo-1 — a case report. *Clinical and Experimental Dermatology*, 19, 146–8.

Moder, K.G., Gaffey, T.A., and Matteson, E.L. (1993). Idiopathic inflammatory myopathy of the antisynthetase (Jo-1) type associated with noncaseating granulomas. *Arthritis and Rheumatism*, 36, 1743–7.

Morgan, O.St.C., Mora, C., Rodgers-Johnson, P., and Char, G. (1989). HTLV-1 and polymyositis in Jamaica. *Lancet*, ii, 1184–7.

Moulds, J.M. *et al.* (1990). C4 Null genes in American whites and blacks with myositis. *Journal of Rheumatology*, 17, 331–4.

Moxley, R.T. (1994). Evaluation of neuromuscular function in inflammatory myopathy. *Rheumatic Disease Clinics of North America*, 20, 827–44.

Nagaraja, D., Taly, A.B., Suresh, T.G., Gourie-Devi, M., Sarala Das, and Rao, B.S.S. (1992). Epidemic of acute inflammatory myopathy in Karnataka, South India: 30 cases. *Acta Neurologica Scandinavia*, 86, 230–36.

Naparstek, Y. and Plotz, P.H. (1993). The role of autoantibodies in autoimmune disease. *Annual Review of Immunology*, 11, 79–104.

Nelson, P.N., Lever, A.M., Bruckner, F.E., Isenberg, D.A., Kessaris, N., and Hay, F.C. (1994). Polymerase chain reaction fails to incriminate exogenous retroviruses HTLV-I and HIV-1 in rheumatological diseases although a minority of sera cross react with retroviral antigens. *Annals of the Rheumatic Diseases*, 53, 749–54.

Nishikai, M. (1994). Coxsackievirus infection and the development of polymyositis/dermatomyositis. *Rheumatology International*, 14, 43–6.

Nishikai, M. and Sato, A. (1991). Human T lymphotropic virus type I and polymyositis and dermatomyositis in Japan. *Arthritis and Rheumatism*, 34, 791–2.

Nishino, H., Engel, A.G., and Rima, B.K. (1989). Inclusion body myositis: the mumps virus hypothesis. *Annals of Neurology*, 25, 260–64.

Oddis, C.V. (1991). Therapy for myositis. *Current Opinion in Rheumatology*, 3, 919–24.

Oddis, C.V. (1993). Therapy for myositis. *Current Opinion in Rheumatology*, 5, 742–8.

Oddis, C.V. (1994). Therapy of inflammatory myopathy. *Rheumatic Disease Clinics of North America*, 20, 899–918.

Oddis, C.V. and Hill, P. (1993). Pregnancy outcome in women with inflammatory myopathy. *Arthritis and Rheumatism*, 36, S255 (Abstract).

Oddis, C.V. and Medsger, T.A., Jr. (1988). Relationship between serum creatine kinase level and corticosteroid therapy in polymyositis-dermatomyositis. *Journal of Rheumatology*, 15, 807–11.

Oddis, C.V. and Medsger, T.A., Jr. (1989). Current management of polymyositis and dermatomyositis. *Drugs*, 37, 382–90.

Oddis, C.V., Conte, C.G., Steen, V.D., and Medsger, T.A., Jr. (1990a). Incidence of polymyositis-dermatomyositis: a 20-year study of hospital diagnosed cases in Allegheny County, PA 1963–1982. *Journal of Rheumatology*, 17, 1329–34.

Oddis, C.V., Medsger, T.A., Jr., and Cooperstein, L.A. (1990b). A subluxing arthropathy associated with the anti-Jo-1 antibody in polymyositis/dermatomyositis. *Arthritis and Rheumatism*, 33, 1640–45.

Oddis, C.V., Okano, Y., Rudert, W.A., Trucco, M., Duquesnoy, R.J., and Medsger, T.A., Jr. (1992). Serum autoantibody to the nucleolar antigen polymyositis-Scl: clinical and immunogenetic associations. *Arthritis and Rheumatism*, 35, 1211–17.

Oddis, C.V., Carroll, P., Abu-Elmagd, K., McCauley, J., Fung, J.J., and Starzl, T.E. (1994). FK 506 in the treatment of polymyositis. *Arthritis and Rheumatism*, 37, S286 (Abstract).

O'Hanlon, T.P., Dalakas, M.C., Plotz, P.H., and Miller, F.W. (1994a). Predominant TCR-alpha beta variable and joining gene expression by muscle-infiltrating lymphocytes in the idiopathic inflammatory myopathies. *Journal of Immunology*, 152, 2569–76.

O'Hanlon, T.P., Dalakas, M.C., Plotz, P.H., and Miller, F.W. (1994b). The alpha beta T-cell receptor repertoire in inclusion body myositis: diverse patterns of gene expression by muscle-infiltrating lymphocytes. *Journal of Autoimmunity*, 7, 321–13.

Okano, Y., Steen, V.D., and Medsger, T.A., Jr. (1992). Autoantibody to U3 Nucleolar ribonucleoprotein (fibrillarin) in patients with systemic sclerosis. *Arthritis and Rheumatism*, 35, 95–100.

O'Neill, T.W. and Maddison, P.J. (1993). Rheumatoid arthritis associated with myositis and anti-Jo-1 antibody. *Journal of Rheumatology*, 20, 141–3.

Orimo, S. *et al.* (1994). Immunohistochemical analysis of perforin and granzyme A in inflammatory myopathies. *Neuromuscular Disorders*, 4, 219–26.

O'Rourke, K.S., Blaivas, M., and Ike, R.W. (1994). Utility of needle muscle biopsy in a university rheumatology practice. *Journal of Rheumatology*, 21, 413–24.

Osterman, P.O., Askmark, H., and Wistrand, P.J. (1985). Serum carbonic anhydrase III in neuromuscular disorders and in healthy persons after a long-distance run. *Journal of Neurological Science*, 70, 347–57.

Pamphlett, R. (1988). Muscle biopsy. In *Inflammatory diseases of muscle* (ed. F.L. Mastaglia), pp. 17–36. Blackwell Scientific, Oxford.

Park, J.H. *et al.* (1990). Dermatomyositis: correlative MR imaging and P-31 MR spectroscopy for quantitative characterization of inflammatory disease. *Radiology*, 177, 473–9.

Park, J.H. *et al.* (1994). Magnetic resonance imaging and P-31 magnetic resonance spectroscopy provide unique quantitative data useful in the longitudinal management of patients with dermatomyositis. *Arthritis and Rheumatism*, 37, 736–46.

Park, J.H. *et al.* (1995). Use of magnetic resonance imaging and P-31 magnetic resonance spectroscopy to detect and quantify muscle dysfunction in the amyopathic and myopathic variants of dermatomyositis. *Arthritis and Rheumatism*, 38, 68–77.

Pierce, L.R., Wysowski, D.K., and Gross, T.P. (1990). Myopathy and rhabdomyolysis associated with lovastatin-gemfibrozil combination therapy. *Journal of the American Medical Association*, 264, 71–5.

Pitt, A.M., Fleckenstein, J.L., Greenlee, R.G., Jr., Burns, D.K., Bryan, W.W., and Haller, R. (1993). MRI-guided biopsy in inflammatory myopathy: initial results. *Magnetic Resonance Imaging*, 11, 1093–9.

Plotz, P.H. (1992). Not myositis: a series of chance encounters. *Journal of the American Medical Association*, 268, 2074–7.

Plotz, P.H., Dalakas, M., Leff, R.L., Love, L.A., Miller, F.W., and Cronin, M.E. (1989). Current concepts in the idiopathic inflammatory myopathies: polymyositis, dermatomyositis, and related disorders. *Annals of Internal Medicine*, 111, 143–57.

Plotz, P.H., Rider, L.G., Targoff, I.N., Raben, N., O'Hanlon, T.P., and Miller, F.W. (1995). Myositis: immunologic contributions to understanding cause, pathogenesis, and therapy. *Annals of Internal Medicine*, 122, 715–24.

Pluschke, G., Rüegg, D., Hohlfeld, R., and Engel, A.G. (1992). Autoaggressive myocytotoxic T lymphocytes expressing an unusual gamma/delta T cell receptor. *Journal of Experimental Medicine*, 176, 1785–9.

Preston, D.C. (1993). Electrophysiology of *Microsporidia* myositis in an AIDS patient. *Muscle and Nerve*, 16, 1420–22.

Raben, N. *et al.* (1994). A motif in human histidyl-tRNA synthetase which is shared among several aminoacyl-tRNA synthetases is a coiled-coil that is essential for enzymatic activity and contains the major autoantigenic epitope. *Journal of Biological Chemistry*, 269, 24277–83.

Ramirez, G., Asherson, R.A., Khamashta, M.A., Cervera, R., D'Cruz, D., and Hughes, G.R.V. (1990). Adult-onset polymyositis-dermatomyositis: description of 25 patients with emphasis on treatment. *Seminars in Arthritis and Rheumatism*, 20, 114–20.

Rechavia, E., Rotenberg, Z., Fuchs, J., and Strasberg, B. (1985). Polymyositic heart disease. *Chest*, 88, 309–11.

Reichlin, M. and Arnett, F.C. (1984). Multiplicity of antibodies in myositis sera. *Arthritis and Rheumatism*, 27, 1150–56.

Reimers, C.D., Fleckenstein, J.L., Witt, T.N., Muller-Felber, W., and Pongratz, D.E. (1993). Muscular ultrasound in idiopathic inflammatory myopathies of adults. *Journal of Neurological Science*, 116, 82–92.

Reimers, C.D. *et al.* (1994). Magnetic resonance imaging of skeletal muscles in idiopathic inflammatory myopathies of adults. *Journal of Neurology*, 241, 306–14.

Reimold, A.M. and Weinblatt, M.E. (1994). Tachyphylaxis of intravenous immunoglobulin in refractory inflammatory myopathy. *Journal of Rheumatology*, 21, 1144–6.

Reveille, J.D., Targoff, I.N., Mimori, T., Nguyen, H.C., Goldstein, R., and Arnett, F.C. (1992). MHC class II alleles associated with myositis. *Arthritis and Rheumatism*, 35, S84 (Abstract).

Rider, L.G. and Miller, F.W. (1995). Laboratory evaluation of the inflammatory myopathies. *Clinical Diagnosis and Laboratory Immunology*, 2, 1–9.

Rider, L.G. *et al.* (1994). Association of autoantibodies to the U5-ribonucleoprotein (U5-RNP) with idiopathic inflammatory myopathy (IIM). *Arthritis and Rheumatism*, 37, S242 (Abstract).

Riminton, D.S., Chambers, S.T., Parkin, P.J., Pollock, M., and Donaldson, I.M. (1993). Inclusion body myositis presenting solely as dysphagia. *Neurology*, 43, 1241–3.

Ringel, S.P., Carry, M.R., Aguilera, A.J., and Starcevich, J.M. (1986). Quantitative histopathology of the inflammatory myopathies. *Archives of Neurology*, 43, 1004–9.

Roberts, L.J. and Fink, C.W. (1988). Childhood polymyositis/dermatomyositis. *Clinics in Dermatology*, 6, 36–46.

Rockerbie, N.R., Woo, T.Y., Callen, J.P., and Giustina, T. (1989). Cutaneous changes of dermatomyositis precede muscle weakness. *Journal of the American Academy of Dermatology*, 20, 629–32.

Rodgers, W.B., Yodlowski, M.L., and Mintzer, C.M. (1993). Pyomyositis in patients who have the human immunodeficiency virus. Case report and review of the literature. *Journal of Bone and Joint Surgery*, 75, 588–92.

Rosenberg, M.J. and Reichlin, M. (1994). Is there an association between injectable collagen and polymyositis/dermatomyositis? *Arthritis and Rheumatism*, 37, 747–53.

Rosenberg, N.L. (1993). Experimental models of inflammatory myopathies. *Baillière's Clinical Neurology*, 2, 693–715.

Rosenberg, N.L., Rotbart, H.A., Abzug, M.J., Ringel, S.P., and Levin, M.J. (1989). Evidence for a novel picornavirus in human dermatomyositis. *Annals of Neurology*, 26, 204–9.

Rosenzweig, B.A., Rotmensch, S., Binette, S.P., and Phillippe, M. (1989). Primary idiopathic polymyositis and dermatomyositis complicating pregnancy: diagnosis and management. *Obstetrics and Gynecology Survey*, 44, 162–70.

Rowe, D., Isenberg, D.A., and Beverley, P.C.L. (1983). Monoclonal antibodies to human leucocyte antigens in polymyositis and muscular dystrophy. *Clinical and Experimental Immunology*, 54, 327–36.

Rubin, R.B. and Neugarten, J. (1989). Cocaine-induced rhabdomyolysis masquerading as myocardial ischemia. *American Journal of Medicine*, 86, 551–3.

Sabina, R.L., Sulaiman, A.R., and Wortmann, R.L. (1990). Reduced transcript availability and myoadenylate deaminase (MAD) activity in polymyositis: implications for acquired MAD deficiency. *Arthritis and Rheumatism*, 33, S70.

Saito, E., Kuroda, K., Yoshimoto, Y., Oshima, H., and Kinoshita, M. (1989). Mechanism of the damaging effect of dermatomyositis mononuclear cells on cultured human skin fibroblasts. *Journal of Rheumatology*, 16, 1055–60.

Sanmarti, R. *et al.* (1994). Reduced activity of serum creatine kinase in rheumatoid arthritis: a phenomenon linked to the inflammatory response. *British Journal of Rheumatology*, 33, 231–4.

Sano, M., Suzuki, M., Sato, M., Sakamoto, T., and Uchigata, M. (1994). Fatal respiratory failure due to polymyositis. *Internal Medicine*, 33, 185–7.

Satoh, M., Ajmani, A.K., Hirakata, M., Suwa, A., Winfield, J.B., and Reeves, W.H. (1994). Onset of polymyositis with autoantibodies to threonyl-tRNA synthetase during pregnancy. *Journal of Rheumatology*, 21, 1564–6.

Sayers, M.E., Chou, S.M., and Calabrese, L.H. (1992). Inclusion body myositis: analysis of 32 cases. *Journal of Rheumatology*, 19, 1385–9.

Schulman, P., Kerr, L.D., and Spiera, H. (1991). A reexamination of the relationship between myositis and malignancy. *Journal of Rheumatology*, 18, 1689–92.

Schwarz, M.L., Matthay, R.A., Sahn, S.A., Stanford, R.E., Marmorstein, B.L., and Scheinhorn, D.J. (1976). Interstitial lung disease in polymyositis and dermatomyositis: analysis of six cases and review of the literature. *Medicine*, 55, 89–104.

Seidman, R., Peress, N.S., and Nuovo, G.J. (1994). *In situ* detection of polymerase chain reaction-amplified HIV-1 nucleic acids in skeletal muscle in patients with myopathy. *Modern Pathology*, 7, 369–75.

Sigurgeirsson, B., Lindelof, B., Edhag, O., and Allander, E. (1992). Risk of cancer in patients with dermatomyositis or polymyositis: a population-based study. *New England Journal of Medicine*, 326, 363–7.

Simpson, D.M. and Bender, A.N. (1988). Human immunodeficiency virus-associated myopathy: Analysis of 11 patients. *Annals of Neurology*, 24, 79–84.

Sinoway, P.A. and Callen, J.P. (1993). Chlorambucil. An effective corticosteroid-sparing agent for patients with recalcitrant dermatomyositis. *Arthritis and Rheumatism*, 36, 319–24.

Sintani, S., Murase, H., Tsukagoshi, H., and Shiigai, T. (1992). Glycyrrhizin (licorice)-induced hypokalemic myopathy: report of 2 cases and review of the literature. *European Neurology*, 32, 44–51.

Soueidan, S.A. and Dalakas, M.C. (1993). Treatment of inclusion-body myositis with high-dose intravenous immunoglobulin. *Neurology*, 43, 876–9.

Steinberg, A.D. (1993). Chlorambucil in the treatment of patients with immune-mediated rheumatic diseases. *Arthritis and Rheumatism*, 36, 325–8.

Stiglbauer, R. *et al.* (1993). Polymyositis: MRI-appearance at 1.5 T and correlation to clinical findings. *Clinics in Radiology*, 48, 244–8.

Stommel, E.W., Parsonnet, J., and Jenkyn, L.R. (1991). Polymyositis after ciguatera toxin exposure. *Archives of Neurology*, 48, 874–7.

Stonecipher, M.R., Jorizzo, J.L., White, W.L., Walker, F.O., and Prichard, E. (1993). Cutaneous changes of dermatomyositis in patients with normal muscle enzymes: dermatomyositis sine myositis? *Journal of the American Academy of Dermatology*, 28, 951–6.

Stonecipher, M.R., Jorizzo, J.L., Monu, J., Walker, F., and Sutej, P.G. (1994). Dermatomyositis with normal muscle enzyme concentrations. A single-blind study of the diagnostic value of magnetic resonance imaging and ultrasound. *Archives of Dermatology*, 130, 1294–9.

Strongwater, S.L., Dorovini-Zis, K., Ball, R.D., and Schnitzer, T.J. (1984). A murine model of polymyositis induced by coxsackievirus B1 (Tucson strain). *Arthritis and Rheumatism*, 27, 433–42.

Takahashi, K., Ogita, T., Okudaira, H., Yoshinoya, S., Yoshizawa, H., and Miyamoto, T. (1986). D-Penicillamine-induced polymyositis in patients with rheumatoid arthritis. *Arthritis and Rheumatism*, 29, 560–64.

Tam, P.E., Schmidt, A.M., Ytterberg, S.R., and Messner, R.P. (1994). Duration of virus persistence and its relationship to inflammation in the chronic phase of coxsackievirus B1-induced murine polymyositis. *Journal of Laboratory and Clinical Medicine*, **123**, 346–56.

Tami, L.F. and Bhasin, S. (1993). Polymorphism of the cardiac manifestations in dermatomyositis. *Clinics in Cardiology*, **16**, 260–64.

Taneja, V., Mehra, N., Singh, Y.N., Kumar, A., Malaviya, A., and Singh, R.R. (1990). HLA-D region genes and susceptibility to D-penicillamine-induced myositis. *Arthritis and Rheumatism*, **33**, 1445–7.

Tanimoto, K. *et al.* (1995). Classification criteria for polymyositis and dermatomyositis. *Journal of Rheumatology*, **22**, 668–74.

Taniyama, M., Yoh, S., Asaba, Y., Maruyama, T., Takei, I., and Kataoka, K. (1987). Elevated serum creatine kinase level in diabetic patients with nephrotic syndrome: a role of fluid retention. *Annals of Internal Medicine*, **106**, 711–12.

Targoff, I.N. (1988). Laboratory manifestations of polymyositis/dermatomyositis. *Clinics in Dermatology*, **6**, 76–92.

Targoff, I.N. (1990). Inflammatory muscle disease. In *The lung in rheumatic diseases* (ed. G.W. Cannon and G.A. Zimmerman), pp. 303–28. Marcel Dekker, Inc., New York.

Targoff, I.N. (1991). Polymyositis. In *Systemic autoimmunity* (ed. P.E. Bigazzi and M. Reichlin), pp. 201–46. Marcel Dekker Inc., New York.

Targoff, I.N. (1994). Immune manifestations of inflammatory muscle disease. *Rheumatic Disease Clinics of North America*, **20**, 857–80.

Targoff, I.N. and Arnett, F.C. (1990). Clinical manifestations in patients with antibody to PL-12 antigen (alanyl-tRNA synthetase). *American Journal of Medicine*, **88**, 241–51.

Targoff, I.N., Arnett, F.C., Berman, L., O'Brien, C.A., and Reichlin, M. (1989). Anti-KJ: a new antibody associated with the myositis/lung syndrome that reacts with a translation-related protein. *Journal of Clinical Investigation*, **84**, 162–72.

Targoff, I.N., Johnson, A.E., and Miller, F.W. (1990). Antibody to signal recognition particle in polymyositis. *Arthritis and Rheumatism*, **33**, 1361–70.

Targoff, I.N., Trieu, E.P., Plotz, P.H., and Miller, F.W. (1992). Antibodies to glycyl-transfer RNA synthetase in patients with myositis and interstitial lung disease. *Arthritis and Rheumatism*, **35**, 821–30.

Targoff, I.N., Trieu, E.P., and Miller, F.W. (1993). Reaction of anti-OJ autoantibodies with components of the multi-enzyme complex of aminoacyl-tRNA synthetases in addition to isoleucyl-tRNA synthetase. *Journal of Clinical Investigation*, **91**, 2556–64.

Taylor, A.J., Wortham, D.C., Burge, J.R., and Rogan, K.M. (1993). The heart in polymyositis: a prospective evaluation of 26 patients. *Clinics in Cardiology*, **16**, 802–8.

Tazelaar, H.D., Viggiano, R.W., Pickersgill, J., and Colby, T.V. (1990). Interstitial lung disease in polymyositis and dermatomyositis. *American Review of Respiratory Diseases*, **141**, 727–33.

Tymms, K.E. and Webb, J. (1985). Dermatopolymyositis and other connective tissue diseases: a review of 105 cases. *Journal of Rheumatology*, **12**, 1140–48.

Uncini, A., Lange, D.J., Lovelace, R.E., Solomon, M., and Hays, A.P. (1990). Long-duration polyphasic motor unit potentials in myopathies: a quantitative study with pathological correlation. *Muscle and Nerve*, **13**, 263–7.

Urbano-Marquez, A., Casademont, J., and Grau, J.M. (1991). Polymyositis/dermatomyositis: the current position. *Annals of the Rheumatic Diseases*, **50**, 191–5.

Varga, J., Heiman-Patterson, T., Munoz, S., and Love, L.A. (1993). Myopathy with mitochondrial alterations in patients with primary biliary cirrhosis and antimitochondrial antibodies. *Arthritis and Rheumatism*, **36**, 1468–75.

Wada, K. *et al.* (1983). Radioimmunoassay for antibodies to human skeletal muscle myosin in serum from patients with polymyositis. *Clinical and Experimental Immunology*, **52**, 297–304.

Wei, N., Pavlidis, N., Tsokos, G., Elin, R.J., and Plotz, P.H. (1981). Clinical significance of low creatine phosphokinase values in patients with connective tissue diseases. *Journal of the American Medical Association*, **246**, 1921–3.

Whitmore, S.E., Rosenshein, N.B., and Provost, T.T. (1994). Ovarian cancer in patients with dermatomyositis. *Medicine*, **73** 153–60.

Wiley, C.A., Nerenberg, M., Cros, D., and Soto-Aguilar, M.C. (1989). HTLV-I polymyositis in a patient also infected with the human immunodeficiency virus. *New England Journal of Medicine*, **320**, 992–5.

Wolf, P.L. (1991). Abnormalities in serum enzymes in skeletal muscle diseases. *American Journal of Clinical Pathology*, **95**, 293–6.

Wolf, R.E. and Baethge, B.A. (1990). Interleukin-1a, interleukin-2, and soluble interleukin-2 receptors in polymyositis. *Arthritis and Rheumatism*, **33**, 1007–14.

Wolf, R.F., Sprenger, H.G., Mooyaart, E.L., Tamsma, J.T., Kengen, R.A., and Weits, J. (1990). Nontropical pyomyositis as a cause of subacute, multifocal myalgia in the acquired immunodeficiency syndrome. *Arthritis and Rheumatism*, **33**, 1728–32.

Woo, T.Y., Callen, J.P., Voorhees, J.J., Bickers, D.R., Hanno, R., and Hawkins, C. (1984). Cutaneous lesions of dermatomyositis are improved by hydroxychloroquine. *Journal of the American Academy of Dermatology*, **10**, 592–600.

Wright, G.D., Wilson, C., and Bell, A.L. (1994). D-penicillamine induced polymyositis causing complete heart block. *Clinics in Rheumatology*, **13**, 80–82.

Yousef, G.E., Isenberg, D.A., and Mowbray, J.F. (1990). Detection of enterovirus specific RNA sequences in muscle biopsy specimens from patients with adult onset myositis. *Annals of the Rheumatic Diseases*, **49**, 310–15.

Ytterberg, S.R. (1994). The relationship of infectious agents to inflammatory myositis. *Rheumatic Disease Clinics of North America*, **20**, 995–1016.

Ytterberg, S.R., Mahowald, M.L., and Messner, R.P. (1987). Coxsackievirus B1-induced polymyositis: lack of disease expression in nu/nu mice. *Journal of Clinical Investigation*, **80**, 499–506.

Ytterberg, S.R., Roelofs, R.I., and Mahowald, M.L. (1993). Inclusion body myositis and renal cell carcinoma: report of two cases and review of the literature. *Arthritis and Rheumatism*, **36**, 416–21.

Zantos, D., Zhang, Y., and Felson, D. (1994). The overall and temporal association of cancer with polymyositis and dermatomyositis. *Journal of Rheumatology*, **21**, 1855–9.

Zieglschmid-Adams, M.E., Pandya, A.G., Cohen, S.B., and Sontheimer, R.D. (1995). Treatment of dermatomyositis with methotrexate. *Journal of the American Academy of Dermatology*, **32**, 754–7.

Zuckner, J. (1994). Drug-related myopathies. *Rheumatic Disease Clinics of North America*, **20**, 1017–32.

5.9.2 Polymyositis and dermatomyositis in children

Lauren M. Pachman

Introduction

The range of inflammatory muscle disease in children includes acute viral or bacterial myositis, and chronic myositis—juvenile dermatomyositis, polymyositis, and inflammatory myopathy associated with other autoimmune rheumatic diseases or with parasitic infection. Worldwide, most of the inflammatory myopathies accompany bacterial or parasitic infections, but in North America and Europe a viral aetiology is seen more commonly.

The major advances in the study of these diseases include more definite clinical characterization of subsets and an emerging appreciation of their epidemiology as shown by their specific as well as their shared clinical and laboratory features. Recent evidence suggests that

This work was supported in part by Grant NIH/NIAMS P60-AR-30692 from the National Institutes of Health and grants from the Illinois Chapter of the Arthritis Foundation.

Table 1 Criteria for diagnosis of juvenile dermatomyositis and polymyositis in childhood[a]

	Juvenile dermatomyositis	Polymyositis
Characteristic rash	+	–
Symmetrical proximal muscle weakness[b]	+	+
Elevated muscle-derived enzymes	+	+
Muscle histopathology[c]	+	+
Electromyographic changes; inflammatory myopathy	+	+

[a]In addition to presence (or absence) of characteristic rash and exclusion of other rheumatic diseases, three of four criteria must be met to confirm diagnosis.
[b]Exclusion of other rheumatic diseases.
[c]The histology of childhood polymyositis is different from juvenile dermatomyositis. Definite JDMS: rash plus three or four criteria; Probable JDMS: rash plus two criteria; possible JDMS: rash plus one criteria.
Modified from Bohan and Peter (1975). *New England Journal of Medicine*, **292**, 344–7.

genetic and infectious factors may play a part in disease susceptibility. The primary clinical feature of both juvenile dermatomyositis and polymyositis is chronic and progressive weakness of proximal muscles. In juvenile dermatomyositis the vasculopathy and distinctive skin manifestations are associated commonly with muscle involvement; in polymyositis the skin is spared. Fulfilment of the criteria of Bohan and Peter (1975) is needed to establish the diagnosis of either type of myopathy (Table 1). The diagnosis of definite juvenile dermatomyositis is made if, in addition to the typical rash, three of the four criteria are present; of definite polymyositis, if three of the four criteria are found. Myositis is often a part of other autoimmune rheumatic diseases and, therefore, it is essential to exclude such conditions as systemic lupus erythematosus, mixed connective tissue disease, juvenile chronic arthritis (especially of systemic onset), the spondylarthropathies, and Sjögren's syndrome.

Epidemiology

Demographic data

The bimodal age distribution of populations of combined polymyositis/dermatomyositis is well known with a childhood peak (at 5 to 9 years of age, 3.7 cases/million per year and at 10 to 14 years of age, 4.3 cases/million per year) and an adult peak (at 45 to 64 years or age, 10 cases/million per year) (Medsger et al. 1970). Children of African or Asian origin may be at increased risk for chronic myositis (Benbassat et al. 1980), but in the United States, Caucasian children with juvenile dermatomyositis are reported more frequently, and twice as many girls as boys are affected; in the United Kingdom and Ireland, five times as many girls were diagnosed as boys, with a incidence of 1.9/million children under the age of 16 years (Symmons et

al. 1995). A similar trend is found in China (Wang et al. 1993), in contrast to Japan where a ratio of 1.3 boys to 1 girl was identified; none had associated malignancy or interstitial lung disease (Hiketa et al. 1992). In children, dermatomyositis occurs at least 10 to 20 times more often than polymyositis. In marked contrast to earlier reports of one-third mortality and one-third morbidity (Bitnum et al. 1964), both of these adverse outcomes have decreased in childhood since the advent of steroid therapy (Hochberg 1988; Ansell et al. 1990). In Japan, during a 10-year period (1973 to 1983) there was a 2.9 per cent mortality rate (Hidano et al. 1986).

Although an increased frequency of malignancy may be associated with adult dermatomyositis within 2 years of disease onset (Masi and Hochberg 1988), this does not appear to be the case in children with either juvenile dermatomyositis or polymyositis (Hidano et al. 1986); only sporadic cases of children with both an inflammatory myopathy and malignancy have been cited (Sherry et al. 1993), and a population-based survey did not find malignancy in any patient less than 16 years of age (Sigurgeirsson et al. 1992).

There is some data to suggest that in the United States children are more likely to have onset of disease in the early months of the year. A comparison of disease onset of juveniles with dermatomyositis and adults with polymyositis–dermatomyositis living in Memphis, Tennessee, revealed a seasonal onset (February to April) in 55 per cent of the children but not in the adults (Medsger et al. 1970). In contrast, a case–control study (all paediatric inflammatory myopathy, numbers of juvenile dermatomyositis unknown) conducted in a different region of the country did not document a specific season of onset (Koch et al. 1976). In the next decade, in north central region, children with definite juvenile dermatomyositis (diagnosed within 4 months of onset) were more likely to have their first symptoms in the months of January to June than at other periods of time in each of 7 years (1974 to 1980) (Christensen et al. 1983); in Canada clustering was observed as well, suggesting an environmental influence (Rosenberg 1994). In the United Kingdom and Ireland, several clusters of disease onset were identified, the largest of which was in April and May in 1992; the timing of these clusters appeared to vary from year to year (Symmons et al. 1995). In Athens, Greece, of those adults (children were not included) with polymyositis–dermatomyositis who were admitted to hospital, 39 per cent were in March, April, or May with onset of symptoms in the same months (Manta et al. 1989). It is not yet firmly established if prevalence for season of onset is the same for both adults and children living in the same region or if the peak onset of polymyositis is in the same period as that of dermatomyositis in either age group. A national study is ongoing in the United States to determine if there is in fact seasonality or symptoms of antecedent illness in children with juvenile dermatomyositis.

Infectious agents and juvenile dermatomyositis

Several agents have been associated with the onset (and on occasion, flare) of juvenile dermatomyositis, of which the most prominent have been the RNA picornaviruses, group A β-haemolytic streptococci, and *Toxoplasma gondii*. Coxsackievirus B (CVB) 2 was isolated from the stool, and the titre of CF (complement fixing) antibody rose in a child with chronic myositis (Schiraldi and Iandolo 1978); others have measured rise in B4 antibodies (Travers et al. 1977). As noted above, there may be temporal, seasonal, and regional differences in agents associated with disease onset. Sera from newly diagnosed children during 1974 to 1980 from the Chicago area had an increased frequency of antibody (both neutralizing and complement fixing) to coxsackievirus B, as well as increased frequency of the histocompatibility antigens HLA B8/DR3 (Christensen *et al.* 1986) (see Genetics below), which was not reproduced by the same group of investigators in a study of 20 children with dermatomyositis from the same region with onset of disease in the years 1987 to 1992 (Pachman *et al.* 1995*b*). Enteroviral RNA was identified in the muscle of English patients with polymyositis/dermatomyositis (Bowles *et al.* 1987; Yousef *et al.* 1990), but other investigators have not found viral RNA in cases from the United States, either in Jo-1 positive adults (Leff *et al.* 1992), or in MRI-directed muscle biopsies of 20 newly diagnosed, untreated, children with active dermatomyositis (Pachman *et al.* 1995*b*). Other infectious agents have been thought to play a role in juvenile dermatomyositis, including toxoplasmosis (Schroter *et al.* 1987; Lapetina 1989) and hepatitis B (Peters *et al.* 1991), but antibody titres to these agents were not increased either in a regional study (Christensen *et al.* 1983) or in a case–control national study of new onset juvenile dermatomyositis spanning the years 1987 to 1992 (Pachman *et al.* 1992*a*; Pachman *et al.* 1995*b*). Although Theiler's murine encephalomyelitis virus (TMEV) was identified in adult polymyositis, none of the children with dermatomyositis were positive for this agent (Rosenberg *et al.* 1989). Taken together, the above data suggests that the aetiology of juvenile dermatomyositis is multifactorial, perhaps permitting a role for molecular mimicry. Evidence that may support this hypothesis is found in a report of skeletal myosin (which has sequence homology with the streptoccal type 5 M protein) stimulating lymphocytes from a child with recurrent dermatomyositis following streptococcal infections (Martini *et al.* 1992).

Clinical presentation

Cutaneous findings

In juvenile dermatomyositis, the rash may predate or follow the onset of symmetrical weakness in proximal muscles. Periorbital erythema and oedema, and/or eyelid telangiectasia, are seen in 50 to 90 per cent of affected children. The eyelid telangiectasia (as well as that elsewhere) may persist long after other signs and symptoms of disease activity have resolved. The rash has a violaceous or heliotrope hue, and is often most prominent on the eyelid, where small infarctions may be seen (Fig. 1). The rash may also cross the bridge of the nose and be precipitated by even a brief unprotected exposure to the sun. Sunlight may simply exacerbate the skin manifestations or may activate symptoms of myositis. Other areas of erythema involving the upper torso, the extensor surfaces of the arms and legs, medial malleoli of the ankles, as well as the buttocks may occur in the absence of raised serum concentrations of muscle-derived enzymes (see below). The skin over the knuckles is often either hypertrophic or pale red, evolving into colourless bands of atrophic skin (Gottron's sign). Similar patches can occur in a variety of places including over the metacarpal phalangeal joints, the extensor aspect of the elbows or knees, or the medial canthus of the eyelid. Lipoatrophy which is not tender despite a lymphohistiocytic panniculitis (Commens *et al.* 1990), as well as acanthosis nigricans, associated with insulin-resistant diabetes, have also been seen in children with juvenile dermatomyositis. Diffuse vasculopathy (nailbed telangiectasia, infarction of oral epithelium and skin folds, or digital ulceration) associated clearly with more severe disease, is correlated

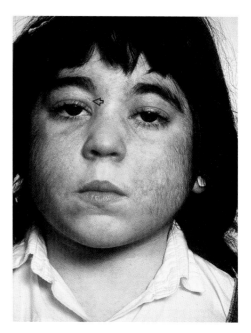

(a)

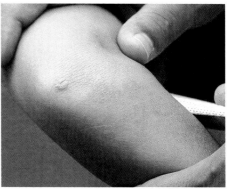

(b)

Fig. 1 (a) This young girl has the typical rash of juvenile dermatomyositis. Erythema and oedema involving the eyelids are seen, with healed microinfarcts at the medial aspect of the right upper eyelid (open arrow). The rash crosses the bridge of the nose and has areas of relative decreased vascularity as well as erythema. (b) Gottron's papules on the elbow of a 4-year-old child with recurrent juvenile dermatomyositis.

with the child's clinical course (Silver and Maricq 1989), and can be quantified to aid in diagnosis and in monitoring response to therapy (Pachman *et al.* 1995*d*). Although calcinosis without known antecedent muscle disease has been reported as a presenting sign of dermatomyositis in childhood (Martini *et al.* 1987), it may be considered to be related to disease severity and duration (Pachman *et al.* 1985). Delay in diagnosis by 6 months, which may be a consequence of difficulty in identification of the rash on pigmented skin, was associated with an increased incidence of calcinosis (Pachman *et al.* 1992*b*). None of 20 recently diagnosed and treated children with juvenile dermatomyositis developed calcinosis, suggesting that aggressive therapy early in the disease course may be of substantial benefit (Callen *et al.* 1994).

Musculoskeletal symptoms

Proximal muscle weakness as evidenced by difficulty in climbing stairs, getting up from a chair, combing hair, or using the hands to push off the body in an attempt to stand (Gower's sign) is common; weakness of the neck flexors is a particularly sensitive indicator of muscular impairment. Complaints of pain on compression of the muscles are found in over 60 per cent of cases, but are less severe than in the bacterial-related myopathies. Fatigue is common, and also expressed by children with the dystrophies (most commonly those of Duchenne and Becker). The most common symptoms are listed in Table 2. Usually the child is more comfortable when the limbs are held in the flexed position, promoting the development of flexion contractures. Inflammation can be detected by electromyography or muscle biopsy despite the appearance of clinical quiescence (Miller *et al.* 1987). The use of MRI-directed biopsies minimizes error in sampling uninvolved areas in this focal disease (Pitt *et al.* 1993), and can monitor a child's response to therapy (Yanagisawa *et al.* 1983; Keim *et al.* 1991; Hernandez *et al.* 1993). The MRI may become normal several months after the muscle enzymes return to the normal ranges (Huppertz and Kaiser 1994). P-32 spin MRI has been in use for the past few years and gives useful information about the child's muscle strength and performance (Park *et al.* 1994). Decreased bone density (associated with a depressed serum osteocalcin) is frequent in untreated juvenile dermatomyositis and places the child at risk of bony fracture (Reed *et al.* 1990), which is further augmented by steroid administration.

Gastrointestinal involvement

One of the most troubling prognostic indicators is impairment of the flow of secretions associated with decreased oesophageal motility, which can be documented by radiographic contrast studies showing retained barium in a widened atonic, pyriform sinus. The swallowing of liquids may also be impaired; oesophageal reflux may result in aspiration pneumonia and appropriate precautions should be taken to prevent this (e.g. using thickened foods, raising the bed head, and bronchial drainage). Smooth muscle dysfunction can also result in decreased lower-gastrointestinal dysmotility, making constipation an annoying symptom. Involvement of the masseter may result in difficulty in chewing; chronic masseter atrophy is often apparent once the disease has become quiescent, and may endow the child with a characteristic chipmunk appearance. Vasculopathy affects any part of the gastrointestinal tract; in severe disease there is weight loss and mucosal ulceration with life-threatening perforation. In the young child, development of normal speech patterns can be disturbed; soft palate involvement is often revealed by nasal, high-pitched speech (for example by saying the alphabet) and usually resolves with a decrease in the inflammatory component of the myositis.

Cardiorespiratory abnormalities

The ECG is abnormal at disease onset in over half the children with definite juvenile dermatomyositis. Asymptomatic conduction abnormalities predominate, with an occasional complete block of the right bundle branch (Pachman and Cooke 1980), which usually resolves with decrease in disease activity. In the absence of respiratory complaints, a decrease in ventilatory capacity, with a normal diffusion of carbon dioxide was found in 78 per cent of children with juvenile dermatomyositis whose sera were subsequently found to be negative for antibody to the tRNA synthetase, Jo-1 (Pachman and Cooke 1980). The decrease in ventilatory capacity can be associated with diminished speech volume; several of our children have developed

Table 2 Juvenile dermatomyositis symptoms at diagnosis

Symptoms	Percentage at diagnosis
Weakness	100
Rash	100
Muscle pain	72
Fever	65
Difficulty swallowing	45
Abdominal pain	37
Arthritis	36
Calcifications	22

vocal cord nodules, presumably as a result of the stress of trying to be heard. Pulmonary fibrosis may occur in both adults and children with inflammatory myopathy, but it is more commonly found in individuals who carry antibody to the tRNA synthetases, of which anti-Jo-1 is the most common in adults (see Pathophysiology). Myositis-specific antibodies (MSA) are rare in children and are just starting to be identified (Rider *et al.* 1994). A young woman with Jo-1-positive myositis with onset in childhood has been recently described; her initial complaints included a reactive airway component (were called 'asthma'), but progressed to include arthritis and were accompanied by pulmonary fibrosis and a markedly decreased diffusion of carbon dioxide. The severe myopathy occurred 7 years after onset of respiratory symptoms (Bowles *et al.* 1987). In general, the few children with Jo-1 who have been identified recently are similar to adults with antisynthetase antibodies and are characterized by dyspnoea on exertion, a pulmonary perfusion deficit with evidence of pulmonary fibrosis on both histological and radiographical examination, and disease flares with the reduction of therapy. Most have severe arthritis; some have 'mechanic's hands' (Rider *et al.* 1995), which is much more common in adults, and rarely seen in children.

Genitourinary involvement

Massive breakdown of muscle elements as well as primary compromise of the renal parenchyma itself, may occur in children with an active myopathic process requiring prompt hydration and monitoring of renal function. If unchecked, renal failure can occur. On histochemical examination, cytoplasmic tubular arrays (may be a correlate of α-interferon production) are found in the renal glomerular endothelium as well as cutaneous fibroblastic cells (Pachman and Maryjowski 1984). Necrosis of the ureter has been reported, involving the middle one-third (iliac) segment, which is more vulnerable to vascular compromise as a consequence of inflammation. This vulnerability occurs because of the relatively sparse blood supply to this region compared with the upper (lumbar) or lower (pelvic) segments (Borrelli *et al.* 1988).

Eye signs

The most common finding is persistent thrombosis of dilated vessels at the margin of the upper eyelid, which may persist years after other clinical signs of inflammation have disappeared. In active disease, transient retinal exudates and 'cotton wool' spots may occur after the occlusion of small vessels, leading to intraretinal oedema with injury to retinal nerve fibres, optic atrophy, and sustained visual loss. Neovascularization of the retina with spontaneous regression has also been reported (Fong and Yeung 1990). Disease of conjunctival vessels can also lead to an avascular zone with a potential for infarction. Children treated with steroids should be monitored for both glaucoma and for the development of sublenticular cataracts, which are related to the dose of corticosterids given (Callen *et al.* 1994). If there is a family history of red–green colour blindness, the use of hydroxychloroquine should be avoided.

Other disease manifestations

Vasculopathy involving the central nervous system may be associated with depression and/or wide mood swings, which may be exacerbated by steroid therapy (see below). It is not usual for a child with juvenile dermatomyositis to present with Raynaud's phenomenon; these symptoms are found more frequently in overlap syndromes.

Differential diagnosis of juvenile dermatomyositis

General

The differential diagnosis of this inflammatory myopathy includes many of the major neuromuscular disorders of infancy and childhood as well as metabolic and infectious diseases which can be symptomatic at any age. Table 3 presents most of the potential candidates for consideration.

Skin

Many of the other autoimmune diseases exhibit some of the cutaneous signs of juvenile dermatomyositis. As in systemic lupus, exposure to sun can exacerbate both the malar rash as well as the systemic complaints in children with dermatomyositis. Gottron's sign can be mimicked by psoriatic lesions, accompanied by healing foci of hypopigmentation found in areas usually unaffected in juvenile dermatomyositis, such as the pretibial region. These rashes may clear with sun exposure, rather than becoming more prominent. A description of a child with psoriatic arthritis and myopathy underlines the differences in clinical presentation (Thompson *et al.* 1990). Telangiectasia, a prominent feature of scleroderma, also occurs in overlap syndromes in which myositis is a component. Capillary destruction with resulting avascularity and healing can be monitored using nailfold capillary microscopy, which can help to differentiate juvenile dermatomyositis from some of the other vasculopathies (Pachman 1995). For example, a 2-year-old child had progressive unilateral focal calcinosis since the age of 5 months, as well as elevated muscle enzymes, but no muscle weakness or rash. Her capillary microscopy was abnormal, but not in the pattern seen in juvenile dermatomyositis, ultimately leading to the correct diagnosis of progressive osseous heterotopia (Sachrison *et al.* 1995).

Muscle-derived enzymes

Skeletal muscle is rich in enzymes which can be released from the sarcoplasm to the peripheral circulation as a consequence of reduced vascular supply, trauma, or immunological cytotoxicity. Increased serum concentrations of enzymes result from either tissue necrosis or leakage through damaged cell membranes; sera to be analysed must be free of haemolytic products. Functional myopathies and those that result from denervation are accompanied by decreased muscle mass, weakness, pain, and loss of function or, in severe cases, paralysis. In these diseases, the serum creatine kinase, its muscle and brain isoenzymes, as well as the pyruvate kinase, lactate dehydrogenase, and aldolase are normal. In contrast, in some of the dystrophies, creatine kinase and aldolase may be increased by as much as 30 times the normal level; creatine kinase muscle isoenzymes are elevated after an acute myocardial infarction and after back surgery, and may also be raised in Duchenne's as well as Becker's muscular dystrophy. Increases are also seen in myocardial and skeletal muscle disease or trauma ranging from vigorous physical exercise (e.g. marathon runners) and surgical and accidental crush injuries to intramuscular injections. Drugs that enhance the permeability of muscle membranes, also result in elevated concentrations of the muscle isoenzyme form of creatine kinase; for example, aminocaproic acid, D-penicillamine, halothane (hyperpyrexia), and quinidine. Overdose with amphetamines, barbiturates, ethanol, or heroin results in a massive increase in creatine kinase (Lott and Landesman 1984). Disorders of calcium metabolism such as hypocalcaemia (either isolated or associated with rickets, hypoparathyroidism) or chronic renal failure can be accompanied by increased creatine kinase. Once the low levels of ionized calcium become normal, the rise in creatine kinase usually resolves. Aldolase has a short half-life and can be increased in viral hepatitis, metastatic liver disease, some prostate tumours, and in some of the leukaemias and anaemias (Lott and Landesman 1984). Lactate dehydrogenase has five isoenzymes: the anodal forms are increased in cardiac and renal disease, and in some diseases of skeletal muscle, while the cathodal forms are elevated in skeletal muscle and liver dysfunction. Other less specific enzymes that may also be found in higher concentrations in muscle damage are aspartate aminotransferase and alanine aminotransferase. Myoglobin is present only in skeletal and cardiac muscle. This oxygen-binding haem protein is elevated in serum from children with myopathies; persistent or massive myoglobinuria can result in renal failure, which should be prevented by infusion of adequate intravenous hydration.

Muscle complaints

Children with juvenile dermatomyositis may complain of pain on compression of the proximal muscles, or of muscle cramps, but weakness of symmetrical proximal muscles is still the predominant symptom. Other conditions associated with muscle cramps and contractures include hypothyroidism, uraemia, and electrolyte imbalance such as hypokalemia (either iatrogenic or in conjunction with familial periodic paralysis). Pretibial tenderness is seen with erythema nodosum, but is not a feature of juvenile dermatomyositis. Pain that awakens the child at night should be investigated for another cause such as malignancy, osteoid osteoma, or osteomyelitis. Muscle weakness can be see in hormonal derangements, either endogenous or iatrogenic, such as in adrenal dysfunction, or after long-term high-dose steroid administration. In addition, thyroid, pituitary, and parathyroid dysfunction may be accompanied by skeletal complaints. Metabolic muscle diseases include defects of glycolysis (e.g. phosphofructokinase deficiency) and are associated with contractures, exercise

Table 3   Classification of the major neuromuscular disorders of infancy and childhood

I. Primary myopathies
   A. The muscular dystrophies
      1. Sex-linked recessive
         (a) Duchenne muscular dystrophy
         (b) Becker's muscular dystrophy
         (c) Variants
      2. Autosomal dominant
         (a) Facioscapulohumeral
         (b) Distal myopathy
         (c) Ocular myopathy
         (d) Oculopharyngeal muscular dystrophy
      3. Autosomal recessive
         (a) Limb-girdle
   B. Congenital myopathies
      1. Congenital muscular dystrophy
         (a) Arthrogrypsosis multiplex congenita (myopathic form)
      2. Benign congenital myopathy
      3. Central core disease
      4. Nemaline myopathy
      5. Myotubular myopathy
   C. Myotonic disorders
      1. Myotopia congenita
      2. Dystrophia myotonia
   D. Metabolic disorders
      1. Glycogen storage disease
         (a) Type II: acid maltase deficiency
         (b) Type III; amylo-1,6-glucosidase deficiency (brancher
            enzyme)
         (c) Type IV: amylo-(1,4→1,6) transglucosidase
            deficiency (brancher enzyme)
         (d) Type V: phosphorylase deficiency
         (e) Type VII: phosphofructokinase deficiency
      2. Familial periodic paralysis
         (a) Hyperkalaemic
         (b) Hypokalaemic
         (c) Normokalaemic
      3. Carnitine deficiency
      4. Carnitine palmityl transferase deficiency
      5. Secondary to endocrinopathies
         (a) Addison's disease
         (b) Cushing's syndrome
         (c) Hypopituitarism
         (d) Hypothyroidism
      6. Myoadenylate deaminase deficiency
      7. Chronic haemodialysis

E. Inflammatory diseases
   1. Postinfectious
      (a) Viral syndromes
         (i) Influenza B
         (ii) Coxsackievirus B
         (iii) Echovirus
         (iv) Poliomyelitis
         (v) HIV/HTLV-1
      (b) Toxoplasmosis, sarcosporidiosis
      (c) Trichinosis, cysticercosis
      (d) Septic (staphylococci and other pyogenic organisms)
      (e) Tetanus
      (f) Gas gangrene
   2. Autoimmune rheumatic diseases
      (a) Juvenile rheumatoid arthritis
      (b) Dermatomyositis
      (c) Systemic lupus erythematosus
      (d) Scleroderma
      (e) Polyarteritis
F. Genetic abnormalities
   1. Osteogenesis imperfecta
   2. Ehlers–Danlos syndrome
   3. Mucopolysaccharidoses
G. Trauma
   1. Physical
      (a) Crush syndrome
      (b) Exhaustive physical exertion (rhabdomyloysis)
   2. Toxic
      (a) Snakebite
   3. Drugs
      (a) Glucocorticoids
      (b) Hydroxychloroquine
      (c) Diuretics, liquorice
      (d) Amphotericin B
      (e) Alcohol
      (f) Vincristine
      (g) D-Penicillamine
      (h) Cimetidine
II. Neurogenic atrophies
   A. Spinal muscular and anterior horn-cell dysfunction
      1. Infantile and juvenile muscle atrophy
         (a) Type I: acute infantile
         (b) Type II: infantile spinal muscular atrophy, chronic variant
         (c) Type III: Juvenile spinal muscular atrophy
      2. Arthrogrypsosis multiplex congenita
      3. Amyotrophic lateral sclerosis
   B. Peripheral nerve dysfunction
      1. Peroneal muscular atrophy
      2. Neurofibromatosis
      3. Acute infectious polyneuritis
   C. Disorders of neuromuscular transmission
      1. Congenital myasthenia gravis
      2. Botulism
      3. Tick paralysis
      4. Organophosphate poisoning

Adapted from the Research Group on Neuromuscular Diseases (1968). Classification of the neuromuscular disorders. *Journal of Neurological Science*, **6**, 165.

intolerance, myoglobinuria, and a positive ischaemic lactate test. There may be a defect in lipid metabolism such as a carnitine deficiency state (Breningstall 1990), which may be exacerbated by non-steroidal anti-inflammatory drugs; or a myalgia syndrome, which can be detected by a positive ischaemic ammonia test. Inclusion-body myositis, which often runs a steroid-resistant course, has also been described in children (Serratrice *et al.* 1989).

Acute infectious viral myositis in children, most frequently attributed to influenza A or B, is differentiated clinically from chronic myositis by its localization to the muscles of the calf, severe pain, and rapid resolution in 1 to 4 weeks (Mejlszenkier *et al.* 1973). The agent of this acute myositis has been isolated from cultures of muscle biopsy, accompanied by rise in complement-fixing antibody titres to influenza and by myoglobinuria, electomyographic changes, and elevated creatine kinase. As in adults with HIV or HTLV-1, children with these illnesses may also have muscle complaints.

Other autoimmune rheumatic disorders may also be accompanied by inflammatory muscle disease. For example, children with systemic-onset juvenile arthritis may have spiking fevers and an evanescent rash. Often they do not wish to be held and have increased concentrations of muscle enzymes, making the appropriate diagnosis of the specific connective tissue disease imperative. Confusion may be created by a child who has classical Gottron's papules, elevated muscle enzymes, and muscle biopsy evidence of perifascicular atrophy in the presence of antibody to RNP or PM/Scl. Such children with overlap syndrome are less likely to have complete resolution of their disease, requiring long-term therapy.

Electromyogram

Evidence of an inflammatory myopathy on electromyography is not specific to juvenile dermatomyositis and is similar in other autoimmune rheumatic disorders which have a myopathic component. Selection of a site of active involvement is facilitated by MRI identification of focally involved muscles. Once the location of the electrodes has been chosen (not the site of a future biopsy), insertional irritability, followed by spontaneous electrical activity at rest is often observed. This pattern can be also seen in the muscular dystrophies and in early acute myositis. Abnormal early full recruitment of muscle fibres with moderate effort occurs in about 45 per cent of patients with juvenile dermatomyositis, and bizarre, high-frequency discharges occur in 15 to 20 per cent of patients tested. Reduced motor unit activity is seen in Duchenne muscular dystrophy as well as in juvenile dermatomyositis. Myasthenia gravis can coexist with an inflammatory myopathy, resulting in a greater degree of instability of motor-unit potential than is found in the uncomplicated inflammatory myopathies.

Pathophysiology of juvenile dermatomyositis

Vascular findings

The vasculopathy of this disease may occur in the absence of a prominent inflammatory component, and is a characteristic of children with dermatomyositis (Banker and Victor 1966); vascular occlusion in the absence of an inflammatory infiltrate in adults with early lesions of dermatomyositis has also been well described (Emslie-Smith and Engel 1990). In juvenile dermatomyositis, damage to capillaries,

venules, and small arteries causes loss of the capillary network resulting in structural change in the nailfold capillary bed as well as in muscle, with a subsequent decrease in the capillary/fibre ratio. Appropriate controls must be age, gender, and activity related, for there is a progressive increase in mean fibre diameter, capillary/fibre ratio, and number of capillaries surrounding a single fibre, together with a decrease in capillary density (capillaries/mm² of muscle fibre) which was documented when data from normal infants, children, and teenagers were compared (Carry *et al.* 1986). In adults with dermatomyositis, both large and small vessels (less than 20 µm in diameter) are involved (Kalovidouris *et al.* 1988).

Muscle pathology

The muscle pathology in juvenile dermatomyositis reflects vascular compromise and capillary dropout, with perifascicular atrophy of both type I and type II fibres (Fig. 2). Multiple satellite cells are frequently seen in atrophic fibres; focal repair takes place concomitantly with fibre atrophy (Woo *et al.* 1988). In muscle biopsies from children aged 3 to 11 years with juvenile dermatomyositis, mitochondria in muscle appeared to be increased in number, but were reduced in size and in the total content of cytochrome C oxidase as measured both histochemically and biochemically. The biochemical changes were physically associated with perifascicular atrophy, suggesting that ischaemia could lead to structural change (Woo *et al.* 1988). Low-grade ischaemia may also be related to expression of class I and class II major histocompatibility complex gene products, which also were found primarily in the perifascicular area (Karpati *et al.* 1988). In some children with juvenile dermatomyositis who despite normal serum levels of muscle-derived enzymes have elevated levels of von Willebrand-factor antigen and/or neopterin (see below), the muscle biopsy can reveal active foci of inflammation (Pachman *et al.* 1996). In contrast, in polymyositis there appears to be less primary involvement of vessels — they may be normal in number and structure. It is not known if dermatomyositis in the adult has the identical pathophysiology as in the child, but comprehensive national studies in the United States are under way which should clarify this issue. In adult dermatomyositis, the infiltrate is composed of DR+ B cells and there is an increased CD4/CD8 ratio (it should be noted that few children have been extensively studied). It appears that informed discussion of specific immunohistopathology must include classification of the patients with respect to myositis-specific antibodies, as well as the duration of inflammatory disease, the presence of previous therapy at the time of biopsy, verification that the biopsy site was appropriate (for example, positive on MRI or ultrasound), data concerning the child's HLA phenotype with respect to the presence or absence of DQA1*0501, and the specific anatomic site of the biopsy under consideration (perivascular, endomesial, perifascicular, etc.). Overall, in dermatomyositis, there appears to be a close relationship between CD4+ cells and B cells as well as macrophages, suggesting a cytotoxic mechanism, perhaps directed against immune complex-modified endothelial cells (Engel and Arahata 1986; Hohlfeld and Engel 1994). The relationship of the tissue localization of cells from the immune system to those that are circulating is just beginning to be understood (see below). The various possible mechanisms of immunological injury have been discussed in Chapter 5.9.1, but this information is poorly defined for children at different stages of disease duration and activity.

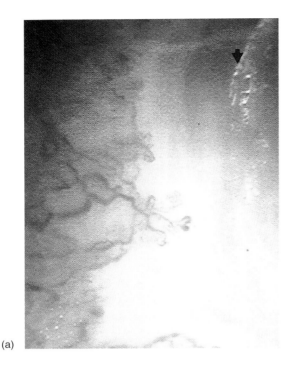

(a)

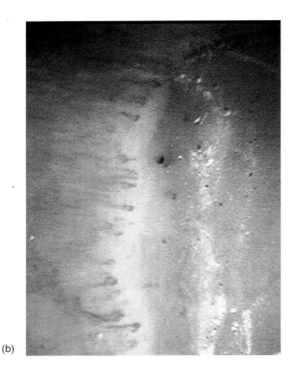

(b)

Fig. 2 (a) Nailfold capillary studies of a child with dermatomyositis of 2 years duration with severe active disease (not able to walk, flexion contractures) referred for evaluation. Her nailfolds display a prominent subcapillary venous plexus and marked avascularity with decreased numbers of end capillary loops. The few end capillaries that are present are tortuous and show terminal bushing characteristic of this disease. The black arrow indicated the edge of the nail. (b) The same nailfold 2 years and 4 months later: the child is now walking, attending school, but still requires intensive therapy. The prominent subcapillary venous plexus has been replaced by new capillary formation which has decreased the areas of avascularity. The end capillary loops are still not normal: there is increased dilation and open loop formation.

Calcification in soft tissues

The aetiology of the calcinosis must be determined and clearly differentiated from other syndromes in which calcinosis occurs, such as in heterotopic calcinosis or following trauma. In juvenile dermatomyositis, calcification in soft tissue may be a correlate of disease severity and duration (Pachman *et al.* 1985) Delay in diagnosis (Pachman *et al.* 1992*b*) and/or insufficient therapy (Callen *et al.* 1994) appears to be correlated with the development of calcinosis. Therefore, early recognition of the disease and institution of appropriate therapy can prevent the development of calcinosis (Callen *et al.* 1994). The therapeutic dilemma for the physician is to identify indicators of disease activity that are useful for an individual child. Those children with juvenile dermatomyositis who do develop calcifications may have one of several outcomes. The calcifications may resolve spontaneously, draining as a white, cheesy or serosanguinous exudate, and leaving dry pitted, scars. The calcifications do not decrease when chelating agents are given. In some children with persistent, active disease, the calcifications progress to become a sheath, impairing flexion and function, braking the barrier of the skin to form a site of entry of infection. Sepsis is not uncommon in this event and contributes to morbidity and mortality from this disease.

Calcinosis is accompanied by increased urinary excretion of γ-carboxyglutamic acid (**GLA**), which is a component of the vitamin K-dependent coagulation pathway. This increased excretion of GLA (when compared with age-/sex-matched controls) was present both in children with juvenile dermatomyositis who had no clinical or radiological evidence of calcinosis (whose mean values for GLA excretion were twice normal) and in those who did have calcinosis (whose mean values were three time normal) (Lian *et al.* 1982). Routine measures of coagulation, including the prothrombin and activated partial thromboplastin times were normal (Lian *et al.* 1982). Calcifications are not correlated with antinuclear antibody, immune complexes, or class II HLA antigens (Pachman *et al.* 1985).

Immunological, genetic, and haematological data

Immunological data

Children with active untreated juvenile dermatomyositis are lymphopenic (O'Gorman *et al.* 1995). Despite this lymphopenia, there is a relative increase in the percentage of B cells (defined by anti-CD19 monoclonal antibody), which is correlated with a clinical disease activity score (in contrast, the percentages of CD4, CD8, and CD25 are not correlated with disease activity) (Eisenstein *et al.* 1995). This increased percentage of B cells may reflect response to medical therapy by returning to normal ranges at a time when other serological indicators of disease activity have already become normal (Pachman 1994). The CD4:CD8 cell ratio is increased, suggesting that there is a decrease in circulating CD8+ cells in the periphery (O'Gorman *et al.* 1995). Efforts to identify clonal expansion of T cells in the muscle of children with new-onset untreated juvenile dermatomyositis have not yet demonstrated a specific increase in T-cell receptor variable gene expression (V) as determined by polymerase chain reaction and sequencing of the CDR3 region in six children positive for the HLA antigen DQA1*0501 (Pachman *et al.* 1995*a*).

Humoral immunity may be abnormal in a minority of patients: in early disease, IgM (Pachman and Cooke 1980) or IgG (O'Gorman *et al.* 1995) may be elevated or IgA deficiency may be present (Pachman and Cooke 1980). Peripheral blood lymphocytes from children with juvenile dermatomyositis appear to have a high spontaneous rate of immunoglobulin synthesis *in vitro* (Cambridge 1990). Tests for an array of antibodies with tissue or organ specificity were negative when comparing sera from 89 patients with newly diagnosed juvenile dermatomyositis with 105 age-/sex-matched controls. Only the antinuclear antibodies (ANA) and antibody to the polymyositis antigen 1 (PM-1) were more frequent in patients than controls ($p < 0.005$, $p < 0.001$ respectively) (Pachman *et al.* 1985; Montecucco *et al.* 1990). The ANA is speckled and cytoskeletal in pattern in 60 to 70 per cent of children (often in high titres), but negative for Jo-1 (Pachman *et al.* 1984). A similar speckled ANA was found in sera from children with a primary cardiomyopathy (who were positive on culture for CVB) and in CVB type-specific mouse monoclonal antibody, suggesting that a response to a viral antigen may play a role in juvenile dermatomyositis (Patterson *et al.* 1989). Other unconfirmed investigations identified an antibody specificity for heat shock protein 60 in the juvenile dermatomyositis sera (Patterson *et al.* 1993).

As in adults, identification of the ANA specificity in a person with an inflammatory myopathy may allow greater understanding of the aetiology and pathogenesis of theses heterogenous diseases (Love *et al.* 1991). Five children have been identified with Jo-1, the most common of the antisynthetases (Rider *et al.* 1995); in addition nine out of eleven other children had antibody to Mi-2 and their disease onset and course was the same as other ANA-positive, MSA-negative children; seven out of the nine were Hispanic, one was Asian, the other child was black. They had no obvious pattern in the season of onset of their weakness; fevers and joint contractures without associated arthritis were frequent in this group, but cardiopulmonary symptoms were uncommon (Rider *et al.* 1994). This was in contrast to the child with anti-SRP who had a sudden onset in the autumn of proximal and distal muscle weakness without the rashes characteristic of dermatomyositis, or cardiac involvement or palpitations prominent in adults with anti-SRP disease. Once her specific inflammatory myopathy was recognized, she was switched from corticosteroids (which worsened her disease) to cytotoxic agents and intravenous immunoglobulin to achieve remission (Rider *et al.* 1994).

Complement activation has been implicated in several studies which included children with juvenile dermatomyositis: the C5b–9 membrane-attack complex was localized to the intramuscular microvasculature in 10 of 12 patients (Kissel *et al.* 1986); the duration of the clinical disease was correlated with this finding (Kissel *et al.* 1991). Immune complexes appear to participate in the pathophysiology of this disease: there is data demonstrating complement activation (despite normal levels of total complement, C3 and C4) accompanied by increased levels of fibrinopeptide A and von Willebrand factor antigen (Scott and Arroyave 1987).

Another useful indicator of disease activity is neopterin, a member of the pteridine family derived from GTP via guanosinetriphosphate cyclohydrolase and released from macrophages as a consequence of T-cell dependent interactions (Barak *et al.* 1989) involving interferon-γ. Early reports of increased neopterin levels in active dermatomyositis in children (Myones *et al.* 1989) were confirmed (DeBenedetti *et al.* 1993). Further studies demonstrated that neopterin levels were a correlate of a clinical disease activity score in over 65 per cent of cases (Pachman *et al.* 1995*c*).

Genetic studies

Records of juvenile dermatomyositis in more than one family member are sporadic, but the disease has been reported in monozygotic twins, who developed muscle-related abnormalities 2 weeks after an upper respiratory tract infection (Harati *et al.* 1986). In a large, cross-sectional study of children with juvenile dermatomyositis and their families, there was a marked increase in Caucasians with HLA B8 (relative risk 2.8, $p < 0.01$) (Friedman *et al.* 1983*a*) and DR3 (relative risk 3.8, $p < 0.01$); in Latin Americans, the relative risk for HLA DR3 was 18.5 ($p < 0.05$) (Friedman *et al.* 1983*b*). The association of the supratypes A1, Cw7, B8, and DR3 suggests that there might be a genetic component to disease susceptibility or expression. Further examination showed that there was an increased association of HLA DQA1*0501 but not C4a when 30 Caucasian children with juvenile dermatomyositis were compared with regional controls matched for HLA DR3 (Reed *et al.* 1991). This observation was sustained when other racial groups in the United States were studied (Reed and Stirling 1995), but did not appear to be true for Czech children with this disease (Vavrincova *et al.* 1993).

Haematological data

In children with juvenile dermatomyositis, the usual indicators of an acute-phase reaction are often within normal range, although children with acute severe disease or infected sites of calcinosis may have elevated values. The lymphopenia is not commonly accompanied by an abnormal platelet count, although a mild microcytic anaemia may be present. A sensitive indicator of inflammatory disease is an elevated von Willebrand factor antigen (Bowyer *et al.* 1989; Guzman *et al.* 1994) which may precede a disease flare (when muscle enzyme data is normal), or remain elevated once the enzymes have returned to normal (Scott and Arroyave 1987). The von Willebrand factor antigen is correlated with disease activity in some but not all children (Bloom *et al.* 1995). In over 50 per cent of children, levels of this antigen correlate with a clinical score of disease activity; analysis of the multimers confirms that it is endothelial in origin, reflecting endothelial cell damage (Miller *et al.* 1995).

These clues to disease activity — the MRI, neopterin, von Willebrand factor antigen, and percentage of B cells — are still imperfect guides to therapy (Pachman 1995), but may be of substantial aid in the characterization of the severity of the immunologically mediated inflammatory process (Pachman 1994).

Course and therapy

Course

The outcome of juvenile dermatomyositis has improved greatly since the 1960s when one-third of the children died, one-third were crippled, and the remainder recovered (Bitnum *et al.* 1964). Several types of disease course have been described — monocyclic, recurrent, and continuous (Spencer *et al.* 1984) — but they may be attenuated by early diagnosis and aggressive therapy. The frequency of calcinosis (which was associated with loss of mobility) has decreased from over 60 per cent of cases (Bowyer *et al.* 1983) to none (Callen *et al.* 1994). Late disease recurrence after years of apparent inactivity has been reported (Lovell and Lindsley 1986), suggesting the need for periodic monitoring with more sensitive indicators of disease activity. It is difficult to predict outcome at the onset of illness, although the magnitude of the initial creatine kinase appears

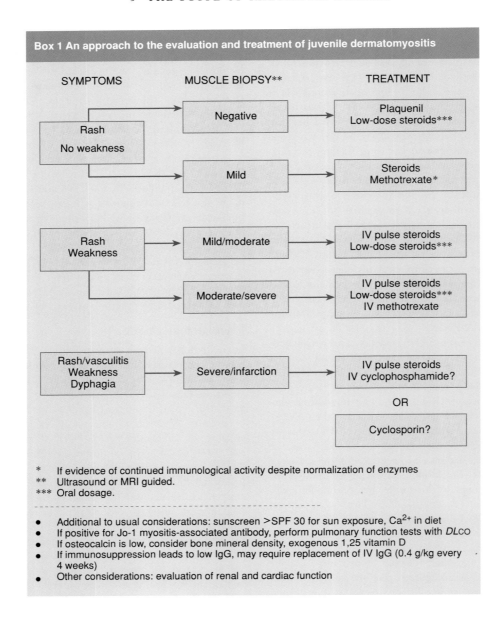

Box 1 An approach to the evaluation and treatment of juvenile dermatomyositis

*   If evidence of continued immunological activity despite normalization of enzymes
**   Ultrasound or MRI guided.
***   Oral dosage.

- Additional to usual considerations: sunscreen >SPF 30 for sun exposure, Ca^{2+} in diet
- If positive for Jo-1 myositis-associated antibody, perform pulmonary function tests with DL_{CO}
- If osteocalcin is low, consider bone mineral density, exogenous 1,25 vitamin D
- If immunosuppression leads to low IgG, may require replacement of IV IgG (0.4 g/kg every 4 weeks)
- Other considerations: evaluation of renal and cardiac function

to be a direct correlate of disease severity (Van Rossum *et al*. 1994). Several groups have found that prognosis is related directly to the degree of vascular involvement (Crowe *et al*. 1982; Bowyer *et al*. 1983).

Therapy

There is continuing controversy over the type, duration, and route of medication to be instituted (Malleson 1990). Recommendations are impaired because of lack of long-term outcome data; medical practices have changed in the recent past, and it is not known how this will affect the children's course in the future—both the consequences of the autoimmune disease and its therapy. Given these caveats, there is sparse data on long-term outcome. A summary of the treatment of juvenile dermatomyositis is given in Box 1.

Several investigators have observed the utility of high-dose intravenous intermittent (pulse) methylprednisolone for the treatment of juvenile dermatomyositis over the past 2 decades (Miller

1980; Yanagisawa *et al*. 1983; Laxer *et al*. 1987). When children with similar clinical disease activity scores were compared, one group had been given 2 mg/kg per day of prednisone to treat their active disease, and required about 4 years until all therapy was discontinued. The other group was given intravenous intermittent high-dose methylprednisone at 30 mg/kg, supplemented with vitamin D and a calcium-sufficient diet, and low daily doses of about 0.5 mg/kg on days when they did not receive intravenous methylprednisolone. The children receiving the intravenous therapy had a shorter disease course with respect to persistence of rash (1.5 years compared with 3.9 years), weakness (1.5 years compared with 2.7 years), and did not have calcinosis or growth retardation, although the frequency of cataracts was the same in both groups (Pachman *et al*. 1994). When a subset of this group, who had a monocyclic disease course, was subjected to a cost analysis, the intravenously treated group had 2 disease-free years, but their bill was about $US10 000 higher than those given oral therapy (Klein-Gitelman *et al.* 1996). Cost differences associated with long-term outcomes are not known.

In our centre, the child with active juvenile dermatomyositis is thoroughly evaluated on admission, using the parameters appropriate to the child. Adequate hydration lessens the possibility of renal damage. If there is evidence of dysphagia or difficulty in handling secretions, then serious consideration is given to the immediate use of weekly intravenous methotrexate at a starting dose of 15 mg/m^2, to be administered immediately following the administration of high-dose intermittent pulse methylprednisolone at 30 mg/kg per day in 100 ml D5W to be given over at least 30 min with monitoring of vital signs every 15 min for 30 min after the infusion is completed. The frequency of the intravenous steroid administration is determined by the rate of response of the child, using the parameters that reflect that child's inflammatory response. Low-dose oral steroids, at 0.5 mg/kg per day are given in the morning on the days that the intravenous methylprednisolone is not infused. The protocol for each child is individual. In general, an intensive course of intravenous methylprednisolone is used until the laboratory tests become normal, with gradual reduction in therapy. The use of high-dose methylprednisolone is not without some side-effects. In an analysis of the drug usage over a 5-year period in which 213 children with various types of serious rheumatic disease were given over 2622 doses, 46 children (22 per cent) experienced an adverse reaction of which 21 had behavioural changes ranging from euphoria to emotional lability. There was one case of anaphylaxis (Klein-Gitelman and Pachman 1995).

When there is severe skin involvement, hydroxychloroquine (7 mg/kg per day) is given if there is no family history of red–green colour blindness. With milder involvement, the cutaneous symptoms often resolve within several weeks, making the use of this drug unnecessary. Topical agents to lessen dryness help the occasional pruritis as do topical steroids, which should be used sparingly (Stonecipher *et al.* 1993). For breaks in the integument, a 'skin substitute' (e.g. 'Second skin', duoderm) should be considered. Sepsis secondary to infected calcinosis must be treated aggressively.

Children who have severe onset, or who do not respond to steroids, have been treated with methotrexate for the past 2 decades (Jacobs 1977). More recently, earlier use of this drug at doses of 15 mg/m^2 per week has reduced the morbidity of the disease (Miller *et al.* 1992), and permits the use of lower doses of steroids. In active disease, intravenous administration of methotrexate assures drug absorption; as the disease becomes quiescent, oral administration is tolerated. Complaints of nausea can be circumvented by dividing the dose but giving the full amount in a 24-h period. The function of the liver and bone marrow must be monitored. If it appears that a child remains severely ill (sometimes despite the muscle enzymes becoming normal), evaluation of the immune system may help to guide therapy (e.g. the percentage of B cells remains elevated in 40 to 60 per cent) (Eisenstein *et al.* 1995). Intravenous cyclophosphamide therapy, starting at 500 mg/m^2 every 3 weeks (following adequate hydration), with mesna for bladder protection, is instituted and the methotrexate is discontinued (Pachman 1994). As with most modes of immunosuppression, levels of IgG must be checked on a periodic basis to ensure that they are adequate; if not, replacement therapy (0.4 g/kg every 3 to 4 weeks) is needed to prevent recurrent infections.

When considering therapies other than steroids, high-dose (not replacement) intravenous gammaglobin may initially dampen the inflammatory process, especially the rash (Roifman *et al.* 1987; Lang *et al.* 1991) if given early in the disease course (Basta and Dalakas 1994), but it is unclear if prolonged control of disease activity can be achieved with this modality alone. Plasmapheresis alone does not appear to be effective in adults (Miller *et al.* 1992) and no data is available for children. Evaluation of the efficacy of cyclosporin has been proposed (Heckmatt *et al.* 1989) but has been hampered by coexisting therapies (Pistoia *et al.* 1993). FK506 has been useful in the therapy of adults with Jo-1 myopathy (Oddis *et al.* 1994), but no published data are available for children.

At the moment there are no successful therapies for long-standing calcinosis in children with inactive disease. In those children who do have calcinosis and residual evidence of an active immunological process, an MRI may reveal more inflammation than expected, permitting more aggressive therapy, which may result in regression (and occasionally radiological resolution) of the calcinosis. Treatment with low-dose warfarin early in the disease has been suggested (Berger *et al.* 1987), but is a considerable hazard for the active child, is not useful in advanced disease (Lassoued *et al.* 1988), and has not yet been proved effective in a case–control study.

The progression of osteopenia, a consequence of disease activity as well as therapy, can be slowed with a calcium-sufficient diet, and the addition of thrice-weekly (Monday, Wednesday, Friday) 1,25-vitamin D (20 µg under 30 kg; 50 µg over 30 kg) in conjunction with disease control. Administration of vitamin D and increasing the calcium intake may aid in calcium absorption from the gastrointestinal tract in the face of steroid therapy (which inhibits calcium absorption), and diminishes the occurrence of one of the most serious consequences of steroid therapy, osteopenia, which can progress to spinal cord compression fractures (Callen *et al.* 1994).

Combined drug treatment (to suppress inflammation) and physiotherapy (gentle, passive stretching) are required in the early phase of the disease, and more intensive, graded physiotherapy is effective later in the disease, once the inflammation has abated. Prevention of sunburn, both by avoidance and barriers (clothing, UVA/UVB PABA-free sunblocks over SPF 30) helps keep the disease in remission.

In summary, juvenile dermatomyositis, characterized by genetically restricted and immunologically mediated vasculopathy, is under intense investigation. It is axiomatic that as more knowledge of the specific pathophysiology of the disease(s) is accrued, more effective therapeutic interventions will be devised.

References

Ansell, B.A., Miller, J.J., III, Pachman, L.M., and Sullivan, D.B. (1990). Controversies in juvenile dermatomyositis. *Journal of Rheumatology*, **17** (Suppl. 22), 1–6.

Banker, B.Q. and Victor, M. (1966). Dermatomyositis (systemic angiopathy) of childhood. *Medicine*, **45**, 261–89.

Barak, M., Merzback, D., and Gruener, N. (1989). The effect of immunomodulators on PHA or IFN- gamma induced release of neopterin from purified macrophages and peripheral blood mononuclear cells. *Immunology Letters*, **21**, 317–22.

Basta, M. and Dalakas, M.C. (1994). High-dose intravenous immunoglobulin exerts its beneficial effect in patients with dermatomyositis by blocking endomysial deposition of activated complement fragments. *Journal of Clinical Investigation*, **95**, 1729–35.

Benbassat, J., Geffel, D., and Zlotnick, A. (1980). Epidemiology of polymyositis–dermatomyositis in Israel. *Israel Journal of Medical Science*, **16**, 197–200.

Berger, R.G., Featherstone, G.L., Raasch, R.H., McCartney, W.H., and Handler, N.M. (1987). Treatment of calcinosis universalis with low-dose warfarin. *American Journal of Medine*, **83**, 72–6.

Bitnum, C., Dawschnor, C.W., and Travis, L.B. (1964). Dermatomysitis. *Journal of Pediatrics*, **64**, 101–31.

Bloom, B.J., Tucker, L.B., Miller, L.C., and Schaller, J.G. (1995). Von Willebrand factor in juvenile dermatomyositis. *Journal of Rheumatology*, **22**, 320–5.

Bohan, A. and Peter, J.B. (1975). Polymyositis and dermatomyositis (parts 1 and 2). *New England Journal of Medicine*, **292**, 344–7, 403–7.

Borrelli, M.P. *et al.* (1988). Ureteral necrosis in dermatomyositis. *Journal of Urology*, **139**, 1275–7.

Bowles, N.E., Dubowitz, V., Sewry, C.A., and Archand, L.C. (1987). Dermatomyositis, polymyositis, and coxsackie-B-virus infection. *Lancet*, **ii**, 1004–7.

Bowyer, S.L., Blane, C.E., and Sullivan, D.B. (1983). Childhood dermatomyositis: factors predicting functional outcome and development of dystrophic calcification. *Journal of Pediatrics*, **103**, 882–8.

Bowyer, S.L., Ragsdale, C.G., and Sullivan, D.B. (1989). Factor VIII related antigen and childhood rheumatic diseases. *Journal of Rheumatology*, **16**, 1093–7.

Breningstall, G.N. (1990). Carnitine deficiency syndromes. *Pediatric Neurology*, **6**, 75–81.

Callen, A.M., Pachman, L.M., Hayford, J.R., Chung, A., and Ramsey-Goldman, R. (1994). Intermittent high-dose intravenous methylprednisolone (IV pulse) therapy prevents calcinosis and shortens disease course in juvenile dermatomyositis (JDMS). *Arthritis and Rheumatism*, **37**, R10.

Cambridge, G. (1990). What is the role of the immune system in juvenile dermatomyositis. In *Pediatric rheumatology update* (ed. P. Woo, P. White, and B. Ansell), p.182. Oxford University Press.

Carry, M.R., Ringel, S.P., and Starcevich, J.M. (1986). Distribution of capillaries in normal and diseased human skeletal muscle. *Muscle and Nerve*, **9**, 445–54.

Christensen, M.L., Pachman, L.M., and Maryjowski, M.L. (1983). Antibody to coxsackie-B virus: increased incidence in sera from children with recently diagnosed juvenile dermatomyositis. *Arthritis and Rheumatism*, **26**, S24.

Christensen, M.L., Pachman, L.M., Schneiderman, R., Patel, D.C., and Friedman, J.M. (1986). Prevalence of coxsackie B virus antibodies in patients with juvenile dermatomyositis. *Arthritis and Rheumatism*, **29**, 1365–70.

Commens, C., O'Neill, P., and Walker, G. (1990). Dermatomyositis associated with multifocal atrophy. *Journal of the American Academy of Dermatology*, **22**, 966–9.

Crowe, W.E., Love, K.E., Levinson, J.E., and Hilton, P.K. (1982). Clinical and pathogenetic implications of histopathology in childhood polydermatomyositis. *Arthritis and Rheumatism*, **25**, 126–39.

DeBenedetti, F., DeAmici, M., Aramini, L., Ruperto, N., and Martini, A. (1993). Correlations of serum neopterin concentrations with disease activity in juvenile dermatomyositis. *Archives of Diseases in Childhood*, **69**, 232–5.

Eisenstein, D.E., O'Gorman, M.R.G., and Pachman, L.M. (1995*a*). Peripheral blood lymphocyte (PBLn) subsets in patients with juvenile dermatomoysitis (JDMS). *Arthritis and Rheumatism*, **38**, S361.

Eisenstein, D.M., O'Gorman, M.R.G., Donovan, M., and Pachman, L.M. (1995*b*). Percentage of B cells in peripheral blood of patients with JDMS. *Arthritis and Rheumatism*, **38**, R15.

Emslie-Smith, A.M. and Engel, A.G. (1990). Microvascular changes in early and advanced dermatomyositis: a quantitative study. *Annals of Neurology*, **27**, 343.

Engel, A.G. and Arahata, K. (1986). Mononuclear cells in myopathies: quantitation of functionally distinct subsets, recognition of antigen-specific cell-mediated cytotoxicity in some diseases, and implications for the pathogenesis of the different inflammatory myopathies. *Human Pathology*, **17**, 704–21.

Fong, L.P. and Yeung, J. (1990). Spontaneous regression of retinal neovascularization in juvenile dermatomyositis. *Australian and New Zealand Journal of Ophthalmology*, **18**, 107–8.

Friedman, J.M. *et al.* (1983*a*). Immunogenetic studies of juvenile dermatomyositis: HLA antigens in patients and their families. *Tissue Antigens*, **21**, 45–9.

Friedman, J.M. *et al.* (1983*b*). Immunogenetic studies of juvenile dermatomyositis: HLA-DR antigen frequencies. *Arthritis and Rheumatism*, **26**, 214–16.

Guzman, J., Petty, R.E., and Malleson, P.N. (1994). Monitoring disease activity in juvenile dermatomyositis: the role of von Willebrand factor and muscle enzymes. *Journal of Rheumatology*, **21**, 739–43.

Harati, Y., Niakan, E., and Bergman, E.W. (1986). Childhood dermatomyositis in monozygotic twins. *Neurology*, **36**, 721–3.

Heckmatt, J.Z. *et al.* (1989). Effectiveness of cyclosporin for dermatomysitis. *Lancet*, **i**, 1063–6.

Hernandez, R.J., Sullivan, D.B., and Chenevert, T.L. (1993). MR imaging in children with dermatomyositis: musculoskeltal findings and correlation with clinical and laboratory findings. *American Journal of Roentgenology*, **161**, 359–66.

Hidano, A., Keneka, K., and Arai, Y. (1986). Survey of the prognosis for dermatomyositis with special reference to its associated malignancy and pulmonary fibrosis. *Journal of Dermatology*, **13**, 233–41.

Hiketa, T., Matsumoto, Y., Ohashi, M., and Sakaki, R. (1992). Juvenile dermatomyositis: a statistical study of 114 patients with dermatomyositis. *Journal of Dermatology*, **19**, 470–6.

Hochberg, M.C. (1988). Epidemiology of polymyositis/dermatomyositis. *Mount Sinai Journal of Medicine*, **55**, 447–52.

Hohlfeld, R. and Engel, A.G. (1994). The immunobiology of muscle. *Immunology Today*, **15**, 269–74.

Huppertz, H.I. and Kaiser, W.A. (1994). Serial magnetic resonance imaging in juvenile dermatomyositis — delayed normalization. *Rheumatology International*, **4**, 127–9.

Jacobs, J.C. (1977). Methotrexate and azathioprine treatment of childhood dermatomyositis. *Pediatrics*, **59**, 212–18.

Kalovidouris, A.E., Stoesz, E., Muller, J., and Kimes, T. (1988). Relationships between clinical features and distribution of mononuclear cells in muscle of patients with polymyositis. *Journal of Rheumatology*, **15**, 1401–6.

Karpati, G., Pouliot, Y., and Carpenter, S. (1988). Expression of immunoreactive major histocompatibility complex products in human skeletal muscles. *Annals of Neurology*, **23**, 64–72.

Keim, D.R., Hernandez, R.J., and Sullivan, D.B. (1991). Serial magnetic resonance imaging in juvenile dermatomyositis. *Arthritis and Rheumatism*, **34**, 1580–4.

Kissel, J.T., Mendell, J.R., and Rammohan, K.W. (1986). Microvascular deposition of complement membrane attack complex in dermatomyositis. *New England Journal of Medicine*, **314**, 329–34.

Kissel, J.T., Halterman, R.K., Rammohan, K.W., and Mendell, J.R. (1991). The relationship of complement-mediated microvasculopathy to the histologic features and clinical duration of disease in dermatomyositis. *Archives of Neurology*, **48**, 26–30.

Klein-Gitelman, M. and Pachman, L.M. (1995). IV pulse corticosteroids (CS): adverse reactions are more variable than expected in children. *Arthritis and Rheumatism*, **38**, S338.

Klein-Gitelman, M., Waters, T., and Pachman, L.M. (1996). A comparison of the cost effectiveness of IV and PO corticosteroids in the treatment of juvenile dermatomyositis (JDMS). *Arthritis and Rheumatism*, **39**, R13.

Koch, M.J., Brody, J.A., and Gillespie, M.M. (1976). Childhood polymyositis: a case-controlled study. *American Journal of Epidemiology*, **104**, 627–31.

Lang, B.A., Laxer, R.M., Murphy, G., Silverman, E.D., and Roifman, C.M. (1991). Treatment of dermatomyositis with intravenous gammaglobulin. *American Journal of Medicine*, **91**, 169–72.

Lapetina, F. (1989). Toxoplasmosis and dermatomyositis: a causal or casual relationship. *Pediatrica Medica e Chirurgica*, **11**, 197–203.

Lassoued, K., Saiag, P., Anglade, M., Roujeau, J., and Touraine, R.L. (1988). Failure of warfarin in treatment of calcinosis universalis. *American Journal of Medicine*, **84**, 795–6.

Laxer, R.M., Stein, L.D., and Petty, R.E. (1987). Intravenous pulse methylprednisolone treatment of juvenile dermatomyositis. *Arthritis and Rheumatism*, **30**, 328–34.

Leff, R.L., Miller, F.W., Greenberg, S.J., Klein, E.A., Dalakas, M.C., and Plotz, P.H. (1992). Viruses in idiopathic inflammatory myopathies: absence of candidate viral genomes in muscle. *Lancet*, **339**, 1192–5.

Lian, J.B., Pachman, L.M., Gundberg, C.M., Partridge, R.E.H., and Maryjowski, M.L. (1982). Gamma-carboxyglutamate excretion and calcinosis in juvenile dermatomyositis. *Arthritis and Rheumatism*, **25**, 1094–100.

Lott, J.A. and Landesman, P.W. (1984). The enzymology of skeletal muscle disorders. *Critical Review in Clinical Laboratory Sciences*, **20**, 153–90.

Love, L.A. *et al.* (1991). A new approach to the classification of idiopathic inflammatory myopathy: myositis-specific autoantibodies define useful homogeneous patient groups. *Medicine (Baltimore)*, **70**, 360–74.

Lovell, H.B. and Lindsley, C.B. (1986). Late recurrence of childhood dermatomyositis. *Journal of Rheumatology*, **13**, 821–2.

Malleson, P.N. (1990). Controversies in juvenile dermatomyositis. *Journal of Rheumatology*, **17** (Suppl. 22), 1.

Manta, P., Kalfakis, N., and Vassilopoulos, D. (1989). Evidence for seasonal variation in polymyositis. *Neuroepidemiology*, **8**, 262–5.

Martini, A., Ravelli, A., Viola, S., Sambugaro, R., and De Benedette, F. (1987). Calcinoisis as the presenting sign of juvenile dermatomyositis in a 14-month-old boy. *Helvetia Paediatrica*, **42**, 181–4.

Martini, A., Ravelli, A., Albani, S., Viola, S., Scotta, S., Magrini, U., and Burgio, G.R. (1992). Recurrent juvenile dermamtomyositis and cutaneous necrotizing arteritis with molecular mimicry between streptoccal type 5 protein and human skeletal myosin. *Journal of Pediatrics*, **121**, 739–42.

Masi, A.T. and Hochberg, M.C. (1988). Temporal association of polymyositis–dermatomyositis with malignancy: methodologic and clinical considerations. *Mount Sinai Journal of Medicine*, **55**, 471–8.

Medsger, T.A., Jr., Dawson, W.N., and Masi, A.T. (1970). The epidemiology of polymyositis. *American Journal of Medicine*, **48**, 715–23.

Mejlszenkier, J.D., Safran, A.E., and Healy, J.J. (1973). The myositis of influenza. *Arcives of Neurology*, **29**, 441–3.

Miller, C.H., Donovan, J.M., Maduzia, L., Chung, A., and Pachman, L.M. (1995). Relationship of von Willebrand factor antigen to disease activity in juvenile dermatomyositis. *Arthritis and Rheumatism*, **39**, R13.

Miller, F.W. *et al.* (1992). Controlled trial of plasma exchange and leukapheresis in polymyositis and dermatomyositis. *New England Journal of Medicine*, **326**, 1380–4.

Miller, J.J., III (1980). Prolonged use of large intravenous steroid pulses in the rheumatic diseases of children. *Pediatrics*, **65**, 989–94.

Miller, L.C., Michael, A.F., and Kim, Y. (1987). Childhood dermatomyositis. *Clinical Pediatrics*, **26**, 561–8.

Miller, L.C., Sisson, B.A., Tucker, L.B., DeNardo, B.A., and Schaller, J.G. (1992). Methotrexate treatment of recalcitrant childhood dermatomyositis. *Arthritis and Rheumatism*, **35**, 1143–9.

Montecucco, C., Ravelli, A., Caporali, R., Viola, S., De Gennerao, F., Albani, S., and Martini, A. (1990). Autoantibodies in juvenile dermatomyositis. *Clinical and Experimental Rheumatology*, **8**, 193–6.

Myones, B.L., Luckey, J.P., Hayford, J.R., and Pachman, L.M. (1989). Increased neopterin levels in juvenile dermatomyositis correlate with disease activity and are indicative of macrophage activation. *Arthritis and Rheumatism*, **52**, S83.

Oddis, C.V., Carroll, P., Abu-Elmagd, K., McCauley, J., Fung, J.J., and Starzl, T.E. (1994). FK506 in the treatment of polymyositis. *Arthritis and Rheumatism*, **37**, S286.

O'Gorman, M.R.G., Corrochano, V., Roleck, J., Donovan, M., and Pachman, L.M. (1995). Flow cytometric analysis of the lymphocyte subsets in pheripheral blood of children with untreated active juvenile dermatomyositis. *Clinical, Diagnostic and Laboratory Immunology*, **2**, 205–8.

Pachman, L.M. (1994). Juvenile dermatomyositis (JDMS): new clues to diagnosis and pathogenesis. *Clinical and Experimental Rheumatology*, **12**, S69–S73.

Pachman, L.M. (1995). Imperfect indications of disease activity in juvenile dermatomyositis. *Journal of Rheumatology*, **2**, 193–7.

Pachman, L.M. and Cooke, N. (1980). Juvenile dermatomyositis: a clinical and immunologic study. *Journal of Pediatrics*, **96**, 226–34.

Pachman, L.M. and Maryjowski, M.L. (1984). Juvenile dermatmyositis and polymyositis. In *Inflammatory diseases of muscle* (ed. B.A. Ansell), p.95. W.B. Saunders, Philadelphia, PA.

Pachman, L.M., Hardin, J.A., Cobb, M.A., and Arroyave, C.M. (1984). The antinuclear antibody (ANA) in juvenile dermatomyositis (JDMS) is not Jo-1, suggesting that JDMS and polymyositis (PM) are different diseases. *Arthritis and Rheumatism*, **27**, S45.

Pachman, L.M. *et al.* (1985). Immunogenetic studies of juvenile dermatomyositis. III. Study of antibody to organ-specific and nuclear antigens. *Arthritis and Rheumatism*, **28**, 151–7.

Pachman, L.M. *et al.* (1992a). Seasonal onset in juvenile dermatomyositis (JDMS): an epidemiological study. *Arthritis and Rheumatism*, **35**, S88.

Pachman, L.M., Hayford, J.R., Sinacore, J., Bowyer, S.L., and Hochberg, M.C. (1992b). New onset juvenile dermatomyositis (JDMS): a clinical description. *Arthritis and Rheumatism*, **35**, S88.

Pachman, L.M., Callen, A.M., Hayford, J.R., Chung, A., Sinacore, J., and Ramsey-Goldman, R. (1994). Juvenile dermatomyositis (JDMS): decreased calcinoisis (Ca++) with intermittant high-dose intravenous methylprednisolone (IV pulse) therapy. *Arthritis and Rheumatism*, **37**, S429.

Pachman, L.M., Lawton, T.P., Litt, D.L., Corvera, J.S., and Pope, R.L. (1995a). Lack of oligoclonality of T cell receptor (TCR) V 8 in muscle obtained by MRI directed biopsy of six children positive for HLA DQA1*0501 with active untreated juvenile dermatomyositis (JDMS). *Arthritis and Rheumatism*, **39**, R14.

Pachman, L.M. *et al.* (1995b). Lack of detection of enteroviral RNA or bacterial DNA in MRI directed muscle biopsies from twenty children with active untreated juvenile dermatomyositis. *Arthritis and Rheumatism*, **38**, 1513–18.

Pachman, L.M., Maduzia, L., Chung, A., Donovan, M., and Ramsey-Goldman, R. (1995c). Juvenile dermatomyositis (JDMS): disease activity scores are correlated with levels of neopterin in serum. *Arthritis and Rheumatism*, **38**, R16.

Pachman, L.M., Sundberg, J., Maduzia, L., Daugherty, C., and Litt, D. (1995d). Sequential studies of nailfold capillary vessels (NFC) in 10 children with juvenile dermatmyositis (JDMS): correlation with disease activity score (DAS) but not von Willebrand factor antigen (vWF:Ag). *Arthritis and Rheumatism*, **38**, S361.

Pachman, L.M., Crawford, S., Morello, F., Maduzia, L., Caliendo, J., and Heller, S. (1996). MRI directed needle biopsy for the assessment of juvenile dermatomyositis (JDMS) response to therapy: comparison of intitial and follow-up biopsies using a histological rating scate evaluating disease severity/chronicity. *Arthritis and Rheumatism*, **39**, R14.

Park, J.H. *et al.* (1994). Magnetic resonance imaging and P-31 magnetic resonance spectroscopy provide unique quantitative data useful in the longitudinal management of patients with dermatomyositis. *Arthritis and Rheumatism*, **37**, 736–46.

Patterson, B., Jacobitz, J., Pachman, L.M., Christensen, M., and Pallansch, M. (1989). A study of autoantibodies in coxsackievirus group B (COXB) infected children and in juvenile dermatomyositis (JDMS). *Clinical Research*, **30**, 964A.

Patterson, B.K. *et al.* (1993). Antinuclear antibody (ANA) positive sera from juvenile dermatomyositis (JDMS) has specificity for heat shock protein 60 (HSP-60). *Pediatric Research*, **33**, 157A.

Peters, A.M. *et al.* (1991). Renal haemodynamics of cyclosporin A nephrotoxicity in children with juvenile dermatomyositis. *Clinical Science*, **81**, 153–9.

Pistoia, V. *et al.* (1993). Cyclosporin A in the treatment of juvenile chronic arthritis and childhood polymyositis–dermatomyositis. Results of a preliminary study. *Clinical and Experimental Rheumatology*, **11**, 203–8.

Pitt, A.M., Fleckenstein, J.L., Greenlee, R.G., Jr., Burns, D.K., Bryan, W.W., and Haller, R. (1993). MRI-guided biopsy in inflammatory myopathy: initial results. *Magnetic Resonance Imaging*, **11**, 1093–9.

Reed, A.M. and Stirling, J.D. (1995). Association of the HLA-DQa1*0501 allele in multipe racial groups with juvenile dermatomysitis. *Human Immunology*, **44**, 131–5.

Reed, A.M., Haugen, M., Pachman, L.M., and Langman, C.B. (1990). Abnormalities in serum osteocalcin values in children with chronic rheumatic diseases. *Journal of Pediatrics*, **116**, 574.

Reed, A.M., Pachman, L.M., and Ober, C. (1991). Molecular genetic studies of major histocompatibility complex genes in children with juvenile dermatomyositis: increased risk associated with HLA-DQA1*0501. *Human Immunology*, **32**, 235–40.

Rider, L.G. *et al.* (1994). A broadened spectrum of juvenile myositis: myositis-specific autoantibodies in children. *Arthritis and Rheumatism*, **37**, 1534–8.

Rider, L.G. *et al.* (1995). Anti-Jo-1 autoantibodies define a clinically homogenous subset of childhood idiopathic inflammatory myopathy (IIM). *Arthritis and Rheumatism*, **38**, S362.

Roifman, C.M., Schaffer, F.M., Wachsmuth, S.E., Murphy, G., and Gelfand, E.W. (1987). Reversal of chronic polymyositis following intravenous immune serum globulin therapy. *Journal of the American Medical Association*, **258**, 513–15.

Rosenberg, A.M. (1994). Geographical clustering of childhood dermatomyositis in Saskatchewan. *Arthritis and Rheumatism*, **37**, S402.

Rosenberg, N.L., Rotbart, H.A., Abzug, M.J., Ringel, S.P., and Levin, M.J. (1989). Evidence for a novel picornavirus in human dermatomyositis. *Annals of Neurology*, **26**, 204–9.

Sachrison, B.T., Pachman, L.M., Kaplan, F.S., and Gannon, G.H. (1995). A 5 months old with progressive osseus heteroplasia (POH). *Arthritis and Rheumatism*, 38, R16.

Schiraldi, E. and Iandolo, E. (1978). Polymyositis accompanying coxsackievirus B2 infection. *Infection*, 6, 32–4.

Schroter, H.M., Sarnet, H.B., Matheson, D.S., and Seland, T.P. (1987). Juvenile dermatomyositis induced by toxoplasmosis. *Journal of Child Neurolology*, 2, 101–4.

Scott, J.P. and Arroyave, C. (1987). Activation of complement and coagulation in juvenile dermatomyositis. *Arthritis and Rheumatism*, 30, 572–6.

Serratrice, G., Schiano, A., Pellissier, J.F., and Desnuelle, C. (1989). Les expressions anatomocliniques des pollymyosites chez l'enfant. *Annals Pediatrie (Paris)*, 36, 237–43.

Sherry, D.D., Haas, J.E., and Milstein, J.M. (1993). Childhood polymyositis as a paraneoplastic phenomenon. *Pediatric Neurology*, 9, 155–6.

Sigurgeirsson, B., Lindelöf, B., Edhag, O., and Allander, E. (1992). Risk of cancer in patients with dermatomyositis or polymyositis. A population-based study. *New England Journal of Medicine*, 326, 363–7.

Silver, R.M. and Maricq, H.R. (1989). Childhood dermatomyositis: serial microvascular studies. *Pediatrics*, 83, 278–83.

Spencer, C.H., Hanson, V., Singsen, B.H., Bernstein, B.H., Kornreich, H.K., and King, K.K. (1984). Course of treated juvenile dermatomyositis. *Journal of Pediatrics*, 105, 399–408.

Stonecipher, M.R., Callen, J.P., and Jorizzo, J.L. (1993). The red face: dermatomyositis. *Clinical Dermatology*, 11, 261–73.

Symmons, D.P.M., Sills, J.A., and Davis, S.M. (1995). The incidence of juvenile dermatomyositis: results from a nation-wide study. *British Journal of Rheumatology*, 43, 732–5.

Thompson, G.T.D., Johnston, J.L., Barager, F.D., and Toole, J.W.P. (1990). Psoriatic arthritis and myopathy. *Journal of Rheumatology*, 17, 395–8.

Travers, R.L., Hughes, G.R.V., Cambridge, G., and Sewell, J.R. (1977). Coxsackie B neutralization titers in polymyositis/dermatomyositis. *Lancet*, i, 1268.

Van Rossum, M.A.J., Hiemstra, I., Prieur, A.M., Rijkers, G.T., and Kuis, W. (1994). Juvenile dermato/polymositis: a retrospective analysis of 33 cases with special focus on initial CPK levels. *Clinical and Experimental Rheumatology*, 12, 339–42.

Vavrincova, P., Havelka, S., Cerna, M., and Stastny, P. (1993). HLA class II alleles in juvenile dermatomyositis. *Journal of Rheumatology*, 20 (Suppl. 37), 17–18.

Wang, Y.-J., Lii, Y.-P., Lan, J.-l., Chi, C.-S., Mak, S.-C., and Scian, W.-J. (1993). Juvenile and adult dermatomyositis among the Chinese: a comparative study. *Chinese Medical Journal (Taipei)*, 52, 285–92.

Woo, M., Chung, S.J., and Nonaka, I. (1988). Perifascicular atrophic fibres in childhood dermatomyositis with particular reference to mitochondrial changes. *Journal of Neurological Science*, 88, 133–43.

Yanagisawa, T. *et al.* (1983). Methylprednisolone pulse therapy in dermatomyositis. *Dermatologica*, 167, 47–51.

Yousef, G.E., Isenberg, D.A., and Mowbray, J.F. (1990). Detection of enterovirus specific RNA sequences in muscle biopsy specimens from patients with adult onset myositis. *Annals of the Rheumatic Diseases*, 49, 310–15.

5.10 Sjögren's syndrome

Athanasios G. Tzioufas, Pierre Youinou, and H. M. Moutsopoulos

Introduction

Sjögren's syndrome is a chronic autoimmune disease of unknown aetiology, characterized by lymphocyte infiltration of exocrine glands resulting in xerostomia and keratoconjunctivitis sicca. This syndrome is particularly interesting among the autoimmune diseases for two reasons. First, it has a broad clinical range extending from autoimmune exocrinopathy to extraglandular (systemic) disease affecting the lungs, kidneys, blood vessels, and muscles; it may occur alone (primary Sjögren's syndrome) or in association with other autoimmune diseases (secondary Sjögren's syndrome) (Table 1). Secondly, it is a disorder in which a benign autoimmune process can terminate in a lymphoid malignancy. Thus, Sjögren's syndrome is a 'cross-roads disease' that offers potential insight into the mechanisms whereby immunological dysregulation may predispose to malignant transformation of B cells that are already involved in an autoimmune process.

Historical review (Moutsopoulos *et al.* 1980)

The clinical features of the disorder were first described by Hadden in 1888. Four years later, Mikulicz described the case of a German farmer who suffered from bilateral enlargement of the parotid glands. A biopsy of the parotid showed an intense, focal, lymphocytic infiltrate that is known today as the hallmark of the disease. In the 1920s Gougerot described the disease in France and in 1933, Sjögren, a Swedish ophthalmologist, wrote the classic monograph on the disease in which he emphasized that the eye manifestations are local findings of a systemic disorder. In 1953, Morgan and Castleman showed that the histopathological findings in Sjögren's syndrome and Mikulicz disease are identical. In the 1960s the diverse clinical range of the syndrome was recognized and the study of its autoantibodies was initiated. The genetic predisposition to the disease was substantiated with the study of HLA in the 1970s; in the 1980s, with progress in molecular biology, the specificity of autoantibodies to the cellular components Ro(SSA) and La(SSB), and the composition of the focal lymphocytic infiltration of the exocrine glands, were dissected.

Epidemiology

The syndrome primarily affects women (nine women to every one man), mainly in the fourth and fifth decades of life (Pavlidis *et al.* 1982). However, it can occur in people of all ages, including children and elderly persons (Drosos *et al.* 1988; Siamopoulou-Mavridou *et al.* 1989). Autopsy studies revealed that approximately 2 to 3 per cent of individuals without connective tissue disease had unexplained focal lymphocytic infiltrates of the minor labial salivary glands compatible with Sjögren's syndrome (Scott 1980). On the other hand, clinical studies from Great Britain and Greece have found that Sjögren's syndrome occurs in 3 to 5 per cent of geriatric populations (Whaley *et al.* 1972; Drosos *et al.* 1988).

In an epidemiological study of 705 Swedish adults the calculated prevalence for the disease was 2.7 per cent (Jacobsson *et al.* 1989). Symptoms of dry eyes and dry mouth were correlated with elevated levels of anti-Ro/SSA and anti-La/SSB antibodies (Jacobsson *et al.* 1992). In another study, using as a tool the recently proposed questionnaire and diagnostic criteria for Sjögren's syndrome, as suggested by the European Union concerted action (Vitali *et al.* 1992*a*), it was found that among 837 females (age range from 18 to 90 years), the prevalence of definite and probable Sjögren's syndrome was 0.6 per cent and 3 per cent, respectively (Tzioufas *et al.* 1994).

Aetiology and pathogenesis

Over the past two decades, research in immunopathology, autoantibodies, immunogenetics, and viruses has further refined the concepts of the pathophysiology and pathogenesis of Sjögren's syndrome. One may speculate that the disease develops in three

Table 1 Association of Sjögren's syndrome with other autoimmune diseases

Rheumatoid arthritis

Systemic lupus erythematosus

Systemic sclerosis

Mixed connective tissue disease

Primary biliary cirrhosis

Myositis

Vasculitis

Thyroiditis

Chronic active hepatitis

Mixed cryoglobulinaemia

steps: first, autoimmunity may be triggered by a given environmental factor that acts on a particular genetic background; second, the autoimmune reactivity becomes chronic through abnormal immune regulatory mechanisms; and third, the lesion occurs as a consequence of the continuing inflammatory process.

The triggering of autoimmunity

Environment

Autoimmune reactions against host tissue following viral infection have been reported in both man and experimental animals. Viruses are therefore suspected as being major contributing factors in certain autoimmune disorders. One chronic infection that is especially emphasized is with cytomegalovirus. This involves many organs; among them the salivary glands are prime targets (Hudson et al. 1979). Antibodies to cytomegalovirus of both IgG and IgM classes have been found in the serum of patients with primary Sjögren's syndrome, using an enzyme-linked immunosorbent assay (Shillitoe et al. 1982). However, no controls were used in that study and Venables et al. (1985) were not able to confirm those observations.

Epstein–Barr virus (EBV), another herpesvirus, could well be a better candidate than cytomegalovirus. Its replication also occurs in the salivary glands during primary infection (Wolf et al. 1984). The virus remain latent at this site in immunologically intact adults. Expression of EBV-associated antigens in the salivary glands of some patients with Sjögren's syndrome and increased content of EBV-DNA in their saliva (Fox et al. 1986a) have been demonstrated. However, EBV reactivation may arise as a consequence rather than as a cause of lymphoproliferation in these patients.

Hepatitis C virus may produce a chronic lymphocytic sialadenitis, which mimics that observed in Sjögren's syndrome, since more than 50 per cent of patients infected with hepatitis C virus have been reported, in one study, to present with histological changes compatible with Sjögren's syndrome in their minor salivary glands (Haddad et al. 1992). On the other hand, patients with Sjögren's syndrome do not usually have antibodies to hepatitis C virus in their sera (Vitali et al. 1992b).

The retroviruses are another group of viruses that should be seriously considered in the pathogenesis of autoimmune diseases in general and Sjögren's syndrome in particular. Antibodies to the p24 capsid glycoprotein of human immunodeficiency virus have been detected in approximately 30 per cent of patients with Sjögren's syndrome, whilst the frequency of these antibodies in the serum of healthy, age-matched controls is 1 to 4 per cent (Talal et al. 1990). Transgenic mice bearing the tax gene of the human T-lymphotrophic virus type 1 develop an autoimmune exocrinopathy resembling that of Sjögren's syndrome: an initial increase and proliferation of the acinar epithelial cells is followed by a gradual infiltration of lymphocytes and plasma cells, leading to destruction of the acini (Green et al. 1989). Furthermore, a type A retroviral particle has been identified in extracts from labial gland biopsies in two out of six patients with Sjögren's syndrome after coculture with the lymphoblastoid cell line, RH9: this was distinguishable from the human immunodeficiency virus particles by several physicochemical and ultrastructural criteria (Garry et al. 1990).

The c-myc proto-oncogene is involved in the pathogenesis of B-cell malignancies and especially Burkitt's lymphoma caused by EBV. Increased expression of c-myc mRNA has been found in peripheral mononuclear cells of patients with Sjögren's syndrome as well as in those of normal people after stimulation (Boumpas et al. 1990). Skopouli et al. (1992), using in situ hybridization with specific c-myc probes, have demonstrated the expression of c-myc mRNA in minor salivary glands of patients with Sjögren's syndrome. The minor labial salivary glands of normal individuals and of patients with rheumatoid arthritis and sarcoidosis did not show this picture. Immunostaining of the hybridized tissue with monoclonal antibodies and correlation with the clinicoserological and histological findings showed that the proto-oncogene is expressed on the acinar epithelial cells and its appearance is correlated strongly with the duration of disease as well as with the intensity of the T-cell infiltration. It is not known yet whether this aberrant c-myc expression in the epithelial cells is a primary phenomenon resulting from a viral infection or an epiphenomenon attributable to the action of cytokines or cytokine-like molecules.

All the above data suggest viral involvement in Sjögren's syndrome. Transient or persistent infection of the epithelial cells by a putative virus may be the initiating event; accumulation of the helper/inducer memory T cells and B cells may be the second step; and monoclonal expansion of B cells under selective antigenic or T-cell-induced pressures the final step.

Genetic background (immunogenetics)

It is well known that members of the family of patients with Sjögren's syndrome have a higher prevalence of the syndrome and a higher incidence of serological autoimmune abnormalities than age- and sex-matched controls.

Numerous investigators have shown associations between primary Sjögren's syndrome and factors encoded by the major histocompatibility complex; HLA-DR3 has been reported in 50 to 80 per cent of patients with Sjögren's syndrome. The association, however, of HLA-DR3 and Sjögren's syndrome has been reported to be weaker than that of HLA-DR3 with Sjögren's syndrome and anti- Ro/SSA antibody positivity (Mann 1987).

As shown in Table 2 the ethnic origin of the patients, studied so far, influences the association with the HLA-DR phenotype. Given the linkage disequilibrium that exists between alleles of HLA loci, it is unclear whether the disease susceptibility is dependent on the associated allele or on a closely related gene. HLA-DQ, and to a lesser extent HLA-DP, alleles are tightly linked to HLA-DR (Navarrette et al. 1985). Thus, common amino acid sequences of the hypervariable region of these genes may be shared between different HLA-DR specificities, hence influencing disease susceptibility (shared epitope hypothesis) (Gregerson et al. 1987). The application of molecular biological techniques has made possible an understanding of the association of autoimmune diseases with different HLA haplotypes in various patient populations. In this regard, a DNA sequence-specific, oligonucleotide probe typing and a sequence analysis of Israeli Jewish and Greek non-Jewish patients with Sjögren's syndrome has been carried out (Tambur et al. 1993). It was found that the majority of patients in both groups presented either DRBI* 1101 or DRBI* 1104 alleles that were linked in a linkage disequilibrium with DRBI*0301 and DQA1*0501. Molecular analysis of DQB1 and DQA1 alleles found in American Caucasian and American black patients with Sjögren's syndrome revealed high frequencies of DQB1*0201 and DQA1*0501 (Reveille et al. 1991). Therefore, the majority of patients with Sjögren's syndrome, independent of their racial and ethnic background, carry a common

Table 2 Ethnic variations in the association between antigens encoded by the major histocompatibility complex and Sjögren's syndrome

Ethnic group	HLA association	Reference
Caucasoid	HLA-B8	Fye et al. (1976)
	HLA-DW3	Chused et al. (1977)
	HLA-DR3	Mann (1987)
	HLA-DR3 and extraglandular features	Vitali et al. (1986)
	HLA-DRw52	Mann (1987)
Greeks	HLA-DR5	Papasteriades et al. (1988)
Israelis	HLA-DR11 (subtype of DR5) in Israelis	Brautbar (personal communication)
Japanese	HLA-DRw53	Moriuchi et al. (1986)

allele, the *DQA1*0501* allele. Furthermore, it has been shown that a glutamine residue at position 34 of the outermost domain of the *DQA1* and/or leucine at position 26 of the outermost domain of the *DQB1* chain have a 'gene dosage' role in the anti-Ro/SSA and anti-La/SSB antibody response. The *DQA1*0501* gene is one of the genes that possess glutamine at position 34 and is found in the majority of patients with anti-Ro/SSA and anti-La/SSB. Taken together, it appears that the DQA1*0501 molecule is probably an important determining factor for the predisposition of certain individuals to primary Sjögren's syndrome.

Development and continuation of the autoimmune process

The two major autoimmune phenomena observed in Sjögren's syndrome are the B-lymphocyte hyper-reactivity and the focal lymphoplasmacytic infiltrates in the exocrine glands. Numerous studies have sought to describe and delineate (a) the nature of these phenomena and (b) the mechanisms involved in their perpetuation.

Humoral studies

Polyclonal hyper-reactivity
The most common serological finding in Sjögren's syndrome is hypergammaglobulinaemia. The increased amount of immunoglobulins in these patients often contains a number of autoantibodies directed against non-organ-specific antigens such as other immunoglobulins (rheumatoid factor), antinuclear antibodies (which usually give a speckled pattern on immunofluorescence), cellular antigens [Ro(SSA), La(SSB), RANA], and organ-specific antigens such as salivary ductal cells, thyroid gland cells, and gastric mucosa (Harley 1987). The most common autoantibodies to cellular antigens in patients with Sjögren's syndrome are directed against two ribonucleoprotein antigens known as Ro or SSA and La or SSB. These autoantibodies are not specific for the syndrome and may be found in other autoimmune diseases, especially systemic lupus erythematosus (see Chapter 5.7.1). Anti-Ro and anti-La are detected by immunodiffusion in approximately 45 and 20 per cent, respectively, of patients with Sjögren's syndrome but in up to 95 and 85 per cent, respectively, by more sensitive techniques such as enzyme-linked

immunosorbent assay. Characterization of these ribonucleoproteins has led to the observation that the fine specificity of antibodies to the polymorphic forms of Ro differs in Sjögren's syndrome and systemic lupus (reviewed in Chapter 4.5). Thus, autoantibodies to the 52-kDa Ro protein are frequently found in serum from patients with the syndrome, while antibodies to a 60-kDa Ro protein are found more often in serum from patients with systemic lupus (Ben Chetrit et al. 1990).

The presence of anti-Ro(SSA)/La(SSB) autoantibodies is associated with certain clinical manifestations of primary Sjögren's syndrome: they are correlated with earlier onset and longer duration of disease, recurrent enlargement of the parotids, and with splenomegaly/lymphadenopathy and vasculitis. In addition, the incidence of these antibodies correlates with the intensity of the infiltration of minor salivary glands (Manoussakis et al. 1986).

Oligomonoclonal hyper-reactivity
Several patients with primary Sjögren's syndrome have been shown to have circulating monoclonal immunoglobulins. In a study of serum and urine from unselected patients with the primary syndrome, using high-resolution agarose electrophoresis combined with immunofixation, approximately, 80 per cent of those with extraglandular (systemic) disease had monoclonal light chains or immunoglobulins in the serum. Furthermore, all patients excreted monoclonal light chains in the urine. In contrast, only one-quarter of patients with disease limited to the exocrine glands had monoclonal light chains or immunoglobulins in their serum, while only 43 per cent of these excreted light chains in the urine (Moutsopoulos et al. 1983a; Moutsopoulos et al. 1985).

Subsequent analysis of cryoglobulins from patients with Sjögren's syndrome by high-resolution agarose gel electrophoresis combined with immunofixation demonstrated that these are mixed monoclonal cryoglobulins (type II), containing an IgM-κ monoclonal rheumatoid factor (Tzioufas et al. 1986) (Fig. 1). The above data suggest that patients with Sjögren's syndrome express circulating monoclonal immunoglobulins very early in the disease, together with the polyclonal B-cell activation. Monoclonality is observed more often in those patients with systemic, extraglandular disease. This is of particular interest, as patients with extraglandular manifestations are at higher risk for developing lymphoid malignancy. In this regard,

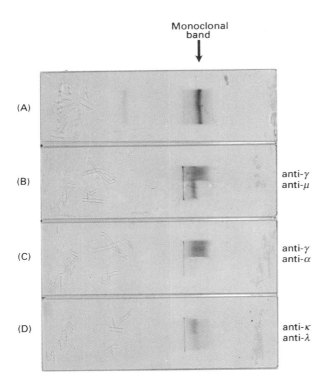

Fig. 1 High-resolution agarose gel electrophoresis of the cryoglobulins of a Sjögren's syndrome patient reveals a monoclonal band (A). Immunofixation, using anti-human κ, λ light and α, γ, μ heavy chains, identified the monoclonal bands as an IgM-κ monoclonal immunoglobulin (B, C, and D).

serial follow-up studies have shown that the presence of mixed mono-clonal (type II) cryoglobulinaemia correlates with lymphoma in patients with primary Sjögren's syndrome (Tzioufas *et al*. 1996).

Schmidt *et al*. (1982) suggested that the benign lymphoepithelial lesion of salivary glands in Sjögren's syndrome, which has areas of confluent lymphoid proliferation and contains plasma cells that have monoclonal IgM-κ immunoglobulins in their cytoplasm, represents an '*in situ*' malignant lymphoma. This suggestion was further substantiated by immunogenotypic and immunophenotypic studies (Fishleder *et al*. 1987; Moutsopoulos *et al*. 1990), which showed that in the lymphoepithelial lesion there were rearrangements of oligo- or monoclonal immunoglobulin genes. In one study, three patients with benign lymphoepithelial lesion developed non-Hodgkin's lymphoma 2 to 8 years after the initial biopsy (Freimark *et al*. 1989). The presence of circulating monoclonal immunoglobulins is asso-ciated with a monoclonal B-cell expansion in the salivary glands. This has been demonstrated by a peroxidase–antiperoxidase bridge technique for the detection of intracytoplasmic immunoglobulins in the salivary lymphocytic infiltrates. Seven of 12 patients with Sjögren's syndrome with cryoprecipitable IgM-κ monoclonal immunoglobulins had a predominance of κ-positive plasma cells in the minor salivary glands, while patients without cryoglobulins or with polyclonal cryoglobulins had almost equal numbers of κ- and λ-positive cells (Moutsopoulos *et al*. 1990).

Monoclonal rheumatoid factors share cross-reactive idiotypes. Monoclonal rheumatoid factors from patients with Waldenström's macroglobulinaemia have been divided into three groups (Wa, Po, and Bla) (Kunkel *et al*.1973; Agnello *et al*. 1980). The light chains of the monoclonal rheumatoid factor that reacted with anti-Wa anti-bodies belong to the $V_{\kappa IIIb}$ subgroup (Kipps *et al*. 1987). The 17.109 monoclonal antibody reacted with half of the monoclonal rheumatoid factors. The 17.109 idiotype is associated with the expression of the Humkv325 germ-line gene (Kipps *et al*. 1989). Cross-reactive idio-types are shared by rheumatoid factors from autoimmune diseases. Some of them are shared by patients with Sjögren's syndrome and rheumatoid arthritis, while others (such as 17.109), have been found only in rheumatoid factors from patients with Sjögren's syndrome (Fox *et al*. 1986*b*). In fact, 12 out of 15 monoclonal rheumatoid factors from patients with Sjögren's syndrome reacted with the 17.109 mono-clonal antibody. Furthermore, B cells containing immunoglobulin, bearing the 17.109 idiotype, were detected in the salivary gland biop-sies of 11 out of 12 patients with Sjögren's. Further analysis of the B cells bearing the 17.109 idiotype in the salivary glands of patients with primary Sjögren's syndrome has shown that these are of multi-clonal origin, in which somatic mutations accumulate in a non-random fashion, strongly suggesting an antigen- or T-cell-driven process in the expansion of these cells (Kipps *et al*. 1989). Two-thirds of patients with primary Sjögren's share a common idiotype, detected with a polyclonal anti-idiotype antibody directed against an IgM-κ monoclonal rheumatoid factor from patients with Sjögren's syndrome. The presence of this idiotype is correlated with extra-glandular manifestations, autoantibodies, and monoclonal immunoglobulins (Katsikis *et al*. 1990).

Comparative studies of three cross-reactive idiotypes in patients with primary Sjögren's syndrome have shown that these are expressed very early in the clinical spectrum of the syndrome and that their prevalence increases as the disease evolves. The presence of 17.109 and G6 (a VH1-associated cross-reactive idio-type), were found mainly in patients with Sjögren's syndrome with lymphoma, suggesting that these idiotypic determinants may serve as markers for lymphoma development in the syndrome (Tzioufas *et al*. 1996).

Lymphocyte studies

Peripheral blood lymphocytes
The absolute number of the total lymphocytes as well as T and B cells in peripheral blood does not differ substantially from that observed in normal individuals. Studies of T-lymphocyte subsets in Sjögren's syndrome were inconclusive (Fauci and Moutsopoulos 1981). Although decreased numbers of CD4+ and CD8+ T cells have been reported, this finding has not been substantiated by other investiga-tors (Moutsopoulos and Manoussakis 1989). Peripheral blood B lymphocytes from patients with Sjögren's syndrome and normal controls, unlike lymphocytes from patients with systemic lupus, did not spontaneously secrete increased amounts of immunoglobulins. Thus, the activated B cells in patients with systemic lupus are distrib-uted widely but in patients with Sjögren's syndrome they are probably localized to, and infiltrate, organs such as the minor labial salivary glands or the spleen.

Tissue lymphocytes
During the 1970s there some efforts were made to determine the composition of the lymphocytic infiltrates in the salivary glands but the results were controversial (Moutsopoulos and Talal 1987).

The application of molecular biological techniques, including the use of monoclonal antibodies and nucleic acid probes, heralded a more precise understanding of the immunopathological lesion in the exocrine glands of patients with Sjögren's syndrome. Several studies using monoclonal antibodies against specific lymphocyte markers have evaluated the composition of round-cell infiltrates in the labial salivary glands of primary Sjögren's syndrome. It was shown that the majority of the infiltrating lymphocytes are T cells, while B lymphocytes constitute 20 to 25 per cent of the round cells. Monocytes, macrophages, as well as natural killer cells, are less that 5 per cent (Moutsopoulos and Talal 1987). Studies of T-lymphocyte subpopulations have shown that 60 to 70 per cent of the T lymphocytes bear the CD4 phenotype and that the majority of them exhibit the memory/inducer marker (CD45 Ro). Almost all infiltrating T cells express the α T-cell receptor (**TCR**) (Skopouli *et al.* 1991). Analysis of the receptor repertoire of the infiltrating T lymphocytes from minor salivary-gland biopsies of patients with Sjögren's syndrome by a quantitative polymerase chain reaction revealed that the repertoire of the *TCR V* gene was not restricted, although $V_{\beta 2}$ and $V_{\beta 13}$ were predominantly expressed in the inflammatory infiltrates (Sumida *et al.* 1992). Interestingly, $V_{\beta 2}$- and $V_{\beta 13}$-positive T cells can be stimulated by minor lymphocyte determinants of bacterial toxins, the so-called superantigens (Kappler *et al.* 1989). Thus, exposure to these molecules (e.g. after a bacterial infection) may lead to the stimulation and expansion of T cells expressing these two genes. In this regard, the junctional sequences of cDNA encoding the $V_{\beta 2}$ and $V_{\beta 13}$ genes of TCR from T lymphocytes infiltrating the minor salivary glands of patients with Sjögren's syndrome were investigated (Yonaha *et al.* 1992). Despite the fact that $V_{\beta 2}$- and $V_{\beta 13}$-positive T cells were polyclonal, the junctional usage was found to be restricted, supporting the notion that autoreactive T cells that contribute to the immunopathological lesion in Sjögren's syndrome are of oligoclonal origin.

The activation status of T cells was evaluated by searching for membrane expression of HLA class II molecules, interleukin-2 (**IL-2**) receptor (**r**), the lymphocyte function-associated antigen 1, and IL-2 production (Moutsopoulos and Talal 1987; Skopouli *et al.* 1991). Although none of the tissue lymphocytes was positive for IL-2 and IL-2r when monoclonal antibodies were used, studies using *in situ* hybridization with oligonucleotide mRNA probes demonstrated both IL-2 and its receptor in the infiltrating lymphocytes of the labial salivary glands of patients with primary Sjögren's syndrome (Boumba *et al.* 1995).

B lymphocytes infiltrating the labial salivary glands are activated, since they are able to produce increased amount of immunoglobulins with autoantibody activity (Anderson *et al.* 1972). In addition, evaluation with an immunoperoxidase technique of the isotypes of intracytoplasmic immunoglobulins of the plasma cells infiltrating the salivary glands of patients with Sjögren's syndrome showed that the IgG and IgM isotype predominates, in contrast to the plasma cells of the normal salivary glands, where the IgA isotype is dominant (Lane *et al.* 1983). This observation prompted some investigators to support the notion that quantitation of cells containing IgA and IgG intracytoplasmic immunoglobulins may serve as diagnostic criterion with high specificity and sensitivity for Sjögren's syndrome (Bodeuitsch *et al.* 1992).

B-cell activation is one of the most prominent immunoregulatory aberrations in patients with Sjögren's syndrome. This aberration can follow various stages of evolution. It begins as polyclonal activation, evolves to polyclonal–oligoclonal–monoclonal activation, and ends up as malignant monoclonal proliferation.

Immunopathology

As clearly shown in the previous sections, both the B and the T lymphocytes that contribute to the tissue lesion of primary Sjögren's syndrome are activated. This is of particular interest since the classic antigen-presenting cells, monocytes/macrophages, are poorly represented in this lesion. These findings suggest that possibly another cell may play the part of the antigen presenter in the immunopathological lesion of Sjögren's syndrome. Several recent studies suggest that the glandular or acinar epithelial cells may be play that part; these are summarized in the following list.

1. Histopathological studies in newly diagnosed cases of Sjögren's syndrome reveal that the focal lymphocytic infiltrates start around the ducts.

2. Staining of the labial salivary glands with anticlass-II HLA monoclonal antibodies showed that the ductal and acinar epithelial cells inappropriately express these molecules (Skopouli *et al.* 1991). Interferon-γ and tumour necrosis factor-α have been shown to up-regulate the expression of both histocompatibility antigen classes on the surface of epithelial and other cells. These cytokines are produced locally by the activated T cell. Therefore it is not known whether the HLA-DR expression and possible antigen presentation by epithelial cells predates, or is a consequence of, the lymphocytic infiltration.

3. Studies on the expression of proto-oncogene mRNA in the minor salivary glands of patients with Sjögren's syndrome revealed that c-*myc*, in contrast to c-*fos* and c-*jun*, is selectively expressed by the epithelial glandular cells (Skopouli *et al.* 1992). Since the expression of the c-*myc* is so restricted, this phenomenon cannot be attributed to microenvironmental factors. The expression of HLA class II antigen and c-*myc* by epithelial cells may indicate a specific way of activating these cells.

4. Acinar epithelial cells coexpress accessory adhesion molecules and autoantigens, which in conjunction with the expression of class II antigen may potentially prime an autoimmune response. In fact, translocation and membrane localization of the nuclear antigen La/SSB has been observed in conjunctival epithelial cells of patients with Sjögren's syndrome (Yannopoulos *et al.* 1992). In addition, the infiltrating lymphocytes express a diverse array of cell adhesion molecules (lymphocyte function-associated antigen 1 and 3, CD2), while the intercellular adhesion molecule 1 was expressed on acinar epithelial cells adjacent to sites of intense inflammation (St Clair *et al.* 1992).

5. In recent years, cytokine production in the immunopathological lesion of Sjögren's syndrome has been studied extensively by *in situ* hybridization and reverse-transcriptase, quantitative, polymerase chain reaction (Fox *et al.* 1994; Boumba *et al.* 1995). Both techniques demonstrated the presence of proinflammatory cytokines IL-1 and IL-6 in the labial salivary glands of patients with Sjögren's syndrome. These cytokines were produced by both infiltrating and epithelial cells, which reinforces the concept that epithelial cells are active counterparts in the inflammatory response rather than targets of the immune-mediated injury.

Pathology

The common finding in all affected organs in patients with Sjögren's syndrome is a potentially progressive lymphocytic infiltration. These infiltrates cause functional disability of the affected organs, producing the various clinical manifestations.

So far, the salivary glands are the best-studied organs, because (i) they are affected in almost all patients and (ii) they are readily accessible. Microscopic examination of the enlarged major salivary glands reveals a benign lymphoepithelial lesion, characterized by lymphocytic replacement of the salivary epithelium and the presence of epimyoepithelial islands, which are composed of keratin-containing epithelial cells. Sometimes, the salivary gland biopsy does not show benign lymphoepithelial lesions, but instead contains various degrees of focal lymphocytic infiltration [defined as focal aggregates of 50 or more lymphocytes and histiocytes (Daniels et al. 1987)]. It is not known whether the focal lymphocytic infiltration is a precursor of the benign lymphoepithelial lesion.

The need for a practical and easy way to assess the salivary component of Sjögren's syndrome led to the introduction of labial gland biopsy. The histopathological characteristics of the biopsy of the minor salivary glands include (i) focal aggregates of at least 50 lymphocytes/plasma cells and macrophages, adjacent to and replacing the normal acini, and (ii) the consistent presence of these foci in all or most of the glands in the specimen (Fig. 2). Larger foci often show the formation of germinal centres but epimyoepithelial islands are very uncommon. These pathological lesion are, in fact, typical findings for a chronic lymphocytic sialadenitis (Batsakis and Howard 1982). However, a biopsy of minor salivary glands can be very specific for Sjögren's syndrome if it is obtained through normal-appearing mucosa, includes 5 to 10 glands, separated from the surrounding connective tissue, and shows focal lymphocytic infiltrates in all or most of the glands in the specimen, with a focus score above a chosen diagnostic threshold. Therefore, several methods of scoring the number of foci have been applied. Chisholm and Mason (1968) used a semiquantitative method to assess inflammation in salivary gland biopsies from 40 patients with several autoimmune diseases;

only in patients with Sjögren's syndrome was there more than one focus of lymphocytes per 4 mm^2 of gland. Using a modification of this method, Greenspan et al. (1974) enumerated scores from 1 to 12 foci/4 mm^2 and found a significant positive correlation between a higher score and larger foci in biopsies of minor salivary glands of patients with Sjögren's syndrome. In another study, grading of 86 biopsies from primary and secondary Sjögren's syndrome showed, by qualitative criteria, larger lymphocytic foci in the primary syndrome (Tarpley et al. 1974). Biopsies from labial and sublingual salivary glands have been compared: there was a better correlation between infiltration of the ductal structure and the focus score in the sublingual glands (Pennec et al. 1990).

In a recent study, comparison of patterns in the minor salivary gland biopsy taken from 618 patients with keratoconjunctivitis sicca and suspected Sjögren's syndrome showed that suspected Sjögren's syndrome was better associated with focal lymphocytic sialadenitis rather than chronic sialadenitis or even xerostomia (Daniels and Whitcher 1994).

Although there is no perfect diagnostic criterion for the salivary component of Sjögren's syndrome, the finding of the characteristic focal sialadenitis in biopsies of minor salivary glands is the best single criterion in terms of its disease specificity, convenience, availability, and low risk.

Animal models

There are several animals in which clinical manifestations resembling Sjögren's syndrome can be experimentally or spontaneously induced. Experimental models of sialoadenitis have been produced in rats, guinea-pigs, and mice using salivary gland extracts, adjuvants, and allogeneic antisera (Hoffman and Walker 1987). Infection of rats with a specific coronavirus results in swelling of the neck and ophthalmic lesions (Innes and Stanton 1961). Several days after exposure, the affected rats present with necrosis of ductal epithelial cells and infiltrates consisting of histiocytes, lymphocytes, and polymorphonuclear leucocytes. These findings are more prominent in lacrimal glands; submaxillary and parotid salivary glands are less commonly affected. Viral particles can be found by electron microscopy in ductal epithelial cells.

Spontaneously induced disease with features resembling those of human Sjögren's syndrome has been recognized in autoimmune strains of mice that develop a lupus-like syndrome. These include the NZB, NZB/NZW, and MRL/1pr, MRL/n (lacking the *lpr* gene) strains. All experimental animals have various degrees of lymphoplasmacytic infiltration in the lacrimal and salivary glands, with the milder form in the NZB mice and the more severe form in the MRL/n mice. Antibodies to Ro(SSA) and/or La(SSB) autoantigens were not detected in their sera.

Other experimental models of 'Sjögren's-like disease' include the canine keratoconjunctivitis sicca and the chicken dysgammaglobulinaemia that is associated with Coombs'-positive haemolytic anaemia, cryoglobulins, rheumatoid factor and infiltration of several parenchymal organs with mononuclear cells (Hoffman and Walker 1987).

In the last few years, the lymphoproliferation in Sjögren's syndrome has been studied in **SCID** (severe combined immunodeficient) mice. The CB17 scid/scid mice are born with severe combined immunodeficiency, lacking mature T and B lymphocytes. Injection of peripheral blood mononuclear cells from anti-La(SSB)-positive patients with Sjögren's syndrome into

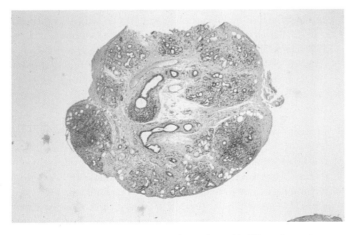

Fig. 2 Minor salivary gland biopsy of a patient with Sjögren's syndrome, showing moderate and large focal lymphocytic infiltrates around the acini and ducts.

these mice resulted in the development of lymphoid infiltrates in several tissues consistent with disseminated lymphoid neoplasia (Whittingham *et al.* 1991).

In another study, after implantation of minor salivary gland biopsies under the kidney capsules of SCID mice, the proportion of human CD4+ T cells gradually decreased while the number of CD19+ B cells increased. The animals died after 6 to 12 weeks with human lymphoid tumours (Kang *et al.* 1991). These results suggest that, in an immunoincompetent environment, B cells of patients with Sjögren's syndrome tend to proliferate and develop malignancy.

Clinical picture

Sjögren's syndrome can occur alone (primary) or in association with other autoimmune diseases (secondary). In most patients the primary syndrome runs a rather slow and benign course. The initial manifestation can be non-specific (Table 3) and usually 8 to 10 years elapse from the initial symptoms to the full-blown development of the syndrome (Pavlidis *et al.* 1982).

Glandular manifestations

Oral component

Symptoms and signs

The principal oral symptom of Sjögren's syndrome is dryness (xerostomia). Patients describe this as difficulty in swallowing dry food, inability to speak continuously, changes in sense sensation, a burning sensation, an increase in dental caries (Fig. 3), and problems in wearing complete dentures. Examination shows a dry, erythematous, sticky oral mucosa and often dental caries, while saliva from the major glands is either not expressible or is cloudy. Atrophy of the filiform papillae of the tongue is apparent (Fig. 4) and in some cases overgrowth of *Candida* is observed.

Enlargement of the parotids or other major salivary glands occurs in two-thirds of patients with the primary syndrome, but is uncommon in those with Sjögren's syndrome and rheumatoid arthritis (see below). In many patients the salivary gland enlargement is episodic, but some have chronic enlargement. The swelling of the parotids may begin unilaterally but often becomes bilateral (Fig. 5). In Table 4, conditions other than Sjögren's syndrome causing parotid enlargement are depicted.

Diagnosis

A variety of medical conditions other than Sjögren's syndrome can cause xerostomia (Table 5). To evaluate the oral component of the syndrome, various tests are used with different specificity and sensitivity for the disease.

Sialometry

Salivary flow rates can be measured clinically for whole saliva or for separate secretions from the parotid or submandibular and sublingual glands, with or without stimulation. Patients with clinically overt Sjögren's syndrome have reduced flow. However, flow rates depend on many factors such as age, sex, medication, and time of day. Therefore, setting a cut-off point between the normal and abnormal is difficult because of the wide range of flow rates among normal individuals (Skopouli *et al.* 1989).

Table 3 Initial manifestations of primary Sjögren's syndrome (data from 132 Greek patients with Sjögren's syndrome)

	n	%
Sicca manifestations:		
Subjective xerophthalmia	63	47.0
Subjective xerostomia	56	42.5
Parotid gland enlargement	24	24.0
Dyspareunia	7	5.0
Fever/fatigue	13	10.0
Arthralgias, arthritis	37	28.0
Raynaud's phenomenon	28	21.0
Lung involvement	2	1.5
Kidney involvement	2	1.5

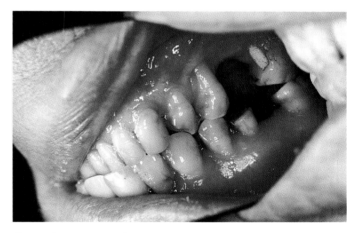

Fig. 3 Dental caries in Sjögren's syndrome; note also the remarkable periodontitis in both lower and upper teeth.

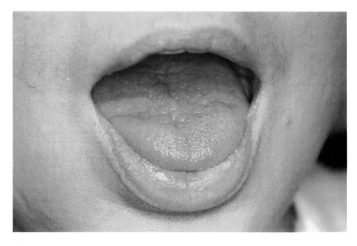

Fig. 4 Dry tongue of a patient with Sjögren's syndrome. Note the remarkable atrophy of filiform papillae.

Table 4 Differential diagnosis of parotid gland enlargement

Unilateral

Salivary gland neoplasm

Bacterial infection

Chronic sialadenitis

Bilateral

Viral infection (mumps, influenza, Epstein–Barr, coxsackie A, cytomegalovirus, HIV)

Sjögren's syndrome

Sarcoidosis

Miscellaneous (diabetes mellitus, hyperlipoproteinaemia, hepatic cirrhosis, chronic pancreatitis, acromegaly, gonadal hypofunction)

Recurrent parotitis of childhood

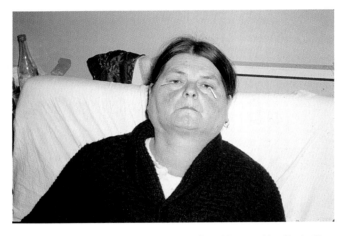

Fig. 5 Bilateral parotid-gland enlargement in a 65-year-old patient with Sjögren's syndrome.

Table 5 Causes of xerostomia

Drugs:
  Psychotherapeutic
  Parasympatholytic
  Antihypertensive

Viral infections

Dehydration:
  Diabetes mellitus
  Trauma

Psychogenic

Irradiation

Congenital (absent or malformed glands)

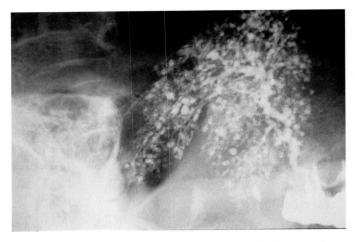

Fig. 6 Sialography of the parotid gland of a patient with Sjögren's syndrome. The retention of the sialographic medium at the end-points of the duct system reveals several degrees of sialectasis.

Sialography

This is a radiocontrast method of assessing anatomical changes in the salivary ductal system. It has been widely used in patients with Sjögren's syndrome, in whom various degrees of sialectasis have been found (Fig. 6). Sialography with oil-based contrast material shows an increased incidence of sialectasis in these patients (Daniels *et al.* 1987).However, sialography causes pain and swelling of the parotid glands and sometimes allergic reactions to the radiopaque material. In addition, some have suggested that sialography is insensitive and non-specific (Moutsopoulos and Talal 1989). However, Vitali *et al.* (1988) described sialography with water-soluble media in 84 patients with primary and secondary Sjögren's syndrome and compared it with the findings of minor salivary gland biopsy, as well as with the patients' clinical and the serological picture. They reported that sialography was as sensitive and specific as the biopsy. Furthermore, hypergammaglobulinaemia, anti-Ro(SSA) antibodies, extraglandular manifestations, and parotid swelling were all correlated with both sialographic and histological abnormalities, suggesting that both tests are necessary for the evaluation of salivary gland involvement in Sjögren's syndrome.

Scintigraphy

Isotope scanning provides a functional evaluation of all the salivary glands by observing the rate and density of uptake of the [^{99}Tc^{m}]-pertechnetate and the time taken for it to appear in the mouth during a 60-min period after intravenous injection. In patients with Sjögren's syndrome the uptake of the label by the glands and the secretion of labelled saliva is delayed or absent. An abnormal scan was found to correlate with the presence of reduced salivary flow, the sialographic picture, and the intensity of lymphocytic infiltrates in minor salivary glands (Daniels *et al.* 1987).

In a study of 320 patients with oral dryness who had primary or secondary Sjögren's syndrome, graft-versus-host disease and other autoimmune diseases, scanning had high sensitivity but no well-established disease specificity (Parrago *et al.* 1987).

Sialochemistry

Chemical and immunological factors in saliva of patients with Sjögren's syndrome have been examined extensively in the past. So far, the results are conflicting and controversial (Baum and Fox 1987), offering very limited diagnostic value.

Ocular component

Ocular involvement is a major glandular manifestation of Sjögren's syndrome. Diminished secretion of tears leads to the destruction of the corneal and bulbar conjunctival epithelium termed keratoconjunctivitis sicca. The patients usually complain of a burning, foreign-body sensation, a sandy or scratchy sensation under the lids, itchiness, redness, and photosensitivity. Clinical signs include dilation of the bulbar conjunctival vessels, pericorneal injection, irregularity of the corneal image, and sometimes enlargement of the lacrimal glands. All tests for the evaluation of this condition are very sensitive but not specific for Sjögren's syndrome, as keratoconjunctivitis sicca may occur in a number of other conditions.

The Schirmer's test is used for the evaluation of tear secretion. The test is made with strips of filter paper 30 mm in length. The strip is slipped beneath the inferior lid, with the remainder of the paper hanging out (Fig. 7). After 5 min the length of paper wetted is measured. Wetting of less than 5 mm is a strong indication of diminished secretion. The presence of decreased tear secretion is not diagnostic of keratoconjunctivitis sicca. In contrast, it can easily be diagnosed using rose bengal staining. Rose bengal is an aniline compound that stains the devitalized or damaged epithelium of both the cornea and conjunctiva. Slit-lamp examination after rose bengal staining shows a punctate pattern of filamentary keratitis (Fig. 8).

The break-up time of tears is another useful measure. A drop of fluoroscein is instilled in the eye and the time between the last blink and appearance of dark, non-fluorescent areas in the tear film is measured. An overly rapid break-up of the tear film indicates an abnormality of either the mucin or the lipid layer (Kincaid 1987).

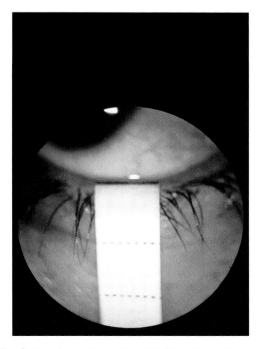

Fig. 7 The Schirmer's test in a patient with Sjögren's syndrome: the filter-paper strip is slipped under the lid, with part hanging out; the length of paper wetted, measured after 5 min, is less than 5 mm in this case.

Systemic (extraglandular) manifestations

Extraglandular (systemic) manifestations are seen in one-third of patients with primary Sjögren's syndrome (Moutsopoulos *et al.* 1980) (Table 6). These patients complain most often of being easily fatigued, of low-grade fever, and of myalgias and arthralgias.

Arthritis

Seventy per cent of patients with primary Sjögren's syndrome experience an episode or episodes of arthritis during the course of their disease. In some cases it can precede the sicca manifestations. Joint symptoms and signs include arthralgias, myalgias, morning stiffness, intermittent synovitis, and chronic polyarthritis that sometimes lead to Jacoub's arthropathy (Maini 1987). In contrast to rheumatoid arthritis, radiographs of the hand usually do not reveal pathological

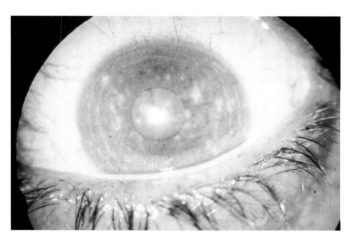

Fig. 8 Slit-lamp examination of the eye of a patient with Sjögren's syndrome after rose bengal staining. The retention of the stain in the corneal conjunctiva shows damaged epithelium and filaments, which are diagnostic of keratoconjunctivitis sicca.

Table 6 Incidence of extraglandular manifestations in primary Sjögren's syndrome (data from 132 Greek patients)

Clinical manifestation	n	%
Arthralgias/arthritis	79	60
Raynaud's phenomenon	49	37
Lymphadenopathy	19	14
Vasculitis	15	11
Lung involvement	18	14
Kidney involvement	12	9
Liver involvement	8	6
Splenomegaly	4	3
Peripheral neuropathy	3	2
Myositis	1	1
Lymphoma	8	6

changes (Castro-Poltronieri and Alarcon-Segovia 1983; Tsampoulas *et al*. 1990).

Raynaud's phenomenon

This occurs in 35 per cent of patients with primary Sjögren's and usually precedes sicca manifestations by many years. Patients with the primary syndrome and Raynaud's phenomenon present with swollen hands, but, in contrast to those with scleroderma, they do not experience digital ulcers and telangiectasias are not seen. Radiographs of the hands of these patients may show small tissue calcifications (Skopouli *et al*. 1990). Non-erosive arthritis has also been shown to be significantly more frequent in patients with Raynaud's phenomenon than in those without (Youinou *et al*. 1990*a*).

Skin involvement

Cutaneous lesions are seen frequently in patients with primary Sjögren's syndrome. Patients with dry skin complain of dermal stinging and itching. Nasal dryness with crusting, vaginal dryness syndrome with dyspareunia, and cheilitis have also been described. Other cutaneous manifestations include skin hyper- or hypopigmentation, patchy alopecia, and hypersensitivity vasculitis (Fye and Talal 1984). Some patients with Sjögren's syndrome may present with annular erythema affecting mainly the face and the trunk; it extends centrifugally and fades without leaving pigmentation (Teramoto *et al*. 1989).

Pulmonary involvement

Manifestations from the trachea to the pleura have been described in patients with Sjögren's syndrome. These are frequent but rarely important clinically. They can present with a range of symptoms from dry cough secondary to dryness of the tracheobronchial mucosa (xerotrachea) to dyspnoea from interstitial disease or even airway obstruction (Constantopoulos and Moutsopoulos 1987).

Interstitial lung disease in Sjögren's syndrome was thought to be a very common manifestation, since chest radiographs revealed an interstitial pattern in approximately half of patients with Sjögren's syndrome studied. High-resolution CT scanning of the lungs performed in 21 patients with the most prominent abnormalities, however, demonstrated that in 14 patients the main findings were either thickened bronchial walls at the segmental level or a mild interstitial pattern distributed around the bronchi. Transbronchial biopsy performed in 12 of these patients disclosed bronchiolar lymphoid infiltrates and follicular bronchiolitis (bronchus-associated lymphoid tissue hyperplasia). Fibrosing alveolitis was absent from all tissue specimens (Papiris *et al*. 1994).

Pseudolymphoma or frank lymphoma should always be suspected when lung nodules or hilar and/or mediastinal lymphadenopathy are found on chest radiographs (Constantopoulos and Moutsopoulos 1987).

There are differences in respiratory manifestations between the primary and secondary syndrome. In the latter, the respiratory involvement is a reflection of the primary rheumatic disorders. In fact, pleural effusions are usually found in Sjögren's syndrome associated with other rheumatic disorders and not in the primary syndrome.

Gastrointestinal and hepatobiliary features

Patients with Sjögren's syndrome often complain of dysphagia, owing to dryness of the pharynx and oesophagus, or to abnormal oesophageal motility. Nausea and epigastric pain are also common complaints. Biopsies of gastric mucosa show chronic atrophic gastritis and lymphocytic infiltrates (Buchanan *et al*. 1966), similar to those described in minor salivary glands. In addition, patients with Sjögren's syndrome have hypopepsinogenaemia, an elevated serum gastrin, low serum vitamin B_{12}, and antibodies to parietal cells (Trevino *et al*. 1987).

Acute or chronic pancreatitis has been reported rarely. In contrast, subclinical pancreatic involvement is a rather common finding, as illustrated by the fact that hyperamylasaemia is found in one-quarter of patients with the syndrome (Tsianos *et al*. 1984).

The prevalence and nature of liver involvement was studied in 300 patients with Sjögren's syndrome (Skopouli *et al*. 1994). Seven per cent had antimitochondrial antibodies and 5 per cent had elevated liver enzymes. Patients with antimitochondrial antibodies had elevated liver enzymes and no evidence of hepatitis B and C viral infection. Eleven out of 17 patients with antimitochondrial antibodies underwent liver biopsy. The histopathological picture disclosed in seven specimens was an 'autoimmune cholangiitis', that is a chronic granulomatous cholangiitis affecting small and medium-sized bile ducts and a mild periportal inflammation, without, however, evidence of 'piecemeal' necrosis (Fig. 9). These histological features are similar with those observed in stage I of primary biliary cirrhosis.

There is also a high incidence of Sjögren's syndrome in patients with primary biliary cirrhosis: sicca manifestations have been described in approximately half of a group of patients with primary biliary cirrhosis; among these, 10 per cent had severe clinical features of dryness (Tsianos *et al*. 1990).

Renal involvement

Overt kidney disease is found in approximately 10 per cent of patients with Sjögren's syndrome (Kassan and Talal 1987), while approximately 35 per cent have an abnormal urine acidification test. Interstitial disease is the most common renal finding. Most of the patients present with hyposthenuria and hypokalaemic, hyperchloraemic distal tubular acidosis. Distal tubular acidosis can be silent or can present with recurrent renal colic and/or hypokalaemic muscular weakness. Untreated renal tubular acidosis leads to renal stones, nephrocalcinosis, and compromised renal function (Moutsopoulos *et al*. 1991) (Fig. 10). Less commonly, these patients have proximal tubular acidosis with Fanconi syndrome (Kassan and Talal 1987);

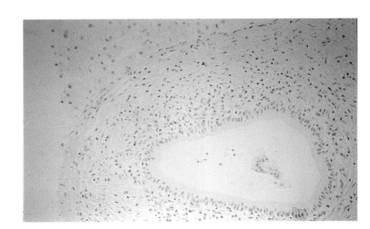

Fig. 9 Periportal inflammation in liver biopsy of a patient with Sjögren's syndrome.

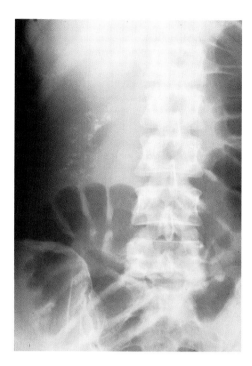

Fig. 10 Abdominal radiograph of a patient with Sjögren's syndrome reveals nephrocalcinosis of the right kidney.

renal biopsy reveals interstitial lymphocytic infiltration. Glomerunophritis in Sjögren's syndrome has been described in few patients (Moutsopoulos *et al.* 1978); the histological type may be membranous or membranoproliferative. In all cases a consistent serological finding was cryoglobulinaemia associated with hypocomplementaemia.

Vasculitis

Vascular involvement is found in approximately 5 per cent of patients with Sjögren's syndrome. It affects small and medium-sized vessels. The most common manifestations are purpura (Fig. 11), recurrent

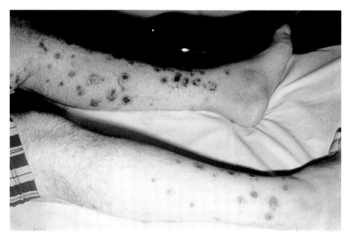

Fig. 11 The lower extremities of a patient with Sjögren's syndrome with hypergammaglobulinaemia and cryoglobulins show diffuse, palpable purpura.

urticaria, skin ulcerations, and mononeuritis multiplex. However, cases of systemic vasculitis with visceral involvement affecting kidney, lung, gastrointestinal tract, spleen, breast, and the reproductive tract have been described (Alexander 1987*a*; Tsokos *et al.* 1987). There are two histopathological types of vasculitis, according to the type of the infiltrating cell — the mononuclear and the neutrophil type. The latter is associated with hypergammaglobulinaemia, high titres of rheumatoid factor, antibodies to Ro(SSA) cellular antigen, and hypocomplementaemia (Alexander 1987*a*). In another classification of vascular involvement (Tsokos *et al.* 1987), the small-vessel vasculitis was of the hypersensitivity type, that is leucocytoclastic and lymphocytic, while the medium-vessel vasculitis was acute necrotizing and simulated polyarteritis nodosa but without the formàtion of aneurysms. Endarteritis obliterans was seen in patients with a long-standing history of vasculitis.

Neuromuscular involvement

Neurological manifestations of Sjögren's syndrome include peripheral sensory or sensorimotor neuropathy as a consequence of vascular involvement. Cranial neuropathy, usually affecting single nerves such as the trigeminal or the optic, has been well documented. Involvement of the central nervous system in the syndrome is a matter of considerable controversy. Over the last decade some investigators have described a high proportion of such involvement, which before had been unrecognized internationally. They found that this disease was multifocal, recurrent, and progressive. The clinical signs included hemiparesis, hemisensory deficits, seizures, movement disorders, and transverse myelopathy. Some patients presented with diffuse brain injury expressed as encephalopathy, aseptic meningitis, and dementia (Alexander 1987*b*). On the other hand, others have failed to demonstrate severe central involvement in 55 patients with primary and 50 with secondary Sjögren's syndrome (Binder *et al.* 1988). Eighteen of these patients had mild neurological abnormalities confined to the secondary syndrome; all were characteristics of the underlying rheumatic disorders. A study of 63 consecutive patients with primary Sjögren's syndrome revealed that 17 had a mild sensory or sensorimotor neuropathy while one patient with past history of hypertension had had a mild episode (Andonopoulos *et al.* 1990*a*), suggesting that peripheral neuropathy is a rather common finding in Sjögren's syndrome whereas central nervous disease must be rare.

Many patients with the primary syndrome complain of myalgia, but muscle enzymes are usually normal or slightly elevated. Severe polymyositis with extensive necrosis of muscle fibres and invasion of macrophages into the affected muscle has been described in Sjögren's syndrome (Leroy *et al.* 1990). This kind of myositis seems to respond well to pulse cyclophosphamide therapy.

Other manifestations

Autoimmune thyroid disease has been described in some patients with primary Sjögren's syndrome. In a study by Karsh *et al.* (1980), half of the patients with Sjögren's syndrome presented with antithyroid antibodies and signs of altered thyroid function as evaluated by a basal thyroid-hormone stimulation test.

Sjögren's syndrome may also associated with interstitial cystitis (Van de Merwe *et al.* 1993), which is a non-bacterial disease of the bladder producing constant or intermittent, long-lasting symptoms, such frequent micturition, nocturia, and suprapubic or perineal pain. Bladder biopsy discloses intense inflammation in the mucosa and submucosa with lymphoid cells and mast cells. Lymphoid cell infiltrates contain CD4+ T cells as well as B-cell nodules with germinal centres. Detrusor fibrosis can be seen in the later stages of the disease (Harrington *et al.* 1990).

Mild normochromic and normocytic anaemia is a common finding; leucopenia and thrombocytopenia are relatively rare features. An elevated erythrocyte sedimentation rate is found in approximately 70 per cent of patients (Moutsopoulos *et al.* 1980). In contrast, C-reactive protein is not detected in patients with primary Sjögren's syndrome but is found in those with Sjögren's syndrome and rheumatoid arthritis (Table 7) (Moutsopoulos *et al.* 1983*b*).

Lymphoproliferative disease

Patients with Sjögren's syndrome have a 44 times higher relative risk of developing lymphoma, compared with age-, sex-, and race-matched normal controls (Kassan *et al.* 1978). Immunohistological studies in biopsies of such patients with lymphoma show that these are primarily of B-cell origin, usually expressing IgM-κ in their cytoplasm (Zulman *et al.* 1978). The lymphomas are of two major types, either of highly undifferentiated B cells or well-differentiated immunocytomas.

Lymphomas may differ by location and grading. In our patients, among eight lymphomas in patients with Sjögren's syndrome, six were low-grade immunocytomas and two intermediate-grade non-Hodgkin's lymphomas. Five of the immunocytomas were diagnosed from biopsies of minor salivary or lacrimal glands. Two of the patients with immunocytomas showed spontaneous regression, while the other two developed high-grade lymphoma 3 and 5 years later (Pavlidis *et al.* 1992). Therefore, the clinical picture of Sjögren's syndrome-associated lymphoma appears to be diverse, suggesting that the therapeutic approach should be guided by the stage and the grade of the disease.

Table 7 Laboratory findings in Greek patients with primary Sjögren's syndrome (data tabulated from 132 patients)

	n	%
Anaemia (Hb <35)	27/130	21
Leucopenia (WBC <3500 cells/mm³)	8/130	6
Thrombocytopenia (PLT <10 000)	2/132	2
ESR (>25 mm/h)	76/125	61
C-reactive protein (<8 mg/l)	8/130	6
Cryoglobulinaemia	34/111	28
ANA (>1:80)[a]	119/132	92
Rheumatoid factor (>1:40[b])	80/131	61
Antimitochondrial antibodies	8/132	6
Anti-Ro (SSA)	75/131	57
Anti-La (SSB)	49/131	38
Anti-nRNP	4/131	3
Anti-Sm	2/131	2

[a]Hep-2 cells as substrate.
[b]Latex fixation.

Other organs that may be affected by the lymphomas are the reticuloendothelial system, lungs, kidneys, and the gastrointestinal tract.

The diagnostic interpretation of a tissue with lymphoproliferative infiltration is sometimes very difficult. The term pseudolymphoma describes lesions that show tumour-like clusters of lymphoid cells but do not meet criteria for malignancy. Despite the use of modern molecular techniques, such as immunogenotyping (Cleary *et al.* 1987), pseudolymphoma remains in ill-defined clinicopathological entity and lymphoma should always be suspected in a patient with lymphadenopathy, organomegaly, or enlargement of major salivary glands.

Secondary Sjögren's syndrome

The association of Sjögren's syndrome with rheumatoid arthritis was first described by Henrik Sjögren in 1939. During the following years it became evident that sicca manifestations can also be found in other autoimmune rheumatic diseases, such as systemic lupus erythematosus and progressive systemic sclerosis. In addition, manifestations of Sjögren's syndrome have been described in polymyositis, polyarteritis nodosa, and primary biliary cirrhosis (see Table 1) (Moutsopoulos *et al.* 1980).

The incidence of clinically overt Sjögren's syndrome in patients with rheumatoid arthritis is around 5 per cent. Using a special questionnaire, however, 20 per cent of patients with rheumatoid arthritis registered complaints of dry eyes and/or xerostomia (Andonopoulos *et al.* 1987). The diagnosis of rheumatoid arthritis usually preceded that of Sjögren's syndrome by many years. Patients with the arthritis and the syndrome usually present with keratoconjunctivitis sicca, while enlargement of the parotids or other major salivary glands is less common than in primary Sjögren's syndrome. In addition, extra-glandular features of the primary syndrome, such as lymphadenopathy, renal involvement, and Raynaud's phenomenon, are uncommon in Sjögren's syndrome associated with rheumatoid arthritis. Such clear differences in the natural history and the clinical manifestations of the syndrome in the presence and absence of rheumatoid arthritis are not usually found in other autoimmune diseases associated with sicca manifestations. In fact, patients with primary Sjögren's syndrome and those with systemic lupus may have similar disease manifestations such as arthralgias, rash, peripheral neuropathy, and glomerulonephritis. These observations prompted Heaton (1959) to conclude that Sjögren's syndrome was a benign form of systemic lupus. The diagnosis is usually obtained histologically; approximately 20 per cent of patients with systemic lupus have lymphocytic infiltrates in biopsies from their minor salivary glands (Andonopoulos *et al.* 1990*b*).

Dry eyes and mouth are found in approximately 20 per cent of unselected patients with scleroderma (Medsger 1987). Subjective xerostomia could be due to fibrosis of the exocrine glands. In fact, in biopsies from minor salivary glands of 44 unselected patients with scleroderma, 38 per cent had fibrosis while only 22 per cent had lymphocytic infiltration compatible with Sjögren's syndrome (Andonopoulos *et al.* 1989).

Diagnosis and differential diagnosis

Since the initial definition and the proposed criteria of Sjögren's syndrome by Bloch *et al.* (1965), several sets of criteria have been used by different groups for the diagnosis of Sjögren's syndrome. As a result, patients with Sjögren's syndrome had often been missed at diagnosis, or classified incorrectly due both to the great variability at disease presentation and to the lack of well-defined and commonly accepted diagnostic criteria.

Recently, a prospective concerted action involving 26 centres in 12 European countries led to a study with the goal of obtaining validated criteria for the diagnosis of Sjögren's syndrome. The study resulted in: (i) the validation of a simple 6-item questionnaire for determination of dry eyes and mouth, useful in the initial screening for Sjögren's syndrome, and (ii) the definition of a new set of criteria for Sjögren's syndrome. The sensitivity and specificity of both questionnaire and diagnostic criteria were determined, exhibiting good discrimination between patients and controls. Hence, using this set of criteria, a general agreement can be reached on the diagnosis of Sjögren's syndrome (Vitali *et al*. 1992*a*).

Differential diagnosis must be, of course, from other diseases responsible for dry eyes, xerostomia, and parotid enlargement. Sarcoidosis in one disease that can mimic the clinical picture of Sjögren's syndrome (Drosos *et al*. 1989). However, the biopsy of minor salivary glands reveals non-caseating granulomas in sarcoidosis, while there is a lack of autoantibodies to Ro(SSA) or La(SSB).

Other medical conditions that can mimic the syndrome are lipoproteinaemias (types II, IV, and V), chronic graft-versus-host disease, amyloidosis, and, more recently, patients with human immunodeficiency virus (**HIV**) infection (Moutsopoulos and Talal 1989). In fact, sicca manifestations, with parotid enlargement, pulmonary involvement and lymphadenopathy, have been reported in 12 patients with HIV infection. These patients has an increased prevalence of HLA-DR5 alloantigen. The virus has been detected in lymphocytes from labial salivary glands in two of six patients with HIV infection, but the two diseases seem to be different, as patients with HIV infection have no autoantibodies to Ro(SSA) and La(SSB) autoantigens, and the lymphocytic infiltrates in their salivary glands are not as prominent as in Sjögren's syndrome and consist of CD8+ T cells (Youinou *et al*. 1990*b*).

Therapy — prognosis (Box 1)

Sjögren's syndrome is a chronic, multisystem disease. Therefore, patients with Sjögren's syndrome should be followed regularly for significant functional deterioration, signs of complications and significant changes in the course of the disease. The patient should

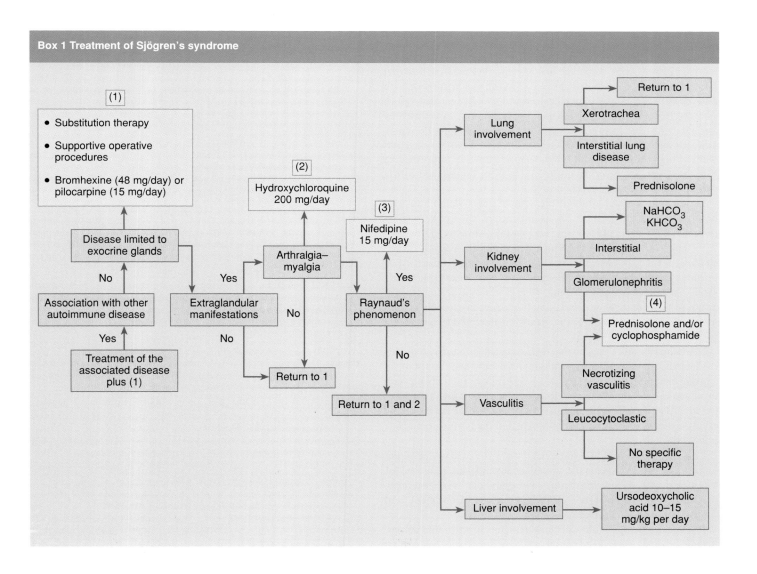

Box 1 Treatment of Sjögren's syndrome

be informed that regular outpatient visits, and close collaboration with the outpatient clinics for rheumatology, ophthalmology, and oral medicine, give the most satisfactory results.

Sicca manifestations are of unknown aetiology. Hence, treatment of Sjögren's syndrome is aimed at symptomatic relief and limiting the damaging local effects of chronic xerostomia and keratoconjunctivitis sicca by substitution of the missing secretions (Moutsopoulos and Vlachoyiannopoulos 1993).

Keratoconjunctivitis sicca is treated with fluid replacement supplied as often as necessary. To replace deficient tears, there are several readily available ophthalmic preparations (Tearisol; Liquifilm; 0.5 per cent methylcellulose; Hypo Tears). In severe cases, it may be necessary for patients to use these as often as every 30 min. If corneal ulceration is present, eye-patches and boric acid ointment are recommended. Certain drugs that may cause further deterioration of lacrimal and salivary function, such as diuretics, antihypertensive drugs and antidepressants, should be avoided. The low levels of humidity in air-conditioned environments, as well as windy or dry climates, must be avoided. Soft contact lenses may help to protect the cornea, especially in the presence of filaments. However, the lenses themselves require wetting and the patients must be followed very carefully due to the increased risk of infection.

Treatment of xerostomia is difficult. Stimulation of salivary flow by sugar-free, highly flavoured lozenges has been found to be rather helpful. Most patients carry water and use sugarless lemon drops or chewing-gum. These must be sugar free, because of the risk of rampant dental caries. Adequate oral hygiene after meals is essential for the prevention of dental disease. Topical oral treatment with fluoride enhances dental mineralization and retards damage to tooth surfaces. In rapidly progressive dental disease, fluoride can be directly applied to the teeth from plastic trays that are used at night. Propionic acid gels may be used to treat vaginal dryness. Bromhexine given orally at high doses (48 mg/day) has been suggested to improve sicca manifestations. However, frequent ingestion of fluids, particularly with meals, is often the best solution.

Pilocarpine hydrochloride (5 mg, three times daily) can also improve sicca manifestations, via its muscarinic, cholinergic activity (Fox 1992). Flushing and sweating are possible side-effects.

Patients with Sjögren's syndrome often complain of parotid gland swelling. If the gland becomes tender with permanent enlargement, infection should be ruled out and treatment with tetracycline orally should be recommended (500 mg, four times daily). Local moist heat and non-steroidal anti-inflammatory drugs are usually helpful in resolving this problem. If the gland remains tender, lymphoma should be ruled out by biopsy.

Preliminary studies showed that hydroxychloroquine, which is efficacious and safe in other autoimmune diseases, may be useful in treating Sjögren's patients. A dose of 200 mg/day partially corrects hypergammaglobulinaemia and decreases the titre of IgG antibodies to La/SSB antigen. Furthermore, hydroxychloroquine decreased the erythrocyte sedimentation rate and increased the haemoglobin (Fox et al. 1988).

Corticosteroids (prednisolone 0.5–1 mg/kg per day) or other immunosuppressive agents (i.e. cyclophosphamide) are indicated for the treatment of life-threatening extraglandular manifestations, particularly when renal or severe pulmonary involvement and systemic vasculitis are present.

In conclusion, Sjögren's syndrome remains an incurable disease without a single therapeutic approach that can change its natural course. The prognosis of the disease depends on the extension and type of the systemic features, and the appearance of a lymphoma. The treatment and prognosis of malignant lymphoma depends on the histological type, the location, and the extension. Decisions about chemotherapy and/or radiotherapy should be guided by experienced oncologists.

References

Agnello, V. et al. (1980). Evidence for a subset of rheumatoid factors that cross react with DNA-histone and have a distinct cross-idiotype. *Journal of Experimental Medicine*, **151**, 1514–27.

Alexander, E. L. (1987a). Inflammatory vascular disease in Sjögren's syndrome. In *Sjögren's syndrome: clinical and immunological aspects* (ed. N. Talal, H. M. Moutsopoulos, and S. S. Kassan), pp. 102–24. Springer, Berlin.

Alexander, E. L. (1987b). Neuromuscular complications of primary Sjögren's syndrome. In *Sjögren's syndrome: clinical and immunological aspects* (ed. N. Talal, H. M. Moutsopoulos, and S. S. Kassan), pp. 61–82. Springer, Berlin.

Anderson, L. G. et al. (1972). Salivary gland immunoglobulin and rheumatoid factor synthesis in Sjögren's syndrome: natural history and response to treatment. *American Journal of Medicine*, **49**, 49–54.

Andonopoulos, A. P., Drosos, A. A., Skopouli, F. N., Acritidis, N. C., and Moutsopoulos, H. M. (1987). Secondary Sjögren's syndrome in rheumatoid arthritis. *Journal of Rheumatology*, **1**, 1098–103.

Andonopoulos, A. P., Drosos, A. A., Skopouli, F. N., and Moutsopoulos, H. M. (1989). Sjögren's syndrome in rheumatoid arthritis and progressive systemic sclerosis: a comparative study. *Clinical and Experimental Rheumatology*, **7**, 203–5.

Andonopoulos, A. P., Lagos, G., Drosos, A. A., and Moutsopoulos, H. M. (1990a). The spectrum of neurological involvement in Sjögren's syndrome. *British Journal of Rheumatology*, **29**, 21–3.

Andonopoulos, A. P., Skopouli, F. N., Dimou, G. S., Drosos, A. A., and Moutsopoulos, H. M. (1990b). Sjögren's syndrome in systemic lupus erythematosus. *Journal of Rheumatology*, **17**, 201–4.

Batsakis, J. G. and Howard, D. R. (1982). Sjögren's syndrome: an immune response associated disorder. *Clinical Laboratory Annals*, **1**, 171–88.

Baum, B. J. and Fox, P. C. (1987). Chemistry of saliva. In *Sjögren's syndrome: clinical and immunological aspects* (ed. N. Talal, H. M. Moutsopoulos, and S. S. Kassan), pp. 25–34. Springer, Berlin.

Ben-Chetrit, E., Fox, R. I., and Tan, E. M. (1990). Dissociation of immune response to the SSA (Ro) 52 kD and 60 kD polypeptides in systemic lupus erythematosus and Sjögren's syndrome. *Arthritis and Rheumatism*, **33**, 349–55.

Binder, A., Snaith, M. L., and Isenberg, D. (1988). Sjögren's syndrome: a study of its neurological complications. *British Journal of Rheumatology*, **27**, 275–80.

Bloch, K. J., Buchanan, W. W., Wohl, M. J., and Bunim, J. J. (1965). Sjögren's syndrome: a clinical, pathological and serological study of sixty-two cases. *Medicine (Baltimore)*, **44**, 187–231.

Bodeuitsch, C. et al. (1992). Quantitative immunohistologic criteria are superior to the lymphocytic focus score criterion for the diagnosis of Sjögren's syndrome. *Arthritis and Rheumatism*, **35**, 1075–87.

Boumba, D., Skopouli, F. N., and Moutsopoulos, H. M. (1995). Cytokine mRNA expression in the labial salivary gland tissues from patients with primary Sjögren's syndrome. *British Journal of Rheumatology*, **34**, 326–33.

Boumpas, D. T. et al. (1990). c-myc, proto-oncogene expression in peripheral blood mononuclear cells from patients with primary Sjögren's syndrome. *Arthritis and Rheumatism*, **33**, 49–56.

Buchanan, W. W., Cox, A. G., Harden, R. M. G., Glen, A. I. M., Anderson, J. R., and Gray, K. G. (1966). Gastric studies in Sjögren's syndrome. *Gut*, **7**, 351–9.

Castro-Poltronieri, A. and Alarcon-Segovia, D (1983). Articular manifestation of primary Sjögren's syndrome. *Journal of Rheumatology*, **10**, 485–90.

Chisholm, D. M. and Mason, D. K. (1968). Labial salivary gland biopsy in Sjögren's syndrome. *Journal of Clinical Pathology*, **21**, 656–60.

Chused, T. M., Kassan, S. S., Opelz, G., Moutsopoulos, H. M., and Terasaki, P. I. (1977). Sjögren's syndrome associated with HLA DW3. *New England Journal of Medicine*, **296**, 895–7.

Cleary, M. L., Calini, N., Levy, N., Talal, N., and Sklar, J. (1987). Detection of lymphoma by analysis of immunoglobulin gene rearrangements. In *Sjögren's syndrome: clinical and immunological aspects* (ed. N. Talal, H. M. Moutsopoulos, and S. S. Kassan), pp. 137–43. Springer, Berlin.

Constantopoulos, S. H. and Moutsopoulos, H. M. (1987). The respiratory system in Sjögren's syndrome. In *Sjögren's syndrome: clinical and immunological aspects* (ed. N. Talal, H. M. Moutsopoulos, and S. S. Kassan), pp. 83–9. Springer, Berlin.

Daniels, T. E. and Whitcher, J. P. (1994). Association of patterns of labial salivary gland inflammation with keratoconjunctivitis sicca. *Arthritis and Rheumatism*, 37, 869–77.

Daniels, T. E., Aufdemorte, T. B., and Greenspan, J. S. (1987). Histopathology of Sjögren's syndrome. In *Sjögren's syndrome: clinical and immunological aspects* (ed. N. Talal, H. M. Moutsopoulos, and S. S. Kassan), pp. 266–86. Springer, Berlin.

Drosos, A. A., Antonopoulos, A. P., Costopoulos, J. S., Papadimitriou, C., and Moutsopoulos, H. M. (1988). Prevalence of primary Sjögren's syndrome in an elderly population. *British Journal of Rheumatology*, 27, 123–7.

Drosos, A. A., Constantopoulos, S. H., Phsychos, D., Stefanou, D., Papadimitriou, C. S., and Moutsopoulos, H. M. (1989). The forgotten cause of sicca complex; sarcoidosis. *Journal of Rheumatology*, 16, 1548–51.

Fauci, A. S. and Moutsopoulos, H. M. (1981). Polyclonally triggered B-cells in the peripheral blood of normal individuals and in patients with SLE and primary Sjögren's syndrome. *Arthritis and Rheumatism*, 24, 577–84.

Fishleder, A., Tubbs, R., Hesse, B., and Levine, H. (1987). Uniform detection of immunoglobulin gene rearrangements in benign lymphoepithelial lesions. *New England Journal of Medicine*, 316, 1118–21.

Fox, R. I. (1992). Treatment of patients with Sjögren's syndrome. *Rheumatic Disease Clinics of North America*, 18, 699–709.

Fox, R. I., Pearson, G., and Vaughan, J. H. (1986a). Detection of Epstein–Barr virus-associated antigens and DNA in salivary gland biopsies from patients with Sjögren's syndrome. *Journal of Immunology*, 137, 3162–7.

Fox, R. I., Chen, P., Carson, D. A., and Fong, S. (1986b). Expression of a cross-reactive idiotype on rheumatoid factor in patients with Sjögren's syndrome. *Journal of Immunology*, 136, 477–83.

Fox, R. I., Chan E., Bentol, L., Fong, S., Freidlaender, M., and Howell, F. W. (1988). Treatment of primary Sjögren's syndrome with hydroxychloroquine. *American Journal of Medicine*, 85 (Suppl. 4A), 62–7.

Fox, R. I. et al. (1994). Cytokine mRNA expression in salivary biopsies of Sjögren's syndrome. *Journal of Immunology*, 152, 5532–9.

Freimark, B., Fantozzi, R., Bone, R., Bordin, G., and Fox, R. (1989). Detection of clonally expanded salivary gland lymphocytes in Sjögren's syndrome. *Arthritis and Rheumatism*, 32, 859–69.

Fye, K. H. and Talal, N. (1987). Skin manifestations of Sjögren's syndrome. In *Dermatology in general medicine* (ed. T. B. Fitzpatrick, A. Z. Eisen, K. Walff, I. M. Freedberg, and K. F. Austen), pp. 1883–7. McGraw-Hill, New York.

Fye, K. H., Terasaki, P. I., Moutsopoulos, H. M., Daniels, T. E., Michalski, J. P., and Talal, N. (1976). Association of Sjögren's syndrome with HLA-B8. *Arthritis and Rheumatism*, 19, 883–6.

Garry, R. F., Fermin, C. D., Hart, D. J., Alexander, S. S., Donehower, L. A., and Luo-Zhang, H. (1990). Detection of a human intracisternal A-type retroviral particle antigenically related to HIV. *Science*, 250, 1127–9.

Green, J. E., Hinricks, S. H., Vogel, J., and Jay, G. (1989). Exocrinopathy resembling Sjögren's syndrome in HTLV-1 *tax* transgenic mice. *Nature*, 341, 72–4.

Greenspan, J. S., Daniels, T. E., Talal, N., and Sylvester, R. A. (1974). The histopathology of Sjögren's syndrome in labial salivary gland biopsies. *Oral Surgery, Oral Medicine, Oral Pathology*, 37, 217–19.

Gregerson, P. K., Silver, J., and Winchester, R. J. (1987). The shared epitope hypothesis. An approach to understanding the molecular genetics of susceptibility to rheumatoid arthritis. *Arthritis and Rheumatism*, 30, 1205–13.

Haddad, J. et al. (1992). Lymphocytic sialadenitis of Sjögren's syndrome associated with chronic hepatitis C virus liver disease. *Lancet*, 339, 321–3.

Harley, J. B. (1987). Autoantibodies in Sjögren's syndrome. In *Sjögren's syndrome: clinical and immunological aspects* (ed. N. Talal, H. M. Moutsopoulos, and S. S. Kassan), pp. 218–34. Springer, Berlin.

Harrington, D. S., Fall, M., and Johanson, S. E. (1990). Interstitial cystitis: bladder mucosa lymphocyte immunophenotyping and peripheral blood flow cytometry analysis. *Journal of Urology*, 144, 868–71.

Heaton, J. M. (1959). Sjögren's syndrome and systemic lupus erythematosus. *British Medical Journal*, 1, 466–9.

Hoffman, R. W and Walker, S. E. (1987). Animal models of Sjögren's syndrome. In *Sjögren's syndrome: clinical and immunological aspects* (ed. N. Talal, H. M. Moutsopoulos, and S. S. Kassan), pp. 266–86. Springer, Berlin.

Hudson, J., Chanther, J., Lok, L., Misra, V., and Muller, M. (1979). Model systems for analysis of latent CMV infections. *Canadian Journal of Microbiology*, 25, 245–50.

Innes, J. R. M. and Stanton, M. F. (1961). Acute disease of the submaxillary and harderian glands (sialodacryoadenitis) of rats with cytomegaly and no inclusion bodies. *American Journal of Pathology*, 38, 455–68.

Jacobsson, L. et al. (1989). Dry eyes or mouth—an epidemiological study in Swedish adults with special reference to primary Sjögren's syndrome. *Journal of Autoimmunity*, 2, 521–7.

Jacobsson, L., Hansen, B. U., Manthrope, R., Hardgrave, K., Neas, B., and Harley, J. B. (1992). Association of dry eyes and dry mouth with anti Ro/SSA and anti La/SSB autoantibodies in normal adults. *Arthritis and Rheumatism*, 35, 1492–501.

Kang, H., Pisa, P., Moore, K., Abrams, J., and Fox, R. I. (1991). Sjögren's syndrome pseudolymphoma induced in Scid/hu mice chimeras. *Clinical and Experimental Rheumatology*, 9, 334 (Abstr.).

Kappler, J. et al. (1989). VB specific stimulation of human T cells by staphylococcal toxins. *Science*, 244, 811–13.

Karsh, J., Pavlidis, N., Neintraub, B. D., and Moutsopoulos, H. M. (1980). Thyroid disease in Sjögren's syndrome. *Arthritis and Rheumatism*, 23, 1326–9.

Kassan, S. S. and Talal, N. (1987). Renal disease with Sjögren's syndrome. In *Sjögren's syndrome: clinical and immunological aspects* (ed. N. Talal, H. M. Moutsopoulos, and S. S. Kassan), pp. 96–102. Springer, Berlin.

Kassan, S. S. et al. (1978). Increased risk of lymphoma in sicca syndrome. *Annals of Internal Medicine*, 89, 888–92.

Katsikis, P. D., Youinou, P. Y., Galanopoulou, V., Tzioufas, A. G., and Moutsopoulos, H. M. (1990). Monoclonal process in primary Sjögren's syndrome and rheumatoid factor associated cross reactive idiotype. *Clinical and Experimental Immunology*, 82, 509–14.

Kincaid, M. C. (1987). The eye in Sjögren's syndrome. In *Sjögren's syndrome: clinical and immunological aspects* (ed. N. Talal, H. M. Moutsopoulos, and S. S. Kassan), pp. 25–34, Springer, Berlin.

Kipps, T. J., Fong, S., Tomhave, E., Chen, P. P., Goldfien, R. D., and Carson, D. A. (1987). High-frequency expression of a conserved kappa light-chain variable region gene in chronic lymphocytic leukemia. *Proceedings of the National Academy of Sciences (USA)*, 84, 2916–20.

Kipps, T. J., Tomhave, E., Chen, P. P., and Fox, R. I. (1989). Molecular characterization of a major autoantibody associated cross-reactive idiotype in Sjögren's syndrome. *Journal of Immunology*, 142, 4261–8.

Kunkel, H. G., Agnello V., Joslin, F. G., Winchester, R. J., and Capra, J. D. (1973). Cross-idiotypic specificity among monoclonal IgM proteins with anti-gamma-globulin activity. *Journal of Experimental Medicine*, 137, 331–42.

Lane, H. C., Callahay, T. R., Jaffe, E. S., Fauci, A. S., and Moutsopoulos, H. M. (1983). The presence of intracytoplasmic infiltrates of the minor salivary glands of patients with primary Sjögren's syndrome. *Clinical and Experimental Rheumatology*, 1, 237–9.

Leroy, J. P., Drosos, A. A., Yannopoulos, D. I., Youinou, P., and Moutsopoulos, H. M. (1990). Intravenous pulse cyclophosphamide therapy in myositis and Sjögren's syndrome. *Arthritis and Rheumatism*, 33, 1579–81.

Maini, R. N. (1987). Relationship of Sjögren's syndrome to rheumatoid arthritis. In *Sjögren's syndrome: clinical and immunological aspects* (ed. N. Talal, H. M. Moutsopoulos, and S. S. Kassan), pp. 165–77. Springer, Berlin.

Mann, D. (1987). Immunogenetics of Sjögren's syndrome. In *Sjögren's syndrome: clinical and immunological aspects* (ed. N. Talal, H. M. Moutsopoulos, and S. S. Kassan), pp. 235–43. Springer, Berlin.

Manoussakis, M. N., Tzioufas, A. G., Pange, P. J. E., and Moutsopoulos, H. M. (1986). Serological profiles in subgroups of patients with Sjögren's syndrome. *Scandinavian Journal of Rheumatology*, 61 (Suppl.), 89–92.

Medsger, T. A., Jr (1987). Sjögren's syndrome and systemic sclerosis (scleroderma). In *Sjögren's syndrome: clinical and immunological aspects*, (ed. N. Talal, H. M. Moutsopoulos, and S. S. Kassan), pp. 182–7. Springer, Berlin.

Moriuchi, J. *et al.* (1986). Association between HLA and Sjögren's syndrome in Japanese patients. *Arthritis and Rheumatism*, **29**, 1518–21.

Moutsopoulos, H. M. and Manoussakis M. N. (1989). Immunopathogenesis of Sjögren's. Facts and fancy. *Autoimmunity*, **5**, 17–24.

Moutsopoulos, H. M. and Talal, N. (1987). Immunologic abnormalities in Sjögren's syndrome. In *Sjögren's syndrome: clinical and immunological aspects*, (ed. N. Talal, H. M. Moutsopoulos, and S. S. Kassan), pp. 258–65. Springer, Berlin.

Moutsopoulos, H. M. and Talal, N. (1989). New developments in Sjögren's syndrome. *Current Opinion in Rheumatology*, **1**, 332–8.

Moutsopoulos, H. M. and Vlachoyiannopoulos, P. G. (1993). What would I do if I had Sjögren's syndrome. *Rheumatology Review*, **2**, 17–23.

Moutsopoulos, H. M., Ballow, J. E., Lawley, T. J., Stahl, N. I., Antonovych, T. T., and Chused, T. M. (1978). Immune complex glomerulonephritis in sicca syndrome. *American Journal of Medicine*, **64**, 955–60.

Moutsopoulos, H. M. *et al.* (1980). Sjögren's syndrome (sicca syndrome): current issues. *Annals of Internal Medicine*, **92**, 212–26.

Moutsopoulos, H. M., Steinberg, A. D., Fauci, A. S., Lane, H. C., and Papadopoulos, N. M. (1983*a*). High incidence of free monoclonal λ light chains in the sera of patients with Sjögren's syndrome. *Journal of Immunology*, **130**, 2263–5.

Moutsopoulos, H. M., Elkon, K. B., Mavridis, A. K., Acritidis, N. C., Hughes, G. R. V., and Pepys, M. B. (1983*b*). Serum C-reactive protein in primary Sjögren's syndrome. *Clinical and Experimental Rheumatology*, **1**, 57–8.

Moutsopoulos, H. M., Costello, R., Drosos, A. A., Mavridis, A. K., and Papadopoulos, N. M. (1985). Demonstration and identification of monoclonal proteins in the urine of patients with Sjögren's syndrome. *Annals of the Rheumatic Diseases*, **44**, 109–12.

Moutsopoulos, H. M., Tzioufas, A. G., Bai, M. K., Papadopoulos, N. M., and Papadimitriou, C. S. (1990). Serum IgMκ monoclonicity in patients with Sjögren's syndrome is associated with an increased proportion of κ-positive plasma-cells infiltrating the labial minor salivary glands. *Annals of the Rheumatic Diseases*, **49**, 929–31.

Moutsopoulos, H. M., Cledes, J., Skopouli, F. N., Elisaf, M., and Youinou, P. (1991). Nephrocalcinosis in Sjögren's syndrome. *Journal of Internal Medicine*, **230**, 187–91.

Navarette, C. *et al.* (1985). Genetic and functional relationships of the HLA-DR and HLA-DQ antigens. *Immunogenetics*, **21**, 97–101.

Papasteriades, C., Skopouli, F. N., Drosos, A. A., Andonopoulos, A. P., and Moutsopoulos, H. M. (1988). HLA alloantigen association in Greek patients with Sjögren's syndrome. *Journal of Autoimmunity*, **1**, 85–90.

Papiris, S. A., Skopouli, F. N., Maniati, M. A., Constantopoulos, C. H., and Moutsopoulos, H. M. (1994). Bronchiolitis in primary Sjögren's syndrome. In *Sjögren's syndrome. State of the art* (ed. M. Homma, S. Sugai, T. Tojo, N. Miyakaka, and M. Akizuki), pp. 431–2. Kugler Publications, Amsterdam.

Parrago, G., Rain, G. D., Brochierion, C., and Rocher, F. (1987). Scintigraphy of the salivary glands in Sjögren's syndrome. *Journal of Clinical Pathology*, **40**, 1463–7.

Pavlidis, N. A., Karsh, J., and Moutsopoulos, H. M. (1982). The clinical picture of primary Sjögren's syndrome. *Journal of Rheumatology*, **40**, 1463–7.

Pavlidis, N. A. *et al.* (1992). Lymphoma in Sjögren's syndrome. *Medical Pediatric Oncology*, **20**, 279–83.

Pennec, Y. L., Leroy, J. P., Jouquan, J., Lelong, A., Katsikis, P., and Youinou, P. (1990). Comparison of labial and subclinical salivary gland biopsies in the diagnosis of Sjögren's syndrome. *Annals of the Rheumatic Diseases*, **49**, 37–9.

Reveille, J. D., Macleod, M. J., Whittington, K., and Arnett, F. C. (1991). Specific amino acid residues in the second hypervariable region of HLA-DQA1 and DQB1 chain genes promote the Ro(SSA)/La(SSB) autoantibody responses. *Journal of Immunology*, **146**, 3871–5.

Schmidt, U., Helbron, D., and Lennert, K. (1982). Development of malignant lymphoma in myoepithelial sialadenitis (Sjögren's syndrome). *Virchow's Archives*, **395**, 11–43.

Scott, J. (1980). Quantitative observations on the histology of human salivary glands obtained post mortem. *Journal of Biologie Buccale*, **8**, 187–92.

Shillitoe, E. J., Daniels, T. E., Whitcher, J. P., Strand, D. V., Talal, N., and Greenspan, J. S. (1982). Antibody to cytomegalovirus in patients with Sjögren's syndrome as detected by enzyme-linked immunosorbent assay. *Arthritis and Rheumatism*, **25**, 260–5.

Siamopoulou-Mavridou, A., Drosos, A. A., and Andonopoulos, A. P. (1989). Sjögren's syndrome in childhood: report of two cases. *European Journal of Pediatrics*, **18**, 523–4.

Skopouli, F. N., Siouna-Fatourou, H. I., Ziciadis, C., and Moutsopoulos, H. M. (1989). Evaluation of unstimulated whole saliva flow rate and stimulated parotid flow as confirmatory tests for xerostomia. *Clinical and Experimental Rheumatology*, **7**, 127–9.

Skopouli, F. N. *et al.* (1990). Raynaud's phenomenon in primary Sjögren's syndrome. *Journal of Rheumatology*, **17**, 618–20.

Skopouli, F. N., Fox, P. C., Galanopoulou, V., Atkinson, J. C., Jaffe, E. C., and Moutsopoulos, H. M. (1991). T-cell subpopulation in the labial minor salivary gland histopathologic lesion of Sjögren's syndrome. *Journal of Rheumatology*, **18**, 210–14.

Skopouli, F. N., Kousvelari, E., Mertz, P., Jaffe, E. S., Fox, P. C., and Moutsopoulos, H. M. (1992). c-*myc* mRNA expression in minor salivary glands of patients with Sjögren's syndrome. *Journal of Rheumatology*, **19**, 693–9.

Skopouli, F. N., Barbatis, C., and Moutsopoulos, H. M. (1994). Liver involvement in primary Sjögren's syndrome. *British Journal of Rheumatology*, **33**, 745–8.

St Clair, E. W., Angellilo, J. C., and Signer, K. H. (1992). Expression of cell adhesion molecules in the salivary gland microenvironment of Sjögren's syndrome. *Arthritis and Rheumatism*, **35**, 62–6.

Sumida, T. *et al.* (1992). T-cell receptor repertoire of infiltrating T-cells in lips of Sjögren's syndrome patients. *Journal of Clinical Investigation*, **89**, 681–5.

Talal, N., Dauphinee, M. J., Dang, H., Alexander, S. S., Hart, D. J., and Garry, R. F. (1990). Detection of serum antibodies to retroviral proteins n patients with primary Sjögren's syndrome (autoimmune exocrinopathy). *Arthritis and Rheumatism*, **33**, 774–81.

Tambur, A. R. *et al.* (1993). Molecular analysis of HLA class II genes in primary Sjögren's syndrome: a study of Israeli and Greek non-Jewish patients. *Human Immunology*, **36**, 235–42.

Tarpley, T. M., Anderson, L. G., and White, C. L. (1974). Minor salivary gland involvement in Sjögren's syndrome. *Oral Surgery, Oral Medicine, Oral Pathology*, **37**, 64–74.

Teramoto, N. *et al.* (1989). Annular erythema: a possible association with primary Sjögren's syndrome. *Journal of the American Academy of Dermatology*, **20**, 596–601.

Trevino, H., Tsianos, E. B. and Schenkers, S. (1987). Gastrointestinal and hepatobiliary features in Sjögren's syndrome. In *Sjögren's syndrome. Clinical and immunological aspects* (ed. N. Talal, H. M. Moutsopoulos, and S. S. Kassan), pp. 89–95. Springer, Berlin.

Tsampoulas, C. G. *et al.* (1990). Hand radiographic changes in patients with primary and secondary Sjögren's syndrome. *Scandinavian Journal of Rheumatology*, **15**, 333–9.

Tsianos, E. B., Tzioufas, A. G., Kita, M. D., Tsolas, O., and Moutsopoulos, H. M. (1984). Serum isoamylases in patients with autoimmune rheumatic diseases. *Clinical and Experimental Rheumatology*, **2**, 235–8.

Tsianos, E. B. *et al.* (1990). Sjögren's syndrome in patients with primary biliary cirrhosis. *Hepatology*, **11**, 730–4.

Tsokos, M., Lazarou, S. A., and Moutsopoulos, H. M. (1987). Vasculitis in primary Sjögren's syndrome: histologic classification and clinical presentation. *American Journal of Clinical Pathology*, **88**, 26–31.

Tzioufas, A. G., Manoussakis, M. N., Costello, R., Silis, M., Papadopoulos, N. M., and Moutsopoulos, H. M. (1986). Cryoglobulinemia in autoimmune rheumatic diseases: evidence of circulating monoclonal cryoglobulins in patients with primary Sjögren's syndrome. *Arthritis and Rheumatism*, **29**, 1098–104.

Tzioufas, A. G., Boumba, D. S., Skopouli, F. N., and Moutsopoulos, H. M. (1996). Mixed monoclonal cryoglobulinemia and monoclonal rheumatoid factor cross-reactive idiotypes as predicting factors for lymphoma development in primary Sjögren's syndrome. *Arthritis and Rheumatism*, **39**, 767–72.

Tzioufas, A. G., Staikos, P., and Moutsopoulos, H. M. (1994). Epidemiology of Sjögren's syndrome in Greece. In *Sjögren's syndrome. State of the art* (ed. M. Homma, S. Sugai, T. Tojo, N. Miyakaka, and M. Akizuki), pp. 395–6. Kugler Publications, Amsterdam.

Van de Merwe, J. P., Kamerling, R., Arendsen, H. S., Mulder, A. H., and Hooijkaas, H. (1993). Sjögren's syndrome in patients with interstitial cystitis. *Journal of Rheumatology*, **20**, 962–6.

Venables, P. J. W., Ross, M. G. R., Charles, P. J., Melson, R. D., Griffith, P. D., and Maini, R. N. (1985). A seroepidemiological study of cytomegalovirus and Epstein–Barr virus in rheumatoid arthritis and sicca syndrome. *Annals of the Rheumatic Diseases*, **44**, 742–6.

Vitali, C. *et al.* (1986). HLA antigens in Italian patients with primary Sjögren's syndrome. *Annals of the Rheumatic Diseases*, **45**, 412–16.

Vitali, C. *et al.* (1988). Parotid sialography and minor salivary gland biopsy in the diagnosis of Sjögren's syndrome: a comparative study of 84 patients. *Journal of Rheumatology*, **15**, 262–7.

Vitali, C. *et al.* (1992*a*). Preliminary criteria for the classification of Sjögren's syndrome. Results of a prospective concerted action supported by the European Community. *Arthritis and Rheumatism*, **36**, 340–8.

Vitali, C. *et al.* (1992*b*). Anti hepatitis C virus antibodies in primary Sjögren's syndrome: false positive results are related to hyper-γ-globulinemia. *Clinical and Experimental Rheumatology*, **10**, 103–4.

Whaley, K. *et al.* (1972). Sjögren's syndrome and autoimmunity in a geriatric population. *Age and Ageing*, **1**, 197–200.

Whittingham, S., Nasseli, G., Hicks, J. D., O'Brien C., and Sculley, T. B. (1991). Studies on Sjögren's syndrome in Scid mice. *Clinical and Experimental Rheumatology*, **9**, 332 (Abstr.).

Wolf, H., Haus, M., and Wilmes, E. (1984). Persistence of Epstein–Barr virus in the parotid gland. *Journal of Virology*, **51**, 795–8.

Yannopoulos, D. I. *et al.* (1992). Conjunctival epithelial cells from patients with Sjögren's syndrome inappropriately express major histocompatibility complex molecules, La/SSB antigen and heat shock proteins. *Journal of Clinical Immunology*, **12**, 259–65.

Yonaha, F., Sumida, T., Maeda, T., Tomioka, H., Koike, T., and Yoshioda, S. (1992). Restrictive junctional usage of T-cell receptor Vβ2 And Vβ13 genes, which are overpresented on infiltrating T-cells in the lips of patients with Sjögren's syndrome. *Arthritis and Rheumatism*, **35**, 1362–6.

Youinou, P., Pennec, Y. L., Katsikis, P., Jouquan, J., Faugment, P., and Le Goff, P. (1990*a*). Raynaud's phenomenon in primary Sjögren's syndrome. *British Journal of Rheumatology*, **29**, 205–7.

Youinou, P., Moutsopoulos, H. M., and Pennec, Y. L. (1990*b*). Clinical features of Sjögren's syndrome. *Current Opinion in Rheumatology*, **2**, 687–93.

Zulman, J., Jaffe, R., and Talal, N. (1978). Evidence that the malignant lymphoma of Sjögren's syndrome is a monoclonal B-cell neoplasm. *New England Journal of Medicine*, **299**, 1215–20.

5.11 Primary vasculitides

5.11.1 Classification of vasculitis

David G. I. Scott and Richard A. Watts

Introduction

Vasculitis means inflammation of blood vessels. Implicit in this definition is that the blood vessel is the primary site of inflammation. The blood vessel wall is thus infiltrated with inflammatory cells and perivascular cuffing does not equate with vasculitis. The consequence of such inflammation is often destruction of the vessel wall which is seen on histology as fibrinoid necrosis (Fig. 1). It is for this reason that many use the term 'necrotizing vasculitis'.

The vasculitides are a heterogeneous group of relatively uncommon diseases which can arise *de novo* (e.g. polyarteritis nodosa, Wegener's granulomatosis) or as a secondary feature of an established clinical disease such as rheumatoid arthritis or systemic lupus erythematosus.

The consequences of such vascular inflammation depend upon the size, site, and the number of blood vessels involved. Vasculitis can occasionally be localized and clinically insignificant but more commonly is generalized and potentially life threatening, especially

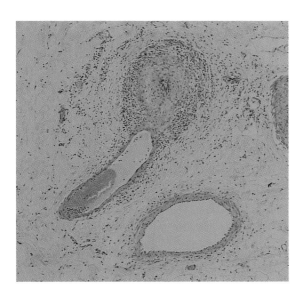

Fig. 1 Histology showing typical necrotizing vasculitis

when small muscular arteries are involved. Muscular arteries may develop focal or segmental lesions. The former (affecting part of the vessel wall) may lead to aneurysm formation and possibly rupture; segmental lesions (affecting the whole circumference) are more common and lead to stenosis or occlusion with distal infarction. Haemorrhage or infarction of vital internal organs are the most serious problems of systemic vasculitis and explain the poor prognosis of untreated polyarteritis nodosa (Frohnert and Sheps 1967) or of arteritis complicating rheumatoid arthritis (Schmid *et al.* 1961; Bywaters and Scott 1963; Scott *et al.* 1981). Small vessel vasculitis, by contrast, most commonly affects the skin and rarely causes dysfunction of internal organs. Widespread small-vessel vasculitis may cause problems, especially in the kidney, when sufficient numbers of adjacent vessels are affected with significant release of inflammatory mediators or where overall perfusion is threatened.

Epidemiology

The epidemiology of the systemic vasculitides is documented poorly. Many studies have been from tertiary referral centres with the problems of referral bias and uncertainty of denominator population or have involved small populations. We have estimated the incidence of the major forms of systemic vasculitis in a stable, ethnically homogeneous population — the Norwich (United Kingdom) Health Authority (414 000 adults) over a 6-year period between 1988 and 1994 (Watts *et al.* 1995). The overall annual incidence of systemic vasculitis (excluding giant cell arteritis) was 38.6 per million (95 per cent confidence intervals 31.3 to 47.2). The commonest systemic vasculitides were systemic rheumatoid vasculitis — 12.5 per million per year (95 per cent confidence intervals 8.5 to 17.7) and Wegener's granulomatosis — 8.5 per million per year (95 per cent confidence intervals 5.2 to 12.9). Details of the incidence of this and the other commoner systemic vasculitides are shown in Table 1. These data suggest that the overall incidence of systemic vasculitis is significantly greater than previously thought (estimated at 10 per million per year). Whether this represents a genuine increased incidence with time or increased physician awareness, especially in association with the introduction of the antineutrophil cytoplasmic antibody (**ANCA**) test is uncertain.

Classification of vasculitis

Classification means distribution in classes or groups according to a method or system. Classification of vasculitis is confusing because of the considerable overlap between the different vasculitic syndromes and because the cause of the vasculitis is usually unknown.

Table 1 Estimated annual incidence of the commoner vasculitides in the Norwich Health Authority 1988 to 1994

	Number of patients	Annual incidence (per million; 95% confidence intervals)
Systemic rheumatoid vasculitis	31	12.5 (8.5–17.7)
Wegener's granulomatosis	21	8.5 (5.2–12.9)
Churg–Strauss syndrome	6	2.4 (0.9–5.3)
Microscopic polyangiitis	6	2.4 (0.9–5.3)
Henoch–Schönlein purpura	3	1.2 (0.3–3.5)
Systemic lupus erythematosus[a]	9	3.6 (1.7–6.9)
Miscellaneous[b]	8	
Unclassified	12	
Systemic vasculitis (overall)[c]	96	38.6 (31.3–47.2)

The adult population of the Norwich Health Authority is 414 000
[a]Arteritis diagnosed on clinical or histological evidence.
[b]Infection, carcinoma, cryoglobulinaemia.
[c]Overall figure excludes giant cell arteritis and localized cutaneous vasculitis.

Historical

Kussmaul and Maier (1866) are credited with the first description of 'periarteritis nodosa' in 1866 when they described a 'new disease' characterized by numerous nodules along the course of small muscular arteries. Earlier descriptions by Rokitansky (1852), Pelletan (1810), and possibly by Michaelis and Matani (1755) referenced by Lamb (1914), suggest that formal recording of the disease is at least 200 years old.

In the early part of the twentieth century there were large numbers of reports of vasculitis labelled as periarteritis nodosa, including patients with rheumatic fever (von Glahn and Pappenheimer 1926), hypersensitivity states in animals and man (Rich 1942; Rich and Gregory 1943), and most cases with histological evidence of vasculitis affecting any size of vessel, leading to considerable confusion.

In 1952, Zeek reviewed the literature relating to vasculitis and periarteritis nodosa and used the generic term 'necrotizing angiitis' to indicate the specific damage to the blood vessel wall rather than the presence of anti-inflammatory cells alone (see above); she classified these into five distinct entities: (i) hypersensitivity angiitis, (ii) allergic granulomatous angiitis, (iii) rheumatic arteritis, (iv) periarteritis nodosa, and (v) temporal arteritis. Almost all modern classifications are based on this system, which essentially combined histological changes and clinical features. Refinements included use of the term polyarteritis nodosa in the 1950s, the identification of patients with and without lung involvement (Rose and Spencer 1957), and the relationship between vasculitis and granuloma formation discussed by Alarcon-Segovia and Brown (1964), who considered the vasculitides to represent 'a continuous spectrum of tissue changes ranging from pure necrosis and granuloma formation to pure angiitis'. Two notable omissions from Zeek's classification were Wegener's granulo-

matosis and Takayasu's arteritis; these were not fully described in the English literature until after 1953 (Lie 1988).

1970 to 1990

In the 1970s it was realized that there was a considerable overlap in the size of arteries involved (Gilliam and Smiley 1976). At this time Fauci advocated a classification scheme which, apart from including more conditions, also included Churg–Strauss syndrome in an overlapping group of systemic necrotizing vasculitides (Fauci *et al.* 1978).

During the 1980s, classification schemes developed based on the histopathological changes, in particular the size of the predominant vessel involved (e.g. Scott 1988; Lie 1988; Lie 1994). Lie also included a group of infectious vasculitides and vasculitis 'look-alikes'. The latter group includes atheroembolism which can present with clinical features very similar to polyarteritis nodosa. Furthermore he divided the vasculitides into primary and secondary vasculitis, that is vasculitis of unknown aetiology and that occurring secondary to either an infection or some other disease process, typically an autoimmune rheumatic disease.

Current classifications

In 1993 an international consensus conference was convened in Chapel Hill (**CHCC**) which developed definitions for the nomenclature of the systemic vasculitides based on clinical and laboratory features (Table 2) and a new classification scheme based on vessel size (Jeanette *et al.* 1994).

This and other current classification schemes have not addressed pathogenic mechanisms, in particular the relationship between ANCA and systemic vasculitis. Antibodies directed against proteinase 3 are associated strongly with Wegener's granulomatosis and those against myeloperoxidase with microscopic polyangiitis.

All previous studies required either histopathological or angiographic evidence of vasculitis. The increasing use of tests for ANCA, in particular, has resulted in some patients having a diagnosis of vasculitis made without biopsy or angiographic confirmation and this has resulted in changes in diagnostic emphasis. For example the increase in Wegener's granulomatosis seen in Leicester (United Kingdom) during the 1980s was attributed partly to increased diagnostic awareness following introduction of assays for ANCA (Andrews *et al.* 1990). If a classification system is to be useful then it should reflect aetiopathogenesis and/or approaches to treatment.

We feel that because of these developments the CHCC system is inadequate and we have developed a modification (Table 3) which reflects not only dominant vessel size but also ANCA (Scott and Watts 1994). Unlike the CHCC classification we have split Wegener's granulomatosis, Churg–Strauss syndrome, and microscopic polyangiitis from the rest because: (i) they often involve small arteries; (ii) they are diseases most commonly associated with ANCA; (iii) they are associated with a high risk of glomerulonephritis; and (iv) they are diseases which respond best to immunosuppresion with cyclophosphamide. The aetiology of these diseases is probably unrelated to immune complex formation, in contrast to pure small-vessel vasculitis such as Henoch–Schönlein purpura and essential mixed cryoglobulinaemia. Our classification also reflects broad therapeutic strategies (Table 4), with the medium and small vessel group responding best to immunosuppression with cyclophosphamide in addition to corticosteroids, the large vessel group requiring

Table 2 Names and definitions of vasculitides adopted by the Chapel Hill Consensus conference on the nomenclature of systemic vasculitis[a]

Large vessel vasculitis Giant cell (temporal) arteritis	Granulomatous arteritis of the aorta and its major branches, with a predilection for the extracranial branches of the carotid artery. *Often involves the temporal artery. Usually occurs in patients older than 50 and often is associated with polymyalgia rheumatica.*
Takayasu's arteritis	Granulomatous inflammation of the aorta and its major branches. *Usually occurs in patients younger than 50.*
Medium-sized vessel vasculitis Polyarteritis nodosa[b] (classic polyarteritis nodosa)	Necrotizing inflammation of medium-sized or small arteries without glomerulo-nephritis or vasculitis in arterioles, capillaries, or venules.
Kawasaki disease	Arteritis involving large, medium-sized, small arteries, and associated with mucocutaneous lymph node syndrome. *Coronary arteries are often involved. Aorta and veins may be involved. Usually occurs in children.*
Small vessel vasculitis Wegener's granulomatosis[c]	Granulomatous inflammation involving the respiratory tract, and necrotizing vasculitis affecting small to medium-sized vessels (e.g. capillaries, venules, arterioles, and arteries). *Necrotizing glomerulonephritis is common.*
Churg–Strauss syndrome[c]	Eosinophil-rich and granulomatous inflammation involving the respiratory tract, necrotizing vasculitis affecting small to medium-sized vessels, and associated with asthma and eosinophilia.
Microscopic polyangiitis[b] (microscopic polyarteritis)[c]	Necrotizing vasculitis, with few or no immune deposits, affecting small vessels (i.e. capillaries, venules, or arterioles). *Necrotizing arteritis involving small and medium-sized arteries may be present. Necrotizing glomerulonephritis is very common. Pulmonary capillaritis often occurs.*
Henoch–Schönlein purpura	Vasculitis, with IgA-dominant immune deposits, affecting small vessels (i.e. capillaries, venules, or arterioles). *Typically involves skin, gut, and glomeruli, and is associated arthralgia or arthritis.*
Essential cryoglobulinaemic vasculitis	Vasculitis, with cryoglobulin immune deposits, affecting small vessels (i.e. capillaries, venules, or arterioles), and associated with cryoglobulins in serum. *Skin and glomeruli are often involved.*
Cutaneous leucocytoclastic vasculitis	Isolated cutaneous leucocytoclastic angiitis without systemic vasculitis or glomerulonephritis.

[a]Large vessel refers to the aorta and the largest branches directed towards the major body regions (e.g. to the extremities and the head and neck); medium-sized vessel refers to the main visceral arteries (e.g. renal, hepatic, coronary, and mesenteric arteries); small vessel refers to venules, capillaries, arterioles, and the intraparenchymal distal arterial radicals that connect with arterioles. Some small and large vessel vasculitides may involve medium-sized arteries, but large and medium-sized vessel vasculitides do not involve vessels smaller than arteries. Essential components are represented by normal type; italicized type represents usual, but not essential, components.
[b]Preferred term.
[c]Strongly associated with antineutrophil cytoplasmic antibodies.
Reproduced from Jeanette *et al.* (1994) with permission.

moderate- to high-dose corticosteroids, usually alone, and the small vessel group only sometimes requiring corticosteroids at a low dose.

Despite these developments in classification and definition of the vasculitides a number of problems still remain. There is still considerable overlap between the groups (Fig. 2). For example palpable purpura due to leucocytoclastic vasculitis of small vessels affects up to 20 per cent of patients with 'polyarteritis nodosa' as defined in studies by Cohan and Adu (Cohan *et al.* 1980; Adu *et al.* 1987), but the CHCC definition of polyarteritis nodosa specifically excludes such microscopic/small vessel involvement. Necrotizing arteritis can involve the temporal arteries, mimicking giant cell arteritis (Morgan and Harris 1978; Fraha and Abu-Haider 1979). Giant cell arteritis itself can affect smaller vessels in the breast (Potter *et al.* 1981) and mimic carcinoma, and also involve the posterior ciliary artery resulting in blindness. Classification should thus be based on dominant vessel size and not be over-restrictive. The CHCC classification

has not received universal acceptance because of these problems (Lie 1994).

Localized vasculitis produces particular problems in classification. It is important to exclude systemic symptoms and so confirm the benign nature of the vasculitis with long-term follow-up studies. Localized 'polyarteritis nodosa' has been described in a number of sites, including the gall bladder, uterus, and skin (Remigo and Zaino 1970; Borrie 1972; Diaz-Perez and Winkelmann 1974; Scott *et al.* 1982). Whether any of the described cases represents vasculitis truly localized to an individual vessel is debatable, but the lack of progression of cutaneous polyarteritis in long-term studies emphasizes that these cases should be classified and treated differently to their systemic counterparts.

The concept of localized giant-cell arteritis is more difficult. Most cases have arteritis restricted to the head and neck, but there are sporadic reports of giant cell arteritis at other sites, including the

Table 3 Classification of systemic vasculitis

Dominant vessel involved	Primary	Secondary
Large arteries	Giant cell arteritis Takayasu's arteritis Isolated CNS angitis	Aortitis associated with RA Infection (e.g. syphilis)
Medium arteries	Classical PAN Kawasaki disease	Infection (e.g. hepatitis B) Hairy cell leukaemia
Small vessels and medium arteries	Wegener's granulomatosis[a] Churg–Strauss syndrome[a] Microscopic polyangiitis[a]	Vasculitis 2° to RA, SLE, SS Drugs, malignancy Infection (e.g. HIV)
Small vessels (leucocytoclastic)	Henoch–Schönlein purpura Essential mixed cryoglobulinaemia Cutaneous leucocytoclastic angiitis	Drugs[b], malignancy Infection (e.g. hepatitis B,C)

[a]Diseases most commonly associated with ANCA (antimyeloperoxidase and antiproteinase 3 antibodies), a significant risk of renal involvement, and which are most responsive to immunosuppression with cyclophosphamide.
[b]e.g. sulphonamides, penicillins, thiazide diuretics, and many others.
CNS, central nervous system; HIV, human immunodeficiency virus; PAN, polyarteritis nodosa; RA, rheumatoid arthritis; SLE, systemic lupus erythematosus; SS, Sjögren's syndrome.
From Scott and Watts (1994).

Table 4 Relationship between vessel size and response to treatment

Dominant vessel involved	Corticosteroids alone	Cyclophosphamide + corticosteroids	Others
Large arteries	+++	−	+
Medium arteries	+	++	++[a]
Small vessels and medium arteries	+	+++	−
Small vessels	+	−	++

[a]Includes plasmapheresis, antiviral therapy for hepatitis B associated vasculitis, and intravenous immunoglobulin for Kawasaki disease.
Reproduced from Scott and Watts (1994) with permission.

aorta, breast, and skin (Klein *et al.* 1975; Potter *et al.* 1981; Goldberg *et al.* 1987; Smith *et al.* 1988). The most convincing case of localized giant-cell arteritis was a mesenteric arteritis leading to bowel perforation; there was no evidence of giant cell arteritis at other sites and the patient remained well after surgery, requiring no drug therapy during an 18 month follow-up (Smith *et al.* 1988). Such cases stress the importance of the word 'systemic' in classification of arteritis, and the importance of detailed investigations, including histology, before embarking on potentially harmful drug treatment.

Rheumatoid vasculitis also causes problems with classification (see Table 3). A wide range of vessels may be involved, from digital capillaries to medium-sized arteries. Aortitis involving the aortic arch has been described in a few cases, so classification can involve all four groups. Aneurysms have been described rarely (indicating true involvement of medium-sized arteries) but we have seen arteritic changes on angiograms in four patients with severe systemic rheumatoid vasculitis.

Classification criteria for individual vasculitides

The American College of Rheumatology (**ACR**) has now published criteria for the classification of vasculitis (Fries *et al.* 1990). This series of papers describes 807 patients with seven different vasculitic diseases—polyarteritis nodosa, Wegener's granulomatosis,

Churg–Strauss vasculitis, hypersensitivity vasculitis, Henoch–Schönlein purpura, giant cell arteritis and Takayasu's arteritis, seen in 48 medical centres in North America. These patients have been analysed to look for classification criteria for each specific disease; that is, those clinical findings that both identify the disease and separate it from others. The authors stress the classification criteria provide a standard way of evaluating and describing groups of patients in therapeutic, epidemiological, or other studies. A list of the proportion of patients in a group that fulfils the criteria gives considerable information about the clinical status of the patients included. The ACR criteria were presented in two forms: a traditional table and a tree format. The sensitivity and specificity rates varied considerably: 71.0 to 95.3 per cent for sensitivity and 78.7 to 99.7 per cent for specificity (Fries *et al.* 1990; Hunder *et al.* 1990). The most sensitive and specific criteria were found in Churg–Strauss syndrome, giant cell arteritis and Takayasu's arteritis; hypersensitivity vasculitis was the least well-defined condition. The criteria were not tested against the general population or against patients with other autoimmune rheumatic diseases or rheumatic conditions. These papers are important as for the first time they enable comparison of patients reported in an uniform manner—a problem which hitherto has bedevilled the study of vasculitis.

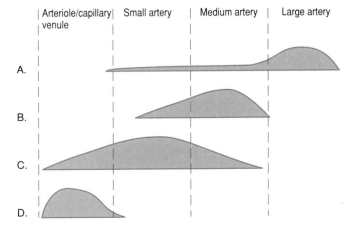

Fig. 2 Relationship between vessel size and classification.

Polyarteritis nodosa and microscopic polyangiitis

Polyarteritis nodosa is a multisystem disease characterized by inflammation and necrosis of medium-sized muscular arteries leading to aneurysm formation and organ infarction (Kussmaul and Maier 1866). Davson in 1948 showed that in some patients who at autopsy had extrarenal vasculitis involving small and medium arteries, the only detectable renal lesion was capillary inflammation (Davson *et al.* 1948). These patients have been said to have 'microscopic' polyarteritis. The main clinical feature in these patients is rapidly progressive renal failure. This is in contrast to patients in whom the dominant involvement is of medium-sized arteries, the condition now called 'classical' polyarteritis nodosa, with organ infarction as the main clinical feature (e.g. gut, nerve, or renal infarction). Microscopic polyarteritis is associated with ANCA, usually of myeloperoxidase specificity, unlike classical polyarteritis nodosa which is usually ANCA negative.

The ACR (1990) described criteria for classical polyarteritis nodosa but not for microscopic polyarteritis. The classification criteria for polyarteritis nodosa are given in Table 5 and have greater than 80 per cent specificity and sensitivity (Lightfoot *et al.* 1990). A classification tree was also constructed using the following six criteria: angiographic abnormality (Fig. 3), biopsy-proven granulocyte or mixed leucocyte infiltrate in arterial wall, neuropathy, sex, weight loss greater than 6.5 kg, and elevation of serum hepatic enzymes. This gave a sensitivity of 87.3 per cent and specificity of 89.3 per cent. These ACR criteria do not have an absolute requirement for a tissue diagnosis or arteriographic abnormality to make the diagnosis of polyarteritis nodosa.

The CHCC specifically addressed the definition of both classical and microscopic polyarteritis (Table 2) (Jeanette *et al.* 1994). They

defined classical polyarteritis nodosa as a disease of medium- and small-sized arterites without glomerulonephritis or vasculitis in arterioles, capillaries, or venules. This complete exclusion of small vessel disease has caused controversy because some patients show considerable overlap. A segmental necrotizing glomerulonephritis can occur in some patients with aneurysms of medium arteries. More commonly segmental necrotizing glomerulonephritis occurs without evidence of interlobar or interlobular arteritis and this explains why the concept of microscopic polyarteritis nodosa was introduced (Wainwright and Davson 1950). The glomerulonephritis in microscopic polyangiitis and Wegener's granulomatosis is similar to other vasculitic diseases, including systemic lupus erythematosus and Henoch–Schönlein purpura, except for the very low levels of immunoglobulin or complement deposition. The term 'pauci-immune' glomerulonephritis is sometimes used. The CHCC defined microscopic polyarteritis as a necrotizing vasculitis predominately affecting small vessels but small- and medium-sized arteries may be involved. They prefer, as we do, the term microscopic polyangiitis for this pattern of disease, emphasizing the difference between it and classical polyarteritis nodosa.

Polyarteritis nodosa has always been a rare disease with an estimated annual incidence of 2 to 10 per million (Sack *et al.* 1975; Scott *et al.* 1982; Kurland *et al.* 1984). Detailed analysis of the patients in these studies suggests that they included some patients with microscopic polyangiitis and Churg–Strauss syndrome, and hence that the annual incidence may be less than they reported. Using the CHCC definition of classical polyarteritis nodosa we have not seen a single case since 1988, suggesting that it has become a very rare disease. However, comparing the ACR criteria for polyarteritis nodosa with the CHCC definitions we have seen five patients with microscopic polyangiitis who fulfil the ACR criteria for polyarteritis nodosa and a further five with microscopic polyangiitis who do not.

Table 5 ACR 1990 criteria for the classification of polyarteritis nodosa (traditional format)

Criterion	Definition
1. Weight loss ≥ 4 kg	Loss of 4 kg or more of body weight since illness began, not due to dieting or other factors
2. Livedo reticularis	Mottled retricular pattern over the skin of portions of the extremities or torso
3. Testicular pain or tenderness	Pain or tenderness of the testicles, not due to infection, trauma, or other causes
4. Myalgias, weakness, or leg tenderness	Diffuse myalgias (excluding shoulder and hip girdle) or weakness of muscles or tenderness of leg muscles
5. Mononeuropathy or polyneuropathy	Development of mononeuropathy, multiple mononeuropathies, or polyneuropathy
6. Diastolic BP > 90 mmHg	Development of hypertension with the diastolic BP higher than 90 mmHg
7. Elevated blood area or creatinine	Elevation of BUN > 40 mg/dl or creatinine > 1.5 mg/dl, not due to dehydration or obstruction
8. Hepatitis B virus	Presence of hepatitis B surface antigen or antibody in serum
9. Arteriographic abnormality	Arteriogram showing aneurysms or occulsions of the visceral arteries, not due to arteriosclerosis, fibromuscular dysplasia, or other non-inflammatory causes
10. Biopsy of small or medium-sized artery containing PMN	Histological changes showing the presence of granulocytes or granulocytes and mononuclear leucocytes in the artery wall

For classification purposes, a patient shall be said to have polyarteritis nodosa if at least three of these ten criteria are present. The presence of any three or more criteria yields a sensitivity of 82.2% and a specificity of 86.6%. BP, blood pressure; BUN, blood urea nitrogen; PMN, polymorphonuclear neutrophils.
Reproduced from Lightfoot *et al.* (1990) with permission.

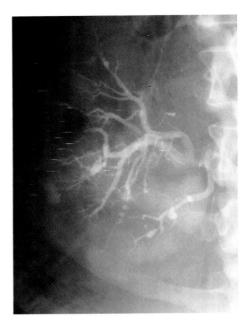

Fig. 3 Renal angiogram showing typical small aneurysms.

Seven of these ten patients with microscopic polyangiitis are ANCA positive.

The annual incidence of microscopic polyangiitis in Leicester (United Kingdom) increased from 0.5 to 3.3 per million following the introduction of the ANCA test in 1987 (Andrews *et al.* 1990). Data from our epidemiological studies in Norwich suggest that the annual incidence of microscopic polyangiitis is very similar at 2.4 per million (Watts *et al.* 1995) Whether these changes in incidence represent a true change or reflect changes in diagnostic patterns is uncertain.

Wegener's granulomatosis (see also Chapter 5.11.2)

Wegener first described this form of granulomatous necrotizing vasculitis in 1936 (Wegener 1936). The disease is characterized by necrotizing granulomata of the upper and lower respiratory tract, a necrotizing systemic vasculitis, and a focal glomerulonephritis (Godman and Churg 1954). A more limited form of the disease has been described with lesions restricted to the upper and lower respiratory tract (Carrington and Liebow 1966). This was thought to represent a more benign form of the disease because of the absence of overt renal disease, although 5 out of 16 patients died from non-renal disease within 1 year of diagnosis. Respiratory tract disease may precede systemic and renal vaculitis by many months or years. DeRemee classified Wegener's granulomatosis on the basis of the organs involved (ELK) — E standing for ear, nose, throat; L for lung involvement; and K for kidney involvement (DeRemee *et al.* 1976). This classification has proved useful in staging patients with the disease, but presupposes a progression from E–L–K, which does not always occur. Patients may present with pulmonary or renal involvement. More recently this progression has been viewed as a continous spectrum which may be entered at any point (Luqmani *et al.* 1994a).

The ACR 1990 classification criteria for the diagnosis of Wegener's granulomatosis are shown in traditional format in Table 6 (Leavitt *et al.* 1990). A classification tree was also constructed with five criteria: the same four criteria plus haemoptysis. This gave a sensitivity of 87.1 per cent and specificity of 93.6 per cent.

The CHCC definition restricts the term Wegener's granulomatosis to patients with necrotizing granulomatous inflammation (Table 2) (Jeanette *et al.* 1994). In the earlier stages of disease there may be overlap between Wegener's granulomatosis and microscopic polyangiitis, and subsequently the illness may evolve with development of new inflammatory lesions. Neither the CHCC nor the ACR classification scheme address the issue of limited disease.

The incidence of Wegener's granulomatosis appears to be increasing. In 1980 to 1986 in Leicester (United Kingdom) the annual incidence of Wegener's granulomatosis was estimated to be 0.7 per million, while in 1987 to 1989 the incidence was 2.8 per million (Andrews *et al.* 1990). In Norwich during the period 1988 to 1994 the estimated annual incidence was 8.5 per million (Carruthers *et al.* 1996). This does not appear to be due to changing diagnostic criteria as we have compared the clinical features of our patients to those seen at the National Institutes of Health (**NIH**, United States; 1962 to 1983) and Birmingham (United Kingdom;

Table 6   ACR 1990 criteria for the classification of Wegener's granulomatosis (traditional format)

Criterion	Definition
1. Nasal or oral inflammation	Development of painful or painless oral ulcers, or purulent or bloody nasal discharge
2. Abnormal chest radiograph	Chest radiograph showing the presence of nodules, fixed infiltrates, or cavities
3. Urinary sediment	Microhaematuria (>5 red blood cells per high power field) or red cell casts in urine sediment
4. Granulomatous inflammation on biopsy	Histological changes showing granulomatous inflammation within the wall of an artery or in the perivascular or extravascular area (artery or arteriole)

For purposes of classification, a person shall be said to have Wegener's granulomatosis if at least two of these four criteria are present. The presence of any two or more criteria yields a sensitivity of 88.2% and a specificity of 92.0%.
Reproduced from Leavitt *et al.* (1990) with permission.

1981 to 1991) and did not find any significant differences between the three groups. The Leicester group used the same diagnostic criteria as the NIH. It is, however, noteworthy that as the annual incidence of Wegener's granulomatosis has apparently increased that of classical polyarteritis nodosa has decreased, suggesting that some patients formerly labelled as polyarteritis nodosa may now be reclassified as Wegener's granulomatosis.

Churg–Strauss syndrome

In 1951, Churg and Strauss described the postmortem features of 13 patients who died following an illness characterized by asthma, eosinophilia, fever, and a systemic illness (Churg and Strauss 1951). Histologically there is a granulomatous necrotizing vasculitis. Chumbley, in 1977, reported a series of 30 patients with Churg–Strauss syndrome, and stressed the relative infrequent occurrence of renal involvement (Chumbley et al. 1977). Lanham, in 1984, provided a clinical definition of Churg–Strauss syndrome as a triad of asthma, eosinophilia (greater than $1 \times 10^9/l$), and a systemic vasculitis involving two or more extrapulmonary organs (Lanham et al. 1984). In their experience extravascular granulomata were not essential for the diagnosis of Churg–Strauss syndrome. They also noted a triphasic pattern of illness with allergic rhinitis, evolving into asthma; followed by peripheral blood eosinophilia and eosinophilic tissue infiltrates; and finally a systemic vasculitis phase. The granulomata may be localized and associated with a variety of systemic manifestations. Furthermore the necrotizing vasculitis may be indistinguishable from that found in classical polyarteritis nodosa and/or microscopic polyangiitis.

The ACR criteria for the diagnosis of Churg–Strauss syndrome are given in Table 7 (Masi et al. 1990). These criteria do not include some common clinical features of Churg–Strauss syndrome such as rash or cardiac involvement, as they gave poor discrimination. The combination of asthma and eosinophilia are both sensitive and highly specific for the diagnosis of Churg–Strauss syndrome. A classification tree was also constructed using three of six criteria that gave a sensitivity of 95 per cent and a specificity of 99.2 per cent.

The CHCC definition of Churg–Strauss syndrome (Table 2) includes the presence of asthma and eosinophilia (Jeanette et al. 1994). The presence of conspicious eosinophils in inflammatory infiltrates is not alone a discriminating feature as they can occur in other types of vasculitis including Wegener's granulomatosis and microscopic polyangiitis.

The annual incidence of Churg–Strauss syndrome has been estimated to be 2.4 per million (Watts et al. 1995).

Hypersensitivity vasculitis

Vasculitis occurring secondary to allergic or hypersensitivity mechanisms has been considered to be a distinct entity since the late 1940s (Zeek et al. 1948) and was included in Zeek's original classification (Zeek 1952). Distinguishing features were considered to be the prominent cutaneous involvement and frequent precipitation by serum or drugs. Pathologically the disease involves small vessels with leucocytoclasis. The lesions are all of the same age and can be induced experimentally. However, often there is no clear evidence of an inciting agent and a similar picture can be seen in vasculitis associated with connective tissue disease (rheumatoid arthritis, systemic lupus erythematosus, Sjögren's syndrome), malignancy, Henoch–Schönlein purpura, and cryoglobulinaemia.

The ACR 1990 criteria for the diagnosis of hypersensitivity vasculitis were relatively insensitive (71.0 per cent) and non-specific (78.5 per cent). This reflects the occurrence of a hypersensitivity-like picture in other conditions, particularly Henoch–Schönlein purpura and microscopic polyangiitis, and some authorities consider these conditions to represent different forms of hypersensitivity to foreign antigens (Heng 1985).

The CHCC did not use the term hypersensitivity vasculitis but considered that the 'categories of microscopic polyangiitis and cutaneous leucocytoclastic angiitis probably best equate with the

Table 7	ACR 1990 criteria for the classification of Churg–Strauss syndrome (traditional format)
Criterion	**Definition**
1. Asthma	History of wheezing or diffuse high-pitched rales on expiration
2. Eosinophilia	Eosinophilia > 10% on white blood cell differential count
3. History of allergy[a]	History of seasonal allergy (e.g. allergic rhinitis) or other documented allergies, including food, contactants, and others, except for drug allergy
4. Mononeuropathy or polyneuropathy	Development of mononeuropathy, multiple mononeuropathies, or polyneuropathy (i.e. glove/stocking distribution) attributable to a systemic vasculitis
5. Pulmonary infiltrates, non-fixed	Migratory or transitory pulmonary infiltrates on radiographs (not including fixed infiltrates), attributable to a systemic vasculitis
6. Paranasal sinus abnormality	History of acute or chronic paranasal sinus pain or tenderness or radiographic opacification of the paranasal sinuses
7. Extravascular eosinophils	Biopsy including artery, arteriole, or venule, showing accumulations of eosinophils in extravascular areas

[a]History of allergy, other than asthma or drug related, is included only in the tree classification set and not in the traditional format criteria set, which requires four or more of the other six items listed here. The presence of any four or more criteria yields a sensitivity of 85.0% and a specificity of 99.7%.
Reproduced from Masi et al. (1990) with permission.

most common usage of hypersensitivity vasculitis' (Jeanette *et al*. 1994).

Henoch–Schönlein purpura

Schönlein initially described acute purpura and arthritis occurring in children in 1837 (Schönlein 1837). Subsequently Henoch described the additional features of colicky abdominal pain and nephritis in 1874 (Henoch 1874). The classical presentation is with purpura, arthritis, haemorrhagic gastrointestinal involvement, and glomerulonephritis. It occurs most often in children, but rarely, adults of any age may be affected. Significant IgA deposition is usually seen in renal or skin biopsies. Henoch–Schönlein purpura is often considered to be a form of hypersensitivity vasculitis.

The ACR criteria readily distinguish Henoch–Schönlein purpura from other forms of vasculitis, although it was recognized that there were considerable similarities between Henoch– Schönlein purpura and hypertensitivity vasculitis, both in terms of clinical features and the classification criteria (Mills *et al*. 1990). Palpable purpura was a common criterion for both diseases. Also, although arthritis and nephritis are typical features of Henoch–Schönlein purpura, neither

was sensitive for the diagnosis, and haematuria as a sign of nephritis was neither sensitive nor specific. A classification tree was also constructed with similar criteria and yielded a sensitivity of 89.4 per cent and a specificity of 88.1 per cent (Table 8).

The CHCC definition of Henoch–Schönlein purpura is a small vessel vasculitis with IgA-dominant immune deposits (Table 2) (Jeanette *et al*. 1994). These deposits distinguish Henoch–Schönlein purpura from microscopic polyangiitis. The CHCC did not consider other types of immune-complex mediated disease apart from cryoglobulinaemic vasculitis.

The annual incidence of Henoch–Schönlein purpura in children is 135 per million (Stewart *et al*. 1988). Our data from Norwich suggest that the annual incidence in adults is 1.2 per million (Watts *et al*. 1995).

Takayasu's arteritis

Takayasu's arteritis is a chronic, granulomatous large-vessel arteritis which was described in 1908 by Takayasu (Takayasu 1908), but Savory had described the association between the absence of radial pulses and ocular abnormalities in 1856 (Savory 1856).

Table 8 ACR 1990 criteria for the classification of Henoch–Schönlein purpura (traditional format)

Criterion	Definition
1. Palpable purpura	Slightly raised 'palpable' haemorrhagic skin lesions, not related to thrombocytopenia
2. Age < 20 years	Patient 20 years or younger at onset of first symptom
3. Bowel angina	Diffuse abdominal pain, worse after meals, or the diagnosis of bowel ischaemia, usually including bloody diarrhoea
4. Wall granulocytes on biopsy	Histological changes showing granulocytes in the walls of arterioles or venules

For purposes of classification, a patient shall be said to have Henoch–Schönlein purpura if at least two of these four criteria are present. The presence of any two or more criteria yields a sensitivity of 87.1% and a specificity of 87.7%.
Reproduced from Mills *et al*. (1990) with permission.

Table 9 ACR 1990 criteria for the classification of Takayasu's arteritis (traditional format)

Criterion	Definition
1. Age at disease onset < 40 years	Development of symptoms or findings related to Takayasu's arteritis at age < 40 years
2. Claudication of extremities	Development and worsening of fatigue and discomfort in muscles of one or more extremity while in use, especially the upper extremities
3. Decreased brachial artery pulse	Decreased pulsation of one or both brachial arteries
4. BP difference > 10 mmHg	Difference of > 10 mmHg in systolic blood pressure between arms
5. Bruit over subclavian arteries or aorta	Bruit audible on auscultation over one or both subclavian arteries or abdominal aorta
6. Arteriogram abnormality	Arteriographic narrowing or occlusion of the entire aorta, its proximal branches, or large arteries in the proximal upper or lower extremities, not due to arteriosclerosis, fibromuscular dysplasia, or similar causes; changes usually focal or segmental

For purposes of classification, a patient shall be said to have Takayasu's arteritis if at least three of these six criteria are present. The presence of any three or more criteria yields a sensitivity of 90.5% and a specificity of 97.8%. BP, blood pressure.
Reproduced from Arend *et al*. (1990) with permission.

Ishikawa proposed diagnostic criteria for Takayasu's arteritis in 1988 and suggested that an age of less than 40 years should be an obligatory criterion for the diagnosis (Ishikawa 1986). In this study of 96 Japanese patients with Takayasu's arteritis two major criteria were proposed: arteriographic evidence of left or right mid-subclavian artery stenosis or occlusion. In addition minor diagnostic criteria were described: high erthrocyte sedimentation rate, carotid artery tenderness, hypertension, aortic regurgitation, or arteriographic evidence of lesions in other branches of the aorta. The presence of both major, or one major and two minor, or four or more minor criteria suggested a diagnosis of Takayasu's arteritis with a sensitivity of 84 per cent (Ishikawa 1986). These patients were, however, only compared with 12 patients having other aortic disease and not to patients with other forms of vasculitis.

The ACR classification criteria for the diagnosis of Takayasu's arteritis are given in Table 9 (Arend *et al*. 1990). Takayasu's arteritis is clearly distinguished from giant cell arteritis by age. A high erthrocyte sedimentation rate, carotid artery tenderness, and/or hypertension lack specificity and sensitivity to differentiate patients with Takayasu's arteritis from other forms of arteritis. A classification tree was also constructed with five of the same six criteria omitting claudication of a limb. This gave a sensitivity of 92.1 per cent and specificity of 97.0 per cent.

The CHCC considered Takayasu's arteritis to be a granulomatous inflammation of the aorta and its branches 'usually' occurring in patients younger than 50 years (Table 2) (Jeanette *et al*. 1994). They recognized that age is a useful discriminator between Tayakasu's arteritis and giant cell arteritis.

Takayasu's arteritis is rare in the United States with an annual incidence of up to 2.6 per million (Hall *et al*. 1985), but much more common in Japan and the Far East. In the United Kingdom we have not seen a single case from the Norwich Health District in 7 years. However, 7 cases were seen in the West Midlands from a population of 6 million during an 8-year period in the 1990s, suggesting a much lower annual incidence (0.14 per million) (D.G.I. Scott, unpublished data).

Kawasaki disease

Kawasaki disease (mucocutaneous lymph node syndrome) is an acute vasculitis of unknown aetiology that primarily affects infants and young children, and was first described in Japan in 1967 (Kawasaki 1967). Coronary vasculitis is a major cause of morbidity and mortality.

There is no laboratory test for the diagnosis of Kawasaki disease and the diagnosis is therefore based on standard clinical criteria (Table 10) (Rauch and Hurwitz 1985). There are several problems with these criteria. Some patients who do not fulfil the criteria develop coronary artery disease; also the mucocutaneous features are very variable. Burns and colleagues compared 280 patients with acute Kawasaki disease with 42 patients evaluated for Kawasaki disease in whom other diagnoses were eventually made (Burns *et al*. 1991). They found considerable overlap between the two groups with 46 per cent of the control group satisfying the criteria for Kawasaki disease. The most common alternative diagnoses were measles and group A β-haemolytic streptococcal infection.

The ACR did not develop criteria for Kawasaki disease. The CHCC considered Kawasaki disease and felt that the presence of mucocutaneous lymph node syndrome is the defining feature that separates Kawasaki disease from juvenile polyarteritis nodosa

Table 10 Diagnostic criteria for Kawasaki disease

Fever of at least 5 days duration

Presence of at least four of the five following conditions

1. Bilateral non-exudative conjunctival injection
2. One of the following changes in oropharynx:
   injected or fissured lips, injected pharynx, or 'strawberry tongue'
3. One of the following extremity changes:
   erythema of the palms or soles, oedema of the hands or feet, or periungual desquamation
4. Rash, primarily polymorphous but not vesicular
5. Acute non-suppurative cervical lymphadenopathy

Illness not explained by an other known disease process

From Rauch and Hurwitz (1985).

(Jeanette *et al*. 1994). The absence of involvement of vessels smaller than arteries in their view distinguishes Kawasaki disease from microscopic polyangiitis, this is however controversial as involvement of small vessels has been described (Lie 1994).

Other vasculitides

The CHCC also considered essential cryoglobulinaemic vasculitis, cutaneous leucocytoclastic vasculitis, and giant cell arteritis. Classification criteria for giant cell arteritis are considered elsewhere.

Cryoglobulins are plasma proteins which reversibly precipitate in the cold and have been classified on the basis of the type of immunoglobulin contained within the cryoprecipitate. Types II and III contain two types of immunoglobulin (mixed cryoglobulinaemia) and are associated with a small vessel vasculitis. They may occur in the absence of underlying disease (essential mixed cryoglobulinaemia).

Cutaneous leucocytoclastic vasculitis is confined to patients in whom there is no evidence of systemic involvement. These patients have a much better prognosis. Other systemic vasculitides must be excluded rigorously. Those patients with elevated levels of immune complexes are at greater risk of immune-complex mediated disease such as Henoch–Schönlein purpura and cryoglobulinaemic vasculitis, whilst those with ANCA are at risk of developing an ANCA-associated disease (e.g. Wegener's granulomatosis).

The development of the ACR criteria and the CHCC definitions have been important steps in improving the classification and definition of the systemic vasculitides. However, despite the use of these criteria a significant number of patients cannot be classified;. in our experience approximately 10 per cent. It is possible that some of these will evolve into typical forms of systemic vasculitis, but others may represent rarer forms which are currently poorly documented and understood.

Secondary vasculitis

Vasculitis occurring as a consequence of an autoimmune rheumatic disease is relatively common and is in our experience the commonest

Table 11   Classification criteria for systemic rheumatoid vasculitis

The presence in a patient with rheumatoid arthritis of one or more of :

1. Mononeuritis multiplex or acute peripheral neuropathy

2. Peripheral gangrene

3. Biopsy evidence of acute necrotizing arteritis plus systemic illness (e.g. fever, weight loss)

4. Deep cutaneous ulcers or active extra-articular disease (e.g. pleurisy, pericarditis, scleritis) if associated with typical digital infarcts or biopsy evidence of vasculitis

Other causes of such lesions such as diabetes mellitus and atherosclerosis should be excluded. Patients with nailfold or digital infarcts alone are excluded.
From Scott and Bacon (1984).

cause of systemic vasculitis, particularly secondary to rheumatoid arthritis and systemic lupus erythematosus (Table 1). It may also occur in dermatomyositis, scleroderma, overlap syndromes, Sjögren's syndrome, rheumatic fever, and relapsing polychondritis. Classification criteria are not well established except for vasculitis occurring secondary to rheumatoid arthritis.

Rheumatoid arthritis

Vasculitis complicating rheumtoid arthritis was first described in 1898, in a patient with involvement of the vasa nervorum (Bannatyne 1898). The association was clearly established in the 1940s and 1950s (Bywaters 1949; Bywaters 1957). The classical features are peripheral gangrene and mononeuritis multiplex (Hart *et al.* 1957; Pallis and Scott 1965). However, pericarditis, scleritis, nodules, and systemic disease occur frequently, and more recent series have described a wider spectrum of disease (Scott *et al.* 1981; Luqmani *et al.* 1994b). The size of vessel involved ranges from the aorta to capillaries. Small vessel vasculitis can occur in isolation as small nail-edge or nailfold lesions. These lesions are generally considered to be benign but can herald or coexist with major arterial disease (Bywaters 1957; Bywaters and Scott 1963). Systemic rheumatoid vasculitis occurs more commonly in males with longstanding rheumatoid arthritis who are strongly seropositive for rheumatoid factor (Scott *et al.* 1981; Luqmani *et al.* 1994b).

Scott and Bacon proposed criteria for the definition of systemic rheumatoid vasculitis (Table 11) (Scott and Bacon 1984). An obligatory criterion was the presence of established rheumatoid arthritis as defined by the ACR. This should prevent confusion with other forms of either primary or secondary vasculitis as such patients are unlikely to meet the ACR criteria for the diagnosis of rheumatoid arthritis. However, these criteria have not been validated formally.

In our experience systemic rheumatoid vasculitis as defined by the Scott and Bacon criteria is amongst the commonest forms of systemic vasculitis with an annual incidence of 12.5 per million (Watts *et al.* 1994).

Aetiology

The 'best' classification system should involve the aetiological agent responsible for the vascular damage. This is unknown in the majority of cases of vasculitis, but even when it appears to be known there is still considerable confusion. For example, hepatitis B surface antigen has been associated with pure cutaneous vasculitis, cryoglobulinaemic vasculitis, glomerulonephritis, arthritis, and polyarteritis nodosa (Scott 1986). There is also one report of hepatitis B associated with giant cell arteritis (Bacon *et al.* 1975). A similar picture has now emerged with the vasculitis associated with human immunodeficiency virus infection, with descriptions of leucocytoclastic vasculitis, eosinophilic vasculitis, polyarteritis nodosa, granulomatous angiitis, and lymphomatoid granulomatosis (Siefert 1989).

The most frequently postulated pathogenetic mechanism for the production of vasculitis is the deposition of circulating immune complexes. This has been documented particularly in the small vessel vasculitides, though circulating immune complexes have been detected in almost all diseases associated with vasculitis. The activity of these complexes and their relation to pathogenesis is often doubtful; for example complement activation is rare in the group associated with systemic necrotizing arteritis, except in those cases associated with hepatitis B infection. Complement activation is seen much more frequently in small vessel vasculitis (cryoglobulinaemia, Henoch–Schönlein purpura) and vasculitis complicating rheumatoid arthritis and systemic lupus erythematosus.

Other proposed mechanisms include *in situ* formation of immune complexes, direct invasion of the vessel wall by antigen (including virus), antibodies to myelocyte lysosomal enzymes (see below), cytotoxic antibodies to endothelium, and cell-mediated immune reactions to cell-wall antigens. The importance of these mechanisms to classification is as yet undefined, with the possible exception of ANCA.

ANCA

Antineutrophil cytoplasmic antibodies were first described in 1985 as sensitive and specific markers for Wegener's granulomatosis (Van der Woude *et al.* 1985). Since then ANCA have been described in other types of systemic vasculitis (e.g. microscopic polyangiitis) and some non-vasculitic diseases (Gross *et al.* 1993a), and the disease associations and antigenic targets of ANCA have been defined more clearly. Two major staining patterns are seen on indirect immunofluorescence: cytoplasmic (cANCA) and perinuclear (pANCA). Proteinase 3 is the main target antigen of cANCA and is chiefly found in patients with Wegener's granulomatosis, whilst myeloperoxidase is the predominant target antigen of pANCA and is found in microscopic polyangiitis (Falk and Jeanette 1988).

Disease associations of cANCA

cANCA are highly sensitive (81 per cent) and specific for Wegener's granulomatosis (97 per cent) and are directed against proteinase 3 (Gross *et al.* 1993b). The specificity of cANCA for biopsy-proven Wegener's granulomatosis is around 90 per cent (Gross *et al.* 1993b). In limited or initial-phase Wegener's granulomatosis (i.e. upper and lower airways disease only) 55 per cent of patients are cANCA positive, whereas in systemic disease 88 per cent of patients are cANCA positive (Gross *et al.* 1993b). cANCA can be found in types of vasculitis with close clinical and pathological relations to Wegener's granulomatosis, such as microscopic polyangiitis (15 per cent) and Churg–Strauss syndrome (25 per cent), but rarely in classical polyarteritis nodosa (2 per cent) (Hauschild *et al.* 1993). False-positive cANCA (i.e. occurring in non-vasculitic illnesses) are very rare (Gross *et al.* 1993).

Disease association of pANCA

Unlike cANCA, pANCA are not specific for a single disease but are seen in a wide spectrum of disease including: (i) systemic vasculitis, e.g. microscopic polyangiitis, Churg–Strauss syndrome, Wegener's granulomatosis; (ii) necrotizing glomerulonephritis; (iii) rheumatic disease, e.g. rheumatoid arthritis, Still's disease, Felty's syndrome; (iv) autoimmune rheumatic disease, e.g. systemic lupus erythematosus, Sjögren's syndrome; and (v) inflammatory bowel disease. pANCA is present in less than 3 per cent of patients with biopsy-proven Wegener's granulomatosis (Hauschild *et al.* 1993).

The major target autoantigen of pANCA is myeloperoxidase (therefore sometimes called myeloperoxidase-ANCA). Myeloperoxidase-ANCA are found in 70 per cent of patients with microscopic polyangiitis and up to 50 per cent of patients with Churg–Strauss syndrome. pANCA may, however, be targeted against other antigens such as lactoferrin, cathepsin G, human neutrophil elastase, and lysozyme. In these circumstances the immunofluorescence staining pattern may be slightly different from the characteristic pANCA, such a staining pattern is known as atypical or xANCA.

An association between ANCA and extra-articular manifestations of vasculitis in patients with rheumatoid arthritis or Felty's syndrome (Juby *et al.* 1992) has been reported, especially if antibodies to lactoferrin or elastase were present (Coremans *et al.* 1992). Antibodies to cathepsin G have been described in patients with ulcerative colitis (Kallenberg *et al.* 1992). xANCA are detected in sera from patients with an even broader range of diseases including infection and carcinoma (Peter 1993).

Role of ANCA in classification

A classical, cANCA staining pattern strongly suggests a diagnosis of Wegener's granulomatosis in a patient with appropriate clinical findings. However, the presence of ANCA detected by immunofluorescence alone has limited diagnostic value. Indirect immunofluorescence should be followed by antigen-specific assays for proteinase 3 and myeloperoxidase. Proteinase 3 antibodies are associated strongly with Wegener's granulomatosis, myeloperoxidase antibodies less strongly with microscopic polyangiitis. The diagnostic value of a positive ANCA by immunofluorescence which is not directed against proteinase 3 or myeloperoxidase is uncertain. A diagnosis of systemic vasculitis, including Wegener's granulomatosis and necrotizing glomerulonephritis, should not be based on the detection of specific ANCAs alone but should be considered in the correct clinical background. A tissue diagnosis is still frequently needed to confirm the diagnosis.

For broad classification purposes we have grouped Wegener's granulomatosis, microscopic polyangiitis, and Churg–Strauss syndrome together, as they share some clinical and pathological features and are the three diseases most commonly associated with ANCA (Table 3). Using CHCC definitions, other types of vasculitis are much less frequently associated, or have no association, with ANCA.

Prognosis

Twenty years ago, a precise characterization of the different types of vasculitis might have been considered of academic interest only, because of the lack of any specific, effective treatment. Immunosuppressive therapy, particularly with cyclophosphamide, has dramatically changed the outcome of many of the more severe forms of vasculitis, especially Wegener's granulomatosis, polyarteritis nodosa, and systemic rheumatoid vasculitis (Fauci *et al.* 1979; Fauci *et al.* 1983; Scott and Bacon 1984; Hoffman *et al.* 1992; Gordon *et al.* 1993). It is important to diagnose these diseases accurately, not only to instigate early appropriate treatment, but also to avoid using cytotoxic agents (with their potentially severe side-effects) in diseases where their use is unnecessary.

Despite recent therapeutic advances, the vasculitic diseases still have significant morbidity and mortality, reflecting the importance of accurate classification. Prognosis is affected particularly by the size of vessel involved and the presence (or absence) of renal involvement. Up to 40 per cent of patients with polyarteritis nodosa, 20 to 30 per cent with systemic rheumatoid vasculitis, and 10 to 20 per cent with Wegener's granulomatosis, die within a year of diagnosis. Although the terminal event is now more commonly sepsis than uncontrolled vasculitis, the importance of renal involvement in the mortality of systemic vasculitis is shown by comparing those whose serum creatinine is more than 500 mmol/l (47 per cent mortality) with those whose serum creatinine is less than 500 mmol/l (15 per cent mortality) at the time of diagnosis (Adu *et al.* 1987), stressing the danger of any delay in diagnosis. A similar picture is seen in Wegener's granulomatosis, where, in addition, there may be significant morbidity from nasal, laryngeal, or pulmonary involvement. Signifiant renal damage is rare in patients with systemic rheumatoid vasculitis. However, these patients also have a significant morbidity and mortality; the presence of arteritis, either clinically or on biopsy, is associated with a higher mortality (44 per cent) than small vessel disease (20 per cent), where cardiac disease (restrictive pericarditis, aortic regurgitation, etc.) is a common cause of death (Scott and Bacon 1987). All these figures stress the importance of accurate classification, particularly of those patients with vasculitis involving small- or medium-sized arteries.

By contrast the prognosis for small vessel vasculitis is much more favourable. Less than 10 per cent of patients with Henoch–Schönlein purpura develop significant renal involvement and of these only a few develop chronic renal disease. Some patients with essential mixed cryoglobulinaemia develop a polyarteritis-like picture years after presentation (Gorevic *et al.* 1980). Giant cell arteritis and Takayasu's arteritis are rarely fatal but may be associated with significant complications (e.g. blindness and ischaemia).

Conclusion

The systemic vasculitides are a group of important inflammatory conditions resulting in inflammation and necrosis of blood vessel walls. They are somewhat commoner than previously believed with an annual incidence approaching 40 per million. The most common forms of systemic vasculitis are systemic rheumatoid vasculitis (12.5 per million per year) and Wegener's granulomatosis (8.5 per million per year).

Classification criteria and disease definitions are now well established, which should lead to conformity between different centres.

Particular problems still exist with the definition of classical poly-arterits nodosa and microscopic angiitis, and it is important when these terms are employed that the classification criteria used for diagnosis are always given.

Classification systems are still evolving. Recent changes include the recognition of the importance of the dominant blood-vessel size, the distinction between primary and secondary vasculitis, and the incorporation of pathogenetic markers such as ANCA (Table 3).

References

Adu, D., Howi, A.J., Scott, D.G.I., Bacon, P.A., McGonigle, R.J.S., and Michael, J. (1987). Polyarteritis and the kidney. *Quarterly Journal of Medicine*, **62**, 221–37.

Alarcon-Segovia, D. and Brown, A.L. (1964). Classification and aetiologic aspects of necrotising angiitides. *Mayo Clinic Proceedings*, **39**, 205–22.

Andrews, M., Edmunds, M., Campbell, A., Walls, J., and Feehally, J. (1990). Systemic vasculitis in the 1980s — is there an increasing incidence of Wegener's granulomatosis and microscopic polyarteritis? *Journal of the Royal College of Physicians*, **24**, 284–8.

Arend, W.P., Michel, B.A., Block, D.A., *et al.* (1990). The American College of Rheumatology 1990 criteria for the classification of Takayasu's arteritis. *Arthritis and Rheumatism*, **33**, 1129–34.

Bacon, P.A., Doherty, S.M., and Zuckermann, A.J. (1975). Hepatitis-B antibody in poly-myalgia rheumatica. *Lancet*, **ii**, 476–8.

Bannatyne, G.A. (1898). In *Rheumatoid arthritis*, (2nd edn), p. 73. John Wright, Bristol.

Borrie, P. (1972). Cutaneous polyarteritis nodosa. *British Journal of Dermatology*, **87**, 87–95.

Burns, J.C., Mason, W.H., Gode, M.P., *et al.* (1991). Clinical and epidemiological characteristics of possible Kawasaki disease. *Journal of Paediatrics*, **118**, 680–86.

Bywaters, E.G.L. (1949). A variant of rheumatoid arthritis characterized by digital pad nodules and palmar fasciitis, closely resembling palindromic rheumatism. *Annals of the Rheumatic Diseases*, **8**, 2–30.

Bywaters, E.G.L. (1957). Peripheral vascular obstruction in rheumatoid arthritis and its relationship to other vascular lesions. *Annals of the Rheumatic Diseases*, **16**, 84–103.

Bywaters, E.G.L. and Scott, J.T. (1963). The natural history of vascular lesions in rheumatoid arthritis. *Journal of Chronic Diseases*, **16**, 905–14.

Carrington, C.B. and Liebow, A.A. (1966). Limited forms of angiitis and granulo-matosis of Wegener's type. *American Journal of Medicine*, **41**, 497–527.

Carruthers, D., Watts, R.A., Scott, D.G.I., and Symmons, D.P.M. (1996). Wegener's granulomatosis — increased incidence or increased recognition? *British Journal of Rheumatology*, **35**, 142–5.

Chumbley, L.C., Harrison, R.A., and DeRemee, R.A. (1977). Allergic granuloma-tous angiitis (Churg–Strauss syndrome): report and analysis of 30 cases. *Mayo Clinic Proceedings*, **52**, 477–84.

Churg, J. and Strauss, L. (1951). Allergic granulomatosis, allergic angiitis and peri-arteritis nodosa. *American Journal of Pathology*, **27**, 277–301.

Cohan, R.D., Conn, D.L., and Ilstrup, D.M. (1980). Clinical features, prognosis and response to treatment in polyarteritis. *Mayo Clinic Proceedings*, **55**, 146–55.

Coremans, I.E.M., Hagen, E.C., Daha, M.R., *et al.* (1992). Antilactoferrin antibo-dies in patients with rheumatoid arthritis are associated with vasculitis. *Arthritis and Rheumatism*, **35**, 1466–75.

Davson, J., Ball, J., and Platt, R. (1948). The kidney in periarteritis nodosa. *Quarterly Journal of Medicine*, **17**, 175–202

DeRemee, R.A., McDonald, T.J., Harrison, E.G., and Coles, D.T. (1976). Wegener's granulomatosis: anatomic correlates — a proposed classification. *Mayo Clinic Proceedings*, **51**, 777–81.

Diaz-Perek, J.L. and Winkelmann, R.K. (1974). Cutaneous periarteritis nodosa. *Archives of Dermatology*, **110**, 407–14.

Falk, R.J. and Jeanette, J.C. (1988). Antineutrophil cytoplasmic autoantibodies with specificity for myeloperoxidase in patients with systemic vasculitis and idiopathic necrotising and crescentic glomerulonephritis. *New England Journal of Medicine*, **318**, 1651–7.

Fauci, A.S., Haynes, B.F., and Katz, P. (1978). The spectrum of vasculitis: clinical, pathologic, immunologic, and therapeutic considerations. *Annals of Internal Medicine*, **89**, 660–76.

Fauci, A.S., Katz, P., Haynes, B.F., and Wolff, S.M. (1979). Cyclophosphamide therapy of severe systemic necrotizing vasculitis. *New England Journal of Medicine*, **301**, 235–8.

Fauci, A.S., Haynes, B.F., Katz, P., and Wolff, S.M. (1983). Wegener's granuloma-tosis: prospective clinical and therapeutic experience with 85 patients for 21 years. *Annals of Internal Medicine*, **98**, 76–85.

Fraha, R.A. and Abu-Haider, F. (1979). Polyarteritis nodosa masquerading as temporal arteritis. *Journal of Rheumatology*, **6**, 76–9.

Fries, J.F., Hunder, G.G., Bloch, D.A., *et al.* (1990). The American College of Rheumatology 1990 criteria for the classification of vasculitis: summary. *Arthritis and Rheumatism*, **33**, 1135–6.

Frohnert, P.P. and Sheps, S.G. (1967). Long term follow up study of periarteritis nodosa. *American Journal of Medicine*, **43**, 8–14.

Gilliam, J.N. and Smiley, J.D. (1976). Cutaneous necrotising vasculitis and related disorders. *Annals of Allergy*, **37**, 328–39.

Godman, G.C. and Churg, J. (1954). Wegener's granulomatosis: pathology and review of the literature. *Archives of Pathology*, **58**, 533–53.

Goldberg, J.W., Lee, M.L., and Sajjad, S.M. (1987). Giant cell arteritis of the skin simulating erythema nodosum. *Annals of the Rheumatic Diseases*, **46**, 706–8.

Gordon, M., Luqmani, R.A., Adu, D., *et al.* (1993). Relapses in patients with a systemic vasculitis. *Quarterly Journal of Medicine*, **86**, 779–89.

Gorevic, P.D., Kasseb, H.J., Levo, Y., *et al.* (1980). Mixed cryoglobulinaemia: clinical aspects and long-term follow up of 40 patients. *American Journal of Medicine*, **69**, 287–308.

Gross, W.L., Schmitt, W.H., and Csernok, E. (1993*a*). ANCA and associated diseases: immunodiagnostic and pathogenic aspects. *Clinical and Experimental Immunology*, **91**, 1–12.

Gross, W.L., Hauschild, S., and Mistry, N. (1993*b*). The clinical relevance of ANCA in vasculitis. *Clinical and Experimental Immunology*, **91** (Suppl. 1), 7–11.

Hall, S., Barr, W., Lie, J.T., *et al.* (1985). Takayasu arteritis: a study of 32 North American patients. *Medicine (Baltimore)*, **64**, 89–99.

Hart, F.D., Golding, J.R., and Mackenzie, D.H. (1957). Neuropathy in rheumatoid disease. *Annals of the Rheumatic Diseases*, **16**, 471–80.

Hauschild, S., Schmitt, W.H., Csernok, E., *et al.* (1993). ANCA in systemic vasculi-tides, collagen vascular diseases, rheumatic disorders and inflammatory bowel diseases. In *ANCA associated vasculitides: immunodiagnostic and pathogenetic value of anti-neutrophil cytoplasmic antibodies* (ed. W.L. Gross). Plenum Press, London.

Heng, M.C.Y. (1985) Henoch–Schönlein purpura. *British Journal of Dermatology*, **112**, 235–40.

Henoch, E.H. (1874). Über ein eigenthümliche Form von Purpura. *Berliner Klinika Wochenschrift*, **11**, 641–3.

Hoffman, G.S., Kerr, G.S., Leavitt R.Y., *et al.* (1992). Wegener's granulomatosis: an analysis of 158 patients. *Annals of Internal Medicine*, **116**, 488–98.

Hunder, G.G., Arend, W.P., Bloch, D.A., *et al.* (1990). The American College of Rheumatology 1990 criteria for the classification of vasculitis: introduction. *Arthritis and Rheumatism*, **33**, 1065–7.

Ishikawa, K. (1986). Diagnostic approach and proposed criteria for the clinical diagnosis of Takayasu's arteriopathy. *American Journal of Cardiology*, **12**, 964–72.

Jeanette, J.C., Falk, R.J., Andrassy, K., *et al.* (1994). Nomenclature of systemic vasculitides. Proposal of an international consensus conference. *Arthritis and Rheumatism*, **37**, 187–92.

Juby, C., Johnson, C., and Davies, P. (1992). Antinuclear and antineutrophil cyto-plasmic antibodies (ANCA) in the serum of patients with Felty's syndrome. *British Journal of Rheumatology*, **31**, 185–8.

Kallenberg, C.G.M., Mulder, A.H., and Cohen Tervaert, J.W. (1992). Antineutrophil cytoplasmic antibodies: a still growing class of autoantibodies in inflammatory disorders. *American Journal of Medicine*, **93**, 675–82.

Kawasaki, T. (1967). Acute febrile mucocutaneous syndrome with lymphoid involvement with specific desquamation of the fingers and toes in children: clinical observations in 50 cases. *Japanese Journal of Allergology*, **16**, 178–222.

Klein, R.G., Hunger, G.G., Stenson, A.W., and Sheps, S.G. (1975). Large artery involvement in giant cell (temporal) arteritis. *Annals of Internal Medicine*, **83**, 806–9.

Kurland, L.T., Chuang, T.Y., and Hunder, G. (1984). The epidemiology of systemic arteritis. In *The epidemiology of the rheumatic diseases* (ed. R.C. Lawrence and L.E. Shulman), pp. 196–205. Gower Publishing, New York.

Kussmaul, A. and Maier, R. (1886). Über eine bisher nicht beschreibene eigenthümliche Arterienerkrankung (Periarteritis nodosa), die mit Morbus Bright und rapid fortschreitender allgemeiner Muskellhmung einhergeht. *Deutsche Archive Klinical Medizin*, 1, 484–514.

Lamb, A.R. (1914). Periarteritis nodosa — a clinical and pathological review of the disease. *Archives of Internal Medicine*, 14, 481–516.

Lanham, J.G., Elkon, K.B., Pusey, C.D., and Hughes, G.R.V. (1984). Systemic vasculitis in asthma and eosinophilia: a clinical approach to the Churg–Strauss syndrome. *Medicine (Baltimore)*, 63, 65–81.

Leavitt, R.Y., Fauci, A.S., Block, D.A., *et al.* (1990). The American College of Rheumatology 1990 criteria for the classification of Wegener's granulomatosis. *Arthritis and Rheumatism*, 33, 1101–7.

Lie, J.T. (1988). Classification and immunodiagnosis of vasculitis: a new solution or promises unfulfilled? (Editorial). *Journal of Rheumatology*, 15, 5.

Lie, J.T. (1994). Nomenclature and classification of vasculitis: plus ça change, plus c'est la mme chose. *Arthritis and Rheumatism*, 37, 181–6.

Lightfoot, R.W., Michel, A.B., Bloch, D.A., *et al.* (1990). The American College of Rheumatology 1990 criteria for the classification of polyarteritis nodosa. *Arthritis and Rheumatism*, 33, 1088–93.

Luqmani, R.A., Bacon, P.A., Beaman, M., *et al.* (1994a). Classical versus non-renal Wegener's granulomatosis. *Quarterly Journal of Medicine*, 87, 161–7.

Luqmani, R.A., Watts, R.A., Scott, D.G.I., and Bacon, P.A. (1994b). Treatment of vasculitis in rheumatoid arthritis. *Annales de Médecine Interne*, 145, 566–76.

Masi, A.T., Hunder, G.G., Lie, J.T., *et al.* (1990). The American College of Rheumatology 1990 criteria for the classification of Churg–Strauss syndrome (allergic granulomatosis and angiitis). *Arthritis and Rheumatism*, 33, 1094–100.

Mills, J.A., Michel, B.A., Block, D.A., *et al.* (1990). The American College of Rheumatology 1990 criteria for the classification of Henoch–Schönlein purpura. *Arthritis and Rheumatism*, 33, 1114–21.

Morgan, G.J. and Harris, E.D. (1978). Non-giant cell temporal arteritis. *Arthritis and Rheumatism*, 21, 362–6.

Pallis, C.A. and Scott, J.T. (1965). Peripheral neuropathy in rheumatoid arthritis. *British Medical Journal*, i, 1141–7.

Pelletan, P.J. (1810). Aneurismes particuliers. In *Clinique chirugical ou memoires des observations de Chirurgien Clinique*, Vol. 2, p.l. J.G. Dentu, Paris.

Peter, H.H., Metzger, D., Rump, A., and Rother, E. (1993). ANCA in diseases other than systemic vasculitis. *Clinical and Experimental Immunology*, 91 (Suppl. 1), 12–14.

Potter, B.T., Howley, E., and Thomson, D. (1981). Giant cell arteritis mimicking carcinoma of breast. *British Medical Journal*, 282, 1665–6.

Rauch, A. and Hurwitz, E. (1985). Centers for disease control case definition of Kawasaki disease. *Paediatric Infectious Disease Journal*, 4, 702–3.

Remigo, P. and Zaino, E. (1970). Polyarteritis nodosa of the gall bladder. *Surgery*, 67, 427–31.

Rich, A.R. (1942). The role of hypersensitivity in periarteritis nodosa. *Bulletin of the Johns Hopkins Hospital*, 71, 123–40.

Rich, A.R. and Gregory, J.E. (1943). The experimental demonstration that periarteritis nodosa is a manifestion of hypersensitivity. *Bulletin of the Johns Hopkins Hospital*, 72, 65–88.

Rokitansky, K. (1852). Ueber einige der wichtigsten Krankheiten der Arterien. Deukschriften der Kais. *Akademie der Wissenschaften Besonders Abgedrucket*, 4, 49.

Rose, G.A. and Spencer, H. (1957). Polyarteritis nodosa. *Quarterly Journal of Medicine*, 26, 43–81.

Sack, M., Cassidy, J.T., and Bole, G.G. (1975). Prognostic factors in polyarteritis. *Journal of Rheumatology*, 2, 411–20.

Savory, W.S. (1856). Case of a young woman in whom the main arteries of both upper extremities and of the left side of the neck were throughout completely obliterated. *Medical and Chirurgical Transactions (London)*, 39, 205.

Schmid, F.R., Cooper, N.S., Ziff, M., and McEwan C. (1961). Arteritis in rheumatoid arthritis. *American Journal of Medicine*, 30, 56–83.

Schönlein, H. (1837). *Allgemeine und specielle Pathologie und Therapie*, Vol. 2 (3rd edn). Herisau, Würzburg.

Scott, D.G.I. (1986). Vasculitis. In *Copeman's textbook of the rheumatic diseases* (6th edn), (ed. J.T. Scott), pp. 1292–324. Churchill Livingstone, Edinburgh.

Scott, D.G.I. (1988) Classification and treatment of systemic vasculitis (Editorial). *British Journal of Rheumatology*, 27, 251–3.

Scott, D.G.I. and Bacon, P.A. (1984). Intravenous cyclophosphamide plus methyl prednisolone in the treatment of systemic rheumatoid vasculitis. *American Journal of Medicine*, 76, 377–84.

Scott, D.G.I. and Bacon, P.A. (1987). Cardiac involvement in immunological diseases. *Clinics in Immunology and Allergy*, 1, 537–75.

Scott, D.G.I. and Watts, R.A. (1994). Classification and epidemiology of systemic vasculitis. *British Journal of Rheumatology*, 33, 897–99.

Scott, D.G.I., Bacon, P.A., and Tribe, C.R. (1981). Systemic rheumatoid vasculitis: a clinical and laboratory study of 50 cases. *Medicine (Baltimore)*, 60, 288–97.

Scott, D.G.I., Bacon, P.A., Elliott, P.J., Tribe, C.R., and Wallington, T. (1982). Systemic vasculitis in a district general hospital 1972–1980: clinical and laboratory features, classification and prognosis of 80 cases. *Quarterly Journal of Medicine*, 203, 292–311.

Siefert, M. (1989). The rheumatology of HIV infection. *Topical Reviews*, 11.

Smith, J.A.E., O'Sullivan, M., Gough, J., and Williams, B.D. (1988). Small intestine perforation secondary to localized giant cell arteritis of the mesenteric arteries. *British Journal of Rheumatology*, 27, 236–8.

Stewart, M., Savage, J.M., Bell, B., *et al.* (1988). Long term renal prognosis of Henoch–Schönlein purpura in an unselected childhood population. *European Journal of Paediatrics*, 147, 113–15.

Takayasu, M. (1908). Cases with unusual changes of the central vessels in the retina. *Acta Societas Ophthalmologica Japonica*, 12, 554.

van der Woude, F.J., Rasmussen, N., Lobatto, S., *et al.* (1985). Autoantibodies against neutrophils and monocytes: a tool for diagnosis and marker of disease activity in Wegener's granulomatosis. *Lancet*, i, 425–9.

von Glahn, W.C. and Pappenheimer, A.M. (1926). Specific lesions of peripheral blood vessels in rheumatism. *American Journal of Pathology*, 2, 235–50.

Wainwright, J. and Davson, J. (1950). The renal appearances in microscopic form of polyarteritis nodosa. *Journal of Pathology and Bacteriology*, 62, 189–96.

Watts, R.A., Carruthers, D.M., Symmons, D.P.M., and Scott, D.G.I. (1994). The incidence of rheumatoid vasculitis in the Norwich Health Authority. *British Journal of Rheumatology*, 33, 832–3.

Watts, R.A., Carruthers, D.M., and Scott, D.G.I. (1995). Epidemiology of systemic vasculitis — changing incidence or definition. *Seminars in Arthritis and Rheumatism*, 25, 28–34.

Wegener, F. (1936) Uber generalisierte, septische Gefasserkrankungen. *Verhandlungers der Deutschen Gesellschaft für Pathologie*, 29, 202–9.

Zeek, P.M.(1952). Periarteritis nodosa: a critical review. *American Journal of Clinical Pathology*, 22, 777–90.

Zeek, P.M., Smith, C.C., and Weeter, J.C. (1948). Studies on periarteritis nodosa III. The differentiation between the vascular lesions of periarteritis nodosa and hyper-sensitivity. *American Journal of Pathology*, 24, 889–917.

5.11.2 Wegener's granulomatosis

Wolfgang L. Gross

Introduction

Wegener's granulomatosis has been recognized as a distinct clinico-pathological entity for 60 years. Of unknown aetiology, it is a granulomatous disorder associated with systemic necrotizing vasculitis (for review, see Wegener 1990; Wegener 1990b). It involves predominantly the upper airways, the lungs, and the kidneys: 'classical' Wegener's granulomatosis represents a triad of upper airway (= **E**), lung (= **L**) and renal disease (= **K**) according to the **ELK** classification (DeRemee *et al.* 1976). However, since the disease may be confined to E or to E and L as a purely granulomatous process without clinical evidence of systemic vasculitis, these *formes frustes* of Wegener's granulomatosis have been designated 'limited disease' (without kidney involvement), 'limited forms' (E or E and L) or 'initial phase' (locoregional restricted granulomatous process without clinically apparent vasculitis) (Carrington and Liebow 1966; Gross 1989; Nölle *et al.* 1989; DeRemee 1993).

The 'classical' syndrome represents a generalized disease process that usually begins with an initial phase of variable duration characterized by symptoms limited mostly to the upper and/or lower respiratory tract (for review, see Wegener 1990; Wegener 1990b). Since more and more of these limited forms of Wegener's granulomatosis are being detected early, due partly to increased physicians' awareness and partly to more sophisticated diagnostic procedures, it has been learned that most of these 'initial phases' follow a rather subacute or chronic protracted course of unpredictable duration before transforming into the generalized (systemic) phase associated usually with high titres of antineutrophil cytoplasmic antibodies (**ANCA**). This is the well-recognized, full-blown disease characterized by systemic necrotizing vasculitis, usually with renal and pulmonary involvement. If untreated, it can turn into the fulminant form of the disease (e.g. renal–pulmonary syndrome), which carries a devastating prognosis (for review, see Gross 1989). Rheumatic complaints, and eye or peripheral nerve involvement, are frequently an ominous herald of the onset of the generalized vasculitic phase, which is usually also associated with constitutional symptoms such as malaise, weight loss, fever, and night sweats (Noritake *et al.* 1987; Gross 1989; Alcalay *et al.* 1990; Gross *et al.* 1991). In this phase, non-specific markers of inflammation, for example the erythrocyte sedimentation rate and C-reactive protein, are usually elevated. cANCA (proteinase 3 ANCA; **PR3-ANCA**), which has a 90 per cent specificity for Wegener's granulomatosis, is detectable in 95 per cent of sera from patients with generalized Wegener's granulomatosis, but in only about half of patients in the initial phase (Nölle *et al.* 1989).

Because of the potentially life-threatening course of many of the major necrotizing vasculitides, such as generalized Wegener's granulomatosis or microscopic polyangiitis, 'standard' treatment (United States National Institutes of Health standard therapy/Fauci's scheme) consisting of daily 'low-dose' (2–4 mg/day) cyclophosphamide plus glucocorticoids is generally considered to be of most benefit to the majority of patients (for review, see Hoffman 1990). This view has been challenged in recent years by data indicating (i) the variability of clinical course and aggressiveness in the same disease entity, (ii) continued morbidity despite therapy with cyclophosphamide plus glucocorticoids, (iii) a high incidence of relapse among patients thought to be 'cured', and (iv) the alarming range of toxic effects induced by the 'standard protocol' (Anderson *et al.* 1992; Frankel *et al.* 1992; Hoffman *et al.* 1992a).

Improved diagnostic procedures, including computed tomographic (**CT**) imaging of the lung and magnetic resonance imaging (**MRI**) of the head (Greenan *et al.* 1992; Muhle *et al.* 1993), immunodiagnostic methods such as ANCA assays, and the detection of cytokine/cytokine-receptor molecules such as the soluble interleukin-2 receptor, have enhanced diagnostic precision by clarifying the anatomical distribution of involvement and the clinical activity

of the disease (Nölle *et al.* 1989; Salvarani *et al.* 1992; Schmitt *et al.* 1992; Stegemann *et al.* 1993). Consequently, it is now possible to design stage-adapted and disease-activity related therapeutic protocols instead of adhering to the rather rigid standard regimen developed 20 years ago.

Definition and classification

In spite of substantial efforts by many investigators, the nomenclature of the various subsets of Wegener's granulomatosis remains enigmatic (for review, see Gross 1996). A major problem is the lack of standardized terms and definitions. Thus different names are used (e.g. Wegener's granulomatosis; Wegener's vasculitis; microscopic polyarteritis of Wegener's type, etc.) for various forms of the same disease, and different interpretations of the same term (e.g. 'limited' Wegener's granulomatosis) can be found in the literature. In a first attempt to address this problem, an International Consensus Conference held in Chapel Hill in 1992 presented a proposal for both the nomenclature and definitions of vasculitides (see Table 2 of Chapter 5.11.1).

Usually, generalized ('full-blown', classical) Wegener's granulomatosis (Fig. 1) is described as a distinct clinicopathological entity characterized by lesions induced by necrotizing granulomatous inflammation in the upper (ear, nose, and throat) and the lower respiratory tract (including the lung), and by vasculitis (including kidney: glomerulonephritis) involving various additional organs (Wegener 1939). According to the original criteria of Godman and Churg (1954), Wegener's granulomatosis characteristically involves a triad of airway, lung, and renal disease.

The 'ELK classification' proposed by DeRemee *et al.* (1976) has proved to be useful in clinical practice. Patients are classified according to the extent of the organ system involvement observed

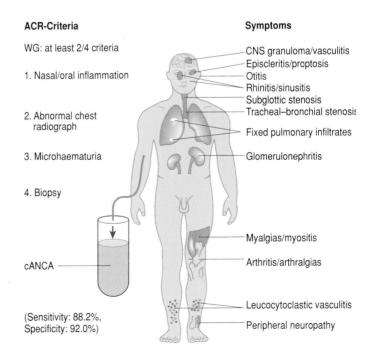

ACR-Criteria

WG: at least 2/4 criteria

1. Nasal/oral inflammation

2. Abnormal chest radiograph

3. Microhaematuria

4. Biopsy

cANCA

(Sensitivity: 88.2%, Specificity: 92.0%)

Symptoms

CNS granuloma/vasculitis
Episcleritis/proptosis
Otitis
Rhinitis/sinusitis
Subglottic stenosis
Tracheal–bronchial stenosis
Fixed pulmonary infiltrates
Glomerulonephritis
Myalgias/myositis
Arthritis/arthralgias
Leucocytoclastic vasculitis
Peripheral neuropathy

Fig. 1 Schematic representation of the characteristic clinical symptoms of Wegener's granulomatosis and the ACR 1990 classification criteria.

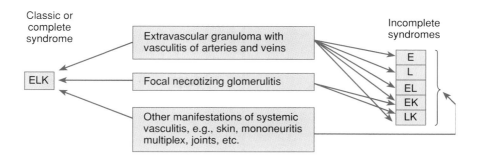

E – Upper respiratory tract (nose, throat, trachea, paranasal sinuses)
L – Lower respiratory tract (lung and bronchi)
K – Kidney

Fig. 2 Scheme for Wegener's granulomatosis in the ELK classification according to DeRemee *et al.* (1976) (with permission).

Table 1 ACR 1990 criteria for the classification of Wegener's granulomatosis

Criteria	Definition
1. Nasal or oral inflammation	Development of painful or painless oral ulcers or purulent or bloody nasal discharge.
2. Abnormal chest radiograph	Radiograph of the chest showing the presence of nodules, fixed infiltrates, or cavities.
3. Urinary sediment	Microhaematuria (over 5 red blood cells/hpf) or red cell casts in the urine sediment.
4. Granulomatous inflammation on biopsy	Histological changes showing granulomatous inflammation within the wall of an artery or in the peri- or extravascular area (artery or arteriole)

Number of criteria present rule: for classification purposes, a patient shall be said to have Wegener's granulomatosis if he/she has satisfied any two or more of these four criteria; this rule is associated with a sensitivity of 88.2 per cent and a specificity of 92.0 per cent.
From Leavitt *et al.* (1990) with permission.

during the disease course (see Introduction; Fig. 2). The 'extended' ELK classification is now the basis for the 'Disease Extension Index' used in clinical studies (Nölle *et al.* 1989; Reinhold-Keller *et al.* 1994; Gross 1996) and, sometimes, in everyday practice.

The American College of Rheumatology 1990 criteria for the classification of Wegener's granulomatosis (**ACR 1990** classification criteria) were developed by comparing 85 patients with Wegener's granulomatosis with 722 control patients with other forms of vasculitis (Leavitt *et al.* 1990). For the traditional format classification, four criteria were selected (Table 1). A classification tree was also constructed, based on the selection of five criteria. These criteria were the same as for the traditional format, plus haemoptysis. The classification tree had a sensitivity of 87.1 per cent and a specificity of 93.6 per cent.

The Chapel Hill Consensus Conference on the Nomenclature of Systemic Vasculitis (**CHC 1992** definitions; Jennette *et al.* 1994) defined Wegener's granulomatosis as follows: granulomatous inflammation involving the respiratory tract, and necrotizing vasculitis affecting small to medium-sized vessels (e.g. capillaries, venules, arterioles, and arteries). Necrotizing glomerulonephritis is common. The disease is often associated with ANCA (see Table 2 of Chapter 5.11.1).

Neither the CHC definitions nor the ACR 1990 classification criteria addressed *formes frustes* of Wegener's granulomatosis. The criteria for definition and classification proposed for Wegener's

granulomatosis (as part of the nomenclature for the vasculitides) require the presence of systemic vasculitis — but Wegener's granulomatosis may also occur as an inflammatory granulomatous process without apparent vasculitis! It must be borne in mind that neither the ACR 1990 nor the CHC 1992 constitute actual diagnostic criteria.

Epidemiology and natural history

Wegener's granulomatosis is a worldwide disease (Malaviya *et al.* 1990). New diagnostic tests (especially for ANCA) have led to an increased awareness of Wegener's granulomatosis (Andrews *et al.* 1990). Studies in the United States suggest an annual incidence of 4 per million population, while studies in England report an incidence of 8.5 per million (95 per cent confidence interval: 5.2–12.9), with an incidence for males of 10.8 and for females of 6.2 per million (Scott and Watts 1994). Wegener's granulomatosis has been observed in children and in elderly people; the peak incidence is in the fourth and fifth decades (Fauci *et al.* 1983; Hall *et al.* 1985; Weiner *et al.* 1986; McHugh *et al.* 1991; Rottem *et al.* 1993; Chakravarty *et al.* 1994).

Although, until the last decade, Wegener's granulomatosis was generally regarded as an invariably serious and fatal disease (Fauci *et al.* 1983), perceptions of it have since changed (Gross 1989; Hoffman *et al.* 1993a). As with systemic lupus erythematosus, improved diagnostic procedures, including CT imaging of the lung and MRI of the head, as well as immunodiagnostic methods, such as ANCA assays, have enhanced diagnostic precision by identifying unclear clinical manifestations in the E or L region, and by clarifying the anatomical distribution of involvement (disease extension) and clinical disease activity (Luqmani *et al.* 1994; Reinhold-Keller *et al.* 1994). So, in addition to full-blown forms of Wegener's granulomatosis with possibly fatal outcome, indolent and/or less aggressive and life-threatening variants have been found to occur more frequently than once thought. In addition, the introduction of immunosuppressive drugs, dialysis, and renal transplantation have led to a dramatic improvement in survival rates in serious cases.

Prognosis

In their updated analysis of 158 patients with Wegener's granulomatosis, Hoffman *et al.* (1992a) emphasized the variability of the disease before diagnosis: the disease followed a confusing and indolent course in many cases (particularly in patients without renal manifestations) for up to 16 years before a definite diagnosis was established. The median and mean periods from onset of symptoms to diagnosis of Wegener's granulomatosis were 4.7 and 15 months, respectively. Diagnosis was made within 3 months after the onset of symptoms in only 42 per cent of patients; this is surprising because earlier studies had reported a median survival of only 5 months (Walton 1958). In Great Britain, 265 patients with Wegener's granulomatosis were observed between 1975 and 1985 (Anderson *et al.* 1992). The mean intervals from onset of symptoms to presentation and from presentation to diagnosis were both approximately 7 months; correct diagnosis was often missed for many years (range: less than 1–188 months). The mean survival of 4.2 years (shorter if renal disease was present) in patients receiving no drug treatment (10 per cent) indicates that these variants must have been very mild. Furthermore, it is striking that the median survival of 72 patients treated with glucocorticoids alone exceeded 12 years. Unfortunately, the investigators did not indicate the number of patients in the different treatment groups nor their disease activity and extent. Similar observations were published earlier and are reviewed elsewhere (Gross 1996).

Clinical features

Although Wegener's granulomatosis is a systemic disease with characteristic features reflected in the involvement of multiple organ systems (Table 2), it is essentially a true respiratory–renal syndrome. These two organ systems are largely responsible for the clinical course of the disease.

Along with the well-known triad of necrotizing granulomas of the upper (E) and lower respiratory tract (L), plus glomerulonephritis (i.e. renal vasculitis; K), generalized Wegener's granulomatosis may also involve joints (A), skin (S), peripheral nerves (P), skeletal muscle (A), heart (H), brain (C) and eyes (EY), mostly via vasculitis of the small vessels (Fig. 1).

In Wegener's granulomatosis, involvement characteristically begins in the upper respiratory tract and precedes symptoms of generalized disease for a long period of time. These and pulmonary features may evolve over several months and even years, and can be followed by the overt presentation of systemic vasculitis, including glomerular disease. Because of the sometimes slow evolution, the diagnosis 'Wegener's granulomatosis' may not be made until some time after respiratory presentation.

Table 2 Organ system involvement in Wegener's granulomatosis

Organ or system	Patients			
	(number)		(%)	
	Group 1[a]	Group 2[b]	Group 1[a]	Group 2[b]
Lung	80	100	94	64
Paranasal sinuses	77	124	91	80
Kidney	72	104	85	67
Joints	57	120	67	77
Nose or nasopharynx	54	142	64	92
Ear	52	65	61	42
Eye	49	94	58	61
Skin	38	51	45	33
Nervous system	19	74	22	48
Heart	10	35	12	23

[a]From Fauci *et al.* (1983) (*n*=85); [b]from Lübeck/Bad Bramstedt (*n*=155).

On the other hand, Wegener's granulomatosis may sometimes start without obvious granulomatous lesions as a 'purely' small-vessel vasculitis (generalized phase). It is important to realize that there are overlapping features shared by Wegener's granulomatosis and microscopic polyangiitis, combined with the subsequent development over time of inflammatory lesions (for example, glomerulonephritis followed by skin vasculitis followed by pulmonary vasculitis—and, lastly, followed by obvious granulomatous lesions in the respiratory tract).

In any case, a strict diagnosis of Wegener's granulomatosis depends on (i) characteristic clinical symptoms, (ii) the demonstration of characteristic granulomas in biopsy material, and/or (iii) the detection of characteristic cANCA (PR3-ANCA) in the serum. It is noteworthy that each of these 'characteristics' can be observed in similar disorders, and that 'diagnosis' should not rely on any one of these variables alone.

Initial phase

['Initial stage'; E, L, EL according to the ELK classification, 'purely' granulomatous Wegener's granulomatosis; for review, see Gross (1989), DeRemee (1993), Boudes (1990).]
In most instances the ENT region (upper respiratory tract including the nose, sinuses, ears, and throat) is affected first. Characteristically, there are no clinical signs of systemic vasculitis. Patients with initial-phase Wegener's granulomatosis account for 10 per cent of those with vasculitis in a rheumatological unit.

The earliest nasal manifestations (E) usually include nasal obstruction (mucosal swelling), serosanguineous discharge, and epistaxis.

Examination reveals granulation (Fig. 3), and there may be thick crusts that upon removal reveal friable mucosa or even septal perforation. In many patients the clinical diagnosis can be confirmed by the characteristic histological appearances obtained from nasal biopsy (Devaney *et al.* 1990; Del Bueno and Flint 1991). In addition to the symptoms described, facial pain, nosebleeds, nasal chondritis, saddling of the nose (Fig. 4), and involvement of paranasal sinuses (chronic sinusitis) typically occur.

In the oral cavity and oropharynx (E), gingival involvement can lead to ulcerative stomatitis, frank ulcerations (Fig. 5), or hyperplastic gingivitis (Fig. 6). Laryngeal symptoms such as hoarseness and/or increasing stridor are frequently due to reddish, friable, circumferential narrowing just below the cords and extending for 3 to 5 cm.

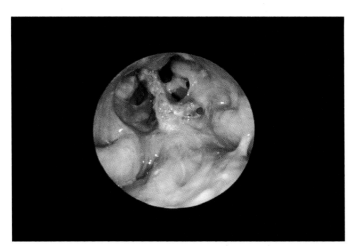

Fig. 3 Intranasal bilateral and septal mucosal disease with granulations and crusts leading to permanent serosanguinous discharge.

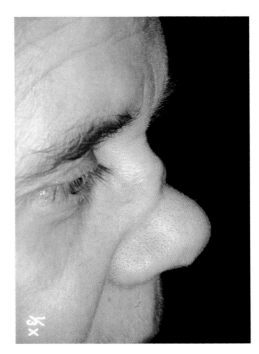

Fig. 4 Saddling of the nose due to destruction of the septal cartilage is a common finding in Wegener's granulomatosis.

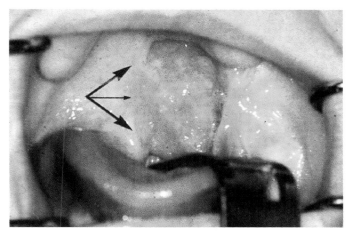

Fig. 5 Ulceration of the palate (an unusual site of manifestation for Wegener's granulomatosis) whose characteristic histological appearances led to the correct diagnosis in a patient with cavitating round nodules of the lung (see Fig. 11).

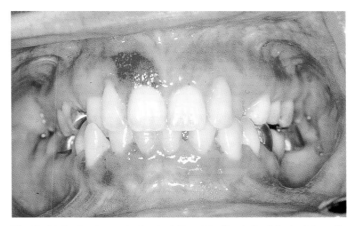

Fig. 6 Distinctive hyperplastic gingivitis originating in the interdental papilla area (biopsy-proven Wegener's granulomatosis).

Otological manifestations

The otological manifestations (E) of Wegener's granulomatosis include involvement of the external ear (chondritis, sometimes with secondary atrophy of the ear lobe), or middle ear (serous otitis media; suppurative otitis media, mastoiditis). Sometimes peripheral facial-nerve palsy occurs (D'Cruz *et al.* 1989; Murty 1990).

Eye symptoms

The eye symptoms (EY) — excluding those arising from small-vessel vasculitis seen only in generalized Wegener's granulomatosis, and which do lead to 'red eye' — derive from the granulomatous lesions (obstruction of the nasolacrimal duct) and masses developing retro-orbitally (protrusio bulbi; compression of the optic nerve; Figs 7 and 8). Less frequently, orbital involvement may result from the spread of a purulent sinusitis, for example due to secondary bacterial infection (Charles *et al.* 1991; Satorre *et al.* 1991; Duncker *et al.* 1993).

Three types of involvement of the peripheral nervous system (P) have been described: disseminated vasculitis (see below: generalized Wegener's granulomatosis), contiguous granulomatous lesions, and

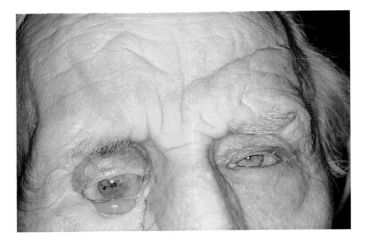

Fig. 7 Eye disease in Wegener's granulomatosis usually manifests itself in one of two ways: retro-orbital granuloma masses leading to proptosis (etc.), and small-vessel vasculitis leading to 'red eye' (see Fig. 18).

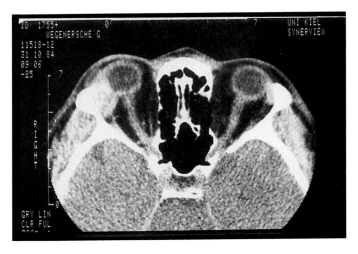

Fig. 8 Protrusio bulbi induced by retro-orbital granulomatous masses (CT scan).

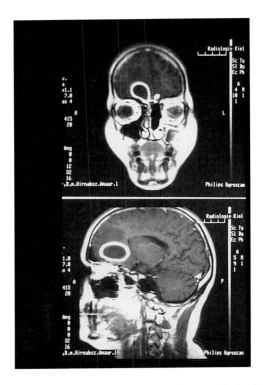

Fig. 9 Intracerebral spread of contiguous granulomatous lesion (frontal lobe) from the sinuses.

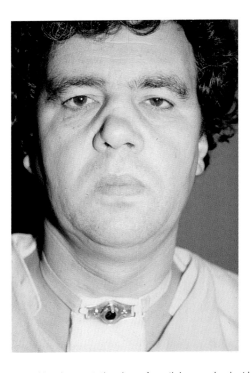

Fig. 10 Laryngeal involvement: the circumferential narrowing just below the cords led to subglottic stenoses requiring tracheostomy (see also: saddle nose deformity).

disseminated, multicentric granulomatous lesions. The contiguous granulomatous lesion originates from the sinuses (Fig. 9) and middle ear, and spreads to the retropharyngeal area and base of the skull. This can lead to involvement of cranial nerves (I, II, III, VI, VII, VIII), and to proptosis (see above), or to diabetes insipidus, meningitis, etc. (Rosete *et al*. 1991; Greenan *et al*. 1992, Asmus *et al*. 1993; Nishino *et al*. 1993).

The tracheobronchial tree including the lung may also be involved in this locoregionally restricted and not yet generalized process of granulomatous inflammation: subglottic pseudotumour and/or stenosis leading to stridor and dyspnoea (Fig. 10); bronchial stenosis, which may cause atelectasis and/or obstructive pneumonia. Single or multiple nodules with or without cavitation (Fig. 11) are found incidentally in the lung of thus far asymptomatic persons (Specks and DeRemee 1990; Travis *et al*. 1991; Hoffman *et al*. 1992a).

Because of the locoregionally restricted symptoms (mostly confined to the ENT region: E or lower respiratory tract including lung), the initial stage is puzzling to the diagnostician. It often takes years for Wegener's granulomatosis to be suspected and a histological

diagnosis finally made. Fever can occur, perhaps caused by the underlying inflammatory disease, although it appears to be more commonly associated with secondary bacterial infection (mostly caused by *Staphylococcus aureus*) of the involved paranasal sinus (Fig. 12).

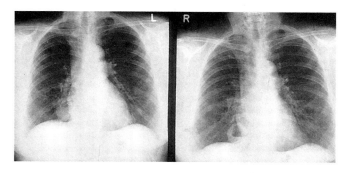

Fig. 11 Nodules in the lung usually consist of rounded lesions with well-defined margins (a); they tend to cavitate (b).

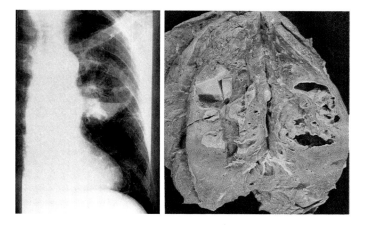

Fig. 12 Cavitary air-space consolidation initially thought to represent necrotizing bacterial pneumonia (radiographic findings and autopsy material).

Generalized Wegener's granulomatosis

['Systemic' Wegener's granulomatosis; E, L, K stage according to the ELK classification; for review, see Gross (1989), DeRemee (1993).]
The transition from the initial stage to the active generalized phase with its not infrequent fulminant course is heralded by the indirect symptoms of systemic vasculitis: weight loss, fever, night sweats (constitutional symptoms; similar to 'B-symptomatology' in Hodgkin's disease). Clinically, this combination of fatigue, malaise, and anorexia, together with uncharacteristic rheumatic complaints (polymyalgia, arthralgia; see below) and the striking laboratory abnormalities typical of this phase (erythrocyte sedimentation rate and C-reactive protein maximally elevated, leucocytosis, thrombocytosis), warrant close scrutiny to ensure early recognition of the imminent complications, which, if untreated, lead to the life-threatening conditions described below. Direct signs of the small-vessel vasculitis characteristically found in generalized Wegener's granulomatosis are 'red eye' (due to episcleritis, scleritis), palpable purpura of the lower extremities (due to leucocytoclastic vasculitis of the skin), peripheral neuropathy (due to the vasculitis of the vasa nervorum) and, most dangerous of all, renal involvement, which ranges from mild focal and segmental glomerulonephritis with minimal haematuria and little diminution of the glomerular filtration rate, to fulminant diffuse necrotizing and crescentic glomerulonephritis (rapidly progressive glomerulonephritis) with haematuria, pyuria,

and red-cell casts, leading within several days or a few weeks to oligoanuria and dialysis. Additionally — or separately — pulmonary symptoms can arise, which may ultimately lead to pulmonary haemorrhage and severe respiratory insufficiency. In fulminant Wegener's granulomatosis, all of the symptoms described here can occur together (for example, in the form of a pulmonary–renal syndrome) or separately (alveolar haemorrhage syndrome without glomerulonephritis; rapidly progressive glomerulonephritis without alveolar haemorrhage, etc.). In these, only rapid diagnosis and immediate immunosuppressive treatment can restrain this life-threatening condition and prevent endstage renal failure or death.

Most patients suffering from Wegener's granulomatosis, however, follow a clinical course lying between these extremes (initial-phase and fulminant generalized disease).

Otological manifestations in generalized Wegener's granulomatosis — in addition to those described for initial-phase Wegener's granulomatosis — characteristically include hearing loss due to sensorineural deafness, usually induced by the small-vessel vasculitis of the cochlear vessels and/or the vasa nervorum of the acoustic nerve. Vestibular impairment as manifested by vertigo can also occur. Similarly, peripheral facial nerve palsy can be induced by the otitis media (including mastoiditis) and the vasculitis (D'Cruz *et al.* 1989; Murty 1990).

Eye manifestations in the generalized stage of Wegener's granulomatosis are episcleritis ('red eye') (Fig. 13), vasculitis of the optic nerve, and occlusion of retinal arteries, all due to the now prominent vasculitic process, and in addition to the granulomatous lesions described above (Charles *et al.* 1991).

The bronchial tree and lung (L) are involved usually in the systemic phase of Wegener's granulomatosis. In addition to the stenotic processes and nodules (this kind of pulmonary involvement itself is more typical of the initial phase of Wegener's granulomatosis and rather asymptomatic), localized or diffuse infiltrates should alert to the possibility of an alveolar haemorrhage resulting from the predominantly alveolar capillaritis. The three most consistent features for clinical recognition of alveolar haemorrhage are haemoptysis, infiltrates on the chest radiograph, and anaemia. The radiograph typically shows an alveolar or mixed alveolar–interstitial pattern. A distribution like that in pulmonary oedema is most common, but focal and sometimes migratory shadows are also observed (Fig. 14).

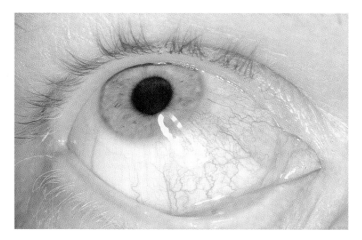

Fig. 13 Episcleritis as a characteristic clinical sign of disease activity in Wegener's granulomatosis.

However, the clinical and radiographic manifestations of immune alveolar haemorrhage are similar regardless of their aetiology. Such patients usually also have a rapidly progressive glomerulonephritis (Fig. 15) and thus typically present a pulmonary–renal vasculitic syndrome. Immunohistochemical tests on lung biopsies (e.g. via bronchoscopy) or kidney specimens reveal only a few or no immune deposits, thus excluding immune complex-mediated and antibasement membrane antibody-mediated pulmonary and pulmonary–renal vasculitic syndromes. Most patients with such 'pauci-immune' pulmonary–renal vasculitic syndromes have either cANCA (PR3-ANCA) or pANCA induced by myeloperoxidase antibodies (**myeloperoxidase-ANCA**) (Specks *et al.* 1989; Aberle *et al.* 1990; Cordier *et al.* 1990; Lombard *et al.* 1990; Dreisin 1993; Nishino *et al.* 1993).

Abnormalities of pulmonary function include obstruction to airflow, reduced lung volumes, and abnormalities of diffusing capacity.

Kidney involvement (K) in generalized Wegener's granulomatosis shows considerable variation. At an extreme lies rapidly progressive glomerulonephritis, which is a major indicator of poor prognosis (see above). The most common manifestation of renal disease, however, is asymptomatic (micro-)haematuria with a nephritic urinary sediment and little if any renal functional impairment; this erythrocyturia is due to focal segmental glomerulonephritis. Immunohistologically, the glomeruli typically have no deposits of immunoglobulin; similarly, there is little ultrastructural evidence for immune-complex deposits. This has led to the term 'pauci-immune necrotizing and crescentic glomerulonephritis'. It is noteworthy that very similar lesions due to 'microscopic' vessel inflammation are seen in other 'ANCA-associated vasculitides' (e.g. microscopic polyangiitis) (Weiss and Crissman 1984; Wegener 1990; Falk and Jennette 1993; Jennette and Falk 1994a).

Clinical manifestations in the heart (**H** = heart involvement in the extended ELK classification) are not common in generalized Wegener's granulomatosis. However, asymptomatic pericardial effusions frequently occur and frank peri- (pan) carditis, severe granulomatous giant-cell myocarditis, and cardiomyopathy have been described (Weidhase *et al.* 1990).

Rheumatic complaints (**A** = arthralgia and/or myalgia, etc. in the extended ELK classification) ranging from mild myalgias and/or arthralgias to frank arthritis and/or myositis represent the second most frequent symptom complex (after ENT region symptoms) in generalized Wegener's granulomatosis. Musculoskeletal involvement, particularly arthralgia and arthritis, was reported decades ago. More recently, these rheumatic manifestations were described in two-thirds of patients in a large series of cases of Wegener's granulomatosis. Twenty-eight per cent had non-erosive and non-deforming polyarthritis. Sacroiliitis was found in 3 of 50 and relapsing polychondritis in 2 of 50 patients with Wegener's granulomatosis. Rheumatoid factor was present in half of the patients with generalized Wegener's granulomatosis tested. In our own series of 186 patients with Wegener's granulomatosis (148 biopsy-proven), we found episodes of arthralgia, myalgia, or arthritis in two-thirds of cases as the presenting symptom and in three-quarters of all cases over time. Thus rheumatic complaints have been found to belong to the main symptom complex (Fig. 16). They are more frequent than symptoms of the eye, skin, or nervous system. The most common is myalgia (45 per cent), followed by frank arthritis (21 per cent), mainly in the larger joints (monoarthritis, 10 patients; oligoarthritis, 5; polyarthritis, 6). Approximately 90 per cent of patients with Wegener's granulomatosis suffering from rheumatic symptoms have a generalized form of the disease and the rheumatic symptoms usually occur together with the constitutional symptoms typically associated with active vasculitis (Noritake *et al.* 1987; Alcalay *et al.* 1990; Gross *et al.* 1991; Hoffman *et al.* 1992a) Wegener's granulomatosis can be associated with secondary relapsing polychondritis (Handrock and Gross 1993).

Skin involvement (**S** = skin in the extended ELK classification) in systemic Wegener's granulomatosis usually occurs as palpable

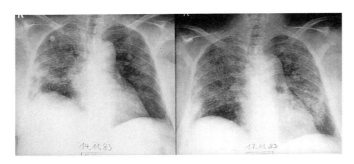

Fig. 14 Radiographic manifestation of alveolar haemorrhage in Wegener's granulomatosis.

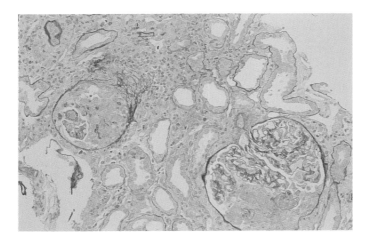

Fig. 15 Histopathology of a necrotizing and crescentic glomerulonephritis from a patient with rapidly progressive glomerulonephritis in Wegener's granulomatosis.

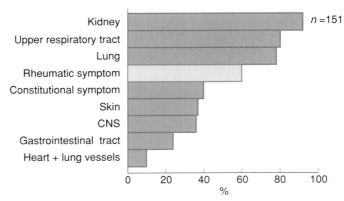

Fig. 16 Clinical symptoms in Wegener's granulomatosis.

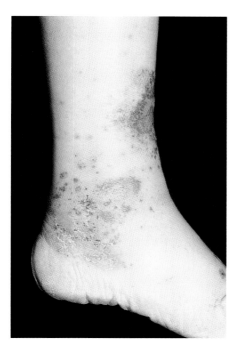

Fig. 17 Palpable purpura in a patient with fulminant Wegener's granulomatosis.

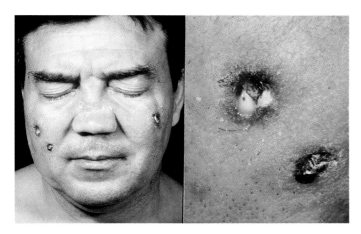

Fig. 18 Necrotic papules (and saddle-nose deformity) in Wegener's granulomatosis.

purpura due to leucocytoclastic vasculitis (Fig. 17). Less frequent are necrotic papules (Fig. 18) due to necrotizing vasculitis. Livedo reticularis and pyoderma gangrenosum are occasionally seen, sometimes as the presenting feature (Dreisin 1993; Frances *et al.* 1994).

About one-third of patients with Wegener's granulomatosis have involvement of the nervous system (**C** = nervous system in the extended ELK classification). Peripheral neuropathy (excluding cranial neuropathy) occurs in about 30 per cent of patients; mononeuropathy multiplex and distal sensorimotor polyneuropathy are the leading lesions. Cerebrovascular events, seizures, and cerebritis are less frequent findings (Nishino *et al.* 1993).

In addition to this broad spectrum of symptoms, a wide variety of other manifestations, including involvement of the breast, ovaries,

prostate, urethral duct, have been described, mostly in the form of case reports.

Laboratory investigations

Up to the mid-1980s, no disease-specific laboratory index for Wegener's granulomatosis existed. Disease activity was evaluated according to the clinical picture and general indices of inflammation (erythrocyte sedimentation rate, C-reactive protein) in the blood (Hoffman *et al.* 1992). In addition, the degree of normochromic normocytic anaemia, leucocytosis (usually with no or only moderate eosinophilia: less than 10 per cent), and thrombocytosis was correlated with the disease activity: all of these variables are only slightly elevated in the initial phase of Wegener's granulomatosis, and, by contrast, maximally elevated in the fulminant generalized stage, sometimes with 'leukaemoid' reactions (Gross 1996).

In contrast to the family of autoimmune rheumatic diseases (e.g. systemic lupus), generalized Wegener's granulomatosis is associated with no or only mild hypergammaglobulinaemia (minor elevations of all immunoglobulins in serum), no or only low-titre antinuclear antibody, no complement consumption (rather slight elevations), but with a rheumatic factor in up to 50 per cent of patients. In addition, cryoglobulins are characteristically absent. Indices for organ lesions, for example kidney involvement, have to be monitored by their typical tests, as for example by urine analysis (haematuria, seldom gross proteinuria), serum creatinine, etc.

Recently, cytokines, cytokine-receptor molecules, and adhesion molecules were shown to be associated with clinical disease activity when measured in serum and/or plasma (Schmitt *et al.* 1992; Stegemann *et al.* 1993; Mrowka and Sieberth 1994). Soluble interleukin-2 receptor (**sIL2-R**) is higher in patients with generalized and active disease than in those with limited and inactive disease. Surprisingly, amounts of sIL2-R are significantly elevated in patients with complete clinical remission. Further, high, amounts of sIL2-R are associated with a high probability of relapse in this group. Serum levels of soluble cell-adhesion molecules (**CAM**) (sICAM-1, sVCAM-1, sE-selectin) were found to be significantly higher in Wegener's granulomatosis than controls; in addition, sICAM-1 and sVCAM-1 decreased with clinical remission. Surface-antigen expression of LAM-1 on granulocytes was decreased in patients with low disease activity (Riecken *et al.* 1994).

Markers of endothelial perturbation and damage (Blann *et al.* 1992; Pearson 1993; Ohdama *et al.* 1994) have been shown to be useful indicators of disease activity or progression. von Willebrand factor in plasma is secreted from endothelial cells and is widely used as one of the best markers for vasculitic disease activity. However, as with other markers (e.g. C-reactive protein), von Willebrand factor is transiently elevated during any acute-phase response to infection. Thrombomodulin, an endothelial cell-specific glycoprotein that is an important regulator of activated thrombin (converting thrombin from a procoagulant to an anticoagulant by altering its substrate specificity so that it no longer cleaves fibrinogen but activates protein C), has been found in the circulation of patients with vasculitis, including Wegener's granulomatosis. The levels of elevated soluble thrombomodulin correlate well with disease activity. In addition, autoantibodies recognizing endothelial-cell antigens are present in the serum of patients with Wegener's granulomatosis. However, they do not play a major part in the routine analysis of disease activity.

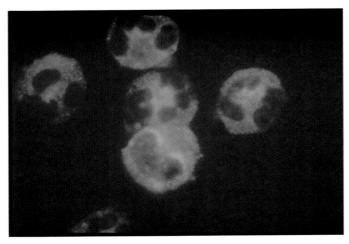

(a)

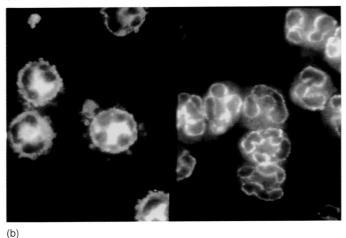

(b)

Fig. 19 Antineutrophil cytoplasmic autoantibodies: (a) cANCA and (b) pANCA fluorescence patterns.

Antineutrophil cytoplasmic autoantibodies represent a class of antibodies directed not only against various constituents of neutrophil granules but even against monocytic and endothelial antigens (for review, see Jennette and Falk 1993; Gross and Csernok 1995; Kallenberg *et al*. 1994). ANCA are routinely detected by indirect immunofluorescence on ethanol-fixed neutrophils (Wiik *et al*. 1993). At least three different patterns of fluorescence can be distinguished: the (*c*)lassic) cytoplasmic pattern (Fig. 19(a)) with accentuated fluorescence intensity in the area within the nuclear lobes (cANCA), the *p*erinuclear pattern (pANCA) (Fig. 19(b)), and a more diffuse cytoplasmic staining pattern (atypical ANCA). In vasculitis, cANCA is a seromarker for Wegener's granulomatosis and pANCA is a marker for microscopic polyangiitis; the cytoplasmic pattern associated with Wegener's granulomatosis is characteristically induced by PR3-ANCA, and the perinuclear pattern seen in microscopic polyangiitis is typically induced by myeloperoxidase-ANCA. However, the associations are not absolute and PR3-ANCA is sometimes seen in microscopic polyangiitis and myeloperoxidase-ANCA in Wegener's granulomatosis.

Three major studies on cANCA comprising a total of more than 200 patients with Wegener's granulomatosis have found a 90 per cent sensitivity of the test for generalized (systemic) Wegener's granulomatosis and 75 per cent for limited Wegener's granulomatosis. It should be mentioned that these data concern patients with active disease only; during remission, cANCA were detected in a far lower percentage of the patients. However, few patients with active generalized Wegener's granulomatosis have been found to be cANCA-negative.

Various longitudinal studies have shown that titres of ANCA rise before a relapse of Wegener's granulomatosis. The rise proved to be a sensitive indicator for ensuing relapse and was detectable a mean of 49 days before the clinical manifestations. Moreover, rising titres may not only predict a relapse but can also help to differentiate relapses from the superinfections occurring not infrequently during immunosuppressive therapy. Since cANCA titres do not follow disease activity in a considerable number of patients, titres alone should not be used as a criterion for changing treatment protocols.

The specificity of cANCA for Wegener's granulomatosis has been found to be as high as 98 per cent. The application of cANCA screening to identify oligosymptomatic Wegener's granulomatosis (e.g. E, L, K, or EL, or K in the ELK classification) has led to a rise in the frequency of diagnosis of this disease. 'Initial phase' Wegener's granulomatosis can now be diagnosed using the ACR 1990 classification criteria, the definition developed by the Chapel Hill Conference in 1992, and ANCA serology. Detection of ANCA allows for the recognition (and treatment) of the underlying disease in cases presenting as Tolosa–Hunt syndrome, facial nerve paralysis, polyneuritis cranialis, peripheral neuropathy, secondary relapsing polychondritis, idiopathic necrotizing–crescentic glomerulonephritis, or renal failure of unknown origin requiring haemodialysis. It does not, however, enable recognition of acute renal failure following infectious vasculitis due to leptospirosis, as has been reported in the literature (see Gross and Csernok 1995 for review).

cANCA are found infrequently in vasculitides closely related to Wegener's granulomatosis, for example microscopic polyarteritis, Churg–Strauss syndrome, classical polyarteritis nodosa, and only exceptionally in giant-cell arteritides and Takayasu arteritis, Henoch–Schönlein purpura, cutaneous leucocytoclastic angiitis, and cryoglobulinaemic vasculitis.

A homogeneous 'cANCA' fluorescence pattern has been observed in symptomatic patients who are human immunodeficiency virus-positive and, more recently, in patients with amoebic liver abscess. In general, though, the findings of cANCA is rare in infectious disorders and one should always be aware of the possibility of a concomitant (secondary) vasculitis. Numerous recent studies, however, have shown that 'ANCA' are far from specific for Wegener's granulomatosis and have challenged the diagnostic potential of these autoantibodies. Therefore, a multinational group of experts sponsored by the European Community has attempted to work out a standardization of assays (Hagen *et al*. 1993a; Hagen *et al*. 1993b). Using their technique, one can be sure that the detection of cANCA (and/or PR3-ANCA) will help in diagnosing and evaluating disease activity in Wegener's granulomatosis.

Monitoring disease activity and disease extension

Because generalized Wegener's granulomatosis is a multisystem disease with a high rate of relapse (Hoffman *et al*. 1992a; Gordon *et al*. 1993), it is especially important that the clinical aspect of disease activity and disease extension be monitored on a regular and controlled basis by an interdisciplinary team of physicians, ear, nose, and throat surgeons, ophthalmologists, neurologists, and radiologists (Gross 1996).

At the biochemical level, the value of the erythrocyte sedimentation rate and C-reactive protein as — admittedly non-specific — indices of disease activity is accepted generally. In the initial phase of disease, both can be normal, although secondary and opportunistic infections can lead to elevated levels. cANCA titers seem to correlate with disease activity in most patients (Nölle *et al.* 1989). Consequently, changes in cANCA titre remain one of the most important laboratory markers for changes in disease activity, and the only one specific for Wegener's granulomatosis. In contrast to the erythrocyte sedimentation rate and C-reactive protein, the cANCA titre does not rise in a secondary infection. Greatly increased amounts of sIL-2R are found in patients with increased disease activity and may be an indicator of imminent relapse in those in complete clinical remission (Schmitt *et al.* 1992).

The value of MRI of the head in determining disease extension is now widely recognized (Greenan *et al.* 1992; Asmus *et al.* 1993; Muhle *et al.* 1993; Heller *et al.* 1995). MRI can demonstrate not only extensions of the granulomatous lesions within the upper respiratory tract not detectable by nasal endoscopy or conventional radiographs, but it can also disclose intracerebral granulomas (Fig. 9) and/or infarcts of grey and white matter following vasculitis.

In patients with obvious lung involvement or in those under immunosuppression who have suspected opportunistic infection, bronchoalveolar lavage can help in obtaining a histological diagnosis from transbronchial biopsy specimens (Lombard *et al.* 1990) and in demonstrating Wegener's granulomatosis-specific disease activity (marked increase in neutrophils) or *Pneumocystis carinii* (or cytomegalovirus etc.) infection (Hoffman *et al.* 1991; Sen *et al.* 1991; Barth *et al.* 1991; Jarrousse *et al.* 1993).

For patients in whom cytotoxic agents have been employed previously, continued surveillance must include the evaluation of signs and symptoms that suggest toxicity (haemorrhagic cystitis, bladder cancer, myelodysplasia, lymphoma, etc.). Because of the occurrence of 'silent' relapses, especially in the kidneys and lungs, urinalysis (sediment) and chest radiographs should be performed at close intervals if there are even minor clinical symptoms.

Pathology and pathogenesis

Wegener's granulomatosis is a clinicopathological entity closely associated with cANCA, particularly those induced by the PR3 antibodies, whose diagnosis requires the fulfilment of specific clinical and pathological criteria and/or the presence of ANCA (PR3-ANCA) in the serum.

Until fairly recently, autopsy pathology had provided most of the tissue for morphological investigations that led to the model of the classic pathological triad of granulomatous inflammation, necrosis, and vasculitis (Godman and Churg 1954). As a matter of fact, however, only tissue from open lung biopsies exhibits this triad. More commonly, only one or two elements of the triad are seen in biopsies not of the airway. Therefore, a pathological study was performed on 126 head-and-neck biopsies from 70 patients with Wegener's granulomatosis to work out criteria for the diagnosis of Wegener's granulomatosis based on such biopsies (Devaney *et al.* 1990). The following criteria were proposed:

1. If all three major pathological criteria are present, it may be considered diagnostic if there is clinical involvement of E, L, K or either L or K.

2. If two major pathological criteria are met, it may be considered diagnostic if there is typical clinical involvement of the lung and kidney as well (E, L, K); however, if only one of these sites is involved (E, L, or K), the diagnosis may be considered as probable and further biopsies should be performed.

3. If only one of the major pathological criteria is present, it may be considered as suggestive of Wegener's granulomatosis if the patient has typical clinical evidence of Wegener's granulomatosis (E, L, K) or as suspicious for Wegener's granulomatosis if the patient has only one additional site of disease (E and L or E and K).

The diagnostic value and limitations of orbital biopsy in Wegener's granulomatosis were recently delineated (Kalina *et al.* 1992).

Wegener's granulomatosis begins with granulomatous changes, as Fienberg's group was able to establish after decades of research (for review, see Wegener 1990). More recently, open lung biopsies have been studied to determine the histogenesis of pulmonary lesions and to identify early lesions (Mark *et al.* 1988). The earliest microscopic lesion is a small focus of necrosis of collagen. This is followed by an accumulation of histiocytes and their aggregation around the necrosis to form a palisading granuloma. Progression continues from micronecrosis (usually with neutrophils: 'microabscesses') to macronecrosis (wide-spread necrosis), and later to fibrosis.

Collagen in many structures of the lung was seen to have become necrotic. This included walls of blood vessels and conducting airways, alveolar walls and pleura. The primary process, therefore, is not restricted to blood vessels, although Wegener's granulomatosis is often described as a primary vasculitis.

In this study the major criteria for the histological diagnosis of Wegener's granulomatosis based on lung biopsies were outlined. The major discriminating features are palisading granulomas or palisading histiocytes in vascular walls and in extravascular tissue, microabscesses or fibrinoid necrosis in vascular walls, leucocytoclastic capillaritis, diffuse granulomatous tissue, and granulomatous bronchiolitis. Granulomatous inflammation must be found in any case.

Palisading granuloma should be distinguished from a compact, circumscribed, rounded granuloma of tuberculoid or sarcoid type. Palisading granuloma is virtually pathognomonic of Wegener's granulomatosis; by contrast, the observation of a granuloma of the tuberculoid or sarcoid type is strong evidence against Wegener's granulomatosis. Analogous to chronic granulomatous inflammation in response to a known cause (e.g. tuberculosis), palisading histiocytes and diffuse granulomatous tissue may constitute signs of a good host response in Wegener's granulomatosis. Fibrinoid necrosis of collagen within scars suggests active disease in the face of repair and preceding a host response.

From the morphological point of view, the second major feature of Wegener's granulomatosis, vasculitis, is even more polymorphic. Vasculitis generally originates in granulomas of the respiratory tract. In many cases, the anatomical picture is dominated by a necrotizing vasculitis similar to the microscopic form of polyarteritis. Vessels of many types can be affected in Wegener's granulomatosis, resulting in various clinical expressions. Less frequently, the histological picture resembles that seen in classic polyarteritis nodosa, giant-cell or Horton's arteritis, and other vasculitic disorders.

Characteristically, the acute vasculitis exhibits segmental necrotizing lesions in the walls of arteries, arterioles, capillaries, and venules. Commonly involved vessels include arteries and arterioles in skeletal and cardiac muscle as well as in liver and kidneys, post-capillary venules and arterioles in the skin, and capillaries in the pulmonary alveoli and renal glomeruli.

The third feature of the classical triad, involvement of the kidneys (for review, see Ritz *et al.* 1991; Jennette and Falk 1994b; Gross *et al.* 1995), is also characterized by a variety of clinical and anatomical pictures. As in other affected organs, the kidneys exhibit scattered granulomas in addition to variably disseminated vasculitic processes and often marked interstitial inflammatory infiltration. Glomerular involvement is frequent and is characterized histologically by segmental fibrinoid necrosis and crescent formation. No ultrastructural evidence of immune-complex localization can be found ('pauci-immune necrotizing and crescentic glomerulonephritis). Glomerular basement membranes and Bowman's capsule are often disrupted in areas of necrosis. Injury to the glomerular capillary wall is an important initiating event in the formation of glomerular crescents. Thus, the extent of renal capillaritis determines the number of crescents that ultimate lead to rapidly progressive glomerulonephritis.

Immunopathology

The aetiology of Wegener's granulomatosis is still completely unknown. In recent years, microbial infections, drugs, and tumours have been described as the 'triggering events'; in case reports viral infections (coxsackie B3, parvovirus B19) have appeared to precipitate Wegener's granulomatosis. Furthermore, an association between chronic nasal carriage of *S. aureus* and higher relapse rates in Wegener's granulomatosis has been reported (Stegemann *et al.* 1994). It has also been speculated that *S. aureus* may produce proteases with antigenic cross-reactivity with PR3 ('Wegener's autoantigen'). Sequencing of the genome of *S. aureus* will certainly be helpful in the search for possible candidates displaying molecular mimicry of PR3 and *S. aureus*.

Hydralazine, propylthiouracil, and a few other medications can induce side-effects similar to vasculitis. Both drugs have been reported to precipitate Wegener's granulomatosis (or microscopic polyarteritis). Transformation of these drugs into cytotoxic products by activated neutrophils has been described. Cytotoxicity may induce autoimmunity by exposing autoreactive lymphocytes to abnormal forms of self-material released during premature cell death (Jiang *et al.* 1994).

Recently, an association between Wegener's granulomatosis and malignancy was observed: 6.1 per cent (29/477) in a large series of patients with malignant disease. In 23 patients the tumour was diagnosed before or simultaneously with the Wegener's granulomatosis. Nearly one-third of these patients suffered from renal-cell carcinoma. Since PR3 has been found in a renal cancer cell line, autoimmunity could be induced via this pathway (for review, see Gross and Csernok 1995).

Predisposing factors are far less well accepted in Wegener's granulomatosis than in the group of collagen vascular diseases. Infrequently, Wegener's granulomatosis occurs in several members of one family (Muniain *et al.* 1986; Knudsen *et al.* 1988; Hay *et al.*

1991; Stoney *et al.* 1991; Rottem *et al.* 1993). The association between Wegener's granulomatosis and certain HLA antigens (B8, DR2) is weak. Interestingly, the persistence of ANCA in treated Wegener's granulomatosis is associated with HLA-DQw7 (Elkon *et al.* 1983; Murty *et al.* 1991). An association of severe and moderate deficiencies in protease inhibitor phenotypes with PR3-ANCA-associated vasculitis has been observed (Esnault *et al.* 1993; Elzouki *et al.* 1994). In addition, Fcγ-receptor alleles may represent inheritable disease risk factors influencing the magnitude of this process, which is probably induced by neutrophil activation via ANCA (Porges *et al.* 1994).

Autoantibodies against PR3-ANCA are highly specific for Wegener's granulomatosis and since their titre often follows clinical disease activity it is believed that PR3-ANCA are of immunopathogenic relevance in this disorder. This has been extensively reviewed in recent years: for example Jennette and Falk (1992); Gross *et al.* (1993a); Gross *et al.* (1993b); Hagen *et al.* (1993); Wiik (1993); Jennette and Falk (1994a). It has been shown that the autoantibody interferes with the biological functions (e.g. by inhibition of elastinolytic activity), and with enzyme inhibitors (e.g. α_1-antitrypsin) of PR3. It can also activate neutrophils when PR3 is accessible on the cytoplasmic membrane by engaging the FcγRIIa receptors to produce reactive oxygen species and to degranulate. The latter event has led to the ANCA–cytokine sequence theory: As a unifying construct, it was proposed that priming doses of proinflammatory cytokines (such as those produced during infection) induce surface expression of ANCA target antigens. Binding of ANCA to these antigens leads to neutrophil degranulation and endothelial cell injury with subsequent vascular damage.

ANCA can activate primed [tumour necrosis factor-α-(**TNF-α**) pretreated] polymorphonuclear neutrophils to produce reactive oxygen species to release lysosomal enzymes (Falk *et al.* 1990) and to cause endothelial cell injury (Ewert *et al.* 1990; Savage *et al.* 1993). Proinflammatory cytokines and/or their receptors are found in serum (plasma) in active systemic vasculitis (Kekow *et al.* 1993; Roux-Lombard *et al.* 1994).

The activation pathway was once unrecognized, since PR3 (and myeloperoxidase) were thought to be located only within the azurophilic granules (Calafat *et al.* 1990). Then PR3 was detected on the plasma membrane of neutrophils using the monoclonal antibody WG M1 and electron microscopy (Csernok *et al.* 1990). Later, *in vitro* and *ex vivo* studies using flow cytometric analysis revealed that TNF-α and interleukin (**IL**) 8 act synergistically and induce a translocation of PR3 from the intragranular loci to the cell surface of neutrophils (Csernok *et al.* 1994). Apart from studies revealing upregulation of PR3 and the ability of ANCA-positive F(ab)₂ preparations to bind to the surface of neutrophils, to stimulate a respiratory burst, and to modulate neutrophil migration (Keogan *et al.* 1993), more recent investigations on the pathway of full neutrophil activation have shown that murine monoclonal ANCA IgG (but not IgM) binds to PR3 and stimulates the FcγRIIa ligand to activate human neutrophils via the receptor-mediated signal transduction system (Porges *et al.* 1994). Thus, ANCA-mediated neutrophil activation may occur mostly as a consequence of engagement of FcγRIIa by the Fc region of ANCA and, at least in part, via F(ab)₂ binding. The sum of *in vitro* and *in vivo* experimental findings supports the pathophysiological model of ANCA-mediated vasculitis depicted in Fig. 20.

Mayet *et al.* (1993a) have added exciting observations to the sparse data on ANCA–endothelial cell interactions. They were able to show

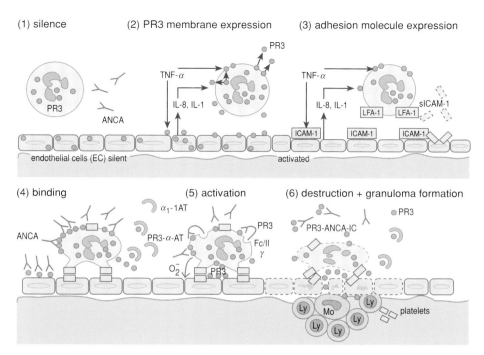

(1) silence   (2) PR3 membrane expression   (3) adhesion molecule expression

(4) binding   (5) activation   (6) destruction + granuloma formation

Fig. 20 Pathophysiological model of ANCA-mediated vasculitis (ANCA–cytokine sequence theory).

that TNF-α, IL-1α/β, and interferon-γ lead to increased PR3 expression in the cytoplasm of endothelial cells, with translocation of PR3 to the cell membrane. Thus, PR3 located directly on the inner surface of the vessel wall becomes accessible for ANCA binding. Adhesion of polymorphonuclear neutrophils occurs via the induction of endothelial leucocyte adhesion molecule-1 (**ELAM-1**) expression on the endothelial cell surface (Mayet and Meyer zum Büschenfelde 1993). On the other hand, ANCA can bind to endothelial cells incubated with myeloperoxidase or PR3 via charge differences (cationic lysosomal proteins bind to anionic structures such as the surface of endothelial cells) and can, *in vitro*, induce complement-dependent endothelial cell lysis (Savage *et al.* 1993). Although these *in vitro* studies have demonstrated that ANCA can interact with endothelial cells, direct immunocytochemistry on lesional tissue has failed to demonstrate the binding of PR-ANCA to (Brouwer *et al.* 1994; Mrowka *et al.* 1995), or the deposition of IgG on, endothelial cells (Noronha *et al.* 1993), thus casting doubt on the immunopathological relevance of these *in vitro* findings.

PR3/myeloperoxidase deposits in tissue from ANCA-associated vasculitis have been studied by several groups (Brouwer *et al.* 1994; Mrowka *et al.* 1994; Gross *et al.* 1995). Cytokine-induced expression of adhesion molecules (e.g. LFA-1, ICAM-1, ELAM-1) facilitate close contact between neutrophils and endothelial cells, with subsequent shielding of these aggressive enzymes from their natural inhibitors (α_1-antitrypsin, elafin, etc.; Fig. 20). Immunohistological studies of vasculitic tissue have demonstrated that both kinds of molecules are up-regulated: among the active (ANCA-associated) resident cells in glomerulonephritis, endothelial and infiltrating mononuclear cells express a variety of cytokines (IL-1, -2 and -3, TNF-α, interferon-γ, platelet-derived growth factor, and transforming growth factor-β), cytokine and growth-factor receptors (**R**) (TNF-R, IL-1R type II, IL-2R, interferon-γR, and platelet-derived growth factorβ-R) as well as the adhesion molecules described above (Waldherr *et al.* 1993). ICAM-1 was most abundantly present in renal

lesions of Wegener's granulomatosis and the intensity of its expression correlated with the presence of glomerular crescents and the number of LFA-1 (CD11a) leucocytes. Serum levels of soluble adhesion molecules (e.g. sICAM-1) correlated with disease activity and renal functional impairment (Hauschild *et al.* 1992; Kekow *et al.* 1993; Brouwer *et al.* 1994; Mrowka and Sieberth 1994).

Activated neutrophils and the extracellular localization of lysosomal enzymes were recently observed in renal biopsies from Wegener's granulomatosis (Brouwer *et al.* 1994; Gross *et al.* 1995). Activation of neutrophils was assessed by measuring hydrogen peroxide production *in situ*; the number of activated cells in the biopsy correlated with the extent of renal functional impairment. Accordingly, PR3, myeloperoxidase, and human leucocyte elastase were localized extracellularly in renal tissue. Using a plastic embedding method, the binding of these enzymes to negatively charged structures such as endothelial cells and the glomerular basement membrane was well demonstrated, but the expression of PR3 was not found within endothelial cells. This observation was recently confirmed by Mrowka *et al.* (1995), who studied the distribution of PR3 and human leucocyte elastase in 120 renal biopsies from patients with glomerulonephritis and found these ANCA antigens expressed in ANCA-positive and -negative glomerulonephritis.

A growing body of evidence indicates that autoantibody activity in autoimmune diseases might be regulated by idiotype–anti-idiotype reactions. Observations on the clinical and *in vitro* effects of pooled human immunoglobulin and ANCA interactions (Jayne *et al.* 1993; Richter *et al.* 1993; Pall *et al.* 1994) suggest that a defect in the regulation of the idiotypic network could be involved in the production of these autoantibodies. Furthermore, network interactions can be used to develop important experimental and therapeutic agents. Our group recently generated a murine monoclonal antibody directed against a human monoclonal anti-PR3 antibody (Csernok and Gross 1993). This antibody (type Ab2β, designated 5/7) inhibits the anti-PR3 activity of cANCA in serum from patients with Wegener's granulomatosis. The anti-idiotype 5/7 is a powerful tool for studying the organization of the idiotypic network in Wegener's granulomatosis and can be used for therapeutic immunoabsorption. Furthermore, the binding of PR3-ANCA to cytokine-treated endothelial cells was blocked by the 5/7 idiotype (Mayet *et al.* 1993b). These data indicate that regulation of the idiotypic network may play an important apart in the interaction between ANCA and vascular endothelium.

Granuloma formation usually indicates a state of T-cell hyperactivity and immunohistological studies have revealed a predominance of CD4+ cells in renal biopsies of patients with Wegener's granulomatosis (Brouwer *et al.* 1991). In cellular crescents of rapidly progressive glomerulonephritis and in the peripheral blood of patients with Wegener's granulomatosis, the number of activated (CD25+) T cells is also increased. An increase in concentrations of serum cytokines (e.g. TNF-α, IL-6) during the acute phase of the disease is an indirect indicator of T-cell activation (for review, see Kekow *et al.* 1993). Elevated concentrations of sIL-2R have been detected in serum from patients with Wegener's granulomatosis, and were shown to correlate with disease activity. It has been demonstrated that even in complete remission, sIL-2R tends to be increased in Wegener's granulomatosis (Schmitt *et al*, 1992). However, T-cell responses to neutrophil extract did not differ between patients with vasculitis and controls: both showed only low levels of antigen-specific proliferation, and these could not be amplified by *in vitro* selection (Mathieson *et al.* 1992). In contrast to these findings, T cells from patients with Wegener's granulomatosis (PR3-ANCA positive) have been found to proliferate after exposure to highly purified PR3; however, 33 per cent of samples from healthy controls also reacted *in vitro* to PR3. In any case, the above noted extracellular localization of lysosomal proteins in renal biopsies (or elsewhere in tissue lesions in Wegener's granulomatosis) could induce the accumulation and activation of monocytes, and transform them to epithelioid and/or multinucleated giant cells characteristic of granulomas, as delineated in Fig. 20.

The IgG subclass distribution of cANCA shows a high prevalence of IgG4 antibody (Brouwer *et al.* 1991), together with increased total IgG4. This suggests repeated antigen stimulation in a T-cell response and contrasts with the IgG subclass distribution of, for example, antinuclear antibodies, which are mainly restricted to IgG1 and IgG3 (Kallenberg *et al.* 1991). Recently, a reduced CD4/CD8 T-cell ratio was reported, but this has not yet been confirmed by others (Ikeda *et al.* 1992).

Necrotizing vasculitis occurs in a number of experimental conditions involving animal models, but none of these closely resembles human systemic vasculitis (for review, see Mathieson *et al.* 1993). Brown Norway rats treated with HgCl develop a number of autoantibodies, including myeloperoxidase-ANCA, resulting in tissue injury in a number of organs, with necrotizing vasculitis especially prevalent in the gut (Mathieson *et al.* 1993). Despite similarities with human systemic vasculitis, the lack of nephritis in particular reveals the weakness of this model. The typical renal lesion of the ANCA-associated vasculitides is a pauci-immune glomerulonephritis that lacks any prominent deposition of immunoglobulin or complement, but often has extracapillary proliferation forming 'crescents' (Falk *et al.* 1990).

Brouwer *et al.* (1993) immunized Brown Norway rats with human myeloperoxidase. Five weeks after immunization the left kidney was perfused with various injurious agents, including hydrogen peroxidase plus myeloperoxidase or other products of activated neutrophils. The rats developed necrotizing crescentic glomerulonephritis and vasculitis. Since myeloperoxidase, IgG, and C3 could be detected along the glomerular basement membrane 24 h after perfusion, the 'pauci-immune' character of this vasculitis model is questionable, even when immune deposits were generally absent 4 and 10 days after perfusion. In addition, others have consistently found immune deposits along the glomerular basement membrane in both rat strains (Brown Norway and spontaneously hypertensive) used by Brouwer (Yang *et al.* 1993).

Inflammation of the vessel wall has been elicited by direct gene transfer of a foreign class I major histocompatibility complex gene, HLA-B7, to specific sites in porcine arteries. Transfer and expression of this recombinant gene was confirmed by polymerase chain reaction and immunohistochemistry, and cytolytic T cells specific for HLA-B7 were detected. This model demonstrates that vessel damage can be induced by cell-mediated immune injury (Nabel *et al.* 1992).

Treatment

Because of the possibly life-threatening course of generalized Wegener's granulomatosis there has been general agreement that the 'standard' treatment (Fauci *et al.* 1983) consisting of daily 'low-dose' (2–4 mg/day) cyclophosphamide plus glucocorticoids — undoubtedly an extremely effective therapy — is of most benefit to the majority of patients (Cupps 1990; Hoffman 1993b). This view has been challenged recently by data indicating (i) the variability of clinical course in Wegener's granulomatosis, (ii) continued morbidity despite treatment with cyclophosphamide plus glucocorticoids, (iii) a high incidence of relapse, and (iv) an alarming range of toxic effects induced by this protocol (for review, see Gross 1994).

Although the introduction of therapy with cyclophosphamide plus glucocorticoids 30 years ago improved the prognosis in Wegener's granulomatosis from a mean survival of 5 months (Walton 1958)) to a 93 per cent chance of remission (Fauci *et al.* 1983), an updated analysis (Hoffman *et al.* 1992a) now presents less favourable data on both the efficacy of the protocol (remission rate, 75 per cent) and its side-effects (serious infectious complications, 46 per cent; cyclophosphamide-induced haemorrhagic cystitis, 43 per cent; bladder cancer, 2.8 per cent; myelodysplasia, 2 per cent). These side-effects were noted earlier and are alarming because of their high rate of induced morbidity and mortality (Conn *et al.* 1988; Stillwell *et al.* 1988; Bradley *et al.* 1989; Ettinger *et al.* 1989; Anderson *et al.* 1992; Jarrousse *et al.* 1993). In addition, immediate hypersensitivity reactions to cyclophosphamide and mesna have also been observed (Knysak *et al.* 1994).

Glucocorticoids alone have failed to produce satisfactory results (Hoffman *et al.* 1992, Briedigkeit *et al.* 1993). On the other hand, high doses of glucocorticoids (in combination with daily cyclophosphamide; standard protocol in Wegener's granulomatosis) given over prolonged periods (several months) are accompanied by serious infectious complications: 50 per cent of all infections due to bacteria, pneumocystis, and fungi occurred during daily glucocorticoid therapy, 21 per cent during alternate-day therapy, 16 per cent under single-agent cytotoxic therapy, and 12 per cent during periods of no therapy (Hoffman *et al.* 1992). Such infections can contribute to vascular occlusion (Conn *et al.* 1988). Therefore glucocorticoids should be used only in conjunction with cyclophosphamide (or see below: methotrexate, azathioprine) and high initial doses of glucocorticoids should be tapered more vigorously (see Table 3) than recommended in the original report (Fauci *et al.* 1983).

The knowledge that Wegener's granulomatosis follows a two-phase course, together with the increasing identification of cases during the initial phase due to the diagnostic use of ANCA, provide a rationale for stage-adapted treatment (for review, see Hoffman 1993b; Gross and Rasmussen 1994; Gross 1996). The recognition of the toxicity and the newly discovered aspects of the disease course have led investigators to study other types of therapy for this disorder.

Trimethoprim–sulphamethoxazole

While trimethoprim–sulphamethoxazole may have the capacity to induce remission in the 'initial phase' of Wegener's granulomatosis (DeRemee *et al.* 1985; DeRemee *et al.* 1993; Reinhold-Keller *et al.* 1996), the possibility that it may actually prolong the initial phase is currently being investigated in double-blind, controlled studies. Recent experience does not indicate that trimethoprim–sulphamethoxazole can prevent relapse of generalized Wegener's granulomatosis in remission and thus it does not appear suited for treatment of classical Wegener's granulomatosis (Reinhold-Keller *et al.* 1996). Despite the lack of prospective, controlled studies, the available data on trimethoprim–sulphamethoxazole have led to its more widespread use (2 × 1 tablet, double strength) in patients in the initial stage of Wegener's granulomatosis, as described above.

Pulse cyclophosphamide

Inconsistent results were obtained in 12 patients with generalized Wegener's granulomatosis treated with pulse cyclophosphamide (Steppat and Gross 1989). Similarly, the National Institutes of Health reported only temporary benefit in 13 of 14 patients treated with the same pulse cyclophosphamide regimen; lack of response and failure to sustain improvement or tolerate continued treatment were noted in 79 per cent of patients (Hoffman *et al.* 1990). By contrast, two nephrological groups reported that the outcome after pulse cyclophosphamide therapy was similar to that following the 'standard protocol' (Falk *et al.* 1990; Haubitz *et al.* 1991). These differences may be ascribed to the fact that all of the nephrological patients had renal involvement, whereas only 50 per cent and 32 per cent of the patients investigated in the former studies showed signs of renal disease. In addition, the group studied in Chapel Hill (Falk *et al.* 1990) was mixed: only 19 of 37 patients with Wegener's granulomatosis had cANCA and a majority of the other patients had pANCA, suggesting that cases of microscopic polyangiitis had been included. Therefore, in order to determine for ourselves the clinical and/or immunological markers affecting response to pulse cyclophosphamide, we studied its efficacy in 43 patients with cANCA-positive and biopsy-proven Wegener's granulomatosis. Fifty-eight per cent of our patients did not respond to pulse cyclophosphamide treatment. Collectively, a poor response was seen in patients with generalized disease involving more than four organ systems (mainly the heart, nervous system, eyes, skin) and with constitutional symptoms and a high cANCA titre (Reinhold-Keller *et al.* 1994). We conclude, therefore, that pulse cyclophosphamide should be used in order to reduce the total amount of cyclophosphamide. Pulse cyclophosphamide can also be applied in generalized Wegener's granulomatosis with less extensive disease and a lower ANCA titre (according to the disease extension index) or in generalized Wegener's granulomatosis with formerly extensive and/or fulminant disease in partial remission (Table 3).

Table 3 Recommendations for drug usage in generalized Wegener's granulomatosis with respect to disease activity and extension

Disease activity	Drugs	Doses		Glucocorticoids
Active and extended	Daily CP[1]	2 mg/kg	*plus*	low-dose GC[4]
Progressive	Daily CP[1]	2–4 mg/kg	*plus*	GC 1 mg/kg[4]
Fulminant (e.g. AH[5], RPGN[6], PRS[7])	Daily CP[1]	2–4 kg/kg	*plus*	Methyl-prednisolone pulse[4]
Partial remission and/or mild active/less extended	Bolus CP[1] *or*	15 mg/kg every 3 weeks	*plus*	low-dose GC (daily)
	weekly MTX[2] *or*	0.2–0.3 mg/kg	*plus*	low-dose GC
	daily AZA[3]	2 mg/kg	*plus*	low-dose GC

[1]CP (cyclophosphamide): a reduction of the dose may be required in the setting of significant impairment of renal function (adjust to leucocyte count) and in the elderly (>60 years). Adequate fluid intake to main a 3 litre output/day will decrease the risk of bladder toxicity.
[2]MTX (methotrexate): *avoid* in the setting of impairment of renal function. *Avoid* additional co-trimoxazole.
[3]AZA (azathioprine): *avoid* additional allopurinol.
[4]GC (glucocorticoids): 'low-dose' ⩽7.5 mg prednisolone/day; initiate GC at 1 mg/kg per day in divided dose (every 8 h) for the first week, consolidate the dose of GC to single daily dose over the second week, then GC can be gradually tapered within the next 4–8 weeks to 'low-dose' GC. GC pulse will be performed for 3 days (methyl-prednisolone: 250 mg/day).
[5]Alveolar haemorrhage syndrome.
[6]Rapidly progressive glomerulonephritis.
[7]Pulmonary renal syndrome.
[8]Under conventional standard treatment (e.g. daily CP plus GC).

Methotrexate

Hoffman *et al.* (1992b) recently used 'low-dose' methotrexate (20–30 mg weekly) plus glucocorticoids in 29 patients with Wegener's granulomatosis without 'immediately life-threatening disease', although 12 (41 per cent) did have active glomerulonephritis. Treatment produced a marked improvement in 76 per cent and remission in 69 per cent. However, 3 of the 29 patients (10 per cent) suffered from *Pneumocystis carinii* pneumonia during the first month of treatment (including prednisone 60 mg/day). These data have been confirmed by Handrock *et al.* (1994). In conclusion, weekly low-dose methotrexate can be used to maintain (partial) remission in cases of Wegener's granulomatosis without renal function impairment.

Cyclosporin

Until now cyclosporin has been used only as a back-up treatment in Wegener's granulomatosis. In four patients with poor response to (oral) cyclophosphamide or with intolerable side-effects, cyclosporin was able to control disease activity at dosages between 5 and 10 mg/kg per day (Schollmeyer *et al.* 1990). Recently, Allen *et al.* (1993) presented data on patients with active Wegener's granulomatosis undergoing combined therapy with cyclosporin and low-dose glucocorticoids. Cyclosporin was effective at initial doses of up to 5 mg/kg per day, but mild flare-ups occurred when this was lowered to 2 mg/kg per day.

Schmitt *et al.* (1993) reported on 20 patients who received renal transplants between 1982 and 1993. Treatment before transplant consisted of oral cyclophosphamide and glucocorticoids in 18 patients, and of pulse cyclophosphamide and glucocorticoids or azathioprine plus glucocorticoids in one patient each. At the time of transplant, 6 patients had symptoms of active disease. Nevertheless, 18 patients are still alive with functioning grafts (mean creatinine, 1.7 mg/per cent) and 16 are in complete remission. These results demonstrate that the rate of survival and graft function in patients with Wegener's granulomatosis is similar to that of other transplant recipients, so patients with active Wegener's granulomatosis need not be excluded from transplantation.

These data indicate that immunosuppressive therapy after transplantation must not necessarily include cyclophosphamide and that cyclosporin is effective under such circumstances.

High-dose intravenous immunoglobulin

The ability of intravenous immunoglobulin to diminish vasculitic features was described quite recently (Jayne *et al.* 1991; Tuso *et al.* 1992). Intravenous immunoglobulin was applied to 26 patients (14 with Wegener's granulomatosis, 11 with polyarteritis nodosa, 1 with rheumatoid vasculitis) requiring an intensification of therapy but mostly refractory or intolerant to glucocorticoids and cytotoxic drugs. They received a total dosage of 2 g/kg Sandoglobulin over 5 days. All patients appeared to improve after intravenous immunoglobulin, with 13/26 achieving full remission; the benefit was sustained in 18/26 at 12 months. Allowing for changes in other medications, 19/26 were in full remission after 1 year, six in partial remission, while one had died of septic complications.

In another study, intravenous immunoglobulin was given to nine patients with Wegener's granulomatosis and one with systemic pANCA-associated vasculitis, none of whom had attained complete remission under 'standard therapy' (Richter *et al.* 1995). The response

was measured by blind interdisciplinary clinical assessment, cranial MRI, and immunodiagnostic analyses. All 15 patients were treated with Venimmune (0.4 g/kg per day) for 5 days. Sixty per cent of the patients responded to therapy with improvement of single disease manifestations, but none experienced complete remission. In conclusion, intravenous immunoglobulin may play a part in Wegener's granulomatosis as an adjuvant to conventional therapy in patients with progressive disease.

Monoclonal-antibody therapy

This was introduced in 1990 for treatment of vasculitis (Mathieson *et al.* 1990). A case of severe vasculitis treated several times with an anti-CDw52 antibody (Campath 1H) responded with significant but only transient improvement. Remission lasted for more than 2 years, but this was achieved by following anti-CD52 with injection of an anti-CD4 antibody. The same group has since reported on four patients (two each with microscopic polyangiitis, Sjögren's syndrome, and Behçet's disease) who were unresponsive to immunosuppressive drugs but who received 'substantial and sustained benefit' from Campath 1H and hIgG1 anti-CD4 antibody (Lockwood *et al.* 1993). Similar results have been obtained in a few patients with systemic Wegener's granulomatosis (C. M. Lockwood, personal communication). Two other groups have reported on the successful treatment of two severe and intractable cases of relapsing polychondritis with vasculitis using a mouse and chimerical anti-CD4 monoclonal antibody (Choy *et al.* 1991; van der Lubbe *et al.* 1991).

In conclusion, preliminary studies have achieved encouraging results in patients with severe Wegener's granulomatosis refractory or intolerant to standard immunosuppressive therapy. Because such patients have a poor prognosis, these protocols appear suited as rescue regimens and should only be undertaken at experienced centres familiar with the side-effects or in trials already underway.

Azathioprine

Azathioprine has been used in the treatment of Wegener's granulomatosis and microscopic polyangiitis for many years. It has been found to be clearly less effective than cyclophosphamide for the induction of remission in generalized disease, but it seems to be valuable for maintenance of remission (Bouroncle *et al.* 1967; Fauci *et al.* 1983; Gaskin and Pusey 1992; Gordon *et al.* 1994).

Therapeutic recommendations

Recent long-term studies have revealed considerable variation in the clinical severity of Wegener's granulomatosis, while 'standard' therapy (e.g. daily cyclophosphamide plus glucocorticoids), as outlined above, is associated with considerable treatment-related morbidity, mortality, and a high incidence of relapses. On the other hand, less toxic therapeutic strategies (e.g. methotrexate) are being pursued with remarkable success. For the future, therefore, stage- and activity-dependent therapy protocols have to be developed and strategies for inducing remission must be differentiated from strategies for desperate situations (compassionate regimens). At present, many centres follow the procedures described below (see Table 3).

In initial-phase Wegener's granulomatosis, treatment can start with daily co-trimoxazole (2 × 1 double-strength tablet) if the patient can be followed easily.

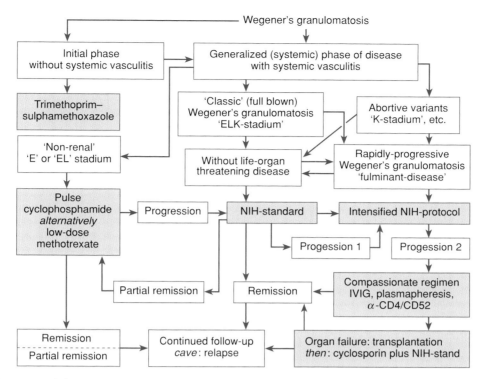

Fig. 21 Flow chart of recommended management.

In active and extended (generalized phase) Wegener's granulomatosis, most centres still begin treatment with the National Institutes of Health standard protocol (daily 2 mg/kg cyclophosphamide plus glucocorticoids). However, in contrast to the originally described concept (treatment should be continued for 1 year after the induction of remission), the therapeutic strategy is usually changed when partial remission is achieved (e.g. within the first year of treatment) to a less toxic protocol, such as pulse cyclophosphamide or weekly low-dose methotrexate (if there is no renal insufficiency) or to azathioprine (see Table 3). In addition, glucocorticoids should be tapered more vigorously (Table 3).

In the setting of (slowly) progressive Wegener's granulomatosis, by contrast, higher daily doses of cyclophosphamide (2–4 mg/kg) and glucocorticoids have to be used. The dose of cyclophosphamide will then be adjusted to maintain a total leucocyte count between 3000 and 4000/l ('intensified' National Institutes of Health protocol) for several weeks in order to stop disease progression. In addition to an adequate fluid intake (3–4 l/day), mesna can be used to decrease the risk of cyclophosphamide-induced bladder toxicity.

In more rapidly progressive Wegener's granulomatosis (including fulminant disease), methylprednisolone pulses (250 mg/day for 3 days) are used in addition to the 'intensified' National Institutes of Health protocol. Plasmapheresis is recommended only if rapidly progressive glomerulonephritis could lead to oligoanuria and dialysis.

In cases of generalized Wegener's granulomatosis without life- or organ-threatening disease activity, especially in the 'non-renal' variants, therapy can begin with milder protocols, for example pulse cyclophosphamide treatment every 3 weeks or weekly low-dose methotrexate, if the patient can be closely followed-up.

The adverse effects of cyclophosphamide therapy are significant (for review, see Cupps 1990). During the initial phase the leucocyte

and platelet counts should be monitored at least 2 to 3 times per week. The dose of cyclophosphamide necessary to maintain a specific leucocyte count decreases as the total dose of glucocorticoids is reduced. The dose of both agents should be adapted to the age of the patient (complications arise in elderly people). The use of cyclic oestrogens may decrease the cyclophosphamide-associated toxicity in the ovary. Patients should be encouraged to maintain a fluid intake of about 3 l/day. The toxicity of glucocorticoids can be minimized by vigorous tapering (see above) and, in the event of pre-existing osteopenia, by supplementary vitamin D. A flow chart of recommended management is shown in Fig. 21.

It would be a grave error to assume that the available pharmacological options are enough to provide sufficient treatment. Wegener's granulomatosis obviously involves many organs and requires multi-disciplinary care. Patients frequently need, for example, tympanostomies, drainage tubes for otitis media, subglottic and thoracic surgery for stenosis in the lower respiratory tract, ophthalmic surgery for obstruction of the nasolacrimal ducts, cytoscopy for cyclophosphamide-induced cystitis or bladder cancer, and renal transplantation. In addition, because of its relapsing nature, the physician treating Wegener's granulomatosis is obliged to maintain constant surveillance. This is especially true for those organs in which relapse may be asymptomatic (kidneys, lungs).

References

Aberle, D. R., Gamsu, G., and Lynch, D. (1990). Thoracic manifestations of Wegener's granulomatosis: Diagnosis and course. *Radiology*, **174**, 703–9.

Alcalay, M. *et al.* (1990). Les manifestations articulaires de la maladie de Wegener. *Revue du Rhumatism*, **57**, 845–53.

Allen, N. B., Caldwell, D. S., Rice, J. R., and McCullum, R. M. (1993). Cyclosporin A therapy for Wegener's granulomatosis. In *ANCA-associated vasculitides* (ed. W. L. Gross), pp. 473–6). Plenum, New York.

Anderson, G. *et al.* (1992). Wegener's granuloma. A series of 265 British cases seen between 1975 and 1985. A report by a sub-committee of the British Thoracic Society Research Committee. *Quarterly Journal of Medicine*, **302**, 427–38.

Andrews, M., Edmunds, M., Campbell, A., Walls, J., and Feehally, J. (1990). Systemic vasculitis in the 1980s — is there an increasing incidence of Wegener's granulomatosis and microscopic polyarteritis? *Journal of the Royal College of Physicians of London*, **24**, 284–8.

Asmus, R. *et al.* (1993). MRI of the head in Wegener's granulomatosis. In *ANCA-associated vasculitides* (ed. W. L. Gross), pp. 319–22. Plenum, New York.

Barth, J., Petermann, W., Zemke, F., Kreipe, H., and Gross, W. L. (1991). Bronchoalveolar Lavage bei Wegener'scher Granulomatose. *Pneumologie*, **45**, 570–4.

Blann, A. D., Hopkins, J., Winkles, J., and Wainwright, A. C. (1992). Plasma and serum von Willebrand factor antigen concentrations in connective tissue disorders. *Annals of Clinical Biochemistry*, **29**, 67–71.

Boudes, P. (1990). Purely granulomatous Wegener's granulomatosis: a new concept for an old disease. *Seminars in Arthritis and Rheumatism*, **19**, 365–70.

Bouroncle, B. A., Smith, E. J., and Cuppage, F. E. (1967). Treatment of Wegener's granulomatosis with Imuran. *American Journal of Medicine*, **42**, 314–18.

Bradley, J. D., Brandt, K. D., and Katz, B. P. (1989). Infectious complications of cyclophosphamide treatment for vasculitis. *Arthritis and Rheumatism*, **32**, 45–53.

Briedigkeit, L., Ulmer, M., Reinhold-Keller, E., Göbel, U., Natusch, R., and Gross, W. L. (1993). Die Therapie der Wegener'scher Granulomatose: Erfahrungen mit der konventionellen und der stadienadaptierten Behandlung bei 111 Patienten während 24 Jahren. *Innere Medizin*, **48**, 183–9.

Brouwer, E. *et al.* (1991). Immunohistology of renal biopsies in Wegener's granulomatosis (WG): clues to its pathogenesis. *Kidney International*, **39**, 1055.

Brouwer, E., Cohen Tervaert, J. W. C., van Goor, H., Huitema, M. G., Weening, J. J., and Kallenberg, C. G. M. (1993). Activated neutrophils in renal biopsies from patients with Wegener's granulomatosis. *Clinical and Experimental Immunology*, **93** (Suppl. 1), 20 (Abstr.).

Brouwer, E. *et al.* (1994). Neutrophil activation *in vitro* and *in vivo* in Wegener's granulomatosis. *Kidney International*, **45**, 1120–31.

Calafat, J., Goldschmeding, R., Ringeleing, P. L., Janssen, H., and van der Schoot, C. E. (1990). *In situ* localization by double-labeling immunoelectron microscopy of anti-neutrophil cytoplasmic autoantibodies in neutrophils and monocytes. *Blood*, **75**, 242–50.

Carrington, C. B. and Liebow, A. A. (1966). Limited forms of angiitis and granulomatosis of Wegener's type. *American Journal of Medicine*, **41**, 497–527.

Chakravarty, K., Scott, D. G. I., Blyth, J., and Courteney-Harris, R. G. (1994). Wegener's granulomatosis in the elderly — unusual presentations and misdiagnosis. *Journal of Rheumatology*, **21**, 1157–9.

Charles, S. J., Meyer, P. A. R., and Watson, P. G. (1991). Diagnosis and management of systemic Wegener's granulomatosis presenting with anterior ocular inflammatory disease. *British Journal of Ophthalmology*, **75**, 201–7.

Choy, E. H. S., Chikaza, I. C., Kingsley, G. H., and Panayi, G. S. (1991). Chimaeric anti-CD4 monoclonal antibody for relapsing polychondritis. *Lancet*, **338**, 450.

Conn, D. L., Tompkins, R. B., and Nichols, W. L. (1988). Glucocorticoids in the management of vasculitis — a double edged sword?. *Journal of Rheumatology*, **15**, 1181–2.

Cordier, J-F., Valeyre, D., Guillevin, L., Loire, R., and Brechot, J-M. (1990). Pulmonary Wegener's granulomatosis. A clinical imaging study of 77 cases. *Chest*, **97**, 906–12.

Csernok, E. and Gross, W. L. (1993). Production and characterization of an antiidiotypic monoclonal antibody that inhibits the anti-proteinase 3 activity of cANCA. *Clinical and Experimental Immunology*, **93** (Suppl. 1), 19.

Csernok, E., Lüdemann, E., Gross, W. L., and Bainton, D. F. (1990). Ultrastructural localization of proteinase 3, the target antigen of anti-cytoplasmic antibodies circulating in Wegener's granulomatosis. *American Journal of Pathology*, **137**, 1113–20.

Csernok, E., Ernst, M., Schmitt, W. H., Bainton, D. F., and Gross, W. L. (1994). Activated neutrophils express proteinase 3 on their plasma membrane *in vitro* and *in vivo*. *Clinical and Experimental Immunology*, **95**, 244–50.

Cupps, T. R. (1990). Cyclophosphamide: to pulse or not to pulse. *American Journal of Medicine*, **89**, 399–402.

D'Cruz, D. P., Baguley, E., Asherson, R. A., and Hughes, G. R. V. (1989). Ear, nose, and throat symptoms in subacute Wegener's granulomatosis. *British Medical Journal*, **299**, 419–22.

Del Buono, E. A. and Flint, A. (1991). Diagnostic usefulness of nasal biopsy in Wegener's granulomatosis. *Human Pathology*, **22**, 107–10.

DeRemee, R. A. (1993). The nosology of Wegener's granulomatosis utilizing the ELK format augmented by c-ANCA. In *ANCA-associated vasculitides* (ed. W. L. Gross), pp. 209–16. Plenum, New York.

DeRemee, R. A., McDonald, T. J., Harrison, E. G. J. R., and Coles, D. T. (1976). Wegener's granulomatosis. Anatomic correlates, a proposed classification. *Mayo Clinic Proceedings*, **51**, 777–81.

DeRemee, R. A., McDonald, T. J., and Weiland, L. H. (1985). Wegener's granulomatosis: observations on treatment with antimicrobial agents. *Mayo Clinic Proceedings*, **60**, 27–32.

Devaney, K. O., Travis, W. D., Hoffman, G., Leavitt, R., Lebovics, R., and Fauci, A. S. (1990). Interpretation of head and neck biopsies in Wegener's granulomatosis. *American Journal of Surgical Pathology*, **14**, 555–64.

Duncker, G., Nölle, B., Asmus, R., Koltze, H., and Rochels, R. (1993). Orbital involvement in Wegener's granulomatosis. In *ANCA-associated vasculitides* (ed. W. L. Gross), pp. 315–18. Plenum, New York.

Elkon, K. B., Sutherland, D. C., Rees, A. J., Hughes, G. R. V., and Batchelor, J. R. (1983). HLA antigen frequencies in systemic vasculitis: increase in HLA-DR2 in Wegener's granulomatosis. *Arthritis and Rheumatism*, **26**, 102–5.

Elzouki, A-N.Y., Segelmark, M., Wieslander, J., and Eriksson, S. (1994). Strong link between the alpha1-antitrypsin PiZ allele and Wegener's granulomatosis. *Journal of Internal Medicine*, **236**, 543–8.

Esnault, V. L. M. *et al.* (1993). Alpha1-antitrypsin genetic polymorphism in ANCA-positive systemic vasculitis. *Kidney International*, **43**, 1329–32.

Ettinger, J., Feiden, W., Hübner, G., and Schreiner, M. (1989). Progressive multifokale Leukoenzephalopathie bei Wegener'scher Granulomatose unter Therapie mit Cyclosporin A. *Klinische Wochenschrift*, **67**, 260–4.

Ewert, B. H. *et al.* (1990). Antimyeloperoxidase antibodies stimulate neutrophils to adhere to human umbilical vein endothelial cells. Abstract book of 3rd International Workshop of ANCA, Washington DC, p. 28.

Falk, R. J., Hogan, S. L., Carey, T. S., and Jennette, C. J. (1990). Clinical course of antineutrophil cytoplasmic autoantibody-associated glomerulonephritis and systemic vasculitis. *Annals of Internal Medicine*, **113**, 656–63.

Fauci, A. S., Haynes, B. F., Katz, P., and Wolff, S. M. (1983). Wegener's granulomatosis: prospective clinical and therapeutic experience with 85 patients for 21 years. *Annals of Internal Medicine*, **98**, 76–85.

Frances, C. *et al.* (1994). Wegener's granulomatosis: dermatological manifestations in 75 cases with clinicopathologic correlation. *Archives of Dermatology*, **130**, 861.

Frankel, A. H., Singer, D. R. J., Winearls, C. G., Evans, D. J., Rees, A. J., and Pusey, C. D. (1992). Type II essential mixed cryoglobulinaemia: Presentation, treatment and outcome in 13 patients. *Quarterly Journal of Medicine*, **82**, 101–24.

Gaskin, G. and Pusey, C. D. (1992). Systemic vasculitis. In *Oxford textbook of clinical nephrology* (1st edn) (ed. J. S. Cameron, A. M. Davison, J. Grunfeld, D. N. S. Kerr, and E. Ritz), pp. 612–36. Oxford University Press.

Godman, G. C. and Churg, J. (1954). Wegener's granulomatosis. *Archives of Pathology*, **58**, 533–53.

Gordon, M. *et al.* (1993). Relapses in patients with a systemic vasculitis. *Quarterly Journal of Medicine*, **86**, 779–89.

Gordon, M. *et al.* (1994). Necrotizing vasculitis — relapse despite cytotoxic therapy. *Advances in Experimental Medicine and Biology*, **336**, 477–82.

Greenan, T. J., Grossman, R. I., and Goldberg, H. I. (1992). Cerebral vasculitis: MR imaging and angiographic correlation. *Radiology*, **182**, 65–72.

Gross, W. L. (1989). Wegener's granulomatosis. New aspects of the disease course, immunodiagnostic procedures and stage-adapted treatment. *Sarcoidosis*, **6**, 15–29.

Gross, W. L. (1994). New developments in the treatment of systemic vasculitis. *Current Opinion in Rheumatology*, **6**, 11–19.

Gross, W. L. (1996). New concepts in Wegener's granulomatosis. In *The vasculitides* (ed. B. M. Ansell, P. A. Bacon, J. T. Lie, and Y. Shoenfeld), pp. 145–70. Chapman and Hall, London.

Gross, W. L. and Csernok, E. (1995). Antineutrophil cytoplasmic autoantibodies (ANCA). Immunodiagnostic and pathophysiological aspects. *Current Opinion in Rheumatology*.

Gross, W. L. and Rasmussen, N. (1994). Treatment of Wegener's granulomatosis: the view from two non-nephrologists. *Nephrology Dialysis Transplantation*, **9**, 1219–25.

Gross, W. L., Schmitt, W. H., and Csernok, E. (1991). Antineutrophil cytoplasmic autoantibody-associated diseases: a rheumatologist's view. *American Journal of Kidney Diseases*, **18**, 175–9.

Gross, W. L., Csernok, E., and Flesch, B. (1993*a*). 'Classic' anti-neutrophil cytoplasmic autoantibodies (cANCA), 'Wegener's autoantigen' and their immunopathogenic role in Wegener's granulomatosis. *Journal of Autoimmunity*, **6**, 171–84.

Gross, W. L., Schmitt, W. H., and Csernok, E. (1993*b*). ANCA and associated diseases: immunodiagnostic and pathogenetic aspects. *Clinical and Experimental Immunology*, **91**, 1–12.

Gross, W. L., Csernok, E., and Helmchen, U. (1995). Antineutrophil cytoplasmic antibodies, autoantigens and systemic vasculitis. *Acta Pathologica Microbiologica et Immunologica Scandinavica (Copenhagen)*, **103**, 81–97.

Hagen, E. C. *et al.* (1993*a*). The value of indirect immunofluorescence and solid phase techniques for ANCA detection. A report on the first phase of an international cooperative study on the standardization of ANCA assays. *Journal of Immunological Methods*, **159**, 1–16.

Hagen, C., Baillieux, B. E. P. B., van Es, L., Daha, M. R., and van der Woude, F. J. (1993*b*). Antineutrophil cytoplasmic autoantibodies: a review of the antigens involved, the assays, and the clinical and possible pathogenetic consequences. *Blood*, **81**, 1996–2002.

Hall, S. L., Miller, L. C., Duggan, E., Mauer, S. M., Beatty, E. C., and Hellerstein, S. (1985). Wegener granulomatosis in pediatric patients. *Journal of Pediatrics*, **106**, 739–44.

Handrock, K. and Gross, W. L. (1993). Relapsing polychondritis as a secondary phenomenon of primary systemic vasculitis. *Annals of Rheumatic Diseases*, **52**, 895–7.

Handrock, K., Reinhold-Keller, E., Heller, M., Duncker, G., Rudert, H., and Gross, W. L. (1994). Beneficial effects of low-dose methotrexate (MTX) in Wegener's granulomatosis (WG). *Arthritis and Rheumatism*, **37** (Suppl.), 1152 (Abstr.).

Haubitz, M., Frei, U., Rother, U., Brunkhorst, R., and Koch, K. M. (1991). Cyclophosphamide pulse therapy in Wegener's granulomatosis. *Nephrology Dialysis Transplantation*, **6**, 531–5.

Hauschild, S., Schmitt, W. H., and Kekow, J. (1992). Hohe Serumspiegel von ICAM-1 bei der aktiven generalisierten Wegener'schen Granulomatose. *Immunität und Infektion*, **20**, 84–5.

Hay, E. M., Beaman, M., Ralston, A. J., Ackrill, P., Bernstein, R. M., and Holt, P. J. L. (1991). Wegener's granulomatosis occurring in siblings. *British Journal of Rheumatology*, **30**, 144–5.

Heller, M., Muhle, C., Reuter, M., and Schubert, F. (1995). MRI and CT in vasculitis. In *The vasculitides* (ed. B. M. Ansell, P. A. Bacon, J. T. Lie, and Y. Shoenfeld). Chapman and Hall, London.

Hoffman, G. S. (1993*a*). Wegener's granulomatosis. *Current Opinion in Rheumatology*, **5**, 11–17.

Hoffman, G. S. (1993*b*). Treatment of chronic idiopathic systemic vasculitides. In *ANCA-associated vasculitides* (ed. W. L. Gross), pp. 227–34. Plenum, New York.

Hoffman, G. S., Leavitt, R. Y., Fleisher, T. A., Minor, J. R., and Fauci, A. S. (1990). Treatment of Wegener's granulomatosis with intermittent high-dose intravenous cyclophosphamide. *American Journal of Medicine*, **89**, 403–10.

Hoffman, G. S. *et al.* (1991). Bronchoalveolar lavage analysis in Wegener's granulomatosis. *American Review of Respiratory Disease*, **143**, 401–7.

Hoffman, G. S. *et al.* (1992*a*). Wegener granulomatosis: an analysis of 158 patients. *Annals of Internal Medicine*, **116**, 488–98.

Hoffman, G. S., Leavitt, R. Y., Kerr, G. S., and Fauci, A. S. (1992*b*). The treatment of Wegener's granulomatosis with glucocorticoids and methotrexate. *Arthritis and Rheumatism*, **35**, 1322–9.

Ikeda, M., Tsuru, S., Watanabe, Y., Kitahara, S., and Inouye, T. (1992). Reduced CD4–CD8 T cell ratios in patients with Wegener's granulomatosis. *Journal of Clinical and Laboratory Immunology*, **38**, 103–9.

Jarrousse, B. *et al.* (1993). Increased risk of Pneumocystis carinii pneumonia in patients with Wegener's granulomatosis. *Clinical and Experimental Rheumatology*, **11**, 615–21.

Jayne, D. R. W., Davies, M. J., Fox, C. J., Black, C. M., and Lockwood, C. M. (1991). Treatment of systemic vasculitis with pooled intravenous immunoglobulin. *Lancet*, **337**, 1137–9.

Jayne, D. R. W., Esnault, V. L. M., and Lockwood, C. M. (1993). ANCA anti-idiotype antibodies and the treatment of systemic vasculitis with intravenous immunoglobulin. *Journal of Autoimmunity*, **6**, 207–19.

Jennette, J. C. and Falk, R. J. (1992). Disease associations and pathogenic role of antineutrophil cytoplasmic autoantibodies in vasculitis. *Current Opinion in Rheumatology*, **4**, 9–15.

Jennette, J. C. and Falk, R. J. (1993). Pathogenic potential of anti-neutrophil cytoplasmic autoantibodies. In *ANCA-associated vasculitides* (ed. W. L. Gross), pp. 7–15. Plenum, New York.

Jennette, J. C. and Falk, R. J. (1994a). Pathogenic potential of anti-neutrophil cytoplasmic autoantibodies. *Laboratory Investigation*, **70**, 135–7.

Jennette, J. C. and Falk, R. J. (1994b). The pathology of vasculitis involving the kidney. *American Journal of Kidney Disease*, **24**, 130–41.

Jennette, J. C. *et al.* (1994). Nomenclature of systemic vasculitides. Proposal of an International Consensus Conference. *Arthritis and Rheumatism*, **37**, 187–92.

Jiang, X., Khursiga, G., and Rubin, R. L. (1994). Transformation of lupus-inducing drugs to cytotoxic products by activated neutrophils. *Science*, **266**, 810–13.

Kalina, P. H., Lie, J. T., Campbell, R. J., and Garrity, J. A. (1992). Diagnostic value and limitations of orbital biopsy in Wegener's granulomatosis. *Ophthalmology*, **99**, 120–4.

Kallenberg, C. G. M. *et al.* (1991). Autoimmunity to lysosomal enzymes: new clues to vasculitis and glomerulonephritis. *Immunology Today*, **12**, 61–4.

Kallenberg, C. G. M., Brouwer, E., Weening, J. J., and Cohen Tervaert, J. W. (1994). Antineutrophil cytoplasmic antibodies: current diagnostic and pathophysiological potential. *Kidney International*, **46**, 1–15.

Kekow, J., Szimkowiak, C. H., Sticherling, M., Schröder, J. M., Christophers, E., and Gross, W. L. (1993). Pro- and anti-inflammatory cytokines in primary systemic vasculitis. In *ANCA-associated vasculitide* (ed. W. L. Gross), pp. 341–4. Plenum, New York.

Keogan, M. T., Rifkin, I., Ronda, N., Lockwood, C. M., and Brown, D. L. (1993). Anti-neutrophil cytoplasmic antibodies (ANCA) increase neutrophil adhesion to cultured human endothelium. In *ANCA-associated vasculitides* (ed. W. L. Gross), pp. 115–19. Plenum, New York.

Knudsen, B. B., Juergensen, T., and Munch-Jensen, B. (1988). Wegener's granulomatosis in a family. *Scandinavian Journal of Rheumatology*, **17**, 225–7.

Knysak, D. J., McLean, J. A., Solomon, W. R., Fox, D. A., and McCune, W. J. (1994). Immediate hypersensitivity reaction to cyclophosphamide. *Arthritis and Rheumatism*, **37**, 1101–4.

Leavitt, R. Y. *et al.* (1990). The American College of Rheumatology 1990 criteria for the classification of Wegener's granulomatosis. *Arthritis and Rheumatism*, **33**, 1101–7.

Lockwood, C. M., Thiru, S., Isaacs, J. D., Hale, G., and Waldmann, H. (1993). Long-term remission of intractable systemic vasculitis with monoclonal antibody therapy. *Lancet*, **341**, 1620–2.

Lombard, C. M., Duncan, S. R., Rizk, N. W., and Colby, T. V. (1990). The diagnosis of Wegener's granulomatosis from transbronchial biopsy specimens. *Human Pathology*, **21**, 838–42.

Luqmani, R. A. *et al.* (1994). Birmingham Vasculitis Activity Score (BVAS) in systemic necrotizing vasculitis. *Quarterly Journal of Medicine*, **87**, 671–8.

McHugh, K., Manson, D., Eberhard, B. A., Shore, A., and Laxer, R. M. (1991). Wegener's granulomatosis in childhood. *Pediatric Radiology*, **21**, 552–5.

Malaviya, A. N. *et al.* (1990). Wegener's granulomatosis in India: not so rare.. *British Journal of Rheumatology*, **29**, 499–500.

Mark, E. J., Matsubara, O., Tan-Liu, N. S., and Fienberg, R. (1988). The pulmonary biopsy in the early diagnosis of Wegener's (pathergic) granulomatosis: a study based on 35 open lung biopsies. *Human Pathology*, **19**, 1065–71.

Mathieson, P. W. *et al.* (1990). Monoclonal-antibody therapy in systemic vasculitis. *New England Journal of Medicine*, **323**, 250–4.

Mathieson, P. W., Lockwood, C. M., and Oliveira, D. B. G. (1992). T and B cell responses to neutrophil cytoplasmic antigens in systemic vasculitis. *Clinical Immunology and Immunopathology*, **63**, 135–41.

Mathieson, P. W., Quasim, F. J., Esnault, V. L. M., and Oliveira, D. B. G. (1993). Animal models of systemic vasculitis. *Journal of Autoimmunity*, **6**, 251–64.

Mayet, W. J. and Meyer zum Büschenfelde, K. H. (1993). Antibodies to proteinase 3 increase adhesion of neutrophils to human endothelial cells. *Clinical and Experimental Immunology*, **94**, 440–6.

Mayet, W. J., Csernok, E., Szymkowiak, C., Gross, W. L., and Meyer zum Büschenfelde, K. H. (1993*a*). Human endothelial cells express proteinase 3, the target antigen of anticytoplasmic antibodies in Wegener's granulomatosis. *Blood*, **82**, 1221–9.

Mayet, W. J., Csernok, E., Gross, W. L., and Meyer zum Büschenfelde, K. H. (1993*b*). Inhibition of cANCA binding to human endothelial cells by an anti-idiotypic anti-PR3 antibody. *Clinical and Experimental Immunology*, **93** (Suppl. 1), 19.

Mrowka, C. and Sieberth, H. G. (1994). Circulating adhesion molecules ICAM-1, VCAM-1 and E-selectin in systemic vasculitis: marked differences between Wegener's granulomatosis and systemic lupus erythematosus. *Clinical Investigator*, **72**, 762–8.

Mrowka, C. H., Csernok, E., Gross, W. L., Feucht, H. E., Bechtel, U., and Thoenes, G. H. (1995). Distribution of the granulocyte serine proteinases proteinase 3 and elastase in human glomerulonephritis. *American Journal of Kidney Diseases*.

Muhle, C. *et al.* (1993). MRI of the head in Wegener's granulomatosis — result of a prospective study. *Clinical and Experimental Immunology*, **93** (Suppl. 1), 36 (Abstr.).

Muniain, M. A., Moreno, J. C., and Gonzalez Campora, R. (1986). Wegener's granulomatosis in two sisters. *Annals of Rheumatic Diseases*, **45**, 417–21.

Murty, G. E. (1990). Wegener's granulomatosis: otorhinolaryngological manifestations. *Clinical Otolaryngology*, **15**, 385–93.

Murty, G. E., Mains, B. T., Middleton, D., Maxwell, A. P., and Savage, D. A. (1991). HLA antigen frequencies and Wegener's granulomatosis. *Clinical Otolaryngology*, **16**, 448–51.

Nabel, E. G., Plautz, G., and Nabel, G. S. (1992). Transduction of a foreign histocompatibility gene into the arterial wall induces vasculitis. *Proceedings of National Academy of Sciences (USA)*, **89**, 5157–61.

Nishino, H., Rubino, F. A., DeRemee, A., Swanson, J. W., and Parisi, J. E. (1993). Neurological involvement in Wegener's granulomatosis: an analysis of 324 consecutive patients at the Mayo Clinic. *Annals of Neurology*, **33**, 4–9.

Nölle, B., Specks, U., Lüdemann, J., Rohrbach, M. S., DeRemee, R. A., and Gross, W. L. (1989). Anticytoplasmic autoantibodies: their immunodiagnostic value in Wegener's granulomatosis. *Annals of Internal Medicine*, **111**, 28–40.

Noritake, D. T., Weiner, S. R., Bassett, L. W., Paulus, H. E., and Weisbart, R. (1987). Rheumatic manifestations of Wegener's granulomatosis. *Journal of Rheumatology*, **14**, 949–51.

Noronha, I. L., Kruger, C., Andrassy, K., Ritz, E., and Waldherr, R. (1993). *In situ* production of TNF-alpha, IL-1 and IL-2R in ANCA-positive glomerulonephritis. *Kidney International*, **43**, 682–92.

Ohdama, S., Takano, S., Miyake, S., Kubota, T., Sato, K., and Aoki, N. (1994). Plasma thrombomodulin as a marker of vascular injuries in collagen vascular diseases. *American Journal of Clinical Pathology*, **101**, 109–13.

Pall, A. A., Varagunam, M., Adu, D., Smith, N., Richards, N. T., Taylor, C. M., and Michael, J. (1994). Anti-idiotypic activity against anti-myeloperoxidase antibodies in pooled human immunoglobulin. *Clinical and Experimental Immunology*, **93** (Suppl. 1), 12–14.

Pearson, J. D. (1993). Markers of endothelial perturbation and damage. *British Journal of Rheumatology*, **32**, 651–2.

Porges, A. J., Redecha, P. B., Kimberley, W. T., Csernok, E., Gross, W. L., and Kimberley, R. P. (1994). Anti-neutrophil cytoplasmic autoantibodies engage and activate human neutrophils via FcγRIIa.. *Journal of Immunology*, **153**, 1271–80.

Reinhold-Keller, E. *et al.* (1994). Influence of disease manifestation and antineutrophil cytoplasmic antibody titer in the response to pulse cyclophosphamide therapy in patients with Wegener's granulomatosis. *Arthritis and Rheumatism*, **37**, 919–24.

Reinhold-Keller, E., de Groot, E., Rudert, H., Nölle, B., Heller, M., and Gross, W. L. (1996). Response to trimethoprim/sulfamethoxazole in Wegener's granulomatosis depends on the phase of the disease. *Quarterly Journal of Medicine*, **89**, 15–23.

Richter, C., Schnabel, A., Csernok, E., Reinhold-Keller, E., and Gross, W. L. (1995). Treatment of Wegener's granulomatosis with intravenous immunoglobulin. In *ANCA-associated vasculitides* (ed. W. L. Gross), pp. 487–90. Plenum, New York.

Riecken, B., Gutfleisch, J., Schlesier, M., and Peter, H. H. (1994). Impaired granulocyte oxidative burst and decreased expression of leucocyte adhesion molecule-1 (LAM-1) in patients with Wegener's granulomatosis. *Clinical and Experimental Immunology*, **96**, 43–7.

Ritz, E., Andrassy, K., Küster, S., and Waldherr, R. (1991). Wegener's granulomatosis, microscopic polyarteritis and pauciimmune crescentic necrotizing glomerulonephritis. *Contributions to Nephrology*, **94**, 1–12.

Rosete, A., Cabral, A. R., Kraus, A., and Alarcon-Segovia, D. (1991). Diabetes insipidus secondary to Wegener's granulomatosis: report and review of the literature. *Journal of Rheumatology*, **18**, 761–5.

Rottem, M., Fauci, A. S., Hallahan, C. W., Kerr, G. S., Lebovics, R., Leavitt, R. Y., and Hoffman, G. S. (1993). Wegener granulomatosis in children and adolescents: Clinical presentation and outcome. *Journal of Pediatrics*, **122**, 26–31.

Roux-Lombard, P., Lin, J. M., Peter, J. B., and Dayer, J. M. (1994). Elevated serum levels of TNF soluble receptors in patients with positive anti-neutrophil cytoplasmic antibodies. *British Journal of Rheumatology*, **33**, 428–31.

Salvarani, C. *et al.* (1992). Soluble interleukin-2 receptors in polymyalgia rheumatica/giant cell arteritis. Clinical and laboratory correlations. *Journal of Rheumatology*, **19**, 1100–6.

Satorre, J., Antle, M., O'Sullivan, R., White, V. A., Nugent, R. A., and Rootman, J. (1991). Orbital lesions with granulomatous inflammation. *Canadian Journal of Ophthalmology*, **26**, 174–95.

Savage, C., Gaskin, G., Pusey, C. D., and Pearson, J. D. (1993). Myeloperoxidase binds to vascular endothelial cells, is recognized by ANCA and can enhance complement dependent cytotoxicity. In *ANCA-associated vasculitides* (ed. W. L. Gross), pp. 121–3. Plenum, New York.

Schmitt, W. H., Heesen, C., Csernok, E., Rautmann, A., and Gross, W. L. (1992). Elevated serum levels of soluble interleukin-2 receptor in patients with Wegener's granulomatosis. *Arthritis and Rheumatism*, **35**, 1088–96.

Schmitt, W. H., Haubitz, M., Mistry, N., Brunkhorst, R., Erbslöh-Möller, B., and Gross, W. L. (1993). Renal transplantation in Wegener's granulomatosis. *Lancet*, **342**, 860.

Schollmeyer, P. and Grotz, W. (1990). Cyclosporin in the treatment of Wegener's granulomatosis (WG) and related diseases. *Acta Pathologica Microbiologica et Immunologica Scandinavica (Copenhagen)*, **19** (Suppl.), 54–5.

Scott, D. G. I. and Watts, R. A. (1994). Classification and epidemiology of systemic vasculitis. *British Journal of Rheumatology*, **33**, 897–900.

Sen, R. P., Walsh, T. P., Fisher, W., and Brock, N. (1991). Pulmonary complications of combination therapy with cyclophosphamide and prednisone. *Chest*, **99**, 143–6.

Specks, U. and DeRemee, R. A. (1990). Granulomatous vasculitis: Wegener's granulomatosis and Churg–Strauss syndrome. *Rheumatic Diseases Clinics of North America*, **16**, 377–97.

Specks, U., DeRemee, R. A., and Gross, W. L. (1989). Die Wegener'scher Granulomatose: Systemerkrankung mit bevorzugtem Befall des Respirationstrakts. *Pneumologie*, **43**, 648–59.

Stegemann, C., Tervaert, J. W. C., Huitema, M. G., and Kallenberg, C. G. M. (1993). Serum markers of T-cell activation in relapses of Wegener's granulomatosis. In *ANCA-associated vasculitides* (ed. W. L. Gross), pp. 389–92. Plenum, New York.

Stegemann, C., Cohen Tervaert, J. W., Sluiter, W. J., Manson, W. L., de Jong, P. E., and Kallenberg, C. G. M. (1994). Association of chronic nasal carriage of *Staphylococcus aureus* and higher relapse rates in Wegener's granulomatosis. *Annals of Internal Medicine*, **120**, 12–17.

Steppat, D. and Gross, W. L. (1989). Stage-adapted treatment of Wegener's granulomatosis. *Klinische Wochenschrift*, **67**, 666–71.

Stillwell, T. J., Benson, R. C., DeRemee, R. A., McDonald, T. J., and Weiland, L. H. (1988). Cyclophosphamide-induced bladder toxicity in Wegener's granulomatosis. *Arthritis and Rheumatism*, **31**, 465–70.

Stoney, P. J., Davies, W., Ho, S. F., Paterson, I. C., and Griffith, I. P. (1991). Wegener's granulomatosis in two siblings: a family study. *Journal of Laryngology and Otology*, **105**, 123–4.

Travis, W. D., Hoffman, G. S., Leavitt, R. Y., Pass, H. I., and Fauci, A. S. (1991). Surgical pathology of the lung in Wegener's granulomatosis. *American Journal of Surgical Pathology*, **15**, 315–33.

Tuso, P., Moudgil, A., Goodman, D., Kamil, E., Koyyana, R., and Jordan, S. C. (1992). Treatment of antineutrophil cytoplasmic autoantibody-positive systemic vasculitis and glomerulonephritis with pooled intravenous gammaglobulin. *American Journal of Kidney Diseases*, **5**, 504–8.

van der Lubbe, P. A., Miltenburg, A. M., and Breedveld, F. C. (1991). Anti-CD4 monoclonal antibody for relapsing polychondritis. *Lancet*, **337**, 1349.

Waldherr, R., Noronha, I. L., Niemir, Z., Krüger, C., Stein, H., and Stumm, G. (1993). Expression of cytokines and growth factors in human glomerulonephritides. *Pediatric Nephrology*, **7**, 471–8.

Walton, E. W. (1958). Giant-cell granuloma of the respiratory tract (Wegener's granulomatosis). *British Medical Journal*, 265–9.

Wegener, F. (1939). Über eine eigenartige rhinogene Granulomatose mit besonderer Beteiligung des Arteriensystems und der Nieren. *Beiträge zur Pathologie*, **102**, 36–68.

Wegener, F. (1990). Wegener's granulomatosis. Thoughts and observations of a pathologist. *European Archives of Otorhinolaryngology*, **247**, 133–42.

Weidhase, A., Gröne, H-J., Unterberg, C., Schuff-Werner, P., and Wiegand, V. (1990). Severe granulomatous giant cell myocarditis in Wegener's granulomatosis. *Klinische Wochenschrift*, **68**, 880–5.

Weiner, S. R., Paulus, H. E., and Weisbart, R. H. (1986). Wegener's granulomatosis in the elderly. *Arthritis and Rheumatism*, **29**, 1157–9.

Weiss, M. A. and Crissman, J. D. (1984). Renal biopsy findings in Wegener's granulomatosis: Segmental necrotizing glomerulonephritis with glomerular thrombosis. *Human Pathology*, **15**, 943–56.

Wiik, A. (1993). Antineutrophil cytoplasmic antibodies in Wegener's granulomatosis. *Clinical and Experimental Rheumatology*, **11**, 191–201.

Wiik, A., Rasmussen, N., and Wieslander, J. (1993). Methods to detect autoantibodies to neutrophilic granulocytes. *Manual of Biological Markers of Disease*, **A9**, 1–14.

Yang, J., Tuttle, R., Jenette, C., and Falk, R. J. (1993). Glomerulonephritis in rats immunized with myeloperoxidase (MPO). *Clinical and Experimental Immunology*, **93** (Suppl. 1), 22.

5.11.3 Classical polyarteritis nodosa, microscopic polyarteritis, and Churg–Strauss syndrome

D. Adu and Paul A. Bacon

Introduction and historical background

The aetiology and pathogenesis of most forms of systemic necrotizing vasculitis remain obscure. Few areas are more contentious than the classification of the necrotizing vasculitides. The difficulties are in part due to the clinical overlap within these disorders and in part because we know so little about their aetiology. Our levels of description are based on histopathology, clinical presentation, immunology, and behaviour either spontaneous or in response to treatment, and these are inexact tools for classification (see Chapter 5.11.1).

The simplest classification is into three groups of diseases based on vessel size — giant-cell arteritis of large arteries; necrotizing vasculitis of medium and small muscular arteries; and small vessel disease involving arterioles, capillaries, and venules. The necrotizing arteritis group contains both vasculitis as a complication of connective tissue disorders, such as rheumatoid arthritis, and idiopathic disease. The latter ranges from pure arteritis (classical polyarteritis nodosa) to granulomatous vasculitis (Wegener's).

In the 19th century, following Kussmaul and Maier's (1866) classical description onwards, periarteritis nodosa was considered as a rare distinct disease entity. It was characterized by visible nodular lesions at autopsy involving the muscular arteries. However in the 20th century cases were described in which the diagnosis was made microscopically, with consequent changes in emphasis of disease descriptions. In her classic review Zeek (1952) divided the necrotizing vasculitides into five main groups. The first of these was hypersensitivity angiitis which typically involved capillaries, arterioles, and the small arteries as well as the venules and which she differentiated from periarteritis nodosa, allergic granulomatous angiitis, rheumatoid arteritis, and temporal arteritis. The organs involved were the kidney in particular, often with necrotizing glomerulonephritis, but the angiitis was usually widespread and pulmonary vessels were frequently involved. The term hypersensitivity angiitis is now used for clinical syndromes in which cutaneous manifestations predominate and in which visceral involvement is uncommon.

Pulmonary disease is a prominent feature of systemic vasculitis and studies in the 1930s separated off firstly Wegener's granulomatosis with predominant respiratory tract granuloma formation but also complicated by a vasculitis as an entity that was distinct from polyarteritis (Wegener 1936). In 1951, Churg and Strauss described the clinical syndrome of asthma, eosinophilia, and systemic vasculitis with extravascular granulomata that bears their name.

Renal lesions have been associated with polyarteritis since the comprehensive description by Kussmaul and Maier (1866). Most classic reviews have found an incidence of renal involvement in approximately 80 per cent. The morphological changes of polyarteritis nodosa — a term first used by Ferrari (1903) — were described in detail by Arkin (1930). He pointed out that in cases without aneurysms the vasculitis may only be seen microscopically, and referred to such cases as microscopic polyarteritis nodosa. This theme was taken up and expanded in a detailed clinicopathological study by Davson *et al.* (1948). They linked the presence of the primary systemic vasculitis with the occurrence of segmental necrotizing glomerulonephritis in a subgroup of patients. They again suggested that such patients had a microscopic form of polyarteritis, which they thought was distinct from the periarteritis (or polyarteritis) nodosa described by Kussmaul and Maier. They divided their patients into two groups, those with severe and widespread glomerular disease (9 out of 14) and those with minimal or no glomerular disease. Half of the first group had arterial (arcuate artery) involvement in addition to glomerular disease. These presented with a rather uniform clinical picture with pyrexia, leucocytosis, and uraemia in the presence of a normal

Acknowledgement: We are grateful to Dr A.J. Howie for the photomicrographs used in Chapter 5.11.3.

blood pressure. The second group had variable clinical symptoms including elevated blood pressure, locomotor symptoms, abdominal pain, heart and lung involvement. Pathology here showed lesions typical of classical periarteritis and of malignant hypertension. Davson *et al.* concluded that the microscopic form of polyarteritis was different from the classical aneurysmal type. Importantly, they stated clearly that it was possible to separate microscopic polyarteritis from other forms of diffuse nephritis on both clinical and pathological grounds, establishing that the nephritis was not a coincidental or unrelated feature.

Definition of microscopic polyangiitis (polyarteritis)

It is now widely accepted on both sides of the Atlantic that the microscopic form of necrotizing angiitis with predominant involvement of the renal and pulmonary capillaries is a separate disease entity from the original descriptions of periarteritis or polyarteritis nodosa. The main question is that of nomenclature, and we favour that proposed by the Chapel Hill consensus conference (Jennette *et al.* 1994) (Table 1) but many would disagree (Lie 1994). The preferred name is now microscopic polyangiitis (microscopic polyarteritis) which has to be distinguished from classical polyarteritis nodosa. The most important distinguishing feature is the presence of vasculitis in small vessels (arterioles, venules, and capillaries) in microscopic polyangiitis and its absence in the latter. It has to be emphasized that some overlap of the size of vessel involved is seen. By definition microscopic polyangiitis must have involvement of microscopic vessels, but it is recognized that it can also involve small or medium-sized arteries. In contrast classical polyarteritis nodosa must have no involvement of microscopic vessels and therefore no glomerulonephritis. Microscopic polyangiitis and classical polyarteritis nodosa are thus differentiated by the presence or absence of small vessel involvement, rather than by the involvement of medium-sized arteries which can occur in either. The precise definitions and the question of whether involvement at all sites carry the same diagnostic weight, are still matters of discussion. For example the occurrence of small vessel involvement of the skin in classical polyarteritis nodosa with otherwise typical arterial involvement at all other sites would not change the diagnosis in our view. The definition of microscopic polyangiitis also requires few or no immune deposits in the blood vessels, in order to allow differentiation from those variants of small vessel vasculitis that do have well-defined immune complexes. This is particularly important to allow distinction from Henoch–Schönlein purpura and cryoglobulinaemic vasculitis, both with predominant cutaneous involvement. It also differentiates other forms of immune complex-mediated small vessel vasculitis such as that seen in systemic lupus erythematosus. The most frequent, clinically important aspect of microscopic polyangiitis is the glomerular lesion; similar small vessel lesions may occur in the lung. It is recognized that identical glomerular lesions may be seen in Wegener's granulomatosis but there are other important distinctions from that condition examined below.

Comparison with classical polyarteritis nodosa

The clinical distinction between the microscopic and the classical aneurysmal form of polyarteritis is not always easy. The overlapping vessel size which occurs in microscopic polyangiitis confuses interpretation of older series and makes the interrelationship of the two

Table 1 Nomenclature of vasculitis proposed by the Chapel Hill consensus conference

Size of vessel	Syndrome	Granuloma	ANCA
Large	Takayasu's arteritis	+	+
	Temporal arteritis	+	−
Medium	Polyarteritis nodosa	−	+C
	Churg–Strauss syndrome	+	+P
	Kawasaki disease	−	−
Small	Wegener's granulomatosis	+	+C
	Microscopic polyangiitis	−	+P
	Leucocytoclastic vasculitis	−	−

From Jennette *et al.* 1994.

syndromes difficult to interpret. For example 25 per cent of renal patients in our series (Adu *et al.* 1987), all of whom had glomerulonephritis, also had renal arteritis. There is a similarity in the clinical symptoms. Even in the renal series, the majority of patients first present with non-renal symptoms. However, previous experience in a District General Hospital had emphasized the wide spectrum of severe organ involvement in classical polyarteritis nodosa (Scott *et al.* 1982). A comparison of several series of patients from renal units with those from general or overlapping departments confirmed that there are real differences (Adu *et al.* 1987). The general series, which contained many cases of classical polyarteritis nodosa, showed a higher incidence of fever, heart and lung, gastrointestinal, and peripheral nerve involvement. The difference in vessel size involved appears to dictate not just the clinical pattern of organ damage but also the prognosis. Thus visceral infarction or haemorrhage in classical polyarteritis nodosa contributes prominently to the overall outcome. The overt clinical symptoms often also contribute to an earlier diagnosis and thus institution of therapy in classical polyarteritis nodosa.

In microscopic polyangiitis there is an increase in both renal and lung disease. Pulmonary involvement in this disease has been noted in previous series and contributes to a poor prognosis (Savage *et al.* 1985; Adu *et al.* 1987). Patients may present with overt or even massive pulmonary haemorrhage in association with renal failure—so-called pulmonary renal syndrome—and these patients tend to fair badly. Less dramatic pulmonary involvement is even more frequent. The pathological lesion, a necrotizing vasculitis in small alveolar vessels, is essentially the same as in the kidney. The most striking difference between the two conditions in our series is the frequency of presentation. Eight microscopic polyangiitis cases have been seen for every classical polyarteritis nodosa case. This is not due to a biased collection from a renal centre, since the Birmingham Vasculitis Group collects cases from rheumatological as well as renal clinics and from general physician referrals. It reflects the widespread experience in Europe now that microscopic polyangiitis is common (and perhaps increasing in incidence) while classical polyarteritis nodosa is rare (and perhaps decreasing). There is also a difference in outcome. Relapse rates are high in vasculitis and this was seen in two-fifths of our classical polyarteritis nodosa cases, but only in a quarter of the microscopic polyangiitis group. However, the overall prognosis is much worse in microscopic polyangiitis, which in our series showed a 40 per cent overall mortality over the decade, largely related to renal failure often associated with delayed referrals. In contrast classical polyarteritis nodosa responded well to therapy, with a 100 per cent survival in our hands despite the relapses (Gordon *et al.* 1993).

The advent of testing for antineutrophil cytoplasmic antibodies (ANCA) has provided another way to compare the two forms of angiitis (reviewed by Kallenberg *et al.* 1994). In microscopic polyangiitis the majority of patients (80 per cent) are ANCA positive. Specificity is directed predominantly towards myeloperoxidase and to a lesser extent against proteinase 3. In contrast, in our patients with classical polyarteritis nodosa a positive ANCA was found in 14 per cent. Others have also concluded that classical polyarteritis nodosa, without evidence of small vessel involvement, is usually ANCA negative (Cohen Tervaert *et al.* 1991; Guillevin *et al.* 1993).

Comparison with Wegener's granulomatosis

Although patients with Wegener's granulomatosis have, by definition, disease of the upper and lower respiratory tract and histological evidence of necrotizing granulomata often with an accompanying vasculitis, biopsies of lesions often show only a non-specific inflammation. A particular feature of respiratory disease in Wegener's granulomatosis is that even with treatment it is persistent and often relapsing and this helps to differentiate this disease from microscopic polyangiitis where the respiratory disease, for example pulmonary haemorrhage or epistaxis, is usually acute and transient. Wegener's granulomatosis is the classical disease which is ANCA positive, with an antibody specificity directed primarily to proteinase 3. An identical, pauci immune, necrotizing glomerulonephritis also occurs in this condition, but there is little to support the concept that microscopic polyangiitis represents a renal-limited form of Wegener's granulomatosis (Adu *et al.* 1987; Gordon *et al.* 1993).

Treatment

Therapy in these previously incurable disorders with a very high mortality has been revolutionized in the past two decades by the introduction of cytotoxic/immunosuppressive regimes. The dramatic effect of cyclophosphamide together with steroids in Wegener's granulomatosis was first established in 1971 (Novack and Pearson 1971) and these observations were later confirmed (Fauci and Wolff 1973) and extended to polyarteritis (Fauci *et al.* 1979). Recent controlled data support this beneficial effect.

Specific diseases

Classical polyarteritis

Classical polyarteritis nodosa is a systemic illness characterized by necrotizing inflammation of medium-sized arteries leading to aneurysm formation. It affects the viscera and other organs. The clinical presentation is dominated by organ infarction and haemorrhage, a neuropathy, and myalgia in the context of a systemic illness.(Frohnert and Sheps 1967; Sack *et al.* 1975; Leib *et al.* 1979; Cohen *et al.* 1980; Scott *et al.* 1982)

Age, sex, and race

In most studies there is a consistent predominance of males (male: female ratio, 1.9–2:1). The majority of patients have been Caucasian although the disease has been described in black and Asian groups. The age range is from 14 to 80 years with a peak frequency of onset in the 40s and 50s.

Clinical presentation

The clinical presentation in these patients is summarized in Fig. 1 and compared with those of patients with microscopic polyangiitis. Patients with classical polarteritis nodosa often present with systemic features comprising malaise, fever, and weight loss. About 60 per cent of patients have an arthralgia (or less commonly an arthritis) and 50 per cent of patients have a rash that is erythematous, purpuric, or vasculitic. Punched-out ulcers may occur, often around the ankles. A prominent feature in these patients is a peripheral neuropathy in 40 per cent of patients, often presenting as a mononeuritis multiplex. Gastrointestinal involvement is frequent, found in 45 per cent of our series, and carries a high morbidity and mortality. Presenting features include gut infarction, bleeding, pancreatitis, and infarction of the gallbladder, as well as non-specific abdominal pain. Renal disease in the form of an abnormal urinary sediment occurs in 55 per cent of patients, although only 24 per cent of patients have renal impairment and it is often mild. Myalgia is a prominent symptom and biopsy of affected muscles often shows a vasculitis. Rarely, testicular pain is a presenting feature of polyarteritis.

Hepatitis B and classical polyarteritis nodosa

Positive hepatitis B serology has been noted in between 5 and 40 per cent of different series of patients with classical polyarteritis nodosa (Frohnert and Sheps 1967; Sack *et al.* 1975; Leib *et al.* 1979; Cohen *et al.* 1980). Its prevalence appears to reflect the incidence of hepatitis B carriage in the population. It also suggests that polyarteritis nodosa is not a disease with a single aetiological agent or mechanism. In England less than 10 per cent of patients have positive hepatitis B serology (Scott *et al.* 1982) but this is considerably higher in studies from some parts of Europe (Guillevin *et al.* 1988). Clinically these patients appear more likely to have a nephrotic syndrome, which is otherwise rare in polyarteritis (Guillevin *et al.* 1988).

Localized polyarteritis

Isolated organ involvement in polyarteritis is rare. Involvement of the skin, testes, epididymis, breasts, uterus, appendix, and gallbladder have all been reported and we have seen arteritis localized to one kidney. It is not yet clear how these patients should be managed, especially if there are no systemic signs of vasculitis. The risk of progression to systemic disease in such cases is not known, although one study suggested that on long-term follow-up, the majority of patients progressed to systemic disease (Minkowitz *et al.* 1991). Close long-term follow-up is clearly important.

Microscopic polyangiitis

These patients have predominant involvement of glomerular capillaries but without granuloma formation, such as is seen in Wegener's granulomatosis. Unlike classical polyarteritis nodosa most patients with microscopic polyangiitis present with or develop severe renal disease, particularly if the diagnosis is delayed, and most studies of

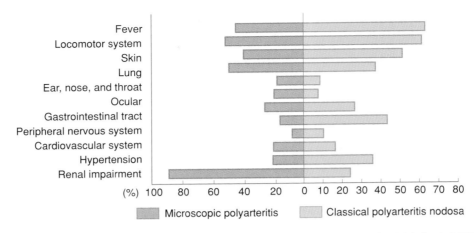

Fig. 1 Clinical features at presentation in classical polyarteritis nodosa (Frohnert and Sheps 1967; Sack *et al.* 1975; Leib *et al.* 1979; Cohen *et al.* 1980; Scott *et al.* 1982) and microscopic polyarteritis (Serra *et al.* 1984; Savage *et al.* 1985; Adu *et al.* 1987).

this disorder emanate from renal units (Serra *et al.* 1984; Savage *et al.* 1985; Coward *et al.* 1986; Adu *et al.* 1987). There may be little evidence of multisystem disease but diagnosis is aided by the detection of ANCA. In microscopic polyangiitis a perinuclear pattern of staining (**p-ANCA**) is usually seen, in contrast with the diffuse granular cyto-plasmic staining (**c-ANCA**) seen in Wegener's granulomatosis (Falk and Jennette 1988; Lee *et al.* 1990). P-ANCA detects a much wider range of antigens than c-ANCA but in microscopic polyangiitis the frequent antigenic specificity is to myeloperoxidase.

Age, sex, and race

Most studies show a male predominance (male:female ratio, 1.2–1.8:1) and the overwhelming majority of patients reported are Caucasian, with only a few Negroid patients and Asians from the Indian subcon-tinent (Serra *et al.* 1984; Savage *et al.* 1985; Adu *et al.* 1987). The mean age at presentation is around 50 years.

Clinical features of microscopic polyangiitis

Much of the initial clinical presentation of microscopic polyangiitis is non-specific. The symptoms of microscopic polyangiitis are compared with those of classical polyarteritis nodosa in Fig. 1 (Serra *et al.* 1984; Savage *et al.* 1985; Adu *et al.* 1987). Systemic symptoms such as malaise, anorexia, fever, and weight loss predominate initially and these are accompanied by often asynchronous episodes of rash, arthralgia, myalgia, and conjunctivitis. These symptoms have often been present for months before there is a clinical suspicion of a multi-system disorder. A rash is present in approximately 40 per cent of cases, usually purpuric or vasculitic, and occurs most commonly on the limbs, in particular the hands and feet (Fig. 2). Skin ulceration is uncommon, being found in less than 5 per cent of patients, most commonly around the ankles (Fig. 2). Arthralgia or myalgia is present in about a half of patients and a quarter of these develop an asymmetric large joint arthritis.

Renal disease

The clinical presentation of renal disease is with microscopic haema-turia (80 per cent of patients), frank haematuria (6 per cent of patients) and proteinuria (80 per cent of patients). Over 90 per cent of patients have renal impairment, and in most series no fewer than 30 per cent of patients were oliguric by the time the diagnosis was

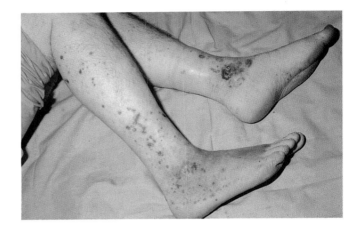

Fig. 2 Vasculitic rash and 'punched-out' ulcer on the leg of a patient with microscopic polyangiitis.

made. Hypertension is infrequent, being found in 21 per cent of patients, and usually mild.

Pulmonary disease

Symptoms of lung disease are found in about 50 per cent of patients and usually take the form of haemoptysis, pleurisy, and asthma. Frank pulmonary haemorrhage develops in 5 per cent of patients (Fig. 3) and this can be severe enough to require mechanical ventilation. The importance of diffuse pulmonary haemorrhage in both microscopic polyangiitis and Wegener's granulomatosis has been emphasized (Haworth *et al.* 1985).

Churg–Strauss syndrome

Clinical features

In 1951, Churg and Strauss described autopsy features in 13 patients who died following an illness characterized by asthma, eosinophilia, fever, and a systemic illness. All 13 patients had had asthma for up to 10 years prior to the onset of other symptoms. Fever was a universal finding, as was eosinophilia, although the levels varied considerably within individuals over time. Anaemia, weight loss, heart failure,

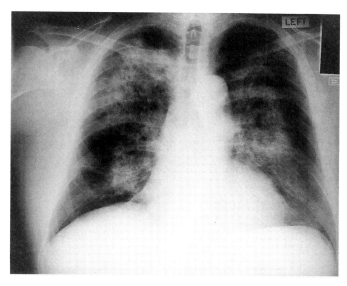

Fig. 3 Diffuse reticulonodular pulmonary shadowing in the chest radiograph of a patient with microscopic polyangiitis and pulmonary haemorrhage.

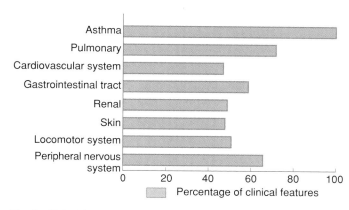

Fig. 4 Clinical features of Churg–Strauss syndrome (Lanham *et al.* 1984).

recurrent pneumonia, and bloody diarrhoea were common. Hypertension was seen in patients with more long-standing disease. Skin lesions were usually present, varying from purpura to nodules (biopsy of which revealed granulomata). Central and peripheral nerve involvement were common, especially peripheral neuropathy (in 8 out of 13 cases). Significant renal involvement was unusual in their patients, although mild urinary sediment abnormalities were often seen.

The spectrum of clinical features of this disorder are summarized in Fig. 4. Lanham *et al.* (1984) provided a clinical definition of Churg–Strauss syndrome as a triad of asthma, eosinophilia (more than 1.5×10^9), and a systemic vasculitis involving two or more extrapulmonary organs. From their experience and a review of the literature they concluded that extravascular granulomas were not essential for the diagnosis of Churg–Strauss syndrome. In their study, asthma or an allergic rhinitis often preceded by years the development of a peripheral blood eosinophilia and pulmonary shadowing resembling Löffler syndrome, and this in turn was followed by a systemic vasculitis. However, these manifestations may occur simultaneously (Chumbley *et al.* 1977). Although infrequently reported, renal involvement does occur and usually presents with microscopic haematuria plus proteinuria and less commonly with renal failure or a nephrotic syndrome (Clutterbuck *et al.* 1990).

Differential diagnosis of Churg–Strauss syndrome

The prominence of asthma, an allergic rhinitis, and persistent elevation of the eosinophil count as well as the predominance of eosinophils in areas of inflammation help to differentiate Churg–Strauss syndrome from Wegener's granulomatosis, classical polyarteritis nodosa, and microscopic polyangiitis. Clinically this differentiation is not always easy (Guillevin *et al.* 1988) and the American College of Rheumatology had difficulty in classifying some of their patients with Wegener's granulomatosis, polyarteritis nodosa, and Churg–Strauss syndrome according to well-defined criteria (Masi *et al.* 1990).

Approach to the diagnosis of vasculitis

Difficulties in the classification of vasculitis often lead to delays in diagnosis. This delay is particularly marked in the elderly when it is often asociated with the rapid development of renal failure, which in turn carries a high mortality.

Clinical

The initial diagnosis is often clinical, and a high index of suspicion is required in patients with a multisystem disease, especially with a fever, skin, or renal involvement. A particular feature of systemic vasculitis is that the symptoms may be separated in time and also often fluctuate in severity. Thus for example an individual may have had an episode of arthritis followed by a uveitis and then renal disease before the possibility of a vasculitis is considered. The clinical suspicion should be pursued aggressively and with urgency in order to establish a diagnosis quickly. The overwhelming need at this stage to establish a diagnosis of a vasculitis which then requires therapy is greater than the need to establish a precise syndrome diagnosis. This may not be apparent at first presentation but subsequent progress often clarifies that. Usually there is an otherwise unexplained acute phase response with a high white blood-cell count, C-reactive protein, and erythrocyte sedimentation rate. A biopsy of clinically involved tissue is often helpful, for example skin, muscle, sural nerve, or kidney. Where there is no specific organ involvement, renal and coeliac axis angiograms should be considered.

Immunological investigations in microscopic polyangiitis, classical polyarteritis nodosa, and Churg–Strauss syndrome

Antineutrophil cytoplasmic antibodies (reviewed by Kallenberg *et al.* 1994; see also Chapter 5.11.2)

ANCA were first described by Davies *et al.* (1982) and Hall *et al.* (1984) in patients with a segmental necrotizing glomerulonephritis, some of whom had features consistent with a systemic vasculitis. The report of Van der Woude *et al.* (1985) showed that antineutrophil cytoplasmic antibodies were found commonly in the sera from patients with Wegener's granulomatosis. Subsequently these observations were extended to patients with microscopic polyangiitis (Savage *et al.* 1987). Two broad patterns of cytoplasmic staining have been recognized. In the first there is granular staining of the cytoplasm of ethanol-fixed neutrophils (c-ANCA). This pattern of staining is commonly seen in the sera of patients with Wegener's granulomatosis (Van der Woude *et al.* 1985). The target antigen for this antibody is almost entirely restricted to a 29 kDa serine proteinase, neutrophil serine proteinase 3 (Goldschmeding *et al.* 1989). The second pattern is of perinuclear staining (p-ANCA) which is seen in the sera of patients with microscopic polyangiitis and also idiopathic segmental necrotizing glomerulonephritis. A wider range of specificities is seen with p-ANCA, although the majority of these antibodies are directed against myeloperoxidase (Falk and Jennette 1988; Lee *et al.* 1990) and in a few cases against elastase and lactoferrin.

Approximately 80 per cent of patients with active, systemic Wegener's granulomatosis have c-ANCA antibodies in their sera (reviewed by Van der Woude *et al.* 1989; Specks and De Remee 1990). P-ANCA are found in the sera of approximately 80 per cent of patients with microscopic polyangiitis and about 75 per cent of patients with Churg–Strauss syndrome (Cohen Tevaert *et al.* 1991; Guillevin *et al.* 1993). P-ANCA is less disease specific as well as less sensitive. Elevated titres are reported in Kawasaki's syndrome, rheumatoid vasculitis, and idiopathic segmental necrotizing glomerulonephritis. Between 14 and 20 per cent of patients with classical polyarteritis nodosa have a positive ANCA (Adu *et al.* 1993; Guillevin *et al.* 1993) and in patients with polyarteritis nodosa that is positive for hepatitis B, 11 per cent are reported to have a positive ANCA (Guillevin *et al.* 1993). It is important to recognize that ANCA have also been described in systemic lupus erythematosus (rarely), rheumatoid arthritis, inflammatory bowel disease, and in some infectious diseases (reviewed by Kallenberg *et al.* 1994).

ANCA in pathogenesis
The pathogenesis of vascular inflammation in systemic vasculitis is unknown. ANCA have recently been postulated to have a major role in this (reviewed by Kallenberg *et al.* 1994). Proinflammatory cytokines induce the surface expression of PR3 and MPO on neutrophils where they are accesible to react with ANCA (Falk *et al.* 1990a). Recent studies have shown that neutrophils primed with tumour necrosis factor-α are activated by ANCA to produce reactive oxygen products as well as to degranulate by the cross-linking of surface-expressed ANCA antigen with FcγR11 (Porges *et al.* 1994) and this can lead to bystander injury to endothelial cells (Ewert *et al.* 1992; Savage *et al.* 1992). MPO and PR3 bind to endothelial cells of cultured human umbilical vein by a charge mechanism and can then react with ANCA, with the potential for subsequent endothelial cell damage through complement activation or neutrophil adhesion and activation (Savage *et al.* 1992; Varagunam *et al.* 1992a). Further, it has been reported that ANCA can increase neutrophil adhesion to cultured endothelial cells, although the mechanism of this is unclear.

ANCA-negative vasculitis
The majority of patients with classical polyarteritis nodosa (more than 80 per cent) and a minority of patients with microscopic polyangiitis (20 per cent) have a negative ANCA. This means that

whilst ANCA are a useful non-invasive test in the diagnosis for vasculitis they are not essential for diagnosis. Serial studies suggest that while rising ANCA titres may predict a later flare, this is not always the case (Jayne *et al.* 1995). Strictly ANCA appear to be neither necessary nor sufficient for either diagnosis or flares of vasculitis, emphasizing the complex interactions which lead to disease expression.

Antiendothelial cell antibodies
Several studies have reported the presence of antibodies to endothelial cells (AECA) in the sera of patients with both Wegener's granulomatosis and polyarteritis (Frampton *et al.* 1990; Varagunam *et al.* 1992b). It has been suggested that AECA are important in the pathogenesis of vasculitis and inferred that they might cause endothelial injury. Alternatively they may be a reaction to endothelial damage and thus useful in assesment. It is as yet unclear whether these antibodies are going to be useful in diagnosis or management of these disorders.

Renal and coeliac angiograms

The value of arteriography in the diagnosis of classical polyarteritis nodosa has been reviewed by Travers *et al.* (1979). The radiological findings include aneurysms and also segmental narrowing and variation in the calibre of arteries, together with pruning of the peripheral vascular tree. Interpretation of the significance of such findings requires a radiologist with special experience. Aneurysms are most found commonly in the hepatic and renal arterial tree (Fig. 5) but can also occur in cerebral and pulmonary arteries. In the kidneys, wedge-shaped areas of infarction may be seen. Angiography is helpful both for confirming the presence and for documenting the extent of a necrotizing vasculitis. It is less useful in establishing the precise disease label. Aneurysms may also occur infrequently in other vasculitic disorders such as Wegener's granulomatosis and systemic lupus erythematosus. Where there is a clinical suspicion of classical polyarteritis nodosa it is sensible to do renal and coeliac angiograms and only to proceed to a renal biopsy if no aneurysms are found.

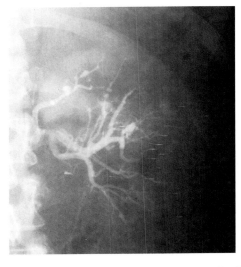

Fig. 5 Renal arteriogram in classical polyarteritis nodosa showing multiple aneurysms on renal vessels.

Pathology

Classical polyarteritis nodosa

Histology shows an arteritis with endothelial damage, fibrinoid necrosis affecting both intima and media (Fig. 6) and an inflammatory infiltrate of intima and media consisting predominantly of neutrophils but also of mononuclear cells. Often there is destruction of the internal elastic lamina. In some lesions the media and adventitia are surrounded by an infiltrate of mononuclear leukocytes and neutrophils. Immunofluorescent studies are in general negative for immunoglobulins and complement (Spargo *et al.* 1980; Cupps and Fauci 1981; Ronco *et al.* 1983).

Microscopic polyangiitis — renal pathology

The characteristic renal lesion is a focal, segmental necrotizing glomerulonephritis with fibrinoid necrosis and thrombosis of segments of the glomerular tufts surrounded by neutrophils (Fig. 7) (Davson *et al.* 1948; Serra and Cameron 1985; D'Agati *et al.* 1986; Adu *et al.* 1987). Often there is rupture of the glomerular basement membrane with adjacent extracapillary proliferation. Between 15 and 20 per cent of biopsies show extensive extracapillary proliferation

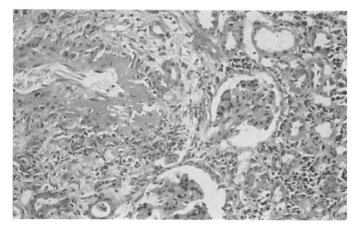

Fig. 6 Photomicrograph of a renal biopsy showing fibrinoid necrosis of an interlobular artery. Haematoxylin and eosin, original magnification × 25.

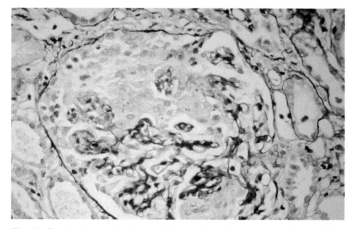

Fig. 7 Photomicrograph of a renal biopsy showing a segmental necrotizing glomerulonephritis with thrombosis and disruption of glomerular capillary loops and overlying extracapillary proliferation (crescents). Periodic acid–methenamine silver, original magnification × 100.

(crescent formation). Healed glomerular lesions are characterized by sharply defined segmental scars in which disrupted glomerular capillary loops can be seen. Glomerular immune deposits of immunoglobulin and complement are sparse and this is of value in differentiating the glomerular lesions of microscopic polyangiitis from those of other vasculitic disorders such as systemic lupus erythematosus and Henoch–Schönlein purpura. In about 20 per cent of the patients there is an acute vasculitis affecting arterioles as well as arteries. This often takes the form of endothelial damage, with fibrinoid necrosis disrupting the internal elastic lamina, and an infiltrate of neutrophils plus mononuclear cells in the media, the adventitia, and surrounding the vessel.

Most biopsies show a tubulointerstitial infiltrate with lymphocytes and eosinophils often around affected glomeruli. The severity of renal impairment correlates more closely with the severity of tubular damage than with the extent of glomerular disease.

Electron microscopy (D'Agati et al. *1986)*

Electron microscopy of glomeruli and also of arteries and arterioles shows that the earliest changes are of endothelial swelling and degeneration with focal detachment of the endothelium and subendothelial deposits of fibrin. With more advanced lesions there is more widespread denudation of endothelium with intraluminal fibrin deposits and occasional thrombi. At this stage polymorphonuclear leucocytes and monocytes are found both in the vessel lumen and within and around the walls.

Leucocyte infiltrate

Studies of renal histology in patients with Wegener's granulomatosis and microscopic polyangiitis have shown infiltrating monocytes/macrophages and neutrophils within glomeruli and in crescents. CD3 and IL-2R positive T cells were also identified in crescents, in the periglomerular area, and in the interstitium (Noronha *et al.* 1993; Brouwer *et al.* 1994)

Cell adhesion molecules

Cell adhesion molecules (**CAMs**) play a critical role in the migration of leucocytes to sites of inflammation, in selecting the types of leucocytes that accumulate, and in modifying leucocyte function, thus providing a mechanism by which leucocytes accumulate in renal tissues leading to glomerular and interstitial inflammation. CAMs expressed by the human kidney include the glycoproteins, intercellular adhesion molecule-1 (ICAM-1, CD54), and vascular cell adhesion molecule-1 (**VCAM-1**), which belong to the immunoglobulin supergene family, and the selectin, E-Selectin. The glomerular endothelium in biopsies from patients with Wegener's granulomatosis and microscopic polyangiitis expresses VCAM-1, which was not seen in any of the normal biopsies studied (Bruijn and Dinklo 1993; Pall *et al.* 1996). VCAM-1 expression by the glomerular endothelium may be important in selectively recruiting monocytes/macrophages and T lymphocytes that express VLA-4 (CD49d/CD29). It is possible that this adhesion molecule is involved in the genesis of this type of glomerular inflammation.

Churg–Strauss syndrome

The histological lesions described by Churg and Strauss included extravascular necrotic lesions which were widespread but most commonly seen in the epicardium. Acute lesions showed a predominant eosinophilic infiltrate whilst more chronic lesions comprised of giant-cell granulomata. In addition there was often a necrotizing arteritis with an infiltrate comprising eosinophils and giant-cell granulomata. Subsequent studies by Chumbley et al. (1977) and Lanham et al. (1984) suggest that a granulomatous vasculitis and extravascular granulomata were not essential for the diagnosis of Churg–Strauss syndrome. As with microscopic polyangiitis, the predominant renal lesion found in 85 per cent of cases is a focal, segmental necrotizing glomerulonephritis, often with extracapillary proliferation. Eosinophil infiltration and granulomata in the renal interstitium and a necrotizing arteritis are uncommon and found in less than 10 per cent of cases (Clutterbuck et al. 1990).

Other investigations in patients with a vasculitis

These provide evidence of an acute phase response with anaemia, high white blood-cell count, erthrocyte sedimentation rate, C-reactive protein, platelets, and serum complement levels, and a low serum albumin (reviewed by Serra and Cameron 1985). Serum levels of factor VIII-related antigen are raised in patients with vasculitis (Woolf et al. 1987). An eosinophilia (more than $1.5 \times 10^9/l$) is a characteristic feature of Churg–Strauss syndrome, although lesser degrees of eosinophilia may be seen in patients with classical polyarteritis nodosa who usually also have pulmonary disease (Frohnert and Sheps 1967). Microscopic haematuria and proteinuria are common presenting abnormalities in patients with renal disease. Abnormal liver function tests with a raised serum alkaline phosphatase are found in approximately 50 per cent of patients with microscopic polyangiitis (Savage et al. 1985; Adu et al. 1987). Low titres of rheumatoid factor are found in both Wegener's granulomatosis (Fauci et al. 1983) and classical polyarteritis nodosa (Leib et al. 1979; Scott et al. 1982). Low titres of antinuclear antibodies are found in a minority of patients with classical polyarteritis nodosa (Cohen et al. 1980; Scott et al. 1982). Immune complexes, usually in low titre, have been reported in the sera of some patients with a vasculitis (Scott et al. 1982; Ronco et al. 1983; Serra et al. 1984) but their significance is uncertain.

Therapy and prognosis of vasculitis

Overview of treatment

There is now a general consensus of opinion that the prognosis of idiopathic systemic necrotizing vasculitis (Wegener's granulomatosis, classical polyarteritis nodosa, and microscopic polyangiitis) has been greatly improved by the addition of cyclophosphamide to steroid treatment as originally reported by Fauci et al. (1979; Fauci et al. 1983). The only controlled study in patients with classical polyarteritis nodosa confirmed this (Guillevin et al. 1991). Before the use of steroids and immunosuppressive therapy the 1-year survival rate in Wegener's granulomatosis was 20 per cent and the 2-year survival 7 per cent (Walton 1958). In classical polyarteritis nodosa the overall 5-year survival was less than 15 per cent (Frohnert and Sheps 1967; Leib et al. 1979). There are no historical data on the treatment of microscopic polyangiitis. Most published clinical series are relatively recent and include a large proportion of patients with renal failure. Recent studies show that over 80 per cent of patients with Wegener's granulomatosis and classical polyarteritis nodosa and over 70 per cent

of patients with microscopic polyangiitis now survive for more than 5 years (reviewed by D'Amico and Sinico 1990).

Treatment of these vasculitides is essentially the same; the sole exception to this is antiviral treatment in polyarteritis nodosa induced by hepatitis B. The aims of treatment of systemic vasculitis are first to induce remission of active disease, thereby limiting the consequences of vascular injury so as to improve survival and limit disease-related morbidity. Second, to maintain remission thereby preventing organ damage from relapses. Third, to limit the consequences of the toxicity of treatment with cyclophosphamide and steroids. Now that most patients with a systemic vasculitis survive their acute illness this is an important additional aim. This makes choice of remission maintenance regimes a key issue (see Box 1).

Treatment of classical polyarteritis nodosa and microscopic polyangiitis

There is still uncertainty as to how much cyclophosphamide and prednisolone should be given, whether they should be given continuously and orally, or as intermittent intravenous pulses, and for how long treatment should be given.

Continuous oral prednisolone and cyclophosphamide
This has been used in most studies (Fauci et al. 1979; Fauci et al. 1983; Adu et al. 1987). Prednisolone is used at an initial dose of 0.6 to 1 mg/kg per day and the dose tapered to around 0.15 mg/kg per day at 4 to 6 months. Cyclophosphamide is started at a dose of 1.5 to 2 mg/kg per day and the dose adjusted to avoid a leucocyte count of less than $4 \times 10^9/l$.

Intermittent bolus prednisolone and cyclophosphamide
Our current intermittent regime, initially intravenous and then switched to oral pulses, has been described in detail elsewhere (Bacon 1987; Bacon et al. 1992) and is summarized in the appendix. Following evidence of the benefits of this regime in rheumatoid vasculitis (Scott and Bacon 1984) and lupus nephritis (Austin et al. 1986), we have successfully used a similar regime in patients with Wegener's granulomatosis, classical polyarteritis nodosa, and microscopic polyangiitis (Bacon et al. 1992; Adu et al. 1993). Previous studies in lupus nephritis showed that pulse cyclophosphamide was as effective in improving and stabilizing renal function and was associated with a lower incidence of cyclophosphamide toxicity than the continuous oral regime (Austin et al. 1986). Haemorrhagic cystitis or malignancy was not seen in patients treated with pulse cyclophosphamide and amenorrhoea appeared to be less common in patients treated with pulse cyclophosphamide compared with those receiving continuous oral cyclophosphamide. Uncontrolled studies of pulse cyclophosphamide in systemic vasculitis have yielded contradictory findings. Falk et al. (1990b) showed that monthly intravenous cyclophosphamide plus continuous oral prednisolone for 6 months was as effective as continuous oral cyclophosphamide plus prednisolone in patients with ANCA-positive glomerulonephritis and systemic vasculitis in terms of renal improvement and patient survival. Likewise, Haubitz et al. (1991) found that all eight patients with Wegener's granulomatosis treated with monthly intravenous cyclophosphamide and oral prednisolone went into remission and that drug toxicity was less than in 15 patients treated with continuous oral cyclophosphamide and prednisolone. By contrast Hoffman et al. (1990) found that only 2 out of 11 (18 per cent) patients with Wegener's granulomatosis treated with monthly pulse

cyclophosphamide and oral prednisolone achieved sustained remission. We use a pulse regime with only a 2-week gap between the initial three doses. In our ongoing controlled study, we found that pulse cyclophosphamide and steroids were equally as effective in inducing remission (Adu *et al.* 1993) and improving renal function as continuous cyclophosphamide and steroids. With both treatment regimes survival was comparable, with 90 per cent of patients with a systemic vasculitis surviving their first year of treatment. It is unlikely that this can be improved significantly. Relapses in the short term were comparable in the two treatment regimens.

Dose adjustments for renal failure and age
The metabolites of cyclophosphamide are excreted by the kidneys and accumulate in renal failure (Juma *et al.* 1981). In our experience this can lead to marrow suppression (Adu *et al.* 1987). The dose of cyclophosphamide must, therefore, be reduced in patients with renal impairment. A similar dose reduction is also advised in patients over the age of 70 years as they appear to be more sensitive than younger patients to marrow suppression with cyclophosphamide.

Duration of treatment
There is no agreed view on how long treatment should be continued. The duration of treatment is important as cyclophosphamide and steroids have substantial side-effects that have become more important as more patients survive their acute disease. On the one hand an inadequate duration of treatment might be accompanied by relapses, organ damage from vasculitis, and the consequences of this; and on the other hand overtreatment leads to a high drug toxicity. With the improved survival with current treatment, morbidity from haemorrhagic cystitis, bladder carcinoma, and lymphoma has become a major clinical problem. In Wegener's granulomatosis Fauci *et al.* (1983) recommended that treatment with cyclophosphamide should be continued for a year after remission is induced, after which the dose of cyclophosphamide and prednisolone should be tapered over several months. In patients on continuous oral prednisolone and cyclophosphamide we currently change from cyclophosphamide to azathioprine when remission is induced, usually after 4 to 6 months of treatment. Azathioprine and low-dose prednisolone is then continued with a low-dose alternative-day regime. Fuiano *et al.*

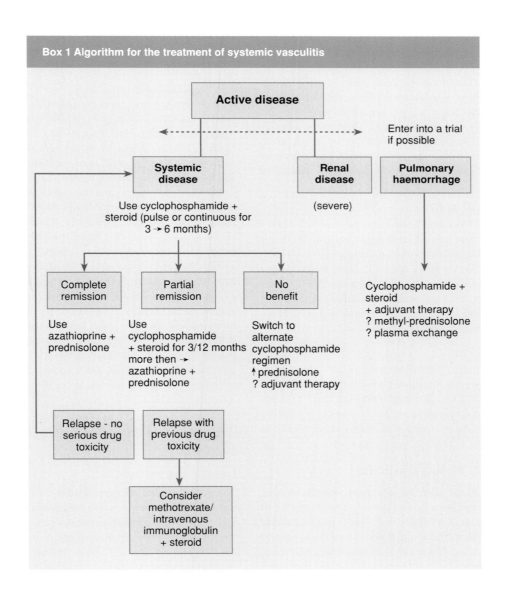

Box 1 Algorithm for the treatment of systemic vasculitis

(1988) also recommended keeping the patient on long-term prednisolone and azathioprine once cyclophosphamide has been discontinued. With the intermittent prednisolone and cyclophosphamide regime, cyclophosphamide is currently discontinued at 18 months and the patient changed to azathioprine and low-dose alternate-day prednisolone. The total dose of cyclophosphamide with the intermittent regime is considerably lower than with the continuous regime but we are currently studying shorter pulse regimes.

Intravenous methylprednisolone

This has been used in patients with active disease, especially when there is a crescentic glomerulonephritis. There is no compelling evidence that this confers any additional benefits when given in conjunction with continuous oral prednisolone and cyclophosphamide.

Plasmapheresis

Data from the Hammersmith Hospital suggest that plasma exchange may be of benefit in patients with a vasculitis who are also dialysis dependent (Hind et al. 1983; Pusey et al. 1991). We reserve the use of plasma exchange for patients with severe vasculitis, unresponsive to cytotoxics and steroids, or for patients with diffuse pulmonary haemorrhage or a diffuse crescentic glomerulonephritis.

Pooled, human intravenous immunoglobulin

Jayne et al. (1990) have suggested a beneficial effect of intravenous, pooled, normal human immunoglobulin in patients with ANCA-positive vasculitis. In vitro studies have shown that intravenous immunoglobulin contains anti-idiotypic antibodies to ANCA and AECA, capable of inhibiting the binding of these autoantibodies to their autoantigens. The possible mechanisms by which intravenous immunoglobulin works are still unclear. The treatment must be regarded as experimental until data from controlled studies are available.

Anti-T-lymphocyte antibodies

In a recent case report, Mathieson et al. (1990) successfully used a genetically engineered monoclonal antibody, Campath-1H (anti-CDw52) directed against lymphoid cells and monocytes specifically, together with an anti-CD4 antibody against T-helper cells, to treat one patient with intractable systemic vasculitis that was ANCA negative. A subsequent study confirmed and extended these observations to four patients (Lockwood et al. 1993). This treatment may be of use in systemic vasculitis that is resistant to conventional treatment.

Other treatments

There are anecdotal reports that cyclosporin may be of benefit in patients with Wegener's granulomatosis resistant to cyclophosphamide (Borleffs et al. 1987; Gremmel et al. 1988) but these have not been confirmed. There appears to be no good reason at present for using this drug to treat patients with a vasculitis in preference to cyclophosphamide.

Treatment of Churg–Strauss syndrome

Lanham et al. (1984) found that steroids alone were beneficial, although 4 of their 16 cases were given cytotoxic agents, and 3 had additional plasma exchange. Chumbley et al. (1977) also found that steroids alone were useful, although the 5-year survival was only 62 per cent, suggesting that the long-term prognosis might have been improved by the addition of cytotoxic agents. In patients with renal involvement, additional cyclophosphamide has been reported to be of benefit (Clutterbuck et al. 1990). We and others (Guillevin et al. 1991) routinely add cyclophosphamide to steroids if renal or neurological disease occurs.

Side-effects of treatment

A prominent complication of treatment with steroids and cyclophosphamide is sepsis and in our earlier study this was a major cause of death (Adu et al. 1987). We routinely use prophylactic oral amphotericin to reduce the risk of oral candidiasis and an H_2-receptor antagonist to reduce peptic ulceration. Cystitis is a well-recognized complication of cyclophosphamide therapy with an incidence varying from 15 to 34 per cent (Stillwell and Benson 1988; Fauci et al. 1983). We have not seen this complication in patients on intermittent intravenous cyclophosphamide. We routinely give Mesna. By binding the acrolein metabolites of cyclophosphamide, Mesna reduces the urothelial toxicity of cyclophosphamide (Bryant et al. 1980). With prolonged treatment this toxicity can lead to the development of bladder tumours (Stillwell et al. 1988). Other malignancies associated with long-term use of cyclophosphamide include leukaemia and lymphoma (Green et al. 1986). Cyclophosphamide may also lead to the development of azoospermia (Fairley et al. 1972) and ovarian dysfunction (Miller et al. 1971) and, when indicated, storage of gametes may be advised. Rarely cyclophosphamide can lead to the development of an interstitial pulmonary fibrosis (Cooper et al. 1986).

Consequences of drug toxicity

In their follow-up report of patients with Wegener's granulomatosis treated with long-term cyclophosphamide, Hoffman et al. (1992) found that drug-related toxicity had become a major cause of morbidity, being found in 42 per cent of patients. On long-term follow-up, 43 per cent of their patients developed cyclophosphamide-induced haemorrhagic cystitis, 2.8 per cent a bladder cancer, 2 per cent lymphomas, 2 per cent myelodysplasia, and 57 per cent of the women ovarian failure. Overall there was a 2.4-fold increase in malignancies, a 33-fold excess risk of bladder cancer and an 11-fold excess risk of lymphoma compared with age-matched controls. Despite this very significant treatment toxicity from cyclophosphamide, the patients had active disease for 54 per cent of the total time of follow-up. A clear conclusion of these data and our own is that whilst cyclophosphamide is effective in inducing remission it appears to be relatively ineffective in maintaining remission. As more patients survive their acute illness this burden of serious drug-related toxicity becomes unacceptably high, prompting a search for safer and at least equally effective ways of maintaining remission. There are now real anxieties about the appropriateness of using long-term oral cyclophosphamide in patients with a systemic vasculitis.

Monitoring disease activity in systemic vasculitis

Clinical disease activity

Accurate assesment of disease activity makes it possible to differentiate disease activity from the effects of chronic damage with dysfunction and infection. This is important as a guide to increasing or reducing the doses of potentially toxic drugs. Several disease activity scores have been developed. These include the Kallenberg score (Kallenberg et al. 1990), the vasculitis activity index (Olsen et al.

1992), and the Birmingham vasculitis activity score (**BVAS**) (Luqmani *et al.* 1994). In our study there was reasonable correlation between these three scores. In clinical practice the BVAS score appeared to provide a precise assessment of organ involvement in vasculitis compared with a physician's global assessment (Luqmani *et al.* 1994). For longer-term follow-up, assessment of damage (accumulating, non-healing scars) and the patient's functional status are also important. In the European Community collaborative studies, a protocol combining all these aspects has been devised (Bacon *et al.* 1995).

ANCA and disease activity

There is now good evidence that ANCA titres correlate with disease activity, tending to fall in remission and rise with relapse (Cohen Tervaert *et al.* 1989; Nolle *et al.* 1989). Sequential titres of antibodies to proteinase 3 and myeloperoxidase are useful in monitoring disease activity and predicting relapses but do not always provide correct predictions (Jayne *et al.* 1995) and thus should be used with other markers of activity. The correlation with disease activity is not sufficiently close (Kerr *et al.* 1993) to justify an increase in immunosuppressant therapy with rises in ANCA titre as has been suggested (Cohen Tervaert *et al.* 1989). Some of our patients with a positive ANCA or a rise in ANCA titre have remained free of active disease for several years.

Non-specific markers of disease activity

C-reactive protein
C-reactive protein is an acute phase protein and several studies have reported that the serum levels correlate closely with disease activity in patients with Wegener's granulomatosis and microscopic polyangiitis (Hind *et al.* 1984). The serum levels of C-reactive protein rise with sepsis and both this and factor VIII-related antigen may be persistently elevated in infarction. This can limit its usefulness in monitoring disease activity in vasculitis. In addition they do not predict relapse.

Factor VIII-related antigen
Factor VIII-related antigen is a glycoprotein that is present in endothelial cells and megakaryocytes and synthesized by both cell types. It plays a role in platelet adhesion to the subendothelium, and serum levels are raised in endothelial injury. Recent studies have reported that serum levels of factor VIII-related antigen are raised in patients with vasculitis (Woolf *et al.* 1987). Our own observations are that the serum levels of this antigen rise after the onset of vascular injury and that this rise persists for several months after clinical improvement. This limits its usefulness as a marker of disease activity.

Circulating soluble adhesion molecules
Cell adhesion molecules circulate in a soluble form from proteolytic cleavage of the membrane-bound CAMs. Significantly raised serum levels of sICAM-1 and sE-selectin are found in patients with active Wegener's granulomatosis and microscopic polyangiitis and these probably reflect the extent of endothelial activation and injury (Pall *et al.* 1994). It is as yet unclear whether this is going to be useful in predicting disease activity.

Outcome

Short-term outcome

Survival has improved in all of the vasculitides and in excess of 80 per cent of patients now survive their acute illness. Although our current treatment regimes are effective in inducing remission, current strategies for maintaining remission are inadequate. We have not achieved disease- and treatment-free remission for our patients.

Relapses

With an increasing proportion of patients surviving their acute illness, it has become important to define the risks and consequences of relapses, and to balance this against the potential toxicity of continued treatment with cyclophosphamide and prednisolone. The study of Gordon *et al.* (1993) reported a high rate of relapses of up to 70 per cent over a 10-year period in patients with Wegener's granulomatosis, classical polyarteritis, and microscopic polyangiitis. In that study the tendency of the survival curves to flatten out with time (Fig. 8) contrasted markedly with the cumulative relapse rate with time (Fig. 9). Relapses occurred for up to 68 months and there was no suggestion from the actuarial curves that the rate at which relapses are occurring decreased with time. There have been suggestions that classical polyarteritis nodosa may be a self-limiting disease which tended not to recur once remission was induced. In the study of Fauci *et al.* (1979) no relapses occurred whilst patients were on cyclophosphamide and steroids. Leib *et al.* (1979), however, found that 12 per cent of patients ran a chronic course and Gordon *et al.* (1993) found that 42 per cent of patients with classical polyarteritis nodosa relapsed. Few series report on relapses in patients with microscopic polyangiitis. Savage *et al.* (1985) reported that 12 out of 33 patients with microscopic polyangiitis had 19 relapses. Serra *et al.* (1984) described 18 patients with microscopic polyangiitis who had a chronically active course which they described as a 'smouldering' vasculitis. These patients had a worse prognosis than long-term survivors with 'stable' inactive vasculitis. In the study of Gordon *et al.* (1993) relapses in microscopic polyangiitis occurred least frequently of all the vasculitides at a rate of 25.3 per cent and this compares with the rate of 36.4 per cent reported by Savage *et al.* (1985) 10 years earlier. The median time to relapse was shorter in microscopic polyangiitis (24 months) than in classical polyarteritis nodosa (33 months). A significant proportion of patients who relapsed, microscopic polyangiitis (33 per cent) and classical polyarteritis nodosa (40 per cent), did so once all treatment had been discontinued, although patients with microscopic polyangiitis had more relapses whilst on treatment albeit in a reducing dose. The clinical pattern of relapse does not necessarily mimic the original presentation, in that entirely new organs could be involved at relapse. The clinical features at relapse were in general less severe than at initial presentation in patients with microscopic polyangiitis who had significantly less systemic, renal, and pulmonary symptoms probably because they were under close supervision. Most patients at relapse had a rash and arthralgia. Patients with classical polyarteritis nodosa had more systemic symptoms at relapse. While relapse was generally a mild, non-systemic phenomenon, it may carry serious consequences including the development of renal failure and death.

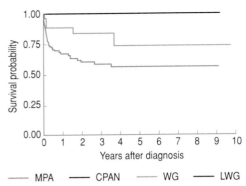

Fig. 8 Kaplan-Meier curve of the probability of survival of patients with microscopic polyangiitis (MPA), classical polyarteritis (CPAN), Wegener's granulomatosis (WG), and limited Wegener's granulomatosis (LWG). (From Gordon *et al.* 1993, with permission.)

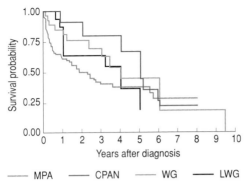

Fig. 9 Kaplan-Meier curve of the probability of surviving in terms of remaining free of relapse or of dying in patients with microscopic polyangiitis (MPA), classical polyarteritis (CPAN), Wegener's granulomatosis (WG), and limited Wegener's granulomatosis (LWG). (From Gordon *et al.* 1993, with permission.)

The vasculitides are not curable with our current treatment strategies. The implications of this are that these patients require long-term follow-up and possibly treatment.

One group of patients who had a low relapse rate were patients with microscopic polyangiitis who were on chronic dialysis and it seems either that patients with endstage renal failure have 'burned out' their disease or that renal failure is in itself immuno-suppressive.

Whilst current drug treatments for inducing remission seem fairly successful it is clear that our regimes for maintaining remission are inadequate. The likelihood that relapse is a consequence of the way in which treatment modifies these diseases means that any future trial considering the efficacy of different treatments should measure not only survival as an endpoint, but also the rate of relapse and toxicity as a means of assessing the impact of treatment on patients with these diseases. There is clearly a need for prolonged follow-up in patients with a vasculitis as relapses can occur unpredictably after many years of remission.

Long-term prognosis (Fig. 8)

Overall the prognosis in patients with a vasculitis has improved over the past few years. Nevertheless, these disorders still carry a substantial mortality and morbidity.

Classical polyarteritis nodosa

The 5-year survival in classical polyarteritis nodosa ranges from 63 per cent (Guillevin *et al.* 1988) to 80 per cent (Leib *et al.* 1979) and in our own studies was 100 per cent (Gordon *et al.* 1993). Adverse prognostic factors include increasing age (Sack *et al.* 1975; Leib *et al.* 1979; Guillevin *et al.* 1988), renal failure, and gastrointestinal disease (Guillevin *et al.* 1988).

Microscopic polyangiitis

The overall prognosis in microscopic polyangiitis is much worse and in our series showed a 40 per cent mortality over a decade, largely related to renal failure often associated with delayed referrals. In other studies the 5-year survival in patients with microscopic polyangiitis ranges from 38 to 80 per cent (reviewed

by D'Amico and Sinico 1990). Adverse prognostic factors include age (Adu *et al.* 1987; Fuiano *et al.* 1988) and the severity of renal failure before institution of therapy (Serra *et al.* 1984; Adu *et al.* 1987).

Churg–Strauss syndrome

The overall 5-year survival in Churg–Strauss syndrome is reported to be 62 per cent (Chumbley *et al.* 1977).

Conclusion

Progress in therapy will be linked to an increased understanding of the aetiology of disease and pathogenetic mechanisms, which probably vary from one syndrome to another despite almost identical histopathology of necrotizing vasculitis. Only when these have been defined will more specific, and hopefully less toxic, therapy be available. Nevertheless, the prognosis in vasculitis has improved enormously, so that aggressive therapy is rewarding. At present the main aim must be earlier diagnosis, since therapy is both more successful and less toxic before advanced renal impairment develops; together with the development of less-toxic long-term maintenance regimes.

Appendix

Protocol for the treatment of vasculitis with intermittent pulses of cyclophosphamide and prednisolone

Table 2 sets out the protocol for the treatment of vasculitis with intermittent pulses of cyclophosphamide and prednisolone, and should be used in conjunction with the following notes.

The induction regimen is used for up to 6 months. It can be shorter if clinical remission is achieved early but is continued for at least 3 months of treatment.

The remission regimen commences immediately after the end of the induction regimen, and is continued for up to 1 year from the start of induction.

The consolidation regimen is normally for a further 6 months, but may be continued for longer if disease activity is still apparent.

Table 2 Protocol for the treatment of vasculitis

Phase	Time (week)	Pulse number	Route	Dose	
				Cyclophosphamide	Prednisolone
Induction	0, 2, 4,	1–3	IV	15 mg/kg × 1	10 mg/kg
	7, 10, 13, 17, 21, 25	4–9	Oral	5 mg/kg × 3	3.3 mg/kg × 3
Remission	30, 35, 40, 46, 52	10–14	Oral	5 mg/kg × 3	3.3 mg/kg × 3
Consolidation	58, 64, 70, 76	15–21	Oral	5 mg/kg × 3	3.3 mg/kg × 3
Maintenance	Oral prednisolone, 0.15 mg/kg alternate days				

The maintenance phase is continued probably indefinitely.

In patients who are already being treated with immunosuppressive agents, the pulse therapy should not be started until 2 weeks has elapsed off cytotoxics to avoid severe marrow toxicity. All patients should be prescribed ordinary (not enteric coated) prednisolone in view of potential problems of variable absorption of active compound. During the pulse week, all patients are prescribed ranitidine, 150 mg at night, and amphotericin lozenges, 10 mg four times daily as prophylaxis. Further use is at the discretion of the physician. If patients develop infections during the course of treatment, then immunosuppression will be stopped until the infection has been adequately treated. If there is evidence of renal impairment or marrow suppression, or the patient is over the age of 70 years, the dose of cyclophosphamide and steroid will be adjusted accordingly (see dose adjustments below).

Tests before each pulse

Full blood count should be measured before each pulse is given, and the values should be in the normal range. If they are not, the pulse should be deferred until they are. Creatinine should be measured before each pulse, and if abnormal the dose of the pulse should be adjusted according to Table 3.

Escalation protocol

At any stage as decided by the clinician, the following may be given:

1. Additional bolus methylprednisolone intravenously, 1 g/day × 3 days;

2. Additional bolus cyclophosphamide intravenously, 5 mg/kg.day × 3 days;

3. Plasma exchange (optional).

Mesna is to be given in three oral doses totalling 75 per cent of the dose of cyclophosphamide for every dose of intravenous cyclophosphamide.

Dose adjustments are devised for the following reasons:

1. Maximum doses: the maximum bolus dose of cyclophosphamide, regardless of weight, will be 1000 mg. The maximum bolus dose of prednisolone regardless of weight will be 1000 mg.

2. Cytopenia prior to bolus therapy: delay bolus until count restored to above lower limit of normal (white cell count > 3.5 or

Table 3 Bolus therapy

Serum creatinine	Cyclophosphamide dose	Prednisolone dose
<150	15 mg/kg	10 mg/kg
150–250	10 mg/kg	10 mg/kg
251–500	7.5 mg/kg	10 mg/kg
>500	5 mg/kg	7 mg/kg

neutrophil count > 2.0, platelets > 140). If cytopenia recurs, reduce cyclophosphamide bolus by 25 per cent.

3. Renal failure on bolus therapy: reduce as shown in Table 3.

4. Bolus therapy in the elderly (defined as over the age of 70 years): reduce the cyclophosphamide dose to 10 mg/kg, steroid dose unchanged.

References

Adu, D., Howie, A.J., Scott, D.G.I., Bacon, P.A., McGonigle, R.J.S., and Michael, J. (1987). Polyarteritis and the kidney. *Quarterly Journal of Medicine*, **62**, 221–37.

Adu, D., Pall, A., Luqmani, R.A., *et al.* (1993). Controlled trial of treatment of vasculitis. *Clinical and Experimental Immunology*, **93** (Suppl.1), 38.

Arkin, A. (1930). A clinical and pathological study of periarteritis nodosa. *American Journal of Pathology*, **6**, 401–26.

Austin, H.A., Klippel, J.H., Balow J.E., *et al.* (1986). Therapy of lupus nephritis: controlled trial of prednisolone and cytotoxic drugs. *New England Journal of Medicine*, **314**, 614–19

Bacon, P.A. (1987). Vasculitis — clinical aspects and therapy. *Acta Medica Scandinavica*, **715** (Suppl.), 157–63.

Bacon, P.A., Luqmani, R.A., Scott, D.G.I., and Adu, D. (1992). Immunopharmacology of vasculitic syndrome. In *Immunopharmacology in autoimmune disease and transplants* (ed. H.E. Rugstad), pp. 273–89. Plenum Publishing Corporation, New York.

Bacon, P.A., Moots, R.J., Exley, A., Luqmani, R.A., and Rasmussen, N. (1995). Vital assessment of vasculitis. *Clinical and Experimental Rheumatology*, **13**, 275–8.

Borleffs, J.C., Derksen, R.H., and Hene, R.J. (1987). Treatment of Wegener's granulomatosis with cyclosporin. (Letter.) *Annals of the Rheumatic Diseases*, **46**, 175.

Brouwer, E., Huitema, M.G., Mulder, A.H.L., *et al.* (1994). Neutrophil activation in vitro and in vivo in Wegener's geanulomatosis. *Kidney International*, **45**, 1121–311.

Bruijn, J.A. and Dinklo, N.J.C.M. (1993). Distinct patterns of expression of intercellular adhesion molecule-1, vascular cell adhesion molecule-1, and endothelial-leukocyte adhesion molecule-1 in renal disease. *Laboratory Investigation*, **69**, 329–35.

Bryant, B.M., Jarman, M., Ford, H.T., and Smith, I.E. (1980). Prevention of isophosphamide-induced urothelial toxicity with 2-mercaptoethane-sulphanate sodium (mesnum) in patients with advanced carcinoma. *Lancet*, **ii**, 657–9.

Chumbley, L.C., Harrison, R.A., and DeRemee, R.A. (1977). Allergic granulomatous angiitis (Churg–Strauss syndrome). Report and analysis of 30 cases. *Mayo Clinic Proceedings*, **52**, 477–84.

Churg, J. and Strauss, L. (1951). Allergic granulomatosis, allergic angiitis, and periarteritis nodosa. *American Journal of Pathology*, **27**, 277–301.

Clutterbuck, E.J., Evans, D.J., and Pusey, C.D. (1990). Renal involvement in Churg–Strauss syndrome. *Nephrology Dialysis Transplantation*, **5**, 161–7.

Cohen, R.D., Conn, D.L., and Ilstrup, D.M. (1980). Clinical features, prognosis and response to treatment in polyarteritis. *Mayo Clinic Proceedings*, **55**, 146–55.

Cohen Tervaert, J.W., Van Der Wonde, F.J., Fauci, A.S., *et al.* (1989). Association between active Wegener's granulomatosis and anti-cytoplasmic antibodies. *Archives of Internal Medicine*, **149**, 2461–5.

Cohen Tervaert, J.W., Limburg, P.C., Elema, J.D., *et al.* (1991). Detection of auto-antibodies against myeloid lysosomal enzymes: a useful adjunct to classification of patients with biopsy-proven necrotizing arteritis. *American Journal of Medicine*, **91**, 59–66.

Cooper, J.A.D., White, D.A., and Matthay, R.A. (1986). Drug-induced pulmonary disease. 1. Cytotoxic drugs. *American Review of Respiratory Diseases*, **133**, 321–40.

Coward, R.A., Handy, N.A.T., Shortland, J.S., and Brown, C.B. (1986). Renal microscopic polyarteritis: a treatable condition. *Nephrology Dialysis Transplantation*, **1**, 31–7.

Cupps, T.R. and Fauci, A.S. (1981). *The vasculitides*. Saunders, Philadelphia.

D'Agati, V., Chander, P., Mash, M., and Mancilla-Jimenez, R. (1986). Idiopathic microscopic polyarteritis nodosa: ultrastructural observations on the renal, vascular and glomerular lesions. *American Journal of Kidney Diseases*, **8**, 95–110.

D'Amico, G. and Sinico, R.G. (1990). Treatment and monitoring of systemic vasculitis. *Nephrology Dialysis Transplantation*, **1** (Suppl.), 53–7.

Davies, D.J., Moran, J.E., Niale, J.F., and Ryan, G.B. (1982). Segmental necrotising glomerulonephritis with antineutrophil antibody: possible arbovirus aetiology. *British Medical Journal*, **285**, 606.

Davson, J., Ball, J., and Platt, R. (1948). The kidney in periarteritis nodosa. *Quarterly Journal of Medicine*, **17**, 175–202.

Ewert, B.H., Jennette, J.C., and Falk, R.J. (1992). Anti-myeloperoxidase antibodies stimulate neutrophils to damage human endothelial cells. *Kidney International*, **41**, 375–83.

Fairley, K.F., Barrie, J.U., and Johnson, W. (1972). Sterility and testicular atrophy related to cyclophosphamide therapy. *Lancet*, **i**, 568–9.

Falk, R.L. and Jennette, J.C. (1988). Antineutrophil cytoplasmic auto-antibodies with specificity for myeloperoxidase in patients with systemic vasculitis and idiopathic necrotising and crescentic glomerulonephritis. *New England Journal of Medicine*, **318**, 1651–7.

Falk, R.J., Terrell, R.S., Charles, L.A., and Jennette, J.C. (1990*a*). Anti-neutrophil cytoplasmic autoantibodies induce neutrophils to degranulate and produce oxygen radicals in vitro. *Proceedings of the National Academy of Sciences USA*, **87**, 4115–19.

Falk, R.J., Hogan, S., Carey, T.S., and Jennette, C. (1990*b*). Clinical course of antineutrophil cytoplasmic autoantibody-associated glomerulonephritis and systemic vasculitis. *Annals of Internal Medicine*, **113**, 656–63.

Fauci, A.S. and Wolff, S.M. (1973). Wegener's granulomatosis: studies in eighteen patients and a review of the literature. *Medicine (Baltimore)*, **52**, 535–61.

Fauci, A.S., Katz, P., Haynes, B.F., and Wolff, S.M. (1979). Cyclophosphamide therapy of severe systemic necrotizing vasculitis. *New England Journal of Medicine*, **301**, 235–8.

Fauci, A.S., Haynes, B.F., Katz, P., and Wolff, S.M. (1983). Wegener's granulomatosis: prospective clinical and therapeutic experience with 85 patients for 21 years. *Annals of Internal Medicine*, **98**, 76–85.

Ferrari, E. (1903). Ueber Polyarteritis acuta nodosa (sogenannte Periarteritis nodosa) und ihre Beziehungen zur Polymyositis und Polyneuritis acuta. *Beitraege zur Pathologischen Anatomie und Allgemeinen Pathologie*, **34**, 1–25.

Frampton, G., Jayne, D.R.W., Perry, G.J., Lockwood, C.M., and Cameron, J.S. (1990). Auto-antibodies to endothelial cells and neutrophil cytoplasmic antigens in systemic vasculitis. *Clinical and Experimental Immunology*, **82**, 227–32.

Frohnert, P.P. and Sheps, S.G. (1967). Long term follow up study of periarteritis nodosa. *American Journal of Medicine*, **43**, 8–14.

Fuiano, G., Cameron, J.S., Raftery, M., Hartley, B.H., Williams, D.G., and Ogg, C.S. (1988). Improved prognosis of microscopic polyarteritis in recent years. *Nephrology Dialysis Transplantation*, **3**, 383–91.

Goldschmeding, R., Van Der Shoot, C.E., and ten Bokkel Huinink, D. (1989). Wegener's granulomatosis autoantibodies identify a novel diisopropylfluorophosphate-binding protein in the lysosomes of normal human neutrophils. *Journal of Clinical Investigation*, **84**, 1577–87.

Gordon, M., Luqmani, R.A., Adu, D., *et al.* (1993). Relapses in patients with a systemic vasculitis. *Quarterly Journal of Medicine*, **86**, 779–89.

Green, M.H., Harris, E.L., Gershenson, D.M., and Malkasian, G.D. (1986). Melphalan may be a more potent leukemogen than cyclophosphamide. *Annals of Internal Medicine*, **105**, 360–7.

Gremmel, F., Druml, W., Schmidt, P., and Graninger, W. (1988). Cyclosporin in Wegener's granulomatosis. *Annals of Internal Medicine*, **108**, 491.

Guillevin, L., Le Thi Huong Du, Godeau, P., Jais, P., and Wechsler, B. (1988). Clinical findings and prognosis of polyarteritis nodosa and Churg–Strauss angiitis: a study of 165 patients. *British Journal of Rheumatology*, **27**, 258–64.

Guillevin, L., Jarousse, B., Lok, C., *et al.* (1991). Longterm followup after treatment of polyarteritis nodosa and Churg–Strauss angiitis with comparison of steroids, plasma exchange and cyclophosphamide to steroids and plasma exchange. A prospective randomized trial of 71 patients. *Journal of Rheumatology*, **18**, 567–74.

Guillevin, L., Visser, H., Noel, L.H., *et al.* (1993). Antineutrophil cytoplasm antibodies in systemic polyarteritis nodosa with and without hepatitis B virus infection and Churg–Strauss syndrome. *Journal of Rheumatology*, **20**, 1345–9.

Hall, T.B., Wadham, B., McN., and Wood, C.J. (1984). Vasculitis and glomerulonephritis — a subgroup with an antineutrophil cytoplasmic antibody. *Australian and New Zealand Journal of Medicine*, **14**, 277–8.

Haubitz, M., Frei, U., Rother, U., Brunkhorst, R., and Koch, K.M. (1991). Cyclophosphamide pulse therapy in Wegener's granulomatosis. *Nephrology Dialysis Transplantation*, **6**, 531–5.

Haworth, S.J., Savage, C.O.S., Carr, D., Hughes, J.M.B., and Rees, A.J. (1985). Pulmonary haemorrhage complicating Wegener's granulomatosis and microscopic polyarteritis. *British Medical Journal*, **290**, 1775–8.

Hind, C.R.K., Paraskevakou, H., Lockwood, C.M., Evans, D.J., Peters, D.K., and Rees, A.J. (1983). Prognosis after immunosuppression of patients with crescentic nephritis requiring dialysis. *Lancet*, **1**, 263–5.

Hind, C.R.K., Winearls, C.G., Lockwood, C.M., Rees, A.J., and Pepys, M.B. (1984). Objective monitoring or activity in Wegener's granulomatosis by measurement of C-reactive protein concentration. *Clinical Nephrology*, **21**, 341–5.

Hoffman, G.S., Leavitt, R.Y., Fleischer, T.A., Minor, J.R., and Fauci, A.S. (1990). Treatment of Wegener's granulomatosis with intermittent high-dose intravenous cyclophosphamide. *American Journal of Medicine*, **89**, 403–10.

Hoffman, G.S., Kerr, G.S., Leavitt, R.Y., Hallahan, C.W., Lebovics, R.S., and Travis, W.D. (1992). Wegener's granulomatosis: an analysis of 158 patients. *Annals of Internal Medicine*, **116**, 488–98.

Jayne, D.R.W., Davies, M.J., Fox, C.J.V., Black, C.M., and Lockwood, C.M. (1990). Treatment of systemic vasculitis with pooled intravenous immunoglobulin. *Lancet*, **337**, 1137–9.

Jayne, D.R.W., Gaskin, G., Pusey, C.D., and Lockwood, C.M. (1995). ANCA and predicting relapse in systemic vasculitis. *Quarterly Journal of Medicine*, **88**, 127–33.

Jennette, J.C., Falk, R.J., Andrassy, K., *et al.* (1994). Nomenclature of systemic vasculitides: the proposal of an international consensus conference. *Arthritis and Rheumatism*, **37**, 187–92.

Juma, F.D., Rogers, H.J., and Trounce, J.R. (1981). Effect of renal insufficiency on the pharmacokinetics of cyclophosphamide and some of its metabolites. *European Journal of Clinical Pharmacology*, **19**, 443–51.

Kallenberg, C.G.M., Cohen Tervaert, J.M., and Stegeman, C.A. (1990). Criteria for disease activity in Wegener's granulomatosis: a requirement for longtitudinal studies. *APMIS Suppl*, **19**, 37–9.

Kallenberg, C.G.M, Brouwer, E., Weening, J.J., and Cohen Tervaert, J.W. (1994). Anti-neutrophil cytoplasmic antibodies: current diagnostic and pathophysiological potential. *Kidney International*, **46**, 1–15.

Kerr, G.S., Fleisher, T.A., Hallahan, C.W., Leavitt, R.Y., Fauci, A.S., and Hoffman, G.S. (1993). Limited prognostic value of changes in antineutrophil cytoplasmic antibody titer in patients with Wegener's granulomatosis. *Arthritis and Rheumatism*, **36**, 365–71.

Kussmaul, A. and Maier, R. (1866). Über eine bisher nicht beschreibene eigenthümliche Arteriener Krankung (periarteritis nodosa): die mit Morbus Brightii und rapid fortschreitender allgemeiner Muskellahmung einhergeht. *Deutsches Archiv für Klinische Medizin*, **1**, 484–517.

Lanham, J.G., Elkon, K.B., Pusey, C.D., and Hughes, G.R.V. (1984). Systemic vasculitis with asthma and eosinophilia: a clinical approach to the Churg–Strauss syndrome. *Medicine (Baltimore)*, **63**, 65–81.

Lee, S.S., Adu, D., and Thompson, R. (1990). Anti-myeloperoxidase antibodies in systemic vasculitis. *Clinical and Experimental Immunology*, **79**, 41–6.

Leib, E.S., Restivo, C., and Paulus, H.E. (1979). Immunosuppressive and corticosteroid therapy of periarteritis nodosa. *American Journal of Medicine*, **67**, 941–7.

Lie, J.T. (1994). Nomenclature and classification of vasculitis: plus ça change, plus c'est la mme chose. *Arthritis and Rheumatism*, **37**, 181–6.

Lockwood, C.M., Thiru, S., Isaacs, J.D., Hale, G., and Waldmann, H. (1993). Long term remission of intractable systemic vasculitis with monoclonal antibody therapy. *Lancet*, **341**, 1620–2.

Luqmani, R.A., Bacon, P.A., Moots, R.J., *et al.* (1994). Birmingham Vasculitis Activity Score in systemic necrotizing vasculitis. *Quarterly Journal of Medicine*, **87**, 671–8.

Masi, A.T., Hunder, G.G., Lie, J.T., Michel, B.A., Bloch, D.A., and Arend, W.P. (1990). The American College of Rheumatology 1990 criteria for the classification of Churg–Strauss syndrome (allergic granulomatosis and angiitis). *Arthritis and Rheumatism*, **33**, 1094–110.

Mathieson, P.W., Cobbold, S.P., Hale, G., *et al.* (1990). Monoclonal antibody therapy in systemic vasculitis. *New England Journal of Medicine*, **323**, 250–4.

Miller, J.J., III, Williams, G.F., and Leissring, J.C. (1971). Multiple late complications of therapy with cyclophosphamide including ovarian destruction. *American Journal of Medicine*, **50**, 530–5.

Minkowitz, G., Smoller, B.R., and McNutt, N.S. (1991). Benign cutaneous polyarteritis nodosa. *Archives of Dermatology*, **127**, 1520–3.

Nolle, B., Specks, V., Ludeman, J., Rohrbach, M.S., De Remee, R.A., and Gross, W.L. (1989). Anticytoplasmic autoantibodies: their immunodiagnostic value in Wegener's granulomatosis. *Annals of Internal Medicine*, **111**, 28–40.

Noronha, I.L., Krüger, C., Andrassy, K., Ritz, E., and Waldherr, R. (1993). *In situ* production of TNFα, IL-1β and IL-2R in ANCA-positive glomerulonephritis. *Kidney International*, **43**, 682.

Novack, S.N. and Pearson, C.M. (1971). Cyclophosphamide therapy in Wegener's granulomatosis. *New England Journal of Medicine*, **285**, 1493–6.

Olsen, T.L., Whiting O'Keefe, Q.E., and Hellman, D.B. (1992). Validity and precision of a vasculitis activity index (VAI). *Arthritis and Rheumatology*, **35**, S164.

Pall, A.A., Adu, D., Drayson, M., Taylor, C.M., Richards, N.T., and Michael, J. (1994). Circulating soluble adhesion molecules in systemic vasculitis. *Nephrology Dialysis Transplantation*, **9**, 770–4.

Pall, A.A., Howie, A.J., Adu, D., *et al.* (1996). Glomerular VCAM-1 expression in renal vasculitis. *Journal of Clinical Pathology*, **49**, 238–42.

Porges, A.J., Redecha, P.B., Kimberly, W.T., Csernok, E., Gross, W.L., and Kimberly, R.T. (1994). Anti-neutrophil cytoplasmic antibodies engage and activate human neutrophils via FcγR11a. *Journal of Immunology*, **153**, 1271–80.

Pusey, C.D., Rees, A.J., Evans, D.J., Peters, D.K., and Lockwood, C.M. (1991). Plasma exchange in focal necrotizing glomerulonephritis without anti-GBM antibodies. *Kidney International*, **40**, 757–63.

Ronco, P., Verroust, P., Mignon, F., *et al.* (1983). Immunopathologic studies of polyarteritis nodosa and Wegener's granulomatosis: a report of 43 patients with 51 renal biopsies. *Quarterly Journal of Medicine*, **52**, 212–23.

Sack, M., Cassidy, J.T., and Bole, G.G. (1975). Prognostic factors in polyarteritis. *Journal of Rheumatology*, **2**, 411–20.

Savage, C.O.S., Winearls, C.G., Evans, D.J., Rees, A.J., and Lockwood, S.M. (1985). Microscopic polyarteritis: presentation, pathology and prognosis. *Quarterly Journal of Medicine*, **56**, 467–83.

Savage, C.O.S., Jones, S., Winearls, C.G., Marshall, P.D., and Lockwood, C.M. (1987). Prospective study of radio-immunoassay for antibodies against neutrophil cytoplasm in diagnosis of systemic vasculitis. *Lancet*, **i**, 1389–93.

Savage, C.O.S., Pottinger, B.E., Gaskin, G., Pusey, C.D., and Pearson, J.D. (1992). Autoantibodies developing to myeloperoxidase and proteinase 3 in systemic vasculitis stimulate neutrophil cytotoxicity towards cultured endothelial cells. *American Journal of Pathology*, **141**, 335–42.

Scott, D.G.I. and Bacon, P.A. (1984). Intravenous cyclophosphamide plus methyl-prednisolone in the treatment of systemic rheumatoid vasculitis. *American Journal of Medicine*, **76**, 377–84.

Scott, D.G.I., Bacon, P.A., Elliott, P.J., Tribe, C.R., and Wallington, T.B. (1982). Systemic vasculitis in a district general hospital 1972–1980: clinical and laboratory features, classification and prognosis of 80 cases. *Quarterly Journal of Medicine*, **51**, 292–311.

Serra, A. and Cameron, J.S. (1985). Clinical and pathological aspects of renal vasculitis. *Seminars in Nephrology*, **5**, 15–33.

Serra, A., Cameron, J.S., Turner, D.R., *et al.* (1984). Vasculitis affecting the kidney: presentation, histopathology and long term outcome. *Quarterly Journal of Medicine*, **53**, 181–207.

Spargo, B.H., Seymour, A.E., and Ordenez, N.G. (1980). Vasculitis. In *Renal biopsy pathology with diagnostic and therapeutic implications*, pp. 205–18. Wiley, New York.

Specks, U. and De Remee, R.A. (1990). Granulomatous vasculitis: Wegener's granulomatosis and Churg–Strauss syndrome in vasculitic syndromes. *Rheumatic Disease Clinics of North America*, **16**, 377–97.

Stillwell, T.J. and Benson, R.C., Jr. (1988). Cyclophosphamide-induced haemorrhage cystitis. A review of 100 patients. *Cancer*, **61**, 451–7.

Stillwell, T.J., Benson, R.C., Jr., De Remee, R.A., McDonald, T.J., and Weiland, L.H. (1988). Cyclophosphamide-induced bladder toxicity in Wegener's granulomatosis. *Arthritis and Rheumatism*, **31**, 465–70.

Travers, R.L., Allison, D.J., Brettle, R.P., and Hughes, G.R.V. (1979). Polyarteritis nodosa: a clinical and angiographic analysis of 17 cases. *Seminars in Arthritis and Rheumatism*, **8**, 184–99.

Van der Woude, F.J., Rasmussen, N., Lobatto, S., *et al.* (1985). Auto-antibodies against neutrophils and monocytes: tool for diagnosis and marker of disease activity in Wegener's granulomatosis. *Lancet*, **ii**, 425–9.

Van der Woude, F.J., Daha, M.R., and Vanes, L.A. (1989). Review: the current status of neutrophil cytoplasmic antibodies. *Clinical and Experimental Immunology*, **78**, 143–8.

Varagunam, M., Adu, D., Taylor, C.M., *et al.* (1992*a*). Endothelium myeloperoxidase-antimyeloperoxidase interaction in vasculitis. *Nephrology Dialysis Transplantation*, **7**, 1077.

Varagunam, M., Nwosu, Z., Adu, D., *et al.* (1992*b*). Little evidence for anti-endothelial cell antibodies in microscopic polyarteritis and Wegener's granulomatosis. *Nephrology Dialysis Transplantation*, **8**, 113.

Walton, E.W. (1958). Giant cell granuloma of the respiratory tract (Wegener's granulomatosis). *British Medical Journal*, **1**, 265–70.

Wegener, F. (1936). Über generalisierte, septische Gefasserkrankungen. *Verhandlungens der Deutschen Gesellschaft für Pathologie*, **29**, 202–9.

Woolf, A.D., Wakerley, J., Wallington, T.B., Scott, D.J.I., and Dieppe, P.A. (1987). Factor VIII related antigen in the assessment of vasculitis. *Annals of the Rheumatic Diseases*, **46**, 441–4.

Wuthrich, R.P. (1992). Intercellular adhesion molecules and vascular cell adhesion molecule-1 and the kidney. *Journal of the American Society of Nephrology*, **3**, 1201–11.

Zeek, P.M. (1952). Perarteritis nodosa: a critical review. *American Journal of Clinical Pathology*, **22**, 777–90.

5.11.4 Small vessel vasculitis

Clive E. H. Grattan and Victoria A. Jolliffe

Introduction

Small vessel vasculitis is characterized by inflammation centred on damaged capillaries and postcapillary venules. Muscular arteries are not usually involved although, confusingly, a recent international consensus on the classification of vasculitis (Jennette *et al.* 1994) includes patterns of vasculitis involving small and medium-sized arteries (Wegener's granulomatosis, Churg–Strauss syndrome, and microscopic polyangiitis) within the spectrum of small vessel vasculitis. It is however clear that there is a range of clinical and pathological features within defined diagnostic groups depending on the organ and size of vessel affected. The cutaneous lesions of Wegener's granulomatosis, for instance, may show the typical clinical and histological features of small vessel vasculitis as part of the wider spectrum of this systemic granulomatous disorder (Daoud *et al.* 1994; Francès *et al.* 1994). Small vessel vasculitis usually presents in the skin although the microvasculature of any tissue may be affected, especially the joints and kidneys. The most widely recognized clinicopathological patterns of small vessel vasculitis are listed in Table 1. Henoch–Schönlein purpura is regarded by many as a special form of allergic vasculitis. The division into leucocytoclastic and non-leucocytoclastic patterns of vasculitis is not absolute since skin biopsies may show a spectrum of pathological changes ranging from predominantly neutrophilic to predominantly mononuclear cell infiltrates in Sjögren's syndrome, drug-induced vasculitis, urticarial vasculitis, and nodular vasculitis. There is some evidence that cellular infiltrates

Table 1 Clinicopathological classification of small vessel vasculitis

1. Leucocytoclastic vasculitis

   Allergic vasculitis (synonym: hypersensitivity angiitis)

   Drugs, infections, autoimmune diseases, inflammatory diseases, malignancy, idiopathic

   Henoch–Schönlein purpura (synonym: anaphylactoid purpura)

   Urticarial vasculitis (synonym: hypocomplementaemic vasculitis)

   Cryoglobulinaemia

   Hypergammaglobulinaemic purpura (of Waldenström)

   Erythema elevatum diutinum and granuloma faciale

2. Non-leucocytoclastic vasculitis

   Drug-related vasculitis

   Nodular vasculitis

   Livedo vasculitis

   Pityriasis lichenoides acuta and chronica

may evolve from neutrophilic to mononuclear as lesions mature, but in many patients the pattern of inflammation remains unchanged throughout the course of their illness.

The definition of small vessel vasculitis is open to different interpretations. Some authors restrict it to lesions with a clearly defined leucocytoclastic histology showing neutrophils within and around blood vessel walls, leucocytoclasis (fragmentation of neutrophils), fibrin in and around the damaged blood vessels, and swelling, hypertrophy, or necrosis of endothelial cells. Others will accept the presence of inflammatory cells within vessel walls and at least one of the above features as being sufficient for diagnosis. Evidence of vessel wall damage should be the key feature for diagnosis whether the predominant cell type is neutrophilic, eosinophilic, mononuclear, or mixed. Red cells may be seen in the surrounding tissue and intraluminal fibrin thrombi may form as a result of it. Of 98 cases of cutaneous vasculitis diagnosed on skin biopsy over a 5-year period in an adult population of around 400 000, 49 had definite leucocytoclastic vasculitis, 13 showed some features of it, and 12 had a predominantly lymphocytic vasculitis (unpublished data).

The clinical presentation of cutaneous leucocytoclastic vasculitis can vary considerably even though the underlying pathological changes may be indistinguishable. Conversely, the appearance of skin lesions may be similar even though the nature of the inflammatory infiltrate may differ. The full-blown picture of small vessel vasculitis with systemic features can be very similar to other patterns of vasculitis, including polyarteritis nodosa. This overlap may cause difficulty in distinguishing one form of vasculitis from another with complete certainty.

A management flow chart is given in Box 1. Although skin biopsy is essential to confirm the diagnosis of small vessel vasculitis, clinical decisions should not be delayed until the result is available in an unwell patient.

Leucocytoclastic vasculitis

Pathogenesis

Immune complex deposition appears to be important in the pathogenesis of most, if not all, forms of leucocytoclastic vasculitis. Experimental immune complex disease in animals is accompanied by leucocytoclastic vasculitis. Immune complex deposits were demonstrated by tissue immunofluorescence as early as 20 min after the onset of experimental Arthus reactions in guinea-pig skin and had disappeared by 18 h (Cream *et al.* 1971). Cochrane (1971) showed that soluble factors from sensitized rabbit basophils caused platelet clumping when reacted with antigen, this in turn caused release of vasoactive amines leading to permeability of the blood vessel and subsequent deposition of immune complexes. Immunofluorescence studies have demonstrated immunoglobulins and C3 within small blood vessels of lesional and adjacent normal skin in patients with leucocytoclastic vasculitis (Sams *et al.* 1975). Immune complexes can be demonstrated in a subendothelial location by electron microscopy and direct immunofluorescence of histamine-induced vasculitis lesions and clinically normal skin of patients with leucocytoclastic vasculitis (Braverman and Yen 1975; Gower *et al.* 1977). Serial biopsies of cold-induced urticaria in a patient with cold urticaria and vasculitis demonstrated C3 deposition within 5 min of ice application, preceding the deposition of fibrin, immunoglobulin, or obvious mast cell degranulation (Eady *et al.* 1981). An antibody raised against

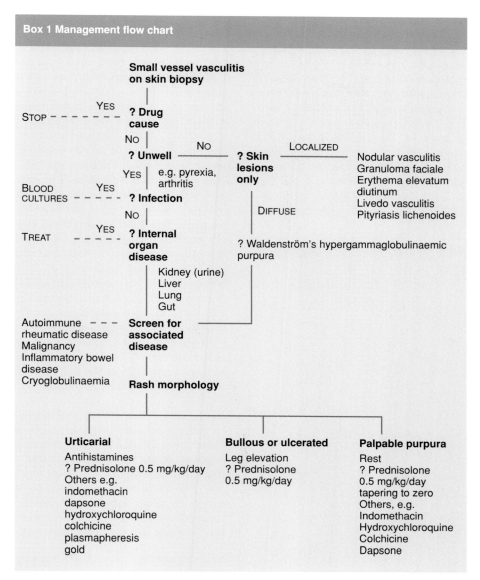

Box 1 Management flow chart

Small vessel vasculitis on skin biopsy

STOP — — — — YES **? Drug cause**

NO

? Unwell — NO — **? Skin lesions only** — LOCALIZED — Nodular vasculitis / Granuloma faciale / Erythema elevatum diutinum / Livedo vasculitis / Pityriasis lichenoides

YES | e.g. pyrexia, arthritis

BLOOD CULTURES — — — YES **? Infection**

NO

DIFFUSE

TREAT — — — YES **? Internal organ disease**

? Waldenström's hypergammaglobulinaemic purpura

Kidney (urine) / Liver / Lung / Gut

Autoimmune — — — **Screen for associated disease**
rheumatic disease
Malignancy
Inflammatory bowel disease
Cryoglobulinaemia

Rash morphology

Urticarial
Antihistamines
? Prednisolone 0.5 mg/kg/day
Others e.g.
indomethacin
dapsone
hydroxychloroquine
colchicine
plasmapheresis
gold

Bullous or ulcerated
Leg elevation
? Prednisolone
0.5 mg/kg/day

Palpable purpura
Rest
? Prednisolone
0.5 mg/kg/day
tapering to zero
Others, e.g.
Indomethacin
Hydroxychloroquine
Colchicine
Dapsone

the terminal components of the complement pathway (C5b to C9) stained 13 of 15 lesional biopsies from patients with leucocytoclastic vasculitis (Boom *et al.* 1987) indicating that activation of the terminal complement components may contribute to local tissue damage. Antigens of candida, *Mycobacterium tuberculosis*, and streptococci have been identified in skin lesions of patients with neutrophilic vasculitis, together with IgG (Parish 1971), suggesting that bacterial antigen–antibody complexes formed *in vivo* may trigger the subsequent inflammatory events. In a series of 53 patients with cutaneous vasculitis 77 per cent showed two or more positive serological tests for circulating immune complexes (Andrews *et al.* 1979).

The following sequence of pathogenetic events may occur: (1) the endothelium of postcapillary venules becomes more permeable due to release of vasoactive factors, including histamine; (2) circulating immune complexes, formed in response to infections, foreign haptens, or self-antigens lodge beneath the endothelium; (3) local complement activation initiates adherence of neutrophils to endothelium through adhesion molecule expression; (4) they release lysosomal enzymes that damage the vessel wall and surrounding tissues; (5) newly generated C3a and C5a anaphylatoxins degranulate

mast cells, releasing neutrophil and eosinophil chemotactic factors and vasoactive mediators, thereby amplifying the tissue reaction; (6) the acute response is followed by an influx of mononuclear cells and macrophages (Zax *et al.* 1990) which promote resolution of the reaction through recruitment of suppressor T lymphocytes and phagocytosis of the cellular debris.

Clinical

Clinical features, laboratory abnormalities, treatment, and prognosis are considered below.

Allergic vasculitis

Allergic vasculitis corresponds approximately to 'hypersensitivity angiitis' in Pearl Zeek's original classification of necrotizing vasculitis (Zeek 1952). The term allergic is a little contentious since it implies an immunological aetiology, which may be an oversimplification. Leucocytoclastic vasculitis is sometimes used synonymously as a clinicopathological term but this usage is better avoided because it may lead to confusion with the histological reaction pattern.

Allergic vasculitis is the commonest pattern of leucocytoclastic vasculitis in adults. It is characterized by purpuric or necrotic skin lesions, with or without systemic features. Men and women are affected equally. The onset may be from childhood to old age. Skin lesions tend to be distributed maximally over the lower legs. The buttocks, trunk, and upper extremities may also be affected. There is often a mixture of haemorrhagic papules that do not blanche on pressure (palpable purpura) (Fig. 1), erythematous or purpuric macules, urticarial plaques, vesicles, pustules, haemorrhagic bullae (Fig. 2), erosions, and ulcers. One or more systemic features occur in at least 50 per cent of patients. Arthralgia and arthritis, microscopic haematuria, abdominal symptoms (pain, nausea, diarrhoea, or bleeding), low-grade fever or malaise are the commonest. Pulmonary involvement (cough, dyspnoea, or haemoptysis) and neurological manifestations (peripheral neuropathy, benign intracranial hypertension, aseptic meningitis, and uveitis) have been reported. The erythrocyte sedimentation rate (**ESR**) is usually raised, in the region of 50 mm/h, and there may be mild to moderate anaemia. Complement consumption and immune complex formation tend to reflect disease severity. Hypocomplementaemia was found in patients showing neutrophilic rather than predominantly mononuclear infiltrates in lesional skin biopsies (Soter *et al.* 1976). Non-organ-specific autoantibodies, including antinuclear antibody, rheumatoid factor, and extractable nuclear antigen antibodies may be detectable. It is important to perform frequent urinalysis. Renal function should be monitored carefully if persistant haematuria or proteinuria are found and a renal biopsy performed where indicated.

Some important precipitants and disease associations are summarized in Table 2. Allergic vasculitis has been reported with many classes of drugs including antibiotics, thiazide diuretics, non-steroidal anti-inflammatory drugs, and recombinant human granulocyte colony stimulating factor (Jain 1994). There have been case reports of many others, including additives in a drug formulation (Lowry *et al.* 1994). Human immunodeficiency virus (**HIV**) antigen has been found in lesional skin biopsies of symptomatic HIV-infected individuals with granular immune deposits in small vessel walls (Gherardi *et al.* 1993). Embolic lodging of bacteria and microthrombi in the skin microvasculature may account for the vasculitic lesions seen in infective endocarditis and septicaemia. Small vessel vasculitis may occur in autoimmune rheumatic disorders (rheumatoid arthritis, Sjögren's syndrome, and systemic lupus erythematosus). Rheumatoid arthritis was the commonest association in a series of 88 patients presenting with cutaneous leucocytoclastic vasculitis (Ekenstam and Callen 1984). The presence of antibodies to Ro and rheumatoid factor in Sjögren's syndrome was associated closely with skin lesions showing leucocytoclastic vasculitis on histology (Molina *et al.* 1985). Various other inflammatory disorders have been associated, including inflammatory bowel disease, chronic active hepatitis, and sarcoidosis (Aractingi *et al.* 1993). Greer *et al.* (1988) have reviewed the association with malignancy. However, despite

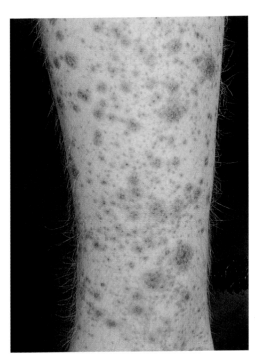

Fig. 1 Palpable purpura on the lower leg of a patient with allergic vasculitis.

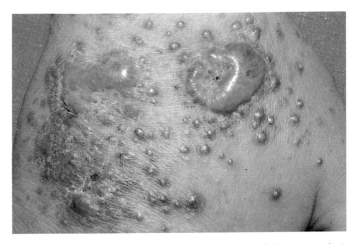

Fig. 2 Haemorrhagic blisters on the back of the hand of the same patient shown in Fig. 1.

Table 2 Causes of allergic vasculitis
Precipitants
Drugs, e.g. sulphonamides, penicillins, thiazides, and many others
Infections
Viral, e.g. hepatitis B, human immunodeficiency virus
Bacterial, e.g. β-haemolytic streptococcus
Foreign protein, e.g. serum sickness
Associations
Autoimmune diseases, e.g. rheumatoid arthritis, Sjögren's syndrome (anti-Ro positive), systemic lupus erythematosus
Inflammatory diseases, e.g. chronic active hepatitis, ulcerative colitis, Crohn's disease, sarcoidosis
Malignancy, e.g. myelo- and lymphoproliferative disorders, solid tumours

thorough clinical evaluation and laboratory investigation over 50 per cent of cases remain unexplained (idiopathic) in most reported series.

The condition is often acute and self-limiting but may pursue a relapsing or chronic course. Occasionally death may occur from a number of causes, including renal failure, gastrointestinal haemorrhage, or perforation. In a review of lesional skin biopsies Hodge *et al.* (1987) found that the overall histological severity correlated with a clinical severity score based on cutaneous and visceral involvement but did not predict the presence or absence of systemic vasculitis. Deeper infiltrates were associated with a higher frequency of pulmonary involvement.

Identifiable causes should be removed or treated whenever possible. Bed rest seems to reduce the appearance of new skin lesions but probably does not alter the long-term outcome. The legs should be elevated and bandaged to reduce oedema. Analgesia may be required. Although encouraging responses have been claimed with indomethacin (Millns *et al.* 1980), hydroxychloroquine (Lopez *et al.* 1984), colchicine (Callen 1985), and dapsone (Fredenberg and Malkinson 1987) for control of the underlying disease, systemic steroids are often required and may have to be used at high doses, especially for progressive renal involvement. Immunosuppressive agents, such as azathioprine, may be appropriate for patients with refractory disease.

Henoch–Schönlein purpura

This tends to be regarded as a special form of allergic vasculitis. It is also known as 'anaphylactoid purpura'. The classical presentation is with purpura, arthritis, haemorrhagic gastrointestinal involvement, and glomerulonephritis. It occurs most often in children but adults of any age may be affected. IgA is usually detectable in biopsies of skin, gut, and kidney. Complement appears to be activated by the alternative rather than the classical pathway. It is not clear whether the cases originally described as peliosis rheumatica by Schönlein (1837) and those of Henoch (1874) would have fitted the current concept of a predominantly IgA-associated small vessel vasculitis, because immunological investigations, including direct immunofluorescence, were not available at the time. The paediatric aspects of Henoch–Schönlein purpura are discussed in Chapter 5.11.8.

The skin lesions are often indistinguishable from those seen in allergic vasculitis. The appearance of palpable purpuric plaques on the lower legs with multifocal areas of haemorrhage or necrosis and reticulated borders has been emphasized as a distinctive sign of Henoch–Schönlein purpura in adults (Piette and Stone 1989). Systemic involvement is common but not invariable. Cream *et al.* (1970) found evidence of renal involvement in 50 per cent of 77 adults, presenting with urinary abnormalities alone, acute nephritis, or as slowly progressive renal failure without an initial acute nephritic syndrome. Gastrointestinal involvement (abdominal pain, melaena stool, haematemesis, diarrhoea, or constipation) occurred in 44 per cent, arthralgia or arthritis in 56 per cent, and oedema of legs and ankles in 57 per cent of their series.

Corticosteroids given during the acute illness appear to relieve abdominal pain and arthralgia but there is little convincing evidence that they prevent progression of renal disease or influence the eventual prognosis (Roth *et al.* 1985).

Urticarial vasculitis

Urticarial skin lesions and arthritis are the commonest presentation of this systemic disorder. Females outnumber males in most reported series by over 2:1. Patients are usually middle-aged. Morphologically, the urticarial wheals resemble those of chronic (ordinary) urticaria (Fig. 3) but may also show central purpura or rarely resemble erythema multiforme. They can occur at sites of pressure and be associated with facial and laryngeal angio-oedema. As a general rule, the wheals of urticarial vasculitis last from 24 to 72 h and tend to have a burning or painful quality, whereas those of chronic urticaria are pruritic and last less than 24 h. The commonest systemic features are musculoskeletal. Malaise and low-grade fever may accompany the attacks of urticaria. Renal damage (evidenced by haematuria, proteinuria), gastrointestinal symptoms (abdominal pain, nausea, vomiting, diarrhoea), and pulmonary disease (cough, dyspnoea, haemoptysis) may occur. Other less common manifestations include lymphadenopathy, uveitis, and benign intracranial hypertension.

A rare variant of urticarial vasculitis (Schnitzler's syndrome) is characterized by chronic urticaria-like lesions, arthralgia, lymphadenopathy, bone pain, intermittent fever, high ESR, leucocytoclastic vasculitis, and IgM macroglobulinaemia (Schnitzler *et al.* 1974). Interleukin-α antibodies found in some of these patients may play a part in its pathogenesis (Saurat *et al.* 1991).

The term 'hypocomplementaemic vasculitis' has been used for urticarial vasculitis because some early reports described cases in which the early components of complement were reduced (McDuffie *et al.* 1973), but complement abnormalities are by no means invariable and many cases are normocomplementaemic. Hypocomplementaemia and circulating immune complexes were detected in just under half the patients studied in one large series (Sanchez *et al.* 1982). Reduced levels of C1q have been linked with the presence of immunoglobulin G C1q precipitins in some patients (Zeiss *et al.* 1980) but they are not specific for urticarial vasculitis. The most consistent laboratory abnormality is an elevated ESR (Soter *et al.* 1974). Non-organ-specific antibodies are uncommon. Lesional skin

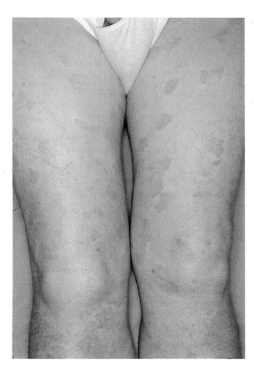

Fig. 3 The wheals of urticarial vasculitis resemble those of chronic urticaria but last longer and may show bruising.

biopsies show a range of histological changes from typical leucocytoclastic vasculitis to dense or sparse mixed perivascular infiltrates (Russell Jones *et al.* 1983). Interstitial dermal neutrophilic infiltrates were found in addition to perivascular infiltrates in patients with hypocomplementaemic urticarial vasculitis (Mehregan *et al.* 1992).

Patients with hypocomplementaemia tend to have more systemic manifestations than those with normocomplementaemia. However, the majority of patients with urticarial vasculitis, including those with systemic involvement, follow a chronic but benign course. Glomerulonephritis and chronic obstructive airways disease are potentially the most serious complications. The relationship between urticarial vasculitis and systemic lupus erythematosus is not entirely clear as urticarial lesions showing histological leucocytoclastic vasculitis have been reported in 7 per cent of patients with systemic lupus erythematosus (Provost *et al.* 1980). Progression of urticarial vasculitis to systemic lupus erythematosus appears to be rare but has been described (Bisaccia *et al.* 1988).

The treatment of urticarial vasculitis has been reviewed by Berg *et al.* (1988). Systemic antihistamines are used widely but tend to be disappointing. Indomethacin, hydroxychloroquine, dapsone, colchicine, plasmapheresis, and gold (Handfield-Jones and Greaves 1991) have been reported to be helpful in small series or anecdotal reports. Systemic steroids often have to be given in high doses to achieve control and tapered to the lowest maintenance level to prevent relapse.

Cryoglobulinaemia

Cryoglobulins are immunoglobulins which precipitate when cold. They have been divided into three types: in type I the cryoglobulin fraction is a single monoclonal immunoglobulin; type II has mixed monoclonal and polyclonal components, usually consisting of IgM rheumatoid-like factor combined with polyclonal IgG; type III has exclusively mixed polyclonal components. Mixed cryoglobulins are associated with autoimmune rheumatic diseases, lymphoproliferative disorders, and infections. The prefix 'essential' is used if no underlying disorder can be found. Hepatitis B virus infection should always be excluded as the virus or its antibody were found in a high proportion of patients previously thought to have essential mixed cryoglobulinaemia when cryoprecipitates were examined as well as sera (Levo *et al.* 1977).

Mixed cryoglobulinaemia presents with purpuric skin lesions showing leucocytoclastic vasculitis on biopsy, polyarthralgia, weakness, and progressive renal disease. It is uncommon. Women are affected about twice as frequently as men, usually in their sixth decade. Gorevic *et al.* (1980) have summarized an 18-year experience of 40 patients with mixed cryoglobulinaemia and reviewed the literature: recurrent palpable purpura were present in all their patients, polyarthralgias in 72 per cent, and renal disease in 55 per cent. Hepatic involvement (hepatomegally, abnormal liver function tests, or mild to severe inflammation on biopsy) was present in 70 per cent of their series. Oedema, hypertension, leg ulcers, Raynaud's phenomenon, abdominal pain, and susceptibility to bacterial pneumonia also occurred in descending order of frequency. A more recent report describes similar skin changes with type I cryoglobulinaemia (Cohen *et al.* 1991). Peripheral neuropathy may occur. Accompanying laboratory abnormalities include reductions in the early components of complement, a raised ESR, and anaemia.

The prognosis is much worse in patients with renal disease. The main causes of death are renal failure, systemic vasculitis, and infec

tion. Necropsy findings showed widespread arteritis in some patients (Gorevic *et al.* 1980) indicating that the vasculitis is not always confined to small vessels.

Treatment of symptomatic mixed cryoglobulinaemia is generally unsatisfactory. High-dose steroids, chemotherapy, plasmapheresis, or a combination of all three (Geltner *et al.* 1981) may bring about limited improvement in renal function, leg ulcers, and purpura. Anecdotal success has been reported with high-dose intravenous gammaglobulin (Boom *et al.* 1988).

Hypergammaglobulinaemic purpura

Waldenström (1943) described three female patients with hyperglobulinaemia, long-standing purpura, and an elevated ESR. This benign disorder should not be confused with Waldenström's macroglobulinaemia which is a lymphoma characterized by a monoclonal IgM paraproteinaemia. Histology of the purpuric skin lesions shows a leucocytoclastic vasculitis. The similarity between hypergammaglobulinaemic purpura and the cutaneous features of some patients with Sjögren's syndrome has been emphasized (Alexander and Provost 1983).

Erythema elevatum diutinum and granuloma faciale

Erythema elevatum diutinum and granuloma faciale are rare but distinctive forms of localized chronic cutaneous leucocytoclastic vasculitis. There is no systemic involvement. The aetiology of these disorders is unknown but erythema elevatum diutinum has been associated with myeloma.

Erythema elevatum diutinum is characterized by slowly enlarging oedematous purplish-brown plaques over the backs of hands, elbows, or knees which heal slowly over months or years with fibrosis. Early lesions may blister (Fig. 4). The clinical and laboratory features have been reviewed by Gibson and Su (1990).

Granuloma faciale presents with single or multiple pink to brown, well-defined smooth papules and plaques on the face (Fig. 5) which persist for years. It is distinguished histologically from erythema elevatum diutinum by the presence of numerous eosinophils and a zone of normal collagen beneath the epidermis.

The chronicity of both erythema elevatum diutinum and granuloma faciale is surprising in view of the histology which would suggest an acute pattern of inflammation. Erythema elevatum

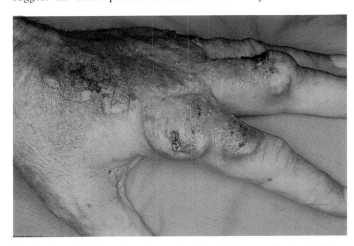

Fig. 4 An early lesion of erythema elevatum diutinum on the back of the hand showing bullous changes.

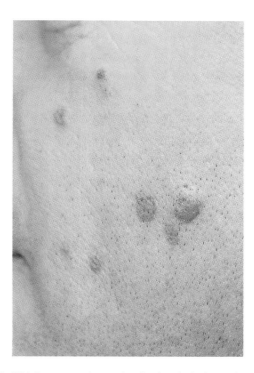

Fig. 5 Reddish-brown papules on the cheek typical of granuloma faciale.

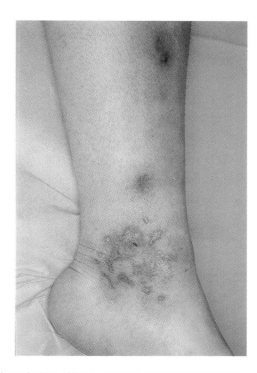

Fig. 6 Acute lesions of livedo vasculitis heal with pigmentation and 'atrophie blanche' scarring.

diutinum may respond well to dapsone. Intralesional steroids can help granuloma faciale.

Non-leucocytoclastic vasculitis

Drug-related vasculitis

Cutaneous and systemic vasculitis showing mononuclear infiltrates and eosinophils in vessel walls without fibrin deposition or necrosis, have been attributed to a variety of drugs, including penicillins and thiazides (Mullick *et al*. 1979).

Nodular vasculitis

The differential diagnosis of nodular forms of cutaneous vasculitis embraces a wide range of disorders, including erythema nodosum and other inflammatory diseases of the subcutaneous fat (Ryan 1992).

Nodular vasculitis is regarded as a distinct subgroup characterized by recurrent subcutaneous nodules usually occurring on the legs of young or middle-aged women. Patients are otherwise healthy. The histological changes range from perivascular lymphocytic infiltrates and granulomatous changes to leucocytoclastic vasculitis with fibrinoid necrosis. The aetiology is uncertain. Associated streptococcal infection may occasionally be found and should be treated. Tuberculosis does not appear to be associated, as with erythema induratum (Bazin's disease). The condition tends to resolve spontaneously but may persist for many years. Individual lesions may respond to intralesional triamcinolone. High doses of potassium iodide have been reported to be beneficial (Schulz and Whiting 1976).

Livedo vasculitis

Ischaemic damage may result from vascular occlusion rather than primary vessel wall inflammation. Livedo vasculitis (segmental hyalinizing vasculitis) is characterized histologically by endothelial proliferation and intraluminal thrombosis. Elevated fibrinopeptide levels, normal complement, and absence of immune complexes on serological studies favour a thrombogenic vasculopathy (McCalmont *et al*. 1992).

Clinically there is a livedo-like pattern of purpura, ulcers, and white atrophic scars known as *atrophie blanche* (Bard and Winkelmann 1967) (Fig. 6). The relevance of antiphospholipid antibodies to the pathogenesis of this disorder and others characterized by vaso-occlusion, including Degos' disease, has been reviewed (Grattan and Burton 1991).

Pityriasis lichenoides

The acute form of this relatively uncommon skin disorder is characterized by crops of oedematous pink papules which enlarge rapidly, and may become haemorrhagic before developing necrotic centres which heal over several weeks with scarring (Fig. 7). Although the eruption may be accompanied by mild constitutional symptoms, such as fever and arthralgia, there are no systemic complications and the disorder is usually self-limiting. Histology shows a lymphocytic perivascular infiltrate. While the endothelial cells are often blurred or swollen, fibrinoid necrosis is seen very rarely and some authorities believe that the changes do not amount to true vasculitis. However, the presence of IgM and C3 deposition in the walls of superficial blood vessels of fresh lesions in both acute and chronic forms of the disease support an immune complex aetiology (Clayton and Haffenden 1978).

Pityriasis lichenoides chronica may succeed the acute form or arise *de novo*. The early pink lesions mature into reddish-brown papules with adherent scale which usually heal without scars. Successive

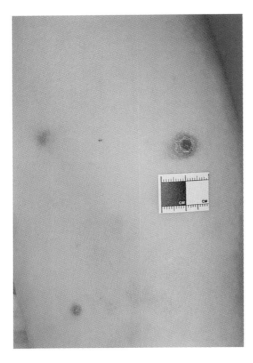

Fig. 7 Oedematous papules on the upper arm of a patient with pityriasis lichenoides acuta showing early central necrosis which will heal with scarring.

crops of lesions may erupt consecutively for months or years. Treatment with ultraviolet B irradiation is often helpful.

References

Alexander, E.L. and Provost, E.L. (1983). Cutaneous manifestations of primary Sjögren's syndrome: a reflection of vasculitis and association with anti-Ro (SSA) antibodies. *Journal of Investigative Dermatology*, 80, 386–91.

Andrews, B.S., Cains G., McIntoch, J., Petts, J., and Penny, R. (1979). Circulating and tissue immune complexes in cutaneous vasculitis. *Journal of Clinical and Laboratory Immunology*, 1, 311-20.

Aractingi, S., Cadranel, J., Milleron, B., Saiag, P., Malepart, M.J., and Dubertet, L. (1993). Sarcoidosis associated with leucocytoclastic vasculitis. *Dermatology*, 187, 50–3.

Bard, J.W. and Winkelmann, R.K. (1967). Livedo vasculitis. Segmental hyalinizing vasculitis of the dermis. *Archives of Dermatology*, 96, 489–99.

Berg, R.E., Kantor, G.R., and Bergfeld, W.F. (1988). Urticarial vasculitis. *International Journal of Dermatology*, 27, 468–72.

Bisaccia, E., Adamo, V., and Rozan, S.W. (1988). Urticarial vasculitis progressing to systemic lupus erythematosus. *Archives of Dermatology*, 124, 1088–90.

Boom, B.W., Out–Luiting, C.J., Baldwin, W.M., Westedt, M–L., Daha, M.R., and Vermeer, B–J. (1987). Membrane attack complex of complement in leukocytoclastic vasculitis of the skin. *Archives of Dermatology*, 123, 1192–5.

Boom, B.W., Brand, A., Bavinck, J–N.B., Eernisse, J.G., Daha, M.R., and Vermeer, B–J. (1988). Severe leukocytoclastic vasculitis of the skin in a patient with essential mixed cryoglobulinaemia treated with high-dose γ-globulin intravenously. *Archives of Dermatology*, 124, 1550–3.

Braverman, I.M. and Yen, A. (1975). Demonstration of immune complexes in spontaneous and histamine-induced lesions and in normal skin of patients with leukocytoclastic vasculitis. *Journal of Investigative Dermatology*, 64, 105–12.

Callen, J.P. (1985). Colchicine is effective in controlling chronic cutaneous leukocytoclastic vasculitis. *Journal of the American Academy of Dermatology*, 13, 193–200.

Clayton, R. and Haffenden, G. (1978). An immunofluoresence study of pityriasis lichenoides. *British Journal of Dermatology*, 99, 491–3.

Cochrane, C.G. (1971). Mechanisms involved in the deposition of immune complexes in tissues. *Journal of Experimental Medicine*, 134, 75–89.

Cohen, S.J., Pittelkow, M.R., and Su, W.P.D. (1991). Cutaneous manifestations of cryoglobulinaemia: clinical and histopathological study of seventy two patients. *Journal of American Academy of Dermatology*, 25, 21–7.

Cream, J.J., Gumpel, J.M., and Peachey, R.D.G. (1970). Schönlein–Henoch purpura in the adult. A study of 77 adults with anaphylactoid or Schönlein–Henoch purpura. *Quarterly Journal of Medicine*, 156, 461–84.

Cream, J.J., Bryceson, A.D.M., and Ryder, G. (1971). Disappearance of immunoglobulin and complement from the Arthus reaction and its relevance to studies of vasculitis in man. *British Journal of Dermatology*, 84, 106–9.

Daoud, M.S., Gibson, L.E., DeRemee, R.A., Specks, U., el-Azhary, R.A., and Su, W.P.D. (1994). Cutaneous Wegener's granulomatosis: clinical, histopathologic, and immunopathologic features of thirty patients. *Journal of American Academy of Dermatology*, 31, 605–12.

Eady, R.A.J., Keahey, T.M., Sibbald, R.G., and Kobza Black, A. (1981). Cold urticaria with vasculitis: report of a case with light and electron microscopic, immunofluorescence and pharmacological studies. *Clinical and Experimental Dermatology*, 6, 355–66.

Ekenstam, E. and Callen, J.P. (1984). Cutaneous leukocytoclastic vasculitis. *Archives of Dermatology*, 120, 484–9.

Francès, C. *et al.* (1994). Wegener's granulomatosis. Dermatological manifestations in 75 cases with clinicopathologic correlation. *Archives of Dermatology*, 130, 861–7.

Fredenberg, M.F. and Malkinson, F.D. (1987). Sulphone therapy in the treatment of leukocytoclastic vasculitis. *Journal of the American Academy of Dermatology*, 16, 772–8.

Geltner, D., Kohn, R.W., Gorevic, P., and Franklin, E.C. (1981). The effect of combination therapy (steroids, immunosuppressives, and plasmapheresis) on 5 mixed cryoglobulinaemia patients with renal, neurologic, and vascular involvement. *Arthritis and Rheumatism*, 24, 1121–7.

Gherardi, R. *et al.* (1993). The spectrum of vasculitis in human immunodeficiency virus-infected patients. *Arthritis and Rheumatism*, 36, 1164–74.

Gibson, L.E. and Su, W.P.D. (1990). Cutaneous vasculitis. *Rheumatic Disease Clinics of North America*, 16, 309–24.

Gorevic, P.D. *et al.* (1980). Mixed cryoglobulinemia: clinical aspects and long-term follow-up of 40 patients. *American Journal of Medicine*, 69, 287–308.

Gower, R.G., Sams, W.M., Thorne, E.G., Kohler, P.F., and Claman, H.N. (1977). Leukocytoclastic vasculitis: sequential appearance of immunoreactants and cellular changes in serial biopsies. *Journal of Investigative Dermatology*, 69, 477–84.

Grattan, C.E.H. and Burton, J.L. (1991). The antiphospholipid syndrome and cutaneous vasocclusive disorders. *Seminars in Dermatology*, 10, 152–9.

Greer, J.M., Longley, S., Edwards N.L., Elfenbein, G.J., and Panush, R.S. (1988). Vasculitis associated with malignancy. Experience with 13 patients and literature review. *Medicine*, 67, 220–30.

Handfield-Jones, S.E. and Greaves, M.W. (1991). Urticarial vasculitis-response to gold therapy. *Journal of the Royal Society of Medicine*, 84, 169–70.

Henoch, E. (1874). Ueber eine eigenthümliche Form von Purpura. *Berliner Klinische Wochenschrift*, 51, 641–3.

Hodge, S.J., Callen, J.P., and Ekenstam, E. (1987). Cutaneous leukocytoclastic vasculitis: correlation of histopathological changes with clinical severity and course. *Journal of Cutaneous Pathology*, 14, 279–84.

Jain, K.K. (1994). Cutaneous vasculitis associated with granulocyte colony stimulating factor. *Journal of American Academy of Dermatology*, 31, 213–15.

Jennette, J.C. *et al.* (1994). Nomenclature of systemic vasculitides. Proposal of an international consensus conference. *Arthritis and Rheumatism*, 37, 187–92.

Levo, Y., Gorevic, P.D., Kassab, H.J., Zucker-Franklin, D., and Franklin, E.C. (1977). Association between hepatitis B virus and essential mixed cryoglobulinemia. *New England Journal of Medicine*, 296, 1501–4.

Lopez, L.R., Davis, K.C., Kohler, P.F., and Schocket, A.L. (1984). The hypocomplementaemic urticarial-vasculitis syndrome: therapeutic response to hydroxychloroquine. *Journal of Allergy and Clinical Immunology*, 73, 600–3.

Lowry, M.D., Hudson, C.F., and Callen J.P. (1994). Leukocytoclastic vasculitis. *Journal of the American Academy of Dermatology*, 30, 854–5.

McCalmont, C.S., McCalmont, T.H., Jorizzo, J.L., White, W.L., Leshin, B., and Rothberger, H. (1992). Livedo vasculitis: vasculitis or thrombotic vasculopathy? *Clinical and Experimental Dermatology*, 17, 4–8.

McDuffie, F.C., Sams, W.M., Maldonado, J.E., Andreini, P.H., Conn, D.L., and Samayoa, E.A. (1973). Hypocomplementemia with cutaneous vasculitis and arthritis. Possible immune complex syndrome. *Mayo Clinic Proceedings*, 48, 340–8.

Mehregan, D.R., Hall, M.J., and Gibson, L.E. (1992). Urticarial vasculitis. *Journal of the American Academy of Dermatology*, 26, 441–8.

Millns, J.L., Randle, H.W., Solley, G.O., and Dicken, C.H. (1980). The therapeutic response of urticarial vasculitis to indomethacin. *Journal of the American Academy of Dermatology*, 3, 349–55.

Molina, R., Provost, T.T., and Alexander, E.L. (1985). Two types of inflammatory vascular disease in Sjögren's syndrome. Differential association with seroreactivity to rheumatoid factor and antibodies to Ro (SS-A) and with hypocomplementaemia. *Arthritis and Rheumatism*, 28, 1251–8.

Mullick, F.G., McAllister, H.A., Wagner, B.M., and Fenoglio, J.J. (1979). Drug related vasculitis. Clinicopathological correlations in 30 patients. *Human Pathology*, 10, 313–25.

Parish, W.E. (1971). Studies on vasculitis I. Immunoglobulins, β1C, C-reactive protein, and bacterial antigens in cutaneous vasculitis lesions. *Clinical Allergy*, 1, 97–109.

Piette, W.W. and Stone, M.S. (1989). A cutaneous sign of IgA-associated small dermal vessel leukocytoclastic vasculitis in adults (Henoch–Schönlein purpura). *Archives of Dermatology*, 125, 53–6.

Provost, T.T., Zone, J.J., Synkowski, D., Maddison, P.J., and Reichlin, M. (1980). Unusual cutaneous manifestations of systemic lupus erythematosus: I. Urticaria-like lesions. Correlation with clinical and serological abnormalities. *Journal of Investigative Dermatology*, 75, 495–9.

Roth, D.A., Wilz, D.R., and Theil, G.B. (1985). Schönlein–Henoch syndrome in adults. *Quarterly Journal of Medicine*, 55, 145–52.

Russell Jones, R., Bhogal, B., Dash, A., and Schifferli, J. (1983). Urticaria and vasculitis: a continuum of histological and immunopathological changes. *British Journal of Dermatology*, 108, 695–703.

Ryan, T.J. (1992). Cutaneous vasculitis. In *Rook/Wilkinson/Ebling Textbook of Dermatology*, Vol. 3, (5th edn) (ed. R.H. Champion, J.L. Burton, and F.J.G. Ebling), Ch. 45, pp. 1893–961. Blackwell Scientific Publications, Oxford.

Sams, W.M., Claman, H.N., Kohler, P.F., McIntosh, R.M., Small, P., and Mass, M.F. (1975). Human necrotizing vasculitis: immunoglobulins and complement in vessel walls of cutaneous lesions and normal skin. *Journal of Investigative Dermatology*, 64, 441–5.

Sanchez, N.P., Winkelmann, R.K., Schroeter, A.L., and Dicken, C.H. (1982). The clinical and histopathologic spectrums of urticarial vasculitis: study of forty cases. *Journal of the American Academy of Dermatology*, 7, 599–605.

Saurat, J-H., Schifferli, J., Steiger, G., Dayer, J-M., and Didierjean, L. (1991). Anti-interleukin-1α autoantibodies in humans: characterisation, isotype distribution, and receptor-binding inhibition—higher frequency in Schnitzler's syndrome (urticaria and macroglobulinaemia). *Journal of Allergy and Clinical Immunology*, 88, 244–56.

Schnitzler, P.L., Schubert, B., Boasson, M., Gardais, J., and Tourmen, A. (1974). Urticaire chronique, lésions osseuses, macroglobulinémie IgM: maladie de Waldenström? *Bulletin de la Société Française de Dermatologie et Syphiligraphie* 81, 363.

Schönlein, J.L. (1837). Peliosis rheumatica. *Allgemeine und specielle Pathologie und Therapie, Freyburg*, 2, 48–9.

Schulz, E.J. and Whiting, D.A. (1976). Treatment of erythema nodosum and nodular vasculitis with potassium iodide. *British Journal of Dermatology*, 94, 75–8.

Soter, N.A., Austen, K.F., and Gigli, I. (1974). Urticaria and arthralgias as manifestations of necrotizing angiitis (vasculitis). *Journal of Investigative Dermatology*, 63, 485–90.

Soter, N.A., Mihm, M.C., Gigli, I., Dvorak, H.F., and Austen, K.F. (1976). Two distinct cellular patterns in cutaneous necrotizing angiitis. *Journal of Investigative Dermatology*, 66, 344–50.

Waldenström, J. (1943). Kliniska metoder för pÅvisande av hyperproteinämi och deras praktiska värde för diagnostiken. *Nordisk Medicin*, 20, 2288–95.

Zax, R.H., Hodge, S.J., and Callen, J.P. (1990). Cutaneous leukocytoclastic vasculitis. Serial histopathological evaluation demonstrates the dynamic nature of the infiltrate. *Archives of Dermatology*, 126, 69–72.

Zeek, P.M. (1952). Periarteritis nodosa: a critical review. *American Journal of Clinical Pathology*, 22, 777–90.

Zeiss, C.R., Burch F.X., Marder R.J., Furey, N.L., Schmid, F.R., and Gewurz, H. (1980). A hypocomplementemic vasculitic urticarial syndrome. Report of four new cases and definition of the disease. *The American Journal of Medicine*, 68, 867–75.

5.11.5 Polymyalgia rheumatica

G. S. Panayi

Definitions
Polymyalgia rheumatica

Since both polymyalgia rheumatica and giant cell arteritis are clinical syndromes it is important that agreed definitions of the conditions are employed not only for uniformity of diagnosis but also for epidemiological and investigational studies. The criteria of Jones and Hazleman (Table 1) are succinct and easily applied in practice for the diagnosis of polymyalgia rheumatica. Some comments are necessary. There may be apparent weakness on testing the shoulder and pelvic girdle muscles but this is due to pain rather than intrinsic muscle weakness. Investigations to exclude inflammatory arthritis, malignant disease, or muscle diseases should be carried out objectively but with restraint as discussed under 'diagnosis' below.

Giant cell arteritis

The criteria for diagnosis of giant cell arteritis according to Jones and Hazleman (1981) are shown in Table 2, whilst those by Ellis and Ralston (1983) are shown in Table 3. The advantages of the criteria of Ellis and Ralston (1983) are that they do not include the erythrocyte sedimentation rate (**ESR**) and have a more inclusive description of the clinical features of giant cell arteritis compared with the criteria

Table 1 The diagnostic criteria for polymyalgia rheumatica

1. Shoulder and pelvic girdle pain which is primarily muscular in the absence of true muscle weakness
2. Morning stiffness
3. Duration of at least 2 months unless treated
4. ESR over 30 mm/h or C-reactive protein over 6 µg/ml
5. Absence of rheumatoid or inflammatory arthritis or malignant disease
6. Absence of objective signs of muscle disease
7. Prompt and dramatic response to systemic corticosteroids

From Jones and Hazleman (1981).

Table 2 The Jones and Hazleman (1981) diagnostic criteria for giant cell arteritis

1. Positive temporal artery biopsy or cranial artery tenderness noted by a physician
2. One or more of the following: visual disturbance, headache, jaw pain, cerebrovascular insufficiency
3. ESR over 30 mm/h or C-reactive protein over 6 μg/ml
4. Response to systemic corticosteroids

Table 3 The Ellis and Ralston (1983) diagnostic criteria for giant cell arteritis

1. Age greater than 55 years
2. Positive response within 48 h to corticosteroid therapy
3. Length of history greater than 2 weeks
4. Positive temporal artery biopsy
5. Proximal, symmetrical girdle, or upper arm muscle pain+ stiffness+tenderness
6. Jaw claudication
7. Clinical abnormality of the temporal artery (tenderness, thickening, redness)
8. Systemic symptoms or signs (malaise, anorexia, weight loss, anaemia, pyrexia)
9. Temporal headache
10. Visual disturbance (loss, diplopia, blurring)

Positive diagnosis present if criteria 1 to 3 present plus any three of criteria 5 to 10 *or* criterion 4.

Table 4 ACR 1990 criteria for the classification of giant cell arteritis (traditional format)

1. Age at disease onset ≥ 50 years
2. New headache
3. Temporal artery tenderness or decreased pulsation
4. Elevation of ESR ≥ 50 mm/h
5. Abnormal artery biopsies showing necrotizing arteritis with mononuclear infiltrate or granulomatous inflammation usually with multinucleated giant cells

Diagnosis of giant cell arteritis, if three of five criteria are present.

from controls better than any other criteria. The tree classification defines giant cell arteritis in fairly simple terms as a vasculitis with onset above 50 years of age, abnormal temporal arteries, or claudication of jaw and/or tongue upon deglutition, and arterial biopsy showing vasculitis with predominantly mononuclear cells or granulomatous inflammation. One hundred and ninety-six of 214 patients with giant cell arteritis had biopsies showing arteritis and 18 lacked biopsy proof. Fifteen out of 18 had negative biopsies and in three biopsy was not performed.

It should be noted that several controls with other types of vasculitis, such as Wegener's granulomatosis and polyarteritis nodosa, had biopsies of lung or other tissues showing chronic granulomatous arteritis together with enough additional criteria to misclassify them as giant cell arteritis. Biopsies of a temporal artery was not specified because few controls had this procedure. If temporal artery biopsy was specified, few controls would have been misclassified.

The ACR criteria are easy to apply and do not require exclusions other than the presence of a autoimmune rheumatic disease. In the tree classification the use of scalp tenderness and headache as surrogates for temporal artery abnormality and positive biopsy provide flexibility when some clinical data are not available.

Relationship between polymyalgia rheumatica and giant cell arteritis

Patients with features of both polymyalgia and giant cell arteritis are seen and this raises the question of the relationship between the two. Polymyalgia rheumatica is a more common condition than giant cell arteritis. One-half of the patients with giant cell arteritis have polymyalgic symptoms and 15 to 22 per cent of patients with polymyalgia rheumatica have been shown to have giant cell arteritis by either temporal artery biopsy or clinical symptoms (Huston *et al.* 1978; Chuang *et al.* 1982). In other studies the proportion of patients with a myalgic presentation who have positive arterial biopsies but no clinical features of giant cell arteritis varies from 6 per cent (Hunder and Allen 1973), to 40 per cent (Fauchald *et al.* 1972), to 50 per cent, which is the highest recorded (Malmvall and Bengston 1978). It used to be thought that polymyalgia rheumatica was always a manifestation of giant cell arteritis but most patients with the former, even if followed for many years, do not develop clinical or biopsy-proven giant cell arteritis. This was true even in the days before the use of systemic corticosteroids. There are, undoubtedly, patients with polymyalgia rheumatica who have a positive biopsy for giant cell arteritis but

of Jones and Hazleman (1981). However, the diagnostic criteria of the latter have the advantage of brevity. It should be remembered that although up to one-quarter of patients can present with normal ESR, before being treated with corticosteroids, they are still liable to serious complications including visual loss. This can happen even during treatment when there is a normal ESR. The biopsy is classifically taken from the temporal artery but other sites have included practically all vessels arising from the arch of the aorta.

The American College of Rheumatology (**ACR**) has developed criteria for the classification of giant cell arteritis by comparing a group of 214 patients with the condition and 593 controls with other forms of vasculitis (Hunder *et al.* 1990) (Table 4). In the traditional format a patient shall be said to have giant cell arteritis if at least three out of five criteria listed in the Table are present. The presence of three or more criteria yielded a sensitivity of 93.5 per cent and a specificity of 91.2 per cent. A classification tree was also constructed using six criteria. Elevated ESR was excluded in the tree format due to low specificity (48 per cent) and claudication of jaw and/or tongue on deglutition was included. In the classification tree the presence of temporal artery tenderness of decreased pulsation separated cases whose clinical picture is identical to patients with polymyalgia rheumatica without the lesions of giant cell arteritis (Fauchald *et al.* 1972). Conversely, there are patients with giant cell arteritis who also have clinical evidence of polymyalgia rheumatica. Thus, polymyalgia rheumatica and giant cell arteritis may be considered as components of a single syndrome, the expression of which depends on unknown factors; genetic factors may be the most important of these.

Genetic and epidemiological studies

Genetic studies

A genetic basis for polymyalgia rheumatica/giant cell arteritis has long been suspected because of the occurrence of the disease within families and in sib pairs (Moss and Soukop 1988). However, their mode of inheritance remained unknown until studies on possible HLA associations were undertaken. The study of Hansen *et al.* (1985) has been the only one to show an association with a class I major histocompatibility antigen, HLA Cw3. The increased occurrence of HLA A31, HLA B40 and, of greater importance, HLA DR4 was ascribed as being secondary and due to their linkage disequilibria with HLA Cw3. Armstrong *et al.* (1983) showed a link between polymyalgia rheumatica and giant cell arteritis and HLA Cw6 with a relative risk of 9.0. This is the only reported association with a C locus antigen. However, most studies agree that the true link is with HLA DR4. Richardson *et al.* (1987) found an association between polymyalgia rheumatica or polymyalgia rheumatica plus giant cell arteritis with HLA DR4, whilst giant cell arteritis alone did not show this association. By contrast, Ninet *et al.* (1987) found that it was giant cell arteritis, whether alone or associated with polymyalgia rheumatica, which was linked to HLA DR4. Whether this discrepancy can be accounted for by the racial differences in the two studies, Anglo–Saxon in the former and French in the latter, is not known, but it should be emphasized that Armstrong *et al.* (1983) found a link with polymyalgia rheumatica or giant cell arteritis while Cid *et al.* (1988), in a Spanish population, found a link of HLA DR4 with polymyalgia rheumatica alone. It may be that differences in the population of patients being studied may account for some of the discrepancies. The studies by Sakkas *et al.* (1990) have used restriction fragment length polymorphism (**RFLP**) with DRβ, DQα, and DQβ probes and appropriate restriction endonucleases in order to investigate the class II MHC association at the molecular level. In this study the link between polymyalgia rheumatica and HLA DR4 was confirmed whilst the DQ specifities DQw7 and DQw8 (previously DQ3.1 and DQ3.2 respectively) were found in similar frequency to the controls. Rheumatoid arthritis is linked to the third hypervariable region of HLA DR4. Whilst polymyalgia rheumatica and giant cell arteritis are also linked to HLA DR4, molecular analysis has shown that this is with the second hypervariable region of the HLA DRB1 gene (Weyand *et al.* 1994a). Two conclusions can be drawn from these findings. First, the reported association of rheumatoid arthritis with polymyalgia rheumatica/giant cell arteritis is probably due to chance or to misdiagnosis. Second, HLA-DRB1 alleles are not predictive for progression of polymyalgia rheumatica to giant cell arteritis.

Demaine *et al.* (1983) have reported that the immunoglobulin allotypic marker G1m(2) was significantly increased in patients with giant cell arteritis but not with polymyalgia rheumatica. The increase in G1m(2) in the group with giant cell arteritis was not accompanied by a corresponding rise in the number of patients homozygous for G1m(2), i.e. all the increase could be attributed to patients with the G1m(1, 2, 3): G3M (5, 10, 21) phenotype. Using a DNA probe for the switch region of Igμ and α1 heavy chain genes and RFLP analysis, Sakkas *et al.* (1990) were unable to pinpoint these Gm polymorphisms further. However, these findings suggest that genes outside the MHC and probably residing in the region of the immunoglobulin heavy chain on chromosome 14q are also involved in the genetics of polymyalgia rheumatica/giant cell arteritis. It is these additional genetic factors which may modify the clinical expression of disease.

The T-cell receptor genes are highly polymorphic and intimately involved in the genetics of the immune response. No RFLP association was found with T-cell receptor α, β, or γ genes (Sakkas *et al.* 1990).

Epidemiological studies

The prevalence of giant cell arteritis/polymyalgia rheumatica has strikingly different rates in different racial groups with Scandinavians having the highest and black and Hispanic races the lowest (Gonzalez *et al.* 1989). Furthermore, only 12 to 25 per cent of black patients with giant cell arteritis have polymyalgia rheumatica compared with 40 to 60 per cent in white patients (Love *et al.* 1986) and this may be related to the low frequency of HLA DR4 in the black population. There may be geographical variation in the expression of clinical features as a Japanese study has reported a higher frequency of fever and involvement of the pelvic girdle than the Western reports (Nishioka *et al.* 1986).

Ninety-six patients with polymyalgia rheumatica were identified in a 10-year survey (1970 to 1979) at the Olmstead County Hospital, Minnesota (Chuang *et al.* 1982) leading to an average annual incidence of 11.1/100 000 persons (53.7/100 000 in persons over 50 years of age). Polymyalgia rheumatica is more common in older age groups with age-specific incidence increasing from 19.8/100 000 in persons aged 50 to 59 years to 112.2/100 000 in those aged 70 to 79 years. Giant cell arteritis was found in 15 out of 96, i.e. 18 per cent of those surveyed. Bengtsson and Malmvall (1982) surveyed the incidence of polymyalgia rheumatica over 3 years at Goteborg, Sweden which has a population of 400 000. The annual incidence was lower with an incidence rate of 6.7/100 000 persons or 20.4/100 000 in those 50 years or older. In the Swedish study the incidence of giant cell arteritis was 41 out of 90 patients with polymyalgia rheumatica, i.e. 46 per cent. The differences in data between the two studies may be partly due to the difference in diagnostic criteria and methods of data collection. A 9-year study of polymyalgia rheumatica/giant cell arteritis in Reggio Emilia, Italy, from 1980 to 1988 revealed an annual incidence of 6.9/100 000 in persons over 50 years of age (Salvarani *et al.* 1991).

The incidence of polymyalgia rheumatica/giant cell arteritis, at least amongst the white races in the northern hemisphere, lies between 1.7 and 7.7 per 1000 of the elderly population. However, it is obvious that these figures derive from studies using different diagnostic criteria, prospective or retrospective design, and different catchment populations. Properly controlled, large, and prospective studies in different racial groups from different parts of the world are urgently required. Such data may enhance our understanding of the genetic and environmental factors contributing to the development and expression of polymyalgia rheumatica/giant cell arteritis.

The frequent acute influenza-like onset has stimulated interest in the search for an environmental agent in polymyalgia rheumatica/

giant cell arteritis. Polymyalgia rheumatica has been reported as being preceded by viral infection, vaccination for influenza or typhoid fever, and by *Yersinia enterocolitica* infection. The finding of antibodies to hepatitis B antigen (Bacon *et al.* 1975) has not been verified (Bridgeford *et al.* 1980). The higher prevalence and titre of antibodies to adenovirus and respiratory syncytial virus in patients with polymyalgia rheumatica compared with controls is intriguing (Cimmino *et al.* 1993). Case reports of polymyalgia rheumatica and giant cell arteritis in conjugal pairs also suggest as environmental agent (Kyle *et al.* 1984). Antibodies to intermediate filaments have been described in high concentrations in polymyalgia rheumatica/giant cell arteritis (Dasgupta *et al.* 1987). These antibodies are typically found in viral infections and may suggest a viral aetiology. Polymyalgia rheumatica has been reported following a tick bite in an 84-year-old woman with serological evidence of *Borrelia burgdorferi* injection. Sixty-three per cent of patients (12 of 19) with polymyalgia rheumatica/giant cell arteritis were found to have elevated or borderline IgG antibody titres (Vaith *et al.* 1988) to this pathogen.

Arterial biopsy

In diagnosis

The histological proof of granulomatous change in the temporal artery or in an artery arising from the aorta or in the aorta itself is generally considered diagnostic proof of giant cell arteritis even if the symptoms are those of incomplete giant cell arteritis or even polymyalgia rheumatica alone (Table 5). An adequate biopsy requires a segment of artery 2- to 3-cm long. Many centres recommend biopsy of the opposite artery if histology is negative in the selected artery. Granulomatous giant cell arteritis is seen in approximately 50 per cent of positive biopsies, showing panarteritis with a mixed cellular infiltrate that is predominantly lymphomononuclear (Lie *et al.* 1990) (Fig. 1). Occasionally a circumferential band of fibrinoid necrosis may also be seen. There is no correlation between histological and clinical features in individual patients (Lie 1987). Pretreatment biopsies give the most successful diagnostic rate (80 per cent) which falls to 60 per cent after 1 week of treatment and becomes much lower after longer periods of treatment (Lie 1987), although others have found that up to 14 days of glucocorticoid treatment does not alter the biopsy positivity rate (Achkar *et al.* 1994).

The presence of skip lesions and of differential involvement means that histological proof of giant cell arteritis can vary from 11 to 44 per cent of temporal artery biopsies depending on various selection factors. Efforts have been made to improve the positive biopsy rate by means of arteriographic or Doppler ultrasound examination of the temporal artery but to no avail. There can be large artery involvement with a variety of symptoms including intermittent claudication of an extremity, paraesthesia, Raynaud's phenomenon, and aortic rupture. Clinical examination may reveal absent or decreased pulsation of large arteries with bruits over them. The angiographic findings are characteristic and help to distinguish it from atheromatous stenosis (Klein *et al.* 1975). Angiography reveals (1) long segments of smooth arterial stenoses alternating with those of normal or an increased calibre, (2) smoothly tapered occlusions of affected large arteries, (3) absence of irregular plaques and ulceration, which is characteristic of atheromatous involvement, and (4) anatomic distribution with major involvement of subclavian, axillary, or brachial arteries.

For understanding the pathogenesis

The pathogenesis of polymyalgia rheumatica/giant cell arteritis is not known. Since there is obvious vascular involvement in giant cell arteritis and since giant cell arteritis and polymyalgia rheumatica frequently coexist, it has been assumed that polymyalgia rheumatica also has a vascular basis but direct proof of this supposition is difficult to find. Although evidence of endothelial damage or activation can be found in elevated levels of circulating von Willebrand factor and factor VIII, this observation is common to many inflammatory conditions. Immune complexes have been conspicuous by their absence. Antineutrophil cytoplasmic antibodies (**ANCA**), which are elevated in many forms of macroscopic and microscopic vasculitides, are not found in polymyalgia rheumatica/giant cell arteritis, although Cats and colleagues have found high titres of ANCA, but of unknown specificity, in the serum of patients with giant cell arteritis (Cats *et al.* 1993). Antibodies to intermediate filaments may reflect underlying disease activity (Monteagudo *et al.* 1994).

However, patients with of polymyalgia rheumatica/giant cell arteritis have low numbers of circulating CD8 T cells which are activated, as shown by their high positivity for HLA-DR antigen, which is normally absent from the surface of resting T cells. The relationship

Table 5   Recent studies on the value of temporal artery biopsy in the diagnosis of polymyalgia rheumatica (PMR)/giant cell arthritis (GCA)

Disease	Artery	Positive biopsy (%)	Year	Author
GCA	Temporal	30/98 (31)	1992	Chmelewski *et al.*
PMR/GCA	Temporal	14/75 (14)	1989	Stuart
PMR/GCA	Temporal	21/81 (25.9)	1988	Robb-Nicholson *et al.*
GCA	Temporal	29/107 (27.1)	1988	Fernandez-Herlihy
GCA	Temporal	42/200 (21)	1988	Ponge *et al.*
GCA	Temporal	5/45 (11.1)	1988	Mashiah *et al.*
GCA	Temporal	43/103 (43.7)	1987	Vilaseca *et al.*

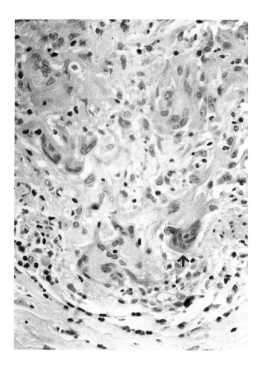

Fig. 1 Typical arterial histology from a patient with giant cell arteritis showing granulomatous inflammation with giant cells (arrow points to a giant cell).

of these findings to the pathogenesis of polymyalgia rheumatica/giant cell arteritis is not known but they are similar to those found in the blood of children with Kawasaki's syndrome in which arterial damage is very prominent. Activated CD8 T cells can be cytotoxic and also produce a variety of proteolytic enzymes, especially granzymes, which have cytotoxic and inflammatory potential. A temporal artery with positive histological appearance shows infiltration of mononuclear cells, T cells, and macrophages, and disruption of the elastic lamina of the artery. The lesion may contain deposits of IgG, IgM, IgA, complement, and fibrinogen and the use of immunofluorescence to detect these deposits may be more sensitive and specific than light microscopy alone, although this has not been adopted for routine clinical use (Wells *et al.* 1989). There is also a marked accumulation of fibronectin, fibrin, fibrinogen, and their degradation products, as well as factor VIII, but none of these findings is characteristic (Chemnitz *et al.* 1987).

The T cells infiltrating the temporal artery in giant cell arteritis are CD4+: these are activated as shown by their positivity for HLA DR and the interleukin-2 receptor but, interestingly, show little or no surface expression of the transferrin receptor which is another T-cell activation marker (Andersson *et al.* 1987; Cid 1989). The reason for this discrepancy is unknown but it is worth remarking that although CD4+ T cells in the rheumatoid synovium are HLA-DR positive, few of them express the interleukin-2 receptor. Thus T-cell activation in different chronic inflammatory foci may be at different stages. The elevated serum levels of soluble interleukin-2 receptor provide systemic evidence for T-cell activation but are not useful for disease monitoring (Salvarani *et al.* 1992). Analysis of the T-cell receptor genes used by CD4 T cells expanded from the temporal artery biopsies suggests that they are of limited heterogeneity. This implies that

locally present antigen may be driving the granulomatous reaction (Schaufelberger *et al.* 1993; Weyand *et al.* 1994b).

CD8+ T cells form the minority T-cell population and there are few or no B cells and no natural killer cells. The paucity of B cells in the lesions correlates with the lack of a systemic hypergammaglobulinaemia. Although corticosteroids do not influence the cellular distribution within the lesion, a finding similar to that in the rheumatoid synovium, they nevertheless induce functional changes in T cells since within 4 days of starting corticosteroid therapy there is a dramatic fall in the number of T cells positive for interleukin-2 receptors from 87.5 to 14 per cent (Cid 1989).

Macrophages are found in increased numbers in all lesions and are activated as shown by their high expression of HLA DR and transferrin receptor (Andersson *et al.* 1987). Macrophages in the arterial biopsies have been shown to produce interleukin 6, interleukin 1β, and a 72-kDa type IV collagenase. Monocytes from the peripheral blood of patients with giant cell arteritis or polymyalgia rheumatica express interleukins 6 and 1β. These findings suggest that these diseases have local as well as systemic inflammation (Wagner *et al.* 1994). Studying the bone marrow might be rewarding. Macrophages could also act as antigen-presenting cells. The additional cells present are interdigitating cells, which are a form of antigen-presenting cell, found in 41 per cent of temporal artery biopsies; these patients have a significantly shorter disease duration before presentation (mean 1.5 months compared with 3.8 months) (Cid 1989). Arterial smooth muscles are HLA-DR negative so it is unlikely that they are serving as antigen-presenting cells (Andersson *et al.* 1988).

Clinical features

Polymyalgia rheumatica and giant cell arteritis are rare in patients less than 50 years old and the mean age at onset is approximately 70 years. Women are affected more than men (ratio 2:1). The onset is frequently abrupt with pain and stiffness in the neck and shoulder girdle. Hips and thighs are involved less often. Prolonged and severe morning stiffness is a characteristic feature. There may be asymmetry at onset although symptoms become quickly bilateral. Systematic symptoms such as malaise, anorexia, weight loss, low-grade fever, and depression are present frequently. Active joint mobility is often restricted by pain and stiffness whereas passive movements are full. There is no objective muscle weakness although severe muscle pain and stiffness may give this misleading impression

Arthralgia and even synovitis is not uncommon (Chou and Schumacher 1984). Synovitis of the knees and sternoclavicular joints may be evident clinically. Shoulder and hip joint involvement may be more difficult to detect due to the overlying muscles. Synovial fluid examination, arthroscopic synovial biopsies, and joint scintiscanning (O'Duffy *et al.* 1976) have confirmed joint inflammation. Indeed, it has even been proposed that the prominence of shoulder and pelvic girdle symptoms is due to axial synovitis involving the glenohumoral and hip joints (Koski 1992). Arthroscopic synovial biopsies have revealed a lymphocytic inflammatory infiltrate. However, florid synovitis is uncommon in true polymyalgia rheumatica and a clinically significant, chronic, erosive arthropathy suggests an alternative diagnosis of rheumatoid arthritis as this may have a polymyalgic onset in the elderly.

There are case reports of polymyalgia rheumatica associated with underlying malignancy, although it is unclear whether the incidence of neoplasm is increased truly compared with age and sex-matched controls. A retrospective study of case notes reported a high incidence of hypothyroidism in polymyalgia rheumatica/giant cell arteritis (Wiseman *et al.* 1989) but a subsequent study failed to confirm these findings (Dasgupta *et al.* 1990).

Giant cell arteritis

Presenting symptoms may vary widely but headache is the most common initial symptom, being present in two-thirds of patients. The pain is often severe and usually localized to arteries of the scalp (superficial, temporal, and occipital) though it may be more diffuse. The artery involved may be tender or exhibit reduced pulsations. Frequently there is diffuse scalp tenderness.

Visual symptoms are said to occur in 25 to 50 per cent of cases and include diplopia, ptosis (transient or permanent), and partial or total blindness. The symptoms are caused by ischaemia of the optic nerve secondary to involvement of branches of the ophthalmic or posterior ciliary arteries. Recent reports suggest that visual complications may be less frequent than previously reported in pure polymyalgia rheumatica (Myles *et al.* 1992). Unfortunately there are no predicative features for when these may occur and such complications have occurred in patients with quiescent disease and normal erythrocyte sedimentation rates.

Laboratory features

A marked acute-phase response is characteristic of both polymyalgia rheumatica and giant cell arteritis. There is a mild to moderate normochromic anaemia, thrombocytosis is common, and the white cell count is usually normal. The erythrocyte sedimentation rate (ESR) is elevated and frequently much raised, over 100 mm/h, although in occasional cases it may be completely normal. C-reactive protein is often raised and some studies have claimed it is more sensitive than ESR. Long-term studies have shown that ESR is as good an indication of the acute-phase response (Kyle and Hazleman 1989). There may be a decrease in albumin concentration and increase in α_2-globulins, fibrinogen, and other acute-phase reactants.

Serum immunoglobulins are usually normal although they may be raised in severe cases. Complement levels are normal. Tests for auto-antibodies and rheumatoid factor are negative. Antibodies to intermediate filaments and to neutrophil cytoplasmic antigens have been described (see above).

Increases in alkaline phosphatase can occur and less frequently there is increase in transaminases with prolonged prothrombin time, Liver biopsies are generally normal although granulomatous hepatitis has been described. Muscle enzymes and electromyography are normal. Muscle histology is normal, although ultrastructural studies of muscle have shown crystalline inclusions in the mitochondria. Thyroid function tests are usually normal although they may reflect changes due to non-thyroidal illness. Synovial fluid analysis is compatible with an inflammatory state with poor mucin clot and leucocyte counts ranging from 1000 to 20 000/mm^3 with a majority of polymorphonuclear leucocytes. Biopsies have shown a lymphocytic synovitis.

Levels of factor VIII/von Willebrand factor have been found to be elevated in polymyalgia rheumatica/giant cell arteritis. Values are highest in giant cell arteritis but do not closely parallel the ESR and may reflect endothelial damage. Nordberg *et al.* (1991) studied 53 patients with giant cell arteritis by serial analysis of von Willebrand

factor antigen and plasminogen activator inhibitor. The concentration of von Willebrand factor slowly decreased and reached control range 18 months after diagnosis. However, levels failed to correlate with clinical features and results of temporal biopsy, and failed to predict flare-up of disease and vascular complications. The activity of plasminogen activator inhibitor was no different from levels in age-matched controls. Von Willebrand factor antigen is present along the lamina elastica of the arterial wall in giant cell arteritis but absent from arterial biopsy in pure polymyalgia rheumatica (Olsson *et al.* 1990). Fibrinolysis has also been described in these conditions (Grau *et al.* 1984). Plasma fibronectin was not significantly different from controls in a study by Puccetti *et al.* (1987).

Interleukin 6 (**IL-6**) is a multifunctional cytokine responsible for secretion of acute-phase proteins by hepatocytes. The level of serum IL-6 was raised in 15 patients with untreated polymyalgia rheumatica/giant cell arteritis and declined following therapy (Dasgupta *et al.* 1990; Roche *et al.* 1993). However, in seven patients it remained elevated above baseline at 6 months despite optimum treatment and remission of symptoms. This suggests ongoing disease activity despite suppression of acute-phase response and symptoms. As stimulated endothelial cells are a potent source of IL-6, elevated IL-6 levels may reflect endothelial damage. However, immunohistochemistry and in situ hybridization have shown that IL-6 is produced predominantly by macrophages and some fibroblasts in the media of the inflamed artery and by endothelial cells (Emilie *et al.* 1994). Paradoxically, the very effectiveness of glucocorticoids in returning the acute-phase response to normal pose a problem in deciding how quickly and by how much steroids should be decreased. Serial estimation of α_1-antichymotrypsin may be helpful as it does not return to normal until some 18 months after institution of glucocorticoid therapy (Pountain *et al.* 1994).

A study of T-cell subsets in peripheral blood showed selective depletion of CD8+ cells, which remained depressed after 1 year of treatment and only becomes normal after 2 years of treatment (Dasgupta *et al.* 1989).

Blood flow has been studied in temporal arteries (Brunholz and Mullen 1988) and in the central retinal, short posterior ciliary, and ophthalmic arteries (Ho *et al.* 1994) by Doppler ultrasonography. Abnormal flow (reduced, reversed, or alternating flow) was seen. This procedure may be useful in diagnosis and management as some of the waveforms were not seen in non-arteritic optic neuropathy.

Diagnosis

The diagnosis of polymyalgia rheumatica is based essentially on clinical symptoms and signs and it is significant that on follow-up in two large series the diagnosis was revised in 20 to 25 per cent of cases. Thus, even after the diagnosis has been made and treatment started, the possibility of other diseases should be kept in mind. Table 6 lists the conditions which can present with polymyalgic symptoms. The following conditions cause greatest difficulty.

1. Rheumatoid arthritis. It may be impossible to distinguish polymyalgic onset of rheumatoid arthritis from true polymyalgia rheumatica. High titres of rheumatoid factor, prominent articular symptoms, and partial response to low-dose steroids may distinguish the former, while polymyalgia rheumatica is associated with low-grade synovitis and low titre or, more commonly, absent rheumatoid factor.

2. Neoplasia. Although it is still debatable whether there is true association of neoplasia with polymyalgia rheumatica, it is important not to mistake the generalized musculoskeletal aching, systemic symptoms, weight loss, and raised ESR of occult cancer for polymyalgia rheumatica. A thorough physical examination is mandatory and although it is not necessary to embark on detailed investigation, tests such as a protein electrophoretic strip and a chest radiograph should be carried out.

3. Inflammatory myopathies may present with muscle pains. However, in polymyalgia rheumatica there should be no objective muscle weakness. In addition creatine kinase levels and electromyography are normal.

4. Chronic sepsis may simulate polymyalgia rheumatica especially if associated with low-grade pyrexia. Blood cultures should be obtained if fever is present.

5. Hypothyroidism and less frequently hyperthyroidism may present with muscle pain and generalized stiffness. Thyroid function should be checked although abnormalities may merely reflect changes from a non-thyroidal illness.

6. Parkinsonian rigidity can occasionally mislead the unwary, although the condition is easily distinguished once it is considered and sought.

7. Bilateral capsulitis of shoulders, such as is seen in diabetes, can mimic polymyalgia rheumatica but should easily be differentiated by the restriction of passive movements. Similarly, osteoarthritis of hips and shoulders can cause difficulty but can be excluded by radiographs.

8. Depressive illnesses can frequently present with myalgic symptoms and should therefore be considered.

The limitations to the diagnosis of polymyalgia rheumatica are that there are no specific clinical features or any specific laboratory tests for this disease. The acute-phase response and its response to steroids is helpful but should be interpreted with caution as a raised ESR, whatever the cause, is likely to decrease with high-dose steroids (e.g. 20 mg or more daily). What distinguishes polymyalgia rheumatica is a complete and quick response (within 4 days) to low-dose steroids (e.g. 10 to 15 mg daily).

CD8+ lymphocytes in the peripheral blood may help in providing a marker of disease activity that is independent of the acute-phase response. We have found that even after a year CD8 cell numbers were low, probably reflecting disease activity. Most other conditions with similar presentations are accompanied by normal levels of CD8 so this test may help in distinguishing the condition, although further comparative studies are required to establish the specificity and sensitivity. A study of CD8 levels in 108 patients undergoing temporal artery biopsies suggests a positive predictive value of 85 per cent for either biopsy-positive giant cell arteritis or polymyalgia rheumatica while the likelihood of absence of giant cell arteritis or giant cell arteritis syndrome with normal CD8+ values was 60 per cent (Elling *et al.* 1990).

Treatment (Boxes 1, 2)

Polymyalgia rheumatica and giant cell arteritis are indications for corticosteroid treatment. Dramatic symptomatic response usually occurs within 48 h of introducing steroids. Despite this early gratifying response, continuing skilled supervision is necessary for several reasons, including the need to monitor for disease complications and the complications of steroid therapy. Correct assessment of disease activity is paramount in preventing steroid-related morbidity.

Polymyalgia rheumatica responds to low-dose steroids and treatment should be started with prednisolone at 15 mg daily as a single morning dose. There are no universal guidelines to tapering steroid dosage although, according to a recent report, prednisolone at 10 mg/day is required in the second month to prevent an unacceptable relapse rate (Kyle and Hazleman 1990). Further reductions below 10 mg are recommended in 1 mg decrements every 4 to 6 weeks.

Behn *et al.* (1983) in a prospective study of 176 patients reported that 10 mg of prednisolone is sufficient for control of symptoms of polymyalgia rheumatica. Others (Healey and Wilske 1977; Spiera and Davison 1978) have concurred but Kyle and Hazleman (1989), in a controlled prospective study, found that 13 of 20 patients with polymyalgia rheumatica relapsed on an initial dose of 10 mg/day, and 15 to 20 mg of prednisolone was required for adequate disease control.

The rationale for a lower dose of steroids than used hitherto in polymyalgia rheumatica/giant cell arteritis is based on several studies showing that major and minor steroid side-effects are quite common and their occurrence is related to initial dose, treatment duration, and, most critically, to cumulative dose. It is important to use the lowest satisfactory dose which contains symptoms and not merely be guided by the ESR. It is wrong to use the ESR as a chief guide to therapy since active disease may exist with a normal ESR and, on the other hand, it may be impossible to attain a normal ESR without an excessively high steroid dosage. Laboratory measures independent of the acute-phase response, such as the percentage of circulating CD8+ T cells and serum α_1-antichymotrypsin, may be helpful in long-term disease monitoring.

Other routes of steroid therapy may also be useful in polymyalgia rheumatica. In a pilot study, 120 mg of intramuscular methylprednisolone acetate administered initially for 3 weeks and then monthly at

Table 6 Conditions that can present with polymyalgic symptoms

1. Rheumatic disease in the elderly
   Rheumatoid arthritis
   Systemic lupus erythematosus

2. Inflammatory myopathies

3. Endocrinopathy
   Hypothyroidism
   Hyperthyroidism

4. Neoplasia
   Carcinoma
   Multiple myeloma

5. Occult sepsis

6. Bilateral shoulder capsulitis especially with diabetes

7. Osteoarthritis

8. Depressive illness

9. Parkinsonism

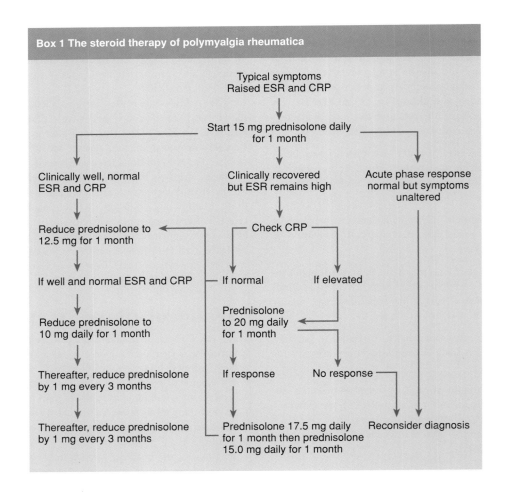

Box 1 The steroid therapy of polymyalgia rheumatica

Typical symptoms
Raised ESR and CRP

Start 15 mg prednisolone daily
for 1 month

Clinically well, normal
ESR and CRP

Clinically recovered
but ESR remains high

Acute phase response
normal but symptoms
unaltered

Reduce prednisolone to
12.5 mg for 1 month

Check CRP

If well and normal ESR and CRP — If normal   If elevated

Reduce prednisolone to
10 mg daily for 1 month

Prednisolone
to 20 mg daily
for 1 month

Thereafter, reduce prednisolone
by 1 mg every 3 months

If response   No response

Thereafter, reduce prednisolone
by 1 mg every 3 months

Prednisolone 17.5 mg daily
for 1 month then prednisolone
15.0 mg daily for 1 month

Reconsider diagnosis

reducing doses was successful in induction and maintenance of disease remission (Dasgupta *et al.* 1991). Cumulative steroid dosage was 40 to 60 per cent lower than in a conventional regimen. This route has the advantage of ensuring compliance, and may not suppress the hypothalamic–pituitary axis. Further controlled

Box 2 Summary

Elevated ESR in the face of a normal CRP
suggests that inflammation is controlled

Give calcium and vitamin D supplements
to prevent osteoporosis

Only some 50% of patients have
ceased prednisolone by 2 years

Follow same schedule for giant cell arteritis but
start therapy at 30 mg prednisolone daily

studies are needed to compare the efficacy of this steroid regimen with that of oral prednisolone, as well as incidence of steroid side-effects with particular emphasis on bone mineral density.

Other agents such as dapsone, azathioprine, and D-penicillamine have been used in polymyalgia rheumatica/giant cell arteritis. Use of dapsone has been associated with very serious haematological complications such as agranulocytosis and haemolytic anaemia. Azathioprine has been anecdotally reported to have been of benefit and a controlled study showed a small but significant response (De Silva 1986).

Non-steroidal anti-inflammatory drugs have been used in polymyalgia rheumatica but should not be the first choice unless there is a major contraindication to steroid therapy.

References

Achkar, A.A., Lie, J.T., Hunder, G.G., O'Fallon, W.M., and Gabriel, S.E. (1994). How does previous corticosteroid treatment affect the biopsy findings in giant cell (temporal) arteritis? *Annals of Internal Medicine*, **120**, 987–92.

Andersson, R., Jonsson, R., Tarkowski, A., Bengtsson, B., and Malmvall, B.E. (1987). T cell subsets and expression of immunological activation markers in the arterial walls of patients with giant cell arteritis. *Annals of the Rheumatic Diseases*, **46**, 915–23.

Andersson, R., Hansson, G.K., Soderstrom, T., Jonsson, R., Bengtsson, B.A., and Hordborg, E. (1988). HLA-DR expression in the vascular lesion and circulating T lymphocytes of patients with giant cell arteritis. *Clinical and Experimental Immunology*, **73**, 82–7.

Clinical features

The clinical features of Takayasu's arteritis have been reviewed recently in a series of patients from the United States (Table 4) and are broadly similar to previous series (Lupi-Herrera *et al.* 1977). The spectrum of presentation, disease severity, and pace of progression can often lead to a delay in diagnosis. The classic description of Takayasu's arteritis is of a triphasic illness characterized by pre-pulseless inflammation, followed by painful ischaemic vessels, and ending

Table 4 Clinical features of Takayasu's arteritis

	Onset	Total
Vascular (100%)		
Carotid bruit	20	70
Claudication	33	70
Decreased/absent pulse	22	58
Asymmetric BP	12	48
Hypertension	18	33
Carotidynia	18	31
Subclavian bruit	5	20
CNS (57%)		
Light headed/dizziness	18	35
Visual disturbance	10	28
Visual loss	2	8
Stroke	6	8
TIA	0	8
Musculoskeletal (53%)		
Chest wall	8	30
Arthralgia	10	30
Myalgia	5	15
Constitutional (43%)		
Malaise	22	32
Fever	20	25
Weight loss	12	16
Night sweats	1	1
Cardiac (38%)		
Aortic incompetence	8	20
Angina	2	12
Palpitations	0	8
Cardiac failure	1	7
Pericarditis	3	3
Myocardial infarction	0	1

From Kerr *et al.* (1994).
BP = blood pressure; CNS = central nervous system; TIA = transient ischaemic attacks.

in 'burnt out disease' (Lupi-Herrera *et al.* 1977; Hall *et al.* 1985). More recent studies suggest that 20 per cent of patients have a monophasic illness not requiring therapy and that 57 per cent of patients never have constitutional symptoms (Kerr *et al.* 1994).

The hallmark of the disease is vascular ischaemic symptoms with bruit, claudication, or diminished pulses. Disease is often extensive involving the aorta and its branches. The most common vascular abnormality (more than 90 per cent of cases) is a bruit occurring most frequently in the carotid vessels (70 per cent) and in multiple sites in a third of cases. Claudication and a diminished or absent pulse is more common in the arms than legs. Carotidynia occurs in a third of patients and a similar proportion complain of lightheadedness or dizzyness. Hypertension occurs in 30 to 70 per cent of patients as a consequence of renal artery stenosis, which may be either unilateral or bilateral (Lupi-Herrera *et al.* 1977; Ishikawa 1988; Kerr *et al.* 1994).

Musculoskeletal symptoms occur in half of patients, with arthralgias in one third to one half of patients. Peripheral synovitis is less common occurring in 18 per cent of patients. Myalgia is found infrequently but can be severe.

Cardiac lesions occur in 40 per cent with aortic incompetence (20 per cent) resulting from aortitis, which may also involve the proximal coronary arteries. Congestive cardiac failure may result from aortic incompetence or systemic hypertension and accounts for the majority of fatal outcomes. Hypertension contributes to left ventricular hypertrophy and myocardial failure, but coronary arteritis results in myocardial infarction and fibrosis. Pulmonary artery involvement is common (50 per cent) with lesions localized to large and medium pulmonary vessels (Lupi-Herrera *et al.* 1977).

Cutaneous manifestations include erythema nodosum (8 per cent) which responds to treatment of the disease and probably reflects vasculitis rather than panniculitis. Leg ulcers, hypocomplementaemic vasculitis and pyoderma gangrenosum have all been described occurring in association with Takayasu's arteritis.

Neurological features occur in all stages of the disease and reflect carotid artery involvement. Non-specific symptoms such as headache and vertigo are seen in up to 90 per cent of cases (Churg 1993), but sensory loss and aphasia occur infrequently. Strokes are an important contributor to mortality. Visual disturbance occurs in 30 per cent of patients with either blurring of vision, which may be posturally dependent, diplopia or amaurosis fugax. Retinal disease with arteriovenous anastomosis occurs late in the disease. Visual disturbances are often related to systemic hypertension and 40 per cent of cases have fundal changes consistent with hypertension. Cataracts and neovascularization as described by Takayasu is now uncommon (Hall *et al.* 1985; Kerr *et al.* 1994).

Takayasu's arteritis may develop during childhood. In Eastern countries presentation is often with cardiac failure and hypertension in association with renal artery stenosis. Comparison of paediatric with adult onset patients in the United States suggests that systemic features are more common, whilst claudication is less common in childhood cases (Kerr *et al.* 1994).

Takayasu's arteritis should be considered in any young patient with limb or organ ischaemia, hypertension, or systemic illness. These patients should be investigated with full angiography (see below).

Assessment

Objective assessment of disease activity in systemic vasculitis is difficult and differentiation must be made between new lesions and scars from previous active disease. Generic assessment schemes such as the Birmingham Vasculitis Assessment Score (BVAS) may be utilized (Luqmani *et al.* 1994). Active disease was defined by Kerr and colleagues as new or worsening of two or more characteristic features. (Kerr *et al.* 1994). Complete resolution of all clinical features or their stabilization, in the setting of fixed vascular lesions, was indicative of remission. Clinical assessment of involved vessels may be difficult as symptoms of ischaemia will depend on the degree of stenosis and the adequacy of any collateral circulation. Measurement of blood pressure may be difficult in patients with diminished or absent pulses in several limbs.

Laboratory investigation

The erythrocyte sedimentation rate is often elevated in active disease. Serial measurements may correlate with disease activity, but not with histological extent (Kerr *et al.*, 1994). Other surrogate measures such as von Willebrand factor and endothelin-1 have been reported to reflect disease activity, but have not been established as reliable markers (Woolf *et al.* 1987). Antineutrophil cytoplasmic antibodies are not associated with Takayasu's arteritis (Churg 1993). Levels of soluble adhesion molecules such as soluble intracellular adhesion molecule-1 (sICAM-1), soluble vascular adhesion molecule-1 (sVCAM-1), and soluble E-selectin may reflect endothelial activation and damage, and hence be used as markers of vascular damage. Levels of sICAM-1, sVCAM-1 and sELAM are elevated in other forms of systemic vasculitis (e.g. Wegener's granulomatosis and giant cell arteritis) (Carson *et al.* 1993) but there have not yet been any systematic studies in Takayasu's arteritis.

The diagnosis of Takayasu's arteritis has depended on arteriography to demonstrate the characteristic changes in the aorta and its major branches; long stenotic lesions occur in almost all patients (Figs 1 and 2). Total arteriography is essential for angiographic diagnosis of the extent of the disease. Irregularity of the vessel wall occurs in one-third and aneurysms in 27 per cent of patients (Kerr *et al.* 1994). The distribution of lesions has been classified to reflect

disease above and below the diaphragm — type I disease is localized to the aortic arch and its branches; type II involves the thoracic descending aorta and abdominal aorta but not the aortic arch; type III is a mixture of types I and II; type IV features aspects of types I, II, or III together with involvement of the pulmonary artery (Lupi-Herrera *et al.* 1977).

High resolution B-mode ultrasonography is more sensitive in detecting carotid lesions than angiography and correlates with the presence of bruits (Maeda *et al.* 1991). The ultrasonographic hallmark of Takayasu's arteritis is a diffuse thickening of the intima–media complex, the 'Macaroni sign'. Ultrasonography is limited by its inability to image the thoracic aorta and pulmonary arteries.

The role of magnetic resonance angiography (MRA) is still being evaluated. MRA is able to image the aorta and its major branches and demonstrate aortic wall thickening, stenosis and aneurysms. Improving resolution and newer scanning techniques are improving rapidly the ability of MRA to evaluate blood vessels and it is likely that it will become the technique of choice, replacing conventional contrast angiography (Link *et al.* 1993).

Aetiology and immunopathogenesis

The aetiopathogenesis of Takayasu's arteritis is not well understood. The association with mycobacterial infection has not been confirmed (Lupi-Herrera *et al.* 1977). Occasional examples of multicase families have been published, suggesting a common genetic or environmental factor. Immunopathological findings include hypergammaglobulinaemia, the presence of rheumatoid factors, anti-aorta antibodies, immune complexes (Lupi-Herrera *et al.* 1977) and anti-endothelial cell antibodies in peripheral blood (Sima *et al.* 1994). Antineutrophil cytoplasmic antibodies are not present. Elevated numbers of CD4+ T

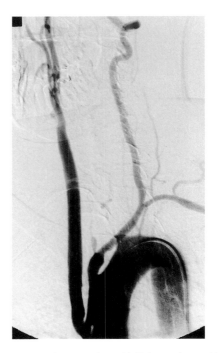

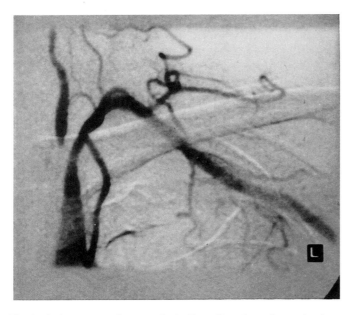

Fig. 1 Arch aortogram from a patient with aortic arch syndrome showing a long tapering stenosis of the left subclavian artery.

Fig. 2 Arch aortogram from a patient with Takayasu's arteritis. This shows (i) occlusion of the left subclavian at its origin, (ii) absence of the left common carotid artery, (iii) grafts *in situ* between the origin of the left common carotid and the left subclavian/vertebral artery and also between the aortic arch and right common carotid artery.

cells in peripheral blood, together with a decrease in CD8+ T cells and B cells have been reported but the significance of this finding is uncertain (Sagar *et al.* 1992). The inflammatory infiltrate conversely has an excess of CD8+ T cells, which are cytotoxic to endothelial cells in vitro (Scott *et al.* 1986).

In Japanese patients there is an association with the HLA haplotypes Bw52, Dw12, DR2, and DQW 1 (Dong *et al.* 1992; Kasuya *et al.* 1992) but this association has not been found in American patients (Hall *et al.* 1992). HLA-Bw52 positive Japanese patients have an association with heart disease and a worse prognosis with a higher incidence of aortic incompetence and left ventricular perfusion abnormalities (Kasuya *et al.* 1992)

A single case of Takayasu's arteritis following hepatitis B vaccination has been reported (Castrenasa-Isla *et al.* 1993). The patient developed erythema nodosum, arthralgia and upper limb claudication after receiving plasma-derived hepatitis B vaccine. Hepatitis B infection has not otherwise been associated with Takayasu's arteritis, unlike the well recognized association with polyarteritis nodosa.

Management

Medical treatment

Initial medical treatment for patients with active Takayasu's arteritis is with corticosteroids (prednisolone, 60 to 80 mg/day) and response rates of 20 to 100 per cent have been reported, with subsequent resolution of symptoms and stabilization of vascular abnormalities (Sen *et al.* 1963; Fraga *et al.* 1972; Lupi-Herrera *et al.* 1977; Kerr *et al.* 1994). However, 40 per cent of patients require additional cytotoxic agents, and 23 per cent have chronic unremitting disease (Kerr *et al.* 1994). The median time to remission in this study was 22 months (Kerr *et al.* 1994). Our experience of 7 patients confirms this data, with 3 patients requiring cytotoxic therapy in addition to corticosteroids (2, cyclophosphamide; 1, azathioprine). Continuous oral cyclophosphamide has been shown to induce remission in patients with corticosteroid-resistant disease in 4 of 6 patients treated (Shelhamer *et al.* 1985). The toxicity of cyclophosphamide in the treatment of systemic vasculitis can be reduced with the use of pulse intravenous regimens. There is little experience in the use of pulse cyclophosphamide in Takayasu's arteritis, although we have used such a regimen with good results in a small number of patients. Methotrexate is being used increasingly as a steroid sparing agent in the vasculitides. Hoffman and colleagues recently reported their experience of low-dose oral methotrexate in 18 patients with Takayasu's arteritis (Hoffman *et al.* 1994). Sixteen patients were followed up for an average of 2.8 years. The mean dose of methotrexate was 17.1 mg per week, which together with corticosteroids, resulted in remission in 13 patients; however, 7 patients relapsed on reduction of corticosteroid dose. Reintroduction of methotrexate resulted in a further remission. Sustained remissions of 4 to 34 months have been observed. Methotrexate is an effective method of inducing disease remission, permits reduction in the total corticosteroid dose and is therefore an alternative to cyclophosphamide in patients with disease that is difficult to control with corticosteroids alone. A flow diagram illustrating the managment of Takayasu's arteritis is given in Fig. 3.

Hypertension can be difficult to manage in patients with Takayasu's arteritis, particularly in those individuals with involvement of subclavian and femoral arteries, making measurement of blood pressure difficult. Wherever possible hypertension should be controlled by

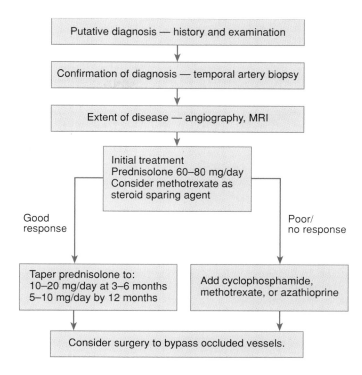

Fig. 3 Flow diagram illustrating the immunosuppresive treatment of large vessel involvement in Takayasu's arteritis and giant cell arteritis.

angioplasty or surgery. Medical control of hypertension must be cautious because of the risk to organs perfused by stenosed arteries from a fall in blood pressure. Angiotensin converting enzyme (ACE) inhibitors must be used with caution in patients with renal artery stenosis, because such patients have elevated renin levels and may be especially sensitive to the first dose of an ACE inhibitor. Beta-blockers may be used as an alternative. Vasodilators are potentially dangerous in the presence of fixed stenotic lesions (Ito 1992).

Anticoagulation is not currently recommended for Takayasu's arteritis. The role of anticoagulation and/or antiplatelet drugs in patients with no evidence of a hypercoagulable state has not been evaluated, but low dose aspirin may be sensible.

Surgical treatment

Surgery has an important adjunctive role in the management of patients with Takayasu's arteritis. Hypertension secondary to renal artery stenosis is a common mode of presentation, particularly in South-East Asia. Percutaneous transluminal angioplasty has been reported to restore patency in up to 80 per cent of cases (Sharma *et al.* 1992), but restenosis can occur within 1 to 2 years (Kumar *et al.* 1990). This can be managed with repeated angioplasty but formal bypass surgery may be necessary.

Elective bypass procedures are best performed during the inactive phase of the disease. Operative procedures include bypass of stenosed segments of arteries, resection of aneurysms and replacement of aortic valves (Ohtecki *et al.* 1992; Robbs *et al.* 1994). Anastomotic sites should be chosen in areas unaffected by inflammation, and autologous grafts perform better than synthetic grafts (Kerr *et al.* 1994). Overall operative mortality is 3 to 4 per cent and is associated with surgery for aneurysm rupture (Robbs *et al.* 1994).

Prognosis

The majority of patients (74 per cent) have some impairment of activities of daily living, and 47 per cent are permanently disabled (Kerr *et al.* 1994). Mortality is, however, low and 5- and 10-year survival rates of 80 to 90 per cent have been reported (Hall *et al.* 1985; Ishikawa 1988; Subramayan *et al.* 1989). Hypertension, cardiac involvement, aortic or arterial aneurysms, and severe functional disability predict greater morbidity and mortality in these studies. Ishikawa recently reported the long-term outcome in 120 patients followed for a median of 13 years (Ishikawa and Maetani 1994). The survival rate at 15 years was 82.9 per cent. The major determinants of outcome were the presence of complications (retinopathy, hypertension, aortic regurgitation and aneurysm) and the pattern of previous disease.

Pregnancy does not appear to exacerbate the inflammatory process, but if pregnancy is considered then it may be safer in a quiescent phase (Kerr *et al.* 1994). Hypertension, aneurysms and extent of disease are associated with an increased risk of maternal or fetal death (Wong *et al.* 1983). The increases in intravascular volume during pregnancy may exacerbate hypertension, aortic regurgitation and congestive cardiac failure. Moderate doses of corticosteroids have not had a detrimental effect on the fetus. Normal vaginal delivery is possible and caesarean section should be considered on obstetric merits and not because of coexistence of Takayasu's arteritis (Kerr *et al.* 1994).

Giant cell arteritis

Giant cell arteritis is a granulomatous arteritis of the aorta and its major branches, with a predilection for the extracranial branches of the carotid artery (Jeanette *et al.* 1994). The main features of the disease and its relation to polymyalgia rheumatica (PMR) are described elsewhere (Chapter 5.11.5). This section will review large vessel involvement in giant cell arteritis.

The inflammatory process of giant cell arteritis may involve the aorta and its major branches; this involvement may be minimal and clinically silent, however, extensive inflammation may lead to aortic incompetence, aneurysm formation, aortic rupture and death. Postmortem studies have demonstrated the extensive nature of the inflammatory process in giant cell arteritis, but many lesions are clinically silent (Cooke *et al.* 1946; Wilkinson and Russell 1972; Ostberg 1973). In a prospective study of 889 postmortem cases in which the temporal arteries and two transverse sections of the aorta were examined, giant cell arteritis was found in 1.7 per cent (Ostberg 1973).

Hamrin found that the aortic arch syndrome was present in 14 out of 93 cases of giant cell arteritis (Hamrin *et al.* 1972), whilst Klein and colleagues reviewed 248 patients with this disease and found that 34 (13.7 per cent) had definite or possible clinical evidence of involvement of the aorta and its major branches (Klein *et al.* 1975). At presentation of giant cell arteritis, 5 per cent of patients have large vessel involvement (Klein *et al.* 1975). Upper limb involvement is present in 6.3 per cent of patients with giant cell arteritis/polymyalgia rheumatica (Ninet *et al.* 1990). Our experience suggests that large vessel involvement in giant cell arteritis is less common. We have seen 3 cases over a 6 year period compared with approximately 100 cases of uncomplicated giant cell arteritis/polymyalgia rheumatica.

Clinical features

Systemic manifestations are present in a majority of patients with large vessel involvement, with malaise, fever, anorexia, sweats and weight loss. There is no difference in the frequency of polymyalgic symptoms and permanent visual loss between patients with large artery involvement and those without (Klein *et al.* 1975).

Intermittent claudication is the most common symptom occurring in 75 per cent of patients (Table 5) (Hunder 1990). Raynaud's phenomenon occurs in 20 per cent and may be unilateral. Physical examination reveals bruits over large arteries and/or decreased pulses. Bruits may be audible over long sections of artery. The arms alone were involved in 50 per cent of cases, legs alone in 12 per cent and arms and legs in 24 per cent (Klein *et al.* 1975). The remaining 12 per cent were either asymptomatic or had symptoms related to the chest or abdomen. Lie reviewed 72 cases with histologically proven extracranial giant cell arteritis: the ascending and aortic arch were most frequently involved (39 per cent), subclavian and axillary arteries (26 per cent), and femoropopliteal arteries (18 per cent) (Lie 1995). Evans and colleagues from the Mayo clinic identified 41 patients with giant cell arteritis and thoracic aortic aneurysms seen between 1950 and 1991 (Evans *et al.* 1994). During this period 1330 cases of biopsy-proven giant cell arteritis were seen. Laboratory investigations were similar in patients with and without aortic involvement. In 8 patients thoracic aorta involvement was diagnosed before or simultaneously with giant cell arteritis. The median interval in the remaining 33 patients was 7 years (3 months to 20 years). In only half of the patients was there evidence of active or recurrent giant cell arteritis at the time of development of thoracic involvement.

Large vessel involvement can become clinically apparent at any stage of the disease, either at initial presentation, when corticosteroid dose is being reduced or after corticosteroids have been withdrawn (Hunder 1990). Development of intermittent claudication of the arms may be the first manifestation of giant cell arteritis in a patient without symptoms suggestive of either polymyalgia rheumatica or temporal artery tenderness.

Table 5 Clinical features of large vessel arteritis occurring in giant cell arteritis

Symptom/sign	%
Intermittent claudication	74
Upper limb	40
Lower limb	13
Both	22
Raynaud's phenomenon	22
Paraesthesia	9
Decreased/absent pulses	91
Upper limb	61
Lower limb	17
Both	13

From Hunder (1990).

Diagnosis of large vessel involvement requires careful examination of arteries for tenderness, decreased pulses and bruits. Angiography is necessary to demonstrate the extent of arterial disease.

The differential diagnosis of patients with large vessel involvement due to giant cell arteritis includes Takayasu's arteritis and atherosclerosis. Takayasu's arteritis involves a younger age group (less than 50 years), different ethnic communities (giant cell arteritis is rare in non-Caucasians, whilst Takayasu's arteritis is common in Asians), the disease is usually more extensive and temporal artery biopsy is negative. Atherosclerosis, like giant cell arteritis, affects the population over 60 years of age, but is a more common cause of claudication than giant cell arteritis; however, the presence of claudication with evidence of a systemic illness (fever, malaise, weight loss, raised erythrocyte sedimentation rate) should suggest the possibility of an underlying vasculitic process. The diagnosis can be confirmed by angiography or temporal artery biopsy.

Laboratory investigations

The erythrocyte sedimentation rate is usually elevated at the time of diagnosis of large vessel involvement, but cases have been reported of large vessel disease developing at a time of apparent disease quiescence. The diagnosis should be considered in patients with an elevated erythrocyte sedimentation rate and limb, especially upper limb, ischaemia. In these patients temporal artery biopsy should be performed even if the temporal arteries are clinically normal.

Histology of large arteries is similar to that seen in the temporal artery with disruption of the elastic lamina, mononuclear cell infiltrate, giant cells and granulomata. Fibrosis occurs in longstanding lesions and results in luminal narrowing.

The demonstration of the extent of large vessel involvement in giant cell arteritis is dependent on imaging of the vessels involved. Doppler ultrasonography will demonstrate diminution of blood flow in an extremity and allow localization of lesions. Angiography has been the key to diagnosis of large vessel involvement (Fig. 4). The angiographic features most suggestive of arteritis are: (i) long segments of smooth arterial stenosis alternating with areas of normal or increased calibre, (ii) smooth tapered occlusions of affected large arteries, (iii) absence of irregular plaques and ulceration, and (iv)

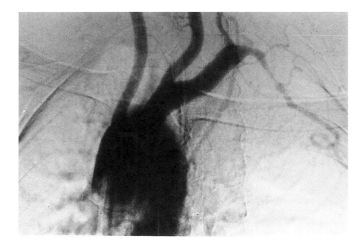

Fig. 4 Arch aortogram from a patient with giant cell arteritis showing dilatation of the right subclavian artery terminating in a long stricture distal to the origin of the vertebral artery (from Watts *et al.* 1989 with permission).

anatomical distribution of these changes with major involvement of subclavian, axillary and brachial arteries (Klein *et al.* 1975). The role of magnetic resonance imaging is uncertain at present, but as with Takayasu's arteritis will undoubtedly become more important.

Treatment and prognosis

Improvement in blood flow through extremities rapidly occurs following treatment with high-dose corticosteroids (45 to 60 mg/day), rendering reconstructive surgery unnecessary. Evolution of arterial stenosis can be serially monitored using Doppler ultrasonography. Vessels that are occluded on the angiogram rarely recanalize and in these cases clinical improvement is due to collateral formation. Surgery should be considered in patients with persistent limb ischaemia. This should be after the inflammatory phase has subsided to prevent early thrombosis of the graft (Ninet *et al.* 1990).

Large vessel involvement in giant cell arteritis is potentially fatal following rupture of an inflammatory aortic aneurysm, stroke or myocardial infarction (Save-Söderburgh *et al.* 1986). All patients with giant cell arteritis should be assessed carefully for large artery lesions.

Cytotoxic agents (methotrexate or cyclophosphamide) should be considered for those patients with persistent disease activity.

The vasculitides in general, although well recognized as a cause of coronary ischaemia, are rarely considered in the assessment of patients with ischaemic heart disease.

Infection-related arteritis

Infection-related aortitis was first described by Ambrose Paré in the sixteenth century, who associated syphilis with aortic aneurysms. During the nineteenth century, syphilis was recognized as the most common cause of aortitis, but pyogenic organisms and tuberculosis were increasingly recorded. A wide variety of organisms have since been recognized as causing a large vessel arteritis, including bacteria, fungi and spirochaetes (Table 6). Viral infections are not known to be associated with a large vessel arteritis.

Table 6	Causes of infective large vessel arteritis
Bacterial	Staphylococcus
	Streptococcus
	Pneumococcus
	Klebsiella
	Pseudomonas
	Brucella
	Salmonella
	Haemophilus
	Serratia
Mycobacterial	Mycobacterium tuberculosis
Fungal	Candida
	Cryptococcus
	Aspergillus
	Coccidioides
	Histoplasma
	Mucor
	Blastomyces
Spirochaetal	Syphilis

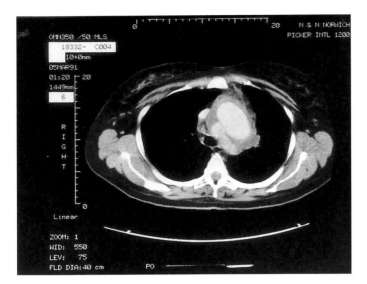

Fig. 5 Thoracic CT scan showing an aneurysm of the descending aorta. *Pneumococcus pneumoniae* was cultured from the resected vessel (from Chakravarty and Scott 1992 with permission).

The vascular reaction to direct infection depends on the organism and the site of infection. Two mechanisms for infection-related vasculitis have been proposed: first, direct microbial toxicity either by endothelial invasion or the effect of microbial toxins on endothelium; or second, immune-mediated either via immune complexes or cellular responses. Large vessel vasculitis secondary to infection occurs as a result of direct microbial endothelial invasion and leads to an erosive arteritis with mycotic aneurysm formation (Fig. 5).

Bacterial infective arteritis

Infective arteritis occurring as a result of direct endothelial invasion by bacteria or fungi results in formation of a mycotic aneurysm. Such aneurysms may develop in several ways, by septic embolization from a focus of infection such as a cardiac valve, by direct extension from a neighbouring abscess or by haematogenous spread of organisms from a portal of entry. Previously damaged or atherosclerotic vessel walls are very susceptible to bacterial seeding. Predisposing factors for development of a mycotic aneurysm include immunodeficiency, malignancy, diabetes mellitus, intravenous drug abuse and malignancy.

A wide variety of bacteria have been reported as causing infective large vessel arteritis including *Staphylococcus*, *Streptococcus*, *Klebsiella*, *Pneumococcus*, and *Pseudomonas* spp. (Table 6). Recently vasculitis has been described in association with more unusual organisms: *Salmonella* (Oskoui *et al.* 1993), *Haemophilus* (Chakravarty and Scott 1992) and *Brucella* (Aguado *et al.* 1987). *Staphylococcus* and *Salmonella* were the most frequently identified organisms in a 10-year study of 21 patients (Oz *et al.* 1989).

Aortic mycotic aneurysms may be clinically silent until they reach a massive size and rupture, with fatal haemorrhage occurring before a clinical diagnosis is made. Clinical symptoms are usually related to the systemic manifestations of infection (fever, leucocytosis), and if the aneurysm is large enough it may cause pressure effects—cough, chest pain, hoarseness and dysphagia with thoracic aneurysms, and epigastric or lumbar pain and a palpable mass with abdominal aneur-

ysms. In the limbs mycotic aneurysms usually present with pain, tenderness and fever associated with a pulsatile mass, which may be palpable when present in the extremities. They are associated with a high mortality from sepsis and haemorrhage. The source of the infection is often from infected heart valves (80 per cent), though rarely it may be the result of direct microbial arteritis. Transient bacteraemia occurs frequently in intravenous drug abusers and results in direct vessel wall infection. *Salmonella*, *Staphylococcus*, and *E. coli* are the usual organisms. The presentation may be insidious and diagnosis delayed until haemorrhage occurs.

Diagnosis is based on a high level of suspicion particularly in patients with fever, leucocytosis, abdominal pain and positive blood cultures. The aorta may appear normal on plain radiographs and a CT scan may be required to demonstrate aortic infection

The mortality of bacterial aortitis is still high. In a series of 21 cases seen over 10 years, there were 8 disease-related deaths, but no graft infections were seen in the survivors (Oz *et al.* 1989).

Spirochaetal infection

Treponema pallidum is a well recognized cause of aortitis, with aneurysm formation and development of aortic incompetence. The primary histological changes are in the vasa vasorum with endarteritis, and perivascular infiltration with lymphocytes and plasma cells. Infection occurs early in the disease and organisms lie dormant in the aortic wall. Spirochaetes can, however, only rarely be detected in tissue. Symptomatic aortic disease occurs as a feature of tertiary disease. The majority of syphilitic aneurysms are located in the thoracic aorta with the following distribution: sinus of Valsalva less than 1 per cent, ascending aorta 36 per cent, aortic arch 24 per cent, descending aorta 24 per cent, and multiple locations 4 per cent (Berkman 1986). Presentation is with aortic incompetence (60 per cent of cases) or coronary ostial stenosis. Coronary arteritis may occur independently of aortitis. Diagnosis is based on the radiographic appearances and serological tests. Treatment is with antibiotics and surgical resection. The differential diagnosis of syphilitic aortitis includes Takayasu's arteritis, extracranial giant cell arteritis, and the aortitis of rheumatic diseases.

Borrelia burgdorferi infection causes a small vessel vasculitis which does not involve large vessels.

Fungal infections

Fungal infections of the endothelium are rare. *Candida*, *Aspergillus*, and *Histoplasma* are the most common organisms; however, *Blastomyces*, *Coccidioides*, *Cryptococcus*, and *Mucor* have been described rarely (Berkman 1986; Leavitt and Kauffman 1988). Infection results in formation of a mycotic aneurysm, similar to that seen with bacterial arterial infections. Direct infection is rare. Most cases of fungal aortitis occur in patients who are already severely immunocompromised from other diseases, those who have received multiple courses of intravenous antibiotics, or intravenous drug abusers. These patients have a high mortality (70 per cent) and require aggressive antifungal therapy.

Mycobacterial infection

Mycobacterial infection may involve blood vessels of any size, with veins being more vulnerable than arteries. Large vessel tuberculous arteritis is uncommon, with an equal division between thoracic and abdominal aneurysms (Silbergleit *et al.* 1965; Berkman 1986). The aorta may be infected by the tubercle bacillus by haematogenous dissemination in miliary disease, lymphangitic spread and direct extension from contiguous structures. Aneurysm formation occurs in half of the cases. Clinical presentation is non-specific with fever, chest pain, haemoptysis, dysphagia, abdominal pain and a palpable mass. Tuberculous vasculitis results in granuloma formation and a panarteritis. Acid-fast bacilli may be detectable in macrophages of the inflammatory infiltrate. Treatment is with antituberculous drugs, combined with surgical resection.

Mycobacterium leprae may cause vasculitis but this typically involves small arteries. Other atypical mycobacteria have not been described as causing a large vessel aortitis.

Rheumatoid arthritis

Systemic rheumatoid vasculitis was first described by Bywaters in 1949 and the clinical features delineated over the next decade (Bywaters 1957). The annual incidence of this disease is 12.6 per million, making it one of the most common forms of systemic vasculitis (Watts *et al.* 1994). All sizes of vessel from large arteries to capillaries may be involved. Large vessel involvement with aortitis or aortic regurgitation is rare in patients with rheumatoid arthritis and was only first clearly described by Zvaifler and Weintraub (1963). In a large comparative series seen between 1970 and 1994 from three centres in the United Kingdom comprising nearly 150 cases of systemic rheumatoid vasculitis, large vessel involvement was seen in 5 per cent (Luqmani *et al.* 1995). Aortitis was identified in 10 cases in a series of 180 postmortems performed on patients with rheumatoid vasculitis (Gravallese *et al.* 1989). As with other forms of systemic rheumatoid vasculitis, the typical patient with large vessel disease has long-standing seropositive erosive rheumatoid vasculitis. In most cases there is multiorgan involvement (Gravallese *et al.* 1989) including a coronary arteritis. Aortitis is rarely diagnosed antemortem, but may be the cause of death, particularly in cases with associated coronary arteritis. Aortitis and aortic incompetence may result in haemodynamic compromise with congestive cardiac failure.

Histological features of rheumatoid aortitis include necrosis of medial smooth muscle and elastica, with an inflammatory infiltrate comprising lymphocytes and plasma cells. A panmural aortitis can occur. Rheumatoid granulomata are seen in half of the cases (Gravallese *et al.* 1989).

Systemic rheumatoid vasculitis responds well to corticosteroids and cyclophosphamide (Luqmani *et al.* 1995). There is however no data on the response of rheumatoid aortitis or aortic incompetence to immunosuppressive therapy, however this treatment should be considered in patients presenting with active aortitis since prevention or delay in the necessity for surgery may be achieved.

Spondylarthopathies

Aortitis may complicate the seronegative spondylarthropathies in particular ankylosing spondylitis (Buckley and Roberts 1973) and Reiter's syndrome (Morgan *et al.* 1986). The aortic ring and ascending aorta are the typical sites of involvement but distal aortitis has been described (Morgan *et al.* 1984). Aortic incompetence occurs in up to 5 per cent of cases of ankylosing spondylitis, 2.5 per cent of cases of Reiter's syndrome and probably less frequently in the other seronegative spondylarthropathies (Townend *et al.* 1991).

The seronegative spondylarthropathies are associated with the HLA-B27 haplotype. Inflammatory diseases associated with this haplotype have been found in 15 to 20 per cent of patients with lone aortic regurgitation, suggesting that lone aortic regurgitation may reflect an inflammatory valvulitis or aortitis (Bergfeldt *et al.* 1988)

Echocardiography shows thickening of the aortic leaflets, subaortic echodense bumps and aortic root densities (Labresh *et al.* 1985). Histologically there is thickening of the aortic valve cusps and aorta, together with lymphocytic infiltration in the aortic wall and fibrosis of the aortic root (Buckley and Roberts 1973). These changes can be difficult to distinguish from lesions occurring in syphilitic aortitis.

Treatment of the inflammatory process with immunosuppressive agents has been suggested, but no controlled data exists as to their benefit in this situation, in particular whether the need for aortic valve replacement can be delayed or prevented (Townend *et al.* 1991).

Systemic lupus erythematosus

The typical vascular lesion of systemic lupus erythematosus involves small vessels, large vessels are rarely involved. Saxe and Altman reviewed 19 reported cases of Takayasu's arteritis associated with systemic lupus erythematosus, and pointed out that the diseases have a similar age of onset and female preponderance (Saxe and Altman 1992). However, the absence of specific markers for systemic lupus erythematosus in patients with Takayasu's arteritis who subsequently develop systemic lupus erythematosus suggests that the coexistence of these two conditions may be coincidental. Some of these cases are incompletely reported and would not be considered necessarily to be either of the diseases using current diagnostic criteria. Patients with systemic lupus erythematosus who develop large vessel thrombosis as part of the antiphospholipid antibody syndrome, may mimic the obstructive vasculopathy seen in Takayasu's arteritis.

Relapsing polychondritis

Relapsing polychondritis is a systemic disease of unknown aetiology with inflammation of cartilaginous structures. Vasculitis occurs in 11 to 56 per cent of cases with involvement of large and medium-sized vessels (Michet 1990). Large artery involvement is uncommon (less than 15 per cent of cases) and present as an aortic arch syndrome, thoracic or abdominal aortic aneurysm with rupture, or aortic regurgitation. Small vessel vasculitis and a segmental necrotizing glomerulonephritis may occur simultaneously. The vasculitis may present at the same time as other manifestations of relapsing polychondritis or many years afterwards. The aortitis of relapsing polychondritis results in loss of glycosaminoglycans from the aortic wall, particularly in the media with loss of elastic tissue.

Treatment is with corticosteroids, and the role of cytotoxic agents is uncertain. Surgical repair is required for valvular and artery occlusions.

Behçet's syndrome

Behçet's syndrome is a chronic relapsing condition characterized by a triad of aphthous stomatitis, genital ulceration, and uveitis. A large vessel arteritis is well described (Little and Zarins 1982; Lakhanpal *et al.* 1985). Major arterial occlusions were present in 36 per cent and there was evidence of vasculitis in 18 per cent of cases at autopsy (Lakhanpal *et al.* 1985). Shimizu and colleagues described 81 patients with Behçet's disease in whom occlusion of large arteries was present in 17 and aneurysms in 24 patients (Shimizu *et al.* 1979). Aortitis is uncommon and is represented histologically by inflammation in the media and adventitia, particularly around the vasa vasorum. Multiple pulmonary aneurysms occur which may communicate with the bronchi and present as massive haemoptysis.

Cogan's syndrome

Cogan's syndrome is a rare condition characterized by recurrent episodes of acute sensorineural hearing loss and non-syphilitic keratitis (Cogan 1945). Systemic features occur and vascular involvement is common (Vollertsen *et al.* 1986).

Vasculitis occurs early in the disease, within the first year in two-thirds of patients, but can occur up to 8 years after onset (Vollertsen *et al.* 1986). The clinical manifestations will depend on the vessel involved.

Cardiac involvement occurs in 15 to 25 per cent of patients (Cheson *et al.* 1976; Vollertsen *et al.* 1986), manifesting mainly as aortic regurgitation which may be rapidly progressive over a period of months. It is associated with either a valvulitis or an aortitis. Aortic regurgitation may occur at diagnosis or up to 12 years after diagnosis (Vollertsen *et al.* 1986). Aortitis may lead to narrowing of the coronary ostia and arteries arising from the aortic arch; a distal coronary arteritis may also occur.

Angiography demonstrates arterial occlusion of large and medium vessels with scattered stenosis, and a diffuse irregular narrowing can also be seen (Vollertsen *et al.* 1986).

Histological examination of the aorta reveals neutrophils, mononuclear cells, giant cells, destruction of the elastic lamina, neovascularization, necrosis, scarring and fibrotic hypertrophy (Cheson *et al.* 1976). Similar findings are observed in other vessels.

Treatment of Cogan's syndrome is with corticosteroids, and clinical improvement occurs in most cases. The role of cytotoxic drugs in undetermined. Treatment of aortic regurgitation is by valve replacement (Cochrane and Tatoulis 1991). Arterial bypass grafting may be required.

Kawasaki disease

Kawasaki disease is a inflammatory vascular disease of childhood which typically results in the formation of coronary artery aneurysms. Systemic artery aneurysms occur in 4 per cent of patients with Kawasaki disease, the most common site being the axillary and iliac arteries (Inioue *et al.* 1988). Aortitis and consequent aneurysm formation is rare. Fibrosis and arterial luminal stenosis is a late sequelae of acute Kawasaki disease. Treatment of acute disease is with aspirin and intravenous immunoglobulin.

Wegener's granulomatosis

Wegener's granulomatosis is a disease of predominately small and medium vessels. The clinical features and management of Wegener's granulomatosis is described in Chapter 5.11.2. Coronary and large artery involvement has only rarely been described in patients with Wegener's granulomatosis (Davenport *et al.* 1994;

Logar *et al.* 1994). Two patients had clinically significant aortic valve incompetence. Histology of the resected valve showed myxoid degeneration due to previous vasculitis affecting the vessels of the aortic wall, together with valvular necrosis (Davenport *et al.* 1994). Carotid arteritis has been described in a patient with ANCA-positive crescentic glomerulonephritis (Logar *et al.* 1994).

Rheumatic fever

Rheumatic fever occurs as part of the immune response to Group A streptococci. During acute rheumatic fever arteritis can develop in different sized arteries, and Aschoff bodies may develop in the adventitia of the aorta and other large arteries. An acute vasculitis may involve the vasa vasorum, with endothelial cell swelling, luminal leucocytes, and a perivascular infiltrate of lymphocytes, macrophages, and leucocytes (Virmani and McAllister 1986).

Sarcoidosis

Sarcoidosis is a systemic granulomatous disease of unknown aetiology. Cardiac involvement is well recognized in patients who die suddenly. Sarcoid granulomata have been described rarely in the aorta and its large branches. The granulomata are found in the adventitia (Virmani and McAllister 1986).

Central nervous system angiitis

Primary angiitis of the central nervous system is a rare disease of unknown aetiology, occasionally it involves large vessels but more typically medium or small arteries (Calabrese and Mallek 1988; Abu-Shakra *et al.* 1994). The clinical features are non-specific and entirely neurological. Presentation may be acute with severe headache, stroke, neurocognitive defect, or seizure. There may be evidence of systemic illness with elevation of acute phase proteins. The diagnosis is made by the presence of characteristic histological findings, with a granulomatous vasculitis in the leptomeninges or cortex. Angiography demonstrates beading or ectasia alternating with stenosis. These changes are typically distal to the termination of the carotid arteries. Treatment is with corticosteroids with or without cyclophosphamide.

References

Abu-Shakra, M., Khraisha, M., Grosman, H., Lewtas, J., Cividino, A., and Keystone, E.C. (1994). Primary angiitis of the CNS diagnosed by angiography. *Quarterly Journal of Medicine*, **87**, 351–8.
Achar, K.N. and Al-Nahib, B. (1986). Takayasu's arteritis and ulcerative colitis. *American Journal of Gastroenterology*, **81**, 1215–7.
Aguado, J.M., Barros, C., Gomez Garces, J.L., and Fernandez-Geurrero, M.L. (1987). Infective aortitis due to *Brucella melitensis*. *Scandinavian Journal of Infectious Disease*, **19**, 483–4.
Arend, W.P. *et al.* (1990). The American College of Rheumatology 1990 criteria for the classification of Takayasu arteritis. *Arthritis and Rheumatism*, **33**, 1129–34.
Baldursson, O., Steinsson, K., Bornsson, L., and Lie, J.T. (1994). Giant cell arteritis in Iceland. An epidemiologic and histopathologic analysis. *Arthritis and Rheumatism*, **37**, 1007–12.
Bengtsson, B-Å. and Malmvall, B.E. (1981). The epidemiology of giant cell arteritis including temporal arteritis and polymyalgia rheumatica: incidences of different clinical presentations and eye complications. *Arthritis and Rheumatism*, **24**, 899–904.
Bergfeldt, L., Insulander, P., Lindblom, D., Möller, E., and Edhag, O. (1988). HLA-B27: an important genetic risk factor for lone aortic regurgitiation and severe conduction abnormalities. *American Journal of Medicine*, **85**, 12–18.

Berkman, Y. (1986). Medical aspects of infectious aortitis. In *Aortitis* (ed. A. Lande, Y.M. Berkman, and H.A. McAllister), pp. 161–72. Raven Press, New York.

Buckley, B.H. and Roberts, W.C. (1973). Ankylosing spondylitis and aortic regurgitation. Description of the characteristic lesion from study of eight necropsy cases. *Circulation*, 48, 1014–27.

Bywaters, E.G.L. (1957). Peripheral vascular obstruction in rheumatoid arthritis and its relationships to other vascular lesions. *Annals of the Rheumatic Diseases*, 16, 84–103.

Calabrese, L. and Mallek, J.A. (1988). Primary angiitis of the central nervous system. *Medicine*, 67, 20–39.

Carson, C.W., Beall, L.D., Hunder, G.G., Johnson, C.M., and Newman, W. (1993). Serum ELAM-1 is increased in vasculitis, scleroderma, and systemic lupus erythematosus. *Journal of Rheumatology*, 20, 809–14.

Castrenasa-Isla, C.J., Herrera-Martinez, G., and Vega-Molin, J. (1993). Erythema nodosum and Takayasu arteritis after immunisation with plasma derived hepatitis B vaccine. *Journal of Rheumatology*, 20, 1417–8.

Chakravarty, K.C. and Scott, D.G.I. (1992). Mycotic aneurysm of the aortic arch masquerading as systemic lupus erythematosus. *Annals of the Rheumatic Diseases*, 51, 1079–81.

Cheson, B.D., Bluming, A.Z., and Alroy, J. (1976). Cogan's syndrome and systemic vasculitis. *American Journal of Medicine*, 60, 549–55.

Churg, J. (1993). Large vessels arteritis. *Clinical and Experimental Immunology*, 93 (Suppl.), 11–12.

Cochrane, A.D. and Tatoulis, J. (1991). Cogan's syndrome with aortitis, aortic regurgitation, and aortic arch vessel stenoses. *Annals of Thoracic Surgery*, 52, 1166–7.

Cogan, D.G. (1945). Syndrome of nonsyphilitic interstitial keratitis and vestibulo-auditory symptoms. *Archives of Ophthalmology*, 33, 144–9.

Cooke, W.T., Cloake, P.C.P., and Govan, A.D.T. (1946). Temporal arteritis: a generalised disease. *Quarterly Journal of Medicine*, 15, 47–76.

Davenport, A., Goodfellow, J., Goel, S., MacIver, A.G., and Walker, P. (1994). Aortic valve disease in Wegener's granulomatosis. *American Journal of Kidney Diseases*, 24, 205–8.

DiGiacomo, V. (1984). A case of Takayasu's disease occurred over two hundred years ago. *Angiology*, 35, 750–4.

Dong, R-P., Kimur, A., Numamno, F., Nishimura, Y., and Sasazuki, T. (1992). HLA-linked susceptibility and resistance to Takayasu arteritis. *Heart Vessels*, 7, 73–81.

Evans, J.M., Bowles, C., Bjornsson, J., Mullany, C.G., and Hunder, G.G. (1994). Thoracic aortic aneurysm and rupture in gaint cell arteritis. *Arthritis and Rheumatism*, 37, 1539–47.

Fraga, A., Mintz, G., Valle, L., and Flores-Izquierd, G. (1972). Takayasu's arteritis: frequency of systemic manifestations (study of 22 patients) and favourable response to maintenance steroid therapy with adrenocorticosteroids. *Arthritis and Rheumatism*, 15, 617–24.

Gravallese, E.M. *et al.* (1989). Rheumatoid aortitis: a rarely recognised but clinically significant entity. *Medicine (Baltimore)*, 68, 95–106.

Hall, S. and Nelson, A.M. (1986). Takayasu's arteritis and juvenile rheumatoid arthritis. *Journal of Rheumatology*, 13, 431–3.

Hall, S. *et al.* (1985). Takayasu arteritis: a study of 32 North American patients. *Medicine (Baltimore)*, 64, 89–99.

Hall, S., Saga, S., Ganguly, N.K., Koicha, M., and Sharma, B.K. (1992). Immunopathogenesis of Takayasu's arteritis. *Heart Vessels*, 7, 85–90.

Hamrin, B. (1972). Polymyalgia arteritica. *Acta Medica Scandinavica*, 533 (Suppl.), 1–131.

Hoffman, G.S., Leavitt, R.Y., Kerr, G.S., Rottem, M., Sneller, M.C., and Fauci, A.S. (1994). Treatment of gluco-corticoid resistant or relapsing Takayasu arteritis with methotrexate. *Arthritis and Rheumatism*, 37, 78–82.

Hunder, G.G. (1986). Giant cell arteritis and giant cell aortitis. In *Aortitis* (ed. A. Lande, Y.M. Berkman, and H.A. McAllister), pp. 193–204. Raven Press, New York.

Inioue, O. *et al.* (1988). Systemic artery involvement in Kawasaki disease. In *Proceedings of the 3rd International Kawasaki disease symposium*, Tokyo, 29 November to 2 December 1988, p. 23.

Ishikawa, K. (1986). Pattern of symptoms and prognosis in occlusive thromboaortopathy (Takayasu's disease). *Journal of the American College of Cardiology*, 8, 1041–6.

Ishikawa, K. (1988). Diagnostic approach and proposed criteria for the clinical diagnosis of Takayasu's arteriopathy. *Journal of the American College of Cardiology*, 12, 964–72.

Ishikawa, K. and Maetani, S. (1994). Long term outcome for 120 Japanese patients with Takayasu's disease. Clinical and statistical analyses of related prognostic factors. *Circulation*, 90, 1855–60.

Ito, I. (1992). Medical treatment of Takayasu's arteritis. *Heart Vessels*, 7 (Suppl.), 133–7.

Jeanette, J.C. *et al.* (1994). Nomenclature of systemic vasculitides. Proposal of an international consensus conference. *Arthritis and Rheumatism*, 37, 187–92.

Jonasson, F., Cullen, J.F., and Elton, R.A. (1979). Temporal arteritis: a 14 year epidemiological, clinical and prognostic study. *Scottish Medical Journal*, 24, 111–7.

Kasuya, K., Hashimoto, Y., and Numano, F. (1992). Left ventricular dysfunction and HLA Bw5z antigen in Takayasu arteritis. *Heart Vessels*, 7, 116–9.

Kerr, G.S. *et al.* (1994). Takayasu's arteritis. *Annals of Internal Medicine*, 120, 919–29.

Klein, R.G., Hunder, G.G., Stanson, A.W., and Sheps, S.G. (1975). Large artery involvement in giant cell (temporal) arteritis. *Annals of Internal Medicine*, 83, 806–12.

Kumar, S. *et al.* (1990). Percutaneous transluminal angioplasty in non-specific aortoarteritis (Takayasu's disease): experience of 16 cases. *Cardiology Interventional Radiology*, 12, 321–5.

Labresh, K.A., Lally, E.V., Sharma, S.C., and Ho, G. (1985). Two dimensional echocardiographic detection of preclinical aortic root abnormalities in rheumatoid variant diseases. *American Journal of Medicine*, 78, 908–12.

Lakhanpal, S. *et al.* (1985). Pathological features of Behçet's disease. A review of Japanese autopsy registry data. *Human Pathology*, 16, 790–5.

Lande, A. and Berkman, M.Y. (1976). Aortitis: pathological, clinical and arteriographic review. *Radiological Clinics of North America*, 14, 219–40.

Leavitt, A.D. and Kauffman, C.A. (1988). Cryptococcal aortitis. *American Journal of Medicine*, 85, 108–10.

Lie, J.T. (1995). Aortic and extra-cranial large vessel giant cell arteritis. *Seminars in Arthritis and Rheumatism*, 24, 422–31.

Link, K.M., Loehr, S.P., Baker, D.M., and Lesko, N.M. (1993). Magnetic resonance imaging of the thoracic aorta. *Seminars in Ultrasound, CT and MRI*, 14, 91–105.

Little, A.G. and Zarins, C.K. (1982). Abdominal aortic aneurysm and Behçet's disease. *Surgery*, 91, 359–62.

Logar, D., Rozman, B., Vizjak, A., Ferluga, D., Mulder, A.H., and Kallenberg, C.G. (1994). Arteritis of both carotid arteries in a patient with focal crescentic glomerulonephritis and anti-neutrophil cytoplasmic antibodies. *British Journal of Rheumatology*, 33, 167–9.

Lupi-Herrera, E., Sanchez-Torres, G., Marcushamer, J., Mispireta, J., Horwitz, S., and Vela, J.E. (1977). Takayasu's arteritis. Clinical study of 107 cases. *American Heart Journal*, 93, 94–103.

Luqmani, R.A. *et al.* (1994). Birmingham vasculitis activity score (BVAS) in systemic vasculitis. *Quarterly Journal of Medicine*, 87, 671–8.

Luqmani, R.A., Watts, R.A., Scott, D.G.I., and Bacon, P.A. (1994). Treatment of vasculitis in rheumatoid arthritis. *Annals de Medicine Interne*, 145, 566–76.

Maeda, H. *et al.* (1991). Carotid lesions detected by B-mode ultrasonography in Takayasu's arteritis: 'macaroni sign' as an indicator of disease. *Ultrasound Medicine and Biology*, 17, 695–701.

Magaro, M., Altomonte, L., Mirone, L., Zoli, A., and Corvino, G. (1988). Seronegative spondarthritis associated with Takayasu's arteritis. *Annals of the Rheumatic Diseases*, 47, 595–7.

Michet, C.J. (1990). Vasculitis and relapsing polychondritis. *Rheumatic Disease Clinics of North America*, 16, 441–4.

Morgan, S.H., Asherson, R.A., and Hughes, G.R.V. (1984). Distal aortitis complicating Reiter's syndrome. *British Heart Journal*, 52, 115–6.

Ninet, J.P., Bachet, P., Dumontet, C.M., Du Colombier, P.B., Stewart, M.D., and Pasquier, J.H. (1990). Subclavian and axillary involvement in temporal arteritis and polymyalgia rheumatica. *American Journal of Medicine*, 88, 13–20.

Ohtecki, H. *et al.* (1992). Aortic valve replacement for Takayasu's arteritis. *Journal of Thoracic Cardiovascular Surgery*, 104, 482–6.

Oskoui, R., Davis, R.A., and Gomes, M.N. (1993). Salmonella aortitis. *Archives of Internal Medicine*, 153, 517–25.

Ostberg, G. (1972). Morphological changes in the large arteries in polymyalgia arteritica. *Acta Medica Scandinavia*, 533 (Suppl.), 135–64.

Oz, M.C. *et al.* (1989). A ten year experience with bacterial aortitis. *Journal of Vascular Surgery*, 10, 439–49.

Rijbroek, A., Moll, F.L., van-Dijk, H.A., Meijer, R., and Jansen, J.W (1994). Inflammation of the abdominal aortic aneurysm wall. *European Journal of Vascular Surgery*, 8, 41–6.

Robbs, J.V., Abdool-Carrim, A.T., and Kadwa, A.M. (1994) Arterial reconstruction for non-specific arteritis (Takayasu's disease). *European Journal of Vascular Surgery*, 8, 401–7.

Rush, P.J., Inman, R.,and Reynolds, W.J. (1986). Rheumatoid arthritis after Takayasu's arteritis. *Journal of Rheumatology*, 13, 427–30.

Sagar, S., Ganguly, N.K., Koicha, M., and Sharma, B.K. (1992) Immunopathogenesis of Takayasu arteritis. *Heart Vessels*, 7, 85–90.

Säve-Söderburgh, J., Malmvall, B-E., Andersson, R., and Bengtsson, B-Å. (1986). Giant cell arteritis as a cause of death. *Journal of the American Medical Association*, 255, 493–6.

Saxe, P.A., and Altman, R.D. (1992). Takayasu's arteritis syndrome associated with systemic lupus erythematosus. *Seminars in Arthritis and Rheumatism*, 21, 295–305.

Scott, D.G.I. and Watts, R.A. (1994). Classification and epidemiology of systemic vasculitis. *British Journal of Rheumatology*, 33, 897–9.

Scott, D.G.I. *et al.* (1986). Takayasu's arteritis: a pathogenic role for cytotoxic T lymphocytes? *Clinical Rheumatology*, 5, 517–22.

Sen, P.K., Kinare, S.G., Engineer, S.D., and Parulkar, G.B. (1963). The middle aortic arch syndrome. *British Heart Journal*, 35, 610–8.

Sharma, S. *et al.* (1991). Non-specific aorto-arteritis (Takayasu's disease) in children. *British Journal of Radiology*, 64, 690–8.

Sharma, S. *et al.* (1992). Renal artery stenosis caused by non-specific arteritis (Takayasu disease): results of treatment with percutaneous transluminal angioplasty. *American Journal of Roentgenology*, 158, 417–22.

Shelhamer, J.H, Volkman, D.J., Parrillo, J.E., Lawley, T.J., Johnston, M.R., and Fauci, A.S. (1985). Takayasu's arteritis and its therapy. *Annals of Internal Medicine*, 103, 121–6.

Shimizu, T., Ehrlich, G.E., and Hayashi, K. (1979). Behçet disease (Behçet syndrome). *Seminars in Artritis and Rheumatism*, 8, 223–60.

Silbergleit, A. *et al.* (1965). Tuberculous aortitis—surgical resection of ruptured false aneurysms. *Journal of the American Medical Association*, 193, 333–5.

Sima, D. *et al.* (1994). Anti-endothelial cell antibodies in Takayasu arteritis. *Arthritis and Rheumatism*, 37, 441–2.

Subramayan, R., Joy, J., and Balakrishan, K.G. (1989). Natural history of aortoarteritis (Takayasu's disease). *Circulation*, 80, 429–37.

Takayasu, M. (1908). Case with unusual changes of the central vessels of the retina. *Acta Societatis Ophthalmologica Japonica*, 21, 554.

Townend, J.N., Emery, P., Davies, M.K., and Littler, W.A. (1991). Acute aortitis and aortic incompetence due to systemic rheumatological disorders. *International Journal of Cardiology*, 33, 253–8.

Virmani, R. and McAllister, H.A. (1986). Pathology of the aorta and major arteries. In *Aortitis* (ed. A. Lande, Y.M. Berkman, and H.A. McAllister), pp. 7–53. Raven Press, New York.

Vollertsen, R.S., McDonald, T.J., Younge, B.R., Banks, P.M., Stanson, A.W., and Ilstrup, D.M. (1986). Cogan's syndrome: 18 cases and a review of the literature. *Mayo Clinic Proceedings*, 61, 344–61.

Waern, A.U., Andersson, P., and Hemmingsson, A. (1983). Takayasu's arteritis: a hospital- region based study on occurrence, treatment and prognosis. *Angiology*, 34, 311–20.

Watts, R.A,. Bhalla, A.K., Binder, A.I., and Coppen, M. (1989). Giant cell arteritis presenting as limb claudication. *Journal of the Royal Society of Medicine*, 82, 51–2.

Watts, R.A., Carruthers, D.M., Symmons, D.P.M., and Scott, D.G.I. (1994). The incidence of rheumatoid vasculitis in the Norwich Health Authority. *British Journal of Rheumatology*, 33, 832–3.

Watts, R.A., Carruthers, D.M., and Scott, D.G.I. (1995). Epidemiology of systemic vasculitis changing incidence or definition? *Seminars in Arthritis and Rheumatism*, 25, 28–34.

Wilkinson, I.M.S. and Russell, R.W.R. (1972). Arteritis of the head and neck in giant cell arteritis. *Archives of Neurolology*, 27, 378–91.

Wilson, W.A., Morgan, O.S., Bain, B., and Taylor, J.E. (1979). Takayasu's arteritis association with Still's disease in an adult. *Arthritis and Rheumatism*, 22, 684–8.

Wong, V.C.W., Yang, R.Y.C., and Tse, T.F. (1983). Pregnancy and Takayasu's arteritis. *American Journal of Medicine*, 75, 597–601.

Woolf, A.D., Wakerley, G., and Wallington, T.B. (1987). Factor VIII related antigen in the assessment of vasculitis. *Annals of the Rheumatic Diseases*, 46, 441–7.

Zvaifler, N.J. and Weintraub, A.M. (1963). Aortiitis and aortic insufficiency in the chronic rheumatic disorders—a reappraisal. *Arthritis and Rheumatism*, 6, 241–5.

5.11.7 Behçet's syndrome

Hasan Yazıcı, Sebahattin Yurdakul, and Vedat Hamuryudan

Introduction

Behçet's syndrome is a systemic vasculitis (Lie 1992) of unknown aetiology with a definite and peculiar geographic distribution. Most cases are clustered around the countries of the Mediterranean basin, the Middle East, and the Far East. Its most dreaded complication, eye disease, is one of the leading causes of blindness in these areas.

Beginning with Hippocrates many have written about patients with disorders that today are considered elements of Behçet's syndrome. In 1937 Hulusi Behçet, professor of dermatovenereology in Istanbul, described in detail three patients with oral and genital ulceration and hypopyon uveitis, and proposed that this was a distinct entity. Subsequently it was realized that many other clinical manifestations were part of this syndrome (Shimizu *et al.* 1979). Table 1 gives the most important of these manifestations.

Epidemiology

The usual onset of the syndrome is in the third or fourth decade. The onset is rare in children and after the age of 45. Recently there has been an increased awareness of childhood cases (Özdoğan 1994).

Table 1 Clinical findings in Behçet's syndrome

Lesion	Prevalence (%)
Aphthous ulcerations	97–100
Genital lesions	80–90
Skin lesions	80
Eye lesions	50
Arthritis	40–50
Thrombophlebitis	25
Neurological involvement	1–15
Gastrointestinal involvement	0–25

The male:female ratio is approximately equal but the syndrome has a more severe course in men. Large scale epidemiological studies are lacking. Based on case registries, the prevalence is about 1:300 000 in Northern Europe and 1:10 000 in Japan. The prevalence may be higher in Mediterranean countries. In Turkey, based on two spot surveys among the adult population, the prevalence rates were 8 and 38:10 000 (Yurdakul *et al.* 1988). For unexplained reasons, few cases are reported from the United States and Australia.

Genetics

The syndrome is associated with HLA B5, specifically with HLA B51 (Ohno *et al.* 1982), however there is geographical variation. Patients from the Mediterranean countries and Japan show this association whereas those from the United States and United Kingdom, perhaps with the exception of those with eye disease, do not (Yazıcı *et al.* 1980). The association with HLA B5 is primarily with those patients attending hospital and therefore with more severe disease (Yurdakul *et al.* 1988).

In a syndrome associated with an HLA allele, one would expect a more pronounced familial occurrence than one ordinarily sees in Behçet's syndrome. In general there is no consistent inheritance pattern (Bird Stewart 1986). We have seen two monozygotic brothers concordant for the syndrome (Hamuryudan *et al.* 1991a). There is also an increased prevalence of lymphocytotoxic antibodies among the healthy children of patients with Behçet's syndrome (Günaydın *et al.* 1992).

Clinical features
Skin and mucosal involvement

Oral aphthae (Fig. 1)

These are almost always present. However, 1 to 3 per cent of patients can have several of the other features of the syndrome without ever having aphthae. Aphthae are frequently the first manifestation of the syndrome. It is not uncommon for some patients to have only aphthae for many years before other features appear. The majority of oral ulcers in Behçet's syndrome are indistinguishable from those seen in recurrent oral ulceration, but tend to be multiple and occur more frequently. Large (major) ulcers are less frequent and herpetiform

ulcers are rare. Major ulcers, however, can be very troublesome because they heal with scarring, which can even occlude the oropharynx. The minor ulcers do not as a rule leave scars. The histology reveals non-specific ulceration with necrotic material. There is evidence of vasculitis with an increase in mast cells.

Genital ulceration (Fig. 2)

In the male, 90 per cent of the genital ulcers occur on the scrotum and almost always leave scars. They are less frequent on the shaft and on the glans penis. Urethritis is not observed unless there is an associated meatal ulcer.

In the female the labia (major and minor) are affected commonly. Ulcers are less frequent in the more proximal part of the genital tract and cervical lesions are rarely seen. Histologically, they are indistinguishable from oral aphthae.

Skin lesions (Fig. 3)

The skin lesions of Behçet's syndrome can be divided into three main types: (i) nodular lesions resembling erythema nodosum, (ii) papulopustular lesions also called acneiform or simply acne, (iii) others (palpable purpura, ulcerations, Sweet's syndrome, etc.) all representing various forms of vasculitis. The lesions resembling erythema

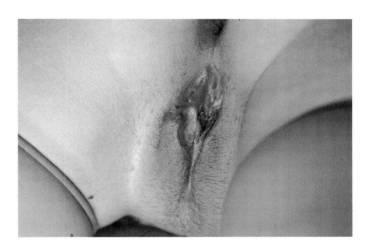

Fig. 2 Fresh genital ulceration.

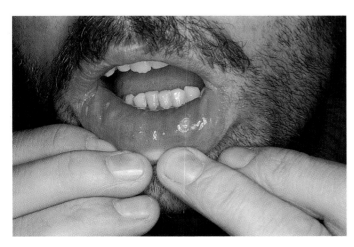

Fig. 1 Oral aphthae.

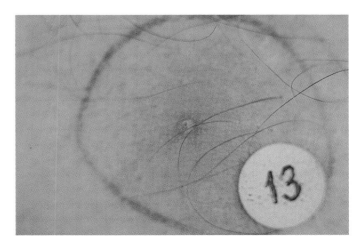

Fig. 3 The pathergy reaction in the form of a pustule.

nodosum are similar to idiopathic erythema nodosum and those due to other conditions (e.g. sarcoidosis). Their tendency to leave a pigmented area after the acute period is a somewhat distinguishing feature, and one which is explained by the erythrodiapedesis observed histologically. Sometimes superficial thrombophlebitis can be clinically indistinguishable from erythema nodosum. The papulo-pustular lesions, when present in intertrigenous areas like axillae and the inguinal folds, tend to erode and ulcerate. Most papulopustular lesions are histologically very similar to ordinary acne. However, they differ from the latter in their propensity to occur also in the extremities. The other forms of skin lesions are leucocytoclastic vasculitis, necrotizing arteritis of the small and medium arteries, superficial thrombophlebitis, and unclassifiable papules and pustules (Azizlerli *et al.* 1992). Painful papules, which histologically show a neutrophilic infiltration of the skin without fibrinoid necrosis (Sweet's syndrome) are also seen (Lakhanpal *et al.* 1988).

The pathergy reaction (Fig. 3), a curious hyperreactivity of the skin to a needle prick, is peculiar to this syndrome (Gilhar *et al.* 1989). The only other condition in which it is known to be positive with any consistency is pyoderma gangrenosum. After a skin puncture with a needle a papule or a pustule forms in 24 to 48 h.

There is some debate as to the true prevalence of this reaction. It is seldom found among patients in Northern Europe or the United States. In patients from Japan and Turkey it is positive in around 60 to 70 per cent when tested repetitively. It is, however, possible that its prevalence may be decreasing in recent years (Dilşen *et al.* 1993). Whether this is a matter of patient selection, the recent use of disposable needles, or a true decline in prevalence is a matter of debate.

The mechanism of the pathergy reaction is still obscure. Surgical cleaning of the skin considerably dampens this reaction (Fresko *et al.* 1993), which suggests that more than disrupting the integrity of the epidermis and dermis is required.

The reaction shows an initial accumulation of neutrophils followed by mast cells and mononuclear cells. The pathergy phenomenon in Behçet's syndrome is not confined to the skin: various tissues are known to be hyperreactive to surgical trauma, and it is not uncommon to have attacks of uveitis after eye surgery and synovitis after an arthrocentesis.

The propensity for inflammation in Behçet's syndrome can also be observed in the response these patients have to intradermal injections of sodium monourate crystals (Çakır *et al.* 1991). Patients with Behçet's syndrome have an augmented response to these crystals and it is interesting to note that British patients show a similar heightened response even though they are, as noted above, generally pathergy negative.

Eye involvement (Fig. 4)

This is one of the most serious manifestations. Males and those with younger age of onset, i.e. less than 25 years of age, have an increased prevalence. While the overall prevalence is about 50 per cent, in the younger male it is approximately 70 per cent. Females are affected less severely. Disease is bilateral in 90 per cent of the patients with ocular involvement. The onset of eye disease is usually within 2 to 3 years of the development of the syndrome.

Eye disease in Behçet's syndrome consists of a chronic relapsing posterior and anterior uveitis. Isolated anterior uveitis is found in only 10 per cent of those with ocular involvement. Conjunctivitis is rare. Occasionally episcleritis and conjunctival ulceration are seen.

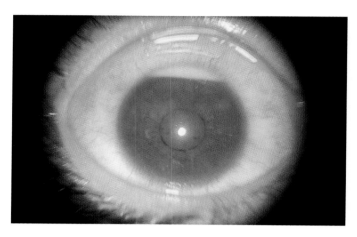

Fig. 4　Hypopyon uveitis.

Hypopyon uveitis (Fig. 4) is very typical of Behçet's syndrome, although occasionally it can be observed in Reiter's syndrome. It is an accumulation of white cells and debris in the anterior chamber that precipitates to form a layer due to gravity. Hypopyon is seen in 20 per cent of patients with eye disease and as rule is almost always associated with severe retinal disease.

The basic retinal lesion is a vasculitis, which can lead to exudates, haemorrhages, venous thrombosis, papilloedema, and macular disease that frequently results in a hole. The pars plana is also involved. During an acute flare there is a marked influx of fibrin, inflammatory cells, and cellular debris into the vitreous. After each flare there is usually some residual structural damage in the form of retinal changes, vitreal opacities, posterior synechiae, and cataracts. Secondary glaucoma frequently develops. The extent of these structural changes determinates the course of eye disease in Behçet's syndrome.

Musculoskeletal system

Behçet himself, as early as 1938, described 'rheumatoid' involvement in Behçet's syndrome. It can occasionally be the initial manifestation. Involvement of the joints (Table 2) is seen in about one-half of the

Table 2　Features of arthritis in Behçet's syndrome

Seen in 50 per cent of the patients either as arthritis or arthralgia

Non-deforming and short lasting (few weeks)

Knees, ankles, wrists, and elbows are involved most commonly

Sacroiliac joint involvement is not prevalent in controlled studies

Usually mono- or oligoarticular but can be symmetrical with a potential for confusion with rheumatoid arthritis

Synovial fluid is commonly inflammatory but a good mucin clot is usual

Synovial histology is non-diagnostic; paucity of plasma cells and superficial-layer ulceration are the most outstanding features

Aseptic necrosis of the bone not related to steroid use can be seen patients in the form of arthritis or arthralgia (Yurdakul *et al.* 1983). It is mono- or oligoarticular but can be symmetrical. It is quite common to have symmetrical disease of the wrist or elbow, which can be confused with rheumatoid arthritis. Usually lasting a few weeks it seldom leads to deformity. Erythema of the overlying skin is not seen. Erosions are uncommon. Chronic synovitis lasting months to years with deformity and erosions are seen, but rare. The synovial fluid is inflammatory (see below). The histological changes are non-specific.

Knees are the most commonly affected joints, followed in frequency by ankles, wrists, and elbows. There has been much debate about the involvement of the sacroiliac joints in Behçet's syndrome, but an increased prevalence has not been found in controlled studies. Furthermore there is considerable interobserver variation in interpretation of the sacroiliac joint on a plain radiograph of the pelvis (Yazıcı *et al.* 1987a). Regardless of the presence or absence of involvement of this joint, back pain is quite rare in Behçet's syndrome. The main debate about sacroiliac involvement centres around the erroneous inclusion of Behçet's syndrome among the seronegative spondylarthropathies (Moll *et al.* 1974). Other reasons why Behçet's syndrome is not a spondylarthritis include the lack of familial association with the spectrum of spondylarthritides, the association with HLA B51 and, most importantly, the presence of widespread vasculitis. In addition, the nature of the 'shared' clinical features in Behçet's syndrome is very different from that in this group of diseases. The genital ulceration is usually scrotal, urogenital infection is absent, nail changes are not seen, and the nature and course of eye involvement are totally different (Yazıcı 1987).

Myositis is occasionally found in Behçet's syndrome. It is usually local but generalized forms can also be seen. The muscle enzymes are not raised in the local forms and the histological features are indistinguishable from those of polymyositis.

Another musculoskletal manifestation associated with Behçet's syndrome is aseptic necrosis of the bone. This is possibly related to vasculitis and not necessarily to steroid use.

Neurological involvement (Fig. 5)

There is much variation in the reported prevalence rates of neurological involvement. In a prospective survey a prevalence rate of 5 per cent was found (Serdaroğlu *et al.* 1989). Pyramidal signs are the most common, followed by cerebellar and sensory symptoms and signs. Symptoms of increased intracranial pressure and meningeal irritation are also observed. Dementia can develop in an occasional patient. In the majority of the cases, headaches can be related to the basic pathology only if there are other associated signs and symptoms in the central nervous system. Papilloedema usually indicates occlusion of a venous sinus (Wechsler *et al.* 1992). As is true with eye involvement, the most severe forms of central nervous involvement are seen in the male.

The findings in cerebrospinal fluid are non-specific. Opening pressures and protein content are usually increased. Pleocytosis is present. Glucose can be low. Computed tomographic scans are of limited value unless localizing symptoms are present. Magnetic resonance imaging may prove to be more sensitive and specific.

The most common site of involvement is the brainstem. Hemispheric, meningeal, and spinal cord lesions are also seen. In contrast to the other vasculitides, peripheral nerve disease is unusual.

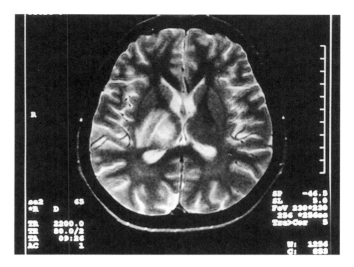

Fig. 5 Involvement of the central nervous system (T_2-weighted MRI showing a hyperintense lesion in the right thalamus, capsula interna, and nucleus lentiformis in a 28-year-old male patient).

The histological appearances of the central nervous lesions in Behçet's syndrome are non-specific. There are inflammatory and degenerative changes. Frank vasculitis is not seen. The usual vascular change is a perivascular infiltration, sometimes with perivascular lamellar fibrosis. Microabscesses can also be observed.

Some patients develop psychiatric problems. Reliable prevalence rates are lacking. As in systemic lupus some of the psychiatric problems in Behçet's syndrome may be the result of a situational response to a chronic disease and occasionally of steroid use.

Cardiovascular and pulmonary involvement

Cardiac involvement

Endocarditis, myocarditis, and pericarditis can all occur but are rare. Cases with coronary vasculitis and ventricular aneurysms have also been documented. In a prospective controlled survey among 64 patients we failed to find an increased prevalence of cardiac disease (Özkan *et al.* 1992).

Venous lesions

Involvement of the veins is one of the main manifestations of Behçet's syndrome. In fact, Behçet's syndrome, together with systemic lupus and Buerger's disease, is one of the few vasculitides that can involve the venous side of the circulatory system together with the arterial side. Furthermore, in contrast to the other two, it can involve the vena cavae.

Thrombophlebitis occurs in 25 per cent of all patients. More frequent in the calf, it is also seen in veins of the upper extremity. There is a propensity to develop venous thromboses after venepunctures. A frequent outcome of thrombosis in the lower extremities is dermatitis of chronic stasis associated with recurring skin ulcers. Thrombosis of the iliac veins and both vena cavae is less frequent and seen almost only in male patients. This is usually less associated with the formation of collateral vessels. Occlusion of the suprahepatic veins can cause a Budd–Chiari syndrome, which carries a high mortality.

In the common variety of thrombophlebitis, for example of the pelvic veins in the postoperative state, only a short segment of the vessel wall is diseased. The thrombus is adherent to the wall at this site and has a long, non-adherent tail. This is not so in Behçet's syndrome. Here large segments of the vessel wall are diseased and consequently the thrombus formed is adherent to the wall at all places. Sometimes the entire length of the inferior vena cava is thus affected. This explains, we believe, why pulmonary embolism is rare in Behçet's syndrome even though thrombophlebitis is seen in one-quarter of the patients.

Arterial lesions (Figs 6 and 7)

Starting with the aorta, all the arterial tree can be afflicted (Hamza 1987; Koç *et al.* 1992). Aneurysms of the abdominal aorta, carotid, femoral, popliteal, and less commonly coronary arteries can be seen (Fig. 6). The rupture of these aneurysms is frequently fatal. The basic pathology is thought to be a vasculitis of the vasa vasorum. There is a high recurrence rate after reconstructive surgery of the aneurysms of the peripheral vessels. This complication is thought to be related to the pathergy phenomenon.

The basic pulmonary pathology in Behçet's syndrome is also related to vasculitis. Pulmonary vascular changes in the form of arterial aneurysms, arterial and venous thromboses, and pulmonary infarcts are found (Efthimiou *et al.* 1986; Hamuryudan *et al.* 1994a). The classic radiographic finding is the non-cavitating mass lesion (Fig. 7). Computed tomographic scans are usually adequate for diagnosis.

Pulmonary arterial aneurysms in Behçet's syndrome carry a grave prognosis. Among our patients the mortality was 50 per cent despite treatment, the terminal event usually being the rupture of an aneurysm into a bronchus.

Pleural effusions are seldom in Behçet's syndrome. They may be associated with the pulmonary vascular disease or may be present independently.

Gastrointestinal involvement

While gastrointestinal involvement is seen in about one-third of patients from Japan (Shimizu *et al.* 1979), it is quite rare among patients reported from the Mediterranean basin. The basic pathology is that of mucosal ulceration. This is seen most commonly in the ileum, followed by the caecum and other parts of the colon. Occasionally oesophageal ulceration can occur. Histologically the ulcers are indistinguishable from those found in ulcerative colitis. Intestinal lymphangiectasia have also been reported. The course of intestinal Behçet's syndrome is that of exacerbations and remissions. The usual symptoms are abdominal pain and melaena. A mass is often palpable in the abdomen. The ileocaecal ulcers have the worst prognosis, with a distinct tendency to perforate.

Hepatic problems are not common in Behçet's syndrome except when an associated Budd–Chiari syndrome is present. A slightly enlarged spleen is noticed in 20 per cent of the male patients (Soysal *et al.* 1990), not necessarily related to portal hypertension secondary to venous thrombosis.

Other clinical features

Renal involvement is seen much less frequently than one would expect in a systemic vasculitis. There are occasional reports of

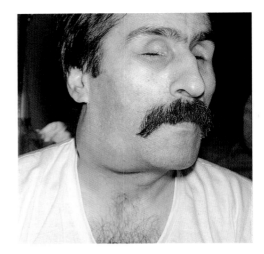

Fig. 6 Carotid artery aneurysm.

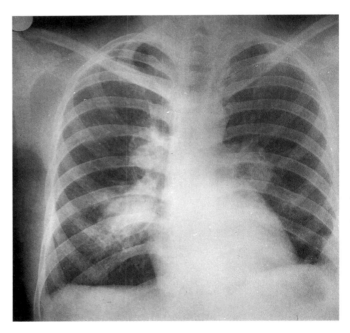

Fig. 7 Pulmonary artery aneurysms.

glomerulonephritis (Hamuryudan *et al.* 1991b). Epididymitis is seen around 5 per cent of the patients.

Amyloidosis is seen sporadically and when present usually presents with a nephrotic syndrome. It is of the AA type and carries a grave prognosis. In a rectal biopsy survey of non-symptomatic patients without any proteinuria, no cases of silent amyloidosis could be identified (Yurdakul *et al.* 1990).

Diagnosis

The full-blown syndrome is easy to identify; the so-called incomplete forms sometimes cause problems. Reiter's and Stevens–Johnson syndromes can also be problems in differential diagnosis for the uninitiated. However, an occasional patient with inflammatory bowel disease associated with oral ulcers, skin lesions, and episcleritis may be impossible to differentiate from Behçet's syndrome. Another difficult aspect is a patient with multiple sclerosis with one or two features of Behçet's syndrome.

Many criteria have been proposed to diagnose Behçet's syndrome. Recently a set of classification criteria have been proposed by a computer analysis of clinical features of 914 cases collected around the globe (International Study Group for Behçet's Disease 1990). Diseased controls with features that may be confused with Behçet's syndrome were also included in the analysis. Using the presence of recurrent aphthous ulceration as mandatory, together with proper exclusions, these criteria require involvement of two other organ systems. In this scheme a positive pathergy test can replace involvement of an organ system.

Laboratory investigations

There are no laboratory findings specific for Behçet's syndrome. A moderate anaemia of chronic disease and leucocytosis are seen in 15 per cent of the patients. Neither reflects the clinical activity. The erythrocyte sedimentation rate is only mildly elevated, as is the C-reactive protein. Again neither correlates well with disease activity (Müftüoğlu et al. 1986).

The synovial fluid is usually inflammatory. The cell count is between 5 000 and 50 000/mm³ with neutrophils predominating. Despite this high cell count the mucin clot is usually good (Yurdakul et al. 1983).

Serum immunoglobulins are sometimes elevated, while autoantibodies are absent. Complement levels may be high. Despite the pauci-immune nature of the basic disease process, antineutrophilic antibodies are not a feature of Behçet's syndrome.

Pathogenesis

The prevailing opinion is that Behçet's syndrome is caused by a defect in immunoregulation and this defect in turn is triggered by an infectious agent(s) (Lehner et al. 1991). Among the candidates for the infectious agents are herpes simplex type 1 (Denman et al. 1980; Eglin et al. 1982) and some strains of streptococcus (Mizushima et al. 1988). Microbial and human heat shock proteins (HSP) show marked amino acid homology. Behçet's syndrome patients have both lymphocytes and antibodies which recognize certain synthetic peptides derived from mycobacterial HSP. Likewise a similar recognition exists to human mitochondrial HSP peptides that are homologous to mycobacterium HSP peptides. Finally these peptides are uveitogenic in rats (Stanford et al. 1994). These observations indicate that multiple agents, through molecular mimicry of their HSP peptides to the human tissues, can initiate an immune response and organ disease in Behçet's syndrome.

The evidence for immunological aberration is abundant (Arbesfeld and Kurban 1988). Antibodies to oral mucosa, circulating immune complexes, lymphocytotoxins in serum, a decrease in the OKT4:OKT8 ratio and in natural killer cells during disease exacerbations are among these. Increased levels of soluble interleukin-2 receptors, a common finding in autoimmune disease, also occur in Behçet's syndrome (Hamzoui and Ayed 1989). There is also an increased in vivo accumulation of activated lymphocytes expressing γ T-cell receptors at the sites of inflammation (Hamzoui et al. 1994).

In contrast, the lack of autoantibodies, the rarity of associated Sjögren's syndrome (Günaydın et al. 1994), the lack of association with other autoimmune diseases both among the patients and their relatives, the rather poor response to steroids, and finally the more severe disease expression among males are points against an autoimmune mechanism in Behçet's syndrome (Yazıcı 1987).

The heightened inflammatory response, best manifested by the pathergy reaction (Tüzün et al. 1979), prompted research into leucocyte activity. Polymorphonuclear leucocyte activity is certainly increased (Matsumura and Mizushima 1975). A transgenic mice model has also been developed which attempts to provide an explanation for this heightened inflammatory activity (Takeno et al. 1995).

The widespread vascular disease in Behçet's syndrome has justifiably turned attention to endothelial pathology, and the increase in thromboses to problems with coagulation. Increased levels of factor VIII-related antigen are found only in patients with major (i.e. pulmonary artery and its branches; vena cavae) involvement of vessels (Yazıcı et al. 1987b). There is also a defect in prostacyclin production from the vessel wall (Kansu et al. 1986). Two other stigmas of endothelial injury in this syndrome are the presence of the antiendothelial cell antibodies (Aydıntuğ et al. 1993) and increased serum levels of endothelin (Koç et al. 1993). Both observations might obviously be secondary events. Fibrinolytic activity is defective in Behçet's syndrome (Hampton et al. 1991). However, no single abnormality has been shown to account for this. The initial reports of increased levels of antiphospholipid antibodies have not been confirmed in subsequent studies.

Any theory that tries to explain the pathogenesis of Behçet's syndrome should also take into consideration the reasons for the more severe disease seen in the male and the young (Yazıcı et al. 1984). The pathergy reaction is also more strongly positive in the male (Yazıcı et al. 1985). This brings sex hormones into consideration. Serum concentrations of the major sex hormones are normal among the patients; however, this does not negate a possible influence of hormonal effects via metabolic products or alterations of end-organ responsiveness. In this respect the so-called acneiform skin lesion of Behçet's syndrome is clinically and histologically indistinguishable from ordinary acne, an androgen-dependent lesion.

Management (Yazıcı et al. 1995)

There are several important features of Behçet's syndrome that have to be taken into consideration when planning the management: (i) the usual course of the syndrome in any organ system is that of exacerbations and remissions with the overall activity generally abating with the passage of time; thus the principal aim is to prevent irreversible structural damage, which is the outcome of the early stormy course; (ii) being young and male are separate and additive negative prognostic factors; (iii) eye disease usually occurs, if at all, either initially or within the first few years; (iv) the syndrome can be fatal, especially in the young male; and (v) there are many patients with Behçet's syndrome who do not need any treatment but reassurance. Box 1 contains a scheme for the treatment of Behçet's syndrome.

Immunosuppressive drugs are the main line of treatment for eye involvement. Although corticosteroids have been used for a long time, there is no formal evidence that they are effective. In fact there is suspicion that they may be harmful. Their short-term use over a few months, however, may shorten the duration of an attack. Large centres treating Behçet's syndrome are now using steroids less frequently.

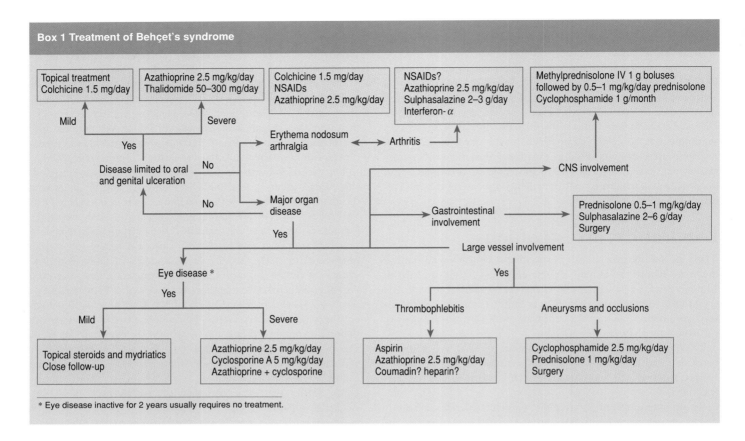

Box 1 Treatment of Behçet's syndrome

* Eye disease inactive for 2 years usually requires no treatment.

In the only controlled, double-blind study of cytotoxic immuno-suppressive agents, azathioprine at 2.5 mg/kg per day was shown to be superior to placebo in maintaining visual acuity and perhaps more importantly in preventing the emergence of new eye disease (Yazıcı et al. 1990). It was not useful in restoring the already compromised vision. It would be unrealistic to expect restoration of impaired visual acuity when this is due to structural changes like synechiae. Thus it is important that treatment is begun well before these changes appear. Other cytotoxic, immunosuppressive agents such as chlorambucil and cyclophosphamide are also used, and extrapolating from the controlled experience with azathioprine their use is justified (O'Duffy 1990).

Cyclosporin is an effective and rapidly acting drug in the uveitis of Behçet's syndrome (Masuda et al. 1989). Problems with cyclosporin are the potential nephrotoxicity, especially at doses greater than 5 mg/kg per day, and the very frequent relapses after cessation of therapy. The high cost is another problem. Eye disease in remission for 2 years or more needs no further treatment. Young males usually need to be treated more vigorously. Once initiated, the usual course for cytotoxic or cyclosporin therapy is a minimum of 2 years, after which attempts at discontinuation are made. In some patients, after a course for 6 to 8 months of combined azathioprine and cyclosporin, treatment is continued with azathioprine only. In more resistant cases azathioprine is used in combination with cyclosporin (both at conventional doses) for extended periods of time. Our uncontrolled experience with this mode of therapy in severe eye disease is quite favourable.

Structural damage to the eye can be managed surgically (i.e. vitrectomy) at specialized centres. However, the results are not

uniformly satisfactory. There is always the problem of new attacks of inflammation in surgically handled tissue in Behçet's syndrome. Also the already established disease in the retina can not be helped by surgery. Local mydriatics should be used in the acute stage to prevent synechiae.

The oral and genital ulcers are usually well controlled by immunosuppressives and steroids. However, these should be reserved for more severe cases. Most of the time, a local steroid preparation that adheres to fresh ulceration (such as triamcinolone acetonide oral paste) is all that is required. Thalidomide in doses ranging from 50 mg on 3 nights a week to 300 mg daily seems to be highly effective in the treatment of the orogenital ulcers of Behçet's syndrome. Limitations for its use are teratogenicity and peripheral neuropathy. The incidence and relationship of the neuropathy to the dose used is a matter of debate (Denman et al. 1993).

Colchicine has been claimed to be beneficial for almost every manifestation of Behçet's syndrome, but without any formal trials. The rationale for its use is the increased chemotaxis of the polymorphonuclear leucocytes found in this syndrome. In the only controlled study with colchicine it was superior to placebo only in the treatment of erythema nodosum and arthralgias (Aktulga et al. 1980). When started the usual practice is to use the colchicine for several years.

Cyclophosphamide, either 2 to 2.5 mg/kg per day orally or 500 to 1500 mg weekly or monthly intravenous boluses, is required to treat those patients with severe cutaneous, arterial, or pulmonary vasculitis or those with arterial aneurysms or vena caval involvement. There is no formal experience with any therapy for central nervous disease; however, steroids and immunosuppressives are again used. Steroids are usually employed in the form of pulsed intravenous

Table 3 Other significant symptoms and findings in Kawasaki disease
The cardiovascular system: heart murmurs, gallop rhythm, ECG changes, cardiomegaly, two-dimensional echo findings of pericardial effusion, coronary artery aneurysms, aneurysms of peripheral arteries, angina pectoris and myocardial infarction
The gastro-intestinal tract: diarrhoea, vomiting, abdominal pain, hydrops of the gallbladder, ileus and jaundice
The blood: leucocytosis, thrombocytosis, increased erythrocyte sedimentation rate, increased C reactive protein, hypo-albuminaemia, and anaemia
The urine: proteinuria, increased leucocytes in sediment
The skin: transverse furrows of finger nails
The respiratory tract: cough and rhinorrhoea
The joints: pain and swelling
The neurological system: pleocytosis in cerebrospinal fluid, convulsions and facial palsy

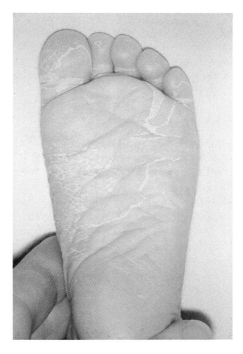

Fig. 4 Kawasaki disease showing membranous desquamation of skin of the foot in convalascent phase.

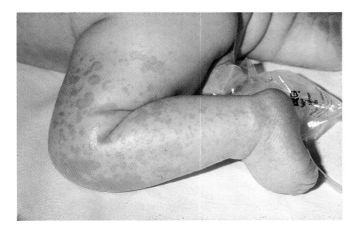

Fig. 3 Kawasaki disease showing characteristic rash, redness of the sole and oedema of the dorsum of the foot.

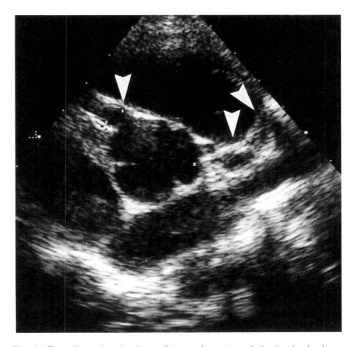

Fig. 5 Two-dimensional echocardiogram (parasternal short-axis view) showing medium-sized aneurysm (6.8 mm) of right coronary artery and smaller aneurysms of left main and left arterior descending coronary arteries (arrows) in child with Kawasaki disease.

Laboratory investigations

In patients with Kawasaki disease a polymorphonuclear leucocytosis and thrombocytosis is seen and circulating platelet-aggregating factors and immune complexes are demonstrable (Levin *et al.* 1985). Both ANCA and anti-endothelial cell antibodies (AECA) have also been determined in acute sera from patients (Leung *et al.* 1986; Savage *et al.* 1989; Tizard *et al.* 1991c; Kaneko *et al.* 1994). The ANCA findings on immunofluorescence were thought to be characteristic with a diffuse cytoplasmic staining and possibly distinct antigens involved (Kaneko *et al.* 1993). However, the diagnostic value of ANCA and AECA in Kawasaki disease has recently been questioned (Guzman *et al.* 1994; Nash *et al.* 1995) in studies showing that these antibodies did not differentiate early Kawasaki disease from other childhood illnesses.

Aetiology

Most workers agree that Kawasaki disease is likely to have an infective basis but the nature of the infective agent and the mechanisms involved remain in doubt. A number of organisms have been considered including *Streptococcus sanguis*, *Propionibacterium acnes*,

Epstein–Barr virus, human herpes virus 6, chlamydia, rickettsia and retroviruses (Shulman 1987; Kawasaki 1989; Takahashi and Taubert 1993). Presently there has been considerable interest in the possibility that the condition is caused by new clones of staphylococci that cause toxic shock syndrome or streptococci that produce pyrogenic exotoxin (Leung *et al.* 1993).

Treatment and prognosis

Therapeutically aspirin and high-dose intravenous gammaglobulin, either as four or five daily doses of 400 mg/kg per day (Newburger *et al.* 1986) or one dose of 2 g/kg (Newburger *et al.* 1991), are recommended. Dipyridamole has also been used by some groups in addition to aspirin. When giant coronary artery aneurysms are present, especially with evidence of ischaemia, intravenous prostacyclin has been utilized (Tizard *et al.* 1991b) and intra-arterial or intravenous urokinase has been advocated in circumstances of coronary artery occlusion with thrombus (Terai *et al.* 1985). Revascularization surgery of the coronary arteries may be indicated for stenotic lesions after the acute phase of the illness is over (Susuki *et al.* 1985). The use of steroids remains controversial. There has been a policy contraindicating their use because of increased risks of coronary artery complications compared with aspirin, but this may need to be reconsidered since they certainly have been of value, given with antiplatelet therapy, in children with severe disease who do not respond to gammaglobulin treatment at The Hospital for Sick Children in London.

The overall outlook for children with Kawasaki disease is good. A 1 to 2 per cent acute mortality rate from myocardial infarction has been reduced further in many countries by alertness of clinicians to the diagnosis and early use of gammaglobulin with antiplatelet therapy. Nonetheless, there is a late morbidity and occasional mortality caused by stenotic lesions of coronary arteries in later life and it has been postulated that adult atheromatous coronary disease in some cases may have its origins in childhood and be due to covert or overt Kawasaki disease (Brecker *et al.* 1988).

Wegener's granulomatosis

Wegener's granulomatosis (Wegener 1936) is a necrotizing granulomatous vasculitis of the upper and lower respiratory tract, associated with glomerulonephritis and variable degrees of small vessel vasculitis elsewhere. It can be a generalized disorder or present in a limited local form, involving, initially at least, the respiratory tract. It is rare in childhood but has been reported (Moorthy *et al.* 1977; Baliga *et al.* 1978; Orlowski *et al.* 1978; Halstead *et al.* 1986; Dillon 1990; Singer *et al.* 1990; Rottem *et al.* 1993) and the association with ANCA showing a cytoplasmic immunofluorescence appearance has created another means of diagnosis as well as a method of monitoring disease activity (Van der Woude *et al.* 1985; Savage *et al.* 1987).

Clinical and laboratory findings

Clinical manifestations are similar to those reported in polyarteritis nodosa. There are, however, particular features that might lead clinicians to the diagnosis including subglottic stenosis due to granulomatous involvement of the trachea (Fig. 6), at times requiring tracheostomy (Halstead *et al.* 1986; Dillon 1990; Tizard *et al.* 1991a; Rottem *et al.* 1993), and other upper airway findings such as sinus opacity, nasal septum disease and lower respiratory tract features

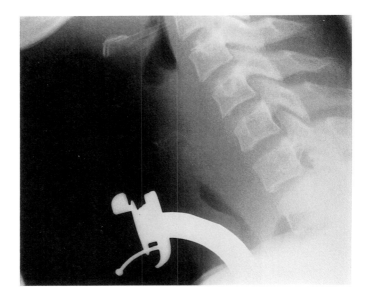

Fig. 6   Subglottic stenosis due to granulomatous involvement of the trachea in Wegener's granulomatosis. Note tracheostomy tube.

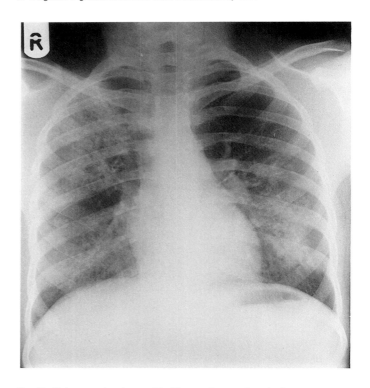

Fig. 7   Pulmonary involvement in Wegener's granulomatosis.

frequently masquerading as infection (Fig. 7). Some of these findings are also seen in relapsing polychondritis, an even rarer condition of childhood, which can cause diagnostic confusion (Blau 1976). Glomerulonephritis, at times taking the form of an aggressive crescentic glomerulonephritis, is seen but is not a prerequisite for the diagnosis. A proportion of children have disease that is limited to the upper and lower respiratory tract (Hall *et al.* 1985b; Rottem *et al.* 1993). Patients' serum usually contains circulating ANCA with the characteristic granular cytoplasmic distribution (C-ANCA) on indirect immunofluorescence and an antibody directed against proteinase 3 (Jennette and Falk 1990; Dillon and Tizard 1991; Gross et al. 1991; Wong et al. 1992).

Treatment and prognosis

Steroids and cyclophosphamide (orally or by pulsed intravenous injection) are the mainstays of treatment, but additionally some use antiplatelet medication and antimicrobials such as cotrimoxazole and, in life-threatening situations, plasma exchange (Gaskin and Pusey 1992; Roberti et al. 1993; Rottem et al. 1993). Response to therapy is variable but the majority of patients need to remain on long-term steroid and immunosuppressive agents. Once remission has been induced, it can be maintained in many children on a combination of steroid and azathioprine or cyclosporin (Dillon 1990; Gaskin and Pusey 1992). Mortality rate amongst The Hospital for Sick Children patients has been of the order of 15 per cent (Tizard et al. 1991a).

Churg–Strauss syndrome

Churg–Strauss syndrome or allergic granulomatosis is extremely rare in childhood (Churg and Straus 1951; Frayha 1982). The clinical picture consists of variable vasculitic features with asthma, eosinophilia, infiltrates on chest radiographs, and extravascular granulomata on biopsy (Chumbley et al. 1977). ANCA may be present with perinuclear or cytoplasmic staining on indirect immunofluorescence. Steroids are the mainstay of therapy but cytotoxic agents such as cyclophosphamide may need to be introduced to control disease activity (Chumbley et al. 1977; Roberti et al. 1993).

Henoch–Schönlein purpura (anaphylactoid purpura)

Henoch–Schönlein purpura is the most common form of systemic vasculitis of childhood and comes into the general category of leucocytoclastic vasculitides, involving small vessels especially in the skin (Gairdner 1948; Allen et al. 1960). Within this general group of conditions there is often an identifiable initiating factor such as a drug or a microorganism, hence the alternative descriptive terms of allergic or hypersensitivity vasculitis. Henoch–Schönlein purpura is chiefly a disease of childhood, more common in males, often preceded by an upper respiratory infection and more common in the winter months (Meadow et al. 1972; Levy et al. 1976).

Clinical characteristics

The salient features are a non-thrombocytopenic palpable purpura, arthritis or arthralgia, abdominal pain, gastrointestinal haemorrhage and glomerulonephritis. The palpable purpura is prominent on dependent and pressure-bearing areas such as the lower limbs and buttocks, but in young children facial involvement and subcutaneous oedema are features. Glomerulonephritis occurs in 50 per cent of patients and in 10 per cent of these it is serious (Kobayashi et al. 1977; Koskimies et al. 1974). The spectrum of renal disease varies from isolated microscopic haematuria to a nephritic/nephrotic syndrome with renal failure.

Laboratory investigations

The majority of affected children have a moderate leucocytosis and thrombocytosis. Thrombocytopenia would raise serious doubts about the diagnosis. Serum IgA and IgM are increased in 50 per cent of patients and a proportion have circulating IgA containing immune complexes and cryoglobulins (Trygstad and Stiehm 1971; Levinsky and Barratt 1979; Knight 1990). In some patients IgA ANCA have been demonstrated (Van den Wall Bake et al. 1987). Haematuria and proteinuria are found frequently. Renal function impairment, with or without hypertension in the presence of nephrotic range proteinuria, would be an indication for a renal biopsy. Histological examination of biopsy material may reveal proliferative glomerulonephritis of variable severity from focal segmental lesions to extensive crescentic glomerulonephritis. Immunofluorescence will often demonstrate mesangial IgA deposits and in some cases C3, fibrin, and IgM.

Treatment and prognosis

Treatment is supportive. Corticosteroids given over a few weeks may help severe gut disease but are not thought to benefit the renal disease except in the context of aggressive rapidly progressive glomerulonephritis when steroid, immunosuppressive and antiplatelet therapy have a therapeutic role. If renal function is rapidly deteriorating pulsed methyl prednisolone and/or plasmapheresis appear to have some beneficial effects.

The prognosis is usually good, but there is some morbidity and occasional mortality associated with gut and kidney disease (Allen et al. 1960). Amongst patients who present with a nephritic, nephrotic or nephritic/nephrotic syndrome, 44 per cent have hypertension or impaired renal function on long-term follow-up, whereas 82 per cent who present with haematuria (with or without proteinuria) are normal (Goldstein et al. 1992). Overall, 2 to 5 per cent of children with Henoch–Schönlein purpura progress to endstage renal failure accounting for approximately 10 per cent of renal failure in childhood (Kobayashi et al. 1977; Koskimies et al. 1981). Renal transplantation is possible and successful in such patients and recurrence in the graft rare.

Hypersensitivity angiitis

The commonest small vessel vasculitis other than Henoch–Schönlein purpura is hypersensitivity vasculitis. This is usually a drug-induced condition but can be associated with other antigens including infectious agents (Kunnamo et al. 1986). The predominant clinical manifestations involve the skin, with palpable nodules or purpura (Fig. 8), although other organs can be affected and it is important to realise that the condition can with time evolve into one of the systemic necrotizing vasculitides (Fauci et al. 1978). Removal of the precipitating agent is usually followed by resolution, but sometimes non-steroidal anti-inflammatory drugs and steroids may be indicated.

Cutaneous polyarteritis

This is another syndrome with some similarities to Henoch–Schönlein purpura with crops of painful skin nodules and livido reticularis often with a story of preceding upper respiratory tract infection (Diaz-Perez and Winklemann 1980; Fink 1991; David et al.

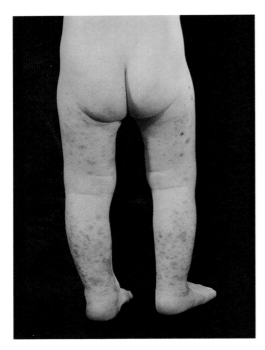

Fig. 8 Palpable purpuric nodules in skin of patient with hypersensitivity vasculitis.

1993). The condition responds to penicillin, non-steroidal anti-inflammatory drugs, and steroids. However, the concern is that the condition may be a manifestation of a systemic necrotizing vasculitis. Should this be the case, additional immunosuppressive therapy will be necessary. David *et al.* (1993) reported that all their patients had an erythematous, nodular, painful rash, often on the medial aspect of the feet, plus an evanescent arthritis affecting the knees and ankles. More than 50 per cent of patients also had brawny oedema of muscles and periorbital oedema. Two of their 12 patients went on to develop angiographically-confirmed polyarteritis nodosa (David *et al.* 1993). Cutaneous vasculitis usually runs a benign course, but relapses, particularly in association with recurrent streptococcal infection, are seen in up to 25 per cent of cases. Clinicians seeing this condition usually advise continuing penicillin prophylaxis throughout childhood to prevent relapses since it is amongst the relapsing group that systemic vasculitis tends to occur.

Vasculitis associated with autoimmune rheumatic disorders

Vasculitis is seen at times in systemic lupus erythematosus, juvenile chronic arthritis, mixed connective tissue disease, dermatomyositis and scleroderma and the concept that some of these disorders may be forms of systemic vasculitis has a degree of support. This is particularly relevant to juvenile dermatomyositis in which necrotizing vasculitis in arterioles, capillaries and venules of striated muscle, skin, subcutaneous tissue and gastrointestinal tract has been identified (Banker and Victor 1966; Dillon and Ansell 1995). Crowe *et al.* (1982) reported a group of children with dermatomyositis in which there was muscle infarction, lymphocytic vasculitis and a non-inflammatory vasculopathy associated with extensive erythematous and ulcerative cutaneous disease and who tended to develop calcinosis.

Clinically, within this group of patients, periungual erythema and telangiectasia of the nail beds are characteristic, as is telangiectasia along the eyelids which may be accompanied by oedema. Occlusive endarteropathy is likely to be responsible for the cutaneous lesions with ulceration and this, at times, occurs in a livido reticular pattern. Infarction of the palate is associated with weakening of palatal movement and retinal exudates can occur as a result of retinal vascular involvement. Vasculitis can cause acute gastrointestinal ulceration with bleeding or perforation and occasionally there can also be myocardial involvement. Therapeutically, bolus intravenous methylprednisolone is recommended for severe gastrointestinal involvement or vasculitic ulcers. Intravenous gammaglobulin may also have a role and plasma exchange has been utilized. Persistence of widespread ulceration in spite of therapy with severe changes in the capillary loops would be an indication for additional immunosuppressive therapy. Methotrexate in recalcitrant dermatomyositis has been generally accepted (Miller *et al.* 1992); however, there is relatively little information as to how effective it is in vasculitis. As with other vasculitides cyclophosphamide may prove effective when other regimens have failed.

Giant cell arteritis (Takayasu disease)

Giant cell arteritis (Takayasu disease) is a segmental inflammatory vasculitis causing stenosis and aneurysm formation in large arteries, especially the aorta and its major branches (Hall *et al.* 1985a). After Henoch–Schönlein purpura and Kawasaki disease it is the third commonest form of childhood vasculitis if considered worldwide (Lee *et al.* 1967; Wiggelinkhuizen and Cremin 1978). Its aetiology is unclear but genetic and infective factors, for example, tuberculosis, may play a part (Wiggelinkhuizen and Cremin 1978).

Clinical features and management

Early disease manifestations include fever, night sweats, anorexia, weight loss, and arthritis (Lupi-Herrera *et al.* 1977). Subsequently features of hypertension, heart failure and pulse deficits become apparent (Lee *et al.* 1967; Wiggelinkhuizen and Cremin 1978; Hall *et al.* 1985a). Leg length inequality can also occur as a result of the aortic pathology compromising lower limb blood supply (Morales *et al.* 1991). The erythrocyte sedimentation rate is increased as are other acute-phase reactants and there may be widening and calcification of the aorta on a plain abdominal radiograph. Doppler ultrasonography, plus magnetic resonance or standard angiography are usually required to establish the diagnosis (Southwood *et al.* 1988). Corticosteroids, plus other immunosuppressives, have been utilized therapeutically in the acute phase (Sunamori *et al.* 1976; Lupi-Herrera *et al.* 1977). A positive tuberculin test may justify antituberculous therapy and hypotensive agents and antiplatelet therapy also have a place. Reconstructive surgery and transluminal angioplasty have been undertaken in older children with inactive disease (Shelhamer *et al.* 1985).

Miscellaneous vasculitides

A number of other conditions in which there is a vasculitic component exist that are too numerous to deal with individually in this chapter. However, there are three that deserve special mention:

5.12 Overlap syndromes in adults and children

Enrique Roberto Soriano and Neil John McHugh

Introduction

Autoimmune rheumatic diseases (connective tissue diseases) are an overlapping group of disorders of unknown aetiology. Their classification depends on identifying clusters of clinical and laboratory features. At least three problems arise when attempting to classify individual patients into one of the defined autoimmune rheumatic diseases early on in their disease or when they present with clinical overlaps: (1) most of the clinical or laboratory features are not exclusive to one disease; (2) many of the symptoms and signs that define the autoimmune rheumatic diseases do not occur concurrently, but rather occur sequentially; (3) as many as 25 per cent of patients with autoimmune rheumatic disease present with an overlap syndrome with typical features of more than one disorder.

The terms undifferentiated connective tissue disease, overlap syndrome, and even mixed connective tissue disease (**MCTD**), have been used for patients who are not comfortably placed within any one of the defined autoimmune rheumatic diseases. These terms are not interchangeable, but unfortunately are often applied loosely. This chapter will describe some of the more common overlap conditions, and what is known concerning environmental triggers. Mixed connective tissue disease is discussed at some length reflecting the large proportion of studies in this area, although there is debate as to whether this disease is a distinct entity or a disease in evolution. Mention will be made of attempts to define more homogeneous subsets of autoimmune rheumatic disease by knowledge of immunogenetic and serological profiles.

Undifferentiated connective tissue disease

The diagnosis of undifferentiated connective tissue disease is best applied to those patients with features strongly suggestive of an autoimmune rheumatic disease but who do not fulfil criteria for any one disorder. The features usually include Raynaud's phenomenon, polyarthritis, rash, and myalgia (Alarcon *et al.* 1991). Undifferentiated connective tissue disease may develop into a well defined autoimmune rheumatic disease, may persist unchanged over time, or the symptoms may even disappear. Outcomes from large multicentre prospective studies are awaited (Alarcon *et al.* 1991). Raynaud's phenomenon is probably the most frequent clinical feature of undifferentiated connective tissue disease. Other factors that may be

---

Table 1	Possible prognostic factors in Raynaud's phenomenon

Scleroderma-like nailfold capillary abnormalities

Positive antinuclear antibody (titre > 1/100)

Anticentromere or antitopoisomerase 1 (Scl-70) antibody

Digital pitting scars

Abnormal erythrocyte sedimentation rate

Adapted from LeRoy and Medsger (1992).

predictive of the development of later autoimmune rheumatic disease are listed in Table 1.

Overlap syndrome

The term overlap syndrome has been used when two or more autoimmune rheumatic diseases, or some of their unique manifestations, occur in the same individual simultaneously. Features that are characteristic of certain defined autoimmune rheumatic diseases are given in Table 2. The overlap may consist of full expression of the features of two or more conditions, or more commonly may be limited to one or more manifestations of each disease. In the latter case, the diagnosis of undifferentiated connective tissue disease may equally apply.

Serological subsets

A characteristic feature of autoimmune rheumatic diseases is the presence of autoantibodies. As autoantibodies are associated with particular clinical features, knowledge of the autoantibody profile may help in diagnosis and prognosis. The best known example is the association of anti-U1RNP antibodies with mixed connective tissue disease which will be further discussed. Other examples include the association of anti-Ro (SS-A) and anti-La (SS-B) antibodies with Sjögren's syndrome, antiphospholipid antibodies with the antiphospholipid syndrome, and antibodies to tRNA synthetases with the antisynthetase syndrome. There are less common

Table 2 Features usually restricted to one conneective tissue disease, and less common in others

Systemic lupus erythematosus	Systemic sclerosis	Poly/dermatomyositis	Rheumatoid arthritis
Malar rash	Scleroderma	Myositis	Erosive arthritis
Photosensitivity	Oesophageal hypomobility	Heliotrope rash	Subcutaneous nodules
Glomerulonephritis		Gottron's papules	Rheumatoid factor
Central nervous system disease	Telangiectasia	Antisynthetase antibodies	
Anti-Sm antibodies		Anti-Mi-2 antibodies	
Anti-double-stranded DNA	Antitopoisomerase 1 antibodies		

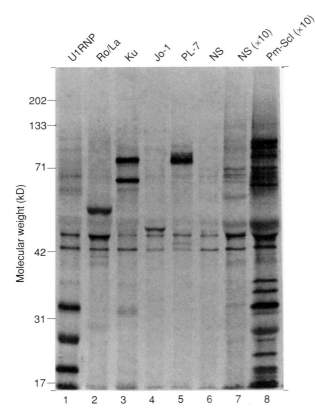

Fig. 1 Proteins immunoprecipitated using sera containing autoantibodies that are associated with overlap syndromes; anti-U1RNP with MCTD, anti-Ro/La antibodies with systemic lupus erythematosus (**SLE**)/Sjögren's syndrome, anti-Ku with systemic lupus erythematosus or scleroderma, anti-Jo-1 (histidyl-tRNA synthetase) and anti-PL-7 (threonyl- tRNA synthetase) with the antisynthetase syndrome, and anti-Pm-Scl with polymyositis/scleroderma/arthritis. NS, normal serum.

autoantibodies such as anti-Pm-Scl (Fig. 1) which may identify patients with other overlap features. Also, in most cases there are strong associations between autoantibody-defined subsets of disease and HLA genes that may explain the genetic basis for disease susceptibility (Table 3).

Mixed connective tissue disease

Definition

Mixed connective tissue disease was first described by Sharp and co-workers (Sharp *et al.* 1971; Sharp *et al.* 1972) as an 'apparently distinct rheumatic disease syndrome' in which the clinical characteristics included a combination of features similar to those of systemic lupus erythematosus, scleroderma, and polymyositis. The spectrum has been broadened by some to include features of rheumatoid arthritis (Hench *et al.* 1975; Sullivan *et al.* 1984). Mixed connective tissue disease was considered unique as it was associated with autoantibodies to a ribonuclease-sensitive component of extractable nuclear antigen, now known as U1RNP.

There remains debate as to whether mixed connective tissue disease is a distinct disease, a disease in evolution, or a subset of another autoimmune rheumatic disease such as systemic lupus erythematosus (LeRoy *et al.* 1980; Lazaro *et al.* 1989; McHugh *et al.* 1990; Black and Isenberg 1992). Diagnosis that is dependent on a single serological finding may suffer from ascertainment bias. Many patients with the clinical features 'characteristic' of mixed connective tissue disease do not have anti-U1RNP antibodies (Ginsburg *et al.* 1983; Lazaro *et al.* 1989), and conversely anti-U1RNP antibodies may appear in other conditions (McHugh *et al.* 1990). None the less, mixed connective tissue disease is considered by some to be a syndrome that has a core of manifestations associated with a serological marker (Alarcon-Segovia 1994). Three substantially revised and distinct sets of diagnostic criteria have been proposed (Table 4).

Epidemiology

Mixed connective tissue disease is a disease of the second to fourth decades of life with a mean age of onset of 35 years in adults (Sharp *et al.* 1972; Prakash *et al.* 1985), and 10 years in children (Singsen *et al.* 1977; Savouret *et al.* 1983). Women are affected more often than men at all ages, and represent around 80 per cent of patients. The incidence of mixed connective tissue disease in adults remains unknown. A hospital-based retrospective study of children under 15 in Sweden, reported an incidence of 0.13/100 000 per year, compared with an incidence of 0.43/100 000 per year for systemic lupus erythematosus and 0.28/100 00 per year for polymyositis/dermatomyositis (Magnusson 1993). In a nationwide, prospective, hospital-based

Table 3 Recognized clusters of clinical overlaps, autoantibodies, and HLA class II alleles

Overlap syndrome	Autoantibody specificity	HLA class II allele
Mixed connective tissue disease	U1RNP	HLA-DR4 (DRB1*0401) HLA-DQ3 (DQB1*0301) (Kuwana, et al. 1995)
Polymyositis, interstitial lung disease, Raynaud's, arthritis	Jo-1 (histidyl-tRNA synthetase) and less often other tRNA synthetases	HLA-DR3, DRw52 (Goldstein et al. 1990)
Systemic sclerosis, polymyositis	PM-Scl Ku U2-RNP	HLA-DR3 (Marguerie et al. 1992)

Table 4 Diagnostic criteria for mixed connective tissue disease (MCTD)

Sharp (1987)	Kasukawa et al. (1987)	Alarcon-Segovia et al. (1987)

Major criteria
1. Myositis, severe
2. Pulmonary invovement
  (a) CO diffusing capacity<%
  or
  (b) Pulmonary hypertension
  (c) Proliferative vascular lesions on biopsy
3. Raynaud's phenomenon or oesophageal hypomotility
4. Swollen hands
5. Highest observed anti-ENA> 1:10 000 and anti-U1RNP positive and anti-Sm negative
	I Common symptoms
	  1. Raynaud's phenomenon
	  2. Swollen fingers or hands
	
	II Anti-nRNP antibodies
	
	III Mixed findings
	  A. SLE-like findings
	    1. Polyarthritis
	    2. Lymphadenopathy
	    3. Facial erythema
	    4. Pericarditis or pleuritis
	    5. Leucocytopenia (<4000/mm^3) or thrombocytopenia (<100 000/mm^3)
	  B. PSS-like findings
	    1. Sclerodactyly
	    2. Pulmonary fibrosis, restrictive change of lung (% VC<80%) or reduced diffusion capacity (DLCO<70%)
	    3. Hypomobility or dilatation of oesophagus
	  C. PM-like findings
	    1. Muscle weakness
	    2. Increased serum level of myogenic enzymes (CPK)
	    3. Myogenic pattern in EMG
		1. Serological
		Positive anti-nRNP at a haemagglutination titre of 1:1600 or higher
		
		2. Clinical
		Oedema of hands
		Synovitis
		Myositis (laboratory or biopsy proven)
		Raynaud's phenomenon
		(2 or 3 colour phase)
		Acrosclerosis (with or without proximal scleroderma)

	Requirements for MCTD	
Definite=four majors	1. Positive in either one or two common symptoms 2. Positive anti-nRNP antibodies 3. Positive in one or more findings in two or three disease categories of A, B, and C	1. Serological 2. At least three clinical findings 3. Association of oedema of the hands, Raynaud's phenomenon, and acrosclerosis requires at least one of the other two criteria

PN, polymyositis; PSS, progressive systemic sclerosis; SLE, systemic lupus erythematosus

Table 5 Frequent clinical features in adults and children with mixed connective tissue disease

Feature	Adults (%)					Children (%)	
	Bennett and O'Connell (1980) (n=20)	Sullivan et al. (1984) (n=34)	Prakash et al. (1985) (n=81)	Kitridou et al. (1986) (n=30)	Haamenkorpi et al. (1993) (n=22)	Singsen et al. (1977) (n=14)	Tiddens et al. (1993) (n=14)
Raynaud's	75	91	79	83	100	78	93
Arthritis	100	85[b]	62	97	68	93	71
Swollen hands	75	85[b]	–	60	100	14	78
Sclerodactyly	20	85	54	60	23[e]	78	86
Myositis	35	79	48[c]	53	36	50	43
Oesophageal dysmotility	47	74	49[d]	60	43	678	–
Lymphadenopathy	50	50	26	17	–	50	14
Pleuritis	–	35	6	33	5	14	21
Renal[a]	20	26	–	40	14	50	7
Cardiac	35	26	–	–	–	64	21
Neurological	55	6	–	20	36	21	–

[a]Clinical and/or histological evidence of renal involvement;
[b]Swollen hands and sclerodactyly were considered together;
[c]Defined as muscle weakness; 44/55 patients had abnormal electromyograms;
[d]Only 39/81 patients were studied;
[e]Acrosclerosis;
[f]12/14 patients were studied.

study for 4 years in Finland in children aged 0 to 15 years, the annual incidence rate for mixed connective tissue disease (diagnosed according to Sharp's criteria) was 0.10/100 000 compared with 0.37 for systemic lupus erythematosus, 0.30 for polymyositis/dermato-myositis, and 0.05 for scleroderma (Pelkonen *et al.* 1994).

Clinical features (Table 5)

General symptoms

The typical patient is a 20- to 30-year-old female presenting with Raynaud's phenomenon, arthralgias/arthritis, swollen hands and/or puffy fingers, in association with a high titre, speckled pattern, anti-nuclear antibody (ANA) (Fig. 2). Other presenting symptoms may include fatigue, fever, serositis, mild myositis, aseptic meningitis or unexplained lymphadenopathy.

Vascular involvement

Raynaud's phenomenon is present in 75 to 100 per cent of adults and children (Table 5), and is often the first symptom to appear. Ischaemic necrosis and ulcerations of the fingertips are rare but may occur (Sharp *et al.* 1972; Gilliam and Prystowsky 1977; Peller *et al.* 1985). Nailfold capillaroscopy shows capillary dilatation and capillary loss (avascular areas) in 50 to 90 per cent of patients with mixed connec-tive tissue disease (Maricq *et al.* 1980; Peller *et al.* 1985; Granier *et al.* 1986) and may be associated with pulmonary disease (Sullivan *et al.*

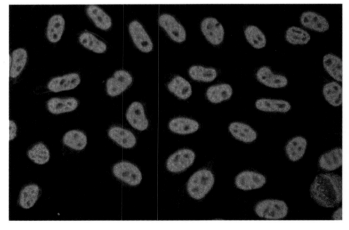

Fig. 2 Typical coarse speckled pattern of ANA detected by indirect immunofluorescence in serum from a patient with mixed connective tissue disease. Note the relative sparing of staining of the nucleolus within the cell nucleus.

1984; Pallis *et al.* 1991). Dystrophic, branched 'bushy' capillaries may be especially characteristic for mixed connective tissue disease (Granier *et al.* 1986). Angiographic studies have shown evidence of vasculopathy of both small and medium-sized vessels in the hands (Peller *et al.* 1985).

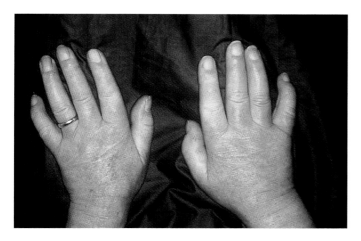

Fig. 3 Typical 'sausage-shaped' swollen fingers of a patient with mixed connective tissue disease.

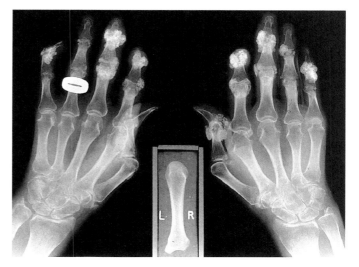

Fig. 4 Prominent periarticular calcification in a patient with mixed connective tissue disease.

Skin

Swelling of the hands, particularly of the fingers leading to a sausage appearance (Fig. 3), occurs more frequently in adults than in children. The skin of the hands may be taut and thick and histologically resembles scleroderma. Scleroderma extending more proximally is not usually a feature of mixed connective tissue disease. Other less frequent cutaneous manifestations are alopecia, depigmentation, telangiectasia, erythema nodosum, and chronic discoid lesions. A malar rash, suggestive of systemic lupus erythematosus, and dermatomyositis–like skin are more frequent in children than in adults.

Joints

Polyarthralgia is an early symptom and occurs in most patients. A symmetrical polyarthritis most often involving hands and wrists may mimic rheumatoid arthritis but is less deforming and erosive. None the less ulnar deviation, swan neck changes, and flexion contractures are not rare and atlantoaxial subluxation has been reported (Stuart and Maddison 1991). Erosions are found in about 60 per cent of the patients (Udoff *et al.* 1977; Bennett and O'Connell 1980; Catoggio *et al.* 1983), and are usually small, punched-out, and asymetrically distributed (O'Connell and Bennett 1977). Prominent periarticular calcification is not uncommon (Fig. 4) and arthritis induced by hydroxyapatite crystal has been reported (Hutton *et al.* 1988). Avascular necrosis of bone may occur in children (Tiddens *et al.* 1993) and adults (O'Connell and Bennett 1977). Minute, multiple peritendinous nodules may be found adjacent to the flexor tendons of the forearms and the extensor tendons of the hands (Babini *et al.* 1985). Arthritis may be more frequent and destructive in children in whom the initial diagnosis may be juvenile chronic arthritis.

Muscle

Myalgias are common and about two-thirds of patients develop an inflammatory myopathy that is identical clinically and histologically to polymyositis (Sharp *et al.* 1972; Bennett and O'Connell 1980). Very often myositis may occur acutely in a patient who has other mild features (Bennett and O'Connell 1980; Lundberg *et al.* 1992a), and prompts the diagnosis of mixed connective tissue disease. The prognosis seems more favourable than in polymyositis/dermatomyositis with less corticosteroid treatment needed (Nimelstein *et al.* 1980; Lundberg *et al.* 1992a). In children, vasculitis and inflammatory infiltration of skeletal muscle has been reported at autopsy, without clinical or laboratory evidence of muscle disease (Singsen *et al.* 1977).

Gastrointestinal tract

Gastrointestinal involvement is similar to that in systemic sclerosis, with heartburn and dysphagia the most common symptoms (Table 6). Oesophageal manometry is abnormal in up to 85 per cent of patients (Marshall *et al.* 1990; Doria *et al.* 1991). Corticosteroid treatment may improve oesophageal dysfunction (Marshall *et al.* 1990) but is needed rarely. Extensive gastrointestinal tract involvement with malabsorption (Norman and Fleischmann 1978), colonic and small bowel perforations due to vasculitis, acute pancreatitis (Marshall *et al.* 1990), duodenal haemorrhage (Hirose *et al.* 1993),

Table 6 Gastrointestinal symptoms in 61 patients with mixed connective tissue disease

Symptom	Number of patients	Frequency
Asymptomatic	16	26
Heartburn or regurgitation	29	48
Dysphagia	23	38
Dyspepsia	12	20
Diarrhoea	2	8
Constipation	3	5
Vomiting	2	3

Adapted from Marshall *et al.* (1990).

pneumatosis intestinalis and pneumoperitoneum (Bennett and O'Connell 1980; Pun *et al.* 1991), haemobilia due to vasculitis of the gallbladder (Kuipers *et al.* 1991), protein-losing enteropathy (Furuya *et al.* 1992), and secretory diarrhoea (Thiele and Krejs 1985) have all been reported. Hepatomegaly and splenomegaly are found in about 25 per cent of patients but major liver involvement is uncommon. The spectrum of gastrointestinal involvement is similar in children with mixed connective tissue disease.

Keratoconjunctivitis sicca

Sicca symptoms are not uncommon in adults and children with mixed connective tissue disease, depending on the bias of patients selected for study. Sialectasia was found in 82 per cent of 39 adults with mixed connective tissue disease studied by parotid sialography (Ohtsuka *et al.* 1992), although 50 per cent of these patients also fulfilled criteria for Sjögren's syndrome.

Neurological involvement

Trigeminal sensory neuropathy may occur in up to 10 per cent of patients and may be an early manifestation of the disease (Bennett *et al.* 1978; Searles *et al.* 1978; Sullivan *et al.* 1984; Hagen *et al.* 1990). Involvement of the central nervous system is rare in adults although an aseptic meningitis-like syndrome has been reported (Bennett and O'Connell 1980). Other occasional findings are headaches, seizures, peripheral neuropathy (Bennett *et al.* 1978), spinal cord involvement (Kappes and Bennett 1982), transverse myelitis (Weiss *et al.* 1978), hypertrophic cranial pachymeningitis (Fujimoto *et al.* 1993), and demyelination (Nitsche *et al.* 1991). Three of the 14 children reported by Singsen *et al.* had cerebral involvement (Singsen *et al.* 1977).

Heart

Major cardiovascular abnormalities are uncommon (Table 7). Pericarditis may occur in up to 20 per cent of patients and pericardial tamponade has been reported (Bennett and O'Connell 1980; Langley and Treadwell 1994). Electrocardiogram abnormalities are more common (Alpert *et al.* 1983; Oetgen *et al.* 1983),and cardiac conduction defects have been described (Emlen 1979; Rakovec *et al.* 1982). Echocardiographic changes including pericardial effusions, mitral valve prolapse, and right ventricle enlargement have been found in 38 to 60 per cent of patients (Alpert *et al.* 1983; Oetgen *et al.* 1983). Abnormal left ventricular diastolic filling has been documented by Doppler studies in the absence of myocardial disease (Leung *et al.* 1990). Intimal hyperplasia of coronary arteries and inflammatory cell infiltrates of the myocardium may be found in both adults and children (Singsen *et al.* 1977; Alpert *et al.* 1983).

Lungs

Pleuropulmonary involvement is common and may be clinically inapparent. The most common clinical findings are dyspnoea, pleuritic pain, and bibasilar rales (Table 8). Children may present with reduced exercise tolerance. Chest radiograph abnormalities include basal interstitial fibrosis, pleural effusion, pneumonic infiltrates, and pleural thickening (Sullivan *et al.* 1984; Prakash *et al.* 1985). Abnormalities of pulmonary function test are very common and may include a restrictive pattern, small airway involvement and respiratory muscle weakness (Izumiyama *et al.* 1993; Lazaro *et al.* 1993). Interstitial lung disease usually responds to corticosteroids but rapidly progressive cases have been reported (Weiner-Kronish *et al.* 1981).

Table 7 Cardiac involvement in adults with mixed connective tissue disease

Symptom	Alpert *et al.* (1983) (*n*=38) (%)	Oetgen *et al.* (1983) (*n*=16) (%)	Prakash *et al.* (1985) (*n*=81) (%)
Dyspnoea	63[a]	38[a]	16
Pericardial chest pain	6	19	7[b]
Angina pectoris	8	19	7[b]
Palpitations	16	25	–

[a]Dyspnoea could be attributed to pulmonary origin in all but one patient in each series.
[b]Cause of chest pain not stated.

Table 8 Pulmonary involvement in adults with mixed connective tissue disease

Feature	Sullivan *et al.* (1984) (*n*=34) (%)	Prakash *et al.* (1985) (*n*=81) (%)
Asymptomatic	33	75
Dyspnoea	58	16
Pleuritic pain	40	7
Bibasilar rales	42	–
Cough	24	5
Abnormal chest radiograph	30	21
Restrictive pulmonary function tests	41	69
Decreased diffusing capacity	72	69

Pulmonary hypertension is frequent in mixed connective tissue disease, may be difficult to detect and is a major cause of death (Table 9). The presence of scleroderma-type capillary changes on nailfold capillary microscopy may be predictive of the development of pulmonary hypertension (Sullivan *et al.* 1984). Anticardiolipin antibodies and/or a lupus anticoagulant may be more frequent in this group of patients (Hainaut *et al.* 1986; Miyata *et al.* 1992). Histological findings show proliferative vascular abnormalities resembling those found in the **CREST** (calcinosis, **R**aynaud's phenomenon, (o)esophageal dysmotility, sclerodactly, telangiectasia) syndrome. Patients with post-sternal pain, pulmonary diastolic

Table 9 Reported causes of death in mixed connective tissue disease		
Presumed cause of death	Death (*n*=31)	Frequency (%)
Pulmonary hypertension	11	35
Septicaemia	3	10
Sudden death	3	10
Myocardial infarction	2	6
Pulmonary embolus	1	3
Pulmonary vasculitis	1	3
Scleroderma-like renal crisis	1	3
Others, possibly unrelated	8	26
Unknown	2	6

Data taken from Bennett and O'Connell 1980, Nimelstein *et al.* 1980, Grant *et al.* 1981, Sullivan *et al.* 1984, Prakash *et al.* 1985, and Kitridou *et al.* 1986.

murmur, right ventricular hypertrophy on ECG, and higher mean pulmonary artery pressure have a poor prognosis (Kasukawa *et al.* 1990). Pulmonary hypertension seems less frequent in children.

Kidney

In their initial report Sharp *et al.* (1972) stressed the paucity of renal involvement but later reports have found a prevalence of up to 50 per cent in adults and children (Table 5, and Hench *et al.* 1975; Bennett and Spargo 1977; Grant *et al.* 1981). Nephrotic syndrome associated with membranous nephropathy is the most common presentation and may respond to high-dose corticosteroid therapy (Kitridou *et al.* 1986). The characteristic renal lesion is an immune- deposit nephritis. Renal crisis is a rare manifestation but should be suspected in a patient with accelerated hypertension as the treatment with angiotensin-converting enzyme inhibitor may be effective (Satoh *et al.* 1994). Glomerular and vascular deposition of amyloid material have been reported (Piirainen 1989; Kessler *et al.* 1992). As in systemic lupus erythematosus, renal lesions may be found in adults and children without clinically evident renal disease (Bennett and Spargo 1977; Singsen *et al.* 1977; Singsen *et al.* 1980).

Laboratory findings

The most common laboratory features in adults and children are listed in Table 10. A moderate anaemia of chronic inflammation is usually present. Frank haemolytic anaemia and severe thrombocytopenia requiring splenectomy may occur but are rare complications. Thrombocytopenia may be associated with anticardiolipin antibodies (Doria *et al.* 1992a). Hypergammaglobulinaemia is more frequent than in systemic lupus erythematosus. Hypocomplementaemia and cryoglobulins are present in about a third of patients but neither seem specifically associated with renal or other organ involvement. An elevated creatine phosphokinase may be associated with aseptic meningitis and trigeminal neuropathy in addition to myositis (Bennett and O'Connell 1980).

Autoantibodies

The presence of autoantibodies to the ribonuclease-sensitive component of extractable nuclear antigen (**ENA**) by a haemagglutination test is a characteristic serological feature of mixed connective tissue disease. The autoantibodies are now termed anti-U1RNP antibodies. The presence of these autoantibodies is suggested by a high titre, coarse speckled, nuclear pattern on an indirect immunofluorescence screen for antinuclear antibodies (Fig. 2). Immunodiffusion tests are now more commonly used than haemagglutination to confirm the presence of anti-U1RNP antibodies. The ribonuclease-resistant component of ENA is recognized by anti-Sm antibodies which frequently coexist with anti-U1RNP antibodies. The absence of anti-Sm antibodies and anti-DNA antibodies in sera positive for anti-U1RNP is also felt to be an important discriminatory finding (Table 4) as anti-Sm and anti-DNA antibodies are more specific for systemic lupus erythematosus.

Anti-U1RNP and anti-Sm antibodies recognize polypeptides on small ribonucleoproteins which participate in the formation of spliceosomes and process RNA. Anti-U1RNP antibodies selectively immunoprecipitate the U1RNA by recognition of 70 kDa, A and C polypeptides which are unique to the U1RNP particle, whereas anti-Sm antibodies immunoprecipitate the abundant uridine-rich small RNAs U1, U2, U5, and U4/U6 by recognition of core polypeptides found on all these RNAs. These core proteins common to each snRNP are B' (29 kDa), B (28 kDa), D1 to D3 (16 kDa), E (12 kDa), F (10 kDa) and G (9 kDa), of which B'/B and D are the major targets for anti-Sm antibodies. Precise characterization of the autoantibody specificity may be obtained by the technique of western blotting (Fig. 5). Although there is no clear-cut association between the titre of anti-U1RNP antibodies and activity of disease, the profile of autoantibody recognition to the U1RNP particle may change over time, and in some cases has been related to changes in features of the disease (Fisher *et al.* 1985).

Pathogenesis

It is likely that environmental factors trigger mixed connective tissue disease in genetically susceptible individuals. Various environmental agents have been reported including drugs such as procainamide, toxins such as polyvinyl chloride (Kahn *et al.* 1989), and silicone implants (Kumagai *et al.* 1984). Familial cases are rare but autoimmune conditions including mixed connective tissue disease may cluster in families, suggesting the inheritance of a common autoimmune diathesis. There appears to be a link with MHC class II genes (Table 3).

Histopathology

Proliferative vascular changes may be widespread and involve organs not clinically affected (Singsen *et al.* 1980). The vascular changes are similar to systemic sclerosis but accompanied by less fibrosis. There is a predilection for intimal thickening of large arteries including coronary, pulmonary, renal, and aortic arteries (Singsen *et al.* 1980; Alpert *et al.* 1983; Sullivan *et al.* 1984). Skin biopsies show dermal thickening with hypertrophy of collagen bundles, thickening of blood vessel walls and a perivascular mononuclear cell infiltration. Immunofluorescence studies of non-involved skin have shown a particulate epidermal nuclear staining pattern and granular dermo–epidermal junction deposits of immunoglobulin (Gilliam and

Table 10 Laboratory features in adults and children with mixed connective tissue disease

Feature	Adults (%)			Children (%)	
	Bennett and O'Connell (1980) (n=20)	Sullivan et al. (1984) (n=34)	Prakash et al. (1985) (n=81)	Singsen et al. (1977) (n=14)	Tiddens et al. (1993) (n=14)
Anaemia	75	24	–	(most)	64
Leucopenia	75	21	–	64	43
High ESR	100	–	–	100	–
Hypergammaglobulinaemia	75	53	73	60	–
High creatine kinase	43	–	–	–	50
Positive direct Coombs'	60	–	–	–	–
Positive rheumatoid factor	25	59	49	64	57
Low complement	–	32	5	–	–
Positive LE cell	–	18	–	–	–
Thrombocytopenia	–	–	–	50	21
Positive ANA	100[a]	100	93	100	100
Anti-U1RNP	100[a]	100	100	100	100
Anti-dsDNA	0	23	4	0	21

[a]By definition patients had positive ANA, RNPase-sensitive ENA haemagglutination test, negative anti-Sm, and negative anti-dsDNA.
NA, antinuclear antibodies; ESR, erythrocyte sedimentation rate; LE, lupus erythematosus.

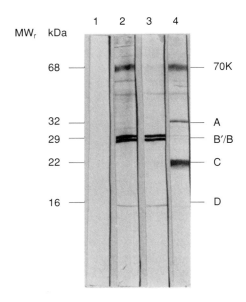

Fig. 5 Immunoblot showing the U1RNP and Sm antigenic peptides. Lane 1, normal serum; Lane 2, anti-U1RNP and anti-Sm serum; Lane 3, anti-Sm serum; Lane 4, anti-U1 RNP and anti-Sm serum.

Prystowsky 1977; Reimer *et al.* 1983). High levels of circulating anti-endothelial antibodies (Bodolay *et al.* 1989), factor VIII-related antigen (James *et al.* 1990) and ristomycin-cofactor activity (Udvardy *et al.* 1991) point to endothelial cell injury and alteration of platelet function.

Immunoregulatory abnormalities

B-cell hyperactivity is evident by polyclonal hypergammaglobulin-aemia, and spontaneous *in vitro* production of immunoglobulins (Kallenberg *et al.* 1988). However the autoantibody response to the U1RNP particle appears antigen-driven rather than as a result of non-specific polyclonal activation. Recognition of one protein on the snRNP particle may allow processing and presentation of other proteins on the same complex by B cells (Fatenjad *et al.* 1993). Under conditions in which T cell tolerance to snRNPs is overcome, such a mechanism may lead to affinity maturation of a high-titre autoanti-body response to the U1RNP particle. The initial autoantibody response may be initiated by molecular mimicry. Indeed, there are several regions of homology between U1RNP proteins and infectious agents such as human retroviral proteins (Query and Keene 1987). Antibodies to native HIV-1 and HTLV-I have been reported in mixed connective tissue disease (Ranki *et al.* 1992), although retroviral genomic material was not isolated in these patients.

T cells reactive to snRNPs have been isolated from patients with mixed connective tissue disease as well as healthy individuals (Hoffman *et al.* 1993). T-cell clones reactive to the snRNP A protein show restricted usage of TCR-β chain genes (Okubo *et al.* 1994). Therefore, snRNP-reactive oligoclonal T cells may accumulate in patients with mixed connective tissue disease. Rapidly dividing cells randomly accumulate gene mutations including mutations in the hypoxanthine-guanine phosphoribosyl transferase (**HPRT**) gene. An increased frequency of mutations in the HPRT gene in T cells isolated from patients with mixed connective tissue disease has been found, which may suggest a role for activated T cells in pathogenesis (Holyst *et al.* 1994). Prolonged survival of autoreactive cells by defects in apoptosis accounts for accelerated autoimmunity including the generation of autoantibodies to snRNPs in certain inbred strains of mice (Watanabe-Fukunaga *et al.* 1992). The role of molecules which regulate apoptosis such as Fas receptor and Fas ligand in human autoimmune disease is currently unknown.

Diagnosis

The presence of anti-U1RNP antibodies is a major criteria for diagnosis (Table 4), but should not be used alone to make the diagnosis. Only the criteria proposed by Sharp (1987) (Table 4) allow for the diagnosis of mixed connective tissue disease without the presence of anti-U1RNP antibodies. All sets of criteria had similar sensitivity when applied to a large population with autoimmune rheumatic disease (Alarcon-Segovia and Cardiel 1989), and although the criteria of Alarcon-Segovia (Alarcon-Segovia and Villarreal 1987) appeared more specific, the findings need validation in a less selected series of patients. An advantage of Alarcon-Segovia's criteria is their simplicity, but a disadvantage is the need for a haemagglutination test which is now seldom used in clinical practice. The Japanese diagnostic criteria for mixed connective tissue disease (Kasukawa *et al.* 1987) was highly specific and sensitive in a group of Italian patients (Doria *et al.* 1991), and seems useful in children (Tiddens *et al.* 1993).

Longitudinal studies in mixed connective tissue disease

Long-term follow-up studies have shown that after many years of disease, features of only one autoimmune rheumatic disease (mainly scleroderma or systemic lupus erythematosus) predominate over the 'overlap' features present earlier in the course of the disease, which has cast doubt on mixed connective tissue disease being a separate entity. However, many of the patients that fulfil carefully selected criteria for mixed connective tissue disease at the time of diagnosis, will still fulfil them at long-term follow-up. Most of the patients originally described by Sharp *et al.* (1972) developed either systemic sclerosis or systemic lupus erythematosus of variable severity on long-term follow-up, although 5 of 25 patients were virtually asymptomatic (Nimelstein *et al.* 1980). In a series of 14 children with mixed connective tissue disease followed for nearly 10 years, features of systemic lupus erythematosus and polymyositis became less prominent, but scleroderma-like symptoms and joint abnormalities persisted (Tiddens *et al.* 1993).

Scleroderma-like skin abnormalities in adults and children are less responsive to treatment than initially thought and in most cases will persist, or may develop in patients who are initially diagnosed as having seronegative rheumatoid arthritis (Bennett and O'Connell 1980; Catoggio *et al.* 1993). Therefore the clinical features of mixed connective tissue disease do appear to evolve with time; skin and pulmonary lesions persist in adults whereas skin and joint involvement are prominent in children. The differentiation of mixed connective tissue disease into systemic lupus erythematosus or systemic sclerosis may be determined by the immunogenetic background (Gendi *et al.* 1995).

Studies in patients with anti-U1RNP antibodies

About 50 per cent of patients with anti-U1RNP antibodies do not have mixed connective tissue disease, even with extended follow-up (Table 11), although sometimes long periods of time are needed for the development of overlap manifestations (Lemmer *et al.* 1982). High titres of anti-U1RNP antibodies are associated more strongly with the development of mixed connective tissue disease than low titres (Lundberg and Hedfors 1991). Virtually all patients with mixed connective tissue disease will fulfil criteria for another autoimmune rheumatic disease at some stage in their illness. In our experience, patients with anti-U1RNP antibodies who fulfil criteria for mixed connective tissue disease without fulfilling criteria for systemic lupus erythematosus or systemic sclerosis are extremely rare (McHugh *et al.* 1990). None the less, studies that exclude mixed connective tissue disease once another autoimmune rheumatic disease is diagnosed (Calderon *et al.* 1984; Van Den Hoogen *et al.* 1994) may be misleading, as such patients may still be said to have the former disease. In the context of systemic lupus erythematosus, the presence of anti-U1RNP antibodies is associated with Raynaud's phenomenon, swollen fingers, myositis, pulmonary involvement, and less renal disease (Reichlin and Mattioli 1972; Maddison *et al.* 1978; McHugh *et al.* 1990). In patients with an overlap syndrome, the presence of anti-U1RNP antibodies may be associated with Raynaud's phenomenon and pulmonary hypertension (Ginsburg *et al.* 1983; Lazaro *et al.* 1989).

Prognosis

The prognosis is not as favourable as originally reported. The major cause of mortality appears to be pulmonary hypertension (Table 9). One-third of the 34 patients followed by Sullivan *et al.* (1984) had very severe disease requiring repeated courses or sustained high doses of corticosteroids, and 4 patients died. The mortality rate in some of the larger series is shown in Table 12. The 5- and 10-year survival rate was 90.5 per cent and 82.1 per cent in a Japanese series of patients, which was similar to that for systemic lupus erythematosus (Miyawaki and Onodera 1987). In children the presence of reactivity to the Sm D polypeptide is associated with a poorer prognosis (Hoffman *et al.* 1993).

Management

Management of mixed connective tissue disease depends on manifestations of the disease. A suggested approach to management is outlined in Fig. 6. The scleroderma-like features are not as responsive to corticosteroids as originally reported. Raynaud's phenomenon is managed as in scleroderma, with emphasis on the patient keeping warm, avoiding trauma to the fingers, and discouragement of cigarette smoking. Vasodilators such as calcium channel blockers,

Table 11 Outcome in patients with anti-U1RNP antibodies

	Method of detection	n	Follow-up (years)	Disease duration (years)	Definitive diagnosis						
					MCTD	SLE	UCTD	PSS	RA	PM	Others
Sharp et al. (1976)	Haemagglutination	100	NS	NS	74	12	6	8	–	–	–
Maddison et al. (1978)	Immunodiffusion	43	1–12	NS	5	30	4	1	1	–	2
Rasmussen et al. (1987)	Haemagglutination	97	mean 9	NS	42	22	11	7	9	6	–
Lemmer et al. (1982)	Immunodiffusion haemagglutination	44	NS	1–16	11	10	20	1	–	2	–
Lundberg et al. (1992)	CIE	32	mean 5.4	mean 10.1	17	5	5	–	1	–	4
Catoggio et al. (1993)	Immunodiffusion	37	median 4	median 9	17	11	3	2	4	–	–
Van Den Hoogen et al. (1994)	CIE immunoblot	46	mean 15	mean 17	24	11	–	7	4	–	–
Total		399			190	101	49	26	19	8	6
(%)					(47)	(25)	(12)	(6.5)	(5)	(2)	(1.5)

MCTD mixed connective tissue disease; SLE systemic lupus erythematosus. UCTD undifferentiated connective tissue disease; PSS progressive systemic sclerosis; RA rheumatoid arthritis; PM polymyositis; CIE counterimmunoelectrophoresis.

Table 12 Reported mortality in mixed connective tissue disease

	Number of patients	Follow-up (years)	Disease duration (years)	Number of deaths (%)
Bennett and O'Connell (1980)	20	4	–	4 (20)
Nimelstein et al. (1980)	22	3.75	12	8 (36)
Grant et al. (1981)	23	–	–	5 (22)
Sullivan et al. (1984)	34	6.26	11	4 (12)
Prakash et al. (1985)	81	5	–	6 (7)
Kitridou et al. (1986)	30	9.4	13	4 (13)
Total	210			31 (15)

angiotensin-converting enzymes, pentoxifylline and ketanserin are effective in some patients. Intravenous prostacyclin may be used for acute ischaemic digital lesions.

Oesophageal involvement may respond to corticosteroids, although such treatment is rarely justified. More often, antacids, H_2-antagonists and omeprazole are required. Fatigue, fever, lymphadenopathy, arthralgia, and myalgia may respond to non-steroidal anti-inflammatory drugs in conventional doses. The addition of antimalarial agents early in the course of the disease is becoming a more widespread practice. Low-dose corticosteroids (less than 20 mg of prednisolone per day) may be needed if general symptoms do not respond to other measures. The development of an erosive polyarthritis may warrant the introduction of methotrexate or azathioprine. Myositis in mixed connective tissue disease may

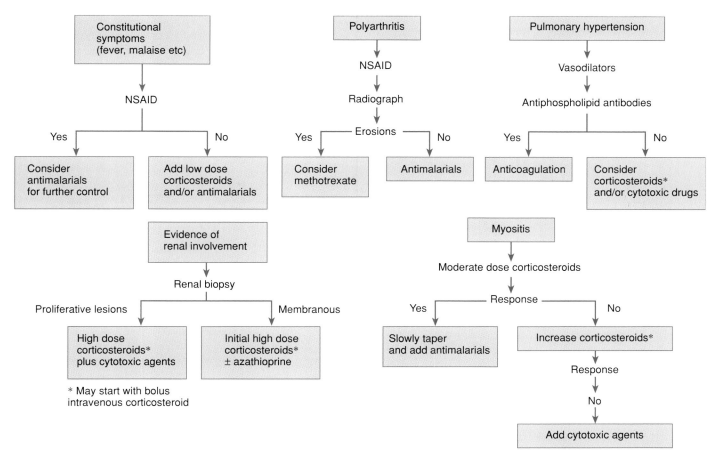

Fig. 6 Management of overlap syndrome.

respond to lower doses of corticosteroids than polymyositis (Lundberg *et al.* 1992).

The management of renal disease remains controversial, although knowledge of histology may help in the decision. High-dose corticosteroids were effective for nephrotic syndrome and proteinuria in about two-thirds of patients described by Kitridou *et al.* (1986). However, cytotoxic drugs are probably indicated for those patients with more proliferative lesions, or those patients that require large corticosteroid doses for long periods of time.

Antiphospholipid antibodies should be sought in patients with pulmonary hypertension, and anticoagulation therapy considered when these antibodies are present (Ueda *et al.* 1991). Corticosteroids and cytotoxic drugs should be considered at an early phase because of the poor prognosis associated with pulmonary hypertension in mixed connective tissue disease and its usually rapid progression (Weiner-Kronish *et al.* 1981; Alpert *et al.* 1992). There are reports of patients responding to chlorambucil (Weiner-Kronish *et al.* 1981), cyclophosphamide (Friedman *et al.* 1992), and cyclophosphamide and cyclosporin A (Dahl *et al.* 1992). Recurrent episodes of pulmonary vasoconstriction may contribute to the development of pulmonary hypertension in patients with diffuse systemic sclerosis, the CREST syndrome and mixed connective tissue disease (Alpert *et al.* 1992). Nifedipine, hydralazine, prazosin, phenotolamine, ketanserin, prostacyclin, and captopril are all capable of acute and sustained reduction of pulmonary vascular resistance in such patients and therefore may be of additional therapeutic value.

Polymyositis overlap syndromes

Anti-tRNA synthetases syndrome

Autoantibodies are found in the majority of patients with polymyositis and dermatomyositis (Reichlin and Arnett 1984). The most frequent autoantibody is anti-Jo-1 which is directed against histidyl-tRNA synthetase, one of the 20 different enzymes that attaches the tRNA with its specific amino acid (Mathews and Bernstein 1983; Wasicek *et al.* 1984). Antibodies to five of these synthetases have been identified in patients with inflammatory myopathy (Targoff 1992). Anti-Jo-1 is found in 15 to 20 per cent of all myositis patients, and is found very rarely in dermatomyositis (Nishikai and Reichlin 1980).

A characteristic group of clinical features is associated with this group of autoantibodies. The 'antisynthetase syndrome' is characterized by myositis (100 per cent), interstitial lung disease (50 to 75 per cent), arthritis (60 to 100 per cent), and Raynaud's phenomenon (60 per cent) (Targoff 1992). A particular cutaneous feature is the presence of hyperkeratosis and fissuring along the lateral aspects of the fingers, so-called 'mechanic's (or machinist's) fingers' (Fig. 7).

Interstitial lung disease is one of the characteristic findings in the antisynthetase syndrome. Interstitial lung disease is found in 50 to 75 per cent of myositis patients with anti-Jo-1, compared with only 10 to 20 per cent of myositis overall (Bernstein *et al.* 1984; Hochberg *et al.* 1984; Love *et al.* 1991; Targoff 1992). The interstitial lung disease

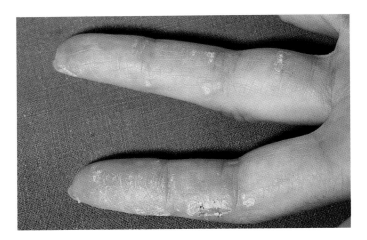

Fig. 7 Mechanic's finger.

is indistinguishable from idiopathic interstitial lung disease, and it may persist despite response of the myositis to treatment and become a greater clinical problem than the myositis itself (Targoff and Arnett 1990). Arthritis is more frequent in patients with anti-Jo-1 antibodies (Bernstein *et al.* 1984; Plotz *et al.* 1989; Oddis *et al.* 1990; Targoff 1992). It is usually non-erosive, but deforming arthritis may be seen in one-third of patients. The wrist and finger joints are the most commonly involved joints.

Almost all patients with anti-Jo-1 antibodies have myositis at some stage in the course of their disease. However, antisynthetase antibodies may be found in patients with 'idiopathic' lung disease without clinical myositis (Bernstein *et al.* 1984; Targoff and Arnett 1990). Subclinical or absent myositis is more common with other non-Jo-1 antisynthetase antibodies (Targoff 1992). The myositis is indistinguishable from that of patients without antisynthetase antibodies, although patients with the autoantibodies may develop myositis at a younger age and have a more rapid form of onset (Plotz *et al.* 1989).

Rhupus

The existence of patients with a clinical picture resembling both rheumatoid arthritis and systemic lupus erythematosus has long been recognized. The description of lupus erythematosus cells by Hargraves in 1948 allowed a more precise segregation of patients with systemic lupus erythematosus, although a number of patients with 'true' rheumatoid arthritis, usually with more severe disease and extra-articular manifestations, were positive for lupus erythematosus cells. Conversely, there are patients with systemic lupus erythematosus who have a prominent synovitis associated with rheumatoid factor.

The appearance of nodules or an erosive arthropathy in patients with systemic lupus erythematosus (Cohen and Webb 1987) suggests a genuine overlap between the two conditions. The term 'rhupus' has been used to describe such patients (Panush *et al.* 1988). Although numerous case reports have appeared documenting a true coexistence of diffuse glomerulonephritis with nodules or erosive polyarthritis, 'rhupus' does not seem to occur more frequently than expected than the chance concurrence of systemic lupus erythematosus and rheumatoid arthritis (Panush *et al.* 1988). Some of the patients described in these earlier studies had overlap features and if

serological techniques had been available for detecting anti-U1RNP antibodies, they may have fulfilled criteria for mixed connective tissue disease. Immunogenetic factors may determine which clinical features become most prominent (Brand *et al.* 1992).

Scleroderma overlap syndromes

Scleroderma and primary biliary cirrhosis

The association between systemic sclerosis and primary biliary cirrhosis is well recognized (Murray-Lyon *et al.* 1970; Reynolds *et al.* 1971). Scleroderma occurs in 4 to 17 per cent of patients with primary biliary cirrhosis according to large series (Clarke *et al.* 1978). Scleroderma in primary biliary cirrhosis is usually the CREST syndrome, now better referred to as limited cutaneous systemic sclerosis. Conversely, up to 5 per cent of patients with scleroderma have clinical evidence of primary biliary cirrhosis (Reimer 1990).

Antimitochondrial antibodies, the serological hallmark of primary biliary cirrhosis, are found in 15 to 25 per cent of sera from patients with systemic sclerosis, with a minority of the latter patients having overt evidence of primary biliary cirrhosis (Reimer 1990). Anticentromere antibodies, the serological hallmark of the CREST syndrome, are found in up to 30 per cent of sera from patients with primary biliary cirrhosis (Reynolds *et al.* 1971; Bernstein *et al.* 1982), and more than half of these patients have at least some features of CREST (Bernstein *et al.* 1982). The serological overlap between primary biliary cirrhosis and systemic sclerosis is more prevalent than the clinical overlap, although subclinical hepatic involvement may not be evident without liver biopsy. The serological overlap is not because of cross-reactivity between mitochondrial and centromere-associated antigens, which are independent antigenic targets (Whyte *et al.* 1994).

Patients with primary biliary cirrhosis also have a high prevalence of Sjögren's syndrome or keratoconjunctivitis sicca (Culp 1985). While evaluating 17 patients with primary biliary cirrhosis keratoconjunctivitis sicca was found in 76 per cent and a positive lip biopsy compatible with Sjögren's in 62 per cent of patients (Soriano *et al.* unpublished data)

Scleroderma–polymyositis overlap

Muscle involvement was recognized early in the description of the systemic sclerosis. Two different types of myopathy may occur. The more common myopathy is characterized by mild or no proximal muscle weakness, mild elevation of muscle enzymes, polyphasic motor unit potentials of normal amplitude and duration on electromyograms, and interstitial fibrosis and variation in diameter of muscle fibres without active inflammation on biopsy. This form has been classified as 'simple myopathy' (Clements *et al.* 1978) and does not appear to change significantly over long periods of time. A less frequent form resembles polymyositis with more proximal muscle weakness, very high muscle enzyme concentrations, inflammatory changes on biopsy, and polyphasic motor unit potentials of short duration and small amplitude on electromyography. The latter form requires active therapy and has been labelled inflammatory myopathy or 'complicated myopathy' (Clements *et al.* 1978).

In the series of patients with polymyositis reported by Bohan and co-workers (Bohan *et al.* 1977), 21 per cent of 153 patients had another autoimmune rheumatic disorder and were classified as type V polymyositis. The most frequently associated autoimmune rheumatic disease was scleroderma (36 per cent). The diagnosis of mixed connective tissue disease was not considered, especially as detailed serological investigation was not available. However, anti-U1RNP antibodies were present in 25 to 33 per cent of a later series of similar patients (Hochberg *et al.* 1986; Love *et al.* 1991). Of 34 patients studied in Argentina with polymyositis/dermatomyositis, 14 (41 per cent) had type V polymyositis. Anti-U1RNP was present in 67 per cent of cases, and one-half fulfilled Alarcon Segovia's criteria for mixed connective tissue disease (Imamura *et al.* 1993).

Other autoantibody specificities may also be associated with the scleroderma–polymyositis overlaps. Anti-Ku antibodies are associated with polymyositis–scleroderma overlap syndrome in Japan, but are less frequent in the United States; conversely anti-Pm-Scl antibodies are more frequent in polymyositis–scleroderma overlap in the United States but not in Japan (Targoff 1992). In general anti-Pm-Scl antibodies are found in 8 per cent of myositis patients and 3 per cent of scleroderma patients (Targoff 1992). Among 22 patients with anti-Pm-Scl antibodies, polymyositis/dermatomyositis alone was present in 55 per cent, scleroderma without polymyositis/ dermatomyositis in 5 per cent, and myositis–scleroderma overlap in 41 per cent (Reichlin *et al.* 1984).

The prognosis of patients with type V polymyositis is no different from that in polymyositis alone (Bohan *et al.* 1977). It is possible that lower doses of corticosteroids may be sufficient to control myositis in association with mixed connective tissue disease (Lundberg *et al.* 1992).

Eosinophilia–myalgia syndrome, toxic oil syndrome, eosinophilic fasciitis

The eosinophilia–myalgia syndrome was first defined in 1989 (Centers for Disease Control 1989) as a new epidemic in association with the ingestion of L-tryptophan preparations (Belongia *et al.* 1990; Eidson *et al.* 1990), traced to a single Japanese manufacturer. (Belongia *et al.* 1990; Carr *et al.* 1994). The clinical picture and the pathological features, strongly resemble those of the Spanish toxic oil syndrome. Toxic oil syndrome was another epidemic that occurred in Spain in 1981 and was associated with the ingestion of adulterated rapeseed cooking oil. The presence of eosinophilia and fasciitis, link these two epidemics with eosinophilic fasciitis. However, no toxin has been associated with eosinophilic fasciitis.

Eosinophilia–myalgia syndrome and toxic oil syndrome

Epidemiology

The use of L-tryptophan was widespread in the United States in 1989 for the treatment of insomnia, premenstrual syndrome, and depression. Tryptophan was available to consumers without a prescription; thus a very large section of the population were at risk. As of 1 August 1992, the Centers for Disease Control had received a total of 1511 reports, including 38 deaths (Nightingale 1992). The surveillance case definition of eosinophilia–myalgia syndrome was as follows: eosinophil count greater than 1000/mm^3, incapacitating myalgia,

and exclusion of other infectious or neoplastic illnesses that could account for the other two findings (Kilbourne *et al.* 1990). However, the actual number of individuals in whom some type of eosinophilia– myalgia syndrome had developed was estimated to be several times higher (Nightingale 1992).

National surveillance data from the United States in 1990 showed that 84 per cent of affected patients were female, 97 per cent were non-Hispanic white, and 87 were aged 35 years or older (median: 48; range: 4 to 85) (Swygert *et al.* 1990). The female preponderance is more likely due to ingestion patterns rather than gender susceptibility (Silver 1993). The usual daily dose ranged from 10 to 15 000 mg (median: 1500), and the median time between beginning use of tryptophan and the onset of symptoms was 127 days (range: 1 to 3668). Twenty-two per cent of those affected with eosinophilia–myalgia syndrome had taken tryptophan for more than 1 year before becoming ill, and 12 per cent had discontinued tryptophan a median of 15 days (range: 1 to 2858) before onset of symptoms (Swygert *et al.* 1990). Two risk factors for developing eosinophilia–myalgia syndrome were older age and the quantity of tryptophan consumed. The latter risk factor was not associated with the syndrome in a recent epidemiological study in Germany (Carr *et al.* 1994), possibly because of batch variations of quantities of the contaminants in the L-tryptophan (Mayeno and Gleich 1994). The occurrence rate of eosinophilia–myalgia syndrome in Germany was estimated as 40 per 100 000 users of the implicated source (Carr *et al.* 1994).

Toxic oil syndrome occurred in Spain in 1981 affecting more than 20 000 individuals with about 500 deaths (Mayeno and Gleich 1994). Epidemiological investigations implicated the use of aniline-denatured rapeseed oil that was sold and reprocessed illegally (Kilbourne *et al.* 1988).

Clinical features and histology

Symptoms at presentation

The more common clinical and laboratory manifestations of eosinophilia–myalgia syndrome and toxic oil syndrome are summarized in Table 13. The majority of patients with eosinophilia–myalgia syndrome presented with a flu-like syndrome characterized by myalgia and arthralgia, associated with profound weakness and fatigue (Kaufman *et al.* 1990). By definition all patients had severe myalgia with an elevated peripheral eosinophil count. Myalgia was generally diffuse, although could be localized, and accompanied by severe episodic muscle cramps (Kaufman *et al.* 1990; Hedberg *et al.* 1992). By contrast, patients with toxic oil syndrome presented as an atypical pneumonia, with non-productive cough, pleuritic chest pain, headache, fever, and bilateral pulmonary infiltrates. Gastrointestinal findings and striking eosinophilia became prominent within the first month.

Neuromuscular involvement

The clinical and pathological manifestations of neuromuscular involvement were qualitatively similar in both diseases, although more severe in toxic oil syndrome (Hertzman and Abaitua Borda 1993). In the acute and intermediate phases myalgia, muscle cramps, weakness, arthralgia, paraesthesia, and dysaesthesia were reported (Table 13). Late severe sensorimotor polyradiculopathy, with progressive weakness and occasional respiratory muscle involvement, and neuropathic contractures of the hands and wrist more commonly occurred in patients with toxic oil syndrome (30 per cent compared with less than 5 per cent) (Hertzman and Abaitua Borda 1993;

Table 13 Prevalence of selected clinical and laboratory findings in eosinophilia–myalgia syndrome (EMS) and toxic oil syndrome (TOS)

Feature	EMS (Swygert et al. 1990) n=1075 (%)	TOS (Kilbourne et al. 1983) n=121 (%)
Myalgia	100	55.5
Arthralgia	73	8.4
Rash	60	64.7
Peripheral oedema	59	64.7
Cough	59[b]	68.1
Dyspnoea	59[b]	42
Fever	36	68.1
Scleroderma-like skin	32	–
Alopecia	28	5
Neuropathy	28	39.5
Hepatomegaly	5	37
Leucocytosis	85	71.1
Eosinophilia ($>500 \, mm^3$)	100[a]	77.7
Elevated ESR	33	38.8
Elevated aldolase	46	55.4
Elevated creatine kinase	10	–
Abnormal chest radiograph	21	87.6
Abnormal liver function test	43	41.3

[a]By definition all patients had incapacitating myalgia and eosinophil count of more than 1.0×10^9 cells (Swygert et al. 1990)
[b]Cough and dyspnoea taken together (Swygert et al. 1990)

Bolster and Silver 1994). In toxic oil syndrome the presence of severe initial systemic findings was associated with progression to neuromuscular illness (Kilbourne et al. 1983).

The most prominent histological feature in both conditions was a perimysial and epimysial inflammatory infiltrate consisting of mononuclear cells, histiocytes, and eosinophils (Kaufman et al. 1990; Varga et al. 1993; Lin et al. 1992). The degree of inflammatory infiltrate appeared to correlate with the extent of clinical symptoms (Kaufman et al. 1990). Myofibril atrophy, regeneration, and necrosis were almost absent in all biopsies, despite the severe and incapacitating myalgia (Lin et al. 1992). Later in the course of the disease, muscle fibre atrophy consistent with denervation was observed in both conditions (Hertzman and Abaitua Borda 1993).

Lungs
Pulmonary involvement was a major feature in both conditions. Toxic oil syndrome was characterized by an acute onset of cough and dyspnoea. Radiographic and pathological changes in toxic oil syndrome were consistent with a non-inflammatory non-cardiogenic

pulmonary oedema, and 250 deaths occurred from this complication (Hertzman and Abaitua Borda 1993). Acute respiratory involvement in eosinophilia–myalgia syndrome occurred less frequently and was characterized by an interstitial pneumonitis that resolved spontaneously or was highly responsive to corticosteroids (Hertzman and Abaitua Borda 1993). Dyspnoea in eosinophilia–myalgia syndrome was related to parenchymal involvement of the lungs and to respiratory muscle weakness (Read et al. 1992).

Pulmonary hypertension developed in the intermediate stage of both conditions (1 to 12 months) in 8 per cent of patients with toxic oil syndrome (Cheg 1993) and in 5 per cent of patients with eosinophilia–myalgia syndrome (Martin et al. 1990). Cardiac involvement was rare and usually occurred as a result of pulmonary hypertension. However, primary involvement of the heart and coronary arteries has been reported in eosinophilia–myalgia syndrome (Berger et al. 1994) and in toxic oil syndrome (James et al. 1991).

Skin
The most frequent cutaneous manifestations in the acute phase of eosinophilia–myalgia syndrome and toxic oil syndrome were diffuse erythematous macules over the trunk and extremities. Oedema associated with cutaneous induration in the arms and legs was found in 28 to 60 per cent of patients with eosinophilia–myalgia syndrome (Kaufman et al. 1990; Swygert et al. 1990), and in 90 per cent of those with toxic oil syndrome. The oedema was due to fascial inflammation and was often accompanied by venous furrowing and the 'peau d'orange' induration characteristic of eosinophilic fasciitis (Kaufman et al. 1990). Histologically the changes could not be distinguished from eosinophilic fasciitis, with an inflammatory infiltrate of the fascial layers, a chronic perivascular infiltrate in the dermis in early cases, and thickening and homogenization of collagen bundles in later cases (Lin et al. 1992). Active skin lesions had disappeared in biopsy specimens at late follow-up (Hertzman and Abaitua Borda 1993), with oedema replaced by scleroderma-like changes. Non-necrotizing vascular lesions were more common in toxic oil syndrome than in eosinophilia–myalgia syndrome (Bolster and Silver 1994).

Gastrointestinal tract
Hepatomegaly, abdominal pain, nausea, diarrhoea, odynophagia, and dysphagia were particularly prominent during the first month in patients with toxic oil syndrome. Gastrointestinal symptoms have been reported in 64 per cent of patients who died of causes related to eosinophilia–myalgia syndrome (Swygert et al. 1993). Clinical evidence of pancreatic disease was rare in both entities, but 30 per cent of autopsies on patients with toxic oil syndrome showed marked atrophy of the pancreas (Hertzman and Abaitua Borda 1993).

Central nervous system
Cognitive symptoms and significant impairments of verbal and visual memory, conceptual reasoning, and motor speed were reported in 62 per cent of patients with eosinophilia–myalgia syndrome (Krupp et al. 1993) and 20 to 30 per cent of patients with toxic oil syndrome (Hertzman and Abaitua Borda 1993). Most patients with eosinophilia–myalgia syndrome were taking L-tryptophan because of insomnia and depression, and the use of antidepressive drugs may have contributed to some of these features. (Krupp et al. 1993). Electroencephalograms, computed tomography scans, and magnetic resonance imaging studies were normal (Hertzman and Abaitua Borda 1993; Krupp et al. 1993).

Laboratory findings

The laboratory findings are shown in Table 13. The most characteristic finding was the presence of eosinophilia in peripheral blood, usually within the first week. The eosinophilia was responsive to corticosteroid treatment and in eosinophilia–myalgia syndrome to discontinuation of L-tryptophan. The serum IgE levels were characteristically normal in eosinophilia–myalgia syndrome but were elevated in nearly half of patients with toxic oil syndrome (Belongia *et al.* 1990). Antinuclear antibodies were found in 40 per cent of patients with eosinophilia–myalgia syndrome and in a minority of patients with toxic oil syndrome. Normal creatine kinase levels were seen in almost all patients, although isolated elevation of serum aldolase was reported in 58 per cent of patients with eosinophilia–myalgia syndrome (Kaufman *et al.* 1990)

Aetiology and pathogenesis

Eosinophilia–myalgia syndrome

The epidemic nature of eosinophilia–myalgia syndrome, and its association with batches of L-tryptophan originating from a single manufacturer, suggested a contaminant (Varga *et al.* 1993). High-performance liquid chromatography analysis of L-tryptophan revealed more than 60 contaminants (Belongia *et al.* 1990). A single absorbance peak labelled 'peak E', or peak 97, and later identified as 1,1'-ethylidene bis[tryptophan] (**EBT**), was found consistently in L-tryptophan lots associated with eosinophilia–myalgia syndrome (Belongia *et al.* 1990). Lewis rats treated with EBT and/or case-associated L-tryptophan for 6 weeks developed significant increases in the thickness of the myofascia, compared with animals treated with vehicle or L-tryptophan not associated with the case. However, only animals treated with case-associated L-tryptophan (and not those receiving EBT) showed evidence of immune activation. Although these results demonstrated the pathological effect of EBT, they did not rule out the possibility that other impurities in the L-tryptophan associated with eosinophilia–myalgia syndrome may have contributed to some of the features of the syndrome (Love *et al.* 1993). Another murine model of eosinophilia–myalgia syndrome induced by intraperitoneal administration of EBT was reported recently (Silver *et al.* 1994). A second contaminant (peak UV-5) has been identified as 3-(phenylamino)alanine (**PAA**) and related to L-tryptophan associated with cases of eosinophilia–myalgia syndrome (Mayeno *et al.* 1992). Of interest, PAA is chemically similar to 3-phenylamino-1,2-propanediol, an aniline derivative implicated in the development of toxic oil syndrome. The fact that many patients had ingested tryptophan for long periods (10 years or more) before becoming ill makes the existence of an inborn error of tryptophan metabolism an unlikely cause of eosinophilia–myalgia syndrome (Carr *et al.* 1994; Mayeno and Gleich 1994). However, several studies have found abnormal tryptophan metabolism in patients with eosinophilia–myalgia syndrome and toxic oil syndrome, with a shunting of L-tryptophan metabolism to the kynurenine pathway (Silver *et al.* 1992; Varga *et al.* 1993; Bolster and Silver 1994). These abnormalities could play a role in the pathogenesis of eosinophilia–myalgia syndrome, but more probably are a consequence of inflammation (Varga *et al.* 1993).

Both cellular and humoral autoimmune mechanisms have been implicated in the pathogenesis of eosinophilia–myalgia syndrome (Varga *et al.* 1993). A hypothetical model is that the initial trigger (tryptophan contaminant or metabolite) activates inflammatory cells, which are induced to secrete cytokines (IL-5, GM-CSF, transforming growth factor-β) that cause activation of eosinophils, and fibroblasts. Activated eosinophils may release cytokines and toxic granule proteins (including major basic protein), that may contribute to tissue injury. Activated fibroblasts produce increased amounts of collagen and other extracellular matrix components resulting in the characteristic fibrosis (Varga *et al.* 1993).

Toxic oil syndrome

Fatty acid anilides have been proposed as the aetiological agents in toxic oil syndrome. Fatty acid anilides may alter arachidonic acid metabolism or impair fibrinolytic activity in endothelial cells leading to the early intimal lesions seen in these patients (Bolster and Silver 1994).

Prognosis

The disease-related mortality rate for the first year was 2.7 per cent for eosinophilia–myalgia syndrome and 1.5 to 3.6 per cent for toxic oil syndrome (Alonso-Ruiz *et al.* 1993; Kaufman 1993; Swygert *et al.* 1993). It is likely that the incidence rate of eosinophilia–myalgia syndrome was underestimated, and toxic oil syndrome was more severe than eosinophilia–myalgia syndrome in its acute stages (Kaufman 1993). Progressive polyneuropathy and myopathy accounted for 67 per cent of deaths in patients with eosinophilia–myalgia syndrome. Older age and involvement of more than one organ system, in particular neuromuscular, pulmonary, and cardiovascular sequelae, suggested a poor prognosis (Swygert *et al.* 1993).

Long-term morbidity was frequent in both syndromes. Persistent symptoms such as myalgia (50 to 94 per cent), muscle cramping (43 to 90 per cent), and neuropathy (30 to 91 per cent) were reported up to 36 months after the onset of eosinophilia–myalgia syndrome (Kaufman 1993). The consumption of multivitamin supplements before the appearance of eosinophilia–myalgia syndrome was associated with reduced severity of subacute symptoms (Hatch and Goldman 1993). In an 8-year follow-up study of 332 patients with toxic oil syndrome, only 9 per cent achieved full remission (Alonso-Ruiz *et al.* 1993). The severity of the chronic manifestations was variable, but was mild in most of the cases (Alonso-Ruiz *et al.* 1993). Muscle cramps and chronic musculoskeletal pain were the most common symptoms.

Management

A variety of medical regimens, mainly non-steroidal anti-inflammatory agents and corticosteroids, have been used to treat patients with eosinophilia–myalgia syndrome and toxic oil syndrome. Although acute symptoms such as oedema, acute pulmonary disease, and eosinophilia responded to corticosteroid treatment, such treatment was not associated with long-term improvement in symptoms. Corticosteroids may have been life saving in cases of acute respiratory failure due to non-cardiogenic pulmonary oedema in toxic oil syndrome.

Eosinophilia–myalgia syndrome in children

Eosinophilia–myalgia syndrome occasionally has been identified among children, including a neonate with persistent eosinophilia whose mother ingested tryptophan during pregnancy (Hatch *et al.* 1991). More recently a case of eosinophilia–myalgia syndrome was reported in a child with phenylketonuria who developed the syndrome after ingesting a specialized infant formula containing contaminated tryptophan (Springer *et al.* 1992).

Eosinophilic fasciitis

Eosinophilic fasciitis is a relatively uncommon idiopathic disease, first described by Shulman (1974), and characterized by fasciitis and peripheral blood eosinophilia. It shares similar clinical and histological features with eosinophilia–myalgia syndrome and toxic oil syndrome, but significant internal organ involvement is uncommon. Also, there are differences that distinguish eosinophilic fasciitis from systemic sclerosis: the absence of Raynaud's phenomenon, normal nailfold capillaries, sparing of the dermis, infrequent visceral involvement, absence of the serological features characteristic of systemic sclerosis, and the development of haematological complications, such as aplastic anaemia and thrombocytopenia, seldom reported in typical systemic sclerosis (Michet *et al.* 1981; Maddison 1991). The age of onset is 30 to 40 years (mean: 47; range: 11 to 72), and in half of the patients a history of recent strenuous exertion can be recalled (Lakhampal *et al.* 1988).

Cutaneous manifestations are the most common presenting feature and usually evolve through three stages: pitting oedema, 'peau d'orange', and induration. These stages are often present simultaneously in different areas of the body (Maddison 1991). The arms and legs are affected most commonly and simultaneous involvement of hands and feet is not uncommon. Localized morphoea may occur in other areas, especially in children (Miller 1992). Synovitis is not uncommon and may be the presenting feature. Low-grade myositis may be present, although serum creatine kinase levels are usually normal.

Eosinophilic fasciitis has been associated with malignancy and may present as a paraneoplastic syndrome (Naschitz *et al.* 1994), which remits with successful cancer surgery. Haematological malignancies are overrepresented, and aplastic anaemia in particular has a high associated mortality (Hoffman *et al.* 1982). Eosinophilic fasciitis associated with malignancy has a female predominance and usually fails to respond to corticosteroids (Naschitz *et al.* 1994).

Peripheral eosinophilia, sometimes impressive, is the most striking laboratory feature. Eosinophilia may be transient and the diagnosis should not be dismissed because of its absence. Diagnosis is confirmed by a cutaneous biopsy to include tissue extending from the epidermis to skeletal muscle and the deep fascia. Characteristic histological findings are a widespread inflammatory infiltrate involving the deep fascia and septae of the subdermal fat as well as the dermal layer and a normal epidermis.

The cause of eosinophilic fasciitis is unknown. Of interest is the association with strenuous exertion, especially in men. After the description of eosinophilia–myalgia syndrome associated with L-tryptophan, some retrospective studies have found an association of eosinophilic fasciitis with the consumption of L-tryptophan (Freundlich *et al.* 1990; Martin *et al.* 1991), while others have not (Varga *et al.* 1991). Recently two cases of diffuse fasciitis with peripheral eosinophilia were described in which *Borrelia burgdoferi* was identified on biopsy specimens. The term borrelial fasciitis was used to describe such lesions (Granter *et al.* 1994).

More than half of patients with eosinophilic fasciitis respond to corticosteroids, although complete remission is achieved in only 15 per cent. There may be spontaneous remissions. Other agents such as cimetidine, hydroxychloroquine, colchicine, D-penicillamine, and cyclosporin (Laneuville 1992) have been used with variable results. In children, two-thirds of patients developed cutaneous fibrosis (Farrington *et al.* 1993).

References

Alarcon, G.S. *et al.* (1991). Early undifferentiated connective tissue disease. I. Early clinical manifestation in a large cohort of patients with undifferentiated connective tissue diseases compared with cohorts of well established connective tissue disease. *Journal of Rheumatology*, **18**, 1332–9.

Alarcon-Segovia, D. (1994). Mixed connective tissue disease and overlap syndromes. *Clinics in Dermatology*, **12**, 309–16.

Alarcon-Segovia, D. and Villarreal, M. (1987) Classification and diagnostic criteria for mixed connective tissue diseases. In *Mixed connective tissue diseases and antinuclear antibodies* (ed. R. Kasukawa and G.C. Sharp), pp. 33–40. Excerpta Medica, Amsterdam.

Alarcon-Segovia, D. and Cardiel, M.H. (1989). Comparison between 3 diagnostic criteria for mixed connective tissue disease. Study of 593 patients. *Journal of Rheumatology*, **16**, 328–34.

Alonso-Ruiz, A., Calabozo, M., Perez-Ruiz, F., and Mancebo, L. (1993). Toxic oil syndrome: a long-term follow-up of a cohort of 332 patients. *Medicine (Baltimore)*, **72**, 285–95.

Alpert, M.A. *et al.* (1983). Cardiovascular manifestations of mixed connective tissue disease in adults. *Circulation*, **68**, 1182–93.

Alpert, M.A., Pressly, T.A., Mukerji, V., Lambert, C.R., and Mukerji, B. (1992). Short-and long-term hemodynamic effects of captopril in patients with pulmonary hypertension and selected connective tissue disease. *Chest*, **102**, 1407–12.

Babini, S.M., Maldonado-Cocco, J.A., Barcelo, H.A., and Garcia-Morteo, O. (1985). Peritendinous nodules in overlap syndrome. *Journal of Rheumatology*, **12**, 160–4.

Belongia, E.A. *et al.* (1990). An investigation of the cause of the eosinophilia–myalgia syndrome associated with tryptophan use. *New England Journal of Medicine*, **323**, 357–65.

Bennett, R.M. and O'Connell, D.J. (1980). Mixed connective tissue disease: a clinicopathologic study of 20 cases. *Seminars in Arthritis and Rheumatism*, **10**, 25–50.

Bennett, R.M. and Spargo, B.H. (1977). Immune complex nephropathy in mixed connective tissue disease. *American Journal of Medicine*, **63**, 534–41.

Bennett, R.M., Bong, D.M., and Spargo, B.H. (1978). Neuropsychiatric problems in mixed connective tissue disease. *American Journal of Medicine*, **65**, 955–62.

Berger, P.B., Duffy, J., Reeder, G.S., Karon, B.L., and Edwards, W.D. (1994) Restrictive cardiomyopathy associated with the eosinophilia–myalgia syndrome. *Mayo Clinic Proceedings*, **69**, 162–5.

Bernstein, R.M., Callender, M.E., Neuberger, J.M., Hughes, G.R.V., and Williams, R. (1982). Anticentromere antibody in primary biliary cirrhosis. *Annals of the Rheumatic Diseases*, **41**, 612–14.

Bernstein, R.M. *et al.* (1984). Anti Jo-1 antibody: a marker for myositis with interstitial lung disease. *British Medical Journal*, **289**, 151–3.

Black, C. and Isenberg, D.A. (1992). Mixed connective tissue disease — goodbye to all that. *British Journal of Rheumatology*, **31**, 695–700.

Bodolay, E., Bojan, F., Szegedi, G., Stenszky, V., and Farid, N.R. (1989). Cytotoxic endothelial cell antibodies in mixed connective tissue disease. *Immunology Letters*, **20**, 163–7.

Bohan, A., Peter, J.B., Bowman, R.L., and Pearson, C.M. (1977). A computer-assisted analysis of 153 patients with polymyositis and dermatomyositis. *Medicine (Baltimore)*, **56**, 255–86.

Bolster, M.B. and Silver, R.M. (1994). Eosinophilia–myalgia syndrome, toxic-oil syndrome, and diffuse fasciitis with eosinophilia. *Current Opinion in Rheumatology*, **6**, 642–9.

Brand, C.A., Rowley, M.L., Tate, B.D., Muirden, K.D., and Whittingham, S.F. (1992). Coexistent rheumatoid arthritis and systemic lupus erythematosus. Clinical, serological and phenotypic features. *Annals of the Rheumatic Diseases*, **51**, 173–6.

Calderon, L., Rodriguez-Valverde, V., Sanchez-Andrade, S., Riestra, J.L., and Gomez-Reyno, J. (1984). Clinical profiles of patients with antibodies to nuclear ribonucleoprotein. *Clinical Rheumatology*, **8**, 483–92.

Carr, L., Ruther, E., Berg, P.A., and Lehnert, H. (1994). Eosinophilia–myalgia syndrome in Germany: an epidemiologic review. *Mayo Clinic Proceedings*, **69**, 620–5.

Catoggio, L.J., Evison, G., Harkness, J.A.L., and Maddison, P.J. (1983). The arthropathy of systemic sclerosis (scleroderma); comparison with mixed connective tissue disease. *Clinical and Experimental Rheumatology*, **1**, 101–12.

Catoggio, L.J., Soriano, E.R., Imamura, P., Almeida, V., Gonzales Salas, P., and Mayorga, L.M.(1993). Caracteristicas y evolucion de 52 pacientes con anti U1 RNP. *Revista Argentina de Reumatologia*, **4**, 138 (abstract).

Centers for Disease Control (1989). Eosinophilia–myalgia syndrome New Mexico. *Morbidity and Mortality Weekly Report*, **38**, 765–7.

Cheg, T.O. (1993). Pulmonary hypertension in patients with eosinophilia–myalgia syndrome or toxic oil syndrome. *Mayo Clinic Proceedings*, **68**, 823–4.

Clarke, A.K., Galbraith, R.M., Hamilton, E.B.D., and Williams, R. (1978). Rheumatic disorders in primary biliary cirrhosis. *Annals of the Rheumatic Diseases*, **37**, 42–7.

Clements, P.J. *et al.* (1978). Muscle disease in progressive systemic sclerosis. *Arthritis and Rheumatism*, **21**, 62–71.

Cohen, M.G. and Webb, J. (1987). Concurrence of rheumatoid arthritis and systemic lupus erythematosus: report of 11 cases. *Annals of the Rheumatic Diseases*, **46**, 853–8.

Culp, K.S. (1985). Autoimmune associations in primary biliary cirrhosis. *Mayo Clinic Proceedings*, **57**, 365.

Dahl, M., Chalmers, A., Wade, J., Calverley, D., and Munt, B. (1992). Ten year survival of a patient with advanced pulmonary hypertension and mixed connective tissue disease treated with immunosuppressive therapy. *Journal of Rheumatology*, **19**, 1807–9.

Doria, A., Bonavina, L., Anselmino, M., Ruffatti, A., Favaretto, M., and Gambari, P. (1991). Esophageal involvement in mixed connective tissue disease. *Journal of Rheumatology*, **18**, 685–90.

Doria, A., Ghirardello, A., Zambiasi, P., Ruffatti, A., and Gambari, P. (1992). Japanese diagnostic criteria for mixed connective tissue disease in Caucasian patients. *Journal of Rheumatology*, **19**, 259–64.

Doria A. *et al.* (1992). Antiphospholipid antibodies in mixed connective tissue disease. *Clinical Rheumatology*, **11**, 48–50

Eidson, M., Philen, R.M., Sewell, C.M., Voorhees, R., and Kilbourne, E.M. (1990). L-tryptophan and eosinophilia–myalgia syndrome in New Mexico. *Lancet*, **335**, 645–8.

Emlen, W. (1979). Complete heart block in mixed connective tissue disease. *Arthritis and Rheumatism*, **22**, 679–80.

Farrington, M.L., Haas, J.E., Nazar-Stewart, V., and Mellins, E.D. (1993). Eosinophilic fasciitis in children frequently progress to scleroderma-like cutaneous fibrosis. *Journal of Rheumatology*, **20**, 128–32.

Fatenjad, S., Mamula, M.J., and Craft, J. (1993). Role of intermolecular/intrastructural B- and T-cell determinants in the diversification of autoantibodies to ribonucleoprotein particles. *Proceedings of the National Academy of Sciences (USA)*, **90**, 12010–14.

Fisher, D.E., Reeves, W.H., Wisniewolski, R., Lahita, R.G., and Chiorazzi, N. (1985). Temporal shifts from Sm to ribonucleoprotein reactivity in systemic lupus erythematosus. *Arthritis and Rheumatism*, **28**, 1348–55.

Freundlich, B. *et al.* (1990). L-tryptophan ingestion associated with eosinophilic fasciitis but not progressive systemic sclerosis. *Annals of Internal Medicine*, **112**, 758–62.

Friedman, D.M., Mitnick, H.J., and Danilowicz, D. (1992). Recovery from pulmonary hypertension in an adolescent with mixed connective tissue disease. *Annals of the Rheumatic Diseases*, **51**, 1001–4.

Fujimoto, M., Kira, J., Murai, H., Yoshimura, T., Takizawa, K., and Goto, I.(1993). Hypertrophic cranial pachymeningitis associated with mixed connective tissue disease; a comparison with idiopathic and infectious pachymeningitis. *Internal Medicine*, **32**, 510–12.

Furuya, T. *et al.* (1992). Mixed connective tissue disease associated with protein losing enteropathy, successful treatment with intravenous cyclophosphamide therapy. *Internal Medicine*, **31**, 1359–62.

Gendi, N.S.T., Welsh, K.I., Van Venrooij, W.J., Vancheeswaran, R., Gilroy, J., and Black, C. (1995). HLA type as a predictor of mixed connective tissue disease differentiation. Ten-year clinical and immunogenetic followup of 46 patients. *Arthritis and Rheumatism*, **38**, 259–66.

Gilliam, J.N. and Prystowsky, S.D. (1977). Mixed connective tissue disease syndrome. Cutaneous manifestations of patients with epidermal nuclear staining and high titer serum antibody to ribonuclease-sensitive extractable nuclear antigen. *Archives of Dermatology*, **113**, 583–7.

Ginsburg, W.W., Conn, D., Bunch, T.W., and McDuffie, F.C. (1983). Comparison of clinical and serologic markers in systemic lupus erythematosus and overlap syndrome: a review of 247 patients. *Journal of Rheumatology*, **10**, 235–41.

Goldstein, R. *et al.* (1990). HLA-D region genes associated with autoantibody responses to histidyl-transfer RNA synthetase (Jo-1) and other translation-related factors in myositis. *Arthritis and Rheumatism*, **33**, 1240–8.

Granier, F., Vayssairat, M., Priollet, P., and Housset, E. (1986). Nailfold capillary microscopy in mixed connective tissue disease. Comparison with systemic sclerosis and systemic lupus erythematosus. *Arthritis and Rheumatism*, **29**, 189–95.

Grant, K.D., Adams, L.E., and Hess, E.V. (1981). Mixed connective tissue disease—a subset with sequential clinical and laboratory features. *Journal of Rheumatology*, **8**, 587–98.

Granter, S.R., Barnhill, R.L., Hewins, M.E., and Duray, P.H. (1994). Identification of *Borrelia burgdorferi* in diffuse fasciitis with peripheral eosinophilia: borrelial fasciitis. *Journal of the American Medical Association*, **272**, 1283–5.

Hagen, N.A., Stevens, J.C., and Michet, C.J., Jr. (1990). Trigeminal sensory neuropathy associated with connective tissue diseases. *Neurology*, **40**, 891–6.

Hainaut, P., Lavenne, E., Magy, J.M., and Lebacq, E.G. (1986). Circulating lupus type anticoagulant and pulmonary hypertension associated with mixed connective tissue disease. *Clinical Rheumatology*, **5**, 96–101.

Hameenkorpi, R., Ruuska, P., Forsberg, S., Tiilikainen, R., Makitalo, R., and Hakala, M. (1993). More evidence of distinctive features of mixed connective tissue disease. *Scandinavian Journal of Rheumatology*, **22**, 63–8.

Hatch, D.L. and Goldman, L.R. (1993). Reduced severity of eosinophilia–myalgia syndrome associated with the consumption of vitamin-containing supplements before illness. *Annals of Internal Medicine*, **153**, 2368–73.

Hatch, D.L., Garona, J.E., Goldman, L.R., and Walker, K.O. (1991). Persistent eosinophilia in an infant with probable intrauterine exposure to L-tryptophan-containing supplements. *Pediatrics*, **88**, 810–13.

Hedberg, K., Urbach, D., Slutsker, L., Matson, P., and Fleming, D. (1992). Eosinophilia–myalgia syndrome. Natural history in a population-based cohort. *Archives of Internal Medicine*, **152**, 1889–92.

Hench, P.K., Edgington, T.S., and Tan, E.M. (1975). The evolving clinical spectrum of mixed connective tissue disease (MCTD). *Arthritis and Rheumatism*, **18**, 404.

Hertzman, P.A. and Abaitua Borda, I. (1993). The toxic oil syndrome and the eosinophilia–myalgia syndrome: pursuing clinical parallels. *Journal of Rheumatology*, **20**, 1707–10.

Hirose, W. *et al.* (1993). Duodenal hemorrhage and dermal vasculitis associated with mixed connective tissue disease. *Journal of Rheumatology*, **20**, 151–4.

Hochberg, M.C., Feldman, D., Stevens, M.B., Arnett, F.C., and Reichlin, M. (1984). Antibody to Jo-1 in polymyositis/dermatomyositis. Association with interstitial pulmonary disease. *Journal of Rheumatology*, **11**, 663–5.

Hochberg, M.C., Feldman, D., and Stevens, M.B. (1986). Adult onset polymyositis/dermatomyositis: an analysis of clinical and laboratory features and survival in 76 patients with a review of the literature. *Seminars in Arthritis and Rheumatism*, **15**, 168–78.

Hoffman, R., Young, N., Ershler, W.B., Mazur, E., and Gewirtz, A. (1982). Diffuse fasciitis and aplastic anemia: a report of four cases revealing an unusual association between rheumatologic and hematologic disorders. *Medicine*, **61**, 373–81.

Hoffman, R.W. *et al.* (1993). Human T cell clones reactive against U-small nuclear ribonucleoprotein autoantigens from connective tissue disease patients and healthy individuals. *Journal of Immunology*, **151**, 6460–9.

Holyst, M.M., Hill, D.L., Sharp, G.C., and Hoffman, R.W. (1994). Increased frequency of mutations in the hprt gene of T cells isolated from patients with anti-U1-70 kD-autoantibody-positive connective tissue disease. *International Archives of Allergy and Immunology*, **105**, 234–7.

Hutton, C.W., Maddison, P.J., Collins, A.J., and Berriman, J.A. (1988). Intra-articular apatite deposition in mixed connective tissue disease: crystallographic and technetium scanning charcacteristics. *Annals of the Rheumatic Diseases*, **47**, 1027–30.

Imamura, P.M., Catoggio, L.J., Soriano, E.R., Baruzzo, C., and Mayorga, L.M. (1993). Clinical and serological characteristics of 34 Argentine patients with dermato-polymyositis. *Revista Argentina de Reumatologia*, **4**, 90–8.

Izumiyama, T. *et al.* (1993). Small airway involvement in mixed connective tissue disease. *Tokyo Journal of Experimental Medicine*, **170**, 173–83.

James, J.P. *et al.* (1990). Factor VIII-related antigen in connective tissue disease patients and relatives. *British Journal of Rheumatology*, **29**, 6–9.

James, T.N. *et al.* (1991). Cardiac abnormalities in the toxic oil syndrome, with comparative observations on the eosinophilia–myalgia syndrome. *Journal of the American College of Cardiology*, **18**, 1367–79.

Kahn, M.F., Bourgeois, P., Aeschlimann, A., and de Truchis, P. (1989). Mixed connective tissue disease after exposure to polyvinyl chloride. *Journal of Rheumatology*, **16**, 533–5.

Kallenberg, C.G., Van-Dissel Emiliani, F., Huitema, M.G., Limburg, P.C., and The, T.H. (1988). B-Cell proliferation and differentiation in systemic lupus erythematosus and mixed connective tissue disease. *Journal of Clinical Laboratory and Immunology*, **26**, 55–61.

Kappes, J. and Bennett, R.M. (1982). Cauda equina syndrome in a patient with high titer anti-RNP antibodies. *Arthritis and Rheumatism*, **25**, 349–52.

Kasukawa, R. *et al.* (1987). Preliminary diagnostic criteria for classification of mixed connective tissue diseases. In *Mixed connective tissue diseases and antinuclear antibodies* (ed. R. Kasukawa and G.C. Sharp), pp. 41–7. Excerpta Medica, Amsterdam.

Kasukawa, R., Nishimaki, T., Takagi, T., Miyawaki, S., Yokohari, R., and Tsunematsu, T. (1990). Pulmonary hypertension in connective tissue disease. Clinical analysis of sixty patients in a multi-institutional study. *Clinical Rheumatology*, **9**, 56–62.

Kaufman, L.D. (1993). Eosinophilia–myalgia syndrome: morbidity and mortality. *Journal of Rheumatology*, **20**, 1644–6.

Kaufman, L.D., Seidman, R.J., and Gruber, B.L. (1990). L-tryptophan-associated eosinophilic perimyositis, neuritis, and fasciitis. A clinicopathologic and laboratory study of 25 patients. *Medicine (Baltimore)*, **69**, 187–99.

Kessler, E., Halpern, M., Chagnac, A., Zevin, D., Hammel, I., and Ben-Bassat, M. (1992). Unusual renal deposit in mixed connective tissue disease. *Archives of Pathology and Laboratory Medicine*, **116**, 261–4.

Kilbourne, E.M. *et al.* (1983). Clinical epidemiology of toxic-oil syndrome. *New England Journal of Medicine*, **309**, 1408–14.

Kilbourne, E.M. *et al.* (1988). Chemical correlates of pathogenicity of oils related to the toxic oil syndrome epidemic in Spain. *American Journal of Epidemiology*, **127**, 1210–27.

Kilbourne, E.M. *et al.* (ed.) (1990). Interim guidance on the eosinophilia–myalgia syndrome. *Annals of Internal Medicine*, **112**, 85–6.

Kitridou, R.C., Akmal, M., Turkel, S.B., Ehresmann, G.R., Quismorio, F.P., Jr., and Massry, S.G. (1986). Renal involvement in mixed connective tissue disease: a longitudinal clinicopathologic study. *Seminars in Arthritis and Rheumatism*, **16**, 135–45.

Krupp, L.B., Masur, D.M., and Kaufman, L.D. (1993). Neurocognitive dysfunction in the eosinophilia–myalgia syndrome. *Neurology*, **43**, 931–6.

Kuipers, E.J., Van-Leeuwen, M.A., Nillels, P.G., Jager, J., and Van Rijswijk, M.H. (1991). Hemobilia due to vasculitis of the gall bladder in a patient with mixed connective tissue disease. *Journal of Rheumatology*, **18**, 617–18.

Kumagai Y., Shiokawa Y., Medsger T.A., and Rodnan G.P. (1984). Clinical spectrum of connective tissue disease after cosmetic surgery. *Arthritis and Rheumatism*, **27**, 1–12.

Kuwana, M., Okano, Y., Kaburaki, J., Tsuji, K., and Inoko, H. (1995). Major histocompatibility complex class II gene associations with anti-U1 small nuclear ribonucleoprotein antibody. *Arthritis and Rheumatism*, **38**, 396–405.

Lakhampal, S., Ginsburg, W.W., Michet, J.J., Doyle, J.A., and Breanndan Morre, S. (1988). Eosinophilic fasciitis: clinical spectrum and therapeutic response in 52 cases. *Seminars in Arthritis and Rheumatism*, **17**, 221–31.

Laneuville, P. (1992). Cyclosporin A induced remission of CD4+ T CLL, associated with eosinophilia and fasciitis. *British Journal of Haematology*, **80**, 252–4.

Langley, R.L. and Treadwell, E.L. (1994). Cardiac tamponade and pericardial disorders in connective tissue diseases: case report and literature review. *Journal of the National Medical Association*, **86**, 149–53.

Lazaro, M.A. *et al.* (1989). Clinical and serologic characteristics of patients with overlap syndrome: is mixed connective tissue disease a distinct clinical entity? *Medicine (Baltimore)*, **68**, 58–65.

Lazaro, M.A., Gomez Tejada, R., Berenstein, T., Gene, R., Citera, G., and Maldonado Cocco, J.A. (1993). Pulmonary hypertension in overlap syndrome. *Arthritis and Rheumatism*, **36** (Suppl.), S276 (abstract).

Lemmer, J.P., Curry, N.H., Mallory, J.H., and Waller, M.V. (1982). Clinical characteristics and course in patients with high titer anti-RNP antibodies. *Journal of Rheumatology*, **9**, 536–42.

LeRoy, E.C. and Medsger, T.A., Jr. (1992). Raynaud's phenomenon: a proposal for classification. *Clinical and Experimental Rheumatology*, **10**, 485–8.

LeRoy, E.C., Mariq, H.R., and Kahaleh, M.B. (1980). Undifferentiated connective tissue syndromes. *Arthritis and Rheumatism*, **23**, 341–3.

Leung, W.H., Wong, K.L., Lau, C.P., Wong, C.K., Cheng, C.H., and Tai, Y.T. (1990). Doppler-echo evaluation of left ventricular diastolic filling in patient with mixed connective tissue disease. *Cardiology*, **77**, 93–100.

Lin, J.D. *et al.* (1992). Pathologic manifestations of the eosinophilia–myalgia syndrome: analysis of 11 cases. *Human Pathology*, **23**, 429–37.

Love, L.A. *et al.* (1991). A new approach to the classification of idiopathic inflammatory myopathy: myositis-specific autoantibodies define useful homogenous patient groups. *Medicine (Baltimore)*, **70**, 360–74.

Love, L.A. *et al.* (1993). Pathological and immunological effects of ingesting L-tryptophan and 1,1'-ethylidenebis(L-tryptophan) in Lewis rats. *Journal of Clinical Investigation*, **91**, 804–11.

Lundberg, I. and Hedfors, E. (1991). Clinical course of patients with anti-RNP antibodies. A prospective study of 32 patients. *Journal of Rheumatology*, **18**, 1511–9.

Lundberg, I., Nennesmo, I., and Hedfors, E. (1992). A clinical, serological, and histopathological study of myositis patients with and without anti-RNP antibodies. *Seminars in Arthritis and Rheumatism*, **22**, 127–38.

Lundberg, I., Nyman, U., Pettersson, I., and Hedfors, E. (1992). Clinical manifestations and anti-(U1)sn RNP antibodies: a prospective study of 29 anti-RNP antibody positive patients. *British Journal of Rheumatology*, **31**, 811–17.

Maddison, P.J. (1991). Mixed connective tissue disease, overlap syndromes, and eosiniphilic fasciitis. *Annals of the Rheumatic Diseases*, **50**, 887–93.

Maddison, P.J., Mogavero, H., and Reichlin, M. (1978). Patterns of clinical disease associated with antibodies to nuclear ribonucleoprotein. *Journal of Rheumatology*, **5**, 407–11.

Magnusson, B. (1993). Collagen diseases in children 0–15 years of age in Sweden 1984–88. *Journal of Rheumatology*, **20** (Suppl.), 61 (abstract).

Marguerie, C. *et al.* (1992). The clinical and immunogenetic features of patients with autoantibodies to the nucleolar antigen PM-Scl. *Medicine (Baltimore)*, **71**, 327–36.

Maricq, H.R. *et al.* (1980). Diagnostic potential of in vivo capillary microscopy in scleroderma and related disorders. *Arthritis and Rheumatism*, **23**, 183–9.

Marshall, J.B. *et al.* (1990). Gastrointestinal manifestations of mixed connective tissue disease. *Gastroenterology*, **98**, 1232–8.

Martin, R.W. *et al.* (1990). The clinical spectrum of the eosinophilia–myalgia syndrome associated with L-tryptophan ingestion. *Annals of Internal Medicine*, **113**, 124–34.

Martin, R.W., Duffy, J., and Lie, J.T. (1991). Eosinophilic fascitis associated with use of L-tryptophan: a case control study and comparison of clinical and histopathologic features. *Mayo Clinic Proceedings*, **66**, 892–8.

Mathews, M.B. and Bernstein, R.M. (1983). Myositis autoantibody inhibits histidyl-tRNA synthetase: a model for autoimmunity. *Nature*, **304**, 177–9.

Mayeno, A.N. and Gleich, G.J. (1994). The eosinophilia–myalgia syndrome: lessons from Germany. *Mayo Clinic Proceedings*, **69**, 702–4.

Mayeno, A.N., Belongia, E.A., Lin, F., Lundy, S.K., and Gleich, G.J. (1992). 3-(Phenylamino)alanine, a novel aniline-derived amino-acid associated with the eosinophilia–myalgia syndrome: a link to the toxic oil syndrome? *Mayo Clinic Proceedings*, **67**, 1134–9.

McHugh, N., James, I., and Maddison, P. (1990). Clinical significance of antibodies to a 68 kDa U1RNP polypeptide in connective tissue disease. *Journal of Rheumatology*, **17**, 1320–8.

Michet, C.J., Doyle, J.A., and Ginsburg, W.W. (1981). Eosinophilic fascitis. Report of 15 cases. *Mayo Clinic Proceedings*, **56**, 27–34.

Miller, J.J., 3rd. (1992). The fasciitis–morphea complex in children. *American Journal of Diseases of Children*, **146**, 733–6.

Miyata, M. *et al.* (1992). Pulmonary hypertension in MCTD: report of two cases with anticardiolipin antibody. *Clinical Rheumatology*, **11**, 195–201.

Miyawaki, S. and Onodera, H. (1987). Clinical course and prognosis of patients with mixed connective tissue disease. In *Mixed connective tissue disease and antinuclear antibodies* (ed. R. Dasukawa and G. Sharp), pp. 331–6. Excerpta Medica, Amsterdam.

Murray-Lyon, I.M., Thompson, R.P.H., Ansell, I.D., and Williams, R. (1970). Scleroderma and primary biliary cirrhosis. *British Medical Journal*, **iii**, 258–9.

Naschitz, J.E. *et al.* (1994). Cancer associated fasciitis panniculitis. *Cancer*, **73**, 231–5.

Nightingale, S.L. (1992). From the Food and Drug Administration. *Journal of the American Medical Association*, **268**, 1828.

Nimelstein, S.H., Brody, S., Mcshane, D., and Holman, H.R. (1980). Mixed connective tissue disease: a subsequent evaluation of the original 25 patients. *Medicine (Baltimore)*, **59**, 239–48.

Nishikai, M. and Reichlin, M. (1980). Heterogeneity of precipitating antibodies in polymyositis and dermatomyositis: characterization of the Jo-1 antibody system. *Arthritis and Rheumatism*, **23**, 881–8.

Nitsche, A., Leiguarda, R.C., Maldonado Cocco, J.A., Lazaro, M.A., and Garcia Morteo, O. (1991). Neurological features in overlap syndrome. *Clinical Rheumatology*, **10**, 5–9.

Norman, D.A. and Fleischmann, R. (1978). Gastrointestinal systemic sclerosis in serologic mixed connective tissue disease. *Arthritis and Rheumatism*, **21**, 811–9.

O'Connell, D.J. and Bennett, R.M. (1977). Mixed connective tissue disease—clinical and radiological aspects of 20 cases. *British Journal of Radiology*, **50**, 620–5.

Oddis, C.V., Medsger, T.A., Jr, and Cooperstein, L.A. (1990). A subluxing arthropathy associated with the anti-Jo 1 antibody in polymyositis/dermatomyositis. *Arthritis and Rheumatism*, **33**, 1640–5.

Oetgen, W.J., Mutter, M.L., Lawless, O.J., and Davia, J.E. (1983). Cardiac abnormalities in mixed connective tissue disease. *Chest*, **83**, 185–8.

Ohtsuka, E., Nonaka, S., Shingu, M., Yasuda, M., and Nobunaga, M. (1992). Sjögren syndrome and mixed connective tissue disease. *Clinical and Experimental Rheumatology*, **10**, 339–44.

Okubo, M., Kurokawa, M., Ohto, H., Nishimaki, T., Nishioka, K., and Kasukawa, R. (1994). Clonotype analysis of peripheral blood T cells and autoantigen-reactive T cells from patients with mixed connective tissue disease. *Journal of Immunology*, **153**, 3784–90.

Pallis, M., Hopkinson, N., and Powell, R. (1991). Nailfold capillary density as a possible indicator of pulmonary capillary loss in systemic lupus erythematosus but not in mixed connective tissue disease. *Journal of Rheumatology*, **18**, 1532–6.

Panush, R.S., Edwards, L., Longley, S., and Webster, E. (1988). 'Rhupus' syndrome. *Archives of Internal Medicine*, **148**, 1633–6.

Pelkonen, P.M. *et al.* (1994). Incidence of systemic connective tissue diseases in children: a nationwide prospective study in Finland. *Journal of Rheumatology*, **21**, 2143–6.

Peller, J.S., Gabor, G.T., Porter, J.M., and Bennett, R.M. (1985). Angiographic findings in mixed connective tissue disease. Correlation with fingernail capillary photomicroscopy and digital photoplethysmography findings. *Arthritis and Rheumatism*, **28**, 768–74.

Piirainen, H.I., Helve, A.T., Tornroth, T., and Pettersson, T.E. (1989). Amyloidosis in mixed connective tissue disease. *Scandinavian Journal of Rheumatology*, **18**, 165–8.

Plotz, P.H., Dalakas, M., Leff, R.L., Love, L.A., Miller, F.W., and Cronin, M.E. (1989). Current concepts in the idiopathic inflammatory myopathies: polymyositis, dermatomyositis, and related disorders. *Annals of Internal Medicine*, **111**, 143–57.

Prakash, U.B.S., Luthra, H.S., and Divertie, M.B. (1985). Intrathoracic manifestations in mixed connective tissue disease. *Mayo Clinic Proceedings*, **60**, 813–21.

Pun, Y.L., Russell, D.M., Taggart, G.J., and Barraclough, D.R. (1991). Pneumatosis intestinalis and pneumoperitoneum complicating mixed connective tissue disease. *British Journal of Rheumatology*, **30**, 146–9.

Query, C.C. and Keene, J.D. (1987). A human autoimmune protein associated with U1 RNA contains a region of homology that is cross-reactive with retroviral p30[gag] antigen. *Cell*, **51**, 211–20.

Rakovec, P., Kenda, M.F., Rozman, B., Zemva, A., and Cibic, B. (1982). Panconductional defect in mixed connective tissue disease. Association with Sjögren's syndrome. *Chest*, **81**, 257–9.

Ranki, A., Kurki, P., Riepponen, S., and Stephansson, E. (1992). Antibodies to retroviral proteins in autoimmune connective tissue disease. Relation to clinical manifestations and ribonucleoprotein autoantibodies. *Arthritis and Rheumatism*, **35**, 1483–91.

Rasmussen, E.K., Ullman, S., Horer-Madsen, M., Sorensen, S.F., and Halberg, P. (1987). Clinical implications of ribonucleoprotein antibody. *Archives of Dermatology*, **123**, 601–5.

Read, C.A., Clauw, D., Weir, C., Da-Silva, A.T., and Katz, P. (1992). Dyspnea and pulmonary function in the L-tryptophan-associated eosinophilia–myalgia syndrome. *Chest*, **101**, 1282–6.

Reichlin, M. and Arnett, F.C. (1984). Multiplicity of antibodies in myositis sera. *Arthritis and Rheumatism*, **27**, 1150–6.

Reichlin, M. and Mattioli, M. (1972). Correlation of a precipitin reaction to an RNA protein antigen and a low prevalence of nephritis in patients with systemic lupus erythermatosus. *New England Journal of Medicine*, **286**, 908–11.

Reichlin, M. *et al.* (1984). Antibodies to a nuclear/nucleolar antigen in patients with polymyositis-overlap syndrome. *Journal of Clinical Immunology*, **4**, 40–4.

Reimer, G. (1990). Autoantibodies against nuclear, nucleolar, and mithochondrial antigens in systemic sclerosis (scleroderma). *Rheumatic Disease Clinics of North America*, **16**, 169–83.

Reimer, G., Huschka, U., Keller, J., Kammerer, R., and Hornstein, O.P. (1983). Immunofluorescence studies in progressive systemic sclerosis (scleroderma) and mixed connective tissue disease. *British Journal of Dermatology*, **109**, 27–36.

Reynolds, T.B., Denison, E.K., Frankl, H.D., Lieberman, F.L., and Peters, R.L. (1971). Primary biliary cirrhosis with scleroderma, Raynaud's phenomena, and telangiectasis. *American Journal of Medicine*, **67**, 302–12.

Satoh, K., Imai, H., Yasuda, T., Wakui, H., Miura, A.B., and Nakamoto, Y. (1994). Sclerodermatous renal crisis in a patient with mixed connective tissue disease. *American Journal of Kidney Diseases*, **24**, 215–8.

Savouret, J.F., Chudwin, D.S., Wara, D.W., Ammann, A.J., Cowan, M.J., and Miller, W.L. (1983). Clinical and laboratory findings in childhood mixed connective tissue disease: presence of antibody to ribonucleoprotein containing the small nuclear ribonucleic acid U1. *Journal of Pediatrics*, **102**, 841–6.

Searles, R.P., Mladinich, E.K., and Messner, R.P. (1978). Isolated trigeminal sensory neruopathy: early manifestation of mixed connective tissue disease. *Neurology*, **28**, 1286–9.

Sharp, G.C. (1987). Diagnostic criteria for classification of MCTD. In *Mixed connective tissue diseases and anti-nuclear antibodies* (ed. R. Kasukawa and G.C. Sharp), pp. 23–32. Excerpta Medica, Amsterdam.

Sharp, G.C. *et al.* (1971). Association of autoantibodies to different nuclear antigens with clinical patterns of rheumatic disease and responsiveness to therapy. *Journal of Clinical Investigation*, **50**, 350–9.

Sharp, G.C., Irvin, W.S., Tan, E.M., Gould, R.G., and Holman, H.R. (1972). Mixed connective tissue disease—an apparently distinct rheumatic disease syndrome associated with a specific antibody to an extractable nuclear antigen (ENA). *American Journal of Medicine*, **52**, 148–59.

Sharp, G.C. *et al.* (1976). Association of antibodies to ribonucleoprotein and Sm antigens with mixed connective-tissue disease, systemic lupus erythematosus and other rheumatic diseases. *New England Journal of Medicine*, **295**, 1149–54.

Shulman, L.E. (1974). Diffuse fasciitis with hypergammaglobulinaemia and eosiniphilia in a new syndrome. *Journal of Rheumatology*, **1** (Suppl.), 46.

Silver, R.M. (1993). Eosinophilia–myalgia syndrome, toxic-oil syndrome, and diffuse fasciitis with eosinophilia. *Current Opinion in Rheumatology*, **5**, 802–8.

Silver, R.M., Sutherland, S.E., Carreira, P., and Heyes, M.P. (1992). Alterations in tryptophan metabolism in the toxic oil syndrome and in the eosinophilia–myalgia syndrome. *Journal of Rheumatology*, **19**, 69–73.

Silver, R.M., *et al.* (1994). A murine model of the eosinophilia-myalgia syndrome induced by 1,1'-ethylidenebis(L-tryptophan). *Journal of Clinical Investigation*, **93**, 1473–80.

Singsen, B.H., Bernstein, B.H., Kornreich, H.K., Koster King, K., Hanson, V., and Tan, E.M. (1977). Mixed connective tissue disease in childhood. A clinical and serologic survey. *Journal of Pediatrics*, **90**, 893–900.

Singsen, B.H., Swanson, V.L., Bernstein, B.H., Heuser, E.T., Hanson, V., and Landing, B.H. (1980). A histologic evaluation of mixed connective tissue disease in childhood. *American Journal of Medicine*, **68**, 710–17.

Springer, M.A., Bock, H.G., Philen, R.M., Hill, R.H., Jr., and Crawford, L.V. (1992). Eosinophilia–myalgia syndrome in a child with phenylketonuria. *Pediatrics*, **90**, 630–3.

Stuart, R.A. and Maddison, P.J. (1991). Atlantoaxial subluxation in a patient with mixed connective tissue disease. *Journal of Rheumatology*, **18**, 1617–20.

Sullivan, W.D. *et al.* (1984). A prospective evaluation emphasizing pulmonary involvement in patients with mixed connective tissue disease. *Medicine (Baltimore)*, **63**, 92–107.

Swygert, L.A., Maes, E.F., Sewell, L.E., Miller, L., Falk, H., and Kilbourne, E.M. (1990). Eosinophilia–myalgia syndrome. Results of national surveillance. *Journal of the American Medical Association*, **264**, 1698–703.

Swygert, L.A., Back, E.E., Auerbach, S.B., Sewell, L.E., and Falk, H. (1993). Eosinophilia–myalgia syndrome: mortality data from the US national surveillance system. *Journal of Rheumatology*, **20**, 1711–17.

Targoff, I.N. (1992). Autoantibodies in polymyositis. *Rheumatic Disease Clinics of North America*, **18**, 455–82.

Targoff, I.N. and Arnett, F.C. (1990). Clinical manifestatioins in patients with antibody to PL-12 antigen (alanyl-tRNA synthetase). *American Journal of Medicine*, **88**, 241–51.

Thiele, D.L. and Krejs, G.J. (1985). Secretory diarrhea in mixed connective tissue disease. *American Journal of Gastroenterology*, **80**, 107–10.

Tiddens, H.A.W.M. *et al.* (1993). Juvenile-onset mixed connective tissue disease: longitudinal follow-up. *Journal of Pediatrics*, **122**, 191–7.

Udoff, E.J., Genant, H.K., Kozin, F., and Ginsberg, M. (1977). Mixed connective tissue disease: the spectrum of radiographic manifestations. *Radiology*, **124**, 613–18.

Udvardy, M., Bodolay, E., Szegedi, G., Harsfalvi, J., Boda, Z., and Rak, K. (1991). Alterations of primary haemostasis in mixed connective tissue disease (MCTD). *Thrombosis Research*, **63**, 281–6

Ueda, Y. *et al.* (1991). Successful treatment of acute right cardiac failure due to pulmonary thromboembolism in mixed connective tissue disease. *Japanese Journal of Medicine*, **30**, 568–72.

Van Den Hoogen, F.H.J. *et al.* (1994). Long-term follow-up of 46 patients with anti-(U1)snRNP antibodies. *British Journal of Rheumatology*, **33**, 1117–20.

Varga, J., Griffin, R., Newman, J.H., and Jimenez, S.A. (1991). Eosinophilic fasciitis is clinically distinguishable from the eosinophilia–myalgia syndrome and is not associated with L-tryptophan use. *Journal of Rheumatology*, **18**, 259–63.

Varga, J., Jimenez, S.A., and Uitto, J. (1993). L-tryptophan and the eosinophilia–myalgia syndrome: current understanding of the etiology and pathogenesis. *Journal of Investigative Dermatology*, **100**, 97S–105S.

Wasicek, C.A., Reichlin, M., Montes, M., and Raghu, G. (1984). Polymyositis and interstitial lung disease in a patient with anti-Jol prototype. *American Journal of Medicine*, **76**, 538–44.

Watanabe-Fukunaga, R., Brannan, C.I., Coopeland, N.G., Jenkins, N.A., and Nagata, S. (1992). Lymphoproliferation disorder in mice explained by defects in Fas antigen that mediates apoptosis. *Nature*, **356**, 314–17.

Weiner-Kronish, J.P., Solinger, A.M., Warnock, M.L., Gurg, A., Ordonez, N., and Golden, J.A. (1981). Severe pulmonary involvement in mixed connective tissue disease. *American Review of Respiratory Dziseases*, **124**, 499–503.

Weiss, T.D., Nelson, J.S., Woolsey, R.M., Zuckner, J., and Baldasare, A.R. (1978). Transverse myelitis in mixed connective tissue disease. *Arthritis and Rheumatism*, **21**, 982.

Whyte, J., Hough, D., Maddison, P.J., and McHugh, N.J. (1994). The association of primary biliary cirrhosis and systemic sclerosis is not accounted for by cross reactivity between mitochondiral and centromere antigens. *Journal of Autoimmunity*, **7**, 413–24.

5.13 Miscellaneous inflammatory conditions

5.13.1 Amyloidosis

Gunnar Husby

Definition of amyloid and amyloidosis

The term amyloidosis relates to a heterogeneous group of disorders (rather than a single disease entity) characterized by extracellular deposition of a proteinaceous, fibrillar material — amyloid — in various tissues and organs (Glenner 1980; Husby and Sletten 1986; Husby 1992). The unique amyloid fibril is the principal component of all amyloids irrespective of the clinical expression, tissues, or species involved, or whether they arise spontaneously or are induced in experimental animals.

Amyloid fibrils as seen in the electron microscope are rigid and non-branching with a diameter of 10 to 15 nm, of indefinite length, and consist of polypeptide chains arranged in a twisted β-pleated sheet (Glenner 1980). This specific structure of the fibril proteins determines the tinctorial and optical properties of amyloid, i.e. the affinity for Congo red and the typical green/yellow birefringence seen when amyloid stained with Congo red is viewed in a polarizing microscope (Cooper 1974). The low solubility and relative resistance to proteolytic digestion of the amyloid fibrils contribute to the irreversible and often progressive course of amyloidosis, in many cases leading to death within months or a few years of diagnosis (Husby 1985).

Benditt and Eriksen (1964) observed that in spite of the morphological similarities between amyloids in different clinical settings, amyloid is heterogeneous also with respect to the nature of the amyloid fibrils. Subsequent studies of amyloid extracted from different affected tissues (Pras *et al.* 1968) have revealed that they may be composed of a variety of different protein subunits (Husby and Sletten 1986).

In addition, an extrafibrillar protein called the amyloid-P component or protein **AP**, derived from a normal plasma glycoprotein, termed **SAP**, is invariably present in amyloid, regardless of the type of fibril protein (Pepys 1988). A carbohydrate moiety in the form of glycosaminoglycans and proteoglycans has also been demonstrated in all amyloids deposits so far examined (Kisilevski 1987; Magnus *et al.* 1989; Husby *et al.* 1994b; Stenstad *et al.* 1994).

Amyloid fibril proteins

The chief component of amyloid fibrils is a distinct protein subunit with a relatively small molecular mass — 3000 to 30 000 Da in different fibril preparations (Glenner 1980; Husby and Sletten, 1986). Several, apparently non-related proteins can constitute this amyloid fibril subunit in different cases of amyloidosis, a common feature being the ability to assume the β-pleated sheet typical of amyloid (Glenner 1980). A steadily increasing number of such proteins (17 at the present time) have been characterized by their amino acid sequence (Table 1), and in many cases complementary DNA has also been established. The different amyloid proteins are often related to distinct clinical forms of amyloidosis. Indeed, many types of amyloid disease can now be defined and classified by structural analysis of the fibril proteins and/or the genes coding for them (Benditt and Eriksen 1971; Glenner 1980; Husby and Sletten 1986; Husby 1994).

Certain serum proteins are precursors of the different fibril proteins in the various systemic forms of amyloidosis (Glenner 1980; Husby and Sletten 1986). Two important types of fibril protein related to systemic amyloidosis are the amyloid-L (**AL**) and amyloid-A (**AA**) proteins (Table 1). Protein AL, which consists of homogeneous (monoclonal) immunoglobulin light chains or their aminoterminal fragments is seen in idiopathic and myeloma-associated amyloidosis (AL amyloidosis) (Glenner 1980; Husby 1983). Protein AA (Table 2), which is derived from the serum amyloid-A protein (Husebekk *et al.* 1985), is associated with reactive amyloidosis, familial Mediterranean fever, familial nephropathic amyloidosis with febrile urticaria — the Muckle–Wells syndrome (Muckle 1979; Linke *et al.* 1983) — and spontaneous or experimental amyloidosis in animals (Glenner 1980; Husby and Sletten 1986). These forms of amyloidosis could therefore also be called AA. Serum amyloid A (**SAA**), an apolipoprotein present on high-density lipoprotein in serum, is one of the most sensitive acute-phase proteins described (Marhaug *et al.* 1986). However, its function is largely unknown except for its association with AA amyloidosis and an active role in the metabolism and transport of cholesterol (Meek *et al.* 1994). An extensive review of the histology of SAA/AA proteins and genes and their relation to AA amyloidosis has recently been published (Husby *et al.* 1994a).

Different genetic variants of transthyretin (Table 1), previously termed prealbumin (Husby *et al.* 1990), are associated with the autosomal-dominant familial amyloid polyneuropathies and cardiomyopathies (Nordlie *et al.* 1988; Benson and Wallace 1989). Normal transthyretin makes up systemic senile amyloid (Westermark *et al.* 1986).

Table 1 Nomenclature and classification of human amyloid and amyloidosis[a]

Amyloid protein	Protein precursor	Protein type or variant	Clinical
AA	SAA		Reactive (secondary)
			Familial Mediterranean fever
			Familial amyloid nephropathy with urticaria and deafness
			(Muckle–Wells' syndrome)
AL	κ, λ e.g. κIII	AκAλ e.g. AκIII	Idiopathic (primary), myeloma- or macroglobulinaemia-associated
AH	IgH, e.g. λ_1	$A\lambda_1$	
ATTR	Transthyretin	e.g. Met 30	Familial amyloid polyneuropathy, Portuguese
		e.g. Met 111 TTR	Familial amyloid cardiomyopathy, Danish
$AApoA_1$	$apoA_1$	e.g. Arg 26	Familial amyloid polyneuyropathy, Iowa
		Arg 60	Hereditary non-neuropathic systemic amyloidosis
			(Ostertag-type)
AGel	Gelsolin	Asn 187 (15)	Familial amyloidosis, Finnish
ACys	Cystatin C	Gin 68	Hereditary cerebral haemorrhage with amyloidosis, Icelandic
ALys	Lysozyme	e.g. Thr 56	Hereditary non-neuropathic systemic anyloidosis
			(Ostertag-type)
AFib	Fibrinogen	Leu 554	Hereditary renal anyloidosis
Aβ	β protein precursor, e.g. βPP 695		Alzheimer's disease
			Down's syndrome
		Gin 618(22)	Hereditary cerebral haemorrhage with amyloidosis, Dutch
Aβ2M	β_2Microglobulin		Associated with chronic dialysis
AScr	Scrapie protein precursor 33–35, cellular form	Scrapie protein 27–30	Creutzfeldt–Jakob disease etc.
		e.g. Leu 102	Gerstmann–Straüssler–Scheinker syndrome
ACal	(Pro)calcitonin	(Pro)calcitonin	In medullary carcinomas of the thyroid
AANF	Atrial natriuretic factor		Isolated atrial amyloid
AIAPP	Islet amyloid polypeptide		In islets of Langerhans, diabetes type II, insulinoma

[a]See Husby *et al.* (1990) and Husby (1994) for more details.

Three other serum proteins are also associated with hereditary amyloidosis (Table 1). A variant of apolipoprotein **AI** represents the fibril protein in familial amyloid polyneuropathy from Iowa (Nichols *et al.* 1988), whereas a variant gelsolin, an actin-modulating protein, plays the same role in familial amyloid polyneuropathy of Finnish origin (Maury 1990a). Recently a molecular variant of fibrinogen (Uemichi *et al.* 1994) was found to be associated with hereditary renal amyloidosis, the first form of inherited amyloidosis to be described by Ostertag (1932). A variant of the bacteriolytic enzyme, lysozyme (a product of macrophages and polymorphs normally present in various body secretions), is the amyloid fibril protein found in cases of systemic amyloidosis with predominant renal effects (Pepys *et al.* 1993).

A variant of cystatin C, an enzyme inhibitor, is the fibril protein precursor in inherited cerebral haemorrhage with amyloidosis, Icelandic type (Ghiso *et al.* 1986). The cerebral vessels of members of a Dutch family with a similar clinical picture are affected by amyloid made up by the amyloid β-protein, a 42-amino acid fragment of a variant β-protein precursor (Levy *et al.* 1990). Amyloid β-protein derived from normal β-protein precursor (a cell membrane protein) makes up the cerebral amyloid in Alzheimer's disease and Down's syndrome (Glenner and Murphy 1989).

β_2-Microglobulin, which represents a part of class I histocompatibility molecules, makes up the fibrils in amyloidosis associated with long-term dialysis treatment for renal failure (Gejyo *et al.* 1985). β_2-Microglobulin-derived amyloid affects mainly structures of the

Table 2 Partial aminoterminal amino acid sequence of serum amyloid-A (SAA) and amyloid-A (AA) proteins from man, mouse, mink, and horse, numbered according to human SAA. Alignment is done to maximize homology. Only the amino acid residues that differ from those of human SAA and AA are shown for mouse, mink, and horse. Those amino acid residues that specify amyloidogenic SAA molecules are underlined.

	1	2	3	4	5	6	7	8	9	10	11	12	13	14	15	16	17	18
Human SAA	Arg	Ser	Phe	Phe	Ser	Phe	Leu	Gly	Glu	Ala	Phe	Asp	Gly	Ala	Arg	Asp	Met	Trp
Human AA	–	–	–	–	–	–	–	–	–	–	–	–	–	–	–	–	–	–
Mouse SAA1		Gly	–	–	–	–	Val	His	–	–	–	Gln	–	–	Gly	–	–	–
Mouse SAA2		Gly	–	–	–	–	<u>Ile</u>	<u>Gly</u>	–	–	–	Gln	–	–	Gly	–	–	–
Mouse AA		Gly	–	–	–	–	<u>Ile</u>	<u>Gly</u>	–	–	–	Gln	–	–	Gly	–	–	–
Mink SAA1	PCA	Trp	Tyr	–	–	Phe	–	–	–	Ile	Gln	–	–	Trp	–	–	Tyr	
Mink SAA2	PCA	Trp	Tyr	–	–	Phe	–	–	–	<u>Val</u>	Gln	–	–	Trp	–	–	Tyr	
Mink AA	PCA	Trp	Tyr	–	–	Phe	–	–	–	<u>Val</u>	Gln	–	–	Trp	–	–	Tyr	
Horse SAA1	–	–	Leu	Leu	–	–	–	–	–	–	Ala	Arg	–	Thr	Trp	–	–	Ile
Horse SAA2		Leu	Leu	–	–	–	–	–	–	–	Ala	Arg	–	Thr	Trp	–	–	<u>Leu</u>
Horse AA	NH₂	Leu	Leu	–	–	–	–	–	–	–	Ala	Arg	–	Thr	Trp	–	–	<u>Leu</u>

Sources of sequences: human SAA — Sletten *et al.* (1983); human AA — Sletten and Husby (1974); mouse AA — Eriksen *et al.* (1976); mouse SAA — Anders *et al.* (1977), Yamomoto *et al.* (1985); mink AA Waalen *et al.* (1980); mink SAA — Syversen *et al.* (1987), Marhaug *et al.* (1990).

locomotor system, like the carpal tunnel, joints, and bone, but systemic distribution is also seen (Kay 1993).

Several hormones are known to form amyloid. The first to be demonstrated was a calcitonin-like molecule in amyloid deposited locally in medullary carcinomas of the thyroid and their metastases (Sletten *et al.* 1976). Atrial natriuretic factor makes up amyloid in isolated atrial amyloidosis of the heart (Johansson *et al.* 1987), and islet amyloid polypeptide plays the same role in amyloid localized to the islets of Langerhans in association with diabetes type II and insulinomas (Westermark *et al.* 1986).

It is thus clear that amyloidosis is heterogeneous not only with respect to clinical expression and protein composition, but also to the functional aspect of the various amyloid precursors.

Pathogenesis

The mechanisms by which the various soluble precursor proteins are converted to insoluble protein aggregates with the unique morphology of amyloid fibrils, and are then deposited in the different target tissues, are not clarified. Also, the predilection of certain amyloid fibrils for particular tissues or organs, often distant from the cells actually producing the fibril protein precursor, remains a mystery.

It is generally accepted that the aetiology and pathogenesis of amyloidosis are multifactorial. Furthermore, the relative importance of the various amyloid-promoting factors may differ in the different types of amyloidosis. Best studied are the pathogenetic mechanisms in the reactive AA type of amyloidosis, as this type is readily induced

in experimental animals, and spontaneous AA amyloidosis has been demonstrated in a variety of warm-blooded species, ranging from birds to primates (Husby 1989; Husby 1992).

Amyloidosis may be caused by amyloidogenic precursor protein present in excess amounts, either as a consequence of increased production or decreased clearance. AA amyloid is prevalent in those of the chronic inflammatory diseases that are known to stimulate the acute phase response and thereby production of serum amyloid-A protein (e.g. rheumatoid arthritis), but not in those that are not (e.g. scleroderma). However, AA amyloidosis affects only a minority of patients with rheumatoid arthritis, although most such patients have raised serum amyloid A (Husby 1992). Additional pathogenetic factors are obviously required. Serum amyloid A is polymorphic, which means that more than one gene codes for the protein. There is convincing experimental evidence that serum amyloid-A molecules (Table 2) genetically determined to have particular amyloidogenic structures are important in AA amyloidosis (Meek *et al.* 1986; Husby *et al.* 1994b). The same is probably the case in the inherited amyloidoses related to genetic variants of transthyretin, apo-AI, gelsolin, and β-protein precursor (Table 1).

In most instances, the different amyloid proteins comprise a smaller or larger fragment of their precursors, pointing to an incomplete degradation (Glenner 1980). Defective proteolysis may therefore be implicated in amyloidosis (Fuks and Zucker-Franklin 1985; Husby *et al.* 1994a; Husby *et al.* 1994b).

Amyloid-enhancing factor, a poorly defined material probably consisting of both protein and carbohydrate, is produced by reticuloendothelial cells during persistent inflammation (Hol *et al.* 1986;

Kisilevski and Young 1994). This factor precedes the occurrence of amyloid in affected organs in experimental amyloidosis (Kisilevski and Young 1994) and has been shown to shorten the induction time of experimental amyloidosis from weeks to between 24 and 48 h.

Glycosaminoclycans occur in the tissues in close temporal and morphological relationship to amyloid deposition (Snow *et al.* 1987; Stenstad *et al.* 1994) and have been proposed to account for the carbohydrate moiety in amyloid-enhancing factor (Snow *et al.* 1987). The large negative charge of the glycosaminoglycans indicates an effect on the folding of precursor proteins to form fibrils (Snow *et al.* 1987). Glycosaminoglycans may also protect amyloid proteins or their precursors against proteolysis and stabilize the structure of the fibrils in the extracellular milieu. (Husby *et al.* 1994b).

Protein AP, of which SAP is the precursor, is also invariably present in amyloid deposits as an extrafibrillar constituent (Pepys 1988). AP has also been thought to protect amyloid proteins against proteolysis (Husby *et al.* 1994b). A DNA polymorphic site, 5′ to the SAP gene, was significantly associated with AA amyloidosis in juvenile rheumatoid arthritis, suggesting an active role in amyloidogenesis (Woo *et al.* 1987). Experiments in our laboratory (Husby *et al.* 1994b) strongly suggest a close interaction between the fibril proteins, glycosaminoglycans, and AP *in vivo*, often mediated by calcium-dependent bindings. Chemical manipulation of this may prove to have therapeutical implications in amyloidosis.

Clinical amyloidosis syndromes

A large number of partly overlapping amyloidosis syndromes have been described, and they have been difficult to classify by their clinical expression, although many attempts at this have been made during the last 150 years (Glenner 1980; Kyle 1982; Husby and Sletten 1986; Pepys 1988). The classification of amyloid and amyloidosis based on the nature of the fibril proteins (Table 1) is therefore of great help for clinical practice as well as scientific work (Husby 1994). Under the following headings, the most important amyloidosis syndromes are described in relation to their protein correlates.

Idiopathic and myeloma-associated AL amyloidosis

The mean age at diagnosis of AL amyloidosis is approximately 60 years. The organ distribution of amyloid is similar in idiopathic and myeloma-associated amyloidoses (Kyle 1982; Kyle *et al.* 1986). The most severe clinical features of AL amyloidosis are caused by accumulation of amyloid in the heart and kidneys (Kyle 1982; Janssen *et al.* 1986; Kyle *et al.* 1986; Stone 1990). Interstitial and vascular amyloidosis of the heart leads to congestive heart failure, conduction disturbances or angina pectoris, sometimes myocardial infarction, and causes about one-half of the deaths associated with this condition (Table 3). Decreased voltage on ECG is common. The patients are hypersensitive to digitalis, which, when given, may cause fatal arrhythmias. The extent of cardiac involvement is the most important predictor for survival in AL amyloidosis (Kyle *et al.* 1986).

Glomerular and vascular amyloidosis of the kidneys with consequent nephrosis and/or renal failure causes one-third of the deaths. Pulmonary amyloidosis with cough and dyspnoea is common. Amyloidosis of the skin with purpura, amyloid papules, or tumours is seen in nearly one-half of the patients. Some patients develop peripheral neuropathy (10 per cent) and carpal tunnel syndrome

Table 3 Clinical features of AL and AA amyloidoses

Characteristic of AL amyloidosis

Heart: cause of death in approximately 50% of AL amyloidosis; restrictive cardiomyopathy; congestive heart failure; conduction disturbances; angina pectoris — myocardial infarction; low voltage on ECG; digitalis hypersensitivity

Lungs (90%): cough, dyspnoea

Skin (40%): purpura, papules, tumours

Peripheral neuropathy (10%)

Carpal tunnel syndrome (20%)

Autonomic disturbances: orthostatic hypotension, etc.

Macroglossia (20%)

Bleeding due to vasculopathy and coagulation factor-X deficiency

Amyloid arthropathy: mainly large joints (e.g. 'shoulder-pad sign')

Common to AL and AA amyloidoses

Weakness, fatigue, and loss of weight (most prominent in AL amyloidosis)

Kidneys: cause of death in the majority of AA amyloidosis and in one-third of AL amyloidosis; nephrosis and/or renal failure

Gastrointestinal tract: malabsorption, malnutrition, obstruction, diarrhoea (disturbed motility), bleeding

Liver: mainly enlargement, rare functional disturbance

Spleen, endocrine glands: severe symptoms infrequent

(20 per cent) in addition to autonomic disturbances, for example orthostatic hypotension (Kyle 1982).

Characteristic, but not so common features of AL amyloidosis are macroglossia, seen in 20 per cent of the patients, and amyloid arthropathy affecting mainly large joints. The 'shoulder pad sign' due to amyloid infiltration of the shoulder joint (Fig. 1) is almost pathognomonic. Purpura is a frequent and characteristic finding (Fig. 1). The coagulation factor-X deficiency seen in AL amyloidosis appears to be due to the high affinity of AL-type fibrils for factor X, which may therefore be trapped in the amyloid substance (Furie *et al.* 1981). Together with increased fibrinolysis and amyloid infiltration of the blood vessels, the factor-X deficiency may lead to severe haemorrhages (Kyle 1982).

Gastrointestinal amyloidosis may be associated with malabsorption, malnutrition, obstruction, diarrhoea (disturbed motility), and bleeding. Amyloidosis of the liver causes enlargement rather than functional disturbances. Amyloid is often present in the spleen, lymph nodes, and endocrine glands but severe symptoms are infrequent.

Localized, so-called tumour-forming, AL has been reported to be present in various organs, of which the respiratory and genitourinary tracts and the skin are most frequent (Husby 1992).

The patients with idiopathic AL amyloidosis regularly have increased numbers of plasma cells in the bone marrow; M

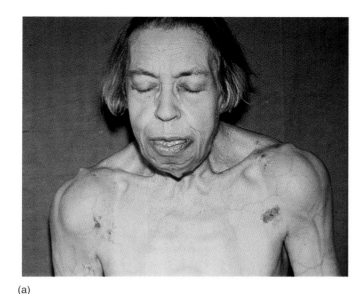

(a)

(b)

Fig. 1 (a) Amyloidosis with purpura around the eyelids, lips, and anterior thorax. Macroglossia with inability to close the mouth and amyloid arthropathy with bilateral shoulder pad sign are also present. (Reprinted from the Revised Clinical Collection on the Rheumatic Diseases 1981; used by permission of the American College of Rheumatology). (b) A 14-year-old girl suffering from severe, seropositive juvenile chronic arthritis with onset at 5 years of age, complicated by AA amyloidosis verified by rectal biopsy 6 years later. The clinical picture is dominated by malabsorption and gastrointestinal bleeds with severe weight loss, anaemia, renal failure, hepatosplenomegaly, hormonal disturbances with dwarfism/infantilism, and severe polyarthritis. These manifestations are caused by the underlying arthritic disorder, its treatment with corticosterioids and cytotoxic drugs, and the systemic AA amyloidosis.

components in serum and Bence-Jones proteinuria are also frequent findings, illustrating that this disorder belongs to the immunocyte dyscrasias with the same basic pathogenetic mechanisms as myelomatosis. The major difference between them is that the osteolytic lesions of myelomatosis are not present in idiopathic AL amyloidosis.

Another difference is that the κ to λ ratio, which is approximately 2:1 in myelomatosis, is reversed (1:2) in AL amyloidosis, thus reflecting the greater amyloidogenic potential of λ-light chains (Husby and Sletten 1986).

Reactive AA amyloidosis

Reactive AA amyloidosis is mainly associated with long-standing infectious or non-infectious inflammation, and less frequently with cancer, mainly renal cell carcinoma or Hodgkin's disease (Husby 1992). In areas where the incidence of chronic infections like tuberculosis and leprosy has declined, reactive amyloidosis is mostly caused by chronic rheumatic diseases, mainly adult rheumatoid arthritis and juvenile chronic arthritis, and ankylosing spondylitis, with frequencies in living patients of about 3 to 10 per cent, and by occasional cases of Reiter's disease and psoriatic arthropathy (Husby 1985). AA amyloidosis is also seen in some cases of Crohn's disease. Interestingly, this form of amyloidosis is extremely rare in systemic autoimmune rheumatic diseases like systemic lupus erythematosus, dermatomyositis, systemic sclerosis, and Sjögren's syndrome, and these diseases are associated with minimal acute-phase protein responses and hence low concentrations of serum amyloid A.

A marked geographic difference in the prevalence of AA amyloidosis in juvenile chronic arthritis, high (5 to 10 per cent) in European countries and low (0.1 per cent) in the United States, has been attributed to a more frequent occurrence of urinary tract infections caused by *Escherichia coli* in Europe (Filipowicz-Sosnowska *et al.* 1978). *E. coli* endotoxin is a highly potent inducer of the acute phase response as well as of experimental amyloidosis.

Arthritic patients with highly systemic disease are more prone to develop amyloidosis than those with milder disease; however, it is hard to predict individual cases at risk (Husby 1985). HLA studies have failed to disclosed markers for reactive amyloidosis.

Amyloid of the AA type has a tendency to localize in small vessels and parenchymal organs (Table 3). Renal disease (Fig. 2), often with the nephrotic syndrome and/or renal failure, is the chief manifestation and the major cause of death. In a series of 189 patients with rheumatoid arthritis and AA amyloidosis reported by Wegelius *et al.* (1980) only seven (3.7 per cent) lacked demonstrable clinical signs of renal involvement, and all patients with juvenile chronic arthritis in a series of 51 who developed amyloidosis had proteinuria at the time of diagnosis (Schnitzer and Ansell 1977). Proteinuria in rheumatoid arthritis should always be associated with possible amyloidosis until its cause is eventually disclosed. Haematuria occurs, but less often. Hypertension is uncommon in adult-onset rheumatoid arthritis with amyloidosis, but is found in about half of the patients with amyloidosis associated with juvenile chronic arthritis (Schnitzer and Ansell 1977; Woo 1994). Renal vein thrombosis is frequently found at autopsy.

Infiltration of blood vessels by amyloid, particularly in the gastrointestinal tract, can result in severe bleeding, sometimes life threatening, and malabsorption. AA amyloidosis of the liver is frequent and causes organ enlargement rather than functional disturbance. This type of amyloid may also affect the spleen, endocrine glands, and heart, but without causing severe symptoms. Interestingly, amyloid arthropathy and carpal tunnel syndrome are not features of AA amyloidosis, but are characteristic of both AL and β_2-microglobulin-associated amyloidoses.

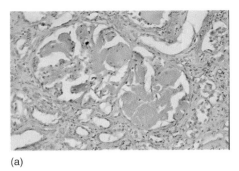 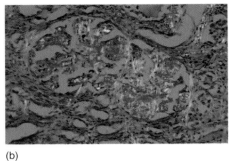 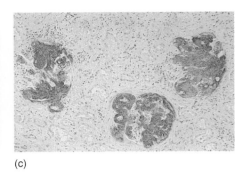

(a)   (b)   (c)

Fig. 2 Renal AA amyloidosis: (a)light microscopy of Congo red-stained glomerular amyloid (original magnification, × 160); (b) polarization microscopy of the same view field revealing the typical green/yellow birefringence of amyloid (× 160); (c) glomerular AA amyloid stained with peroxidase-labelled antiserum to protein AA and examined by light microscopy — no staining was obtained with antisera to other amyloid proteins (× 160).

No routine laboratory test (except biopsy) can distinguish between arthritic patients with and without AA amyloidosis. The high affinity of protein SAP for amyloid fibrils has recently been utilized in the diagnosis of AS and other systemic amyloidoses for research purposes. Radiolabelled SAP injected intravenously produces scintigraphic images quite accurately demonstrating the distrbution of amyloid *in vivo* (Hawkins 1994). So far, this procedure has been used for research purposes.

Familial Mediterranean fever with AA amyloidosis (see Chapter 5.13.2)

Amyloidosis associated with familial Mediterranean fever is the only form of systemic amyloidosis known to be inherited largely as a recessive trait (Pras 1986). Like other forms of AA amyloidosis, nephropathy is the most important feature and a significant cause of death. Familial Mediterranean fever itself is characterized by attacks of fever, peritonitis, pleuritis, and synovitis with onset during childhood, affecting mainly Sephardic Jews, Anatolian Turks, and Armenians with origin in the Mediterranean area. The prevalence as well as the disease course of amyloidosis in Mediterranean fever are highly heterogeneous in the different ethnic groups (Pras 1986). It appears that the febrile attacks and amyloidosis are inherited independently, and marked heterogeneity with regard to the serum amyloid-A genes has also been observed among patients with this fever syndrome (Sack 1988). A substitution of threonine for phenylalanine at position 69 of amyloid protein A involving all three bases of the codon has been observed in one case of amyloidosis in familial Mediterranean fever (Levin *et al.* 1972), but not confirmed in others.

The causal gene for familial Mediterranean fever has been located to the short arm of chromosome 16 (Pras *et al.* 1992), apparently not related to the human SAA gene family on chromosome 11 (Husby *et al.* 1990), and there is no link between this gene locus and that coding for human SAA present on chromosome 11 (Husby *et al.* 1994b)

Inherited autosomal-dominant amyloidosis

Point mutations causing single amino-acid substitutions in various amyloid protein precursors are associated with a heterogeneous group of familial amyloidoses inherited as autosomal dominants (Table 1) (Benson and Wallace 1989; Glenner and Murphy 1989). The majority of cases are related to different genetic variants of transthyretin. Neuropathy, cardiopathy, nephropathy, and vitreous

opacities are the most important clinical problems and occur in a variety of combinations, but also as more or less single clinical entities. Amyloid made up by genetic variants of other proteins (Table 1) may show similar clinical characteristics in addition to causing cerebral amyloid angiopathy and lattice corneal dystrophy. Some examples of inherited, autosomal-dominant amyloidoses, the geographic origin, and protein correlations are listed next (the syndromes are described in more detail by Glenner and Murphy (1989) and Benson (1991)):

(1) familial amyloid polyneuropathy related to transthyretin-methionine 30 — Portuguese, Swedish, Japanese, and others (Andrade 1952);

(2) familial amyloid polyneuropathy, transthyretin–serine 84 — Indiana/Swiss, Maryland/German (Benson and Wallace 1989);

(3) familial amyloid polyneuropathy, transthyretin–histidine 58 — Maryland/German (Nichols *et al.* 1989);

(4) familial amyloid cardiomyopathy and neuropathy, transthyretin–alanine 60 — Appalachian Indians, (Benson and Wallace 1989);

(5) familial amyloid cardiomyopathy (Fig. 3), transthyretin–methionine 111 — Danish (Frederiksen *et al.* 1962; Nordlie *et al.* 1988; Nordvåg *et al.* 1992);

(6) familial amyloid polyneuropathy, apolipoprotein AI–arginine 26 — Iowa (Nichols *et al.* 1988);

(7) familial amyloidosis with lattice corneal dystrophy, gelsoline–aspartic acid 187 — Finnish (Meretoja 1969; Maury 1990a);

(8) hereditary cerebral haemorrhage with amyloidosis, cystatin C–glutamic acid 58 — Icelandic (Ghiso *et al.* 1986) and amyloid β-protein–glutamic acid 618 — Dutch (Levy *et al.* 1990);

(9) the Muckle–Well's syndrome (nephropathy, nerve deafness, and urticaria) related to amyloid protein A (Muckle 1979; Linke *et al.* 1983);

(10) hereditary, non-neuropathic systemic amyloidosis with predominant renal involvement (Ostertag 1932) is related to various substitutions in apolipoprotein A1 (Soutar *et al.* 1992), lysozyme (Pepys *et al.* 1993), or the α-chain of fibrinogen (Table 1) — south or north America, the latter being of Irish or Scandinavian descent (Uemichi *et al.* 1994).

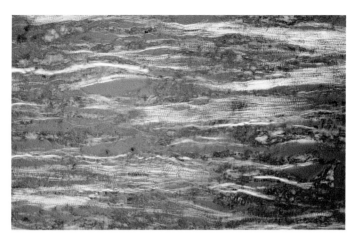

Fig. 3 Cardiac amyloidosis. Polarization microscopy of amyloid-laden myocardium stained with Congo red from a patient with transthyretin–methionine 111 familial amyloid cardiomyopathy of Danish origin; massive infiltration of green birefringent amyloid displacing muscle cells is seen (× 250).

Alzheimer's disease

The presenile dementia described by Alzheimer is probably the most common form of amyloidosis (Glenner and Murphy 1989). Amyloid is deposited extracellularly as Alzheimer's plaques and in the wall of cerebral vessels; even the intraneuronal neurofibrillary tangles are made up by paired helical filaments with the typical β-pleated sheet characteristic of amyloid. The amyloid β-protein in Alzheimer's disease derives from the β-protein precursor whose gene resides on chromosome 21.

The same manifestations of cerebral amyloid composed of the amyloid β-protein is seen in people with Down's syndrome over 40 years of age (Glenner and Murphy 1989). Down's syndrome is associated with trisomy of chromosome 21, and it is conceivable that this leads to an overproduction of β-protein precursor. Altered processing of the amyloid β-protein precursor has been proposed as a pathogenetic factor, and genetic variants of the protein are associated with familial occurrence of Alzheimer's disease. Another risk factor is the type 4 allele of apolipoprotein E (Corder *et al.* 1993). The same type of amyloid is occasionally seen in senile dementia (Glenner and Murphy 1989).

Organ manifestations

Heart

Cardiac amyloidosis manifesting mainly as cardiomyopathy, but also with conduction disturbances and coronary heart disease (Table 3), is a particularly severe manifestation of AL (Kyle 1982; Husby 1983; Janssen *et al.* 1986) and certain forms of inherited amyloidosis (Benson and Wallace 1989). Among the last, the Danish transthyretin–methionine 111 (Nordlie *et al.* 1988) and the Appalachian transthyretin–alanine 60 (Benson and Wallace 1989) are the most important forms (Fig. 3). Cardiac amyloidosis is also a major manifestation of senile systemic amyloidosis related to normal transthyretin (Westermark *et al.* 1990), and senile isolated atrial amyloidosis related to the polypeptide-hormone atrial natriuretic factor (Johansson *et al.* 1987). In general the senile cardiac

amyloidoses are benign. AA amyloidosis of the heart localizes mainly to the vasculature without causing major problems.

The respiratory tract

Amyloid may be deposited in any part of the respiratory system, from the nasal cavity to the pulmonary parenchyma and hilar glands. The clinical consequences are most severe in AL amyloidosis (Kyle 1982). Localized (nodular) AL amyloidosis is quite frequent and has a much more favourable prognosis, but may sometimes require surgical removal (Glenner 1980; Husby 1983).

Kidney and urinary tract

The most severe manifestation is renal amyloidosis, the major cause of death in AA amyloidosis (Glenner 1980; Husby 1985; Woo 1994), and frequently also in AL and hereditary amyloidoses related to variants of transthyretin and apo-AI (Glenner 1980; Kyle 1982; Glenner and Murphy 1989). Affected patients present with proteinuria and/or nephrotic syndrome, and frequently develop fatal renal failure. Hypertension and haematuria are less common. Renal biopsy reveals deposition of amyloid in glomeruli, in addition to its peritubular, vascular, and interstitial localization (Fig. 2).

The gastrointestinal tract

The entire gastrointestinal tract is a common target of amyloid deposition, making it an accepted site for diagnosis biopsy (Fig. 4). Intestinal amyloid causes motility disturbances with diarrhoea or constipation, malabsorption, bleeds, and perforation (Table 3) (Glenner 1980; Kyle 1982; Husby 1992). Nutritional disturbance due to macroglossia in AL amyloidosis (Fig. 1) or altered intestinal motility in the inherited neuropathies are quite common causes of death. Fatal gastrointestinal bleeds due to AA amyloidosis has been observed in several patients with rheumatic disease (Husby 1985).

The endocrine system

Fibrils made up by hormone-related or -derived polypeptides are seen locally in some endocrine tumours. Calcitonin-related amyloid in medullary carcinoma of the thyroid and islet amyloid polypeptide in diabetes type II and insulinomas are best known (Table 1). Endocrine glands are also affected by systemic AA and AL amyloidoses (Husby 1992).

Skin

Amyloid deposits are generally present in subcutaneous fat in both AL and AA, as well as inherited systemic amyloidoses, and thin-needle aspirates of abdominal fat (Fig. 5) have become a useful material for histological diagnosis (Westermark and Stenkvist 1973). In addition, cutaneous amyloid is a common feature of AL amyloidosis in the form of papules, nodules, or purpura (Kyle 1982). The skin is also the site of localized amyloid, e.g. lichen amyloidosus (Black 1976).

The locomotor system

The deposition of amyloid in the locomotor system is perhaps most common in β₂-microglobulin-related amyloidosis affecting patients on long-term dialysis for renal failure, who develop carpal tunnel syndrome, arthropathy, and cystic bone lesions, sometimes with

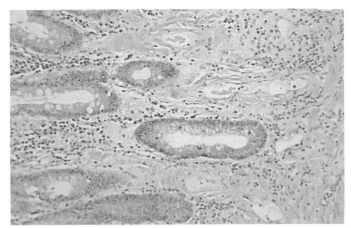

(a)

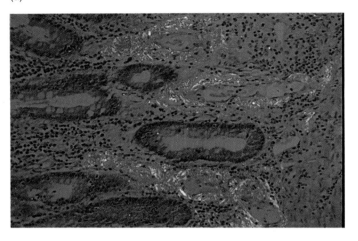

(b)

Fig. 4 Light (a) and polarization (b) microscopy of a Congo red-stained section from a rectal biopsy containing vascular and interstitial amyloid in the submucosal layer (× 160). (Photomicrographs kindly provided by Dr Michael Kearney, Tromsø, Norway.)

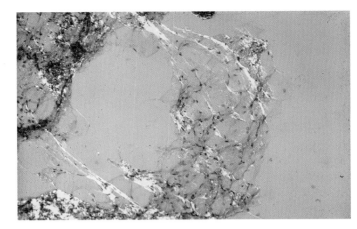

Fig. 5 Polarization microscopy of a subcutaneous, abdominal fat stained with Congo red showing marked deposition of amyloid compatible with the diagnosis of systemic amyloidosis. (Photomicrograph kindly provided by Professor Per Westermark, Linköping, Sweden.)

As amyloid arthropathy often has an inflammatory appearance, it may mistakenly be diagnosed as a rheumatic disorder. However, the joint fluid is generally non-inflammatory, sometimes with amyloid-containing synovial debris (Husby 1983).

Localized 'microdeposits' of amyloid in structures of the locomotor system occur with increasing frequency in aged people, mostly in menisci of the knee, joint capsules, and intervertebral discs, sometimes associated with the deposition of calcium pyrophosphate or with osteoarthrosis. The clinical significance of such amyloids, which possibly originate from local tissue proteins, is not clear (Husby and Sletten 1986).

Inclusion body myositis is a subset of chronic polymyositis characterized by muscle fibres with inclusion bodies containing amyloid fibrils. Very interestingly, the same β_2-amyloid protein as that seen in Alzheimer's disease and its precursor have recently been demonstrated to be constituents of these intramuscular amyloid deposits. This shows that β-amyloid can accumulate also outside the central nervous system. (For review see Askanas and Engel 1993)

Diagnosis

The diagnosis of amyloidosis is based on the demonstration of tissue deposits of amyloid. An absolute prerequisite for diagnosis is therefore that the clinician suspects amyloidosis in relevant clinical states. It is a regrettable fact, however, that the diagnosis of amyloidosis is far too often missed during life and is not evident until autopsy. The clinician should realize that AL amyloidosis may occur without an underlying predisposing disorder or in association with monoclonal gammopathies; that rheumatic disorders, long-standing or recurrent infections, and certain malignancies predispose for reactive, AA amyloidosis; and that a family history of amyloidosis may point to inherited disease. Unexplained manifestations that should alert the clinician to consider amyloidosis are: loss of weight (Fig. 1(a) and (b)), fatigue, proteinuria with or without renal failure, restrictive cardiomyopathy, gastrointestinal or respiratory problems, hepatomegaly, cutaneous conditions including purpura, and neuropathy/carpal tunnel syndrome.

It is established that rectal tissue (Fig. 4) which includes the submucosal vessels is a highly representative biopsy in systemic

pathological fractures, particularly when dialysed for more than 8 years. Ordinary haemodialysis is not able to remove β_2-microglobulin from plasma. Patients with this form of amyloidosis reportedly have abnormally glycosylated β_2-microglobulin capable of inducing inflammation with expression of cytokines and collagenase, which may contribute to destruction of bone and connective tissue (Miyata *et al*. 1994). Although β_2-microglobulin related amyloidosis is undoubtedly of systemic nature, structures of the locomotor system are of marked predilection for amyloid deposition in these patients (Maury 1990b; Kay 1993).

Characteristic of AL amyloidosis, though not so frequent, are the carpal tunnel syndrome (20 per cent), peripheral neuropathy (10 per cent), arthropathy (Fig. 1), or myopathy (less than 5 per cent) (Kyle 1982; Husby 1983). Another infrequent complaint is jaw claudication, which should be considered in the differential diagnosis of temporal arthritis/polymyalgia rheumatica (Gertz *et al*. 1986).

Erosive arthritis occurs in some patients with hereditary amyloidosis, i.e. of the Indiana and Iowa kindreds (Benson and Wallace 1989).

amyloidosis (Husby 1985). There may be bleeding after this procedure, but severe blood loss is infrequent.

In recent years, needle aspirates of abdominal subcutaneous fat (Fig. 5), which are less invasive than rectal biopsy, have increasingly been used for diagnosis (Westermark and Stenkvist 1973). Affected or suspected organs or tissues in the actual case under examination, such as kidneys (Fig. 2), liver, spleen, peripheral nerves, or skin, may be appropriate sites of biopsy but the risk of complications must be considered.

The amyloid carpal tunnel syndrome may be the initial finding in systemic amyloidoses. All tissues removed at surgery for carpal tunnel syndrome should therefore be examined for the presence of amyloid.

Examination of alkaline Congo red-stained tissue sections or aspirated fat smears in a polarizing microscope revealing the apple-green/yellow birefringence characteristic of amyloid deposits is the histochemical method of choice (see Figs 2, 3, 4, and 5) (Glenner 1980; Kyle 1982; Hawkins 1994). Immunohistochemical methods with specific antisera to classify the various amyloid fibril proteins (Fig. 2) are increasingly used, but are not available for routine diagnostic purposes. Electron microscopy may confirm the diagnosis.

The strong calcium-dependent affinity of protein AP/SAP for amyloid fibrils of any protein type can be utilized diagnostically (Hawkins 1994). Radiolabelled SAP injected intravenously will rapidly and specifically localize to the amyloid deposits to yield high resolution scintigraphic images. This technique is currently at the experimental stage in humans, but is a highly promising diagnostic measure in clinical practice.

Other laboratory tests include analysis of DNA or its protein product to detect genetic variants of proteins known to make up amyloid in the hereditary amyloidoses (Benson and Wallace 1989; Nordvåg et al. 1992). Indeed, the use of restriction fragment-length polymorphism combined with in vitro amplification of genes using polymerase chain reaction is an extremely sensitive tool for detecting gene carriers and thereby individuals at risk—even before birth (Nichols et al. 1989; Nordvåg et al. 1992).

Radionuclide imaging using calcium-seeking isotopes, for example $^{99}Tc^m$, echocardiography, bone marrow examination, and demonstration of monoclonal immunoglobulins in serum or urine are examples of laboratory methods used in the clinical work-up of patients with amyloidosis (Hazenberg and van Rijswijk 1994).

Therapeutic aspects

In general, amyloidosis is a progressive disease for which there is no cure. As the aetiology and pathogenesis are multifactorial, there are problems with therapy. Prospective, controlled studies of intervention are sparse. The marked prognostic heterogeneity of patients with hereditary amyloidosis makes genetic counselling difficult (Sequeiros and Saraiva 1987). With these problems in mind, the following therapeutic approaches are suggested:

(1) reduce the availability of precursor protein to prevent or slow down amyloid formation;

(2) attempts at dissolving amyloid deposits in vivo;

(3) treatment directed towards affected organs.

These are now considered in more detail.

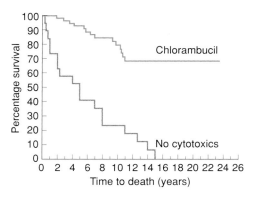

Fig. 6 Survival of juvenile chronic arthritis with amyloidosis with and without treatment using the cytotoxic drug chlorambucil. Although historical controls are used, the markedly improved survival strongly indicates that this can be attributed to treatment. (From Woo (1990) with kind permission from author, editors, and publisher.)

Reduction of amyloid precursor

In reactive AA amyloidosis the synthesis of the precursor serum amyloid A can be reduced by turning down the stimulated hepatic production of acute phase proteins (Husby 1992). This is achieved by effective treatment of the underlying inflammatory or neoplastic disorder, whenever possible. In the face of the poor prognosis of amyloidosis, rather drastic therapeutic intervention may be considered. Cytotoxic drugs have convincingly been shown to improve the prognosis of amyloidosis associated with both adult rheumatoid arthritis (Ahlmen et al. 1987; Berglund et al. 1993) and juvenile chronic arthritis (Fig. 6) (Woo 1994). Any use of cytotoxic drugs must, however, be weighed against the risk of potentially hazardous adverse effects such as leukaemia. Treatment of familial Mediterranean fever with colchicine prevents the occurrence of febrile attacks as well as AA amyloidosis, and is also effective in the treatment of established amyloidosis in such patients (Zemer et al. 1986). A recent review of the literature (Livneh et al. 1993) also concluded that colchicine may be added to any therapeutic regimen of AL or AA amyloidosis.

In controlled trials, treatment with the cytotoxic drug melphalan in combination with corticosteroids has been shown (Kyle et al. 1990) to improve the symptoms and signs, and possibly also survival, in AL amyloidosis. Studies using historical controls shows that colchicine may exert some additional effect on AL amyloidosis when combined with melphalan and prednisolone (Cohen et al. 1987; Kyle et al. 1990; Gertz et al. 1991). These treatments are thought to work by reducing the number of cells producing the monoclonal immunoglobulin light-chain precursor of amyloid, or to hamper their protein production or secretion. High-dose cytotoxic drugs in combination with stem cell transfusion appears promising (Majolino et al. 1993).

A diet where the only source of fat was fish oil high in ω-3 polyunsaturated fatty acids has been shown to retard the progression of azocasein-induced AA amyloidoses in mice (Cathcart et al. 1987). As fish-oil diets may also suppress the activity of chronic inflammation, a prophylactic or retardant effect on human AA amyloidosis associated with arthritis is an interesting possibility.

Plasmapheresis has been tried in those amyloidoses related to genetic variants of transthyretin, but without documented effect. Of more interest are the recently performed liver transplantations in such patients, which remove the site of production of the variant transthyretin and replace it by a liver harbouring only normal transthyretin genes (Holmgren *et al.* 1993).

Renal transplantation improves the articular complaints and retards the development of amyloid bone cysts in β_2-microglobulin-associated amyloidosis (Jadoul *et al.* 1989). A restoration of the normal clearance of β_2-microglobulin may explain the therapeutic effect.

Dissolution of amyloid deposits in vivo

Dimethyl sulphoxide partially dissolves amyloid fibrils *in vitro*, and treatment of amyloidotic mice with this compound reduces the amount of amyloid (Isobe and Osserman 1976). It has therefore been tried in the treatment of human AA, AL, and transthyretin-related amyloidoses. A beneficial effect has been reported in occasional patients (Hazenberg and van Rijswijk 1994), but there are no reports of controlled studies. Many patients refuse to take dimethyl sulphoxide because it gives a bad body odour.

Organ-directed therapy

Renal transplantation is increasingly used in amyloid nephropathy, particularly of AA background (Stone 1990). A series of patients had increased survival as well as improvement of quality of life (Hartmann *et al.* 1992). Although the results of renal transplantation are not as good as in non-amyloid nephropathies, more patients should probably be given the chance to receive renal transplant also in AL, transthyretin, and β_2-microglobulin-associated amyloidoses (Kay 1993).

The effect of heart transplantation for amyloidosis have been reported in a few patients, most of them with AL type (see Stone 1990); five of six such patients were reportedly alive 21 plus or minus 12 months after transplantation.

Other therapeutic considerations

Patients with cardiac amyloid may have increased sensitivity to digitalis, and calcium-channel blocking agents may aggravate heart failure in such patients. Amyloid appears to bind such agents *in vitro* and possibly also *in vivo* (Stone 1990), and they should be used with caution in amyloidosis patients.

Comprehensive reviews of the clinical and therapeutic aspects of adult (Hazenberg and van Rijswijk 1994) and childhood amyloidoses (Woo 1994) of particular interest in rheumatology have recently been published.

Prognosis

The prognosis of amyloidosis depends on the localization and progress of the tissue deposition of amyloid. Survival time is largely dependent on the time of diagnosis, which varies significantly. It is clear, however, that systemic amyloidosis must be regarded as a severe condition with a high risk of death. AA amyloidosis has been estimated to be the cause of up to 47 per cent of deaths in European patients with juvenile chronic arthritis (Baum and Gutowska 1977). A Finnish report concluded that amyloidosis was the cause of death in 8 per cent of patients with adult rheumatoid arthritis coming to autopsy (Koota *et al.* 1975). On the other hand, the outcome of reactive AA amyloidosis is more favourable than many physicians have

previously thought. Reports from Finland and the United States indicate that survival time after diagnosis of amyloidosis associated with rheumatoid arthritis is 4 to 5 years (Wegelius *et al.* 1980; Kyle 1982). In juvenile chronic arthritis with amyloidosis, survival may be even better when treated with cytotoxic drugs for 8 to 9 years (Baum and Gutowska 1977; Schnitzer and Ansell 1977) or longer (Fig. 6) (Woo 1990). There is a large individual variation in survival time for AA amyloidosis, in one report (Tribe *et al.* 1980) ranging from a few weeks up to 20 years.

The prognosis of AL amyloidosis is less favourable. Reported survival rates are less than 2 years for idiopathic type, and 7 months or even less in AL amyloidosis with myeloma (Janssen *et al.* 1986; Kyle 1990). Again, there is a wide range in survival time of individual patients, from weeks up to 5 years or more (Kyle *et al.* 1986). Cardiac amyloid is the most common cause of death and the major determinant of prognosis among patients with AL (Kyle 1990). Urinary excretion of monoclonal λ-light chains is associated with inferior survival in AL amyloidosis compared with monoclonal κ-chains or no monoclonal protein (Gertz and Kyle 1990)

In the hereditary amyloid polyneuropathies and cardiomyopathies related to variants of transthyretin, there are also wide variations in the course and prognosis among the different affected families as well as between individual gene carriers in the same families. Some patients may die with cachexia before the age of 40 years, whereas others may be in good health at 90 years (Sequeiros and Saraiva 1987).

References

Ahlmen, M., Ahlmen, J., Svalander, C., and Bucht, H. (1987). Cytotoxic drug treatment of reactive amyloidosis in rheumatoid arthritis with special reference to renal insufficiency. *Clinical Rheumatology*, **6**, 27–38.

Anders, R.F., Natvig, J.B., Sletten, K., Husby, G., and Nordstoga, K. (1977). Amyloid-related serum protein SAA from three animal species: comparison with human SAA. *Journal of Immunology*, **118**, 229–34.

Andrade, C. (1952). A peculiar form of peripheral neuropathy. Familiar atypical generalized amyloidosis with special involvement of the peripheral nerves. *Brain*, **75**, 408–27.

Askanas, V. and Engel, W.K. (1993). New advances in inclusion-body myositis. *Current Opinion in Rheumatology*, **5**, 732–41.

Baum, J. and Gutowska, G. (1977). Death in juvenile rheumatoid arthritis. *Arthritis and Rheumatism*, **20** (Suppl.), 253–5.

Benditt, E.P. and Eriksen, N. (1964). Starch gel electrophoretic analysis of some proteins extracted from amyloid. *Archives of Pathology*, **78**, 325–30.

Benditt, E.P. and Eriksen, N. (1971). Chemical classes of amyloid substance. *American Journal of Pathology*, **65**, 231–52.

Benson, M.D. (1991). Inherited amyloidosis. *Journal of Medical Genetics*, **28**, 73–8.

Benson, M.D. and Wallace, M.R. (1989). Amyloidosis. In *The metabolic basis of inherited disease*, Vol. 2 (6th edn) (ed. C.R. Scriver, A.L. Beaudet, W.S. Sly, and D. Valle), pp. 2439–60. McGraw-Hill, New York.

Berglund, K., Thysell, H., and Keller C. (1993). Results, principles and pitfalls in the management of renal AA-amyloidosis; a 10–21 year followup of 16 patients with rheumatic disease treated with alkylating cytostatics. *Journal of Rheumatology*, **20**, 2051–7.

Black, M.M. (1976). Primary localised amyloidosis of the skin: clinical variants, histochemistry and ultra-structure. In *Amyloidosis* (ed. O. Wegelius and A. Pasternack), pp. 479–511. Academic Press, London.

Cathcart, E.S., Crystal, A.L., Meydani, S.N., and Hayes, K.C. (1987). A fish oil diet retards experimental amyloidosis, modulates lymphocyte function, and decreases macrophage arachidonate metabolism in mice. *Journal of Immunology*, **139**, 1850–4.

Cohen, A.S., Rubinow, A., Anderson, J.J., Skinner, M., Mason, J.H., and Kayne, L.C. (1987). Survival of patients with primary (AL) amyloidosis: colchicine-treated cases from 1976 to 1983 compared with cases seen in previous years (1961 to 1973). *American Journal of Medicine*, **82**, 1182–90.

Cooper, J.H. (1974). Selective amyloid staining as a function of amyloid composition and structure. Histochemical analysis of the alkaline Congo red, standardized toluidine blue, and iodine methods. *Laboratory Investigation*, **31**, 232–8.

Corder, E.H. *et al.* (1993). Gene dose of apolipoprotein E type 4 allele and the risk of Alzheimer's disease. *Science*, **261**, 921-3.

Eriksen, N., Ericsson, L.H., Pearsall, N., Lagunoff, D., and Benditt, E.P. (1976). Mouse amyloid protein AA: homology with non-immunoglobulin protein of human and monkey amyloid substance. *Proceedings of the National Academy of Sciences (USA)*, **73**, 964–7.

Filipowicz-Sosnowska, A.M., Rostropowicz-Denisiewicz, K., Rosenthal, C.J., and Baum, J. (1978). The amyloidosis of juvenile rheumatoid arthritis. Comparative studies in Polish and American children. *Arthritis and Rheumatism*, **21**, 699–703.

Frederiksen, T., Gøtzsche, H., Harboe, N., Kiaer, W., and Mellangaard, K. (1962). Primary familial amyloidosis with severe amyloid heart disease. *American Journal of Medicine*, **33**, 328–48.

Fuks, A. and Zucker-Franklin, D. (1985). Impaired Kupffer cell function precedes development of secondary amyloidosis. *Journal of Experimental Medicine*, **161**, 1013–28.

Furie, B., LiAnn Voo, B.S., McAdam, K.P.W.J., and Furie, B.C. (1981). Mechanism of factor X deficiency in systemic amyloidosis. *New England Journal of Medicine*, **304**, 827–30.

Gejyo, F. *et al.* (1985). A new form of amyloid protein associated with chronic hemodialysis was identified as β_2-microglobulin. *Biochemical and Biophysical Research Communications*, **129**, 701–6.

Gertz, M.A. and Kyle, R.A. (1990). Prognostic value of urinary protein in primary systemic amyloidosis (AL). *American Journal of Pathology*, **94**, 313–7.

Gertz, M.A., Kyle, R.A., Griffing, W.L., and Hunder, G.G. (1986). Jaw claudication in primary systemic amyloidosis. *Medicine*, **65**, 173–9.

Gertz, M.A., Kyle, R.A., and Greipp, P.R. (1991). Response rates and survival in primary systemic amyloidosis. *Blood*, **77**, 257–62.

Ghiso, J., Jensson, O., and Frangione, B. (1986). Amyloid fibrils in hereditary cerebral hemorrhage with amyloidosis of Icelandic type is a variant of γ-trace basic protein (cystatin C). *Proceedings of the National Academy of Sciences (USA)*, **83**, 2974–8.

Glenner, G.G. (1980). Amyloid deposits and amyloidosis. *New England Journal of Medicine*, **302**, 1283–92.

Glenner, G.G. and Murphy, M.A. (1989). Amyloidosis of the nervous system. *Journal of the Neurological Sciences*, **94**, 1–28.

Hartmann, A. *et al.* (1992). Fifteen years' experience with renal transplantation in systemic amyloidosis. *Transplant International*, **5**, 15–8.

Hawkins, P.N. (1994). Diagnosis and monitoring of amyloidosis. In *Reactive amyloidosis and the acute phase response* (ed. G. Husby), *Baillière's Clinical Rheumatology*, **8**, pp. 635–59.

Hazenberg, B.P.C. and van Rijswijk, M.H. (1994). Clinical and therapeutic aspects of AA amyloidosis. In *Reactive amyloidosis and the acute phase response* (ed. G. Husby), *Baillière's Clinical Rheumatology*, **8**, pp. 661–90.

Hol, P.R., Snel, F.W.J.J., Niewold, T.A., and Gruys, E. (1986). Amyloid enhancing factor (AEF) in the pathogenesis of AA-amyloidosis in the hamster. *Virchows Archive B. Cell Pathology*, **52**, 273–81.

Holmgren, G. *et al.* (1993). Clinical improvement and amyloid regression after liver transplantation in hereditary transthyretin amyloidosis. *Lancet*, **341**, 1113–6.

Husby, G. (1983). Immunoglobulin-related (AL) amyloidosis. *Clinical and Experimental Rheumatology*, **1**, 353–8.

Husby, G. (1985). Amyloidosis and rheumatoid arthritis. *Clinical and Experimental Rheumatology*, **3**, 173–80.

Husby, G. (1989). Pathogenesis of AA amyloidosis. In *Acute phase proteins in the acute phase response*, Argenteul Symposium, (ed. M. Pepys), pp. 169–85. Springer-Verlag, London.

Husby, G. (1992). Amyloidosis. *Seminars in Arthritis and Rheumatism*, **22**, 67–82.

Husby, G. (1994). Classification of amyloidosis. In *Reactive amyloidosis and the acute phase response* (ed. G. Husby), *Baillière's Clinical Rheumatology*, **8**, pp. 503–54.

Husby, G. and Sletten, K. (1986). Clinical and chemical classification of amyloidosis 1985. *Scandinavian Journal of Immunology*, **23**, 253–65.

Husby, G. *et al.* (1990). The 1990 guidelines for nomenclature and classification of amyloid and amyloidosis. In *Amyloid and amyloidosis* (ed. J.B. Natvig *et al.*). Kluwer Academic Publishers, Dordrecht.

Husby, G., Marhaug, G., Dowton, B., Sletten, K., and Sipe, J.D. (1994a). Serum amyloid A (SAA): biochemistry, genetics and the pathogenesis of AA amyloidosis. *International Journal of Experimental and Clinical Investigation*, **1**, 119–37.

Husby, G., Stenstad, T., Magnus, J.H., Sletten, K., Nordvåg, B.Y., and Marhaug, G. (1994b). Interaction between circulating amyloid fibril protein precursors and extracellular tissue matrix components in the pathogenesis of systemic amyloidosis. *Clinical Immunology and Immunopathology*, **70**, 2–9.

Husebekk, A., Skogen, B., Husby, G., and Marhaug, G. (1985). Transformation of myloid precursor SAA to protein AA and incorporation in amyloid fibrils in vivo. *Scandinavian Journal of Immunology*, **21**, 283–7.

Isobe, T. and Osserman, E.F. (1976). Effects of dimethyl sulfoxide (DMSO) on Bence-Jones proteins, amyloid fibrils and casein-induced amyloidosis. In *Amyloidosis* (ed. O. Wegelius and A. Pasternack), pp. 247–57. Academic Press, London.

Jadoul, M., Malghem, J., Pirson, Y., Maldague, B., and van Ypersele de Strihou, C. (1989). Effect of renal transplantation on the radiological signs of dialysis amyloid osteoarthropathy. *Clinical Nephrology*, **32**, 194–7.

Janssen, S., van Rijswijk, M.H., Meijer, S., Ruinen, L., and van der Hem, G.K. (1986). Systemic amyloidosis: a clinical survey of 144 cases. *Netherlands Journal of Medicine*, **29**, 376–85.

Johansson, B., Wernstedt, C., and Westermark, P. (1987). Atrial natriuretic peptide deposited as atrial amyloid fibrils. *Biochemical and Biophysical Research Communications*, **148**, 1087–92.

Kay, J. (1993). β_2-microglobulin amyloidosis. *Rheumatology Review*, **2**, 22–8.

Kisilevski, R. (1987). From arthritis to Alzheimer's disease: current concepts on the pathogenesis of amyloidosis. *Canadian Journal of Physiology and Pharmacology*, **65**, 1805–15.

Kisilevski, R. and Young, I.D. (1994). Pathogenesis of amyloidosis. In *Reactive amyloidosis and the acute phase response* (ed. G. Husby), *Baillière's Clinical Rheumatology*, **8**, pp. 613–26.

Koota, K., Isomäki, H.A., and Mutru, O. (1975). Death rate and causes of death in patients with rheumatoid arthritis. *Scandinavian Journal of Rheumatology*, **4**, 205–8.

Kyle, R.A. (1982). Amyloidosis. *Clinical Haematology*, **11**, 151–80.

Kyle, R.A. (1990). Primary systemic amyloidosis (AL). In *Amyloid and amyloidosis* (ed. J.B. Natvig *et al.*), pp.147–52. Kluwer Academic Publishers, Dordrecht.

Kyle, R.A., Greipp, P.R., and O'Fallon, W.M. (1986). Primary systemic amyloidosis: multivariate analysis for prognostic factors in 168 cases. *Blood*, **68**, 220–4.

Kyle, R.A., Gertz, M.A., Garton, J.P., and Greipp, P.R. (1990). Primary systemic amyloidosis (AL): a randomized trial of colchicine vs. melphalan and prednisone vs. melphalan, predinisone, and colchicine. In *Amyloid and amyloidosis* (ed. J.B. Natvig *et al.*), pp. 231–4, Kluwer Academic Publishers, Dordrecht.

Levin, M., Franklin, E.C., Frangione, B., and Pras, M. (1972). The amino acid sequence of a major non-immunoglobulin component of some amyloid fibrils. *Journal of Clinical Investigation*, **51**, 2773–6.

Levy, E. *et al.* (1990). Mutation of the Alzheimer's disease amyloid gene in hereditary cerebral hemorrhage, Dutch type. *Science*, **248**, 1124–6.

Linke, R.P., Heilmann, K.L., Nathrath, W.B.J., and Eulitz, M. (1983). Identification of amyloid A protein in a sporadic Muckle–Wells syndrome. N-terminal amino acid sequence after isolation from formalin-fixed tissue. *Laboratory Investigation*, **48**, 698–704.

Livneh, A., Zemer, D., Langevitz, P., Shemer, J., Sohar, E., and Pras M. (1993). Colchicine in the treatment of AA and AL amyloidosis. *Seminars in Arthritis and Rheumatism*, **23**, 206–14.

Magnus, J.H., Stenstad, T., and Husby, G. (1989). Proteoglycans, glycosaminoglycans and amyloid deposition. In *Reactive amyloidosis and the acute phase response* (ed. G. Husby), *Baillière's Clinical Rheumatology*, **8**, pp. 575–97.

Majolino, I. *et al.* (1993). High-dose therapy and autologous transplantation in amyloidosis-AL. *Haematologica*, **78**, 68–71.

Marhaug, G., østensen, M., Husby, G., and Husebekk, A. (1986). Serum amyloid A protein, a sensitive inflammation marker. In *Marker proteins in inflammation*, Vol. 3, (ed. J. Bienvenu, J.A. Grim, and P. Laurent), pp. 139–43. Walter de Gryuter, Berlin.

Marhaug, G., Husby, G., Nordstoga, K., and Dowton, S.B. (1990). Mink serum amyloid A protein. Expression and primary structure based on cDNA sequences. *Journal of Biological Chemistry*, **265**, 10049–54.

Maury, C.P.J. (1990a). Complete primary structure of amyloid fibril protein in Finnish hereditary amyloidosis: identification of a new type of amyloid protein derived from variant gelsolin. In *Amyloid and amyloidosis* (ed. J.B. Natvig et al.). Kluwer Academic Publishers, Dordrecht.

Maury, C.P.J. (1990b). β₂-Microglobulin amyloidosis. A systemic amyloid disease affecting primarily synovium and bone in long-term dialysis patients. *Rheumatology International*, **10**, 1–8.

Meek, R.L., Hoffmann, J.S., and Benditt, E.P. (1986). Amyloidogenesis. One serum amyloid A isotype is selectively removed from the circulation. *Journal of Experimental Medicine*, **163**, 499–510.

Meek, R.L., Urieli-Shoval, S., and Benditt, E.P. (1994). Expression of apolipoprotein serum amyloid A mRNA in human atherosclerotic lesions and cultured vascular cells: implications for serum amyloid A function. *Proceedings of the National Academy of Sciences (USA)*, **91**, 3186–90.

Meretoja, J. (1969). Familial systemic paraamyloidosis with lattice dystrophy of the cornea, progressive cranial neuropathy, skin changes and various internal symptoms. A previous unrecognized heritable syndrome. *Annals of Clinical Research*, **1**, 314–24.

Miyata, T. et al.(1994). Involvement of β₂-microglobulin modified with advanced glycation end products in the pathogenesis of hemodialysis-associated amyloidosis. *Journal of Clinical Investigation*, **93**, 521–8.

Muckle, T.J. (1979). The 'Muckle–Wells' syndrome. *British Journal of Dermatology*, **100**, 87–92.

Nichols, W.C., Dwulet, F.E., Liepnieks, J., and Benson, M.D. (1988). Variant apolipoprotein A1 as a major constituent of a human hereditary amyloid. *Biochemical and Biophysical Research Communications*, **156**, 762–8.

Nichols, W.C., Padilla, L.-M., and Benson, M.D. (1989). Prenatal detection of a gene for hereditary amyloidosis. *American Journal of Medical Genetics*, **34**, 520–4.

Nordlie, M., Sletten, K., Husby, G., and Ranløv, P.J. (1988). A new prealbumin variant in familian amyloid cardiomyopathy of Danish origin. *Scandinavian Journal of Immunology*, **27**, 119–22.

Nordvåg, B.Y., Husby, G., Ranløv, I., and El-Gewely, M.R. (1992). Molecular diagnosis of the transthyretin (TTR) Met111 mutation in familial amyloid cardiomyopathy of Danish origin. *Human Genetics*, **89**, 459–61.

Orstertag, B. (1932). Demonstration einer eigenartigen familiaren 'Paramyliodose'. *Zentralblat für Allgemeine Pathologie und Pathologische Anatomie (Jena)*, **56**, 253–4.

Pepys, M.B. (1988). Amyloidosis: some recent developments. *Quarterly Journal of Medicine*, **67**, 283–98.

Pepys, M.B. et al. (1993). Human lysozyme gene mutations cause hereditary systemic amyloidosis. *Nature*, **362**, 553–7.

Pras, M. (1986). The hereditary amyloidoses. In *Amyloidosis* (ed. J. Marring and M.H. van Rijswijk), pp. 185–93. Martin Nijhoff Publishers, Dortrecht.

Pras, M., Schubert, M., Zucker-Franklin, D., Rimon A., and Franklin, E.C. (1968). The characterization of soluble amyloid prepared in water. *Journal of Clinical Investigation*, **47**, 924–33.

Pras, M. et al. (1992). Mapping of a gene causing familial Mediterranean fever to the short arm of chromosome 16. *New England Journal of Medicine*, **326**, 1509–13.

Sack, G.H. Jr. (1988). Serum amyloid A (SAA) gene variation in familial Mediterranean fever. *Molecular Biology and Medicine*, **5**, 61–7.

Schnitzer, T.J. and Ansell, B.M. (1977). Amyloidosis in juvenile chronic polyarthritis. *Arthritis and Rheumatism*, **20**, 245–52.

Sequeiros, J. and Saraiva, M.J.M. (1987). Onset in the seventh decade and lack of symptoms in heterozygotes for the TTR^{Met30} mutation in hereditary amyloid neuropathy-type I (Portuguese, Andrade). *American Journal of Medical Genetics*, **27**, 345–57.

Sletten, K. and Husby, G. (1974). The complete aminoacid sequence of non–immunoglobulin amyloid fibril protein AS in rheumatoid arthritis. *European Journal of Biochemistry*, **41**, 117–25.

Sletten, K., Westermark, P., and Natvig, J.B. (1976). Characterization of amyloid fibril proteins from medullary carcinoma of the thyroid. *Journal of Experimental Medicine*, **143**, 993–7.

Sletten, K., Marhaug, G., and Husby, G. (1983). The covalent structure of amyloid related serum protein SAA from two patients with inflammatory disease. *Hoppe–Seyler's Zeitschrift für Physiologische Chemie*, **364**, 1039–46.

Snow, A.D., Willmer, J., and Kisilevsky, R. (1987). A close structural relationship between sulfated proteoglycans and AA amyloid fibrils. *Laboratory Investigation*, **57**, 687–98.

Soutar, A.K. et al.(1992). Apolipoprotein A1 mutation Arg-60 causes autosomal dominant amyloidosis. *Proceedings of the National Academy of Sciences (USA)*, **89**, 7349–93.

Stenstad, T., Magnus, J.H., and Husby, G. (1994). Characterization of proteoglycans in mouse splenic AA amyloidosis. *Biochemical Journal*, **303**, 663–70.

Stone, M.J. (1990). Amyloidosis: a final common pathway for protein deposition in tissues. *Blood*, **75**, 531–45.

Syversen, V., Sletten, K., Marhaug, G., Husby, G., and Lium, B. (1987). The amino acid sequence of serum amyloid A (SAA) in mink. *Scandinavian Journal of Immunology*, **26**, 763–7.

Tribe, C.R., Bacon, P.A., and Mackenzie, J.C. (1980). Experience with an amyloid clinic. In *Amyloid and amyloidosis* (ed. G.G. Glenner, P.P. Costa, and A. Falcao de Freitas), pp. 179–82. Excerpta Medica, Amsterdam.

Uemichi, T., Liepniks, J.J., and Benson, M.D. (1994). Hereditary amyloidosis with a novel variant fibrinogen. *Journal of Clinical Investigation*, **93**, 731–6.

Waalen, K., Sletten, K., Husby, G., and Nordstoga, K. (1980). The primary structure of amyloid fibril protein AA in endotoxin induced amyloidosis of the mink. *European Journal of Biochemistry*, **104**, 407–12.

Wegelius, O., Wafin, F., Falck, H.M., and Tornroth, T. (1980). Follow-up study of amyloidosis secondary to rheumatid disease. In *Amyloid and amyloidosis* (ed. G.G. Glenner, P.P. Costa, and A. Falcao de Freitas) pp. 183–90, Excerpta Medica, Amsterdam.

Westermark, P. and Stenkvist, B. (1973). A new method for the diagnosis of systemic amyloidosis. *Archives of Internal Medicine*, **132**, 522–3.

Westermark, P., Wernstedt, C., Wilander, E., and Sletten, K. (1986). A novel peptide in the calcitonin gene related peptide family as an amyloid fibril protein in the endocrine pancreas. *Biochemical and Biophysical Research Communication*, **140**, 827–31.

Westermark, P., Sletten, K., Johansson, B., and Cornwell, G.G. (1990). Fibril in senile systemic amyloidosis is derived from normal transthyretin. *Proceedings of the National Academy of Sciences (USA)*, **87**, 2843–5.

Woo, P. (1990). Complications of juvenile arthritis. In *Paediatric rheumatology update* (ed. P. Woo, P.H. White, and B. Ansell), pp. 38–46. Oxford University Press, Oxford.

Woo, P. (1994). Amyloidosis in children. In *Reactive amyloidosis and the acute phase response*. *Baillière's Clinical Rheumatology*, **6**, 613–26.

Woo, P., O'Brien, Robson, M., and Ansell, B.M. (1987). A genetic marker for systemic amyloidosis in juvenile arthritis. *Lancet*, **ii**, 767–9.

Yamamoto, K.-I. and Migita, S. (1985). Complete primary structures of two major murine serum amyloid A proteins deduced from cDNA sequences. *Proceedings of the National Academy of Sciences (USA)*, **82**, 2915–9.

Zemer, D., Pras, M., Sohar, E., Modan, M., Cabili, S., and Gafni, J. (1986). Colchicine in the prevention and treatment of the amyloidosis of familial Mediterranean fever. *New England Journal of Medicine*, **314**, 1001–5.

5.13.2 Familial Mediterranean fever

Pnina Langevitz, Avi Livneh, Deborah Zemer, and Mordechai Pras

History

A genetic disease with a gene frequency as high as that of familial Mediterranean fever in Sephardi Jews must have existed for hundreds or thousands of years. Nevertheless, in the first half of the twentieth century only a few isolated characteristic cases could be traced in medical publications (Janeway and Mosenthal 1908; Alt and Barker 1930). The reason why a disease with such dramatic manifestations has only recently been recognized may be connected with the geographical distribution of its sufferers, who resided mainly in areas where modern medical facilities were not available at the time. This changed in the 1940s and 1950s when the population affected became exposed to advanced medical facilities and research, partly due to migrations.

Siegal (1945) was the first to describe the abdominal attacks as a separate disease entity. Later, many typical cases were included in the heterogeneous case collection termed 'periodic disease' by Reimann (1949). French physicians described many typical cases of familial Mediterranean fever in Jewish patients deriving from North Africa (Mamou and Cattan 1952; Siguier *et al.* 1953; Benhamou *et al.* 1954). They were the first to perceive the familial nature and the fatal renal lesion of the disease.

Tel Hashomer Hospital in Israel served in the early 1950s as a referral centre for the new immigrants who came mainly from Mediterranean countries. Enigmatic cases who appeared on the wards with recurrent, short-lived episodes of fever accompanied by peritoneal, pleural, or arthritic inflammation caught the attention of the group led by Professor Harry Heller. In a series of publications (Heller *et al.* 1958; Heller *et al.* 1961a; Heller *et al.* 1961b; Sohar *et al.* 1961; Sohar *et al.* 1967) they defined the clinical features of the disease and its diagnostic criteria, established its genetic nature, mode of transmission, and ethnic distribution, emphasized the role of amyloidosis, and coined the name 'familial Mediterranean fever'.

Diagnostic criteria

Despite many attempts at elucidation in the last 35 years the mechanisms leading to the clinical manifestations of the disease are still unknown, as is the underlying basic error of metabolism and the location of the gene. There is no specific diagnostic laboratory test. The diagnostic criteria are based on clinical manifestations.

1. Short attacks of fever recurring at irregular intervals. In most cases the temperature rises to 39–40 °C.

2. Painful inflammatory manifestations in the abdomen, chest, joints, or skin, associated with the fever.

3. Nephropathic amyloidosis leading to terminal renal failure early in life.

4. Autosomal-recessive inheritance.

5. Virtual ethnic restriction to Mediterranean stock (Sephardi Jews, Armenians, Anatolian Turks, Arabs, and Ashkenazi Jews).

6. Dramatic response to continuous colchicine treatment in abolishing or reducing febrile attacks.

The inheritance of familial Mediterranean fever

The disease may become manifest as early as during the first year of life, although in most cases onset is later. In two-thirds of our patients the first manifestations appeared during the first decade of life; by the end of the second decade 90 per cent are affected. Only rarely is the onset delayed beyond the age of 40 (Sohar *et al.* 1967). Among our 4000 patients there are only about 100 Ashkenazi Jews and the disease is rare in other Jewish ethnic groups (Yemenite and Iranian). Table 1 shows the prevalence and gene frequency of familial Mediterranean fever, calculated by the number of patients and the size of the total population in each ethnic subgroup.

The peculiar ethnic restriction and the familial aggregation in familial Mediterranean fever suggests a genetic aetiology. Analysis of 229 of our families led us to conclude that the disease is due to a single, recessive autosomal gene (Sohar *et al.* 1967).

In about 90 affected families, out of several hundreds, the disease occurred in more than one generation. Although in most of these families the inheritance could be considered to be autosomal-recessive, in two the transmission could not be explained by recessive inheritance and must be assumed to be dominant (Yuval *et al.* 1995).

The clinical picture

Attacks

The febrile, painful attacks that are the hallmark of the disease are characterized by marked elevation of body temperature, acute inflammation of the peritoneum, synovia, or pleura, a duration of 12 to 48 h, and complete health between attacks (Sohar *et al.* 1967).

Repeated attacks at irregular intervals and in an unpredictable sequence are typical of the disease: periods of one febrile attack a week can vary with remissions of weeks, months, or even years, with no apparent cause. During the illness a patient will probably encounter several forms of attacks, but the recurrence of one type over many years is not uncommon.

The most frequent manifestation is the abdominal attack, experienced by 90 per cent of patients; in 68 per cent of these it is the presenting sign. As the most dramatic manifestation, these attacks attract attention and extensive diagnostic efforts (Sohar *et al.* 1967). They are marked by the sudden onset of fever (often with chills) and pain spreading over the entire abdomen from variable points of origin. As the attack gains in intensity, guarding, rebound tenderness, board-like rigidity, distension, and absence of peristalsis appear. Multiple, small fluid levels in the small bowel on radiography combine to suggest an acute abdominal catastrophe. After 6 to 12 h the signs and symptoms recede, and within 24 to 48 h the attack is usually over, leaving the patient as well as before.

Organization of the exudate may result in fibrous adhesions, which in rare cases may give rise to mechanical ileus (Michaeli *et al.* 1966). This may be responsible for chronic subileus in some patients and

Table 1 Prevalence and gene frequency of familial Mediterranean fever (FMF)

Ethnic origin	Total population	Number of FMF patients	Prevalence of FMF[a]	FMF gene frequency
Algeria, Morocco, Tunis	613 500	866	1:700	1:26
Libya	76 900	310	1:250	1:16
Turkey	91 100	87	1:1000	1:32
Iraq	266 300	261	1:1000	1:32
Ashkenazi Jews	867 500	22+	1:40 000	1:200

[a]This prevalence approximates to the frequency of homozygosity, q^2, of the familial Mediterranean fever gene, q.

ascites in others (Zemer *et al*. 1977). It is probably the cause of sterility in some affected women (Ismachovich *et al*. 1973).

The pleural attack has been experienced by 45 per cent of our patients, and in 5 per cent it was the presenting sign (Sohar *et al.* 1967). It assumes the picture of an acute febrile pleuritis, resembling the peritoneal attacks in its abrupt onset, rapid resolution, and unpredictable recurrence. The pleuritic attack may be limited to the chest or may shift to the abdomen. Breathing is painful and breath sounds are diminished on the affected side. There may be radiological evidence of a small exudate in the costophrenic angle, which is difficult to aspirate and which resolves within 48 h. No sequelae of clinical significance have been noted.

Pericarditis is a rare feature of familial Mediterranean fever. We observed clinical attacks of pericarditis in 20 of our patients (A. Livneh, unpublished data). On M-mode echocardiography, pericardial involvement was reported to be more common than in the general population (Dabestani *et al.* 1982). No permanent sequelae have been reported.

The articular attack is the second most common form of attack. It was experienced by 75 per cent of the patients in our series, and was the presenting symptom in 16 per cent of them. Arthritic attacks may recur for years as the only feature of the disease, before other forms appear (Sohar *et al.* 1967).

As a rule, large joints are involved, particularly those of the lower extremities. Arthritic attacks of familial Mediterranean fever may present in two forms: acute, or chronic and protracted. In the acute form the onset is abrupt, fever ranges from 38 to 40 °C, and the affected single joint is tender, swollen, and held immobile because of the severe pain. Redness and local heat are frequently less marked than would be expected in so acute a process. The signs and symptoms usually peak in 1 to 2 days and then gradually subside, leaving no residue. The attacks can sometimes be precipitated by minor trauma or effort, such as prolonged walking. Synovial effusion is often demonstrable. The synovial fluid is sterile and varies in appearance from cloudy to purulent, depending upon the acuteness and severity of the synovitis. Resolution of a short attack can occur in as soon as 2 to 3 days, but more commonly takes a week and sometimes nearly a month.

About 5 per cent of patients experience protracted attacks, which persist for more than a month. Usually the hip or knee are involved (Sohar *et al.* 1967; Sneh *et al.* 1977), but episodes in other joints, such

as the ankle and, rarely, the temporomandibular or the sternoclavicular, may also assume a protracted course. Rather than recovering after several days, the joint remains markedly swollen and painful, presenting a picture of chronic monoarthritis or in rare cases, chronic oligoarthritis. The affected knee joint, in extreme cases, resembles a fluid bag from which up to 200 ml can be drained (Fig. 1). After several weeks or months, sometimes even after a year or more, the pain subsides spontaneously. During such protracted attacks in a joint, short attacks involving other joints, the abdomen, or chest may occur (Sohar *et al.* 1967).

In some protracted cases, especially in the hips, damage to the joints can be so severe as to cause permanent deformity, which ultimately may require joint replacement (Fig. 2). In 27 of our patients, there was residual incapacity in the affected joint (21 in the hips).

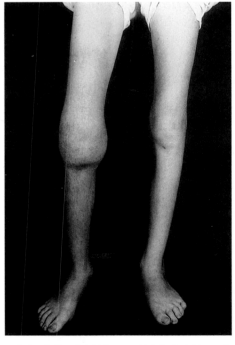

Fig. 1 Protracted arthritis of right knee, which lasted 11 months, in a 15-year-old patient (before colchicine was introduced for treatment).

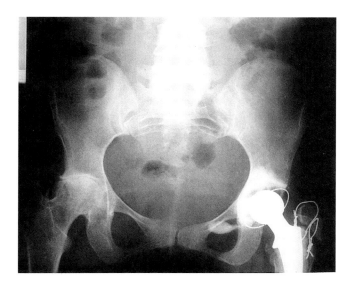

Fig. 2 Results of protracted arthritis of both hips in a 17-year-old girl. State following hip arthroplasty of left hip. Narrowing of the joint space, sclerosis, and aseptic necrosis of the lateral aspect can be seen in the right hip.

Seven hips showed radiologically typical aseptic necrosis of the femoral head, and in 14 sclerosis and narrowing of the joint space was observed. Most of these hips eventually required total prosthetic replacement (Sneh *et al.* 1977). In a summary of 22 total hip replacements performed in 18 patients with familial Mediterranean fever between 1971 and 1985 a relatively high percentage of aseptic loosening of the cemented hip prosthesis was noted. This finding led us to recommend cementless hip prostheses in such patients (Salai *et al.* 1993).

Among 160 patients with protracted arthritis we found a small group of 11 in whom the HLA-B27 was negative, who fulfilled the criteria for seronegative spondylarthropathy. Most of these patients responded to therapy with non-steroidal anti-inflammatory drugs, but some of them required the addition of disease-modifying antirheumatic drugs (Langevitz *et al.* 1994a).

Muscle pains occur in about 20 per cent of patients with familial Mediterranean fever. Usually the pain is not severe, appears in the lower extremities after physical exertion, lasts from a few hours to 1 to 2 days, and subsides with rest or non-steroidal anti-inflammatory drugs. In 12 per cent of patients with familial Mediterranean fever a syndrome of protracted febrile myalgia developed, characterized by severe, debilitating myalgia accompanied by fever, abdominal pain, a high erythrocyte sedimentation rate, leucocytosis, and hyperglobulinaemia. In a few patients a mild, short-lasting, vasculitic, nonthrombocytopenic purpura with a deposition of IgA was noted. In patients that were treated by non-steroidal anti-inflammatory drugs the attacks lasted 6 to 8 weeks, but they subsided promptly after a high dose of prednisone (Langevitz *et al.* 1994b). Since colchicine is known to induce neuropathy and myopathy in rare cases, especially in transplanted patients treated with cyclosporin (Yussim *et al.* 1994), it is important to differentiate colchicine-induced myopathy from an attack of protracted febrile myalgia.

Erysipelas-like erythema is one of the most characteristic manifestations of familial Mediterranean fever. It was reported in 11 per cent of affected children, usually combined with arthritis. Rather sharply bordered red patches, hot, tender, and swollen, and 10 to 35 cm^2 in area, appear on the skin of the lower extremities. They are usually located between the knee and ankle, or on the dorsum of the foot or ankle region, and are also accompanied by abrupt elevation of body temperature and last about 24 to 48 h (Sohar *et al.* 1967).

Orchitis (an acute, unilateral, painful swelling and redness of the testis due to inflammation of the tunica vaginalis) has been recognized as a form of attack in children or young adults; it subsides spontaneously after 12 to 24 h, without anatomical residue (Eshel *et al.* 1988).

Elevation of body temperature, sometimes to 40°C for a few hours, occurs frequently, especially in children, as the only expression of an attack (Sohar *et al.* 1967). This phenomenon is often falsely attributed to viral infection, pharyngitis, or tonsillitis.

One-third of our patients complained of pain in the heels or soles of the feet related to mild exertion such as walking or prolonged standing, which subsides after night rest. There are no objective signs of inflammation or elevation of temperature.

Mild splenomegaly of 1 to 4 cm, unrelated to amyloidosis, was found in many patients. In some patients the liver was also palpable. None showed clinical or laboratory malfunction of these organs.

Haematuria, sometimes only microscopic, has been observed in several patients during and between attacks. Mild anaemia with a low serum iron is common. Low levels of haemoglobin (7–10 g per cent) were found in some patients.

Allied conditions

Henoch–Schönlein purpura occurred in over 40 of our patients admitted to our hospital. Most of the patients were children and young adults, and in most of them the disease was characterized by a prolonged and severe course that required steroid therapy in many cases.

Polyarteritis nodosa has been reported in 15 cases of familial Mediterranean fever (Sachs *et al.* 1987; Glikson *et al.* 1989). All 15 were young patients, while polyarteritis nodosa generally occurs in the fifth or six decade of life. Polyarteritis nodosa is a rare disease with an incidence of 5 to 6 per million and the 15 cases recorded in about approximately 10 000 cases of familial Mediterranean fever are more than would be expected by chance (Pras *et al.* 1996).

A relatively high incidence of fibromyalgia (30 per cent) was found in patients with familial Mediterranean fever, especially in those who suffers from back and leg/foot pain (Langevitz *et al.* 1994c).

Various types of glomerulonephritis were reported in few patients with familial Mediterranean fever, including post-streptococcal glomerulonephritis, diffuse mesangial proliferative glomerulonephritis with IgA and IgM deposits and also rapidly progressive glomerulonephritis (Said *et al.* 1992).

Amyloidosis

A genetically determined, AA-type amyloidosis, clinically manifested as nephropathy (Sohar *et al.* 1967; Levine *et al.* 1972) is the fatal lesion in patients with familial Mediterranean fever.

The role of amyloidosis in the natural history of the disease was studied in an untreated group of 470 patients and revealed some typical features. Its clinical presentation occurs at an early age; 90 per cent of the patients who died from amyloidosis were under 40 and six were under 10 (Sohar *et al.* 1967). Subsequent evaluation showed a lower incidence of amyloidosis in some Jewish ethnic

Table 2   Extrarenal amyloidosis in familial Mediterranean fever
Amyloid cardiomyopathy
Giant hepatomegaly
Amyloid goitre
Addison's disease
Fatal malabsorption

groups (Pras *et al.* 1982) and in Armenians (Schwabe and Peters 1974). The onset of the clinical signs of amyloidosis does not correlate with the frequency or intensity of the febrile attacks.

Recent studies showed that pregnancy may have possible deleterious effect on amyloid nephropathy in patients with more advanced renal failure at conception (Livneh *et al.* 1993).

Clinically, the amyloid nephropathy passes through several stages. There is a preclinical stage but since it can only be diagnosed by repeated rectal and renal biopsies or is inadvertently found in an occasional Congo red-stained appendectomy specimen, no attempt was made to determine its duration. Persistent proteinuria in an otherwise healthy patient with familial Mediterranean fever has proved to be a certain indication of renal amyloidosis.

Clinical evidence of extrarenal amyloidosis was scant when patients died from renal failure before chronic dialysis was introduced as a routine treatment for chronic renal failure. Adrenal insufficiency is not apparent despite the severe involvement observed at autopsy (Sohar *et al.* 1967). Some patients show clinical and laboratory evidence of intestinal malabsorbtion (Ravid and Sohar 1974). Following prolongation of life by chronic dialysis and renal transplantation, amyloid deposition in other organs has become more pronounced. In recent years we have observed extrarenal amyloid deposition that interfered with the normal function of certain organs (Table 2). The deposition of amyloid in the small bowel is a particularly grave consequence that caused the death of six patients.

The amyloidosis of familial Mediterranean fever is not directly related to the recurrent inflammatory attacks. In some patients it occurs before the appearance of the febrile attacks and in a few it is the only manifestation of the disease (Blum *et al.* 1962). Thirteen per cent of our patients who succumbed to amyloidosis were below 15 years of age, and the youngest died at 5 years after amyloidosis had been manifest for 3 years (Sohar *et al.* 1967; Gafni *et al.* 1968).

Amyloidosis is prevalent mainly in Jewish patients of North African origin. Before the time of colchicine treatment only 11 patients of 418 of North African origin (2.5 per cent) survived and reached 40 years of age without demonstrating clinical signs of amyloidosis (Pras *et al.* 1982). The incidence of amyloidosis in untreated patients is very much higher than in the inflammatory and infectious diseases that predispose to reactive ('secondary') amyloidosis.

Laboratory tests

Laboratory findings are meagre and non-specific. The erythrocyte sedimentation rate is accelerated and acute-phase proteins such as α_2-globulin and fibrinogen are increased, especially during attacks,

but also in between (Sohar *et al.* 1967). The special attention accorded to serum amyloid A is due to the fact that its N-terminal fragment is AA protein, which is part of the AA amyloid fibril. Serum amyloid A is raised considerably in amyloidotic patients with familial Mediterranean fever. During attacks, very high concentrations of serum amyloid A are observed, which decrease gradually in the days following an attack. However, even during remissions the serum amyloid A in patients with familial Mediterranean fever is usually two or three times normal (Knecht *et al.* 1985). Since serum amyloid A is a universal acute-phase protein it is found to be elevated in other inflammatory febrile diseases and cannot therefore be used as a diagnostic measure for familial Mediterranean fever. The absence of LE cells, antinuclear factor, and rheumatoid factor, or the elevation of antistreptolysin-O titres, are relevant in patients with joint involvement.

It has recently been found that the familial Mediterranean fever (*FMF*) gene in our Sephardi families is located on the short arm of chromosome 16 (Pras *et al.* 1992a; Pras *et al.* 1992b). Cloning of the *FMF* gene will elucidate the abnormal biochemical product and the pathogenesis of the febrile inflammatory episodes of this disease.

Treatment (Table 3)

Until 1973 therapeutic measures were restricted to alleviating pain. Daily prophylactic treatment with colchicine was suggested by Goldfinger (1972) and assessed by double-blind studies (Zemer *et al.* 1974). The dose required to prevent attacks is not body weight-dependent. Treatment is started with 1 mg colchicine/day, regardless of age or severity of attacks. This dose is increased if necessary to 1.5 to 2 mg, until remission from attacks is achieved. Doses larger than 1 mg must be divided in two. Our experience has shown that if doses of 2 mg/day do not produce remission, further elevation of the dose not improve responsiveness. Omission of a daily dose may be followed promptly by an attack.

Sixty-five per cent of patients enjoy complete remission of attacks if they adhere to their daily dose of colchicine. Partial remission, defined as either a significant decrease in the frequency and severity of all forms of attacks or the remission of one form (usually abdominal) but not of another (usually arthritic), is experienced by an additional 30 per cent. In 5 per cent of treated patients the attack rate remains unchanged. They are maintained on 2 mg/day to prevent amyloidosis.

Our experience showed that continuous prophylactic treatment with colchicine in patients inhibits the development of nephropathic amyloidosis (Zemer *et al.* 1986). Colchicine even reversed the nephrotic syndrome in some patients with amyloidosis (Zemer *et al.* 1992). None of the patients who started treatment without proteinuria has developed amyloidosis during the follow-up period of 21 years, while a control group of non-compliant patients showed the same rate of amyloidosis as would be expected in the natural history of the disease.

Side-effects of colchicine are generally mild. Diarrhoea and nausea are the most common, and usually prove transient and easily controllable.

In 1973, when prophylactic colchicine treatment in familial Mediterranean fever was introduced, we were worried about its possible effects on children, because of its well-known antimitotic action. It is now clear, after hundreds of children have been taking the drug daily for more than 18 years, that in none of the treated patients, including children in their first decade of life, has colchicine

Table 3 Approach to the management of familial Mediterranean fever

Clinical characteristics	Colchicine	Additional therapies
To control febrile attacks and prevention of amyloidosis	Continuous 1–2 mg daily	
Amyloid nephropathy:		
Normal blood creatinine	2 mg daily	
Abnormal creatinine	1 mg daily	
Acute arthritis	Increase the usual dose by 0.5 mg	NSAIDs for 1–2 weeks
Protracted arthritis	1.5–2 mg	NSAIDs for months, intra-articular corticosteroids
Seronegative spondylarthropathy	1.5–2 mg	NSAIDs, DMARDs
Protracted febrile myalgia	1.5–2 mg	Corticosteroids 1 mg/kg per day

DMARD, disease-modifying antirheumatic drug; NSAID, non-steroidal anti-inflammatory drug.

caused any deviation from normal in physical examination, routine laboratory tests, linear growth, or sexual development (Zemer *et al.* 1991). The data on the effect of colchicine on fertility in patients with familial Mediterranean fever are controversial (Ehrenfeld *et al.* 1986; Ehrenfeld *et al.* 1987). It is known that a high temperature may cause transient azoospermia. In many of our patients who had suffered from frequent febrile attacks, colchicine treatment improved spermatogenesis by preventing the inflammatory febrile attacks. Fertility is sometimes apparently impaired in women with familial Mediterranean fever, probably due to the induction of early miscarriages or to pelvic adhesions that develop after frequent abdominal attacks. Colchicine, by preventing the abdominal attacks, may lessen the rate of early miscarriages and the development of pelvic adhesions. Four pregnancies producing infants with Down syndrome were reported in colchicine-treated patients (Ravia *et al.* 1991; Rabinovitch *et al.* 1992; and our unpublished data). So, routine amniocentesis to exclude chromosomal aberrations in colchicine-treated patients is recommended.

A daily dose of 1.5 to 2.0 mg colchicine appears to protect the renal graft from amyloidosis (Livneh *et al.* 1992). Although several live kidney transplantations have been successfully performed in some of our patients, cadaver kidney transplant is the treatment of choice in the endstage disease of familial Mediterranean fever.

References

Alt, H. L. and Barker, H. (1930). Fever of unknown origin. *Journal of the American Medical Association*, **94**, 1457–61.

Benhamou, E., Albou, A., and Griguer, P. (1954). Remarques cliniques biologiques et therapeutiques sur la maladie periodique (a propos de 24 cas personels). *Bulletin et Memoires de la Societe Medical des Hopitaux de Paris*, **70**, 254–8.

Blum, A., Gafni, J., Sohar E., Shibolet, S., and Heller, H. (1962). Amyloidosis as the sole manifestation of familial Mediterranean fever (FMF). *Annals of Internal Medicine*, **57**, 795–9.

Dabestani, A., Noble, L. M., Child, J. S., Krivokapich, M. D., and Schwabe, M. D. (1982). Pericardial disease in familial Mediterranean fever. *Chest*, **81**, 592–5.

Ehrenfeld, M., Levy, M., Margalioth, E. J., and Eliakim, M. (1986). The effects of long-term colchicine therapy on male fertility in patients with familial Mediterranean fever. *Andrology*, **18**, 420–6.

Ehrenfeld, M., Bzezinski, A., Levy, M., and Eliakim, M. (1987). Fertility and obstetric history in patients with familial Mediterranean fever on long-term colchicine therapy. *British Journal of Obstetrics and Gynaecology*, **94**, 1186–91.

Eshel, G., Zemer, D., and Bar-Yochai. A (1988). Acute orchitis in familial Mediterranean fever. *Annals of Internal Medicine*, **109**, 164–5.

Gafni, J., Ravid, M., and Sohar, E. (1968). The role of amyloidosis in familial Mediterranean fever. A population study. *Israel Journal of Medical Sciences*, **4**, 995–9.

Glikson, M., Galun, E., Schlezinger, M., Cohen, D., Haskell, L., Rubinow, A., and Eliakim, M. (1989). Polyarteritis nodosa and familial Mediterranean fever. A report of two cases and review of the literature. *Journal of Rheumatology*, **16**, 536–9.

Goldfinger, S. E. (1972). Colchicine for familial Mediterranean fever. *New England Journal of Medicine*, **287**, 1302.

Heller, H., Sohar, E., and Sherf, L. (1958). Familial Mediterranean fever. *Archives of Internal Medicine*, **102**, 50–71.

Heller, H., Sohar, E., and Gafni, J. (1961a). Amyloidosis in familial Mediterranean fever. *Archives of Internal Medicine*, **107**, 539–50.

Heller, H., Sohar, E., and Pras M. (1961b) Ethnic distribution and amyloidosis in familial Mediterranean fever (FMF). *Pathologia et Microbiologica*, **24**, 718–32.

Ismachovich, B., Zemer, D., Revach, M., Serr, D. M., and Sohar, E. (1973) The causes of sterility in females with familial Mediterranean fever. *Sterility and Fertility*, **24**, 844–7.

Janeway, T. C. and Mosenthal, H. D. (1908). An unusual paroxysmal syndrome probably allied to recurrent vomiting with a study of the nitrogen metabolism. *Transactions of the Association of American Physicians*, **23**, 504–18.

Knecht, A., De Beer, F. C., and Pras, M. (1985). Serum amyloid A protein in familial Mediterranean fever. *Annals of Internal Medicine*, **102**, 71–2.

Langevitz, P., Livneh, A., Zemer, D., Shemer, J., and Pras M. (1994a). Seronegative spondyloarthropathy (SNSA) in familial Mediterranean fever (FMF). *Arthritis and Rheumatism*, **37**, S203 (Abstr.).

Langevitz, P., Zemer, D., Livneh, A., Shemer, J., and Pras, M. (1994b). Protracted febrile myalgia in patients with familial Mediterranean fever. *Journal of Rheumatology*, **21**, 1708–9.

Langevitz, P. *et al.* (1994c). Fibromyalgia in familial Mediterranean fever. *Journal of Rheumatology*, **21**, 1335–7.

Levine, M., Franklin, E. C., Frangione, B. and Pras M. (1972). The amino acid sequence of a major non-immunoglobulin component of some amyloid fibrils. *Journal of Clinical Investigation*, **51**, 2773–6.

Livneh, A., Zemer, D., Siegal, B., Laor, A., Sohar, E., and Pras, M. (1992). Colchicine prevents kidney transplant amyloidosis in familial Mediterranean fever. *Nephron*, **60**, 418–22.

Livneh, A., Cabili, S., Zemer, D., Rabinovitch, O., and Pras, M. (1993). Effect of pregnancy on renal function in amyloidosis of familial Mediterranean fever. *Journal of Rheumatology*, **20**, 1519–23.

Mamou, H. and Cattan R. (1952). La maladie periodique (sur 14 cas personnels dont 8 compliques de nephropaties). *La Semaine des Hopitaux de Paris*, **28**, 1062–70.

Michaeli, D., Pras, M., and Rosen, N. (1966). Intestinal strangulation complicating familial Mediterranean fever (FMF). *British Medical Journal*, **2**, 30–2.

Pras, M., Bronshpigel, N., Zemer, D., and Gafni, J. (1982). Variable incidence of amyloidosis in familial Mediterranean fever among different ethnic groups. *Johns Hopkins Medical Journal*, **150**, 22–6.

Pras, M., Zemer, D., Langevitz, P., and Sohar E. (1992*a*). Familial Mediterranean fever: a genetic disorder prevalent in Sepharadi Jews. In *Genetic diversity among Jews. Diseases and markers at the DNA level* (ed. B. Bonne-Tamir and A. Adam), pp. 223–7. Oxford University Press.

Pras, M. *et al.* (1992*b*). Mapping of a gene causing familial Mediterranean fever to the short arm of chromosome 16. *New England Journal of Medicine*, **326**, 1509–13.

Pras, M., Langevitz, P., Livneh, A., and Zemer, D. (1996). Vasculitis in familial Mediterranean fever. In *The vasculitides* (ed. B. Ansell, P. A. Bacon, J. T. Lie, and H. Yazici), pp. 412–16. Chapman and Hall, London.

Rabinovitch, O., Zemer, D., Kukia, E., Sohar, E., and Mashiach, S. (1992). Colchicine treatment in conception and pregnancy: two hundred thirty-one pregnancies in patients with familial Mediterranean fever. *American Journal of Reproductive Immunology*, **28**, 245–6.

Ravia, Y., Aviram, A., Marom, M., Chaki, R., Bat-Miriam, M., Barkai, G., and Goldman, B. (1991). Increased rate of meiotic and somatic nondisjunction in FMF patients and their fetuses. *American Journal of Medical Genetics*, **49**, 1245.

Ravid, M. and Sohar, E. (1974). Intestinal malabsorption: first manifestation of amyloidosis in familial Mediterranean fever. *Gastroenterology*, **66**, 446–9.

Reimann, H. A. (1949) Periodic disease. Periodic fever, periodic abdominalgia, cyclic neutropenia, intermittent arthralgia, angioneurotic edema, anaphylactoid purpura and periodic paralysis. *Journal of the American Medical Association*, **141**, 175–82.

Rogers, D. B. *et al.* (1989). Familial Mediterranean fever in Armenians. *American Journal of Medical Genetics*, **34**, 168–72.

Sachs, D., Langevitz, P., Morag B., and Pras, M. (1987). Polyarteritis nodosa in familial Mediterranean fever. *British Journal of Rheumatology*, **26**, 139–41.

Said, R., Hamzeh, Y., Said, S., Tarawneh, M., and Al-Khateeb, M. (1992). Spectrum of renal involvement in familial Mediterranean fever. *Kidney International*, **41**, 414–19.

Salai, M., Langevitz, P., Blankstein, A., Zemer, D., Chechick, A., Pras, M., and Horoszowski, H. (1993). Total hip replacement in familial Mediterranean fever. *Bulletin of the Hospital for Joint Diseases*, **53**, 25–8.

Schwabe, A. D. and Peters, R. S. (1974). Familial Mediterranean fever in Armenians, analysis of 100 cases. *Medicine*, **53**, 453–62.

Siegal, S. (1945). Benign paroxysmal peritonitis. *Annals of Internal Medicine*, **22**, 1–21.

Siguier, F., Zara, M., Funck-Bretano, J. L., and Lagrue, G. (1953). Maladies periodiques a formes degradees evoluant chez plusieurs membres d'une meme famille. *Bulletin et Memoires de la Societé Medical de Hopitaux des Paris*, **69**, 679–84.

Sneh, E., Pras, M., Michaeli D., Shain, N., and Gafni J. (1977). Protracted arthritis in familial Mediterranean fever. *Rheumatology and Rehabilitation*, **16**, 102–6.

Sohar, E., Pras, M., Heller, J., and Heller H. (1961). Genetics of familial Mediterranean fever. *Archives of Internal Medicine*, **107**, 529–38.

Sohar, M., Gafni, J., Pras, M., and Heller, H. (1967). Familial Mediterranean fever. A survey of 470 cases and review of literature. *American Journal of Medicine*, **43**, 227–53.

Yussim, A. *et al.* (1994). Gastrointestinal, hepatorenal and neuromuscular toxicity caused by cyclosporine-colchicine interaction in renal transplantation. *Transplantation Proceedings*, **26**, 2825–6.

Yuval, Y., Hemo-Zisser, M., Zemer, D., Sohar, E., and Pras, M. (1995). Dominant Inheritance in two families with familial Mediterranean fever. *American Journal of Medical Genetics*, **57**, 455–7.

Zemer, D. *et al.* (1974). A controlled trial of colchicine in preventing attacks of familial Mediterranean fever. *New England Journal of Medicine*, **291**, 932–4.

Zemer, D., Cabili, S., Revach, M., and Shain, N. (1977). Constrictive pericarditis in familial Mediterranean fever. *Israel Journal of Medical Sciences*, **13**, 55–8.

Zemer, D., Pras, M., Sohar, E., Modan, B., Cabili, S., and Gafni, J. (1986). Colchicine in the prevention and treatment of the amyloidosis of familial Mediterranean fever. *New England Journal of Medicine*, **314**, 1001–5.

Zemer, D., Livneh, A., Danon Y. L., Pras M., and Sohar E. (1991). Long-term colchicine treatment in children with familial Mediterranean fever. *Arthritis and Rheumatism*, **34**, 973–7.

Zemer, D., Livneh, A., and Langevitz, P. (1992). Reversal of the nephrotic syndrome by colchicine in amyloidosis of familial Mediterranean fever. *Annals of Internal Medicine*, **116**, 426.

5.13.3 Panniculitis

Jeffrey P. Callen

Panniculitis refers to inflammation within the subcutaneous fat (Patterson 1983). Panniculitis is probably a dynamic process that progresses through inflammation with neutrophils to lymphocytes to histiocytes and ends with fibrosis (Thiers 1988). The panniculitis can become granulomatous when in the histiocytic phase. The exact nature of the infiltrate perhaps depends upon when the biopsy is taken in relation to the age of the lesion being sampled. The panniculitides have been divided into four categories based on histopathological criteria: (i) septal panniculitis, (ii) lobular panniculitis, (iii) mixed with septal and lobular components, and (iv) panniculitis with vasculitis. Table 1 presents one of the currently accepted classifications for the panniculitides. Frequently the panniculitides are associated with systemic disease. Often the separation of one syndrome from another is possible only after a period of observation.

Clinical features

The prototypic septal panniculitis is erythema nodosum (Soderstrom 1982). A relatively common process, erythema nodosum is usually acute and self-limited. Erythema nodosum occurs most commonly in young adult women, but any age or sex can be affected. The typical clinical presentation is the sudden onset of one or more tender, erythematous nodules on the anterior tibial surface (Fig. 1). The nodules are deep and are better palpated than visualized. As the lesions age they may soften and develop an ecchymotic appearance. Over a 4- to 6-week period, the lesions eventually heal without scar formation. Ulceration of the primary process is extremely rare. While other symptoms may be present, they are usually those of an associated condition.

Although erythema nodosum is usually an acute process, many patients with chronic or recurrent disease have been described. Terms such as chronic erythema nodosum, erythema nodosum migrans, subacute nodular migratory panniculitis (Vilanova's disease), or septal granulomatous panniculitis have been used to characterize these patients (Prestes *et al.* 1990). The patient with erythema nodosum migrans tends to be a middle-aged (mean 45 to 50 years) woman. The disease is often present for several years, and is most common on the legs. As with acute erythema nodosum, accompanying symptoms may be present, but are usually a result of the associated condition.

Table 1 Classification of the panniculitides

I. Septal panniculitis

  A. Erythema nodosum

  B. Vilanova's disease — subacute nodular migratory panniculitis

II. Lobular panniculitis

  A. Weber-Christian disease — relapsing febrile nodular non-suppurative panniculitis

  B. Rothman–Makai syndrome — lipogranulomatosis subcutanea

  C. Subcutaneous fat necrosis of the newborn

  D. Post-steroid panniculitis

  E. Enzymatic panniculitis

    1. Pancreatic

    2. α_1-Antitrypsin deficiency

  F. Calcifying panniculitis (calciphylaxis) associated with renal failure

  G. Physical or factitial panniculitis

  H. Cytophagic panniculitis

  I. Lipodystrophy syndromes

  J. Connective tissue panniculitis — scleroderma or myositis

  K. Sclerosing panniculitis (lipodermatosclerosis)

III. Mixed panniculitis

  Lupus profundus — lupus erythematosus panniculitis

IV. Panniculitis with vasculitis

  A. Small vessel vasculitis (postcapillary venule), leucocytoclastic vasculitis

  B. Medium-sized vessel vasculitis (arterioles or small arteries)

    1. Polyarteritis nodosa

    2. Erythema induratum

Causative or associated conditions are present in about 50 per cent of patients with acute, recurrent, or chronic variants of erythema nodosum. The associated conditions can be broken into three broad categories: infectious diseases, therapeutic agents, or systemic diseases (usually inflammatory). Some of the known associations are listed in Table 2.

The infectious agents associated with erythema nodosum primarily tend to affect the respiratory or gastrointestinal tracts and are most often bacterial or fungal in origin. The most common drugs linked with the disease are antibiotics and oral contraceptives. Pregnancy, particularly in its second trimester, is a known association; and erythema nodosum will recur with subsequent pregnancies or with oral contraceptive use. A specific variant of sarcoidosis is associated with erythema nodosum, known as Löfgren's syndrome. This is an acute, often self-resolving variant in which erythema nodosum occurs in association with asymptomatic bilateral hilar lymphadenopathy, arthritis, and anterior uveitis. Crohn's disease (granulomatous colitis and regional enteritis) and ulcerative colitis have been associated with erythema nodosum. Patients with these inflammatory bowel diseases develop erythema nodosum that parallels the activity of the bowel disease. Panniculitis can occur with the collagen-vascular diseases (Winkelmann 1983), but it may not be best to classify the process as erythema nodosum (see below).

Table 2 Some aetiological causes of or associations with erythema nodosum

Infections:

  Streptococcal pharyngitis

  Tuberculosis

  Valley fever (coccidioidomycosis)

  Blastomycosis

  Histoplasmosis

  Psittacosis

  Yersinia colitis

  Salmonella gastroenteritis

  Cat scratch fever

  Leprosy

Drugs:

  Antibiotics — penicillins, sulphonamides

  Birth control pills

Systemic processes or diseases:

  Pregnancy

  Sarcoidosis

  Inflammatory bowel disease

  Collagen–vascular disorders — dermatomyositis, lupus erythematosus, scleroderma

  Malignancy (rare)

  Sweet's syndrome

Idiopathic

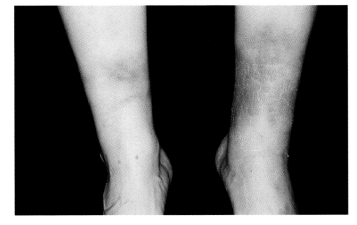

Fig. 1 Erythema nodosum — multiple tender subcutaneous erythematous nodules.

Weber-Christian disease

This is characterized by multiple recurrent subcutaneous nodules (Fig. 2), with accompanying fever (Panush *et al.* 1985). Histopathologically, the disease is characterized by a lobular panniculitis with an early neutrophilic infiltrate, fat degeneration, foamy histiocytes, and giant-cell formation. Eventually fibrosis occurs, and this, in addition to the destruction of fat, results in the clinical finding of an atrophic scar. Other clinical features that commonly occur are arthralgias and myalgias. Some patients also have recurrent abdominal pain. In addition to the skin lesions, any area of the body containing fat can be affected by Weber-Christian disease. Several cases of mesenteric panniculitis have been reported, as has involvement of the heart, lungs, liver, and/or kidneys (Lemley *et al.* 1991). The disease is chronic, but can result in death in 10 to 15 per cent of cases. Some of the patients with Weber-Christian disease have had multiple surgical procedures because of an acute inflammatory lesion in the presence of fever.

The laboratory abnormalities associated with Weber-Christian disease include an elevated sedimentation rate, anaemia, leucopenia or leucocytosis, depression of complement components, and evidence of circulating immune complexes. There have been several reports of α_1-antitrypsin deficiency in patients with Weber-Christian disease (Breit *et al.* 1983), however, the meaning of this finding is not clear. In addition, patients who have lupus erythematosus or pancreatic disease have been diagnosed with this form of panniculitis; however, their accompanying laboratory abnormalities would be those associated with the primary process.

Panniculitis associated with α_1-antitrypsin deficiency

Several groups of patients with a lobular or septal panniculitis have been found to have a deficiency of α_1-antitrypsin (Smith *et al.* 1987).

In a study of 96 patients with panniculitis, Smith *et al.* (1989) found 15 patients with α_1-antitrypsin deficiency. There were differences in the clinical and histopathological manifestations, but very little difference in the associated conditions present in either group. Specifically, the group with α_1-antitrypsin deficiency was more likely to have ulceration and drainage, and correspondingly had greater amounts of fat necrosis and destruction of elastic tissue. Geller and Su (1994) have suggested that the finding of splaying of neutrophils between collagen bundles is highly suggestive of this form of panniculitis. Furthermore, Smith *et al.* (1987) believed that induction of lesions by trauma was more likely in the enzyme deficient group. The recognition of these patients may be important on several grounds. First, debridement of the lesion should be avoided; second, in patients felt to have factitial panniculitis, α_1-antitrypsin deficiency should be considered; third, these patient should be evaluated for pulmonary disease and should be counselled to avoid smoking; and fourth, therapy with α_1-proteinase inhibitor concentrate may be helpful. A recent report documented the effectiveness of doxycycline and postulated that its effects were mediated through anticollagenase properties (Humbert *et al.* 1991).

Pancreatic panniculitis

Some patients with pancreatic diseases develop subcutaneous fat necrosis (lobular panniculitis) (Fig. 3), with accompanying polyarthritis and osseous intramedullary fat necrosis (Wilson *et al.* 1983). A variety of changes have been implicated in the development of this process including pancreatitis, pancreatic carcinoma (acinar cell), pancreatitis secondary to cholelithiasis, post-traumatic lesions, pancreatic ischaemia, pancreatic pseudocyst (Zimmerman-Gorska *et al.* 1986), and a pancreatic difusum (a congenital pancreatic abnormality) (Huber and Asaad 1986). It is not clear whether the

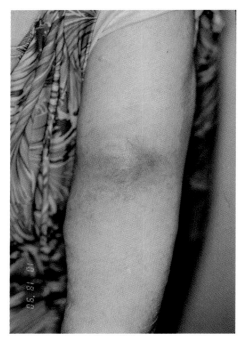

Fig. 2 Weber-Christian disease — this patient developed multiple recurrent subcutaneous lesions with accompanying fever and arthritis.

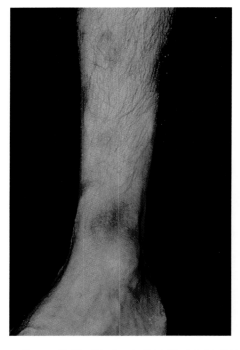

Fig. 3 Pancreatic panniculitis. Tender, erythematous subcutaneous nodules in a patient with pancreatitis (by courtesy of Robert Schosser, MD of Lexington, KY, USA).

Table 1 Non-infectious neutrophilic dermatoses

I. *Non-angiocentric*

    Psoriasis

    Reiter's syndrome

    Subcorneal pustular dermatosis

    Acne fulminans

    Blastomycosis-like pyoderma (pyoderma vegetans)

II. *Angiocentric*

    A. Vessel wall destruction

        1. Leucocytoclastic vasculitis

        2. Polyarteritis nodosa

    B. No vessel wall destruction

        1. Acute febrile neurtrophilic dermatosis (Sweet's syndrome)

            (a) typical

            (b) atypical (cancer-associated) variant

        2. Pyoderma gangrenosum

            (a) typical

            (b) atypical (cancer-associated) variant

        3. 'Pustular vasculitis'

            (a) Behçet's disease

            (b) Bowel-associated dermatosis–arthritis syndrome

        4. Rheumatoid neutrophilic dermatosis

        5. Pyostomatitis vegetans

        6. Pustular eruption of ulcerative colitis

        7. Familial Mediterranean fever

Derived from Jorizzo (1988).

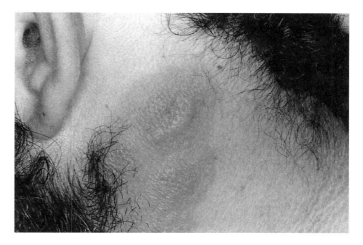

Fig. 1 Sweet's syndrome. This patient developed erythematous plaques with a central mamillated 'microvesicular' surface.

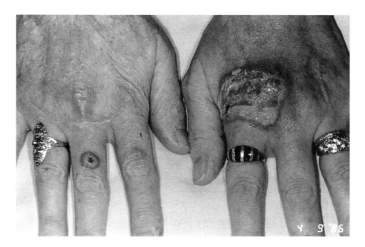

Fig. 2 This patient's pustular lesion on an erythematous base was initiated after a kitchen accident in which boiling water splattered on her hand.

description, more than 500 cases have been reported (von den Driesch *et al.* 1994).

This syndrome is more frequent in women (female:male, 3.7:1) between the ages of 30 and 70 years (mean age 52.6 years). Children with Sweet's syndrome have also been reported (Boatman *et al.* 1994). The disease may be preceded by symptoms suggestive of an upper respiratory tract infection. The skin lesions are felt to be distinctive, but may simulate several other processes. The characteristic lesion is a well defined, erythematous plaque with a mamillated surface, which may give the clinical impression of microvesiculation (Fig. 1). There is rarely any accompanying epidermal change or ulceration, and the lesions usually heal without scar formation. Pustules may stud the surface or may be a major feature of the process. A relatively common clinical variant is a tender, erythematous nodule which clinically resembles erythema nodosum (Cohen *et al.* 1992). Genital lesions have been reported, but are rare (Banet *et al.* 1994). The lesions occur in crops, and may be initiated by a variety of traumatic injuries (pathergy) such as a needle stick, wound debridement, or burn (Fig. 2). The lesions are accompanied by fever and malaise in most patients, and myalgias and/or arthralgias in about half. Headache, nausea, vomiting, diarrhoea, and/or conjunctivitis

may also occur in some patients. Untreated lesions resolve over 6 to 8 weeks, however, many patients continue to produce new lesions chronically or recurrently.

The laboratory findings include a leucocytosis which is composed of mature neutrophils. White blood cell counts generally range from 10 to 20 000 cells/mm³. The remainder of the blood count is within normal limits, except in patients who have leukaemia-associated Sweet's syndrome. The erythrocyte sedimentation rate is frequently elevated. On rare occasions a patient may have proteinuria. Histopathologically there is a dense dermal infiltrate composed of mature polymorphonuclear leucocytes. The infiltrate may be more pronounced in perivascular areas, and leucocytoclasia is frequent, but the vessel walls are spared. Oedema in the papillary dermis may be intense coinciding with the microvesicular lesions observed clinically. Immunofluorescence microscopy has been negative in a small number of cases in which it has been reported.

Sweet's syndrome has been reported with a variety of diseases. Von den Driesch *et al.* (1994) has suggested that Sweet's syndrome can be subdivided into four groups: (i) classic or idiopathic, (ii) parainflammatory, (iii) paraneoplastic, and (iv) pregnancy associated (Cohen *et*

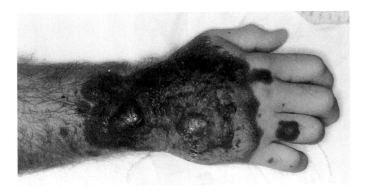

Fig. 3 Sweet's syndrome in a patient with acute myelogenous leukaemia. The purpura is due to bleeding into the lesions associated with thrombocytopenia.

al. 1993). While idiopathic cases are the most frequent, paraneoplastic Sweet's syndrome is the most frequently identified association and myelogenous leukaemia or preleukaemia account for most of the paraneoplastic conditions (Cooper *et al.* 1983; Cohen *et al.* 1988) Sweet's syndrome is not clinically or histopathologically different among the four groups; however, in the presence of leukaemia, the patients more frequently tend to be anaemic or thrombocytopenic and may have haemorrhagic lesions (Fig. 3). Other associated processes in paraneoplastic Sweet's syndrome include benign monoclonal gammopathy, lymphoma, myelodysplastic disorders, and various solid tumours (including breast, stomach, genitourinary, and colon most commonly) (Cohen *et al.* 1993). Parainflammatory Sweet's syndrome has also been reported in conjunction with lupus erythematosus, rheumatoid arthritis (Trentham *et al.* 1976; Haray 1983), Sjögren's syndrome (Prystowsky *et al.* 1978), inflammatory bowel disease (Crohn's disease and ulcerative colitis), Behçet's disease, thyroiditis, various infections (including HIV, hepatitis, mycobacteria, cytomegalovirus, salmonella), and drug hypersensitivity (Johnson and Grimwood 1994; Piette *et al.* 1994). It is not known how frequently paraneoplastic Sweet's syndrome occurs, but most authorities quote a figure ranging from 10 to 20 per cent, with about 40 to 50 per cent of these patients having a haematological malignancy.

The pathogenesis of Sweet's syndrome is not known. Tests for circulating immune complexes, tissue-bound immunoglobulins, or complement have generally been negative. Kemmett and Hunter (1990) reported perinuclear antineutrophil cytoplasmic antibodies (**p-ANCA**) in 6 patients with Sweet's syndrome, but believed this to be an epiphenomenon. Von den Driesch (1994) was unable to demonstrate p- or c-ANCA in any of his 10 patients who were tested. Studies of neutrophil function have not shown a consistent abnormality. Furthermore, abnormalities of T cells and proinflammatory cytokines such as γ-interferon or interleukin 8 have not been reproducibly reported.

Sweet's syndrome is usually an acute, steroid-responsive, self-limited disease. In general, a 2-week tapering course of oral prednisone (40 to 60 mg/day) is effective. One or more exacerbations requiring brief reinstitution of corticosteroids are common. From Sweet's initial report and the many later ones, it appears that the process can follow a chronic course, and the use of steroid-sparing agents should be considered. In reports of individual or small groups of patients, dapsone, potassium iodide, indomethacin, doxycycline, clofazimine, colchicine, metronidazole, isotretinoin, methotrexate,

chlorambucil, cyclosporin, and pulse dosage of methylprednisolone have been successfully used (Hoffman 1977; Horio *et al.* 1980; Subhisa *et al.* 1983; Aram 1984; Case *et al.* 1989; Banet *et al.* 1994; von den Driesch 1994)

Pyoderma gangrenosum

Pyoderma gangrenosum is an uncommon, ulcerative, cutaneous condition with distinctive clinical characteristics (Callen 1990). Frequently there is an associated systemic disease. The diagnosis is made by exclusion of other processes that may cause cutaneous ulcers. Like patients with Sweet's syndrome, patients with pyoderma gangrenosum are often pathergic, with lesions sometimes developing after minor trauma.

The ulcerations of classical pyoderma gangrenosum are frequently clinically characteristic. The border is well defined with a deep erythematous to violaceous colour (Fig. 4). The lesion extends peripherally and often the border overhangs the ulceration (undermined) as the inflammatory process spreads within the dermis, only secondarily causing necrosis of the epidermis. The lesions may be single, or may occur in crops, often beginning as a discrete pustule with a surrounding inflammatory erythema. The lesions may occur on any surface, but are most common on the legs. Pain is a prominent feature and is sometimes so severe that narcotics are required for symptomatic relief. As the lesion heals, scar formation occurs and the resulting scar is often described as cribiform (Fig. 5).

Several variants of pyoderma gangrenosum have been described. The pustular eruption of ulcerative colitis was first reported by O'Loughlin and Perry (1978). In this process the patient is acutely ill with fever and develops multiple sterile pustules (Fig. 6) (Fenske *et al.* 1983; Callen and Woo 1985). The lesions may regress without scarring, or some may progress into a typical lesion of pyoderma gangrenosum. Biopsy of the early lesion reveals sheets of mature polymorphonuclear leucocytes.

Peristomal pyoderma gangrenosum is a recently recognized variant that occurs in patients with ulcerative colitis or Crohn's disease who have had abdominal surgery and have an ileostomy or colostomy (Keltz *et al.* 1993). The ulceration (Fig. 7) may occur as an early or late phenomenon. Perhaps irritation from the ileostomy or colostomy appliance is involved in the induction of this process (pathergy).

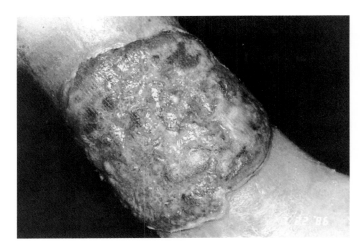

Fig. 4 Pyoderma gangrenosum. Typical large ulceration with an undermined violaceous border.

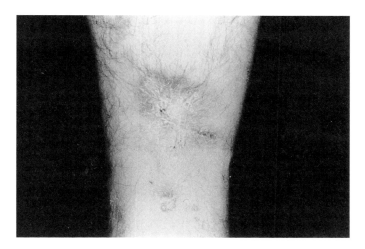

Fig. 5 Healed lesion of pyoderma gangrenosum.

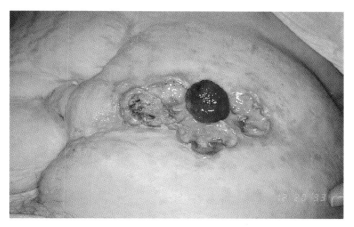

Fig. 7 Peristomal pyoderma gangrenosum in a patient with an ileostomy after bowel surgery for ulcerative colitis.

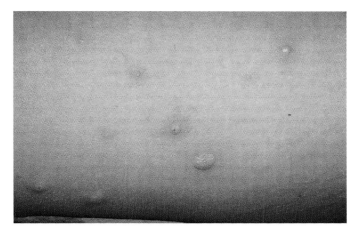

Fig. 6 Vesiculopustular eruption of ulcerative colitis.

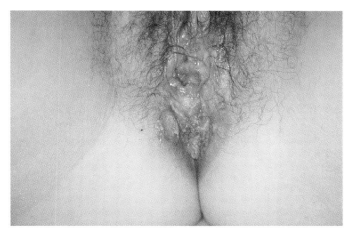

Fig. 8 Vulvar pyoderma gangrenosum.

These ulcerations must be differentiated from infections, dermatitis, or extension of the underlying bowel disease (Crohn's only).

Vulvar pyoderma gangrenosum is another recently recognized variant (McCalmont *et al.* 1991). Except for its location, the ulceration is otherwise typical of pyoderma gangrenosum (Fig. 8). This variant should be differentiated from Behçet's disease.

Another variant is pyostomatitis vegetans. This process is one in which chronic, pustular, eventually vegetative erosions develop on the mucous membranes (Fig. 9), most notably in the oral cavity (Van Hale *et al.* 1985). Most of these patients have had inflammatory bowel disease, and some have had ulcerative skin lesions similar to pyoderma gangrenosum (Storwick *et al.* 1994).

A condition known as malignant pyoderma is distinguished from pyoderma gangrenosum by three features: (i) lesions predominantly on the head and neck (atypical for pyoderma gangrenosum), (ii) lack of associated systemic diseases, and (iii) the absence of undermined borders and surrounding erythema (Perry *et al.* 1968). The distinctiveness of this variant has been questioned (Wernikoff *et al.* 1987; Newman and Frank 1993).

Lastly, there is a variant known as atypical or bullous pyoderma gangrenosum. In this the ulceration is more superficial, there is often a bullous, blue-grey margin (Fig. 10), and the upper extremities and face are more commonly affected (Perry and Winkelmann 1972;

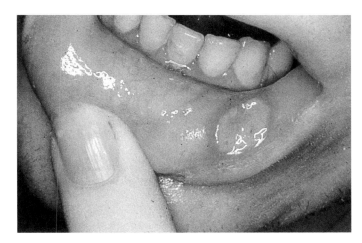

Fig. 9 Pyostomatitis vegetans. This vegetative ulceration occurred in a patient with ulcerative colitis.

Romano and Safai 1979). This variant has been reported with haematological disease, specifically preleukaemic conditions such as myeloid metaplasia (Callen *et al.* 1976), or acute myelogenous leukaemia. At times the separation of atypical pyoderma gangrenosum from leukaemia-associated Sweet's syndrome is difficult.

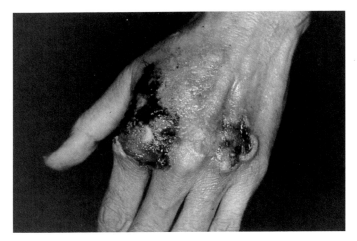

Fig. 10 Atypical pyoderma gangrenosum in a patient with a preleukaemic state. The lesion is a shallow ulcer with a bullous, blue-grey border.

Table 2 Diseases associated with pyoderma gangrenosum

Common associations

Inflammatory bowel disease
  Chronic ulcerative colitis
    Regional enteritis, granulomatous colitis (Crohn's disease)
Arthritis
    Seronegative with inflammatory bowel disease
    Seronegative without inflammatory bowel disease
    Rheumatoid arthritis
Spondylitis
Osteoarthritis
Psoriatic arthritis
Haematological diseases
    Myelocytic leukaemias
    Hairy cell leukaemia
    Myelofibrosis, myeloid metaplasia
    Monoclonal gammopathy (IgA)

Rarely reported associations

Chronic active hepatitis
Myeloma
Polycythaemia rubra vera
Paroxysmal nocturnal haemoglobinuria
Takayasu's arteritis
Primary biliary cirrhosis
Systemic lupus erythematosus
Wegener's granulomatosis
Hidradenitis suppurativa
Acne conglobata
Solid tumours
Thyroid disease
Pulmonary disease
Sarcoidosis
Diabetes mellitus
Deficiency of the seventh component of complement (C7)

The histopathological features of pyoderma gangrenosum are not specific, but are useful in ruling out other causes of cutaneous ulceration. There is controversy over what is the initial histopathological change, with some classifying the process as a neutrophilic dermatosis (Jorizzo 1988), and others believing that the initial changes involve lymphocytic infiltrate, endothelial cell swelling, and fibrinoid necrosis of the vessel wall (a lymphocytic vasculitis) (Su *et al.* 1986). Regardless, the lesion does not involve a leucocytoclastic vasculitis, nor is granuloma formation compatible with a diagnosis of pyoderma gangrenosum.

The aetiology and pathogenesis of pyoderma gangrenosum are not understood, but a variety of abnormalities of the immune system have been described. Although associated conditions are common (Table 2), perhaps a quarter to a half of the patients have 'idiopathic' disease. The most common associated conditions are inflammatory bowel disease, arthritis, paraproteinaemia, and haematological malignancy.

Initial reports of pyoderma gangrenosum emphasized the association with ulcerative colitis (Perry 1959). Eventually, it has become recognized that regional enteritis and Crohn's disease (granulomatous colitis) are found with pyoderma gangrenosum as often as ulcerative colitis (Powell *et al.* 1985, Prystowsky *et al.* 1989). In the most recent accounts, inflammatory bowel disease has constituted about 15 to 20 per cent of the associated phenomena. In addition, early reports stressed the relationship of pyoderma gangrenosum to the activity of the bowel disease, and even suggested that some patients' pyoderma gangrenosum lesions may benefit from surgical resection of the inflamed bowel (ulcerative colitis only). Callen *et al.* (1989) have reported pyoderma gangrenosum in association with inactive terminal ileitis, and Talansky *et al.* (1983) also have reported lack of effect of bowel resection in some patients with pyoderma gangrenosum and ulcerative colitis.

Arthritis is a frequent finding with pyoderma gangrenosum. In some of the later reports, arthritis has been the most frequent associated condition (Powell *et al.* 1985; Prystowsky *et al.* 1989). Five of the nine patients with arthritis reported by Prystowsky *et al.* (1989) had inflammatory bowel disease associated arthritis. In general, the arthritis associated with pyoderma gangrenosum is a symmetrical polyarthritis which may be seronegative or seropositive. Spondylitis, although it may occur in conjunction with inflammatory bowel

disease associated with pyoderma gangrenosum, has not been reported independently with pyoderma gangrenosum.

A variety of malignancies have been reported with pyoderma gangrenosum, most commonly myelogenous leukaemia or preleukaemia. This association may be more common with the atypical variants of pyoderma gangrenosum. Although a variety of solid tumours have been reported, their presence is probably coincidental.

Paraproteinaemia, in general a benign variety, has been reported with pyoderma gangrenosum. With newer techniques of protein

Table 3 Diagnostic evaluation of the patient with pyoderma gangrenosum

Careful history and thorough physical examination

Skin biopsy with tissue taken for cultures
(bacterial, fungal, and/or viral)

Studies of the gastrointestinal tract

Studies for possible abnormal serum proteins, antiphospholipid
antibodies

Complete blood count, examination of the peripheral smear, and
possible bone marrow examination

separation, it appears that 15 per cent of patients with pyoderma gangrenosum may have a benign monoclonal gammopathy, most often of IgA variety (Murray 1983; Prystowsky et al. 1989). The development of myeloma in these patients with pyoderma gangrenosum appears to be very rare.

The diagnostic evaluation (Table 3) of the patient presumed to have pyoderma gangrenosum has two objectives: (i) to rule out other causes of cutaneous ulceration, and (ii) to determine whether there is a treatable, systemic, associated disorder. There is not a specific laboratory or histopathological test that is diagnostic. Moreover, some of the associated disease processes may be clinically silent.

The differential diagnoses of ulcerative cutaneous lesions include: (i) infectious diseases, (ii) halogenodermas, (iii) vasculitis, (iv) insect bites, (v) venous or arterial insufficiency (including occlusive disease associated with antiphospolipid antibodies), and (vi) factitial ulcerations. Cultures should be taken from both exudate and tissues.

To test for the presence of an associated disorder, another series of examinations should be made. A thorough historical evaluation and examination of the gastrointestinal tract should be undertaken in conjunction with a gastroenterologist. Radiographic procedures may include an upper gastrointestinal series and a barium enema. Flexible sigmoidoscopy or colonoscopy, or both, may also be done, with appropriate biopsies being taken. A complete blood count, careful evaluation of the peripheral smear, and possibly a bone marrow aspirate or biopsy will help rule out the presence of an associated haematological malignant process. Serum protein electrophoresis, serum immunodiffusion studies, and possibly, serum and urine immunoelectrophoresis will help to eliminate a diagnosis of an associated monoclonal gammopathy or myeloma. Multiple reports of pyoderma gangrenosum-like leg ulcers in patients with antiphospholipid antibodies have appeared and tests such as VDRL, anticardiolipin antibody, and partial thromboplastin time are now standard in the evaluation of a patient with pyoderma gangrenosum (Babe et al. 1992).

There is not a specific, uniformly effective treatment for pyoderma gangrenosum. Although systemic treatment may affect the underlying disease process in some patients with chronic ulcerative colitis (Mir-Madjlessi 1985), it sometimes becomes necessary to consider colectomy. Some patients' skin lesions will respond to bowel resection, but there are patients in whom total colectomy, including removal of the rectosigmoid colon, does not lead to a remission (Talansky et al. 1983). In one report a patient developed pyoderma gangrenosum 10 years after total colectomy (Cox et al. 1986). In mild

cases, local measures, such as dressings, elevation, rest, topical agents, or intralesional injections may be sufficient to control the disease process. Compresses, wet to dry dressings, or the newer bio-occlusive semipermeable dressings may be useful. Cleansing or therapy with antibacterial agents such as hydrogen peroxide or benzoyl peroxide have been reported to be beneficial in an occasional patient. Hyperbaric oxygen has also been reported, in a small number of cases, to be effective. Superpotent topical corticosteroids and intralesional injections of corticosteroids (Gardner and Archer 1972) may be beneficial in some patients. Care must be taken to avoid introducing an infection and to limit the potential systemic effects of corticosteroids that arise from injecting large doses intralesionally. In general, the periphery of the lesions are injected, but the ulcer base may also be injected. Other topical approaches include the use of sodium cromoglycate, nitrogen mustard, and 5-aminosaliscyclic acid (DeCock and Thorne 1980; Tsele et al. 1992).

In patients who do not respond to topical or local therapies, or whose severe, rapid course warrants the use of a systemic agent, sulphonamides, sulphones, or corticosteroids have been the most commonly used agents. Perry (1959) reported that oral sulphasalazine is effective in patients both with and without inflammatory bowel disease. Dapsone in doses of up to 400 mg per day has often been used as a monotherapy, or as an adjunctive steroid-sparing agent. Usually the drug is administered in lower doses (100 to 150 mg per day), and the usual precautions and pretherapy evaluation are necessary. The mechanism of action of the sulphanomides and sulphones in this process is not understood, but effects on the polymorphonuclear leucocyte may be a factor. Another antileprosy agent, clofazimine, has also been reported to be successful in some patients with pyoderma gangrenosum. Finally, several other antibiotics have been used successfully in individual cases; these include minocycline and rifampicin.

Systemic corticosteroids have been used extensively in patients with pyoderma gangrenosum and its variants and are generally believed to be very effective. Usually, large doses (40 to 120 mg per day) are necessary in order to induce a remission of the disease. These doses, used over the long term, will frequently result in steroid-related side-effects. In the studies by Holt et al. (1980), 6 of their 12 patients treated with corticosteroids developed serious steroid complications, and 4 of these 6 died as a result of the therapy. To avoid the complications of long-term steroid use, Johnson and Lazarus (1982), and subsequently others, have used pulse therapy with 1 g of methylprednisolone given intravenously each day for a period of 5 days. Maintenance of the remission was accomplished with oral corticosteroids every other day. Prystowsky et al. (1989) have reported the experience of Lazarus with a further eight patients. They found that remissions occurred in five of the patients, and that they were usually able to remove oral corticosteroid therapy and often lower the dose of other therapies. Pulse therapy is not without side-effects, which include sudden death. In the hands of Prystowsky et al., and my experience with three patients, this therapy has primarily resulted in transient hyperglycaemia; however, it should only be used with great caution and proper monitoring.

Immunosuppressive agents have been suggested for use in patients who fail to respond to other therapies, particularly systemic corticosteroids, or who develop steroid-related side-effects. Individual reports using oral azathioprine, cyclophosphamide (Newell and Malkinson 1983), chlorambucil (Burruss et al. 1994), cyclosporin (Matis et al. 1992), tacrolimus (FK 506) (Abu-Elmagd et al. 1993), or methotrexate (Teitel 1993) have suggested that, at least in some patients, these agents may be successful. Intravenous pulses of cyclophosphamide (Zonana-Nacach *et al.* 1994) or immunoglobulin (Gupta *et al.* 1995) have also been successful in individual patients. The mode of action of the immunosuppressive agents is not understood.

Rheumatoid neutrophilic dermatitis

Ackerman (1978) described a neutrophilic dermatosis in patients with rheumatoid arthritis. This is apparently a rare manifestation of rheumatoid arthritis, and has only been reported in a small number of patients (Scherbenske *et al.* 1989; Sanchez and Cruz 1990; Lowe *et al.* 1992).The patients are described as having symmetric, erythematous nodules and plaques on the extensor surfaces of the joints (Fig. 11). There is an apparent predilection for the dorsa of the hands and arms. It is not clear whether this condition is clinically or histopathologically distinct, specifically, whether it can be differentiated from Sweet's syndrome. An effective therapy has not been described.

Bowel-associated dermatosis–arthritis syndrome

Patients who had undergone bowel bypass surgery for morbid obesity have occasionally developed scattered pustular lesions (Fig. 12) and arthritis. This became known as the bowel bypass syndrome, and was felt to be an immune-complex disease caused by bacterial overgrowth in the blind loop. Treatment with antibiotics was often effective in clearing the cutaneous lesions and improving the joint symptoms. Later, Jorizzo *et al.* (1983) coined the term 'bowel-bypass syndrome without bowel bypass' or 'bowel-associated dermatosis–arthritis syndrome'. They reported on four patients with this syndrome of whom two had blind loops due to Billroth II procedures, one had ulcerative colitis, and one had Crohn's disease. Dicken (1984) reported two similar patients who had had Roux-en-Y procedures with resultant blind loops. Clinically, these patients present with a widespread eruption characterized by pustules on an erythematous or necrotic base. The lesions may be few in number, or may be extensive. Ulceration is rare. The appearance

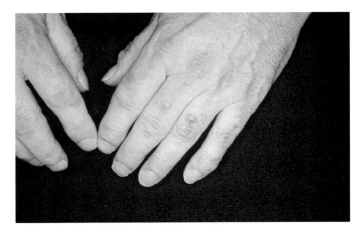

Fig. 11 Rheumatoid neutrophilic dermatosis. This patient developed multiple vesiculopustular plaques on the dorsum of his hands.

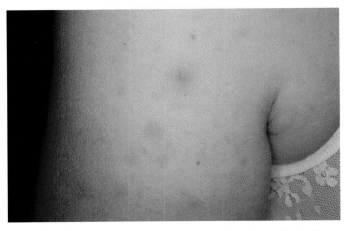

Fig. 12 Scattered pustules on an erythematous base in a patient with a bowel bypass for morbid obesity.

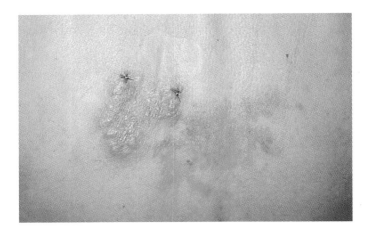

Fig. 13 Vesiculopustular eruption in a patient with previous ulcer surgery (Billroth II) and a blind loop—the so-called 'bowel bypass syndrome without a bowel bypass'.

of the lesions is often accompanied by fever, arthralgias or a true inflammatory arthropathy, and myalgias. The arthritis accompanying this process is generally symmetrical, non-deforming, and most frequently involves the small joints such as the wrists, ankles, metacarpophalangeal, proximal interphalangeal, and metatarsophalangeal joints. Histopathologically, the disease resembles Sweet's syndrome. In fact, only after the report by Jorizzo *et al.* (1983) did we recognize that a patient reported by our group (Bechtel and Callen 1981) probably would have been more correctly diagnosed as having the bowel-associated dermatosis–arthritis syndrome (Fig. 13) rather than Sweet's syndrome, because of his prior Billroth II procedure. This disease is presumed to be due to immune complexes (Jorizzo *et al.* 1984) and while anti-inflammatory therapy is at times helpful, antibiotics frequently control the process, or bowel surgery (to remove 'blind' loops) will reverse it.

References

Abu-Elmagud, K. *et al.* (1993). Resolution of severe pyoderma gangrenosum in a patient with streaking leukocyte factor disease after treatment with tacrolimus (FK 506). *Annals of Internal Medicine*, **119**, 595–8.

Ackerman, A. (1978). *Histologic diagnosis of inflammatory skin diseases: a method by pattern analysis*, pp. 449–50. Lea & Febiger, Philadelphia.

Aram, H. (1984). Acute febrile neutrophilic dermatosis (Sweet's syndrome): response to dapsone. *Archives of Dermatology*, 120, 245–7.

Babe, K.S. Jr., Gross, A., Leyva, W.H., and King, L.E. Jr. (1992). Pyoderma gangrenosum associated with antiphospholipid antibodies. *International Journal of Dermatology*, 31, 588–90.

Banet, D.E., McClave, S.A., and Callen, J.P. (1994). Oral metronidazole, an effective treatment for Sweet's syndrome in a patient with associated inflammatory bowel disease. *Journal of Rheumatology*, 21, 1766–8.

Bechtel, M.A. and Callen JP (1981). Acute febrile neutrophilic dermatosis (Sweet's syndrome). *Archives of Dermatology*, 117, 664–6.

Boatman, B.W., Taylor, R.C., Klein, L.E., and Cohen, B.A. (1994). Sweet's syndrome in children. *Southern Medical Journal*, 87, 193–6.

Burruss, J.B., Farmer, E., and Callen, J.P. (1994). Chlorambucil is an effective corticosteroid-sparing agent for recalcitrant pyoderma gangrenosum. *Arthritis and Rheumatism*, 37, S275 (Abstract).

Callen, J.P. (1990). Pyoderma gangrenosum and related disorders. *Dermatologic Clinics*, 7, 1249–59.

Callen J.P. and Woo T.Y. (1985). Vesiculopustular eruption in a patient with ulcerative colitis. *Archives of Dermatology*, 121, 339–44.

Callen J.P., Dubin H.V., and Gherke, C.F. (1976). Pyoderma gangrenosum and agnogenic myeloid metaplasia. *Archives of Dermatology*, 113, 1585–6.

Callen, J.P., Case, J.D., and Sager, D. (1989). Chlorambucil — an effective, corticosteroid-sparing therapy for pyoderma gangrenosum. *Journal of the American Academy of Dermatology*, 21, 515–9.

Case, J.D., Smith, S.Z., and Callen, J.P. (1989). The use of pulse methylprednisolone and chlorambucil in the treatment of Sweet's syndrome. *Cutis*, 44, 125–9.

Cohen, P.R. (1993). Pregnancy-associated Sweet's syndrome: world literature review. *Obstetrical and Gynecological Survey*, 48, 584–7.

Cohen, P.R., Talpaz, M., and Kuzrock, R. (1988). Malignancy-associated Sweet's syndrome: review of the world literature. *Journal of Clinical Oncology*, 6, 1887–97.

Cohen, P.R., Holder W.R., and Rapini R.P. (1992). Concurrent Sweet's syndrome and erythema nodosum: a report, world literature review and mechanism of pathogenesis. *Journal of Rheumatology*, 19, 814–20.

Cohen, P.R., Holder, W.R., Tucker S.B., Kono, S., and Kurzrock, R. (1993). Sweet syndrome in patients with solid tumors. *Cancer*, 72, 2723–31.

Cooper, P.H., Innes, D.J. Jr., and Greer, K.E. (1983). Acute febrile neutrophilic dermatosis (Sweet's syndrome) and myeloproliferative disorders. *Cancer*, 51, 1518–26.

Cox, N.H., Peebles-Brown, A., and Mackie, R.M.(1986). Pyoderma gangrenosum occurring 10 years after protocolectomy for ulcerative colitis. *British Journal of Hospital Medicine*, 36, 363–5.

DeCock, K.M. and Thorne, M.G. (1980). Treatment of pyoderma gangrenosum with sodium cromoglycate. *British Journal of Dermatology*, 102, 231–3.

Dicken, C.H. (1984). Bowel-associated dermatosis–arthritis syndrome: bowel bypass syndrome without bowel bypass. *Mayo Clinic Proceedings*, 59, 43–6.

Fenske, N.A. *et al.*(1983). Vesiculopustular eruption of ulcerative colitis. *Archives of Dermatology*, 119, 664–9.

Gupta, A.K., Shear, N.H., and Sauder, D.N. (1995). Efficacy of human intravenous immune globulin in pyoderma gangrenosum. *Journal of the American Academy of Dermatology*, 32, 140–2.

Harary, A.M. (1983). Sweet's syndrome associated with rheumatoid arthritis. *Archives of Internal Medicine*, 143, 1993–5.

Hoffman, G.S. (1977). Treatment of Sweet's syndrome (acute febrile neutrophilic dermatosis) with indomethacin. *Journal of Rheumatology*, 4, 201–6.

Holt, P.J.A. *et al.* (1980). Pyoderma gangrenosum. *Medicine*, 59, 114–33.

Horio, T., Immamura, S., Danno, K., Furnkawa, F., and Ofuji, S. (1980). Treatment of acute febrile neutrophilic dermatosis (Sweet's syndrome) with potassium iodide. *Dermatologica*, 160, 341–7.

Johnson, M.L. and Grimwood, R.E. (1994). Leukocyte colony-stimulating factors: a review of associated neutrophilic dermatoses and vasculitides. *Archives of Dermatology*, 130, 77–81.

Johnson, R.B. and Lazarus, G.S. (1982). Pulse therapy. *Archives of Dermatology*, 118, 76–84.

Jorizzo, J.L. (1988). Neutrophilic dermatoses: Sweet's syndrome and pyoderma gangrenosum. In *Inflammation: basic principles and clinical correlates*, (ed. J.I.Gallin, I.M. Goldstein, and R. Syndermoin), pp. 785–802. Raven Press, New York.

Jorizzo, J.L. *et al.* (1983). Bowel bypass syndrome without bowel bypass: bowel-associated dermatosis–arthritis syndrome. *Archives of Internal Medicine*, 143, 457–61.

Jorizzo, J.L. *et al.* (1984). Bowel-associated dermatosis–arthritis syndrome: immune complex-mediated vessel damage and increased neutrophil migration. *Archives of Internal Medicine*, 144, 738–40.

Keltz, M., Lebwohl, M., and Bishop, S. (1993). Peristomal pyoderma gangrenosum. *Journal of the American Academy of Dermatology*, 27, 360–4.

Kemmett, D. and Hunter, J.A.A.(1990). Sweet's syndrome: a clinicopathologic review of twenty-nine cases. *Journal of the American Academy of Dermatology*, 23, 503–7.

Lowe, L., Kornfeld, B., Clayman, J., and Golitz, L.E. (1992). Rheumatoid neutrophilic dermatosis. *Journal of Cutaneous Pathology*, 19, 48–53.

Matis, W.L., Ellis, C.N., Griffiths, C.E.M., and Lazarus, G.S. (1992). Treatment of pyoderma gangrenosum with cyclosporine. *Archives of Dermatology*, 128, 1060–4.

McCalmont, C.S., Leshin, B., White, W.L., Greiss, F.C. Jr., and Jorizzo, J.L. (1991). Vulvar pyoderma gangrenosum. *International Journal of Gynecology and Obstetrics*, 35, 175–8.

Mir-Madjlessi, S.H., Taylor, J.S., and Farmer, R.G.(1985). Clinical course and evolution of erythema nodosum and pyoderma gangrenosum in chronic ulcerative colitis: a study of 42 patients. *American Journal of Gastroenterology*, 80, 615–20.

Murray, J.C. (1983) Pyoderma gangrenosum and IgA gammopathy. *Cutis*, 32, 503–7.

Newell, L.M. and Malkinson, F.D. (1983). Pyoderma gangrenosum: response to cyclophosphamide therapy. *Archives of Dermatology*, 119, 477–86.

Newman, W.P. and Frank, H.J. (1993). Pyoderma gangrenosum of the orbit. *Eye*, 7, 89–94.

O'Loughlin, S. and Perry, H.O. (1978). A diffuse pustular eruption associated with ulcerative colitis. *Archives of Dermatology*, 114, 1061–4.

Perry, H.O. (1959). Pyoderma gangrenosum. *Southern Medical Journal*, 62, 899–908.

Perry, H.O. and Winkelmann, R.K. (1962). Bullous pyoderma gangrenosum and leukemia. *Archives of Dermatology*, 106, 901–5.

Perry, H.O. *et al.* (1968). Malignant pyoderma. *Archives of Dermatology*, 98, 561–74.

Piette, W.W., Trapp, J.F., O'Donnell, M.J., Argenyi, Z., Talbot, E.A., and Burns, C.P. (1994). Acute neutrophilic dermatosis with myeloblastic infiltrate in a leukemia patient receiving all-*trans*-retinoic acid therapy. *Journal of the American Academy of Dermatology*, 30, 293–7.

Powell, F.C. *et al.* (1985). Pyoderma gangrenosum: a review of 86 patients. *Quarterly Journal of Medicine*, 55, 173–86.

Prystowsky, J.H., Kahn, S.N., and Lazarus, G.S. (1989). Present status of pyoderma gangrenosum. *Archives of Dermatology*, 125, 57–64.

Prystowsky, S.D., Fye, K.H., Goette, K.D., and Daniels, T.E. (1978). Acute febrile neutrophilic dermatosis (Sweet's syndrome) associated with Sjögren's syndrome. *Archives of Dermatology*, 114, 1234–5.

Romano, J. and Safai, B. (1979). Pyoderma gangrenosum and myeloproliferative disorders. *Archives of Internal Medicine*, 139, 932–4.

Sanchez, J.L. and Cruz, A.(1990). Rheumatoid neutrophilic dermatosis. *Journal of the American Academy of Dermatology*, 22, 922–5.

Scherbenske, J.M., Benson, P.M., and Lupton, G.P. (1989). Rheumatoid neutrophilic dermatosis. *Archives of Dermatology*, 125, 1105–8.

Storwick, G.S., Prihoda, M.B., Fulton, R.J., and Wood, W.S. (1994). Pyodermatitis–pyostomatitis vegetans: a specific marker for inflammatory bowel disease. *Journal of the American Academy of Dermatology*, 31, 336–41.

Su, W.P.D. *et al.* (1986). Histopathologic and immunopathologic study of pyoderma gangrenosum. *Journal of Cutaneous Pathology*, 13, 323–30.

Subhisa, S. *et al.*(1983). Colchicine in the treatment of acute febrile neutrophilic dermatosis (Sweet's syndrome). *British Journal of Dermatology*, 108, 99–01.

Sweet, R.D. (1964). An acute febrile neutrophilic dermatosis. *British Journal of Dermatology*, 76, 349–56.

Talansky, A.L. *et al.* (1983). Does intestinal resection heal the pyoderma gangrenosum of inflammmatory bowel disease? *Journal of Clinical Gastroenterology*, 108, 580–1.

Teitel, A.D. (1994). Treatment of pyoderma gangrenosum with methotrexate. *Arthritis and Rheumatism*, 36, S163 (Abstract).

Trentham, D.E., Masi, A.T., and Bale, G.F. (1976). Arthritis with an inflammatory dermatoses resembling Sweet's syndrome: report of a unique case and review of the literature on arthritis associated with the inflammatory dermatoses. *American Journal of Medicine*, 61, 424–32.

Tsele, E., Yu, R.C.H., and Chu, A.C. (1992). Pyoderma gangrenosum — response to topical nitrogen mustard. *Clinical and Experimental Dermatology*, 17, 437–40.

Van Hale, H.M. *et al.* (1985). Pyostomatitis vegetans: a reactive mucosal marker for inflammatory disease of the gut. *Archives of Dermatology*, 121, 94–8.

von den Driesch, P. (1994). Sweet's syndrome (acute febrile neutrophilic dermatosis). *Journal of the American Academy of Dermatology*, 31, 535–56.

von den Driesch, P. *et al.* (1994). Sweet's syndrome: therapy with cyclosporin A. *Clinical and Experimental Dermatology*, 19, 274–7.

Wernikoff, S. *et al.* (1987). Malignant pyoderma or pyoderma gangrenosum of the head and neck? *Archives of Dermatology*, 123, 371–5.

Zonana-Nacach, A., Jiménez-Balderas, J., Martínez-Osuna, P., and Mintz, G. (1994). Intravenous cyclophosphamide pulses in the treatment of pyoderma gangrenosum associated with rheumatoid arthritis: report of 2 cases and review of the literature. *Journal of Rheumatology*, 21, 1352–6.

5.13.5 Sarcoidosis

Barry Bresnihan

Sarcoidosis is a multisystem disease of unknown aetiology characterized by the presence of multiple, non-caseating granulomas in involved tissues. Symptoms and signs depend on the severity of disease in the affected organ systems. Tissues that may be involved include joints, bones and muscles.

Aetiology

Environmental factors are important in the aetiology of sarcoidosis. Firstly, the acute form of sarcoidosis presents more frequently during spring months (Poukkula *et al.* 1986), suggesting that an environmental agent with a higher prevalence during the spring may be causative. A number of localized outbreaks of sarcoidosis have suggested the possibility of an infectious agent (Veale and FitzGerald 1990). Others have suggested a relation between sarcoidosis and occupation (Edmondstone 1988).

Genetic factors also appear to be important. There is an increased incidence of sarcoidosis within families. The British Thoracic and Tuberculosis Association (1973) reported 121 patients among 59 families. In one series of 114 patients there was a 9.6 per cent frequency of sarcoidosis in the siblings of index cases (Brennan *et al.* 1984).

A number of studies have examined associations between HLA alleles and sarcoidosis, but no linkages with disease susceptibility have yet been identified (Mehra and Bovornkitti 1988). However, some investigators have suggested associations between HLA-B8 and sarcoid arthropathy (Brewerton *et al.* 1977), and more recently an association between HLA-B8, -DR3 and acute sarcoidosis with arthritis has been demonstrated (Kremer 1986).

Pathology

The characteristic histological feature of sarcoidosis found in all affected tissues is a well-defined, round or oval granuloma composed of compact, radially arranged epithelioid cells, a few multinucleate giant cells and a rim of lymphocytes (Fig. 1). Caseation is absent. A small area of fibrinoid necrosis may be present. Sarcoid granuloma may be divided into early, intermediate, and late stages. The epithelioid cells are derived from circulating monocytes. Giant cells are formed from fusion of epithelioid cells. Their size varies between 150 and 300 μm. Most giant cells are of foreign-body or Langhans type and may contain inclusion bodies, which represent metabolic end-products. The lymphocytes are derived from peripheral blood and consist predominantly of CD4+, T-helper cells (Hunninghake and Crystal 1981). There is evidence to support the suggestion that the accumulation of CD4+ lymphocytes may result from increased production of interleukin 2 (**IL-2**) (Semenzato *et al.* 1993). Soluble IL-2 receptor has been demonstrated in active sarcoidosis (Ina *et al.* 1992). Increased expression of the IL-2 receptor on mononuclear cells and alveolar macrophages correlated positively with serum concentrations of angiotensin-converting enzyme (Pforte *et al.* 1993). Studies of T-cell receptors have suggested that T cells accumulate in sarcoid lesions in response to persistent stimulation by a specific but unidentified antigen (Du Bois *et al.* 1992; Forrester *et al.* 1993).

A number of recent studies have suggested a role for several cytokines, including tumour necrosis factor-α, IL-1β, and IL-6, in disease pathogenesis and granuloma formation (Shakoor and Hamblin 1992; Pueringer *et al.* 1993; Steffen *et al.* 1993).

Epidemiology

Sarcoidosis occurs worldwide, but prevalence, clinical manifestations and outcome vary widely in different areas (Tierstein and Lesser 1983). Sarcoidosis is recognized more often in developed than in

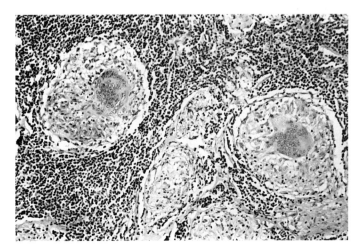

Fig. 1 Sarcoid granuloma. Two, well-formed, non-caseating granulomas are demonstrated in lymph-node tissue. Central multinucleated giant cells are present, surrounded by epithelioid cells and some lymphocytes. (By courtesy of Dr Mary McCabe, St. Vincent's Hospital, Dublin.)

underdeveloped countries, in Western rather than in Far Eastern countries, and in Northern rather than Southern Europe. Moreover, the prevalence within a given region may vary. For example, Sweden and Denmark have prevalence rates of approx. 60 per 100 000 population, while Finland has a prevalence of 7.5 per 100 000. The overall prevalence rate in the United Kingdom has been estimated as 20 per 100 000, and in Ireland as 30 per 100 000. The highest reported prevalence in the United Kingdom (of up to 200 per 100 000) was observed in Irish immigrant women of child-bearing age living in London. In the United States, sarcoidosis is 10 to 17 times more prevalent among black than white individuals.

General clinical features

Sarcoidosis may involve almost any tissue in the body. Approximately half of patients with sarcoidosis will present with pulmonary symptoms such as dyspnoea, cough or chest pain (Sharma 1984a). A further 20 per cent approximately will present with an abnormal routine chest radiograph and minimal or no symptoms. Approximately 1 in 4 patients will present with non-specific constitutional symptoms including fever, weight loss and anorexia. Less than 10 per cent of patients will present with features confined to extrapulmonary systems such as the musculoskeletal system.

Acute sarcoidosis

Acute or subacute sarcoidosis may present as an illness of explosive onset, usually characterized by fever, erythema nodosum, and hilar lymphadenopathy. The association of hilar lymphadenopathy and erythema nodosum is often referred to as Lofgren syndrome (Lofgren 1953). Erythema nodosum appears to be more common among Swedish, Irish, Puerto Rican, and Mexican women of child-

bearing age. This form of sarcoidosis has a high prevalence of spontaneous remission and a good prognosis. The chest radiograph clears within 1 year of presentation in more than 60 per cent of patients with acute sarcoidosis.

Chronic sarcoidosis

Chronic sarcoidosis is less common than acute sarcoidosis and has a subtle onset with an insidious progressive and highly variable clinical course. Chest radiographs demonstrate extensive parenchymal infiltration in more than 90 per cent of patients with chronic sarcoidosis. Pulmonary function tests confirm a restrictive lung defect. Other manifestations are listed in Table 1.

Laboratory investigations

Routine investigations

Most reports are that anaemia is uncommon in sarcoidosis (Sharma 1984b), occurring in approx. 5 per cent of patients. Haemolytic anaemia has been reported, but is rare. Leucopenia occurs in approximately one-third of patients, sometimes in the absence of splenomegaly and may reflect granulomatous infiltration of the bone marrow. Neutrophilia and polycythaemia are rare. There is eosinophilia in approximately one-quarter of patients. Thrombocytopenia has long been recognized as a relatively common complication of sarcoidosis. An elevated erythrocyte sedimentation rate occurs during acute disease episodes, particularly in association with erythema nodosum.

Reports of hypercalcaemia in sarcoidosis vary widely between 2 and 63 per cent. The reasons for such wide variation are unclear. The frequency tends to be higher in North American series. In a worldwide review of more than 3 000 patients, James et al. (1976) reported a frequency of 11 per cent. The serum calcium fluctuates during the course of the disease and may be raised during acute or subacute phases.

Mild elevation of serum bilirubin and alkaline phosphatase are common (Sharma 1984c). Severe jaundice and disturbance of liver function is uncommon, even in the presence of extensive liver involvement.

Urinary hydroxyproline concentrations are considerably increased in acute sarcoidosis, returning to normal as disease manifestations resolve. Hydroxyproline excretion is normal in chronic sarcoidosis. Hypercalcinuria occurs more frequently than hypercalcaemia, and has been reported in 49 per cent of one series where only 13 per cent had hypercalcaemia. Significant proteinuria has been reported in approximately one-third of patients.

Angiotensin-converting enzyme

Angiotensin-converting enzyme catalyses the conversion of angiotensin I to vasoactive angiotensin II and inactivates bradykinin. Increased concentrations of serum angiotensin-converting enzyme were first observed in 83 per cent of patients with active sarcoidosis. The incidence has varied in subsequent series. In one international study of almost 2000 patients, 57 per cent had elevated serum concentrations of this enzyme (Studdy and James 1983). Angiotensin-converting enzyme is produced mainly by the epithelioid cells in the granulomas and enzyme activity reflects the total

Table 1 Clinical manifestations in chronic sarcoidosis

Lung: parenchymal disease

Skin: lupus pernio; skin plaques or nodules

Eye: uveitis; conjunctivitis; keratoconjunctivitis sicca

Lymphatic system: peripheral lymphadenopathy; splenomegaly

Bone marrow infiltration

Liver: hepatic granulomata; portal hypertension; hepatic failure

Kidney: nephrocalcinosis; renal calculi; granulomatous infiltration; glomerular disease; renal arteritis

Heart: cardiomyopathy; conduction abnormalities

Nervous system: cranial and peripheral neuropathy; papilloedema; intracerebral lesions; meningitis; seizures; spinal cord involvement; psychiatric disorders

Endocrine: pituitary; hypothalamus; thyroid; parathyroid; adrenal

Reproductive organs: ovaries; testes

Gastrointestinal tract and pancreas

Salivary and lacrimal glands

Nose, tonsils, larynx

granulomatous 'load' in the body. Serial measurements of this enzyme are useful when monitoring the course of the disease.

Kveim test

The intracutaneous injection of a saline suspension of previously validated human sarcoid spleen or lymph node will give rise to a non-caseating granulomatous reaction after 2 to 6 weeks in approximately three-quarters of patients with sarcoidosis (Kataria *et al.* 1980) The Kveim test is generally regarded as specific for sarcoid, but has a number of disadvantages, including variability of results with different antigen sources, the 2- to 6-week delay and the inability to treat with corticosteroids during the wait, the need for punch biopsy, and variability in histological interpretation. Newer diagnostic procedures yield diagnostic material more rapidly.

Diagnostic imaging

The chest radiograph may be normal, or demonstrate hilar lymph-adenopathy with or without pulmonary infiltration, pulmonary infiltration without adenopathy or advanced and irreversible fibrosis. Computed tomography may demonstrate adenopathy or early granulomatous infiltration that is undetectable on plain radiographs.

Beaumont *et al.* (1982) described [67Ga]citrate scanning of the lungs as a very sensitive method for detecting granuloma formation in sarcoidosis. Several studies have demonstrated that 67Ga scanning of the lungs reflects disease activity and response to therapy (Lawrence *et al.* 1983; Baughmann *et al.* 1984). Lung uptake of 67Ga is greatest in patients with acute disease and high serum concentrations of angiotensin-converting enzyme. Uptake of 67Ga does not correlate with quantitative pulmonary function nor with the clinical course and outcome. It is uncertain why 67Ga accumulates at sites of granulomatous inflammation.

Histology

Sarcoidosis may resemble other diseases such as lymphoma and tuberculosis. Many institutions have a policy of obtaining histological confirmation of the diagnosis in all cases. Transbronchial lung biopsy has become the most widely used biopsy technique and is both highly sensitive and selective (Tierstein 1983). Open lung biopsy and mediastinal lymph-node biopsy are also highly sensitive and selective options, but, being more invasive, have some disadvantages. Other tissues likely to yield positive histological findings include scalene node, liver, skin, muscle, conjunctiva, lacrimal and minor salivary glands, and spleen.

Bronchoalveolar lavage

Bronchoalveolar lavage provides samples of the alveolar secretions for analysis. Lavage fluids may be studied for cellular content and inflammatory mediators. Analysis of bronchoalveolar fluids is a useful aid in the differential diagnosis of some interstitial lung diseases (Hunninghake *et al.* 1979). Patients with acute pulmonary sarcoidosis generally have high lymphocyte counts and high T helper-/T suppressor-cell ratios in bronchoalveolar fluids. Serial analysis of these lavage fluids may provide valuable information on the response to therapy.

Musculoskeletal manifestations

Joint disease

Distinctive patterns of arthropathy are associated with both acute and chronic sarcoidosis (James *et al.* 1976). In acute sarcoidosis, transient flitting arthralgias may precede the emergence of fever, erythema nodosum (Fig. 2), and hilar adenopathy (Fig. 3) (Gumpel *et al.* 1967; Siltzbach and Duberstein 1968; Spilberg *et al.* 1969). The joints most frequently presenting with arthritis after the development of erythema nodosum are the ankles and knees, although others may be involved occasionally. Approximately 65 per cent of patients presenting with acute sarcoidosis will have articular features. Prominent signs of inflammation are present, with marked erythema and tenderness of involved joints causing pain and limited motion. The arthritis is usually symmetrical and migratory, and persists for periods of between 3 to 4 days and 3 to 4 months. It may be difficult on occasion to distinguish features of erythema nodosum from articular and periarticular inflammation of the ankle joints. Ultrasonographic examination may be helpful in this context. In one study, joint effusions were demonstrated in 6 of 24 consecutive patients examined and tenosynovitis was identified in 8 (Kellner *et al.* 1992). Joint effusions in other joints are usually not detectable. When an effusion is present it is usually only mildly inflammatory, with less than 1000 leucocytes/mm³, predominantly lymphocytes and large mononuclear cells. Occasionally an inflammatory effusion is aspirated, with leucocyte counts of greater than 40 000/mm³, predominantly neutrophils. Needle biopsy specimens of synovial membrane in acute sarcoid arthropathy show mild, non-specific synovitis consistent with the clinical impression that much of the inflammation is periarticular. After recovery, acute sarcoidosis only occasionally recurs.

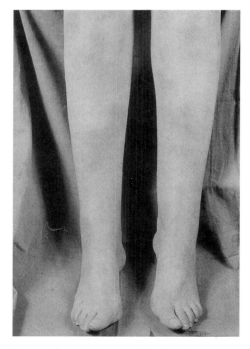

Fig. 2 Erythema nodosum is characteristic of acute sarcoidosis. Tender, red swellings appear on the shins, thighs, and upper limbs. Resolving erythema nodosum resembles painful bruises. Erythema nodosum usually resolves fully within 3 to 6 weeks.

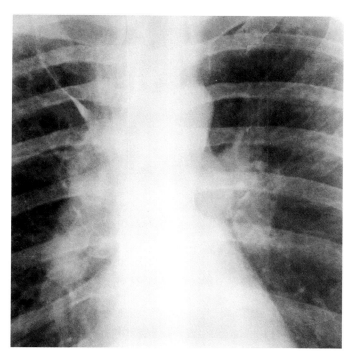

Fig. 3 Bilateral hilar lymphadenopathy due to sarcoidosis may be discovered on routine chest radiographs in asymptomatic individuals. It also frequently presents in acute sarcoidosis with fever, erythema nodosum, and arthritis.

Chronic arthritis is relatively uncommon in sarcoidosis (Gumpel *et al.* 1967; Siltzbach and Duberstein 1968; Spilberg *et al.* 1969; Grigor and Hughes 1976). It usually involves several joints and may appear either early or late in the course of the disease. Chronic monoarticular arthritis is rare. Large joints such as knees and ankles, elbows and wrists are most frequently involved. Hips and shoulders may also be affected. Involvement of spinal and temporomandibular joints has also been reported. Chronic arthritis involving the small joints of hands and feet is rare, except when secondary to osseous disease involving the phalanges (see below). Chronic polyarthritis is more frequently observed in women than men with sarcoidosis. A history of erythema nodosum is unusual in patients with chronic arthritis.

Acute exacerbations may occur over a period of years, especially during periods of generalized disease activity. Chronic sarcoid arthritis is characterized by synovial thickening and effusions. Histological examination of synovial membrane may reveal typical non-caseating granulomas (Fig. 4). However, in some patients with chronic arthritis the histological features in synovial membrane are non-specific (Palmer and Schumacher 1984). Chronic arthritis may progress to joint deformity and destruction.

Bone disease

Bone involvement occurs in approx. 5 per cent of all patients with sarcoidosis. Bone cysts containing characteristic granulomas are most frequently observed in the phalanges of the hands and feet (Gumpel *et al.* 1967; James *et al.* 1976). Bone cysts are occasionally observed in long bones, pelvis, vertebrae, and the bones of the skull. Bone lesions are most frequently found in patients with persistent disease and are particularly frequent in those with lupus pernio (Fig. 5) and other chronic skin lesions (Fig. 6). However, sarcoidosis limited to osseous disease of fingers and toes has been described (Schriber and Firooznia 1975). Bone lesions may be asymptomatic;

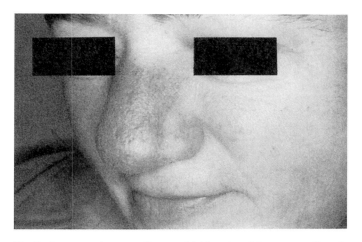

Fig. 5 Lupus pernio, presenting as a bluish-red or violaceous swelling of the nose extending on to the cheek, is a characteristic of chronic sarcoidosis and is frequently associated with bone lesions.

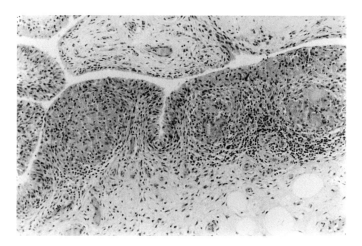

Fig. 4 Chronic arthritis in sarcoidosis showing thickening of the synovial lining layer, mononuclear cell infiltration, and non-caseating granulomas.

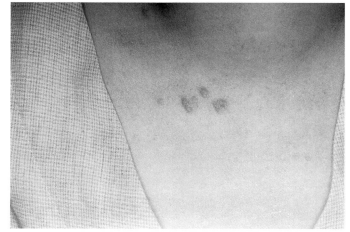

Fig. 6 Chronic cutaneous sarcoidosis, which may accompany bone involvement.

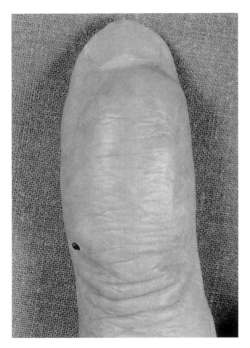

Fig. 7 Sarcoid dactylitis caused by granuloma formation in phalanges and surrounding soft tissue.

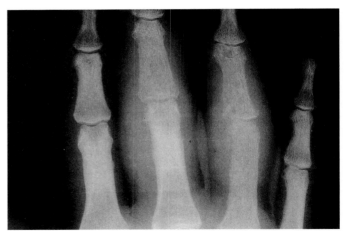

Fig. 8 Bone sarcoidosis presenting as dactylitis of the third and fourth fingers. The radiological changes are relatively early. Note the lacy, reticular pattern in the third middle and the fourth middle and proximal phalanges, associated with prominent soft-tissue swelling.

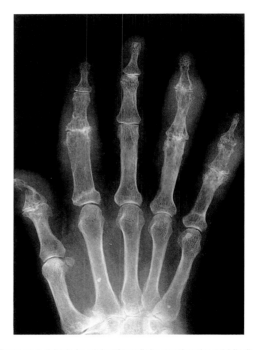

Fig. 9 Bone sarcoidosis involving four digits sparing the middle finger. Soft-tissue swelling, bone cysts and joint-space narrowing are prominent. There is expansion of the second proximal phalanx.

frequently they are identified fortuitously after routine radiographic examination. Bone scanning techniques may be more sensitive than routine radiography in detecting early osseous sarcoidosis. Pain may be absent, even when obvious bone swelling is present.

The most characteristic presentation of osseous sarcoidosis is of swollen, sausage-like digits resulting from cyst formation in the phalanges (Fig. 7). Single or multiple digits may be involved. Radiographic examination will demonstrate lytic lesions of various sizes ranging from minute cortical defects to intraosseous cysts causing diffusely expanded phalanges or cysts in phalangeal or metatarsal heads (Figs 8 and 9). Less frequent radiographic changes include thickening of cortical bone with a fine reticular alteration of the trabecular pattern, acrosclerosis of distal phalanges or, rarely, gross bone destruction. Osseous sarcoidosis may cause secondary articular changes in the joints of the hands and feet.

Vertebral sarcoidosis may present with back pain or with neurological impairment resulting from cord compression. Radiographic examination of the spine will demonstrate extensive lytic or sclerotic changes in one or more vertebrae at any level. Pathological fracture has been reported as a complication of long-bone involvement. Skull involvement may appear as multiple lytic defects associated with overlying soft tissue swellings containing granulomas.

Muscle disease

Sarcoidosis of skeletal muscle is usually asymptomatic. In the early acute stages, especially in the presence of erythema nodosum, asymptomatic granulomatous muscle involvement is common, with a prevalence rate ranging between 50 and 80 per cent. Random muscle biopsy may, therefore, be a useful diagnostic procedure in patients presenting with erythema nodosum. Investigators have emphasized the need for generous sampling and examination of multiple tissue sections.

Muscle sarcoidosis has two clinical types: nodular and myopathic (Hinterbuchner and Hinterbuchner 1964). The nodular type often involves extremities and causes solitary or multiple nodules. The myopathic type involves muscles symmetrically and diffusely without causing an intramuscular mass. Slowly progressive myalgia, weakness and atrophy usually occur. Symptomatic muscular sarcoidosis may accompany the acute disease onset and is characterized by fever and severe pain and tenderness, usually involving the proximal muscles of the upper and lower limb girdles (Douglas *et al.* 1973). The histological appearances in acute symptomatic muscular sarcoidosis are identical to those in asymptomatic patients and consist of characteristic granulomatous lesions located between apparently normal muscle fibres. The electromyographic features are those of idiopathic polymyositis. A number of reports have described patients with isolated sarcoid muscle disease without apparent involvement of other organ systems. It is possible that these patients have granulomas in other tissues without their causing clinical manifestations. In patients who appear to have isolated muscle sarcoidosis, systematic clinical, radiological, and histological evaluation will usually reveal evidence of multisystem disease.

[67]Ga scintigraphy is a useful diagnostic method for demonstrating myopathic disease, whereas abnormalities detected by magnetic resonance imaging may define the nodular type of muscular sarcoidosis (Otake 1994). Computed tomography, ultrasonography, and angiography were less useful in identifying sarcoid muscle disease.

Childhood sarcoidosis

Sarcoidosis is rare in childhood. Chronic arthritis and tenosynovitis have been described (Rosenberg et al. 1983). Arthritis usually affects knees and ankles, and is characterized by boggy thickening of synovia or tendon sheaths and effusion, causing minimal pain and limitation (Fig. 10). Arthritis usually occurs in children with onset of sarcoidosis before the age of 5 years, and is frequently associated with ocular and cutaneous manifestations. Sarcoid arthritis in children usually follows an indolent clinical course, with minimal or absent constitutional symptoms.

Treatment

Acute sarcoidosis with erythema nodosum and hilar lymphadenopathy is usually a self-limiting illness. The arthralgias and arthritis are transient. Symptoms are usually relieved by rest and non-steroidal anti-inflammatory drugs. Occasionally, a short course of corticosteroid therapy may be justified to relieve very acute symptoms. Exacerbations of chronic arthritis are usually associated with active multisystem disease, so that therapeutic decisions usually depend on the severity of the non-articular features. Thus, most patients with chronic arthritis will require corticosteroids for control of systemic disease.

In osseous sarcoidosis, therapy is not indicated for asymptomatic patients. Corticosteroid agents are usually prescribed for symptomatic osseous sarcoidosis, and healing of lytic and destructive lesions has been documented. Similarly, no therapy is required for asymptomatic muscle disease. Corticosteroids are usually recommended for symptomatic patients, although some uncertainties remain about the efficacy of corticosteroid therapy, particularly in chronic sarcoid myopathy.

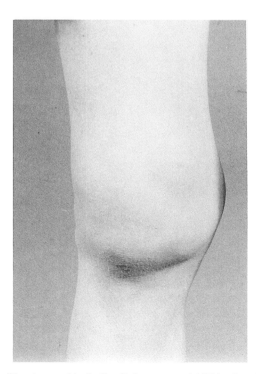

Fig. 10 Chronic sarcoid arthritis with boggy synovial thickening of the knee presenting in a 5-year-old boy who also had uveitis and elevated serum angiotensin-converting enzyme.

References

Baughmann, R. P., Fernandez, M., Bosken, C. H., Mantil, J., and Hurtubise, P. (1984). Comparison of gallium-67 scanning bronchoalveolar lavage and serum angiotensin-converting enzyme levels in pulmonary sarcoidosis: predicting response to therapy. *American Review of Respiratory Diseases*, **129**, 676–81.

Beaumont, D., Herry, S. Y., Sapene, M., Bourguet, P., Larzul, J. J., and De Labarthe, B. (1982). Gallium 67 in the evaluation of sarcoidosis: correlation with serum angiotensin converting enzyme and bronchoalveolar lavage. *Thorax*, **37**, 11–18.

Brennan, J. J., Crean, P., and FitzGerald, M. X. (1984). High prevalence of familial sarcoidosis in an Irish population. *Thorax*, **39**, 14–18.

Brewerton, D. et al. (1977). HL-A antigens in sarcoidosis. *Clinical and Experimental Immunology*, **27**, 277–9

British Thoracic and Tuberculosis Association (1973). Familial association in sarcoidosis. *Tubercle*, **54**, 87–98.

Douglas, A. C., Macleod, J. G., and Matthews, J. D. (1973). Symptomatic sarcoidosis of skeletal muscle. *Journal of Neurology, Neurosurgery and Psychiatry*, **36**, 1034–40.

Du Bois, R. M., Kirby, M., Balbi, B., Saltini, C., and Crystal R. D.(1992). Lymphocytes that accumulate in the lung in sarcoidosis have evidence of recent stimulation of the T-cell antigen receptor. *American Review of Respiratory Diseases*, **145**, 1205–11.

Edmondstone, W. M. (1988). Sarcoidosis in nurses: is there an association? *Thorax*, **43**, 342–3.

Forrester, J. M., Newman, L. S., Wang, Y., King, T. E., Jr, and Kotzin, B. L. (1993). Clonal expansion of lung Vl+ T cells in pulmonary sarcoidosis. *Journal of Clinical Investigation*, **91**, 292–300.

Grigor, R. R. and Hughes, G. R. V. (1976). Chronic sarcoid arthritis. *British Medical Journal*, **2**, 1044.

Gumpel, J. M., Johns, C. J., and Shulman, L. E. (1967). The joint disease of sarcoidosis. *Annals of the Rheumatic Diseases*, **26**, 194–205.

Hinterbuchner, C. N. and Hinterbuchner, L. P. (1964). Myopathic syndrome in muscular sarcoidosis. *Brain*, **87**, 355–66.

Hunninghake, G. W. and Crystal, R. G. (1981). Pulmonary sarcoidosis. A disorder mediated by excess helper T lymphocyte activity at sites of disease activity. *New England Journal of Medicine*, **305**, 429–34.

Hunninghake, G., Gadek, J. E., Kawanami, O., Ferrans, V. J., and Crystal, R. (1979). Inflammatory and immune processes in the human lung in health and disease; evaluation of bronchoalveolar lavage. *American Journal of Pathology*, **97**, 149–206.

Ina, Y., Takada, K., Sato, T., Yamamoto, M., Nodura, M., and Morishita, M. (1992). Soluble interleukin 2 receptors in patients with sarcoidosis: possible origin. *Chest*. **102**, 1128–33.

James, D. G. et al. (1976). A worldwide review of sarcoidosis. *Annals of the New York Academy of Science*, **278**, 321–34.

Kataria, Y. et al. (1980). Kveim antigen Cr-1: its sensitivity and specificity in sarcoidosis, a comparative study. In *Sarcoidosis and other granulomatous diseases* (ed. W. J. Williams and B. H. Davies), p. 660. Alpha Omega, Cardiff.

Kelner, H., Spathling S., and Herzer, P. (1992). Ultrasound findings in Lofgren's syndrome: is ankle swelling caused by arthritis, tenosynovitis or periarthritis? *Journal of Rheumatology*, 19, 38–41.

Kremer, J. M. (1986). Histologic findings in siblings with acute sarcoid arthritis; association with the HLA B8, DR3 phenotype. *Journal of Rheumatology*, 13, 593–7.

Lawrence, E. C., Teague, R. B., Gottlieb, M. S., Jhingran, S. G., and Lieberman, J. (1983). Serial changes in markers of disease activity with corticosteroid treatment in sarcoidosis. *American Journal of Medicine*, 74, 747–56.

Lofgren, S. (1953). Primary pulmonary sarcoidosis. I. Early signs and symptoms. *Acta Medica Scandinavica*, 145, 424–31.

Mehra, N. K. and Bovornkitti, S. (1988). HLA and sarcoidosis. *Sarcoidosis*, 5, 87–9.

Otake, S. (1994). Sarcoidosis involving skeletal muscle: imaging findings and relative value of imaging procedures. *American Journal of Roentgenology*, 162, 369–75.

Palmer, D. G. and Schumacher, H. R. (1984). Synovitis with non-specific histologic changes in synovium in chronic sarcoidosis. *Annals of the Rheumatic Diseases*, 43, 778–82.

Pforte, A. *et al.* (1993). Concomitant modulation of serum-soluble interleukin-2 receptor and alveolar macrophage interleukin-2 receptor in sarcoidosis. *American Review of Respiratory Diseases*, 147, 717–22.

Poukkula, A., Huhti, T., Lilja, M., and Saloheimo, M. (1986). Incidence and clinical picture of sarcoidosis in a circumscribed geographical area. *British Journal of Diseases of the Chest*, 80, 138–47.

Pueringer, R. J., Shwartz, D. A., Dayton, S. C., Gilbert, S. R., and Hunninghake, G. W. (1993). The relationship between alveolar macrophage TNF, interleukin-1 and PGE$_2$ release, alveolitis and disease severity in sarcoidosis. *Chest*, 103, 832–8.

Rosenberg, A. M., Yee, E. H., and MacKenzie, J. W. (1983). Arthritis in childhood sarcoidosis. *Journal of Rheumatology*, 10, 987–90.

Schriber, R. A. and Firooznia, H. (1975). Extensive phalangeal cystic lesions. Sarcoidosis limited to the hands and feet? *Arthritis and Rheumatism*, 18, 123–8.

Semenzato, G., Zambello, P., Trentin, L., and Agostini, C. (1993). Cellular immunity in sarcoidosis and hypersensitivity pneumonitis: recent advances. *Chest*, 103, 138–43.

Shakoor, Z. and Hamblin, A. S. (1992). Increased CD11/CD18 expression on peripheral blood leucocytes of patients with sarcoidosis. *Clinical and Experimental Immunology*, 90, 99–105.

Sharma, O. P. (1984*a*). Clinical Features. In *Sarcoidosis — clinical management*, pp. 22–4, Butterworths, London.

Sharma, O. P. (1984*b*). Laboratory investigations. In *Sarcoidosis — clinical management*, pp. 143–51. Butterworths, London.

Sharma, O. P. (1984*c*). Sarcoidosis of the liver. In *Sarcoidosis — clinical management*, pp. 80–3. Butterworths, London.

Siltzbach, L. E. and Duberstein, J. L. (1968). Arthritis in sarcoidosis. *Clinical Orthopaedics and Related Research*, 57, 31–49.

Spilberg, I., Siltzbach, L. E, and McEwen, C. (1969). The arthritis of sarcoidosis. *Arthritis and Rheumatism*, 12, 126–37.

Steffen, M. *et al.* (1993). Increased secretion of tumor necrosis factor-α, interleukin-1β and interleukin-6 by alveolar macrophages from patients with sarcoidosis. *Journal of Allergy and Clinical Immunology*, 91, 939–49.

Studdy, P. R. and James D. G. (1983). The sensitivity and specificity of serum angiotensin-converting enzyme in sarcoidosis and other diseases. In (Proceedings) *Ninth international conference on sarcoidosis and other granulomatous disorders* (ed. J. Cretien, J. Marsac, and J. C. Saltiel), pp. 679–81. Pergamon, Paris.

Teirstein, A. S. (1983). Fibre-optic bronchoscopy in the diagnosis of sarcoidosis. In *Sarcoidosis and other granulomatous diseases of the lung* (ed. B. L. Fanburg), p 323. Marcel Decker, New York.

Teirstein, A. S. and Lesser, M. (1983). World distribution and epidemiology of sarcoidosis. In *Sarcoidosis and other granulomatous diseases of the lung* (ed. B. L. Fanburg), pp. 101–34. Marcel Decker, New York.

Veale, D. and FitzGerald, O. (1990). Acute sarcoid arthropathy — an infective cause? *British Journal of Rheumatology*, 29, 158–9.

5.13.6 The chronic, infantile, neurological, cutaneous, and articular syndrome (CINCA)

Anne-Marie Prieur

With increasing knowledge in paediatric rheumatology, new inflammatory entities have been more accurately defined. Closer scrutiny of particular sites of joint involvement and long-term follow-up now distinguish certain syndromes from systemic-onset juvenile chronic arthritis. The heterogeneity of so-called systemic-onset juvenile arthritis occurring during the first year of life was stressed several years ago by Prieur and Griscelli (1983). The children in question all had high fever, skin rash, and polyarthritis, but careful analysis of the symptoms allowed us to distinguish various entities. Among these, a group of patients displayed a chronic syndrome that also involved the central nervous system, including the eye and other sensory organs. The autonomy of this syndrome, which in Europe is designated as chronic, infantile, neurological, cutaneous, and articular syndrome (**CINCA**), is now accepted, although its cause remains a mystery.

Clinical presentation

Background

In definitive descriptions of CINCA, the first symptoms occur in early infancy and are often present at birth. The course of the disease is chronic, with intermittent flares associated with fever, and enlargement of lymph nodes and spleen. There have been individual case reports of a disease with these characteristics (Campbell and Clifton 1950; Lorber 1973; Ansell *et al.* 1975, Lampert *et al.* 1975; Fajardo *et al.* 1982), mostly preceding our suggestion that this could be a specific syndrome (Prieur and Griscelli 1981), and others have since confirmed its autonomy (Hassink and Goldsmith 1983; Yarom *et al.* 1985; Kaufman and Lovell 1986). A comprehensive description of the disease is given in Prieur *et al.* (1987). The syndrome is now more easily identified and more fully documented (Torbiak *et al.* 1989).

We have recognized five new cases, in particular a family in which father and daughter, and probably grandmother and great-grandfather, had the disease. The CINCA syndrome tends to be sporadic, but three families where more than one member is affected are known (see also Campbell and Clifton 1950; Ansell *et al.* 1975).

Perinatal events

The frequency of perinatal events is an important feature of this syndrome. These have been identified in half of the neonates in whom details of the perinatal period are known. After generally uneventful pregnancies (except for minor viral infections in a few cases), half of the babies are premature. The average birth weight is 2600 g (range 1700 to 4700 g) after a 38-week pregnancy (range 33 to 42 weeks). Five instances of anomaly in the umbilical cord have been found (umphaloceles or umphalitis). In one case, a histological study of the placenta showed thickened vessel walls with thrombosis and microcalcifications, and infiltration of the umbilical cord by polymorphonuclear cells. There was no evidence of infection in any of

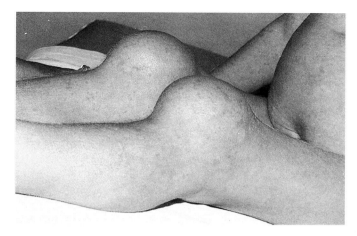

Fig. 1 The skin rash and patella overgrowth with knee deformity. (Reproduced from Prieur *et al.* 1987, with permission.)

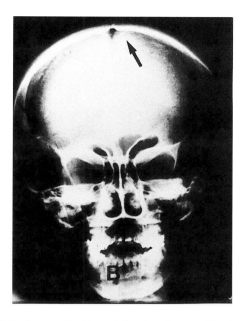

Fig. 2 Calcifications on the falx and dura in a 12-year-old patient. (Reproduced from Prieur *et al.* 1987, with permission.)

the infants, despite the occurrence of respiratory distress in three and icterus in five.

Signs and symptoms

In all cases, the association of skin rash, joint involvement, and central nervous manifestations is present.

Rash

The rash is present at birth in three-quarters of the children or occurs within the first 6 months after birth in the others. In a few patients, it has been noticed later or information on this period of life is lacking. The clinical expression is similar in all patients, although variable in intensity. It resembles the rash of Still's disease but is more intense, often having the appearance of a non-pruritic urticaria (Fig. 1). The rash is exacerbated during flare-ups of other symptoms of the disease. Skin biopsy shows a normal epidermis, mild inflammation in the dermis, and perivascular aggregation of polymorphonuclear cells with some eosinophils. No immunoglobulin or complement deposits have been found by immunofluorescence.

Central nervous and sensory anomalies

These are important manifestations of this syndrome. They are usually discovered at the onset of symptoms that could be related to a chronic meningeal irritation, such as headaches, vomiting, seizures, or transitory episodes of hemiplegia. A chronic meningitis has been identified in 23 of 25 patients investigated; these patients had a mild leucocytosis with polymorphs (and sometimes eosinophils), and/or increased protein concentrations in the cerebrospinal fluid. Anomalies in the cerebrospinal fluid may vary at follow-up. Extensive attempts to demonstrate chronic infection, including electron microscopy of cells in the cerebrospinal fluid, have been negative. Clinical follow-up of the central nervous involvement often shows an increase in the meningeal irritation, with headaches and sometimes seizures. Spasticity of the legs is not uncommon, but to date no persistent neurological defect has been observed. A low IQ has been noticed in several patients.

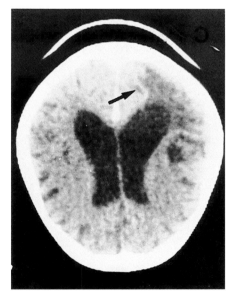

Fig. 3 CT scan: enlargement of ventricles with an area of cerebral change of probable vascular origin. (Reproduced from Prieur *et al.* 1987, with permission.)

The skull has an increased cranial volume and there is delay in the closure of the anterior fontanelle. In some patients, there are calcifications of the falx and dura (Fig. 2). Computed tomography (**CT**) often reveals a mild ventricular dilatation (Fig. 3).

Sensory anomalies are progressive. Varying degrees of perceptive deafness are present in older children, often requiring the use of a hearing aid. Eye involvement can be severe: optic atrophy, papillitis, conjunctivitis, keratitis, uveitis, and chorioretinitis have been observed and can lead to a progressive visual defect (Fig. 4). Hoarseness is frequent.

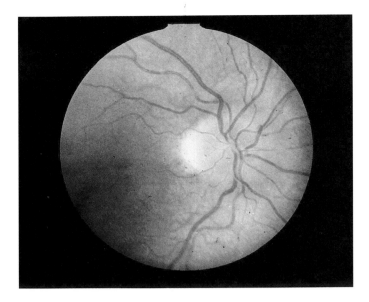

Fig. 4 Papillitis.

Joint involvement

The severity of joint involvement varies among patients. The knees are most frequently affected (see Fig. 1), then elbows, wrists, ankles, and small joints of the hand. In some patients, the joint symptoms are mild, and manifest as transitory inflammation during flare-ups. In this group, the first articular manifestations are generally observed after the age of 2 years. In other patients, the arthropathy may present as early as 10 days of age (Hassink and Goldsmith 1983). The main finding is an overgrowth of the epiphyseal plate of the bone, resulting in hard bony enlargement. The synovial fluid exudate may show a non-specific inflammatory reaction. Progressive contractures and limitation of motion due to patellar and/or epiphyseal overgrowth occur (see Fig. 1).

The radiographic anomalies of affected joints are progressively more characteristic with increasing age in half of the patients. The first finding is swelling of periarticular soft tissues, sometimes with early periosteal reaction of the diaphysis (Kaufman and Lovell 1986). The most characteristic modifications are in the metaphysis and epiphysis of long bones, giving an irregular ossification with abnormal trabeculae. These anomalies may involve growth cartilage plates (Fig. 5); one biopsy showed an irregular metachromasia and completely disorganized columns of cartilaginous cells (Fig. 6). Surprisingly, no inflammatory cells were found in the abnormal cartilage (Fig. 6).

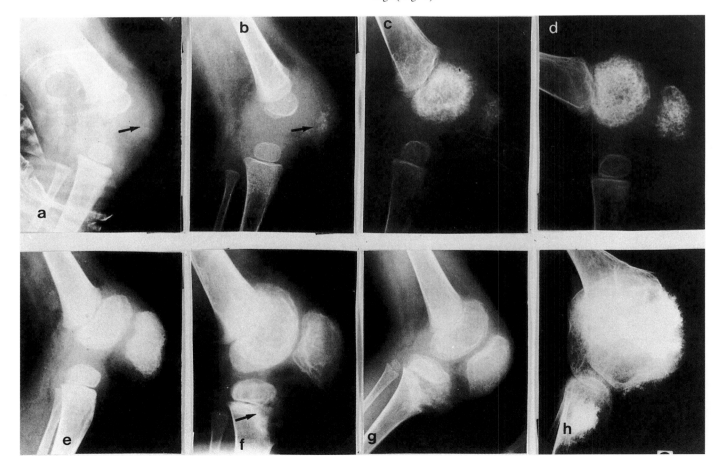

Fig. 5 Follow-up of radiographic anomalies in the knee at various ages: (a) 1 year; (b) 1 year and 6 months; (c) 2 years and 6 months; (d) 3 years and 9 months; (e) 5 years; (f) 6 years (arrow: late modification of tibial growth cartilage); (g) 8 years; (h) 33 years (another patient). (Reproduced from Prieur *et al.* 1987, with permission.)

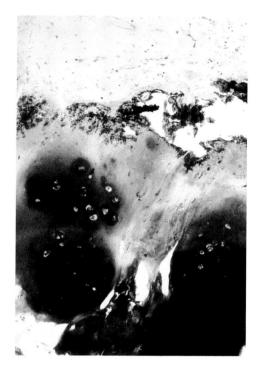

Fig. 6 Biopsy of growth-cartilage overgrowth: irregular metachromasia and disappearance of the normal columns of cartilaginous cells. Note the absence of inflammatory cells in this abnormal cartilaginous tissue. (By courtesy of Giulia Coumot-Witmer.)

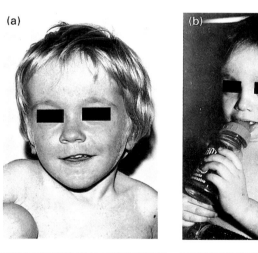
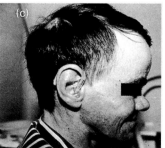
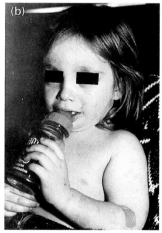
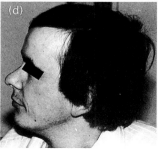

Fig. 7 Morphological aspects of two unrelated children (a) and (b) and two unrelated adults (c) and (d). Patients (b) and (d) are daughter and father.

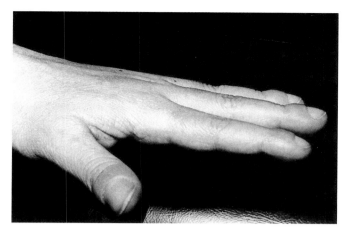

Fig. 8 Clubbing of finger in a 20-year-old girl.

Morphological changes

These patients have morphological changes in common. A progressive growth retardation with height below the third percentile is very frequent, but no defect in growth hormone has been found. The heads of these patients have a similar appearance, with enlargement (often with frontal bossing) and blond hair making these unrelated children look like siblings (Fig. 7(a and b)). The adults also resemble each other, as shown in Fig. 7(c and d). A saddle-back nose is frequent and the patient shown in Fig. 7(c) looks surprisingly like one of the patients in the first published descriptions in 1950 (Campbell and Clifton 1950). There is also clubbing of the fingers and toes (Fig. 8). Hands and feet appear short and thick. In some patients, the palms and soles have a wrinkled appearance.

Adult features

These children may reach adulthood, although eight deaths have been reported in children with this syndrome. The causes of death in five of the children were: secondary amyloidosis (Prieur *et al.* 1987); sepsis (Fajardo *et al.* 1982); leukaemia, possibly related to chlorambucil therapy (Prieur and Griscelli 1981); and subacute necrotizing leucoencephalopathy after head injury (Lampert 1986). An adult died of gangrene of the foot (Warin 1977).

Follow-up

Long-term follow-up reveals a slow worsening of most symptoms despite various therapeutic trials. Non-steroidal anti-inflammatory drugs induce pain relief. Steroids are partially effective for fever and pain, but not for skin lesions or joint disease. Immunosuppressive drugs have no dramatic effect; disease-modifying drugs are ineffective. Physiotherapy improves the functional status in patients with severe arthropathy.

Pathogenesis

The pathophysiology of this syndrome is unknown. There are indications of a non-specific inflammation: hypochromic anaemia, leucocytosis with a predominance of polymorphonuclear neutrophils and eosinophils, high platelet counts, and an increase in erythrocyte sedimentation rate and other acute-phase reactants. A polyclonal stimulation of immunoglobulin synthesis has been found in all patients. Surprisingly, no circulating immune complexes have been detected; no autoantibodies or immunodeficiency have been found. The microscopic architecture of the lymph nodes is preserved except for features of chronic inflammation, with an infiltration of the subcortical T-cell region by polymorphonuclear cells and often eosinophils. Extensive investigations for an infectious agent have been unsuccessful. Evidence of a retroviral infection was sought in leucocytes and cells from cerebrospinal fluid in a recently diagnosed patient, but the outcome was negative (C. Rouzioux, unpublished data).

This disorder is an unremitting inflammatory process that begins at birth. Most of the organs or tissues involved, except cartilage, show chronic inflammation. Cartilage may be the target organ in this syndrome, with the clustering of growth retardation, anomalies of ossification of skull and epiphyses, saddle-back nose, hoarseness suggesting laryngeal localization, and progressive deafness. Indeed, some indications of such a mechanism were suggested by the presence of a toxic effect of the serum from these patients on normal human cartilage cells in culture (Prieur *et al.* 1988). However, the origin of this disease remains unknown, even though one may speculate on an initiating event that takes place before birth. It represents an original and new disorder that must be distinguished from previously described rheumatic diseases of childhood.

References

Ansell, B.M., Bywaters, E.G.L., and Elderkin, F.M. (1975). Familial arthropathy with rash, uveitis and mental retardation. *Proceedings of the Royal Society of Medicine*, 68, 584–5.

Campbell, A.M.G. and Clifton F. (1950). Adult toxoplasmosis in one family. *Brain*, 73, 281–90.

Fajardo, J.E., Geller, T.J., Koenig, H.M., and Kleine, M.L. (1982). Chronic meningitis, polyarthritis, lymphadenitis and pulmonary hemosiderosis. *Journal of Pediatrics*, 101, 738–40.

Hassink, S.G. and Goldsmith T.J. (1983). Neoonatal onset multisystem inflammatory disease. *Arthritis and Rheumatism*, 26, 668–73.

Kaufman, R.A. and Lovell, D.J. (1986). Infantile-onset multisystem inflammatory disease: radiologic findings. *Radiology*, 160, 741–6.

Lampert, F. (1986). Infantile multisystem inflammatory disease: another case of a new syndrome. *European Journal of Paediatrics*, 144, 593–6.

Lampert, F. *et al.* (1975). Infantile chronic relapsing inflammation of the brain, skin and joints. (Letter.) *Lancet*, i, 1250–2.

Lorber, J. (1973). Syndrome for diagnosis: dwarfing; persistently open fontanelle; recurrent meningitis; recurrent subdural effusions with temporary alternate-sided hemiplegia; high tone deafness; visual defect with pseudopapilloedema; slowing intellectual development; recurrent acute polyarthritis; erythema marginatum, splenomegaly and iron resistant hypochromic anemia. *Proceedings of the Royal Society of Medicine*, 66, 1070–1.

Prieur, A.M. and Griscelli, C. (1981). Arthropathy with rash, chronic meningitis, eye lesions and mental retardation. *Journal of Pediatrics*, 99, 79–83.

Prieur, A.M. and Griscelli, C. (1983). Aspect nosologique des formes systémiques de l'arthrite juvénile début très précoce: a propos de dix-sept observations. *Annales de Pediatrie (Paris)*, 30, 565–9.

Prieur, A.M. *et al.* (1987). A chronic, infantile, neurological, cutaneous and articular (CINCA) syndrome: a specific entity analysed in 30 patients. *Scandinavian Journal of Rheumatology*, 66, 57–68.

Prieur, A.M., Cournot-Witmer, G., Plachot, J.J., Griscelli, C., and Corvol, M.T. (1988). *In vitro* study of growth cartilage in children with the infantile onset neurologic, cutaneous and articular syndrome. Inhibitory effect of patient's sera on cultured normal human chondrocyte metabolism. *Arthritis and Rheumatism*, 31, 578.

Torbiak, R.P., Dent, P.B., and Colkshott, W.P. (1989). NOMID–a neonatal syndrome of multisystem inflammation. *Skeletal Radiology*, 18, 359–64.

Warin, R.P. (1977). Familial vasculitis (life-long morbiliform urticaria, neurological changes and arthritis). *British Journal of Dermatology*, 97, 30–1.

Yarom, A., Rennebohm, R.M., and Levinson, J.E. (1985). Infantile multisystem inflammatory disease: a specific syndrome? *Journal of Pediatrics*, 106, 390–6.

5.13.7 Multicentric reticulohistiocytosis

P. J. Maddison

Multicentric reticulohistiocytosis is a rare systemic disease that is recognized clinically by the combination of typical papular and nodular skin lesions and a severe and destructive polyarthritis, although virtually any organ system of the body can be involved. The term 'multicentric reticulohistiocytosis' was introduced by Goltz and Layman (1954) to distinguish the disorder from solitary cutaneous nodules, termed reticulohistiocytomas, which have identical histological appearances but are not associated with systemic disease. There are a number of synonyms, which include lipoid dermato-arthritis, reticulohistiocytosis, giant-cell reticulohistiocytosis, and normocholesterolaemic xanthomatosis. At one time it was thought to be a lipid-storage disease but no consistent abnormality of serum or intracellular lipids has been identified. It is thought generally that the histiocytes and giant cells that characterize the lesions contain a non-specific accumulation of glycoprotein and lipids, and that this disease is a histiocytic granulomatous reaction to an unknown stimulus (Campbell and Edwards 1991). However, in one case, type VI collagen inclusions usually found in lymphohistiocytic neoplasms were demonstrated, supporting the concept of a proliferative rather than an inflammatory background for this condition (Fortier-Beaulieu *et al.* 1993).

Clinical features

Multicentric reticulohistiocytosis is primarily a disorder of adults, being slightly more common in women (Barrow and Holubar 1969), with a mean age of onset in the fifth decade. About 85 per cent of reported cases are caucasoid, but it can also occur in other ethnic groups (Lesher and Allen 1984). Typical cases have been reported in adolescence (Raphael *et al.* 1989), but in most instances the childhood form differs from that in adults in having a familial component, a marked tendency to involve the eye (glaucoma, uveitis, and cataracts), and a lack of giant cells in tissue sections, the last feature being considered an essential feature of multicentric reticulohistiocytosis (Zayid and Farraj 1973).

Skin nodules and a destructive polyarthritis are the most common features (Barrow and Holubar 1969; Chevrant-Breton 1977; Rapini, 1993). Arthritis is frequently the presenting feature. It has a similar distribution to rheumatoid arthritis, including the temporomandibular joints and atlantoaxial involvement (Gold *et al.* 1975), but also affects the distal interphalangeal joints. Commonly involved sites are the hands (75 per cent), knees (70 per cent), shoulders (65 per cent), wrists (65 per cent), hips (60 per cent), ankles (60 per cent), elbows

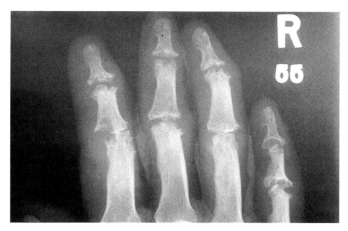

Fig. 1 Radiograph of the hand in multicentric reticulohistiocytosis.

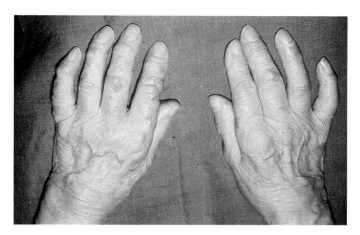

Fig. 2 Multicentric reticulohistiocytosis: nodules involving the hands.

(60 per cent), feet (60 per cent), and spine (50 per cent) Often it has a persistent course with progressive joint destruction, sometimes leading to the picture of arthritis mutilans with 'opera glass' deformities of the hand developing in approximately 20 per cent (Barrow and Holubar 1969). Radiographs of the joints show symmetrical erosions resembling rheumatoid arthritis. However, osteoporosis is not marked (Maki *et al.* 1995) and there is often prominent involvement of the distal interphalangeal joints, and the spread of erosions from the periphery of the joint produces apparent widening of the joint space (Fig. 1). Analysis of joint fluid shows low to moderate cell counts, mostly with a preponderance of mononuclear cells but sometimes of neutrophils. Synovial biopsy shows the presence of lipid-laden giant cells and histiocytes, as found in the involved skin.

Mucocutaneous involvement is apparent in approximately 90 per cent of patients at the time of presentation but may occur in the months following the development of arthritis. Occasionally it is the first feature. Skin lesions consist of numerous, usually non-pruritic, skin-coloured, yellowish or red-brown nodules, ranging from a few millimetres to several centimetres in diameter. Occasionally, however, pruritus is a feature, and can be severe and precede the overt lesions. The nodules mostly involve the hands in a periungual distribution, together with nodules scattered on the fingers and on the face, where lesions develop on the ears, at the corners of the mouth, and the side of the nose adjacent to the alae (Figs 2 and 3). Extensive involvement of the face produces a leonine facies. Lesions can also occur on the forehead, chest, back, and over the olecranon process and knees. Xanthelasma develops in approximately 25 per cent. The oral mucous membranes are involved in approximately half, with, for example, numerous flesh-coloured papules on the buccal mucosa, sides of the tongue, surface of the palate, and gingiva. Occasionally the pharynx and larynx are affected (Katz and Anderson 1988). To date there have been no reports of vaginal or peri-anal involvement.

Although multicentric reticulohistiocytosis usually affects the skin and joints, a large variety of systemic features can occur, reflecting the potential involvement of most tissues and organs of the body. There are also reported associations with various types of malignancy. Constitutional manifestations occur in about one-third of patients, and include fever and weight loss; cases have been reported with peri-carditis, pulmonary involvement, and myositis (Anderson *et al.* 1968; Fast 1976; Lesher and Allen 1984; Widman *et al.* 1988; Gao *et al.* 1990).

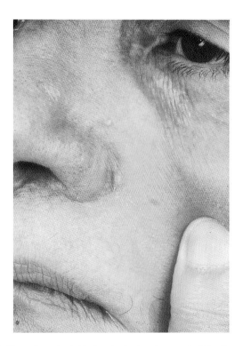

Fig. 3 Multicentric reticulohistiocytosis: involvement of the face.

There have also been case reports of lymph node enlargement, splenomegaly, marrow infiltration resulting in pancytopenia, salivary gland involvement, thyroid infiltration leading to hypothyroidism, and carpal tunnel syndrome (Warin *et al.* 1957; Orkin *et al.* 1964; Ehrlich *et al.* 1972; Furey *et al.* 1983; Finelli *et al.* 1986; Rene *et al.* 1990).

Laboratory abnormalities occur, but are inconsistent, and include a raised erythrocyte sedimentation rate, abnormal liver function tests, and elevated creatine phosphokinase. Paraproteinaemia of γ heavy-chain type has been encountered but serological tests for such as rheumatoid factor are otherwise usually normal. Gallium scintiscans have been used to evaluate multicentric reticulohistiocytosis but the abnormalities are non-specific (Widman *et al.* 1988).

Approximately 25 per cent of patients with multicentric reticulo-histiocytosis have been reported to have malignant disease (Catterall and White 1978). Associations have mostly been with internal carcinomas of the colon, breast, bronchus, cervix, ovary, and stomach.

Cases have also been associated with sarcomas and lymphomas. Patients with malignant melanoma and pleural mesothelioma have also been reported (Coupe *et al.* 1987; Gibson *et al.* 1995). In one review of the literature (Nunnink *et al.* 1985), the onset of both diseases occurred in several patients within 1 year. The onset of multicentric reticulohistiocytosis in adulthood necessitates, therefore, a thorough clinical examination, including a chest radiograph, to look for signs of malignant disease. It is not necessary, however, to embark on invasive procedures to look for occult neoplasms. It should be borne in mind that there may be a bias towards reporting cases with underlying malignancy, especially previously unreported tumours, and some of the associations may be purely coincidental.

Pathology

Histologically, the nodular infiltrates, which have a granular or ground-glass appearance, consist of multinucleate (up to 20 nuclei) giant cells of the foreign-body type and histiocytes of the monocyte–macrophage lineage (Heathcote *et al.* 1985) admixed with small numbers of CD4+ lymphocytes and B cells. Histochemically, the cytoplasm of the giant cells contains diastase-resistant, periodic acid–Schiff-positive material thought to be glycoprotein, neutral fats, phospholipids, and iron (Barrow and Holubar 1969). Ultrastructural studies show the presence of pleomorphic cytoplasmic inclusions (Degas *et al.* 1975; Caputo *et al.* 1981). The giant cells and mononuclear histiocytes express the surface markers of the monocyte–macrophage lineage (Salisbury *et al.* 1990; Zegler *et al.* 1994), and cytokines and enzyme products of activated macrophages have been detected (Lotti *et al.* 1988; Zagala *et al.* 1988). Negative staining with markers such as CD1 and the absence of Birbeck granules helps to confirm that the cells are not derived from Langerhans cells, in contrast to histiocytosis X (Salisbury *et al.* 1990).

Diagnosis

The diagnosis is confirmed by skin or synovial biopsy. Solitary reticulohistiocytomas have identical histological findings but there is no evidence of systemic disease (Zegler *et al.* 1994).

Table 1 Drug treatment for multicentric reticulohistiocytosis

Drug	Comments
Prednisolone	
Taylor (1977)	Single case history with improvement in pruritis and slow resolution of skin lesions
Zeale *et al.* (1985)	High-dose prednisolone effective in one patient
Cytotoxic drugs	
Hanauer (1972)	Remission on cyclophosphamide (one case)
Ehrlich *et al.* (1972)	Response in one patient to combination of azathioprine and prednisolone
Krey *et al.* (1974)	No response to azathioprine (one patient)
Gold *et al.* (1975)	Cyclophosphamide improved skin and joint disease (one case)
Brandt *et al.* (1982)	Improvement on cyclophosphamide with reduction in erosions on hand radiograph (one case); previous improvement of skin lesions with topical nitrogen mustard
Heenan *et al.* (1983)	Good response to chlorambucil before patient died from breast carcinoma
Doherty *et al.* (1984)	Good response first to cyclophosphamide, then to chlorambucil (one case)
Coupe *et al.* (1987)	Skin and joint manifestations responded well to cyclophosphamide until the patient died from associated mesothelioma
Ginsburg *et al.* (1989)	Five patients treated with cyclophosphamide, one with chlorambucil; all improved, five went into remission, one relapsed after treatment stopped
Kenik *et al.* (1990)	Response to cyclophosphamide until the patient died of recurrent melanoma
Other agents	
Davies *et al.* (1968)	Improvement in two patients on combination of hydroxychloroquine and prednisolone
Gold *et al.* (1977)	Improvement on rifampicin plus ethambutol in a patient with coexistent tuberculosis
Doherty *et al.* (1984)	No response to penicillamine (one case)
Giam (1988)	No response to methotrexate (one case)
Gourmelen *et al.* (1991)	Good response to methotrexate resulting in prolonged remission (one case)

Diseases that may possibly be confused with multicentric reticulohistiocytosis on the basis of clinical or histological findings are:

(1) rheumatoid or psoriatic arthritis;

(2) sarcoid dactylitis—associated with discrete tubercles that lack foam cells or giant cells typical of multicentric reticulohistiocytosis;

(3) xanthomas;

(4) fibroxanthoma;

(5) histiocytosis X—usually presents in childhood and proliferating cells are epidermotropic Langerhans cells rather than of true monocyte–macrophage lineage;

(6) generalized eruptive histiocytoma—not associated with arthritis and lesions do not exhibit the typical multinucleate giant cells;

(7) tendon sheath giant-cell tumours—solitary, well-circumscribed nodules in the hands;

(8) Farber's disease—lipogranulomatosis, usually fatal in infancy.

Treatment and course

The disease often runs a waxing and waning course and sometimes it stabilizes. It is difficult to predict the course in the individual case but as a rule the disease 'burns out' after 5 to 8 years, with regression of the cutaneous nodules (Lyell and Carr 1959; Albert *et al.* 1960), leaving the patient with severe joint deformities. Occasionally, systemic involvement can be severe enough to be life threatening (Barrow and Holubar 1969) but otherwise the prognosis is dominated by whether or not there is an associated malignancy.

Various drug treatments have been proposed to suppress the condition, including corticosteroids, adrenocorticotrophic hormone, salicylates, antimalarials, and cytotoxic agents. There are no controlled trials, as the condition is so rare, and therefore reports of efficacy should be interpreted with caution (Table 1).

Corticosteroids are of limited use. Skin infiltration does not usually respond, although there may be relief of troublesome pruritus (Taylor 1977). Joint symptoms sometimes improve (Davies *et al.* 1968).

There is a consensus that alkylating agents are the treatment of choice and there are several reports of improvement in skin, joint, and systemic disease with cyclophosphamide in particular (Ginsburg *et al.* 1989). Patients with long-lasting remission after therapy with cyclophosphamide or chlorambucil have been reported (Hanauer 1972; Brandt *et al.* 1982; Coupe *et al.* 1987; Ginsburg *et al.* 1989; Kenik *et al.* 1990), but some do relapse when treatment is stopped (Ginsburg *et al.* 1989). Methotrexate is also reportedly successful (Gourmelen *et al.* 1991), but not in all cases (Giam 1988).

References

Albert, J., Bruce, W., Allen, A. C., and Blank, M. (1960). Lipoid dermatoarthritis: reticulohistiocytoma of the skin and joints. *American Journal of Medicine*, **28**, 661–7.

Anderson, T. E., Carr, A. J., Chapman, R. J., Downie, A. W., and Maclean, G. D. (1968). Myositis and myotonia in a case of multicentric reticulohistiocytosis. *British Journal of Dermatology*, **80**, 39–45.

Barrow, M. V. and Holubar, K. (1969). Multicentric reticulohistiocytosis: a review of 33 patients. *Medicine (Baltimore)*, **48**, 287–305.

Brandt, F., Lipman, M., Taylor, J. R., and Halprin, K. M. (1982). Topical nitrogen mustard therapy in multicentric reticulohistiocytosis. *Journal of the American Academy of Dermatology*, **6**, 260–2.

Campbell, D. A., and Edwards, N. L. (1991). Multicentric reticulohistiocytosis: systemic macrophage disorder. *Baillières Clinical Rheumatology*, **5**, 301–19.

Caputo, R., Alessi, E., and Berti, E. (1981). Collagen phagocytosis in multicentric reticulohistiocytosis. *Journal of Investigative Dermatology*, **76**, 342–6.

Catterall, M. and White, J. (1978). Multicentric reticulohistiocytosis and malignant disease. *British Journal of Dermatology*, **98**, 221–4.

Chevrant-Breton, J. (1977). La reticulo-histiocytose multicentrique: revue de la litterature recente (depuis 1969). *Annales de Dermatologie et de Venereologie (Paris)*, **104**, 745–9.

Coupe, M. O., Whittaker, S. J., and Thatcher, N. (1987). Multicentric reticulohistiocytosis. *British Journal of Dermatology*, **116**, 245–7.

Davies, M. E., Roenigk, H. H., Hawk, W. A., and O'Duffy, J. D. (1968). Multicentric reticulohistiocytosis: report of a case with histochemical studies. *Archives of Dermatology*, **97**, 543–7.

Degas, R., Civatte, J., Bonvalet, D., and Bouhin, F. (1975). Reticulo-histiocytoma gigantocellulaire. *Annales de Dermatologie et de Syphiligraphie (Paris)*, **102**, 315–17.

Doherty, M., Martin, M. F., and Dieppe, P. A. (1984). Multicentric reticulohistiocytosis associated with primary biliary cirrhosis: successful treatment with cytotoxic agents. *Arthritis and Rheumatism*, **27**, 844–8.

Ehrlich, G., Young, I., Nosheny, S., and Katz, W. (1972). Multicentric reticulohistiocytosis (lipoid dermatoarthritis): a multisystem disorder. *American Journal of Medicine*, **52**, 830–40.

Fast, A. (1976). Cardiopulmonary complications in multicentric reticulohistiocytosis. *Archives of Dermatology*, **112**, 1139–41.

Finelli, L. G., Tenner, L. K., and Ratz, J. L. (1986). A case of multicentric reticulohistiocytosis with thyroid involvement. *Journal of the American Academy of Dermatology*, **15**, 1097–1100.

Fortier-Beaulieu, M., Thomine, E., Boullie, M. C., Le Loet, X., Lauret, P., and Hemet, J. (1993). *American Journal of Dermatopathology*, **15**, 587–9.

Furey, N., DiMauro, J., Eng, A., and Shaw, J. (1983). Multicentric reticulohistiocytosis with salivary gland involvement and pericardial effusion. *Journal of the American Academy of Dermatology*, **8**, 679–84.

Gao, I. K., Goronzy, J. J., and Weyand, C. M. (1990). Ten-year follow-up of a patient with multicentric reticulohistiocytosis associated with myopathy. *Scandinavian Journal of Rheumatology*, **19**, 437–41.

Giam, Y. C. (1988). Multicentric reticulohistiocytosis. *Annals of the Academy of Medicine of Singapore*, **17**, 548–50.

Gibson, G., Cassidy, M., O'Connell, P., and Murphy, G. M. (1995). Multicentric reticulohistiocytosis associated with recurrence of malignant melanoma. *Journal of the American Academy of Dermatology*, **32**, 134–6.

Ginsburg, W. W., O'Duffy, J. D., and Morris, J. L. (1989). Multicentric reticulohistiocytosis: response to alkylating agents in six patients. *Annals of Internal Medicine*, **111**, 384–8.

Gold, R. H., Metzger, A. L., and Mirra, J. M. (1975). Multicentric reticulohistiocytosis (lipoid dermato-arthritis): an erosive polyarthritis and distinctive clinical, roentgenographic and pathological features. *American Journal of Roentgenology, Radiation Therapy and Nuclear Medicine*, **124**, 610–24.

Gold, K. D., Sharp, J. T., Estrada, R. G., Duffy, J., and Person, D. A. (1977). Relationship between multicentric reticulohistiocytosis and tuberculosis. *Journal of the American Medical Association*, **237**, 2213–14.

Goltz, R. W. and Layman, C. W. (1954). Multicentric reticulohistiocytosis of the skin and synovia. *Archives of Dermatology and Syphilology*, **69**, 717–22.

Gourmelen, O. *et al.* (1991). Methotrexate treatment for multicentric reticulohistiocytosis. *Journal of Rheumatology*, **18**, 627–8.

Hanauer, L. B. (1972). Reticulohistiocytosis: remission after cyclophosphamide therapy. *Arthritis and Rheumatism*, **15**, 636–40.

Heathcote, J. G., Guenther, L. C., and Wallace, A. C. (1985). Multicentric reticulohistiocytosis: A report of a case and a review of the pathology. *Pathology*, **17**, 601–8.

Heenan, P. J., Quirk, C. J., and Spagnolo, D. V. (1983). Multicentric reticulohistio-cytosis: a light and electron microscopic study. *Australasian Journal of Dermatology*, **24**, 122–6.

Katz, R. W. and Anderson, K. F. (1988). Multicentric reticulohistiocytosis. *Oral Surgery, Oral Medicine, Oral Pathology*, **65**, 721–5.

Kenik, J.G., Fok, F., Huerter, C.J., Hurley, J.A., and Stanoshek, J.F. (1990). Multicentric reticulohistiocytosis in a patient with malignant melanoma: a response to cyclophosphamide and a unique cutaneous feature. *Arthritis and Rheumatism*, **33**, 1047–51.

Krey, P. R., Comerford, F. R., and Cohen, A. S. (1974). Multicentric reticulohistio-cytosis: fine structural analysis of the synovium and synovial fluid cells. *Arthritis and Rheumatism*, **17**, 615–33.

Lesher, J. L. and Allen, B. S. (1984). Multicentric reticulohistiocytosis. *Journal of the American Academy of Dermatology*, **11**, 713–23.

Lotti, T., Santucci, M., Casigliani, R., Fabbri, P., Bondi, R., and Panconesi, E. (1988). Multicentric reticulohistiocytosis: report of three cases with evalua-tion of tissue proteinase activity. *American Journal of Dermatopathology*, **10**, 497–504.

Lyell, A. and Carr, A. (1959). Lipoid dermato-arthritis (reticulohistiocytosis). *British Journal of Dermatology*, **71**, 12–21.

Maki, D. D., Caperton, E. M., and Griffiths, H. J. (1995). Radiologic case study. Multicentric reticulohistiocytosis. *Orthopedics*, **18**, 77–81.

Nunnick, J. C., Krusinski, P. A., and Yates, J. W. (1985). Multicentric reticulohis-tiocytosis and cancer: a case report and review of the literature. *Medical Pediatric Oncology*, **13**, 273–9.

Orkin, M., Goltz, R. W., Good, R. A., Michael, A., and Fisher, I. (1964). A study of multicentric reticulohistiocytosis. *Archives of Dermatology*, **89**, 640–54.

Raphael, S. A., Cowdery, S. L., Faerber, E. N., Lischner, H. W., Shumacher, R., and Tourtellotte, C. D. (1989). Multicentric reticulohistiocytosis in a child. *Journal of Paediatrics*, **114**, 266–9.

Rapini, R. P. (1993). Multicentric reticulohistiocytosis. *Clinics in Dermatology*, **11**, 107–11.

Rene, J., Starz, T., and Miller, E. B. (1990). Multicentric reticulohistiocytosis and Sjögren's syndrome. *Arthritis and Rheumatism*, **33**, 1870–1.

Salisbury, J., Hall, P. A., Williams, H. C., Mangi, M. H., and Mufti, G. J. (1990). Multicentric reticulohistiocytosis: detailed immunophenotyping confirms macrophage origin. *American Journal of Surgical Pathology*, **14**, 687–93.

Taylor, D. R. (1977). Multicentric reticulohistiocytosis. *Archives of Dermatology*, **113**, 320–2.

Warin, R. P., Evans, C. D., Hewitt, M., Taylor, A. L., Price, C. H., and Middlemiss, J. H. (1957). Reticulohistiocytosis (lipoid dermato-arthritis). *British Medical Journal*, **1**, 1387–91.

Widman, D., Swayne, L. C., and Rozan, S. (1988). Multicentric reticulohistiocy-tosis: Assessment of pulmonary disease by gallium–67 scintigraphy. *Journal of Rheumatology*, **15**, 132–5.

Zagala, A., Guyot, A., Benson, J. C., and Phelip, X. (1988). Multicentric reticulohistiocytosis: a case with enhanced interleukin-1 prostaglandin E_2 and interleukin-2 secretion. *Journal of Rheumatology*, **15**, 136–8.

Zayid, I. and Farraj, F. (1973). Familial histiocytic dermatitis: a new syndrome. *American Journal of Medicine*, **54**, 793–800.

Zeale, P. J., Miner, D., Honig, S., Waxman, M., and Bartfield, H. (1985). Multicentric reticulohistiocytosis: a cause of dysphagia with response to corti-costeroids. *Arthritis and Rheumatism*, **28**, 231–4.

Zegler, B., Soyer, H. P., Misch, K., Orchard, G., and Wilson-Jones, E. (1994). Reticulohistiocytoma and multicentric reticulohistiocytosis. Histopathologic and immunophenotypic distinct entities. *American Journal of Dermatopathology*, **16**, 577–84.

5.13.8 Hyperlipidaemias

*Keng Hong Leong, J. Reckless,
and Neil John McHugh*

Introduction

The relationship of lipid disorders to rheumatic diseases is multifa-ceted. For instance several abnormalities in the lipid and lipoprotein profile (or dyslipidaemia) have been documented in various forms of chronic arthritis. The dyslipidaemia may depend on the type or activity of the joint disease or may be influenced by other factors such as treatment or systemic complications of the disease. Whenever the dyslipidaemia is present, its severity will be influenced by diet and lifestyle factors, and also by the underlying genetic predis-position. Renal involvement in systemic lupus erythematosus is an example where the disease, treatment of the disease, or complications of the disease such as nephrotic syndrome may each have a separate influence on lipid metabolism. The dyslipidaemia may potentially influence disease outcome itself by accelerating atheroma, although the relative contribution of dyslipidaemia to the increased mortality from vascular disease observed in several rheumatic disorders is uncertain.

Musculoskeletal symptoms may be a manifestation of an under-lying hyperlipidaemia and will be described in more detail. There is some evidence that potentially toxic lipid particles, such as oxidized low density lipoprotein (**LDL**), may accumulate within joints (Winyard *et al.* 1993), as well as having more recognized proinflamma-tory effects on other tissues. Oxidized LDL may be a target for potentially pathogenic autoantibodies that cross-react with phospho-lipids (Vaarala *et al.* 1993). Conversely, dietary modification of lipid intake may have beneficial effects on inflammatory disease. Dietary supplementation with polyunsaturated fatty acids of the omega 3 and omega 6 series may be effective therapy for certain rheumatic diseases as it is in animal models of inflammatory arthritis. This chapter will cover some of the above relationships between lipids and rheumatic disease and give an outline of appropriate manage-ment where relevant.

Lipid metabolism

A comprehensive review of lipid metabolism would not be appropriate but a brief reminder of certain aspects relevant to rheumatology is given here.

Lipid composition

Lipoproteins are complex particles that transport lipids such as triglycerides and cholesterol through the plasma. The composition of a typical lipoprotein particle is shown in Fig. 1. Each particle is composed of a non-polar core containing variable proportions of hydrophobic lipids (triglycerides and cholesterol ester) surrounded by a polar coat of phospholipids and free cholesterol, within which there are various apolipoproteins. This outer coat allows the particle to be soluble in aqueous plasma. The apolipoproteins have both structural roles in the lipoproteins and functional roles as enzyme

Table 1 The major classes of lipoproteins

Lipoprotein	Major lipids	Major lipoproteins
Chylomicrons and remnants	Dietary triglycerides	AI, AII, B48, CI, CII, CIII, E
VLDL	Endogenous triglycerides	B48, CI, CII, CIII, E
IDL	Cholesteryl esters, triglycerides	B100, CIII, E
LDL	Cholesteryl esters	B100
HDL	Cholesteryl esters	AI, AII

activators or as ligands with high affinity for specific tissue-cell receptors. There are five main types of lipoprotein, defined by their relative density, that differ in their composition of lipid and the type of apolipoprotein (Table 1). Apolipoprotein A (**apoA**) is the major apolipoprotein in high density lipoprotein (**HDL**) and apolipoprotein B (**apoB**) is the major structural apolipoprotein of the other lipoproteins, chylomicrons, very low dense lipoprotein (**VLDL**), intermediate density lipoprotein (**IDL**), and LDL. The full apoB (apoB100) is found in VLDL, IDL, and LDL, having structural and functional components, but a truncated form, apoB48, having only the structural role, is present in chylomicrons made by gut cells. The main cholesterol-carrying lipoproteins are LDL and HDL while the main triglyceride-carrying lipoproteins are chylomicrons and VLDL. As VLDL is catabolized, remnants are formed known as IDL which are normally rapidly removed from the liver or converted to LDL.

Lipid subclasses

The major lipoproteins are heterogeneous and subclasses can be detected by methods such as precipitation or ultracentrifugation.

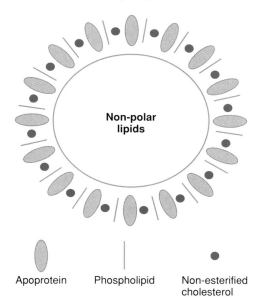

Fig. 1 Composition of typical lipoprotein particle.

HDL can be separated into two main fractions—HDL2 and HDL3. HDL3 accepts cholesterol from cholesterol-replete tissues, converts to larger HDL2, which in turn delivers cholesterol to the liver or other lipoproteins. LDL exists in three main subclasses—LDL1, LDL2, and LDL3—which can be separated by cumulative flotation ultracentrifugation. The normal LDL pattern is predominantly LDL2 with some LDL1 and less LDL3, but under certain circumstances this pattern can shift towards smaller particles with a predominance of small, dense LDL3 which is cholesterol depleted and relatively triglyceride rich. LDL3 is less readily recognized by normal LDL receptors and is more readily recognized (and much more likely to be taken up) by macrophages in the arterial subintimal space which form the foam cells of the fatty streak of early atheroma (Campos *et al.* 1992). VLDL can be separated into three main fractions—VLDL1, VLDL2, and VLDL3. The larger, more buoyant, triglyceride-rich VLDL1 particles, formed especially when there is increased hepatic triglyceride synthesis, are more likely to be precursors for LDL3, while small VLDL particles favour generation of the larger (more normal) LDL subclasses. Changes in the proportion of lipoprotein subclasses will not be apparent on basic lipid screening, yet this has an important bearing on the risk of atherosclerosis and may be influenced by metabolic and systemic alterations that accompany chronic rheumatic disorders. For example triglyceride lipases that have important roles in determining lipoprotein composition are influenced by cytokines that are upregulated in inflammatory conditions (as discussed below).

Exogenous pathway of lipid transport

Chylomicrons carry dietary triglycerides and cholesterol from the intestine to adipose tissue and skeletal muscle. Lipoprotein lipase liberates free fatty acid and monoglycerides which cross the endothelium to the peripheral tissue for further metabolism. The chylomicron remnant is removed by the liver.

Endogenous pathway of lipid transport

Triglycerides are synthesized in the liver and incorporated into VLDL particles. VLDL is a substrate for lipoprotein lipase in peripheral tissue where triglycerides are hydrolysed. VLDL becomes IDL which is either taken back up by the liver or loses further triglyceride and apolipoproteins apart from apoB and becomes cholesterol-rich LDL. Both the liver and extrahepatic tissues that utilize cholesterol recognize LDL via receptor-mediated pathways. Otherwise a variable amount of LDL is scavenged by the reticuloendothelial system and particularly by macrophages. HDL can accept cholesterol from cholesterol-replete tissues. Cholesterol is esterified on the surface of HDL by the enzyme lecithin:cholesterol acyltransferase to become a HDL core cholesterol ester. Subsequently, cholesterol ester in HDL can be exchanged with VLDL and LDL through the action of cholesterol ester transfer protein, or HDL cholesterol can be returned to the liver.

Lipoprotein (a)

ApoA is a complex protein with a protease domain and multiple repeats, called kringles, which have considerable homology with plasminogen. It is linked by a single disulphide bridge to the apoB of a LDL molecule to give lipoprotein (a). The apo (a) gene is highly polymorphic and lipoprotein (a) levels are mainly genetically determined.

Interest in lipoprotein (a) stems from its reported association with the presence, severity, and progression of coronary heart disease (Terres et al. 1995). However, the risk of atherosclerosis may be most when high levels of lipoprotein (a) are associated with concomitant elevation in LDL–cholesterol levels (Maher and Brown 1995). High lipoprotein (a) levels are linked to premature macrovascular disease, but may not be as good a predictor of atheroma in the long term. Recent work in transgenic mice suggests that lipoprotein (a) acts to inhibit plasminogen activation, leading to reduced activation of transforming growth factor-β which has several adverse effects on vessel wall function (Grainger et al. 1994).

Lipids and inflammation

Essential fatty acids and inflammatory mediators

In addition to being core components of complex lipids, fatty acids are either incorporated into cell membranes or serve as precursors for biologically active metabolites, such as prostaglandins and leukotrienes. Essential fatty acids such as linoleic acid cannot be synthesized by mammals and are required in the diet. Polyunsaturated fatty acids contain at least two double bonds in their carbon backbone. Arachidonic acid is the commonest dietary polyunsaturated fatty acids and is a precursor for the potent proinflammatory 2-series prostanoids, via the action of cyclo-oxygenase, and for the 5-series leukotrienes, via the action of 5-lipoxygenase. Metabolites of arachidonic acid are also intimately involved in the early events controlling coagulation and vascular homeostasis. Platelet-derived thromboxane-A_2 is a powerful vasoconstrictor and causes platelet aggregation, whereas endothelial-derived prostacyclin, or PGI_2, causes vasodilatation and opposes platelet aggregation.

Omega-3 fatty acids are essential polyunsaturated fatty acids found in fish oils and include eicosapentaenoic acid. They are precursors of the 3-series prostanoids and the 5-series leukotrienes which competitively inhibit formation of proinflammatory eicosanoids derived from arachidonic acid. Another natural source of essential fatty acids is evening primrose oil which contains predominately gammalinoleic acid. This is a precursor of prostaglandin E_1 and of 15-OH-dihomo-gammalinoleic acid. Prostaglandin E_1 has anti-inflammatory effects and 15-OH-dihomo-gammalinoleic acid inhibits both 5- and 12-lipoxygenases, which generate proinflammatory eicosanoids.

Lipid peroxidation and antioxidants

Polyunsaturated fatty acids are the main target for lipoperoxidative injury by oxygen free radicals. In particular, polyunsaturated fatty acids and their attached phospholipid in plasma LDL can be oxidized by endothelial cells and macrophages. Oxidized LDL may exert several proinflammatory effects by virtue of its chemotactic, cytotoxic, and, possibly, immunogenic properties. LDL is modified by close contact with endothelial cells and becomes a much more ready substrate for scavenger uptake by subintimal macrophages. Hence, endothelially minimally-modified LDL is taken up by receptors on scavenger cells which become lipid-laden foam cells, representing an early event in atheroma formation. LDL3 in particular is more likely to be oxidized, to be immunogenic, to be poorly recognized by the LDL receptor, and more readily taken up by the scavenger pathway.

Therefore, the generation of oxidized LDL may be an important factor in atherosclerosis, in addition to contributing to proinflammatory mechanisms in rheumatological disorders.

Certain micronutrients, such as selenium and vitamins A and E, act as antioxidants by preventing the accumulation of oxygen free radicals (Fox 1996). Levels of antioxidants may also have relevance to the susceptibility of LDL to oxidation. As the fat-soluble, antioxidant vitamins are carried on lipoproteins such as LDL, the antioxidant levels may be reflected in the delay time before oxidation propagation occurs in LDL.

Types of hyperlipidaemia

Various patterns of elevated lipoproteins have been recognized (Table 2). However, most patterns can be caused by several different genetic disorders or they may be secondary to other metabolic disturbances. Many hyperlipidaemias are the result of environmental factors exacerbating an underlying monogenic or, more usually, polygenic hyperlipidaemic tendency or background. Nonetheless it is worth considering a framework to classify the primary inherited hyperlipidaemias, as shown in Table 3, together with what is known about their genetic basis. The pattern of secondary hyperlipidaemia associated with several rheumatic disorders will be discussed.

It is worth mentioning here that several drugs used in the treatment of hyperlipidaemia are known to give rise to rheumatic complaints, although this is extremely rare. Myopathy has been described in patients treated with statins, fibrates, or nicotinic acid (Zuckner 1990; Goldman et al. 1989; Ross Peirce et al. 1990). Rhabdomyolysis is also possible, although rare (Hino et al. 1996). However, early reports included patients on cyclosporin following heart transplantation, where cyclosporin impaired renal clearance of statins. Recently, the Committee on the Safety of Medicines have calculated that the statin or the fibrate use risk of serious myositis is less than one per 100 000 patient years exposure. Use of statin and fibrate together may increase the risk and milder cases of myositis may be missed. There are case reports of drug-induced lupus caused by lovostatin and clofibrate (Ahmad 1991; Howard and Brown 1973).

Table 2 Patterns of dyslipidaemia

Lipoprotein pattern	Lipoprotein	Lipid
Type 1	Chylomicrons	Triglycerides
Type 2a	LDL	Cholesterol
Type 2b	LDL and some VLDL	Cholesterol and triglycerides
Type 3	Chylomicron remnants and IDL	Triglycerides and cholesterol
Type 4	VLDL	Triglycerides
Type 5	VLDL and chylomicrons	Triglycerides (and some cholesterol)

Table 3 Primary hyperlipidaemias

Genetic disorder	Biochemical defect	Lipoproteins elevated (pattern)	Clinical findings
Lipoprotein lipase deficiency	Lipoprotein lipase deficiency	Chylomicrons (1)	Pancreatitis, eruptive xanthomata
Apoprotein CII deficiency	Apoprotein CII deficiency	Chylomicrons and VLDL (1 or 5)	Pancreatitis
Familial type 4 hyperlipoproteinaemia	Abnormal apoprotein E	Chylomicron remnants and IDL (3)	Palmar and tuberous xanthomata, premature atherosclerosis
Familial hypercholesterolaemia	LDL receptor deficiency	LDL (2A)	Tendon xanthomata, premature atherosclerosis
Familial hypertriglyceridaemia	Unknown	VLDL (4)	Eruptive xanthomata
Familial combined hyperlipidaemia	Unknown	LDL and VLDL (2a, 2b, 4)	

Musculoskeletal manifestations of primary hyperlipidaemia

Musculoskeletal symptoms or signs may be the first manifestation of a hyperlipidaemia. A transient polyarthritis is especially common in patients with familial hypercholesterolaemia. Larger rather than smaller peripheral joints tend to be affected. In 1968, Khadchadurian studied 14 families from whom 18 homozygotes with type 2 hyperlipoproteinaemia were identified (Khadchadurian 1968). Ten of these patients experienced a migratory polyarthritis resembling rheumatic fever. A monoarthritis or oligoarthritis may also occur in heterozygotes, commonly affecting the knee or occasionally the first metatarsophalangeal joint. Oligoarthritis and periarticular hyperaesthesia have been described in patients with type 4 hyperlipidaemia (Goldman *et al.* 1972; Buckingham *et al.* 1975). Articular manifestations have not been reported for type 1 or type 3 hyperlipidaemia.

Recurrent tendinitis is a common problem in patients with familial hypercholesterolaemia. Tendinous, tuberous, or periosteal xanthomata may also be present. Common sites for tendon xanthomata are the tendo-Achillis, patellar tendons and extensor tendons of the hands and feet. Sometimes, tenosynovitis may occur without obvious xanthomata. Tendinitis may occur during the early weeks of statin use, usually in patients with very high cholesterol levels. These episodes may result from the mobilization of deposited tissue cholesterol as blood levels fall with treatment, rather analogous to the acute gout that accompanies urate mobilization in the initial weeks of allopurinol treatment. Palmar xanthomata are typically seen in type III, remnant lipidaemia (familial dysbetalipoproteinaemia). Type I, V, and severe IV hyperlipoproteinaemias may be associated with eruptive xanthomatas over the knees, buttocks, shoulders, and back.

In addition to diet and change of lifestyle, for primary hypercholesterolaemia requiring drug therapy, statins (3-hydroxy-3-methylglutaryl coenzyme A, HMG Co-A, reductase inhibitors) are the agents of choice, with or without resins (bile acid sequestrants) where tolerated. For mixed lipidaemia fibrate drugs (fenofibrate, ciprofibrate, bezafibrate, or gemfibrozil) are first choice.

In a recent study of 80 patients with hyperlipidaemia, tendon xanthomatas, particularly of the tendo-Achillis, were found in about 50 per cent of patients with either adult familial hypercholesterolaemia or with mixed hyperlipidaemia (increased cholesterol and triglycerides), often with an associated tendinitis (Klemp *et al.* 1993). Oligoarthritis was seen only in patients with mixed hyperlipidaemia. The manifestations improved with lipid-lowering therapy.

Most cases of acute arthropathy associated with hyperlipidaemia resolve spontaneously. The synovial fluid is usually non-inflammatory. Positively birefringent suspected lipid crystals have been aspirated from a bursitis in a patient with hypercholesterolaemia (Schumaker and Michaels 1989). Subcutaneous cholesterol nodules mimicking rheumatoid nodules and gouty tophi have been described in patients with an apparently normal lipid profile (Szachnowski and Bridges 1994).

Lipids in joints

Lipid microspherules have been found in the joints of patients with rheumatoid arthritis. The mean levels of apoAI, apoB, and cholesterol levels were significantly higher in the synovial fluid of 12 patients with untreated rheumatoid arthritis than in eight patients with degenerative joint disease (Ananth *et al.* 1993). A likely explanation is the increased permeability for these lipoprotein constituents across inflamed synovial membranes. Lazarevic *et al.* did not find concomitant systemic lipid abnormalities nor the presence of antilipoprotein antibodies in such patients (Lazarevic *et al.* 1993a).

Whether synovial lipoproteins are involved in the pathogenesis of rheumatoid arthritis is unclear. Winyard *et al.* have reported positive immunostaining for oxidized LDL in synovial membranes from six patients with rheumatoid arthritis (Winyard *et al.* 1993). The staining was confined to foamy macrophages in the region of synovial blood vessels. The authors point out that inflamed synovial tissue has all the appropriate requirements for enhanced lipid peroxidation, such as macrophage enrichment, extensive iron deposits, and reduced concentrations of antioxidants such as vitamin E. Also, peroxidation products, such as 4-hydroxynonenal, have been detected in synovial fluid (Selley *et al.* 1992). Fairburn *et al.* found reduced levels of the lipid soluble antioxidant α-tocopherol, which terminates the process of lipid peroxidation, suggesting depleted levels may point to increased oxidative activity (Fairburn *et al.* 1992).

The pattern of dyslipidaemia in rheumatic disorders

Low levels of HDL have been found in several chronic inflammatory disorders and seem related to disease activity. Ilowite *et al.* identified such a pattern in a set of paediatric systemic lupus erythematosus patients studied longitudinally (Ilowite *et al.* 1988). The mean HDL–cholesterol and apoA1 were markedly lower in untreated and clinically active systemic lupus erythematosus patients compared to controls. Levels of HDL–cholesterol and apoA1 returned to normal as the systemic lupus erythematosus became less active. In our own patients in Bath, low levels of HDL were found with systemic lupus erythematosus (Leong *et al.* 1995) and psoriatic arthritis (Jones *et al.* 1994) which was most noticeable in those patients with active disease. In rheumatoid arthritis, low levels of HDL–cholesterol have been found, which return to normal with treatment of the arthritis (Lazarevic *et al.* 1992; Svenson *et al.* 1987a; Svenson *et al.* 1987b).

Low levels of HDL are normally associated with high triglycerides epidemiologically. However, there are conflicting results for levels of other lipoprotein components apart from HDL in rheumatic disorders, which may be explained by confounding influences such as corticosteroid treatment, renal disease, and possibly altered catabolic states associated with chronic inflammation. Ilowite *et al.* (Ilowite *et al.* 1988) found an increase in total triglycerides and VLDL–cholesterol in children with systemic lupus erythematosus. Our systemic lupus erythematosus patients selected for absence of renal disease or corticosteroid treatment had lower levels of total cholesterol, triglycerides, and total LDL (although LDL-3 was increased) but VLDL was unchanged (Leong *et al.* 1995). A similar pattern was seen in patients with psoriatic arthritis where only LDL-3 was increased (Jones *et al.* 1994). Svenson *et al.* studied 48 patients with untreated rheumatoid arthritis and 21 with seronegative spondylarthropathy. Compared to healthy controls, the patients with active rheumatic disease had lower levels of VLDL–cholesterol and VLDL–triglyceride, as well as lower HDL–triglyceride and HDL–cholesterol (Svenson *et al.* 1987a). Lazarevic *et al.* also found low levels of LDL–cholesterol in patients with active rheumatoid arthritis or psoriatic arthritis (Lazarevic *et al.* 1992).

In individuals without rheumatic disorders, the usual effect of endogenous steroids (Cushing's syndrome) or of exogenous steroid therapy is predominantly to increase serum cholesterol, due to increased LDL–cholesterol and often VLDL–cholesterol. There is often increased triglycerides but this is less obvious unless there are additional reasons for hypertriglyceridaemia, such as diabetes (Havel *et al.* 1980) or underlying polygenic mixed hyperlipidaemia. HDL–cholesterol may rise with prednisolone treatment (Zimmerman *et al.* 1984).

The use of corticosteroids or nephrotic syndrome contributes to a type 2b hyperlipidaemia (raised cholesterol with moderately raised triglycerides). Ettinger *et al.* compared 46 systemic lupus erythematosus patients with 30 controls and found that systemic lupus erythematosus patients on corticosteroids had higher levels of total cholesterol, total triglyceride, and LDL–cholesterol (Ettinger *et al.* 1987; Ettinger and Hazzard 1988). Those who were not on steroids had levels similar to controls, apart from a lower HDL–cholesterol. Similar results were found in a study of 100 Singaporean Chinese patients with systemic lupus erythematosus (Leong *et al.* 1994). In the latter study, the type 2b pattern was associated with renal involvement and the use of corticosteroids. MacGregor *et al.* found raised concentrations of triglyceride and apoB in systemic lupus erythematosus patients treated with corticosteroids (MacGregor *et al.* 1992).

Evidence for increased mortality from atherosclerosis in rheumatic disorders

Rheumatoid arthritis is associated with an increased mortality. Mortality is higher in those with more severe disease (Wolfe *et al.* 1994). Prior *et al.* studied 489 consecutive patients with classical rheumatoid arthritis followed-up for a mean of 11.2 years and found a three-fold increase in overall mortality compared with age and gender-specific rates in the general population (Prior *et al.* 1984). Cardiovascular deaths were 2.5 times higher than expected values compared to age and gender-matched population figures. Rasker and Cosh followed a cohort of 100 patients for 18 years (Rasker and Cosh 1981). Of the 43 patients who died, 16 deaths were related to rheumatoid arthritis and 27 were unrelated. In the latter group, 14 were cardiac deaths and 8 were cerebrovascular events. However, results from other studies recording causes of death in 2262 rheumatoid arthritis patients from 13 centres, suggests that cardiovascular disease accounts for 40 per cent of deaths in rheumatoid arthritis which was no different from the general population (Pincus and Callahan 1986).

Urowitz *et al.* recognized a bimodal pattern of mortality in systemic lupus erythematosus with early deaths due to active disease or infections and late events related to atherosclerotic complications (Urowitz *et al.* 1976). Further analysis of 665 patients from the same centre largely confirmed the earlier findings, with about a five-fold overall excess death rate in systemic lupus erythematosus (Abu-Shakra *et al.* 1995). The authors concluded that atherosclerosis is a major cause of death and morbidity in patients with systemic lupus erythematosus. It is not clear whether the late cardiovascular disease is related primarily to corticosteroid treatment or to other manifestations of the disease. Petri *et al.* studied prospectively the risk factors for coronary artery disease in 229 systemic lupus erythematosus patients (Petri *et al.* 1992). Nineteen patients (8.3 per cent) had coronary artery disease which was associated with age at systemic lupus erythematosus diagnosis, duration of corticosteroid use, requirement for antihypertensive treatment, maximum cholesterol level, and obesity.

Many studies, including autopsy studies, have shown premature coronary atherosclerosis and myocardial infarction in relatively young patients with systemic lupus erythematosus. Bulkley and Roberts compared necroscopy findings of 36 systemic lupus erythematosus patients on corticosteroids with findings in patients not on corticosteroids (Buckley and Roberts 1975). Subepicardial and myocardial fat was increased in all the former group. In 42 per cent of the 18 patients who received corticosteroids for more than 1 year, the lumen of at least one of the three major coronary arteries was narrowed by more than 50 per cent by atherosclerotic plaques. In contrast, none of the 17 patients who received corticosteroids for less than 1 year, and who were on average 5 years older, had such findings. Systemic hypertension was twice as common in patients who received corticosteroids for longer than 1 year.

A number of other chronic rheumatic disorders are associated with a shortened life expectancy (Callahan and Pincus 1995). Patients with renal involvement and scleroderma, vasculitis, or systemic lupus erythematosus generally have the poorest prognosis. However, conditions thought to have a better outlook, such as ankylosing spondylitis, may also have an excess death rate (Radford et al. 1977; Rigby 1991). Current data suggests that there is a tendency for premature death in patients with rheumatic diseases. One significant contributor is the presence of cardiovascular or cerebrovascular disease. Longer-term, prospective studies with appropriate population controls will help clarify risk factors. As our ability to manage patients improves due to our increasing knowledge, survival of patients will be prolonged, as has already happened with systemic lupus erythematosus. Awareness of potential problems from premature atherosclerosis will become increasingly important.

Mechanisms for dyslipidaemia

Several mechanisms may account for the dyslipidaemia associated with chronic inflammatory disorders. Lipoprotein lipase is a membrane-bound enzyme responsible for liberation of fatty acids from VLDL resulting in formation of LDL. Reduced mass or inhibition of activity of lipoprotein lipase is an attractive hypothesis as it would account for reduced clearance of VLDL–triglyceride and an associated rise in plasma triglycerides. Normal or slightly low LDL–cholesterol would be expected as a result of lower precursor input into LDL — and LDL concentrations in plasma would tend to fall. HDL levels would also tend to fall because there would be a slower reduction in VLDL size, and therefore less VLDL surface coat given up to provide HDL.

Lipoprotein lipase activity is inhibited by several regulatory cytokines such as tumour necrosis factor-α (Fried and Zechner 1989), interleukin-1, and γ-interferon (Querfeld et al. 1990), that are upregulated in inflammation. Furthermore, 24-h infusion of recombinant human tumour necrosis factor-α is associated with a decrease in serum cholesterol and HDL levels (Spriggs et al. 1988). However, tumour necrosis factor-α and other cytokines may also stimulate hepatic lipid secretion and increase de novo fatty acid synthesis (Feingold and Grunfeld 1992). Lipoprotein lipase is also an insulin-dependent enzyme and its synthesis in adipose and muscle is increased by insulin treatment. Whether the dyslipidaemia in active rheumatic disease may be due to a form of insulin resistance is not known. Hypertriglyceridaemia, low HDL, small dense LDL3, and insulin resistance (known as the atherogenic lipid profile) is often accompanied by glucose intolerance or diabetes, hypertension, hyperuricaemia, or gout, and procoagulant changes with high PA1–1 and fibrinogen.

Alternatively, an increased production of acute phase proteins by the liver in inflammation may occur at the expense of lipoprotein production. Also, acute phase reactants may interfere with HDL metabolism. Kumon et al. showed that in patients with rheumatic disease, total HDL cholesterol, apoA-I, and apoA-II were lower than in normal subjects and were inversely correlated with plasma concentrations of serum amyloid A protein (Kumon et al. 1993). It was suggested that serum amyloid A protein may displace apoA-I and apoA-II on HDL particles, and especially on HDL3.

Corticosteroids cause increased hepatic production of VLDL resulting in elevated plasma cholesterol, plasma triglyceride, HDL-C, VLDL-C, and LDL-C. Proteinuria leads to increased generalized hepatic protein synthesis, and hence lipoprotein synthesis which may also be driven by urinary loss of apoA of HDL. Conversely, control of hyperlipidaemia may retard the development of glomerulosclerosis (Kasiske et al. 1988).

Antibody-mediated mechanisms may also be important. Lazarevic et al. found antilipoprotein antibodies against VLDL and LDL in one-third of patients with active rheumatoid arthritis, but not in patients with osteoarthritis, psoriatic arthritis, or healthy blood donors (Lazarevic et al. 1993b). Autoantibodies against LDL have been demonstrated in diabetes mellitus. More recently anti-apoA1 antibodies have been described in systemic lupus erythematosus (Merrill et al. 1995). Rarely, antibodies against apoC-II may be associated with severe hypertriglyceridaemia, due to myeloma and clonal production of the antibody.

Rheumatic disorders

Systemic lupus erythematosus

Mechanisms accounting for vasculopathy

Factors to account for the increase in vascular disease in systemic lupus erythematosus include corticosteroid treatment, renal disease, dyslipidaemia, an underlying coagulopathy, vasculitis, and, possibly, antibody or immune-complex mediated injury. In support of the latter, Kabakov et al. demonstrated that in the presence of lupus sera, lipid accumulation in cultured smooth muscle cells is increased up to six fold compared to cells cultured with normal human sera from healthy donors (Kabakov et al. 1992). Incubation of the smooth muscle cells with circulating immune complexes isolated from lupus sera caused a three to four-fold increase in intracellular cholesterol level. The atherogenic effect was thought to be due to LDL-containing immune complexes.

Lipoprotein (a)

There are conflicting findings concerning the levels of lipoprotein (a) in systemic lupus erythematosus and the risk of thrombosis. Takegoshi reported a case of an 18-year-old systemic lupus erythematosus patient who had severe elevations of lipoprotein (a) associated with myocardial infarction and cerebral infarction (Takegoshi et al. 1990). Elevated levels of lipoprotein (a) levels have been reported in a few studies of patients with systemic lupus erythematosus (Matsuda et al. 1994; Borba et al. 1994) but not in association with thrombosis, which is in accordance with our own unpublished results. However, one recent study found increased lipoprotein (a) levels in systemic lupus erythematosus patients with myocardial and cerebral infarction (Kawai et al. 1995).

Lipids and antiphospholipid antibodies

The interplay between lipid abnormalities and antiphospholipid antibodies may be complex. A plasma cofactor which forms part of the antigenic complex recognized by antiphospholipid antibodies has been identified as β_2-glycoprotein I or apoH. Whether lipoproteins other than β_2-glycoprotein I are involved in the pathogenesis of the antiphospholipid syndrome is unknown. There may be an additive risk of thrombotic clinical events if both antiphospholipid antibodies and hyperlipidaemia are present together (Garrido *et al.* 1994). Lahita *et al.* found an association between anticardiolipin antibodies and low levels of HDL and apoAI, although cholesterol levels were also low in these patients (Lahita *et al.* 1993).

Antibodies to oxidized LDL have been described in patients with systemic lupus erythematosus (Vaarala *et al.* 1993). Monoclonal antibodies to cardiolipin have been derived from a mouse model of the antiphospholipid syndrome that have reactivity against β_2-glycoprotein and cross-react with oxidized LDL (Mizutani *et al.* 1995). In a prospective study of middle-aged dyslipidaemic men, there was a correlation between anticardiolipin levels and antibodies to oxidized LDL and the presence of both had an additive risk for myocardial infarction (Vaarala *et al.* 1995).

Rheumatoid arthritis

Most studies have shown that patients with rheumatoid arthritis have a lipid profile that increases the risk of atherosclerosis, especially when samples are studied during active phases of the disease (Lazarevic *et al.* 1992; Svenson 1987a; Svenson 1987b; Rantapää-Dahlqvist *et al.* 1991). The most consistent abnormality is a reduction in HDL. Magaro *et al.* reported lower levels of apoA1 compared with controls, although apoB was also reduced (Magaro *et al.* 1991). Lipoprotein (a) levels may also be increased (Rantapää-Dahlqvist *et al.* 1991). Therefore, dyslipidaemia associated with active rheumatoid arthritis needs to be considered as a contributing factor to the excess death rate observed in mortality studies.

Psoriatic arthritis

Patients with psoriatic arthritis have a similar pattern of dyslipidaemia to that occurring in rheumatoid arthritis (Lazarevic *et al.* 1992). Jones *et al.* found an atherogenic profile with low total HDL and HDL3, and elevated LDL3 and lipoprotein (a) levels (Jones *et al.* 1994). Elevated LDL3 may be particulary important as this small, dense subclass of LDL is much more likely to be taken up by macrophages in the arterial subintimal space, possibly explaining its association with coronary artery disease (Campos *et al.* 1992).

There may also be an imbalance in fatty acids and antioxidants either contributing to disease pathogenesis or as a secondary metabolic consequence of chronic inflammation. Azzini *et al.* found abnormalities in red blood cell fatty acid composition with increased total fatty acids and decreased ω-6 polyunsaturated fatty acids (Azzini *et al.* 1995). Reduced levels of the antioxidant selenium and increased plasma concentrations of copper were also found (Azzini *et al.* 1995).

Systemic sclerosis

Vascular impairment secondary to reperfusion injury and the formation of free radicals are postulated as disease mechanisms in scleroderma. Bruckdorfer *et al.* reported that LDL in patients with systemic sclerosis are more susceptible to oxidation (Bruckdorfer *et al.* 1995). In addition to its toxic effects on endothelium, oxidized LDL may potentially contribute to the increased matrix synthesis seen in systemic sclerosis by upregulating certain adhesion molecules and growth factors such as platelet-derived growth factor.

Gout

There is a clear association between gout and type 4 hyperlipidaemia. Decreased HDL–cholesterol and increased VLDL levels have been reported (Ulreich *et al.* 1985; Matsubara *et al.* 1989). The association is unlikely to be causal as patients with gout often have other predisposing factors for hyperlipidaemia, such as obesity, increased alcohol consumption, and altered nutritional habit. Furthermore, in the disorder of insulin resistance the syndrome complex includes hyperuricaemia with or without gout, hypertension, mixed dyslipidaemia, glucose intolerance or diabetes mellitus, central obesity, hyperfibrinogenaemia, high PAI-1, and associated coronary heart disease and peripheral vascular disease.

Hyperlipidaemia may also be more directly associated with decreased renal excretion of uric acid. Renal excretion of urate is lower in hyperuricaemic–hyperlipidaemic patients than in hyperuricaemic–normolipidaemic patients. Tinahones *et al.* reported increased VLDL levels, diminished fractional excretion of uric acid, and increased apoCIII/CII ratios in patients with hyperuricaemia and hypertriglyceridaemia (Tinahones *et al.* 1995). ApoCIII inhibits the hydrolysis of triglycerides by lipoprotein and hepatic lipase, whereas apoCII is an activator of lipoprotein lipase. An altered apoCIII/CII ratio would lengthen the time VLDL remains in the plasma. The mechanism is unknown whereby lipids are directly or indirectly associated with altered renal handling of urate.

Management

The use of essential fatty acids in the treatment of rheumatic diseases

The use of essential fatty acids to treat inflammation has a supportive in vivo and biochemical basis, although the clinical efficacy and cost-effectiveness of such treatment in man remains uncertain. In animal models, marine oils have been effective in suppressing inflammation. Eicosapentaenoic acid supplementation prevented renal disease from developing in NZB/NZW mice (Prickett *et al.* 1981). A fish oil diet had a beneficial effect on the severity of collagen-induced arthritis (Cathcart and Gonnerman 1991) and on lupus-like features in MRL-*lpr* mice (Robinson *et al.* 1986).

Prostaglandins are synthesized from essential fatty acids (see above). The addition of omega 3 or omega 6 polyunsaturated fatty acids to the diet may shift the balance of prostaglandin metabolism towards substances that have less of a proinflammatory action. The two most extensively studied therapies have been fish oils and evening primrose oil. The former contains high levels of polyunsaturated fatty acids of the omega-3 series (such as eicosapentaenoic acid and docosahexaenoic acid) and the latter predominantly gammalinoleic acid.

Several studies in rheumatoid arthritis have shown some beneficial effects of diets containing essential fatty acids in fish oils, such as a reduced requirement for non-steroidal anti-inflammatory drugs (Lau *et al.* 1993). In a study of 66 patients randomized to fish oil or corn oil, Kremer *et al.* reported a decreased number of tender joints, morning stiffness, and global arthritis activity and pain in the fish oil group (Kremer *et al.* 1995). Geusens *et al.* studied 90 patients on various dosage regimes of fish versus olive oil and found an improvement in the patients' global evaluation and physicians' assessment of pain in those patients taking the higher dose of fish oil (2.6 g/day)

(Geusens *et al.* 1994). It is worth mentioning that olive oil may also have some active beneficial effects as it contains mainly unsaturated fats. Gammalinoleic acid at a dose of 1.4 g/day was better than placebo in improving joint tenderness and swelling in patients with rheumatoid arthritis (Leventhal *et al.* 1993).

There is some evidence that fish oils may be beneficial in other conditions such as psoriasis and systemic lupus erythematosus. Bittiner reported decreased pruritus, erythema, and scaling of skin psoriasis in 28 patients treated with fish oil compared to a placebo (Bittiner *et al.* 1988). A number of studies have reported an improvement in skin lesions with eicosapentaenoic acid. However, a preparation containing eicosapentaenoic acid, gammalinoleic acid, and decosahexaenoic acid (Efamol) had no significant beneficial effect in patients with psoriatic arthritis despite a fall in leukotriene B4 (Veale *et al.* 1994). It is possible that an insufficient dose of eicosapentaenoic acid was used in the latter study. In a study of 27 patients with active systemic lupus erythematosus, symptoms were favourably affected by an eicosapentaenoic acid enriched diet in 14 patients compared to placebo (Walton *et al.* 1991). Another benefit of a fish oil diet is an alteration of the thromboxane/prostacyclin ratio towards substantially less thrombotic thromboxane and a substantially more antithrombotic prostacyclin.

It is important to note that the amount of essential fatty acids needed to produce clinical effects are often in excess of the dose available in commercial preparation. Also, it may be difficult to achieve such doses by ingestion of natural food substances. Fahrer *et al.* found that 7.5 g of fish oil, the therapeutic dose in many studies, is the equivalent of 700 g of fish (Fahrer *et al.* 1991) and carries a 70 calorie load. This means that four to six meals of fish per week are required in order to induce a potentially useful anti-inflammatory effect.

Longer-term studies with larger numbers of patients are required to help clarify the therapeutic role of essential fatty acids. It is possible that essential fatty acid supplementation may be a reasonable treatment alternative to non-steroidal anti-inflammatory agents, especially when the latter are contraindicated. Fish oils can improve moderate to marked hypertriglyceridaemia in some individuals, but do not alter LDL-cholesterol much — a dose of 10 g of fish oil (as Maxepa) being needed, equivalent to 90 calories daily.

Rationale for lipid-lowering treatment

Rheumatic diseases may well carry an increased risk of morbidity and mortality from premature atherosclerosis, although more evidence is needed. Abnormalities in the LDL subfraction are clearly present in patients on long-term corticosteroid treatment (Ettinger *et al.* 1987; Ettinger and Hazzard 1988; MacGregor *et al.* 1992). Many studies have shown the relationship between hypercholesterolaemia and the risk of coronary artery disease. The Framingham study showed that the risk of myocardial infarction was associated with higher levels of LDL-cholesterol and inversely associated with HDL levels (Castelli *et al.* 1986), as did the study of 362 262 American men screened from the Multiple Risk Factor Intervention Trial (Neaton *et al.* 1992). Therefore the dyslipidaemia present in chronic rheumatic diseases would appear to increase the risk of atheroma.

There is good evidence that the treatment of lipid abnormalities influences outcome, with reduced coronary heart disease deaths and events. In older studies, this was shown for cholesterol lowering with cholestyramine (Lipid Research Clinics Program 1984) or with gemfibrozil where triglyceride was also lowered and HDL cholesterol raised (Frick *et al.* 1987). More recently, the more potent statins have shown reduction in coronary heart disease deaths and events, in coronary artery surgery requirements, and in total mortality, both in primary (West of Scotland Coronary Prevention Study) (Shepherd *et al.* 1995) and in secondary (Scandinavian Simvastatin Survival Study) (Scandinavian Simvastatin Survival Study 1994) prevention studies. Many studies (e.g. Blankenhorn *et al.* 1987) have shown slowing of progression, and some regression, of atheroma in patients actively treated for hyperlipidaemia after coronary artery graft surgery.

Approach to treatment

Risk factors for hyperlipidaemia need to be assessed for the individual patient. A basic fasting lipid profile may be appropriate on any patient with a chronic inflammatory rheumatic disease, although subtle changes in lipid subfraction composition may be missed. Other associated risk factors, such as hypertension, diabetes, and smoking, are important and need to be fully discussed with the patient and managed.

Dietary intervention plays a major role in the management of hyperlipidaemia. While dietary change may produce only modest change in lipid levels, dietary modification may be all that is necessary in moderate hyperlipidaemia. Target levels for treatment of dyslipidaemia have been set in national and international guidelines (National Cholesterol Education Program 1994; Pyorala *et al.* 1994). In systemic lupus erythematosus, benefit of dietary change at 6 months has been shown in patients receiving corticosteroids (Hearth-Holmes *et al.* 1995). In adolescents with systemic lupus erythematosus, dietary modification with fish oil supplementation improved the lipid profile (Ilowite *et al.* 1995). However, a significant number of systemic lupus erythematosus patients might require further pharmacological therapy for persistent dyslipidaemia, with statins, fibrates, or other agents.

The role of hydroxychloroquine

Hydroxychloroquine is often used in the treatment of mild systemic lupus erythematosus and rheumatoid arthritis. Besides its immunomodulatory properties, hydroxychloroquine may have a protective role against hyperlipidaemia induced by corticosteroids. In a case–control study, patients with systemic lupus erythematosus on hydroxychloroquine had 35 to 45 per cent lower levels of total triglyceride, VLDL-triglyceride, LDL-triglyceride, and apoCIII than patients not on treatment (Hodis *et al.* 1993). Wallace *et al.* found that hydroxychloroquine was strongly associated with low levels of cholesterol, triglycerides, and LDL-cholesterol regardless of concomitant corticosteroid use (Wallace *et al.* 1990). In a cohort longitudinal study involving 264 patients with systemic lupus erythematosus (Petri *et al.* 1994) using a regression model for steroid use, a change in prednisolone dose of 10 mg was associated with a change in cholesterol level of 7.5 mg ($\pm$ 1.46 SD) and a weight gain of 2.5 kg ($\pm$ 0.6 SD). On the other hand, hydroxychloroquine at 200 mg or 400 mg/day were both associated with lower serum cholesterol. However, no prospective randomized study of hydroxychloroquine on lipoprotein and lipid levels has been carried out.

Conclusions

There is sufficient evidence to suggest that lipid metabolism is altered in chronic rheumatic diseases in a manner which may promote accelerated atherosclerosis. Further long-term studies are needed to determine the risk more precisely and that contributed by treatments such as corticosteroids. Dietary intervention would seem a sensible first treatment step, and lipid lowering agents may be required, appropriate target levels being cholesterol less than 5.0 mmol/l, triglyceride less than 2 mmol/l, and LDL–cholesterol less than 3.5 mmol/l. A prudent, low-fat diet, partly supplemented by mono- and polyunsaturated fatty acids, with high fibre should be encouraged. Whether dietary supplementaion with marine oils has a place in reducing requirements for anti-inflammatory agents is uncertain, although the dose of fat supplement may be unacceptable.

Lipid peroxidation products such as oxidized LDL may play an important role in promoting endothelial and synovial injury in addition to atheroma and, together with the possible protective role of antioxidants, warrant further study. Where patients have risk factors for coronary heart disease in addition to those from the rheumatic disease itself, for example in patients with systemic lupus erythematosus and hypertension, attention to all possible risk factors may be necessary to help prevent coronary heart disease. Treatment of risk factors is essential in patients who have manifested macrovascular disease, where there is adequate further life expectancy.

References

Abu-Shakra, M., Urowitz, M.B., Gladman, D.D., and Gough, J. (1995). Mortality studies in systemic lupus erythematosus. Results from a single centre. 1.Causes of death. *Journal of Rheumatology*, **22**, 1259–64.

Ahmad, S. (1991). Lovastatin-induced lupus erythematosus. *Archives of Internal Medicine*, **151**, 1667–8.

Ananth, L., Prete, P.E., and Kashyap, M.L. (1993). Apolipoproteins A-I and B and cholesterol in synovial fluid of patients with rheumatoid arthritis. *Clinical and Experimental Metabolism*, **42**, 803–6.

Azzini, M., Girelli, D., Olivieri, O., Guarini, P., Stanzial, A.M., Frigo, A., Milanino, R., Bambara, L.M., and Corrocher, R. (1995). Fatty acids and antioxidant micronutrients in psoriatic arthritis. *Journal of Rheumatology*, **22**, 103–8.

Bittiner, S.B., Tucker, W.F.G., Cartwright, I., and Bleehen, S.S. (1988). A double-blind, randomised, placebo-controlled trial of fish oil in psoriasis. *Lancet*, **i**, 378–80.

Blankenhorn, D.H., Nessim, S.A., and Johnson, R.L. (1987). Beneficial effects of combined colestipol-niacin therapy on coronary atherosclerosis and coronary venous bypass grafts. *Journal of the American Medical Association*, **257**, 3233.

Borba, E.F., Santos, R.D., Bonfa, E., Vinagre, C.G., Pileggi, F.J.C., Cossermelli, W., and Maranhao, R.C. (1994). Lipoprotein(a) levels in systemic lupus erythematosus. *Journal of Rheumatology*, **21**, 220–3.

Bruckdorfer, K.R., Hillary, J.B., Bunce, T., Vancheeswaran, R., and Black, C.M. (1995). Increased susceptibility to oxidation of low-density lipoproteins isolated from patients with systemic sclerosis. *Arthritis and Rheumatism*, **38**, 1060–7.

Buckingham, R.B., Bole, G.G., and Bassett, D.R. (1975). Polyarthritis associated with Type IV lipoproteinemia. *Archives of Internal Medicine*, **135**, 286–90.

Buckley, B.H. and Roberts, W.C. (1975). The heart in systemic lupus erythematosus and the changes induced in it by corticosteroid therapy — a study of 36 necrosopy patients. *American Journal of Medicine*, **58**, 243–63.

Callahan, L.F. and Pincus, T. (1995). Mortality in rheumatic diseases. *Arthritis Care and Research*, **8**, 229–41.

Campos, H., Genest, Jr J.J., Blijlevan, S.E., McNamara, J.R., Jenner, J.L., Ordovas, J.M., Wilson, P.N.F., and Schaefer, E.J. (1992). LDL particle size and coronary artery disease. *Arteriosclerosis and Thrombosis*, **12**, 187–95.

Castelli, W.P., Garrison, R.J., and Wilson, P.W.F. (1986). Incidence of coronary heart disease and lipoprotein cholesterol levels. *Journal of the American Medical Association*, **256**, 2835.

Cathcart, E.S. and Gonnerman, W.A. (1991). Fish oil fatty acids and experimental arthritis. *Rheumatic Disease Clinics of North America*, **17**, 235–42.

Ettinger, W.H. and Hazzard, W.R. (1988). Elevated apolipoprotein-B levels in corticosteroid-treated patients with systemic lupus erythematosus. *Journal of Clinical Endocrinology and Metabolism*, **67**, 425–8.

Ettinger, W.H., Goldberg, A.P., and Apple-Bowden, D., Hazzard, W.R. (1987). Dyslipoproteinemia in SLE — effect of corticosteroids. *American Journal of Medicine*, **83**, 503–8.

Fahrer, H., Hoeflin, F., Lauterberg, B.H., Peheim, E., Levy, A., and Vischer, T.L. (1991). Diet and fatty acids: can fish substitute for fish oil? *Clinical and Experimental Rheumatology*, **9**, 403–6.

Fairburn, K, Grootveld, M., Ward, R.J., Abiuka, C., Kus, M., Williams, R.B., Winyard, P.G., and Blake, D.R. (1992). Alpha-tocopherol, lipids and lipoproteins in knee-joint synovial fluid and serum from patients with inflammatory joint disease. *Clinical Science*, **83**, 657–64.

Feingold, K.R. and Grunfeld, C. (1992). Role of cytokines in inducing hyperlipidaemia. *Diabetes*, **41** (Suppl. 2), 97–101.

Fox, R.I. (1996). Fifth international symposium on Sjögren's syndrome. *Arthritis and Rheumatism*, **39**, 195–6.

Frick, M.H., Elo, O., and Haapa, K. (1987). Helsinki heart study: primary prevention trial with gemfibrozil in middle-aged men with dyslipidaemia. *New England Journal of Medicine*, **317**, 1237–45.

Fried, S.K. and Zechner, R. (1989). Cachetin/tumor necrosis factor decreases human adipose tissue lipoprotein lipase mRNA levels, synthesis, and activity. *Journal of Lipid Research*, **30**, 1917–23.

Garrido, J.A., Peromingo, J.A.D., Sesma, P., and Pia, G. (1994). More about the link between thrombosis and atherosclerosis in autoimmune diseases: Triglycerides and risk for thrombosis in patients with antiphospholipid antibodies. *Journal of Rheumatology*, **21**, 2394.

Geusens, P., Wouters, C., Nijs, J., Jiang, Y., and Dequeker, J. (1994). Long-term effect of omega-3 fatty acid supplementation in active rheumatoid arthritis. A 12-month, double-blind, controlled study. *Arthritis and Rheumatism*, **37**, 824–9.

Goldman, J.A., Glueck, C.J., and Abrams, N.R. (1972). Musculoskeletal disorders associated with Type IV hyperlipoproteinemia. *Lancet*, **2**, 449–52.

Goldman, J.A., Fishman, A.B., and Lee, J.E. (1989). The role of cholesterol-lowering agents in drug-induced rhabdomyolysis and polymyositis. *Arthritis and Rheumatism*, **32**, 358–9.

Grainger, D.J., Kemp, P.R., Liu, A.C., Lawn, R.M., and Metcalfe, J.C. (1994). Activation of transforming growth factor-β is inhibited in transgenic apolipoprotein (a) mice. *Nature*, **370**, 460–2.

Havel, R.J., Goldstein, J.L., and Brown, M.S. (1980). *Metabolic control and disease*, pp. 393–494. WB Saunders, Philadelphia.

Hearth-Holmes, M., Baethge, B.A., Broadwell, L., and Wolf, R.E. (1995). Dietary treatment of hyperlipidemia in patients with systemic lupus erythematosus. *Journal of Rheumatology*, **22**, 450–4.

Hino, I., Akama, H., Furuya, T., Ueda, H., Taniguchi, A., Hara, M., and Kashiwazaki, S. (1996). Pravastatin-induced rhabdomyolysis in a patient with mixed connective tissue disease. *Arthritis and Rheumatism*, **39**, 1259–61.

Hodis, H.N., Quismorio, F.P.Jr, Wickham, E., and Blankenhorn, D.H. (1993). The lipid, lipoprotein, and apolipoprotein effects of hydroxychloroquine in patients with systemic lupus erythematosus. *Journal of Rheumatology*, **20**, 661–5.

Howard, E.J. and Brown, S.M. (1973). Clofibrate-induced antinuclear factor and lupus-like syndrome. *Journal of the American Medical Association*, **226**, 1358–9.

Ilowite, N.T., Samuel, P., Ginzler, E., and Jacobson, M.S. (1988). Dyslipoproteinemia in pediatric systemic lupus erythematosus. *Arthritis and Rheumatism*, **31**, 859–63.

Ilowite, N.T., Copperman, N., Leicht, T., Kwong, T., and Jacobson, M.S. (1995). Effects of dietary modification and fish oil supplementation on dyslipoproteinemia in pediatric systemic lupus erythematosus. *Journal of Rheumatology*, **22**, 1347–51.

Jones, S.M., Lloyd, J.L., Barnes, J., Stirling, C.A., Harris, C.P.D., Reckless, J.P.D., and McHugh, N.J. (1994). Lipoproteins and their subfractions in psoriatic arthritis. *Arthritis and Rheumatism*, **37**, S206.

Kabakov, A.E., Tertov, V.V., Saenko, V.A., Poverenny, A.M., and Orekhov, A.N. (1992). The atherogenic effect of lupus sera: SLE-derived immune complexes stimulate the accumulation of cholesterol in cultured smooth muscle cells from human aorta. *Clinical Immunology and Immunopathology*, 63, 214–20.

Kasiske, B.L., O'Donnell, M.D., Cleary, M.P., and Keane, W.F. (1988). Treatment of hyperlipidemia reduces glomerular injury in obese Zucker rats. *Kidney International*, 33, 667–72.

Kawai, S., Mizushima, Y., and Kaburaki, J. (1995). Increased serum lipoprotein(a) levels in systemic lupus erythematosus with myocardial and cerebral infarctions. *Journal of Rheumatology*, 22, 1210–11.

Khadchadurian, A.K. (1968). Migratory polyarthritis in familial hypercholesterolaemia (type II hyperlipoproteinemia). *Arthritis and Rheumatism*, 11, 385–93.

Klemp, P., Halland, A.M., Majoos, F.L., and Steyn, K. (1993). Musculoskeletal manifestations in hyperlipidaemia: a controlled study. *Annals of the Rheumatic Diseases*, 52, 44–8.

Kremer, J.M., Lawrence, D.A., Petrillo, G.F., Litts, L.L., Mullaly, P.M., Rynes, R.I., Stocker, R.I., Parhami, N., Greenstein, N.S., Fuchs, B.R., Mathur, A., Robinson, D.R., Sperling, R.I., and Bigaouette, J. (1995). Effects of high-dose fish oil on rheumatoid arthritis after stopping nonsteroidal antiinflammatory drugs. Clinical and immune correlates. *Arthritis and Rheumatism*, 38, 1107–14.

Kumon, Y., Suchiro, T., Ikeda, Y., Yoshida, K., Hashimoto, K., and Ohno, F. (1993). Influence of serum amyloid A protein on HDL in chronic inflammatory disease. *Clinical Biochemistry*, 26, 505–11.

Lahita, R.G., Rivkin, E., Cavanagh, I., and Romano, P. (1993). Low levels of total cholesterol, high-density lipoprotein, and apolipoprotein Al in association with anticardiolipin antibodies in patients with systemic lupus erythematosus. *Arthritis and Rheumatism*, 36, 1566–74.

Lau, C.S., Morley, K.D., and Belch, J.J.F. (1993). Effects of fish oil supplementation on non-steroidal anti-inflammatory drug requirement in patients with mild rheumatoid arthritis — a double-blind placebo controlled study. *British Journal of Rheumatology*, 32, 982–9.

Lazarevic, M.B., Vitic, J., Mladenovic, V., Myones, B.L., Skosey, J.L., and Swedler, W.I. (1992). Dyslipoproteinemia in the course of active rheumatoid arthritis. *Seminars in Arthritis and Rheumatism*, 22, 172–80.

Lazarevic, M.B., Skosey, J.L., and Vitic, J. (1993a). Cholesterol crystals in synovial and bursal fluid. *Seminars in Arthritis and Rheumatism*, 23, 99–103.

Lazarevic, M.B., Vitic, J., and Myones, B.L. (1993b). Anti-lipoprotein antibodies in rheumatoid arthritis. *Seminars in Arthritis and Rheumatism*, 22, 385–91.

Leong, K.H., Koh, E.T., Feng, P.H., and Boey, M.L. (1994). Lipid profiles in patients with systemic lupus erythematosus. *Journal of Rheumatology*, 21, 1264–7.

Leong, K.H., Stirling, C.A., Lloyd, J., Reckless, J., Maddison, P.J., and McHugh, N.J. (1995). SLE patients have abnormal lipid profiles compared to age and gender matched controls (abstract). *Lupus*, 4, 149.

Leventhal, L.J., Boyce, E.G., and Zurier, R.B. (1993). Treatment of rheumatoid arthritis with gammalinoleic acid. *Archives of Internal Medicine*, 119, 867–73.

Lipid Research Clinics Program (1984). The Lipid Research Clinics coronary primary prevention trial results. I.Reduction in incidence of coronary heart disease. *Journal of the American Medical Association*, 251, 351–64.

MacGregor, A.J., Dhillon, V.B., Binder, A., Forte, C.A., Knight, B.C., Betteridge, D.J., and Isenberg, D.A. (1992). Fasting lipids and anticardiolipin antibodies as risk factors for vascular disease in systemic lupus erythematosus. *Annals of the Rheumatic Diseases*, 51, 152–5.

Magaro, M., Altomonte, L., Zoli, A., Mirone, L., and Ruffini, M.P. (1991). Serum lipid pattern and apolipoprotein A-I and B100 in active rheumatoid arthritis. *Zeitschrift für Rheumaforschung*, 50, 168–70.

Maher, V.M.G. and Brown, B.G. (1995). Lipoprotein (a) and coronary heart disease. *Current Opinions in Lipidology*, 6, 229–35.

Matsubara, K., Matsuzawa, Y., Jiao, S., Takama, T., Masaharu, K., and Tami, S. (1989). Relationship between hypertriglyceridemia and uric acid production in primary gout. *Metabolism*, 38, 689–701.

Matsuda, J., Gotoh, M., Gohchi, K., Saitoh, N., and Tsukamoto, M. (1994). Serum lipoprotein(a) level is increased in patients with systemic lupus erythematosus irrespective of positivity of antiphospholipid antibodies. *Thrombosis Research*, 73, 83–4.

Merrill, J.T., Rivkin, E., Shen, C., and Lahita, R.G. (1995). Selection of a gene for apolipoprotein Al using autoantibodies from a patient with systemic lupus erythematosus. *Arthritis and Rheumatism*, 38, 1655–9.

Mizutani, H., Kurata, Y., Kosugi, S., Shiraga, M., Kashiwagi, H., Tomiyama, Y., Kanakura, Y., Good, R.A., and Matsuzawa, Y. (1995). Monoclonal anticardiolipin autoantibodies established from the (New Zealand White × BXSB)F_1 mouse model of antiphospholipid syndrome cross-react with oxidised low-density lipoprotein. *Arthritis and Rheumatism*, 38, 1382–8.

National Cholesterol Education Program (1994). Second report of the expert panel on detection, evaluation, and treatment of high blood cholesterol in adults (adult treatment panel II). *Circulation*, 89, 1333–445.

Neaton, J.D., Blackburn, H., Jacobs, D., *et al.* (1992). Serum cholesterol level and mortality findings for men screened in the multiple risk intervention trial. *Archives of Internal Medicine*, 152, 1490–500.

Petri, M., Perez-Gutthann, S., Spence, D., and Hochberg, M.C. (1992). Risk factors for coronary artery disease in patients with systemic lupus erythematosus. *American Journal of Medicine*, 93, 513–19.

Petri, M., Lakatta, C., Magder, L., and Goldman, D. (1994). Effect of prednisone and hydroxychloroquine on coronary artery disease risk factors in systemic lupus erythematosus: A longitudinal data analysis. *American Journal of Medicine*, 96, 254–9.

Pincus, T. and Callahan, L.F. (1986). Taking mortality in rheumatoid arthritis seriously — predictive markers, socioeconomic status and comorbidity. *Journal of Rheumatology*, 13, 841–5.

Prickett, J.D., Robinson, D.R., and Steinberg, A.D. (1981). Dietary enrichment with the polyunsaturated fatty acid eicosapentaenoic acid prevents proteinuria and prolongs survival in NZB × NZW F_1 mice. *Journal of Clinical Investigation*, 68, 556–9.

Prior, P., Symmons, D.P.M., Scott, D.L., Brown, R., and Hawkins, C.F. (1984). Cause of death in rheumatoid arthritis. *British Journal of Rheumatology*, 23, 92–9.

Pyorala, K., de Backer, G., Graham, I., Poole-Wilson, P., and Wood, D. (1994). Prevention of coronary heart disease in clinical practice: recommendations of the task force of the European Society of Cardiology, European Atherosclerosis Society and European Society of Hypertension. *Atherosclerosis*, 110, 121–61.

Querfeld, U., Ong, J.M., Prehn, J., Carty, J., Saffari, B., Jordan, S.C., and Kern, P.A. (1990). Effects of cytokines on the production of lipoprotein lipase in cultured human macrophages. *Journal of Lipid Research*, 31, 1379–86.

Radford, E.P., Doll, R., and Smith, P.G. (1977). Mortality among patients with ankylosing spondylitis not given x-ray therapy. *New England Journal of Medicine*, 297, 572–6.

Rantapää-Dahlqvist, S., Wällberg-Jonsson, S., and Dahlén, G. (1991). Lipoprotein (a), lipids and lipoproteins in patients with rheumatoid arthritis. *Annals of the Rheumatic Diseases*, 30, 366–8.

Rasker, J.J. and Cosh, J.A. (1981). Cause and age of death in a prospective study of 100 patients with rheumatoid arthritis. *Annals of the Rheumatic Diseases*, 40, 115–20.

Rigby, A.S. (1991). Review of UK data on the rheumatic diseases — 5: ankylosing spondylitis. *British Journal of Rheumatology*, 30, 50–3.

Robinson, D.R., Prickett, J.D., Makoul, G.T., Steinberg, A.D., and Colvin, R.B. (1986). Dietary fish oil reduces progression of established renal disease in (NZB × NZW)F1 mice and delays renal disease in BXSB and MRL/I strains. *Arthritis and Rheumatism*, 29, 539–46.

Ross Peirce, L., Wysowski, D.K., and Gross, T.P. (1990). Myopathy and rhabdomyolysis associated with lovastatin gemfibrozil combination therapy. *Journal of the American Medical Association*, 264, 71–5.

Scandinavian Simvastin Survival Study Group (1994). Randomised trial of cholesterol lowering in 4444 patients with coronary heart disease: results of the Scandinavian Simvaastin Survival Study (4S). *Lancet*, 344, 1383–9.

Schumaker, H.R. and Michaels, R. (1989). Recurrent tendinitis and Achilles tendon nodule with positively birefringent crystals in a patient with hyperlipoproteinaemia *Journal of Rheumatology*, 16, 1387–9.

Selley, M.L., Bourne, D.J., and Bartlett, M.R. (1992). Occurrence of (E)-4-hydroxy-2-nonenal in plasma and synovial fluid of patients with rheumatoid arthritis and osteoarthritis. *Annals of the Rheumatic Diseases*, 51, 481–4.

Shepherd, J., Cobbe, S.M., Ford, J., Isles, C.G., Lorimer, A.R., MacFarlane, P.W., McKillop, J.H., and Packard, C.J. (1995). Prevention of coronary heart disease with pravastatin in men with hypercholesterolaemia. West of Scotland Coronary Prevention Study Group. *New England Journal of Medicine*, 333, 1301–7.

Spriggs, D.R., Sherman, M.L., Michie, H., Arthur, K.A., Imamura, K., Wilmore, D., Frei, E., and Kufe, D.W. (1988). Recombinant human tumor necrosis factor administered as a 24-hour intravenous infusion. *Journal of the National Cancer Institute*, 80, 1039–44.

Svenson, K.L.G., Lithell, H., Hällgren, R., and Vessby, B. (1987a). Serum lipoprotein in active rheumatoid arthritis and other chronic inflammatory arthritides. I. Relativity to inflammatory activity. *Archives of Internal Medicine*, 147, 1912–16.

Svenson, K.L.G., Lithell, H., Hällgren, R., and Vessby, B. (1987b). Serum lipoprotein in active rheumatoid arthritis and other chronic inflammatory arthritides. II. Effects of anti-inflammatory and disease-modifying drug treatment. *Archives of Internal Medicine*, 147, 1917–20.

Szachnowski, P. and Bridges, A.J. (1994). Subcutaneous cholesterol nodules. *Journal of Rheumatology*, 21, 2391–2.

Takegoshi. T., Haba, T., Hirai, J., Saga, T., Kitoh, C., and Mabuchi, H. (1990). A case of hyperLp(a)aemia associated with SLE, suffering from myocardial infarction and cerebral infarction. *Japanese Journal of Medicine*, 29, 77–84.

Terres, W., Tatsis, E., Pfalzer, B., Beil, U., Beisiegel, U., and Hamm, C.W. (1995). Rapid angiographic progression of coronary heart disease in patients with elevated lipoprotein (a). *Circulation*, 91, 948–50.

Tinahones, F.J., Collantes, E., C-Soriguer, F.J., González-Ruiz, A., Pineda, M., Anón, J., and Sánchez Guijo, P. (1995). Increased VLDL levels and dimished renal excretion of uric acid in hyperuricaemic-hypertriglycerideaemic patients. *British Journal of Rheumatology*, 34, 920–4.

Ulreich, A., Korner, G.M., Pfeiffer, K.P., Sedlmay, R., and Rainer, F. (1985). Serum lipids and lipoproteins in patients with primary gout. *Rheumatol International*, 5, 73–7.

Urowitz, M.B., Bookman, A.A.M., Koehler, B.E., Gordon, D.A., Smythe, H.A., and Ogryzlo, M.A. (1976). The bimodal mortality pattern of systemic lupus erythematosus. *American Journal of Medicine*, 60, 221–5.

Vaarala, O., Alfthan, G., Jauhiainen, M., Leirisalo-Repo, M., Aho, K., and Palosuo, T. (1993). Crossreaction between antibodies to oxidised low-density lipoprotein and to cardiolipin in systemic lupus erythematosus. *Lancet*, 341, 923–5.

Vaarala, O., Manttari, M., Manninen, V., Tenkanen, L., Puurunen, M., Aho, K., and Palosuo, T. (1995). Anti-cardiolipin antibodies and risk of myocardial infarction in a prospective cohort of middle-aged men. *Circulation*, 91, 23–7.

Veale, D.J., Torley, H.I., Richards, I.M., O'Dowd, A., Fitzsimmons, C., Belch, J.J.E., and Sturrock, R.D. (1994). A double-blind placebo controlled trial of efamol marine on skin and joint symptoms of psoriatic arthritis. *British Journal of Rheumatology*, 33, 954–8.

Wallace, D.J., Metzger, A.L., Stecher, V.J., Turnbull, B.A., and Kern, P.A. (1990). Cholesterol-lowering effect of hydroxychloroquine in patients with rheumatic disease: reversal of deleterious effects of steroids on lipids. *American Journal of Medicine*, 89, 322–6.

Walton, A.J.E., Snaith, M.L., Locniskar, M., Cumberland, A.G., Morrow, W.J.W., and Isenberg, D.A. (1991). Dietary fish oil and the severity of symptoms in patients with systemic lupus erythematosus. *Annals of the Rheumatic Diseases*, 50, 463–6.

Winyard, P.G., Tatzber, F., Esterbauer, H., Kus, M.L., Blake, D.R., and Morris, C.J. (1993). Presence of foam cells containing oxidised low density lipoprotein in the synovial membrane from patients with rheumatoid arthritis. *Annals of the Rheumatic Diseases*, 52, 677–80.

Wolfe, F., Mitchell, D.M., and Sibley, J.T. (1994). The mortality of rheumatoid arthritis. *Arthritis and Rheumatism*, 37, 481–94.

Zimmerman, J., Fainaru, M., and Eisenberg, S. (1984). The effects of prednisone therapy on plasma lipoproteins and apolipoproteins. A prospective study. *Metabolism*, 33, 521–6.

Zuckner, J. (1990). Drug-induced myopathies. *Seminars in Arthritis and Rheumatism*, 19, 259–68.

5.14 Soft-tissue rheumatism

Brian Hazleman

Introduction

Soft-tissue injuries, although commonly overlooked in the planning and provision of health care, are of major and increasing importance. Fortunately there has been an increase in interest in these lesions concomitant with an increase in our understanding of the associated disorders.

When rheumatology first developed as a medical subspeciality its basis was in the articular diseases, a concept that was soon found inadequate as it became apparent that other synovial structures, such as bursal and tendon sheaths, were equally affected by the same conditions. Later, the term 'abarticular rheumatism' was used to distinguish the extra-articular rheumatic complaints from the better-defined articular rheumatism. Because joints are hard and bony, and abarticular rheumatism by definition does not affect joints, the all-embracing term for this group of complaints, now in international usage, is soft-tissue rheumatism. The heterogeneity of soft-tissue rheumatism poses considerable problems in arriving at sensible treatment protocols and systems of management.

Lesions of tendons and their sheaths, fascias, bursae, joint capsules, and the tenoperiosteal junction (the enthesis) cause much illness and loss of productivity. They constitute a significant proportion of the workload of general medical practices and of hospital accident, orthopaedic, and rheumatology departments. As biopsy and surgery are rarely employed in their diagnosis and treatment, histological data are scanty and their pathological backgrounds poorly understood. While there are adequate anatomical and clinical features to allow identification of individual conditions, diagnosis is often imprecise and management remains largely empirical.

Any or all of these lesions may occur in association with overt systemic disease, as, for example, in inflammatory arthritis or infection, but a large proportion occur in its absence. In these circumstances local causes, such as chronic, repetitive, low-grade trauma, excessive and unaccustomed use, either at work or at play, may be responsible. These factors may also cause partial interruption of the blood supply, resulting in incomplete attempts at healing and degeneration, which render the extra-articular structures more vulnerable in the middle-aged and elderly people in whom these lesions predominate.

One feature common to all soft-tissue syndromes is a tendency to spontaneous remission. Many of the lesions take only weeks to improve and few persist with significant symptoms beyond 6 months. Therefore, a clear diagnosis allows the doctor to reassure the patient that arthritis is not present and that the prognosis is good. Failure to resolve is often due to further injury. Few of the lesions require complete rest, but most respond to selective rest of the region involved.

An accurate diagnosis of soft-tissue rheumatism can be made by taking a careful history, considering possible trauma or overuse, and carrying out a systematic examination. For most local lesions, further investigation is unnecessary and radiographs that reveal the expected, age-related degenerative changes can often confuse. It is usually apparent if there is a more generalized condition that requires appropriate investigation.

Classification

Disorders can be classified by clinicopathological process (tendinitis), by anatomical region (shoulder pain), or by aetiology (repetitive strain injury). There is no universally accepted classification. The following is practical and problem-orientated, and divides the conditions into (i) generalized and (ii) localized. The generalized forms may be further divided into those associated or not with inflammation (Table 1). Those that are localized may be regional, involving a few sclerotomes, or affecting a specific site (Table 1).

Fibromyalgia or the 'fibrositis syndrome' is a particular variant of soft-tissue rheumatism. It is characterized by widespread aching and multiple tender sites. The tender sites are central to the definition and our understanding of this condition.

Generalized soft-tissue lesions

These may result from underlying disease, and most of the primary conditions can be diagnosed by careful clinical and laboratory assessment. These conditions will not be discussed here, and polymyalgia rheumatica has been considered elsewhere (Chapter 5.11.5).

The diagnosis of 'psychogenic rheumatism' must be made with caution and after the exclusion of other diseases. Chronic pain may produce psychological overtones. There are several features that will suggest a psychological illness, since overt psychiatric symptoms are not usually present in rheumatic disorders but are common in patients who are unhappy at work or at home. Suggestive features include written lists of symptoms, inconsistent or negative physical findings on repeated examinations, and inappropriate concern with serious future disability.

Localized soft-tissue lesions

The major structures involved and associated lesions are listed in Table 2. Examination should permit accurate localization of the

Table 1   Classification of soft-tissue rheumatism

Generalized

With evidence of inflammation
Polymyalgia rheumatica and cranial arteritis
Prodrome of inflammatory arthopathies and connective tissue
    diseases
Viral and bacterial infections

Without inflammation
Hypothyroidism
Drug-related painful states associated with steroid withdrawal,
    chronic barbiturate abuse, and the contraceptive pill
Dyskinetic phase of Parkinson's disease
Chronic brucellosis
Associated with malignancy, e.g. myeloma, carcinoma
Osteomalacia
Fibrositis, lumbago

Associated with weakness
Prodrome of polymyositis or dermatomyositis
Carcinomatous neuromyopathy (some forms)
Hypokalaemic states

Psychogenic rheumatism

Localized

Regional
Bornholm's disease
Prodrome of herpes zoster
Stitch/cramp

Specific sites
Bursitis and tenosynovitis, e.g. ischial and trochanteric bursitis,
    De Quervain's tenosynovitis
Enthesopathies, e.g. tennis elbow, plantar fasciitis
Entrapment neuropathies, e.g. carpal tunnel syndrome and
    neuralgic paraesthesias
Miscellaneous conditions, e.g. Dupuytren's contracture, Tietze
    syndrome

Table 2   Localized soft-tissue lesions

Structure	Lesion
Tendons, tendon sheaths	Rupture, degeneration tendinitis, peritendinitis, tenosynovitis, ganglia
Tenoperiosteal junction	Enthesopathies, apophysitis
Bursae	Bursitis—acute or chronic
Fascias	Fasciitis, Dupuytren's contracture
Ligaments	Sprain, strain, tear

Table 3   Common soft-tissue lesions and sites

Site	Lesion
Shoulder	Rotator-cuff lesions / Capsulitis of glenohumeral joint
Elbow	Lateral epicondylitis / Medial epicondylitis / Olecranon bursitis
Wrist and hand	Carpal tunnel syndrome / Dupuytren's contracture / De Quervain's tenosynovitis
Trunk	Non-specific neck and low back pain / Trapezius muscle spasm / 'Costochondritis'
Hip	Ischial and trochanteric bursitis / Meralgia paraesthetica
Knee	Bursitis / Ligamentous sprains
Ankle and foot	Achilles tendinitis/peritendinitis / Plantar fasciitis

anatomical structure involved. The conditions frequently encountered in clinical practice are listed in Table 3.

Economic effects and burden on health-care services

Soft-tissue rheumatism is the most commonly encountered rheumatic cause of sickness absences from work, accounting for 44 per cent of medically certified rheumatic spells and 6 per cent of all incapacity spells. As is known from their natural history, however, the amount of time lost from work is comparatively less impressive. Thus the average duration of an incapacity spell for soft-issue rheumatism (21 days), when aggregated, amounts to 2.5 per cent of rheumatic days or 3.5 per cent of all days lost from work. These figures include absences on industrial injury benefit as well as sickness benefit, the former making up about one-fifth of the total. There is an age association in days lost. Traumatic disorders show no very marked trend, but the non-traumatic complaints are associated with an increase in days lost that is progressive with age; the rate is at

least six times greater in the oldest as compared with the youngest quinquennium. This pattern reflects the fact that the average duration of incapacity spells grows longer with age, those occurring in the oldest group being more than twice as long as those in younger people. The overall pattern of spells is generally similar in most of the diagnostic categories, but muscle tendon and fascial lesions are unusual for the undue length of some of their incapacity spells.

In the United Kingdom alone the resultant loss of working days from soft-tissue lesions is likely to cost the country almost a billion pounds a year in lost productivity, apart from the value of social security payments, lost tax revenue, and health and social services applied to this problem. Behind these huge sums is a great deal of pain and misery, and much disruption to family life and work arrangements. The economic effects, loss of time from work, and the load that such patients present to both general practitioners and hospital doctors, are clearly immense. Greater attention needs to be focused on these diseases.

Epidemiology

Studies on the incidence of soft-tissue injuries are sadly inadequate as epidemiological studies have hitherto only infrequently been performed. Indeed, Dixon (1979) has described soft-tissue rheumatism as 'the great outback of rheumatology, a vast frontier land, ill-defined and little explained, its features poorly categorised and far from internationally agreed'. The fact that any or all of these soft-tissue lesions may be associated with overt systemic disease makes the classification and interpretation of data difficult. The lack of universally acceptable, defined criteria for these injuries has been a major obstacle to conducting epidemiological studies.

The absence of specific diagnostic tests for the soft-tissue syndromes highlights the importance of developing diagnostic criteria, based on combinations of the predominant clinical features, that are sensitive enough to exclude those without the syndrome. Most of these syndromes will be covered by the inclusion criteria of pain at a specific site or sites, local tenderness, limitation of movement, and pain on specific resisted movement or movements. There is a need for rigorous diagnostic criteria that take account of the lack of a 'gold standard' reference test, the continuous distribution pattern of the symptoms and signs, the variation in disease expression at differnt times, and the inter- and intraobserver variation in eliciting the specific clinical signs. Diagnostic criteria are required for defining occurrence, measuring outcome, and assessing the effect of intervention, for example in recruitment to clinical trials.

A population survey by the Swedish National Central Bureau of Statistics indicates a prevalence of all forms of soft-tissue rheumatism of 1.6 per cent in men and 3.6 per cent in women (Bjelle *et al.* 1990). Chronic complaints attributed to non-articular rheumatism as well as miscellaneous back disorders were estimated to occur in about 3 per cent of the adult (18–70 years) population of the United States in the 1976 National Health Interview Survey. In comparison, about 3 per cent of symptoms were attributable to rheumatoid arthritis and 8 per cent to degenerative joint disease. Together, soft-tissue lesions comprise one-third of all rheumatic diseases seen by family physicians and 3 to 4 per cent of all ambulatory medical-care visits (Wood *et al.* 1979).

There is considerable confusion in diagnostic terminology and a wide variation in reported incidence between countries, probably reflecting the contrasting, as well as legal, attitudes to these conditions. In general the increased incidence of these disorders appears to be due to new technology leading to advanced automation and mechanization. Occupational disorders are of interest because, theoretically at least, it should be possible to devise methods of working that would prevent their development. Ergonomic and behavioural studies have much to offer. Certainly sufferers are at present at considerable hazard of repeated attendance, as indicated by the reported rates of recrudescence for 'beat' knee (12 per cent), 'beat' elbow (7 per cent), and tenosynovitis of the wrist (6 per cent) (Wood *et al.* 1979). It would be of interest to learn why only some individuals exposed to particular methods of working develop soft-tissue injuries. Automation and mechanization have led to the need for repetitive movements that may produce repetitive strain injuries and associated overuse syndromes; this aspect will be discussed later.

Crude differences in age patterns may be discerned between traumatic and non-traumatic forms of soft-tissue rheumatism. The frequency of spells of strains and sprains tends to reduce after the thirties, whereas non-traumatic conditions show a less marked decline and this does not appear until after the forties. Rates in women tend in general to be less than in men.

Of localized problems, the painful shoulder ranks highest in frequency and consequently has been better documented than most other soft-tissue lesions. Regional shoulder complaints rank fifth amongst the regional rheumatic diseases as a cause of incapacity or of visiting a physician. Data from general medical practices in the United Kingdom (Department of Health and Social Security 1986) suggest that approx. 1 in 170 of the adult population will present to their general practitioner with a new episode of shoulder pain each year. This contrasts with 1 in 30 for back pain.

Elderly people frequently have considerable functional impairment: 20 per cent of the elderly hospital population had shoulder disorders; less than one-fifth of these had sought medical attention (Chard and Hazleman 1987). The association between shoulder pain and occupation was highlighted in a study of the medical outpatient departments of six heavy industries by Bjelle *et al.* (1980). Approximately one-third of the outpatient visits were for non-traumatic musculoskeletal complaints, of which 30 to 50 per cent were neck–shoulder complaints. In the United States, the Health and Nutrition Examination Survey 1971–1975 studied the adult population aged 25 to 74 years. It found that 4.2 per cent had suffered from shoulder complaints and that shoulder abnormalities observed by a physician were present in 1.2 per cent; almost 40 per cent had associated neck complaints. In over 80 per cent the complaints had occurred during the year immediately before the study (Miller 1973). Health-care and insurance data support the influence of age and sex in relation to shoulder complaints amongst workers in production industries. The influence of age may partly be due to the frequent finding of degenerative changes of the rotator cuff that make this tissue highly vulnerable to trauma after the fifth decade. Also, women run a higher risk than men of developing shoulder complaints when working in production industries. Further studies are required to determine whether the age, sex, and occupation pattern seen with shoulder lesions is equally applicable to other soft-tissue injuries.

Tennis elbow or lateral epicondylitis affects 1 to 3 per cent of the population. It occurs mostly between 40 and 60 years of age, and usually affects the dominant arm. Most sufferers experience a recurrence of symptoms within 18 months. While some 40 to 50 per cent of tennis players suffer with tennis elbow, it is more frequent and severe in older players. Less than 5 per cent of cases in total are related to tennis and it is found more often in non-athletes. Labelle *et al.* (1992) report that an average of 62 days is lost from work per patient in industrial workers.

Defining the outcome

There is a very low rate of referral of soft-tissue problems to hospital and thus outcomes from hospital series do not reflect the outcomes from the syndrome as a whole. There is also considerable variation between different hospitals in the case severity of new attendees. This is partly a reflection of waiting-list time, and partly of the interests of general practitioners and hospital clinicians. Also, many conditions are self-limiting: half of patients presenting to general practitioners with soft-tissue back pain are better within a week and 90 per cent by a month.

Pathogenesis

Perhaps one of the biggest hindrances to progress in understanding soft-tissue rheumatism has been a negative attitude to the affected tissues, which are still thought to be inert, homogeneous structures. Their role in joint mechanics and pathology is often considered to be passive and secondary to that of other joint structures such as bone, cartilage, and synovium. These misconceptions are belied by recent studies demonstrating that these tissues are indeed metabolically active, interesting, and worthy of investigation.

As outlined above, many local causes of soft-tissue rheumatism are related to chronic, repetitive, low-grade trauma and excessive and unaccustomed use (both at work and at play), which both may partially interrupt the local blood supply. Incomplete attempts at healing and degeneration will render soft tissues more vulnerable in the older people in whom such lesions are more common. Since the vascular supply to adult tendon is poor, healing of these lesions is slow. Poor tendon repair and degeneration would appear to explain the chronicity of tendon lesions.

Tendon and ligaments: composition and function

Tendons are clusters of parallel collagen fibrils interspersed with a few fibrocytes; the collagen is almost all type I. Larger tendons consist of multiple fascicles separated by loose connective tissue containing nerve fibres and blood vessels. Ligaments may be of a similar structure, but usually exhibit less regular orientation of collagen and contain elastin. They function passively, being structurally superior to tendons for constant tension. Tendons, in contrast, must provide flexibility and resistance to tension, with concentration of force to an attachment area. Loading a tendon causes a brief alignment of fibres, then linear extension to the limit of elasticity. According to Hooke's law this is followed by failure of individual fibres and then rupture. The area of weakness should be the attachment to bone; but the loading is distributed evenly by a mechanism called 'fibre weave'. Therefore, tendons often fail at a distance from the attachment or enthesis.

The fan-shaped point of attachment of tendon to bone (the enthesis) is an area of great stress. It differs histologically from the rest of the tendon. The enthesis is traditionally made up of four zones: tendon, fibrocartilage, mineralized fibrocartilage, and bone. In the zone of mineralized fibrocartilage there is an increase in smooth endoplasmic reticulum, lysosomes, and intracellular lipid, and a more prominent Golgi apparatus.

Blood supply

Arterioles pass between the fascicles in the tendon. These freely communicate and are accompanied by venules and lymphatic vessels. Extensions of vessels from the muscles pass through the tendon and anastomose with those from the periosteum. Studies with radioactive isotopes have demonstrated that the enthesis has a particularly rich blood supply. It is believed that the blood supply to tendon is relatively abundant compared to the metabolic demands. However, there is reduced blood flow when tendons are under tension.

Nerve supply

This is sensory, there being no definite evidence of vasomotor control. Close to the attachment to muscles are found specialized afferent receptors. The nerve fibres from the tendon mainly follow the branch of the motor nerve to the muscle but some fibres form small branches that pass directly into nearby peripheral nerves.

Tensile strength

The tensile strength of normal tendon is greatly in excess of ordinary demands. This strength requires an intact blood supply, even partial interruption leads to a reduction. Normal tendon with a cross-sectional area of 1 cm^2 can support 600 to 1000 kg, which is similar to half that of steel.

Tendon lesions

Rupture

Severe trauma directly to a tendon will result in rupture. Marked strain on a tendon may also do this, although avulsion fracture at site of attachment is more likely. Analyses of spontaneously ruptured tendons have shown degenerative changes that include alterations in the size and orientation of collagen fibres, with increased deposition of proteoglycans between the fibres. The tenocytes have enlarged vacuoles, sometimes containing lipids, and cell necrosis is sometimes found. In some cases calcium is deposited (Kannus and Jozsa 1991).

Similar changes are found in human tendons removed at operation for degeneration of the rotator cuff and lateral epicondylitis (Chard *et al.* 1994).

Tenosynovitis

Inflammation of the synovial lining of the sheath through which a tendon moves may be the result of an inflammatory arthritic condition but is more commonly caused by trauma. It is often the result of unaccustomed exercise or repetitive work action. Tenderness, swelling, and crepitus on palpating the moving tendon are characteristic. When severe and chronic the tendon sheath becomes thickened, especially over bony prominences. Secondary thickening of the tendon distally may occur, producing snapping on movement of the thickened area through the inflamed sheath, for example trigger finger. Sites of tenosynovitis include the thumb (De Quervain's tenosynovitis), finger flexors, flexor carpi radialis, common peroneal sheath, and tibialis posterior tendon. Treatment includes rest, splinting, local steroid injections, and sometimes surgical release.

Tendinitis

This is a poorly defined group of conditions where pain is attributed to strain or injury to tendons and their attachments to bone. In many cases the lesion is believed to be tenoperiosteal, for example lateral humeral epicondylitis (tennis elbow) and jumper's knee, and thus comes under the term enthesopathy. The most important tendon lesions in terms of frequency and severity are those affecting the shoulder, and these produce the majority of cases of shoulder pain.

Pathological studies (Fig. 1)

In vivo work has shown that tendon healing after damage probably involves the reaction of surrounding tissue and adhesion, without participation of the tendon tissue itself. Other studies have revealed that tendons are capable of responding to injury, although it does appear that most actively dividing cells are derived from the superficial part of the tendon.

The majority of cells obtained from tendon that are capable of replication *in vitro* are derived from the superficial layer (epithelium). The growth characteristics of the cell lines have been established by

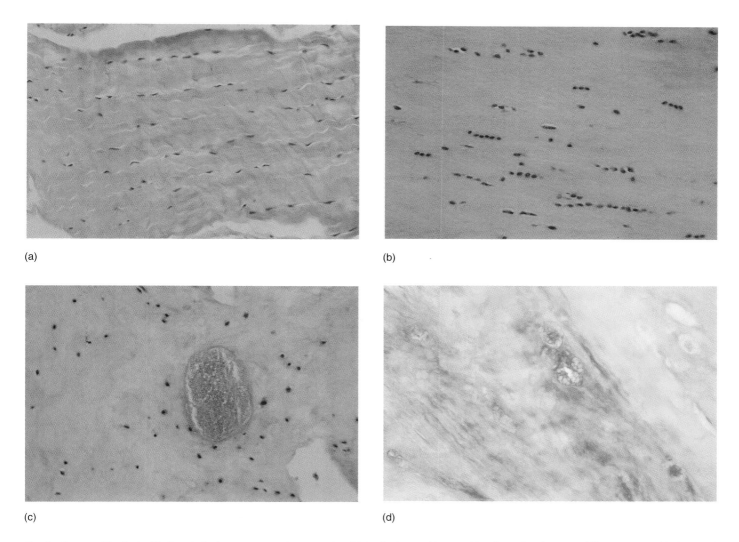

(a)

(b)

(c)

(d)

Fig. 1 Common histological findings in the human supraspinatus tendon: (a) tendon from a 19-year-old cadaver showing normal fibre structure with elongated fibroblasts between parallel fibre bundles (H and E); (b) ruptured tendon from a 65-year-old patient with tendinitis, showing region of fibrocartilage with rows of rounded, chondrocyte-like cells, which may be a pathological change or a normal adaptation to compressive forces acting on the tendon (H and E); (c) ruptured tendon from a 55-year-old patient with tendinitis, showing severe degenerative changes with no distinct fibrillar structure, scattered round cells, and a calcific deposit in the matrix (H and E); (d) specimen from a 76-year-old showing deposition of glycosaminoglycan between collagen fibrils and associated with rounded cells (Alcian blue/periodic acid–Schiff).

investigating DNA synthesis using thymidine incorporation in response to stimulation by fetal calf serum. No significant reduction in growth response with increasing age was found. Initial light-microscopic analyses of normal rotator-cuff tendons (Chard *et al.* 1989) suggest a general thickening of blood vessels, fewer tendon fibroblasts, increased mucopolysaccharide, and increased calcification with increasing age. An increase in cells resembling chondrocytes and hyperplasia of arteriolar intimal are seen (Yamanaka and Fukuda 1991).

Attention has been drawn to the unifying concept of the enthesopathies which suggests that local ischaemia is the common denominator. The enthesis is always at risk because the working muscle takes up most of the blood at the expense of the tendon and insertion. Other contributory factors include overstressing, muscular hypertonus, and excessive cooling. Endogenous factors such as impaired vascularization, metabolic disorders, endocrine disorders,

trophic disorders, toxic damage, and even psychological factors may also influence damage to the enthesis. Tendons without sheaths are better supplied with blood than those with, and dynamic blood-flow studies *in vivo* in these regions may yield valuable information. This section has focused on the tendon and its pathology. Lesions of bursae, fascias, and muscle will be discussed later in the chapter.

Collagen is the basic framework of all soft tissues. Once a tear occurs within the collagen bundles, the defect is replaced by haphazard, loose connective tissue formed in the blood clot that initially fills the torn area. Thus the intrinsic structural strength may be reduced significantly, leading to impaired power, mobility, and skill, and further tears.

Tendon cells are metabolically responsive and capable of repair; they maintain the matrix composition by a balance between anabolic and catabolic processes (Abrahamsson 1991). Biochemical and cell biological studies have shown that diseased tendons have an increased concentration of dermatan and chondroitin sulphates, and a threefold increase in hyaluronan (Riley *et al.* 1994), indicating that a change in proteoglycan synthesis has occurred. There is also an increase in cell numbers, a reduced collagen content, possibly caused by an increase in collagen degradation, and in the majority an increased content of collagen type III. These changes are consistent with inflammation and a fibroproliferative response, presumably in an attempt to repair the tendon defect, although it is not known if this process is primary or secondary to the tendon rupture.

A highly specialized 'fibrocartilage' develops in regions of tendons exposed to compression (Evans *et al.* 1990), which differ biochemically and structurally from tension-bearing regions and have characteristics somewhere between those of classic tendon regions and articular cartilage (Vogel *et al.* 1993). Although type I collagen remains the principal matrix component, the cellular activity in these compressed regions includes the synthesis of both type II collagen and aggrecan.

Growth factors have anabolic effects on tissues, increasing matrix synthesis and reducing matrix breakdown. Cytokines such as interleukin 1 and tumour necrosis factor-α often have the opposite effect, decreasing matrix synthesis and up-regulating the proteinases that promote matrix breakdown. Recent studies have shown that tendons *in vitro* respond to interleukin 1 by altering the synthesis of matrix components and proteinases such as matrix metalloproteinases (Dalton *et al.* 1995). The production of excessive enzyme activity can exceed that of local inhibitors (such as tissue inhibitor of metalloproteinases) and so lead to collagen breakdown.

Recent interest has centred on the role of prostaglandin synthesis and release in response to soft-tissue injury due either to trauma or overuse. Prostaglandins may act synergistically with other inflammatory mediators such as histamine, serotonin, and bradykinin to potentiate both swelling and pain. Muscle injuries are associated with bleeding to a greater or lesser degree, and interstitial haematomas produce marked pain and loss of function. Muscle regeneration is a slow process. Strains affect muscles. With minor strains only fibres are damaged, with the muscle sheath left intact. With more severe strains there is partial or complete rupture of fibres and sheath. A sprain is an overstretch injury of a ligament. It may affect only a few fibres or lead to rupture.

Generalized soft-tissue conditions

Repetitive strain syndrome

Occupational repetition strain injuries have become, particularly in recent years, a significant source of disability at work. There is considerable confusion in diagnostic terminology and a wide variation in reported incidence between countries, perhaps reflecting the contrasting medical and more particularly, legal, attitudes to these conditions. Flexor tenosynovitis, rotator-cuff tendinitis, and lateral epicondylitis have all been described as 'occupationally' induced clinical syndromes; they have high rates of relapse—6 per cent for tenosynovitis of the wrist, for example. Repetitive strain injury has, however, more diffuse clinical features and no clearly defined pathological basis. Two conditions are currently recognized as work-related industrial injuries: PDA4—cramp of the hand or forearm, in people with an occupation entailing prolonged periods of handwriting, typing, or other repetitive movements of the finger, hand, or arm; and PDA8—traumatic inflammation of the tendons of the hand or

forearm or the associated tendon sheaths in any occupation entailing manual labour or frequent or repeated movements of the hand or wrist. In general, as mentioned above, the increased incidence of these disorders appears to be due to new technology with advanced automation and mechanization. This has led to a need for rapid, repetitive movements, often of just the arms or even the hands and wrists alone. Although actual physical workloads may be lighter, it is this increased rate of work concentrated locally on an individual's musculoskeletal system that results in repetitive (repetition) strain injuries, and associated overuse syndromes. The influence of occupation on how we use or overuse parts of our body is striking. This suggests that were alternative ways of accomplishing various activities to be developed, a part of the problem could be controlled. Ergonomic and behavioural studies would seem to have much to offer. Definitions of the association between work and rheumatic complaints have been suggested (World Health Organization 1988). They emphasize the multifactorial nature of work-related musculoskeletal complaints in industrial workers. The load from work may not only be physical; stress factors also are important in some workplaces. Predisposing factors such as age and anthropometric features must also be considered. Repetitive strain syndrome can be defined as follows:

(1) a chronic pain syndrome;

(2) affecting one or both neck–arm regions;

(3) occurs in activities requiring controlled posture, often of a repetitive nature;

(4) psychological factors contribute to the syndrome.

The clinical features consist of:

(1) chronic pain in neck, chest wall, arm, and hand;

(2) inability to achieve previous work performance or carry out full leisure activities;

(3) variable hand–arm–forearm swelling with poor grip strength and taut proximal muscles;

(4) often mild algodystrophy;

(5) poor sleep pattern, often with mood changes.

Terminology

Arm pain associated with work, commonly known as repetitive strain injury, is currently sweeping the developed world. The most recent 'epidemic' began in Australia in the 1980s and has now 'spread' to the United States and United Kingdom. The term repetitive strain injury is perhaps misleading in that it implies that an actual 'injury' has been caused by repetitive movement. This has so far been difficult to establish, given the diffuse clinical features and absence of pathology in most cases. Also, there is no certain pathogenesis for repetitive strain injury that would justify the use of the term 'strain' and many sufferers develop their symptoms as a result of static rather than repetitive or dynamic muscle load (Littlejohn 1986).

Although an association between certain occupations and the incidence of repetitive strain injury has been described, there have been few studies designed to assess the connection properly. In Australia there was a sudden, dramatic increase in reporting symptoms that lasted around 18 months and was followed by an equally rapid reduction to baseline. The rise in cases was mirrored by increasing numbers of media reports on repetitive strain injury. This can be seen in Hocking's study carried out by Telecom Australia (Hocking 1987). Annual reports of repetitive strain injury increased from 109 in 1981 to over 1700 in 1985. Telephonists were most affected and telegraphists least. This order is the inverse of the keystroke rates, which are a few hundred an hour for a telephonist and over 12 000 an hour for a telegraphist. Cleland (1987) has described repetitive strain injury as a model of social iatrogenesis — the treatments, advice, and expectations provided by a wide range of people have provided an environment that has focused attention on discomfort about, and apprehension of, the potentially damaging effects of pain in the workplace. Through this process it is likely that a minor discomfort will be transformed into a protracted, painful, and disabling condition, precluding effective work and degrading quality of life.

The rapid decline in repetitive strain injury in Australia was due to several different factors. Work practices were changed, appropriate work breaks were instituted, and advice given about comfortable work stations. The term repetitive strain injury was also disposed of; if no specific diagnosis could be made, the condition was designated a regional pain syndrome.

Clinical features

Pain is the principal feature; this may be associated with inability to perform routine work or household activities. There may have been an underlying ache in the arm, shoulder or neck for some weeks before the onset of the pain syndrome, or it may follow a specific soft-tissue injury. Usually the symptoms begin around the wrist or forearm or elbow, and within days or weeks spread into the upper arm, shoulder, and neck. They may then involve the opposite side. Up to 20 per cent of patients develop more generalized pain involving the low back, buttock, and leg regions.

Generalized fatigue is common, and pain may fluctuate with activity, emotional stress or temperature change. In addition, patients report disturbance of their usual sleep pattern, with frequent waking and a feeling of tiredness in the morning. Examination shows an altered pain threshold.

Vasomotor changes in the forearm may be apparent and in the minority all the features of an algodystrophy syndrome may occur. The patient describes dysaesthesias in the hand and poor grip strength. There is a sensation of swelling but usually no objective evidence of this. Tender points in such as the first web space in the hand are also present. There is no evidence of synovitis, tenosynovitis, or neurological abnormality.

The syndrome is therefore one of regional pain, but the usual course is of prolonged pain for several months or years, irrespective of treatment or outcome of compensation. Once the regional pain syndrome has developed an exaggeration of tenderness when the patient is assessed for medicolegal purposes may be noted. No racial, social, or professional group has been spared, but the self-employed are not usually affected.

Several psychological factors come into play in occupations requiring rapid, repetitive movements. Indeed a significant body of opinion follows the concept of repetitive strain injury as a largely 'hysterical' or psychogenic illness (Awerbach 1985). A more accurate assessment would seem to be that physical, ergonomic, environmental, and psychological factors are involved in its onset and development.

Treatment

Management is similar to that of other chronic pain syndromes. Prevention and early diagnosis are important. If the full syndrome has developed the patient must be reassured that there is no tissue damage or injury, and that the symptoms are best thought of as a form of' overuse strain' that will recover with suitable modifications of activities.

It is necessary to treat any triggering ergonomic factor, either by modifying work activity or using a cervical collar. The patient should be encouraged to carry out regular exercise that involves stretching of tight, tender regions such as neck and shoulder. Sleep disturbance may require treatment with a hypnotic or low-dose tricyclic antidepressant.

If the syndrome has arisen in connection with paid employment, all the parties involved, including management, trades unions and third-party insurers, should be informed. An early return to work should be encouraged, but modification of work activity may be necessary when the pain is severe. Prolonged rest does not help, nor does the use of anti-inflammatory drugs or extensive physical treatments. Chronic pain is treated by gradually increasing activity under supervision.

Many patients with this problem are involved in disputes over compensation, litigation, or disability assessment. It has been suggested that the occurrence of chronic pain syndromes may be encouraged in those countries where compensation schemes include any symptoms that occur at work. This happened in Australia during the 1980s and is thought to have contributed to the pain syndrome 'epidemic' in that country. Prolonged medicolegal processes counteract any appropriate treatment programme (Littlejohn 1989).

The term repetitive strain injury implies a cause without defining the lesion. Ireland (1988) has emphasized that this condition predominantly affects women employed in low-paid, monotonous, unprestigious jobs. The employees placed the blame on the employment and thus on the employer. However, a small number of patients with this syndrome do present with genuine pain and disability and do not respond to current management. If no specific musculo-skeletal diagnosis can be made, then one should look at social and psychological factors that might promote the pain. These should be addressed and the patient's pain put in its proper context. Occupational issues concerning a constrained and rigid posture, the work cycle, time spent in any one activity, work satisfaction, and social intervention at work are important.

The advice 'if it hurts, stop' runs contrary to all accepted principles of the behavioural management of chronic pain and may lead to chronicity. The involvement of a clinical psychologist in the team, and an active occupational rehabilitation programme, helps most people to return to work.

Hand and arm problems of musicians

Musicians are prone to a variety of problems in the upper limb that produce significant disability; these include overuse syndromes, entrapment neuropathies, and focal motor dystonias. The diagnosis can be difficult as symptoms may be mild and only occur on playing. Episodes may be triggered by changes in repertoire, technique, and instrument, or by increases in daily playing time. The weight of a wind instrument such as the clarinet or oboe frequently leads to pain in the muscles of the first web space. Percussionists have a low prevalence of regional pain syndrome, presumably because their playing is more intermittent.

In reviewing several series of musculoskeletal injuries in musicians, Hoppmann and Patrone (1989) reported that of 179 injured musicians, 62 per cent had overuse syndrome, 18 per cent had nerve-entrapment thoracic-outlet syndrome, and 10 per cent had problems of motor control. Some of the musculoskeletal problems seen in musicians are listed in Table 4. Diagnosis and management are helped by a detailed knowledge of the instruments used and the specific dynamics of music making. Musculoskeletal problems are common in musicians of all ages and levels of skill. Recent research has included attempts to better define overuse, focal dystonia, and the role of hypermobility.

Treatment must take into account the specific injury and the instrument played. Table 5 lists some of the treatments that are generally applicable. Greater consideration is being given to the ergonomics of music making and technique is being assessed as a risk factor.

Musculoskeletal problems in dancers

Overuse injuries are common, and many joints are stressed by ranges of motion exceeding those that anatomy readily permits. The most common problems are back pain, and damage to the ankle and foot. Some 70 to 80 per cent of professional dancers complain of back pain, and the repetitive movements of dance may lead to overuse injuries such as tendinitis, neuritis, and stress fractures (Ramel and Moritz 1994). Pre-existing hypermobility may predispose to injury, and in the case of stress fractures, osteoporosis secondary to eating disorders and amenorrhoea may play a part. In one ballet company 104 dancers sustained 309 injuries over a 3-year period (Garrick and Requa 1993).

Fibromyalgia

The two cardinal features of fibromyalgia are generalized chronic pain and diffuse tenderness at discrete anatomical sites. Fibromyalgia has been found in 2 to 5 per cent of the population, predominantly affecting women in their forties and fifties, and is recognized as the second most common disorder seen in North American rheumatological practice. In some patients the syndrome complicates the illness associated with established rheumatic diseases.

Fibromyalgia is a recognizable syndrome characterized by chronic, diffuse pain, an absence of inflammatory or structural musculoskeletal abnormalities, and a range of symptoms that include fatigue, and sleep and mood disturbances. Physical examination and laboratory testing are unrevealing, except for the presence of pain on palpation of characteristic soft-tissue sites, the tender points.

Despite the recognition of fibromyalgia by the World Health Organization in 1992, it remains a controversial condition and its existence as a distinct entity remains uncertain (Cohen and Quintner 1993). However, the concept of fibromyalgia is a useful one, allowing many investigations to be avoided and appropriate advice on treatment to be given.

Fibromyalgia may overlap with symptoms of, and the patient further impaired by, anxiety and depression; patients with fibromyalgia have high scores on anxiety and depression questionnaires. The term fibromyalgia syndrome does not imply causation and merely describes the most common symptoms. Many patients with

Table 4	Musculoskeletal problems of musicians

Overuse injury:

Specific
    tenosynovitis

Non-specific
    diffuse forearm pain

Entrapment neuropathies

Focal dystonia

Thoracic-outlet syndrome

Hypermobility syndrome

Osteoarthritis

Table 5	Treatment of musculoskeletal injuries in musicians

Rest:

    Complete or incomplete rest periods into practice

Technique:

    Correct problem; noticing posture, muscle tone and
        movements that aggravate injury

Physical or occupational therapy:

    Splints, exercise, adaptive devices

Relaxation techniques:

    May include electromyographic feedback

    Non-steroidal anti-inflammatory drugs or local steroid injections

Surgery:

    Nerve-entrapment release

'chronic fatigue syndrome' fulfil the criteria for fibromyalgia and represent one end of a spectrum of presentation. Evidence for triggering viral infections is lacking in the majority of patients, and, unlike fibromyalgia, most 'postviral' syndromes are self-limiting and are not associated with tender sites. Common presenting symptoms are listed in Table 6.

The only tests required to exclude alternative diagnoses that may present with widespread pain, weakness or fatigue are listed in Table 7.

The tender sites are central to the definition and understanding of this condition. The neck and back show many changes, but the other tender sites reveal no changes sufficient to account for the marked tenderness, and certainly no inflammation. The same sites become tender in regional pain syndromes. The points (Fig. 2) are unknown to the patient, and often quite far from the region of referred pain; so that the pattern cannot be exaggerated for psychological reasons. The tenderness can be quantified, whereas pressure over other sites shows a normal pain threshold.

Table 6 Common symptoms of fibromyalgia

Fatiguability:
    Often extreme, following minimal exertion
    Predominantly axial, often aggravated by stress and cold
    Diffuse and unresponsive to analgesics/NSAIDs
    (all severely (limit daily activities)

Objective swelling of extremities

Paraesthesias, dysaesthesia of hands, feet

Waking unrefreshed

Poor concentration, depressed

Headache, diffuse abdominal pain

Altered bowel habit

Urinary frequency, urgency

NSAIDs, non-steroidal anti-inflammatory drugs.

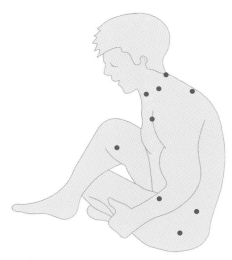

Fig. 2 The 'tender' points.

Table 7 Differential diagnosis and investigation of fibromyalgia

Differential diagnosis	Investigations
Hypothyroidism	Full blood count and ESR
Systemic lupus erythematosus	Calcium, creatine kinase
Inflammatory myopathy	Thyroid function
Hyperparathyroidism	Antinuclear factor
Osteomalacia	Plasma proteins
Parkinsonism	
Myeloma, carcinomatosis	
Polymyalgia rheumatica	

ESR, erythrocyte sedimentation rate.

However, it should be emphasized that the very existence of this condition is a matter of considerable debate. Doubts have been expressed about the validity of both the symptoms reported by patients and the signs observed; some deny the existence of the condition because no objective pathological findings are demonstrable. However, in 1990 the American College of Rheumatology published criteria for the classification (Table 8). According to this set of criteria (American College of Rheumatology 1990), fibromyalgia is a syndrome of widespread pain, by definition affecting both sides of the body and the upper and lower segments. Its symptoms may also include sleep disturbance, fatigue, and stiffness. The most important feature is, however, the 'tender point' count, first described by Smythe (1989). Smythe has suggested that the pain experienced by patients with fibromyalgia is referred pain from mechanical stresses in the lower neck and low back. Studies by

Lewis and Kellgren in the 1930s (Kellgren 1939) demonstrated that irritation of superficial and deep structures in the spine can produced both referred pain and also referred tenderness. Maigne (1972) demonstrated that irritation of posterior branches of spinal nerves could produce referred pain, referred tenderness, skin-rolling tenderness, and reactive hyperaemia in the anatomical distribution of the involved nerves. However, these observations have not been confirmed in patients with fibromyalgia, and the diffuse nature of pain in fibromyalgia suggests that spinal factors alone are not responsible for the clinical syndrome.

In drawing up the criteria for the diagnosis of fibromyalgia syndrome there has been much emphasis on the presence of tender points. It might therefore be asked whether it is possible to distinguish between fibromyalgia and a myofascial trigger-point pain syndrome simply by finding tender points in the former and trigger points in the latter. Myofascial trigger-point pain syndromes usually develop after trauma to the affected muscle or muscles, and the pain is alleviated by deactivating the hyperactive nerve endings at trigger points by one or other of a variety of methods, including the insertion of dry needles. Janet Trowell has written extensively on the subject and shown that each muscle in the body has its own specific pattern of trigger-point pain referral (Travell and Simons 1983).

Rheumatologists in general are not in the habit of looking for trigger points and those that have made a special study of fibromyalgia have never adequately addressed themselves to the question of whether some or perhaps all of the tender points in this condition could be trigger points. It would seem that most rheumatologists simply examine muscles for tender points and do so by applying pressure to them with outstretched fingers rather than by rolling the fingers firmly across them, and because of this tend to overlook the presence of any trigger point containing palpable bands.

It could be argued that tender points and trigger points must be one and the same, as the nociceptive hyperactivity that must be responsible for making the points so tender must also make the nerve endings at these sites at least potentially capable of triggering pain. Recently, it has been suggested that in patients with fibromyalgia, trigger points and tender points many represent the same abnormality. There are no longitudinal studies of myofascial pain to

Table 8 American College of Rheumatology criteria for fibromyalgia

1. *History of widespread pain*

Definition. Pain is considered when all of the following are present:

Pain in the left side of the body, pain in the right side of the body, pain above the waist and pain below the waist. In addition, axial skeletal pain (cervical pain or anterior chest or thoracic spine or low back) must be present. In this definition shoulder and buttock pain is considered as pain for each involved side. 'Low back' pain is considered lower segment pain.

2. *Pain in 11 of 18 tender point sites on digital palpation*

Definition. Pain, on digital palpation, must be present in at least 11 of the following 18 tender point sites:

Occiput: bilateral, at the suboccipital muscle insertions

Low cervical: bilateral; at the anterior aspects of the inter-transverse spaces at C5–C7

Trapezius: bilateral, at the midpoint of the upper border

Supraspinatus: bilateral, at origins, above the scapula spine near the medial border

2nd rib: bilateral, at the second costochondral junctions, just lateral to the junctions on upper surfaces

Lateral epicondyle: bilateral, 2 cm distal to the epicondyles

Gluteal: bilateral, in upper outer quadrants of buttocks in anterior fold of muscle

Greater trochanter: bilateral, posterior to the trochanteric prominence

Knees: bilateral, at the medial fat pad proximal to the joint line

Digital palpation should be performed with an appropriate force of 4 kg. For a tender point to be considered 'positive' the subject must state that the palpation was painful. 'Tender' is not to be considered painful.
*For classification purposes patients will be said to have fibromyalgia if both criteria are satisfied. Widespread pain must have been present for at least 3 months. The presence of a second clinical disorder does not exclude the diagnosis of fibromyalgia.

determine if a subset of patients evolves into a more characteristic fibromyalgia syndrome.

Aggravating factors for fibromyalgia include exhaustion, lack of fitness, disturbed sleep (which may affect the way pain signals are modulated or transmitted), and anxiety. The following are commonly associated: tension headaches, paraesthesiae, subjective swelling of joints, and primary dysmenorrhoea.

In 1975, Smythe and Moldofsky recorded electromyograms and electroencephalograms in 10 patients suffering from so-called 'fibrositis' (Moldofsky et al. 1975). The electroencephalographic changes showed that each patient had a disturbance of stage IV, non-rapid eye movement (**REM**) sleep. This disturbance is brought about by the rapid, 8 to 10 cycles/s α-rhythm, normally found in REM sleep, intruding into the usual slow, 1 to 2 cycles/s δ-rhythm of stage IV deep sleep. Sleep disturbances have subsequently been reported in 60 to 90 per cent of patients with fibromyalgia, but are also recognized as not specific, seen in many other conditions, and in as many as 15 per cent of healthy individuals (Scheuler et al. 1988).

A further study in healthy normal volunteers showed that the same α-intrusion into the δ-wave pattern of deep sleep could be produced experimentally by disturbing the volunteers' sleep by hand contact or a buzzer (Scheuler et al. 1988). When this intrusion occurred the sleepers developed general musculoskeletal pain and tenderness similar to that seen in 'fibrositis'. After a few nights of normal sleep the pain disappeared. These studies led to increasing recognition of fibrositis and the concept of fibrositis as we understand it today.

Some patients have no difficulty in getting off to sleep, consider that they sleep soundly, and yet awake with a general feeling of tiredness, fatigue, and general stiffness. Others experience this feeling after a light, restless sleep. It is not known whether changes in sleep physiology in fibromyalgia are the primary disturbance, with the muscle pains occurring secondary to these, or whether similar electroencephalographic changes develop as a secondary event in those whose sleep is disturbed as a result of pain. There is still insufficient evidence to link fatigue with specific sleep disturbances.

Psychological disturbances are seen only in the minority of people with fibromyalgia. However, emotional upsets and stress seem capable of bringing on the symptoms. Case–control studies on patients with fibromyalgia and matched controls with rheumatic diseases have shown a higher prevalence in fibromyalgia of depression, sexual and physical abuse, and eating disorders preceding the onset of the disease. Psychological stresses are frequent before its onset in adolescents.

There have been studies suggesting a deficiency of the neurotransmitter serotonin in fibromyalgia, with lower concentrations of its metabolites in cerebrospinal fluid. However, if serotonin deficiency was central to the pathophysiology of fibromyalgia, we would expect improvement on treatment with serotonergic drugs such as fluoxetine, which does not appear to be the case. Endorphins and substance P are other neurotransmitters that have been extensively studied in fibromyalgia. Endorphins were found to be normal, whilst substance P was increased in cerebrospinal fluid;

however, healthy controls were used, which prevents firm conclusions (Russell *et al.* 1994).

Treatment

Whether we label sufferers as having fibromyalgia or not, there is no doubt that many have diffuse pain, sleep disturbances, fatigue, and tender points. There is no specific treatment and the prognosis is poor, but individual patients may be helped, by an adequate explanation of the condition, to learn to live better with it and so avoid further unnecessary investigations and drug treatments.

At present, tricyclic antidepressants and aerobic exercises are the treatments that have been most extensively studied. Both have a moderate degree of benefit. Cognitive behavioural approaches and multidisciplinary treatment programmes have also been used in an attempt to help patients gain control over their symptoms, but both are time-consuming and expensive and require fuller study. Aspects of management are summarized in Table 9 and of treatment in Table 10.

As many patients have suffered disappointment, blows to self-confidence and esteem, together with pain and exhaustion, they often find it hard to believe they can recover; they therefore require much encouragement from doctor and therapist. The absence of inflammation in soft tissue is now accepted. This explains the lack of efficacy of non-steroidal anti-inflammatory drugs and corticosteroids. Patients with fibromyalgia are aerobically unfit. There is no evidence to suggest that they have any primary muscle abnormality nor do they suffer from defects in energy metabolism. Aerobic fitness training unfortunately only produces slight benefit.

Tricyclic antidepressants in small doses of 10 to 30 mg are often helpful in improving the quality of sleep, in reducing morning stiffness, and in alleviating pain. However, overall the prognosis is poor and the condition tends to take a protracted course (Felson and Goldenberg 1986).

Conclusions

The opponents of the concept of fibromyalgia consider it a 'non-disease' and suggest that the label is likely to create a population of 'worried well', with adverse social and psychological consequences. The Australian experience with the diagnosis of repetitive strain injury warns us of the possibility of negative disease labelling. The converse argument is that the term fibromyalgia provides the patient with a structure for understanding the condition. Many patients have had numerous diagnoses and investigations, and the average duration of symptoms before the diagnosis of fibromyalgia is made is 5 years. Once it is made and explained, anxiety and frustration often disappear.

Opponents of the fibromyalgia label argue that by labelling a non-disease doctors are legitimizing patients' sickness behaviour. However, the converse is that the term fibromyalgia, put in its proper perspective, provides a health-care professional with the basis to recommend activity rather than inactivity, work modification rather than work termination, and coping strategies.

The clinical syndrome that we now call fibromyalgia has been present for a long time. The facts that it is poorly understood and there are no objective physical and laboratory abnormalities do not mean that the patient is not ill or in distress. Physical and emotional pain may be disabling. We must guide patients away from sickness behaviour; we must also focus on the complicated psychosocial and biological factors that distinguish individuals who cope well with

Table 9	Principal strategies for management of fibromyalgia
Educate patient	
Educate patient's family	
Keep investigations to minimum and stop ineffective drug therapy	
Use interventions to improve sleep disturbance and improve aerobic fitness	

Table 10	Treatment of fibromyalgia
Low-dose amitriptyline:	
Initially give 25 mg at night	
Graded aerobic exercise regimen:	
Individualized for patient	
Encourage frequent but small amounts	
Encourage continuation despite pain	
Set increasing weekly targets	
Coping strategies:	
Behavioural therapy	
Yoga	

their symptoms from those who remain disabled in chronic pain (Goldenberg 1995). Physicians have taken an entity that existed for centuries, given it a new name, and created a major health issue by elevating it in importance and suggesting it deserves disability coverage (Carette 1995).

Hypermobility

The term 'hypermobility syndrome' is used to describe a common disorder in which seemingly otherwise healthy individuals present with articular and/or spinal symptoms for which no explanation is forthcoming, other than their joint hypermobility. The degree of hypermobility relates to the degree of ligamentous laxity. These patients are susceptible to torn muscles and ligaments, and are also predisposed to traumatic and degenerative changes of joints, and prolapsed discs. Dislocation of joints is more likely to occur. Persistent low back pain in the absence of an identifiable anatomical lesion in hypermobile patients is called 'the loose back syndrome'.

Normal individuals have a wide range of joint mobility, apart from the influence of age, sex, and race. Hypermobility diminishes steadily throughout childhood and more slowly during adulthood. Females show a greater range of joint movement than males. Generalized ligamentous laxity, the prerequisite of joint hypermobility, is seen in about 10 per cent of healthy individuals; the majority suffer no ill effects. The diagnosis of joint hypermobility depends on the ability to perform a series of passive joint manoeuvres. The Beighton scale (Beighton *et al.* 1989) is the measurement of choice (Table 11); the maximum score is 9.

The diagnosis is commonly missed, for clinicians are trained to look for loss of range of joint and spinal motion and so fail to recognize an increase in range. Hypermobility syndrome has to be distinguished from the less benign heritable disorders of connective tissues such as the Marfan and Ehlers–Danlos syndromes and osteogenesis imperfecta, with which it shares a number of common features. This distinction is not always easy. Echocardiography, ophthalmic examination, and genetic studies may be required to define the phenotype in individual families.

Tissues that rely for their structural integrity on the tensile strength of collagen may be affected. The skin may be soft and develop striations. An association between mitral-valve prolapse, aortic incompetence, and hypermobility has been reported. There is an increased incidence of abdominal hernia, and rectal and uterine prolapse. Bone fragility may also be present and stress fractures can occur.

Articular features

The clinical effects of hypermobility depend on its degree and are irrespective of its cause. Patients present with a wide variety of traumatic and overuse lesions including joint or tendon-sheath synovitis, friction lesions at insertions of tendons or ligaments, rotator-cuff lesions, or back pain. Others suffer the effects of joint instability, such as flat feet and recurrent dislocation or subluxation. Arthralgia can occur and tends to improve over the years as the joints lose some of their hypermobility. There is also presumptive evidence to suggest that premature osteoarthritis may be a direct consequence of joint hypermobility.

There is a female preponderance of 85 per cent in this syndrome, which reflects the greater laxity of their joints. All patients have a varied pattern of locomotor disorders and it has been suggested that people with hypermobility do not present with different rheumatological problems from other patients; but that they have them in greater variety.

Hypermobility in healthy individuals should not be considered as just a liability. It seems to be an important selection factor enabling them to compete successfully in athletics, music, and ballet. Since inherent joint laxity enables the dancer to achieve impressive ranges of joint movement without effort, hypermobile individuals tend to be selected for ballet schools, upon which their connective tissue abnormality ceases to be an asset and becomes a liability.

Patients with hypermobility syndrome present with an unusual collection of seemingly unconnected locomotor symptoms. Unless the clinical examination is thorough and looks for increased range of joint and spinal movement, the syndrome will be overlooked. It is a common condition and patients are often pleased that someone can explain their symptoms.

Aetiology

Studies of families have provided evidence for a dominant mode of inheritance. Within individual families, females are more frequently and more severely affected than males. Females tend to present with arthralgia and mitral-valve prolapse, while males tend to develop

---

Table 11 The 9-point Beighton scoring system for joint hypermobility

Scoring 1 point on each side

Passive dorsiflexion of the fifth metacarpophalangeal joint to 90°

Apposition of the thumb to the flexor aspect of the forearm

Hyperextension of the elbow beyond 10°

Hyperextension of the knee beyond 10°

Scoring 1 point

Forward trunk flexion placing hands flat on floor with knees extended

---

Table 12 Management of hypermobility

1. Discuss condition and reassure that pain is not imaginary

2. Inform that although children may inherit joint hypermobility they will not necessarily have symptoms

3. Patients with mitral-valve prolapse require antibiotic prophylaxis

4. Anti-inflammatory drugs no more effective than analgesics

5. Stretching exercises aim to restore movement into hypermobile range
   Conventional physiotherapy disappointing

6. Patients should try to avoid activities that provoke or aggravate symptoms

---

dislocations and back pain (Child 1986). The mitral-valve prolapse is usually mild and has no haemodynamic significance.

Skin biopsies show abnormalities in the architecture of the collagen bundles. The normal gradation between the coarser deep and the fine superficial bundles is lost, and a more uniform deposition of the fine bundles prevails throughout the dermis. At the biochemical level there are raised ratios of collagen type III:types II + I, indicating a significant imbalance in the two major collagen types present.

Treatment

Management (Table 12) must first include an explanation of the symptoms. Patients need to know they have a condition that doctors recognize and that they do not have Marfan syndrome with its less favourable prognosis.

Symptoms arising in unstable, weight-bearing joints may be relieved by an appropriate exercise routine, in an attempt to allow muscle to compensate for ligamentous laxity. Many of the complications of hypermobility (osteoarthrosis, ligamentous or muscle tears) are treated along conventional lines. However, the arthralgia and the

Table 13 The painful shoulder

Rotator-cuff lesions

Tendinitis:
  Supraspinatus
  Acute calcific supraspinatus
  Infraspinatus and subscapularis

Rupture:
  Partial
  Complete

Bicipital syndromes

Tenosynovitis of long head

Rupture of long head

Subacromial bursitis

Usually secondary to adjacent pathology

Frozen shoulder (adhesive capsulitis)

Shoulder–hand syndrome and referred pain

'loose back syndrome' can be difficult to treat, apart from noting aggravating factors and trying to avoid them. These pains respond poorly to non-steroidal anti-inflammatory drugs and conventional physiotherapy.

Localized soft-tissue lesions

The painful shoulder

More than 90 per cent of lesions causing the painful shoulder result from extracapsular soft-tissue conditions (Table 13). The glenohumeral joint is a multiaxial joint that permits the greatest freedom of movement of any joint in the body, allowing placement of the hand for optimal function, although this is at the expense of stability. Ligamentous support is important in maintaining the stability of the shoulder joints, and muscles act as prime movers at the shoulders as well as providing some dynamic stability at the glenohumeral joint.

Shoulder pain may be seen in association with several medical conditions and may be referred from cervical, thoracic, or abdominal sources. The mechanism of injury may also help in making a diagnosis. A fall on to an outstretched arm can give rise to glenohumeral instability in the younger person or a rotator-cuff tear in the elderly person. A fall on to the point of the shoulder may result in injury to the rotator cuff or acromioclavicular joint. Throwing injuries tend to stress the capsule and ligaments of the glenohumeral joint, and can also give rise to rotator-cuff or bicipital tendinitis.

Complaints of shoulder pain are frequently related to occupation. Bjelle *et al.* (1979) have documented this association: they monitored the medical departments of six heavy industries and found that approximately one-third of visits were for non-traumatic musculoskeletal complaints, of which 30 to 50 per cent were neck–shoulder complaints.

Hagberg (1981*a*) and Hagberg (1981*b*) studied the relation between task demand and shoulder pain, and assessed endurance and fatigue.

It was found that if the arm is held abducted and in forward flexion at a right angle, the supraspinatus and upper trapezius demonstrate fatigue within 5 min. With a variable workload and repetitive forceful shoulder flexion, the lower trapezius fatigues and there is associated discomfort in the lower neck for as long as 24 h after exertion. Workers were also filmed to gain objective estimates of workload. These physiological insights suggest task modifications that might lead to more comfortable working patterns. Job rotation, shorter exposure times, and job sharing may all lessen shoulder discomfort. These studies suggest that shoulder or neck disorders in industrial workers are multifactorial in origin and that pre-existing disease is important among the causative factors. Workers with chronic shoulder pain were significantly older and women were at higher risk than men of developing shoulder complaints.

A pain history is essential as the location and type of pain varies between conditions. Pain referred from the cervical spine is often maximal over the suprascapular region, with associated paraesthesias or pain in the upper limb. Acromioclavicular and sternoclavicular pain is usually well localized in the involved joint. Pain from the rotator cuff is usually felt at the outer aspect of the upper arm. Capsulitis tends to give rise to an intense aching deep in the shoulder. Night pain tends to be of two main types, either a sharp pain associated with movement indicative of a rotator-cuff tendinitis or acromioclavicular pathology, or pain of a deep, constant aching more suggestive of capsulitis or a rotator-cuff tear.

Examination should include close inspection for deformity, muscle wasting, and abnormalities of scapulohumeral movement. Palpation should assess the presence of tenderness, swelling, and instability as well as trigger points. Active and passive ranges of motion of both shoulders should be assessed in the planes of abduction, forward flexion, and external rotation, both with the arm by the side and at 90° abduction (Table 14).

Periarticular conditions affecting the shoulder can be loosely grouped into those with and without capsulitis. If there is no capsular involvement, then passive joint movement is largely unaffected whereas active movement may be limited by pain or weakness. In capsulitis there is a generalized restriction of movement (Dalton 1989).

Rotator-cuff disorders

As outlined above, these range from mild tendinitis following an episode of glenohumeral instability in the young patient to a complete tear in an older patient. The cuff is subjected to stresses when the arm is in the raised position, and impingement can occur as the supraspinatus tendon is compressed between the humeral head and the overlying acromion, coracoacromial ligament, and the inferior border of the acromioclavicular joint. As the rotator cuff becomes inflamed and thin its function as a depressor of the humeral head is compromised, and migration of the humeral head due to the unopposed action of the deltoid gives rise to further impingement. In the degenerative cuff this can result in a cuff arthropathy with degenerative changes in the subacromial and glenohumeral joints (Neer 1983).

Rotator-cuff tendinitis

While any of the tendons of the rotator cuff may be affected by tendinitis, it most commonly affects the supraspinatus portion of the cuff close to its insertion to the humeral head. Overuse, with resultant

Table 14 Clinical features of some extracapsular shoulder lesions

Lesion	Painful arc	Pain increased by:
Supraspinatus tendinitis, calcific deposit or incomplete tear	Yes	Resisted abduction
Infraspinatus tendinitis	Yes	Resisted external rotation
Acromioclavicular joint disease	Yes; pain begins later in abduction (not below 90°) and increases as full elevation is reached	Local palpation resisted adduction
Subscapularis	No	Resisted internal rotation
Bicipital tendinitis	No	Resisted flexion and supination of the elbow Tender bicipital groove

wear and tear and relative avascularity, may be important in inducing degeneration of the tendon.

In the young adult, rotator-cuff tendinitis usually presents acutely after an activity such as throwing. In middle-aged individuals the onset is more gradual, reflecting the underlying chronic change in the tendon, with pain aggravated by movement into abduction on elevation. Pain at night occurs when lying on the affected side. Active movements may be restricted by pain, but passive range is usually maintained and in the more chronic cases a secondary capsulitis may further restrict the shoulder movement.

Examination shows a painful arc of abduction, usually occurring between 70 and 120°, and then when lowering the shoulder there is often a 'catch' of pain as impingement occurs. Passive movement is usually full and pain-free if there is adequate muscle relaxation. In the older patient there is often involvement of the acromioclavicular joint.

Pain felt in the upper arm may suggest involvement of the cervical root, although this is more likely to present with upper trapezius or suprascapular pain referred down into the arm. Pain on active arm movement and impingement testing helps in confirming a rotator-cuff tendinitis, and the preservation of passive range of movement helps differentiate a tendinitis from a capsulitis. In patients under the age of 25 years, tendinitis is usually due to an underlying instability, which can be confirmed on examination.

Some cases of supraspinatus tendinitis are associated with calcific deposits visible on radiographs (Fig. 3). The exact mechanism responsible for the deposition of the calcium hydroxyapatite crystals in the tendon is unclear (Uthoff and Sarkar 1989). The deposits may remain asymptomatic or produce chronic symptoms with nagging discomfort in the region of the affected tendon. The crystals may also be extravasated into the subacromial bursa, causing acute bursitis with intense shoulder pain, loss of movement, severe tenderness, swelling, and muscle spasm. Fever, sweating, and other systemic symptoms may be present, mimicking gout or septic arthritis.

Infraspinatus and subscapularis lesions
These are less common and do not tend to calcify. While the symptoms are usually similar to those of supraspinatus tendinitis, pain induced by resisted external or internal rotation (Table 14) usually allows the correct diagnosis to be made.

Management
This is often difficult because of the patient's continuing participation in aggravating activities. Rest is necessary to prevent the condition becoming chronic. Initial treatment should aim to reduce inflammation with non-steroidal anti-inflammatory drugs and physical methods such as ultrasound. When there is no response, a subacromial injection of corticosteroid can be used.

In addition to improving pain, treatment should also aim to restore the range of movement and the normal biomechanics of shoulder movement, particularly a normal scapulohumeral rhythm. Then a strengthening programme of exercises should be given, with particular attention to restoring the rotator-cuff muscles to their function of stabilizing and depressing the humeral head.

The younger patient with instability requires a rehabilitation exercise programme and rarely requires injection. The older patient with a degenerative rotator cuff and associated pathology of the acromioclavicular joint may not be helped without surgery. The major indication

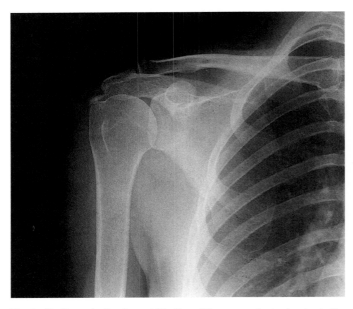

Fig. 3 Radiograph showing calcification of the supraspinatus tendon in the shoulder.

for surgery is pain and, in the presence of an intact rotator cuff, failure to respond to conservative treatment within 1 year. Surgery consists of subacromial decompression by resecting the coracoacromial ligament, and an anterior acromioplasty. If there is pathology of the acromioclavicular joint, this also requires attention. Full-thickness tears can be demonstrated by arthrography, ultrasonography, or magnetic resonance imaging. Arthroscopy is also useful.

Tears of the rotator cuff

Tears of the rotator cuff may be acute or chronic, partial or full thickness, and are most common in patients over the age of 50 years. They usually occur at the enthesis; degenerative changes and alterations in collagen composition may explain the susceptibility to tearing at this site (Kumagai et al. 1994). The mechanism of injury is a fall on to the outstretched arm. Partial tears may occur after trauma at any age and may present as a painful arc syndrome; full active range of movement may be preserved. Complete tears are associated with marked weakness of abduction and external rotation, or of flexion, depending on the tendon involved; passive movement is full. Pain can be severe and there may be no history of injury. Partial tears may be difficult to differentiate from tendinitis, but there is often an inability to maintain the arm in abduction when lowering it from a raised position. Atrophy of supra- and infraspinatus muscles often follows, and weakness of external rotation reflects the size of the tear. Rupture of the tendon of the long head of the biceps is frequently associated with chronic disease of the rotator cuff.

Chronic, full-thickness tears are found in up to 25 per cent of cadavers at autopsy. Cuff arthropathy occurs when there is superior migration of the humeral head against the under surface of the acromion, which happens when the incompetent rotator cuff fails to stabilize and depress the humeral head and therefore counteract the pull of the deltoid.

Radiographs show degeneration and sclerosis of the rotator cuff, and cystic changes at the greater tuberosity. Osteophytes may be present at the inferior margin of the acromioclavicular joint. The subacromial space is narrowed if there is a complete tear.

Treatment

Partial tears of the rotator cuff should initially be managed conservatively in a similar way to tendinitis of the cuff, although corticosteroid injections should be avoided within 6 weeks of injury. Acute ruptures in the young or active patient should have early surgery. In the older or less active patient it is usual to give a trial of conservative treatment. The treatment of large tears is controversial. It now seems that adequate decompression combined with anterior acromioplasty and debridement is preferred over extensive surgical procedures (Burkhart et al. 1994). Surgery should also be considered where there is associated rupture of the biceps tendon, as these patients are more likely to develop a cuff arthropathy.

Bicipital syndromes

The biceps tendon is seldom involved in isolation and involvement usually occurs with tendinitis or impingement of the rotator cuff, or with glenohumeral instability. As with rotator-cuff tendinitis, the young patient should be assessed for joint instability. Acute rupture is usually a result of overuse such as in weight-lifting.

Pain is felt over the anterior aspect of the shoulder, with localized tenderness over the tendon in the bicipital groove. Pain may be reproduced on resisted elbow flexion, although various provocation tests are inconsistently positive. Rupture of the tendon leads to a characteristic increase in the muscle belly of the biceps on resisted elbow flexion.

The tendon of the long head of the biceps tendon may be involved at its attachment to the superior glenoid labrum or as it runs in the bicipital groove.

Treatment

This consists of rest, physical procedures including laser therapy, and non-steroidal anti-inflammatory drugs. Care should be taken not to inject the tendon with corticosteroid. It is essential to assess whether the tendinitis is primary or secondary to pathology or instability of the rotator cuff, as failure to treat these causes will lead to a recurrence.

In chronic resistant cases, surgery may be required; either subacromial decompression or tenodesis, depending on the cause. Rupture of the tendon is usually treated conservatively, except in the occasional young patient where upper-arm strength is essential for their sport.

Subacromial bursitis

In most cases the bursa becomes inflamed as part of the impingement process and coexists with an underlying rotator-cuff tendinitis. In chronic cases the bursa becomes fibrotic and surgical excision or debridement may be necessary.

Acute traumatic bursitis may be differentiated from rotator-cuff tendinitis by the presence of increased tenderness and fluid at the subacromial space. Rest and physical treatment usually result in resolution.

Acromioclavicular syndrome

This is seen as an acute condition following trauma, usually after falls or contact sports. Septic arthritis can also rarely occur. Disruption of the joint may be seen in association with fractures of the clavicle. More common are injuries to the joint itself, which are graded I to III depending on the degree of disruption of the joint capsule and supporting ligaments.

Pain is well localized to the top of the shoulder, and the joint is often tender and swollen. Abduction is often limited. In complete disruption of the joint a visible step deformity is seen.

Treatment

For most injuries treatment is largely symptomatic with analgesics and a sling for a few days. Controversy exists over the management of complete dislocation of the joint. Surgical stabilization is usually unnecessary and has a high failure rate.

Patients with persistent pain at the acromioclavicular joint should be treated with an intra-articular corticosteroid and non-steroidal anti-inflammatory drugs. Long-term treatment is as for osteoarthritis of the joint.

Frozen shoulder (adhesive capsulitis)

This condition may occur spontaneously but can follow other lesions of the rotator cuff or trauma. In addition, conditions that produce pain (e.g. the referred pain of myocardial infarction) or immobility (e.g. from stroke or polymyalgia rheumatica) of the shoulder or arm can predispose to the development of a frozen shoulder. Early arthrography may reveal a small, shrunken, thickened capsule and some insist that these changes need to be present to make a diagnosis of adhesive capsulitis (Neviaser and Neviaser 1987).

Primary capsulitis can be defined as a condition of unknown aetiology in which there is a painful, global restriction of active and passive glenohumeral movement in all planes, in the absence of joint degeneration. Underlying conditions associated with this condition include diabetes mellitus, thyroid disease, and pulmonary disorders such as tuberculosis (Risk and Pinals 1982). Until recently, few pathological studies had been performed; Bunker and Anthony (1995) found features compatible with fibromatosis.

Onset under the age of 40 is uncommon; frozen shoulder is slightly more common in women than men and involvement of the contralateral shoulder occurs in up to 17 per cent of patients over the subsequent 5 years. There is severe night pain and pain on movement; improvement is gradual and spontaneous but may take 1 to 3 years. The extent of the recovery is variable and a clinically detectable limitation of shoulder movement can be seen in up to 15 per cent of patients (Bulgen et al. 1984).

Diagnosis is largely on clinical grounds as few abnormalities are found on investigation. Differentiation from rotator-cuff tendinitis is possible as there is global restriction of passive movement rather than simply loss of abduction and flexion.

Patients with even minor degrees of frozen shoulder may develop a secondary, reflex-sympathetic dystrophy syndrome — the shoulder–hand syndrome. This consists of a symptom complex characterized by an immobile painful shoulder associated with a swollen, painful, cold, and dystrophic-looking hand. The lesion may progress until the patient is left with a painful, tender, useless hand.

Treatment

The emphasis in the early stages should be on pain relief and the prevention of joint restriction. Analgesics are more effective than non-steroidal anti-inflammatory drugs; physiotherapy with interferential can reduce pain and reduce muscle spasm, and exercises within the limits of pain to maintain joint mobility are encouraged.

Intra-articular corticosteroid injections have improved pain and range of movement, although no long-term benefit has been shown. Oral corticosteroids have improved pain but not range of movement. No treatment has been consistently shown to affect rate of recovery or limit restriction of movement.

Distension of the subscapular bursa by arthrography and forced mobilization can result in immediate pain relief (Nobuhara et al. 1994). Manipulation under anaesthetic is sometimes advocated to restore joint movement by rupturing the inferior capsule. Care is required and very active early rehabilitation is necessary in the postmanipulation period to maintain joint mobility. If this treatment is contemplated, it is recommended that it be reserved for the adhesive stage and not the early, painful phase.

This condition is very painful and disability prolonged. It is essential that the patient understands this and for their expectations to be appropriate.

Glenoid labrum tears

There has been considerable recent interest in tears of the glenoid labrum. The labrum is a fibrocartilaginous and fibrous structure attached to the glenoid that supports the stability of the joint by serving as an attachment site for the glenohumeral ligaments. Clinical features of tears include shoulder pain, especially with overhead activities, and snapping and catching on movement. Because the biceps tendon originates at the superioglenoid with its labral attachment, pain may be present in the anterior shoulder on resisted forward flexion with the elbow extended and forearm supinated (Speed's test) (Payne 1994).

The painful elbow

Pain round the elbow is commonly caused by soft-tissue lesions (Table 15), but care must be taken to exclude pain referred from the cervical spine, brachial plexus, and shoulder, and examination of the neck and shoulder is important in the assessment of elbow pain.

Humeral epicondylitis

Lateral involvement (tennis elbow) is much more common than medial involvement (golfer's elbow). In spite of their sporting connotations, both occur more frequently in those performing repetitive movements with their arms, for example operating machinery, using a screwdriver or doing housework, although some 40 per cent of tennis players do suffer from tennis elbow.

In tennis elbow there is pain over the lateral aspect of the elbow with localized tenderness near the lateral epicondyle. In general, tenoperiosteal lesions can be separated from intra-articular conditions because movement of the related joint is full, there is tenderness at the tenoperiosteal junction, and contraction of the muscle attached to the affected tendon reproduces the pain. About 1 to 3 per cent of adults are affected by it; usually they are aged between 40 and 60 years, the dominant arm being most frequently affected (Hamilton 1986). Resisted dorsiflexion of the wrist exacerbates the pain with the elbow in extension, and there is a reduction in grip strength. Tenderness is usually maximal over the lateral epicondyle. Thermography usually shows a discrete 'hot spot' on the side of the elbow. The range of movement of the elbow is usually normal. In golfer's elbow there is a tender spot at the medial epicondyle owing to a lesion of the common flexor tendon, and pain is induced by flexing the wrist against resistance with the elbow fully extended.

Pain on resisted flexion alone indicates the rarer brachialis muscle lesion, with pain and tenderness that is less well localized and found behind the biceps tendon. Although uncommon, such a tear is particularly prone to develop myositis ossificans, which in the early stages

Table 15 The painful elbow

Humeral epicondylitis
Lateral:
  Tennis elbow
Medial:
  Golfer's elbow
  Biceps and triceps tendinitis
  Tear of brachialis muscle
Olecranon bursitis
Traumatic:
  Student's elbow
  Secondary to inflammatory joint disease
Friction neuritis of ulnar nerve

produces a warm, firm mass that can be mistaken for a tumour. It is unusual to have a lesion at the site of the triceps insertion into the olecranon. Lesions usually occur in this tendon at the musculotendinous junction. Ligamentous lesions do not usually occur in isolation; they are usually associated with traumatic synovitis of the joint.

Radial tunnel syndrome or compression of the posterior interosseous nerve can produce lateral elbow and forearm pain. These nerve entrapments are due to compressive lesions caused by fibrous bands in front of the radial head, or an abnormal origin of extensor carpi radialis brevis.

It is thought that the majority of patients have a musculotendinous lesion of the common extensor tendon at the attachment to the lateral epicondyle, especially that portion derived from extensor carpi radialis brevis. Macroscopic tears in the extensor tendon are occasionally found at operation, but these may have been caused by repeated steroid injections. Some cases show mesenchymal transformation suggestive of a chronic traction effect. Age is an important factor since lateral epicondylitis is uncommon before 30 years. Sometimes there may be bilateral involvement, either due to increased stress placed on the unaffected arm or as a general tendency to soft-tissue lesions in that individual.

Management (Table 16)

Reduced activity may result in improvement, particularly in early cases. Corticosteroid injections have been widely used; hydrocortisone is preferable to longer-acting preparations, which may lead to skin atrophy. Approximately 90 per cent of patients respond, but there may be increased pain for up to 48 h following injection and a significant number of cases recur. The injection may be repeated once after 4 weeks.

Non-steroidal anti-inflammatory drugs are often used but there is little evidence of their efficacy. A cock-up wrist splint reduces tension on forearm extensors and may help resolution. Numerous physical forms of treatment have been used but the efficacy of most is unproven (Chard and Hazleman 1989). Ultrasound, by its ability to cross myofascial planes and concentrate near bone, has theoretical advantages; in one study the rate of relapse was less with ultrasound than after corticosteroid injection (Binder *et al.* 1985).

Up to 40 per cent of patients have recurrent symptoms and some minor discomfort can persist for years. Early treatment may improve prognosis; firm strapping of the forearm muscles just distal to the elbow joint or the use of commercial elbow splints may be helpful. Patients should be advised to avoid straining the arm for some 2 months. Graded exercises to strengthen the forearm muscles may be advised, especially in sporting lesions.

Up to 10 per cent of patients fail to respond to physiotherapy. Surgical treatment, which attempts to correct the presumed pathological changes, can be helpful. Excision of tissues around the epicondyle or removal of a synovial fringe of the radiohumeral joint are the most common procedures.

Olecranon bursitis

The superficial bursa over the olecranon process is commonly involved in rheumatoid arthritis (with nodule formation) or gout, but can also be affected by trauma or infection. In the acute stage it distends with fluid, with prominent signs of acute inflammation. If it becomes chronic the wall can be greatly thickened. As the posterior wall of the bursa is so close to the periosteum of the olecranon, pain can be felt down the border of the ulna.

Table 16 Management of lateral epicondylitis

Early/mild	Rest, splinting
	Anti-inflammatory drugs/gels
Persistent	Local corticosteroid injections
	Ultrasound
Resistant	Manipulation?
	Surgery—lateral release

Treatment

Aspiration of the bursa reduces symptoms and allows examination of the fluid to exclude infection and the presence of crystals. If no infection is suspected, local steroid injections are effective; a compressive elastic bandage may help prevent the recurrence of swelling. If recurrent, non-infective bursitis occurs then surgical excision may be necessary. The presence of infection requires appropriate antibiotic treatment and surgical drainage may be necessary.

The painful wrist and hand (Table 17)

Both seropositive and seronegative arthritides have a predilection for inflammatory involvement of the synovial structures of the tendons and joints in the wrist and hand. Tenosynovitis denotes an inflammation of the synovial lining of the tendon sheath, usually accompanied by inflammation of the contained tendon. The clinical manifestations are pain, tenderness, and swelling, with 'crepitus' that is palpable when the tendon moves within the inflamed sheath.

The flexor tendon sheaths enclose the tendons of flexor digitorum superficialis and profundus to their insertions on the middle and distal phalanges, respectively. The tendon sheath of the thumb flexor pollicis longus extends proximally to the carpal tunnel. The flexor sheath of the little finger is often continuous with the common flexor tendon sheath in the wrist. Segmental condensations in the digital flexor sheaths prevent bowstringing of the tendons.

Stenosing tenovaginitis

Stenosing tenovaginitis is primarily a fibrosis of the tendon sheaths with intrathecal narrowing of the lumen, especially involving sites

Table 17 The painful wrist and hand

Dupuytren's contracture

Tenosynovitis—including De Quervain's

Stenosing tenovaginitis

Rupture of tendons

Ganglion

Median nerve compression—carpal tunnel syndrome

Ulnar nerve compression—in Guyon's canal

near bony prominences where tendons pass through fibrous rings. This more commonly affects the flexor than extensor tendons in the hand. If a fibrous nodule develops in the flexor tendons, a 'trigger finger' can result, which further limits function. The finger often locks in flexion. Extension can be forced with difficulty and is often painful. Palpation during muscle action may reveal a mobile nodule within a tendon sheath of a finger or palm. Its incidence as an isolated lesion following overuse is low. The most common cause of a trigger finger or thumb is overuse from repetitive grasping activities.

Management

The management of stenosing tenovaginitis consists of modification of hand activity, gentle exercises, and non-steroidal anti-inflammatory drugs. Extension splinting of the affected digit at night prevents painful flexion during sleep. One or two corticosteroid injections into the affected tendon sheaths are effective in the majority. Surgical transection of the fibrous annular pulley of the finger or thumb flexor sheath is rarely required.

De Quervain's tenosynovitis

This common lesion, caused by repeated minor trauma, results from involvement of the tendon sheaths of abductor pollicis longus and extensor pollicis brevis. The patient complains of pain on using the thumb or wrist. Tenderness is maximal in the 'snuffbox' area between the two tendons, and there is often a visible tender swelling about the radial styloid. Pain can be elicited by forced ulnar deviation after placing the patient's thumb in the palm (Finkelstein's sign).

The tendon sheath, which is normally about 0.75 mm thick, increases in thickness three- or fourfold, and there is cellular infiltration with increased vascularity of the sheath, inflammatory proliferation of the epitendon, and expansion of part of the tendon to form a nodule.

It has been reported for years that De Quervain's is more common in assembly-line workers involved in repeated grasping movements between finger and thumb, and with rapid pronation–supination movements of the forearm, although most studies cannot demonstrate an association with occupation. It is 10 times more prevalent in women.

Treatment

The symptoms often resolve spontaneously with rest, but can be recurrent or persistent. Immobilization of the wrist and thumb by thermoplastic splinting is often helpful. Attention to hand activities with avoidance of tasks that require repetitive thumb movements or pinch grasping is important. In patients with more severe or persistent pain, one or more local corticosteroid injections are often helpful, giving relief in some 70 per cent. Surgical decompression of the first extensor compartment, with or without tenosynovectomy, is indicated in those with persistent or recurrent symptoms for more than 6 months.

Tenosynovitis and peritendinitis crepitans

By definition tenosynovitis is a disorder of the tenosynovium. It has been described after trauma in an industrial context for many years, affecting the long extensors of the fingers at the wrist and less commonly the long flexors. Tenosynovitis occurs after unusually active use of the wrist over a period of days or weeks. Tenosynovitis and peritendinitis crepitans are two distinct syndromes. Both present with pain, particularly on resisted movement, and there is

usually localized swelling, tenderness, and crepitus. The distinguishing feature is the site of the lesion. In tenosynovitis the swelling and tenderness are confined to the synovial sheaths and the wrists, and respond to rest and local steroid injections. Peritendinitis crepitans presents with pain, tenderness, and swelling at the musculotendinous junction above the upper limit of the tendon sheaths in the forearm. It usually responds to rest, and to ultrasound.

Since 1947 tenosynovitis has been a United Kingdom Department of Health (and Social Security) prescribed industrial disease. It was intended to compensate manual workers suffering from tenosynovitis induced by excessively rough or arduous work. More recently, tenosynovitis has come to be used incorrectly as a generic term covering not only traumatic tenosynovitis and paratendinitis crepitans but a wide variety of non-specific aches and pains in the forearm, which trades union health-care advisers and members may often simply call 'teno'. The epidemiological evidence for the accepted overuse syndromes is substantial, although often clouded in recent years by differences in the terms used to describe these disorders and also by the emotional arguments pertaining to repetitive strain disorders (see above).

There is little doubt that the common occupational disorder known as peritendinitis crepitus is related to overuse. Biopsies were first carried out by Von Frisch in 1909; he found oedema with congestion of the peritendinous tissues, mainly at the musculotendinous junction and often around the muscle (Thompson *et al.* 1951). In more recent descriptions it is clear that local anatomical considerations are important (Williams 1977).

Dupuytren's contracture

This condition, of unknown aetiology, produces progressive thickening of the palmar fascia and causes flexion contracture predominantly affecting the ring and little fingers. It is commonly bilateral and can also involve the plantar fascia. The palm of the hand becomes indurated and lines of fibrosis with nodules and skin puckering run along the tendons, causing progressive fixed flexion of the metacarpophalangeal and proximal interphalangeal joints.

The rate of progression is variable and surgical fasciectomy should be performed only when disability is severe, but should be considered before amputation becomes the only alternative.

Management

Treatment depends entirely on the rate of progression and severity of the lesions. In patients with mild disease, local heat, stretching exercises, and the use of protective padded gloves during heavy manual tasks are often helpful. In more severe lesions with pain and inability to straighten the fingers, intralesional steroids may be beneficial. In those with progressive digital contracture of more than 30°, and functional impairment, a palmar fasciectomy with or without a skin graft is indicated. The risk of recurrence is greater in those with a family history or active bilateral disease.

Ganglia

Ganglia are tense, uni- or multilocular, cystic swellings that develop in relation to a joint capsule or tendon sheath and contain a clear, jelly-like substance. They vary in size and can be so tense that they may be mistaken for a bony swelling. They are sometimes provoked by injury or arthritis, but often occur spontaneously.

the various techniques is necessary before reasonable success can be obtained. The correct choice of needle size makes a great deal of difference to the amount of pain experienced, and the amount that is injected varies according to the type of lesion.

The choice of steroid and local anaesthetic varies from user to user but, in practice, preparations differ significantly in their duration of action, and for most purposes the shorter-acting hydrocortisone acetate is suitable. The longer-acting steroids, methyl prednisolone acetate and triamcinolone hexacetonide, may cause skin atrophy when used for superficial lesions such as tennis elbow. After the injection there may be an increase in symptoms for up to 48 h and patients should be warned of this possibility. About 80 per cent of patients gain symptomatic benefit from these injections. It is important not to inject the tendoachilles itself, as this may predispose to rupture. In spite of decades of use of ultrasound in treating a wide spectrum of musculoskeletal disorders, its effectiveness remains unproven. Persistent lesions may require further injections but if conservative measures fail, surgery may be required.

Conclusion

About seven people in every hundred who visit their general medical practitioner seek help with symptoms arising from the soft tissues. The loss of work resulting from these symptoms is of the order of 11 million days annually. However, most soft-tissue lesions are eminently manageable, as discussed above.

References

Abrahamsson, S. O. (1991). Matrix metabolism and healing in the flexor tendon. Experimental studies on rabbit tendon. *Scandinavian Journal of Plastic Surgery of the Hand*, 25 (Suppl. 23), 1–51.

American College of Rheumatology (1990). Criteria for the classification of fibromyalgia: report of the multicentre criteria committee. *Arthritis and Rheumatism*, 33, 160–72.

Awerbach, M. (1985). RSI or 'kangaroo paw'. *Medical Journal of Australia*, 142, 237–328.

Beighton, P. B., Grahame, R., and Bird, H. A. (1989). *Hypermobility of joints*, (2nd edn). Springer, Berlin.

Binder, A., Hodge, G., Greenwood, A. M., Hazleman, B. L., and Page Thomas, D. P. (1985). Is therapeutic ultrasound effective in treating soft tissue lesions? *British Medical Journal*, 292, 512–14.

Bjelle, A., Hagberg, M., and Michaelson, G. (1979). Clinical and ergonomic factors in prolonged shoulder pain among industrial workers. *Scandinavian Journal of Work and Environmental Health*, 5, 205–10.

Bjelle, A., Allander, E., and Magi, M. (1990). Rheumatic disorders in the Swedish population and health care system. *Journal of Rheumatology*, 7, 877–85.

Bulgen, D. Y., Binder, A., and Hazleman, B. L. (1984). Frozen shoulder: prospective clinical study with evaluation of three treatment regimes. *Annals of the Rheumatic Diseases*, 43, 353–60.

Bunker, T. D. and Anthony, P. P. (1995). The pathology of frozen shoulder. *Journal of Bone and Joint Surgery* (B), 77, 677–85.

Burkhart, S. S., Nottage, W. M., Ogilvie-Hans, D. J., Kohn, H. S., and Pacheli, A. (1994). Partial repair of irreparable rotator cuff lesions. *Arthroscopy*, 10, 363–70.

Carette S. (1995). Fibromyalgia 20 years later: What have we really accomplished. *Journal of Rheumatology*, 22, 590–4.

Chard, M. D. and Hazleman, B. L. (1987). Shoulder disorders in the elderly (a hospital study). *Annals of the Rheumatic Diseases*, 46, 684–7.

Chard, M. D. and Hazleman, B. L. (1989). Tennis elbow—a reappraisal. *British Journal of Rheumatology*, 28, 186–90.

Chard, M. D., Gresham, A., and Hazleman, B. L. (1989). Age-related changed in the rotator cuff. *British Journal of Rheumatology*, 28 (Suppl. 1), 19.

Chard, M. D., Cawston, T. E., Riley, G. P., Gresham, G. A., and Hazleman, B. L. (1994). Rotator cuff degeneration and lateral epicondylitis—a comparative histological study. *Annals of the Rheumatic Diseases*, 53, 30–4.

Child, A. H. (1986). Joint hypermobility syndrome: inherited disorders of collagen synthesis. *Journal of Rheumatology*, 13, 239–42.

Cleland, L. G. (1987). RSI: a model of social iatrogenesis. *Medical Journal of Australia*, 147, 236–7.

Clinton, T. and Solcher, B. (1994). Chronic leg pain in the athlete. *Clinical Sports Medicine*, 13, 743–59.

Cohen, M. J. and Quintner, J. L. (1993). Fibromyalgia syndromes a problem of tautology. *Lancet*, 342, 906–9.

Da Cruz, D. J., Geeson, M., Allen, M., and Phair, I. (1988). Achilles paratendinitis: an evaluation of steroid injection. *British Journal of Sports Medicine*, 22, 64–5.

Dalton, S. E. (1989). Clinical examination of the painful shoulder. In *The shoulder joint (Baillière's clinical rheumatology*, Vol. 3, No. 3) (ed. B. L. Hazleman and P. A. Dieppe), pp. 453–74. Baillière Tindall, London.

Dalton, S. E., Cawston, T. E., Riley, G. P., Bayley, I. J. L., and Hazleman, B. L. (1995). Human shoulder tendon biopsy samples in organ culture produce procollagenase and TIMP. *Annals of the Rheumatic Diseases*, 54, 571–7.

Department of Health and Social Security (1986). *Morbidity statistics from general practice. Third national study, 1981–1982*. HMSO, London.

Dixon, A. St. J. (1979). Soft tissue rheumatism. *Clinics in Rheumatic Diseases*, Vol. 5, No. 3, pp. 739–42. WB Saunders, Philadelphia.

Evans, E. J., Benjamin, M., and Pemberton, D. J. (1990). Fibrocartilage in the attachment zones of the quadriceps tendon and patellar ligament of man. *Journal of Anatomy*, 171, 155–62.

Felson, D. T. and Goldenberg, D. L. (1986). The natural history of fibromyalgia. *Arthritis and Rheumatism*, 20, 1522–6.

Garrick, J. G. and Requa, R. K. (1993). Ballet injuries: an analysis of epidemiology and financial outcome. *American Journal of Sports Medicine*, 21, 586–90.

Gelberman, R. H., Aronson, D., and Weisman, M. (1980). Carpal tunnel syndrome. *Journal of Bone and Joint Surgery (A)*, 62, 1181–4.

Goldenberg, D. (1995). Fibromyalgia: why such controversy? *Annals of the Rheumatic Diseases*, 54, 3–5.

Goodchild, J., Kopell, H. P., and Sprelholz, N. I. (1965). The tarsal-tunnel syndrome. *New England Journal of Medicine*, 273, 742–5.

Hagberg, M. (1981a). Muscular endurance and surface electromyogram in isometric and dynamic exercise. *Journal of Applied Physiology*, 51, 1–7.

Hagberg, M. (1981b). Electromyographic signs of shoulder muscle fatigue in two elevated arm positions. *American Journal of Physical Medicine*, 60, 111–21.

Hamilton, P. G. (1986). The prevalence of humeral epicondylitis: a survey in general practice. *Journal of the Royal College of General Practitioners*, 35, 464–5.

Harris, N. H. (1974). Lesions of the symphysis in athletes. *British Medical Journal*, 4, 211–14.

Harter, B. T., McKiernan, J. E., Kirzinger, S. S., Archer, F. W., Peters, C. K., and Harter, K. C. (1993). Carpal tunnel syndrome: surgical and non-surgical treatment. *Journal of Hand Surgery (A)*, 18, 734–9.

Haupt, W. F., Wintzer, G., Schop, A., Lottger, J., and Pawlik, G. (1993). Tunnel decompression. *Journal of Hand Surgery (B)*, 18, 471–4

Hocking, B. (1987). Epidemiological aspects of 'repetitive strain injury' in Telecom. *Medical Journal of Australia*, 147, 218–22.

Hoppmann, R. A. and Patrone, N. A. (1989). A review of musculoskeletal problems in instrumental musicians. *Seminars in Arthritis and Rheumatism*, 19, 117–26.

Ireland, D. C. R. (1988). Psychological and physical aspects of occupational arm pain. *Journal of Hand Surgery (B)*, 13, 5–10.

Kannus, P. and Jozsa, L. (1991). Histopathological changes preceding spontaneous rupture of a tendon. *Journal of Bone and Joint Surgery (A)*, 73, 1507–25.

Kellgren, J. H. (1939). On the distribution of pain arising from deep somatic structures with charts of segmental pain areas. *Clinical Science*, 4, 35–46.

Kumagai, J., Sarkar, K., and Uhthoff, H. K. (1994). The collagen types in the attachment zone of rotator cuff tendons of the elderly: an immunohistological study. *Journal of Rheumatology*, 21, 2096–100.

Labelle, H. *et al.* (1992). Lack of scientific evidence for the treatment of lateral epicondylitis of the elbow. *Journal of Bone and Joint Surgery*, 74, 646–51.

Lester, D. K. and Buchanan, J. R. (1984). Surgical treatment of plantar fasciitis. *Clinical Orthopedics*, **186**, 202–4.

Littlejohn, G. O. (1986). Repetitive strain syndrome: an Australian experience. *Journal of Rheumatology*, **13**, 1004–6.

Littlejohn, G. O. (1989). Medicolegal aspects of fibrositis syndrome. *Journal of Rheumatology*, **16** (Suppl. 19), 169–74.

Maigne, R. (1972). Sémiologie clinique des dérangements intervertébraux mineurs. *Annales de Medecine*, **15**, 175–292.

Miller, H. W. (1973). *Plan and operation of the Health and Nutrition Examination Survey: United States 1973–5. Vital and health statistics*, Series 1, No. 10. Public Health Service, US Department of Health, Washington DC.

Moldofsky, H., Scarisbrick, P., England, R., and Smythe, H. (1975). Musculoskeletal symptoms and non-REM sleep disturbance in patients with 'fibrositis syndrome' and healthy subjects. *Psychosomatic Medicine*, **37**, 341–51.

Neer, C. S. (1983). Rotator cuff athropathy. *Journal of Bone and Joint Surgery (A)*, **65**, 1232–44.

Neviaser, R. J. and Neviaser, T. J. (1987). The frozen shoulder. Diagnosis and management. *Clinical Orthopedics*, **223**, 59–64.

Nobuhara, K., Supapo, A. R., and Himo, T. (1994). Effects of shoulder distension in shoulder disease. *Clinical Orthopedics*, **304**, 25–9.

Payne, L. Z. (1994). Tears of the glenoid labrum. *Orthopedics Review*, **23**, 577–83.

Plattner, P. F. (1989). Tendon problems of the foot and ankle. *Postgraduate Medicine*, **86**, 155–70.

Ramel, E. and Moritz, V. (1994). Self-reported musculoskeletal pain and discomfort in professional ballet dancers in Sweden. *Scandinavian Journal of Rehabilitation Medicine*, **26**, 11–16.

Riley, G. P., Harrall, R. L., Constant, C. R., Chard, M. D., Cawston, T. E., and Hazleman, B. L. (1994). Glycosaminoglycans of human rotator cuff tendons: changes with age and in chronic rotator cuff tendinitis. *Annals of the Rheumatic Diseases*, **53**, 367–76.

Risk, T. E. and Pinals, R. S. (1982). Frozen shoulder. *Seminars in Arthritis and Rheumatism*, **11**, 440–52.

Russell, I. J. *et al.* (1994). Elevated cerebrospinal fluid levels of substance P in patients with fibromyalgia syndrome. *Arthritis and Rheumatism*, **37**, 1593–601.

Scheuler, W. *et al.* (1988). The alpha-sleep pattern: quantitative analysis and functional aspects. In *Sleep* (ed. W. P. Koelta, F. Obal, H. Schultz, and P. Visser). Fischer, Berlin.

Smythe, H. A. (1989). Fibrositis syndrome. A historical perspective. *Journal of Rheumatology*, **16** (Suppl. 19), 1–6.

Thompson, A. R., Pleavis, L. W., and Shaw, E. G. (1951). Peritendinous crepitans and simple tenosynovitis: a clinical study of 544 cases in industry. *British Journal of Industrial Medicine*, **8**, 150.

Travell, J. and Simons, D. G. (1983). *Myofascial pain and dysfunction. The trigger point manual*. Williams and Wilkins, Baltimore.

Uthoff, H. K. and Sarkar, K. (1989). Calcifying tendinitis. In *The shoulder joint* (*Baillière's clinical rheumatology*, Vol. 3, No. 3) (ed. B. L. Hazleman and P. A. Dieppe), pp. 567–81. Baillière Tindall, London.

Vogel, K. G., Ordog, A., Pogany, G., and Olah, J. (1993). Proteoglycans in the compressed regions of human tibialis, posterior tendon and in ligaments. *Journal of Orthopedic Research*, **11**, 68–77.

Wilcox, M. S. and Bilbao, A. (1993). Sensitivity of electrophysiological studies and the carpal tunnel syndrome. *Muscle and Nerve*, **16**, 1265–6.

Williams, J. G. P. (1977). Surgical management of traumatic non- infective tenosynovitis of the wrist extensors. *Journal of Bone and Joint Surgery (B)*, **59**, 408–70.

Wood, P. H., Sturrock, A. W. and Badley, E. M. (1979). Soft tissue rheumatism in the community. In *Soft tissue rheumatism* (*Clinics in Rheumatic Diseases*, Vol. 5, No. 3), pp. 743–53. WB Saunders, Philadelphia.

World Health Organization (1988). *Identification and control of work-related diseases. Report of a WHO expert committee*. World Health Organization Technical Report Series No. 174. WHO, Geneva.

Yamanaka, K. and Fukuda, H. (1991). Ageing process of the human supraspinatus tendon with reference to rotator cuff tears. In *Surgical disorders of the shoulders* (ed. M. S. Watson), pp. 247–58. Churchill Livingstone, Edinburgh.

5.15 Osteoarthritis

Michael Doherty, Adrian Jones, and T. E. Cawston

Introduction

Osteoarthritis is the commonest condition to affect the joints of man. As such it is a major cause of locomotor pain, the single most important rheumatological cause of disability and handicap, and an important health care challenge with major resource implications (Steven 1992; Yelin 1992; Badley *et al.* 1994). Indeed it has been estimated that 15 per cent of the United Kingdom population greater than 55 years of age have symptomatic osteoarthritis of the knee (Fig. 1). Osteoarthritis has, however, only recently become a significant focus of clinical interest and research. Previously considered a boring 'wear and tear', 'degenerative' disease that must be accepted as the inevitable consequence of trauma and ageing, osteoarthritis is increasingly viewed as a dynamic, essentially reparative process with potential for health intervention and prevention.

Historical perspective

At the turn of the century, pathologists and radiologists differentiated two main categories of chronic arthritis — atrophic and hypertrophic. The former was characterized by synovial inflammation with erosion or atrophy of cartilage and bone; it encompassed several disease entities including rheumatoid arthritis. Hypertrophic arthritis, by contrast, was characterized by more focal cartilage loss, minimal evidence of inflammation, and by hypertrophy of adjacent bone and soft tissues; this group became synonymous with osteoarthritis (Goldthwaite 1904) (Fig. 2). Since there were recognized associations with ageing and previous joint trauma, this led to ready acceptance of the alternative term 'degenerative joint disease'. With the major rheumatological interest focusing on inflammatory arthropathies,

osteoarthritis was often used as a 'non-inflammatory' control disease, and even as a surrogate for normal joint tissue, in clinical and laboratory research. The term 'osteoarthrosis' was often used, therefore, to emphasize absence of overt inflammation.

Advances in cartilage biochemistry and the recognition of calcium crystal-associated disease subsets proved important factors in renewing interest in this condition. Although clinical and histological inflammation is not as florid as in rheumatoid arthritis or seronegative spondylarthropathies, it is an undoubted component in many cases. Thus the term osteoarthritis is now generally preferred.

Definition of osteoarthritis

Concepts of osteoarthritis are still changing and there is no universal agreement on its definition. A current working definition of osteoarthritis is:

a condition of synovial joints characterized by cartilage loss (chondropathy) and evidence of accompanying periarticular bone response.

It is noteworthy that chondropathy may occur without hypertrophic bone response (e.g. polychondritis, rheumatoid arthritis), and periarticular new bone may develop without chondropathy (e.g. 'traction'

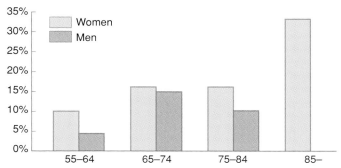

Fig. 1 Prevalence of symptomatic knee osteoarthritis by age group and gender in a United Kingdom community population. (Derived from McAlindon *et al.* 1992).

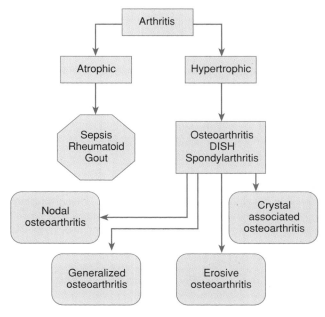

Fig. 2 The increasing differentiation of arthritis subtypes.

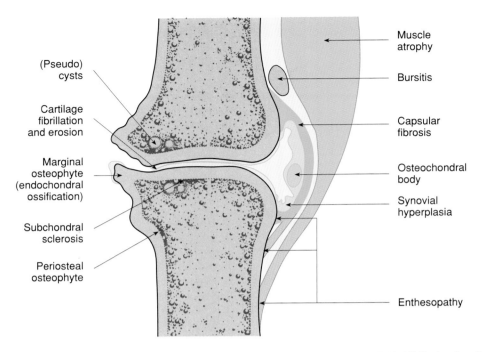

Fig. 3   Joint tissues affected in osteoarthritis. Redrawing from Doherty (ed.) *Color atlas and text of osteoarthritis*. Wolfe, London. (Doherty 1994).

spurs); it is only when the two occur together in synovial joints that the term osteoarthritis is appropriate.

The drawbacks of this working definition include:

(1) exclusion of joints with early (initial) change — the very joints we need to study in order to elucidate aetiopathogenic processes;

(2) emphasis on cartilage and bone — even though all other joint components (synovium, capsule, entheses, muscle) demonstrate change (Fig. 3);

(3) structural rather than physiological emphasis — with no consideration of biological, symptomatic, and functional consequences.

Nevertheless, given these caveats, such a definition is a practicable starting point for examination of existing clinical, epidemiological, and experimental data. The American College of Rheumatology has devised criteria for classification of symptomatic osteoarthritis of knee (Altman *et al.* 1986) (Fig. 4), hand (Altman *et al.* 1990), and hip (Altman *et al.* 1991) that incorporate clinical, laboratory, and/or radiological features. Although these criteria will distinguish osteoarthritis from other painful joint conditions (the basis of their development) there remain questions about their use in other settings. In population studies they may be insensitive and do not detect asymptomatic disease. Many questions thus remain to be resolved. It is likely that future definitions will be critically dependent on the populations and use for which they are intended.

Epidemiology

Current epidemiological data in osteoarthritis is beset by a lack of generally accepted criteria to distinguish a 'case' from a 'non-case'. Histopathological changes are obviously not appropriate for living subjects, and most surveys rely on radiographic features for definition

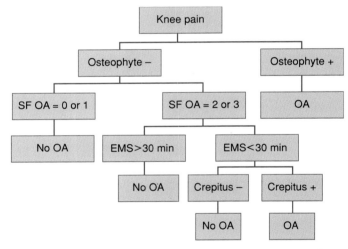

Fig. 4   Decision tree based classification of knee osteoarthritis according to the American College of Rheumatology classification criteria. Derived from Altman *et al.* 1986.

and assessment of severity. Of the various radiographic criteria, the most widely employed are those of Kellgren and Lawrence (Kellgren and Lawrence 1957). Although differing in detail by joint site and by publication, these grade osteoarthritis into four categories depending on the presence and degree of various features (Fig. 5). Although these features purport to measure various pathological changes occurring in cartilage and subchondral bone (Table 1), there are problems with both validity and reproducibility. Particular problems include:

(1) lack of distinction between isolated and chondropathy-associated osteophyte, the aetiological factors for which may vary;

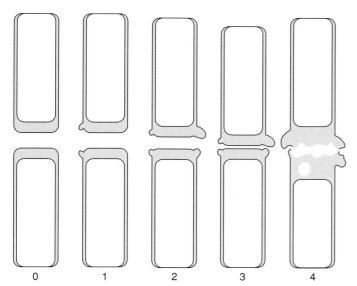

Fig. 5 Basis of Kellgren and Lawrence grading scheme. Grade 0, normal; Grade 1, minimal osteophyte, normal joint space; Grade 2, definite osteophyte, possible joint space narrowing; Grade 3, definite osteophyte and joint space narrowing; Grade 4, definite osteophyte and joint space narrowing with sclerosis and abnormal joint contour.

Table 1 Radiographical—pathological correlates in osteoarthritis	
Pathological change	**Radiographic abnormality**
Cartilage fibrillation, erosion	Decrease in interosseous distance (localized)
Subchondral new bone formation	Sclerosis
New cartilage formation and endochondral ossification	Osteophyte
Fibrous-walled pseudocysts resulting from fluid intrusion or myxoid degeneration	Subchondral cysts
Trabecular compression	Bone collapse/attrition
Fragmentation of osteo-chondral surface; cartilage and bone metaphasia in synovium	Osseous ('loose') bodies

(2) the ignoring of clinical status, symptoms, and function;

(3) inappropriate assumptions about disease progression in grading systems which combine several features, such as that of Kellgren and Lawrence.

Although attempts to define osteoarthritis clinically have been made (Claessens *et al.* 1990; Hart *et al.* 1991; Altman 1991) the lack of a suitable gold standard, poor correlation with currently accepted surrogate 'gold standards' (e.g. radiology), and poor reproducibility have hampered their widespread adoption.

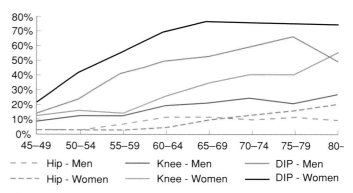

Fig. 6 Prevalence of radiological osteoarthritis by age group and gender in a Netherlands community population. Derived from van Saase *et al.* 1989.

Such problems in the definition of osteoarthritis, radiograph interpretation, and clinical measurement make the epidemiology of osteoarthritis difficult to analyse (Peyron 1979; Spector and Cooper 1993) but several broad conclusions may now be drawn.

Descriptive studies

Autopsy studies suggest that the majority of subjects over age 65 have evidence of osteoarthritis in at least one joint site at the time of death. Prevalence estimates from such studies tend to be higher than those from radiographic surveys, perhaps because the whole joint surface is available for study (Rogers *et al.* 1990).

Radiographic studies also report high prevalence in the middle-aged and elderly. This prevalence varies according to joint site and age, giving different patterns of distribution at different ages. For example hand interphalangeal joints and first metatarsophalangeal joints are affected commonly and at a relatively young age, whereas glenohumeral and shoulder joints are affected less commonly and principally in the elderly. From available large radiographic studies (Mikkelson *et al.* 1970; Lawrence 1977; Felson 1988; Van Saase *et al.* 1989) the following generalizations can be made.

Age

This is a major determinant of prevalence at all important sites including hands, knees, and hips. Prevalence is low under age 45 years. Polyarticular osteoarthritis ($\geqslant 5$ sites involved) is also rare in those aged less than 45 years. Prevalence increases up to age 65, when there is involvement of at least one joint group in at least 50 per cent of the population. Continuing increase in prevalence in those over age 65 is less clear cut, and indeed a plateauing out of prevalence in the very old has been suggested (Bagge *et al.* 1992) (Fig. 6).

Gender

This is important at some, but by no means all, joint sites. Although there is little or no gender difference in the prevalence of mild osteoarthritis, a female preponderance becomes more apparent:

(1) for severe grades of osteoarthritis;

(2) in older age groups;

(3) for osteoarthritis of the hands and knees.

There is also a polyarticular form of hand osteoarthritis that has a predilection for perimenopausal women — so-called nodal generalized osteoarthritis. This is discussed further below.

Ethnic group

Given the difficulties of representative sampling and reproducible assessments, comparison between populations shows surprising similarity in age-specific prevalence by joint site (Van Saase *et al.* 1989). Possible exceptions are:

(1) hip osteoarthritis, which shows substantially lower prevalence among black and Oriental populations than among whites;

(2) polyarticular hand osteoarthritis, which appears to be less common in African and Malaysian populations.

Geographic variation — 'endemic osteoarthritis'

Several forms of disabling polyarticular osteoarthritis occur with high frequency in certain geographical locations (Sokoloff 1985). The best described are Kashin–Beck disease (south-eastern Siberia, northern China, North Korea) and Mselini disease (limited to the Zulu and Tonga tribes of south-east Africa). Other forms of endemic osteoarthritis occur in Malnad and elsewhere in India. These conditions share in common:

(1) onset during the first or second decade;

(2) variable growth restriction;

(3) characteristics of acquired rather than inherited disease;

(4) involvement of impoverished rural communities.

The conditions radiographically most closely resemble those of spondyloepiphyseal dysplasia, and histologically show chondronecrosis as a likely initial event (Fig. 7). The cause(s) of endemic osteoarthritis remain unknown, though mycotoxins elaborated by moulds on local grains and abnormalities of trace elements (e.g. selenium) in soil or water have been investigated.

Analytical studies

Individual risk factors for osteoarthritis may conveniently be viewed as:

(1) those influencing or marking a generalized predisposition to the condition;

(2) those resulting in abnormal biomechanical loading at specific sites (Fig. 8).

Generalized susceptibility

Obesity

This is closely associated with knee osteoarthritis (odds ratio 4.5 for men, 9.0 for women, for those 50 per cent above ideal body weight compared to those at ideal body weight) but interestingly not at the hip (Lawrence *et al.* 1990; Felson *et al.* 1992). At the knee, obesity precedes rather than follows knee osteoarthritis and indeed weight loss may prevent the development of knee osteoarthritis (Felson *et al.* 1992) (Fig. 9). It is associated with radiographic change irrespective of whether symptoms are present or not, arguing against obesity

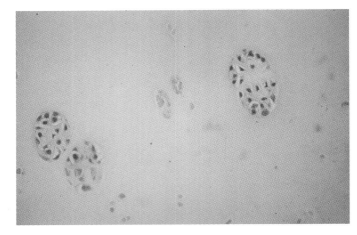

Fig. 7 Radiograph of coronal slab section of femoral head in Mselini hip disease. From Sokoloff (1994) in *Color atlas and text of osteoarthritis* (ed. M Doherty). Wolfe, London.

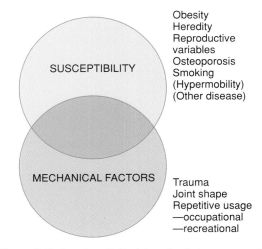

Fig. 8 Susceptibility to osteoarthritis: interaction between generalized and local factors.

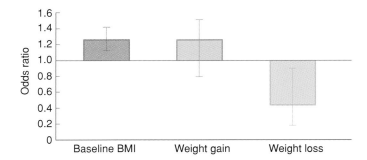

Fig. 9 Risk of symptomatic knee osteoarthritis per 2 units of body mass index (BMI) expressed as odds ratio and 95 per cent confidence interval. Derived from Felson *et al.* 1992).

resulting from more sedentary lifestyle of those with painful knees. It is also true, however, that obesity increases the risk of knee pain for a given degree of structural change. The mechanism relating obesity and osteoarthritis remains speculative although the apparent lack of association with hip osteoarthritis suggests metabolic or systemic factors rather than a purely mechanical explanation.

Genetic factors

A strong familial tendency is recognized for nodal generalized osteoarthritis, a polyarticular form of osteoarthritis occurring mainly in women of perimenopausal age. This is confirmed by family and twin studies (Lawrence 1977). Heberden's nodes appear to be inherited independently as an autosomal dominant trait with greater penetrance in women (Stecher 1953). The genetics and pathogenic mechanism remains unknown but associations have been reported with HLA A1,B8 haplotypes and with the α_1-antitrypsin MZ phenotype (Pattrick *et al.* 1989*a*). In addition, an increased incidence of IgG rheumatoid factors (Hopkinson *et al.* 1992) and a high frequency of immune complexes in cartilage and synovium of hips removed from nodal generalized osteoarthritis compared to pauciarticular osteoarthritis patients (Cooke 1985) has led to speculation of an autoimmune aetiology (Doherty *et al.* 1990). It is hypothesized that an unidentified 'single-shot' insult occurs in a genetically predisposed individual. This triggers an immunological response, leading to polyarticular damage and initiation of the osteoarthritis process (Fig. 10). However, because it is a single temporal insult the repair process wins through, 'compensates', and results in a good outcome, other than for leaving the structurally abnormal joints that we recognize as 'nodal generalized osteoarthritis ' (Doherty *et al.* 1990). These findings have not yet been confirmed.

An association with the COL2A1 gene has been demonstrated for hereditary forms of premature polyarticular osteoarthritis with mild dysplasia (Knowlton *et al.* 1990). It has also been found in some, but not all, forms of hereditary osteo-opthalmoarthropathy (Stickler's syndrome), an hereditary disease with variable ocular and midfacial abnormalities and a premature osteoarthritis-like syndrome (Williams and Jimenez 1993). Similar associations of type II collagen defects with nodal generalized and sporadic osteoarthritis have not been found.

Reproductive variables

Polyarticular osteoarthritis has a strong female predominance, a frequent onset around the menopause, and reported associations with previous hysterectomy, gynaecological surgery, and possible alterations of sex hormone binding globulin. This has led to the suggestion that hormonal factors are important in this subgroup (Spector and Campion 1989). Manipulation of sex hormones in animal models of 'osteoarthritis' and identification of oestrogen receptors on chondrocytes lend some support to a role for hormonal modulation. Similar treatment in humans has been unsuccessful in established osteoarthritis (Kellgren and Moore 1952).

Bone density

A negative association is reported between osteoporosis and osteoarthritis at certain sites (Lane and Nevitt 1994). The strongest evidence relates to the hip, where several studies support a negative correlation between hip osteoarthritis and risk of femoral neck fracture. In patients with polyarticular osteoarthritis, studies of bone density have produced conflicting results, with obesity a frequent confounding factor. One explanation for this negative relationship, if true, is that weak bone may absorb excessive impact loading and thus protect joint cartilage from damage and subsequent osteoarthritis. Certainly, in the converse rare situation of osteopetrosis, where the

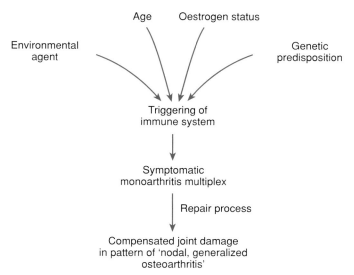

Fig. 10 Hypothesis explaining nodal generalized osteoarthritis as an 'autoimmune' condition.

skeleton is diffusely sclerotic, a high incidence of premature polyarticular osteoarthritis is reported.

Cigarette smoking

A protective influence of smoking on knee osteoarthritis, after correction for possible confounding factors, is reported from the Framingham study (Felson 1988). Other studies have produced both confirmatory and contradictory results and the issue is not yet resolved. The observation is intriguing, however, but the mechanism is unclear. Smoking is a risk factor for osteoporosis, has antioestrogenic properties, and has many effects on cell function. It is unclear which, if any, of these is important.

Other suggested factors

Less definite associations are reported with diabetes, hypertension, and hyperuricaemia, which are independent of obesity. Clearer associations with acromegaly and haemochromatosis are evident (Jones *et al.* 1992). An increased frequency of osteoarthritis in subjects with generalized hypermobility has also been suggested, due either to associated connective tissue abnormality or joint trauma, but rigorous epidemiological support for this is still required.

Local mechanical factors

Trauma

Major direct injury is accepted as a predisposing cause of osteoarthritis (Wright 1990). Intra-articular fracture affecting the articular surface is probably associated with osteoarthritis although much of the evidence is retrospective and uncontrolled. Major injury, particularly fracture, may also alter mechanical loading and predispose to osteoarthritis at distant sites, as with fractures of the femoral shaft (hip osteoarthritis) (Fig. 11), scaphoid (wrist osteoarthritis), tibia (ankle osteoarthritis), or humerus (shoulder osteoarthritis). Although trauma may be a predisposing factor that determines the site of osteoarthritis, mechanical insult alone is usually an insufficient cause for its development. For example following total meniscectomy not everyone develops knee osteoarthritis. Furthermore, the

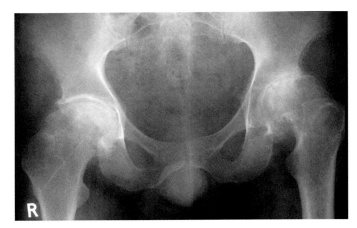

Fig. 11 Asymmetric hip osteoarthritis following previous trauma on the right side in a patient (Ledingham *et al.* 1992).

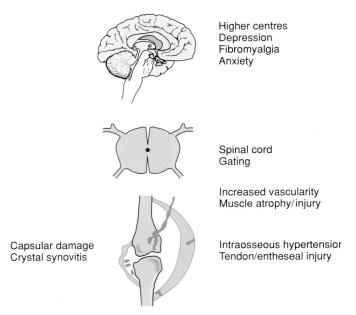

Fig. 12 Potential sites of pain perception and/or modification in osteoarthritis. Redrawn from Jones and Doherty (1992).

increased frequency of postmeniscectomy osteoarthritis in subjects with a generalized predisposition to osteoarthritis (i.e. those with distal interphalangeal joint osteoarthritis) compared to those with no such predisposition supports interaction between generalized (constitutional) and local (mechanical) factors (Doherty *et al.* 1983).

Joint shape
Abnormalities of articular contour, that may lead to abnormal load transmission across the joint, have particularly been linked with predisposition to osteoarthritis at the hip and knee. It is well established that childhood hip disorders such as Perthes' disease, slipped capital epiphysis, and congenital dislocation lead to premature hip osteoarthritis . It has been suggested that lesser degrees of acetabular dysplasia account for a proportion of hip osteoarthritis amongst younger subjects, though the impact of such mild developmental abnormality in causing later hip osteoarthritis is questionable, with a recent study suggesting it is of little importance (Croft *et al.* 1991). Cooke has suggested that mild, often unrecognized, dysplasia of the femoral condyles may similarly predispose to knee osteoarthritis via mechanical effects (Cooke 1985). Abnormal contour following intra-articular fractures may also contribute to premature osteoarthritis.

Occupational and recreational activities
Data in this area were conflicting but a consensus is now emerging (Cooper 1995). For example repetitive impact loading and trauma have been implicated in reported increased frequencies of osteoarthritis in miners (knees, spine), cotton workers (distal interphalangeal joints), and pneumatic drillers (elbows), though conversely parachutists, ballet dancers, and runners show no obvious increased risk of osteoarthritis. It may be that at some sites trauma is more important in selecting the site and severity of the condition than in determining whether osteoarthritis will develop or not. For example examination of patterns of osteoarthritis in the hand suggests that usage may influence distribution of osteoarthritis in the hand (Hadler *et al.* 1977), though evidence for an increase in frequency from repetitive usage is lacking.

At the hip, several studies have now shown a convincing increased incidence of osteoarthritis in farmers. The mechanisms underlying this association are unclear but repetitive trauma is suggested. At the knee there is increasing evidence that repetitive knee bending may be harmful (Felson *et al.* 1991). This association has only been clearly demonstrated in men.

Clinical features

Symptoms and impact of osteoarthritis
The principal clinical features of osteoarthritis are symptoms (pain, stiffness), functional impairment, and signs (primarily anatomical change). Though interrelated, there is often marked discordance between these three.

Symptoms
Although pain is the chief complaint its origin is not at all clear. Hyaline cartilage is aneural and this means that metabolic or structural alteration in this tissue is unlikely to be directly perceived as painful. Several other mechanisms of symptom production have been suggested (Fig. 12). These include:

(1) stimulation of capsular pain fibres and mechanoreceptors by intra-articular hypertension consequent upon synovial hypertrophy, increased fluid production, and decreased joint compliance;

(2) inflammatory mediators stimulating pain fibres in the synovium and capsule;

(3) stimulation of periosteal nerve fibres by intraosseous hypertension accompanying osteoarthritis;

(4) perception of subchondral microfractures, painful enthesopathy, and bursitis that accompany structural alteration, muscle weakness, and altered usage;

(5) maladaptive changes in the spinal cord and brain leading to persistent pain perception.

It has been suggested that these different mechanisms may produce different pain characteristics with, for example, pain predominantly:

(1) on usage — being due to mechanical or enthesopathic problems;

(2) at rest — being inflammatory in origin;

(3) at night — being due to intraosseous hypertension.

The last of these may be a particularly poor prognostic factor and indicates severe damage. Pain in osteoarthritis may, however, be a transient feature and can be absent in spite of severe joint damage (Fig. 13). Correlation between pain and radiographic change varies according to site. It is best at the hip and then knee, with the poorest correlation occurring in the hands and spinal apophyseal joints. Joints with more severe radiographic change are more likely to be symptomatic than those with mild change (Fig. 14) but irrespective of structural change, pain is more common in women (Lawrence *et al.* 1990). As with any locomotor or other pain, the subjective magnitude and perception of pain may be greatly influenced by factors such as personality, anxiety, and/or depression. Indeed, several recent studies have demonstrated that these psychological factors may be much more important in determining symptomatic outcome. One study has even gone further and suggested that factors associated with radiographic outcome may be independent of and distinct from those associated with knee pain and disability (Davis *et al.* 1992). This has led at least one author to question whether we should in fact ignore the entity we try to describe as osteoarthritis and instead concentrate on knee pain (Hadler 1992).

Stiffness is the other chief complaint. This is often described as 'gelling' of the joint after inactivity with difficulty in initiating movement. Prolonged morning or inactivity stiffness, often taken as a reflection of inflammation, is uncommon but may occur, particularly in patients with chronic pyrophosphate arthropathy.

Some patients may complain of joint swelling and deformity (particularly of hands), and coarse crepitus, even in the absence of other symptoms.

Functional impairment

Disability results from reduced range and control of movement and from pain. Handicap, of course, will vary according to individual patient requirements and aspirations. The pain and functional consequences of osteoarthritis are responsible for the huge burden of morbidity in the community. Severe knee and (less commonly) hip disease result in a massive health care problem to a generally older and otherwise fitter population. In addition to morbidity, cumulative mortality rates among subjects aged 55 to 74 in the National Health and Nutrition Examination Survey (NHANES-I) were significantly greater (relative risk 1.1) for women but not men with knee osteoarthritis (Lawrence *et al.* 1990). An increased mortality has also been associated with knee osteoarthritis in Sweden (Danielsson and Hernborg 1970).

Signs

Several features may occur in any combination and primarily reflect altered joint structure. These include:

(1) crepitus, presumed due to an irregular articular surface;

(2) bony enlargement, due to osteophyte and remodelling;

(3) deformity;

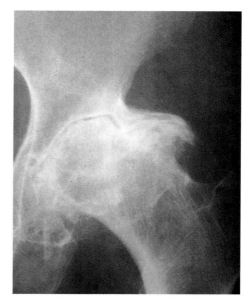

Fig. 13 Radiograph of an asymptomatic individual with severe radiographic osteoarthritis change.

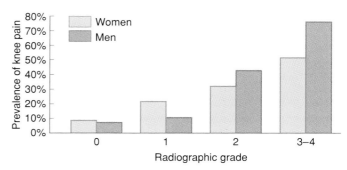

Fig. 14 Prevalence of knee pain by radiographic grade and gender in a United States community population. (Derived from Davis *et al.* 1992.)

(4) instability;

(5) restricted movement;

(6) stress pain.

Varying degrees of synovitis (warmth, effusion, synovial thickening) may accompany joint line tenderness. Muscle weakness and wasting may also be apparent. Periarticular sources of pain, demonstrated by point tenderness away from the joint line and by stress testing, are commonly identified at the knee and hip.

Osteoarthritis 'subsets'

Since osteoarthritis is a process that may be triggered by diverse constitutional and environmental factors, a wide spectrum of clinical expression and outcome is to be expected. Attempts to define and classify osteoarthritis as a single disease entity have not been entirely successful and attempts have been made to separate osteoarthritis into more homogeneous groupings or 'subsets' so as better to define aetiological factors and prognosis.

Osteoarthritis was initially classified as primary (no cause identified) or secondary (an obvious cause identified, such as trauma or dysplasia). Indeed such a distinction is still retained in the American College of Rheumatology criteria (Altman *et al.* 1991). Such artificial separation has often proved unsatisfactory due to:

(1) frequent lack of an identifiable cause, resulting in a large heterogeneous primary group;

(2) overlap between subsets, as shown for example by the influence of predisposition to 'primary' generalized osteoarthritis in determining development of postmeniscectomy 'secondary' osteoarthritis (Doherty *et al.* 1983).

In addition to identifiable predisposing factors, the following more objective features have therefore often been used as a further basis of subset differentiation:

(1) joint site involved (hip, knee, hand);

(2) site within a joint (medial tibiofemoral, lateral tibiofemoral, patellofemoral);

(3) number of joints involved (one, few, many);

(4) presence of associated crystal deposition;

(5) presence of marked clinical inflammation;

(6) radiographic bone response (atrophic, hypertrophic).

A number of 'subsets' have emerged which differ in a number of such characteristics. It is important to note, however, that sharp distinction between subsets does not exist. Many of the above characteristics represent different aspects of the osteoarthritis process (the balance between damage and repair), and may dominate the clinical picture at just one phase in the evolution of the condition. One 'subset' may thus evolve into another, and different 'subsets' may exist at different sites within the same individual. Possibly the most important distinction is simply by site and number of joints involved; predisposing factors are increasingly being associated with specific joint sites, or to polyarticular as opposed to pauciarticular involvement. It follows that knowledge concerning pathogenesis, risk factors, or treatment success of osteoarthritis cannot necessarily be extrapolated from one site to another.

Nodal generalized osteoarthritis

This is perhaps the best recognized subset, characterized by:

(1) polyarticular finger interphalangeal involvement;

(2) Heberden's and Bouchard's nodes;

(3) female preponderance;

(4) peak onset around the menopause;

(5) good functional outcome for hands;

(6) predisposition to osteoarthritis of the knee, hip, and spine;

(7) marked familial predisposition.

The typical patient is a woman in her forties or fifties who develops discomfort followed by swelling of a single finger interphalangeal joint. A few months later another interphalangeal joint becomes painful, then another producing a 'stuttering' onset polyarthritis of distal and proximal interphalangeal joints ('monoarthritis multiplex'). Affected interphalangeal joints may feel very stiff, be tender, and show tight posterolateral swelling with overlying erythema. Aspiration of such swellings may reveal viscous, clear, hyaluronate-rich 'jelly': these cysts represent mucoid transformation of periarticular fibroadipose tissue and may communicate with the joint. Each interphalangeal joint tends to go through a symptomatic phase while swelling and deformity become established, resulting in perhaps 1 to 3 years of episodic discomfort and stiffness. In almost all cases symptoms then subside, leaving the patient with typical posterolateral firm Heberden's (distal interphalangeal joint) and Bouchard's (proximal interphalangeal joint) nodes, characteristic lateral deviations of interphalangeal joints (Fig. 15), and radiographic evidence of osteoarthritis (Fig. 16). In addition to finger interphalangeal joints, the first carpometacarpal, metacarpophalangeal, and interphalangeal joints of the thumb are commonly affected: other joint involvement in the hand and wrist, however, is usually restricted to the index and middle metacarpophalangeal, scaphotrapezoid, and pisiform-triquetral articulations. The prognosis seems to be good.

Nodal generalized hand osteoarthritis is associated with an increased frequency of osteoarthritis at other sites, particularly knees, hips, first metatarsophalangeal joints, and cervical and lumbar apophyseal joints (Kellgren and Moore 1957). This concept of 'generalized osteoarthritis', with hand involvement as the marker for predisposition, was first described by Haygarth in 1805 and is supported by several studies (Roh *et al.* 1973; Acheson and Collart 1975; Solomon 1983). One such survey (Acheson and Collart 1975) suggests division into two groups (although such distinction is not supported by others):

(1) nodal generalized osteoarthritis;
  (a) nodes
  (b) distal interphalangeal joint involved more than proximal interphalangeal joint
  (c) marked female preponderance
  (d) familial aggregation

(2) non-nodal generalized osteoarthritis;
  (a) proximal interphalangeal joint involved more than distal interphalangeal joint
  (b) more equal sex distribution.

The inevitable problem that arises is that one or just a few Heberden's nodes and limited interphalangeal joint osteoarthritis are common, often asymptomatic findings in the elderly, and when should the title 'nodal generalized osteoarthritis' be applied? Although criteria for this have not been defined, some studies suggest that involvement of even a single interphalangeal joint may be important (Croft *et al.* 1992). Polyarticular hand osteoarthritis has been reported to be associated with certain intra-articular patterns of large joint osteoarthritis, for example concentric as opposed to superior pole osteoarthritis of the hip (Marks *et al.* 1979). This evidence supports the notion of nodal generalized osteoarthritis as a distinct condition.

Erosive ('inflammatory') osteoarthritis

This relatively uncommon condition is characterized by the following:

(1) hand interphalangeal joint involvement;

(2) often florid inflammatory component;

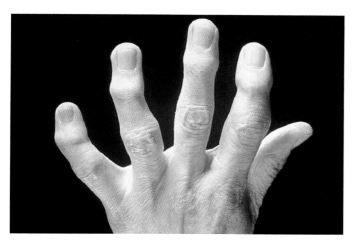

Fig. 15 Typical appearance of multiple Heberden's and Bouchard's nodes in nodal generalized osteoarthritis.

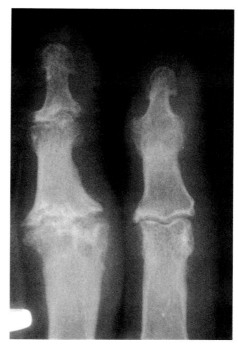

Fig. 17 Subchondral erosive change in erosive osteoarthritis.

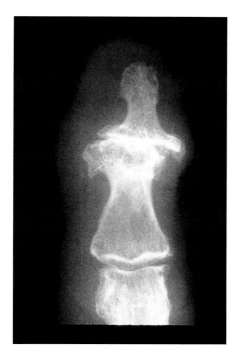

Fig. 16 Radiograph of distal interphalangeal joint showing many of the typical radiographic features of osteoarthritis (joint space narrowing, sclerosis, osteophyte).

(3) radiographic subchondral erosive change;

(4) tendency to interphalangeal joint ankylosis.

The condition clinically resembles nodal generalized osteoarthritis in beginning as an additive polyarthritis of finger joints (Ehlich 1972). Inflammatory symptoms and signs, however, are often marked though episodic. Unlike nodal generalized osteoarthritis, proximal and distal interphalangeal joints are equally involved and, less frequently, index and middle metacarpophalangeal joints. Interphalangeal joint instability, which is rare in nodal generalized osteoarthritis, is common and, since there is also occasional spontaneous ankylosis of one or a few interphalangeal joints, the prognosis

for hand function is less favourable than nodal generalized osteoarthritis (Pattrick *et al.* 1989*b*). The principal hallmark of this condition is the presence of subchondral erosive change (Fig. 17) which may lead to a 'gull's wing' appearance as remodelling occurs (Fig. 18). Early, florid subchondral erosive change is easily recognized, but lesser degrees of erosion, particularly in established cases, may prove difficult to distinguish from cysts and subchondral bony change of nodal generalized osteoarthritis. Indeed, although described as a separate clinical subset, recent data has questioned whether this is really the case or whether erosive osteoarthritis is merely an extreme end of the spectrum of nodal osteoarthritis (Cobby *et al.* 1990) although there is no evidence for predisposition to generalized osteoarthritis in this subset.

Microscopically the synovium is infiltrated with lymphocytes and monocytes, and pannus may be seen. The nature of this inflammatory, destructive condition is unknown although it is of interest that similar hand changes may occur in some patients with Sjögren's syndrome. Of note, perhaps, is that 15 per cent of 170 patients presenting with Sjögren's syndrome and erosive osteoarthritis subsequently developed seropositive rheumatoid arthritis (Ehlich 1975).

Large joint osteoarthritis

Knee osteoarthritis
The knee is a commonly affected site. Involvement is usually bilateral, particularly in women and in the elderly. Although osteoarthritis may affect the knee as a mono- or pauciarticular problem, this site shows strong association with hand osteoarthritis (Kellgren and Moore 1952; Acheson and Collart 1975; Cushnaghan and Dieppe 1991). Population data demonstrates most frequent involvement of the medial tibiofemoral compartment (Fig. 19), severe bone and cartilage attrition at this site giving rise to the characteristic varus deformity (Fig. 20). The patellofemoral compartment, however, is often

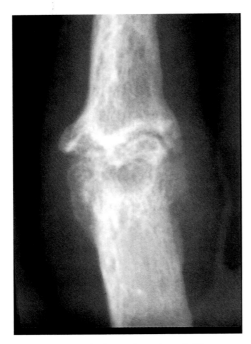

Fig. 18 'Gull's wing' deformity in erosive osteoarthritis.

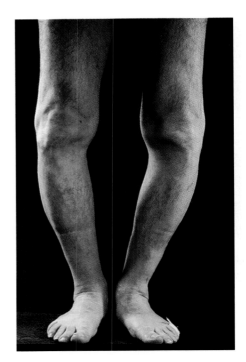

Fig. 20 Typical varus deformity of knee osteoarthritis.

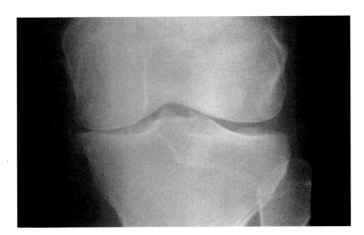

Fig. 19 Predominant medial compartment osteoarthritis at the knee (standing anterioposterior radiograph).

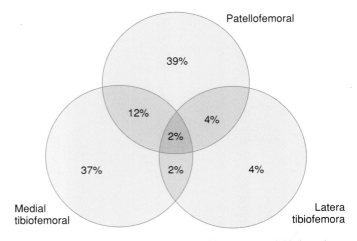

Fig. 21 Sites of radiographic involvement of knee osteoarthritis in patients with radiographic change in a community survey in the United Kingdom. (Derived from McAlindon *et al*. 1992.)

omitted from large studies, but when included it appears to be equally if not more commonly involved than the medial compartment, both symptomatically and radiographically (McAlindon *et al*. 1992) (Fig. 21).

Risk factors for development of knee osteoarthritis include previous trauma (e.g. meniscectomy), obesity (Felson 1988), generalized osteoarthritis, distal femoral dysplasia (Cooke 1985), and female gender and repetitive occupational knee bending (Felson *et al*. 1991). Smoking may be protective at this site (Felson 1988). Prognosis is discussed further below.

Recently, differing patterns of risk factors have been described in different compartments within the same joint. For example in some studies tibiofemoral disease has been more strongly linked to previous trauma and male gender whereas patellofemoral disease is more commonly symmetrical and occurs in women.

Hip osteoarthritis

Study of this joint has been particularly bedevilled by diverse classification systems which have reflected the differing interests of both orthopaedics and rheumatology at this site. Although hip involvement may occur in the context of nodal generalized osteoarthritis or involvement at other large joint sites, subdivision is usually made primarily on the basis of local radiographic patterns. Two groups have particularly been emphasized:

Superior pole osteoarthritis

The commonest pattern, this is characterized by focal cartilage loss in the superior part of the joint (Fig. 22). Osteophyte formation is most prominent at the lateral acetabular and medial femoral margins, often in combination with thickening (buttressing) of the cortex of the

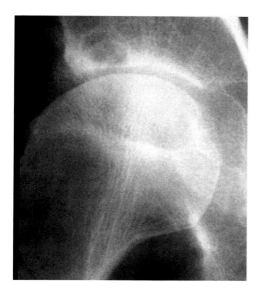

Fig. 22 Superior pole pattern of hip osteoarthritis (early) showing localized reduction in interosseous distance with focal sclerosis at the superior part of the joint, minor femoral osteophyte, and acetabular roof cyst.

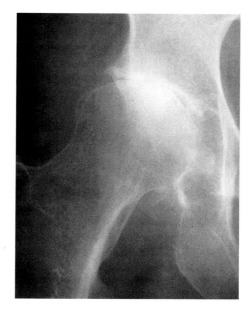

Fig. 23 Superior pole osteoarthritis (late) showing superolateral femoral head migration, bone attrition, and 'buttressing' medial periosteal osteophyte of the femoral neck.

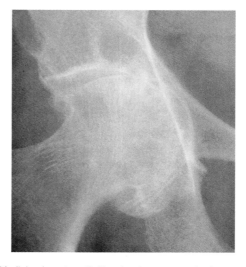

Fig. 24 Medial pole osteoarthritis, showing progression to a protrusio acetabuli deformity.

medial femoral neck (Fig. 23). Subchondral sclerosis and cyst formation on both sides of the narrowed joint may be marked. Originally it was suggested that this pattern is:

(1) more common in men;

(2) mainly unilateral at presentation;

(3) likely to progress, with superolateral (Fig. 13) or superomedial femoral migration;

(4) commonly secondary to local structural abnormality.

Recent studies have questioned whether there is often an underlying structural abnormality (Croft *et al.* 1991). In a hospital based population, progression has been confirmed to be more likely than in other patterns (Ledingham *et al.* 1993).

Central (medial) osteoarthritis
This less common pattern shows more central joint space loss, with less prominent femoral neck buttressing. It is suggested that this pattern is:

(1) more common in women;

(2) commonly bilateral at presentation;

(3) the pattern that particularly associates with nodal generalized osteoarthritis;

(4) less likely to progress (with axial or medial migration) (Fig. 24).

Other patterns are described (e.g. concentric) and many patients have 'indeterminate' radiographic patterns. Most disease is symmetrical unless there is a structural alteration in joint loading (Ledingham *et al.* 1992). Differentiation of these patterns does appear warranted since there may be differences in the association with hand osteoarthritis (Solomon 1976; Marks *et al.* 1979), and in prognosis (Danielsson 1964; Ledingham *et al.* 1992).

Suggested risk factors for development of hip osteoarthritis include previous hip disease (e.g. Perthes', slipped femoral epiphysis),

acetabular dysplasia, avascular necrosis of the femoral head, severe trauma, generalized osteoarthritis, and occupation, particularly farming. The natural history of symptomatic hip osteoarthritis, as with osteoarthritis in general, is poorly documented, and it is impossible to predict outcome for the individual.

Crystal-associated subsets (see also Chapter 5.16)

A number of particles are commonly identified in synovial fluid and other tissues from osteoarthritis joints, most notably calcium pyrophosphate dihydrate and apatite (i.e. carbonated hydroxyapatite and other basic calcium phosphates) (Fig. 25). The origin and role of such particles in the osteoarthritis process remain unknown

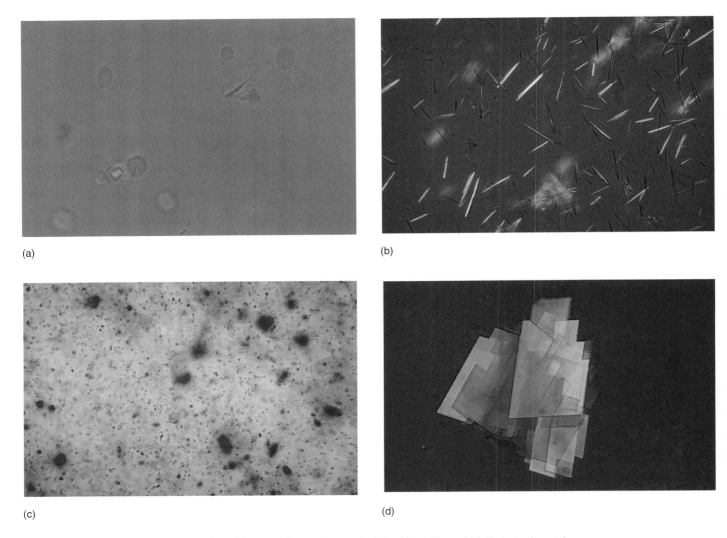

Fig. 25   (a) calcium pyrophosphate dihydrate, (b) monosodium urate monohydrate, (c) apatite, and (d) cholesterol crystals.

(Doherty and Dieppe 1988; Dieppe *et al*. 1988). By analogy with urate crystals in gout, it was initially assumed that such crystals were injurious and the cause of specific 'crystal deposition disease' (McCarty 1976). Certainly calcium pyrophosphate dihydrate and apatite are demonstrably inflammatory agents; being particulate they might also exert deleterious mechanical effects by deposition within cartilage and by acting as wear particles at the surface. However, the not uncommon occurrence of these crystals in asymptomatic, otherwise normal joints, the lack of association with specific locomotor disease, and the critical dependence of crystal identification on the technique used to detect them (Swan *et al*. 1994) has questioned such a direct pathogenic role. Multiple factors may influence deposition of these crystals, and it currently seems that calcium pyrophosphate dihydrate and apatite, in the context of osteoarthritis, most likely reflect underlying metabolic or physical facets of the process, thus potentially acting as markers for differing forms of joint response. In some situations (e.g. pseudogout) the crystals may provoke inflammation; in most others the crystals exert little phlogistic or mechanical effect, and are protected by protein coating from direct interaction with cell membranes and mediators of inflammation.

Pyrophosphate arthropathy

Calcium pyrophosphate dihydrate crystal deposition is the commonest cause of chondrocalcinosis (calcification of fibro- and hyaline cartilage). Although McCarty has proposed a complex clinical classification of 'pseudo-' syndromes (McCarty 1976) (Table 2), the simpler term 'pyrophosphate arthropathy' is often used to encompass those cases with accompanying arthritis. The three common clinical presentations are as:

(1) acute synovitis;

(2) chronic arthropathy;

(3) an incidental finding.

Other presentations are rare.

Table 2 Classification of calcium pyrophosphate dihydrate related 'pseudosyndromes'

Type	Pseudosyndrome	Presentation
A	Pseudogout	Acute or subacute synovitis
B	Pseudorheumatoid	Subacute attacks often with chronic systemic upset
C	Pseudo-osteoarthritis	Osteoarthritic change with superimposed acute synovitis
D	Pseudo-osteoarthritis	Osteoarthritic change without superimposed acute synovitis
E	Asymptomatic chondrocalcinosis	Asymptomatic radiographic finding
F	Pseudoneuropathic	Rapidly destructive often atrophic joint disease

Table 3 Factors that may trigger acute pseudogout

Intercurrent illness (e.g. chest infection)

Direct trauma to joint

Surgery (especially parathyroidectomy)

Blood transfusion, parenteral fluid administration

Institution of thyroxine replacement therapy

Joint lavage

NB Most cases develop spontaneously.

Acute synovitis ('pseudogout')

This is a common cause of acute monoarthritis in the elderly. Acute attacks may be the only manifestation of otherwise asymptomatic calcium pyrophosphate dihydrate deposition but in older patients, particularly women, they may often be superimposed upon a background of chronic symptomatic arthropathy. Any joint may be involved including the first metatarsophalangeal joint, 'pseudopodagra,' but the knee is by far the commonest site, followed by the wrist, shoulder, ankle, and elbow. Concurrent attacks in more than one joint are uncommon, and polyarticular attacks are unusual.

The typical attack develops rapidly with severe pain and swelling which is maximal within 6 to 24 h of onset. Overlying erythema is common and examination reveals a very tender joint with signs of marked synovitis (increased warmth, tense effusion, joint line tenderness, and restricted movement with stress pain). Fever is common, and elderly patients particularly may appear unwell and mildly confused, especially with knee or multiple joint involvement. Aspirated synovial fluid is inflammatory (low viscosity, turbid) and often blood stained. The cell count is usually very high, with predominance of neutrophils (> 90 per cent). The diagnosis is confirmed by demonstration of synovial fluid crystals particularly if these are intracellular. Calcium pyrophosphate dihydrate crystals are poorly visualized by plain light microscopy, but can be seen under compensated polarized light microscopy ($\times 400$). Calcium pyrophosphate dihydrate crystals (Fig. 25) are recognized by:

(1) morphology — predominantly rhomboid or rod-shaped, occasionally needle-shaped;

(2) size — approximately 2 to 10 μm long;

(3) weak positive birefringence;

(4) inclined extinction — 15 to 20°.

'Twinning' of crystals, leaving a chip at one corner, is occasionally seen. Calcium pyrophosphate dihydrate crystals are less easily identified and often less numerous than urate crystals. They may often be missed unless carefully sought. Examination of a spun deposit may increase the detection rate. As with other synovial fluid particles, the use of polarized light microscopy is associated with a false positive and negative rate but identification by more definitive analytical means, such as infra-red spectrophotometry, electron microscopy, and X-ray diffraction, although ideal, is impractical for routine diagnostic purposes. The main differential diagnosis of pseudogout is sepsis and indeed these may coexist. Synovial fluid gram stain and culture should always be undertaken.

Acute attacks are self limiting and usually resolve within 1 to 3 weeks. Most episodes develop spontaneously but several provoking factors are recognized which may precede the attack by 1 to 3 days — the commonest being stress response to intercurrent illness (Table 3). Calcium pyrophosphate dihydrate crystals principally form in fibro- and hyaline cartilage, and it is 'shedding' of preformed, naked (i.e. not protein coated) crystals into the joint space, rather than acute crystallization, that is thought to be the mechanism of the attack. This is the one clear instance where calcium pyrophosphate dihydrate crystals are the likely cause of inflammation and arthritis.

Chronic pyrophosphate arthropathy

This common subset has several characteristics including:

(1) predominance in elderly females;

(2) an often florid inflammatory component possibly with superimposed acute attacks;

(3) particular involvement of the knee;

(4) frequent involvement of joints and joint compartments uncommonly affected by 'sporadic osteoarthritis';

(5) frequent 'hypertrophic' radiographic appearance;

(6) calcification of articular structures;

(7) synovial fluid calcium pyrophosphate dihydrate crystals.

Large- and medium-sized joints are principally involved, with the knees being the most usual and severely affected site, followed by wrists, shoulders, elbows, hips, and midtarsal joints. In the hand, metacarpophalangeal joints (particularly index and middle) are the commonest, most severely affected. Symptoms are usually restricted to just a few joints, though single or multiple joint involvement also occurs; acute attacks may be superimposed upon chronic symptoms. Affected joints show signs of osteoarthritis (bony swelling, crepitus, restricted movement) and varying degrees of inflammation. Synovitis may be marked and is usually most evident at the knee, radiocarpal, or glenohumeral joints. Knees typically demonstrate bi- or tricompartmental involvement, with marked, usually predominant patellofemoral disease. In severe cases fixed flexion with either valgus or varus deformity may occur. Examination often reveals more widespread but asymptomatic joint abnormality; nodal generalized osteoarthritis, for example, is a common accompaniment.

The radiographic changes of this arthropathy are basically those of osteoarthritis with cartilage loss, sclerosis, cysts, osteophyte, and osteochondral bodies. Characteristics which may, however, permit distinction include:

(1) atypical joint and intra-articular distribution compared to uncomplicated osteoarthritis;

(2) often prominent, exuberant osteophyte and cyst formation (particularly at the knee).

These combined features may present a distinctive 'hypertrophic' appearance and distribution that suggest calcium pyrophosphate dihydrate even in the absence of radiographic chondrocalcinosis (Fig. 26). Many cases of pyrophosphate arthropathy, however, appear not dissimilar to 'uncomplicated' osteoarthritis. Furthermore, since nodal generalized osteoarthritis often coexists it is common to find otherwise typical osteoarthritis changes in some joints, with more distinctive changes of pyrophosphate arthropathy at others. It is probable, therefore, that pyrophosphate arthropathy is part of the spectrum of osteoarthritis rather than a truly distinct entity. As discussed further below the presence of crystals may tell us something about the underlying pathophysiological processes at work in the joint.

Radiographic calcification may affect several joint tissues, but need not be present for the diagnosis of pyrophosphate arthropathy. Chondrocalcinosis most commonly affects fibrocartilage, particularly knee menisci, wrist triangular cartilage, and symphysis pubis, but it also occurs in hyaline cartilage, particularly in the knee, glenohumeral joint, and hip. It appears as thick linear deposits parallel to and separate from subchondral bone (Fig. 27). Chondrocalcinosis may be localized, for example to one knee, but usually affects several joints. If absent from knees, wrists, and symphysis pubis it is unlikely to be present elsewhere and thus views of these regions are often recommended for screening for its presence. Capsular and synovial calcification is less common, and usually most obvious at metacarpophalangeal joints (Fig. 28) and the knee. Calcium pyrophosphate dihydrate deposition can occur in tendons, particularly the Achilles, triceps, and obturators, and is typically linear and extensive. This is in comparison to apatite deposition which is typically discrete and nummular. Diffuse calcification of bursae such as the subacromial, olecranon, and retrocalcaneal is an occasional finding. Chondrocalcinosis and calcification are both dynamic features that may increase or decrease with time. Chondrocalcinosis may become less evident particularly if cartilage thickness is lost, or if crystals are 'shed' from cartilage during acute or recurrent inflammatory episodes.

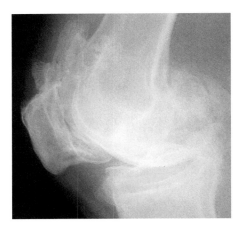

Fig. 26 Exuberant osteophytosis in patellofemoral compartment in pyrophosphate arthropathy.

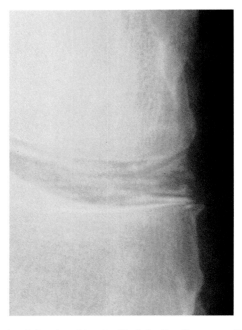

Fig. 27 Isolated chondrocalcinosis of both hyaline (linear, parallel to bone) and fibrocartilage (triangular calcification).

Incidental finding
Isolated chondrocalcinosis is a common age-associated phenomenon and as such is often observed as an incidental radiographic finding in the elderly. The only large population-based radiographic survey to study this is the Framingham study (Felson *et al.* 1989) which in the age range 63 to 93 showed an increasing overall prevalence with age ranging from 3 per cent in those aged 85 years (Fig. 29). A female preponderance was confirmed (relative risk 1.33), but was less pronounced than that derived from patient series. Although less well documented, it is likely that asymptomatic pyrophosphate arthropathy, like uncomplicated osteoarthritis, is common.

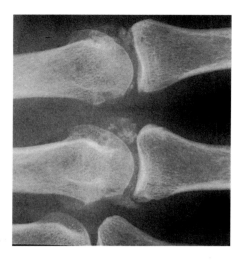

Fig. 28 Metacarpophalangeal joint radiograph in patient with pyrophosphate arthropathy showing calcification of synovium/capsule.

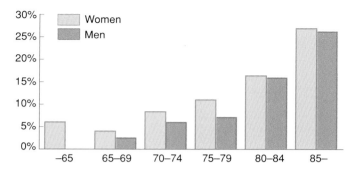

Fig. 29 Prevalence of radiographic chondrocalcinosis by age group and gender in a United States community population. Derived from Felson *et al.* (Felson *et al.* 1989).

Uncommon presentations

Polymyalgia rheumatica
This may be suggested if marked proximal stiffness accompanying glenohumeral and polyarticular involvement occurs.

Ankylosing spondylitis
Severe spinal stiffness, particularly in certain familial forms, may cause 'pseudo-ankylosing spondylitis'. True spinal ankylosis occurs in certain Chilean families.

Meningitis
Acute attacks in axial sites may cause self-limiting meningitic episodes. It is difficult to confirm these episodes although improvements in imaging has led to better recognition of such calcium pyrophosphate dihydrate deposits.

Tendinitis and tendon rupture
Acute inflammatory episodes relating to calcium pyrophosphate dihydrate deposition in tendons are described for triceps, flexor digitorum, and Achilles tendons, and tenosynovitis is reported for hand flexors and extensors. Tendon rupture is a rare complication.

Carpal tunnel syndrome
This may result from flexor tendon involvement or from wrist synovitis. Less frequently, combined median and ulnar nerve entrapment at the wrist may occur.

Bursitis
This may occur in the olecranon, infrapatellar, and retrocalcaneal bursae but is uncommon and is usually associated with widespread pyrophosphate arthropathy.

Tophi
Tophaceous (tumoral) calcium pyrophosphate dihydrate deposition is rare, but has been reported in both intra- and periarticular locations. Such deposits are usually solitary and develop in areas of chondroid metaplasia without predisposing metabolic abnormality or evidence of calcium pyrophosphate dihydrate deposition elsewhere. They produce spotty radiographic calcification and are commonly biopsied as malignant lesions, the diagnosis following histological examination (Fig. 30).

Associations of calcium pyrophosphate dihydrate deposition
A number of associations of calcium pyrophosphate dihydrate crystal deposition are recognized (Table 4). The mechanisms that underpin them are ill understood. Several possible mechanisms may be important for crystal formation including:

(1) changes, usually an increase, in relevant solute concentration;

(2) presence of nucleating factors;

(3) presence or absence of promotors or inhibitors of crystal growth;

(4) the kinetics of crystal removal and dissolution.

In relation to calcium pyrophosphate dihydrate there is evidence to support mechanisms involving an increase in ionic product (calcium × pyrophosphate) and/or influence by promoters or inhibitors of crystal formation/growth in the cartilage matrix, the site of the majority of crystal formation. The precise nature of such matrix factors, however, is not known.

Age
Ageing is perhaps the single major predisposing factor. Indirect association could come from the positive correlation with osteoarthritis, but chondrocalcinosis commonly occurs in otherwise normal cartilage and this association remains unexplained. Inorganic pyrophosphate levels in synovial fluid from normal knees show no increase with age, suggesting that age-related alteration in matrix factors are most likely to be responsible.

Genetic
Chondrocalcinosis is reported from most countries and racial groups but only one study has defined a specific racial predisposition. Genetic predisposition, however, is well described from several countries and different ethnic groups including Czechoslovakia, Chile, Holland, France, Canada, Germany, Sweden, United States, Spain, Japan, Israel, and United Kingdom (Doherty *et al.* 1991*a*). Two main clinical phenotypes have been emphasized:

(1) early onset in the third and fourth decades, florid polyarticular chondrocalcinosis, and varying severity of arthropathy, ranging from mild to severe, destructive;

(2) late-onset oligoarticular chondrocalcinosis and arthritis, mainly affecting the knee, that is indistinguishable from sporadic pyrophosphate arthropathy.

The latter form may be more common than generally recognized

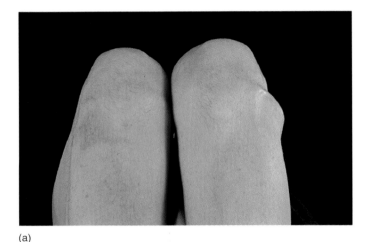

(a)

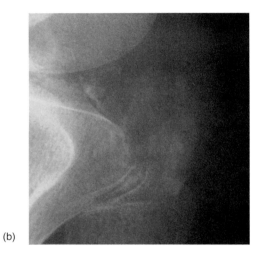

(b)

Fig. 30 Tophaceous pyrophosphate deposition superolateral to the tibiofibular joint; (a) clinical picture and (b) radiograph of the same site.

since the late onset of clinical expression presents difficulties in confirming familial disease. An association with benign childhood fits is reported in one United Kingdom family with early onset polyarticular chondrocalcinosis. Autosomal dominant inheritance occurs in most families but the genetic basis has not been identified. A primary cartilage abnormality is supported by histological study of Swedish and Japanese cases, the former demonstrating proteoglycan depletion that precedes crystal formation, the latter showing hypertrophic lipid-laden chondrocytes in areas of calcium pyrophosphate dihydrate deposition. Conversely a generalized abnormality of pyrophosphate metabolism is suggested by two reports of increased intracellular pyrophosphate concentration (skin fibroblasts or transformed lymphocytes) in French and American kindreds. This finding is not present in five United Kingdom kindreds (Doherty et al. 1991a), thus suggesting differing genetic mechanisms in different kindreds.

Metabolic and endocrine

Although numerous metabolic associations are described, many reflect no more than chance concurrence of common age-related

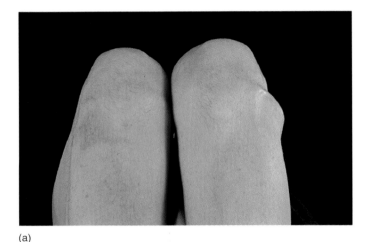
conditions (Table 5). The strongest evidence relates to hyperparathyroidism and haemochromatosis. Less certain evidence implicates hypothyroidism. With rare conditions convincing evidence is provided by occurrence of premature chondrocalcinosis in just a few cases, as with hypophosphatasia and hypomagnesaemia. The status of other previously implicated diseases such as Wilson's disease, ochronosis, and acromegaly remains unclear (Jones et al. 1992). These associations are rationalized through putative effects on pyrophosphate metabolism, extrapolated largely from in vitro data. Suggested mechanisms include:

(1) reduced breakdown of pyrophosphate by alkaline phosphatase due to;
  (a) reduced enzyme levels, in particular hypophosphatasia
  (b) presence of enzyme inhibitors such as calcium, iron, copper
  (c) lack of enzyme cofactors such as magnesium

(2) enhanced crystal nucleation e.g. by iron and copper;

(3) increased calcium concentration e.g. hyperparathyroidism;

(4) increased pyrophosphate production through parathyroid hormone stimulation of adenylate cyclase e.g. hyperparathyroidism;

(5) decreased crystal solubility e.g. hypomagnesaemia;

(6) altered cartilage matrix promoting crystal formation e.g. hypothyroidism.

Effects on pyrophosphate metabolism are certainly supported by elevated synovial fluid pyrophosphate levels in structurally normal knees of patients with hyperparathyroidism, haemochromatosis, or hypomagnesaemia, and elevated urinary pyrophosphate levels in hypophosphatasia (Doherty et al. 1991b). Mechanisms other than effects on pyrophosphate may also operate: bone and cartilage changes may be marked in these disorders, and in those with arthropathy, calcium pyrophosphate dihydrate deposition may be secondary to joint damage, mediated via alterations in matrix factors.

Joint insult

Several observations support a relationship between preceding joint insult and subsequent development of chondrocalcinosis. These include the high frequency of premature chondrocalcinosis localized to knees that have undergone meniscectomy or surgery for osteochondritis dissecans as well as reports of localized pyrophosphate arthropathy as a late complication of juvenile chronic arthropathy, joint instability, and trauma. However, the apparent negative association between calcium pyrophosphate dihydrate deposition and

Table 4 Associations of calcium pyrophosphate dihydrate crystal deposition

Positive	Negative
Ageing	Rheumatoid arthritis
Familial predisposition	
Joint insult, osteoarthritis	
Metabolic disease	

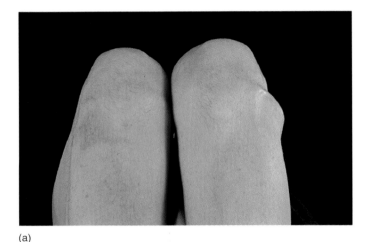

Table 5 Metabolic diseases associated with calcium pyrophosphate dihydrate deposition

	Chondrocalcinosis	Chronic arthritis
Hypophosphatasia	√	×
Hypomagnesaemia	√	×
Hyperparathyroidism	√	×
Haemachromatosis	√	√
Hypothyroidism	√	×
Gout	?	×
Acromegaly	?	×
Familial hypocalciuric hypercalcaemia	?	×
X-linked hypophosphataemic rickets	?	?
Wilson's disease	×	×
Ochronosis	×	×
Diabetes mellitus	×	×

rheumatoid arthritis, suggests that the primary association of calcium pyrophosphate dihydrate is with hypertrophic tissue response/ osteoarthritis rather than with joint damage *per se*. Indeed those few patients with coexistent rheumatoid arthritis and calcium pyrophosphate dihydrate deposition often demonstrate an atypical, hypertrophic response with exuberant osteophytosis and remodelling suggestive of an essentially reparative response (Fig. 31).

Apatite associated arthropathy

This uncommon condition has the following characteristics:

(1) confinement to elderly, predominantly female subjects;

(2) localization to large joints;

(3) rapid progression of arthropathy with instability;

(4) marked attrition of cartilage and bone;

(5) abundant apatite in synovial fluid and synovium.

This condition has a number of synonyms, including 'Milwaukee shoulder','basic calcium phosphate deposition disease', and 'analgesic hip'. Typical patients are elderly women with rapidly progressive arthropathy of the hip, shoulder, or knee. Usually only one or a few joints are affected. Onset is often quite sudden and within a few weeks or months the patient has severe rest and night pain, and shows large, cool effusions, with gross instability. Aspirated synovial fluid is often blood-stained and shows retained, high viscosity and only a modest increased cellularity. Alazarin red S staining at acidic pH shows multiple calcium containing aggregates (Fig. 25), confirmed as apatite, most commonly carbonate substituted hydroxyapatite, by more definitive means. The principal radiographic features are marked attrition of cartilage and bone, with a paucity of osteophyte and sclerosis, that is a markedly 'atrophic' appearance (Fig. 32). The differential diagnosis includes sepsis, an atrophic neuropathic joint, and late avascular necrosis.

The pathogenesis of this condition, particularly as regards the role of the apatite aggregates, is controversial (Halverson and McCarty 1988). McCarty and colleagues have emphasized the presence of activated collagenase in synovial fluid, a proliferative response to crystals in the synovium, and the frequency of accompanying periarticular calcification. They therefore suggest that apatite that has been deposited in capsule and periarticular structures is enzymatically 'strip-mined', the free apatite then interacting with synoviocytes, resulting in further collagenase release, further strip-mining, and progression of arthropathy and instability via an 'amplification loop'. Others, however, have not confirmed increase in collagenase activities, and suggest that the apatite primarily originates from subchondral and marginal bone. The non-specific finding of apatite in varying quantities in other arthropathies, and even in small amounts in normal joints, is consistent with this interpretation. The speed of onset and progression, lack of overt inflammation, marked bone loss, specificity

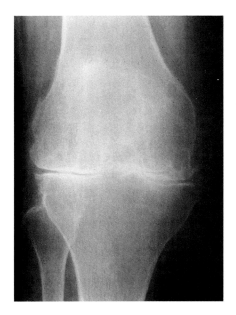
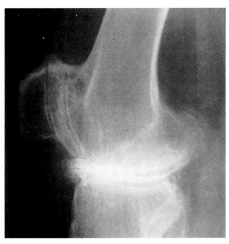

Fig. 31 Rheumatoid arthritis at the knee modified by calcium pyrophosphate dihydrate deposition. There is marked pan-compartmental joint space loss but, in addition, there is marked osteophytosis and little osteopenia.

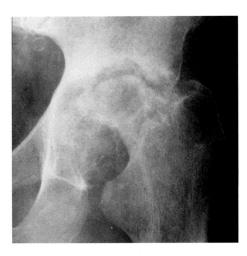

Fig. 32 Radiograph of apatite associated destructive arthritis of the hip, showing apparent increase in joint space (non-loaded film), marked loss of bone (femoral and acetabular components), and minimal bone response.

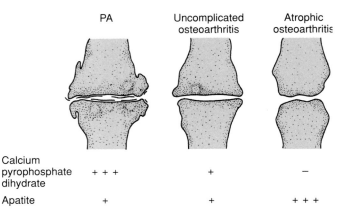

	PA	Uncomplicated osteoarthritis	Atrophic osteoarthritis
Calcium pyrophosphate dihydrate	+ + +	+	−
Apatite	+	+	+ + +

Fig. 33 Diagrammatic representation of calcium pyrophosphate dihydrate and apatite occurring as particulate 'markers' of a tendency to hypertrophic and atrophic osteoarthritis respectively.

to certain anatomic sites, radiographic similarity to late avascular necrosis, and neuropathic joints support the contention that this arthropathy reflects a widespread nutritional catastrophe for the joint, possibly initiated by age-related compromise of subchondral bone blood flow. The large amount of observed apatite may thus simply reflect the rapidity of bone damage.

Other hypotheses seem less plausible; for example the suggestion that this condition results from non-steroidal anti-inflammatory drug usage and is a specific 'iatrogenic Charcot arthropathy', seems unlikely on current evidence (Doherty 1989).

Mixed crystal deposition
Comparison of clinical and radiographic features of typical calcium pyrophosphate dihydrate and apatite associated arthropathies shows marked contrasts, though each clearly falls within the spectrum of 'osteoarthritis'. The finding of both calcium pyrophosphate dihydrate and apatite in the joints of some patients is common although there is little evidence that their combined presence is associated with particular clinical or radiographic characteristics, apart from a possible tendency to a more destructive, widespread osteoarthritis at the knee (Dieppe *et al.* 1988). Rather than classifying joints containing calcium pyrophosphate dihydrate, apatite, or calcium pyrophosphate dihydrate plus apatite as separate conditions it seems more reasonable to view these calcium crystals as markers of varying processes within the osteoarthritis joint, with calcium pyrophosphate dihydrate crystals marking a tendency to hypertrophic response, and plentiful apatite a tendency to atrophic response to insult (Fig. 33). If this is the case and osteoarthritis is regarded as a spectrum with varying balance between chronic injury and repair, frequent concurrence of both calcium crystals (in the same joint, in different joints of the same individual, at the same time or during differing phases) would be expected. In joints showing preponderance of either hypertrophic or atrophic processes (i.e. the two ends of the spectrum) the likelihood of a single crystal species would be higher. Although this may be true for typical cases, several reservations are necessary:

1. Crystal identification is not an all-or-nothing phenomenon and is critically dependent on the experience and diligence of the observer as well as the methods employed (Swan *et al.* 1994).

2. There may not be distinct associations with different crystal types. In a study examining unselected osteoarthritis patients no real distinct characteristics, either clinical or radiographic, could be associated with the presence or absence of different crystal types (Pattrick *et al.* 1993).

Osteoarthritis at other joint sites

Selection of osteoarthritis for certain joint sites is striking. For example compared to osteoarthritis of interphalangeal joints, hips, or knees, involvement of the elbow, glenohumeral joint, or ankle is unusual and principally confined to the elderly.

Osteoarthritis of spinal apophyseal joints (particularly lower cervical and lower lumbar segments), first carpometacarpal, and/or first metatarsophalangeal joints is common and may occur as part of a pattern of generalized osteoarthritis (nodal or non-nodal) or as an isolated feature. In addition to nodal generalized osteoarthritis and trauma, suggested associations include:

(1) metatarsus primus varus and the first metatarsophalangeal joint;

(2) congenital structural anomalies, adjacent spondylosis deformans, and osteoarthritis at the apophyseal joints;

(3) nodal generalized osteoarthritis, pyrophosphate arthropathy, and repetitive (principally occupational) trauma at the elbow, index, and middle metacarpophalangeal joints.

As with other arthropathies, the predilection of osteoarthritis for certain sites, with sparing of others, remains unexplained. However, one intriguing, unifying hypothesis is that human joints most commonly affected by osteoarthritis are in general those that have undergone the most rapid evolutionary change, particularly in regard to bipedal locomotion and oppositional grip (Hutton 1987). Such joints may not have had sufficient evolutionary time to fully adapt to the tasks demanded of them. They therefore have insufficient mechanical reserve, and thus fatigue and 'fail' more commonly than joints that have had longer to adapt to their new function.

Osteoarthritis as part of other disease

If, as we have discussed, osteoarthritis represents the inherent repair process of synovial joints, then osteoarthritic features would be expected to occur during certain phases of other defined arthropathies. For example in rheumatoid arthritis, osteophytosis, sclerosis, and remodelling may become prominent during later, less inflammatory periods of the disease. In such instances 'osteoarthritis' can be seen as an accompanying process of tissue response/repair rather than an acquired second condition.

The same considerations pertain to other inflammatory, metabolic, or structural arthropathies. Ochronosis and spondyloepiphyseal dysplasia, for example, are sometimes included within the umbrella of osteoarthritis since many of their radiographic features are typical of osteoarthritis. Similarly, endemic forms of osteoarthritis need consideration in their own right. For clinical purposes, however, it may still be useful to consider together conditions that may result in non-inflammatory arthropathy with radiographic changes predominantly of osteoarthritis (Table 6). An atypical presentation, however, should lead one to search for a defined, possibly treatable underlying cause. Many are rare, and have distinct clinical and radiographic features. In patients with 'osteoarthritis' one should consider specific predisposing factors when there is:

(1) premature onset osteoarthritis, i.e. less than 45 years;

(2) an atypical joint distribution, e.g. prominent metacarpophalangeal and radiocarpal involvement in haemochromatosis;

(3) premature onset of chondrocalcinosis, i.e. less than 55 years;

(4) florid polyarticular chondrocalcinosis at any age.

Investigations

Osteoarthritis is a diagnosis made on clinical and radiological grounds. To date there are no satisfactory criteria or specific laboratory tests. Furthermore, radiographic changes of osteoarthritis are commonly present but often asymptomatic. The problem is not usually to decide whether osteoarthritis is present but whether it is the cause of the problem. Investigation plays little part in this decision, which should be made by a thorough clinical examination. Some investigations may be necessary to exclude alternative diagnoses or predisposing disease.

Osteoarthritis is not associated with extra-articular disease, synovitis is usually only mild or moderate, and overt immunological abnormality is not a feature. Changes reflecting an acute phase response (anaemia, thrombocytosis, elevated erythrocyte sedimentation rate and/or C-reactive protein) or overt immunological abnormality (autoantibodies, complement breakdown products) are therefore usually absent. However, evidence of a marked acute phase response occurs with pseudogout, and modest elevation of erythrocyte sedimentation rate and C reactive protein may occur in the 'inflammatory' subsets of osteoarthritis, particularly chronic pyrophosphate arthropathy. IgG rheumatoid factor (but not Rose Waaler or Latex) positivity may be more common in nodal generalized osteoarthritis than age-matched controls (Hopkinson *et al.* 1992). Presence of such modest or isolated abnormalities are therefore not against the diagnosis of osteoarthritis, particularly in elderly patients in whom coexistent disease is common. A search for predisposing metabolic or endocrine disease may be undertaken in selected patients with atypical distribution or premature-onset of osteoarthritis, atypical radiographic features, or early-onset or polyarticular chondrocalcinosis; such patients usually have other

Table 6 Principal conditions with presentations and radiographic changes that may simulate osteoarthritis

Generalized 'osteoarthritis'	(Spondylo-) epiphyseal dysplasia Ochronosis Haemochromatosis Wilson's disease Endemic osteoarthritis (e.g. Kashin–Beck disease)

Pauciarticular, large joint 'osteoarthritis'	Neuropathic joints:
	  syringomyelia—shoulders, wrists, elbows
	  diabetes—hindfoot, midfoot
	  tabes—knees, spine
	
	Acromegaly
	
	Avascular necrosis (mainly proximal and distal femur, proximal humerus)

clinical or radiographic clues, and routine 'screening' for all known predisposing diseases is inappropriate.

The only investigations that are of importance in terms of determining the presence of osteoarthritis, the degree of structural and physiological change, and the presence of associated crystal deposition are plain radiographs and other forms of imaging. Synovial fluid analysis may also be useful. Here we shall only discuss selected aspects of imaging, and the potential for future biochemical 'markers' of the osteoarthritic process.

Imaging

Imaging aims to establish the diagnosis, to assess severity, delineate the likely pathology involved, and help exclude alternative diagnoses. Methods include plain radiographs, magnetic resonance imaging, ultrasound and radioisotope scanning. The objective of the user determines the most appropriate modality. Generally techniques that demonstrate structural change do so at the expense of demonstrating current biochemical/physiological activity and vice versa. As discussed below, a possible exception to this may be magnetic resonance imaging.

Plain films

Radiographs give an anatomical picture, that is they demonstrate past structural change rather than current 'disease activity'. Bony structures are readily defined but soft tissue imaging is more difficult. In particular, cartilage is not directly visualized and its thickness has to be inferred by assuming that it comprises the vast majority of the distance between two articulating bones, that is the interosseous distance. Focal cartilage loss is very difficult to detect and the bony changes reflect relatively late pathological abnormalities. Nevertheless, the availability of radiographs and their widespread current and historical use in studying osteoarthritis make them still the principal imaging modality for diagnosis, assessment, and follow-up.

Joint space narrowing, osteophyte, subchondral radiolucencies, and sclerosis are the classic radiological signs of osteoarthritis (Fig. 34). A spectrum of changes exist for each of these signs, there is no fixed correlation between one sign and another, and no one feature has really been shown to have particular discriminatory value, although osteophyte at the knee may be a relatively good predictor of knee pain in epidemiological studies (Spector *et al.* 1993). Additional features and complications may also be visualized including:

(1) effusions;

(2) the osseous component of osteochondral ('loose') bodies;

(3) joint alignment;

(4) subluxation.

Absence of features of other arthritides is expected although the radiographic diagnosis of osteoarthritis does not exclude other co-existing disease. Osteoarthritis may also be secondary to previous bone and joint disease.

Plain films facilitate subsetting of osteoarthritis by:

(1) the distribution of osteoarthritis change within a joint, e.g. superior pole, medial, and concentric patterns of hip; patello-femoral and tibiofemoral knee osteoarthritis;

(2) the emphasis on individual osteoarthritis features, e.g. hyper-trophic versus atrophic appearance;

(3) demonstration of additional features, e.g. calcification of carti-lage and other joint structures in calcium pyrophosphate di-hydrate deposition.

Some of these features may, however, be distorted by overlying structures and magnification effects resulting from the divergence of the X-ray beam. Attempts to improve the reproducibility and interpretability of plain radiographs have been made. Some involve standardization of positioning, the use of multiple observers, the use of different views and specialized radiographic techniques. Aspects of these are discussed further below.

Plain radiography of specific joints

Hand

The pattern of involvement of the interphalangeal joints helps to distinguish osteoarthritis and erosive osteoarthritis from rheumatoid and psoriatic arthropathy. For this purpose a single posteroanterior view of the hand may be satisfactory although it is possible such a view does not detect posterior osteophytes. The distinctive changes are (Fig. 35):

(1) osteoarthritis: bone sclerosis, focal narrowing, and lateral sub-luxation unaccompanied by erosion;

(2) erosive osteoarthritis: changes of osteoarthritis plus erosions which are through the subchondral bone plate;

(3) psoriatic arthritis: marginal erosions associated with a bone response, 'proliferative erosions'.

(4) rheumatoid arthritis: marginal 'bare area' erosions unassociated with bone proliferation;

Knee

Weight-bearing films of the knee show the functional position of the limb and may allow more precise information on the extent of joint space narrowing (Messiah *et al.* 1990). To assess the less involved compartment, or to detect soft tissue laxity, stress views may be

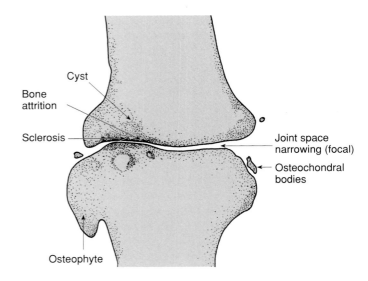

Fig. 34 Major radiographic features of osteoarthritis.

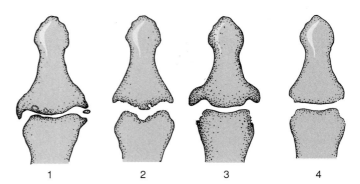

Fig. 35 The radiographic differences between (1) osteoarthritis, (2) erosive osteoarthritis, (3) psoriatic arthritis, and (4) rheumatoid arthritis.

required. However, the changes of fibrillation, cartilage narrowing, and cratering are focal. Attempts to detect early change by using a semiflexed weight-bearing view have been suggested although diffi-culties with precise patient positioning are still evident. Recent evidence has confirmed that the patellofemoral joint is an important site of involvement of osteoarthritis (McAlindon *et al.* 1992). To date there is no consensus on the best plain radiographic method to be used to assess this joint and the choice lies between a lateral view or a 'skyline' view of the patella (Jones *et al.* 1993). Further work is neces-sary to establish the optimum view.

Hip

Traditionally this is taken as a non-weight-bearing anteroposterior view of the pelvis. This has the advantage of incorporating both hips on the same radiograph although gonadal dosage may be a problem. Evidence suggests that at the level of population studies such a view may be satisfactory with minimum joint space the best criteria to define a case. It is possible that this view does not provide full infor-mation of involvement of the hip since early change may be focal and posterior. The role of additional or stressed views is, however, not yet established.

Sacroiliac joints

In the sacroiliac joints, osteophyte and joint space loss may need to be distinguished from inflammatory sacroiliitis. The latter gives erosion and intra-articular ankylosis, whereas osteoarthritis gives more focal joint space narrowing and focal sclerosis with overlying osteophytes. These are usually anterosuperior or inferior, and may be identified by discontinuity of trabecular lines across the joint in contrast to continuous lines of ankylosis (Fig. 36). Usually a single anteroposterior view of the pelvis is obtained as for the assessment of the hip but such a view may be difficult to interpret since the joint margins may overlap. In this situation a coned posteroanterior view of the sacroiliac joints may help.

Foot

A common site of osteoarthritis, this is not usually incorporated in radiographic surveys. A single posteroanterior radiograph of the foot is probably the simplest method required to demonstrate involvement of the first metatarsophalangeal joint. Specialized views would be required to demonstrate involvement of the tarsus and ankle joints but these are not usually employed in studies.

Spine

This can be a difficult area to assess for osteoarthritis. Changes suggestive of osteoarthritis, sclerosis, joint space narrowing, and osteophyte are virtually universal in middle-aged and elderly adults. These are particularly evident in the lower cervical and lower lumbar spine and may involve the facet joints and in the cervical region the uncovertebral joints (the joints of Luschka). In addition, similar changes are seen in the intervertebral discal joints. The precise views necessary to detect spinal osteoarthritis are not clear but lateral lumbosacral and cervical views are probably the most appropriate.

Disease of the spine, particularly if it involves the facet joints with subsequent osteophytosis, may result in either foraminal compression of the nerve roots or canal stenosis. Although plain views, particularly if oblique foraminal views are taken, may demonstrate narrowing (Fig. 37), more specialized techniques such as magnetic resonance imaging or computed axial tomography are usually required.

Standardization of the assessment of plain radiographs

Attempts have been made to standardize and quantitate image analysis. Two approaches have been used. The first has used atlases of standard films against which to compare the study films (Kellgren and Lawrence 1957; Kallman *et al.* 1989; Burnett *et al.* 1994), the second has tried to assess radiographic features using automated approaches. Using an atlas, two further approaches have been employed.

The first has attempted to produce a single a grade of osteoarthritis from a combination of different radiographic features. The use of such a 'global osteoarthritis' grade is attractive since it simplifies statistical analysis and means a joint is assigned to only one of a few radiographic grades. There are dangers with such an approach. Firstly it assumes a hierarchy of change that may not exist. For example in the Kellgren and Lawrence grading system the presence of osteophyte is a *sine qua non* for the diagnosis of osteoarthritis. Yet, histologically and arthroscopically, osteoarthritis, in terms of typical focal cartilage loss, may occur in the absence of detectable osteophyte. Similarly, in moving between grades it is by no means clear that the 'developing' features are indicative of deteriorating osteoarthritis. For example the development of osteophyte has been suggested to be a potentially beneficial process acting to improve joint stability.

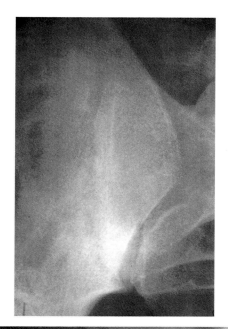

(a)

(b)

Fig. 36 (a) Sacroiliitis compared to (b) sacroiliac osteoarthritis.

The alternative approach which has gained increasing favour is to grade for individual features of osteoarthritis such as osteophyte, joint space narrowing, cysts, and sclerosis. This has the advantage of not assuming a particular hierarchy of change or inter-relationship of features. However, a large amount of descriptive data is generated for each joint which is difficult to combine. Simply summating scores for each feature is probably not valid. No consensus has been reached as to which approach is preferable.

In an attempt to reduce interobserver error, various manual and semiautomated methods have been evaluated particularly in the measurement of joint space. For an individual radiograph such an approach may be very reproducible particularly if an automated computerized method is used. Problems still remain regarding the obtaining of reproducible radiographs upon which to make the measurements (Spector 1995).

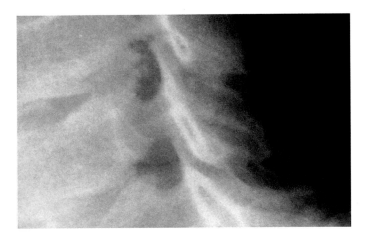

Fig. 37 Foraminal osteophytic encroachment in the neck of a patient who presented complaining of intermittent numbness and paraesthesia of the right arm.

Modified radiographic techniques

Microfocal radiography is a magnification technique that allows higher resolution imaging, with the possibility of stereoscopic reconstruction. This technique appears particularly useful in showing early subchondral bone abnormalities and demonstrating small changes in joint space width over short periods of time (Buckland-Wright *et al.* 1990). Requirements of relatively long exposures and special equipment confine this method to a research tool but one which has particular potential in longitudinal studies (Spector 1995).

Some of the limitations of plain films can be overcome by tomography. This produces cross-sectional images that thus avoid problems of interpreting overlying structures. Images of spinal apophyseal joints are possible, and the pattern of sacroiliac disease is made clearer. In general this technique has been superseded by the newer technique of computed axial tomography.

Arthrography allows cartilage to be coated with contrast and thus be demonstrated, but this is invasive and unsuitable for routine or sequential use. It has a place, however, in demonstrating associated meniscal disease although this role is rapidly becoming superseded by magnetic resonance imaging.

Magnetic resonance imaging (see also Chapter 4.9.1)

This method uses the properties of hydrogen ions, principally those in water. Since cartilage contains a high proportion of water, it can allow cartilage to be imaged. The potential and limitations of this modality in respect to osteoarthritis are still being explored. There are several problems including:

(1) limited resolution, since each image is reconstructed from information from a volume of tissue;

(2) the magnetic effects of bone, particularly when juxtaposed to cartilage;

(3) resolution of synovial fluid from cartilage, since both have a high water content.

However, by using different scan sequences it may be possible to resolve these problems as well as to obtain information on the process involved in osteoarthritis.

Radionuclide studies

Isotope bone scans give information on perfusion and bone activity. The mechanism of bone uptake is non-specific, but is more sensitive than radiographs at identifying involvement. Perhaps its most significant role in assessment of osteoarthritis is its ability to detect abnormalities before radiographic signs are identified, and to identify patients with 'active' disease who may go on to show progression (Hutton *et al.* 1986; Dieppe *et al.* 1993). This may prove useful in evaluation of drugs and other interventions before severe joint damage has occurred.

Ultrasound

This modality requires no radiation exposure and permits imaging of cartilage and tendons. Problems of access and sound distortion mean that its value is restricted and currently it remains a research tool. Nevertheless, it has been shown to give distinction between normal, fibrillated, and thin cartilage at the knee (Aisen *et al.* 1984). It may prove of value in the early detection of cartilage abnormalities.

Potential markers of tissue destruction, inflammation, and repair in osteoarthritis

There is considerable interest in measuring biochemical markers in synovial fluid or serum to allow the diagnosis of diseases, to follow progression of disease and response to treatment, and to determine disease prognosis and mechanism. Osteoarthritis involves active cellular processes of biosynthetic activity and matrix turnover and measurement of these parameters could allow these processes to be monitored. Such studies are based on two assumptions.

1.   When cartilage is damaged there is a loss of matrix components, cytokines, or proteinases into synovial fluid, the lymphatic system, serum, and urine.

2.   This loss is quantitative, with changes in concentration reflecting changes in rates of turnover.

The first of these assumptions is proven but data to support the second are confounded by unknown physiological variables. For example the concentration of fragments in synovial fluid depends not only on the rate of release from cartilage, but also on the volume and turnover of joint fluid and the speed of lymphatic drainage (all difficult to quantify). Similar problems apply to measurements in serum or urine: although they are more readily accessible compartments, the concentrations in them reflect release from all joints (normal and abnormal) and from other cartilage sites; selective, rapid elimination by the lymph nodes or liver, and the possible influence of renal and liver disease complicate interpretation. Finally, it is essential to know what a 'marker' signifies in terms of joint physiology: a reduction in the concentration of a cartilage marker after an intervention may be interpreted as reduced cartilage breakdown, it may signify inhibition of matrix synthesis or reflect the absence of any remaining cartilage within the joint (Fig. 38).

Some of the biochemical products that have been investigated are listed, in Tables 7, 8, and 9 along with the advantages and disadvantages of any particular parameter or method of measurement. The usefulness of these markers is not confined to osteoarthritis, as the principle of joint damage/repair is common to other conditions. At

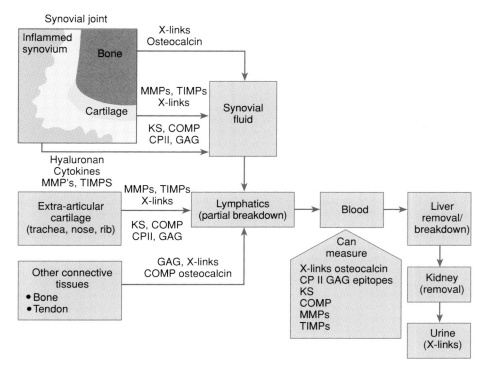

Fig. 38 Physiology of potential 'markers' of the osteoarthritic process.

present there is no marker in biological fluids that can be used for diagnosis or for monitoring of the progression of osteoarthritis (Lohmander 1994).

Cytokines

As little inflammation is present in osteoarthritic joints the measurement of cytokine levels is not helpful in osteoarthritis (Westacott *et al.* 1990).

Matrix components

Proteoglycan and glycosaminoglycan fragments
Because of their relatively rapid turnover many studies have estimated protein and carbohydrate moieties of the large, aggregating proteoglycans (aggrecan) of cartilage. Using immunoassays it has been shown that:

1. Radiographic loss of cartilage in rheumatoid arthritis correlates with a decline in the proteoglycan concentration of synovial fluid (Saxne *et al.* 1985; Poole 1993).

2. High concentrations of proteoglycan in synovial fluid occur in acute reactive arthritis and decline during remission after steroid injection (Saxne *et al.* 1986).

3. Large amounts of proteoglycan fragments occur in synovial fluid with transient synovitis and septic arthritis of the hip in children, and in adults after acute mechanical derangements of the knee (Lohmander *et al.* 1989).

4. Keratan sulphate is raised in synovial fluid in pseudogout and acute Reiter's disease, with significantly lower levels in osteoarthritis and chronic pyrophosphate arthropathy (Ratcliffe *et al.* 1988).

Thus, an increase in proteoglycan fragments in synovial fluid appears to occur only in acute inflammatory conditions, presumably reflecting accelerated breakdown.

Serum keratan sulphate is higher in osteoarthritis, particularly 'hypertrophic' osteoarthritis, than in normal controls (Thonar *et al.* 1987; Sweet *et al.* 1988), but overlap between normal and osteoarthritic individuals is marked. Studies with animal models of osteoarthritis have almost without exception failed to show significant changes in the serum keratan sulphate in early lesions. Nevertheless, the variability of the serum keratan sulphate is less within than between patients. Rather than reflecting the status of cartilage in osteoarthritic joints, elevated levels may thus signify a systemic increase in cartilage matrix turnover and ultimately prove useful in identifying individuals at risk of developing osteoarthritis.

Rather than attempting to detect the increased rate of a normal process (e.g. the release of keratan sulphate from cartilage), it would be preferable to identify a released antigen more distinctive of abnormal tissue. Epitopes that detect changed sequences in sulphation in chondroitin sulphate chains that are found infrequently in normal mature cartilage appear to be increased in experimental models. In experimental canine osteoarthritis, for example, the expression of a chain-terminal chondroitin sulphate epitope (3B3) is greatly increased in proteoglycan from operated joints as part of the pattern of increased synthesis and turnover that also results in longer chondroitin sulphate chains: the distribution of such epitopes varies greatly in chondroitin sulphates of different origin, and their expression is closely controlled during biosynthesis (Caterson *et al.* 1990). The biological significance of the chondroitin sulphate epitopes have yet to be determined. However, they may provide useful markers of processes occurring in cartilage before major joint damage.

Table 7 Physiological correlates of matrix markers of tissue destruction, inflammation, and repair in osteoarthritis and rheumatoid arthritis

Tissue	Markers	Indicates	Osteoarthritis Serum	SF	Rheumatoid arthritis Serum	SF
Synovium	Hyaluronan (hyaluronic acid, hyaluronate, HA)	Synovitis, HA synthesis stimulated by IL-1 and TNF-α	↑	ND	↑	↑
Cartilage	C-propeptide of type II collagen Type II collagen α chain fragments	Synthesis of cartilage type II collagen	↑	↑	↑	↑
		Degradation of cartilage type II collagen	Studies in progress			
	Cartilage oligomeric protein	Synthesis and/or degradation?	ND	↑	↑	ND
	Cartilage matrix protein	Synthesis and/or degradation? only present in non-articular cartilages	ND	ND	↑	ND
Proteoglycan aggrecans	Keratan sulphate	Synthesis/degradation of aggrecan	↑	↑	↓	↑
	Core protein	Degradation	•	↑	•	↑
	Intact chondroitin sulphate epitopes e.g. 846, 3B3	Probably synthesis	↑	•	↑↓[a]	↑
Bone	Bone sialoprotein	Synthesis/degradation	Studies in progress			
	Osteocalcin	Synthesis	↑	↑	•	↑
	3-Hydroxypyridinium (pyridinolone and deoxypyridinoline) cross-links	Degradation	Urine only			

ND=not determined, SF=synovial fluid, [a]acute disease only.

Collagen fragments

The C-terminal propeptide of type II collagen is cleaved off at fibril-logenesis and not retained by interaction with other matrix constituents, and is therefore a molecule with the potential for identifying repair. In urine, the determination of collagen cross-links derived from cartilage (pyridinoline) and bone (pyridinoline and deoxypyridinoline) has provided a sensitive measure of tissue breakdown (Seibel et al. 1989). These cross-links are only present on mature collagen; thus relative amounts may indicate different forms of stages of arthropathy involving the degradation of bone and cartilage. Recent studies using immunoassays have shown that collagen cross-links can also be shown to be raised in osteoarthritis in serum samples (Risteli et al. 1993; Robins et al. 1994).

Little progress has been made in following the release of type II, IX, or XI fragments into synovial fluid as a measure of the dismantling of the collagen fibrillar network. Caution has to be used in synovial fluid studies as often the centrifugation of the fluid to remove any neutrophils or other cells is sufficient to sediment some of the collagen fragments. Further work is needed to establish the usefulness of the measurement of collagen fragments in osteoarthritis.

Proteinases and inhibitors

Measurement of proteinases and inhibitors in serum is often difficult as levels can be low and sometimes below the level of detection (Lohmander et al. 1994). Collagenase, gelatinase, stromelysin, and TIMP are present in synovial fluid but are difficult to measure as the

Table 8 Changes in matrix markers of tissue destruction, inflammation, and repair in osteoarthritis and rheumatoid arthritis

	Osteoarthritis	Rheumatoid arthritis
Hyaluronan	↑	↑
C-propeptide II	↑	↑
Keratan sulphate	↑	↓
Chondroitin sulphate epitopes	↑	?
Cross-links	↑	↑
Matrix metalloproteinases	↑	↑
Tissue inhibitors of metalloproteinases	↑	↑
Cartilage oligomeric protein	↑	↑

fluid has to be fractionated before measurement to allow enzyme activity to be measured whilst inhibitors are also present (Cawston et al. 1984). The development of immunoassays has shown that stromelysin (Lohmander et al. 1993), collagenase, and tissue inhibitor of metalloproteinase (TIMP) (Clark et al. 1994; Shinmei et al. 1992) are elevated in osteoarthritis synovial fluids although there is a large

Table 9 Measurement of matrix markers of tissue destruction, inflammation, and repair (NB low levels may result when most of the cartilage tissue has been destroyed)

Assay	Advantages	Disadvantages
Where?		
Serum	Easy collection All patients	Dilution of marker Contribution from other tissues
Synovial fluid	Local to inflamed joint	Infrequent aspiration Small proportion of patients Low levels may result when large volumes of synovial fluid are produced
Urine		Difficult to collect 24-h urine Final level depends on rate of clearance in other compartments
How?		
Immunoassay	Rapid measurement of total level	Also measure non-functional protein
Activity assay	Measures biological activity	Often inhibitors also present, therefore sample may require fractionation

variation between patients and considerable overlap between disease groups. It is not yet known if high levels of proteinase or low levels of inhibitor correlate with excess joint damage. The results are also difficult to interpret as much of the metalloproteinases present are still in proenzyme form and consequently pose no threat to the joint structures until activated. Some studies have suggested that the measurement of proteinase-inhibitor complexes are more indicative of cartilage breakdown although these results are still to be confirmed in prospective studies. Raised levels of collagenase-TIMP levels in osteoarthritis are infrequent or at least below the level of detection for the immunoassays (Clark *et al.* 1994). Many studies have investigated single samples of synovial fluid from patients. Recently Lohmander *et al.* were able to show that levels of stromelysin and TIMP remained raised for long periods after traumatic injuries in knee joints (Lohmander *et al.* 1994) and this kind of study where individual patients are followed up sequentially with clinical, radiographic, and biochemical markers measured for individual joints represents the best way forward to evaluate these markers.

Diagnosis

The diagnosis of osteoarthritis is essentially clinical and many comments regarding this have already been made in the section on investigations. There are several different clinical problems.

The patient with pain

This is the commonest clinical situation. The priorities in this situation are to determine whether:

(1) 'osteoarthritis' is the cause of the symptoms;

(2) there is an articular or periarticular cause for the pain;

(3) there are predisposing or adverse factors for the development or progression of osteoarthritis;

(4) there is another underlying arthropathy;

(5) how pain is being caused and modified.

Resolving these difficulties depends on a careful clinical history and examination; radiography and laboratory investigations play a relatively minor role. The examination aims to:

(1) localize the site of the pain — joint line or periarticular;

(2) detect the presence of clinical signs of osteoarthritis — crepitus, bony swelling, restricted range of motion;

(3) define any adverse features — obesity, malalignment, abnormal usage (occupational or habitual);

(4) rule out features of other arthropathy — e.g. rheumatoid arthritis, gout, seronegative spondylarthropathy;

(5) determine factors aggravating the pain response — e.g. coexistent fibromyalgia, depression, sleep disturbance.

The radiograph merely serves to confirm the presence of the structural changes of osteoarthritis that may or may not be attributable to the symptoms. Since the radiograph is relatively insensitive, particularly in early disease, a normal radiograph does not rule out a diagnosis of osteoarthritis. Conversely, as has already been discussed, an abnormal radiograph is not necessarily the cause of symptoms.

The radiographic finding

It is not uncommon for patients to have radiographs taken following an acute episode of pain or trauma, particularly of the spine, and for osteoarthritic changes to be discovered. The difficulty then lies in knowing what, if anything to do regarding these findings. Undue emphasis on the structural changes can result in patients being unduly alarmed and adopting inappropriate illness behaviour. Again a careful clinical history and examination is necessary to determine the association between the current clinical problem and any structural change.

Neurological findings

Neurological finding are important, particularly in the lumbar and cervical spine where osteophytosis of the facet or apophyseal joint may lead to foraminal encroachment and subsequent nerve root compression. Peripheral nerve entrapment may also occur as a result of osteophytosis or synovitis. Possible sites for this are the ulnar nerve at the ulnar groove and the median nerve in the carpal tunnel. In such a situation, particularly in the spine, magnetic resonance imaging, computed axial tomography, and, now less commonly, contrast radiculography is necessary to fully elucidate the nature and presence of nerve compression.

As well as direct pressure on a nerve, vascular claudication may also occur, particularly in the lumbar spine, giving rise to the syndrome of spinal claudication. In this situation, exercise results in neurological signs and symptoms in the legs. The diagnosis is essentially based on the history but evidence of canal stenosis is sought, usually with computed axial tomography or magnetic resonance imaging.

In all situations, particularly in the spine, it is essential, in view of the high prevalence of abnormal structural findings in asymptomatic individuals, to ensure that there is a good match between clinical findings and demonstrated structural abnormalities.

Pathogenesis

The nature of osteoarthritis

It has been widely suggested that osteoarthritis is a process, rather than a disease, that shows variability in outcome. Support for this comes from several considerations:

(1) osteoarthritis has accompanied man throughout his evolutionary history;

(2) a similar process occurs in other animals that have fused epiphyses in the adult;

(3) radiographic osteoarthritis is very common in adults, showing increased frequency with age;

(4) in most instances osteoarthritis occurs without symptoms or disability, and its radiographic presence is not necessarily the explanation of locomotor pain;

(5) symptoms relating to osteoarthritis are often phasic and may not necessarily be associated with a poor prognosis.

Such phylogenetic preservation, discordance between symptoms and structural change, and generally good outcome suggest that osteoarthritis reflects the inherent repair process of synovial joints (Fig. 39). In most cases this metabolically active process keeps pace with a variety of triggering insults and is non-progressive. In some, however, it fails to compensate, resulting in 'joint failure' (decompensated osteoarthritis) with perceived symptoms and disability. This interpretation partly explains the marked heterogeneity of osteoarthritis—a wide variety of 'insults' triggering a repair

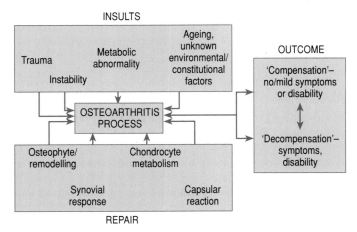

Fig. 39 Diagrammatic representation of osteoarthritis as the inherent repair process of synovial joints.

reaction but each resulting in a different pattern of involvement. As with any biological process, multiple constitutional and environmental factors may further modify the response, leading to variable outcome.

The mechanical, genetic and metabolic factors that may 'insult' the joint and thus trigger the osteoarthritis process have been discussed above. Indeed most evidence regarding the initiation of osteoarthritis in man derives from such studies since diagnosis of the early stages of sporadic osteoarthritis *in vivo* is currently not possible. The response of the joint to these insults has been studied by a variety of methods including *in vivo* animal models, *ex vivo* studies on tissue explants, and from pathological human tissue. The results from such studies and the insights which they give into the nature of osteoarthritis are discussed below.

Structure and metabolism of osteoarthritic tissues

Investigation of human osteoarthritis tissue is problematic: pathological studies often focus on late 'end-stage' osteoarthritis of surgically-derived large joints, whilst cadaveric studies examining 'early' osteoarthritis lack clinical correlates. All such studies are confounded by the heterogeneity of osteoarthritis and by restriction to single time point examination. Much work on pathophysiology therefore derives from animal models and *in vitro* experiments. Animal models often employ small quadrupeds, utilize invasive mechanical or chemical insult to stimulate joint response, or investigate hereditary forms of premature joint failure; the time scale is often short; and immature rather than mature animals may be used. Although some models (e.g. cruciate section in the adult dog) appear closer to human osteoarthritis than others, such contrasts with the clinical situation in man have raised questions as to their relevance. Rather than considering them as models of osteoarthritis, they are probably best viewed as a means of studying, in a well defined and controlled situation, dynamic biochemical and structural events at the earliest stages of joint insult. Thus, while animal models and human studies *in vitro* provide useful insights, caution is required in drawing together the available disparate data to develop a more complete understanding of pathophysiology relevant to human osteoarthritis.

Structural changes

The histological changes characteristic of osteoarthritis cartilage from humans and animal models are well described (Mankin 1974; Brandt 1988) and include:

(1) reduction in stainable proteoglycan;

(2) fibrillation;

(3) collagen crimping;

(4) chondrocyte multiplication or migration (cloning);

(5) loss of cartilage (Fig. 40).

Initially, localized areas of softening present a pebbled texture at the surface, followed by disruption along collagen fibre planes (tangential 'flaking', vertical 'fibrillation'). At the earliest stage of surface erosion and irregularity cartilage appears moderately hypercellular with alteration in staining quality of the matrix; the tidemark may also show irregularities and violation by blood vessels. As increasingly deep clefts form in cartilage, nearby matrix is depleted of metachromatic material indicating loss of proteoglycans. Microscopic changes are also apparent in cells, and necrosis ('ghosting') is often present. More common, however, is focal proliferation producing clumps ('clones') of chondrocytes, often surrounded by intense metachromatic material indicating increased proteoglycan. Such cell proliferation and metabolic activity represents attempted 'intrinsic' repair. With continuing movement fibrillated cartilage in habitually loaded areas may abrade to expose underlying bone, with progression to variable degrees of structural damage. It is noteworthy, however, that fibrillation itself is not necessarily progressive. Indeed, it is a normal finding in adult human joints (e.g. hip, knee, humeroradial joint) in areas of cartilage that are habitually unloaded. In addition to intrinsic repair, 'extrinsic' repair commonly occurs by formation of new cartilage at the joint margin or in subchondral bone; such cartilage is generally more cellular than pre-existing hyaline cartilage and the chondrocytes are evenly distributed throughout the matrix. Extrinsic repair is with fibrocartilage, containing predominently type I collagen. Proliferating nodules of fibrocartilage arising from underlying marrow spaces may protrude through defects in the bone surface, occasionally coalescing to form a near continuous layer of replacement tissue.

In parallel with the cartilage changes, new bone formation occurs in subchondral bone and at the joint margins (central and marginal osteophyte), and occasionally beneath adjacent periosteum (e.g. femoral neck 'buttressing'—periosteal osteophyte). Osteophyte forms through the process of endochondral ossification, either by vascular penetration of existing cartilage or from marginal foci of cartilaginous metaplasia, particularly at capsular and ligamentous insertion sites. The location of osteophyte is characteristic for individual joints. Proliferation of subchondral bone is most apparent beneath areas of cartilage erosion and fibrillation. In such areas the tidemark is generally more irregular, thickened, and reduplicated (showing often three or more parallel tidemarks); new bone and thickening of existing trabeculas gives rise to sclerosis seen radiographically. With gross cartilage loss repeated motion may polish the bone ('eburnation') and, as a result of increased local stress, surface bone additionally may undergo focal pressure necrosis. Subarticular cysts (more correctly 'pseudocysts') predominate where overlying cartilage is thinned or absent. Pathologically, cysts show features of bone necrosis (loss of trabeculas, fibromyxomatous degeneration of marrow), frequently contain dead bone, cartilage, and amorphous material, and are surrounded by a rim of reactive new bone and fibrous tissue. They are thought to result from high intra-articular pressure transmitted through defects (microfractures) in the overlying cortex, or from intraosseous hypertension generated through abnormal loading and force transmission in the mechanically altered joint. As with fibrillation, both marginal osteophyte and cysts may occur in the absence of other features of osteoarthritis, reflecting bone response to mechanical stimulation.

Separated fragments of cartilage and bone may form 'loose bodies', undergo dissolution, or become incorporated into the synovium and proliferate locally. As they grow, their centres necrose and calcify, and periodic extensions give rise to a concentric ringed appearance: endochondral ossification of these bodies may follow vascular invasion. Osteochondral bodies may also arise in synovium by chondroid metaplasia of fibroblastic cells.

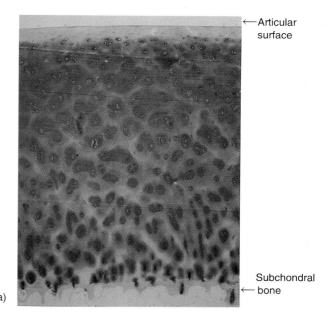

←Articular surface

←Subchondral bone

(a)

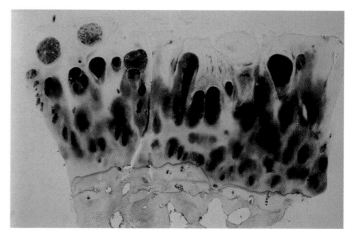

(b)

Fig. 40 (a) normal and (b) osteoarthritic human articular cartilage (toluidine blue). Note the extensive cell clustering, loss of metachromatic staining, fissuring of the tissue, and duplication of the 'tide-mark' in the osteoarthritis specimen.

The synovium becomes both hypertrophic and hyperplastic, and the capsule thickens and contracts. In the synovium lymphoid follicles, as well as more diffuse infiltration by T and B lymphocytes and macrophages (DR positive), may be identified (Revell *et al.* 1988), often with accompanying diffuse and perivascular fibrosis. Synovial extension onto the articular surface (i.e. pannus) is common, particularly at the hip, but both synovitis and pannus are less extensive and aggressive than in rheumatoid arthritis, synovitis usually being confined to synovium rimming the cartilage. Haemosiderin staining of synovium, reflecting previous intra-articular bleeding, is common in large joints, and occasionally is marked. The role of particulate debris (osteochondral fragments, calcium crystals) in producing chronic inflammation is uncertain but, in general, synovitis is regarded more as a secondary, usually late phenomenon than a primary, early event in osteoarthritis.

Calcification is an integral part of new bone formation, and many osteoarthritis joints show evidence of calcium crystal deposition in cartilage, with presumed secondary uptake in synovium. Carbonate-substituted hydroxyapatite is the commonest particulate identified, particularly adjacent to hypertrophic and degenerating chondrocytes (Ohira and Ishikawa 1987). Calcium pyrophosphate dihydrate crystal deposition also associates with osteoarthritis at certain sites, particularly in the elderly (Felson *et al.* 1989). The relationship between calcium crystal formation and osteoarthritis is unclear.

Despite loss of bone and cartilage in some parts of the joint, the net effect of new cartilage and bone formation is an increase in joint size and remodelling of shape. The balance between degradative and reparative features is variable and leads to varying consequences with respect to joint congruity, stability, and load transmission. Associated periarticular abnormalities (muscle atrophy, bursitis, enthesitis) are a common accompaniment to established osteoarthritis. The radiographical–pathological correlations seen in osteoarthritis are outlined in Table 1.

Metabolic changes

Though changes occur in all joint tissues in osteoarthritis, most experimental work has investigated cartilage (Maroudas and Urban 1980; Hardingham and Bayliss 1990). The extracellular matrix of cartilage is complex, and its composition and turnover vary:

(1) in different joints;

(2) at different locations within the same joint;

(3) through the depth of the tissue.

The initiating insult (e.g. mechanical, metabolic) also varies and age-related changes occur. It is sometimes, therefore, difficult to identify common events in osteoarthritis (Table 10).

Analytical studies

The changes in composition of osteoarthritis cartilage, which are markedly different from those due to ageing, include:

(1) an increase in water content;

(2) a loosening of the 'collagen network' with a reduction in collagen fibre size, though the collagen concentration and phenotypes appear normal;

(3) a reduction in proteoglycan concentration with a smaller proportion of total proteoglycan in aggregates, and alteration in proteoglycan structure.

Whereas ageing human cartilage undergoes some degree of dehydration, osteoarthritis cartilage has an increased water content. This increase is one of the earliest changes detected in animal models—initially within loaded regions but eventually involving all of the cartilage. This change probably reflects a defect in the arrangement of collagen fibres that allows proteoglycans to swell. The marked swelling of osteoarthritic cartilage when placed in hypotonic solutions *in vitro* is consistent with a loosening of the collagen network, and ultrastructural studies using animal models confirm early loss of orientation among superficial collagen fibrils, with individual fibrils being more widely spaced than normal. This basic structural change may arise in type II collagen fibres themselves (Maroudas *et al.* 1986), or more likely in cross-link molecules such as type IX collagen, a decrease of which (with little change in production) is reported in

Table 10 Metabolic changes in osteoarthritic cartilage

General	Increased hydration
	Increased swelling
	Loss of tensile strength
	Possible increased biosynthesis of proteoglycan and collagen in early disease and decreased in late disease
	Increased rates of matrix turnover with net loss of proteoglycan and collagen
Specific	
Collagens	Net loss of type II collagen
	Increased damage to collagen fibres
	Loss of tensile strength
	Type III and type X collagen can be synthesized
	Increased content of type VI collagen
Glycosamino-glycan	Chondroitin sulphate (CS) progressively decreases
	CS-4/-6 ratio increased
	CS chain length increases in early disease, decreases later
	Increased expression of native CS epitopes
	Keratan sulphate decreased
	Hyaluronate concentration decreases
Proteoglycans	Increased extractability
	Decreased monomer size
	Diminished/normal aggregation
	Increased rate of maturation of hyaluronate-binding region
	Loss of decorin from surface layers
Proteinases and inhibitors	Increase in matrix metalloproteinases (MMPs) and cathepsins
	Decrease in overall inhibitor levels

the rabbit postmeniscectomy model and in human osteoarthritis. A recent study (Bonassar *et al.* 1995) has shown that this increase in swelling can be mimicked by treatment of cartilage with stromelysin.

A decrease in proteoglycan content is the most consistent feature found in all studies of osteoarthritis. The main finding for glycosaminoglycans in human osteoarthritic cartilage is a decrease in keratan sulphate content. This is a real event, not merely reflecting a decrease in cartilage thickness (the deeper layers of normal cartilage are richer in keratan sulphate than the surface zones). The concomitant decrease in chondroitin-6-sulphate relative to chondroitin-4-sulphate gives an overall composition akin to that of immature cartilage, suggesting that, in osteoarthritis, chondrocytes revert to a chondroblastic state and synthesize fetal-like, immature proteoglycan. Because of the uncertainty over the production of the proteoglycan, however, it remains unclear in established human osteoarthritis if such changes are biosynthetic or arise primarily from catabolic events.

Changes in keratan sulphate:chondroitin-6/-4-sulphate ratios are an inconsistent finding in animal models, and such changes may principally occur late in the pathogenesis. Specific modifications in the sulphation of chondroitin sulphate chains, however, appear early in animal models (at 3 months in Pond–Nuki model) and may relate to larger chain size; in addition, proteoglycans from cartilage with activated chondrocytes react with monoclonal antibodies to novel sequences of sulphation on chondroitin sulphate chains (similar epitopes being detected in proteoglycan from human osteoarthritis and normal immature cartilage). The significance of these structural changes in chondroitin sulphate is unknown, though one function may be to increase matrix binding of growth factors, thereby increasing the local pool of these agents.

There is little evidence from animal or human studies to suggest that proteoglycan is lost from the matrix through any abnormalities in its ability to aggregate. Aggregation of proteoglycan appears to be normal, and although the hyaluronan content of osteoarthritic cartilage is reportedly low, there appears sufficient to accommodate the reduced concentration of proteoglycan (Brocklehurst et al. 1984). The hyaluronan-binding regions of most proteoglycan monomers in osteoarthritic cartilage appear fully functional. In most animal models this also applies to newly synthesized proteoglycans, even though they are often larger than normal. In cartilage from late-stage human osteoarthritis, the assembly of newly synthesized proteoglycans into aggregates in the extracellular matrix appears faster than in normal adult joints, and more similar to that in immature cartilage. This aspect of proteoglycan structure could profoundly affect turnover rates and complicate further our understanding of mechanisms of cartilage repair.

Growth factors and cytokines

Matrix synthesis

The compositional changes occur as chondrocytes respond to a variety of growth factors and cytokines and so alter the rate of proliferation or either synthesis and/or degradation of these matrix components (Goldring 1993). A number of cytokines and growth factors are listed together with the possible effect shown on matrix metabolism (Table 11).

Chondrocytes can increase their biosynthesis to counteract increased loss, particularly early rather than late in the process. For example in the Pond–Nuki model (section of the anterior cruciate ligament in the mature canine stifle joint), chondrocytes from macroscopically normal cartilage show increased incorporation of ^{35}S-sulphate as an early feature that predates fibrillation, and other areas of cartilage that do not proceed to fibrillation may also show this change. In other models early hypermetabolic activity cannot be demonstrated, and whether increased synthesis occurs in early human osteoarthritis remains speculative.

In established human osteoarthritis, the variability in proteoglycan synthesis reported from different centres (i.e. increased or normal) may reflect sampling differences as much as variability of osteoarthritis itself. For example, in reports of increased ^{35}S-sulphate incorporation by human osteoarthritic cartilage, with correlation between synthetic activity and histological grading (Ryu et al. 1984), the high-scoring samples could be mainly mid- and deep-zone cartilage, which in normal tissue contains cells with higher synthetic rates. After 'correcting' for topographical and zonal sampling, no difference in proteoglycan synthesis is apparent between osteoarthritic and normal, age-matched cartilage at the hip or knee (Brocklehurst et al. 1984). There is some evidence that proteoglycan synthesis is decreased in human osteoarthritis and it is also possible that these synthetic rates are affected by the drugs taken by patients. In late human osteoarthritis it is therefore unclear whether chondrocytes

Table 11 Effect of cytokines and growth factors on chondrocyte metabolism

Growth factor	Major function in cartilage
TGFβ	Chondrocyte proliferation, promotes matrix synthesis, modulates IL-1 effects, increases proteinase inhibitors
PDGF	Proliferation of chondrocytes
bFGF	Proliferation and differentiation of chondrocytes, MMP production
IGF-1	Proliferation of chondrocytes, increases GAG synthesis
IL-1	Increases production of MMPs, PGE$_2$, and other cytokines; inhibits GAG synthesis
TNF-α	Similar catabolic effects as IL-1
IL-6	Increases proteinase inhibitor production, proliferation of chondrocytes

TGFβ, Transforming growth factor β; IL-1, interleukin-1; PDGF, platelet derived growth factor; IGF-1, insulin growth factor; TNF-α, tumour necrosis factor α; MMPs, Matrix metalloproteinases; PGE$_2$, prostaglandin E$_2$; GAG, glycosaminoglycans; IL-6, interleukin-6.

are metabolically hyperactive or whether their potential reparative response has been inhibited or lost.

Chondrocytes show an increased rate of synthesis of type II collagen, as with proteoglycans, early in animal models. The long turnover time of type II collagen in adult cartilage might suggest that mature chondrocytes have little chance of even minimal repair of defective collagen network. Nevertheless, an increase in collagen synthesis in human osteoarthritic cartilage has been demonstrated (Lipiello et al. 1977). When type II collagen fibrils form in the extracellular matrix, the N- and C-propeptides are removed by specific proteases and are lost from the matrix. Increased C-propeptide (CP-II) is found in human osteoarthritic compared to normal cartilage, mainly in the lower mid- and deep zones rather than the surface and upper mid zones where collagen degradation is more prevalent (Dodge and Poole 1989). There may thus be the potential for limited repair in deep zones, but an effective response in late osteoarthritis, when major disruption in collagen architecture has occurred, seems less likely.

Type X collagen, with its presumed role in mineralization, is regarded as a unique marker for hypertrophic chondrocytes, which are also rich in alkaline phosphatase activity. In osteoarthritic cartilage the alkaline phosphatase activity is very high, not just in the deep but also in the mid-zones (Fig. 41), and deposition of type X collagen once again becomes evident. Such characteristics are reminiscent of immature cartilage, and suggest that chondrocytes throughout the cartilage are resuming their potential to mineralize.

Matrix degradation

Just as anabolic growth factors can influence matrix synthesis, the proinflammatory cytokines can increase matrix degradation. Both interleukin 1 and tumour necrosis factor are present in cartilage which is degrading extracellular matrix (Table 11) (Hammerman 1989; Goldring 1993). These cytokines when added to cartilage rapidly cause the release of proteoglycan with the later release of collagen fragments (Ellis *et al.* 1994). At the same time the synthesis of matrix components is also down-regulated. It is not known exactly how proteoglycan and collagen turnover is increased in response to these cytokines but the levels of the matrix metalloproteinases are increased (Murphy *et al.* 1991). This family of zinc and calcium dependant proteinases can degrade the proteins of the extracellular matrix at neutral pH and are divided into three main groups—the collagenases, the stromelysins, and the gelatinases (Fig. 42) (Woessner 1992; Brinkerhoff 1991). These enzymes contain common sequences of amino acids; the N-terminal domain contains a characteristic sequence of zinc-binding histidines and contains the catalytic zinc whilst the C-terminal domain determines the differences in substrate specificity. The matrix metalloproteinases can be controlled at different points (Fig. 43) which include stimulation of synthesis and secretion by cytokines, activation of proenzyme forms, and the inhibition by specific inhibitors called TIMPs. These enzymes are found in osteoarthritic cartilage and osteoarthritic cartilage appears deficient in endogenous protease inhibitors (Woessner 1992). This imbalance between matrix metalloproteinases and their inhibitors is likely to play a part in the accelerated breakdown of the matrix (Hammerman 1989; Dean *et al.* 1989). Specific inhibitors of matrix metalloproteinases are able to prevent both proteoglycan and collagen release from resorbing cartilage *in vitro* and in animal models (Andrews *et al.* 1992; Cawston *et al.* 1994). Other proteinases are also implicated in the destruction of cartilage in osteoarthritis (Buttle *et al.* 1993).

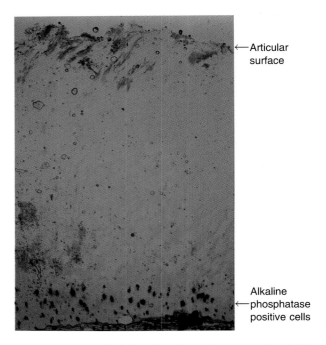

Fig. 41 Localization of alkaline phosphatase in human osteoarthritic cartilage (55-year-old patient).

Recently, the analysis of the fragments released from resorbing cartilage have been studied in order to determine degradative mechanisms. Proteoglycans released from osteoarthritic cartilage during culture *in vitro* cannot interact with hyaluronan and

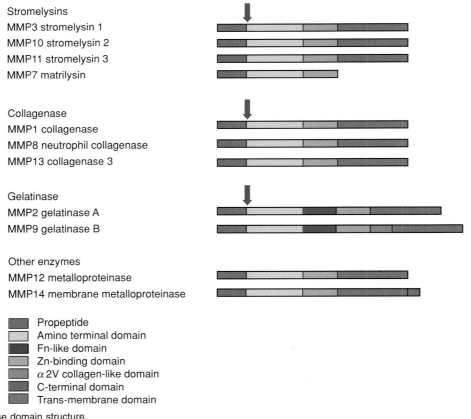

Fig. 42 Metalloproteinase domain structure.

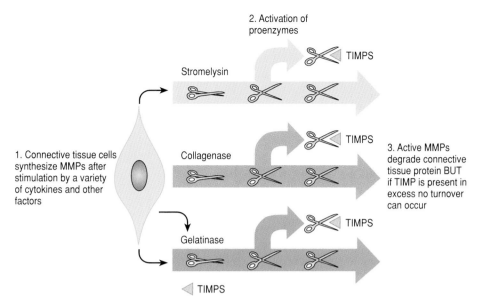

Fig. 43 Control of metalloproteinase activity.

presumably have lost their hyaluronan-binding region. Analysis of the proteoglycan fragments suggest that an unidentified metalloproteinase called aggrecanase is responsible, as the cleavage site in the aggrecan molecule is not cleaved by any known enzyme (Sandy *et al.* 1992). Other studies have used a unique epitope hidden in native collagen but exposed by proteolytic cleavage to follow collagen turnover. In osteoarthritis, cartilage collagen cleavage can be shown by immunohistochemistry in both the superficial and intermediate zones (Hollander *et al.* 1994; Poole 1993).

Debate still continues over the relative importance of cartilage and bone changes in the initiation and progression of osteoarthritis. It is recognized that physiology and structure are initimately linked and that all joint tissues (including synovium, capsule, and periarticular tissues) interact together. Thus 'weakening' of cartilage and surrounding tissues and 'stiffening' of subchondral bone will each be deleterious in all tissues. All locomotor tissues require continuing physical stimulation to sustain normal development, nutrition, and adaptation. Interestingly, many of the metabolic and structural responses of cartilage and bone seen in animal models only develop if joint loading continues, suggesting that the potential repair process of joints is similarly driven by this physiological need. A more pressing question, of course, is what stops all joints progressing once cartilage loss and altered biomechanics have occurred. Articular cartilage has only a limited ability to 'repair' whereas bone is able to remodel and readily adapt to changing biochemical requirements. With respect to progression or non-progression in osteoarthritis, it may be that bone response and less investigated aspects (e.g. neuromuscular control, capsular fibrosis) will also prove to be important.

Management

There is no proven, effective treatment for the osteoarthritis process. Nevertheless, considerable benefit to the patient can be achieved by often very simple interventions, and surgery for severe 'endstage,' particularly large joint, osteoarthritis is excellent. The principal goals of management are:

(1) education of the patient about osteoarthritis;

(2) pain relief;

(3) achieving and maintaining optimal joint and limb function.

A wide variety of modalities are available to realize these goals (Table 12), and an approach to management is outlined in the management summary (Box 1). As with any branch of medicine, an 'holistic' approach is appropriate and more likely to succeed. The frequent discordance between structural change, symptoms, and function is pertinent; since pain and physical handicap are the main clinical problems arising from osteoarthritis, their causes and treatment usually need consideration as independent issues.

General approach

Successful management centres on careful questioning and examination of the patient. The history should yield clear information particularly about:

(1) symptoms and their impact on the patient's life;

(2) functional disability;

(3) functional requirements and thus the level of handicap;

(4) patient expectations both from osteoarthritis and its treatment;

(5) psychological factors including specific concerns and depression.

Careful examination should determine the:

(1) extent of locomotor abnormality;

(2) origin of current pain, either articular and/or periarticular;

Table 12 Current management of osteoarthritis

Goals of management
　Education
　Relief of symptoms
　Optimization of function
Available modalities
　Counselling
　Educational literature
　Physical therapy
　Occupational therapy
　Drugs
　Complementary medicine
　Coping strategies
　Surgery

Box 1 Management summary

- Education concerning osteoarthritis
- Protect compromised joints from excessive loading, e.g.:
　Reduce obesity
　Modify inappropriate daily/occupational activities
　Use a walking stick
　Shock-absorbing insoles
　Correct leg length discrepancy
- Maintain aerobic fitness, e.g., with swimming and/or walking
- Maintain joint motion and stability
　Regular movement - 'little and often'
　Muscle strengthening exercises
- Reduce pain and stiffness, e.g.:
　Physiotherapy
- Intermittent analgesics
　Consider topical NSAIDs
　Consider occasional courses of NSAIDs
　Consider peri- and intra-articular injection
　Consider TENS and nerve blocks for severe pain
- Reduce impact of pain and disability
　Treat depression, anxiety, fibromyalgia
　Consider coping strategies
　Modify patient environment to reduce handicap
- Consider surgery for:
　Persistent severe pain
　Disability

(3) degree of accompanying synovitis;

(4) presence of instability;

(5) local and general muscle condition;

(6) evidence of accompanying fibromyalgia, neurological, or other relevant medical disease.

An accurate diagnosis can thus be made, the extent of the problems assessed, and any associated factors identified. An individual management programme can then be constructed. The results of such interventions need to be reviewed and the programme modified as the patient's characteristics and requirements change. As symptomatic osteoarthritis is a potentially complex problem, it often requires a co-ordinated approach.

Helping the patient understand osteoarthritis

The myth that osteoarthritis is an inevitable, progressive wear and tear disease of old age persists. This leads to negative attitudes in both patients and doctors and may encourage inappropriate action, for example reduced activity for fear of 'wearing the joints out'. It is important that all those involved in patient management have similar concepts so that conflicting information is avoided. It is also important to address the questions that the patient wants answered, and to respond in a manner understandable to the patient. For example most patients want to know about diet, exercise, and factors in their life that may have brought on their arthritis; explanation of cartilage and bone changes may have little relevance for them. Although the natural history of osteoarthritis is poorly documented, available data suggests that it is often considerably better than patients expect. This is not only true for hand involvement in nodal generalized osteoarthritis but also at the hip and knee. A reasonably optimistic, though not unrealistic, approach is therefore justified.

Addressing mechanical factors

Protecting compromised osteoarthritis joints from excessive or unusual loading often reduces pain. Obesity increases loading on many, not just 'weight-bearing', joints during daily activities, and obese patients are best advised to lose weight. Some prospective data

suggest that such weight loss may prevent the development of osteoarthritis (Felson et al. 1991). Its role in established osteoarthritis, though logical, is unproven. An initially reducing, though well balanced and 'healthy' diet should therefore be encouraged. Appropriate use of a walking stick for hip or knee osteoarthritis will help reduce loading through the affected joint, and shock-absorbing footwear (e.g. 'trainers') may reduce impact; both manoeuvres may benefit symptoms. Altered mechanics due to leg length discrepancy may produce pain which is commonly periarticular and correction with a heel raise should be undertaken.

Occupational therapy advice concerning 'joint protection' and appropriate manoeuvres for activities of daily living may markedly reduce unnecessary overloading of upper and lower limb joints. Modification of both workplace and home activities should be considered if appropriate. Appropriate advice regarding sexual activity may also be helpful, particularly for women with hip osteoarthritis and their partners.

The integrity of articular tissues is maintained, and repair of damaged cartilage facilitated, by normal movement and loading of the joint. Patients should therefore be advised to keep active, within the bounds of common sense. 'Little and often' is prudent advice and particular emphasis should be on aerobic exercise since this has been demonstrated to be of symptomatic benefit in osteoarthritis (Minor et al. 1989; Kovar et al. 1992). Bland and Cooper recommend a comprehensive 'rest–exercise programme' based on the rationale that activity aids repair, whereas rest allows rehydration and recovery of cartilage after loading (Bland and Cooper 1984). It is difficult to obtain direct evidence for this in man, but there are considerable experimental data to support this concept. Data on the efficacy of muscle strengthening regimes in improving osteoarthritis are surprisingly sparse and often poorly controlled. The finding, however that quadriceps weakness is closely associated with disability in knee osteoarthritis (McAlindon *et al.* 1993) has led to renewed impetus to explore this area. In contrast, more evidence exists that aerobic exercise that improves fitness as well as improving self-efficacy may be beneficial in osteoarthritis (Minor *et al.* 1989; Kovar *et al.* 1992). All patients with osteoarthritis should be encouraged to maintain activity.

Direct attempts to relieve symptoms

A variety of physical measures, such as local heat, cold, massage, or hydrotherapy, may give temporary pain relief. Such modalities are usually administered initially by physiotherapists, and there is considerable interpatient variability as to which may help.

Simple analgesics and non-steroidal anti-inflammatory drugs are commonly used with good benefit. They should be regarded as an adjunct, rather than substitute, for other treatments. Comparative studies suggest that non-steroidal anti-inflammatory drugs are just marginally, or even no more effective than analgesics (Bradley *et al.* 1992; Williams *et al.* 1993; March *et al.* 1994). Non-steroidal anti-inflammatory drugs are, however, associated with a significant number of side-effects, particularly in the elderly. Simple analgesics should therefore be tried first, including a trial at maximal regular dosage. If unsuccessful, sequential trials of several non-steroidal anti-inflammatory drugs may be considered. There is currently no convincing evidence that one non-steroidal anti-inflammatory drug is superior to another in the symptomatic relief of osteoarthritis. There are, however, emerging differences in the side-effect profiles of different non-steroidal anti-inflammatory drugs (see Chapter 3.5.1). It would therefore seem prudent to begin with a drug with a lower incidence of gastrointestinal side-effects such as ibuprofen or nabumatone before using alternative agents. Due to marked interpatient variability several non-steroidal anti-inflammatory drugs may have to be tried to find which best suits the individual. The patient should be made aware that the aim of these drugs is to reduce, rather than abolish, pain and that they need only be taken when symptoms are bad. Symptoms in osteoarthritis are often phasic: repeat prescribing is to be avoided, and if a patient is taking an non-steroidal anti-inflammatory drug with apparent benefit they should still regularly experiment by stopping the drug to see whether it is still needed. The possibility that non-steroidal anti-inflammatory drugs may affect the osteoarthritis process remains controversial.

Topically applied non-steroidal anti-inflammatory drugs offer considerable theoretical advantage over oral preparations in terms of reduced side-effects. Although there may be benefit for small superficial joints (e.g. hands) and possibly the knee, deep-seated large joints (particularly hip and glenohumeral joints) are less amenable to this approach. It remains unclear whether such agents are any more effective than simple rubefacients.

If pain is thought to be predominantly periarticular in origin, due to enthesopathy or bursitis, then local injection of corticosteroid, possibly with local anaesthetic to the tender site, may prove helpful. Indeed one study has even suggested that peripatellar injection is as effective as intra-articular injection in knee osteoarthritis (Sambrook *et al.* 1987). Even temporary symptom improvement may permit involvement in other aspects of the management programme (e.g. exercise), and engender a more positive approach by the patient.

In patients with symptoms unresponsive to other measures, local injection with corticosteroid may produce temporary benefit, permitting involvement in physiotherapy and exercise, or allowing the patient to undertake a 'special event', for example a holiday or a family occasion. Anecdotally single injection at some sites, notably the thumb base, may provide surprisingly prolonged relief. Intra-articular injection of steroid, however, is controversial. Although studies in knee osteoarthritis show benefit over saline injection this effect is short-lived, probably lasting less than 6 weeks (Gaffney *et al.* 1995). Furthermore, the possibility of steroid-induced cartilage attrition (derived from animal work) is often cited when the issue of injection frequency is raised. The data from animal models is, however, conflicting. Individual patients, often those too infirm or otherwise unsuitable for alternative approaches, undoubtedly derive considerable benefit from occasional injection.

Patients with chronic pyrophosphate arthropathy and persistent synovitis who respond only temporarily to steroid injection may gain more prolonged control of synovitis and symptoms from intra-articular radiocolloid (Doherty and Dieppe 1981). Whether successful control of synovitis alters long term outcome is unclear.

Intra-articular hyaluronate preparations are now available for use in some countries. Their symptomatic benefit has been demonstrated in some but not all clinical trials. Their role is currently unclear. Not all patients derive benefit and most regimens require weekly injections over a period of 3 to 5 weeks. Although putative 'chondroprotective' effects have been demonstrated *in vitro* this has yet to be demonstrated in man. Whether such agents will become more widely available and used is to our minds unclear. Other intra-articular agents, such as the superoxide dismutase inhibitor orgotein, have also undergone promising clinical trials but as yet they remain experimental therapies.

Joint, principally hip, distension with saline is claimed to offer quite prolonged symptomatic benefit. It is a technique used principally in Europe. The proposed rationale is that capsular stretching, with or without rupture, results in reduced intra-articular hypertension.

For patients with troublesome knee synovitis joint lavage with saline either arthroscopically or via percutaneous irrigation may offer benefit, sometimes for several months. The mechanism of this non-specific treatment is unclear.

Local nerve blocks, particularly suprascapular and obturator blocks for glenohumeral and hip osteoarthritis, are also worthy of consideration. These have less side-effects, and are generally more effective than major, centrally acting analgesics. A word of caution has been raised by retrospective studies that have suggested more rapid deterioration in patients treated in this manner. Since these procedures are usually used in patients unfit for or awaiting replacement arthroplasty this fear may be unwarranted.

Coping with osteoarthritis

The ability to cope with chronic pain and disability varies greatly between individuals, and depends on multiple factors. Depression, often unrecognized, is certainly common in patients with osteoarthritis and is perhaps too often overlooked, preventing appropriate treatment. Fibromyalgia (chronic fatigue syndrome) may also be common, and again needs recognition and incorporation into the management programme. Even in the absence of depression, anxiety, or fibromyalgia, 'coping strategies' may improve the individual's response to pain and disability without altering the nature of the condition itself. Certain aspects of complementary medicine (e.g. herbal and dietary additives, magnets, charms) may fall into this category, as can meditation, yoga, psychotherapy (group or individual), and religion. Many patients turn to such supportive activities themselves, though it is apparent that many doctors, whilst perfectly happy with the concept of 'placebo effect', still underestimate and therefore underuse such strategies.

Surgery (see also Chapter 6.1)

The biggest revolution in osteoarthritis therapy undoubtedly has been the treatment of severe disease by surgery. The three principal surgical interventions for hips and knees are osteotomy, arthroplasty, and arthroscopy.

Osteotomy provides immediate pain relief, possibly by reduction in raised intraosseous pressure, and long-term benefit, presumably by alteration of mechanical forces and correction of joint deformity. These observations demonstrate that pain relief can occur without altering joint damage, and that the osteoarthritis joint surface can repair with fibrocartilage, which can function adequately for everyday use. Osteotomy needs careful planning and precision for success, and is still used at the knee, and by enthusiasts at the hip.

The overt success of hip arthroplasty has encouraged widespread use of this procedure. Surgeons, however, now face the growing challenge of revision and salvage operations for failed arthroplasties, and this is one aspect where osteotomy carries major advantage. Given the unpredictable natural history of large joint osteoarthritis, the frequency of the condition, and cost-benefit ratio in relation to non-operative therapy, the indications and timing of replacement surgery present difficulties. As new medical interventions become available the role of surgery will require continual reappraisal.

Arthroscopy is increasingly used for osteoarthritis. It allows direct inspection of the articular surface enabling the detection and assessment of minor degrees of articular cartilage damage. It also allows visualization and surgical correction of ligamentous and meniscal injury. These are increasingly being recognized as important accompaniments and possibly even initiating factors in osteoarthritis. Finally it is also a means whereby joint lavage and removal of 'loose bodies' can be performed. The precise role of arthroscopy in the management of osteoarthritis still remains to be defined (Casscells 1990).

Can we modify osteoarthritis ?— the concept of 'chondroprotection'

The possibility of therapeutic manipulation of the osteoarthritic process (in favour of repair) has gained momentum in the last decade. Much interest focuses on the already available non-steroidal anti-inflammatory drugs, though hyaluronate, sulphated glycosaminoglycans, and cartilage extracts have also been examined in this respect. At present, convincing human data on such compounds are lacking; nevertheless, this is a growing and potentially exciting field that has relevance beyond the sphere of osteoarthritis.

There is considerable *in vitro* and *in vivo* evidence that different non-steroidals may:

(1) variably influence several aspects of cartilage metabolism;

(2) show either detrimental or protective effects in spontaneous or induced animal models of 'osteoarthritis' (Ghosh 1988).

The mechanisms of such actions remain unexplained but appear largely independent of prostaglandin inhibition. They could well affect either the amount of cytokine produced or the response of chondrocytes to cytokines. Interestingly, susceptibility to influence by non-steroidals appears greater for osteoarthritic than for normal cartilage. This could relate to:

(1) increased drug delivery from the hypervascular synovium and breaching of the calcified zone by subchondral vessels;

(2) enhanced drug penetration due to the increased surface area of fissured cartilage and its altered charge characteristics;

(3) increased susceptibility of stimulated chondrocytes.

Notwithstanding certain problems with such experimental data (Doherty 1989), it is apparent that many non-steroidals have suppressive effects on proteoglycan synthesis and other aspects of cartilage metabolism that may be considered potentially detrimental; conversely, others have little or no suppressive effects at concentrations usually attained in man, and may be beneficial to compromised cartilage. Such observations cannot be directly extrapolated to the clinical situation of human osteoarthritis, and unfortunately there are few studies to date that have directly addressed whether non-steroidals influence (beneficially or detrimentally) the process of osteoarthritis in man.

The possibility that non-steroidal anti-inflammatory drugs are detrimental to osteoarthritis of the hip is supported by two studies reporting greater radiographic destructive change in patients taking indomethacin (Ronningen and Langeland 1979) or regular non-steroidals (Newman and Ling 1985) than in those receiving no indomethacin or infrequent non-steroidals. Both studies, however, can be criticized in terms of retrospective design, small numbers, radiographic assessment, and lack of control for factors that may influence progression. Different conclusions were reached in a prospective study of both osteoarthritic and rheumatoid hips, which implicated obesity, but not non-steroidals in the rate of loss of femoral head height (Watson 1976). A more recent prospective study of patients with osteoarthritis of the hip (Rashad *et al.* 1989) found more rapid radiographic progression and a shorter interval before surgery in patients taking indomethacin compared to those taking azapropazone. However, this study is again readily criticized, for example, in terms of radiographic assessment, lack of control for risk factors for progression, questionable criteria for surgical intervention, and lack of blinding in respect to treatments. It is known that several different non-steroidal anti-inflammatory drugs exert profound inhibition of heterotopic new bone formation after hip arthroplasty — an effect that would not be expected to be beneficial to the remodelling of osteoarthritic joints (Doherty 1990).

Some recent progress has been made with the design of low molecular weight inhibitors of the matrix metalloproteinases that have been shown to be effective *in vitro* and in animal models *in vivo* at preventing cartilage breakdown (Cawston 1995). Such compounds are under development and need to be tested in man to determine if cartilage and bone can be protected from degradative enzymes (Vincenti 1994). These trials are likely to be lengthy and costly as the destruction of tissue is relatively slow but such compounds could protect osteoarthritic cartilage.

The problem remains that, because of the heterogeneity of osteoarthritis, the chronicity of the condition, the discordance between anatomical, functional, and symptomatic manifestations, and unresolved difficulties of assessment, studies seeking to demonstrate even marked differences between drugs prove impracticable to organize. An alternative strategy may be to follow two treatment cohorts of patients with unilateral osteoarthritis of the knee (at high risk of developing this condition on the other side) and observe whether one cohort demonstrates less recruitment of osteoarthritis at new sites than the other.

Though cartilage may be the best understood component and the usual focus of interest, it should be remembered that other joint tissues (bone, capsule, synovium, muscle) may also influence the outcome of osteoarthritis. The term 'chondroprotection' is thus misleading; therapeutic modifications (good or bad) of all joint tissues requires consideration.

Prognosis

For such a common disease, the prognosis of osteoarthritis is largely unknown. From the data that is available one can be relatively optimistic about outcome for most patients. Attempts have been made to define the outcome for different subsets of osteoarthritis. By and large this has been difficult to do. The data will now be discussed by joint site and by osteoarthritis subset.

Knee

There is some data available regarding prognosis for knee osteoarthritis. The natural history of knee osteoarthritis may be less favourable than that for hips. Hernborg and Nilsson observed clinical and radiographic deterioration in the majority of cases followed for 10 to 18 years, with varus deformity, earlier age of onset, and being female relating to worse prognosis (Hernborg and Nilsson 1977). Isolated osteophytosis alone was shown not to associate with subsequent development of osteoarthritis change. In a long-term (12-year) study investigating cartilage loss in the general population (Schouten et al. 1992) obesity, presence of generalized osteoarthritis, age and varus/valgus knee deformity were all associated with progressive loss of cartilage. In a study of hospital-referred patients, only the presence of inflammation and calcium pyrophosphate deposition was associated with progression (Ledingham et al. 1995). In addition to increased morbidity, knee osteoarthritis is associated with increased mortality (Danielsson and Hernborg 1970; Lawrence et al. 1990).

Hip

The general view of inevitable progression in the majority of hip osteoarthritis patients may be unwarranted. In a 10-year follow-up study, Danielsson found deterioration in symptoms in only 17 per cent of hip osteoarthritis subjects, symptoms improving over this period in 59 per cent, and completely resolving in 12 per cent; radiographic changes similarly showed progression in only a minority of cases, principally those with initial superolateral migration (Danielsson 1964). Furthermore patients with apparently progressive osteoarthritis who then improve with spontaneous 'healing' on radiographs (remodelling and partial restoration of joint space) are well described (Perry et al. 1972). Possible risk factors for progression (rather than development) include: superior pole pattern (Danielsson 1964); obesity (Watson 1976); presence of chondrocalcinosis at other sites (Menkes et al. 1985); and possibly non-steroidal anti-inflammatory drug usage (Ronningen and Langeland 1979; Newman and Ling 1985; Rashad et al. 1989). Evidence for the latter, however, is far from convincing (Doherty 1989).

Hand

The prognosis for hand osteoarthritis is generally good. Symptoms and hand function of nodal generalized osteoarthritis patients examined two or more decades after onset is no worse than that of similarly aged subjects with no hand osteoarthritis (Pattrick et al. 1989b). In contrast, in erosive osteoarthritis, in which bony ankylosis and instability is more common, long-term functional outcome may be worse (Pattrick et al. 1989b).

Functional outcome for thumb base involvement, carpometacarpophalangeal joint, and scaphotrapezoid disease is less clear-cut but again may be relatively poor.

Spine

Prognosis for osteoarthritis of the spine is unclear. This is largely because of the difficulty of correlating symptoms with structural change. In cases of either cord or nerve root compression prognosis is unclear, with deterioration often being slow.

Chronic pyrophosphate arthropathy

The natural history of chronic pyrophosphate arthropathy is poorly documented. Despite often severe symptoms and structural change at presentation, one 5-year, hospital-based, prospective study (Doherty and Dieppe 1988) suggests that most patients run a benign course, particularly with respect to small and medium-sized joint involvement. As expected symptomatic deterioration occurred mainly in large lower limb joints, but even in severely affected knees (the usual presenting site), two-thirds of patients showed stabilization or improvement of symptoms. The commonest radiographic change is an increase in osteophyte with bone remodelling, rather than progressive cartilage and bone attrition. Nevertheless, severe, progressive 'destructive pyrophosphate arthropathy' may occasionally occur, particularly at the knee, shoulder, and hip. This is virtually confined to elderly women or in association with haemochromatosis and may cause problematic recurrent haemarthrosis and a radiographic appearance of marked destruction resembling a Charcot or neuropathic joint.

Apatite associated destructive arthropathy

The prognosis of this form is seemingly poor with the majority having marked joint destruction requiring joint replacement.

References

Acheson, R.M. and Collart, A.B. (1975). New Haven Survey of joint diseases. XVII. Relationships between some systemic characteristics and osteoarthrosis in a general population. *Annals of the Rheumatic Diseases*, **34**, 379–87.

Aisen, A.M., McCune, W.J., MacGuire, A., Carson, P.L., Silver, T.M., Jafri, S.Z., and Martel, W. (1984). Sonographic evaluation of the cartilage of the knee. *Radiology*, 153, 781–4.

Altman, R.D. (1991). Criteria for classification of clinical osteoarthritis. *Journal of Rheumatology*, 18 (suppl. 27), 10–12.

Altman, R., Asch, E., Block, D., *et al.* (1986). Development of criteria for the classification and reporting of osteoarthritis: classification of osteoarthritis of the knee. *Arthritis and Rheumatism*, 29, 1039–49.

Altman, R., Alarcn, G., Appelrouth, D., *et al.* (1990). The American College of Rheumatology criteria for the classification and reporting of osteoarthritis of the hand. *Arthritis and Rheumatism*, 33, 1601–10.

Altman, R., Alarcn, G., Appelrouth, D., *et al.* (1991). The American College of Rheumatology criteria for the classification and reporting of osteoarthritis of the hip. *Arthritis and Rheumatism*, 34, 505–14.

Andrews, H.J., Plumpton, T.A., Harper, G.P., and Cawston, T.E. (1992). A synthetic peptide metalloproteinase inhibitor, but not TIMP, prevents the breakdown of proteoglycan within articular cartilage *in vitro*. *Agents and Actions*, 37, 147–54.

Badley, E.M., Rasooly, I., and Webster, G.K. (1994). Relative importance of musculoskeletal disorders as a cause of chronic health problems, disability, and health care utilisation: findings from the 1990 Ontario Health Survey. *Journal of Rheumatology*, 21, 505–14.

Bagge, E., Bjelle, A., and Svanborg, A. (1992). Radiographic osteoarthritis in the elderly. A cohort comparison and a longitudinal study of the '70-year old people in Göteborg'. *Clinical Rheumatology*, 11, 486–91.

Bland, J.H. and Cooper, S.M. (1984). Osteoarthritis: a review of the cell biology involved and evidence for reversibility. Management rationally related to known genesis and pathophysiology. *Seminars in Arthritis and Rheumatism*, 14, 106–33.

Bonassar, L.J, Frank, E.H., Murray, J.C., Paguio, C.G., Moore, V.L., Lark, M.W., Sandy, J.D., Wu, J.-J., Eyre, D.R., and Grodzinsky, A.J. (1995). Changes in cartilage composition and physical properties due to stromelysin degradation. *Arthritis and Rheumatism*, 38, 173–83.

Bradley, J.D., Brandt, K.D., Katz, B.P., Kalasinski, L.A., and Ryan, S.I. (1992). Comparison of an anti-inflammatory dose of ibuprofen, an analgesic dose of ibuprofen, and acetaminophen in the treatment of patients with osteoarthritis of the knee. *New England Journal of Medicine*, 325, 87–91.

Brandt, K.D. (1988). Osteoarthritis. *Clinical Geriatric Medicine*, 4, 279–93.

Brinkerhoff, C.E. (1991). Joint destruction in arthritis: metalloproteinases in the spotlight. *Arthritis and Rheumatism*, 34, 1073–5.

Brocklehurst, R., Bayliss, M.T., Maroudas, A., Coysh, H.L., Freeman, M.A.R., Revell, P.A., and Ali, S.Y. (1984). The composition of normal and osteoarthritic articular cartilage from human knee joints. *Journal of Bone and Joint Surgery (America)*, 66A, 95–106.

Buckland-Wright, J.C., MacFarlane, D.G., Lynch, J.A., and Clark, B. (1990). Quantitative microfocal radiographic assessment of progression in osteoarthritis of the hand. *Arthritis and Rheumatism*, 33, 57–65.

Burnett, S., Hart, D.J., Cooper, C., and Spector, T.D. (1994). *A radiographic atlas of osteoarthritis*. Springer-Verlag, London

Buttle, D.J., Handley, C.J., Ilic, M.Z., Saklatvala, J., Murata, M., and Barrett, A.J. (1993). Inhibition of cartilage proteoglycan release by a specific inactivator of cathepsin B and an inhibitor of matrix metalloproteinases; evidence for two converging pathways of chondrocyte-mediated proteoglycan degradation. *Arthritis and Rheumatism*, 36, 1709–17.

Casscells, S.W. (1990). What, if any, are the indications for arthroscopic debridement of the osteoarthritic knee. *Arthroscopy*, 6, 169–70.

Caterson, B., Mahmoodian, F., Sorrell, J.M., *et al.* (1990). Modulation of native chondroitin sulphate structure in tissue development and disease. *Journal of Cell Science*, 97, 411–17.

Cawston, T.E. (1995). Proteinases and connective tissue breakdown. In *Mechanisms and models in rheumatoid arthritis* (ed. Henderson, Edwards, and Pettipher), pp. 333–59. Academic Press.

Cawston, T.E., Mercer, E., De Silva, M., and Hazleman, B.L. (1983). Metalloproteinases and collagenase inhibitors in rheumatoid synovial fluid. *Arthritis and Rheumatism*, 27, 641–6.

Cawston, T.E., Plumpton, T.A., Curry, V.A., Ellis, A., and Powell, L. (1994). The role of TIMP and MMP inhibition in preventing connective tissue breakdown. *Annals of the New York Academy of Science*, 732, 75–83.

Claessens, A., Schouten, J., van den Ouweland, F., and Valkenburg, H. (1990). Do clinical findings associate with radiographic osteoarthritis of the knee? *Annals of the Rheumatic Diseases*, 49, 771–4.

Clark, I.M., Powell, L.K., Ramsey, S., Hazleman, B.L., and Cawston, T.E. (1993). The measurement of collagenase, TIMP and collagenase-TIMP complex in synovial fluids from patients with osteoarthritis and rheumatoid arthritis. *Arthritis and Rheumatism*, 36, 372–9.

Cobby, M., Cushnaghan, J., Creamer, P., Dieppe, P., and Watt, I. (1990). Erosive osteoarthritis: is it a separate disease entity? *Clinical Radiology*, 42, 258–63.

Cooke, T.D.V. (1985). Pathogenic mechanisms in polyarticular osteoarthritis. In *Clinics in rheumatic diseases* (ed. L Sokoloff), Vol. 11 (2), pp. 203–38. WB Saunders, London.

Cooper, C. (1995). Occupational activity and the risk of the osteoarthritis. *Journal of Rheumatology*, 22 (suppl. 43), 10–12.

Croft, P., Cooper, C., Wickham, C., and Coggon, D. (1991). Osteoarthritis of the hip and acetabular dysplasia. *Annals of the Rheumatic Diseases*, 50, 308–10.

Cushnaghan, J. and Dieppe, P. (1991). Study of 500 patients with limb joint osteoarthritis. I. Analysis by age, sex, and distribution of symptomatic joint sites. *Annals of the Rheumatic Diseases*, 50, 8–13.

Danielsson, L.G. (1964). Incidence and prognosis of coxarthrosis. *Acta Orthopaedica Scandinavica*, 66 (suppl.), 1–114.

Danielsson, L.G. and Hernborg, J. (1970). Morbidity and mortality of osteoarthritis of the knee (gonarthrosis) in Malmo, Sweden. *Clinical Orthopaedics and Related Research*, 69, 224–6.

Davis, M.A., Ettinger, W.H., Neuhaus, J.M., Barclay, J.D., and Segal, M.R. (1992). Correlates of knee pain amongst US adults with and without radiographic knee osteoarthritis. *Journal of Rheumatology*, 19, 1943–9.

Dean, D.D., Martel-Pelletier, J., Pelletier, J.P., Howell, D.S., and Woessner, J.F. (1989). Evidence for metalloproteinase and metalloproteinase inhibitor imbalance in human osteoarthritic cartilage. *Journal of Clinical Investigation*, 84, 678–85.

Dieppe, P.A., Campion, G., and Doherty, M. (1988). Mixed crystal deposition. *Rheumatology Disease Clinics of North America*, 14, 415–26.

Dieppe, P., Cushnaghan, J., Young, P., and Kirwan, J. (1993). Prediction of the progression of joint space narrowing in osteoarthritis of the knee by bone scintigraphy. *Annals of the Rheumatic Diseases*, 52, 557–63.

Dodge, G.R. and Poole, A.R. (1989). Immunohistochemical detection and immunochemical analysis of type II collagen degradation in human normal, rheumatoid and osteoarthritic articular cartilages and in explants of bovine articular cartilage cultured with interleukin 1. *Journal of Clinical Investigation*, 83, 647–61.

Doherty, M. (1989). Chondroprotection by NSAIDs. *Annals of the Rheumatic Diseases*, 48, 619–21.

Doherty, M. (ed.). (1994). *Color atlas and text of osteoarthritis*. Wolfe, London.

Doherty, M. and Dieppe, P.A. (1981). Effect of intra-articular yttrium-90 on chronic pyrophosphate arthropathy of the knee. *Lancet*, 2, 1243–6.

Doherty, M. and Dieppe P.A. (1988). Clinical aspects of calcium pyrophosphate dihydrate crystal deposition. *Rheumatology Disease Clinics of North America*, 14, 395–414.

Doherty, M., Watt, I., and Dieppe, P. (1983). Influence of primary generalised osteoarthritis on development of secondary osteoarthritis. *Lancet*, ii, 8–11.

Doherty, M., Pattrick, M., and Powell, RJ. (1990). Hypothesis — nodal generalised osteoarthritis is an auto-immune disease. *Annals of the Rheumatic Diseases*, 49, 1017–20.

Doherty, M., Hamilton, E., Henderson, J., Misra, H., and Dixey, J. (1991*a*). Familial chondrocalcinosis due to calcium pyrophosphate dihydrate crystal deposition in English families. *British Journal of Rheumatology*, 30, 10–15.

Doherty, M., Chuck, A., Hosking, D., and Hamilton, E. (1991*b*). Inorganic pyrophosphate in metabolic diseases predisposing to calcium oyrophosphate dihydrate crystal deposition. *Arthritis and Rheumatism*, 34, 1297–303.

Ehlich, G.E. (1972). Inflammatory osteoarthritis: I. The clinical syndrome. *Journal of Chronic Diseases*, 25, 317–28.

Ehlich, G.E. (1975). Osteoarthritis beginning with inflammation definitions and correlations. *Journal of the American Medical Association*, 232, 157–9.

Ellis, A.J., Curry, V.A., Powell, E.K., and Cawston, T.E. (1994). The prevention of collagen breakdown in bovine nasal cartilage by TIMP, TIMP-2 and a low molecular weight synthetic inhibitor. *Biochemical Biophysical Research Communications*, **201**, 94–101.

Felson, D.T. (1988). Epidemiology of hip and knee osteoarthritis. *Epidemiologic Reviews*, **10**, 1–28.

Felson, D.T., Anderson, J.J., Naimark, A., Kannel, W., Meenan, R.F. (1989). The prevalence of chondrocalcinosis in the elderly and its association with knee osteoarthritis: the Framingham study. *Journal of Rheumatology*, **16**, 1241–5.

Felson, D.T., Hannan, M.T., Naimark, A., Berkely, J., Gordon, G., Wilson, P.W.F., and Anderson, J. (1991). Occupational physical demands, knee bending, and knee osteoarthritis: results from the Framingham study. *Journal of Rheumatology*, **18**, 1587–92.

Felson, D.T., Ahange, Y., Anthony, J.M., Naimark, A., and Anderson, J.J. (1992). Weight loss reduces the risk for symptomatic knee osteoarthritis in women. *Annals of Internal Medicine*, **116**, 535–9.

Gaffney, K., Ledingham, J., and Perry, J.D. (1995). Intra-articular triamcinolone hexacetonide in knee osteoarthritis: factors influencing the clinical response. *Annals of the Rheumatic Diseases*, **54**, 379–81.

Ghosh, P. (1988). Anti-rheumatic drugs and cartilage. *Clinical Rheumatology*, **2**, 309–38.

Goldring, M.B. (1993). Degradation of articular cartilage in culture: regulatory factors In *Joint cartilage degradation* (ed. J.F. Woessner and D.S. Howell). Marcel Dekker, New York.

Goldthwaite, J.E. (1904). The differential diagnosis and treatment of so-called rheumatoid diseases. *Boston Medical Surgery Journal*, **151**, 529–34.

Hadler, N.M. (1992). Knee pain is the malady — not osteoarthritis. *Annals of Internal Medicine*, **116**, 598–9.

Hadler, N.M., Gillings, D.B., Imbus, H.R., Levitin, P.M., Makuc, D., Utsinger, P.D., Yount, W.J., Slusser, D., and Moskovitz, N. (1977). Hand structure and function in an industrial setting. Influence of three patterns of stereotyped, repetative usage. *Arthritis and Rheumatism*, **20**, 1019–25.

Halverson, P.B. and McCarty, D.J. (1988). Clinical aspects of basic calcium phosphate crystal deposition. *Rheumatology Disease Clinics of North America*, **14**, 427–39.

Hammerman, D. (1989). The biology of osteoarthritis. *New England Journal of Medicine*, **320**, 1322–30.

Hardingham, T. and Bayliss, M. (1990). Proteoglycans of articular cartilage: changes in ageing and in joint disease. *Seminars in Arthritis and Rheumatism*, **20** (suppl. 1), 12–33.

Hart, D.J., Spector, T.D., Brown, P., Wilson, P., Doyle, D.V., and Silman, A.J. (1991). Clinical signs of early osteoarthritis: reproducibility and relation to x-ray changes in 541 women in the general population. *Annals of the Rheumatic Diseases*, **50**, 467–70.

Hernborg, J.S. and Nilsson, B.E. (1977). The natural course of untreated osteoarthritis of the knee. *Clinical Orthopaedics and Related Research*, **123**, 130–7.

Hollander, A.P., Heathfield, T.F., Webber, C., Iwata, Y., Bourne, R., Rorabeck, C., and Poole, A.R. (1994). Increased damage to type II collagen in osteoarthritic articular cartilage detected by a new immunoassay. *Journal of Clinical Investigation*, **93**, 1722–32.

Hopkinson, N., Powell, R.J., and Doherty, M. (1992). Auto-antibodies, immunoglobulins and Gm allotypes in nodal generalised osteoarthritis. *British Journal of Rheumatology*, **31**, 605–8.

Hutton, C. (1987). Generalised osteoarthritis: an evolutionary problem. *Lancet*, **i**,1463–5.

Hutton, C.W., Higgs, E.R., Jackson, P.C., Watt, I., Dieppe, P.A. (1986). TcHMDP bone scanning in generalised nodal osteoarthritis. II. The four hour bone scan image predicts radiographic change. *Annals of the Rheumatic Diseases*, **45**, 622–6.

Jones, A.C. and Doherty, M. (1992).The treatment of osteoarthritis. *British Journal of Clinical Pharmacology*.

Jones, A.C., Chuck, A.J., Arie, E.A., Green, D.J., and Doherty, M. (1992). Diseases associated with calcium pyrophosphate deposition disease. *Seminars in Arthritis and Rheumatism*, **22**, 188–202.

Jones, A.C., Ledingham, J., McAlindon, T., Regam, M., Hart, D., MacMillan, P.J., and Doherty, M. (1993). Radiographic assessment of patellofemoral osteoarthritis. *Annals of the Rheumatic Diseases*, **52**, 655–8.

Kallman, D.A., Wigley, F.M., Scott, W.W., Hochberg, M.C., and Tobin, J.D. (1989). New radiographic grading scales for osteoarthritis of the hand. *Arthritis and Rheumatism*, **32**, 1584–91.

Kellgren, J.H. and Lawrence, J.S. (1957). Radiological assessment of osteoarthritis. *Annals of the Rheumatic Diseases*, **16**, 494–502.

Kellgren, J.H. and Moore, R. (1952). Generalised osteoarthritis and Heberden's nodes. *British Medical Journal*, **1**, 181–7.

Knowlton, R.G., Katzenstein, P.L., Moskowitz, R.W., Weaver, E.J., Malemud, C., Pathria, M., Jimenez, S., and Prockop, D.J. (1990). Demonstration of genetic linkage of a polymorphism in the type II procollagen gene (Col2A1) to primary osteoarthritis associated with mild chondrodysplasia. *New England Journal of Medicine*, **322**, 526–30.

Kovar, P.A., Allegrante, J.P., MacKenzie, C.R., Peterson, M.G.E., Gutin, B., and Charlson, M.E. (1992). Supervised fitness walking in patients with osteoarthritis of the knee. *Annals of Internal Medicine*, **116**, 529–34.

Lane, N.E. and Nevitt, M.C. (1994). Osteoarthritis and bone mass. *Journal of Rheumatology*, **21**, 1393–6.

Lawrence, J.S., Bremner, J.M., and Beir, F. (1966). Osteoarthrosis. Prevalence in the population and relationship between symptoms and x-ray changes. *Annals of the Rheumatic Diseases*, **25**, 1–24.

Lawrence, R.C., Everett, D., Hochberg, M.C. (1990). Arthritis. In *Health status and well-being of the elderly: national health and nutrition examination-I Epidemiologic followup survey* (ed. R. Huntley and J. Cornoni-Huntley), pp. 136–51. Oxford University Press, New York.

Ledingham, J., Dawson, S., Preston, B., Milligan, G., and Doherty, M. (1992). Radiographic patterns and associations of osteoarthritis of the hip. *Annals of the Rheumatic Diseases*, **51**, 1111–6.

Ledingham, J., Dawson, S., Preston, B., Milligan, G., and Doherty, M. (1993). Radiographic progression of hospital referred osteoarthritis of the hip. *Annals of the Rheumatic Diseases*, **52**, 263–7.

Ledingham, J., Regam, M., Jones, A., and Doherty, M. (1995). Factors affecting radiographic progression of knee osteoarthritis. *Annals of the Rheumatic Diseases*, **54**, 53–8.

Lipiello, L., Hall, D., and Mankin, H.J. (1977). Collagen synthesis in normal and osteoarthritic human cartilage. *Journal of Clinical Investigation*, **59**, 593–600.

Lohmander, L.S., (1994). Articular cartilage and osteoarthritis. The role of molecular markers to monitor breakdown, repair and disease. *Journal of Anatomy*, **184**, 477–92.

Lohmander, L.S., Dahlberg, L., Ryd, L., and Heinegard, D. (1989). Increased levels of proteoglycan fragments in knee joint fluid after injury. *Arthritis and Rheumatism*, **32**, 1434–42.

Lohmander, L.S., Hoerrner, L.A., and Lark, M.W. (1993). Metalloproteinases, tissue inhibitor and proteoglycan fragments in knee synovial fluid in human osteoarthritis. *Arthritis and Rheumatism*, **36**, 181–9.

Lohmander, L.S., Roos, H., Dahlberg, L., Hoerrner, L.A., and Lark, M.W. (1994). Temporal patterns of stromelysin-1, tissue inhibitor, and proteoglycan fragments in human knee joint fluid after injury to the cruciate ligament or meniscus. *Journal of Orthopaedic Research*, **12**, 21–8.

Mankin, H.J. (1974). The reaction of cartilage to injury and osteoarthritis. Parts I and II. *New England Journal of Medicine*, **291**, 1285–92; 1335–40.

March, L., Irwig, L., Schwarz, J., Simpson, J., Choch, C., and Brooks, P. (1994). N of 1 trials comparing a non-steroidal anti-inflammatory drug with paracetamol in osteoarthritis. *British Medical Journal*, **309**, 1041–6.

Marks, J.S., Stewart, I.M., and Hardinge, K. (1979). Primary osteoarthrosis of the hip and Heberden's nodes. *Annals of the Rheumatic Diseases*, **38**, 107–11.

Maroudas, A. and Urban, J.P.G. (1980). Metabolism of cartilage. In: *Studies in joint disease* (ed. A. Maroudas and E.J. Holborow), pp. 87–116, Vol 1. Pitman Medical, London.

Maroudas, A., Katz, E.P., Wachtel, E.J., *et al.* (1986). Physiochemical properties and functional behaviour of normal and osteoarthritic human cartilage. In *Articular cartilage biochemistry* (ed. K.E. Kuettner, R. Schleyerbach, and V. Hascall), pp. 311–30. Raven Press, New York.

McAlindon, T.E., Snow, S., Cooper, C., and Dieppe, P.A. (1992). Radiographic patterns of osteoarthritis of the knee joint in the community: the importance of the patellofemoral joint. *Annals of the Rheumatic Diseases*, **51**, 844–9.

McAlindon, T.E., Cooper, C., Kirwan, J.R., and Dieppe, P.A. (1993). Determinants of disability in osteoarthritis of the knee. *Annals of the Rheumatic Diseases*, 52, 258–62.

McCarty, D.J. (1976). Calcium pyrophosphate dihydrate crystal deposition disease 1975. *Arthritis and Rheumatism*, 19 (suppl.), 275–86.

Menkes, C.-J., Decraemere, W., Postel, M., and Forest, M. (1985). Chondrocalcinosis and rapid destruction of the hip. *Journal of Rheumatology*, 12, 130–3.

Messiah, S.S., Fowler, P.J., and Munro, T. (1990). Anteroposterior radiographs of the osteoarthritic knee. *Journal of Bone and Joint Surgery (British)*, 72-B, 639–40.

Mikkelsen, W.M., Duff, I.F., and Dodge, H.J. (1970). Age, sex specific prevalence of radiographic abnormalities of the joints of the hands, wrists, and cervical spine of adult residents of the Tecumseh, Michigan community health study area, 1962–1965. *Journal of Chronic Diseases*, 23, 151–9.

Minor, M.A., Hewett, J.E., Webel, R.R., Anderson, S.K., and Kay, D.R. (1989). Efficacy of physical conditioning exercise in patients with rheumatoid arthritis and osteoarthritis. *Arthritis and Rheumatism*, 32, 1396–405.

Murphy, G., Docherty, A.J.P., Hembry, R.M., and Reynolds, J.J. (1991). Metalloproteinases and tissue damage. *British Journal of Rheumatology*, 30, 25–31.

Newman, N.M. and Ling, R.S.M. (1985). Acetabular bone destruction related to non-steroidal anti-inflammatory drugs. *Lancet*, ii, 11–14.

Ohira, T. and Ishikawa, K. (1987). Hydroxyapatite deposition in osteoarthritic articular cartilage of the proximal femoral head. *Arthritis and Rheumatism*, 30, 651–60.

Pattrick, M., Manhire, A., Milford-Ward, A., and Doherty, M. (1989*a*). HLA AB antigens and alpha-1-antitrypsin phenotypes in nodal generalised osteoarthritis and erosive osteoarthritis. *Annals of the Rheumatic Diseases*, 48, 470–5.

Pattrick, M., Aldridge, S., Hamilton, E., Manhire, A., and Doherty, M. (1989*b*). A controlled study of hand function in nodal and erosive osteoarthritis. *Annals of the Rheumatic Diseases*, 48, 978–82.

Pattrick, M., Hamilton, E., Wilson, R., Austin, S., and Doherty, M (1993). Association of radiographic changes of osteoarthritis, symptoms and synovial fluid particles in 300 knees. *Annals of the Rheumatic Diseases*, 52, 97–103.

Perry, G.H., Smith, M.J.G., and Whiteside, C.G. (1972). Spontaneous recovery of the joint space in degenerative hip disease. *Annals of the Rheumatic Diseases*, 31, 440–8.

Peyron, J.G. (1979). Epidemiologic and aetiologic approach to osteoarthritis. *Seminars in Arthritis and Rheumatism*, 8, 288–306.

Poole, R.A. (1993). Immunochemical markers of joint inflammation, skeletal and repair where are we now? *Annals of the Rheumatic Diseases*, 53, 305.

Rashad, S., Revell, P., Hemingway, A., Low, F., Rainsford, K., and Walker, F. (1989). Effect of non-steroidal anti-inflammatory drugs on the course of osteoarthritis. *Lancet*, ii, 519–22.

Ratcliffe, A., Doherty, M., Maini, R.N., and Hardingham, T.E. (1988). Increased levels of proteoglycan components in the synovial fluids of patients with acute but not chronic joint disease. *Annals of the Rheumatic Diseases*, 47, 826–32.

Revell, P.A., Mayston, V., Lalor, P., and Mapp, P. (1988). The synovial membrane in osteoarthritis: a histological study including the characterisation of the cellular infiltrate present in inflammatory osteoarthritis using monoclonal antibodies. *Annals of the Rheumatic Diseases*, 47, 300–7.

Risteli, J., Glorian, I., Nierin, S., Naramo, A., and Risteli, L. (1993). Radioimmunoassay for the pyridinoline cross-linked C terminal telopeptide of type 1 collagen. A new serum marker of bone collagen degradation. *Clinical Chemistry*, 39, 635–40.

Robins, S.P., Woitge, H., Hesley, R., Ju, J., Seyedin, S., and Seibel, M.J. (1994). Direct, enzyme-linked immunoassay for urinary deoxypyridinoline as a specific marker for measuring bone resorption. *Journal of Bone and Mineral Research*, 9, 1643–9.

Rogers, J., Watt, I., and Dieppe, P. (1990). Comparison of visual and radiographic detection of bony changes at the knee joint. *British Medical Journal*, 300, 367–8.

Roh, Y.S., Dequecker, J., and Mulier, J.C. (1973). Osteoarthrosis at the hand skeleton in primary osteoarthrosis of the hip and in normal controls. *Clinical Orthopedics*, 90, 90–4.

Ronningen, H. and Langeland, N. (1979). Indomethacin treatment in osteoarthritis of the hip joint. Does the treatment interfere with the natural course of the disease? *Acta Orthopaedica Scandinavica*, 50, 169–74.

Ryu, J., Treadwell, B.V., and Mankin, H.J. (1984). Biochemical and metabolic abnormalities in normal and osteoarthritic human articular cartilage. *Arthritis and Rheumatism*, 27, 49–56.

Sambrook, P.N., Champion, G.D., Browne, C.D., Cairns, D., Cohen, M.L., Day, R.O., *et al.* (1987). Corticosteroid injection for osteoarthritis of the knee: peripatellar compared to intra-articular route. *Clinical and Experimental Rheumatology*, 7, 609–13.

Sandy, J.D., Flannery, C.R., Neame, P.J., and Lohmander, L.S. (1992). The structure of aggrecan fragments in human synovial fluid: Evidence for the involvment in osteoarthritis of a novel proteinase. *Journal of Clinical Investigation*, 89, 1512–6.

Saxne, T., Heinegard, D., Wollheim, F.A., *et al.* (1985). Difference in cartilage proteoglycan level in synovial fluid in early rheumatoid arthritis and reactive arthritis. *Lancet*, ii, 127–8.

Saxne, T., Heinegard, D., and Wollheim, F.A. (1986). Therapeutic effects on cartilage metabolism in arthritis as measured by release of proteoglycan structures into the synovial fluid. *Annals of the Rheumatic Diseases*, 45, 491–7.

Schouten, J.S.A.G., van den Ouweland, F.A., and Valkenburg, H.A. (1992). A 12 year follow up study in the general population on prognostic factors of cartilage loss in osteoarthritis of the knee. *Annals of the Rheumatic Diseases*, 51, 932–7.

Seibel, M.J., Duncan, A., and Robins, S.P. (1989). Urinary hydroxy-pyridinium crosslinks of collagen reflect cartilage and bone involvement in rheumatic joint diseases. *Journal of Rheumatology*, 16, 964–70.

Shinmei, M., Inamori, Y., Yoshihara, Y., Kikuchi, T., and Hayakawa, T. (1992). The potential of cartilage markers in joint fluid for drug evaluation. In *Articular cartilage and osteoarthritis* (ed. K. Kuettner *et al.*). Raven Press, New York.

Sokoloff, L. (1985). Endemic forms of osteoarthritis. *Clinics in the Rheumatic Diseases*, 11, 187–202.

Sokoloff, L. (1994). In *Color atlas and text of osteoarthritis* (ed. M. Doherty). Wolfe, London.

Solomon, L. (1976). Patterns of osteoarthritis of the hip. *Journal of Bone and Joint Surgery (British)*, 58-B, 176–83.

Solomon, L. (1983). Osteoarthritis, local and generalised: a uniform disease? *Journal of Rheumatology*, 10 (suppl. 9), 13–15.

Spector, T.D. (1995). Measuring joint space in knee osteoarthritis: position or precision? *Journal of Rheumatology*, 22, 807–8.

Spector, T.D. and Campion, G.D. (1989). Generalised osteoarthritis: a hormonally mediated disease. *Annals of the Rheumatic Diseases*, 48, 523–7.

Spector, T.D. and Cooper, C. (1993). Radiographic assessment of osteoarthritis in the general population: whither Kellgren and Lawrence? *Osteoarthritis and Cartilage*, 1, 203–6.

Spector, T.D., Hart, D.J., Byrne, J., Harris, P.A., Dacre, J.E., and Doyle, D.V. (1993). Definition of osteoarthritis of the knee for epidemiological studies. *Annals of the Rheumatic Diseases*, 52, 790–4.

Stecher, R.M. (1953). Heberdens nodes. A clinical description of osteoarthritis of the finger joints. *Annals of the Rheumatic Diseases*, 14, 1–10.

Steven, M.M. (1992). Prevalence of chronic arthritis in four geographical areas of the Scottish Highlands. *Annals of the Rheumatic Diseases*, 51, 186–96.

Swan, A., Chapman, B., Heap, P., Seward, H., and Dieppe, P. (1994). Submicroscopic crystals in osteoarthritic synovial fluids. *Annals of the Rheumatic Diseases*, 53, 467–70.

Sweet, M.B.E., Coelho, A., Schnitzler, C.M., Schnitzer, T.J., Lenz, M.E., Jakin, I., Kuettner, K.E., and Thonar, E.J.M.A. (1988). Serum keratan sulphate levels in osteoarthritis patients. *Arthritis and Rheumatism*, 31, 648–52.

Thonar, E.J.-M.A., Schitzner, T., and Kuettner, K.E. (1987). Quantification of keratan sulphate in blood as a marker of cartilage catabolism. *Journal of Rheumatology*, 14 (suppl. 14), 23–4.

van Saase, J.L.C.M., Van Romunde, L.K.J., Cats, A., Vandenbrouke, J.P., and Valkenburg, H.A. (1989). Epidemiology of osteoarthritis: Zoetermeer survey. Comparison of radiological osteoarthritis in a Dutch population with that in 10 other populations. *Annals of the Rheumatic Diseases*, 48, 271–80.

Vincenti, M.P., Clark, I.M., and Brinkerhoff, C.E. (1994). Using inhibitors of metalloproteinases to treat arthritis. Easier said than done? *Arthritis and Rheumatism*, **37**, 1115–26.

Watson, M. (1976). Femoral head height loss: a study of the relative significance of some of its determinants in hip degeneration. *Rheumatology Rehabilitation*, **15**, 264–9.

Westacott, C.I., Whicher, J.T., Barnes, I.C., Thompson, D., Swan, A.J., and Dieppe, P.A. (1990). Synovial fluid concentrations of five cytokines in rheumatic diseases. *Annals of the Rheumatic Diseases*, **49**, 676–81.

Williams, C.J. and Jimenez, S.A. (1993). Heriditary, genes and osteoarthritis. *Rheumatology Disease Clinics of North America*, **19**, 523–43.

Williams, W.J., Ward, J.R., Eggar, M.J., Neuner, R., Brooks, R.H., Clegg, D.O., et al. (1993). Comparison of naproxen and acetaminophen in a two-year study of treatment of osteoarthritis of the knee. *Arthritis and Rheumatism*, **36**, 1196–206.

Woessner, J. (1991). Matrix metalloproteinases and their inhibitors in connective tissue remodeling. *FASEB Journal*, **5**, 2145–54.

Wright, V. (1990). Post-traumatic osteoarthritis — a medico-legal minefield. *British Journal of Rheumatology*, **29**, 474–8.

Yelin, E. (1992). Arthritis: the cumulative impact of a common chronic condition. *Arthritis and Rheumatism*, **35**, 489–97.

5.16   Crystal arthropathies

Ann K. Rosenthal

The crystal arthropathies include gout, calcium pyrophosphate dihydrate (**CPPD**) deposition disease, the basic calcium phosphate (**BCP**)-associated syndromes, and calcium oxalate arthritis. The most common forms of crystal-associated arthritis are readily diagnosed at the bedside, and yet continue to present many challenges to the clinician.

Gout
History

Gout is one of the oldest known forms of arthritis, and holds a unique place in the history of medicine. Famous physicians such as Hippocrates (1886) and Sydenham (Copeman 1964) made observations about gout which remain true centuries later. Gout has served as a paradigm for the study of other types of crystal-associated arthritis and as a prime example of the way in which understanding the pathophysiology of a disease leads to the development of effective therapy.

Uric acid was first identified in a renal calculus in the late 1700s by Scheele (1776), but it was not until 1899 that Freudweiler (1899) showed that intra-articular injection of uric acid crystals mimicked attacks of gouty arthritis. Decades later, uric acid crystals were identified in synovial fluids (McCarty and Hollander 1961). Based on the prescient work of Garrod (1876) in the 19th century, the link between gout and hyperuricaemia was established. Progress was aided by the discovery that an enzyme involved in purine metabolism was responsible for the Lesch–Nyhan syndrome (Seegmiller et al. 1967). Subsequently, from knowledge of purine and uric acid metabolism, effective drugs for hyperuricaemia were developed.

Definition

The term gout is derived from the latin word 'guta' meaning a drop, and originally may have referred to a drop of poison or evil humor. However, gout remains poorly defined as a clinical descriptor (Simkin 1993). In its most general sense, it is a group of diseases characterized by hyperuricaemia and uric acid crystal formation. These clinical syndromes include gouty arthritis, tophaceous gout, uric acid nephrolithiasis, and gouty nephropathy. In its more narrow and perhaps more commonly used definition, gout refers to arthritis caused by uric acid crystals.

Epidemiology

Gout is not an uncommon disease. Recent statistics from the United States show a self-reported prevalence of 13.6/1000 persons in adult males and 6.4/1000 persons for females (Collins 1988). In older studies utilizing physician diagnoses, gender specific rates were 5 to 6.6/1000 in men and 1 to 3/1000 in women (Lawrence et al. 1989). Similarly, in a study of patients in the Scottish Highlands, the overall prevalence of physician-documented gout was 3.4/1000 (Steven 1992). With an estimated prevalence of 1 per cent among adults in the United States, gout is the most common cause of inflammatory arthritis in men (Lawrence et al. 1989). Despite effective therapy, it is estimated that 37 million working days per year in the United States have been lost to gout (Hochberg 1991).

Incidence rates for gout are more difficult to ascertain. A longitudinal study of American medical students showed an incidence of 1.7 cases per 1000 person-years of follow-up (Roubenoff et al. 1991). Similar results were obtained from the Framingham data (Abbott et al. 1988). Gout may be more common in certain areas of the world such as Java (Darmawan et al. 1992), and among certain races (Lennane et al. 1960).

There is good evidence to suggest that average uric acid levels have been slowly rising over the last two decades (Gresser et al. 1990). Self-reported prevalence studies also show a parallel increase in the prevalence of gout (Lawrence et al. 1989)

The known risk factors for gout are well characterized and mirror risk factors for hyperuricaemia (Table 1). Gout is clearly more common in men and is rare in women prior to menopause. Overall, less than 5 per cent of patients with gout are female (Lally et al. 1986). Mean urate levels rise at puberty in boys and remain 1 to 2 mg/dl higher in men than women until menopause, when gender differences in uric acid levels diminish. Serum urate levels increase with age in both men and women (Becker 1988). The peak incidence of gout in men is between the fourth and sixth decade (Hall et al. 1967). In women, it is between the sixth and seventh decade (Puig et al. 1991).

Primary gout is associated with a variety of medical conditions. Some such as obesity, renal insufficiency, and diuretic use clearly cause hyperuricaemia. Serum urate levels are directly correlated with body weight (Seidell et al. 1986). Obesity is a particularly important risk factor for gout in men (Roubenoff et al. 1991). Similarly, alcohol use increases uric acid levels by providing a dietary source of purines (Gibson et al. 1984). Ethanol increases lactic acidaemia thus interfering with the excretion of uric acid (Lieber et al. 1962), and increases adenine nucleotide catabolism via acetate intermediaries (Puig and Fox 1984) At one time, alcohol (particularly port wine and moonshine or unbonded whisky) was also an excellent source of lead (Ball and Sorenson 1969).

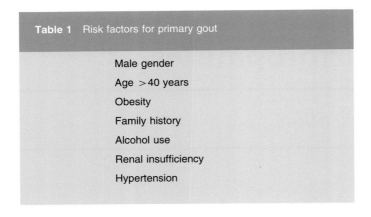

Table 1 Risk factors for primary gout

Male gender
Age >40 years
Obesity
Family history
Alcohol use
Renal insufficiency
Hypertension

Other risk factors for gout such as hypertension, family history, and coronary artery disease may not be causally associated with high uric acid levels. Hypertension occurs in 25 to 50 per cent of gout patients (Grahame and Scott 1970), and a similar percentage of untreated hypertensives will have hyperuricaemia (Wyngaarden and Kelley 1976). Gout is also associated with hypertriglyceridaemia (Scott 1977). The association between gout and coronary artery disease is somewhat controversial (Myers *et al.* 1968; Emmerson 1974; Abbott *et al.* 1988). Gout may be associated with atherosclerosis only because of the high prevalence of obesity and hypertension in gout patients (Abbott *et al.* 1988). Alternatively, gout may be an independent risk factor for coronary artery disease (Gertler *et al.* 1931).

Lastly, between 6 and 18 per cent of patients with gout will have a family history of gout (Neel 1947).

Risk factors for gout in women are not as clearly defined as those for men. As in men, age, renal insufficiency, and diuretic use are certainly linked with gout in women. However, other male risk factors such as body weight and alcohol intake may not play as important a role in gout in women (Puig *et al.* 1991).

Pathophysiology

Delineating the pathophysiology of gout requires an understanding of purine metabolism, as uric acid is an end product of purine biosynthesis. Hyperuricaemia is a necessary but not a sufficient condition for the development of gout; and although the mechanisms of excess uric acid accumulation are well defined, the subsequent phases of crystal formation and release into tissues remain less well characterized.

Purine metabolism

Purines are derived from two sources. They are ingested in food or are generated via a complex *de novo* synthetic pathway (Wyngaarden and Kelley 1976). The synthetic pathway is outlined in Fig. 1. Components of the purine ring are complexed to the donor substrate phosphoribosylpyrophosphate (**PRPP**). These are then taken through a 10-step process culminating in purine nucleotide formation. PRPP is also used as a substrate for pyrimidine and pyridine synthesis. Thus, the first committed step in purine synthesis is catalysed by the enzyme amidophosphoribosyl transferase (**amidoPRT**).

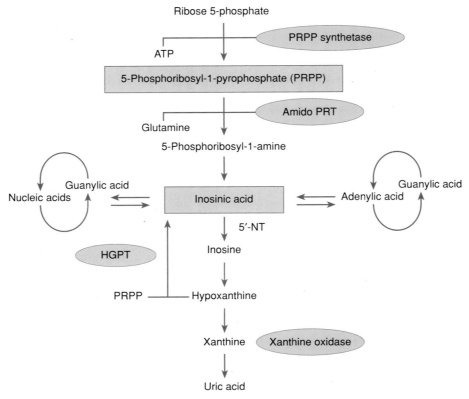

Fig. 1 Simplified scheme of normal purine metabolism in man. PRPP synthetase, phosphoribosylpyrophosphate synthetase; amidoPRT, amidophosphoribosyl transferase; HGPT, hypoxanthine guanine phosphoribosyl transferase; 5′-NT, 5′-nucleotidase.

The *de novo* synthetic pathway requires heavy energy consumption in the form of ATP (Holmes 1978). Consequently, numerous enzymes for salvaging and interconverting premade purines exist to recycle these energy-rich compounds. Two salvage enzymes are particularly important in gout. These are hypoxanthine guanine phosphoribosyl transferase (**HPRT**) and adenine phosphoribosyl transferase (**APRT**).

Control of normal purine metabolism in man is well understood. The first commited step in purine biosynthesis is rate limiting. AmidoPRT is allosterically activated by its substrate PRPP and inhibited by purine nucleotides, its end products (Holmes *et al.* 1973). The enzyme PRPP synthetase is similarly regulated, but is less sensitive to small changes in end-product concentrations (Yen *et al.* 1981; Becker and Kim 1987). Thus, control of purine metabolism is negatively affected by purines themselves and positively influenced by PRPP (Becker and Kim 1987; Itakura *et al.* 1981).

Uric acid metabolism

Uric acid is ultimately formed from purine nucleotides through the intermediate compounds xanthine, hypoxanthine, and guanine by the enzyme xanthine oxidase. It is a terminal product as no mammalian uricase exists. Uric acid is made primarily in the liver. The average pool size is 1200 mg in men and 600 mg in women. In both men and women, about two-thirds of the total uric acid pool is turned over each day (Scott *et al.* 1969). Uric acid pools in patients with gout are always larger than normal, usually in the range of 2000 to 4000 mg. In patients with tophi, uric acid burdens can be as high as 30 000 mg. (Benedict *et al.* 1949; Bishop *et al.* 1951; Sorenson 1959).

Two-thirds of uric acid is renally excreted (Buzzard *et al.* 1955; Sorenson 1960). The remainder is degraded by gut bacteria via the process of 'intestinal uricolysis' (Wyngaarden and Stetten 1953). The renal handling of uric acid is complex and not fully understood. It entails a four-step process beginning with glomerular filtration, followed by active reabsorption in the proximal tubule, tubular secretion at some distal site, and ending with postsecretory tubular reabsorption (Levinson and Sorenson 1980) (Fig. 2).

For the sake of discussion, we will divide the known metabolic causes of hyperuricaemia associated with gout into three catagories: causes of primary gout, defined inborn errors of metabolism, and aetiologies of secondary gout.

Mechanisms of hyperuricaemia in primary gout

Primary gout is simply defined by the absence of any identifiable underlying disease causing hyperuricaemia. This criterion defines the largest group of patients with gout. Most of these patients are older men and 80 to 85 per cent are hyperuricaemic on the basis of underexcretion of uric acid (Wyngaarden and Kelley 1985). There is no difference in rates of intestinal uricolysis in patients with primary gout compared with controls (Sorenson 1962). Thus, the site of the abnormality in patients with primary gout who underexcrete is most likely to be at the kidney. Simkin (1977*b*) has shown that most patients with primary gout have low fractional uric acid excretion rates. The mechanism of underexcretion remains to be elucidated but is most likely a defect in secretion or reabsorption rather than in filtration (Reiselbach *et al.* 1970).

A minority of patients with primary gout have high urinary uric acid levels and excessive *de novo* purine synthesis. The best evidence to date supports a role for increased PRPP availability or decreased purine nucleotide concentrations (thus diminishing feedback

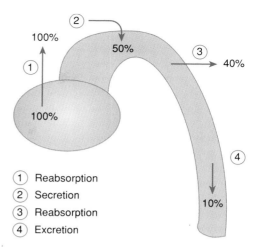

Fig. 2 Simplified scheme of renal excretion of urate. (1) reabsorption after filtration, (2) secretion in the proximal tubule, (3) reabsorption at some distal site, and (4) excretion in the urine.

1. Reabsorption
2. Secretion
3. Reabsorption
4. Excretion

inhibition of the synthetic enzymes) in patients with primary gout who overproduce (Levinson and Becker 1993).

A recent study of purine metabolism in women with primary gout showed similar abnormalities to men with primary gout (Puig *et al.* 1994).

Inborn errors of metabolism causing hyperuricaemia

The enzyme defects associated with gout often present as precocious gout in childhood or early adulthood in the setting of a strong family history of gout. There are three well-characterized enzyme defects causing hyperuricaemia. Together these account for less than 5 per cent of cases of gout. These are summarized in Table 2 and include HPRT deficiency, PRPP synthetase superactivity, and glucose 6-phosphatase (**G6P**) deficiency.

HPRT deficiency produces hyperuricaemia by increasing *de novo* synthesis of purine nucleotides through increased availability of the substrate PRPP, which stimulates synthesis. In its most complete form, HPRT deficiency results in the Lesch–Nyhan syndrome (Lesch and Nyhan 1964). This syndrome presents in early childhood with severe mental retardation, self-mutilation, choreoathetosis, spasticity, hyperuricaemia, and premature gout. Although it is linked to the X chromosome, there are two reported cases in girls (Yukawa *et al.* 1992). Partial defects of HPRT result in hyperuricaemia alone without the severe neurological consequences of complete HRPT deficiency (Kelley *et al.* 1967). Some patients with partial HPRT deficiencies may have subtle neurological impairments (Kelley *et al.* 1969). The diagnosis of HPRT deficiency can be made by measuring HPRT activity in erythrocytes (Kelley *et al.* 1969). In partial deficiencies, activity levels vary from less than 1 to 70 per cent of normal values. Over 26 different genetic mutations have been described in HPRT deficiency (Wilson *et al.* 1983).

Increased PRPP synthetase activity was described by Sperling *et al.* (1972) in two brothers. Overactivity of this enzyme results in increased PRPP levels and causes profound premature hyperuricaemia. The trait is inherited as an X-linked dominant condition (Yen *et al.* 1978). Three kindreds each with a different genetic mutation have been well characterized. Gout and renal stones develop in the second and third decades in affected males.

Table 2 Inherited metabolic disorders causing gout

Syndrome	Pattern of inheritance	Mechanism of hyperuricaemia
HPRT deficiency (Lesch–Nyhan)	X-linked	HPRT deficiency increases PRPP
Increased PRPP synthetase	X-linked	Overactivity of PRPP synthetase
von Gierke's disease (G6P deficiency)	Autosomal recessive	Increased activity of amidoPRT, decreased renal excretion due to acidaemia

The third well-characterized enzyme defect associated with gout is glucose 6-phosphatase deficiency (Alepa *et al.* 1967). This is also known as glycogen storage disease type I, or von Gierke's disease. It presents in childhood with characteristic short stature, hepatomegaly, and recurrent hypoglycaemia. Less frequently, a bleeding diathesis may accompany the syndrome. Affected patients cannot release glucose from premade glycogen stores. Subsequent hypoglycaemia results in ATP catabolism, lactic acidaemia, and elevated levels of free fatty acids, pyruvate, and triglycerides. Hyperuricaemia in this syndrome is due to two effects. Renal excretion of uric acid is diminished because other organic anions compete for transport in the kidney. Overproduction via the *de novo* synthetic pathway due to decreased feedback inhibition of amidoPRT also occurs (Itakura *et al.* 1981). Hyperuricaemia is often present from infancy, with gout occurring as early as 10 years of age. In its classic form, the inheritance is as an autosomal recessive disorder. Some forms of partial enzyme deficiency have been described (Nuki and Parker 1979).

Causes of secondary gout

The causes of secondary gout are well defined. Some may result in hyperuricaemia on the basis of overproduction of uric acid, such as tumour lysis syndrome, myeloproliferative disease, haemolytic anaemia, and psoriasis. All of these conditions are characterized by increased cell turnover with a subsequent increase in purine synthesis and catabolism.

Alternatively, conditions such as renal failure and many drugs produce hyperuricaemia and gout by promoting undersecretion of uric acid. Although mild renal insufficiency from any cause is a risk factor for gout (Berger and Yu 1960), certain forms of kidney disease such as autosomal dominant polycystic kidney disease may be preferentially associated with gout (Mejias *et al.* 1989). Interestingly, endstage renal disease often produces hyperuricaemia, but these patients rarely develop gout (Richet *et al.* 1965; Sarre and Mertz 1965).

Lead exposure is a cause of secondary gout. Saternine gout, which is associated with heavy lead exposures (often from the ingestion of lead-laden whisky), is rare today. Lead interferes with renal excretion of uric acid by altering the tubular transport of urate. It affects purine metabolism by altering purine nucleotide turnover (Ludwig 1957; Forkas *et al.* 1978). Lead levels are increased in gout patients. Whether this phenomenon is primary or secondary to the renal insufficiency that often accompanies gout remains to be determined. Industrial lead exposure occurs in plumbers, pipe fitters, painters, steel workers, battery plant employees, and vehicle mechanics

Table 3 Drugs associated with hyperuricaemia and gout

Drugs causing overproduction	Drugs causing underexcretion
Ethanol	Ethanol
Fructose	Salicylates (<2 g/day)
Cytotoxic drugs	Cyclosporin
Vitamin B_{12}	Diuretics
Warfarin	Ethambutol
	Pyrazinamide
	Levodopa
	Angiotensin
	Vasopressin
	Laxatives
	Nicotinic acid
	Nitroglycerin
	Methoxyflurane

(Hochberg 1991). Recent changes in environmental safety standards may reduce lead exposure in these settings.

Drugs commonly associated with hyperuricaemia are listed in Table 3.

Urate crystal formation (Fig. 3)

We know little about why uric acid crystals form *in vivo*. Yet, because the vast majority of patients with hyperuricaemia never develop gout (Hall *et al.* 1967), it is these processes of crystal formation and release that define clinical gout.

Our current understanding of urate crystal formation is based on knowledge of the biochemistry of urate, *in vitro* studies of crystallogenesis, and the histopathology of gout. Urate is present in two forms in the body. At neutral and alkaline pH, the monosodium salt (MSU) predominates. At acidic pH, such as in urine, the primary form is uric acid. Both forms are relatively insoluble, although uric acid is less soluble than its salt (Peters and Van Slyke 1946). A solution is supersaturated with monosodium urate at 37°C at concentrations

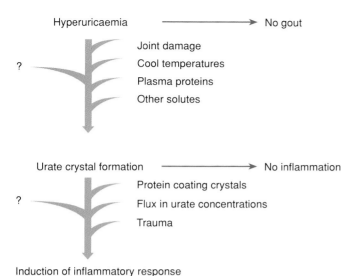

Fig. 3 Overview of factors influencing the development of gouty arthritis.

greater than 6.4 mg/dl (Peters and Van Slyke 1946). Cooler temperatures decrease urate solubility (Loeb 1972), thus predicting the association of gout with distal joints.

In vitro studies of crystallogenesis have yielded conflicting results in regard to the influences of serum, synovial fluid, and many individual plasma proteins, including albumin and proteoglycans, on crystal formation (Katz and Erlich 1986; McGill and Dieppe 1991*b*). Crystal formation is probably enhanced by IgG and type I collagen (McGill and Dieppe 1991*b*). In addition, urate crystals themselves initiate further crystal formation. McGill and Dieppe (1991*a*) and others (Tak *et al.* 1980; Burt and Dutt 1986) demonstrated increased crystallogenesis in the presence of 'particulate-free' synovial fluid from patients with gout compared with those with rheumatoid arthritis or CPPD deposition disease, suggesting the presence of as yet uncharacterized promoters of crystal formation in gouty fluid.

Urate crystals have a unique distribution in the body. They prefer sites rich in connective tissue, such as synovium, cartilage, tendon, skin, and the renal interstitium (Sokoloff 1957). Gouty arthritis often develops in previously damaged joints. Disturbances of proteoglycan metabolism or collagen structure may promote crystal formation and release (Katz and Erlich 1974; Wilcox and Khalaf 1975; Perricone and

Brandt 1978). Joint effusions may also affect urate crystal formation. Because the diffusion of urate through the synovial membrane is less than that of water (Simkin 1977*a*), resorption of water in a joint with an effusion during recumbency would increase the effective urate concentration and promote crystal formation.

Pathogenesis of the acute attack (Fig. 4)

Once monosodium urate crystals form in the joint, they may induce an acute attack of gouty arthritis. Urate crystals clearly cause inflammation (Seegmiller *et al.* 1962); yet we are unable to explain why they are present in synovial fluids from asymptomatic uninflamed joints (Pascual 1991). The type and quantity of protein coating the crystals may affect their ability to induce inflammation. IgG is found in association with MSU crystals and increases cell activation (Russell *et al.* 1983). Terkeltaub *et al.* (1991) demonstrated a role for the lipoprotein apoE in inhibiting crystal-induced inflammation.

The effects of uncoated MSU crystals on cells are well characterized. The cells that urate crystals first encounter in the joint are most probably macrophage-like synovial cells. Here they induce the release of vasoactive prostaglandins, proteases, and proinflammatory cytokines including interleukin 1 (**IL-1**), IL-6, and IL-8 which initiate a vigorous inflammatory response (DiGiovine *et al.* 1987). Recruited polymorphonuclear leucocytes release proteases, superoxides, leukotrienes, and interleukins when exposed to MSU crystals. (Abramson *et al.* 1982; Cheung *et al.* 1983*b*; Bhatt and Spillberg 1988). MSU crystals activate complement via the classical pathway (Giclas *et al.* 1979). They also promote the release of Hageman factor and the subsequent activation of bradykinin, kallikrein, and other coagulation factors (Ginsberg *et al.* 1980).

The mechanisms through which they stimulate these cells remain to be elucidated. Certainly, some crystals are phagocytosed and cause lysis of the phagolysosome, release of its toxic contents, and death of the cell (Schumacher and Phelps 1971). Other effects may be mediated through cell membrane perturbations (Mandel 1976). The highly charged surfaces of MSU crystals may bind to and cross-link membrane receptors, thus mediating some of the crystals' immediate effects (Burt and Jackson 1990).

The factors that terminate an acute attack remain unclear. One hypothesis suggests changes in crystal size and protein coating render the crystals less inflammatory. These changes may be mediated through generation of oxygen free radicals by polymorphonuclear leucocytes (Marcalongo *et al.* 1988).

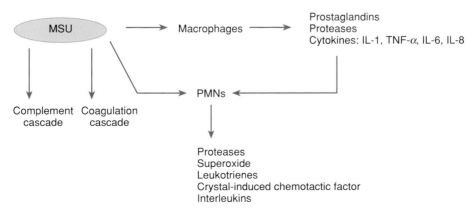

Fig. 4 The mechanisms through which monosodium urate (MSU) crystals cause inflammation in the joint.

Tophus formation

Tophi are soft tissue deposits of urate. We know little about how and why they form. Palmer *et al.* (1989) proposed that tophi are urate-lowering organs. Based on histological studies, they proposed that acini of macrophages develop in areas of high local urate concentrations. These organized cells actively transport urate from the interstitial fluid to the centre of the acinus. They grow to a certain size and then fuse with other acini, eventually forming tophi. Further work is necessary to confirm this theory.

Clinical features

We will discuss the clinical features of acute and chronic gout, and renal syndromes associated with uric acid.

Articular gout is often divided into four clinical stages. The first stage is defined by asymptomatic hyperuricaemia. This is followed by acute gouty arthritis and then by another asymptomatic phase termed intercritical gout. When allowed to proceed untreated, some patients will go on to develop chronic tophaceous gout.

Acute gout

The first clinical symptom of gout is usually an acute, self-limited, monoarticular inflammatory arthritis affecting the joints of the lower extremities. Gout has a predilection for the first metatarsophalangeal joint. As many as 50 to 70 per cent of first gout attacks occur in the big toe (Delbarre *et al.* 1967; Grahame and Scott 1970). Other frequently involved joints include those of the foot, ankle, knee, wrist, elbow, and the small joints of the hands. The large axial joints and those of the spine are uncommon sites for early acute gout attacks.

The onset of an attack occurs suddenly and often late at night or early in the morning. Patients will describe very severe pain, associated with swelling, extreme tenderness, and redness overlying the joint. Without intervention, the attack will usually subside within 5 to 7 days (Bellamy *et al.* 1987). Low-grade fever, malaise, and anorexia may occur. The attack may be preceded by brief twinges of pain (petit attacks) in the affected joint.

Common precipitants of acute attacks include excess alcohol intake, intercurrent illness, surgery (Bartles 1957), starvation, trauma, and the initiation of drugs that alter urate metabolism. All of these precipitants alter serum urate levels.

Physical examination shows signs of inflammation with erythema, warmth, and swelling over the joint, often extending to the overlying skin. There is exquisite tenderness over the affected joint. Not infrequently, an overlying cellulitis or accompanying tenosynovitis occurs. The skin may desquamate in the later days of an attack. Acute gout can also occur in bursas, and gout is a common cause of acute inflammatory olecranon bursitis (Canosa and Yood 1979).

After the attack resolves, the patient will be completely asymptomatic. This phase is referred to as intercritical gout. Most patients will go on to have an additional attack within 2 years of the first attack (Gutman 1973). In one study, 78 per cent had recurrent attacks within 2 years, and after 10 years, 93 per cent had had more than one attack. Untreated, the intercritical phases become shorter. Interestingly, they still present an opportunity for diagnosis, as many joints will still have urate crystals in the synovial fluid during the intercritical phase if they were involved in a previous attack, and urate-lowering therapy has not been initiated (Pascual 1991).

Chronic tophaceous gout

In the later stages of untreated disease, clinical manifestations characteristically change. Acute attacks are more often polyarticular. The intercritical stage shortens, and repeated joint damage results in permanent deformities, loss of motion, chronic pain, and tophi (Nakayama *et al.* 1984).

Polyarticular gout occurs in late stage disease, although some patients present earlier with polyarticular attacks (Raddatz *et al.* 1983; Lawry *et al.* 1988). Intercritical stages are short or non-existent and involvement of atypical sites including the upper extremities, the spine, and axial joints may ensue (Lagier and MacGee 1983; Varga *et al.* 1985). After repeated attacks in a single joint, deformity and loss of motion may occur.

Tophi are deposits of urate embedded in a matrix composed of amorphous urates, lipids, proteins, and calcific debris (Fig. 5). Tophi are usually subcutaneous, but they can occur in bone and other organs including the heart valves and the eye (Ferry *et al.* 1985; Gawoski *et al.* 1985). Classic sites include the pinna of the ear, bursas around elbows and knees, the dorsal surfaces of the metacarpophalangeal joints, and the Achilles tendon. Tophi are not distinguishable on physical examination from rheumatoid nodules or other subcutaneous nodules. There is no accompanying inflammation and they are usually painless. The overlying skin may be taut and shiny. A thick white or whitish-yellow exudate is seen if the skin integrity is compromised.

Tophi or chronic polyarthritis may occur as early as 3 years or as late as 42 years after the first acute attack. In the pretreatment era, 50 per cent of patients with gout had tophi after 10 years of disease (Gutman 1973). Currently, about 5 per cent of patients with gout will have tophi (O'Duffy *et al.* 1975). Their occurrence is directly correlated with serum urate levels, and they identify a group of patients with severe and prolonged hyperuricaemia (Nakayama *et al.* 1984). Another group at risk of developing tophi and polyarticular

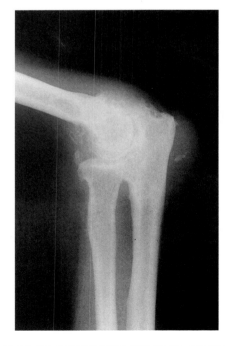

Fig. 5 A tophus in the olecranon bursa appears as a typical soft tissue density with a small amount of calcification.

gout are elderly women with primary nodal osteoarthritis on diuretic therapy (Macfarlane and Dieppe 1985).

Other articular manifestations of gout

Gout has been variably associated with avascular necrosis of the femoral head (Hunder *et al.* 1968; Stockman *et al.* 1980). Patients with gout may also have a higher prevalence of chondrocalcinosis (Dodds and Steinbach 1966).

Renal disease and gout

The relationship between kidney dysfunction and gout remains complex and confusing. Three renal syndromes are associated with gout. Urate crystals can form in the renal interstitium causing urate nephropathy. Uric acid can acutely precipitate in the collecting tubules resulting in uric acid nephropathy. Lastly, uric acid nephrolithiasis may occur.

Urate nephropathy
The pathological changes that define urate nephropathy are common. MSU crystals in the renal medulla are associated with a giant-cell inflammatory reaction (Sokoloff 1957). The clinical significance of these pathological findings, however, remains unclear. Renal insufficiency is unequivocally common in patients with gout, but controversy exists as to the aetiology of this renal dysfunction. Current dogma states that urate crystals themselves produce only a minor amount of renal damage. Most of the renal disease associated with gout is secondary to inadequately controlled hypertension and other comorbidities (Fessel 1967; Berger and Yu 1960).

Uric acid nephropathy
Excluding nephrolithiasis, the renal syndrome most often associated with uric acid today is acute uric acid nephropathy (Reiselbach *et al.* 1962; Frei *et al.* 1963). This often occurs in an acutely ill, dehydrated patient treated with cytotoxic drugs for a lymphoproliferative disorder. An acute obstructive uropathy ensues with oliguric renal failure. Uric acid crystals form in the collecting tubules and are found in the urine. Uric acid/creatinine ratios are often greater than 1.0. This complication can be avoided with adequate hydration and the prophylactic administration of allopurinol prior to initiating chemotherapy.

Uric acid nephrolithiasis
The association between gout and nephrolithiasis is well established (Yu and Gutman 1967). Prevalence figures for renal stones vary between 10 and 42 per cent of patients with gout. Of these stones, 84 per cent are uric acid stones. Risk factors for developing uric acid stones include elevated urinary uric acid levels, and low urine pH (Plante *et al.* 1968; Yu 1981). Half the patients excreting greater than 1100 mg uric acid per day will have stones (Yu and Gutman 1967). Interestingly, however, only 20 per cent of patients with uric acid stones are hyperuricaemic (Talbott 1957). Patients with gout also are at a higher risk for non-urate stones. Of the 16 per cent of stones in patients with gout that do not contain uric acid, 8 per cent are calcium oxalate, 4 per cent are calcium phosphates, and 4 per cent are mixed stones. It is postulated that uric acid serves as a nidus for calcium oxalate crystal growth. Alternatively, or in addition, levels of inhibitors of calcium oxalate stone formation may be decreased in the urine of patients with gout.

Laboratory investigation

Investigation of the patient with an acute attack

Synovial fluid analysis remains the single most important diagnostic study in the patient with suspected gout. Synovial fluid is usually easily obtained from a large joint, while often only a drop of fluid or blood from the joint or adjacent tissues is necessary to provide a sample for definitive diagnosis of gout in a small joint. Synovial fluid is typically inflammatory with a mean white cell count of 20 000 cells/mm^3. Most cells are polymorphonuclear leucocytes. Viscosity is often poor. A definite diagnosis can be made if typical, negatively birefringent, needle-shaped crystals are seen in the fluid with a polarizing light microscope (Fig. 6). They may be extra- or intracellular. Rarely one may see spherules of uric acid in acute gout (Fiechtner and Simkin 1981).

Few other laboratory studies are of significant clinical utility in diagnosing acute gout. Serum uric acid levels during the acute attack may not reflect pre-attack levels and can not be used to make a diagnosis

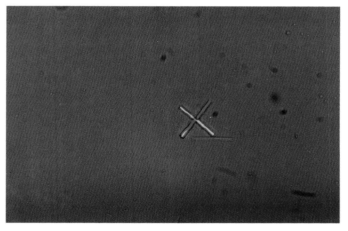

(a)

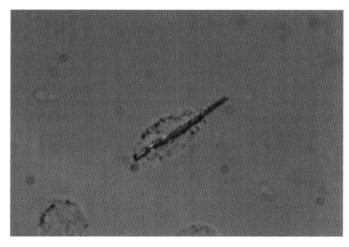

(b)

Fig. 6 Typical, needle-shaped, negatively birefringent crystals are seen under polazing light microscopy in the synovial fluid of patients with gouty arthritis. These crystals may be extracellular (a) or intracellular (b).

of gout in the absence of urate crystals in the synovial fluid. One may see a peripheral leucocytosis, an elevated erythrocyte sedimentation rate, and increased levels of other acute-phase reactants during an acute attack. Synovial fluid cultures and Gram stains may help rule out concurrent infection. Radiographs are often normal during early episodes of gout. They may be useful to differentiate other problems such as fracture or infection from acute gout. Often soft tissue swelling is the sole radiographic finding in early gout.

Evaluation of the patient with recurrent attacks

Serum uric acid levels and 24-h urine collections for creatinine and uric acid may be helpful in evaluating the patient once the acute attack has subsided. Serum urate levels over 7 mg/dl define hyperuricaemia in most laboratories. Values of urinary uric acid over 1000 mg/day on an unrestricted diet define patients that overproduce, and may influence the choice of therapy. Patients suspected of a primary metabolic disorder should have a 24-h urine sample tested for creatinine, protein, and uric acid and a careful family history taken. If urinary uric acid levels are high, levels of enzyme activity for HPRT, PRPP synthetase, and glucose 6-phosphatase can be measured in specialist laboratories.

In later disease, gout has a typical radiographic appearance (Block *et al.* 1980; Barthelemy *et al.* 1984). The hallmarks of radiographic gout are due to the presence of tophi in or near the joint. In the soft tissues, tophi appear eccentric and nodular (Fig. 5). A small percentage of them calcify. Tophi may occur in or near a joint or distant from periarticular tissues. As a soft tissue tophus enlarges, it may encroach on the adjacent bone and produce a cortical erosion with focal periosteal new bone formation. This occurrence results in an erosion with a typical overhanging margin, present in 40 per cent of gouty erosions (Martel 1968) (Fig. 7). When in the joint, tophi produce marginal erosions with a characteristic 'punched out' or sclerotic border (Fig. 8). Erosions are particularly common on the medial and dorsal portions of the first metatarsal head. Similar changes can affect the digits of the hand. Bony abnormalities of the periosteum may occur in association with tophus formation. Specifically, a 'lace pattern' of finely striated periosteal reaction may develop adjacent to a tophus (Fig. 9). Rarely, bony proliferation may occur at the ends or shafts of long bones (mushrooming). Diaphyseal thickening may also occur. The joint space is characteristically well preserved until late in the disease. When joint space narrowing does occur it affects all joint compartments symmetrically, similar to other inflammatory joint disorders (Fig. 10). Bones may be osteopenic from disuse, but are usually well mineralized.

Diagnosis

A definitive diagnosis of gout can only be made by the identification of urate crystals in the synovial fluid of an affected joint. Identification of urate crystals in tophi also allows a definitive diagnosis to be made. In the absence of these findings, other clinical criteria may be used to make a putative diagnosis of gout (Wallace *et al.* 1977). As crystals may be present in the intercritical phase, one may aspirate an asymptomatic but previously affected joint to establish a definite diagnosis.

Many clinical conditions can mimic acute gout (Table 4). These include infectious arthritis, other crystal-associated arthropathies such as pseudogout or BCP-associated periarthritis, or trauma. Patients with palindromic rheumatism may give a similar history of self-limited monoarticular attacks associated with exquisite pain,

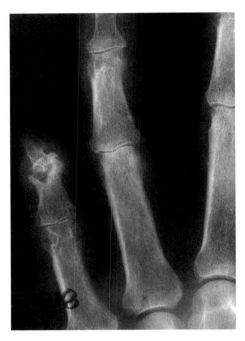

Fig. 7 A typical gouty erosion with overhanging margins is seen on the medial aspect of the proximal interphalangeal joint in this radiograph.

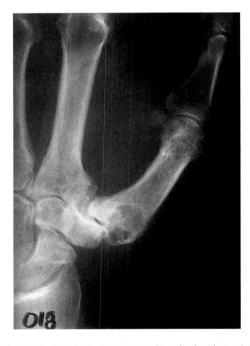

Fig. 8 An interosseus tophus appears as a 'punched out' or sclerotic erosion at the base of the proximal phalanx of the thumb.

tenderness, and erythema near the affected joint. Rarely, other causes of polyarticular inflammatory arthritis, particularly psoriatic arthritis or Reiter's syndrome, may present with monoarticular self-limited attacks of the lower extremities which may be confused with gout. Once tophi and deformities occur, gout can be misdiagnosed as rheumatoid arthritis. As many as 30 per cent of patients with gout will have positive serum rheumatoid factors (Kozin and McCarty 1977).

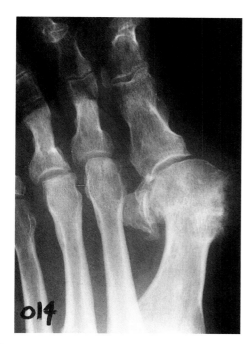

Fig. 9 On the lateral aspect of the distal metatarsal joint, a lace-like periosteal reaction adjacent to a tophus can be seen.

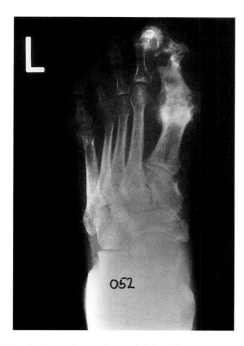

Fig. 10 Extensive bony destruction and deformities are seen with far-advanced gouty arthritis of the foot.

Management of gouty arthritis

Management of gouty arthritis can be divided into three phases: treatment of acute gout, treatment of chronic or tophaceous gout, and preventive measures.

Preventive measures

Gout is a significant public health problem despite our excellent therapy. Hochberg (1991) suggests that we may be able to decrease

Table 4	Clinical conditions that mimic gouty arthritis
CPPD disease (pseudogout)	
BCP arthritis	
Cellulitis	
Erythema nodosum arthritis	
Trauma	
Palindromic rheumatism	
Reiter's syndrome	
Psoriatic arthritis	
Rheumatoid arthritis	

the incidence of gout with preventive measures such as avoiding excess weight gain, reducing risks for hypertension, avoiding diuretic therapy, controlling alcohol intake, and minimizing occupational lead exposures. The efficacy of such interventions remains to be proven.

Management of acute gout

Traditional therapies for acute gout include non-steroidal anti-inflammatory drugs (**NSAIDs**), colchicine, and steroids. Rest and splinting of the affected joint may be helpful adjuncts to any pharmacological therapy. The management of acute gout is summarized in Box 1.

NSAIDs

NSAIDs have replaced colchicine as the most commonly used drugs in the treatment of acute gout (Wallace 1977; Stuart *et al.* 1991). They interfere with the inflammation induced by MSU crystals (Abramson and Weissmann 1989). Traditionally, indomethacin has been the NSAID of choice in acute gout, but probably has no advantage over other NSAIDs (Sterling 1991). Sulindac may be better tolerated in those patients at high risk of renal side-effects from NSAIDs (Ciabottoni *et al.* 1984). In general, drugs with a shorter half-life achieve quicker therapeutic plasma levels and faster relief of pain.. With treatment, symptoms should subside within 3 to 5 days. NSAIDs are contraindicated in patients with significant renal insufficiency, peptic ulcer disease, concurrent warfarin therapy, or liver disease.

Colchicine

Colchicine is the oldest drug for gout, but its safety remains controversial. When used correctly, it can be very effective with a rapid onset of action. Colchicine tends to be much more effective in the early hours of an attack and loses efficacy with time. The mechanism of action of colchicine is unknown. It inhibits polymorphonuclear leucocyte function through its action on microtubules, but may also have very specific effects on crystal-induced inflammation (Roberge *et al.* 1993). Colchicine can be given in intravenous and oral forms.

Current recommendations for intravenous use are cautious (Moreland and Ball 1991) (Table 5). A dose of 1 to 3 mg diluted in 20 ml of normal saline can be slowly instilled into a large vein. Another 1-mg dose can be given 6 h later if the clinical response is

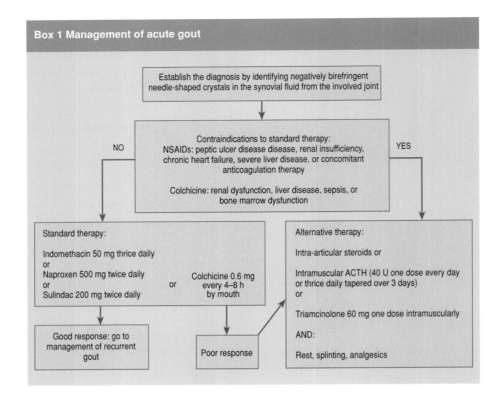

Box 1 Management of acute gout

Establish the diagnosis by identifying negatively birefringent
needle-shaped crystals in the synovial fluid from the involved joint

NO ← Contraindications to standard therapy:
NSAIDs: peptic ulcer disease disease, renal insufficiency,
chronic heart failure, severe liver disease, or concomitant
anticoagulation therapy

Colchicine: renal dysfunction, liver disease, sepsis, or
bone marrow dysfunction → YES

Standard therapy:

Indomethacin 50 mg thrice daily
or
Naproxen 500 mg twice daily   or   Colchicine 0.6 mg
or   every 4–8 h
Sulindac 200 mg twice daily   by mouth

Alternative therapy:

Intra-articular steroids or

Intramuscular ACTH (40 U one dose every day
or thrice daily tapered over 3 days)
or

Triamcinolone 60 mg one dose intramuscularly

AND:

Rest, splinting, analgesics

Good response: go to
management of recurrent
gout

Poor response

incomplete. The maximum dose is 4 mg in 24 h. No additional doses should be given for 7 days after the initial dose. Intravenous colchicine is particularly useful for patients unable to take oral medications. Now that parenteral forms of NSAIDs are available, its use may decline further. Absolute contraindications to the use of intravenous colchicine include significant renal or hepatic compromise, bone marrow suppression, or sepsis. It should be used with great caution in patients with mild renal or hepatic disease, and, for example, those on daily oral colchicine prophylaxis. Side-effects range from venous sclerosis or tissue damage from extravasation of colchicine, to fatal bone marrow failure. Other side-effects include renal or hepatic failure, disseminated intravascular coagulation, and neuromuscular toxicity. Deaths from misuse of intravenous colchicine have been reported (Roberts *et al.* 1987).

Oral colchicine is currently used more frequently than the intravenous form. It is given as an initial 0.5 to 0.6 mg dose which is repeated every 1 to 2 h until gastrointestinal symptoms ensue or pain resolves. Doses should not exceed 5 mg in 24 h. Similar side-effects are reported for oral and intravenous forms. Oral colchicine, however, has a higher incidence of gastrointestinal side-effects and a lower incidence of major toxicities, probably because the tolerated dose is lower.

Corticosteroids

Corticosteroid use in gout has endured much ebb and flow in popularity during recent years. Although ACTH has been used for many years to treat gout, textbooks of the last two decades cautioned against systemic steroids because of concerns about rebound symptoms and inconsistent results (Gutman and Yu 1952). More recently, there has been a resurgence of interest in their use in gout. Regimens for acute gout include intramuscular ACTH (Axelrod and Preston 1989; Ritter *et al.* 1993), intramuscular triamcinolone (Siegel *et al.*

Table 5 Recommendations for the use of colchicine

(1) Intravenous colchicine should not be given in patients with:

Creatinine clearance <10 ml/min

Significant active liver disease or extrahepatic biliary obstruction

Sepsis

Bone marrow depression

(2) Intravenous colchicine should be used cautiously in patients on oral colchicine prophylaxis, with poor venous access, or with any degree of hepatic or renal compromise

(3) Recommended doses should not exceed 3 mg intravenous per 24 h or 5 mg orally per 24 h

1994), and oral steroids (Groff *et al.* 1990) (Table 6). These regimens are safe and well tolerated. Their efficacy remains to be proven. They may be particularly useful for patients in whom NSAIDs and colchicine are contraindicated (Ritter *et al.* 1993). The use of intra-articular steroids is less controversial. Although no studies of the efficacy of intra-articular steroids have been published, they remain a mainstay of therapy in patients unable to tolerate more traditional therapies (Hollander 1953).

Prophylactic therapy

Drugs which reduce serum uric acid levels such as allopurinol and probenecid are the standard therapies available for prophylaxis of

Table 6 Regimens for use of corticosteroids in acute gouty arthritis

Drug	Dose	Route of administration	Length of use
Triamcinolone acetonide	60 mg	Intramuscular	Give once, repeat in 48 h if needed
Prednisone	20–50 mg with daily taper	Oral	3–20 days (mean 10 days)
ACTH	40 IU	Intramuscular	Give once
ACTH	40–80 IU	Intramuscular, intravenous or subcutaneous	Every 8 h then every 12 h then each day on 3 successive days

gout attacks. Colchicine and NSAIDs are less commonly used as prophylactic drugs, but may also decrease attack frequency and severity when used alone or in combination with other therapies. Indications for the use of prophylactic drugs include recurrent attacks, tophi, severe or polyarticular disease, renal disease, or an inborn error of metabolism causing gout. Urate-lowering therapies are traditionally not started during an acute attack and are initiated concurrently with a 2-week course of low-dose colchicine or a NSAID. This regimen may avoid the risk of precipitating an acute attack by rapidly lowering uric acid levels. Goals of therapy are to decrease attack frequency, dissolve tophi, and maintain serum uric acid levels in the normal range. The management of recurrent gout is summarized in Box 2.

Allopurinol

Allopurinol is the drug most commonly used for the prevention of acute gout and the treatment of chronic tophaceous gout (Stuart et al. 1991). It is a xanthine oxidase inhibitor and thus decreases uric acid production. It may also have other actions (Adriani and Naraghi 1985). It is very effective in lowering serum uric acid levels and is the drug of choice for patients with renal insufficiency, a history of nephrolithiasis, or tophi. It is also indicated in patients who clearly overproduce uric acid such as those with tumour lysis syndrome or primary metabolic defects. Allopurinol is usually given as a once daily dose of 300 mg. The dose should be adjusted downward in the presence of significant renal compromise. It may be increased to a maximum of 900 mg/day to achieve normal uric acid levels. The onset of action is rapid and effects can be seen as early as 4 days to 2 weeks (Wyngaarden et al. 1965; Rundle et al. 1966). Allopurinol interferes with the metabolism of azathioprine, potentiating its marrow-suppressive effects (Boston Collaborative Drug Surveillance Program 1974), and may augment anticoagulant effects of warfarin (Self et al. 1957). In general, the incidence of side-effects with allopurinol is low (less than 2 per cent). The most common side-effects include a hypersensitivity syndrome of rash and fever (McInnes et al. 1981; Singer and Wallace 1986). Life-threatening reactions, including fulminant hepatitis, interstitial nephritis, and toxic epidermal necrolysis, are even more unusual (Lupton and Odom 1979). Patients with renal disease may have a greater incidence of drug allergy (Singer and Wallace 1986). Allopurinol can be given cautiously to an allergic patient using available desensitization regimens (Northridge and Almack 1986; Fam et al. 1992).

Uricosurics

Probenecid and sulphinpyrazone are the most commonly used uricosuric drugs. They interfere with the renal handling of urate by altering organic anion transport, thus increasing urate excretion (Gutman and Yu 1957). Usual doses of probenecid are 0.5 to 2 g given in twice daily doses (Boger and Strickland 1955). Sulphinpyrazone is given in doses of 300 to 400 mg/day (Emmerson 1963). Both drugs are well tolerated and effective. Maximum doses of 3 g/day of probenecid and 800 mg/day of sulphinpyrazone are occasionally necessary to return the levels of serum uric acid to normal. Uricosurics are contraindicated in patients with nephrolithiasis and ineffective in patients with significant renal compromise, or those using acetylsalicylates. Side-effects include rare hypersensitivity reactions, rashes, gastrointestinal complaints, and nephrotic syndrome (Reynolds et al. 1957; Hertz et al. 1972).

Benzbromarone is a uricosuric drug available in Europe, that is effective in the presence of renal insufficiency. At doses of 25 to 125 mg/day, it may lower values of serum uric acid in patients with serum creatinine levels as high as 2.0 mg/dl (Zollner et al. 1970).

Colchicine

In patients who are unable to take allopurinol or a uricosuric drug, daily low-dose oral colchicine may be useful in preventing further attacks of gout (Yu and Gutman 1961). It is given in doses of 0.5 to 1.2 mg/day. Unfortunately, serious side-effects have occurred even on this low-dose regimen in patients with renal insufficiency or liver disease (Neuss et al. 1986).

Drug combinations and other therapies

Patients who continue to have gout attacks on a single prophylactic drug can be treated with a combination of medications. The combination of probenecid and colchicine is more effective than probenecid alone (Paulus et al. 1974). Small numbers of patients have been reported to respond to a combination of allopurinol and a uricosuric (Kuzell et al. 1966) when either one alone was ineffective. Other measures such as eliminating the concurrent use of urate-elevating drugs, decreasing alcohol intake, weight reduction, and improving medication compliance may also help achieve control of uric acid levels in refractory patients. Rarely, patients with long-standing uncontrolled disease have permanent joint dysfunction which is best treated surgically. Tophi may occasionally require surgical removal with a low incidence of recurrence (Smyth 1953).

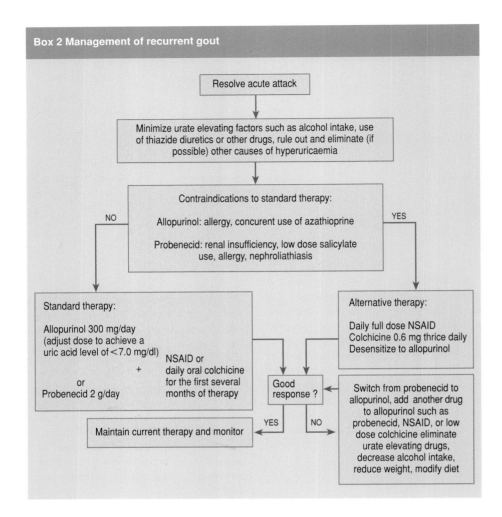

Uricase has been used as a novel approach to gout therapy. This enzyme dissolves uric acid crystals and has been used successfully in a small number of patients (Chua *et al.* 1988; Rozenberg *et al.* 1993). In some cases, polyethylene glycol treatment of the uricase was used to reduce its immunogenicity (Chua *et al.* 1988).

Management of nephrolithiasis

Patients with uric acid stones are best managed with adequate hydration, urinary alkalinization (with bicarbonate or acetozolamide), and allopurinol. Potassium citrate may be used in place of allopurinol if necessary (Pak *et al.* 1986). This regimen is also effective in preventing calcium oxalate stones in patients with hyperuricaemia (Pak *et al.* 1981).

Gout in the transplant recipient

In the late 1980s, it was noted that an unusually large number of cases of gout were occurring in renal transplant patients. This coincided with the popular use of cyclosporin as an immunosuppressant. Hyperuricaemia occurs in 30 to 84 per cent and gout in 7 to 9 per cent of patients with renal transplants who are treated with cyclosporin (Lin *et al.* 1989). The incidence of gout in patients with heart and lung transplants on cyclosporin is also significantly increased (Burak *et al.* 1992). Gout in these patients is often more severe than primary gout. Polyarticular and tophaceous gout occurs earlier in cyclosporin-induced gout than in primary gout (Baethge *et al.* 1993). Post-transplant patients can be particularly difficult to treat because of contraindications to the use of NSAIDs and colchicine, resistance to systemic steroids which they take chronically, and concerns about interactions between allopurinol and azathioprine. These patients are frequently on diuretics, and their risk of infection is high because of their compromised immune status. In the acute management of gout in the transplant patient, an arthrocentesis is usually warranted to eliminate the possibility of infection. Once a diagnosis is established, intra-articular steroids and systemic pain medications may be helpful. Chronically, some of these patients may be treated with uricosurics. If allopurinol is indicated, azathioprine can be reduced to one-third of its usual dose and 50 to 100 mg of allopurinol can be added. Blood counts should be carefully monitored during the initiation of allopurinol therapy.

Prognosis

In the era of antihyperuricaemic therapy, the prognosis for patients with gouty arthritis is excellent. Moreover, despite the association of hyperuricaemia with heart disease, hypertension, and renal insufficiency, there is no evidence that patients with gout have decreased longevity compared with controls who do not have gout.

Calcium pyrophospate dihydrate (CPPD) disease

CPPD disease is the second most common form of the crystal-associated arthritides. Unlike gout, the pathophysiology of CPPD disease remains poorly understood, and consequently no specific therapies for this arthropathy exist.

History

CPPD disease was initially described by McCarty et al. (1962) in the early 1960s. While studying crystals from synovial fluid of patients with presumed gout, it was noted that some crystals were resistant to dissolution by uricase (McCarty et al. 1962). On further characterization, these crystals were composed of calcium pyrophosphate dihydrate (Kohn et al. 1962). Similar crystals were subsequently identified in the synovial fluid from patients with both acute and chronic arthritis (McCarty 1966). They were noted to be associated with advanced age, radiographic chondrocalcinosis, and a characteristic pattern of severe joint degeneration. Our understanding of the pathophysiology of CPPD crystal formation remains rudimentary.

Definition

No concensus as to the proper nomenclature of CPPD disease exists. CPPD disease or CPPD deposition disease are the terms most commonly used to refer to the arthritis caused by CPPD crystals. Other terms used similarly include CPDD disease and pyrophosphate arthropathy (McCarty 1982). The acute form of CPPD disease is commonly referred to as pseudogout. Chondrocalcinosis, a frequent associated finding, is defined by the radiographic presence of finely stippled calcification in articular hyaline and fibrocartilage. Although these deposits are usually composed of CPPD crystals, other mineral forms have been identified in pathological specimens with chondrocalcinosis (McCarty 1966).

Epidemiology

Because the clinical syndromes associated with CPPD crystals are heterogeneous and may mimic other rheumatic diseases, the prevalence and incidence of CPPD deposition disease is difficult to define. Small studies have suggested a prevalence rate as high as 0.9/1000 (O'Duffy 1976), a figure about half that of gouty arthritis. Gender predominance varies from study to study, but symptomatic CPPD disease may be more common in women (Bergstrom et al. 1986a; Bergstrom et al. 1986b; Felson et al. 1989). The average age in the largest collection of symptomatic patients with definite or probable CPPD disease is 72 years (Ryan and McCarty 1993).

Most studies on prevalence have relied on data from autopsies or are based on radiographic chondrocalcinosis. These studies clearly demonstrate that CPPD crystal deposition increases with age. Autopsy studies show prevalence rates of 20 per cent in knee joints from patients over the age of 60 years (Mitrovic et al. 1988). CPPD crystals are unusual in joints of patients under the age of 60, and may be present in about 50 per cent of nonagenarians (Mitrovic et al. 1988). Radiographic studies confirm this pattern. An overall prevalence of chondrocalcinosis of 8.1 per cent in the population between the ages of 63 and 93 was noted in Framingham, Massachusetts. Age-specific rates rose from 3.2 per cent in the 65 to 69 year age group to 27.1 per cent in patients over the age of 85 years (Felson et al. 1989).

Similar results were described in Nottingham. Prevalence rates were 6 per cent in the 55 to 64 age group and 32 per cent in people over 75 years of age (Jones et al. 1992a).

CPPD disease usually occurs sporadically. However, familial cases in the Chiloean Islands of South America (Reginato et al. 1975), France (Gaucher et al. 1977), Spain (Balsa et al. 1990), Mexico, (Richardson et al. 1983), and Canada (Gaudreau et al. 1981) have been well characterized. Familial CPPD occurs prematurely and is often associated with very severe arthritis presenting in the second and third decades. Although the genetics of these kindreds are variable, most show an autosomal dominant pattern of inheritance (Ryan and McCarty 1993). The incidence of familial CPPD disease may be underestimated (Rodriguez-Valverde et al. 1988).

Like gout, CPPD disease is associated with a variety of other medical conditions. Unlike gout, the pathophysiological connections between CPPD disease and these disorders is not always apparent. Associated conditions can be divided into definite and possible associations. Definite associations include hypomagnesaemia (Milazzo et al. 1981; Salvarini et al. 1989), hypophosphatasia (O'Duffy 1970; Whyte et al. 1982; Chuck et al. 1989), haemochromatosis (Hamilton et al. 1981), Wilson's disease (Feller and Schumacher 1972; Golding and Walshe 1977), and hyperparathyroidism (Bywaters et al. 1963; McGill et al. 1984). Possible associations include gout (Stockman et al. 1980), ochronosis (Reginato et al. 1973; Rynes et al. 1975), familial hypocalciuric hypercalcaemia (Marx et al. 1981) and perhaps other causes of sustained hypercalcaemia, diabetes mellitus (Solnica et al. 1966; Boussina et al. 1971), and X-linked hypophosphataemic rickets (Taylor and Hothersall 1991). An association with hypothyroidism is controversial (Jones et al. 1992a). An excellent review of these associated diseases was recently published (Jones et al. 1992a)

Clinical features

CPPD disease is a clinically heterogeneous disorder causing both acute and chronic arthritis. Its presentations have been separated into seven syndromes based on clinical features (Ryan and McCarty 1993) (Table 7).

The most commonly recognized form of CPPD disease is the acute arthritis known as pseudogout (or CPPD disease type A). Pseudogout is often clinically indistinguishable from gout, hence its name. It is characterized by the acute onset of pain, warmth, erythema, and swelling usually affecting a single joint. The knee is most commonly involved. Other large joints such as shoulders, wrists, elbows, and ankles may be affected. Pseudogout occurs only rarely in small joints. Attacks are variable in duration, lasting from 2 to 108 days (O'Duffy 1976). Few other signs or symptoms are present. Precipitants of acute attacks include intercurrent illnesses, stroke, trauma, surgery (particularly parathyroidectomy; Glass and Grahame 1976), and rapid diuresis (O'Duffy 1973; O'Duffy 1976).

In the extremely elderly or ill patient, acute pseudogout may have a dramatic presentation. High fever, hypotension, and delerium may mimic sepsis or other systemic diseases (Bong and Bennett 1981).

CPPD disease may have a rheumatoid-like (type B) presentation. This form of CPPD disease accounts for less than 5 per cent of patients with CPPD disease. Symptoms include generalized joint pain and stiffness. The large joints such as knees, wrists, and elbows are commonly involved. Morning stiffness may be prolonged. Synovitis is noted on physical examination. Features which distinguish CPPD disease from rheumatoid arthritis include the absence

Table 7   Clinical presentations of CPPD disease

Type	Clinical description	Frequency (%)
A	Pseudogout/acute inflammatory monoarthritis	25
B	Pseudorheumatoid/polyarthritis with synovitis	5
C and D	Pseudo-osteoarthritis/joint degeneration with (type C) or without (type D) acute attacks	50
E	Lanthanic/asymptomatic	?
F	Pseudoneurotrophic/severe joint destruction with or without neuropathy	Rare
Others	Tophaceous CPPD deposits Spinal CPPD deposition Crowned dens syndrome Spinal stenosis	Rare

of small joint involvement, negative serum rheumatoid factor, and the presence of CPPD crystals in the synovial fluid of involved joints. In addition, patients with rheumatoid arthritis have polyarthritis which flares in phase, while the patients with pseudorheumatoid disease will have joint flares out of phase with one another (Ryan and McCarty 1993).

More than 50 per cent of patients with CPPD disease present with an osteoarthritis-like syndrome. These patients are classified as having the type C and type D forms of the disease. They have pain, stiffness, and limited range of motion of the affected joints. Joints not commonly involved in osteoarthritis may be affected, such as shoulders, elbows, and wrists. Examination shows little or no synovitis. Radiographs may show severe degenerative joint disease. Patients with the type C disease differ from those with type D in that they have acute attacks superimposed on chronic symptoms. Patients with the type D disease do not have acute attacks.

CPPD disease type E is clinically silent. It is also referred to as lanthanic CPPD disease. It is picked up incidently as radiographic chondrocalcinosis. This may be the most common type of CPPD disease.

Type F (or neuropathic) CPPD disease remains controversial and is rare; although described in patients with tertiary syphilis and severe neurotrophic arthritis (McCarty 1966). A similar clinical picture can be seen even in the absence of significant neuropathy (Menkes et al. 1976).

Although this classification scheme is helpful in describing patients with CPPD disease, not all cases are easily catagorized. The scheme does serve to emphasize the clinical heterogeneity of this disorder and the fact that CPPD disease must be considered as a cause of acute and chronic, inflammatory and non-inflammatory arthritis.

Tophaceous deposits of CPPD crystals have been described, but are not commonly seen (Jones et al. 1992b). In the wrist they can cause median nerve compression (Rate et al. 1992). In the spine, they may involve the ligamentum flavum and have been reported to produce symptoms of central canal stenosis (Delamarter et al. 1993) as well as cervical myelopathy (Berghausen et al. 1987). The crowned dens syndrome involves the deposition of CPPD (or BCP) crystals around the atlantoaxial joint and is a cause of acute neck pain (Bouvet et al. 1985). CPPD deposits rarely occur in tendons, bursas, and bone (Jones et al. 1992b; Kanterewicz et al. 1993).

Laboratory investigation

CPPD disease is defined by the presence of CPPD crystals in the synovial fluid of affected joints. Synovial fluids should be collected in heparin-containing tubes and carefully examined under polarized-light microscopy for the positively birefringent rhomboidal crystals of calcium pyrophosphate dihydrate (Fig. 11). These crystals may be sparse or abundant and can be either intra- or extracellular. Their number is not correlated with the degree of inflammation in the joint (Ryan and McCarty 1993). Synovial fluid from patients with acute pseudogout may have cell counts as low as 500 cells/mm³ or as high as 50 000 cells/mm³. The mean cell counts are similar to those of acute gout (20 000 cells/mm³) with greater than 90 per cent polymorphonuclear leucocytes (Ryan and McCarty 1993). Fluid may be haemorrhagic, particularly early in an attack (Ryan and McCarty 1993). Many synovial fluids will also contain BCP crystals (Rachow et al. 1988). During the acute attack, serum levels of acute-phase reactants may be elevated.

Radiographs of the affected joint may not be helpful in establishing a diagnosis acutely. However, the presence of chondrocalcinosis increases the likelihood of CPPD disease. Chondrocalcinosis is found in both fibrocartilage and hyaline articular cartilage. Common sites for chondrocalcinosis are the menisci of the knee (Fig. 12), the triangular cartilage of the wrist (Fig. 13), and the symphysis pubis (Fig. 14) (Ryan and McCarty 1993). Other radiographic changes may provide helpful supportive data. Typical findings include eburnation, joint space narrowing, and subchondral cyst formation (Resnick et al. 1977). Osteophyte formation is variable, but may be less common than in osteoarthritis. Progressive destruction of the joint with bony collapse and loose body formation occurs frequently in CPPD disease.

The distribution and pattern of radiographic involvement may be helpful in differentiating CPPD disease from osteoarthritis. CPPD disease affects joints not commonly involved in osteoarthritis. Axial involvement with intervertebral disc calcification, sacroiliac erosions, and subchondral cysts of the facet joints occur with CPPD disease. In the knee, tricompartmental involvement or isolated patellofemoral abnormalities are seen with CPPD disease more commonly than with osteoarthritis. Cortical erosions on the femur superior to the patella and osteonecrosis of the medial femoral condyle may also be diagnostic clues to CPPD disease (Lagier 1974; Watt and Dieppe 1983).

Patients with CPPD disease should be screened for one of the unusual metabolic disorders that promotes premature CPPD deposition. Laboratory evaluation should include serum levels of calcium, magnesium, phosphate, iron, and measurement of iron-binding capacity, and alkaline phosphatase.

Diagnosis

A definite diagnosis of CPPD disease can only be made when typical crystals are seen in synovial fluid with polarized-light miscroscopy.

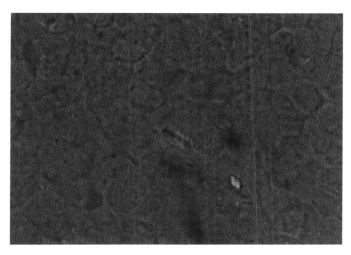

Fig. 11 Typical, positively birefringent crystals of calcium pyrophosphate dihydrate are seen here. Note the rhomboid shape and the weak birefringence.

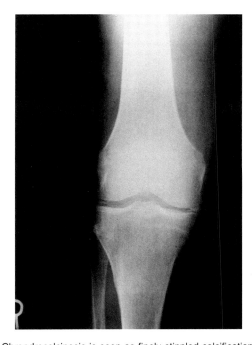

Fig. 12 Chrondrocalcinosis is seen as finely stippled calcification of the cartilage in the knee.

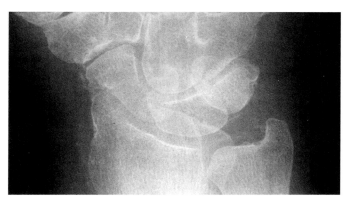

Fig. 13 Chrondrocalcinosis is seen in the triangular cartilage of the wrist.

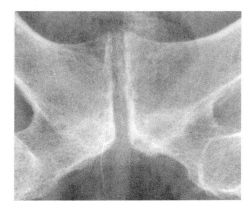

Fig. 14 Chrondrocalcinosis is seen in the pubic symphysis.

Phase-contrast microscopy may be a useful adjunct in detecting crystals. Radiographic changes can be used to establish a probable diagnosis. Diagnostic criteria based on crystal identification and radiological findings have been proposed (Ryan and McCarty 1993).

The differential diagnosis of pseudogout is much the same as that of gout. Infectious arthritis, trauma, and other crystal-associated arthropathies are the conditions that are most often mistaken for pseudogout. The chronic arthritis of CPPD disease can be mistaken for osteoarthritis, any one of the seronegative spondylarthropathies, rheumatoid arthritis, or neurotrophic arthritis.

Pathogenesis (Fig. 15)

The pathogenesis of CPPD disease remains obscure. Conceptually, CPPD crystal deposition, like gout, can be divided into phases of crystal formation, crystal release, and the induction and cessation of an inflammatory response. Using gout as a paradigm, much of the work on the pathophysiology of CPPD deposition rests on the theory that various metabolic abnormalities lead via a final common pathway to CPPD crystal formation. Unlike gout, the nature of this final common pathway remains unclear. Both radiological and histological studies of affected joints implicate cartilage as the primary site of CPPD crystal deposition. Crystals form in both fibrocartilage and the mid-zone of hyaline articular cartilage. The smallest and presumably the earliest crystals are found adjacent to chondrocytes or may replace the chondron (Pritzker *et al.* 1988). Crystals occur less commonly in synovium and tendon and may form in areas of chondroid metaplasia in these tissues (Beutler *et al.* 1993).

In cartilage, crystals are associated with large or 'hypertrophic' chondrocytes which contain unusual inclusions (Masuda *et al.* 1989). These are not seen in osteoarthritic cartilage. Fragmented collagen fibres and histochemical markers associated with degenerated cartilage such as type I collagen, S-100 protein, and the proteoglycan, dermatan sulphate, have been identified near crystal deposits (Masuda *et al.* 1989).

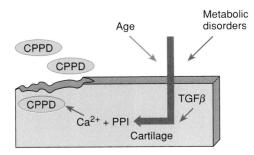

Fig. 15 Scheme of the pathogenesis of CPPD crystal deposition.

Theoretically, three components influence CPPD crystal formation. Changes in local concentrations of calcium and pyrophosphate as well as alterations of cartilage matrix might favour crystallogenesis. Despite the association between sustained hypercalcaemia and CPPD disease, no consistent changes in local calcium concentrations in affected joints have been documented (Ryan and McCarty 1993). Moreover, treatment of hyperparathyroidism, for example, does not usually ameliorate the arthritis (Pritchard and Jessop 1977). Studies of crystal formation in gels implicate a role for matrix in influencing crystal formation (Mandel and Mandel 1985), but in general the influence of matrix changes has been difficult to approach in the laboratory. For these and other reasons, much of the work on CPPD crystal formation has concentrated on pyrophosphate metabolism.

Pyrophosphate levels are elevated in the synovial fluids of patients with CPPD disease when compared with patients with other types of arthritis (Silcox and McCarty 1974). Moreover, skin fibroblasts from patients with familial CPPD disease have higher levels of pyrophosphate than those from normal controls (Lust et al. 1981). In vitro, normal hyaline and fibrocartilage elaborate extracellular pyrophosphate while other joint tissues do not (Ryan et al. 1981).

Thus, disordered pyrophosphate metabolism appears to have a crucial role in CPPD crystal formation. Whether this pyrophosphate is generated extracellularly through the activity of the family of ectoenzymes known as nucleoside triphosphate pyrophosphohydrolases (Huang et al. 1994), or is made inside the chondrocyte (Rosenthal et al. 1991), remains unclear. A role for transforming growth factor-β, a cartilage growth factor involved in repair, is supported by its unique ability to stimulate pyrophosphate elaboration by cartilage (Rosenthal et al. 1991), and to increase articular cartilage vesiculation (Derfus et al. 1994).

Understanding pyrophosphate metabolism may aid in determining the link between CPPD disease and its associated metabolic disorders. For example, magnesium is a cofactor of pyrophosphatase, which hydrolyses pyrophosphate to phospate. Thus, low magnesium would prevent action of this enzyme and favour elevated pyrophosphate concentrations in the joint. Similarly, hypophosphatasia which is characterized by low alkaline phosphatase activity could cause elevation of pyrophosphate levels by decreasing pyrophosphate hydrolysis.

When concentrations of pyrophosphate and calcium as well as matrix conditions are favourable, CPPD crystals form. Clinical symptoms arise when crystals are released into the synovial space. The mechanisms through which crystals are released into the joint space remain unknown. It has been postulated that trauma or sudden changes in crystal solubility may induce crystal release. Like MSU crystals, CPPD crystals are phlogistic and initiate an inflammatory response similar to that initiated by gout crystals (Malawista et al. 1985). The smallest crystals may be the most inflammatory (Ishikawa et al. 1987). Like gout, the factors terminating an acute attack remain speculative.

Management

Because our understanding of the pathophysiology of CPPD disease is inadequate, we have no specific treatments for this disorder. Standard therapies include NSAIDs, intra-articular corticosteroids, and colchicine. The management of acute and chronic CPPD deposition disease is summarized in Boxes 3 and 4.

NSAIDs are the most commonly used therapy for CPPD disease. There are no controlled trials of their efficacy and no single NSAID is preferable over others. Sulindac may be renal sparing (Ciabottoni et al. 1984), and may be safer than other NSAIDs in this elderly population.

Joint aspiration with intra-articular instillation of corticosteroids remains a mainstay of therapy for patients with pseudogout. Although no prospective trials of intra-articular corticosteroids in CPPD exist, two retrospective studies support the their effectiveness in shortening the duration of an acute attack (O'Duffy 1976; Masuda and Ishikawa 1987). As in gout, there has been a resurgence of interest in using parenteral corticosteroids, particularly ACTH, for acute pseudogout. Doses vary between 40 IU and 80 IU given every 8 h with a 3-day taper (Ritter et al. 1993).

Intravenous colchicine is of proven efficacy in acute pseudogout (Spilberg et al. 1980). However, the age and comorbidities of patients with CPPD disease often preclude its use. Low-dose oral colchicine may be useful prophylactically. At doses of 1 mg/day, it reduced the frequency of acute attacks of pseudogout in one small study (Avarellos and Spilberg 1986).

Other less traditional treatments for CPPD disease have been proposed. Magnesium carbonate increases the solubility of CPPD crystals and acts as a cofactor for pyrophosphatases. At a dosage of 10 mEq thrice daily, magnesium carbonate decreased the severity of symptoms in patients with chronic CPPD deposition disease (Doherty and Dieppe 1983). Intra-articular Arteparon, a glycosaminoglycan polysulphate, was demonstrated to decrease pain, stiffness, and immobility in one uncontrolled trial (Sarkozi et al. 1988). Intra-articular yttrium-90 combined with steroids was also effective in patients with chronic knee pain from CPPD diseases (Doherty and Dieppe 1981). Intramuscular gold has been used in patients with a pseudorheumatoid presentation with reportedly good results (Ryan and McCarty 1993). Rest, splinting, and eventual joint replacement may be helpful adjunctive measures.

Prognosis

The prognosis for CPPD disease patients is not known. Most cases of acute pseudogout are alleviated with standard therapy. However, as no good prophylactic treatment exists, and the disease often coexists with severe joint degeneration, many patients have unrelenting symptoms from CPPD disease.

The basic calcium phosphate (BCP)-associated syndromes

BCP crystals include hydroxyapatite, octacalcium phosphate, and tricalcium phosphate. These crystals are often (less accurately)

Box 3 Management of acute CPPD deposition disease

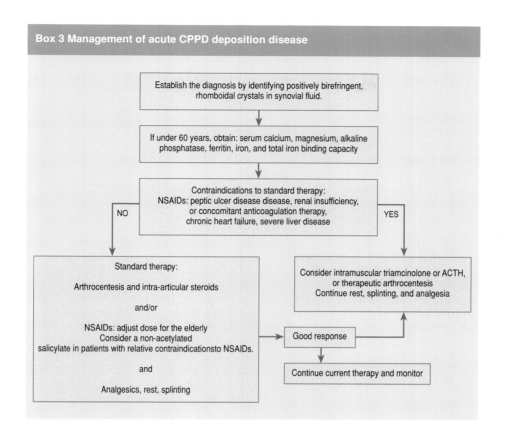

Box 4 Management of chronic CPPD deposition disease

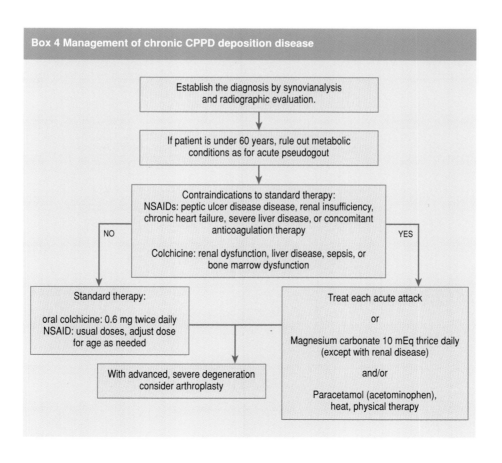

referred to as apatite or hydroxyapatite crystals. They are associated with a wide variety of clinical syndromes as illustrated in Table 8. The management of BCP crystal diseases is summarized in Box 5.

History

Calcific periarthritis and tendinitis have been recognized for many years, and a clinical syndrome similar to Milwaukee shoulder syndrome was described by Robert Adams in 1857 (McCarty 1989). With the identification of BCP crystals in the synovial fluid of patients with arthritis (Dieppe *et al.* 1976), interest in these crystals and their biological effects grew. Although several BCP-associated syndromes have recently been characterized, there is still much to learn about the significance and distribution of BCP crystals.

Arthritis associated with BCP crystals

Milwaukee shoulder syndrome

This unusual form of arthritis is one of the better defined of the BCP crystal-associated syndromes (McCarty *et al.* 1981; Halverson *et al.* 1984; Halverson *et al.* 1990). Milwaukee shoulder syndrome was initially described in 1981 as a severe shoulder arthropathy of elderly women.

Thirty patients with Milwaukee shoulder syndrome have been carefully described. (Halverson *et al.* 1990). The syndrome is more common in women then men. Patients describe a gradual onset of mild to moderate shoulder pain that is often bilateral and worse at night. Symptoms are more severe on the dominant side. Knee pain, stiffness, and swelling may also occur. Instability, large effusions, and loose bodies are noted on examination of the shoulder. A history of

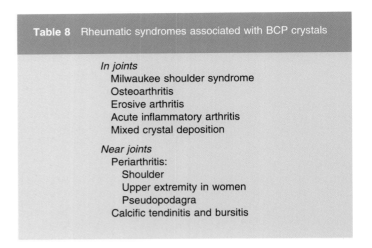

Table 8 Rheumatic syndromes associated with BCP crystals

In joints
  Milwaukee shoulder syndrome
  Osteoarthritis
  Erosive arthritis
  Acute inflammatory arthritis
  Mixed crystal deposition

Near joints
  Periarthritis:
    Shoulder
    Upper extremity in women
    Pseudopodagra
  Calcific tendinitis and bursitis

trauma or overuse may antedate the development of this syndrome. Renal disease may also be a predisposing factor (Halverson *et al.* 1987).

Radiographs show exaggerated joint degeneration (Fig. 16). Glenohumeral joint space narrowing, deformities of the humeral head with focal osteoporosis, small osteophytes, loose bodies, and calcifications are particularly characteristic. Large and extensive rotator cuff tears are commonly seen on arthrograms. Knee involvement is common and differs from primary osteoarthritis in that the lateral compartment is often predominantly involved. Synovial fluids have low white blood-cell counts (less than 500 cells/mm³). Particulate collagens and variable levels of active proteases have been

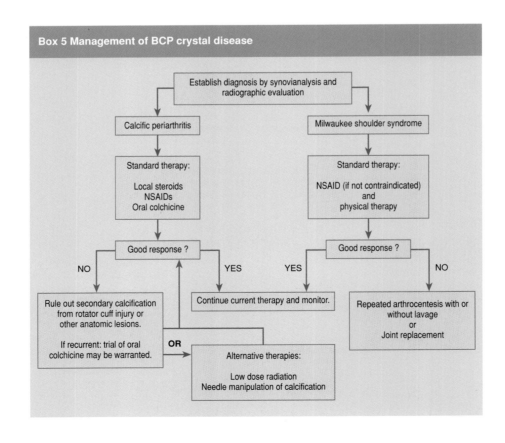

Box 5 Management of BCP crystal disease

Establish diagnosis by synovianalysis and radiographic evaluation

Calcific periarthritis

Standard therapy:
Local steroids
NSAIDs
Oral colchicine

Good response ?

NO — Rule out secondary calcification from rotator cuff injury or other anatomic lesions. If recurrent: trial of oral colchicine may be warranted.

YES — Continue current therapy and monitor.

OR — Alternative therapies:
Low dose radiation
Needle manipulation of calcification

Milwaukee shoulder syndrome

Standard therapy:
NSAID (if not contraindicated) and physical therapy

Good response ?

YES — Continue current therapy and monitor.

NO — Repeated arthrocentesis with or without lavage or Joint replacement identified in effusions from patients with Milwaukee shoulder syndrome. CPPD crystals are present in one-third of patients. There is currently no widely available method for detecting or quantifying BCP crystals. They can not be reliably identified with conventional or polarized-light microscopy. Stains such as Alizarin red are sensitive but not specific for BCP crystals (Halverson and McCarty 1979). Characteristic crystals can be seen under electron microscopy. At certain centres, a semiquantitative radiometric assay based on diphosphonate binding is in use (Halverson and McCarty 1979).

The pathogenesis of Milwaukee shoulder syndrome remains an area of active research. BCP crystals are mitogenic and induce the elaboration of collagenase and other proteases from synovial fibroblasts (Cheung *et al.* 1981) and chondrocytes (Cheung *et al.* 1983*a*). These proteases may be responsible for the extensive destruction of joint structures seen in this syndrome.

No specific therapy is available for Milwaukee shoulder syndrome. Some patients may respond to conservative treatment with analgesics such as NSAIDs and repeated joint aspirations. The utility of intra-articular corticosteroid injections remains unclear. With far-advanced disease or collapse of the humeral head, shoulder arthroplasties may be indicated.

The prognosis for recovery of motion and decreased pain in patients with far-advanced joint degeneration is poor.

BCP crystals in osteoarthritis

BCP crystals are found in 30 to 60 per cent of synovial fluids from patients with osteoarthritis using widely available detection techniques (Dieppe *et al.* 1979; Gibilisco *et al.* 1985). Small or sparse submicroscopic crystals may be found in even higher percentages of osteoarthritic synovial fluids when carefully examined (Swan *et al.* 1994). The quantity of BCP crystal present correlates with the degree of radiographic degeneration. There is no association between synovial fluid cell count (Dieppe *et al.* 1979) or the pattern of radiographic appearance (Halverson and McCarty 1986) and BCP crystals. Thus, the significance of these crystals is unclear.

Erosive arthritis associated with BCP crystals

Several patients with erosive arthritis associated with BCP crystals have been described (Schumacher *et al.* 1981; Zwillich *et al.* 1988). These patients have peripheral or axial arthritis with acute attacks. Pre-existing renal disease, chronic arthritis, and tophus-like subcutaneous nodules have also been described. Radiographs show bony erosions and calcifications. ACTH and colchicine improve symptoms in some patients.

Acute arthritis associated with BCP crystals

A small number of patients with an acute gout-like syndrome associated with BCP crystals in the synovial fluid have been reported (Schumacher *et al.* 1977). These patients have elevated synovial fluid cell counts and normal radiographs. They may represent an early stage of the erosive arthritis described above.

Mixed crystal deposition

BCP and CPPD crystals frequently coexist in a single joint (Dieppe *et al.* 1977; Rachow *et al.* 1988). It is more common to see these crystals together than to identify either one alone. No clear radiographic or clinical syndromes have been characterized on the basis of the co-existence of these two crystals.

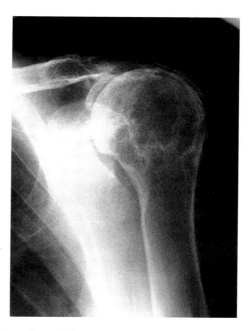

Fig. 16 This radiograph illustrates typical findings in Milwaukee shoulder syndrome. Note the abnormally high position of the humeral head.

Syndromes associated with non-articular BCP crystals

Periarthritis associated with BCP crystals

BCP crystals often cause periarthritis. BCP periarthritis occurs most often around the shoulder joint of people between the ages of 30 and 60 years. Familial forms, involving multiple sites, have been described (Marcos *et al.* 1981). Renal failure may predispose to BCP deposition. Patients usually present with acute pain, warmth, erythema, and swelling in the affected area lasting for several weeks. The diagnosis is suggested by the presence of extrarticular calcium deposits on radiographs.

Two variants of BCP periarthritis have been characterized recently. The first is periarthritis involving the hand and elbow in young women (McCarthy *et al.* 1993; Yosipovitch and Yosipovitch 1993). This occurs in otherwise healthy young women without an antecedent history of trauma. Several patients had recently given birth and were breast feeding. The symptoms are acute and severe and are often misdiagnosed as gout or cellulitis. Sites of involvement include the lateral epicondyle of the elbow, the wrist, and the finger joints. Symptoms respond dramatically to intralesional corticosteroids. Follow-up radiographs demonstrate resolution of the calcific deposits within 7 to 36 days.

The term hydroxyapatite pseudopodagra has been used to refer to BCP periarthritis of the first metatarsophalangeal joint. These patients present with acute pain, swelling, warmth, and erythema of this joint (Fam and Rubenstein 1989). It often occurs in young women and is clinically indistinguishable from gout. Radiographs show amorphous periarticular calcifications. No patients had metabolic abnormalities, although pseudopodagra has been reported in pregnancy (McCarty 1991). Attacks are self-limited, lasting 1 to 3 weeks, and respond to conservative treatment with NSAIDs. Intralesional corticosteroids have also been used with good success (McCarty 1991).

Calcific tendinitis and bursitis

This syndrome frequently involves the shoulder. It is often clinically indistinguishable from traumatic tendinitis or bursitis. Patients present with acute onset of severe pain in the affected area lasting several weeks. The radiographic presence of amorphous calcific deposits and the absence of antecedent trauma suggest this diagnosis. Calcific deposits in the shoulder may also occur with chronic rotator cuff injuries. These deposits occur at the insertion site of the rotator cuff on the humerus and are not reabsorbed with time. In contrast, the calcifications of calcific tendinitis occur in metaplastic fibrocartilage within the rotator cuff and disappear with time (Sakar and Uthoff 1984). The pathophysiology of calcific tendinitis is unknown. Treatment with NSAIDs and intralesional corticosteroids usually results in rapid improvement. Colchicine may also be of some benefit (Swannell *et al.* 1970).

Calcium oxalate arthritis

Calcium oxalate crystals produce an unusual form of arthritis. Although seen most commonly in patients with renal failure on dialysis, calcium oxalate arthritis has also been described in patients with bowel disease and primary oxalosis, a rare inborn error of metabolism.

Epidemiology

There are no good studies of the incidence or prevalence of calcium oxalate arthritis in susceptible populations. Primary oxalosis is quite rare. In contrast, 90 per cent of patients on long-term haemodialysis have pathological evidence of calcium oxalate deposition in kidney and bone tissue (Fayemi *et al.* 1977).

Ascorbic acid supplementation is an added risk factor in patients on dialysis (Balcke *et al.* 1984), although oxalate arthritis has been reported in patients on dialysis who did not receive ascorbic acid supplements (Rosenthal *et al.* 1988). Other risk factors include short bowel syndrome from bowel bypass surgery or inflammatory bowel disease, dietary excesses of unusual foods such as rhubarb, and thiamine and pyridoxine deficiencies (Williams and Smith 1968) (Table 9).

Clinical features

Oxalate arthritis most often occurs in the setting of renal failure. No large-scale studies of affected patients exist. Patients usually present with acute mono- or oligoarticular arthritis involving the small joints of the hands particularly the proximal interphalangeals and the metacarpophalangeals. Oxalate arthritis may be symmetric, and is often accompanied by tenosynovitis. Bursal involvement has also been described. Unlike gout, initial episodes may be prolonged and chronic arthritis may rapidly develop.

Primary oxalosis results from one of two defined enzyme deficiencies (Williams and Smith 1968). It is inherited as a recessive trait. Patients with primary oxalosis succumb to endstage renal disease in their early twenties. They have diffuse oxalate deposits at autopsy which may also involve articular tissues. Acute and chronic arthritis (Hockaday *et al.* 1964) as well as tenosynovitis (Cohen and Reid 1935) have been described in these patients, but identification of crystals in affected joints has been difficult (Hockaday *et al.* 1964).

Table 9 Conditions associated with calcium oxalate arthritis

Endstage renal disease on dialysis
Short bowel syndrome
Unusual diets rich in rhubarb, spinach, or ascorbic acid
Thiamine deficiency
Pyridoxine deficiency
Primary oxalosis

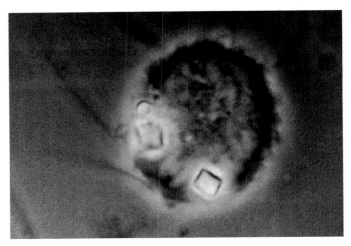

Fig. 17 The typical bipyramidal crystals of calcium oxalate dihydrate are seen here inside a cell.

Diagnosis

The diagnosis of calcium oxalate arthritis is made by identifying characteristic crystals in synovial fluid from affected joints. Calcium oxalate crystals may be of two morphologies (Hoffman *et al.* 1982; Reginato *et al.* 1986). The more commonly identified type is weddelite or calcium oxalate dihydrate. This is a positively birefringent bipyramidal crystal (Fig. 17). Less commonly, calcium oxalate monohydrate (whewellite) occurs. Whewellite is polymorphic and may be seen as chunks, rods, ovals, or microspherules. Scanning electron microscopy and X-ray diffraction are often necessary to confirm the identities of these crystals.

Synovianalysis usually shows clear or bloody fluid with normal viscosity. Cell counts are typically low and often neutrophils predominate, although large mononuclear cells have also been described (Hoffman *et al.* 1982).

Radiographs are not diagnostic but may be helpful. Miliary calcific deposits in the soft tissue can be seen. Similarly, vascular calcification is a common finding. Less commonly, bony abnormalities such as localized or metaphyseal sclerosis, pseudoarthroses, and pathological fractures can be seen (Milgram 1974; Gherardi *et al.* 1980; Nartijn and Thijn 1982).

Pathophysiology

Oxalic acid is a metabolic end product of amino acid synthesis and ascorbic acid metabolism. It is well absorbed from the gut and is

Crystal	Morphology	Setting	Significance
Lipid	Round	Trauma	Uncertain
Cholesterol	Plate-like	Unclear	Uncertain
Steroids	Any shape, very bright	After injection	Recent steroid injection
Cryoglobulin	Polygonal, positively birefringent	Cryoglobulinaemia	
Charcot–Leyden	Bipyramidal or hexagonal	Hypereosinophilia	
Cystine	Hexahedral, weak or bright	Cystinosis	
Xanthine	Rhomboidal or plate-like	Xanthinuria	

Table 10 Other crystals found in synovial fluid

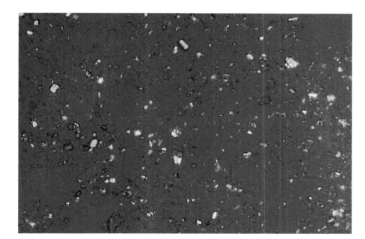

Fig. 18 Steroids crystals can be seen in synovial fluids after intra-articular corticosteroid injections.

renally excreted. Hence oxalate may accumulate in tissues from excess absorption, overproduction, or underexcretion. Renal failure causes underexcretion of oxalate and levels are high in patients on dialysis. Neither haemo- nor peritoneal dialysis adequately clears oxalate from tissues (Op de Hock *et al.* 1980). Causes of overproduction include the enzyme defects of primary oxalosis, and thiamine and pyridoxine deficiencies. Dietary excesses of spinach, rhubarb, and ascorbic acid supplements may also raise oxalate levels. Excess intestinal absorption may be due to short bowel syndrome from any causes. The most common associated bowel disorders are bowel bypass syndrome from obesity surgery and inflammatory bowel disease.

Once oxalate crystals form in articular tissues, they are released by unknown mechanisms and initiate an inflammatory response (Faires and McCarty 1962).

Management

There is no specific treatment for calcium oxalate arthritis. In general, response to conventional therapies including NSAIDs, intra-articular corticosteroids, colchicine, and increased dialysis are poor. The grim outlook for patients with primary oxalosis may be brightened by early liver transplantation before renal failure has developed (Watts *et al.* 1991).

Other crystals

Other types of crystals can be identified in synovial fluid. These crystals are listed in Table 10. Commonly seen crystals are illustrated in Figs 18, 19, and 20.

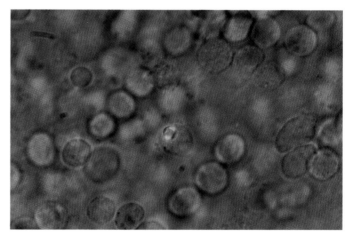

Fig. 19 The typical appearance of lipid crystals in synovial fluid.

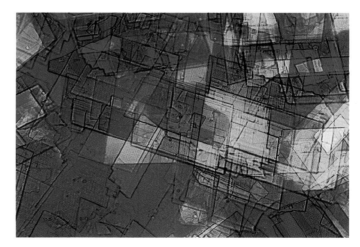

Fig. 20 The typical appearance of cholesterol crystals in synovial fluid.

References

Abbott, R.D., Brand, F.N., Kannel, W.B., and Castelli, W.P. (1988). Gout and coronary heart disease: the Framingham study. *Journal of Clinical Epidemiology*, **41**, 237–42.

Abramson, S.B. and Weissmann, G. (1989). The mechanism of action of nonsteroidal antiinflammatory drugs. *Arthritis and Rheumatism*, **32**, 1–9.

Abramson, S., Hoffstein, S.T., and Weismann, G. (1982). Superoxide anion generated by human neutrophils exposed to monosodium urate. *Arthritis and Rheumatism*, **15**, 174–80.

Adriani, J. and Naraghi, M. (1985). Allopurinol: actions, adverse reaction and drug interactions. *IM*, **6**, 114–23.

Alepa, F.P. *et al.* (1967). Relationship between glycogen storage disease and tophaceous gout. *American Journal of Medicine*, **42**, 58–63.

Avarellos, A. and Spilberg, I. (1986). Colchicine prophylaxis in pseudogout. *Journal of Rheumatology*, **13**, 804–6.

Axelrod, D. and Preston, S. (1989). Comparison of parenteral adrenocorticotropic hormone with oral indomethacin in the treatment of acute gout. *Arthritis and Rheumatism*, **31**, 803–5.

Baethge, B.A., Work, J., Landreneau, M.D., and McDonald, J.C. (1993). Tophaceous gout in patients with renal transplants treated with cyclosporine A. *Journal of Rheumatology*, **20**, 718–20.

Balcke, P. *et al.* (1984). Ascorbic acid aggravates secondary hyperoxalemia in patients on chronic hemodialysis. *Annals of Internal Medicine*, **10**, 344–5.

Ball, G.V. and Sorenson, L.B. (1969). Pathogenesis of hyperuricemia in sauternine gout. *New England Journal of Medicine*, **280**, 1199–202.

Balsa, A. *et al.* (1990). Familial articular chondrocalcinosis in the Spanish population. *Annals of the Rheumatic Diseases*, **49**, 531–5.

Barthelemy, C.R. *et al.* (1984). Gouty arthritis: a prospective radiographic evaluation of sixty patients. *Skeletal Radiology*, **11**, 1–8.

Bartles, E.C. (1957). Gout as a complication of surgery. *Surgical Clinics of North America*, **38**, 845–8.

Becker, M.A. (1988). Clincial aspects of monosodium urate monohydrate crystal deposition disease (gout). *Rheumatic Diseases Clinics of North America*, **14**, 377–94.

Becker, M.A. and Kim, M. (1987). Regulation of purine synthesis *de novo* in human fibroblasts by purine nucleotides and phosphoribosylpyrophosphate. *Journal of Biological Chemistry*, **262**, 14531–5.

Bellamy, K.N., Downie, W.W., and Buchana, W.W. (1987). Observations on spontaneous improvement in patients with podagra; implications for therapeutic trials fo non-steroidal anti-inflammatory drugs. *British Journal of Clinical Pharmacology*, **24**, 33–6.

Benedict, J.D., Forsham, P.H., and Stetten, D.W., Jr (1949). The metabolism of uric acid in normal and gouty human studied with the aid of istopic uric acid. *Journal of Biological Chemistry*, **181**, 183–93.

Berger, L. and Yu, T-F. (1960). Renal function in gout: an analysis of 524 gouty subjects including long-term follow-up studies. *Proceedings of the Royal Society of Medicine*, **53**, 522–6.

Berghausen, E.J. *et al.* (1987). Cervical myelopathy attributable to pseudogout. *Clinical Orthopaedics and Related Research*, **214**, 217–21.

Bergstrom, G. *et al.* (1986a). Joint disorders at ages 70, 75, and 79 years—a cross-sectional comparison. *British Journal of Rheumatology*, **25**, 333–41.

Bergstrom, G. *et al.* (1986b). Prevalence of rheumatoid arthritis, osteoarthritis, choncrocalcinosis and gouty arthritis at age 79. *Journal of Rheumatology*, **13**, 527–34.

Beutler, A., Rothfuss, S., Clayburne, G., Sieck, M., and Schumacher, H.R. (1993). Calcium pyrophosphate dihydrate crystal deposition in synovium: relationship to collagen fibers and chondrometaplasia. *Arthritis and Rheumatism*, **36**, 704–15.

Bhatt, A. and Spliberg, I. (1988). Purification of crystal-induced chemotactic factor from neutrophils. *Clinical Biochemistry*, **21**, 342–5.

Bishop, C., Garne, W., and Talbot, J.H. (1951). Pool size, turnover rate, and rapidity of equilibrium of injected isotopic uric acid in normal and pathological subjects. *Journal of Clinical Investigation*, **30**, 879–88.

Block, C., Hermann, G., and Yu, T.F. (1980). A radiologic re-evaluation of gout: a study of 2000 patients. *American Journal of Roentgenology*, **134**, 781–8.

Boger, W.P. and Strickland, S.C. (1955). Probenecid (Benemid) its use and side effects in 2502 patients. *Archives of Internal Medicine*, **95**, 83–92.

Bong, D. and Bennett, R. (1981). Pseudogout mimicking systemic disease. *Journal of the American Medical Association*, **246**, 1438–40.

Boston Collaborative Drug Surveillance Program (1974). Allopurinol and cytotoxic drugs. Interaction in relation to bone marrow depression. *Journal of the American Medical Association*, **227**, 1036–40.

Boussina, I. *et al.* (1971). Etude de la frequence du diabete sucre dans la chondrocalcinose articulaire. *Schweizerische Medizinische Wochenschrift*, **101**, 1413–17.

Bouvet, J. *et al.* (1985). Acute neck pain due to calcifications surrounding the odontoid process: the crowned dens syndrome. *Arthritis and Rheumatism*, **22**, 928–32.

Burak, D.A., Griffith, B.P., Thompson, M.E., and Kahl, L.E. (1992). Hyperuricemia and gout among heart transplant recipients receiving cyclosporine. *American Journal of Medicine*, **92**, 141–6.

Burt, H.M. and Dutt, Y.C. (1986). Growth of monosodium urate monohydrate crystals: effect of cartilage and synovial fluid components on *in vitro* growth rates. *Annals of the Rheumatic Diseases*, **45**, 858–64.

Burt, H.M. and Jackson, J.K. (1990). Role of membrane proteins in monososium urate crystal-membrane interactions: 2. Effect of pretreatment with membrane permeable and impermeable protein crosslinking agents. *Journal of Rheumatology*, **17**, 1359–63.

Buzzard, J., Bishop, C., and Talbott, J.H. (1955). The fate of uric acid in the normal and gouty human being. *Journal of Chronic Diseases*, **2**, 42–9.

Bywaters, E.G., Dixon, A., St J., and Scott, J.T. (1963). Joint lesion of hyperparathyroidism. *Annals of the Rheumatic Diseases*, **22**, 171–87.

Canosa, J.J. and Yood, R.A. (1979). Acute gouty bursitis: report of 15 cases. *Annals of the Rheumatic Diseases*, **38**, 326–8.

Cheung, H.S., Halverson, P.B., and McCarty, D.J. (1981). Release of collagenase, neutral protease and prostaglandins from cultured mammalian synovial cells by hydroxyapatite and calcium pyrophosphate dihydrate crystals. *Arthritis and Rheumatism*, **24**, 1338–44.

Cheung, H.S., Halverson, P.B., and McCarty, D.J. (1983a). Phagocytosis of hydroxyapatite or calcium pyrophosphate crystals by rabbit articular chondrocytes release of collagenase, neutral protease and prostaglandin E2 and F2. *Proceedings of the Society for Experimental Biology and Medicine*, **173**, 181–9.

Cheung, H.S., Bohon, S., and Kozin, F. (1983b). Kinetics of collagenase and neutral protease release by neutrophils exposed to microcrystalline sodium urate. *Connective Tissue Research*, **2**, 79–85.

Chua, C.C., Greenberg, M.L., Viau, A.T., Nucci, M., Brenchman, W.D., and Hershfield, M.S. (1988). Use of polyethylene glycol-modified uricase (PEG-uricase) to treat hyperuricemia in a patient with non-Hodgkin lymphoma. *Annals of Internal Medicine*, **109**, 114–17.

Chuck, A.J. *et al.* (1989). Crystal deposition in hypophosphatasia: a reappraisal. *Annals of the Rheumatic Diseases*, **48**, 571–6.

Ciabottoni, G. *et al.* (1984). Effects of sulindac and ibuporfen in patients with chronic glomerular disease. *New England Journal of Medicine*, **310**, 279–83.

Cohen, H. and Reid, J.B. (1935). Tenosynovitis crepitans associated with oxaluria. *Liverpool Med Chirurg, J*, **77**, 195–205.

Collins, J.G. (1988). *Prevalence of selected chronic conditions, United States 1983–85*. Advance data from Vital and Health Statistics of the National Center for Health Statistics, No. 155, USDHHS, Washington, DC.

Copeman, W.C.S. (1964). *A short history of the gout*. University of California Press. Los Angeles.

Darmawan, J., Valkenburg, H.A., Muriden, K.D., and Wigley R.D. (1992). The epidemiology of gout and hyperuricemia in a rural population of Java. *Journal of Rheumatology*, **19**, 1595–9.

Delamarter, R.B., Sherman, J.E., and Carr, J. (1993). Lumbar spinal stenosis secondary to calcium pyrophsophate crystal deposition. *Clinical Orthopedics*, **289**, 127–30.

Delbarre, F., Braun, S., and St. George-Chaumet, F. (1967). La Goutte: problems clinique, biologiques et therapeutices. *Semaines des Hopitaux Paris*, **43**, 623–33.

Derfus, B.A., Rosenthal, A.K., and Ryan, L.M. (1994). TGFβ1 and ascorbate each increase mineralizing vesicle elaboration from articular cartilage monolayers. *Arthritis and Rheumatism*, **35**, S75.

Dieppe, P.A. *et al.* (1976). Apatite deposition disease. A new arthropathy. *Lancet*, i, 266–76.

Dieppe, P.A. *et al.* (1977). Mixed crystal deposition disease and osteoarthritis. *British Medical Journal*, **1**, 150–60.

Dieppe, P.A. *et al.* (1979). Synovial fluid crystals. *Quarterly Journal of Medicine*, **192**, 533–53.

DiGiovine, F.S. *et al.* (1987). Interleukin 1(IL1) as a mediator of crystal arthritis. Stimulation of T cell and synovial fibroblast mitogenesis by urate crystal induced IL1. *Journal of Immunology*, **138**, 3213–18.

Dodds, W.J. and Steinbach, H.L. (1966). Gout associated with calcification of cartilage. *New England Journal of Medicine*, **275**, 745–9.

Doherty, M. and Dieppe, P.A. (1981). Effect of intra-articular yttrium-90 on chronic pyrophosphate arthropathy of the knee. *Lancet*, i, 1243–6.

Doherty, M. and Dieppe, P.A. (1983). Double blind placebo controlled trial of magnesium carbonate in chronic pyrophosphate arthropathy. *Annals of the Rheumatic Diseases*, **42** (Suppl), 106–7.

Doherty, M. and Dieppe, P. (1986). Crystal deposition in the elderly. *Clinics in the Rheumatic Diseases*, **12**, 97.

Emmerson, B.T. (1963). A comparison of uricosuric agents in gout, with special reference to sulfinpyrazone. *Medical Journal of Australia*, **1**, 839–44.

Emmerson, B.T. (1974). Atherosclerosis and urate metabolism. *Australian and New Zealand Journal of Medicine*, **3**, 410–12.

Faires, J.S. and McCarty, D.J. (1962). Acute synovitis in normal joints of man and dog produced by injections of microcrystalline sodium urate, calcium oxalate and corticosteroid esters. *Arthritis and Rheumatism*, **5**, 95.

Fam, A.G. and Rubenstein, J. (1989). Hydroxyapatite pseudopodagra: a syndrome of young women. *Arthritis and Rheumatism*, **32**, 741–7.

Fam, A.G., Lewtas, J., Stein, J., and Paton, T.W. (1992). Desensitization to allopurinol in patients with gout and cutaneous reactions. *American Journal of Medicine*, **93**, 299–302.

Fayemi, A.O., Ali, M., and Braun E.V. (1977). Oxalosis in hemodialysis patients. A pathologic study of 80 cases. *Archives of Pathology and Laborarory Medicine*, **103**, 58–62.

Feller, E.R. and Schumacher, H.R. (1972). Osteoarticular changes in Wilson's disease. *Arthritis and Rheumatism*, **15**, 259–66.

Felson, D.T., Anderson, J.J., Naimark, A., Kannel, W., and Meenan, R.F. (1989). The prevalence of chondrocalcinosis in the elderly and its association with knee osteoarthritis: the Framingham study. *Journal of Rheumatology*, **16**, 1241–5.

Ferry, A.P., Safir, A., and Melikian, H.E. (1985). Ocular abnormalities in patients with gout. *Annals of Opthalmology*, **17**, 632–5.

Fessel, J.W. (1967). Renal outcomes of gout and hyperuricemia. *American Journal of Medicine*, **42**, 27–37.

Fiechtner, J.J. and Simkin, P. (1981). Urate spherules in gouty synovia. *Journal of the American Medical Association*, **245**, 1533–6.

Forkas, W.K., Stanawitz, T., and Schneider, M. (1978). Saternine gout: lead-induced formation of guanine crystals. *Science*, **199**, 786–92.

Frei, E. *et al.* (1963). Renal complications of neoplastic diseases. *Journal of Chronic Diseases*, **16**, 757–76.

Freudweiler, M. (1899). Experimentelle Untersuchungen uber das wesen der Gichtnoter. *Deutsche Archiv der Klinische Medizin*, **63**, 266–355.

Garrod, A.B. (1876) *Treatise on gout and rheumatic gout (rheumatoid arthritis)* (3rd edn). Longmans Green and Co., London.

Gaucher, A. *et al.* (1977). Hereditary diffuse articular chondrocalcinosis. *Scandinavian Journal of Rheumatology*, **6**, 217–21.

Gaudreau, A. *et al.* (1981). Familial articular chondrocalcinosis in Quebec. *Arthritis and Rheumatism*, **24**, 611–15.

Gawoski, J.M., Balogh, K., and Landis, W.J. (1985). Aortic valve tophus: identification by X-ray diffraction of urate and calcium phosphates. *Journal of Clinical Pathology*, **38**, 873–6.

Gertler, M., Garn, S.M., and Levine, S.A. (1931). Serum uric acid in relation to age and physique in health and coronary artery disease. *Annals of Internal Medicine*, **34**, 1421–31.

Gherardi, G. *et al.* (1980). Bone oxalosis and renal osteodystrophy. *Archives of Pathology and Laboratory Medicine*, **104**, 105–11.

Gibilisco, P.A. *et al.* (1985). Synovial fluid crystals in osteoarthritis. *Arthritis and Rheumatism*, **28**, 511–15.

Gibson, T., Rodgers, A.V., Simmonds, H.A., and Toseland, P. (1984). Beer drinking and its effect on uric acid. *British Journal of Rheumatology*, **23**, 203–9.

Giclas, P.C., Ginsberg, M.H., and Cooper, N.R. (1979). Immunoglobulin G independent activation of the classical complement pathways by monosodium urate crystals. *Journal of Clinical Investigation*, **63**, 759–765.

Ginsberg, M.H., Jaques, B., Cochrane, C.G., and Griffin, J.H. (1980). Urate crystal-dependent cleavage of Hageman factor in human plasma and synovial fluid. *Journal of Laboratory and Clinical Medicine*, **95**, 497–506.

Glass, J.S. and Grahame, R. (1976). Chondrocalcinosis after parathyroidectomy. *Annals of the Rheumatic Diseases*, **35**, 521–5.

Golding, D.N. and Walshe, J.M. (1977). Arthropathy of Wilson's disease. *Annals of the Rheumatic Diseases*, **36**, 99–111.

Grahame, R. and Scott, J.T. (1970). Clincial survey of 354 patients with gout. *Annals of the Rheumatic Diseases*, **29**, 461–8,

Gresser, U., Gathof, B., and Zollner, N. (1990). Uric acid levels in southern Germany in 1989, a comparison with studies from 1962, 1971, and 1984. *Klinische Wochenschrift*, **68**, 1222–8.

Groff, G.D., Franck, W.A., and Raddatz, D.A. (1990). Systemic steroid therapy for acute gout: a clinical trial and review of the literature. *Seminars in Arthritis and Rheumatism*, **19**, 329–36.

Gutman, A.B. (1973). The past four decades of progress in the knowledge of gout with an assessment of the present status. *Arthritis and Rheumatism*, **16**, 431–45.

Gutman, A.B. and Yu, T-F. (1952). Current principles of management in gout. *American Journal of Medicine*, **13**, 744–59.

Gutman, A.B. and Yu, T-F. (1957). Protracted uricosuric therapy in tophaceous gout. *Lancet*, ii, 1258–60.

Hall, A.P., Barry, P.E., Dawber, T.R., and McNamara, P.M. (1967). Epidemiology of gout and hyeruricemia. *American Journal of Medicine*, **134**, 332–9.

Halverson, P.B. and McCarty, D.J. (1979). Identification of hydroxyapatite crystals in synovial fluid. *Arthritis and Rheumatism*, **22**, 389–95.

Halverson, P.B. and McCarty, D.J. (1986). Patterns of radiographic abnormalities associated with basic calcium phosphate and calcium pyrophosphate dihydrate crystal deposition in the knee. *Annals of the Rheumatic Diseases*, **45**, 603–5.

Halverson, P.B., McCarty, D.J., Cheung, H.S., and Ryan, L.M. (1984). Milwaukee shoulder syndrome: 11 additional cases with involvement of the knee in 7. *Seminars in Arthritis and Rheumatism*, **14**, 36–44.

Halverson, P.B., Cheung, H.S., and McCarty, D.J. (1987). Milwaukee shoulder syndrome (MSS): description of predisposing factors. *Arthritis and Rheumatism*, **30**, S131,

Halverson, P.B., Carrera, G.F., and McCarty, D.J. (1990). Milwaukee shoulder syndrome: fifteen additional cases and a description of contributing factors. *Archives of Internal Medicine*, **150**, 677–82.

Hamilton, E.B.D. *et al.* (1981). The natural history of arthritis in idiopathic haemochromotosis: progression of the clinical and radiologic features over ten years. *Quarterly Journal of Medicine*, **50**, 3321–9.

Hertz, P., Yager, H., and Richardson, J.A. (1972). Probenecid induced nephrotic syndrome. *Archives of Pathology*, **94**, 241–3.

Hippocrates (1886). *The genuine works of Hippocrates.* Vols 1 and 2. (trans. and annotated by F. Adams). Wood, New York.

Hochberg, M.C. (1991). Opportunities for the primary and secondary prevention of gout. *Mediguide to Inflammatory Diseases*, **10**, 1–5.

Hockaday, T.D.R., Clayton, J.E., Frederick, E.W., and Smith, L.H. (1964). Primary hyperoxaluria. *Medicine*, **43**, 315–45.

Hoffman, G.S. *et al.* (1982). Calcium oxalate micro-crystalline-associated arthritis in end stage renal disease. *Annals of Internal Medicine*, **97**, 36–42.

Hollander, J.L. (1953). Intra-articular hydrocortisone in arthritis and allied conditions. *Journal of Bone and Joint Surgery*, **35A**, 983.

Holmes, E.W. (1978). Regulation of purine biosynthesis *de novo*. In *Uric acid: handbook of experimental pharmacology*, Vol 51 (ed. W.N. Kelley and I.M. Weiner). Springer-Verlag, New York.

Holmes, E.W. *et al.* (1973). Human glutamine phosphoribosylpyrophosphate amidotransferase: kinetic and regulatory properties. *Journal of Biological Chemistry*, **248**, 144–50.

Huang, R. *et al.* (1994). Expression of the murine plasma cell nucleotide pyrophoshydrolase PC-1 is shared by human liver, bone and cartilage cells. Regulation of PC-1 expression in osteosarcoma cells by transforming growth factor-β. *Journal of Clinical Investigation*, **94**, 560–7.

Hunder, G.G., Worthington, J.W., and Bickel, W.H. (1968). Avascular necrosis of the femoral head in a patient with gout. *Journal of the American Medical Association*, **203**, 101–3.

Ishikawa, H., Ueba, Y., Isobe, T., and Hirohata, K. (1987). Interaction of polymorphonuclear leukocytes with calcium pyrophosphate dihydrate crystals deposited in chondrocalcinosis cartilage. *Rheumatology International*, **7**, 217–21.

Itakura, M., Sabina, R.L., Heald, P.W., and Holmes, E.W. (1981). Basis for the control of purine biosynthesis by purine ribonucleotides. *Journal of Clinical Investigation*, **67**, 994–1002.

Jones, A.C., Chuck, A.J., Arie, E.A., Green, D.J., and Doherty, M. (1992*a*). Diseases associated with calcium pyrophosphate deposition disease. *Seminars in Arthritis and Rheumatism*, **22**, 188–202.

Jones, A., Baron, N., Pattrick, M., and Doherty, M. (1992*b*). Tophaceous pyrophosphate deposition with extensor tendon rupture. *British Journal of Rheumatology*, **31**, 421–3.

Kanterewicz, E., Sanmarti, R., Panella, D., and Brugues, J. (1993). Tendon calcifications of the hip adductors in chondrocalcinosis: a radiologic study of 75 patients. *British Journal of Rheumatology*, **32**, 790–3.

Katz, W.A. and Ehrlich, G.E. (1968). The solubility of monosodium urate in serum and connective tissue fractions. *Arthritis and Rheumatism*, **11**, 492–7.

Kelley, W.N., Rosenbloom, F.M., Henderson, J.F., and Seegmiller, J.E. (1967). A specific enzyme defect in gout associated with overproduction of uric acid. *Proceedings of the National Academy of Sciences (USA)*, **57**, 1735–9.

Kelley, W.N. *et al.* (1969). Hypoxanthine-guanine phosphoribosyl transferase deficiency in gout. *Annals of Internal Medicine*, **70**, 155–206.

Kohn N.N. *et al.* (1962). The signficance of calcium phosphate crystals in the synovial fluid of arthritis patients: the 'pseudogout syndrome.' II. Identification of crystals. *Annals of Internal Medicine*, **56**, 738–45.

Kozin, F. and McCarty, D.J. (1977). Rheumatoid factors in the serum of gouty patients. *Arthritis and Rheumatism*, **18**, 49–58.

Kuzell, W.C., Seebach, L.M., Glover, R.P., and Jackman, A.E. (1966). Treatment of gout with allopurinol and sulfinpyrazone in combination and with allopurinol alone. *Annals of the Rheumatic Diseases*, **25**, 634–42.

Lagier, R. (1974). Case report: rare femoral erosions and osteoarthritis of the knee associated with chondrocalcinosis. A histological study of this cortical remodeling. *Virchows Archiv* (A), **364**, 215–23.

Lagier, R. and MacGee, W. (1983). Spondylodiscal erosions due to gout: anatomicroradiologic study of a case. *Annals of the Rheumatic Diseases*, **42**, 350–3.

Lally, E.W., Ho, G., Jr, and Kaplan, S.R. (1986). The clinical spectrum of gouty arthritis in women. *Archives of Internal Medicine*, **146**, 2221–5.

Lawrence, R.C. *et al.* (1989). Estimates of the prevalence of selected arthritic and musculoskeletal diseases in the United States. *Journal of Rheumatology*, **16**, 427–41.

Lawry, G.V., Fan, P.T., and Bluestone, R. (1988). Polyarticular versus monoarticular gout: a prospective comparative analysis of clinical features. *Medicine*, **67**, 335–43.

Lennane, G.A.Q., Rose B.S., and Isdale, I.C. (1960). Gout in the Maori. *Annals of the Rheumatic Diseases*, **19**, 120–5.

Lesch, M. and Nyhan, W.L. (1964). A familial disorder of uric acid metabolism and central nervous system funcion. *American Journal of Medicine*, **36**, 561–70.

Levinson, D.J. and Becker, M.A. (1993). Clinical gout and the pathogenesis of hyperuricemia. In *Arthritis and allied conditions* (12th edn) (ed. D.J. MCarty and W.J. Koopman.), pp. 1773–805. Lea and Febiger, Philadelphia.

Levinson, D.J. and Sorenson, L.B. (1980). Renal handling of uric acid in normal and gouty subjects: evidence for a 4-component system. *Annals of the Rheumatic Diseases*, **39**, 173–9.

Lieber, C.S. *et al.* (1962). Interrelation of uric acid and ethanol metabolism in man. *Journal of Clinical Investigation*, **41**, 1863–70.

Lin, H-Y., Rocher, L.L., McQuillan, M.A., Schmaltz, S., Palella, T.D., and Fox, I.H. (1989). Cyclosporine induced hyperuricemia and gout. *New England Journal of Medicine*, **321**, 287–92.

Loeb, J.N. (1972). The influence of temperature on the solubility of monosodium urate. *Arthritis and Rheumatism*, **15**, 189–92.

Ludwig, G.D. (1957). Saternine gout. *Archives of Internal Medicine*, **100**, 802–10.

Lupton, G.P. and Odom, R.B. (1979). The allopurinol hypersensitivity syndrome: unnecessary morbidity and mortality. *Journal of the American Academy of Dermatology*, **1**, 365–74.

Lust, G., Faurem, G., Netter, P., and Seegmiller, J.E. (1981). Increased pyrophosphate in fibroblasts and lymphoblasts from patients with hereditary diffuse articular chondrocalcinosis. *Science*, **214**, 809–10.

Macfarlane, D.G. and Dieppe, P.A. (1985). Diuretic induced gout in elderly women. *British Journal of Rheumatology*, **24**, 155–7.

Malawista, S.E. *et al.* (1985). Crystal-induced endogenous pyrogen production. A further look at gouty inflammation. *Arthritis and Rheumatism*, **28**, 1039–46.

Mandel, N.S. (1976). The structural basis of crystal-induced membranolysis. *Arthritis and Rheumatism*, **19**, 439–55.

Mandel, N.S. and Mandel, G.S. (1985). Nucleation and growth of CPPD crystals and related species in vitro. In *Calcium in biologic systems* (ed. R.P. Rubin, G. Weiss, and J.W. Putner). Plenum, New York.

Marcalongo, R., Calabria, A.A., Lalumera, M., Gerli, R., Alessandrini, C., and Cavallo, G. (1988). The 'switch-off' mechanism of spontaneous resolution of acute gout attack. *Journal of Rheumatology*, **15**, 101–9.

Marcos, J.C. *et al.* (1981). Idiopathic familial chondrocalcinosis due to apatite crystal deposition. *American Journal of Medicine*, **71**, 557–563.

Martel, W. (1968). The overhanging margin of bone: a roentgenologic manifestation of gout. *Radiology*, **91**, 1755–6.

Marx, S.J. *et al.* (1981). The hypocalciuric or benign variant of familial hypercalcemia: clinical and biochemical features in fifteen kindreds. *Medicine*, **60**, 397–412.

Masuda, I. and Ishikawa, K. (1987). Clincial features of pseudogout attack: a survey of 50 cases. *Clinical Orthopaedics and Related Research*, **229**, 173–9.

Masuda, I., Ishikawa, K., and Usuku, G. (1989). A histologic and immunohistologic study of calcium pyrophosphate dihydrate crystal deposition disease. *Clinical Orthopedics and Related Research*, **263**, 272–87.

McCarthy, G.M., Carrera, G.F., and Ryan, L.M. (1993). Acute calcific periarthritis of the finger joints: a syndrome of young women. *Journal of Rheumatology*, **20**, 1077–9.

McCarty, D.J. (1966). Calcium pyrophosphate deposition disease. In *Arthritis and allied conditions* (ed. H.L. Hollander), pp. 947–64. Lea and Febiger, Philadelphia.

McCarty, D.J. (1982). The Hebreden Oration. Crystals, joints and consternation. *Annals of the Rheumatic Diseases*, **42**, 243–53.

McCarty, D.J. (1989). Robert Adams' rheumatic arthritis of the shoulder: Milwaukee shoulder syndrome revisited. *Journal of Rheumatology*, **16**, 668–70.

McCarty, D.J. (1991). Podagra due to calcific periarthritis in a young woman. *Internal Medicine*, **12**, 68, 75–76.

McCarty, D.J. and Hollander, J.L. (1961). Identification of urate crystals in gouty synovial fluid. *Annals of Internal Medicine*, **54**, 454–60.

McCarty, D.J., Kohn, N.N., and Faires, J.S. (1962). The significance of calcium phosphate crystals in the synovial fluid of arthritis patients: the 'pseudogout syndrome' I. Clinical aspects. *Annals of Internal Medicine*, **56**, 711–37.

McCarty, D.J., Halverson, P.B., Carrera, G.F., Brewer, B.J., and Kozin, F.K. (1981). Milwaukee shoulder syndrome: association of microspheroids containing hydroxyapatite crystals, active collagenase, and neutral protease with rotator cuff defects. I: Clinical aspects. *Arthritis and Rheumatism*, **24**, 464–73.

McGill, N.W. and Dieppe, P.A. (1991*a*). Evidence for a promoter of urate crystal formation in gouty synovial fluid. *Annals of the Rheumatic Diseases*, **50**, 558–61.

McGill, N.W. and Dieppe, P.A. (1991*b*). The role of serum and synovial fluid components in the promotion of urate crystal formation. *Journal of Rheumatology*, **18**, 1042–5.

McGill, P.E., Grange, A.T., and Royston, C.S.M. (1984). Chondrocalcinosis in primary hyperparathyroidism. *Scandinavian Journal of Rheumatology*, **13**, 56–8.

McInnes, G.T., Lawson, D.H., and Jick, H. (1981). Acute adverse reactions attributed to allopurinol in hospitalized patients. *Annals of the Rheumatic Diseases*, **40**, 245–9.

Mejias, E., Lluberes, R., and Martinez-Maldanado, M. (1989). Hyperuricemia, gout, and autosomal dominant polycystic kidney disease. *American Journal of the Medical Sciences*, **297**, 145–8.

Menkes, C.J., Simon, F., Delrieu, F., Forest, M., and Delbarre, F. (1976). Destructive arthropathy in chondrocalcinosis articularis. *Arthritis and Rheumatism*, **19**, 329–48.

Milazzo, S.C., Cleland, L.G., and Ahern, M.J. (1981). Calcium pyrophosphate dihydrate deposition disease and familial hypomagnesemia. *Journal of Rheumatology*, **8**, 767–77.

Milgram, J.W. (1974). Chronic renal failure, recurrent secondary hyperparathyroidism, multiple metaphyseal infractions, and secondary oxalosis. *Bulletin / Hospital for Joint Diseases*, **35**, 118–44.

Mitrovic, D.R. *et al.* (1988). The prevalence of chondrocalcinosis in the human knee joint: an autopsy survey. *Journal of Rheumatology*, **15**, 633–41.

Moreland, L.W. and Ball, G.V. (1991). Colchicine and gout. *Arthritis and Rheumatism*, **34**, 782–6.

Myers, A.R. *et al.* (1968). The relationship of serum uric acid to risk factors in coronary heart disease. *American Journal of Medicine*, **45**, 520–8.

Nakayama, D.A. *et al.* (1984). Tophaceous gout: a clincial and radiographic assessment. *Arthritis and Rheumatism*, **27**, 468–71.

Nartijn, A. and Thijn, C.J.P. (1982). Radiologic findings in primary oxaluria. *Skeletal Radiology*, **8**, 21–4.

Neel, J.V. (1947). The clinical detection of the genetic carriers of inherited disease. *Medicine*, **26**, 115–53.

Neuss, M.N., McCallum, R.M., Brenckman, W.D., and Silberman, H.R. (1986). Long-term colchicine administration leading to colchicine toxicity and death. *Arthritis and Rheumatism*, **29**, 448–9.

Northridge, D.B. and Almack, P.M. (1986). Allopurinol desensitisation. *British Journal of Pharmaceutical Practice*, **8**, 200–5.

Nuki, G. and Parker, J. (1979). Clinical and enzymatic studies in a child with type I glycogen storage disease associated with partial deficiency of hepatic glucose-6-phosphatase. *Advances in Experimental Medicine and Biology*, **122A**, 189–202.

O'Duffy, J.D. (1970). Hypophosphatasia associated with calcium pyrophosphate dihydrate deposits in cartilage. *Arthritis and Rheumatism*, **13**, 381–8.

O' Duffy, J.D. (1973). Pseudogout syndrome in hospitalized patients. *Journal of the American Medical Association*, **226**, 42.

O'Duffy, J.D. (1976). Clinical studies of acute pseudogout attacks. Comments on prevalence, predispositions, and treatment. *Arthritis and Rheumatism*, **19** (Suppl.), 349.

O'Duffy, J.D., Hunter, G.G., and Kelly, P.J. (1975). Decreasing prevalence of tophaceous gout. *Mayo Clinic Proceedings*, **50**, 227–8.

Op de Hoch, C.T. *et al.* (1980). Oxalosis in chronic renal failure. *Proceedings of the European Dialysis and Transplantation Association*, **17**, 730–5.

Pak, C.Y.C. *et al.* (1981). Is selective therapy of recurrent nephrolithiasis possible? *American Journal of Medicine*, **71**, 615–22.

Pak, C.Y.C., Sakhaee, K., and Fuller, C. (1986). Successful management of uric acid nephrolithiasis with potassium citrate. *Kidney International*, **30**, 422–8.

Palmer, D.G., Highton, J., and Hessian, P.A. (1989). Development of the gout tophus: a hypothesis. *American Journal of Clinical Pathology*, **91**, 190–5.

Pascual, E. (1991). Persistence of monosodium urate crystals and low-grade inflammation in the synovial fluid of patients with untreated gout. *Arthritis and Rheumatism*, **34**, 141–5.

Paulus, H.E., Schlosstein, L.H., Godfrey, R.G., Klinenberg, J.R., and Bluestone, R. (1974). Prophylactic colchicine therapy of intercritical gout: a placebo-controlled study of probenecid-treated patients. *Arthritis and Rheumatism*, **17**, 609–14.

Perricone, E. and Brandt, K.D. (1978). Enhancement of urate solubility by connective tissue: 1. effect of proteoglycan aggregates and buffer cation. *Arthritis and Rheumatism*, **21**, 453–60.

Peters, J.P. and Van Slyke, K.K. (1946). *Quantitiative clinical chemistry*, Vol 1. (2nd edn), p. 937. Williams and Wilkins Company, Baltimore.

Plante, G.E., Durivage, J., and Lemieux, G. (1968). Renal excretion of hydrogen in primary gout. *Metabolism*, **17**, 377–97.

Pritchard, M.H. and Jessop, J.D. (1977). Chondrocalcinosis in primary hyperparathyroidism. *Annals of the Rheumatic Diseases*, **36**, 146–51.

Pritzker, K.P.H., Cheng, P.T., and Renlund, R.C. (1988). Calcium pyrophosphate crystal deposition in hyaline cartilage. Ultrastructural analysis and implications for pathogenesis. *Journal of Rheumatology*, **15**, 828–35.

Puig, J.G. and Fox, I.H. (1984). Ethanol-induced activation of adenine nucleotide turnover. Evidence for a role for acetate. *Journal of Clinical Investigation*, **74**, 936–41.

Puig, J.G. *et al.* (1991). Female gout: clinical spectrum and uric acid metabolism. *Archives of Internal Medicine*, **151**, 726–32.

Puig, J.G. *et al.* (1994). Purine metabolism in women with primary gout. *American Journal of Medicine*, **97**, 332–8.

Rachow, J.W., Ryan, L.M., McCarty, D.J., and Halverson, P.B. (1988). Synovial fluid inorganic pyrophosphate concentration and nucleotide pyrophosphohydrolase activity in basic calcium phosphate deposition arthropathy and Milwaukee shoulder syndrome. *Arthritis and Rheumatism*, **31**, 408–13.

Raddatz, D.A., Mahowald, M.L., and Bilka, P.J. (1983). Acute polyarticular gout. *Annals of the Rheumatic Diseases*, **42**, 117–22.

Rate, A.J., Parkinson, R.W., Meadows, T.H., and Freemont., A.J. (1992). Acute carpel tunnel syndrome due to pseudogout. *Journal of Hand Surgery* (*British*), **17**, 217–18.

Reginato, A.J., Schumacher, H.R., and Martinez, V.A. (1973). Ochronotic arthropathy with calcium pyrophosphate dihydrate crystal deposition. *Arthritis and Rheumatism*, **16**, 705–14.

Reginato, A.J. *et al.* (1975). Familial chondrocalcinosis in the Chiloe Islands, Chile. *Annals of the Rheumatic Diseases*, **34**, 260–8.

Reginato, A.J. *et al.* (1986). Arthropathy and cutaneous calcinosis in hemodialysis oxalosis. *Arthritis and Rheumatism*, **29**, 1387–96.

Reiselbach, R.E. *et al.* (1962). Uric acid excretion and renal function in the acute hyperuricemia of leukemia. *American Journal of Medicine*, **37**, 872–84.

Reiselbach, R.E., Sorenson, L.B., Selp, W.D., and Steele, T.H. (1970). Diminished renal urate secretion per nephron as a basis for primary gout. *Annals of Internal Medicine*, **73**, 359–66.

Resnick, D. *et al.* (1977). Clinical, radiologic, and pathologic abnormalities in calcium pyrophosphate dihydrate deposition disease (CPPD) pseudogout. *Diagnostic Radiology*, **122**, 1–15.

Reynolds, E.S. *et al.* (1957). Fatal massive necrosis of the liver as a manifestation of hypersensitivity to probenecid. *New England Journal of Medicine*, **256**, 5.

Richardson, B.B. *et al.* (1983). Hereditary chondrocalcinosis in a Mexican–American family. *Arthritis and Rheumatism*, **26**, 1387–96.

Richet, G., Mignon, F., and Ardaillou, R. (1965). Goutte secondaire de nephropathies chroniques. *Presse Médicale*, **73**, 633–8.

Ritter, J., Kerr, L.D., Valeriano-Marcet, J., and Spiera, H. (1993). ACTH revisited: effective treatment for acute crystal induced synovitis in patients with multiple medical problems. *Journal of Rheumatology*, **21**, 696–9.

Roberge, C.J., Gaudry, M., deMedicis, R., Lussier, A., Poubelle, P.E., and Naccache, P.H. (1993). Crystal-induced neutrophil activation. IV. Specific inhibition of tyrosine phosphorylation by colchicine. *Journal of Clinical Investigation*, **92**, 1722–9.

Roberts, W.M., Liang, M.H., and Stern, S.H. (1987). Colchicine in acute gout. *Journal of the American Medical Association*, **257**, 1920–1.

Rodriquez-Valverde, V. *et al.*, (1988). Hereditary articular chondrocalcinosis. *American Journal of Medicine*, **84**, 101–8.

Rosenthal, A.K., Ryan, L.M., and McCarty, D.J. (1988). Arthritis associated with calcium oxalate crystals in an anephric patient treated with peritoneal dialysis. *Journal of the American Medical Association*, **260**, 1290–2.

Rosenthal, A.K., Cheung, H.S., and Ryan, L.M. (1991). Transforming growth factor-β stimulates inorganic pyrophosphate elaboration by porcine cartilage. *Arthritis and Rheumatism*, **34**, 904–10.

Roubenoff, R., Klag, M.J., Mead, L.A., Liang, K-Y., Seidler, A.J., and Hochberg, M.C. (1991). Incidence and risk factors for gout in white men. *Journal of the American Medical Association*, **266**, 3004–7.

Rozenberg, S., Koeger, A-C., and Bourgeois, P. (1993). Urate-oxidase for gouty arthritis in cardiac transplant recipients. *Journal of Rheumatology*, **20**, 2171.

Rundle, R.W., Metz, E.N., and Silberman, H.R. (1966). Allopurinol in the treatment of gout. *Annals of Internal Medicine*, **64**, 842–7.

Russell, I.J. *et al.* (1983). Effects of IgG and C-reactive protein on complement depletion by monosodium urate crystals. *Journal of Rheumatology*, **10**, 425–33.

Ryan, L.M. and McCarty, D.J. (1993). Calcium pyrophosphate crystal deposition disease; pseudogout; articular chondrocalcinosis. In *Arthritis and allied conditions* (12th edn) (ed. D.J. McCarty and W.J. Koopman), pp. 1835–55. Lea and Febiger, Philadelphia.

Ryan, L.M., Cheung, H.S., and McCarty, D.J. (1981). Release of pyrophosphate by normal mammalian hyaline and fibrocartilage. *Arthritis and Rheumatism*, **24**, 1522–7.

Rynes, R.I., Sosman, J.L., and Holdsworth, D.E. (1975). Pseudogout in ochronosis. *Arthritis and Rheumatism*, **18**, 21–5.

Sakar, K. and Uhthoff, H.K. (1984). Rotator cuff tendinopathies with calcification. In *Calcium in biological systems* (ed. R.P. Rubin, G. Weiss, and J.W. Putney). Plenum, New York.

Salvarini, C. *et al.* (1989). Bartter's syndrome and chondrocalcinosis: a possible role for hypomagnesemia in the deposition of calcium pyrophosphate dihyrate (CPPD) crystals. *Clinical and Experimental Rheumatology*, 7, 415–20.

Sarkozi, A.M., Nemeth-Csoka, M., and Bartosiewicz, G. (1988). Effect of glycosoaminoglycan polysulfate in the treatment of chondrocalcinosis. *Clinical and Experimental Rheumatology*, 6, 3–8.

Sarre, H. and Mertz, D.P. (1965). Sekundare Gight bei Neireninsuffizenz. *Klinische Wochenschrift*, 43, 1134–40.

Scheele, K.W. (1776). Examen chemicum calculi urinarii. *Opuscula*, 2, 73.

Schumacher, H.R. and Phelps, P. (1971). Sequential changes in human polymorphonuclear leukocytes after urate crystal phagocytosis. *Arthritis and Rheumatism*, 14, 513–26.

Schumacher, H.R. *et al.* (1977). Arthritis associated with apatite crystals. *Annals of Internal Medicine*, 87, 411–16.

Schumacher, H.R., Miller, J.L., Ludivico, C., and Jessar, R.A. (1981). Erosive arthritis associated with apatite crystal deposition. *Arthritis and Rheumatism*, 24, 31–7.

Scott, J.T. (1977). Obesity and hyperuricaemia. *Clinics in the Rheumatic Diseases*, 3, 25–35.

Scott, J.T. *et al.* (1969). Studies of uric acid pool size and turnover rate. *Annals of the Rheumatic Diseases*, 28, 366–73.

Seegmiller, J.D., Howell, R.R., and Malawista, S. E. (1962). Inflammatory reaction to sodium urate: its possible relationship to genesis of acute gouty arthritis. *Journal of the American Medical Association*, 180, 469–76.

Seegmiller, J.E., Rosenbloom, F.M., and Kelley, W.M. (1967). An enzyme defect associated with a sex-linked neurologic disorder and excessive purine synthesis. *Science*, 155, 1682–4.

Seidell, J.C. *et al.* (1986). Overweight and chronic illness — a retrospective cohort study with a follow-up of 6–17 years in men and women of intially 20–50 years of age. *Journal of Chronic Diseases*, 39, 585–93.

Self, T.H., Evans, W.E., and Ferguson, T. (1957). Drug enhancement of warfarin activity. *Lancet*, ii, 557–8.

Siegel, L.B., Alloway, J.A., and Nashel, D.J. (1994). Comparison of adrenocorticotropic hormone and triamcinolone acetonide in the treatment of acute gouty arthritis. *Journal of Rheumatology*, 21, 1325–7.

Silcox, D.C. and McCarty, D.J. (1974). Elevated inorganic pyrophosphate concentrations in synovial fluid in osteoarthritis and pseudogout. *Journal of Laboratory and Clinical Medicine*, 83, 518–31.

Simkin, P.A. (1977a). The pathogenesis of podagra. *Annals of Internal Medicine*, 86, 230–3.

Simkin, P.A. (1977b). Urate excretion in normal and gouty men. *Developmental and Experimental Medicine and Biology*, 76B, 41–5.

Simkin, P.A. (1993). Towards a coherent terminology of gout. *Annals of the Rheumatic Diseases*, 52, 693–4.

Singer, J.Z. and Wallace, S.L. (1986). The allopurinol hypersenstivity syndrome. Unnecessary morbidity and mortality. *Arthritis and Rheumatism*, 29, 82–7.

Smyth, C.J. (1953). Gout. In *Comroe's arthritis and allied conditions* (5th edn) (ed. J.L. Hollanders). Lea and Febiger, Philadelphia.

Sokoloff, L. (1957). The pathology of gout. *Metabolism*, 6, 230–43.

Solnica, J. *et al.* (1966). Les chondrocalinoses articulaires etude clinique, biologique crystallographique et etiologique. *Revue du Rhumatisme et des Maladies Osteo-Articulaires*, 33, 93–9.

Sorenson, L.B. (1959). Degradation of uric acid in man. *Metabolism*, 8, 687–703.

Sorenson, L.B. (1960). The elimination of uric acid in man studied by means of ^{14}C-labelled uric acid. *Scandinavian Journal of Clinical and Laboratory Investigation*, 12 (Suppl.), 1–14.

Sorenson, L.B. (1962). The pathogenesis of gout. *Archives of Internal Medicine*, 109, 379–90.

Sperling, O. *et al.* (1972). Accelerated erythrocyte 5'-phosphoribosyl-1-pyrophosphate synthesis. A familial abnormality associated with excessive uric acid production and gout. *Biochemical Medicine*, 6, 310–16.

Spilberg, I. *et al.* (1980). Colchicine and pseudogout. *Arthritis and Rheumatism*, 23, 1062–3.

Sterling, L.P. (1991). The clinical management of gout. *American Pharmacy*, (NS) 31, 368–74.

Steven, M.M. (1992). Prevalence of chronic arthritis in four geographical areas of the Scottish Highlands. *Annals of the Rheumatic Diseases*, 51, 186–94.

Stockman, A., Darlington, L.G., and Scott, J.T. (1980). Frequency of chondrocalcinosis of the knee and avascular necrosis of the femoral head in gout. *Annals of the Rheumatic Diseases*, 39, 7–11.

Stuart, R.A., Gow, P.J., Bellamy, N., Campbell, J., and Grigor, R. (1991). A survey of current prescribing practices of antiinflammatory and urate-lowering drugs in gouty arthritis. *New Zealand Medical Journal*, 104, 115–17.

Swan, A., Chapman, B., Heap, P., Seward, H., and Dieppe, P. (1994). Submicroscopic crystals in osteoarthritic synovial fluids. *Annals of the Rheumatic Diseases*, 53, 467–70.

Swannell, A.J., Underweeo, F.A., and Dixon, A.S. (1970). Periarticular calcific deposits mimicking acute arthritis. *Annals of the Rheumatic Diseases*, 29, 380–5.

Tak, H-J., Cooper, S.M., and Wilcox, W.R. (1980). Studies on the nucleation of monosodium urate at 37°C. *Arthritis and Rheumatism*, 23, 574–80.

Talbott, J.S. (1957). *Gout*. Grune and Stratton, New York.

Taylor, H.G. and Hothersall, T.E. (1991). Hypophosphataemic rickets and pyrophosphate arthropathy. *Clinical Rheumatology*, 10, 155–7.

Terkeltaub, R.A. *et al.* (1991). Apolipoprotein E inhibits the capacity of monosodium urate crystals to stimulate neutrophils. *Journal of Clinical Investigation*, 87, 20–6.

Varga, J., Giampaola, C., and Goldenberg, D.L. (1985). Tophaceous gout of the spine in a patient with no peripheral tophi. Case report and review of the literature. *Arthritis and Rheumatism*, 28, 1312–15.

Wallace, S.L. (1977). The treatment of the acute attack of gout. *Clinics in the Rheumatic Diseases*, 3, 133–43.

Wallace, S.L. *et al.* (1977). Preliminary criteria for the classification of the acute arthritis of primary gout. *Arthritis and Rheumatism*, 20, 895–900.

Watt, I. and Dieppe, P. (1983). Medial femoral condyle necrosis and chondrocalcinosis; a causal relationship. *British Journal of Radiology*, 56, 7–22.

Watts, W.E. *et al.* (1991). Combined hepatic and renal transplantation in primary hyperoxaluria type I: clinical report of 9 cases. *American Journal of Medicine*, 90, 179–87.

Whyte, M.P., Murphy, W.A., and Fallon, M.D. (1982). Adult hypophosphatasia with chondrocalcinosis and arthropathy. *American Journal of Medicine*, 72, 631–41.

Wilcox, W.R. and Khalaf, A.A. (1975). Nucleation of monosodium urate crystals. *Annals of the Rheumatic Diseases*, 34, 332–9.

Williams, H.E. and Smith, H.E. (1968). Disorders of oxalate metabolism. *American Journal of Medicine*, 45, 715–35.

Wilson, J.M., Young, A.S., and Kelley, W.N. (1983). Hypoxanthine-guanine phosphoribosyltransferase deficiency: the molecular basis of the clinical syndromes. *New England Journal of Medicine*, 309, 900–10.

Wyngaarden, J.B. and Kelley, W.N. (1976). *Gout and hyperuricemia*. Grune and Sratton, New York.

Wyngaarden, J.B. and Kelley, W.N. (1985). Gout. In *The metabolic basis of inherited disease*. (5th edn) (ed. J.B. Stanbury *et al.*), pp. 1043–114. McGraw-Hill, New York.

Wyngaarden, J.B. and Stetten, D.W., Jr (1953). Uricolysis in normal man. *Journal of Biological Chemistry*, 203, 9–21.

Wyngaarden, J.B., Rundle, R.W., and Metz, E.N. (1965). Allopurinol in the treatment of gout. *Annals of Internal Medicine*, 62, 842–7.

Yen, R.C.K., Adams, W.B., Lazar, C., and Becker, M.A. (1978). Evidence for X-linkage of human phosphoribosylpyrophosphate synthetase. *Proceedings of the National Academy of Sciences (USA)*, 75, 482–5.

Yen, R.C.K., Raivio, K.O., and Becker, M.A. (1981). Inhibition of phosphoribosylpyrophosphate synthesis by 6-methylthionisoinate. *Journal of Biological Chemistry*, 256, 1839–45.

Yosipovitch, G. and Yosipovitch, Z. (1993). Acute calcific periarthritis of the hand and elbows in women. A study and review of the literature. *Journal of Rheumatology*, 20, 1533–8.

Yu, T-F. (1981). Urolithiasis in hyperuricemia and gout. *Journal of Urology*, 126, 424–30.

Yu, T-F. and Gutman, A.B. (1961). Efficacy of colchicine prophylaxis. Prevention of recurrent gout arthritis over a mean period of five years in 208 gouty subjects. *Annals of Internal Medicine*, **55**, 179–85.

Yu, T-F., and Gutman, A.B. (1967). Uric acid nephrolithiasis in gout: predisposing factors. *Annals of Internal Medicine*, **67**, 1133–48.

Yukawa, T., Akazawa, H., Miyake, Y., Takahashi, Y., Nagao, H., and Takeda, E. (1992). A female patient with Lesch–Nyhan syndrome. *Developmental Medicine and Child Neurology*, **34**, 543–6.

Zollner, N., Griebsch, A., and Fink, J.K. (1970). Uber die Wirking von Benzbromarone auf den Serumharnsauerspiegel und die Harnsaureausscheidung des Gichtkranken. *Deutsche Medizinische Wochenschrift*, **95**, 2405–11.

Zwillich, S.H., Schumacher, H.R., Jr., Hoyt, T.S., Luger, A.M., Morrison, G., and Walder, S.E. (1988). Universal spondylodiscitis in a patient with erosive peripheral arthritis and apatite crystal deposition. *Journal of Rheumatology*, **15**, 123–8.

5.17   Diseases of bone and cartilage

5.17.1   Osteoporosis and osteomalacia

A. K. Bhalla

Introduction

Disorders of bone that lead to a reduction in bone mass and strength cause much suffering in the population and often present to the rheumatologist with pain, fractures, and deformity. The most common bone disorder in Western nations is osteoporosis, although globally osteomalacia or rickets secondary to vitamin D deficiencies are more common. Unlike osteomalacia, in osteoporosis the mineralized bone, while reduced, is normal; the disorder can be defined as a reduction in bone mass and strength resulting in an increased risk of fracture with minimal or no trauma. The term 'osteopenia' is sometimes used to delineate a state of reduced bone mass, for example identified during radiological investigation or bone mass measurement, without fracture.

Osteoporosis

Definition

Until recently there was no internationally agreed definition of osteoporosis. A 1991 Consensus Development Conference defined osteoporosis as 'a disease characterised by low bone mass and micro architectorial deterioration of bone tissue, leading to enhanced bone fragility and a consequent increased risk in fracture' (Consensus Development Conference 1991).

This definition of osteoporosis has been accepted by the World Health Organization (**WHO**), which has now also defined osteoporosis on the basis of bone density. The categories of disease as defined by the WHO 1994 criteria based on bone mineral density are shown in Table 1.

These diagnostic criteria for osteoporosis do have some limitations and are likely to be changed in time. It is important to remember that they apply to postmenopausal women and it is not yet agreed what criteria should be applied to men or to young individuals who have yet to attain skeletal maturity, or to special situations such as corticosteroid osteoporosis. Kanis *et al.* (1994*b*) suggest that, since in some populations the risk of fracture in men is substantially lower for bone mineral measurements within their own reference range, diagnostic criteria of 3–4 SD below a young reference mean may be more appropriate. In addition, different cut-off values may be appropriate for different communities since differences in the risk of hip fractures

Table 1   Categories of osteoporosis as defined by WHO based on bone mineral density (after Kanis et al. 1994a)

Disease category	BMD or BMC value
Normal	Not less than 1 SD below young adult mean value
Low bone mass (osteopenia)	More than 1 SD below young adult mean value but not less than 2.5 SD below young adult mean value
Osteoporosis	More than 2.5 SD below young adult mean value
Severe osteoporosis (established osteoporosis)	More than 2.5 SD below young adult mean value in the presence of one or more low-trauma or fragility fractures

BMD, bone mineral density; BMC, bone mineral content.

between communities cannot solely be explained on the basis of bone mineral density.

Epidemiology

In the Western world osteoporosis causes considerable suffering in individuals over the age of 50, and, because it predisposes to skeletal failure and fractures, is responsible for consuming an enormous amount of the budget devoted to health care. The main sites of fracture traditionally thought to be related to osteoporosis are the vertebral body, proximal femur, distal forearm, the proximal humerus, and pelvis, of which the first three are more common (Fig. 1) (Riggs and Melton 1986). The risk of an osteoporotic fracture

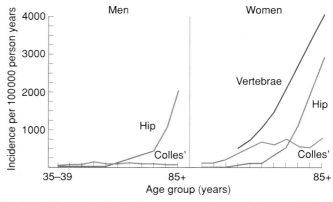

Fig. 1   Incidence rates for the three common osteoporotic fractures (Colles', hip, and vertebral) in men and women, plotted as a function of age at the time of the fracture (reproduced from Riggs and Melton 1986 with permission).

Table 2 Lifetime fracture risk in 50-year-old white men and women (Melton et al. 1992)

Fracture site	Lifetime risk (%)	
	Men	**Women**
Hip	6.0	17.5
Vertebral	5.0	15.6
Distal forearm	2.5	16.0
Any of the above	13.1	39.7

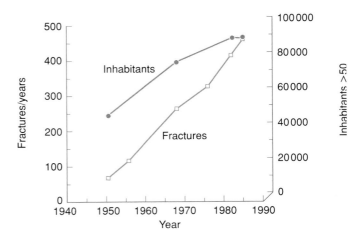

Fig. 2 The relation between the total number of fractures of the hip and the population over 50 years of age in Malmo, Sweden (reproduced from Obront *et al.* 1989 with permission).

is greater in women than men, and in both sexes the risk varies appreciably between countries. In women from the United States and Europe, the lifetime risk of a hip fracture at the age of 50 is 17.5 per cent whilst the lifetime risk of a hip fracture in a male is 6 per cent. The lifetime risk of a vertebral fracture is estimated at 15.6. per cent for women and 5 per cent for men, and the risk of having either a fracture of the femur or the distal forearm is approx. 40 per cent in women aged over 50 years and 13.1 per cent in men (Table 2) (Melton *et al.* 1992).

As discussed below, the three most common fractures have different sex ratios and incidence rates at different decades. The incidence of fractures of the distal forearm in women increases soon after the menopause, with a peak incidence between the ages of 50 and 65 (there is a peak in the risk of falls in women aged 45 to 60 years), while in adult males the incidence rates remain constant. Presumably the attempt to break the fall by stretching out the arm accounts for this fracture. In contrast, fractures of the proximal femur show an exponential increase in incidence much later in life, with a 20-fold increase between the ages of 65 to 85 years (where the incidence of falls increases by only twofold) and a male:female ratio of 1:2. This indicates that the probability of a fall resulting in a fracture of the femoral neck is modulated by other age-related factors. Such factors would include the progressive loss of bone with ageing (Winner *et al.* 1989), and a tendency, with increasing age, for a greater likelihood of a fall on the hip than on the hand, presumably due to neuromuscular impairment making it less likely that he or she has enough time to break the fall by throwing out an arm (Grimley Evans 1990).

Proximal femoral fracture

Hip fracture, the most serious complication of osteoporosis, usually follows a fall from a standing position, although it may occur spontaneously. The occurrence of hip fracture has a seasonal variation in both hemispheres. Hip fractures occur more frequently during the winter months; the majority follow falls indoors and therefore are not related to slipping on ice. In most Western countries the incidence of hip fractures has been rising steadily and not all the increase can be explained by an ageing population (Boyce and Vessey 1985; Obront *et al.* 1989). In Sweden the total number of hip fractures between 1950 and 1985 has increased sevenfold while the number of inhabitants over the age of 50 has doubled during this period (Fig. 2). A large part of the increase in hip fracture is due to an increase in the age-adjusted incidence of hip fractures (Obront *et al.* 1989).

In the United Kingdom the incidence of hip fractures rises exponentially with age in both sexes (Fig. 3) and with an approximate 2:1 female to male incidence. This fact, and because there is a large number of elderly women in the population, results in over 80 per cent of all hip fractures occurring in women over the age of 65.

There were 46 000 hip fractures in England and Wales in 1985 and current estimates suggest that 60 000 occur annually (Advisory Group on Osteoporosis 1994). In 1989 the Royal College of Physicians estimated that if the 1985 age- and sex-specific incidence rates continue to double every 30 years, then by the year 2016 there will be 117 000 hip fractures annually. Using 1985 incidence rates the probability of a woman sustaining a hip fracture before the age of 85 in the United Kingdom is 12 per cent; for a man it is 5 per cent. In the United Kingdom the direct hospital cost for hip fractures in 1985 were about £160 million. The most recent estimate, using 1992/93 prices, suggests that in England alone the acute inpatient costs will be £237 million, and additional costs of long-term and community care could be a further £444 million (Advisory Group on Osteoporosis 1994).

In the United States there were 238 000 hip fractures in 1986 in adults over the age of 50 years, and, assuming that current age-specific incidence rates remain unaltered, then by the year 2020 there will be 347 000 hip fractures. The annual acute-care costs will rise from the current sum of $8 billion by four- to eightfold.

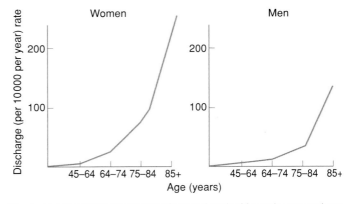

Fig. 3 Hospital discharge rates for fractured neck of femur by age and sex in England, 1985 (derived from Royal College of Physicians 1989).

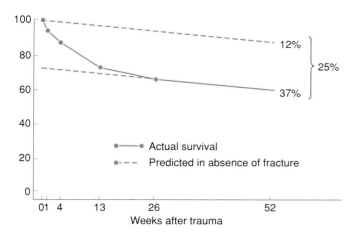

Fig. 4 Relation between survival and passage of time since femoral-neck fracture in women (reproduced from Aitken 1987 with permission).

Table 3	Important risk factors for hip fractures in women

Maternal history of hip fracture
Low body-mass index
Height age 25
Short fertile period
Previous hyperthyroidism
Previous treatment with benzodiazepines or anticonvulsants
Poor mental score
Poor depth perception
Low physical activity

Hip fractures are recognized as major health problems in Western countries, but there is a belief that since most fractures occur in Caucasian populations the problem may not affect the nations of Asia, South America, and Africa. However, using current incidence rates of hip fractures in various parts of the world to projected populations in the year 2050, it has been estimated that the number of hip fractures occurring world-wide each year will rise from 1.6 million in 1990 to 6.26 million by 2050. Whilst in 1990 nearly half the fractures occurred in North America and Europe, with 31 per cent in Asia, by the year 2050 50 per cent of hip fractures will occur in Asia, with 13 per cent in Europe and 12 per cent in North America. Thus osteoporosis, particularly hip fractures, will become a world-wide problem requiring preventative strategies to be developed in regions where currently it is thought not to be a major problem (Cooper *et al.* 1992).

Hip fractures result in considerable mortality. Surveys suggests that between 10 and 40 per cent of all patients who fracture a hip die within 12 months of the fracture (Fig. 4) (Aitken 1987). The excess mortality may, in part, be due to the presence of more coexisting morbidity in patients with fractures than in the age-matched, non-fractured population. In a prospective study, patients admitted with a hip fracture alone has 0 per cent mortality at 1 year compared to 14 per cent and 24 per cent if two or three or more additional medical conditions were present (Svensson *et al.* 1996).

Risk factors for hip fracture

Recently, two large, well-conducted studies have examined the role of risk factors in hip fracture (Table 3) (Cummings *et al.* 1995; Johnell *et al.* 1995). Cummings *et al.* (1995) followed 9516 women aged 65 or over for 4 years and identified 192 incidences of hip fractures. These investigators reported that a maternal history of hip fracture doubled the risk of hip fracture, with a relative risk of 2 falling to 1.8 after adjusting for bone density. Women with a history of any previous fracture since the age of 50 showed an increased risk of hip fracture (relative risk 1.5), confirming previous observations (Cooper *et al.* 1988). Other identifiable risk factors included height at the age of 25 (odds ratio 1.3 per 6 cm), a finding also noted by Meyer *et al.* (1993). The reason for this association may be that tall women have further to fall and that they also have a longer hip axis (the distance from the greater trocanter to

the inner pelvic ring), which has been associated with a greater risk of hip fracture (Faulkner *et al.* 1993).

Johnell *et al.* (1995) found no significant adverse effect of smoking, unlike Cummings *et al.* (1995), who could show a significant effect of smoking in an age-adjusted model only, but not after multivariate adjustment for factors such as weight, poor health, and inadequate exercise, all of which were more pronounced in smokers. The relation between calcium intake and hip fractures remains controversial in view of the inconsistent findings in these two epidemiological studies. Cummings *et al.* 1995 found no relation between dietary calcium intake and hip fracture, while in the European study (Johnell *et al.* 1995) a low intake of milk was associated with a significantly increased risk. The increased risk was, however, confined to that 10 per cent of the population with a calcium intake of less than 240 mg daily.

The incidence of hip fracture rises depending on the number of risk factors present. For example, those with two or less risk factors had an incidence of 1.1 hip fractures per 1000 women years compared to an incidence of 19 in those with five or more risk factors. The risk of fracture is greatly increased if bone density is reduced (see Fig. 5) in association with other risk factors (Cummings *et al.* 1995). In the European study (Johnell *et al.* 1995), risk factors such as late

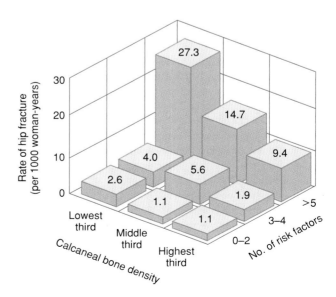

Fig. 5 Annual risk of hip fracture in relation to number of risk factors and calcaneal bone density (after Cummings *et al.* 1995).

menarche, poor mental score, low body mass index, reduced physical activity, low sunshine exposure, and low intake of calcium explained about 70 per cent of the total risk of fracture. Further studies are required to confirm these observations.

Vertebral fractures

The prevalence of vertebral fractures is not accurately known since there is no universally agreed definition of vertebral fracture and they are often asymptomatic so that clinical diagnosis may be delayed until multiple fractures have occurred, leading to spinal deformity and loss of height. The socioeconomic costs of vertebral fracture are therefore unknown.

Epidemiological studies on the prevalence of vertebral fractures have often used differing criteria for defining a fracture and currently there is no accepted definition of vertebral fracture based on the degree of deformation. The criterion for defining a wedge fracture varies from a 20 to 30 per cent reduction in anterior or posterior height of the vertebra compared with adjacent vertebrae, and the lack of agreement may account for the discordant results from studies of drugs, such as fluoride, in established osteoporosis. A clinically significant vertebral fracture requires a deformation of at least 20 to 25 per cent and more minor deformities may reverse spontaneously (Kleerekoper 1992).

The incidence of vertebral fractures increases with age and about 20 to 30 per cent of women aged over 60 may have an asymptomatic vertebral fracture on routine radiography. In cross-sectional studies in the United States, it has been estimated that each year 538 000 postmenopausal women will sustain their first vertebral fracture (Riggs and Melton 1986). The prevalence of vertebral fractures in the United Kingdom has been estimated at 7.8 per cent and the prevalence rises with advancing age from 4.3 per cent at 55 to 59 years to 27.8 per cent at 80 years or over (Cooper et al. 1991). It has recently been estimated that 40 000 clinically diagnosed vertebral fractures occur annually in postmenopausal women in the United Kingdom. Studies of the Scandinavian population show not only an age-related increase in incidence of vertebral fractures, but also a fourfold increase in incidence and prevalence between 1950 and 1980 (Benger et al. 1988). The prevalence of vertebral fracture increases with decreasing bone density and approaches 50 per cent in those with vertebral bone density below 0.6 g/cm^2 as measured by dual-photon absorptiometry (Riggs and Melton 1986). A recent European epidemiological study suggests that the prevalence of vertebral deformities is 12 per cent in women (range 6–21 per cent) and 12 per cent in men (range 8–20 per cent). The prevalence increased with age in both sexes with a steeper rise in women. In women aged 76 to 79 the prevalence was 24.7 per cent compared to 18.1 per cent in men (O'Neill et al. 1996). Using the prevalence figures for the United Kingdom from the study, it is estimated that 900 000 men and 1 million women between the age of 50 and 79 years have vertebral deformity, and, even if only 1 out of 3 is symptomatic, 350 000 more will seek medical advice and help (O'Neill et al. 1996).

Distal radius fractures

The incidence of fracture of the distal radius (Colles' fracture) after a fall increases in women after the age of 40 and continues to rise until age 65, when it reaches a plateau. No such increase is observed in men (Fig. 1). The reason for the plateau in incidence rates in females after the age of 65 is unknown, but may relate to the incidence patterns of fall with advancing age. In older women, impaired neuromuscular coordination is more likely to lead to a fall on the hip than on the wrist whereas a younger woman may be able to break the fall by outstretching her arms. It is assumed that the fracture after trauma is the result of rapid loss of trabecular bone following the menopause. There is a peak in the incidence of falls between the ages of 45 and 60 years in women, which may contribute to the incidence of this fracture (Winner et al. 1989). The occurrence of a Colles' fracture may provide an early warning of osteoporosis in the affected individual.

Classification

There are several causes of osteoporosis and it may be either primary or secondary (Table 4).

Physiological or primary osteoporosis has been divided into two main types by some as type I (postmenopausal) and type II (age-related) osteoporosis. Type I osteoporosis affects predominantly trabecular bone and is associated with an increased risk of wrist and vertebral fractures, while type II affects both trabecular and cortical bone leading to hip fractures. In practice there is considerable overlap between these groups, since patients with vertebral fractures

Table 4 Classification of osteoporosis

Physiological or primary
  Postmenopausal (type I)
  Age-related (type II)

Idiopathic

Juvenile

Secondary
Endocrine
  Cushing syndrome
  Hyperparathyroidism
  Hypogonadism
  Thyroid toxicosis
  Hypopituitarism
  Insulin-dependent diabetes mellitus
Drugs
  Corticosteroids
  Excess thyroxine replacement
  Heparin
  Anticonvulsants
  Methotrexate
Haemopoietic
  Multiple myeloma
  Lymphoma, leukaemia
  Mastocytosis
Immobilization
Idiopathic hypercalciuria
Gastrectomy and other bowel disease
Osteoporosis of pregnancy

Inflammatory disorders
  Rheumatoid arthritis
  Ankylosing spondylitis

Congenital
  Osteogenesis imperfecta

have a greater risk of having a fractured hip and vice versa. In most patients with osteoporosis, distinguishing primary from secondary osteoporosis may be difficult since many factors may be present in one individual, for example a postmenopausal, elderly woman on corticosteroids.

Physiological osteopenia or age-related osteopenia affects all individuals and occurs in cortical and trabecular bone. It leads mainly to hip and vertebral fractures, but other fractures, such as in pelvis or humerus, are also common. Individuals with age-related osteoporosis have reduced bone mass at all sites, with values in the lower half of the distribution range (for further discussion see below under peak bone mass).

Postmenopausal osteoporosis (type I)

Bone loss in women aged between 40 and 65 years is primarily due to loss of ovarian function, as predicted by Albright (Albright *et al.* 1976). Most studies suggest that, in postmenopausal women, bone loss began perimenopausally and will decrease exponentially after 5 to 8 years to match the slower, age-related loss (Krolner and Nielsen 1982). Even though 80 per cent of the skeleton consists of cortical bone, loss occurs predominantly in bones of primarily trabecular structure since the surface area of trabecular bone is four times that of cortical bone. The rapid bone loss is due to increased resorption superimposed on the age-related loss.

The mechanism by which oestrogens protect the skeleton is unknown. An early hypothesis suggested that malabsorption of calcium was the primary event that leads to removal of calcium from the skeleton. This is unlikely since calcium alone cannot reduce post-menopausal bone loss. In addition, reduced absorption of calcium would be expected to activate the release of parathyroid hormone (**PTH**) and increase the production of $1,25(OH)_2D$ (calcitriol), whereas the opposite is usually found in postmenopausal women. An alternative theory suggested that the menopause is accompanied by a relative deficiency in calcitonin reserve or secretion (Reginster *et al.* 1987), leading to a partial removal of the inhibitory effects of this hormone on osteoclastic bone resorption. However, other studies have not observed impaired calcitonin secretion after the menopause, and patients who have been rendered calcitonin-deficient by thyroidectomy do not have an increased risk of osteoporosis, which would strongly argue against a major role for calcitonin in postmenopausal bone loss (Stevenson 1988). Recently, oestrogen receptors have been identified in human osteoblast-like cells (Eriksen *et al.* 1988) and osteocytes (Braidman *et al.* 1995), which suggests that oestrogen can act directly on bone. One effect of oestrogen on bone cells is to increase the release of anabolic cytokines such as transforming growth factor-β (TGF-β), a potent regulator of osteoblast proliferation and a potential coupling agent between bone resorption and formation in the remodelling cycle (Gowen 1991). Peripheral blood monocytes from women with 'high turnover' osteoporosis, histologically defined as having increased bone resorption and bone formation, synthesize higher amounts of the catabolic cytokine interleukin (**IL**) 1 than those from women with 'low turnover' osteoporosis, in whom bone formation is impaired (Pacifici *et al.* 1987). Furthermore, in the early years after ovarian failure, when bone resorption is rapid, the increased synthesis of IL-1 by monocytes can be blocked by oestrogen replacement therapy (Pacifici *et al.* 1989). Similarly, oestrogen decreases the release of tumour necrosis factor (**TNF**)-α from circulating monocytes of postmenopausal but not premenopausal women (Ralston *et al.* 1990). The increased

production of IL-1 and TNF-α by *ex vivo* cultures of monocytes after a surgical oophorectomy was reversed by oestrogen replacement (Pacifici *et al.* 1991). It is likely that IL-1 and TNF play an important part in bone loss associated with oestrogen deficiency.

Two other cytokines, IL-6 and IL-11, may also be targets for the antiresorptive effect of oestrogens (Manolagas and Jilka 1995). To explore the hypothesis that osteoclasts and granulocyte/macrophages arise from common haemopoietic progenitor, the genesis of osteoclasts in animal models of osteoporosis was assessed by using bone marrow culture and counting granulocyte/macrophage colony-forming units. Ovariectomized mice had a high number of granulocyte/macrophage colony-forming units from bone marrow as well as from spleen than normal controls, which correlated with a greater number of osteoclasts present in their bone. This effect was prevented when animals were treated with either oestrogens or antibodies to IL-6 (Jilka *et al.* 1992). The hypothesis generated by this study was that IL-6 directs the genesis of osteoclasts in oestrogen-depleted animals. More recently the same group have also shown that IL-11 may also play a critical part in osteoclast differentiation and development in an oestrogen-depleted state (Girasole *et al.* 1994). Thus, oestrogens may maintain bone mass by inhibiting the release of cytokines that stimulate bone resorption, probably by an effect on osteoclast differentiation, while upgrading the synthesis of other cytokines involved in bone formation. This interrelation between oestrogens, cytokines, and bone resorption may turn out to be much more complicated, but also offers a potential for targeting therapy of osteoporosis.

Age-related ('senile') osteoporosis (type II)

Type II osteoporosis, as defined by Riggs and Melton (1986), affects men and women of 70 years or older, resulting in hip and vertebral fractures, although fractures at other sites are also common. The vertebral fractures are of the wedge variety leading to dorsal kyphosis, and often the deformity is painless, the result of gradual, age-related loss of trabecular bone. Unlike type I osteoporosis, the incidence of hip fractures in type II osteoporosis is only twice as great in women as in men, suggesting that the age-related bone loss is important in the pathogenesis of this disorder (Fig. 1). It has been suggested that the two important factors responsible for the slow phase of bone loss are defective osteoblast function and renal endocrine failure. The impaired production of $1,25(OH)_2D$ by the kidney leads to decreased calcium absorption and secondary hyperparathyroidism. Low concentrations of $1,25(OH)_2D$ have been found in some elderly patients with hip fractures but concentrations of PTH have not been found to be elevated in all studies. However, in a recent trial on the prevention of hip fractures by vitamin D and calcium supplementation, the effect of these two drugs was to reduce the high normal concentrations of PTH in the elderly population and at the same time reduce substantially the risk of hip fractures (Chapuy *et al.* 1992). In some studies, serum 1,25 dihydroxy vitamin D_3 is found to be lower in women with postmenopausal osteoporosis than in age-matched controls, and the density and function of vitamin D receptors in the intestine were also lower in such individuals. Since synthesis of 1,25 dihydroxy vitamin D_3 in response to PTH may be impaired in women with postmenopausal osteoporosis, one can generate a hypothesis that reduced calcium intake and vitamin D synthesis lead to increased activity of PTH, then producing an attempt to correct the deficiency by stimulating the renal 1α-hydroxylase to synthesize more 1,25-dihydroxyvitamin D_3. As this pathway is less efficient, calcium deficiency persists and the increased PTH leads to increased bone resorption.

Idiopathic osteoporosis

This defines the occurrence of osteoporosis in premenopausal women or men under the age of 60 who do not have an obvious secondary cause for the disease. The male:female ratio is usually 10:1 and presentation is usually with vertebral compression fractures. Some individuals may be found to have mild forms of osteogenesis imperfecta. A subgroup of males with idiopathic osteoporosis has 'high bone turnover' osteoporosis with hypercalcuria and may be treated with antiresorption drugs such as calcitonin and bisphosphonates (Perry *et al.* 1982); most of the others have defective osteoblast function with low rates of bone formation (Jackson *et al.* 1987).

Juvenile osteoporosis

This is an uncommon disorder that occurs before, or at the onset of, puberty and affects both sexes equally. The pathophysiology is unknown. The child usually presents with pain in the lower back, hip, and feet, and fractures of weight-bearing joints and collapsed vertebrae. There is no consistent biochemical abnormality, and radiographs may show osteopenia, fracture and vertebral abnormalities, and scoliosis. The differential diagnosis includes osteogenesis imperfecta and osteomalacia, and other secondary causes should be excluded. There is no specific treatment for this disorder and recovery occurs as puberty progresses, with a return of bone mass towards normal. In some patients, however, fractures lead to deformity of the spine or extremity, and it is important that once the condition is diagnosed, non-weight-bearing and supportive physical therapy be made available.

Endocrine causes

Corticosteroids

Endogenous Cushing syndrome or chronic treatment with glucocorticosteroids is a well-recognized cause for severe osteopenia and fractures (especially of the vertebrae and ribs, sites that contain predominantly trabecular bone) and sometimes occurs without other evidence of glucocorticoid excess. In endogenous Cushing syndrome the prevalence of osteoporosis may be as high as 50 per cent and the incidence of spontaneous fractures 19 per cent (Ross and Linch 1982). In iatrogenic disease the prevalence of fractures may vary from 2 to 17 per cent, but the incidence may depend on the dose of drug used and its duration (Reid 1990). Asthmatics on a mean dose of 12 mg prednisolone over 7 years had a 34 per cent prevalence of vertebral fractures (Luengo *et al.* 1991). In a retrospective study of patients with severe asthma on corticosteroids, vertebral fractures were found in 11 per cent of patients admitted to hospital (Adinoff and Hollister 1983). An even higher prevalence was found in a small prospective study of patients with asthma, with 42 per cent having vertebral and hip fractures (Adinoff and Hollister 1983). An increased incidence of fractures has also been noted in patients with rheumatoid arthritis treated with glucocorticoids. Michel *et al.* (1991) reported a 34 per cent prevalence of vertebral fractures in patients with rheumatoid arthritis on corticosteroids. A more recent study using morphometric techniques found a 12 per cent prevalence in postmenopausal women under 65 years of age with rheumatoid arthritis compared to 6 per cent in matched controls, with no

increase in prevalence in those treated with doses of prednisolone below 7.5 mg (Spector *et al.* 1993). Postmenopausal females with rheumatoid arthritis on a mean daily dose of prednisolone 7 mg experienced twice as many vertebral fractures as patients not receiving prednisolone (Laan *et al.* 1992). A case-controlled study suggested a doubling of the risk of hip fractures in patients with rheumatoid arthritis receiving glucocorticoids (Cooper *et al.* 1995).

Individuals at greatest risk of glucocorticoid-induced osteoporosis are postmenopausal women and men over the age of 50 years, as well as prepubertal children, in whom corticosteroids also delay skeletal growth.

Reduced bone mass in patients treated with corticosteroids has been demonstrated at multiple skeletal sites, including primary cortical bone in, for example, the femoral head, using a variety of techniques including quantitative computed tomography and dual-energy X-ray absorptiometry. Trabecular bone with its larger surface area seems particularly prone to loss. Vertebral bone density may be reduced by as much as 40 per cent in patients treated with a moderate dose of corticosteroids (Laan *et al.* 1993*a*). Bone loss from trabecular regions may occur very rapidly, especially in the first year of treatment (Laan *et al.* 1993*b*).

The diagnosis of corticosteroid-induced osteoporosis is relatively easy in a young patient who sustains fractures whilst on corticosteroids. However, it is a more difficult diagnosis to make in an older patient where there may be other risk factors such as postmenopausal osteoporosis. Although osteoporosis has been defined on the basis of bone density using the WHO criteria, the definition of postmenopausal osteoporosis may not be relevant to corticosteroid-induced osteoporosis since there is evidence that fractures in patients treated with corticosteroids occur at higher bone density (Luengo *et al.* 1991). This difference makes it difficult to identify the individual at risk, particularly on the basis of pretreatment measurements of bone density.

The pathogenesis of glucocorticoid-induced osteoporosis is controversial since these drugs may affect calcium and phosphate metabolism, either directly or indirectly through actions on bone, kidney, and intestine (Fig. 6). Corticosteroids may indirectly enhance bone resorption and directly suppress bone formation by decreasing osteoblast function and maturation. The increased osteoclastic bone resorption by corticosteroids is secondary to reduced intestinal absorption of calcium leading to a rise in PTH, and in animals parathyroidectomy abolishes the osteoclastic response to steroids. The hypothesis that secondary hypoparathyroidism plays a part in the osteoporosis which results from glucocorticoid excess leading to a decrease in intestinal calcium absorption and increased urinary excretion of calcium has been put in some doubt by recent studies showing that, when intact PTH is measured, its concentrations do not change with the use of glucocorticoids.

Another mechanism for steroid osteoporosis may be through inhibition of secretion of calcitonin, a hormone whose major effect is to inhibit bone resorption. Decreased intestinal absorption of calcium by glucocorticoids was thought to be due to decreased production of 1,25-dihydroxyvitamin D_3 from its precursor, 25-hydroxyvitamin D_3. This is unlikely, since recent studies indicate that the circulating concentrations of these vitamin D metabolites are unaltered and that the defect in calcium absorption cannot be overcome entirely by dietary supplementation with them. The mechanism of action is probably indirect, and, since glucocorticoid receptors are present in the small intestine, glucocorticoids may interfere with the binding of

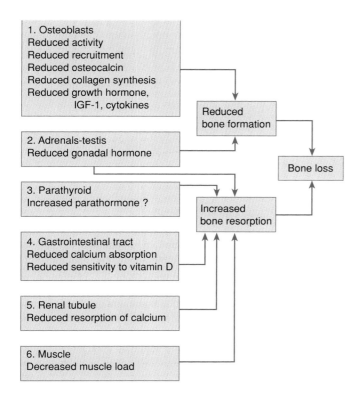

Fig. 6　Pathogenesis of glucocorticoid-induced osteoporosis.

1,25-dihydroxyvitamin D_3 to its receptor in the intestine or affect the function of important enzymes in the mucosal cell needed for calcium absorption and transport.

Excessive exogenous use of corticosteroids may lead to a reduction in testosterone and contribute to bone loss seen in males. In females the adrenal synthesis of androgens may also be reduced due to suppression of endogenous corticosteroid synthesis.

Hyperparathyroidism

Primary hyperparathyroidism is a relatively common disorder with a prevalence in adults estimated at 0.1 to 0.2 per cent. The disease is most common between the fifth and seventh decades of life, and is three times more common in women than men, the female predominance arising entirely from an increased incidence after the menopause (Bhalla 1986). Most patients with mild hyperparathyroidism are asymptomatic, the diagnosis being made during a biochemical screening when a high serum calcium is detected. PTH stimulates osteoclastic bone resorption by an effect primarily on osteoblasts, which in turn release a factor or factors that cause bone resorption or enhance osteoclastic activity. In young individuals, increased bone resorption may be compensated for by increased bone formation, but in older individuals, and in particular postmenopausal females, the compensatory mechanism is less efficient, leading to reduced bone mass in the axial and the appendicular skeleton (Devogelar et al. 1984; Martin et al. 1986), which, however, does not affect all patients. There is conflicting evidence for recovery of bone mass after parathyroidectomy and further studies are necessary (Martin et al. 1986). Since reduced bone mass is a predictor of fractures, parathyroid-mediated bone loss should result in an increased risk of fracture but this possibility remains controversial. Some studies have reported a higher prevalence of spinal fracture

(Dauphine et al. 1975) that others have not been able to confirm (Wilson et al. 1988).

Hypogonadism

All causes of hypogonadism lead to bone loss and may be associated with an increased risk in osteoporotic fractures. Amenorrhoea, whether primary or secondary, is associated with decreased bone mass and increased risk of fracture. Women with endometriosis who are treated with antagonists to luteinizing hormone-releasing hormone develop reversible hypo-oestrogen states in which trabecular bone loss occurs but recovers once treatment is discontinued (Matta et al. 1981). Similarly, women with hyperprolactinaemia and anorexia nervosa accompanied by amenorrhoea develop spinal osteopenia that in some cases leads to vertebral fractures. Amenorrhoea is observed in elite female athletes, who develop a reduced spinal bone destiny compared to that of eumenorrhoeic runners (Drinkwater et al. 1984), indicating that exercise alone cannot protect the skeleton in the face of oestrogen deficiency. The duration of amenorrhoea, from whatever cause, that will lead to irreversible bone loss is unknown, but is thought to be more than 6 months. Testosterone deficiency is present in approx. 30 per cent of men with spinal osteoporosis; they usually present in the sixth decade but most have symptoms of hypogonadism in the preceding 20 to 30 years (Jackson and Kleerekoper 1990). In males, hypogonadism from any cause may be associated with osteoporosis, including those with Klinefelter syndrome, hypogonadotrophic hypogonadism, hyperprolactinaemia, anorexia nervosa, and mumps orchitis.

Hyperthyroidism

In thyrotoxicosis, bone turnover may be significantly increased due to enhanced recruitment and increased resorption. Patient with a past history of thyrotoxicosis when compared with those who have not had thyrotoxicosis have an increased relative risk of hip fractures of 2.4 (Cummings et al. 1992). Thyrotoxicosis causing high-turnover osteoporosis should be thought of in elderly individuals in whom the diagnosis may not be clinically obvious and will be dependent on laboratory testing. Excessive thyroxine replacement in the hyperthyrotoxic individual may also increase bone loss, although the evidence for this is conflicting.

Nutrition

Calcium

While bone mass can may be transiently increased by calcium supplementation in adolescents, there is no evidence to suggest that above-normal intakes of calcium influence the peak bone mass (see 'Management of osteoporosis' below).

Drugs

The effects of glucocorticoids and thyroxine have been discussed above. Chronic heparin therapy can lead to decreased bone mass by enhancing PTH-mediated bone resorption, but warfarin is not associated with this complication despite a low circulating osteocalcin and impaired carboxylation of osteocalcin in warfarin-treated patients. Chronic administration of anticonvulsants lead to disturbance in calcium and vitamin D metabolism. These drugs increase the activity of hepatic microsomal mixed oxidases, leading to increased catabolism of steroid hormones (including vitamin D) and resulting in reduced concentrations of 25-hydroxyvitamin D [**25(OH)D**]. In addition, anticonvulsants directly suppress calcium absorption and antagonize the effects of PTH and vitamin D metabolites on bone. The end result is osteopenia and osteomalacia, particularly if there are other risk factors such as immobility, although not all individuals on chronic therapy are so affected. Methotrexate and other chemotherapeutic agents may affect skeletal metabolism and mass by a direct toxic effect on bone cells or by inducing hypogonadism. The use of antagonists or agonists to luteinizing hormone-releasing hormone to induce ovarian failure in premenstrual tension syndrome and endometriosis results in bone loss that is reversible if treatment is discontinued within 6 months.

Malignancy

Malignant infiltration and replacement of marrow tissue occur in multiple myeloma, lymphoma, leukaemia, systemic mastocytosis, and diffuse bony metastases. Myeloma is usually characterized by focal lytic lesions associated with the accumulation of myeloma cells, but in a small number of patients a diffuse loss of bone that mimics primary osteoporosis occurs. The increased bone resorption is due to the production of osteoclast-activating cytokines such as IL-1 and TNF-α and -β by plasma cells (Garrett *et al.* 1987). In lymphoma a generalized osteoporosis and hypercalcaemia may be the result of local synthesis of 1,25(OH)$_2$D$_3$ by malignant tissue. Mast cells secrete various products (heparin, histamine, prostaglandin) that could lead to increased osteoclastic bone resorption, and increased numbers of mast cells have been reported in the bone marrow in primary osteoporosis (Fallon *et al.* 1983).

Immobilization

Prolonged immobilization leads to disuse osteoporosis affecting trabecular and cortical bone. The rate of bone loss may be as high as 5 per cent per month for the first 6 months, after which it slows down to a new steady-state and some recovery is possible on resuming weight-bearing activities. Immobilization leads to increased bone resorption and decreased bone formation associated with hypercalciuria, and to an increase in plasma calcium, increased risk of renal stone formation, and potential suppression of PTH, 1,25(OH)$_2$D and calcium absorption.

Inflammatory disorders

Rheumatoid arthritis
In rheumatoid arthritis, bone loss can be periarticular, a hallmark of the disease, or a more generalized form, as demonstrated in histological, computed tomographic, and dual-photon absorptiometric studies (Dequeker and Geusens 1990). Increased rates of bone loss have been demonstrated by neutron-activated analysis of total body calcium. The pathogenesis of localized osteoporosis involves the production of numerous cytokines such as IL-1, IL-6, transforming growth factor-β, TNF, other growth factors, prostaglandins, and mast cell products (Dequeker and Geusens 1990). At present it is unclear whether all or only some patients with rheumatoid arthritis are affected by generalized osteoporosis, and when present its clinical significance is debatable. While it is not surprising that patients with long-standing destructive and disabling disease have low bone mass (Verstraeten and Dequeker 1990), population-based epidemiological studies show an increased risk of fracture in patients with rheumatoid

Table 5 Potential factors causing generalized osteoporosis in rheumatoid arthritis

Systemic actions of inflammatory products associated with disease activity
Alterations in circulating sex and calcitropic hormones
Altered calcium metabolism
Changes in load bearing of the skeleton
Effect of drugs used in treatment of arthritis

arthritis, related to age, impaired ambulation, body mass, and corticosteroid use (Hooyman *et al.* 1984; Cooper and Wickham 1990). Factors likely to lead to osteoporosis in rheumatoid arthritis are shown in Table 5. Usually, local factors such as cytokines exert their effect within the local microenvironment. Some cytokines, such as IL-1 and IL-6, may have systemic actions such as the induction of fever and the acute-phase response during inflammation. In rheumatoid arthritis, large amounts of local factors are produced within the joint and have the potential for systemic absorption affecting bone turnover at distant sites. Elevated serum IL-1 that correlates with disease activity has been demonstrated in patients with rheumatoid arthritis (Eastgate *et al.* 1988). However, various inhibitors that may antagonize cytokines have also been found in both serum and synovial fluid (Arend and Dayer 1990) and the net systemic effect on bone turnover of cytokine produced during joint inflammation is unclear. Some studies have demonstrated an association between disease activity and decreased bone mineral content (Sambrook *et al.* 1986) whilst others have not (Rosenspire *et al.* 1980). The difficulty in identifying a correlation between disease activity and bone mineral content is not surprising as almost all the studies involve cross-sectional measurements of the latter, a reflection of long-term accumulation of acute changes in bone turnover, with measurements of disease activity that varies relatively rapidly and may be associated with short-term changes in bone turnover best made by serological and urinary markers of bone metabolism.

During inflammation an alteration in the circulating levels of hormones has the potential for directly affecting bone turnover or modulating the effects of local factors. Various hormonal disturbances have been described in rheumatoid arthritis, such as changes in circulating sex hormone levels, but their significance in terms of disease activity and bone turnover is unclear. Sambrook *et al.* (1988) found a decreased oestrone, dehydroepiandrosterone sulphate (**DHEAS**), and testosterone; they suggested that the reduction in oestrone and testosterone, but not DHEAS, was secondary to the use of prednisolone. They also noted that reduced DHEAS in postmenopausal women with rheumatoid arthritis correlated with reduced bone mineral density of the femoral neck, suggesting that the disease itself may somehow reduce production of adrenal androgens. A decreased free and total testosterone have been found in some males with rheumatoid arthritis but the significance is as yet unclear. There are conflicting results on the effects of rheumatoid arthritis on calcitropic hormones. In most studies, the circulating levels of 25(OH)D, calcitonin, and PTH are reportedly normal but some have shown a low 25(OH)D (Dequeker and Geusens 1990).

Although calcium malabsorption has been described in patients with rheumatoid arthritis, the majority of workers have reported normal serum calcium and phosphate as well as urinary calcium excretion.

Decreased physical activity leads to decreased functional loading of the skeleton resulting in increased bone resorption. Decreased bone mineral content at the femoral neck and lumbar spine of patients with rheumatoid arthritis is significantly correlated with functional activity and is probably one of the major factors responsible for the bone loss associated with rheumatoid arthritis.

Drugs used in the treatment of rheumatoid arthritis may affect bone loss adversely by affecting bone cell activity or favourably by reducing inflammation and indirectly its effect on bone loss. Corticosteroids in high doses result in generalized bone loss and an increased rate of fracture (Hooyman et al. 1984; Cooper et al. 1995). This adverse effect is not as obvious at lower doses and there is conflicting evidence as to whether bone loss occurs with doses of less than 7.5 mg of prednisolone per day (Sambrook et al. 1986; Butler et al. 1991). The effect of intermittent intravenous corticosteroids is unclear, although they are likely to result in an acute suppression of bone metabolism that may be cumulative with frequent treatment. Non-steroidal anti-inflammatory drugs in vitro affect osteoblast and osteoclast function and prostaglandin and cytokine production (Gowen 1991), but an adverse independent effect on bone loss has not been demonstrated. The effect of disease-modifying anti-rheumatic drugs on generalized bone mineral content has not been studied extensively. The rate of generalized bone loss in patients with rheumatoid arthritis on disease-modifying antirheumatic drugs was not different from those not taking them in one study (Reid et al. 1981), but others have shown that the drugs prevent bone loss or increase bone mineral content (Kalla et al. 1991), probably by suppressing disease activity and thereby improving mobility.

Ankylosing spondylitis

Patients with severe ankylosing spondylitis often develop a dorsal kyphosis, and radiological findings of anterior vertebral wedging in the dorsal spine and of biconcave vertebrae suggest moderate osteoporosis (Ralston et al. 1990). Early reports on the prevalence of fractures in ankylosing spondylitis found a low prevalence of vertebral fractures (Wilkinson and Bywater 1958; Hanson et al. 1971; Hunter and Dubo 1978; Hunter and Dubo 1983). These studies also indicated that fractures were related to spinal trauma and correlated directly with the duration of the disease. In contrast, other studies such as by Ralston et al. (1990) found a much higher prevalence of fractures. Ralston et al. (1990) also observed that the development of fractures in their patients correlated directly with disease duration, and noted that vertebral fractures occurred spontaneously and were not related to trauma Cooper et al. (1994) found a significantly increased risk of clinically diagnosed vertebral compression fractures in patients with ankylosing spondylitis, but no increase in the risk of limb fractures.

Reid et al. (1986), using absorptiometry, reported high bone mineral density of the lumbar spine in patients with ankylosing spondylitis, but Will et al. (1989), also using dual X-ray absorptiometry, reported reduced bone mineral density in the lumbar spine and femoral neck of patients with early ankylosing spondylitis when spinal mobility and radiographs were still normal. In patients with more advanced disease there was a further reduction of bone density at the femoral neck and the carpus, suggesting that in ankylosing spondylitis bone loss is progressive and initially involves trabecular bone but later also cortical bone. The same group studied patients with early disease and matched them with same-sex siblings of similar physical activity. The bone density of the femoral neck was reduced in the group with ankylosing spondylitis, indicating that the reduced bone mass is a result of bone loss related to disease rather than failure to achieve adequate bone mass within families with ankylosing spondylitis (Will et al. 1990). The reduction of bone density in early ankylosing spondylitis was confirmed by Devogelar et al. (1992) and Lanyi et al. (1993); in patients with well-established ankylosing spondylitis, both groups of investigators noted increased bone density that was the direct result of syndesmophyte formation. Decreased density of hip bone has also been noted in ankylosing spondylitis (Will et al. 1989; Mullaji et al. 1994). The pathogenesis of reduced bone density in ankylosing spondylitis is unclear. Since reduced bone density has been found in patients with early disease who have normal spinal mobility, it is unlikely that immobilization of the spine is the primary event. Will et al. (1989) suggest that osteoporosis in ankylosing spondylitis is a primary pathological event due to the inflammatory nature of the disease. However, the precise mechanism by which inflammatory mediators are responsible for bone loss remains to be elucidated.

Clinical features

Typically a patient with osteoporosis is a thin Caucasian female aged between 50 and 70 years who presents with back pain resulting from vertebral fractures. Pain is usually of spontaneous onset, well localized, aggravated by movement, and radiates anteriorly to the lower rib cage and around the flank into the abdomen and thigh. Compression of nerve roots is uncommon and the painful episode usually subsides after 4 to 6 weeks. Some patients, particularly after multiple vertebral fractures, develop a constant dull pain in the lower thoracic or lumbar area that shows many of the features associated with mechanical disorders of the spine. Compression of vertebrae, particularly in the lumbar area, is associated with loss of height, which may be the sole complaint in some patients in whom vertebral compression has been painless. Anterior wedging of the vertebrae leads to a dorsal kyphosis (also known as 'dowager's hump'), with downward angulation of the ribs and a reduction in the gap between the ribs and the iliac crest of the pelvis. Contact between the lower ribs and the iliac crest may cause severe pain in the abdomen and inguinal area. Abdominal protuberance results from downward pressure on the abdominal cavity and may be associated with reflux oesophagitis and a feeling of fullness at meal times (Fig. 7).

Patients with appendicular fractures, usually of the wrist and femur, are often seen in emergency departments, although in the elderly individual a diagnosis of a hip fracture may be easily missed as pain may be minimal.

Pathogenesis

Bone growth and peak bone mass

During childhood and adolescence, growth and modelling leads to an increase in the size, shape, strength, and composition of bone. With the closure of the growth plate (also called the epiphyseal cartilage), growth ceases, but the need for mineral homeostasis and skeletal self-repair by removing and replacing effete bone is served by remodelling, a process that continues throughout life. In remodelling, unlike modelling, the sequence of bone formation and resorption is anatomically and quantitatively coupled. The resorption of a given amount of bone is followed by the deposition

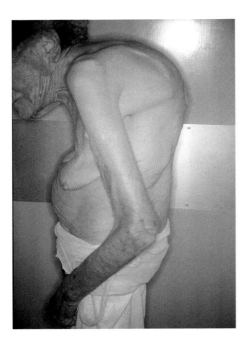

Fig. 7 Severe dorsal kyphosis and protuberant abdomen in a 75-year-old woman with osteoporosis.

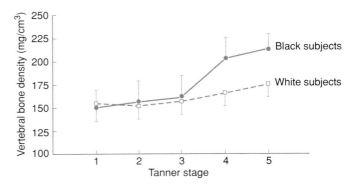

Fig. 8 Vertebral bone density in normal black (●) and white females (□) during different stages of sexual development (adapted from Gilsanz *et al.* 1991).

of an equivalent amount of new bone, but after the age of 35 to 40 years, presumably due to decreased osteoblastic activity, the amount of bone laid down is less than the amount resorbed during each remodelling sequence and leads to the bone loss seen with ageing.

A rapid gain in bone mass occurs in infancy and adolescence in both sexes. In early childhood males and females have similar bone mass, but after puberty males have a greater amount of cortical bone than females. In girls there is a dramatic increase in bone density during puberty and those with low oestrogen concentrations and a history of irregular menses attain a lower bone mass. Bone density in both white and black girls is similar during the early stages of puberty and an increase is observed only in the later stages of puberty, but at a greater rate in black than white girls. Using computed tomography to measure axial bone density, Gilsanz *et al.* (1991) observed that black and white girls have similar bone density in the early stages of puberty; at Tanner stage 4 and 5 of puberty, bone density increased substantially in both races, with black girls achieving a greater increase (39 per cent) than white girls (11 per cent) (Fig. 8).

Peak bone mass, or maximal bone density, is usually achieved in the third decade. Between 85 and 90 per cent of peak bone mass is accumulated during longitudinal growth (i.e. before age 20), but following the closure of the growth plate a further increase in bone mass in the axial and appendicular skeleton occurs between the ages of 20 and 35. Studies by Davies *et al.* (1990) suggest that a gain in bone mass of 3 to 6 per cent per decade may occur from the third decade. Further increases may be possible by changing lifestyle and behavioural patterns (e.g. increased exercise and calcium intake) in adolescence, and it has been suggested, but not yet proven, that increasing the peak bone mass may be an effective means of preventing the consequences of age-related and postmenopausal bone loss. The amount of peak bone mass present at the age of 30 to 35 years is determined by genetic and environmental factors, with the

former accounting for 80 per cent. Females achieve a lower peak mass, which may explain their increased risk of skeletal fractures in later life. The variance in bone mass between monozygotic twins is less than with dizygotic pairs (Pocock *et al.* 1987) (Fig. 9), and daughters of women with spinal crush fractures achieve a lower peak bone mass than age-matched daughters of non-osteoporotic females, indicating the genetic factors behind peak bone mass. Bone density at several sites (spine, hip, and forearm) is more similar between monozygotic twins than dizygotic twins (Pocock *et al.* 1987) (Fig. 10). The intraclass correlation, a measure of the proportion of the total variance in bone density due to variability among twin pairs, is approx. 0.8 in monozygotic twins and 0.3 in dizygotic twins. If bone mass was entirely genetically determined, the intraclass correlation would be 1.0 and 0.5 in monozygotic and dizygotic twins, respectively

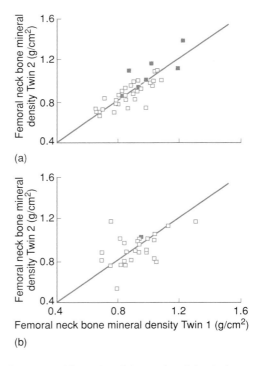

Fig. 9 Correlation of femoral-neck bone mineral density between (a) monozygotic (MZ) twins and (b) dizygotic (DZ) twins showing male (■) and female (□) twin pairs (reproduced from Pocock *et al.* 1987, with permission).

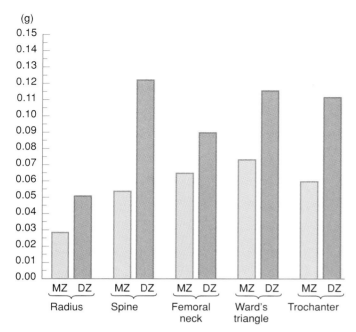

Fig. 10 The mean absolute value of within-pair bone mineral density difference between monozygotic (MZ) and dizygotic (DZ) twins for all skeletal sites (reproduced from Slemenda *et al.* 1991, with permission).

(Pocock *et al.* 1987; Slemenda *et al.* 1990*a*). An alternative way of examining the contribution of the environment to bone mass is to look at the maximum within-pair differences in bone density. At all sites, the mean differences between dizygotic twins are almost twice as great as the mean differences between monozygotic twins (Fig. 10). In monozygotic twins the within-pair difference is due to environmental and behaviour factors, and defines the amount of bone mass that may be changed by altering environmental factors. Further evidence for genetic factors is provided by the finding of greater bone mass in black than white individuals, yet the former may have a less suitable environment for skeletal development. The reason for the greater bone mass in black individuals is unclear, but, at least in girls, the difference is apparent at puberty. The mechanism of this effect remains to be elucidated, with increased resistance to the bone-resorptive effects of the calcitropic hormones, namely PTH and 1,25-dihydroxyvitamin D_3, postulated by some (Bell *et al.* 1985) but not confirmed by others.

Environmental factors have an important influence on peak bone mass, not only during adolescence but also during the consolidation phase when statural growth has ceased. The influence of nutritional factors, particularly calcium, has attracted considerable attention but remains a matter of debate. Matkovic *et al.* (1979) found that metacarpal cortical bone mass was greater and the incidence of hip fractures lower in regions of the former Yugoslavia where calcium intake was higher. However, increased calcium intake may be associated with an improved socioeconomic status and nutrition, so that it is difficult to be certain that calcium intake was the sole factor for improved metacarpal bone mass. Results from a 3-year double-blind, placebo-controlled trial involving 6- to 14-year-old monozygotic twin pairs, in which one twin received 1 g of calcium supplements daily while the other received placebo, suggest that increased calcium intake leads to a more rapid increase in bone mineral density in growing children (Johnston *et al.* 1992). It is too

soon to know whether this early increase leads to a higher peak bone mass or to an earlier establishment of peak bone mass that later does not differ from that of the control twins. Nevertheless, these studies indicate that a population-based strategy for management of osteoporosis may be through improving dietary calcium intake in childhood.

Physical inactivity leads to bone loss and increased physical fitness leads to a greater bone mass in the axial and appendicular skeleton (Pocock *et al.* 1986). In children, weight-bearing physical activity is associated with a moderate increase in bone mass at several sites, which may translate into a greater peak bone mass and a reduced incidence of osteoporotic fractures (Slemenda *et al.* 1991). Excess physical activity, however, is to be avoided, since it may lead to hypothalamic amenorrhoea and bone loss (Drinkwater *et al.* 1984). Although initially the lower bone mass in oligoamenorrhoeic and amenorrhoeic athletes, compared to eumenorrhoeic athletes, was only seen in the lumbar spine, recent studies using improved measurement techniques suggest that bone loss occurs at several sites (Rencken *et al.* 1996). Furthermore, following the return of normal menses, bone mass in these females remains below normal (Drinkwater *et al.* 1990).

Vitamin D receptor gene polymorphism and osteoporosis

Twin studies suggest a strong genetic effect on bone mass, with heritability estimates of 0.5 to 0.9. Higher concentrations of osteocalcin, a marker of increased bone turnover, were reported in twins with a particular vitamin D receptor (*VDR*) gene polymorphism (Morrison *et al.* 1992). Subsequently the same group, using monozygotic and dizygotic twins, noted that 75 per cent of the genetic component of bone density could be attributed to polymorphism of the *VDR* gene (Morrison *et al.* 1994).Similar findings, but with a weaker correlation, were noted in a British population of postmenopausal females (Spector *et al.* 1995). Ferrari *et al.* (1995) suggested that *VDR* gene polymorphism may predict the rate of changes in spinal bone density in elderly people. However, the association between allelic variations in the *VDR* gene and bone mineral density has not been confirmed by others; both sides of the controversy have been discussed recently (Eisman 1995; Peacock 1995). Thus, Hustmyer *et al.* (1994) found no evidence of linkage between *VDR* alleles and bone density at the spine, hip or wrist in white female twins in the United States. Similarly, in French premenopausal women no association was found between *VDR* alleles and bone density or bone turnover (Garnero *et al.* 1995). At present the difference between these studies is difficult to explain. It is possible that *VDR* gene alleles make a much smaller difference than expected to peak bone mass, which might have been missed in some studies. Alternatively, Parfitt (1994) suggests that *VDR* polymorphism may be linked to another gene polymorphism that regulates bone turnover and that this linkage is influenced by environmental factor(s), which in turn may be confined to one geographical area.

Age-related bone loss

Until the age of 35 to 40 years the amount of bone formed equals the amount removed at each remodelling unit. Thereafter there is a slight mismatch, with less bone being formed, and this results in an age-related loss of bone that is universal in humans and affects all skeletal sites. In both sexes, trabecular and cortical bone mass decline by 6 to 8 and 2 to 4 per cent per decade, respectively. In postmenopausal

Table 6 Risk factors for osteoporosis

Race (white or Asian)
Premature loss of ovarian function
Postmenopausal
Short stature and low body-mass index
Positive family history
Nulliparity
Low calcium intake
Inactivity
Excessive alcohol intake
Smoking
Long-term use of corticosteroids

females, further bone loss occurs associated with declining ovarian function, and in the vertebrae the trabecular loss may be as high as 5 to 10 per cent per year (Stevenson 1988), while cortical bone loss may be 2 per cent per year. The rapid rate of bone loss after ovarian failure, a consequence of the decline in circulating oestrogen level, decreases exponentially over 5 to 8 years eventually to match the age-related bone loss (Krolner and Nielsen 1982).

The mechanism of age-related bone loss is unknown but several possibilities exist. Calcium absorption declines with age in both sexes, as does the ability of the intestine to adapt to a reduced calcium intake by improving absorption. Furthermore, the reduced ability to synthesize 1,25-dihydroxyvitamin D, due to reduced activity of the renal 1α-hydroxylase, will affect intestinal calcium absorption. Reduced calcium absorption will lead to chronic stimulation of parathyroid glands and the increased PTH will accelerate bone loss by stimulating osteoclasts and increasing the number of remodelling units at which uncoupling has occurred. Other factors of importance in age-related bone loss include defective osteoblast function, the conversion of haemopoietic marrow into fatty marrow with loss of precursor cells and locally generated growth factors, and impaired reserves and secretion of calcitonin (Stevenson 1988).

Diagnosis

Risk factors

Since it is easier to prevent than to treat established osteoporosis, it has been suggested that assessment for risk factors may be used to select individuals at sufficient risk and offer them further investigation (Riggs and Melton 1986). These risk factors are detailed in Table 6.

The major risk factors are race, loss of ovarian function, and peak bone mass. As mentioned previously, peak bone mass is predominantly genetically determined and racial origin is important in that it is likely that black individuals achieve a greater peak bone mass than white. Loss of ovarian function is associated with bone loss, and premature ovarian failure and amenorrhoea lead to reduced bone mass and are associated with increased risk of osteoporosis. Cigarette smoking may indirectly be harmful to the skeleton because it increases the metabolism of oestrogen, and smokers tend to have a slim build and lower body weight. Obesity may be protective to the skeleton of postmenopausal females by increasing the forces

transmitted through it and by increasing conversion of androstenedione to oestrone in fatty tissue (Schindler et al. 1972). Females of small build tend to have reduced bone mass. Daughters of women with vertebral osteoporosis tend to have reduced bone mass and a positive family history may be regarded as a risk factor. While risk-factor assessment has been useful for epidemiological studies, its ability to predict bone mass and risk of fracture is poor and it cannot be relied upon to estimate the presence or absence of osteoporosis in individual patients (Slemenda et al. 1990b; Cooper et al. 1991).

Bone mass measurement

A high correlation exists between bone mineral density and bone strength and therefore the risk of fragility fracture. Several prospective studies suggest that the best means of assessing risk of fracture is through measurement of bone mineral density (Johnston et al. 1991).

Conventional radiology is a relatively insensitive method of assessing bone mass. Morphological changes, readily assessed semiquantitatively by such methods as the metacarpal index, vertebral body index, and the Singh index for the proximal femur, have been and are still used as a basis for bone mass assay where other techniques are unavailable, but these methods cannot detect early bone loss and also lack sensitivity. Reliable measurements of bone mass can be accurately and precisely obtained by a number of techniques (Table 7). In general these techniques calculate bone mass by measuring tissue absorption of photons obtained from a radioactive or X-ray tube source (Cohn 1991).

Single-photon absorptiometry, available for over 25 years and using low-energy photon beams, measures appendicular bone mass at the forearm and heel. The sites are usually immersed in water to make the soft-tissue thickness constant. The photon beam is directed through the forearm of the patient and detected by a scintillation counter on the other side of the arm. The intensity of the transmitted beam is measured at intervals along the radius and ulna to determine the total bone mineral content. The technique is limited because it can only measure peripheral sites and the position of the beam is critical to avoid errors when doing repeated scans.

Dual-photon absorptiometry uses two photon energies, usually derived from gadolinium, and permits distinction between bone and soft tissue; this allows measurement at sites of fragility fractures in the lumbar spine and proximal femur. The radiation dose is small (50–150 mSv) and precision good (1–4 per cent). The disadvantages are a long scanning time and the need to replace the isotope sources. In many places, dual-photon absorptiometry has been superseded by dual-energy X-ray absorptiometry, which uses X-rays as the source for protons. Its advantages are a reduced scanning time, improved resolution, precision, and accuracy.

Quantitative computed tomography allows volume measurements and also permits distinction between cortical and trabecular bone in the vertebrae. Its main disadvantages are cost and high radiation exposure. Ultrasonography is a non-invasive technique currently under investigation; its use and correlation with bone mineral density measured by dual-energy X-ray absorptiometry is currently being assessed and it cannot as yet be recommended for clinical use.

Bone biopsy

Since the advent of non-invasive techniques to measure bone mass, transiliac bone biopsy is no longer essential to establish the diagnosis of osteoporosis. It may be indicated where osteomalacia is suspected

Table 7 Techniques available for *in vivo* measurement

Technique	Sites	Radiation dose (μSv)	Units of measurement
Radiogrammetry	Carpus Femoral neck Vertebrae	(Skin dose) Carpus 50–900 Lumbar vertebrae 10 000–240 000	Metacarpal index Singh index Vertebral body index
Single-photon absorptiometry	Forearm	50–100	g/cm g/cm^2
Dual-photon absorptiometry	Lumbar spine Femoral neck Forearm Whole body	10–40	g/cm^2
Dual X-ray absorptiometry	Lumbar spine Femoral neck Forearm Whole body	10–40	g/cm^2
Quantitative computed tomography	Lumbar spine Femur Tibia Forearm	100–10 000	g/cm^3 g/cm^3
Ultrasound	Calcaneus Patella	No ionizing radiation	AVU (apparent velocity of ultrasound) (m/s) BUA (broadband ultrasonic attenuation) (db/MHz)

on the basis of abnormal biochemical or radiological features. When undertaken, however, the result often indicates osteoporosis rather than osteomalacia. Bone histomorphometry is of use in quantitating rates of bone formation and resorption, but few centres can undertake this and it is usually done as part of clinical research (Malluche and Faugere 1991).

Biochemical markers

Routine biochemical tests are usually normal in osteoporosis. Biochemical markers of skeletal metabolism are available, but their precise role has not been established. Markers of bone formation include serum alkaline phosphatase (particularly the bone iso-enzyme), osteocalcin (also known as bone gla protein), and type 1 procollagen propeptides. Fasting urinary calcium and hydroxy-proline, and serum tartrate-resistant acid phosphatase, are markers of bone resorption that lack sensitivity. The urinary excretion of the collagen cross-links, pyridinoline and deoxypyridinoline, reflects breakdown of bone and cartilage collagens and appears to be raised in disorders characterized by high bone turnover such as after the menopause and in primary hyperparathyroidism. The biochemical markers may be of help in investigating bone turnover in established osteoporosis by separating individuals with high-turnover from those with low-turnover osteoporosis, and in monitoring the effects of appropriate treatments.

Management

Prevention

Prevention of bone loss appears to be the most effective means of reducing the incidence of fragility fracture. A reduced bone mass in an individual, and therefore the increased risk of fractures, is related to the peak bone mass achieved by that individual, the rate of bone loss with ageing, and, in females, the rate and duration of postmeno-pausal bone loss. The determinants of peak bone mass include genetic factors, which cannot be manipulated, and nutritional and environmental factors, which may be manipulated to the individual's advantage. For pharmacological intervention, particularly hormone replacement therapy, the identification of the individual at risk will help restrict therapy to those who need it and avoid treating those whose risk for fragility fracture is low. At present the only means of achieving this is through bone mass measurement, and prospective studies suggest that a reduction in bone density by 1 SD is associated with a relative risk for fracture that varies from 1.5 to 3.0 with site-specificity. In other words, bone mineral density in the spine and hip is a better predictor for fracture of the respective site than that in the forearm is for fracture of the spine or hip.

Calcium

The role of calcium supplementation in preventing bone loss remains controversial. Matkovic's study (Matkovic *et al*. 1979) is often cited as an important piece of evidence appearing to indicate that the preservation of cortical bone was greater in women living in a community with a high-calcium diet than in one with a low-calcium diet. The study has been criticized in that the association was apparently related to other differences between the two communities: the community with a high-calcium diet was physically more active than the low-calcium (Kanis 1991). In their comprehensive review on calcium, Kanis and Passmore (1989) suggest that the inverse relation between calcium intake and hip fracture rate around the world indicates that calcium intake cannot account for the marked variation in fracture rates and argues against a role for calcium in preventing fractures. Studies by Heaney *et al*. (1978) indicated that increased dietary calcium intake was capable of restoring calcium balance in pre- and postmenopausal women, but others have failed to record the advantages of calcium supplementation in preventing bone loss or acting as an effective substitute for hormone replacement (Nilas *et al.* 1984; Riis *et al.* 1987). There may be a role for increasing calcium intake in the elderly osteoporotic female in preventing cortical bone loss and reducing the incidence of further vertebral fractures. A meta-analysis (Cummings 1990) indicated that the beneficial effects of calcium were greatest when calcium intake is low; the advantages in other situations were small and require further study. Calcium supplementation of prepubertal children enhances the rate of increase in bone mineral density but it is unclear if this gain translates into increased peak bone mass (Johnston *et al.* 1992). It is likely that the benefit may be lost once the supplements are stopped. Recent studies over 4 years have shown that, in postmenopausal women, calcium supplements compared to placebo lead to a reduced rate of loss of total-body bone mineral density (Reid *et al.* 1993; Reid *et al.* 1995). In the lumbar spine and femoral neck the difference between the two groups occurred predominantly in the first year; in the subsequent years the calcium-treated group lost bone but at a lower rate than controls. Although there were significantly fewer symptomatic fractures in the calcium group, the study was not large enough to provide a definite answer, which can only be given by a much larger, prospective study. At present, therefore, calcium supplementation should be restricted to those with definite osteoporosis and with a poor calcium diet (daily calcium intake of less than 400 mg), as supplementary therapy in any anabolic treatment, malabsorption states, and in elderly people. Prophylactic use cannot be justified and would have considerable cost implications.

Exercise

It is generally accepted that skeletal mass at any site is dependent on the stress to which it is subjected (Rubin and Lanyon 1984) and that strenuous physical activity in adults is associated with a greater bone mass (Nilsson and Westlin 1971). There is also some evidence that physical activity may reduce the rate of bone lost due to menopause, although the exact type of exercise needed is unclear (Smith *et al.* 1984). In general, however, the exercise must be weight-bearing in type. Physical activity may also be of importance in children and leads to moderate increases in bone mass at several sites, including the hip. The resultant increase in peak bone mass could lead to a significant decrease in the incidence of osteoporotic fractures in later years (Slemenda *et al.* 1991).

Hormone replacement

The most effective treatment in preventing postmenopausal bone loss is oestrogen replacement therapy, which has been shown to reduce the risk of bone loss and incidence of fractures, particularly those of the hip. Loss of ovarian function is associated with a rapid rate of bone loss over a 5- to 10-year period, after which it gradually slows and returns to the age-related rate of bone loss (Lindsay *et al.* 1987). There is histological evidence of increased osteoclastic bone resorption associated with a relative reduction in osteoblastic activity after the menopause. The administration of oestrogen is associated with a reduced rate of bone resorption and therefore a decreased rate of bone loss (Kanis *et al.* 1990). How oestrogens achieve this effect is unclear but they appear to have a direct action on osteoblast activity (Eriksen *et al.* 1988) with a secondary effect on osteoclast activity mediated by cytokines (McSheety and Chambers 1986). Unfortunately, replacement of oestrogen alone is associated with an increased risk of endometrial cancer, which may persist even after discontinuing oestrogen replacement (Paganini-Hill *et al.* 1989). The endometrial cancers are not aggressive and the 5-year survival was near to 100 per cent. The addition of progestogen allows the shedding of the endometrium, and minimizes the risk of hyperplasia and subsequent neoplasia. In general, 12 days of progestogen with continuous oestrogen use carries a negligible risk of hyperplasia (Whitehead and Fraser 1987) and a relative risk of endometrial cancer of 0.9 compared with 1.4 in women using oestrogen alone (Persson *et al.* 1989). Thus, in women who have a regular scheduled bleed, there is no need for a routine endometrial examination to detect hyperplasia unless the bleed occurs prematurely.

Use of the oral contraceptive pill, early menarche, and a late menopause are risk factors for breast cancer and suggest an oestrogen-related effect. Most studies suggest that oestrogen used in hormone replacement therapy (**HRT**) does not increase the overall risk of breast cancer (Brinton *et al.* 1986). There is, however, some concern over very long-term treatment with oestrogens, especially over 10 years, when there may be a small increase in risk (Bergkvist *et al.* 1989). One study from Sweden has suggested a relative risk of 1.7 in women using HRT for more than 7 years (Bergkvist *et al.* 1989), but a recent large meta-analysis suggests a relative risk of 1.3 (Steinberg *et al.* 1991). The Royal College of Obstetrics and Gynaecology Study Group concluded that there may be a duration-dependent risk of breast cancer with HRT and that there was no evidence that progestogens protect against that risk. More recent evidence from the Nurses Health Study suggests that the risk of breast cancer is significantly increased amongst women taking HRT, the relative risk being 1.32, which is not appreciably different if progestogen is also added to the treatment. The use of HRT for 5 to 9 years led to a relative risk of breast cancer of 1.46, which was greatest amongst women aged 60 to 64 years. The relative risk of death due to breast cancer was also increased, at 1.45 in women who had taken medication for five or more years (Colditz *et al.* 1995). Women who are concerned about the breast cancer risk should be encouraged to participate in the United Kingdom national mammographic screening programme, which offers 3-yearly screening from 50 years of age.

With regard to hypertension, there is no evidence that HRT elevates blood pressure and in some instances it has been found to lower the diastolic pressure. Although oral contraceptives increase blood clotting factors and risk of pulmonary embolism, there is currently no good evidence that postmenopausal oestrogen replacement therapy increases the risk of thromboembolic disease. An increased risk of deep-vein thrombosis and pulmonary emboli has recently been reported in women currently taking HRT (Daly *et al.* 1996; Grodstein *et al.* 1996a; Jick *et al.* 1996). In all three studies, although the relative risk of venous thrombosis was raised to between 2.1 and 3.5, the absolute risks remained low. For example, Daly *et al.* (1996) found an adjusted relative risk of 3.5, but this would yield only one extra case in 5000 users per year.

HRT is associated with decreased mortality from ischaemic heart disease (by 40–50 per cent). A recent prospective study by Stampfer *et al.* (1991) showed a 50 per cent reduction in the risk of major coronary arterial disease or fatal cardiovascular disease, and no increase in the risk of stroke, in women who had ever used oestrogen replacement therapy compared with women who had never used oestrogen. Part of this effect is probably due to the beneficial effects of oestrogen on lipid levels. The addition of a progestogen does not alter the cardioprotective effects of postmenopausal oestrogen

(Grodstein *et al.* 1996*b*). After the menopause, levels of high-density lipoprotein (associated with removing precholesterol from the blood) decline while total cholesterol and low-density lipoprotein increase. Oral oestrogen is associated with a rise in the level of the protective high-density lipoprotein–cholesterol fraction and a decreasing low-density fraction as documented by the Lipid Research Clinic's follow-up study (Bush *et al.* 1983). The effects of combined therapy on ischaemic heart disease are unknown. It is possible, but not proven, that some of the beneficial effects of oestrogen may be reduced by the administration of progestogens (Goldman and Tosteson 1991).

Recently, evidence has also been presented that HRT is associated with an increased risk of deep vein thrombosis and/or pulmonary emboli. The relative risk of venous thrombosis appears to be increased two- to threefold in current users of HRT. The absolute risk in current users remains small, with estimates of 16 and 23 excess cases per 100 000 women per year for all venous thromboembolisms and 6 per 100 000 women per year for pulmonary embolism only. In all three studies presented the risk of venous embolism disappeared on cessation of HRT (Daly *et al.* 1996; Grodstein *et al.* 1996*a*; Jick *et al.* 1996).

Treatment with exogenous oestrogen after the menopause results in a significant reduction in bone resorption as reflected in a fall in the fasting urinary calcium:creatinine and hydroxyproline:creatinine ratios (Lindsay *et al.* 1976). The mechanism of the oestrogen effect is unclear, but is likely to be mediated through the oestrogen-sensitive osteoblast releasing growth factors that inhibit the recruitment and differentiation of osteoclasts from their bone marrow precursors. The minimum oral dose of oestradiol required to prevent bone loss is 2.0 mg/ day, and of conjugated oestrogen 0.625 mg /day. For percutaneous delivery, 3 mg of oestradiol gel, or 50 mg oestradiol implant, or at least 50 mg/24 h of transdermal oestrogen will also be effective. If HRT is discontinued the rate of bone loss is similar to that seen in early years of the menopause. The optimal duration of treatment is unknown, but it should be long-term (from 5 to 10 years) to maximize the benefit to the cardiovascular system and bone without significant risk. Melton (1987) suggests that treatment for 5 years would shift the hip fracture:age curve to the right. Although life expectancy is increased by about 2 years in HRT users, he argued that the shift in the fracture:age curve would still mean that many women would not live beyond the age where the shifted curve is placed (Melton 1987). From findings by Lindsay *et al.* (1987) it is evidently appropriate to start treatment early in the menopause, since it is unlikely that any existing bone loss can be recovered. Although it remains unclear how long the benefits of HRT on bone mass persist after its discontinuation, a Swedish cohort study suggests that the more potent oestrogens gave a 0.37 relative risk of trochanteric fracture in women who had started treatment before the age of 60 years; in contrast the weaker oestrogen did not confer any benefit (Naessen *et al.* 1990). Other data suggest that the use of HRT 14 years after the menopause may still result in reduction of further bone loss and a slight increase in trabecular bone mass in the axial skeleton (Quigley *et al.* 1987; Lindsay and Tomme 1990).

Calcitonin

Calcitonin is a 32-residue peptide hormone produced by the parafollicular cells of the thyroid gland. The hormone binds to high-affinity receptors on osteoclasts, but its precise physiological role in man is uncertain. Preliminary studies suggest that calcitonin may be as effective as oestrogen in abolishing postmenopausal bone loss (Reginster *et al.* 1987). Further studies are necessary to determine optimal dose, route of administration, and long-term effect. If confirmed it may prove an alternative to HRT in individuals in whom oestrogens are contraindicated or unacceptable. At present, calcitonin is given subcutaneously but the development of new formulations means that an effective nasal spray and suppository delivery systems may soon become available.

Treatment of established osteoporosis

For the very elderly individual with osteoporosis-related fractures there is no effective treatment available. However, for postmenopausal women and men aged 50 to 70 years with established disease, available treatments can be grouped into class I agents, which either impair bone resorption and/or reduce activation frequency, or class II agents, which increase bone formation (Table 8).

HRT

As a class I agent, HRT leads to reduced bone turnover and is effective in preventing postmenopausal bone loss. But HRT may also retard bone loss in established osteoporosis: over a 2-year period, a small increase in bone mass may be seen in trabecular rather than cortical bone as formation continues and refilling of the remodelled space occurs. After about 2 years a plateau is achieved and further increases in bone mass are unlikely. A similar plateau for bone mass may occur with other antiresorptive agents such as calcitonin and bisphosphonates. One problem with HRT in older patients is the reluctance to accept the resumption of menstruation. Long-term studies examining the effectiveness of HRT in preventing further vertebral fractures in patients with spinal osteoporosis are not available.

Calcitonin

In patients with vertebral or wrist fractures, treatment with calcitonin leads to a small increase in bone mass over the first 1 to 2 years. The usefulness of this increase in bone mass will become clearer when results become available from prospective studies in progress on the rates of new vertebral fractures. It may be possible to obtain continued increases in bone mass if calcitonin is administered cyclically. At present, synthetic salmon calcitonin is approved for the treatment of postmenopausal osteoporosis but is required to be given parenterally. It is an expensive drug and similar benefits may

Table 8 Potential treatments for established osteoporosis

Class I—impair bone resorption and/or reduce activation frequencies
Hormone replacement therapy
Calcitonin
Bisphosphonates
Anabolic steroids
Calcium
Vitamin D and metabolites

Class II—stimulate bone formation
Sodium fluoride
Intermittent parathyroid injections

1598

5 THE SCOPE OF RHEUMATIC DISEASE

be achieved by giving lower doses every 2 to 3 days, although this must be proved by clinical trials.

The analgesic effect of calcitonin, probably mediated through β-endorphin release, is sometimes useful in controlling pain resulting from vertebral crush fractures and enables early mobilization of the patient.

Bisphosphonates

The bisphosphonates are potent inhibitors of bone resorption and have been successfully used to inhibit osteoclastic activity in Paget's disease of bone and malignant hypercalcaemia. Disodium etidronate has recently been used in the treatment of established vertebral osteoporosis. In two double-blind, placebo-controlled studies, etidronate, given cyclically in a dose of 400 mg daily for 2 weeks every 3 months for 3 years, modestly but significantly increased spinal bone density and reduced the incidence of further vertebral deformity and fractures (Storm *et al.* 1990; Watts *et al.* 1990). There was no significant change in cortical bone mass. In an open-label follow-up of 37 postmenopausal females with osteoporosis treated for 5 years, a further increase in bone density of 1.4 per cent was observed during the last 2 years of study; the reduction in vertebral fracture rate observed in the earlier part of the study was also maintained (Storm *et al.* 1996). Etidronate has been approved for use in established vertebral osteoporosis in the United Kingdom and most European countries, but not in the United States,

The aminobisphosphonate, alendronate sodium (alendronate), increases bone mineral density in the spine, hip and total body, and reduces the incidence of new morphometric vertebral fractures (Liberman *et al.* 1993) (Fig. 11). The results of a randomized trial involving 2027 women with at least one vertebral fracture at baseline and low bone-mass density of the femoral neck, treated with alendronate or placebo, were recently reported; they showed that the relative risk of sustaining a new morphometric vertebral fracture was 0.33 in the treated compared to the control group (Black *et al.* 1996). In addition, there was a reduction in clinically apparent vertebral fractures as well as of any clinical fracture in the hip and wrist. The reduced risk of hip fracture noted in this study of postmenopausal women dwelling in the community suggests that bisphosphonates may be of value in preventing such fractures in women with low bone-mass density of the hip. However, until a formal analysis of cost-effectiveness is made, the expense of using alendronate to prevent such fractures may appear prohibitive.

In general, bisphosphonates are well tolerated but should be used with caution in patients with impaired renal function. Their absorption is impaired by calcium, iron, magnesium, and aluminium, to which they bind. Some unwanted side-effects of etidronate include hypersensitivity reactions, urticaria, and angio-oedema, but these are uncommon. Etidronate should be used cyclically and not daily as this will lead to impaired normal bone mineralization. In contrast, alendronate, because of its high potency, can be given daily. Although the frequency of upper gastrointestinal side-effects with alendronate was similar to placebo in the randomized trial discussed above, the clinical use of alendronate has been associated with oesophagitis, at times severe enough to warrant admission to hospital, and other upper gastrointestinal symptoms. These symptoms may be more common in those with previous upper gastrointestinal problems and in those taking non-steroidal anti-inflammatory drugs. To some extent, these complications can be avoided by asking

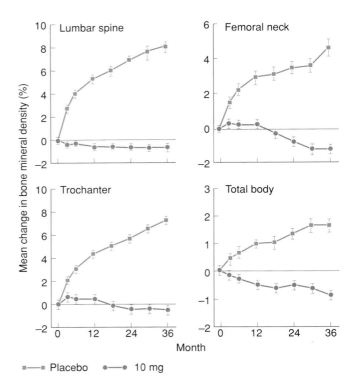

Fig. 11 Changes in bone mineral density from baseline values in women with postmenopausal osteoporosis receiving alendronate 10 mg/day or placebo for 3 years (after Liberman *et al.* 1993)

the patients to take alendronate with at least 100 ml of water and to avoid lying down during the next 30 min.

Testosterone and anabolic steroids

Hypogonadism in males is a well-established cause of osteoporosis and can be prevented by rendering the individual eugonadal with replacement therapy using testosterone, which increases bone mass by stimulating bone formation. The testosterone ester is usually given intramuscularly every 2 weeks. The newer oral testosterone preparations may also be used, but their effects on bone mass have not been fully evaluated. The use of testosterone in osteoporotic male patients with normal gonadal function cannot be recommended until further data become available showing benefit.

The anabolic steroids, stanozolol and nandrolone denoate, appear to reduce bone resorption as determined by hydroxyproline excretion, and lead to an increase in bone mass in both males and females. The reported increases in bone mass with anabolic steroids may in part be due to measurement artefact: these drugs decrease fat mass and increase lean body mass, which leads to a falsely elevated measure of bone mass. Anabolic steroids also cause mild degrees of masculinization, which is unacceptable to many women, and, in addition, they have adverse effects on plasma lipids, raising doubts about their long-term safety.

Vitamin D and metabolites

It has been proposed that circulating 1,25(OH)D (calcitriol) and calcium absorption are decreased in some, especially elderly, osteoporotic patients. A potential therapeutic role for calcitriol is suggested by its ability to stimulate intestinal calcium absorption, reduce secondary hyperparathyroidism, and abolish PTH-mediated bone resorption. Unfortunately, trials of calcitriol treatment for women with osteoporosis have yielded conflicting results. Some found that the bone density of the spine increased with calcitriol (Gallagher and Goldgar 1990) while others found that it decreased by similar amounts in patients and controls (Ott and Chesnut 1989). In all studies the cohorts have not been large enough to evaluate the effects of calcitriol on the rate of new vertebral fractures. More recently, Tilyard *et al.* (1992) have reported their findings on the occurrence of new vertebral fractures in 622 postmenopausal women with spinal fractures entered into a prospective study of calcitriol on calcium. A threefold reduction in the occurrence of new vertebral fractures or deformity was observed over 3 years in women treated with calcitriol. This effect was evident only in women who had five or fewer vertebral fractures on entry into the study. A reduction in the number of peripheral fractures was also noted in those treated with calcitriol. The dose of calcitriol was 0.25 mg twice a day: it was not associated with any major adverse effects, but concerns about the effect of calcitriol on urinary calcium excretion and renal function remain, since these were not estimated in all patients. In elderly women the addition of 800 units of vitamin D_3 and calcium reduced the number of fractures in comparison to a control group; a significant difference in number was apparent only after 12 to 18 months of the 3-year study (Chapuy *et al.* 1992). The incidence of hip fractures showed a marked increase in the placebo group but remained unchanged in the group treated with vitamin D_3, suggesting that vitamin D_3 prevented the exponential increase in the incidence of hip fractures that takes place in this age group.

Vitamin D deficiency is common in elderly persons, owing to reduced exposure to sunlight, decreased synthesis of vitamin D_3 in the ageing skin, and low dietary intake of vitamin D. Ooms *et al.* (1995) noted that supplementation of the elderly with 400 units of vitamin D_3 daily leads to a slight decrease in secondary hyperparathyroidism and an increase in bone density at the femoral neck. Although Chapuy *et al.* (1992) showed a reduction in the incidence of hip fracture following supplementation with 800 units of vitamin D_3, it is not known whether the benefits were due to the supplemental vitamin D or calcium. Supplementation with 400 units of vitamin D_3 administered to elderly men and women dwelling in the community in Amsterdam did not lead to a decrease in the incidence of hip or peripheral fractures (Lips *et al.* 1996). However, this Dutch population differed in many respects to that studied by Chapuy *et al.* (1992): they were younger, fewer had a raised PTH, and evidence for secondary hyperparathyroidism and vitamin D deficiency was less common. In addition, the dose of vitamin D_3 was 400 units not 800 units as in the French study.

The parenteral administration of vitamin D (150 000 to 300 000 units annually) to elderly individuals did not lead to any reduction in fractures of the leg, but fractures of the arms were reduced by half (Heikinheimo *et al.* 1992).

Sodium fluoride

Sodium fluoride stimulates the proliferation and activity of osteoblasts, leading to an increase in osteoid production and trabecular bone volume. It should be given with substantial calcium supplements to allow mineralization to take place, otherwise osteomalacia will develop.

The drug is rapidly absorbed from the gastrointestinal tract if taken in the fasting state; food will impair absorption. Approximately 60 per cent of the drug accumulates in bone and the rest is excreted by the kidneys. Fluoride attaches to apatite in bone, making it more resistant to resorption. In spinal osteoporosis, moderate doses of sodium fluoride (50 mg/day) reduced the incidence of spinal fracture by 25 per cent after 2 years of treatment (Mamelle *et al.* 1988), but others have found it to be less effective. In recent, randomized, placebo-controlled studies of high-dose sodium fluoride (75 mg daily), increases in axial bone-mineral density were found without any reduction in the incidence of fractures, suggesting that the mechanical strength of the newly formed bones may be reduced (Riggs *et al.* 1990; Kleerekoper and Nelson 1992). These studies have been criticized for using excessive doses of fluoride that may have led to the accumulation of unmineralized osteoid. This issue will only be resolved by further, carefully conducted clinical trials, so that at present fluoride remains an investigational drug.

Although slow-release sodium fluoride reportedly prevented new vertebral fractures and increased bone mineral density in the spine and femoral neck (Pak *et al.* 1995), those trials have been criticized for their design and inability to detect any osteotoxic effects of fluoride (Kleerekoper 1996)

Parathyroid hormones

Animals given daily or alternate-day injections of PTH develop increased amounts of trabecular bone that is biologically normal. In man, daily injections of the 1–34 fragments of PTH, when given alone, increased trabecular bone volume but decreased cortical bone mass; the treatment was abandoned because of the potential disadvantage of increasing the risk of limb fractures. Recent studies using PTH 1–34 in combination with HRT (Reeve *et al.* 1990), calcitriol, or calcitonin demonstrated impressive increases in spinal trabecular bone mass, comparable to that seen with fluoride, but achieved within 12 months as compared to 2 years with sodium fluoride. Side-effects were few and the results suggest the need for a randomized control study of PTH in combination with another antiresorptive agent. At present, therefore, PTH, like sodium fluoride, should be regarded as an investigational drug only.

The investigation and management of low-trauma fractures

A low-trauma fracture (i.e., one that follows a fall from standing height or less) should always be investigated to exclude the possibility of osteoporosis. The three most common sites of fracture are the wrist, vertebrae, and hip, and an approach to their management is summarized below.

Wrist fracture

These occur more frequently in younger postmenopausal females than males. The presence of underlying osteoporosis can be confirmed by measuring bone mineral density, although this may not be necessary if the woman elects to go on HRT. If the bone mineral density is consistent with the diagnosis of osteoporosis, treatment suggested in Box 1 should be considered.

Vertebral fracture

Secondary causes such as multiple myeloma and metastases should be excluded where clinically indicated. In those with multiple, atraumatic vertebral fractures, measurement of bone mineral density may be unnecessary, but it should be considered in those with fewer than

Box 1

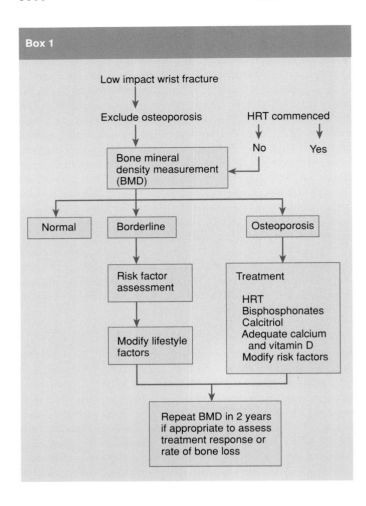

Box 2

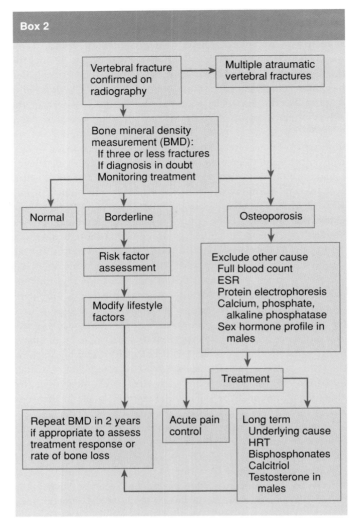

three vertebral fractures. A repeat measurement of bone mineral density should be considered in those whose baseline density is borderline and where a response to treatment is needed (e.g. when using a bisphosphonate, calcitriol, or calcium and vitamin D) (see Box 2).

Hip fracture

The acute treatment of the hip fracture should follow the Royal College of Physicians guidelines. In the frail elderly person, the future management should consist of adequate vitamin D and calcium. In the younger patient and the independently living elderly person, management with other drugs should be considered as outlined in Box 3. The use of hip protectors remains experimental until their benefit in preventing hip fracture can be demonstrated in the community-dwelling elderly person who falls frequently.

Osteomalacia and rickets

Osteomalacia and rickets are characterized by defective mineralization of bone and cartilage leading to an accumulation of unmineralized bone matrix called osteoid. The normal lag between osteoid synthesis and mineralization is prolonged, leading to a decrease in the rate of bone formation. Rickets represents the

occurrence of this defect in growing children before the closure of the epiphyses. Unlike osteoporosis, osteomalacia is characterized by a reduction in the ratio of mineralized bone to matrix.

Although osteomalacia can be caused by many disorders, it mostly results either from a primary disorder of vitamin D metabolism or a primary, and non-PTH-related, defect in renal tubular resorption of phosphate (Table 9).

Clinical and laboratory features

The classic symptoms of osteomalacia are generalized bone pain and tenderness, weakness of proximal muscles, and difficulty in walking. However, symptoms may be vague and of insidious onset, making the diagnosis difficult. The bone pain of osteomalacia is dull, poorly localized, and made worse by weight-bearing. It is usually symmetrical and may involve the back, pelvis, thigh, and ribs, often because of the presence of pseudofractures. Compression of the sternum and rib results in pain. Some patients have no pain, particularly in X-linked hypophosphataemic rickets where, in spite of life-long osteomalacia, pain may occur only in middle age.

Box 3

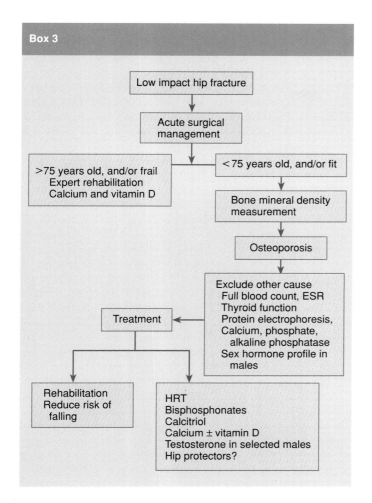

Table 9 Classification of osteomalacia

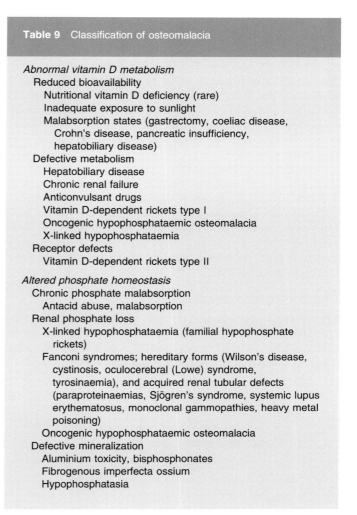

Abnormal vitamin D metabolism
  Reduced bioavailability
    Nutritional vitamin D deficiency (rare)
    Inadequate exposure to sunlight
    Malabsorption states (gastrectomy, coeliac disease,
      Crohn's disease, pancreatic insufficiency,
      hepatobiliary disease)
  Defective metabolism
    Hepatobiliary disease
    Chronic renal failure
    Anticonvulsant drugs
    Vitamin D-dependent rickets type I
    Oncogenic hypophosphataemic osteomalacia
    X-linked hypophosphataemia
  Receptor defects
    Vitamin D-dependent rickets type II

Altered phosphate homeostasis
  Chronic phosphate malabsorption
    Antacid abuse, malabsorption
  Renal phosphate loss
    X-linked hypophosphataemia (familial hypophosphate
      rickets)
    Fanconi syndromes; hereditary forms (Wilson's disease,
      cystinosis, oculocerebral (Lowe) syndrome,
      tyrosinaemia), and acquired renal tubular defects
      (paraproteinaemias, Sjögren's syndrome, systemic lupus
      erythematosus, monoclonal gammopathies, heavy metal
      poisoning)
  Oncogenic hypophosphataemic osteomalacia
  Defective mineralization
    Aluminium toxicity, bisphosphonates
    Fibrogenous imperfecta ossium
    Hypophosphatasia

Muscle weakness, usually proximal, may be of varying severity with only minimal atrophy and no fasciculation. The patient has a waddling gait, and difficulty in climbing stairs and getting out of bed and chair. Muscle biopsy shows no evidence of primary muscle disorder. Proximal weakness is not a feature of X-linked hypophosphataemic rickets.

The features of rickets depend on the age of the child and the underlying syndrome. The child may be hypotonic and apathetic, with growth retardation and delayed walking. Bowing deformities of the long bones will be present when weight-bearing occurs. The epiphyseal plate is widened due to the accumulation of disorganized, unmineralized cartilage, leading to cupping and irregularity at the metaphyseal–epiphyseal junction, usually at the wrist; at the costo-chondral junction this change gives rise to the 'rachitic rosary'. An indentation may develop at the attachment of the diaphragm to the softened ribs (Harrison's groove). In the neonate and young child the rapid growth of the skull leads to softening of the calvarium (cranio-tabes), parietal flattening, and frontal bossing. There is delayed dental eruption and enamel defects. Unfortunately, skeletal deformities often persist, even when the histological defect has been corrected, and may require surgical correction.

In osteomalacia and rickets, hypocalcaemia often causes no symptoms, but it sometimes results in paraesthesias, tetanus, cramps, carpopedal spasm, dysarthria, and cardiac arrhythmias. Hypocalcaemia is infrequently severe enough to lead to depression, psychoses, and convulsions.

Radiological features

The radiological features of rickets are most pronounced at the growth plate, where the epiphyses are widened and the calcification border of the metaphysis becomes cup-shaped. The size and density of the ossification centres are reduced, the cortex is indistinct, and there may be bowing of the long bones. In milder forms there may be no diagnostic radiological features.

The pathognomonic radiological feature of osteomalacia is pseudofracture (also known as Looser's zones and Milkman's fracture). Initially the fracture is incomplete, and extends perpendicularly from the cortex with poor callus formation; radiologically it is seen as a radiolucent line. Pseudofractures, often multiple and bilateral, are mainly found in the pubic rami, femoral neck, ribs, clavicles, the outer border of the scapulae, and the metatarsals. They occur in bones subjected to mechanical stress and may have an anatomical relation to entry sites of blood vessels into bone.

Biochemical features

Vitamin D-deficiency osteomalacia is characterized by a low serum calcium and phosphate with elevated serum alkaline phosphatase, increased urinary phosphate excretion, decreased urinary calcium excretion, low circulating levels of 25(OH)D, and a mild elevation of

PTH (secondary hyperparathyroidism). Levels of 1,25(OH)$_2$D may be normal or elevated, and therefore unhelpful in the diagnosis of osteomalacia. If the serum calcium and 25(OH)D are normal but the phosphate low, a renal phosphate leak syndrome or end-organ resistance should be suspected. A mild hyperchloraemic acidosis, due to renal bicarbonate loss, may accompany vitamin D deficiency and is a consequence of secondary hyperparathyroidism. Severe hyperchloraemic acidosis suggests a renal tubular disorder, which may be confirmed by failure to acidify the urine after loading with ammonium chloride.

When there is doubt about the occurrence of osteomalacia, the diagnosis can be made by bone biopsy. Specific features of osteomalacia are the presence of excess unmineralized matrix (osteoid) over bone trabeculae, and increased thickness of osteoid. If doubt remains, careful histomorphometry may be needed (Malluche and Faugere 1991). In vitamin D deficiency the biopsy will also show features of hyperparathyroidism, which are usually absent in hypophosphataemic disorders.

Metabolism of vitamin D

The two forms of vitamin D, vitamin D$_2$ (ergocalciferol) and vitamin D$_3$ (cholecalciferol), derived from plant and animal tissues respectively, undergo identical metabolism in humans and have similar effects on target tissues. The absence of a subscript often implies a reference to both forms of vitamin D (Fig. 12).

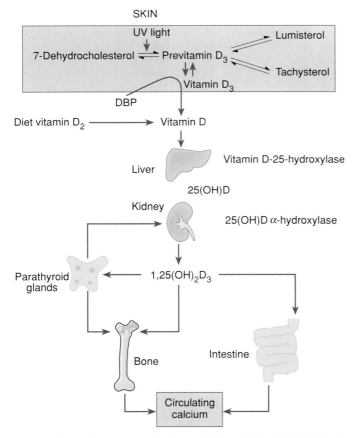

Fig. 12 Schematic representation for metabolism of vitamin D. Previtamin D$_3$ is formed in the skin and isomerizes to vitamin D$_3$ or to other biologically inert isomers. Vitamin D-binding protein (DBP) has affinity only for vitamin D$_3$, which is translocated to the circulation. Vitamin D is then hydroxylated in the liver and kidney to the active metabolite 1,25(OH)$_2$D.

Ultraviolet light converts 7-dehydrocholesterol to previtamin D$_3$. Continued stimulation leads to photoisomerization of previtamin D$_3$ to two biologically inert products (lumisterol and tachysterol). Previtamin D$_3$ undergoes thermal isomerization to vitamin D$_3$, and by binding to vitamin D-binding protein (**DBP**), to which it has a high affinity, it is translocated into the circulation. Dietary vitamin D is absorbed in the jejunum after incorporation into chylomicrons, a process that requires the presence of bile salts, fatty acids, and monoglycerides.

All forms of vitamin D and their metabolites are transported in the circulation through binding to DBP. The protein has a higher affinity for 25(OH)D than vitamin D or 1,25(OH)$_2$D$_3$. The circulating levels of DBP exceed those of vitamin D and its metabolites, so that all but 1 per cent of these metabolites are present in the free, non-bound form to enter into target cells.

Vitamin D is initially transported to the liver where it is hydroxylated on carbon-25, by vitamin D 25-hydroxylase enzyme, to produce 25(OH)D. The production of 25(OH)D is dependent on the supply of substrate; circulating levels of 25(OH)D reflect an individual's vitamin D status. Only in severe liver disorder is the hepatic production of 25(OH)D impaired, and even then the associated intestinal malabsorption is a contributory factor. From the liver, 25(OH)D, bound to DBP, is transported to the kidney, where it is hydroxylated either to 1α,25(OH)$_2$D (calcitriol) by the renal 25(OH)D 1α-hydroxylase or to 24,25 (OH)$_2$D. In mammals the principal source of 1α,25(OH)$_2$D is the kidney, except during pregnancy when the placenta can also synthesize it. It is unclear whether other tissues can produce 1α,25(OH)$_2$D$_3$ in normal humans. Granulomatous tissue may possess 1α-hydroxylase activity and this may be the source of the inappropriately high levels of 1,25(OH)D observed in these disorders (Adams *et al.* 1983). Indeed, macrophages activated by lipopolysaccharide or interferon-α, and human T-cell leukaemia-1 virus-infected cord lymphocytes, can also convert 25(OH)D to 1,25(OH)D. The renal 1α-hydroxylase is tightly regulated by PTH, calcium, phosphate, and calcitriol. A high PTH and low calcium stimulate 1,25(OH)$_2$D production, while a raised 1,25(OH)D inhibits calcitriol production but increases the production of 24,25(OH)$_2$D.

Calcitriol acts by binding to specific intracellular receptors that occur not only in the target tissues of bone, intestine, kidney, and parathyroid glands but also in mononuclear cells, activated T and B lymphocytes, and skin. Calcitriol stimulates calcium and phosphate absorption in the intestine and increases bone resorption to maintain mineral homeostasis. In bone, however, calcitriol also stimulates the osteoblast and is essential for bone formation, an activity that may also be stimulated by 24,25(OH)$_2$D. As mentioned above, receptors for calcitriol are found in tissues that do not have a direct role in mineral homeostasis, including breast cancer cells (Eisman *et al.* 1979), skin keratinocytes and dermal fibroblasts, and haemopoietic cells (Bar-Shavit *et al.* 1983; Bhalla *et al.* 1983). Calcitriol inhibits proliferation and induces differentiation of myeloid cells towards the monocytic lineage (Amento *et al.* 1984; Bhalla *et al.* 1989), perhaps through an early regulation of the c-*myc* gene (Reitsma *et al.* 1983; Kamali *et al.* 1989). *In vivo*, calcitriol, or its 1α analogue, prolong survival of mice inoculated with mouse myeloid leukaemia cells (M1). Calcitriol affects monocyte and T-cell function by influencing the production of cytokines such as IL-1, IL-2, and TNF (Bhalla *et al.* 1986). Since calcitriol can also be synthesized by immune cells it may have an autocrine or paracrine role in the local regulation of immune cell function, but in humans the physiological significance of this needs further elucidated.

Abnormal vitamin D metabolism

Reduced bioavailability

Vitamin D deficiency
Vitamin D deficiency through poor dietary intake is rare unless combined with reduced exposure to sunlight, which occurs especially in elderly people and in the immigrant Asian population of the United Kingdom. Osteomalacia is present in 25 per cent of bone biopsies from elderly patients in the United Kingdom and Scandinavia who have sustained hip fractures, and is likely to be due to insufficient intake of vitamin D and reduced exposure to sunlight. In some countries, dairy products are fortified to prevent nutritional vitamin D deficiency. However, it may still occur in individuals who avoid dairy products and in children who are exclusively breast-fed for prolonged periods.

It is important not to miss a diagnosis of vitamin D-deficiency rickets or osteomalacia, since effective therapy is available and, especially in rickets, limb deformity may be prevented. Bone pain and muscle weakness improve rapidly with replacement therapy, but biochemical and radiological improvements take longer.

The prevention of nutritional vitamin D deficiency is a public-health issue and the deficiency can be eradicated by fortification of certain foods with vitamin D. Simple vitamin D deficiency responds to therapy with oral vitamin D (ergocalciferol) in doses of 2000 to 4000 units (50–100 mg) daily and can be prevented by physiological replacement doses of 200 to 400 units (5–10 mg) daily. In severe vitamin D deficiency it may be better to give a loading dose of 50 000 units (1.25 mg) daily for 1 month followed by physiological replacement. Calcifediol (25(OH)D) can be used instead of vitamin D, where available, and may have fewer problems with accumulation than does vitamin D itself.

Gastrointestinal disorders
Intestinal fat malabsorption due to gastrointestinal, hepatic, or pancreatic disease leads to vitamin D deficiency without the need for other risk factors such as reduced exposure to sunlight. It leads to three distinct types of bone lesions (Rao 1990): (a) increased surface and volume, but not thickness, of osteoid, with normal serum calcium and phosphate but with evidence of secondary hyperparathyroidism — these patients are asymptomatic unless a fracture occurs; (b) increased thickness of osteoid and a prolonged mineralization lag time with reduced concentrations of calcium, phosphate, and elevated alkaline phosphatase — these individuals are symptomatic and have the classical radiological features of osteomalacia; (c) a third group, probably the most common, has low-turnover osteoporosis and is symptomatic only if a fracture occurs. In these disorders and other states of hypovitaminosis it is important to remember that cortical bone loss is irreversible; observe individuals with gastrointestinal disorders regularly to detect vitamin D deficiency. Prevention is best achieved by being aware of the risk and measuring the serum 25(OH)D annually. Treatment of hypovitaminosis D in these situations can be with vitamin D, although larger doses will be needed, or with 25(OH)D or calcitriol. The aim is to keep serum 25(OH)D in the high normal range. In treating established disease, give calcium supplements as well as magnesium if hypomagnesaemia is present.

Defective metabolism

Chronic renal failure
Chronic renal failure leads to reduced production of 1,25(OH)$_2$D and 24,25(OH)$_2$D from 25(OH)D by the kidney. Since a major effect of 1,25(OH)$_2$D on the intestine is to facilitate calcium absorption, in renal failure the intestinal calcium absorption falls, and, in conjunction with skeletal resistance to the calcium-mobilizing action of PTH, leads to hypocalcaemia. The inability of the diseased kidney to excrete phosphate leads to hyperphosphataemia, which aggravates the hypocalcaemia either by decreasing the renal 1α-hydroxylase activity or by impairing the release of calcium from the skeleton. Hypocalcaemia is a large stimulus to the parathyroid glands and leads to parathyroid hyperplasia and secondary hyperparathyroidism. The net result is a complex effect on bone leading to various skeletal disorders described under the term 'renal osteodystrophy'. Patients may have osteitis fibrosa, due to high levels of PTH, osteomalacia, due in part to vitamin D deficiency, or a combination of both. Retention of aluminium, and its deposition at the calcification front, may also play an important part in the development of osteomalacia, which may be refractory to treatment with 1,25(OH)$_2$D (Fig. 13).

Renal osteodystrophy is best managed and prevented by reducing the dietary intake of phosphate, avoiding aluminium-containing phosphate binders, increasing the dietary intake of calcium except when there is marked hyperphosphataemia (because of the risk of extraskeletal calcification), and by supplementation with either 1,25(OH)$_2$D or 1α-OHD$_2$ (alfacalcidol). These treatments usually improve mineral homeostasis, improve clinical symptoms of bone disease, and suppress parathyroid secretion. Occasionally, however, secondary hyperparathyroidism is so severe, with hypercalcaemia, extraskeletal calcification, fractures, and bone pain, that parathyroid surgery may be necessary.

Anticonvulsants
Chronic anticonvulsant therapy induces hepatic microsomal mixed-function oxidases that degrade steroid hormones such as oestrogen

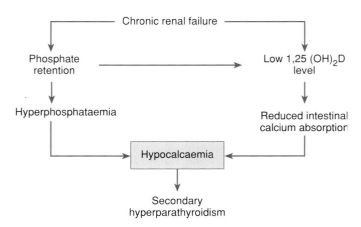

Fig. 13 Pathogenesis of renal bone disease.

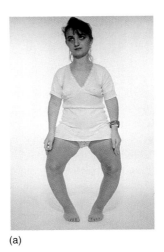 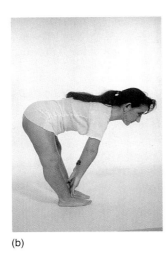

(a)   (b)

Fig. 14 Twenty-one-year-old girl with X-linked hypophosphataemic rickets. (a) Bowing of the femur and tibia due to previous rickets; (b) lumbar flexion is minimal due to spondylitic changes in the spine.

and cortisol. Since the hypothalamic–pituitary axis is intact, feedback regulation helps to maintain normal circulating levels of these hormones. Similarly, the chronic use of anticonvulsants leads to increased metabolic conversion of vitamin D and 25(OH)D to biologically inactive metabolites, which are excreted in the urine and bile. Unlike other steroid hormones, feedback regulation is limited and dependent on dietary intake of vitamin D and sunlight exposure. If dietary intake is defective, vitamin D deficiency may result. Anticonvulsants, however, may also affect calcium homeostasis by inhibiting intestinal calcium transport and the bone-resorbing effects of PTH and 1,25(OH)$_2$D, and by suppressing osteoblastic and osteoclastic activity. There are significant differences between the various anticonvulsant drugs. Phenobarbitone, a more potent inducer of hepatic microsomal enzymes than phenytoin, does not lead to a low 25(OH)D because increased catabolism

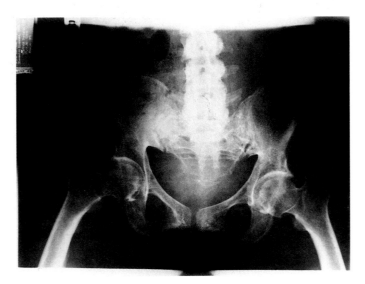

Fig. 15 X-linked hypophosphataemic rickets. Ligamentous calcification of the upper part of the sacroiliac joints and around the hip joints. There is also bridging of the vertebral interspaces.

is matched by increased formation. Phenytoin does not directly affect vitamin D metabolism but causes bone disease more often than phenobarbitone because it impairs intestinal calcium absorption and reduces the release of calcium from bone, leading to hypocalcaemia and secondary hyperparathyroidism. The net effect is that vitamin D requirements are increased by chronic use of anticonvulsants, especially in those on multiple drugs and in institutional care. Such individuals should be given additional vitamin D, but it is unclear whether all patients taking anticonvulsants should receive prophylactic vitamin treatment.

Vitamin D-dependent rickets type I

This is a rare, autosomal-recessive disease, in which a low or undetectable circulating 1,25-(OH)$_2$D is the result of defective renal 25(OH)D 1α-hydroxylase activity, and which manifests itself before the age of 2 years with classical features of rickets. Affected children fail to respond to conventional doses of replacement therapy with vitamin D but do so to large doses of vitamin D and 25(OH)D, or to physiological doses of 1,25(OH)D or 1α(OH)D.

Receptor defects

Vitamin D-dependent rickets type II

This is a rare disorder with rickets and/or osteomalacia but with no biochemical evidence of vitamin D deficiency, hypocalcaemia, secondary hyperparathyroidism, high levels of 1,25(OH)$_2$D, and failure to respond to large doses of vitamin D or its metabolites. About 70 per cent of the cases reported have alopecia (often complete) and absent eyelashes yet the number and morphology of scalp hair follicles is normal. Alopecia is worse in those resistant to treatment with 1,25(OH)D. Affected patients come from consanguineous marriages and the inheritance is most likely to be autosomal-recessive. The disorder is due to defects in the intracellular interaction of 1,25(OH)D with its receptor. Defects include reduced receptor affinity, abnormal numbers of receptors, and impaired ability of the receptor–hormone complex to bind the DNA. In patients with normal hair a clinical remission can be induced with high doses of vitamin D analogues. A 10-fold higher dose is needed in those with alopecia, but even then only one-half will respond.

Altered phosphate homeostasis

Phosphate depletion

Osteomalacia from chronic phosphate depletion is uncommon and is seen in individuals who consume large amounts of phosphate-binding antacids over a number of years (Dent and Winter 1974). The osteomalacia is clinically, radiologically, and histologically similar to that seen in vitamin D deficiency. Biochemically, however, there are differences in that the serum calcium is normal or even increased, serum phosphate may be low or normal, but urinary phosphate excretion is reduced while urinary calcium excretion may be increased. The concentration of calcitriol is increased and may be responsible for increased absorption of calcium. Treatment consists of phosphate supplementation and avoidance of antacids.

Renal phosphate loss

Hypophosphataemic rickets/osteomalacia may result from hereditary or acquired disorders.

X-linked hypophosphataemic rickets

Also known as familial hypophosphataemic rickets, X-linked hypophosphataemic rickets was first described by Albright *et al.* (1937), who noted that in some patients rickets did not improve with normal doses of vitamin D but did when pharmacological doses of vitamin D were used. The disorder was called vitamin D-resistant rickets and later became known as hypophosphataemic (vitamin D-resistant) rickets when it was noted that it occurred in association with a low serum phosphate. The inheritance is usually X-linked dominant, although autosomal forms also occur. The mutant gene in the disease is located in the distal part of the short arm of the X chromosome (Thakker and O'Riordan 1988).

The disease is fully expressed as rickets and short stature in homozygous males, but the expression of the disease in girls is variable, from none to severe rickets and stunted growth (Fig. 14). A low serum phosphate is found soon after birth, but the disease is only clinically manifest soon after the child begins to walk. Bow legs appear first and there is failure of normal growth. There may be a waddling gait. Skull deformities develop from premature closure of the sutures. Unlike vitamin D-deficiency rickets, in X-linked hypophosphataemic rickets there is no proximal myopathy or dental hypoplasia, but tooth eruption is delayed and tooth development poor, leading to dental abscesses and early dental caries.

Radiologically, bone mass is not diminished and may even be above the age-matched normal since there is no secondary hyperparathyroidism. In adults there may be reduced joint mobility, especially at the elbows, shoulders, hip, and spine, due to a widespread enthesopathy (Davies and Stanbury 1981; Polission *et al.* 1985). Spinal enthesopathy may occasionally lead to cord compression. The rigid spine, held straight and with loss of lumbar lordosis, may be confused with ankylosing spondylitis. Indeed, radiographs of the spine may show calcification of the outer fibres of the annulus fibrosus, giving a 'squared-off' appearance to the vertebral bodies, and later complete bridging between vertebrae may lead to a 'bamboo spine'. Ligamentous calcification may obscure the sacroiliac joints, often only in the upper part (Fig. 15). In the long bones, the cortex appears thickened and the trabeculae are coarse and thickened. Pseudofractures may occur. Degenerative changes develop in weight-bearing joints, probably secondary to the limb deformity.

Biochemical tests show a low serum phosphate, a normal calcium and PTH, and normal or low levels of 1,25(OH)₂D. Hypophosphataemia is due to a renal tubular defect, with increased renal loss of phosphate due to lowered renal threshold for phosphate. Renal function is otherwise normal and there are no acidification defects, glycosuria, or aminoaciduria.

It is important to make a correct diagnosis of this disorder as early as possible since proper treatment of the infant will prevent skeletal deformities and allow for normal growth. Although hypophosphataemia is central to the disorder, treatment with phosphate alone leads to secondary hyperparathyroidism and with vitamin D alone to the risk of hypercalcaemia and renal failure. A combination of 1,25(OH)₂D and phosphate is most effective, resulting in a return to normal of serum phosphate and healing of rickets. Hypercalciuria should be avoided; serum phosphate, calcium, and urinary calcium should be monitored regularly (Petersen *et al.* 1992).

Metabolic acidosis

A chronic metabolic acidosis may result from Fanconi syndrome or renal tubular acidosis, and may be associated with rickets and osteomalacia. Fanconi syndrome embraces a number of acquired and hereditary disorders in which there are varying combinations of defects of the renal proximal tubule. The proximal tubular abnormality leads to glycosuria, aminoaciduria, hyperphosphaturia and hypophosphataemia, and a systemic acidosis from failure of bicarbonate reabsorption. The hereditary forms are seen most commonly in cystinosis, Wilson's disease, and Lowe syndrome, while the acquired forms are seen in association with multiple myeloma, light-chain nephropathy, amyloidosis, Sjögren syndrome, heavy metal poisoning, and malignancy. The hereditary form can present with rickets, while rickets or osteomalacia may occur in acquired forms. The mechanism for the rickets/osteomalacia is not fully known. The failure of mineralization is a consequence of hypophosphataemia, hypocalcaemia, and metabolic acidosis. In some forms, e.g. Wilson's disease, hepatic damage may lead to low levels of 25(OH)D, while in other forms levels of 1,25(OH)₂D are reduced due to the proximal renal tubular defect. Treatment of the bone disease is with phosphate supplements and vitamin D metabolites, especially the 1α(OH)D analogue.

Renal tubular acidosis describes disorders in which there is renal loss of bicarbonate resulting in reduced plasma bicarbonate and a systemic acidosis. The pH of the urine is inappropriately high compared to the metabolic acidosis. Renal tubular acidosis exists as two major forms. In the distal tubular form, known as type I, there is failure to secrete protons so that a large pH gradient between blood and the tubular fluid cannot form. In the proximal tubular type (type II) there is bicarbonate wasting but the ability of the distal tubule to excrete protons is intact. Renal tubular acidosis type II is also often associated with Fanconi syndrome and other proximal tubular defects. The development of rickets and osteomalacia in both forms is due to hypophosphataemia and perhaps failure to synthesize 1,25(OH)₂D, a consequence of the systemic acidosis. The treatment consists of correcting the acidosis and using vitamin D if the rickets fails to heal.

Oncogenous hypophosphataemic osteomalacia

Some tumours (usually mesenchymal) lead to rickets or osteomalacia characterized by hypophosphataemia with phosphaturia. The bone disease regresses after removal of the tumour. The biochemical defect is characterized by a low maximum tubular reabsorption of phosphate per volume of glomerular filtrate, suggesting renal phosphate wasting, and, in some patients, by low or inappropriately low levels of 1,25(OH)₂D. While the biochemical abnormalities are similar to those seen in X-linked hypophosphataemic rickets, there are more severe skeletal deformities. Clinical features are predominantly those of bone pain, proximal muscle weakness, sometimes fractures, and, in children, growth retardation (Ryan and Reiss 1984). A similar type of hypophosphataemic osteomalacia may occur in association with fibrous dysplasia and neurofibromatosis. The mechanism responsible for the development of hypophosphataemia is unknown, but the tumour may produce a humoral factor that affects proximal tubular function and leads to phosphate wasting and suppressed production of 1,25(OH)₂D.

The tumour may be small and difficult to locate, but if found and completely removed the bone disorder reverses. Clinical features may return if there is a recurrence of the tumour. If it is not possible to resect the tumour completely, treatment is aimed at correcting the hypophosphataemic osteomalacia by phosphate and 1,25(OH)$_2$D$_3$ supplements.

Defective mineralization

Aluminium

As discussed above, in chronic renal failure aluminium is deposited in bone and impairs mineralization.

Fibrogenesis imperfecta ossium

This is a rare disorder that affects middle-aged men, who develop generalized bone pain and fractures. Approximately 50 per cent of reported cases have an associated monoclonal gammopathy. Radiologically the bones appear dense with loss of normal trabecular pattern; histologically bone shows an increased amount of thick osteoid, reduced mineralization, and decreased birefringence due to the lack of normal lamellar arrangement of collagen. It has been suggested that the disorder is due to an acquired defect of collagen that impairs normal mineralization in lamellar bone, but collagen synthesis elsewhere is normal. Some clinical but not histological improvement may occur with vitamin D. Melphalan reportedly induced a clinical remission, with some improvement in the histological appearances of bone, in a patient with coexistent monoclonal gammopathy (Stamp et al. 1985).

Hypophosphatasia

This is a rare, heritable cause of severe rickets in childhood and recurrent stress fractures in adults, transmitted in an autosomal–recessive manner with an incidence of 1 in 100 000 live births for the severe form. There is a reduction in serum and tissue alkaline phosphatase in association with increased urinary excretion of phosphoethanolamine and increased circulating inorganic pyrophosphate and pyridoxal-5′-phosphate. Infantile forms present before the age of 6 months with growth retardation, rachitic deformities, hypercalcaemia, hypercalciuria, and renal failure. Childhood hypophosphatasia may present with premature loss of deciduous teeth alone or in association with rickets. It may improve spontaneously. Adult hypophosphatasia presents with recurrent stress fractures that heal poorly. Chondrocalcinosis is common and attacks of pyrophosphate arthropathy may occur. The cause for the mineralization defect is unknown but it has been suggested that the accumulation of pyrophosphate, due to failure of alkaline phosphatase to cleave it, leads to deficient skeletal mineralization (Whyte 1989). There is no treatment available for this disorder. Since there is no hypocalcaemia, vitamin D and its metabolites should be avoided; their use may lead to hypercalcaemia and hypercalciuria (Whyte 1989).

References

Adams, J. S., Sharma, O. P., Gacad, M. A., and Singer, F. R. (1983). Metabolism of 25-hydroxyvitamin D$_3$ by cultured pulmonary alveolar macrophages in sarcoidosis. Journal of Clinical Investigation, 72, 1856–60.

Adinoff, A. D. and Hollister, J. R. (1983). Steroid-induced fractures and bone loss in patients with asthma. New England Journal of Medicine, 309, 265–68.

Advisory Group on Osteoporosis. (1994). Report. pp. 5–34. Department of Health, London.

Aitken, M. (1987). Relationship between mortality and femoral neck fracture J and osteoporosis. In Osteoporosis 1987, Vol. 1, (eds. C. Christiansen, J. S. Johnsen, and B. J. Riis), pp. 45–8. Norhaven Press, Viborg, Denmark.

Albright, F., Butler, A. M., and Bloomberg, E. (1937). Rickets resistant to vitamin D therapy. American Journal of Diseases of Children, 54, 529–47.

Albright, F., Bloomberg, F., and Smith, P. H. (1976). Postmenopausal osteoporosis. Transactions of the Association of American Physicians, 55, 298–305.

Amento, E. P. et al. (1984). 1a, 25-dihydroxyvitamin D$_3$ induces the maturation of the human monocyte cell line U937, and, in association with a factor from human T lymphocytes, augments production of the monokine, mononuclear cell factor. Journal of Clinical Investigation, 73, 731–9.

Arend, M. P. and Dayer, J. M. (1990). Cytokines and cytokine inhibitors or antagonists in rheumatoid arthritis. Arthritis and Rheumatism, 33, 305–15.

Bar-Shavit, Z. et al. (1983). Induction of monocyte differentiation and bone resorption by 1,25-dihydroxyvitamin D$_3$. Proceedings of the National Academy of Sciences (USA), 80, 5907–11.

Bell, N. M., Greene, A., Epstein, S., Oexmann, M. J., Shaw, S., and Shary, J. (1985). Evidence for alteration of the vitamin D–endocrine system in blacks. Journal of Clinical Investigation, 76, 470–3.

Benger, V., Johnell, O., and Redlund-Johnell, I. (1988). Changes in incidence and prevalence of vertebral fractures during 30 years. Calcified Tissue International, 42, 293–6.

Bergkvist, L., Adami, H. O., Persson, I., Hoover, R., and Schaiver, C. (1989). The risk of breast cancer after estrogen and estrogen–progestin replacement. New England Journal of Medicine, 321, 293–7.

Bhalla, A. K. (1986). Musculoskeletal manifestations of primary hyperparathyroidism. Clinics in Rheumatic Diseases, 12, 691–705.

Bhalla, A. K., Amento, E. P., Clemens, T. L., Holick, M. F., and Krane, S. M. (1983). Specific high-affinity receptors for 1,25-dihydroxyvitamin D$_3$ in human peripheral blood mononuclear cells: presence in monocytes and induction in T lymphocytes following activation. Journal of Clinical Endocrinology and Metabolism, 57, 1308–10.

Bhalla, A. K., Amento, E. P., and Krane, S. M. (1986). Differential effects of 1,25-dihydroxyvitamin D$_3$ on human lymphocytes and monocyte/macrophages: inhibition of interleukin 2 and augmentation of interleukin 1 production. Cellular Immunology, 98, 311–22.

Bhalla, A. K., Williams, M. M., Lal, S., and Lydyard, P. M. (1989). 1,25 Dihydroxyvitamin D$_3$ but not retinoic acid, induces the differentiation of U937 cells. Clinical and Experimental Immunology, 76, 274–7.

Black, D. M. et al. for the Fracture Intervention Trial Research Group (1996). Randomized trial of effect of alendronate on the risk of fracture in women with existing vertebral fractures. Lancet, 348, 1535–41.

Boyce, W. J. and Vessey, M. P. (1985). Rising incidence of fractures of the proximal femur. Lancet, i, 150–1.

Braidman, I. P., Davenport, L. K., Carter, D. H., Selpy, P. L., Mawer, E. B., and Freemont, A. J. (1995). Preliminary in situ identification of oestrogen target cells in bone. Journal of Bone and Mineral Research, 10, 74–80.

Brinton, L. A., Hoover, R., and Fraumeni, J. F. J. (1986). Menopausal oestrogens and breast cancer risk: an expanded case-control study. British Journal of Cancer, 54, 825–32.

Bush, T. L. et al. (1983). Estrogen uses and all-cause mortality. Preliminary results from the Lipid Research Clinics Program Follow-up Study. Journal of the American Medical Association, 249, 903–6.

Butler, R. C., Pauce, M. W. J., Worsfield, M., and Sharp, C. A. (1991). Bone mineral content in patients with rheumatoid arthritis: relationship to low dose steroid therapy. British Journal of Rheumatology, 30, 86–90.

Chapuy, M. C. et al. (1992). Vitamin D$_3$ and calcium to prevent hip fractures in elderly women. New England Journal of Medicine, 327, 1637–42.

Cohn, S. H. (1991). Noninvasive measurement of bone mass. In Metabolic bone disease and clinically related disorders (eds. L. V. Avioli and S. M. Krane), pp. 264–82. Saunders, Philadelphia.

Colditz, G. A. et al. (1995). The use of oestrogen and progestins and the risk of breast cancer in post-menopausal women. New England Journal of Medicine, 332, 1589–93.

Consensus Development Conference (1991). Prophylaxis and treatment of osteoporosis. American Journal of Medicine, 90, 107–10.

Cooper, C. and Wickham, C. (1990). Rheumatoid arthritis, corticosteroid therapy and hip fracture. In *Osteoporosis 1990* (eds. C. Christiansen and K. Overgaard), pp. 1578–9. Handelstrykkeriet, Aalborg, Denmark.

Cooper, C., Barker, D. J., and Wickham, C. (1988). Physical activity, muscle strength, and calcium intake in fracture of the proximal femur in Britain. *British Medical Journal*, **297**, 1443–6.

Cooper, C. *et al.* (1991). Screening for vertebral osteoporosis using individual risk factors. *Osteoporosis International*, **2**, 48–53.

Cooper, C., Champion, G., and Melton, L. J. (1992). Hip fractures in the elderly: a worldwide projection. *Osteoporosis International*, **2**, 285–9.

Cooper, C., Carbone, L., Michet, C. J., Atkinson, E. J., O'Fallow, W. M., and Melton, L. J., III (1994). Fracture risk in patients with ankylosing spondylitis. A population based study. *Journal of Rheumatology*, **21**, 1877–84.

Cooper, C., Copland, M., and Mitchell, M. (1995). Rheumatoid arthritis, corticosteroid therapy in hip fractures. *Annals of the Rheumatic Diseases*, **54**, 49–52.

Cummings, R. G. (1990). Calcium intake and bone mass: a quantitative review of the evidence. *Calcified Tissue International*, **47**, 194–201.

Cummings, S. R., Tao, J. L., and Browner, W. S. (1992). Hyperthyroidism increases the risk of hip fractures: a perspective study. *Journal of Bone and Mineral Research*, **7** (Suppl. 1), 1–21.

Cummings, S. R. *et al.* (1995). Risk factors for hip fracture in white women. *New England Journal of Medicine*, **332**, 767–73.

Daly, E., Vessey, M. P., Hawkins, M. M., Carson, J. L., Gough, P., and Marsh, S. (1996). Risk of venous embolism in users of HRT. *Lancet*, **348**, 977–80.

Dauphine, R. T., Riggs, B. L., and Scholz, D. A. (1975). Back pain and skeletal crush fractures: an unemphasized mode of presentation for primary hyperparathyroidism. *Annals of Internal Medicine*, **83**, 365–7.

Davies, M. and Stanbury, S. W. (1981). The rheumatic manifestations of metabolic bone disease. *Clinical Rheumatic Diseases*, **5**, 596–646.

Davies, K. M., Recker, R. R., Stegman, M. R., Heaney, R. P., Kimmel, D. B., and Leist, J. (1990). Third decade bone gain in women. In *Calcium regulation and bone metabolism* (ed. D. V. Cohn, F. H. Glorieux, and T. J. Martin). Elsevier Science, Amsterdam.

Dent, C. E. and Winter, C. S. (1974). Osteomalacia due to phosphate depletion from excessive aluminium hydroxide ingestion. *British Medical Journal*, **1**, 551–2.

Dequeker, J. and Geusens, P. (1990). Osteoporosis and arthritis. *Annals of the Rheumatic Diseases*, **49**, 276–80.

Devogelar, J. P., Haux, J. P., and Nagart de Deuxchaisnes, C. (1984). Does mild, asymptomatic, primary hyperparathyroidism require surgery to avoid bone loss in postmenopausal females? In *Osteoporosis* (eds. C. Christiansen *et al.*), p. 365. Aallorg Stiftsbocytykken, Copenhagen.

Devogelar, J. P., Maldague, R., Malghem, J., and de Deuxchaisnes, C. N. (1992) Appendicular and vertebral bone mass in patients with ankylosing spondylitis. *Arthritis and Rheumatism*, **35**, 1062–7.

Drinkwater, B. L., Nilson, K., Chestnut, C. H., Bremner, W. J., Shainholtz, S., and Southwood, M. B. (1984). Bone mineral content of amenorrheic and eumenorrheic athletes. *New England Journal of Medicine*, **311**, 277–81.

Drinkwater, B. L., Bremner, B., and Chesnut, C. H., III (1990). Menstrual history as a determinant of current bone density in young athletes. *Journal of the American Medical Association*, **263**, 545–48.

Eastgate, J. A., Symons, J. A., Woods, N. R., Grinlinton, F. M., di Givoine, F., and Duff, G. W. (1988). Correlation of plasma interleukin 1 levels with disease activity in rheumatoid arthritis. *Lancet*, **ii**, 706–9.

Eisman, J. A. (1995). Vitamin D receptor gene alleles and osteoporosis: an affirmative view. *Journal of Bone and Mineral Research*, **10**, 1289–93.

Eisman, J. A., Martin, T. J., McIntyre, I., and Mosley, J. M. (1979). 1,25-dihydroxyvitamin D receptors in breast cancer cells. *Lancet*, **ii**, 1335–6.

Eriksen, E. F. *et al.* (1988). Evidence of estrogen receptors in normal human osteoblast cells. *Science*, **241**, 84–6.

Fallon, M. D., Whyte, M. P., Craig, R. B., Jr, and Teitelbaum, S. L. (1983). Mast-cell proliferation in postmenopausal osteoporosis. *Calcified Tissue International*, **35**, 29–31.

Faulkner, K. G., Cummings, S. R., Black, D., Palermo, L., Glüer, C. C., and Gerant, H. K. (1993). Simple measurement of femoral geometry predicts hip fracture: the study of osteoporotic fracture. *Journal of Bone and Mineral Research*, **8**, 1211–17.

Ferrari, S., Rizzoli, R., Chevalley, D., Slosman, D., Eisman, J. A., and Bonjour, J-P. (1995). Vitamin D receptor gene polymorphism and change in lumbar spine mineral density. *Lancet*, **345**, 423–4.

Gallagher, J. C. and Goldgar, D. (1990). Treatment of postmenopausal osteoporosis with high doses of synthetic calcitriol: a randomized controlled trial. *Annals of Internal Medicine*, **113**, 649–55.

Garnero, P., Borel, O., Sornay-Rendu, E., and Delman, P. D. (1995). *Journal of Bone and Mineral Research*, **10**, 1283–9.

Garrett, I. R. *et al.* (1987). Production of lymphotoxin, a bone resorbing cytokine by cultured human myeloma cells. *New England Journal of Medicine*, **317**, 526–32.

Gilsanz, V., Roe, T. F., Mora, S., Costin, G., and Goodman, A. G. (1991). Changes in vertebral bone density in black girls and white girls during childhood and puberty. *New England Journal of Medicine*, **325**, 1597–600.

Girasole, G., Passeri, G., Jilka, R. L., and Manolagas, S. C. (1994). Interleukin-11: a new cytokine critical for osteoclast development. *Journal of Clinical Investigation*, **93**, 1516–24.

Goldman, L. and Tosteson, A. N. A. (1991). Uncertainty about postmenopausal estrogen. Time for action not debate. Editorial. *New England Journal of Medicine*, **325**, 800–2.

Gowen, M. (1991). Cytokines regular bone cell function. *Rheumatology Review*, **1**, 43–50.

Grimley Evans, J. (1990). The significance of osteoporosis. In *Osteoporosis 1990* (ed. R. Smith), pp. 1–8. Royal College of Physicians, London.

Grodstein, F. *et al.* (1996a). Prospective study of exogenous hormones and risk of pulmonary embolism in women. *Lancet*, **348**, 983–7.

Grodstein, F. *et al.* (1996b). Postmenopausal estrogen and progestin use and the risk of cardiovascular disease. *New England Journal of Medicine*, **335**, 453–61.

Hanson, C. A., Shagrin, J. W., and Duncan, H. (1971). Vertebral osteoporosis in ankylosing spondylitis. *Clinical Orthopedics*, **74**, 59–64.

Heaney, R. P., Recker, R. R., and Saville, P. D. (1978). Menopausal changes in calcium balance performance. *Journal of Laboratory and Clinical Medicine*, **92**, 953–63.

Heikinheimo, R. J. *et al.* (1992). Annual injection of vitamin D and fractures of aged bones. *Calcified Tissue International*, **51**, 105–10.

Hooyman, J. R., Melton, J. R., Nelson, A. M., O'Fallon, N. M., and Riggs, B. L. (1984). Fractures of rheumatoid arthritis. A population based study. *Arthritis and Rheumatism*, **27**, 1353–61.

Hunter, T. and Dubo, M. I. C. (1978). Spinal fracture complicating ankylosing spondylitis. *Annals of Internal Medicine*, **88**, 546–9.

Hunter, T. and Dubo, M. I. C. (1983). Spinal fracture complicating ankylosing spondylitis: a long term study. *Arthritis and Rheumatism*, **26**, 751–9.

Hustmyer, F. G., Peacock, M., Hui, S., Johnston, C. C., and Christian, J. (1994). Bone mineral density in relation to polymorphism at the vitamin D receptor gene locus. *Journal of Clinical Investigation*, **94**, 2130–4.

Jackson, J. A. and Kleerekoper, M. D. (1990). Osteoporosis in men: diagnosis, pathophysiology and prevention. *Medicine*, **69**, 137–52.

Jackson, J. A., Kleerekoper, M., Parfitt, A. M., Rao, D. S., Villanoeva, A. R., and Frame, B. (1987). Bone histomorphometry in hypogonadal and eugonadal men with spinal osteoporosis. *Journal of Clinical Endocrinology and Metabolism*, **65**, 53–8.

Jick, H., Derby, L. E., Myers, M. W., Vasilakis, C., and Newton, K. M. (1996). Risk of hospital admission for idiopathic venous thromboembolism among users of postmenopausal oestrogen. *Lancet*, **348**, 981–3.

Jilka, R. L. *et al.* (1992). Increased osteoclast development after oestrogen loss: mediation by interleukin-6. *Science*, **257**, 88–91.

Johnell, O. *et al.* (1995). Risk factors for hip fracture in European women: the Medos Study. *Journal of Bone and Mineral Research*, **10**, 1802–15.

Johnston, C. C., Slemenda, C. W., and Melton, J. L. (1991). Clinical use of bone densitometry. *New England Journal of Medicine*, **324**, 1105–9.

Johnston, C. C., Jr *et al.* (1992). Calcium supplementation and increases in bone mineral density in children. *New England Journal of Medicine*, **327**, 82–7.

Kalla, A. A., Meyers, O.L., Chalton, D., *et al.* (1991). Increased metacarpal bone mass following 18 months of slow acting anti-rheumatic drugs for rheumatoid arthritis. *British Journal of Rheumatology*, **30**, 91–100.

Kamali, R., Bhalla, A.K., Farrow, S.M., *et al.* (1989). Early regulation of c-*myc* mRNA by 1,25-dihydroxyvitamin D_3 in human myelomonocytic U937 cells. *Journal of Molecular Endocrinology*, **3**, 43–8.

Kanis, J. A. (1991). Requirement of calcium for optimal skeletal health in women. *Calcified Tissue International*, **49** (Suppl.), 533–41.

Kanis, J. A. and Passmore, R. (1989). Calcium supplementation of the diet. *British Medical Journal*, **296**, 137–40; 205–8.

Kanis, J. A. *et al.* (1990). Osteoporosis: causes and therapeutic implications. In *Osteoporosis 1990* (ed. R. Smith), pp. 46–56. Royal College of Physicians, London.

Kanis, J. A., Melton J, Christiansen, C., Johnston, C.C., and Khaltaev, N. (1994*a*). The diagnosis of osteoporosis. *Journal of Bone and Mineral Research*, **9**, 1137–41.

Kanis, J. A. *et al.* (1994*b*). *Assessment of fracture risk and its application to screening for postmenopausal osteoporosis: report of a WHO study group* (WHO Technical Report Series 843). WHO, Geneva

Kleerekoper, M. (1992). Vertebral fracture or vertebral deformity? *Calcified Tissue International*, **50**, 50–6.

Kleerekoper, M. (1996). Fluoride: the verdict is in, but the controversy lingers. *Journal of Bone and Mineral Research*, **11**, 565–7.

Kleerekoper, M. and Nelson, D.A. (1992). A randomized trial of sodium fluoride as a treatment for postmenopausal osteoporosis. *Osteoporosis International*, **1**, 155–61.

Krolner, B. and Nielsen, S. P. (1982). Bone mineral content of the lumbar spine in normal and osteoporotic women: cross-sectional and longitudinal studies. *Clinical Science*, **62**, 329–36.

Laan, R. E. J. M., van Riel, P. L. C. M., and van Erning, L. J. T. O. (1992). Vertebral osteoporosis in rheumatoid arthritis patients: effects of low dose prednisolone therapy. *British Journal of Rheumatology*, **31**, 91–6.

Laan, R. E. J. M. *et al.* (1993*a*). Differential effects of glucocorticoids on cortical, appendicular and cortical vertebral bone mineral content. *Calcified Tissue International*, **52**, 5–9.

Laan, R. E. J. M. *et al.* (1993*b*). Low dose prednisolone induces rapid reversible axial bone loss in patients with rheumatoid arthritis. *Annals of Internal Medicine*, **119**, 963–8.

Lanyi, E., Ratko, I., and Gomor, B. (1993). On the diagnostic value of DEXA for osteoporosis in case of patients with ankylosing spondylitis. In *Osteoporosis* (Proceedings 4th International Symposium on Osteoporosis and Consensus Development Conference), pp. 192–4. Bath Institute for Rheumatic Diseases, Bath, UK.

Liberman, V. A. *et al.* (1993). Effects of oral alendronate on bone mineral density and the incidence of fractures in postmenopausal osteoporosis. *New England Journal of Medicine*, **333**, 1437–8.

Lindsay, R. and Tomme, J. F. (1990). Estrogen treatment of patients with established postmenopausal osteoporosis. *Obstetrics and Gynecology*, **76**, 290–5.

Lindsay, R., Hart, D. M., Aitken, J. M., MacDonald, E. B., Anderson, J. B., and Clark, A. C. (1976). Long term prevention of postmenopausal osteoporosis by oestrogen. *Lancet*, **i**, 1038–41.

Lindsay, R., Hart, D. M., Abdalla, H., and Al-Azzawi, F. (1987). Inter-relationship of bone loss and its prevention, and fracture expression. In *Osteoporosis 1987* (eds. C. Christiansen, J. S. Johansen, and B. J. Riis), pp. 508–9. Osteoporosis, Copenhagen.

Lips, P., Graafman, W. C., Ooms, M. E., Bezemer, D., and Bouter, L. M. (1996). Vitamin D supplementation and fracture incidence in elderly persons. A randomised, placebo-controlled clinical trial. *Annals of Internal Medicine*, **124**, 400–6.

Luengo, M., Picado, C., Rio, L. D., Guanbons, N., Monserrat, J. M., and Setoain, J. (1991). Vertebral fractures in steroid dependent asthma and involutional osteoporosis. *Thorax*, **46**, 803–6.

McSheety, P. M. J. and Chambers, T. J. (1986). Osteoblastic cells mediate osteoclastic responsiveness to parathyroid hormones. *Endocrinology*, **118**, 824–8.

Malluche, H. H. and Faugere, M-C. (1991). Bone biopsies: histology and histomorphometry of bone. In *Metabolic bone disease and clinically related disorders* (eds. L. V. Avioli and S. M. Krane), pp. 283–328. Saunders, Philadelphia.

Mamelle, N. *et al.* (1988). Risk–benefit ratio of sodium fluoride treatment in primary vertebral osteoporosis. *Lancet*, **ii**, 361–5.

Manolagas, S. C. and Jilka, R. L. (1995). Bone marrow, cytokines, and bone remodelling. Emerging insights into the pathophysiology of osteoporosis. *New England Journal of Medicine*, **332**, 305–11.

Martin, P., Bergmann, P., Gillet, C., *et al.* (1986). Partial reversible osteopenia after surgery for primary hyperparathyroidism. *Archives of Internal Medicine*, **146**, 689–91.

Matkovic, V., Kostial, K., Simonovic, I., Buzina, R., Brodarec, A., and Nordin, B. E. C. (1979). Bone status and fracture rates in two regions of Yugoslavia. *American Journal of Clinical Nutrition*, **32**, 540–9.

Matta, W. M., Shaw, R. W., Hesp, R., and Katz, D. (1981). Hypogonadism induced by luteinising hormone releasing hormone against analogues: effects on bone density in premenopausal women. *British Medical Journal*, **294**, 1523–4.

Melton, L. J. (1987). Postmenopausal bone loss and osteoporosis. In *The climacteric and beyond* (eds. L. Zochella, M. Whitehead, and P. A. van Keep), pp. 125–35. Parthenon, Carnforth.

Melton, L. J., Chrischilles, E. A., Cooper, C., Lane, A. W., and Riggs, B. L. (1992). How many women have osteoporosis? *Journal of Bone and Mineral Research*, **7**, 1005–10.

Meyer, H. E., Tverdal, A., and Falch, J. A. (1993). Risk factors for hip factors for hip fracture in middle-aged Norwegian women and men. *American Journal of Epidemiology*, **137**, 1203–11.

Michel, B. A, Bloch, D. A., and Fries, J. F. (1991). Predictors of fracture in early rheumatoid arthritis. *Journal of Rheumatology*, **18**, 804–8.

Morrison, N. A., Yeoman, R., Kelley, P. J., and Eisman, J. A. (1992). Contribution to trans-acting factor alleles to normal physiological variability: vitamin D receptor gene polymorphism and circulating osteocalcin. *Proceedings of the National Academy of Sciences (USA)*, **89**, 6665–9.

Morrison, N. A. *et al.* (1994). Prediction of bone density from vitamin D receptor alleles. *Nature*, **367**, 284–7.

Mullaji, A. B., Upadhay, S. S., and Ho, E. K. W. (1994). Bone mineral density in ankylosing spondylitis. *Journal of Bone and Joint Surgery* (B), **76**, 660–5.

Naessen, T., Persson, I., Adami, H. O., Bergstrom, R., and Bergkvist, L. (1990). Hormone replacement therapy and the risk for hip fracture. A prospective, population-based cohort study. *Annals of Internal Medicine*, **113**, 95–103.

Nilas, L., Christiansen, C., and Rodbro, P. (1984). Calcium supplementation and postmenopausal bone loss. *British Medical Journal*, **7**, 1103–6.

Nilsson, B. E. and Westlin, N. E. (1971). Bone density in athletes. *Clinical Orthopaedics*, **77**, 177–82.

Obront, K. J., Bengner, U., Johnell, O., Nilsson, B. E., and Sernbo, I. (1989). Increasing age-adjusted risk of fragility fractures: a sign of increasing osteoporosis in successive generations? *Calcified Tissue International*, **44**, 157–67.

O'Neill, T. W., Felsenberg, D., Varlow, J., Cooper, C., and Kanis, J. A. (1996). The prevalence of vertebral deformity in European men and women: The European Vertebral Osteoporosis Study. *Journal of Bone and Mineral Research*, **11**, 1010–17.

Ooms, M. E., Roos, J. C., Bezemer, D., van der Vijgh, W. J., Bouter, L. M., and Lips, P. (1995). Prevention of bone loss by vitamin D supplementation in elderly women: a randomised double-blind trial. *Journal of Clinical Endocrinology and Metabolism*, **80**, 1052–8.

Ott, S. M. and Chesnut, C. H. (1989). Calcitriol treatment is not effective in postmenopausal osteoporosis. *Annals of Internal Medicine*, **110**, 267–74.

Pacifici, R. *et al.* (1987). Spontaneous release of interleukin 1 from human blood monocytes reflects bone formation in idiopathic osteoporosis. *Proceedings of the National Academy of Sciences (USA)*, **84**, 4616–20.

Pacifici, R. *et al.* (1989). Ovarian steroid treatment blocks a postmenopausal increase in blood monocyte interleukin-1 release. *Proceedings of the National Academy of Sciences (USA)*, **86**, 2398–402.

Pacifici, R. *et al.* (1991). Effect of surgical menopause and estrogen replacement on cytokine release from human mononuclear cells. *Proceedings of the National Academy of Sciences (USA)*, **88**, 5134–8.

Paganini-Hill, A., Ross, R. K., and Henderson, B. E. (1989). Endometrial cancer and pattern of use of oestrogen replacement therapy: a cohort study. *British Journal of Cancer*, **59**, 445–7.

Pak, C. Y. C., Sakmaee, K., Adams-Huct, B., Pziak, V., Peterson, R. O., and Poindexter, J. R. (1995). Treatment of postmenopausal osteoporosis with slow release sodium fluoride. *Annals of Internal Medicine*, **112**, 401–8.

Parfitt, A.M. (1994). Vitamin D receptor genotypes in osteoporosis. *Lancet*, **334**, 1580.

Peacock, M. (1995). Vitamin D receptor gene alleles and osteoporosis: a contrasting view. *Journal of Bone and Mineral Research*, **10**, 1294–7.

Perry, H. M., Fallon, M. D., Bergfeld, M., Teitelbaun, S. L., and Avioli, L. V. (1982). Osteoporosis in young men. A syndrome of hypercalciuria and accelerated bone turnover. *Archives of Internal Medicine*, **142**, 1295–8.

Persson, I. *et al.* (1989). Risk of endometrial cancer after treatment with oestrogen alone or in conjunction with prostagens: results of a prospective study. *British Medical Journal*, **298**, 147–51.

Petersen, D. J., Boniface, A. M., Schranck, F. W., Rupich, R. C., and White, M. P. (1992). X-linked hypophosphatemic rickets: a study (with literature review) of linear growth response to calcitriol and phosphonate therapy. *Journal of Bone and Mineral Research*, **7**, 583–97.

Pocock, N. A., Eisman, J. A., Yeates, M. G., Sambrook, P. N., and Eberl, S. (1986). Physical fitness is a major determinant of femoral neck and lumbar spine bone mineral density. *Journal of Clinical Investigation*, **78**, 618–21.

Pocock, N. A., Eisman, J. A., Hooper, J. L., Yeates, M. G., Sambrook, P. N., and Eberl, S. (1987). Genetic determinants of bone mass in adults. *Journal of Clinical Investigation*, **80**, 706–10.

Polission, R. P., Martinez, S., and Khoury, M. (1985). Calcification of entheses associated with X-linked hypophosphataemic osteomalacia. *New England Journal of Medicine*, **313**, 1–6.

Quigley, M. E., Martin, P. L., Burnier, A. M., and Brooks, P. (1987). Estrogen therapy arrests bone loss in elderly women. *American Journal of Obstetrics and Gynecology*, **156**, 1516–23.

Ralston, S. M., Urquhart, G. D., Brezeski, M., and Sturrock, R. D. (1990). Prevalence of vertebral compression fractures due to osteoporosis in ankylosing spondylitis. *British Medical Journal*, **285**, 563–5.

Rao, D. S. (1990). Metabolic bone disease in gastrointestinal and biliary disorders. In *Primer on the metabolic bone diseases and disorders of mineral metabolism* (ed. M. J. Favus). American Society for Bone and Mineral Research, California.

Reeve, J., Davies, U. M., Hesp, R., McNally, E., and Katz, D. (1990). Treatment of osteoporosis with human parathyroid peptide and observations on effect of sodium fluoride. *British Medical Journal*, **301**, 314–18.

Reginster, J. Y. *et al.* (1987). 1-year controlled randomized trial of prevention of early postmenopausal bone loss by intranasal calcitonin. *Lancet*, **ii**, 1481–3.

Reid, D. M. (1990). Corticosteroid-induced osteoporosis. In *Osteoporosis 1990* (ed. R. Smith), pp. 99–117. Royal College of Physicians, London.

Reid, D. M. *et al.* (1981). Bone loss in rheumatoid arthritis and primary generalized osteoarthritis. Effects of corticosteroids, suppressive antirheumatic drugs and calcium supplements. *British Journal of Rheumatology*, **25**, 253–9.

Reid, D.M., Nicoll, J.J., Kennedy, N.S., Smith, M.A., Tothill, P., and Nuki, G. (1986). Bone mass in ankylosing spondylitis. *Journal of Rheumatology*, **13**, 932–5.

Reid, I. R., Ames, R. W., Evans, M. C., Gamble, G. D., and Sharpe, S. J. (1993). Effect of calcium supplementation on bone loss in postmenopausal women. *New England Journal of Medicine*, **328**, 460–4.

Reid, I. R., Ames, R. W., Evans, M. C., Gamble, G. D., and Sharpe, S. J. (1995). Long term effects of calcium supplementation on bone loss and fractures in postmenopausal women: a randomised controlled trial. *American Journal of Medicine*, **98**, 331–5.

Reitsma, P. H. *et al.* (1983). Regulation of *myc* gene expression in HL-60 leukaemic cells by a vitamin D metabolite. *Nature*, **306**, 492–4.

Rencken, M. L., Chesnut, C. H., III, and Drinkwater, B. L. (1996). Bone density at multiple skeletal sites in amenorreic athletes. *Journal of the American Medical Association*, **276**, 238–40.

Riggs, B. L. and Melton, I. J. (1986). Involutional osteoporosis. *New England Journal of Medicine*, **314**, 1676–86.

Riggs, B. L. *et al.* (1990). Effect of fluoride treatment on the fracture rate in postmenopausal women with osteoporosis. *New England Journal of Medicine*, **322**, 802–9.

Riis, B., Thomsen, K., and Christiansen, C. (1987). Does calcium supplementation prevent postmenopausal bone loss? *New England Journal of Medicine*, **316**, 173–7.

Rosenspire, K. C., Kennedy, A. C., Steinbeck, J., Blau, M., and Green, F. A. (1980). Investigation of the metabolic activity of bone in rheumatoid arthritis. *Journal of Rheumatology*, **7**, 469–73.

Ross, E. J. and Linch, D. C. (1982). Cushing's syndrome-killing disease: discriminatory value of signs and symptoms aiding early diagnosis. *Lancet*, **ii**, 646–9.

Royal College of Physicians (1989). *Fractured neck of femur: prevention and management*. Royal College of Physicians, London.

Rubin, C. T. and Lanyon, L. E. (1984). Regulation of bone formation by applied dynamic levels. *Journal of Bone and Joint Surgery*, **66**, 397–402.

Ryan, E. A. and Reiss, E. (1984). Oncogenous osteomalacia: review of the world literature of 42 cases and report of two new cases. *American Journal of Medicine*, **77**, 501–12.

Sambrook, P. N., Eisman, J. A., Yeates, M. G., Pocock, N. A., Eberl, S., and Champion, G. D. (1986). Osteoporosis in rheumatoid arthritis, safety of low dose corticosteroids. *Annals of the Rheumatic Diseases*, **45**, 950–3.

Sambrook, P. N., Eisman, J. A., Champion, G. D., and Pocock, N. A. (1988). Sex hormone status and osteoporosis in postmenopausal women with rheumatoid arthritis. *Arthritis and Rheumatism*, **31**, 973–8.

Schindler, A. E., Ebert, A., and Friedrich, E. (1972). Conversion of androstanedione to estrone by human fat tissue. *Journal of Clinical Endocrinology and Metabolism*, **35**, 627–30.

Slemenda, C., Hui, S. L., and Johnston, C. C., Jr (1990*a*). Patterns of bone loss and physiologic growing: prospects for prevention of osteoporosis by attainment of greater peak bone mass. In *Osteoporosis 1990* (eds. C. Christiansen and K. Overgaard), pp. 948–58. Handelstrykkenel, Aalborg, Denmark.

Slemenda, C. W., Hui, S. L., Longcope, D., Wellman, H., and Johnston, C. C., Jr (1990*b*). Predictors of bone mass in perimenopausal women: a prospective study of clinical data using photon absorptiometry. *Annals of Internal Medicine*, **112**, 96–101.

Slemenda, C.W., Miller, J. Z., Hui, S. L., Reister, T. K., and Johnston, C. C. (1991). Role of physical activity in the development of skeletal mass in children. *Journal of Bone and Mineral Research*, **11**, 1227–33.

Smith, E. L., Smith, P. E., Ensign, C. J., and Shea, M. M. (1984). Bone involution decreases in exercising middle aged women. *Calcified Tissue International*, **36**, 129–38.

Spector, T. D., Hall, G. M., McCloskey, E. V., and Kanis, J. A. (1993). Risk of vertebral fractures in women with rheumatoid arthritis. *British Medical Journal*, **1**, 558.

Spector, T. D. *et al.* (1995). Influence of vitamin D receptor genotype on bone mineral density in postmenopausal women: a twin study in Britain. *British Medical Journal*, **310**, 1357–60.

Stamp, T. C. B., Byers, P. D., Ali, Y., and Jenkins, M. V. (1985). Fibrogenesis imperfecta ossium: remission with melphan. *Lancet*, **i**, 582–3.

Stampfer, M. J. *et al.* (1991). Postmenopausal estrogen therapy and cardiovascular disease. Ten-year follow-up from the Nurses' Health Study. *New England Journal of Medicine*, **325**, 756–62.

Steinberg, K. K. *et al.* (1991). A meta-analysis of the effect of estrogen replacement therapy and the risk of breast cancer. *Journal of the American Medical Association*, **264**, 2648–53.

Stevenson, J. C. (1988). Osteoporosis. Pathogenesis and risk factors. In *Bailliere's clinical endocrinology and metabolism*, Vol. 2, (ed. T. J. Martin), pp. 87–101. Saunders, London.

Storm, T., Thamsborg, G., Steiniche, T., Gerant, H. K., and Sorenson, O. H. (1990). Effect of intermittent cyclical etidronate therapy on bone mass and fracture rate in women with postmenopausal osteoporosis. *New England Journal of Medicine*, **322**, 1265–71.

Storm, T., Kollerup G, Thamsborg, G., Gerant, H. K., and Sorenson, O. H. (1996). Five years of clinical experience with intermittent cyclical etidronate for postmenopausal osteoporosis. *Journal of Rheumatology*, **23**, 1560–4.

Svensson, O., Stromberg, L., Ohlen, G., and Lindgren, U. (1996). Prediction of the outcome after hip fracture in elderly patients. *Journal of Bone and Joint Surgery* (B), **78**, 115–18.

Thakker, R. V. and O'Riordan, J. L. H. (1988). Inherited forms of rickets and osteomalacia. In *Bailliere's clinical endocrinology and metabolism*, Vol. 2, (ed. T. J. Martin), pp. 157–92. Saunders, London.

Tilyard, M. W., Spears, G. F. S., Thompson, J., and Dovey, S. (1992). Treatment of postmenopausal osteoporosis with calcitriol or calcium. *New England Journal of Medicine*, **326**, 357–62.

Verstraeten, A. and Dequecker, J. (1990). Vertebral and peripheral bone mineral content and fracture incidence in postmenopausal patients with rheumatoid arthritis: effect of low dose corticosteroids. *Annals of the Rheumatic Diseases*, **45**, 852–7.

Watts, N. B. *et al.* (1990). Intermittent cyclical etidronate in postmenopausal osteo-porosis. *New England Journal of Medicine*, **323**, 73–9.

Whitehead, M. I. and Fraser, D. (1987). Controversies concerning the safety of estrogen replacement therapy. *American Journal of Obstetrics and Gynecology*, **156**, 1315–22.

Whyte, M. P. (1989). Hypophosphatasia. In *The metabolic basis of inherited disease* (6th edn) (eds. C. R. Scriver, A. L. Beaudet, W. S. Sly, and D. Valle), pp. 2843–56. McGraw-Hill, New York.

Wilkinson, M. and Bywaters, E. (1958). Clinical features and course of ankylosing spondylitis. *Annals of the Rheumatic Diseases*, **17**, 209–28.

Will, R., Palmer, R., Bhalla, A. K., Ring, F., and Calin, A. (1989). Osteoporosis in early ankylosing spondylitis: a primary pathological event? *Lancet*, ii, 1483–5.

Will, R., Palmer, R., Elvins, D., Ring, F., and Bhalla, A. K. (1990). A lower femoral neck BMD occurs in patients with ankylosing spondylitis (AS) compared with same six siblings. In *Osteoporosis 1990* (eds. C. Christiansen and K. Overgaard), pp. 1672–4. Handelstrykkenel, Aalborg, Denmark.

Wilson, R. J., Rao, D. S., Ellis, B., Kleerekoper, M., and Parfitt, M. (1988). Mild asymptomatic primary hyperparathyroidism is not a risk factor for vertebral fractures. *Annals of Internal Medicine*, **109**, 959–62.

Winner, S. J., Morgan, C. A., and Grimley Evans, J. (1989). Perimenopausal risk of falling and the incidence of distal forearm fractures. *British Medical Journal*, **298**, 1486–8.

5.17.2 Paget's disease of bone

Adrian J. Crisp

Introduction and epidemiology

On 14 November 1876 Sir James Paget gave the first comprehensive account of 'osteitis deformans' to the Medical and Chirurgical Society (Paget 1877). Paget's disease is a chronic disorder character-ized by accelerated resorption and production of bone, resulting in deformity and fragility, and, in Paget's phrase, by 'change of size, shape and direction'. A radiological survey in Britain of hospital patients of 55 years and over in 31 towns concluded that 4 to 5 per cent had Paget's disease, with a focus in Lancashire of 7 to 8 per cent (Barker 1984). The male:female ratio is 3:2. About 10 to 30 per cent of patients have a single pagetic lesion (monostotic disease) and the rest polyostotic disease. There have been many reports of the disease affecting more than one family member and of its recurrence in successive generations. The disease is most common in Britain, North America, Australia, and New Zealand but rare in Eire, Scandinavia, Asia, and in non-white races (Barker 1984). This remarkable geographical distribution compels speculation about a genetically determined disorder disseminated by the migration of populations. Paget's disease is not only a cause of bone and joint pain but also of chronic disability; in one study, 42 per cent of middle-aged patients were forced into premature retirement from work by the disease (Harinck *et al.* 1986).

Pathophysiology

Histopathology

The striking histological feature of the disease is the increased number and size of both osteoclasts and osteoclast nuclei, with

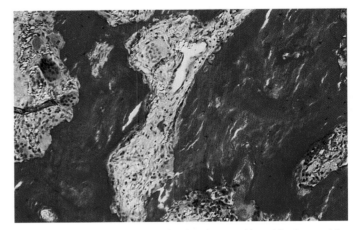

Fig. 1 A section of pagetic bone showing the anarchic architecture and the exaggerated resorption lacunae occupied by multinucleated osteoclasts.

active bone resorption. There is a compensatory increase in the number and size of osteoblasts, leading to exuberant new bone forma-tion. This considerable increase in bone turnover disrupts the normal lamellar structure of the matrix collagen, with increased intraosseous fibrosis, hypervascularity, and enlarged haversian canals. This bone consists of a variable mixture of immature ('woven') bone and irre-gular mature lamellar bone (without haversian systems) separated by deeply staining cement lines in the characteristic mosaic pattern of the disease (Fig. 1).

Aetiology

The weight of evidence argues that Paget's disease is caused by a slow-virus infection of bone cells. Polyclonal antibodies reveal paramyxo-virus antigens in pagetic osteoclasts compatible with measles and respiratory syncytial virus infections. Studies with monoclonal antibo-dies implicate measles, simian virus, and human parainfluenza. *In situ* hybridization with DNA probes specific for measles nucleocapsid protein detects measles sequences in osteoclasts, but probes also hybri-dize with osteoblasts, fibroblasts, and lymphocytes (Basle *et al.* 1987).

Impressive evidence has also come from the demonstration of virus-like particles in osteoclast nuclei (Fig. 2) with a similarity to

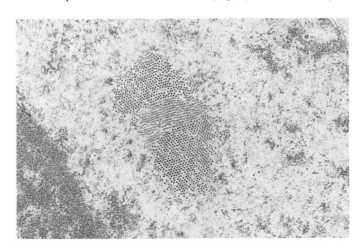

Fig. 2 An electron micrograph of bone tissue from a patient with Paget's disease showing viral microcylindrical elements. (Reproduced with the kind permission of Professor Andre Rebel of Angers, France and of *The Lancet*.)

the measles virus inclusions observed in the brains of patients with subacute sclerosing panencephalitis, a known outcome of measles (Basle *et al.* 1987).

There is some evidence, based on history of exposure of patients with Paget's disease to dogs in early life, implicating canine distemper, a closely related paramyxovirus (O'Driscoll and Anderson 1985). The same Manchester group has also reported the presence of RNA from canine distemper virus in pagetic bone (Gordon *et al.* 1991). The pattern of disease spread also points to infection, perhaps in early life. Paget's disease is characterized by the concurrent appearance of lesions in one or several bones rather than by the sequential recruitment or spread of new bone involvement in each patient.

However, not all studies have found paramyxovirus particles or RNA in pagetic bone (Ralston *et al.* 1991). There has been no convincing recovery of virus from pagetic cells or pagetic osteosarcoma so far, and it has not been possible to passage the disease to uninfected cell cultures and animals. In addition the antiviral agent, inosiplex, which has successfully treated subacute sclerosing panencephalitis, has been ineffective in Paget's disease in preliminary studies.

Kahn (1990) has suggested that the target cell for viral infection may not be the osteoclast but the osteoblast, which can also contain viral RNA. The structure of the osteoblast is also more deranged in Paget's disease than in any other high-turnover states such as renal hyperparathyroidism. Common progenitor cells give rise to osteoclasts, granulocytes, and monocytes and distribute their progeny widely throughout the circulation; one might then expect that new bone involvement would be 'metastatic' in each patient, which is incorrect. Osteoblasts, which are modified fibroblasts, proliferate locally, and this would be more compatible with the pattern of bone involvement in Paget's disease. We know very little of the molecular basis of Paget's disease. Growth factors are likely to influence the anarchic processes in pagetic bone, which are characterized by bone destruction without respect for the existing architecture and with generous formation of new vessels. Non-transforming growth factors, as well as transforming growth factors secreted by some osteosarcoma cells, are convincing candidates for control of the cellular processes in Paget's disease, which has often been considered a benign tumour of the bone (Krane 1986).

Clinical features (Tables 1, 2)

Many patients with Paget's disease are unaware of it. Infection may occur in early life and require many years before bone lesions are detectable. The diagnosis is often made incidentally during radiological or biochemical investigations of other systems. The pagetic vertebra seen on a plain abdominal radiograph or a raised serum alkaline phosphatase are very common presenting features. Although long-term prospective studies of outcome in asymptomatic patients with Paget's disease have not been made, perhaps only a minority of patients will eventually develop clinical symptoms or signs clearly attributable to the disease.

Pain

Bone pain

Typically the bone pain of Paget's disease is constant, deep, and boring, sometimes worse at night and at rest. The cause of the pain is not well understood but is likely to be related to increased internal and periosteal blood flow in metabolically active bone increasing

Table 1 Distribution of Paget's disease in the skeleton

	Percentage
Pelvis	72–76
Lumbar spine	33–58
Thoracic spine	24–45
Femur	25–55
Sacrum	29–44
Skull	28–42
Tibia	22–35
Radius	16
Feet	10
Hands	9
Ribs	3

Table 2 Clinical features of Paget's disease

Pain

Bone expansion and deformity

Fractures

Heat

Neurological syndromes:

    Deafness

    Tinnitus

    Headache

    Spinal cord and root compression

    Brainstem/cerebellar compression

    Blindness

    Other cranial nerve involvement

Malignant osteosarcoma and benign giant-cell tumour

Immobilization hypercalcaemia and hypercalciuria

High-output cardiac failure

Hyperuricaemia and gout

Angioid streaks of retina

intraosseous pressure and stimulating bone pain fibres, which may lie in canaliculi. Long before there is any biochemical evidence of disease control there is often a correlation between pain relief and reduction of bone blood flow, as indicated by thermography, when rapidly acting drugs such as mithramycin (plicamycin) are used (Crisp *et al.* 1989). Compression fractures of verebrae also occur in weakened pagetic bone.

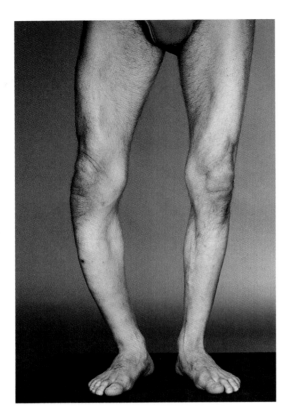

Fig. 3 A patient with Paget's disease of the right femur and tibia causing external rotation of the right leg and secondary osteoarthritis of the knee. A psoriatic patch is also noted on the right knee.

Adjacent joint pain

Bone deformity commonly alters force transmission through the adjacent joint causing premature loss of articular cartilage and secondary osteoarthritis, especially at hip and knee (Fig. 3). Patients can also develop osteoarthritis in an unaffected knee as a result of favouring the contralateral, non-pagetic knee. Metabolically active, hyperaemic, subchondral bone may also be toxic to articular cartilage. Osteoarthritic pain is usually associated with exercise and relieved by rest and sleep. In practice it is often difficult to dissect pagetic bone pain from osteoarthritic pain. Protrusio acetabuli occurs in about one-quarter of hip joints involved by Paget's disease and sacroiliac joint obliteration occurs rarely (Guyer 1980).

Bone expansion and deformity

Bowing long-bone deformity causes effective inequality of leg length, leading to lumbar scoliosis and accelerated degenerative lumbar spondylosis as well as secondary osteoarthritis. Adaptation to slow, insidious deformity may cause remarkably few symptoms.

Fractures

Pain may arise from incomplete fissure fractures involving only cortex on usually the convex side of a bowed long bone. The pain may settle with rest and medical treatment, but the fissure fracture can extend into a completed fracture. Mild injuries may cause pathological fractures in weakened pagetic bone. In a large series of 180 patients, 15 per cent suffered fractures (Harinck *et al.* 1986). Avulsion

fractures, for example, of the patella, can occur after sudden muscular contraction. Non-union may be more common at sites of fracture in pagetic bone.

Heat

Palpation of affected bones near to skin surfaces is often helpful, although bone tenderness is unusual. Auscultation of tibia or skull can sometimes reveal bruits. Temperature may be correlated with both metabolic activity of bone and with bone pain.

Neurological syndromes

Common symptoms of cranial Paget's disease includes non-specific headaches, possibly due to vascular changes in bone and meninges, impaired hearing, and tinnitus. About half the patients with skull involvement will develop deafness, which may be sensineural, conductive, or mixed. Nerve entrapment by the expanded petrous temporal bone is partly responsible, but subtle toxic effects on the inner ear mediated by hypervascularity are also likely. Less commonly the optic nerve and other cranial nerves may be affected with predictable results.

Skull expansion may cause frontal or occipital prominence but if the base of the skull is involved, softened bone may lead to platybasia — the descent of the cranium on to the cervical spine — which may cause dizziness and syncope, owing to kinking of the vertebrobasilar blood vessels, or even cerebellar or brainstem compressive syndromes.

Dysfunction of the spinal cord may rarely result from vertebral expansion and compression but both skull-base and cord dysfunction may follow ill-understood, 'steal' phenomena: increased blood flow in bone 'steals' blood away from neural structures causing ischaemic damage. Hence incipient paraparesis may improve rapidly with intensive medical therapy reducing bone blood flow.

Neoplastic complications

Almost all cases of osteogenic sarcoma in adults arise from pagetic bone but conversely osteosarcoma is a very rare complication of Paget's disease occurring in less than 0.1 per cent of affected patients. The sarcoma is highly malignant and usually rapidly fatal. This diagnosis is worth considering in a patient who develops intense pain in an affected bone, with a progressive lytic lesion and a rising alkaline phosphatase against a background of stable symptoms (Fig. 4). There may be genetic factors: three brothers, who all developed Paget's disease in early life, later died from pagetic osteosarcomas (Brenton *et al.* 1980).

Over 100 cases of the benign giant-cell tumour arising from pagetic bone have been reported. These commonly involve facial bones and mandible, and some cases have been linked by a common family background in Avellino, a small town in Italy (Jacobs *et al.* 1979; Bhambhani *et al.* 1992).

Immobilization, hypercalcaemia, and hypercalciuria

The serum calcium is usually normal but during immobilization for an unrelated illness or orthopaedic surgery, hypercalcaemia and hypercalciuria can occur. Bone formation is inhibited but resorption continues unchecked. Rarely both abnormalities can occur without immobilization, but this can often be traced to coincidental

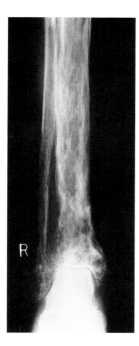

Fig. 4 A radiograph of the right lower leg of a patient with Paget's disease. Just above the ankle joint the markedly lytic region contains an osteosarcoma.

hyperparathyroidism. Hypercalciuria alone is more common, occurring in 21 out of 180 patients, nine of whom described a history of renal calculi (Harinck *et al.* 1986).

Hyperuricaemia

Increased bone-cell turnover might be expected to increase urate synthesis: 13 out of 101 (12.9 per cent) patients without an independent cause had raised urate values. Only three patients suffered from clinical gout (Harinck *et al.* 1986).

High-output cardiac failure

Cardiac index (cardiac output corrected for surface area) is increased in the majority of pagetic patients, especially those with widespread disease. High-output cardiac failure has only rarely been reported when more than one-third of the skeleton is involved.

Other clinical associations

Angioid streaks in the retina caused by disruption of Bruch's membrane may be associated but are also more firmly linked with another condition of abnormal connective tissue, pseudoxanthoma elasticum. Associations with Hashimoto's thyroiditis, Dupuytren's contracture, and chondrocalcinosis have all been proposed but none is firmly based.

Investigations and assessment
Biochemical

Serum alkaline phosphatase

This osteoblastic enzyme, a measure of new bone formation and not resorption, is the most useful and widely available marker and may be elevated by as much as 30 times above the upper limit of the reference range. Analysis of isoenzymes or measurement of alternative liver enzymes help to exclude a significant hepatic contribution to the total alkaline phosphatase. Occasionally, this enzyme is normal with limited Paget's disease but one should not be deterred from treating a painful pagetic lesion by a normal result.

Urine hydroxyproline

Increased osteoclastic bone resorption parallels increased bone formation and may be assessed by assay of urine hydroxyproline excretion, a breakdown product of collagen. Only 20 to 30 per cent of the total hydroxyproline is derived from bone resorption. Ideally the patient should have followed a gelatin (denatured collagen)-free diet for 48 h before the urine collection to exclude a dietary contribution but this is often impractical. The urinary hydroxyproline/creatinine ratio may be determined on a 2-h collection after an overnight fast or on a 24-h specimen.

Urinary pyridinoline collagen cross-links

The recent development of an assay to measure the excretion of bone-specific collagen cross-links offers the prospect of accurate measurement of current osteclastic bone resorption. This is likely to replace measurement of urinary hydroxproline when more widely available (Beardsworth *et al.* 1990).

Serum osteocalcin

Osteocalcin, which is specifically produced by osteoblasts, might in theory be of benefit in the assessment of Paget's disease. However, only one-half of patients with raised alkaline phosphatase have raised osteocalcin and values can be increased by treatment via interactions between parathyroid hormone and 1,25-dihydroxyvitamin D_3. Thus, osteocalcin is unlikely to be a valuable marker of disease activity in Paget's disease.

Serum total acid phosphatase

This osteoclastic enzyme can be raised in active Paget's disease but is of little value. Occasionally metastatic prostatic carcinoma is incorrectly diagnosed in the presence of sclerotic vertebrae and a raised concentration. The two conditions can coexist.

Serum α_2HS glycoprotein

This liver-derived protein is taken up by active bone and levels tend to be lower than normal in active Paget's disease.

Radiological

Plain radiographs

There is a wide variety of appearances in Paget's disease but the key features are lytic areas, especially early in the disease, sclerotic areas, and bone expansion with coarse and disorganized trabecular structures (Figs. 5 and 6).

Isotope bone scanning

In one study (Meunier *et al.* 1987), scanning demonstrated 8.3 per cent more pagetic sites than did plain radiography and is therefore the most sensitive investigation for defining the extent of lesions (Fig. 7). A scan and then plain radiographs of affected sites should be performed at first diagnosis for future comparisons. The percentage

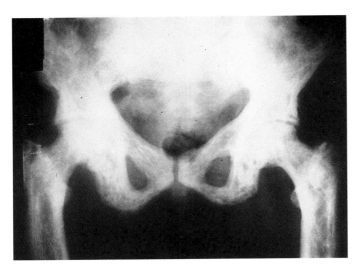

Fig. 5 A radiograph of the pelvis showing typical widespread Paget's disease.

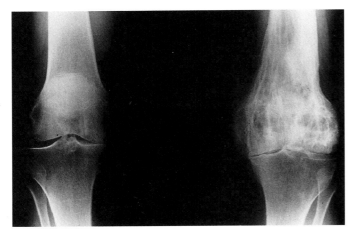

Fig. 6 A radiograph of both knees showing typical pagetic involvement of the left distal femur and worse osteoarthritis of the affected knee when compared with the knee uninvolved by Paget's disease.

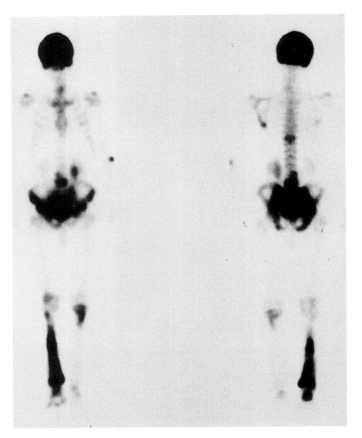

Fig. 7 A scintigram showing a typical pagetic distribution of lesions in skull, vertebrae, pelvis, and both legs.

retention of the isotope after 24 h — less than 40 per cent in normal subjects in our laboratory — provides an index of total pagetic bone activity. During aggressive advance of the resorption front, scanning may underestimate disease activity, suggesting active osteoclastic activity with a poor osteoblastic response — a situation comparable with many lytic lesions in multiple myeloma. Quantitative bone scintigraphy comparing the area of increased uptake with the same area on the contralateral (unaffected) side can be very useful in the assessment of the monostotic lesion when alkaline phosphatase is often normal.

Thermography

Increased bone and periosseous blood flow is demonstrated effectively in superficial bones and is reduced after effective treatment (Fig. 8). Thermographic improvement and pain reduction seem to be linked (Crisp *et al.* 1989).

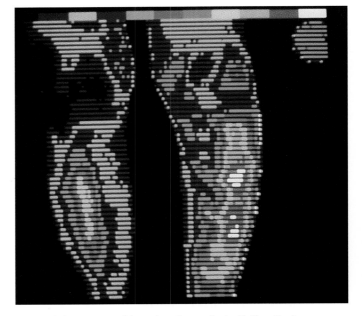

Fig. 8 A thermogram of lower legs in a patient with Paget's disease showing a focus of increased temperature (white and red areas) at the site of active Paget's disease (by kind permission of Dr Brian Hazleman).

Differential diagnosis of Paget's disease

The combination of physical signs, including a warm deformed bone with characteristic radiographs and a raised serum alkaline phosphatase, usually leaves no doubt about the diagnosis of Paget's disease. Consider also:

1. Other causes of raised serum bone alkaline phosphatase:

    (a) metastatic bone disease;
    (b) osteomalacia;
    (c) hyperparathyroidism, with osteitis fibrosa cystica: this may accompany Paget's disease and may be more than co-incidental;
    (d) idiopathic hyperphosphatasia: characterized by bone deformity in childhood and a probably recessive inheritance—its relationship with adult Paget's disease is not known.

2. Other causes with similar radiographic appearances:

    (a) metastatic bone disease; osteolytic and osteoblastic disease, e.g. prostatic secondaries;
    (b) fibrous dysplasia;
    (c) chronic osteomyelitis;
    (d) metaphyseal dysplasia (Engelmann's disease);
    (e) sternocostoclavicular hyperostosis.

Treatment

Attitudes towards treating Paget's disease vary considerably from the therapeutic nihilist, who attributes most of the pain to secondary osteoarthritis and considers specific treatment as an expensive superfluity to the tyro who chooses to treat all patients. The criteria of the present author are listed in Table 3. With the advent of safe effective drugs for Paget's disease there is a firm trend towards early, aggressive

treatment with the objective of maintaining serum alkaline phosphatase within the normal range. Although remission after treatment is related to the degree of biochemical control (Harinck et al. 1987; Kanis and Gray 1987), and there is strong histological evidence that effective suppression promotes more normal bone remodelling, we lack evidence that intensive treatment inhibits the development of long-term complications.

Pagetic and related osteoarthritic pain may be reduced by simple analgesics and non-steroidal anti-inflammatory drugs but pure pagetic bone pain often responds poorly to these. Physical treatment to improve muscle function and correct any inequality in leg length with shoe raises may be very helpful. More effective control will be achieved by drugs that suppress bone turnover. All primarily inhibit osteoclast activity, as reflected by an early decrease in urine hydroxyproline excretion followed by a later fall in serum alkaline phosphatase. Intravenous mithramycin (plicamycin), $15\,\mu g/kg$ per day for 7 to 10 days is highly effective, giving rapid pain relief within 3 days and biochemical improvement, but it has an unacceptable toxicity to bone marrow, liver, and kidneys and is on the verge of obsolescence since the availability of later generation bisphosphonates. It may still be of value for the urgent treatment of acute neurological deterioration, most commonly spinal cord compression, when the rapid control of bone blood flow and perhaps periosteal oedema can lead to impressive improvement.

In most patients the choice of treatment now falls between the bisphosphonates (previously called diphosphonates) and the calcitonins.

The bisphosphonates (Fig. 9)

This family of pyrophosphate analogues share a common P–C–P backbone replacing the P–O–P of pyrophosphate. Side-chain variations confer differing properties but they are all effective for pagetic pain and disease activity. Oral etidronate and more recently oral tiludronate and intravenous pamidronate are licensed for use in Paget's disease in the United Kingdom. There has been additional experience with oral and intravenous clodronate, which is at present licensed only for use in malignant hypercalcaemia.

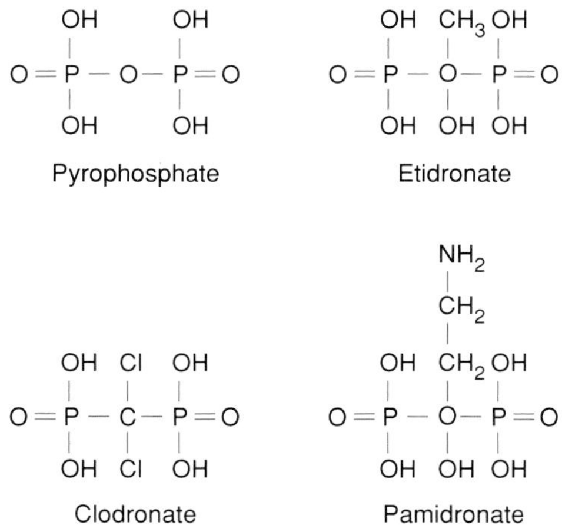

Table 3	Indications for treatment of Paget's disease

Pain arising from a site of known Paget's disease

Early, potentially deforming disease

Osteolytic lesions especially in weight-bearing bones

Skull disease

Complications:

    Progressive neurological syndromes

    Fissure fractures (avoid etidronate)

    Immobilization hypercalcaemia

    High-output cardiac failure

Disease in patients aged under 55 years

Serum alkaline phosphatase and/or urine hydroxyproline concentration more than twice upper limit of normal

Patients likely to undergo joint replacement at involved sites wihtin 6 months

Fig. 9 The structures of pyrophosphate and bisphosphonates in common clinical use.

Calcitonins only partially suppress the disease while treatment continues. Bisphosphonates can achieve prolonged remissions following a course of treatment and are therefore now first choice.

Etidronate disodium

The recommended regimen for oral etidronate is 5 mg/kg per day for up to 6 months, although a month's course of 20 mg/kg per day is probably as effective, without added toxicity (Preston *et al*. 1986; Heath 1987). To achieve maximal gut absorption all oral bisphosphonates should be taken at least 2 h after food. Mild gastrointestinal symptoms and transient increased bone pain are occasional side-effects. Etidronate even at low doses can cause a reversible mineralization defect, which may be minimized by vitamin D supplements, and may increase the risk of fracture. This bisphosphonate is contraindicated for lytic lesions in weight-bearing long bones (Krane 1982). Courses of etidronate should always be followed by a minimum treatment-free period of 3 months to permit recovery of the mineralization defect.

Newer bisphosphonates

The newer bisphosphonates are not completely free of the risk of causing a mineralization defect but the safe therapeutic window is much wider. Clodronate is about 10 times less potent than pamidronate and there has been far less clinical experience with it (Yates *et al*. 1985). Oral tiludronate 400 mg daily for 3 months has been recently licensed for the treatment of Paget's disease in the United Kingdom. Very poor absorption and a high incidence of mild gastrointestinal side-effects with pamidronate effectively limits its use to the intravenous route but absolute compliance with a precise dose is achieved.

The optimal dosage regimen for pamidronate in Paget's disease remains to be determined. Anderson *et al*. (1994) have induced a full biochemical remission (serum alkaline phosphatase falling to normal) in 90 per cent of patients in whom this enzyme was initially raised, with one or more complex courses. Such courses typically induce a remission of about 2 years and Anderson *et al*. claim that a permanent remission can be achieved in 10 to 15 per cent of patients. If the alkaline phosphatase level is below 500 i.u./l they advocate a 30 mg infusion over 2 h followed by three infusions of 60 mg each over 4 h. If the alkaline phosphatase level exceeds 500 i.u./l, six 60 mg infusions are recommended administered at 2-week intervals.

Other groups have argued that a single infusion of a dose large enough to saturate all of the binding sites of bone affected by Paget's disease should achieve as much as complex recurrent regimens (Fig. 10). Watts *et al*. (1993) studied the effect of a single infusion of 105 mg of pamidronate in 14 patients with mean levels of serum alkaline phosphatase about three times the normal upper limit. The alkaline phosphatase level returned to normal (the goal of successful treatment and likely to produce prolonged remission) in 71 per cent of patients with a mean nadir of the enzyme at 5.9 months. Excellent symptomatic control was achieved for 1.5 to 2 years. Four patients received a second infusion of 105 mg of pamidronate, a mean interval of 19 months after the first dose. This resulted in a similar clinical and biochemical response to the first. One patient had a 4-year remission before treatment was required.

Further support for a single dose regimen was reported by Chakravarty *et al*. (1994) who treated 36 patients, with mean levels of serum alkaline phosphatase about four times the normal upper limit, with 60 mg of pamidronate. Alkaline phosphatase levels were returned to normal in 78 per cent of patients at 6 months and 77 per

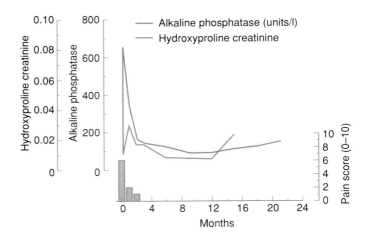

Fig. 10 The effect of a single intravenous infusion of pamidronate (APD) at a dose of 105 mg in one patient with Paget's disease. An early rapid fall in urine hydroxyproline excretion is followed by a slower fall in serum alkaline phosphatase. Pain is abolished after 3 months and the patient is still pain free after 21 months.

cent of patients at 1 year. The efficacy of the two single-dose regimens using pamidronate at 60 to 105 mg therefore is similar, but is marginally inferior to the complex regimen advocated by Anderson *et al*. (1994) which achieves a normal level in 90 per cent of patients.

The author's current practice is to treat pagetic patients with a single infusion of pamidronate 90 mg over 6 hours. Patients are followed up every 3 months with a clinical assessment and measurement of alkaline phosphatase. If this is supranormal at 6 months, a second infusion of 90 mg is administered. Only a small minority of patients do not achieve normal alkaline phosphatase levels with this regimen. This 'resistant' subgroup is treated with 90 mg infusions every 3 months until remission occurs.

Intravenous pamidronate is usually well tolerated but the following side-effects have been reported: transient pyrexia after the first but not usually after later infusions; mild leucopenia and mild hypocalcaemia; myalgia; transient increased bone pain; acute anterior uveitis, which may recur if the patient is rechallenged (unpublished observation).

The calcitonins

Subcutaneous or intramuscular calcitonin (salmon, porcine, or human) is safe and effective but has many disadvantages. It is so far only widely available by injection. It commonly causes mild side-effects such as nausea, flushing, and diarrhoea. After successful initial treatment, patients may relapse while continuing treatment, because of down-regulation of calcitonin receptors. Early relapse after ceasing treatment is also common, and calcitonin is very expensive.

If salmon calcitonin (salcatonin) is chosen, the starting dose after a 10 i.u. test dose is 50 to 100 i.u. daily reducing to 50 i.u. two or three times weekly once the symptomatic response has been achieved. Patients usually notice decreasing pain after 1 to 2 months but if there has been no response by 3 months, then calcitonin treatment should cease. Effective treatment has been claimed to reverse disease progression and, until the advent of the newer bisphosphonates, calcitonin was the treatment of choice for lytic disease of long bones and fissure fractures. Many patients learn to give their own injections but to condemn them to many years of injections 2 to 3 times weekly is becoming increasingly unacceptable when alternative short courses of bisphosphonates can achieve prolonged clinical and biochemical remissions.

It is possible that new formulations of calcitonin given by nasal spray, for example salmon calcitonin at 200 to 400 i.u. daily, when available might be useful but the typical therapeutic effect is weaker than that of the newer bisphosphonates (Reginster *et al.* 1988).

Surgery

There is still no consensus as to whether patients requiring total hip or knee replacement for joints ravaged by the combination of Paget's disease and osteoarthritis should receive specific medical treatment before surgery. There is some evidence that effective treatment — a newer bisphosphonate or calcitonin rather than the demineralizing etidronate — reduces bone blood flow, improves the quality of bone in which the prosthesis will be sited, and facilitates the adhesion of cement to bone. Certainly orthopaedic surgeons should not be deterred from replacement arthroplasty by the presence of Paget's disease, as the risks of prosthetic loosening are only slightly increased. It would seem logical to time surgery to coincide with a phase of clinical and biochemical pagetic remission induced by medical treatment. Prospective studies are awaited.

References

Anderson, D.C. *et al.* (1994). Intravenous pamidronate: evolution of an effective treatment strategy. *Seminars in Arthritis and Rheumatism*, **23** (4), 273–5.

Barker, D.J.P. (1984). The epidemiology of Paget's disease of bone. *British Medical Bulletin*, **40**, 396–400.

Basle, M.F., Rebel, A., Fournier, J.G., Russell, W.C., and Malkani, K. (1987). On the trail of paramyxoviruses in Paget's disease of bone. *Clinical Orthopaedics*, **217**, 9–15.

Beardsworth, L.J., Eyre, D.R., and Dickson, I.R. (1990). Changes with age in the urinary excretion of lysyl- and hydroxy-lysylpyridinoline, two new markers of bone collagen turnover. *Journal of Bone and Mineral Research*, **5**, 671–6.

Bhambhani, M.M., Lamberty, B.G.H., Clements, M.R., Skingle, S.J., and Crisp, A.J. (1992). Giant cell tumours in mandible and spine — a rare complication of Paget's disease of bone. *Annals of the Rheumatic Diseases*, **51**, 1335–7.

Brenton, D., Isenberg, D.A., and Bertram, J. (1980). Osteosarcoma complicating familial Paget's disease. *Postgraduate Medical Journal*, **56**, 238–43.

Chakravarty, K., Merry, P., and Scott, D.G.I. (1994). A single infusion of pamidronate AH Pr BP in the treatment of Paget's disease of bone. *Journal of Rheumatology*, **21**, 2118–21.

Crisp, A.J., Smith, M.L., Skingle, S.J., Smith, M., Page Thomas, D.P., and Hazleman, B.L. (1989). The localisation of the bone lesions of Paget's disease by radiographs, scintigraphy and thermography: pain may be related to bone blood flow. *British Journal of Rheumatology*, **28**, 266–8.

Gordon, M.T., Anderson, D.C., and Sharpe, P.T. (1991). Canine distemper virus localised in bone cells of patients with Paget's disease. *Bone*, **12**, 195–201.

Guyer, P.B. (1980). Radiology in Paget's disease: clinical and aetiological significance. *Hospital Update*, **6**, 1079–91.

Harinck, H.I.J., Bijvoet, O.L.M., Vellenga, C.J.L.R., Blanksma, H.J., and Frijlink, W.B. (1986). Relations between signs and symptoms in Paget's disease of bone. *Quarterly Journal of Medicine*, **226**, 133–51.

Harinck, H.I.J., Papapoulos, S.E., Blanksma, H.J., Moolenaar, A.J., Vermeij, P., and Bijvoet, O.L.M. (1987). Paget's disease of bone: early and late responses to three different modes of treatment with APD. *British Medical Journal*, **295**, 1301–5.

Heath, D.A. (1987). Treating Paget's disease. *British Medical Journal*, **294**, 1048–50.

Jacobs, T.P., Michelsen, J., Polay, J.S., D'Adamo, A.C., and Canfield, R.E. (1979). Giant cell tumor in Paget's disease of bone. *Cancer*, **44**, 742–7.

Kahn, A.J. (1990). The viral etiology of Paget's disease of bone: a new perspective. *Calcified Tissue International*, **47**, 127–9.

Kanis, J.A. and Gray, R.E.S. (1987). Long term follow up observations on treatment in Paget's disease. *Clinical Orthopaedics*, **217**, 99–125.

Krane, S.M. (1982). Etidronate disodium in the treatment of Paget's disease of bone. *Annals of Internal Medicine*, **96**, 619–25.

Krane, S.M. (1986). Paget's disease of bone. *Calcified Tissue International*, **38**, 309–17.

Meunier, P.J. *et al.* (1987). Skeletal distribution and biochemical parameters of Paget's disease. *Clinical Orthopaedics*, **217**, 37–44.

O'Driscoll, J.B. and Anderson, D.C. (1985). Past pets and Paget's disease. *Lancet*, ii, 919–21.

Paget, J. (1887). On a form of chronic inflammation of bones (osteitis deformans). *Transactions of the Medical and Chirurgical Society*, **60**, 37–63.

Preston, C.J. *et al.* (1986). Effective short term treatment of Paget's disease with oral etidronate. *British Medical Journal*, **292**, 79–80.

Ralston, S.H., Digiovine, F.S., Gallacher, S.J., Boyle, I.T., and Duff, G.W. (1991). Failure to detect paramyxovirus sequences in Paget's disease of bone using the polymerase chain reaction. *Journal of Bone and Mineral Research*, **6**, 1243–8.

Reginster, J.Y., Jeugmans-Huynen, A.M., Albert, A., Denis, D., and Franchimont, P. (1988). One year's treatment of Paget's disease of bone by synthetic salmon calcitonin as a nasal spray. *Journal of Bone and Mineral Research*, **3**, 249–52.

Watts, R.A., Skingle, S.J., Bhambhani, M.M., Pountain, G., and Crisp, A.J. (1993). Treatment of Paget's disease of bone with single dose intravenous pamidronate. *Annals of Rheumatic Diseases*, **52**, 616–18.

Yates, A.J.P. *et al.* (1985). Intravenous clodronate in the treatment and retreatment of Paget's disease of bone. *Lancet*, i, 1474–7.

5.17.3 Diseases of bone, cartilage, and synovium

P. J. Maddison

In this chapter, a miscellaneous group of disorders affecting components of the joint and periarticular structures is described. They can present a challenge to the clinician in diagnosis and management. There is often a delay in diagnosis causing pain and disability. Frequently this is due to insufficient clinical suspicion, partly because of the rarity of most of these conditions. Their diagnosis generally depends on recognizing a combination of clinical, laboratory, and histological features, but the advent of techniques such as magnetic resonance imaging (**MRI**) facilitates earlier diagnosis. This is particularly important for conditions such as osteonecrosis where the institution of treatment at an earlier stage in the course of the process may prevent joint destruction.

Osteoid osteoma

Skeletal neoplasms are discussed in Chapters 1.2.1.2 and 5.19.1. Only rarely do they cause problems for the experienced clinician in being mistaken for systemic rheumatic diseases. An exception is hypertrophic osteoarthropathy (Chapter 5.19.1); another is osteoid osteoma. This is a benign osteoid-forming tumour, which can be an elusive cause of bone pain, 'radiculopathy', or 'arthritis' in children and young adults, depending on its site. It is uncommon and accounts for 10 to 12 per cent of benign bone neoplasms (Dahlin and Unni 1986).

The maximum age incidence is in the second and third decades, but this tumour can occur in all age groups, and is two or three times more common in boys than girls. More than two-thirds of the lesions occur in long bones, mostly in the lower extremity and especially involving the femur and tibia. The neck of the femur and the inter-trochanteric region are a particularly characteristic location in the femur (Resnick and Niwayama 1988).

The lesion consists of a small core or nidus of cellular, highly vascularized tissue, with an interlacing network of immature bone and osteoid in varying proportions. The nidus is surrounded by a zone of reactive bone, especially in cortical bone. Very rarely, the osteoid osteoma is multifocal with more than one nidus. High levels of prostaglandins are produced within the lesions (Makley and Dunn 1982). Intra-articular lesions, which are rare and arise at the end of a long bone within the insertion of the joint capsule, are accompanied by a synovitis characterized by a hyperplastic synovium and a prominent lymphocytic infiltrate.

Clinical features

Almost without exception the initial symptom is pain. This may be vague and intermittent at first but becomes increasingly intense. Often, though not invariably, it is worse at night, and typically it is relieved by aspirin and other non-steroidal anti-inflammatory drugs. Although pain is usually felt in the region of the bone lesion, the presentation can be much less characteristic and the diagnosis is often delayed for many months. For example pain can sometimes be referred or radicular, accompanied by muscle atrophy and diminished or absent tendon reflexes in the affected limb, thus mimicking a spinal lesion (Kiers et al. 1990). Intra-articular lesions can also present a confusing picture, with joint pain, stiffness, effusion, muscle atrophy, and loss of function. Osteoid osteomas that arise in the posterior elements of the spine can present with scoliosis or torti-collis.

Diagnosis

A typical lesion (Fig. 1(a)) in the cortex of a long bone is seen on a plain radiograph as a well-defined area of sclerosis, 0.5 to 1.0 cm in diameter, surrounding a radiolucent nidus, which may contain speckled areas of calcification. However, lesions in cancellous bone and neural arch and intra-articular lesions are often difficult to locate with plain radiographs. A bone scan using $^{99}Tc^m$ hydroxymethylene diphosphonate is a highly sensitive technique to screen for an osteoid osteoma, as these lesions avidly accumulate isotope (Fig. 1(b)). Helms et al. have described the 'double density sign' as characteristic for osteoid osteoma (Helms et al. 1984) but it is often not seen and the bone scan is then non-specific for differentiating an osteoid osteoma from lesions such as a stress fracture, synovitis, and a Brodie's abscess. Computed tomography (CT) is also valuable for imaging lesions difficult to locate on plain radiographs, especially those in the spine and proximal femur, and for precisely locating the nidus before surgical resection (Swee et al. 1979). MRI effectively demonstrates the associated intramedullary and soft tissue changes but the resulting image can lead to diagnostic confusion and CT is generally considered to be the better imaging modality for the diagnosis of osteoid osteoma (Assoun et al. 1994).

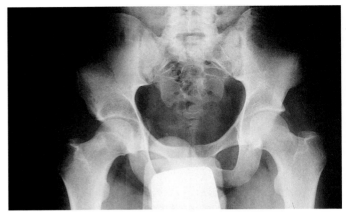
(a)

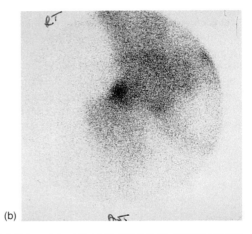
(b)

Fig. 1 (a) Plain pelvic radiograph showing an osteoid osteoma of the femoral neck in an 18-year-old male who presented with a 3-month history of progressively worsening pain. (b) Radionuclide bone scan showing increased uptake of isotope by the lesion.

Treatment

Surgery is curative, provided the nidus is excised completely. If this is not achieved, the osteoid osteoma may recur, up to 10 years afterwards. Many surgeons use an *en bloc* excision but some use CT- or radio-isotope-guided excision of osteomas, mainly of those located in the extremities (Ward et al. 1993; Musculo et al. 1995). Radiofrequency ablation (Rosenthal et al. 1995) or thermocoagulation (De Berg et al. 1995) have been reported as promising and less invasive alternatives to surgery in selected patients.

Synovial chondromatosis

This is a disorder of unknown aetiology that affects synovium-lined joints, tendon sheaths, and bursas. It is characterized by chondro-metaplasia of the subsynovial connective-tissue cells. The joint cavity becomes filled with a thickened synovium containing pearly-white to blue nodules. Some of these lie free in the joint as loose bodies. The histological appearance is of double-nucleated chondro-cytes exhibiting moderate hyperchromasia, arranged in clusters with abundant intervening matrix.

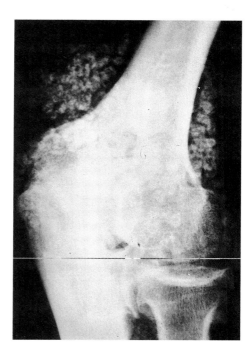

Fig. 2 Anteroposterior view of the elbow demonstrating multiple osteochondral bodies, regularly shaped and uniform in size. This is typical of synovial chondromatosis. (By courtesy of Dr P. Renton, University College London.)

The disorder is uncommon and generally occurs in middle-aged men. It has never been reported before puberty. Most commonly it affects the knee (one-half of cases) or hip, but can also involve other large joints such as the elbow, shoulder, and wrist. Extra-articular involvement of tendons occurs, predominantly in the hands and feet.

Clinically, it resembles pigmented villonodular synovitis (see below). The presenting symptoms are mild, but progressive, pain and locking. Aspirated joint fluid is always yellow or straw-coloured. Plain radiographs (Fig. 2) show small, punctate calcifications outlining the joint margin and sometimes bony erosions due to raised intra-articular pressure. Large osteochondral fragments can be seen but this is not a specific feature. Loss of articular cartilage does not occur. If the cartilaginous nodules are not calcified or ossified, the diagnosis can only be confirmed by arthroscopy.

This is a benign condition. During the active phase it is very slowly progressive but it becomes self-limiting and regression can be observed. In rare cases there is transformation to chondrosarcoma.

Treatment is surgical and most authorities suggest that this should consist of removal of loose bodies and excision of the synovial membrane (Christensen and Poulsen 1975), which can be done via the arthroscope (Coolican and Dandy 1989). Removal of loose bodies without an extensive synovectomy has been reported to give similar results (Shpitzer *et al.* 1990).

Pigmented villonodular synovitis

The term pigmented villonodular synovitis was first coined by Jaffe *et al.* in 1941 to encompass a group of conditions, previously known by a variety of other terms, characterized by exuberant proliferation of synovial cells and mesenchymal supporting tissue affecting joints, tendons, and bursas (Jaffe *et al.* 1941; Flandry and Hughston 1987;

Goldman and DiCarlo 1988). In their seminal paper, Jaffe and colleagues emphasized the villous and nodular proliferation, the deposition of iron and fat, and the non-malignant nature of these conditions. The terminology subsequently was expanded to distinguish localized lesions (sharply localized or pedunculated lesions involving tendon sheaths or part of the joint lining) from diffuse lesions of the joint synovial membrane, which, although similar histologically, are more progressive and tend to recur after treatment.

Aetiological factors

The aetiology is unknown and there are still various hypotheses based on different interpretations of the histological changes. Although once considered to be neoplastic, pigmented villonodular synovitis does not behave like a malignancy and does not metastasize. In contrast, a benign neoplastic process of synovial, vascular, or fibrohistiocytic origin is proposed by some (Rao and Vigorita 1984). This view is supported by some cytogenetic evidence of clonality (Ray *et al.* 1990). Most favour a non-neoplastic aetiology; suggestions include a response to blood and blood products from trauma. An epidemiological study (Myers *et al.* 1980), while showing no evidence of a genetic basis for pigmented villonodular synovitis, demonstrated a history of chronic repetitive trauma and repeated haemarthroses in approximately 50 per cent of cases. However, there has been a general failure to reproduce typical histological changes in experimental models with injection of various substances from whole blood to colloidal iron. Furthermore, clinical experience from haemophiliacs and others with bleeding disorders points away from a reaction to trauma and haemorrhage *per se*. A commonly held, but rather unhelpful, view is that pigmented villonodular synovitis is an inflammatory response to an as yet unknown trigger.

Pathology

The striking pathological feature is the proliferation of synovial lining cells at the surface and invading the subsynovial stroma. The result in diffuse pigmented villonodular synovitis is a greatly thickened synovial membrane bristling with big, long villi, which may be interspersed with nodules of various size. The tissue is often stained red-brown from repeated haemorrhage, with mottled areas of yellow-orange from lipid deposition. Histologically (Schumacher *et al.* 1982), there is marked proliferation of surface lining cells, together with an invasion of the subsynovial stroma by large epithelioid histiocytic cells that electron-microscopic studies show to be a mixture of proliferating synovial fibroblasts and type B synovial lining cells. The stroma also contains multinucleate giant cells and lipid-laden macrophages. In addition, there are a few lymphocytes and plasma cells. Capillary hyperplasia resulting in numerous thin-walled vascular channels is another characteristic feature. Haemosiderin is deposited in the lining and epithelioid cells, and in the stroma. Another typical feature is the ability of pigmented villonodular synovitis to invade subchondral bone. This is thought to be through erosion into the osteocartilaginous junction, by extension into vascular foramina, and from the effect of increased intra-articular pressure causing focal osteopenia in the subchondral bone.

Clinical features

Pigmented villonodular synovitis is rare, with an estimated annual incidence of around 1.8 cases/million population (Myers *et al.* 1980).

Typically it affects adults of both sexes in their third or fourth decade, but there is a wide age range and cases have been reported in children (Docken 1979) and even infants (Curtin *et al.* 1993). Classically, it presents as a monoarthritis. In 80 per cent of cases the knee is involved, followed in order by the hip, ankle, and shoulder; very rarely, multiple joints are involved and there are case reports of involvement at sites such as the spine (Clark *et al.* 1993) and temporo-mandibular joint (Franchi *et al.* 1994). The onset is usually insidious, with pain the most common complaint (Flandry *et al.* 1994a); this is mild at first but progressive. Rarely, there may be sudden exacerbation of pain due to torsion or infarction of a nodule of abnormal tissue. Sometimes there are features of internal derangement, such as locking, especially with localized forms of pigmented villonodular synovitis. Occasionally, an affected knee joint becomes unstable. On examination, there is often swelling and sometimes one or more palpable masses of synovium. There may be local warmth and points of tenderness.

Joint aspiration gives fluid that ranges in colour from yellow or straw, with deep xanthochromia from previous haemorrhage, to brown-stained or frankly bloody. Reports of synovial fluid analysis are sparse but findings point to inflammation and include a slight elevation of protein, reduced glucose, and a low to moderate leucocyte count. The results of other laboratory tests are otherwise normal.

Plain radiographs may be normal or only show the soft tissue outline of synovial swelling, which is made more radiodense by haemosiderin deposition. However, calcification, which occurs in malignant lesions such as synovial sarcoma, is absent. In approximately 50 per cent there are osteoarticular changes corresponding to invasion of bone by the lesion. These include multiple subchondral cysts, which can occur on non-weight-bearing surfaces, and well-demarcated erosions due to increased intra-articular pressure. These changes occur earlier in joints with a tight articular capsule, such as the hip, than in the knee in which a more distensible capsule accommodates a greater degree of soft tissue proliferation. In the knee, bony lesions often develop first in the patellofemoral compartment, where intra-articular soft tissue is more likely to be entrapped (Smith and Pugh 1962). Preservation of joint space is reported to be a typical feature of pigmented villonodular synovitis, but, in fact, loss of joint space can occur as a late feature. Juxta-articular osteoporosis and osteophyte formation are not seen. MRI is very characteristic if there is sufficient haemosiderin and fat deposition in the lesion. Haemosiderin deposition produces a low signal intensity on T_1-weighted images, which decreases even further on T_2-weighted images. In contrast, areas with high fat content have high signal intensity. Consequently, an MRI study demonstrating a multinodular intra-articular lesion with patchy areas having characteristics of fat and haemosiderin deposition is highly suggestive of pigmented villonodular synovitis. However, in practice both false positives and false negatives occur. Techniques such as arthrography and arteriography have been used, but the results are rather non-specific.

Diagnosis

The diagnosis is based on a combination of clinical, radiological, and histological findings and the gross appearance of the lesion. The presence of serosanguinous synovial fluid in a young adult in the absence of a history of recent trauma is highly suggestive of the diagnosis of pigmented villonodular synovitis. The definitive diagnosis, however, often rests on the interpretation of a synovial biopsy. Histological criteria for the diagnosis have not been defined. Although features such as epithelioid cells, multinucleate giant cells, and deposition of fat and haemosiderin are highly characteristic, interpretation of the histological features by a specialist in osteo-articular pathology is required.

Conditions to be considered in the differential diagnosis of pigmented villonodular synovitis include:

(1) malignant synovioma;

(2) synovial haemangioma;

(3) synovial chondromatosis;

(4) tuberculous arthritis;

(5) amyloidosis;

(6) haemophilia;

(7) lipoma arborescens.

Treatment

Localized forms of pigmented villonodular synovitis are treated by marginal excision of the lesion and have a good prognosis. The diffuse form, however, tends to be progressive and recurrence is not uncommon. Treatment suggestions are largely based on anecdotal experience, the published series are small, and post-treatment follow-up is limited. A range of techniques, which include radiation, wide synovectomy, synovectomy combined with radiation, arthrodesis, bone grafting, primary arthroplasty, and radiation synovectomy, has been used. No single method has a uniformly high proportion of good results.

The most commonly reported treatment is surgical synovectomy. There are recent reports of good results (Flandry *et al.* 1994b), although in previous series there have been a high percentage of recurrences, with persistent joint pain and stiffness as common sequelae (Johansson *et al.* 1982). The use of radiation therapy as an adjunct does not improve the outcome. Radiation synovectomy using intra-articular yttrium-90 silicate has been reported, with promising results (Franssen *et al.* 1989). There are several advantages over surgical synovectomy including technical simplicity and fewer complications. There is limited experience, however, and not much long-term follow-up. In advanced cases with joint destruction (especially in the hip), it may be necessary to resort to a total arthroplasty.

Chronic focal osteomyelitis (Brodie's abscess)

This usually follows an acute haematogenous infection in an adolescent male (Boriani 1980). Three-quarters of Brodie's abscesses develop in the lower extremity, most often in the tibia. The acute episode of infection may have been successfully treated with antibiotics from a clinical point of view, only to be followed by a focus of chronic infection that can persist for years if not surgically drained.

Typically, the infection occurs in the metaphyseal side of the growth plate, where it remains localized. In rare cases, the infection extends through the growth plate into the epiphysis. Usually it is unifocal but multiple abscesses have been reported. Approximately 80 per cent involve *Staphylococcus aureus*, although almost any organism can be implicated.

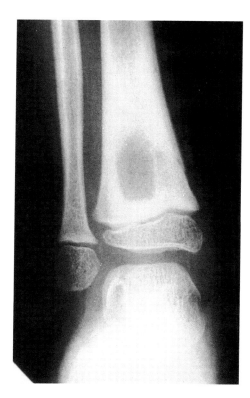

Fig. 3 Anteroposterior view showing a sharply demarcated Brodie's abscess surrounded by reactive sclerosis in the distral diaphysis of the tibia of a child presenting with chronic pain. (By courtesy of Dr P. Renton, University College London.)

Pain is the main complaint, described as aching or boring, and may have been present for months or even years. This is accompanied by localized tenderness and sometimes swelling. Occasionally, the abscess dissects through spongy bone and erodes through the cortex to drain into a joint, or through a sinus to the skin surface. The symptoms and signs of systemic illness that generally accompany acute osteomyelitis are conspicuously absent. Laboratory tests may also be normal, although there can be slight leucocytosis or elevation of the erythrocyte sedimentation rate. Radiographs show a sharply demarcated and irregular area of bone destruction surrounded by sclerosis (Fig. 3). Cultures from the abscess are positive in 50 to 80 per cent of cases.

Treatment is by surgical drainage and appropriate antibiotics. The prognosis is good.

Osteonecrosis

Osteonecrosis is a major reason for orthopaedic surgery to the hip, particularly in younger patients. There are several synonyms: avascular necrosis, aseptic necrosis, ischaemic necrosis, steroid necrosis, segmental subchondral infarction. Osteonecrosis at certain sites is associated with eponyms such as Legg–Perthes' disease (hip), Freiberg's disease (metatarsal), and Kienboch's disease (lunate).

In 1860, James Paget described the gross appearance of osteonecrosis in his lectures on surgical pathology (Bullough and DiCarlo 1990). Necrosis of the femoral head was associated with Caisson's disease in 1888, with corticosteroids in 1957 (Pietrogrande and Mastromarino 1957), and the association with systemic lupus erythematosus was reported in 1960 (Dubois and Cozen 1960). Before the 1960s, most reported cases were associated with fracture. The current prevalence of osteonecrosis is difficult to assess because many cases are clinically silent. Different forms of osteonecrosis affect children, young adults, or elderly people. However, most of those with atraumatic osteonecrosis are relatively young, with a peak incidence in the fifth decade of life. One group reports that about 18 per cent of femoral heads removed in total hip-replacement procedures for non-traumatic causes show evidence of osteonecrosis (Bullough and DiCarlo 1990). Approximately 60 per cent are bilateral, women are slightly more affected (1.2:1), and the mean age of presentation is 55 years compared with 67 years for patients with primary osteoarthritis.

Osteonecrosis, like infarction anywhere, results from a reduction or the obliteration of the blood supply to the affected area. Subchondral bone has a limited collateral circulation and the perfusion pressure and blood flow of epiphyses and fatty marrow is low compared with red diaphyseal marrow. Therefore, ends of bones such as the femoral head are more susceptible to ischaemia. Various mechanisms have been implicated (Mankin 1992):

(1) interruption of extraosseous arterial blood supply (e.g. trauma, vasculitis);

(2) interruption of intraosseous sinusoidal circulation (e.g. nitrogen bubbles, sickled erythrocytes, thrombi, fat emboli);

(3) extravascular compression of sinusoidal circulation (e.g. nitrogen bubbles, intramedullary lipocyte hypertrophy, accumulation of Gaucher's or malignant cells).

Often a combination of factors is involved. A final common pathway appears to be increased bone-marrow pressure, which can be demonstrated in the very earliest stages of the process (Zizic et al. 1986) and which further contributes to the impaired intraosseous microcirculation and progression of necrosis.

The pathology of osteonecrosis is well defined. The first phase is necrosis of bone and bone marrow. A cut section of bone shows a wedge-shaped necrotic zone in the subchondral region, which is demarcated from the normal bone marrow by a hyperaemic border. Granulation tissue develops and then advances from the margin of the infarct and necrotic bone is resorbed. Behind this, a second front of osteoblasts lays down new bone. If articular stress exceeds the structural integrity of the altered bone, there will be collapse of the articular surface and disruption of the joint.

Aetiological factors (Zizic 1990; Mankin 1992; Chang et al. 1993)

Some of the causes of osteonecrosis are:

(1) trauma;

(2) sepsis;

(3) radiation, thermal, and electrical injury;

(4) Caisson's disease;

(5) haemoglobinopathies;

(6) haemophilia;

(7) coagulopathies;

(8) Gaucher's disease;

(9) alcoholism;

(10) Cushing's syndrome;

(11) corticosteroid usage;

(12) systemic lupus erythematosus;

(13) rheumatoid arthritis;

(14) systemic sclerosis;

(15) vasculitis;

(16) organ transplantation (kidney, heart, marrow);

(17) chronic dialysis;

(18) human immunodeficiency virus infection;

(19) pancreatitis;

(20) chronic liver disease;

(21) hypertriglyceridaemia;

(22) pregnancy (especially in the third trimester);

(23) (idiopathic).

The major cause is a fracture that interferes with the blood supply to areas such as the femoral or humeral head, talus, and scaphoid. Osteonecrosis is a major complication of intracapsular fracture of the femoral neck, which is accompanied by disruption of the circulation in approximately 20 per cent of cases. Osteonecrosis occurs in 18 per cent of compressed-air workers and 4 per cent of divers; it appears to be the result of the development of intravascular and extravascular nitrogen gas bubbles during decompression, effectively occluding the circulation to sites such as the femoral and humeral heads. Lesions are frequently multiple and bilateral; involvement of the humeral heads is particularly characteristic. In Caisson's disease, for some reason, the subchondral bone of the knee and the ankle are not involved.

Depending on the genotype, sickle cell haemoglobinopathies have a 5 to 14 per cent prevalence of radiographically detectable osteonecrosis. As in Caisson's disease, the femoral and humeral heads are involved.

The two most common causes of non-traumatic osteonecrosis are alcoholism and hypercortisolism, which account for two-thirds of the cases. A feature they have in common is alteration in systemic fat metabolism. Osteonecrosis may be produced as a result of fatty emboli, or of intramedullary lipocyte hypertrophy and consequent intraosseous sinusoidal compression. Osteonecrosis in rheumatoid arthritis and systemic lupus is mostly associated with corticosteroid treatment. However, as in systemic lupus (see below), osteonecrosis is described as a complication of rheumatoid arthritis in the absence of steroids (Wollheim 1984), although there is little information about the prevalence of this. Osteonecrosis has been reported after repeated intra-articular injections of long-acting corticosteroids (Laroche et al. 1990).

Osteonecrosis in systemic lupus

This is a relatively common and disabling complication of lupus (Cronin 1988). The prevalence of the symptomatic, radiographic lesion in adults with systemic lupus is reported to be between 5 and 10 per cent. However, asymptomatic lesions detected by MRI are more common and present in up to 35 per cent (Nagasawa et al. 1994). Although some become apparent on plain radiographs, present in up to 25 per cent of adult systemic lupus erythematosus patients (Klippel et al. 1979) and possibly in even more children (Bergstein et al. 1974), in only a minority of lesions is the necrosis extensive enough to cause clinical problems. The major risk factor for osteonecrosis is corticosteroid therapy, but there are reports of the complication before the steroid era (Leventhal and Dorfman 1974). Suggested additional risk factors present in the analysis of some studies, but not in others, include younger age, vasculitis, Raynaud's phenomenon, and leucopenia. Osteonecrosis has been reported in association with antiphospholipid antibodies in patients with the 'primary antiphospholipid syndrome' but others (Alarcon-Segovia et al. 1989; Migliaresi et al. 1994) have found no correlation between anticardiolipin antibodies and osteonecrosis in their lupus population. It appears that it is the use of large doses of corticosteroids (e.g. prednisolone, 60 mg daily), sustained over a period of months, that is important for the development of osteonecrosis, rather than the duration of corticosteroids or the accumulative dose per se. Giving pulses of megadose corticosteroids either once or repeated after intervals of several weeks does not independently predispose to osteonecrosis. A meta-analysis reported by Felson and Anderson suggests that this relationship to dose and duration of corticosteroids applies to patients with a variety of clinical conditions (Felson and Anderson 1987). It is worth remembering that a number of malpractice suits have been brought against physicians for failing to inform patients of this complication of corticosteroids.

The onset of localized pain, particularly in a weight-bearing joint, should give rise to a high index of suspicion. The femoral head is most commonly involved, but other sites include the femoral condyle, tibial plateau, humeral head, talus, scaphoid, and lunate. Simultaneous involvement of multiple sites is not infrequent.

Diagnosis

Pain is the principal symptom. In about two-thirds of the patients it occurs at rest and may be troublesome at night (due to increased intraosseous pressure). It is well established that once radiographic changes occur in osteonecrosis the natural history is generally subchondral bone collapse and severe disability. The Arlet and Ficat classification of osteonecrosis is based on the plain radiographic appearance (Ficat and Arlet 1980), as follows:

Stage I: normal appearance;

Stage II: early changes consisting of diffuse osteoporosis, sclerosis, and cyst formation producing a mottled appearance (Fig. 4(a));

Stage III: subchondral bone collapse (crescent sign) with normal joint space;

Stage IV: abnormal contour of bone with joint-space loss.

This has been extended by Steinberg et al. to provide a more sensitive method of following the progress of osteonecrosis in the femoral and humeral heads (Steinberg et al. 1984).

In early stages the plain radiograph is normal. The imaging technique currently combining the greatest sensitivity and specificity for the diagnosis of early cases is MRI (Zizic 1990) (Fig. 4(b) and (c)). The

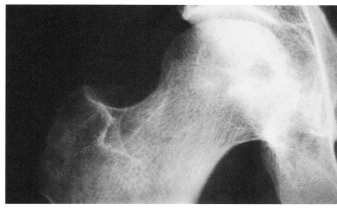

(a)

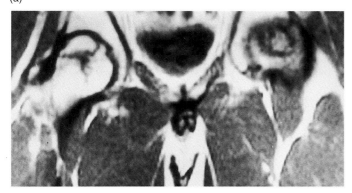

(b)

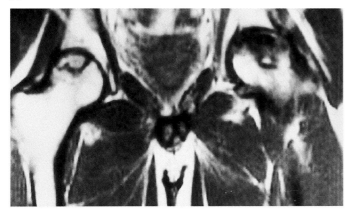

(c)

Fig. 4 (a) Early changes of osteonecrosis of the femoral head shown on plain radiograph (Arlet and Ficat stage II). (b) MRI clearly detects osteonecrosis at an early stage in T_1-weighted and (c) T_2-weighted images. (By courtesy of Dr P. Renton, University College London.)

presence of a low intensity band on T_1-weighted images is an early specific finding of osteonecrosis and MRI has the advantage of identifying early changes in necrotic bone marrow before other changes in bone have taken place (Halland *et al.* 1993; Sugano *et al.* 1994). If MRI is not available, an isotope bone scan with $^{99}Tc^m$ diphosphonate is indicated (Tawn and Watt 1989). This is also helpful in early diagnosis but it is less specific, anatomical resolution is often poor, and false negatives commonly occur, especially when there is bilateral disease. Other methods used for early diagnosis have included CT with multiplanar reconstruction (Sartoris *et al.* 1986). This is reported to be more sensitive than bone scan but the significant radiation exposure makes MRI a more attractive option. Measurement of intramedullary bone pressure and intraosseus venography proposed by Zizic *et al.* is probably also redundant as a routine procedure since the advent of MRI (Zizic *et al.* 1986). However, bone biopsy of the affected site is sometimes necessary, as local infection can be associated with osteonecrosis (Habermann and Friedenthal 1978).

Osteonecrosis at specific sites

Vertebral

This is uncommon but compared with compression fractures of osteoporosis is more often associated with neurological complications (Feldmann *et al.* 1988). This mainly happens in elderly people; the lesions are usually single, and at the thoracolumbar junction. It is not usually associated with malignancy and MRI is helpful in early diagnosis. The intravertebral vacuum cleft is the characteristic feature on the plain radiography.

Keinbock's disease

This describes osteonecrosis of the lunate. It may occur after a fracture but in most cases there is no specific history of this. Often it happens in the dominant hand and is thought to be the result of chronic repetitive trauma. It is associated with a short ulna, which probably reinforces the effects of repeated trauma.

Preiser's disease

This is spontaneous osteonecrosis of the scaphoid, usually affecting the proximal pole. Involvement of the scaphoid is usually post-traumatic and in idiopathic cases the trauma may have been minor and unrecognized.

Hegemann's disease

This describes osteonecrosis of the humeral trochlear. This is rare and happens mainly in preadolescent and adolescent boys, who present with a swollen elbow; this has reduced movement but is not particularly painful. Usually it resolves spontaneously.

Legg–Perthes' disease

This is osteonecrosis of the femoral head, which occurs in children between the age of 4 and 12 years and affects one or both hips. The aetiology is unknown but the condition is associated with increased intraosseous pressure and venous hypertension (Liu and Ho 1991). There may be spontaneous resolution, especially in younger patients, in whom conservative management is indicated.

Osteonecrosis of the femoral condyle

This occurs spontaneously in older people, predominantly affecting the medial condyle.

Kohler's disease

This is the rare involvement of the tarsal navicular, which primarily occurs in male children between the ages of 4 and 10 years. It is usually self-limiting.

Freiberg's disease

This is osteonecrosis of the metatarsal head, usually the second. It mainly affects adolescent females and is usually self-limiting.

Treatment

Advanced osteonecrosis of weight-bearing surfaces, such as the femoral head, leads to secondary osteoarthritis and severe disability. Total joint replacement may be the only solution in such cases. The results are satisfactory, giving a long period of good function. However, one still hesitates to recommend total joint replacement in young people and the failure rate may be higher in operations for osteonecrosis, especially when associated with corticosteroids, than in arthroplasties for other conditions (Cornell *et al.* 1985). Attempts have therefore been made to treat the condition at an earlier stage in order to preserve the integrity of affected bone.

Osteonecrosis of the femoral condyle in elderly people can often be treated conservatively with initial limitation of weight-bearing, non-steroidal anti-inflammatory drugs, hydrotherapy, and muscle strengthening exercises (Motohashi *et al.* 1991).

There is little evidence from retrospective studies that bed rest, modified weight bearing, analgesics, or non-steroidal anti-inflammatory drugs are of much benefit in other cases, at least for osteonecrosis of the hip in adults. Because increased intraosseous pressure is a common feature in early stages, core decompression has been recommended. Encouraging results with prevention of progression in early stages of osteonecrosis of the hip (Hungerford 1989) and the shoulder (Mont *et al.* 1993) have been reported by some groups. However, this is a controversial topic and not all studies have been so encouraging (Learmonth *et al.* 1990). The use of MRI to assess the extent of osteonecrosis may be a way of selecting those most likely to respond to this procedure (Holman *et al.* 1995).

Other ways of preserving the femoral head include bone grafting using a variety of procedures (Rosenwasser *et al.* 1994; Urbaniak *et al.* 1995), the use of electrical stimulation, and sometimes a combination of these (Steinberg *et al.* 1985). In addition, various techniques of osteotomy, such as the transtrochanteric osteotomy of the femoral head, have been used to alter the weight-bearing surface away from the involved area. These techniques are still being refined and evaluated.

Osteochondritis dissecans

Osteochondritis dissecans is usually a solitary lesion of the medial femoral condyle in which a fragment composed of articular cartilage and subchondral bone becomes demarcated from the surrounding bone and cartilage and may form an intra-articular loose body (Green and Banks 1990). Occasionally, it may involve the elbow, hip, and talus. The aetiology is unknown but anomalies of ossification and low-grade trauma appear to be important.

It predominantly affects adolescent males and should be suspected in a child or teenager who, after minor trauma, develops a relatively sudden onset of knee pain followed by mechanical dysfunction. There may be a hereditary component and familial occurrence has been reported (Paes 1989). This is characterized by multiple articular lesions, particularly affecting the hips and knees, and an autosomal dominant inheritance. Sometimes there is associated dwarfism and a generalized epiphyseal abnormality.

Symptoms are mainly pain, reduced joint movement, effusion, and limp. A plain radiograph shows a well-circumscribed, sclerotic lesion demarcated by a radiolucent line from surrounding bone (Fig. 5).

In young patients before skeletal maturity there is a good chance of healing, and treatment is consequently conservative. Once the

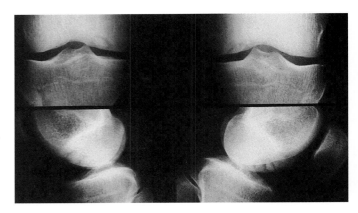

Fig. 5 Anteroposterior and lateral views showing typical lesions of osteochondritis dissecans in both medial femoral condyles. A radiolucent line separates the oval-shaped, *in situ* body from the femoral condyle. (By courtesy of Dr P. Renton, University College London.)

epiphyses have closed, osteochondritis dissecans is more likely to cause intra-articular loose bodies and subsequent symptoms of internal derangement, and eventually secondary osteoarthritis. Arthroscopy can be helpful in assessing the extent of the lesion. A variety of surgical procedures have been recommended, from drilling of the lesion to promote ingrowth of fibrocartilage to replacement of a large deficit with an osteochondral allograft.

Relapsing polychondritis

This is an uncommon, multisystem disorder of unknown aetiology characterized by episodic and sometimes progressive inflammation of cartilaginous structures and tissues rich in glycosoaminoglycans. The characteristic clinical syndrome, with involvement of the pinna of the ears, nose, larynx and upper airways, joints, heart, blood vessels, inner ear, cornea, and sclera, was first described by Jaksch-Wartenhorse (Jaksch-Wartenhorse 1923). In about 30 per cent of cases it is associated with other systemic rheumatic or autoimmune diseases such as rheumatoid arthritis, systemic lupus, Sjögren's syndrome, thyroiditis, ulcerative colitis, psoriasis, and Behçet's syndrome (Kitridou *et al.* 1987; Tishler *et al.* 1987; Orme *et al.* 1990; Harisdangkul and Johnson 1994).

Aetiology and pathogenesis

The most specific lesion is inflammation of cartilage. This leads to cartilage destruction and fibrosis. The lesion is characterized by a dense inflammatory infiltrate of neutrophils, lymphocytes, macrophages, and plasma cells. Initially this involves the perichondral region. There is loss of proteoglycans, destruction of the collagen matrix, and chondrocyte death. Destroyed cartilage is replaced by granulation tissue and there is subsequent fibrosis (Fig. 6). Cartilage matrix proteins, such as cartilage oligomeric matrix protein (COMP), are released and raised levels are present during disease activity (Saxne and Heinegard 1995).

The cause is unknown but, on the basis of circumstantial evidence, it is thought that there is an immunological pathogenesis. Components of cartilage, such as collagen, elastin and proteoglycan, express multiple antigenic determinants but these are normally sequestered from the immune system. A breach of the integrity of

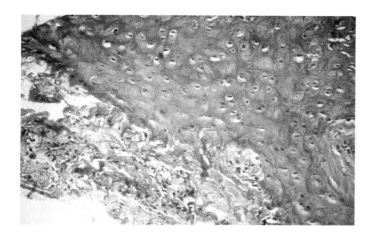

Fig. 6 Acute inflammation of the perichondral region of the external ear with infiltration of neutrophils, mononuclear cells, and plasma cells with destruction of underlying cartilage (haematoxylin and eosin). (By courtesy of Dr A. Balsa, La Paz Hospital, Madrid.)

Table 1 Extent of organ involvement in relapsing polychondritis

Organ	Percentage involvement
External ear	85
Arthritis	75
Nose	60
Eye	50
Respiratory tract	50
Internal ear	40
Skin	25
Kidney	20
Heart	10
Blood vessels	8
Central nervous system	Rare

cartilaginous structures could potentially stimulate an immune response to these constituents. The ubiquitous nature of matrix components such as elastin and proteoglycans could explain the pattern of involvement, which includes respiratory tract cartilage, structures of the eye, and the cardiovascular system.

Antibodies, predominantly IgG, which react specifically with collagens type II, IX, and XI (forming the major fibrillar scaffold in cartilage), can be detected in some but not all patients with relapsing polychondritis (Yang *et al.* 1993). The highest titres are found in the early phase of the disease and the titre may relate to disease activity (Ebringer *et al.* 1981). These antibodies are not disease specific and occur, for example, in rheumatoid arthritis, although possibly they are directed to different epitopes on the collagen molecule (Terato *et al.* 1990). The possibility that humoral factors are involved in the pathogenesis is suggested by the report of polychondritis occurring in the newborn infant of an affected mother and the subsequent recovery of the baby (Arundell and Haserick 1960). Granular deposits of immunoglobulin and complement have been observed at the chondrofibral junction in biopsies from affected ears (Valenzuela *et al.* 1980), suggesting the involvement of immune complexes. Collections of fluid in the middle ear have been reported to be hypo-complementaemic, suggesting complement consumption (McKenna *et al.* 1976). Thus, there is evidence for humoral immune mechanisms being involved in cartilage injury. In addition, earlier reports of cellular immune reactions to proteoglycan and other matrix components (Herman and Dennis 1973) have been supported by the more recent demonstration of cell-mediated immunity to collagens type II, IX, and XI paralleling the humoral response to these structural proteins (Alsalameh *et al.* 1993).

A significant increase in DR4 antigen frequency has been found (Lang *et al.* 1993) but, in contrast to rheumatoid arthritis, there is no predominance of any DR4 subtype.

Clinical features

The disease predominantly affects middle-aged white subjects, with a peak incidence in the fourth to fifth decades, although it has been reported in all races and age groups. The patient typically presents with recurrent swelling and pain of the external ear and/or nose, or with uveitis, or with an arthropathy. The cumulative involvement of various organ systems is summarized in Table 1.

Episodes of inflammation of the cartilaginous portion of one or both ears and the nose are often sudden and last several days. Repeated episodes of protracted inflammation, leading to cartilage destruction, produce deformity such as saddle nose (Fig. 7(a) and (b)).

Joint involvement is also common and occurs independently of other manifestations. The typical clinical picture is episodic, asymmetrical inflammation of both large and small joints, including the parasternal and sacroiliac joints, lasting several days to weeks. Generally it is non-deforming, non-erosive, and seronegative for rheumatoid factor (O'Hanlan *et al.* 1976; Balsa *et al.* 1995). Radiographs have demonstrated narrowing of the joint space without erosion, presumably reflecting the pathological process of

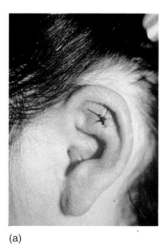
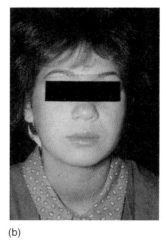

(a)   (b)

Fig. 7 Clinical features of relapsing polychondritis. (a) Acute inflammation of the external ear. (b) Saddle nose deformity. (By courtesy of Dr A. Balsa, La Paz Hospital, Madrid.)

loss of hyaline cartilage only (Booth *et al*. 1989). Aspirated synovial fluid is non-inflammatory. Mitchell and Shepard reported that, in addition to non-specific proliferation of lining cells, a unique feature was the presence in the middle and deeper layers of the synovium of large, clear spaces with projecting multinucleate bodies surrounding chondrocytes (Mitchell and Shepard 1972). In contrast to the 'pure' polyarthritis of relapsing polychondritis, the condition can develop against the background of a well-defined, erosive polyarthritis such as rheumatoid arthritis.

A wide range of rather non-specific ocular manifestations occur in relapsing polychondritis. The most common is episcleritis but more severe involvement includes scleritis and peripheral corneal thinning, both of which can lead to perforation, uveitis, retinal vasculitis, and optic neuritis, any of which can lead to blindness (Hoang-Xuan *et al*. 1989). Also reported are palsy of ocular muscles, orbital inflammation, and papilloedema.

The disease affects the respiratory tract in at least one-half of the patients. This can lead to the breakdown of tracheal and bronchial cartilage, with resulting airway collapse during the respiratory cycle (Crockford and Kerr 1988). The larynx and upper trachea are frequently involved first, and symmetrical subglottic narrowing is a common finding. Eventually the process can involve the distal trachea and main bronchi. Symptoms of respiratory tract involvement include dysphonia, cough, stridor, and dyspnoea; this involvement can dominate the clinical picture. During the active phase there may be tenderness over the thyroid cartilage and trachea. Young patients presenting with involvement of the upper respiratory tract early in the course of the disease tend to be rather resistant to treatment and have a poor prognosis (Neilly *et al*. 1985).

Involvement of the inner ear tends to occur later in the course of the disease and leads to vestibular and auditory dysfunction. A wide range of non-specific skin lesions has been reported, including erythema nodosum and leucocytoclastic vasculitis. The MAGIC (mouth and genital ulcers with inflamed cartilage) syndrome describes an overlap with Behçet's syndrome characterized by prominent orogenital ulceration (Orme *et al*. 1990). Renal manifestations have been reported in as many as 20 per cent of cases (Chang-Miller *et al*. 1987). On renal biopsy the predominant lesions are reported to be mesangial proliferation and segmental, necrotizing glomerulonephritis with crescents. Immunofluorescence and electron-microscopic studies show faint deposition of immunoglobulin and complement, and small amounts of electron-dense deposits, respectively, mainly in the mesangium. Patients with renal involvement tend to have more severe disease with extrarenal vasculitis and worse prognosis.

The heart is involved in about 10 per cent of patients. Aortic incompetence, either from dilatation of the aortic root or valvular destruction, is the most common manifestation. It is often severe, progressing even when other aspects of the disease are in remission (Buckley and Ades 1992), and requires valve replacement in at least a third (Manna *et al*. 1985). Even when valve replacement is successful, there is the possibility of future dehiscence of the prosthetic valve because of continuing inflammation of perivalvular tissues (Lang-Lazdunski *et al*. 1995). Other cardiovascular manifestations include pericarditis, myocarditis, heart block, coronary vasculitis leading to myocardial infarction, and aneurysms of the aorta and other large arteries. Vasculitis involving large and medium-sized arteries may occur independently of cardiac involvement and often carries a poor prognosis. Meningoencephalitis has been reported in association

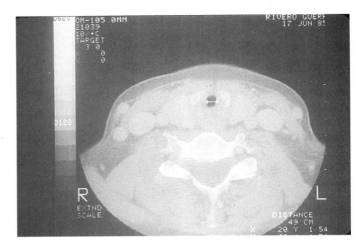

Fig. 8 A CT scan showing cartilage destruction and marked narrowing of the trachea. (By courtesy of Dr A. Balsa, La Paz Hospital, Madrid.)

with polychondritis but central nervous system involvement is rare (Hanslik *et al*. 1994)

Laboratory abnormalities are non-specific and for the most part reflect chronic inflammation. Common features are an acute-phase response, anaemia of chronic disease, and thrombocytosis. There may be a moderate leucocytosis. The development of a myelodysplastic syndrome has been reported (Diebold *et al*. 1995). Serological tests demonstrate anti-type II collagen antibodies in up to one-half of patients, circulating immune complexes in the majority, and antinuclear antibodies in approximately 20 per cent. ANCA have been reported in 24 per cent of patients with polychondritis, mainly during the acute phase of the disease, and in some patients in association with vasculitis (Papo *et al*. 1993; Handrock and Gross 1993). Various imaging techniques are useful for assessing complications of the disease. For example plain radiographs of the respiratory tract should include a soft tissue exposure of the neck in the lateral projection to demonstrate the larynx and upper trachea, together with penetrated frontal views of the trachea and major bronchi in the chest (Crockford and Kerr 1988). CT scanning is an accurate method for assessing the upper and lower airways (Mendelson *et al*. 1985; Davis *et al*. 1989) (Fig. 8). The value of MRI in assessing disease involvement, especially of the upper respiratory tract, is also reported (Fornadely *et al*. 1995).

The clinical course of this disease is highly variable. It is probable that the literature emphasizes the worst end of the spectrum and that many milder cases go unrecognized. It has been suggested that the 5-year and 10-year survival after diagnosis are 74 and 55 per cent (Michet *et al*. 1986). The most common causes of death are infection, cardiac and respiratory involvement, and systemic vasculitis.

Diagnosis

Early diagnosis is important in an attempt to prevent potentially life-threatening complications. There are no universally accepted diagnostic criteria but McAdam *et al*. proposed that the presence of three of the six following clinical features should be diagnostic (McAdam *et al*. 1976):

(1) recurrent chondritis of both auricles;

(2) non-erosive polyarthritis;

(3) chondritis of the nasal cartilage;

(4) ocular inflammation including conjunctivitis, keratitis, scleritis/episcleritis, uveitis;

(5) involvement of laryngeal and/or tracheal cartilage;

(6) cochlear and/or vestibular involvement.

These were modified slightly by Damiani and Levine (Damiani and Levine 1979) to include:

(1) three or more of the above criteria;

(2) at least one clinical criterion plus histological confirmation;

(3) chondritis in two or more separate anatomical locations with a response to treatment.

Treatment

The rarity of relapsing polychondritis, the diversity of its presentation, and the unpredictability of recurrences make it difficult to recommend a particular treatment protocol. There are no controlled trials therefore the following is based on anecdotal experience.

Mild symptoms of joint involvement and inflammation of ear and nose cartilages can sometimes be controlled by non-steroidal anti-inflammatory drugs alone. Dapsone has been reported to be effective for systemic manifestations not controlled with symptomatic treatment alone (Barranco et al. 1976). Corticosteroids can be effective in suppressing acute, severe manifestations. High doses (at least 1 mg/kg per day of prednisolone or equivalent) are required. Alternate-day regimens are not recommended but there are reports of bolus parenteral methylprednisolone being effective for manifestations such as acute airways' obstruction (Lipnick and Fink 1991). It appears that corticosteroids are more effective in treating disease in cartilage of the respiratory tract than, for example, involvement of the joints and eyes. Also, there is no evidence that corticosteroids influence long-term outcome, and in some patients the disease undoubtedly progresses despite giving corticosteroids (Kilman 1978).

In severe cases, the addition of an immunosuppressive agent is required to control disease activity and to be steroid sparing. Successful responses have been reported using agents such as azathioprine and cyclophosphamide. The latter is the drug of choice for features such as necrotizing scleritis and systemic vasculitis. In refractory cases there have been anecdotal reports of success with cyclosporin A (Svenson et al. 1984) and monoclonal antibodies to CD4 (Van der Lubbe et al. 1991).

Additional supportive measures may be needed for those with severe respiratory, cardiac, and renal complications. For example whereas only 14 per cent of patients with this disease present initially with respiratory tract involvement, 80 per cent of these will require tracheostomy. Initially, this is usually for glottic, laryngeal, and subglottic inflammation and oedema producing airways' obstruction (McAdam et al. 1976). Later, the indication for tracheostomy is often the collapse of laryngeal or tracheal cartilages. The recent introduction of expandable metal stents represents an important development in managing patients with major airway stenosis and collapse (Shah et al. 1995).

References

Alarcon-Segovia, D. et al. (1989). Antiphospholipid antibodies and the antiphospholipid syndrome in systemic lupus erythematosus: a prospective study of 500 consecutive patients. Medicine, 68, 353–65.

Alsalameh, S., Mollenhauer, J., Scheuplein, F., Stoss, H., Kalden, J.R., Burkhardt, H., and Burmester, G.R. (1993). Preferential cellular and humoral immune reactivities to native and denatured collagen types IX and XI in a patient with fatal relapsing polychondritis. Journal of Rheumatology, 20, 1419–24.

Arundell, F.W. and Haserick, J.R. (1960). Familial chronic atrophic polychondritis. Archives of Dermatology, 82, 439–41.

Assoun, J., Richardi, G., Railhac, J.J., Baunin, C., Fajadet, P., Giron, J., Maquin, P., Haddad, J., and Bonnevialle, P. (1994). Osteoid osteoma: MR imaging versus CT. Radiology, 191, 217–23.

Balsa, A., Espinosa, A., Cuesta, M., MacLeod, T.I., Gijon-Banos, J., and Maddison, P.J. (1995). Joint symptoms in relapsing polychondritis. Clinical and Experimental Rheumatology, 13, 425–30.

Barranco, V.P., Minor, D.P., and Solomon, H. (1976). Treatment of relapsing polychondritis with dapsone. Archives of Dermatology, 112, 1286–8.

Bergstein, J.M., Wiens, C., Fish, A.J., Vernier, R., and Michael, A. (1974). Avascular necrosis of bone in systemic lupus erythematosus. Journal of Pediatrics, 85, 31–6.

Booth, A., Dieppe, P.A., Goddard, P.L., and Watt, I. (1989). The radiological manifestations of relapsing polychondritis. Clinical Radiology, 40, 147–9.

Boriani, S. (1980). Brodie's abscess: a study of 181 cases with special reference to radiographic diagnostic criteria. Italian Journal of Orthopaedic Traumatology, 6, 373–83.

Buckley, L.M., and Ades, P.A. (1992). Progressive aortic valve inflammation occurring despite apparent remission of relapsing polychondritis. Arthritis and Rheumatism, 35, 812–14.

Bullough, P.G. and DiCarlo, E.F. (1990). Subchondral avascular necrosis: a common cause of arthritis. Annals of the Rheumatic Diseases, 49, 412–20.

Chang, C.C., Greenspan, A., and Gershwin, M.E. (1993). Osteonecrosis: current perspectives on pathogenesis and treatment. Seminars in Arthritis and Rheumatism, 23, 47–69.

Chang-Miller, A. et al. (1987). Renal involvement in relapsing polychondritis. Medicine (Baltimore), 66, 202–17.

Christensen, J.H. and Poulsen, J.O. (1975). Synovial chondromatosis. Acta Orthopaedica Scandinavica, 46, 919–25.

Clark, L.J., McCormick, P.W., Domenico, D.R., and Savory, L. (1993). Pigmented villonodular synovitis of the spine. Journal of Neurosurgery, 79, 456–9.

Coolican, M.R. and Dandy, D.J. (1989). Arthroscopic management of synovial chondromatosis of the knee. Findings and results in 18 cases. Journal of Bone and Joint Surgery, 71B, 498–500.

Cornell, C.N., Salvati, E., and Pincus, P.M. (1985). Longterm followup of total hip replacement in patients with osteonecrosis. Orthopaedic Clinics of North America, 16, 757–69.

Crockford, M.P. and Kerr, I.H. (1988). Relapsing polychondritis. Clinical Radiology, 39, 386–90.

Cronin, M.E. (1988). Musculoskeletal manifestations of systemic lupus erythematosus. Rheumatic Disease Clinics of North America, 14, 99–116.

Curtin, W.A., Lahoti, O.P., Fogarty, E.E., Dowling, F.E., and Regan, B.F. (1993). Pigmented villonodular synovitis arising from the sheath of the extensor hallucis longus in an eight-month-old infant. Clinical Orthopaedics and Related Research, 292, 282–4.

Dahlin, D.C. and Unni, K.K. (1986). Bone tumours: general aspects and data on 8542 cases (4th edn), pp. 88–102. Thomas, Springfield, IL.

Damiani, J.M. and Levine, H.L. (1979). Relapsing polychondritis: report of ten cases. Laryngoscope, 89, 929–44.

Davis, S.D., Berkmen, Y.M., and King, T. (1989). Peripheral bronchial involvement in relapsing polychondritis: demonstration by thin-section CT. American Journal of Roetgenology, 153, 953–4.

De Berg, J.C., Pattynama, P.M., Obermann, W.R., Bode, P.J., Vielvoye, G.J., and Taminiau, A.H. (1995). Percutaneous computed-tomography-guided thermo-coagulation for osteoid osteomas. Lancet, 346, 350–1.

Diebold, L., Rauh, G., Jager, K., and Lohrs, U. (1995). Bone marrow pathology in relapsing polychondritis: high frequency of myelodysplastic syndromes. British Journal of Haematology, 89, 820–30.

Docken, W.P. (1979). Pigmented villonodular synovitis: a review with illustrative case reports. *Seminars in Arthritis and Rheumatism*, 9, 1–22.

Dubois, E.L. and Cozen, L. (1960). Avascular (aseptic) bone necrosis associated with systemic lupus erythematosus. *Journal of the American Medical Association*, 174, 966–84.

Ebringer, R., Rook, G., Swana, G.T., Botazzo, G.F., and Doniach, D. (1981). Autoantibodies to cartilage and type II collagen in relapsing polychondritis and other rheumatic diseases. *Annals of the Rheumatic Diseases*, 40, 473–9.

Feldmann, J.L., Alcalay, M., Queinnec, J.Y., and De Bray, J.M. (1988). Spinal cord compression related to vertebral osteonecrosis. *Clinical Experimental Rheumatology*, 6, 297–300.

Felson, D.T. and Anderson, J.J. (1987). A cross-study evaluation of association between steroid dose and bolus steroids and avascular necrosis of bone. *Lancet*, i, 902–5.

Ficat, R.P. and Arlet, J. (1980). *Ischaemia and necrosis of bone*. Williams and Wilkins, Baltimore.

Flandry, F. and Hughston, J.C. (1987). Pigmented villonodular synovitis. *Journal of Bone and Joint Surgery*, 69A, 942–9.

Flandry, F.C., Hughston, J.C., McCann, S.B., and Kurtz, D.M. (1994a). Diagnostic features of diffuse pigmented villonodular synovitis of the knee. *Clinical Orthopaedics and Related Research*, 298, 212–20.

Flandry, F.C., Hughston, J.C., Jacobson, K.E., Barrack, R.L., McCann, S.B., and Kurtz, D.M. (1994b). Surgical treatment of diffuse pigmented villonodular synovitis of the knee. *Clinical Orthopaedics and Related Research*, 300, 183–92.

Fornadely, J.A., Seibert, D.J., Ostrov, B.E., and Warren, W.S. (1995). The role of MRI when relapsing polychondritis is suspected but not proven. *International Journal of Pediatric Otorhinlaryngology*, 31, 101–7.

Franchi, A., Frosini, P., and Santoro, R. (1994). Pigmented villonodular synovitis of the temporomandibular joint. *Journal of Laryngology and Otology*, 108, 166–7.

Franssen, M.J.A.M., Boerbooms, A.M.Th., Karthaus, R.P., Buijs, W.C.A.M., and van de Putte, L.B.A. (1989). Treatment of pigmented villonodular synovitis of the knee with yttrium-90 silicate: prospective evaluations by arthroscopy, histology, and ^{99m}Tc pertechnetate uptake measurements. *Annals of the Rheumatic Diseases*, 48, 1007–13.

Goldman, A.B. and DiCarlo, E.F. (1988). Pigmented villonodular synovitis. Diagnosis and differential diagnosis. *Radiologic Clinics of North America*, 26, 1327–47.

Green, W.T. and Banks, H.H., (1990). The classic osteochondritis dissecans in children. *Clinical Orthopaedics and Related Research*, 255, 3–12.

Habermann, E.T. and Friedenthal, R.B. (1978). Septic arthritis associated with avascular necrosis of the femoral head. *Clinical Orthopaedics*, 134, 325–31.

Halland, A.M., Klemp, P., Botes, D., Van Heerden, B.B., Loxton, A., and Scher, A.T. (1993). Avascular necrosis of the hip in systemic lupus erythematosus: the role of magnetic resonance imaging. *British Journal of Rheumatology*, 32, 972–6.

Handrock, K. and Gross, W.L. (1993). Relapsing polychondritis as a secondary phenomenon of primary systemic vasculitis. *Annals of the Rheumatic Diseases*, 52, 895–6.

Hanslik, T., Wechsler, B., Piette, J.C., Vidailhet, M., Robin, P.M., and Godeau, P. (1994). Central nervous system involvement in relapsing polychondritis. *Clinical and Experimental Rheumatology*, 12, 539–41.

Harisdangkul, V. and Johnson, W.W. (1994). Association between relapsing polychondritis and systemic lupus erythematosus. *Southern Medical Journal*, 87, 753–7.

Helms, C.A., Hattner, R.S., and Vogler, J.B. (1984). Osteoid osteoma: radionuclide diagnosis. *Radiology*, 151, 779–84.

Herman, J.H. and Dennis, M.V. (1973). Immunopathological studies in relapsing polychondritis. *Journal of Clinical Investigation*, 52, 549–58.

Hoang-Xuan, T., Foster, C.S., and Rice, B.A. (1989). Scleritis in relapsing polychondritis: response to therapy. *Ophthalmology*, 97, 892–8.

Holman, A.J., Gardner, G.C., Richardson, M.L., and Simkin, P.A. (1995). Quantitative magnetic resonance imaging predicts clinical outcome of core decompression for osteonecrosis of the femoral head. *Journal of Rheumatology*, 22, 1929–33.

Hungerford, D.S. (1989). Response: the role of core decompression in the treatment of ischaemic necrosis of the femoral head. *Arthritis and Rheumatism*, 32, 801–6.

Jaffe, H.L., Lichtenstein, L., and Sutro, C.J. (1941). Pigmented villonodular synovitis, bursitis and tenosynovitis. *Archives of Pathology*, 31, 731–65.

Jaksch-Wartenhorse, R. (1923). Polychondropathia. *Wiener Archiv für Innere Medizin*, 6, 93–4.

Johansson, J.E., Ajjoub, S., Coughlin, L.P., Wener, J.A., and Cruess, R.L. (1982). Pigmented villonodular synovitis of joints. *Clinical Orthopaedics*, 163, 159–66.

Kiers, L., Shield, L.K., and Cole, W.G. (1990). Neurological manifestations of osteoid osteoma. *Archives of Disease in Childhood*, 65, 851–5.

Kilman, W.J. (1978). Narrowing of the airway in relapsing polychondritis. *Radiology*, 126, 373–6.

Kitridou, R.C. Wittmann, A-L., and Quismorio, F.P. (1987). Chrondritis in systemic lupus erythematosus: clinical and immunopathological studies. *Clinical and Experimental Rheumatology*, 5, 349–53.

Klippel, J.H., Gerber, L.H., and Pollak, I. (1979). Avascular necrosis in systemic lupus erythematosus: silent symmetric osteonecrosis. *American Journal of Medicine*, 67, 83–8.

Lang, B., Rothenfusser, A., Lanchbury, J.S., Rauh, G., Breedveld, F.C., Urlacher, A., Albert, E.D., Peter, H.H., and Melchers, I. (1993). Susceptibility to relapsing polychondritis is associated with HLA-DR4. *Arthritis and Rheumatism*, 36, 660–4.

Lang-Lazdunski, L., Hvass, U., Paillole, C., Pansard, Y., and Langlois, J. (1995). Cardiac valve replacement in relapsing polychondritis. A review. *Journal of Heart Valve Disease*, 4, 227–35.

Laroche, M., Arlet, J., and Mazieres, B. (1990). Osteonecrosis of the femoral and humeral heads after intraarticular corticosteroid injection. *Journal of Rheumatology*, 17, 549–51.

Learmonth, I.D., Maloon, S., and Dall, G. (1990), Core decompression for early atraumatic osteonecrosis of the femoral head. *Journal of Bone and Joint Surgery (British volume)*, 72, 387–90.

Leventhal, G.H. and Dorfman, H.D. (1974). Aseptic necrosis of bone in systemic lupus erythematosus. *Seminars in Arthritis and Rheumatism*, 4, 73–93.

Lipnick, R.N. and Fink, C.W. (1991). Acute airway obstruction in relapsing polychondritis: treatment with pulse methylprednisolone. *Journal of Rheumatology*, 18, 98–9.

Liu, S-L. and Ho, T-C. (1991). The role of venous hypertension in the pathogenesis of Legg-Perthes disease. *Journal of Bone and Joint Surgery*, 73A, 194–200.

McAdam, L.P., O'Hanlan, M.A., Bluestone, R., and Pearson, C.M. (1976). Relapsing polychondritis: prospective review of 23 patients and review of the literature. *Medicine (Baltimore)*, 55, 193–215.

McKenna, C.H., Luthra, M.S., and Jordan, R.E. (1976). Hypocomplementaemic ear effusion in relapsing polychondritis. *Mayo Clinic Proceedings*, 51, 495–8.

Makley, J.T. and Dunn, M.G. (1982). Prostaglandin synthesis by osteoid osteoma. *Lancet*, ii, 42–5.

Mankin, H.J. (1992). Nontraumatic necrosis of bone (osteonecrosis). *New England Journal of Medicine*, 326, 1473–9.

Manna, R. *et al.* (1985). Relapsing polychondritis with severe aortic insufficiency. *Clinical Rheumatology*, 4, 474–80.

Mendelson, D.S., Son, P.M., Crane, R., Cohen, B.A., and Spiera, H. (1985). Relapsing polychondritis studied by computed tomography. *Radiology*, 157, 489–90.

Michet, C.J. Jr., McKenna, C.H., Luthra, H.S., and O'Fallen, W.M. (1986). Relapsing polychondritis: survival and predictive roles of early disease manifestations. *Annals of Internal Medicine*, 104, 74–8.

Migliaresi, S., Picillo, U., Ambrosone, L., Di Palma, G., Mallozzi, M., Tesone, E.R., and Tirri, G. (1994) Avascular osteonecrosis in patients with SLE: relation to corticosteroid therapy and anticardiolipin antibodies. *Lupus*, 3, 37–41.

Mitchell, N. and Shepard, N. (1972). Relapsing polychondritis: an electron microscopic study of synovium and articular cartilage. *Journal of Bone and Joint Surgery*, 54, 1235–45.

Mont, M.A., Maar, D.C., Urquhart, M.W., Lennox, D., and Hungerford, D.S. (1993). Avascular necrosis of the humeral head treated by core compression. A retrospective review. *Journal of Bone and Joint Surgery (British volume)*, 75, 785–8.

Motohashi, M., Morii, T., and Koshino, T. (1991). Clinical course of roentgenographic changes of osteonecrosis on the femoral condyle under conservative treatment. *Clinical Orthopedics*, 266, 156–61.

Musculo, D.L., Velan, O., Pineda-Acero, G., Ayerza, M.A., Calabrese, M.E., and Santini Araujo, E. (1995). Osteoid osteoma of the hip. Percutaneous resection guided by computed tomography. *Clinical Orthopaedics and Related Research*, **310**, 170–5.

Myers B.W., Masi, A.T., and Feigenbaum, S.L. (1980). Pigmented villonodular synovitis and tenosynovitis. A clinical epidemiologic study of 166 cases and literature reivew. *Medicine*, **59**, 223–38.

Nagasawa, K., Tsukamoto, H., Tada, Y., Mayumi, T., Satoh, H., Onitsuka, H., Kuwabara, Y., and Niho, Y. (1994). Imaging study on the mode of development and changes in avascular necrosis of the femoral head in systemic lupus erythematosus: long-term observations. *British Journal of Rheumatology*, **33**, 343–7.

Neilly, J.B., Wister, J.H., and Stevenson, R.D. (1985). Progressive tracheo-bronchial polychondritis: need for early diagnosis. *Thorax*, **40**, 78–9.

O'Hanlan, M., McAdam, L.P., Bluestone, R., and Pearson, C.M. (1976). The arthropathy of relapsing polychondritis. *Arthritis and Rheumatism*, **19**, 191–4.

Orme, R.L. Nordlund, J.J., Barich, L., and Brown, T. (1990). The MAGIC syndrome (mouth and genital ulcers with inflamed cartilage). *Archives of Dermatology*, **126**, 940–4.

Paes, R.A. (1989). Familial osteochondritis dissecans. *Clinical Radiology*, **40**, 501–4.

Papo, T., Piette, J.C., Du, L.T.H., Godeau, P., Meyer, O., Kahn, M.F., and Bougeous, P. (1993). Antineutrophil cytoplasmic antibodies in polychondritis. *Annals of the Rheumatic Diseases*, **52**, 384–6.

Pietrogrande, V. and Mastromarino, R. (1957). Osteopat da prolongata trattamento cortisonico. *Ortopedia e Traumatologia dell'Apparato Matore*, **25**, 791–810.

Rao, A.S. and Vigorita, V.J. (1984). Pigmented villonodular synovitis (giant cell tumour of tendon sheath and synovial membrane): a review of 81 cases. *Journal of Bone and Joint Surgery*, **66A**, 76–94.

Ray, R.A., Morton, C.A., Lipinski, K.K., Corson, J.M., and Fletcher, J.A. (1990). Cytogenetic evidence of clonality in a case of pigmented villonodular synovitis. *Cancer*, **67**, 121–5.

Resnick, D. and Niwayama, G. (1988). *Diagnosis of bone and joint disorders* (2nd edn), Vol. 6. W. B. Saunders, Philadelphia.

Rosenthal, D.I., Springfield, D.S., Gebhardt, M.C., Rosenberg, A.E., and Mankin, H.J. (1995). Osteoid osteoma: percutaneous radio-frequency ablation. *Radiology*, **197**, 451–4.

Rosenwasser, M.P., Garino, J.P., Kiernan, H.A., and Michelsen, C.B. (1994). Long term followup of thorough debridement and cancellous bone grafting of the femoral head for avascular necrosis. *Clinical Orthopaedics and Related Research*, **306**, 17–27.

Sartoris, D.J. (1986). Computed tomography with multiplanar reformation and 3-dimensional image analysis in the preoperative evaluation of ischaemic necrosis of the femoral head. *Journal of Rheumatology*, **13**, 153–60.

Saxne, T., and Heinegard, D. (1995). Serum concentrations of two cartilage matrix proteins reflecting different aspects of cartilage turnover in relapsing polychondritis. *Arthritis and Rheumatism*, **38**, 294–6.

Schumacher, H.R., Lotke, P., Athreya, B., and Rothfuss, S. (1982). Pigmented villonodular synovitis: light and electron microscopic studies. *Seminars in Arthritis and Rheumatism*, **12**, 32–43.

Shah, R., Sabanathan, S., Mearns, A.J., and Featherstone, H. (1995). Self-expanding tracheobronchial stents in the management of major airway problems. *Journal of Cardiovascular Surgery*, **36**, 343–8.

Shpitzer, T., Ganel, A., and Engelberg, S. (1990). Surgery for synovial chondromatosis: 26 cases followed up for 6 years. *Acta Orthopaedica Scandinavica*, **61**, 567–9.

Smith, J.H. and Pugh, D.G. (1962). Roentgenographic aspects of articular pigmented villonodular synovitis. *American Journal of Roentgenology*, **87**, 1146–56.

Steinberg, M.E., Hayken, G.D., and Steinberg, D.R. (1984). A new method for evaluation and staging of avascular necrosis of the femoral head. In *Bone circulation*, (ed. J. Arlet, R.P. Ficat, and D.S. Hungerford), pp. 398–403. Williams and Wilkins, Baltimore.

Steinberg, M.E., Brighton, C.T., Hayken, G.D., Tooze, S.E., and Steinberg, D.R. (1985). Electrical stimulation in the treatment of osteonecrosis of the femoral head. *Orthopedic Clinics of North America*, **16**, 747–56.

Sugano, N., Ohzono, K., Masuhara, K., Takaoka, K., and Ono, K. (1994). Prognostication of osteonecrosis of the femoral head in patients with systemic lupus erythematosus by magnetic resonance imaging. *Clinical Orthopaedics and Related Research*, **305**, 190–9.

Svenson, K.L.G. *et al.* (1984). Cyclosporin A treatment in a case of relapsing polychondritis. *Scandinavian Journal of Rheumatology*, **13**, 329–31.

Swee, R.G., McLeod, R.A., and Beabout, J.W. (1979). Osteoma detection, diagnosis, and localization. *Radiologic Diagnosis*, **13**, 117–23.

Tawn, D.J. and Watt, I. (1989). Bone marrow scintigraphy in the diagnosis of post traumatic avascular necrosis of bone. *British Journal of Radiology*, **62**, 790–5.

Terato, K. *et al.* (1990). Specificity of antibodies to type II collagen in rheumatoid arthritis. *Arthritis and Rheumatism*, **33**, 1493–1500.

Tishler, M., Caspi, D., and Yaron, M. (1987). Classical rheumatoid arthritis associated with nondeforming relapsing polychondritis. *Journal of Rheumatology*, **14**, 367–8.

Urbaniak, J.R., Coogan, P.G., Gunneson, E.B., and Nunley, J.A. (1995). Treatment of osteonecrosis of the femoral head with free vascularized fibular grafting. A long-term follow-up study of one hundred and three hips. *Journal of Bone and Joint Surgery (American volume)*, **77**, 681–94.

Valenzuela, R., Cooperrider, P.A., Gogate, P., Deodhar, S.D., and Berfeld, W.F. (1980). Relapsing polychondritis: immunomicroscopic findings in cartilage of ear biopsy specimens. *Human Pathology*, **11**, 19–24.

Van der Lubbe, P.A., Multenberg, A.M., and Breedveld, F.C. (1991). Anti-CD4 monoclonal antibody for relapsing polychondritis. *Lancet*, **337**, 1349.

Ward, W.G., Eckardt, J.J., Shayestehfar, S., Mirra, J., Grogan, T., and Oppenheim, W. (1993). Osteoid osteoma diagnosis and management with low morbidity. *Clinical Orthopaedics and Related Research*, **291**, 229–35.

Wollheim, F.A. (1984). Acute and long term complications of corticosteroid pulse therapy. *Scandinavian Journal of Rheumatology*, **54**, (Suppl.), 27–32.

Yang, C.L., Brinckmann, J., Rui, H.F., Vehring, K.H., Lehmann, H., Kekow, J., Wolff, H.H., Gross, W.L., and Muller, P.K. (1993). Autoantibodies to cartilage collagens in relapsing polychondritis. *Archives of Dermatological Research*, **285**, 245–9.

Zizic, T.M. (1990). Avascular necrosis of bone. *Current Opinion in Rheumatology*, **2**, 26–37.

Zizic, T.M., Marcoux, C., Hungerford, D.S., and Stevens, M.B. (1986). The early diagnosis of ischaemic necrosis of bone. *Arthritis and Rheumatism*, **29**, 1177–86.

5.17.4 Diseases of bone and cartilage in children

Barbara M. Ansell

The developmental skeletal disorders are difficult to classify and depend largely on radiological examination (Poznanski 1974; Wynne-Davies *et al.* 1985; Spranger 1992). Their importance lies in that they can present with musculoskeletal pain, alterations in joint movement and growth disturbances, so it is necessary for paediatricians and rheumatologists to be able to recognize such conditions.

The osteochondrodysplasias

There are more than 160 osteochondrodysplasias, divided into three groups: (i) defects of tubular and flat bone, (ii) disorganized development of cartilagenous and fibrous components of the skeleton, and

(iii) idiopathic osteolyses. Features of some of the more common ones which give rise to problems follow.

Achondroplasia

This is the most common form of short-limbed dwarfism. Although inherited as an autosomal dominant trait, many cases represent new mutations. Arms and legs are short and such children usually have hypotonia, and with the head normal in size, may have difficulty in supporting it. There is an increased lumbar lordosis; spinal stenosis may result in neurological complications in adolescence or adult life. Hypochondroplasia resembles achondroplasia but lacks the facial characteristics.

Diatrophic dwarfism

This is characterized not only by short stature but also by cleft palate, thickening of the ear pinnas, severe club feet and thumb deformation, as well as joint dysplasia and scoliosis. It is thought to be inherited as an autosomal recessive trait.

Metatrophic dysplasias

In this, not only are short limbs present at birth and increasing loss of joint mobility, but there is also a kyphoscoliosis which is severe and progressive and cord compression is not uncommon. This disorder is an autosomal dominant one.

Epiphyseal dysplasias
Multiple epiphyseal dysplasia

One of the most common skeletal dysplasias which is inherited as an autosomal dominant trait (Maudsley 1955; Amir et al. 1985). It presents in childhood with pain and stiffness in affected limbs and is characterized by shortening and contractures and occasionally scoliosis. It can easily be confused with chronic arthritis (Patroni and Kredich 1985), but absence of inflammatory signs is important in its differentiation. Radiologically there are progressive irregularities of the end plates of the mid-thoracic vertebral bodies, short metacarpals and terminal phalanges and flattening, sclerosis, and fragmentation of the epiphyses of the hips, (Fig. 1) knees and other joints.

Spondyloepiphyseal dysplasia

This is characterized by short stature with a disproportionately short trunk. Epiphyses of the hips and shoulders are the most severely affected early, and there may be platyspondyly.

Three forms are presently recognized—congenita, pseudoachondroplasia and tarda. The congenita form is inherited as an autosomal dominant; it is present at birth and is associated with myopia and retinal detachment (Anderson et al. 1990a). The pseudoachondroplasia may be inherited as an autosomal dominant or recessive and presents in early childhood (Hall et al. 1987). The patient's stature is short but with a normal face. There is marked irregularity of the epiphyses of the long bones which are late in maturing, and progressive scoliosis (Maroteaux et al. 1980). The tarda form may be inherited as an X-linked recessive (Iceton and Horne 1986) or be dominant, but it can be seen as a new mutation in two or three sibs (Szpiro-Tapio et al. 1988). There is little difference between these forms clinically as

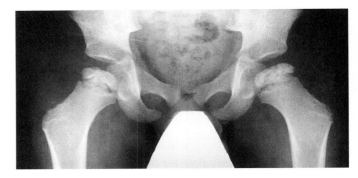

Fig. 1   A 10-year-old boy presenting with recurrent hip problems over 1 year; he had mild epiphyseal dysplasia, but fragmentation of the femoral heads is obvious.

most look the same, however radiological changes may differ and a tentative classification has been suggested by Maroteaux and Spranger (1991).

There are a growing number of mutations in the gene for type II collagen (Col 2 A1), which include point mutations, deletions, insertions and splicing defects (Williams et al. 1993; Reginato et al. 1994). Unrelated families have been reported with Ang[75]Cys or Ang[519]Cys mutation (Williams et al. 1993). Late-onset spondyloepiphyseal dysplasia is associated with precocious osteoarthritis, but in tall patients, has also been shown to be associated with type II procollagen gene (Col 2 A1) mutation in exon 11; recurrent mutations at a few specific sites of Col 2 A1 suggest there may be susceptibility 'hot spots' (Bleasel et al. 1995). However, not all cases are associated with primary defects of type II collagen (Anderson et al. 1990b).

Late-onset spondoepiphyseal dysplasia usually presents between the age of 3 and 10 years, but can be later, with pain in the knees and fingers followed by deformity and can simulate juvenile arthritis (Lewkonia and Beck-Hansen 1992); such children are noted to tire easily on activity and from an early age tend to find stairs difficult, presumably due to the poor development of the hips (Fig. 2). From time to time there may be acute episodes of pain, sometimes associated with swelling. It is not uncommon to have a family history of 'similar arthritis'. Clinically such children are usually of short stature; initially there is a suggestion of bony enlargement of the finger joints which becomes more obvious as deformity progresses (Fig. 3). This is followed by enlargement of the knee joints, particularly the patellas, with gradual loss of function of knees and hips (Wynne-Davies et al. 1982). All the acute phase reactants are normal as is the blood count, there are no immune complexes present; rheumatoid factor, antinuclear antibodies (ANA) and DNA, are negative. Radiological changes are characteristic and diagnostic (Figs 4 and 5). Spranger (1983) described this condition as a progressive 'pseudo-juvenile rheumatoid arthritis'. Pseudogout has also been noted (Bradley 1987). Spinal stenosis as a sequel is not uncommon, while total replacement arthroplasty of the hips for secondary degenerative changes may be required at an early age (Fig. 6). Hypoplasia of the odontoid process can also predispose the patient to cervical cord injury as a result of minor trauma.

Cartilage–hair hypoplasia

This is inherited as an autosomal recessive trait and can usually be diagnosed at birth as these children have achondroplastic features,

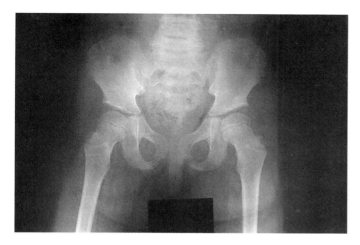

Fig. 2 This girl was described as normal at birth, but at about the age of 3 was noticed to have difficulty climbing up and down stairs; the hip radiographs revealed these poorly developed acetabula and persistence of anteversion of the hips: shortly after this, hand function became impaired and she was diagnosed as spondyloepiphyseal dysplasia.

the hands are short and fat, there is hyperextensibility of the joints with the exception of the elbows and the hair is fine and sparse. Radiographs show widened metaphyses with scalloping, irregular sclerosis and cystic defects (McKusick 1964). These children tend to have a T-cell immunodeficiency which predisposes them to infection (Harris *et al.* 1981; Polmar and Pierce 1986).

Dyggve–Melchior–Clausen syndrome

This appears late in an initially normal child and manifests as dwarfism, claw hands, sternal problems, lumbar lordosis and progressive mental retardation (Dyggve *et al.* 1962; Beighton 1990). Clinically it mimics Morquio's disease, but in addition there is mental retardation. This condition is probably heterogeneous since

both autosomal recessive and X-linked recessive forms have been described.

Acro/acromesomelic dysplasia

Trichorhinophalangeal dysplasia

This is characterized by enlargement of the interphalangeal joints in particular (Fig. 7) which may cause confusion with juvenile chronic arthritis (Noltorp *et al.* 1986). Clinically the bulbous nose with hyperplastic nares, large ears, short brittle hair and short stature suggest the correct diagnosis (Gieodron *et al.* 1973). All acute phase reactants are normal and radiographs show cone-shaped epiphyses with short metacarpals and metatarsals and there may be fragmentation of femoral epiphyses. Many families have shown autosomal dominant inheritance. The chromosome 8q deletion is subtle in that only the very narrow 9-positive band 24.12 is missing (Fryns and Van den Berghe 1986; Bühler *et al.* 1987). There are considerable similarities to the Langer–Gieodron syndrome (TRP II) in which exostoses occur as well as mental retardation and in these children 8q 24.13 is deleted as well.

Storage diseases

The deficiency of a lysosomal degradative enzyme causes an accumulation of its substrate within the lysosomes of the cell; the tissue distribution of the enzyme deficiency determines its expression. Classification is still not entirely satisfactory.

Mucopolysaccharidoses

These are due to deficiency of enzymes involved in the metabolism of glycosaminoglycans (Table 1) (Beck *et al.* 1986; Whitley 1993). All are autosomal recessive disorders (Stanbury *et al.* 1989). A prominent feature is a progressive skeletal dysplasia affecting particularly the hands, hips and vertebrae. It is important to be aware that all these syndromes can present as joint problems, and the first clue to

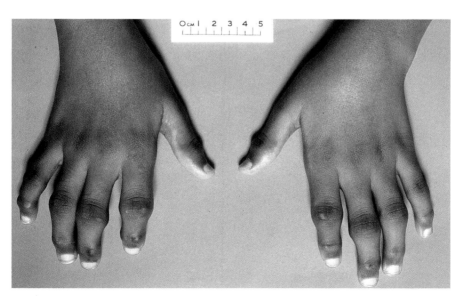

Fig. 3 This shows the clinical appearance of the hands in another case of spondyloepiphyseal dysplasia commencing at the age of 4. By the age of 12, there is obvious bony enlargement of the proximal interphalangeal joints associated with some loss of movement and slight bony enlargement at terminal interphalangeal joints.

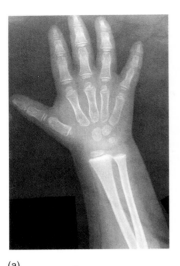
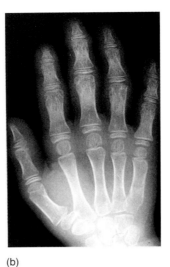

(a)   (b)

Fig. 4 (a) The initial hand radiograph of the patient in Fig. 2 was regarded as normal, although bony changes are starting in the phalanges. By the time bony enlargement was obvious (b) the radiograph shows marked widening of the phalanges at the proximal and distal interphalangeal joints, as well as alteration in texture and epiphyseal changes.

diagnosis may be a claw hand (Fisher *et al.* 1974), but other problems include stiffness of the shoulders, general stiffening and clumsiness in using joints and occasionally dislocation of the hips. In the more severe types such as Hurler's syndrome, there is a gradual coarsening of the facial features associated with dwarfism, mental retardation and clouding of the cornea. There is no difficulty in diagnosis when the fully developed features of Hurler's syndrome are present, but it may take up to 2 years for these to become obvious; flexion deformities of the fingers allow suspicion early, so that prenatal diagnosis of future sibs can be made.

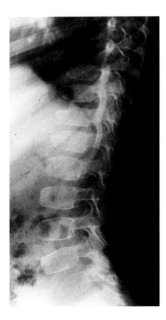

Fig. 5 Lateral radiograph of the spine of a 6-year-old presenting with lumbar lordosis, difficulty in using the hands and limited walking ability. Note the characteristic beaking in vertebral bodies, particularly in the lower thoracic spine, in this child with spondyloepiphyseal dysplasia, which had also affected his father.

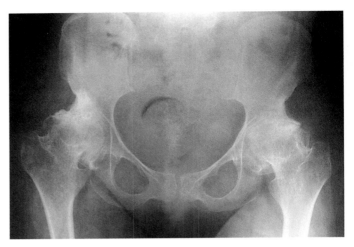

Fig. 6 The shape of the femoral heads, and the avascular necrosis and secondary degenerative changes that have occurred by 16 years of age in the patient illustrated in Fig. 2; this was just prior to bilateral total replacement arthroplasties.

The two conditions that warrant special mention are Scheie and the Morquio–Brailsford syndrome, as these children are of normal intelligence and develop symptoms after the age of 2 or 3 years. In Scheie syndrome, where the disease is caused by a deficiency of the enzyme α-L-iduronidase (Scott *et al.* 1990), the stature is well preserved, but there is progressive stiffening of the joints of the hands (Fig. 8), elbows and knees without swelling and pain and with no evidence of inflammatory indices. Urinary excretion of dermatan sulphate is increased. Clouding of the cornea may mimic iridocyclitis. Later carpal tunnel compression and atlantoaxial subluxation can cause problems; cardiac difficulties involving the aortic and mitral valves are also seen (Butman *et al.* 1989).

A phenotype described by Roubicek *et al.* (1985), intermediate between Hurler and Scheie, has the coarse facial features and corneal clouding, skeletal changes are mild to severe, but mental retardation is mild.

In the Hunter–Scheie syndrome, stiffening of the shoulders associated with some degree of dwarfism occurs early as well as moderate skeletal involvement, but intellectual impairment of varying degree does not develop until later.

In the Morquio–Brailsford syndrome, two different enzyme deficiencies have been noted (Table 1), but symptoms and signs are similar. There is progressive musculoskeletal stiffening which usually begins about the age of 3 or 4 years and is associated with dwarfing. The hands tend to enlarge, valgus deformity of the knees gradually develops and the gait becomes stiff and waddling with some kyphosis and protrusion of the sternum. Initially as the joints enlarge they are hypermobile, but later become stiff. Characteristic radiological findings include platyspondyly and odontoid hypoplasia, and dysplastic hips with poorly developed acetabula. Radiologically they are distinct from the various forms of spondyloepiphyseal dysplasia. Progressive cervical spinal cord damage can occur (Lipson 1977). Clouding of the cornea is mild initially, but deafness may be an early problem. Rarely echocardiographic changes occur and aortic regurgitation develops in a proportion (John *et al.* 1990).

All these children need, not only to be protected against unnecessary therapy with long-acting drugs such as gold, penicillamine, or

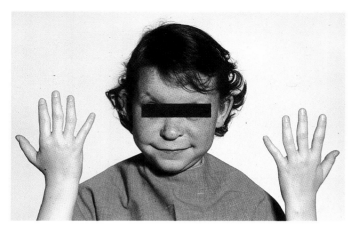

Fig. 7 Trichorhinophalangeal dysplasia; note the bony enlargement of proximal interphalangeal joints together with facies. (By courtesy of Dr Alan Craft, Newcastle.)

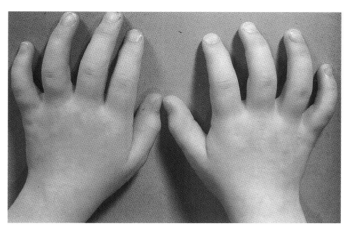

Fig. 8 Hands of child with Hunter–Scheie syndrome which had progressively stiffened from the age of 1 year.

methotrexate, but also to be watched for complications such as carpal tunnel compression (Wraith and Alani 1990), atlantoaxial subluxation (Lipson 1977), and spinal cord compression (Blaw and Langer 1969).

Mucolipidoses

The term mucolipidosis is applied to a group of disorders that are characterized by the intracellular accumulation of both glycosaminoglycans and sphingolipids, but without excess urinary excretion of glycosaminoglycans. Progressive ocular and neurological abnormalities are common to all these disorders, which are autosomal recessive.

Mucolipidosis type I

Isolated neuraminidase deficiency (sialidase) produces a Hurler-like syndrome. The urinary excretion of sialated urinary oligosaccharides is markedly elevated.

Table 1 Mucopolysaccharidoses

Type	Urinary excretion	Enzyme deficiency	Gene	Locus
I Hurler	Dermatan sulphate Heparan sulphate	α-L-Iduronidase	4p	16.3
I Scheie	Dermatan sulphate	α-L-Iduronidase		
I Hurler/Scheie	Dermatan sulphate Heparan sulphate			
II Hunter	Dermatan sulphate Heparan sulphate	Iduronate-L-sulphatase	Xq	27.3
II Hunter/Scheie	Dermatan sulphate Heparan sulphate			
III Sanfilippo A	Heparan sulphate	Heparan		
B		α-N-Acetylglucosaminidase		
C	Heparan sulphate	Acetyl-CoA-α-glucosaminide		
D	Heparan sulphate	N-Acetyl-glucosamine-6-sulphatase	12q	14
IV Morquio-Brailsford A	Keratan sulphate Chondroitin-6 sulphate	Galactose-6-sulphatase		
B		β-Galactosidase		
VI Maroteaux–Lamy	Dermatan sulphate	N-Acetyl-galactosamine-4-sulphatase		
VII Sly	Dermatan sulphate Heparan sulphate Chondroitin sulphate	β-Glucuronidase		

Mucolipidosis type II

Sometimes called 'I cell disease', also causes a Hurler-like syndrome with progressive loss of joint movement. There are prominent intra-cytoplasmic (I) inclusions in lymphocytes and skin fibroblasts. Biochemically there is a deficiency of Glc-*N*-acetylglucosaminyl-phosphotransferase in fibroblasts and leucocytes (Cipolloni *et al.* 1980).

Mucolipidosis type III

This is sometimes known as pseudo-Hurler polydystrophy and is characterized by restriction of joint mobility, which does not become apparent until the second or third year of life. Such patients have presented to us as juvenile arthritis starting with difficulty in raising the shoulders (Fig. 9) and problems with grip (Fig. 10), and atypical carpal tunnel syndrome (Starreveld 1975), or with thickening in the hands and some tightening of the skin mimicking scleroderma. No inflammatory arthritis is present and routine blood tests are all normal. Mentality may be normal or slightly below standard. Radiographic findings are those of a dysotosis multiplex. The condition tends to stabilize in the teens. Ocular features include cloudy cornea, astigmatism, abnormalities of the retina and optic nerve, and visual field defects (Traboulsi and Maumence 1986). Aortic incompetence is not uncommon. The basic defect is in the enzyme that specifically phosphorylates mannose residues of lysosomal glycoproteins. Characteristic inclusions are found in cultured fibroblasts.

Sphingolipidoses

Here there is an accumulation of lipid in the cell as a result of specific enzyme deficiencies; only three of the many different sphingolipidoses have musculoskeletal signs and symptoms, notably Farber's lipogranulomatosis, Gaucher's disease, and Fabry's disease.

Farber's lipogranulamatosis

This is due to deficiency of acid ceramidase and is an autosomal recessive sphingolipidosis. Usually it begins in the neonatal period with a hoarse cry and irritability. Painful red masses develop along tendon sheaths and around joints, followed by the development of contractures. Delayed motor development and mental retardation are prominent. Epiglottal and laryngeal swelling cause repeated pulmonary infections, usually leading to death early in life. It has been suggested that there are milder types of this defect, and recent descriptions of older children presenting with joint deformity and some mental retardation are appearing (Jameson *et al.* 1987). These may confuse the rheumatologist.

Gaucher's disease

This results from a deficiency in the enzyme acid glucosidase and is characterized by an accumulation of glucosyl ceramide in reticulo-endothelial cells in the bone marrow, spleen, liver, lymph nodes and other internal organs. Three clinical forms are now recognized. The most common, type 1, is the chronic non-neuropathic adult form, more prevalent in Ashkenazi Jews. Type 2 is the infantile or active neuropathic form, and death occurs before the age of 2 years. Type 3 is the juvenile or subacute neuropathic form, which occurs particularly among the Swedish, and is thought to be caused by a single

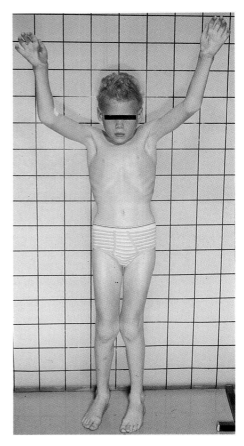

Fig. 9 This boy, who proved to have mucolipidosis type III, presented with difficulty in using his hands; he was found to have very limited shoulder movement, contractures at the elbow and the beginning of contractures at the knees, hips and feet.

mutation in exon 10 of the glucocerebrosidase gene (Dahl *et al.* 1990). Osteoarticular complaints are an important feature, particularly in type 3, where they may be the earliest manifestation of the disease and result from infiltration of the marrow of the subchondral bone. A common complaint is polyarthralgia affecting the large peripheral joints, pathological fracture of a long bone or compression of a vertebra which gives rise to pain. Severe degenerative hip disease as a result of avascular necrosis and collapse of the femoral head is not

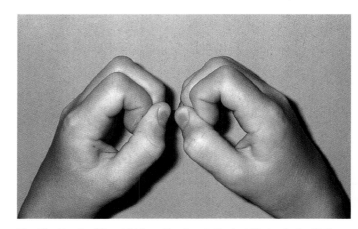

Fig. 10 Hands of the child from Fig. 9; note the inability to pinch with finger and thumb, and the thickening of the tissues due to deposition.

uncommon. The most frequent early radiological finding is widening of the distal portion of the femur just above the medial condyle, the Erlenmeyer flask deformity. Similar flaring may be present in the tibia and humerus (Peters *et al.* 1977; Stowens *et al.* 1985).

Fabry's disease (angiokeratoma corporis diffusum)

This is an X-linked recessive disorder characterized by the progressive accumulation of birefringent deposits of triglycosylceramide in the endothelial and smooth muscle cells of blood vessels and in ganglions and perineural cells of the autonomic nervous system. It results from a deficiency of ceramide trihexoside-α-galactosidase and ceramide trihexosidase, the gene for which has been localized to the Xq 22–23 region of the X chromosome (Sakuraba *et al.* 1990). The affected boys have recurrent attacks of fever and a severe arthritis with a burning and tingling pain in the extremities. This is aggravated by hot weather or exercise. The fingers and elbows may become swollen with difficulty in extending the fingers. The typical rash consists of purple papules — angiokeratoma diffusum universale. Ocular signs include opacification of the cornea in a whirl-like configuration. Secondary osteonecrosis may become increasingly important in weight-bearing joints such as the hips. Female heterozygotes may have a milder form of the disease, as did the mother in a case presenting with fever and lymphadenopathy (Mayou *et al.* 1989). Renal, cardiac and cerebral disease tend to cause death in the mid-adult years (Kramer *et al.* 1985; Sakuraba *et al.* 1986; Morgan *et al.* 1990).

Other rare disorders

Multicentric reticulohistiocytosis (see Chapter 5.13.7)

A disease sometimes referred to as 'lipoid dermatoarthritis'. As yet no biochemical abnormality has been defined, but foamy giant cells and histiocytes are found on biopsy of the skin, synovium and mucous membranes. It causes a mutilating, destructive arthropathy with cutaneous nodules often on the face as well as other sites (Zayid and Farroj 1973).

Winchester syndrome

This begins after the age of a few weeks up to one year with swelling of the proximal interphalangeal joints and enlargement of the wrists; later corneal clouding, coarsening of the face, and joint contractures appear (Winchester *et al.* 1969). Patchy thickening of skin with pigmentation are found over the back, flanks and lateral aspects of the arms. Other features are corneal opacities in mid-childhood, retarded growth, carpal-tarsal osteolysis and destruction of the small joints. Increased urinary oligosaccharide excretion is found (Lambert *et al.* 1989; Winter 1989).

Kniest syndrome

This is associated with congenital short limbs, and with a large head, round face and depressed nasal bridge. It is inherited usually as an autosomal dominant disorder, but sporadic cases have been seen (Kim *et al.* 1975). Stiffness of the fingers, dislocation of the hips and kyphoscoliosis develop; later enlargement of the joints and severe contractures occur (Fraya *et al.* 1979). The cartilage has hypertrophic chondrocytes surrounded by a loose matrix that contains large holes resembling Swiss cheese, hence the name. Other abnormalities, notably cleft palate, vitreo-retinal degeneration and retinal detachment, deafness and hernia are characteristic. Other chondro-dysplasias may have a similar appearance (Sconyers *et al.* 1985).

Moore–Federman disease

Small hands with brachydactyly are noted early, followed by contractures of the hand joints (Fig. 11) and dwarfism (Moore and Federman 1965). This may be the same condition as acromicric dysplasia (Winter *et al.* 1989).

Thiemann's disease

This tends to commence at about the age of 10 or 11 years and is characterized by progressive enlargement of the proximal interphalangeal joints of the hands, the interphalangeal joints of the great toe and occasionally other toes, followed by slight flexion of the enlarged joints. Clinically there is bony swelling but no evidence of soft-tissue swelling and the erythrocyte sedimentation rate is normal. Radiologically there is irregularity of the epiphyses of the phalanges. This condition can be familial (Molloy and Hamilton 1978).

Idiopathic acro-osteolysis

Although destruction and disappearance of bone as a primary condition is rare, a number of different types have been described (Brown *et al.* 1976). Hereditary osteolysis is an autosomal dominant; it usually begins about the age of 3 years and affects children of both sexes (Naranjo *et al.* 1992). The bones of the carpus and tarsus (Urlus *et al.* 1993) are particularly affected, and to a lesser extent the hands and feet as well as elbows and knees. It presents with tender, swollen, limited wrists and ankles closely mimicking juvenile chronic arthritis, but there is no obvious synovitis and the erthrocyte sedimentation rate is usually normal (Beals and Bird 1975). Initially the radiographs are normal, but after a time there is porosis of the carpal bones followed by localized destruction (Fig. 12) and finally complete disappearance

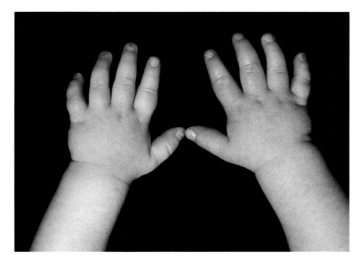

Fig. 11 This 7-year-old presented with some difficulty in gripping and possible swelling of the fingers. She was noted to be short. Her grandfather had very similar hands.

of the bone. This condition tends to stabilize spontaneously in early adult life. The Haydu–Cheney acro-osteolysis is characterized by facial as well as skeletal changes. The eyes slope downwards, the philtrum is long and the nostrils anteverted. The skull radiograph shows wormian bones, an elongated pituitary fossa and a thickened cranium with persistent sutures; the classical acro-osteolysis only develops later in childhood. Inheritance is likely to be autosomal dominant, although most cases are sporadic (Macpherson and Pai 1989). Multicentric osteolysis has also been reported as an autosomal recessive trait with symptoms developing between the age of 2 and 5 years (Torg *et al.* 1969).

The Thieffry–Kohler form is similar to idiopathic multicentric osteolysis, but with a facial appearance characterized by frontal bossing, micrognathia, a small mouth and protruding eyes. It is usually inherited as an autosomal dominant trait. The joint manifestations begin in the wrists and ankles, leading to progressive deformity. It is not certain whether the form associated with progressive nephropathy resulting in hypertension and renal failure in early adult life is the same as Thieffry–Kohler (Shurtleff *et al.* 1964; Carnevale *et al.* 1987).

Phantom bone disease (Gorham's disease)

This is a non-hereditary form which occurs usually between the ages of 5 and 10 years (Gorham and Stout 1955). Any bone can be affected and there are usually multiple sites which are asymmetrical in distribution; histologically there is proliferation of thin-walled blood vessels.

Distal osteolysis

Thought to be inherited as an autosomal dominant trait, it is characterized by progressive osteolysis of the phalanges, metatarsals and metacarpals. It tends to occur in children of 8 years and upwards and often heals spontaneously, although sometimes part of a finger or toe may be lost (Elias *et al.* 1978).

Other oddities

Not all children who present with joint deformities can be characterized, for example the patient shown in Figs 13 and 14, and all skeletal disorders mimicking arthritis have not been covered here, so cross-reference to other chapters is essential. Readers are also referred to Wynne-Davies *et al.* (1985) and Spranger (1992).

Arthrogryposis

This is a symptom complex characterized by stiffness and contractures of the joints at birth. It can affect both the upper and lower limbs in about 50 per cent of cases, while in 40 per cent it is only the lower limbs and 10 per cent the upper limbs. Distal joints are often severely affected with the feet showing talipes equinovarus and the wrists severe flexion deformities. These are frequently associated with flexion contractures of the knees and fixed extended elbows (Lloyd-Roberts and Lettin 1970). The normal contours of the joints are lost as are the skin creases over them; there is absence or underdevelopment of surrounding muscles. The rigidity of joints is thought to be due to fibrosis. In addition, there may be congenital defects of the skeleton. The patients that give rise to problems in differentiation from juvenile arthritis are those with isolated

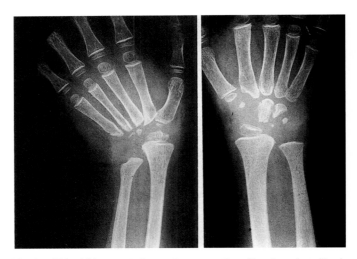

Fig. 12 This child presented some 3 years earlier with pain and swelling in the wrists and feet; note the tapering of the bases of the metacarpals, and absorption of carpal bones at a different rate on the two sides, together with the early absorption of the ulnar head on the left, due to idiopathic acro-osteolysis.

limitation of movement, particularly at the hips, knees, or elbows (Fig. 15). It is important to recognize them early as improvement can be achieved by manipulation and splinting, while soft-tissue release of ligaments and tendons around the joints will help fixed deformities, but should be carried out in relatively young patients.

Kashin–Beck disease

This endemic arthritis with systemic or visceral manifestations has been reported from Eastern Russia, Siberia, Northern China, and Korea and appears to result from eating bread baked from fungus-

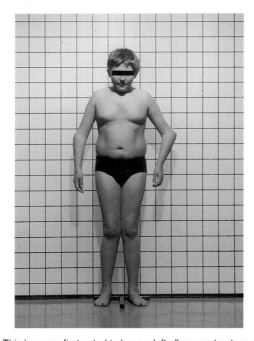

Fig. 13 This boy was first noted to have a left elbow contracture as a baby; this progressed and deformities were noted in the other elbow, wrists, knees, ankles and feet. The only relevant history was that his mother had had mumps during the pregnancy.

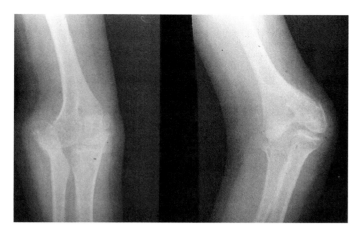

Fig. 14 Unusual bony abnormalities in the elbow radiograph from the patient shown in Fig. 13. The radial head on the left in particular is grossly abnormal.

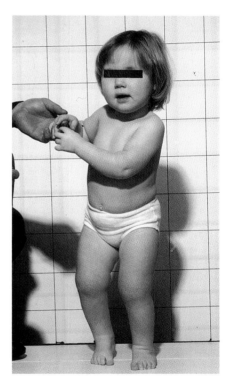

Fig. 15 Although well covered, it was considered that this baby, who had presented with contractures of the hips, knees and ankles at birth, was suffering from a limited form of arthrogryposis.

infected grain (Nesterov 1964). Unknown toxic products cause an epiphyseal and metaphyseal dysplasia of the bones of the interphalangeal, wrist, knee, and ankle joints. This disorder continues to become more severe as long as the child lives in the endemic area eating such products, and will ultimately cause symmetric progressive limitation of movement involving multiple joints. The initial symptoms are in school-aged children and consist of aching and muscle weakness. Laboratory indices of inflammation are absent. The eventual dwarfing, bony dysplasia, and short digits resemble those seen in the lysosomal stores diseases. Experimental animals fed grain infected

with *Fusarium* species have been shown to develop a similar form of dysplasia.

Mseleni disease

The population of the Mseleni area of Northern Zululand has a high incidence of a chronic polyarthritis, commencing in childhood or adolescence and characterized by a restriction of movement and limitation of mobility, with the hips, knees, and ankles as the predominant sites of involvement; mild stunting of growth is common (Lockitch *et al.* 1973). The characteristic radiograph abnormalities include irregularities on the surface of the epiphyses, change in shape and, ultimately, progress to osteoarthritis in the hips, often with protrusio acetabulae; short metacarpals and deformity at the distal end of the ulna may also occur. The aetiology is thought to involve a nutritional deficiency or toxin similar to the Kashin–Beck disease.

References

Amir, D., Mogle, P., and Weinberg, H. (1985). Multiple epiphyseal dysplasia in one family; a further review of seven generations. *Journal of Bone and Joint Surgery*, **67B**, 809–13.

Anderson, I.J. *et al.* (1990*a*). Spondyloepiphyseal dysplasia congenita: genetic linkage to type II collagen (COL2 A1). *American Journal of Human Genetics*, **46**, 896–901.

Anderson, I.J. *et al.* (1990*b*). Spondyloepiphyseal dysplasia, mild autosomal is not due to primary defects of type II collagen. *American Journal of Medical Genetics*, **37**, 272–6.

Beals, R.F. and Bird, G.B. (1975). Carpal and tarsal osteolysis: a case report and review of the literature. *Journal of Bone and Joint Surgery*, **57A**, 681–6.

Beck, M., Glossi, J., Grubisic, A., and Spranger, J. (1986). Heterogeneity of Morquio disease. *Clinical Genetics*, **29**, 325–31.

Beighton, P. (1990). Syndrome of the mouth. Dyggve–Melchior–Clausen syndrome. *Journal of Medical Genetics*, **27**, 512–15.

Blaw, M. and Langer, L.O. (1969). Spinal cord compresssion Morquio–Brailsford disease. *Journal of Pediatrics*, **74**, 593–600.

Bleasel, J.F. *et al.* (1995). Type II procollagen gene (COL 2A1) mutation in exon 11 associated with spondylo-epiphyseal dysplasia tarda. Tall stature and precocious osteoarthritis. *Journal of Rheumatology*, **22**, 255–61.

Bradley, J.D. (1987). Pseudo gout in progressive pseudo-rheumatoid arthritis. *Annals of the Rheumatic Diseases*, **46**, 709–12.

Brown, D.M. *et al.* (1976). The acro-osteolysis syndrome, morphologic and biochemical studies. *Journal of Pediatrics*, **88**, 573–80.

Bühler, E.M., Bühler, U.K., Beutler, L., and Fessler, R. (1987). A final word on the trichorhino-phalangeal syndromes. *Clinical Genetics*, **31**, 273–5.

Butman, S.M., Karl, L., and Copeland, J.S. (1989). Combined aortic and mitral valve replacement in an adult with Scheie's disease. *Chest*, **96**, 209–10.

Carnevale, A. *et al.* (1987). Idiopathic multicentral osteolysis with facial anomalies and nephropathy. *American Journal of Medical Genetics*, **26**, 877–86.

Cipolloni, C. *et al.* (1980). Neonatal mucolipidosis II (I cell disease) clinical, radiological and biochemical studies in a case. *Helvetica Paediatrica Acta*, **35**, 85–95.

Dahl, N., Lagerstrom, M., Erikson, A., and Petterson, U. (1990). Gaucher disease type III (Norbottnian type) is caused by a single mutation in exon 10 of the glucocerebrosidase gene. *American Journal of Human Genetics*, **47**, 275–8.

Dyggve, H.V., Melchoir, J.C., and Clausen, J. (1962). Morquio–Ullrich's disease. *Archives of Disease in Childhood*, **37**, 525–34.

Elias, A.N. *et al.* (1978). Hereditary osteodysplasia and acro-osteolysis. *American Journal of Medicine*, **65**, 627–36.

Fisher, R.C., Horner, R.L., and Wood, V.E. (1974). The hand in mucopolysaccharide disorders. *Clinical Orthopaedics and Related Research*, **104**, 191–9.

Fraya, R., Malheim, R., and Idriss H. (1979). The Kniest (Swiss cheese cartilage) syndrome; description of a distinct arthropathy. *Arthritis and Rheumatism*, **22**, 286–9.

Fryns, J.P. and Van den Berghe, H. (1986). Bq 24.12 interstitial deletion in tricho-phalangeal syndrome type 1. *Human Genetics*, **74**, 188–9.

Gieodron, A. *et al.* (1973). Autosomal dominant transmission of the tricho-rhino-phalangeal syndrome. *Helvetica Paediatrica Acta*, **28**, 249–59.

Gorham, L.V. and Stout, A.P. (1955). Massive osteolysis (acute spontaneous absorption of bone, phantom bone, disappearing bone) in relationship to haemangiomatosis. *Journal of Bone and Joint Surgery*, **37A**, 985–1004.

Hall, J.G., Dorst, J.P., Rotta, J., and McKusick, Y.A. (1987). Gonadal mosaicus in pseudo-achondroplasia. *American Journal of Medical Genetics*, **28**, 143–52.

Harris, R.E. *et al.* (1981). Cartilage–hair hypoplasia, defective T cell function and Diamond–Blackfan anaemia in an Amish child. *American Journal of Medical Genetics*, **8**, 291–7.

Iceton, J.A. and Horne, G. (1986). Spondylo-epiphyseal dysplasia tarda — the X-linked variety in three brothers. *Journal of Bone and Joint Surgery*, **68B**, 616–19.

Jameson, R.A., Holt, P.J.L., and Keen, J.H. (1987). Farber's disease (lysosomal acid ceramidase deficiency). *Annals of the Rheumatic Diseases*, **46**, 559–61.

John, R.M., Hunter, D., and Swanton, R.H. (1990). Echocardiographic abnormalities in type IV mucopolysaccharidoses. *Archives of Disease in Childhood*, **65**, 746–9.

Kim, H.J. *et al.* (1975). Kniest syndrome with dominant inheritance and muco-polysaccharidosis. *American Journal of Human Genetics*, **27**, 755–64.

Kramer, W., Thormann, J., Meuller, K., and Frenzel, H. (1985). Progressive cardiac involvement by Fabry's disease despite successful renal allotransplantation. *International Journal of Cardiology*, **7**, 72–5.

Lambert, J.C. *et al.* (1989). Biochemical and ultrastructural studies of two familial cases of Winchester syndrome. *Journal de Genetique Humaine*, **37**, 231–6.

Lewkonia, R.M. and Beck-Hansen, N.T. (1992). Spondylo-epiphyseal dysplasia tarda simulating juvenile arthritis: clinical and molecular genetic observations. *Clinical and Experimental Rheumatology*, **10**, 411–14.

Lipson, S.J. (1977). Dysplasia of the odontoid process in Morquio's syndrome causing quadriparesis. *Journal of Bone and Joint Surgery*, **59A**, 340–44.

Lloyd-Roberts, G.C. and Lettin, A.W.F. (1970). Arthrogryposis multiplex congenita. *Journal of Bone and Joint Surgery*, **52B**, 494–508.

Lockitch, G. *et al.* (1973). Mseleni joint disease: a pilot study. *South African Medical Journal*, **1**, 2283–93.

Macpherson, R.J. and Pai, G.S. (1989). The Haydu–Cheney syndrome. Case report and review of the literature. *Dysmorphic Clinical Genetics*, **3**, 70–78.

Maroteaux, R. and Spranger J. (1991). The spondylometaphyseal dysplasias: a tentative classification. *Pediatric Radiology*, **21**, 293–7.

Maroteaux, R. *et al.* (1980). The mild form of pseudo-achondroplasia. *European Journal of Pediatrics*, **133**, 227–31.

Maudsley, R.H. (1955). Dysplasia epiphysialis multiplex: a report of 14 cases in 3 familes. *Journal of Bone and Joint Surgery*, **37B**, 228–40.

Mayou, S.C., Kirby, J.D., and Morgan, S.H. (1989). Anderson–Fabry disease: an unusual presentation with lymphadenopathy. *Journal of the Royal Society of Medicine*, **82**, 555–6.

McKusick, V.A. (1964). Metaphyseal dysostosis and thin hair; a new recessively inherited syndrome? *Lancet*, **i**, 832–3.

Molloy, M.G. and Hamilton E.B.D. (1978). Thiemanns disease. *Rheumatology and Rehabilitation*, **17**, 179–80.

Moore, W.T. and Federman, D.D. (1965). Familial dwarfism and stiff joints. *Archives of Internal Medicine*, **115**, 398–404.

Morgan, S.H. *et al.* (1990). The neurological complication of Anderson–Fabry disease (α-galactosidse A deficiency) investigation of symptomatic and presymptomatic patients. *Quarterly Journal of Medicine*, **75**, 491–507.

Naranjo, A. *et al.* (1992). Primary idiopathic osteolysis: description of a family. *Annals of the Rheumatic Diseases*, **51**, 1074–8.

Nesterov, A.L. (1964). The clinical course of Kashin–Beck disease. *Arthritis and Rheumatism*, **7**, 29–40.

Noltorp, S., Kristoffersson, U., and Mardahl N. (1986). Trichorhinophalangeal syndrome type I: symptoms and signs, radiology and genetics. *Annals of the Rheumatic Diseases*, **45**, 31–6.

Patroni, N.A. and Kredich, D.W. (1985). Arthritis in children with multiple epiphy-seal dysplasia. *Journal of Rheumatology*, **12**, 145–9.

Peters, S.P., Lee, R.E., and Glue, R.H. (1977). Gaucher's disease — a review. *Medicine*, **56**, 425–42.

Polmar, S.H. and Pierce, G.F. (1986). Cartilage hair hypoplasia: immunological aspects and their clinical implications. *Clinical Immunology and Immunopathology*, **40**, 87–93.

Poznanski, A.K. (1974). *The hand in radiologic diagnosis*. W.K. Saunders, Philadelphia.

Reginato, A.J. *et al.* (1994). Familial spondyloepiphyseal dysplasia tarda, brachydac-tyly and precocious osteoarthritis associated with an argenine 75→cysteine mutation in the procollagen type II gene in a kindred of Chilue Iolander. *Arthritis and Rheumatism*, **37**, 1078–86.

Roubicek, M., Gehler, J., and Spranger, J. (1985). The clinical spectrum of α-L-iduronidase deficiency. *American Journal of Medical Genetics*, **20**, 471–8.

Sakuraba, H. *et al.* (1986). Cardiovascular manifestations in Fabry's disease. A high incidence of mitral valve prolapse in hemizygotes and heterozygotes. *Clinical Genetics*, **29**, 276–83.

Sakuraba, H. *et al.* (1990). Identification of point mutations in the α-galactosidase A gene in classical and atypical hemizygotes with Fabry disease. *American Journal of Human Genetics*, **47**, 784–9.

Sconyers, S.M. *et al.* (1985). A distal chondrodysplasia resembling Kniest dysplasia. Clinical, roengenographic, histologic and ultrastructural findings. *Journal of Pediatrics*, **103**, 898–904.

Scott, H.A. *et al.* (1990). Chromosomal localisation of the human α-L-iduronidase gene (IUDA) to 4p 236.3. *American Journal of Human Genetics*, **47**, 802–7.

Shurtleff, D.B. *et al.* (1964). Hereditary osteolysis with hypertension and neuro-pathy. *Journal of the American Medical Association*, **188**, 363–8.

Spranger, E.J.P. (1992). International classification of osteochondro dysplasias. (For the International working group on constitutional diseases of bone). *European Journal of Paediatrics*, **151**, 407–15.

Spranger, J. *et al.* (1983). Progressive pseudo-rheumatoid arthropathy of child-hood. A hereditary disorder simulating juvenile rheumatoid arthritis. *European Journal of Paediatrics*, **140**, 34–40.

Stanbury, J.B. *et al.* (1989). *The metabolic basis of disease*, (6th edn). McGraw-Hill, New York.

Starreveld, E. (1975). Bilateral carpal tunnel syndrome in childhood. A report of two sisters with mucolipidosis. *Neurology*, **25**, 234–8.

Stowens, D.W. *et al.* (1985). Skeletal complications of Gaucher's disease. *Medicine*, **64**, 310–22.

Szpiro-Tapiaa, S. *et al.* (1988). Spondyloepiphyseal dysplasia tarda: linkage with genetic markers from the distal short arm of the X chromosome. *Human Genetics*, **81**, 61–3.

Torg, J.S. *et al.* (1969). Hereditary multicentre osteolysis with recessive transmis-sion: a new syndrome. *Journal of Pediatrics*, **75**, 243–52.

Traboulsi, E.I. and Maumence, I.H. (1986). Ophthalmologic findings in muco-lipidosis III (pseudo Hurler's polystrophy). *American Journal of Ophthalmology*, **102**, 592–7.

Urlus, M. *et al.* (1993). Carpo-tarsal osteolysis. Case report and review of the litera-ture. *Genetic Counseling*, **4**, 25–36.

Whitley, C.B. (1993). The mucopolysaccharidoses. In *McKusick's heritable disorders of connective tissue*, (5th edn) (ed. P. Beighton), pp. 367–499. Mosby, London.

Williams, C.J. *et al.* (1993). Spondyloepiphyseal dysplasia and precocious osteo-arthritis in a family with an Arg[75]Cys mutation in the precollagen type II gene (COL 2A1). *Human Genetics*, **92**, 499–505.

Winchester, P.H. *et al.* (1969). A new acid mucopolysaccharidosis with skeletal deformities simulating rheumatoid arthritis. *American Journal of Roentgenology*, **106**, 121–8.

Winter, R.M. (1989). Syndrome of the month — Winchester's syndrome. *Journal of Medical Genetics*, **26**, 772–5.

Winter, R.M. *et al.* (1989). Moore–Federman syndrome and acromicric dysplasias: are they the same entity? *Journal of Medical Genetics*, **26**, 320–25.

Wraith, J.E. and Alani, S.M. (1990). Carpal tunnel syndrome in the muco-polysac-charidoses and related disorders. *Archives of Disease in Childhood*, **65**, 962–6.

Wynne-Davies, R., Hall, C., and Ansell, B.M. (1982). Spondylo-epiphyseal dysplasia tarda with progressive arthropathy. *Journal of Bone and Joint Surgery*, **64B**, 442–5.

Wynne-Davies, R., Hall, C., and Apley, A.(ed.) (1985). *Atlas of skeletal dysplasias*. Churchill Livingstone, Edinburgh.

Zayid, I. and Farroj, J. (1973). Familial histiocytic dermato-arthritis. *American Journal of Medicine*, **54**, 793–800.

5.18 Disorders of the spine

5.18.1 Intervertebral disc disease and other mechanical disorders of the back

Malcolm I. V. Jayson

Introduction

The primary roles of the human spine are to bear the weight of the upper structures of the body, provide flexibility for movements, and protect the vital structures—in particular the spinal cord and the nerves that emerge through the intervertebral foramina. The stresses associated with a lifetime's use, combined with ageing and degenerative changes and the effects of individual and repeated traumatic episodes, are commonly associated with mechanical problems so that back pain due to structural change of the spine is almost a universal experience. However, although mechanical and degenerative changes of the lumbar spine are common, the correlation with back pain is weak (Lawrence 1977). Some patients have minor evidence of damage to the spine yet experience major problems; others may show degenerative change and yet be symptom free. Moreover, structural changes in the spine are permanent but the symptoms of back pain are commonly transient. Acute episodes of pain are separated by periods in which symptoms are minimal or absent. This complicates our understanding of the pathogenesis of back problems. The remitting course of individual episodes emphasizes the need for controlled studies of various treatment programmes.

Epidemiology

Back pain is an extremely common problem. Recent population studies in Britain show a point prevalence of 14 per cent at any one time (Mason 1994), 39 per cent in the last month (Croft and Jayson 1994), 37 per cent in the last year (Mason 1994), and lifetime prevalence of between 58 per cent (Croft and Jayson 1994) and 80 per cent (Waddell 1987). The peak prevalence is between 45 and 59 years although it is common in the young and in the elderly (Papageorgiou et al. 1995). True sciatica appears to be much less frequent. With strict diagnostic criteria, the overall prevalence in studies by Heliovaara et al. was estimated to be 5.3 per cent in men and 3.7 per cent in women (Heliovaara et al. 1987).

Despite a dramatic increase in recent years in disability due to back problems, there is no clear evidence of an increase in the number of back-related injuries (Troup and Edwards 1985). In a recent survey (Mason 1994), 11 per cent of the population (that is 30 per cent of those with back pain in the last year) reported their activities limited by back pain during the previous 4 weeks; 1.9 per cent of all employed people and 6 per cent of employed people with back pain had lost at least 1 day off in the last month. In Britain in 1993, the total work loss was estimated as approximately 150 000 000 days (Clinical Standards Advisory Group 1994). The prevalence of back disability is increasing rapidly with the number of working days lost now running at some four times the figures for 20 years ago, and similar changes are found in most countries. Cats-Baril and Frymoyer estimated the costs in the United States to be between $25 and 100 billion in 1990 (Cats-Baril and Frymoyer 1991). There is, however, little evidence of increase in the numbers of work-related injuries (Health and Safety Executive 1993). We see a dramatic increase in the morbidity associated with back problems but there does not seem to be any change in the nature of the back injuries. It is likely that social, psychological, and employment problems are playing the major role in this dramatic increase in disability.

There is little difference in the prevalence of back pain and disability between men and women. There is an increased prevalence of low back pain and disability with lower social class; the relationship being stronger in males than females (Walsh et al. 1992; Mason 1994). Many patients report the development of back problems in relationship to an accident or injury although commonly this is difficult to evaluate (Mason 1994). Most are work related injuries (Health and Safety Executive 1993) with the highest incidence rate in the construction industry and agricultural sector. There appears to be an association between low back problems and heavy manual work. Videman et al. found that vertebral osteophytes were associated with heavy physical work (Videman et al. 1990). However, symmetrical disc degeneration was associated with sedentary work. A number of studies have shown an increased lifetime prevalence of back problems in those involved in heavy occupations as compared with light work (Biering-Sorenson 1985; Riihimaki et al. 1989) but it is difficult to know whether this is due to the direct effects of overloading the spine or to repeated minor trauma. Mitchell found that people performing heavy manual work had no increase in the number of spells off work with back pain but they were of increased duration (Mitchell 1985). There also appears to be an association between back pain and long-term exposure to driving and vibration (Hulshof and van Zanten 1987).

Epidemiological studies show associations of back pain with neck pain (Porter and Hibbert 1986), chronic musculoskeletal pains (Makela 1993), smoking, psychological distress, and depression (Wright et al. 1995).

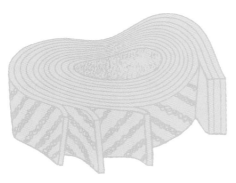

Fig. 1 The collagen fibres of the annulus fibrosus spiralling obliquely around the margins of the intervertebral disc. (By courtesy of Dr J.B. Weiss.)

Structure and function of the lumbosacral spine

The five lumbar and first sacral vertebrae form the principal load carrying structure for the back. Each pair of vertebrae is joined by the intervertebral disc anteriorly and the two apophyseal joints posteriorly. These joints cannot move in isolation and all movements between vertebrae necessarily affects all three. For this reason each pair of vertebrae and the connecting three joints are known as a spinal unit.

The intervertebral disc in the adult consists of a central gelatinous nucleus pulposus surrounded by the tough fibres of annulus fibrosus. The annular fibres spiral obliquely in fascicles between the vertebral rims, lying at about 60° to the spinal axis and interdigitating with each other (Fig. 1). This arrangement makes the intervertebral disc an effective shock absorber which accommodates vertical loads by slight squashing of the disc and bulging of the periphery, and flexion, extension, and lateral flexion movements by alteration of the angles of the crossing fascicles. However, torsion of the lumbar spine is less readily accommodated as twisting of one vertebra on that below means that some collagen fibres of the annulus will be stretched. This is one of the reasons why twisting movements of the lumbar spine are more likely to be associated with annular damage.

There is a lumbar lordosis that is most marked at L4/5 and L5/S1. The associated increase in pressures in the posterior part of the disc, together with the lower lumbar discs carrying higher loads than the upper discs, account for the greater prevalence of lumbar problems at these sites.

The gel-like nucleus of the normal disc consists of a matrix of water and glycosaminoglycan in a random meshwork of Type II collagen fibres (McDevitt 1988). With ageing and disc degeneration there is alteration of the glycosaminoglycan, with a reduction of its molecular size (Adams and Muir 1976), and the nucleus becomes more fibrous. There is loss of water content, the gel-like character of nucleus is lost, and, as a result, it is no longer able to redistribute pressures in an isotropic fashion. Localized areas of pressure concentration appear and may be associated with focal damage and an increase in proportion of the body load is borne by the annulus fibrosus. The normal annulus primarily consists of Type I collagen fibres at its outer periphery but with a gradual change to Type II fibres at its inner margin with the nucleus (Eyre and Muir 1976). Type I collagen is characteristic of collagens involved in resisting tensile loads, which is the primary function of the outer annulus, whereas the inner annular and nuclear Type II collagen is more typical of cartilage collagen and

has to withstand compressive loads. There is clearly an appropriate, functional adaptation of collagen structure within the disc. In degenerative disease this pattern is lost. There is an excess of Type I collagen in both the annulus and nucleus (Herbert *et al.* 1975) interfering with the biomechanical efficiency of the disc. There are alterations in the patterns of degradative enzymes with disc degeneration and herniation (Ng *et al.* 1986) but it is not clear whether these changes play a fundamental role in degeneration of the disc or are secondary to disc damage. Experimental induction of disc prolapse shows that extensive vascular ingrowth is followed by more florid evidence of internal disc disruption (Vernon Roberts 1992). Angiogenic factors associated with the proliferation of new blood vessels are capable of activating degradative enzymes (Weiss and McLaughlin 1993), so providing a possible mechanism for the initiation of disc degeneration.

Measurements of pressures within the intervertebral disc show the increase associated with the upright posture and load bearing (Nachemson 1992). The load on the lumbar spine is increased by contraction of the paravertebral muscles, which stabilize the spine, and reduced by the lumbar lordosis. The design of car seats is largely related to information about the stresses on the disc with varying degrees of lumbar support and back rest inclination.

In contrast to the discs, the apophyseal joints are true synovial joints with fibrous capsules lined by synovium. They lie in an antero-posterior direction although their centres of rotation are behind the disc. Rotation of the lumbar spine is therefore limited and will produce sheer stresses on the disc—again accounting for the risks associated with torsion of the lumbar spine.

Pain is commonly experienced in the back and lower limbs. It may arise from stimulation of the nerve roots or nociceptive receptors (Wyke 1987). These are distributed in:

(1) the skin and subcutaneous tissues;

(2) the fibrous capsules of the apophyseal and sacroiliac joints;

(3) the outer layers of the annulus fibrosus;

(4) the longitudinal ligaments of the spine and, in particular, the posterior longitudinal ligaments;

(5) the periostium and attached fascias, aponeuroses, and tendons;

(6) walls of blood vessels in and around the spine;

(7) the dura mata and epidural adipose tissues.

There is a complex anastomotic network of sensory fibres around the vertebral column and, in particular, around the margins of the intervertebral disc, penetrating the outer annulus and encircling blood vessels (Ashton *et al.* 1994). Substance P immunoreactive fibres can be demonstrated in these areas (Coppes *et al.* 1990). As a result, back pain is often diffuse and it can be difficult to locate the source of the problem from the distribution of symptoms.

Afferent impulses pass through the sensory neurones and the dorsal horn ganglion into the spinal cord. Complex neuropharmacological changes involving substance P, vasoactive intestinal peptide, and other neuropeptides are modulated after nociceptive stimulation of the spine (Weinstein 1986). As a result, pain felt in the back and in the lower limbs can arise due to a wide variety of different reasons. These include:

(1) radicular pain from direct nerve or nerve root compression;

(2) referred pain from damage of nociceptive receptors in the various spinal tissues with referral of symptoms into the lower limb;

(3) deafferentation pain resulting from a loss of the afferent connections of the spinal neurones;

(4) dysregulatory or reactive pain involving the pathophysiology of the afferent motor system with resulting hypertonus of postural muscles;

(5) psychosomatic pain such as pain enhanced by emotion, depression, or social distress.

In addition, recent work suggests central mechanisms by which the perception of pain is modulated. In particular, following nociceptive damage neuromorphological and neurochemical changes occur within the dorsal horn which may be long lasting so the sensation of pain may persist despite the lack of peripheral cause. The cells may be sensitized with increased sensitivity to minor stimulation and the message may spread within the spinal cord so that symptoms are perceived over a wide area (Dubner and Basbaum 1994).

The sympathetic chain runs alongside the vertebral column with multiple anastamosing sympathetic fibres and the peripheral sympathetic system accompanies blood vessels extending into the lower limbs. Many patients with chronic lower limb pain showed evidence of a sympathetic dysfunction syndrome. Most often this follows surgery to the lumbar spine although it can occur in association with mechanical problems (Sachs et al. 1993).

Pathological changes in the spine
Herniated intervertebral disc

Nuclear material can burst through the annulus fibrosus displacing and damaging the surrounding structures. Most often this occurs at the level of the L4/5 and L5/S1 intervertebral discs and the prolapse is usually in a posterolateral position, although sometimes it can be much nearer or in the midline. As a result, the prolapse may damage nerve roots in addition to ligaments, periostium, blood vessels, dura, and other tissues. The degrees of herniation are known as protrusion, extrusion, and sequestration according to their extent and whether the herniated material retains contact with the disc. Herniation most often develops after heavy load bearing with the spine in a flexed and twisted position. However, there is evidence that compression of a healthy lumbar disc will usually cause vertebral end plate fracture and that posterior and posterolateral herniation only occur when there is previous disc degeneration and fissure producing weakening of the annulus fibrosus (Jayson et al. 1973). The particular stress may have acted solely as the final precipitating cause of the problem.

The herniated material is often surrounded by an area of erythema and oedema. Usually it will gradually heal with fibrosis and shrinkage so that eventually the symptoms will improve. However, the annulus will be damaged and there is considerable risk of recurrent disc herniation and later development of secondary degenerative changes. The herniated material may press directly on nerves or compress the epidural veins producing venous obstruction and ischaemia over the relevant nerve. It may be complicated by thickening of the neural sheaths with perineural and intraneural fibrosis, and in turn by neuronal atrophy (Hoyland et al. 1989).

A more central, posterior prolapse can damage the posterior longitudinal ligament, which is innervated by the sinuvertebral nerve, and produce central back pain. A large, central posterior prolapse can compress the cauda equina leading to multiple nerve root damage in the lower limbs and sphincter disturbance.

There seems to be some predisposition towards development of herniation. Pathological studies in cadavers (Jayson and Barks 1973) and magnetic resonance scanning in life (Powell et al. 1986) show that when disc degeneration is present there is an increased risk of changes at multiple levels. There may be familial factors predisposing towards the development of this prolapse although no specific immunogenetic pattern has been identified (Postacchini et al. 1988). Environmental factors clearly play a part. Moderate amounts of physical activity are good for the back but lack of exercise and excessive spinal loads are both associated with increased risks of back pain, disc herniation, and degenerative disease of the spine (Videman et al. 1990).

The classical presentation of a herniated intervertebral disc is the acute onset of back pain followed by radicular pain, numbness, and paraesthesiae in one or other lower limb. The problem may develop after some stress and in particular bending, twisting, and lifting which, when combined, seem to produce the greatest risk. Most patients, however, will give a history of some preceding aching and stiffness in the back over the previous few days.

Clinical pattern

Direct damage to the nerve root will produce pain, numbness, and paraesthesiae as shown in Table 1. A small lateral herniation of the L4/5 disc will commonly affect the L5 nerve and herniation of the L5/S1 disc will affect the S1 root. However, a large prolapse, particularly if it is more central, may affect several nerve roots with widespread neurological symptoms and signs, and perhaps sphincter disturbance. There is considerable overlap in the distributions of the various nerve roots and the symptoms and physical signs only act as approximate guides to which disc has been damaged. In addition, pressure on ligaments and other soft tissues will produce referred pain felt in the buttock and lower limb. This is often confused with radicular symptoms due to nerve root damage. Referred pain is poorly defined and patients commonly have difficulty in describing its distribution. The symptoms of disc herniation are made worse by spinal movements and also by Valsalva manoeuvres such as coughing, sneezing, micturition, and defecation, which raise the cerebrospinal fluid pressure. Examination may show a sciatic scoliosis due to unilateral spasm of the paraspinal muscles. There may be severe limitation of spine movements but often in only one or two directions and in particular movements, including flexion. Palpation of the spine may show local areas of tenderness over the spine or sometimes elsewhere, such as the sacroiliac joints. Straight leg raising is limited with a positive Lasegue's test. The specific neurological signs of nerve root damage should be sought (Table 1).

Investigations

The blood sedimentation rate, plasma viscosity, and routine haematological and biochemical tests are normal. The cerebrospinal fluid obtained by lumbar puncture is usually normal but when there is a large prolapse with a spinal block the protein may be elevated.

Imaging techniques commonly used include:

Plain radiography
In an acute prolapse the spine is normal except perhaps for a scoliosis. When followed over several years, disc narrowing may develop and later on there may be secondary spondylotic changes.

Table 1 Principal changes used for identifying the sites of lumbar nerve root lesions (note that this table does not list the total distribution of each root)

Root	Superficial paraesthesiae and sensory change	Muscle weakness	Tendon reflex changes
L2	Upper thigh: anterior, medial, and lateral surfaces	Flexion and adduction of hip	None
L3	Anterior surface of lower thigh Anterior and medial surfaces of knee	Adduction of hip; extension of knee	Knee jerk possibly decreased
L4	Anteromedial surface of leg	Extension of knee; dorsiflexion and inversion of foot	Knee jerk decreased
L5	Anterolateral surface of leg, dorsum and medial surface of foot, especially dorsal surface of hallux	Extension and abduction of hip Flexion of knee; dorsiflexion of foot and toes, especially hallux	None
S1	Lateral border and sole of foot, back of heel, and lower calf	Flexion of knee; plantar flexion and eversion of foot	Ankle jerk decreased

Radiculography

Water-soluble radio-opaque dye is injected into the subarachnoid space at lumbar puncture. The dye penetrates along the nerve roots and obstruction to flow produced by a prolapse can be clearly identified (Fig. 2).

Discography

Direct injections may be made into an intervertebral disc. A normal, healthy disc will accept about 0.5 ml of fluid without producing significant symptoms. Larger volumes will be accepted by herniated discs with reproduction of symptoms. The pain may be relieved by injection of local anaesthetic. The radiographic appearances of disc herniation may be identified (Fig. 3).

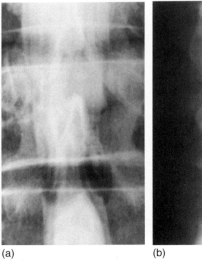
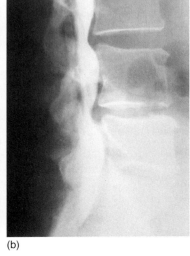

(a)   (b)

Fig. 2 Radiculogram showing (a) left sided L4/5 disc herniation and (b) smaller disc protrusion at L3/4.

Computed tomography (CT)

Herniation of a disc and the size and extent of nerve root involvement can be determined. This technique is sometimes use to complement radiculography when the details of nerve root damage may be clarified.

Magnetic resonance imaging (MRI)

This technique is becoming the investigation of choice. It has the advantage of avoiding the use of X-rays. It will demonstrate the size and extent of a disc herniation as well as degenerative change in the disc by loss of signal on the T_2 image and reduction of disc height (Fig. 4).

Lumbar spondylosis

Degenerative changes in the spine are common. Pathological studies have demonstrated their first appearance to be often around 25 years and they are almost universal in older people. Although patients with severe degrees of spondylosis more commonly develop back pain than those without, the correlation between back pain and radiographic evidence of lumbar spondylosis (Lawrence 1977) and MRI evidence of disc bulging and protrusion (Jensen *et al.* 1994) is poor. Because they are so common it may be better to call these appearances 'ageing change' rather than 'degenerative change' as the latter term conveys a perjorative image to patients and an implication of long-term problems, which is frequently not the case.

There is disorganization of the internal structure of the disc with the loss of the clear distinction between the nucleus pulposus and the annulus fibrosus. Cleft formation within the disc is common. The disc becomes narrowed with osteophytosis around the vertebral margins. Osteoarthritic changes may also develop in the apophyseal joints and it is commonly not clear whether such changes preceded or followed degeneration in the disc. Lumbar spondylosis with osteophytes and often minor degrees of disc herniation can directly impinge upon nerve roots and other structures. More commonly,

pathology. Guidelines for classifying these three groups have been published (Clinical Standards Advisory Group 1994).

Simple backache

Clinical criteria

Patients aged 20 to 55 years;

pain in the lumbosacral region, buttock, and thighs;

pain mechanical in nature varying with physical activity and with time;

patient is well.

Blood tests and lumbar spine radiographs are not indicated unless there is doubt about the diagnostic triage.

Such patients should be managed with simple analgesics such as paracetamol (aminocetophen). Occasionally they may require non-steroidal anti-inflammatory drugs. Narcotics should be avoided and never given for more than 2 weeks. Bed rest should only be prescribed if essential and then normally for only 1 to 3 days. This produces less disability than more prolonged periods of bed rest (Deyo *et al.* 1986).

It is always important to provide ergonomic advice on posture while standing, working, sitting, and lifting in order to protect the back against excessive loads.

Early physical activity is encouraged and reduces pain (Malmivaara *et al.* 1995). Indeed, continuing ordinary activities whenever possible seems to produce the best outcome (Malmivaara *et al.* 1995). Patients should be advised that exercise is not harmful and reduces pain, and that physical fitness is beneficial. The patient should be encouraged to return to work as soon as possible. Simple analgesic, or perhaps anti-inflammatory drugs, may be required and narcotics should be avoided if possible. With a regimen such as this, most patients will return to normal function rapidly.

The role of the therapist is restoration of function and encouraging the patient to be mobile. Physical exercise has an important role. The actual type of exercise is relatively unimportant. The benefits seem to lie in the quantity of exercise rather than in its specific nature. A positive attitude to activity and encouragement to return to work as soon as possible is all important. Early identification of psychosocial problems is important as they predict both the development of back pain (Croft, P., Papageorgiou, A.C., Ferry, S., Thomas, P., Jayson, M.I.V., and Silman, A.C., in press) and of acute back pain becoming chronic (Burton *et al.* 1995).

In order to remobilize the patient there is a wide variety of forms of physiotherapy and manual treatments. There is no evidence that heat, cold, ultrasound, or massage provide any benefit other than comfort at the time they are administered. Exercises and physical fitness are important and an incremental aerobic fitness programme of physical reconditioning is advised.

With this programme the vast majority of patients will recover within 6 weeks. If the pain still persists at 6 weeks, the diagnostic triage should be reviewed and investigations such as erythrocyte sedimentaion rate and a radiograph of the lumbar spine should be requested, if specifically indicated. For the patient with persistent back ache an active rehabilitation programme is necessary and at this stage referral may be required for a second opinion, rehabilitation, additional assessment, pain management, and, occasionally, surgery.

Manipulation is practised by physiotherapists, osteopaths, chiropractors, physicians, and surgeons. Although there has been some conflicting evidence from various trials, overall it appears that manipulation accelerates the rate of recovery in recent onset back pain, although not making any long-term difference to the outcome (Twomey and Taylor 1995). There is no evidence distinguishing the effects of manipulation by the various practitioners except that manipulation under general anaesthesia carries significant risk of neurological damage to the cauda equina (Haldeman and Rubinstein 1992).

Nerve root pain

Clinical criteria

Unilateral leg pain greater than back pain with the pain radiating to the feet or toes;

there may be numbness and paraesthesias in the same distribution;

reduced straight leg raising indicating nerve irritation;

motor sensory or reflex changes limited to one nerve root.

The management of such patients is similar to simple backache but undertaken more slowly. The recovery rate is not as good. If they fail to improve within 6 weeks, they may need more detailed assessment. Such patients may require scans and may be considered for surgery.

Possible serious spinal pathology

Clinical criteria

Aged under 20 or over 55 years;

previous trauma;

constant, progressive non-mechanical pain;

gradual onset —morning stiffness, limitation of movements in all directions and peripheral joint involvement, and other features suggesting ankylosing spondylitis or related disorders;

systemically unwell;

widespread neurological signs and cauda equina syndrome;

weight loss;

significant medical history such as previous carcinoma, steroid therapy, etc.

In such circumstances the patient will require intensive and appropriate investigations.

Recurrent back pain

Many patients have recurrent episodes of back pain which may be precipitated by lifting, twisting, and bending. A detailed understanding of the structure and function of the spine and the appropriate ways to protect it in a variety of physical activities combined with simple exercises to increase physical fitness and strengthen the abdominal and paraspinal muscles seem helpful in preventing further recurrences of back problems. The role of the physiotherapist is back education and the training may be formalized as a series of lessons in a 'back school' (Andersson 1992). The results of such training programmes are at least as good and probably better than conventional physiotherapy treatments.

Chronic back pain

Many patients suffer persistent pain in the back which may spread into the lower limbs. They may become very severely and permanently disabled. Many have previously undergone one or more spinal operations. Detailed assessments are required to elucidate the pathogenesis of the pain in individual subjects and to plan a treatment programme.

Chronic back pain may be due to:

(1) chronic disc herniation with persistent nerve root damage;

(2) severe degenerative change in the intervertebral discs;

(3) non-mechanical pathologies such as inflammatory spondylarthropathies, neoplasms, infections, Paget's disease, etc;

(4) incomplete discectomy or nerve decompression;

(5) recurrent or new disc prolapse;

(6) scar tissue forming around the nerves, perhaps as a reaction to surgery. Retained microscopic cotton debris from the swabs and patties used at operations may be of direct relevance here (Hoyland et al. 1988);

(7) arachnoiditis due to previous oil based myelography (Fig. 8);

(8) sympathetic syndromes with referred symptoms felt in the lower limb (Sachs et al. 1993);

(9) fibromyalgia;

(10) psychological factors—these play an important part in many patients, perpetuating the chronic nature of back pain. They include depression, anxiety, and compensation factors. Operant conditioning refers to the psychological reinforcement of pain behaviour and may include not only financial benefits but also sympathy and concern expressed by relatives, friends, medical, and paramedical staff;

(11) central nervous system modulation.

Assessment of the chronic back pain patient requires a very careful history and examination. The findings suggestive of a substantial non-organic component to the problem (Waddell et al. 1990) include:

(1) pain behaviour;

(2) pain reproduction on simulated movements of the spine such as pressure on the skull, rotation of the pelvis;

(3) restricted straight leg raising on formal testing but unrestricted distracted straight leg raising such as being able to sit up with the lower limbs extended;

(4) regional weakness or sensory disturbance in a non-neurological distribution;

(5) widespread superficial tenderness over the back.

Adequate management can only be undertaken after a thorough evaluation of each individual patient. This should include a very careful review of the medical history together with physical and psychological assessments. When specific pathologies can be identified they may be amenable to the appropriate therapy. For many patients this is not possible. Forms of treatment which may be beneficial include:

1. The use of appropriate medication—pure analgesics such as paracetamol, or perhaps codeine or its derivatives, or dextropropoxyphene are adequate for most patients. For some, particularly if there is a pain pattern suggestive of a secondary vascular/fibrotic/inflammatory element with pain aggravated by rest, non-steroidal anti-inflammatory drugs could be very helpful. Muscle relaxants, such as chlormezanone and baclofen, may be helpful when there is a major element of muscle spasm. Some patients describe a neuralgic element to the pain with electric shock sensations radiating down the lower limbs. This may be relieved by antiepileptic drugs such as carbamezepine or sodium valproate. Others have widespread, superficial paraesthesiae and tenderness and may respond to tricyclic antidepressant drugs such as amitriptyline. In the spinal stenosis syndrome there is some evidence (Porter and Hibbert 1983) that calcitonin may provide relief, perhaps by altering blood flow dynamics within the vertebral column.

2. Physiotherapy and ergonomic advice—this teaches the patients how to perform tasks within their physical capabilities and helps to give them confidence.

3. Local injections may be helpful for some people. They include:

   (a) Trigger point and local injections, usually of steroid and anaesthetic. Although commonly used, the evidence for their value is in doubt. Garvey et al. compared lignocaine alone, lignocaine plus steroid, needle insertion with no injection of material, and application of a vapour coolant spray followed by acupressure and found no differences between these treatments (Garvey et al. 1989).

   (b) Facet joint injections. No study has demonstrated any benefit from this technique.

   (c) Epidural injections. There have been a number of controlled studies with conflicting results. My opinion is that the technique is of value for the patient with radicular pain which has failed to resolve completely. Major adverse effects are rare but they are principally associated with dural puncture and intrathecal injection (Bogduk 1995).

   (d) Acupuncture. Although some studies suggest that needling has advantages over control treatment, all had major methodological flaws. There do not appear to be any differences in outcome with needling in the Chinese meridians compared with misplaced needling. The TENS machines are an alternative method of providing acupuncture.

4. Acupuncture and transcutaneous electrical nerve stimulation is believed to stimulate large afferent fibres blocking pain transmission through nociceptive small fibres. Despite widespread claims that this is of value, no trial has convincing demonstrated significant advantage to these techniques.

5. Patient education. Failure to provide an explanation of the problems leads to patient dissatisfaction (Deyo and Diehl 1986). The back education programme may be structured as a back school. Although appreciated by the patients, their specific value with regard to outcome is in doubt.

6. Lumbar corsets and belts. The evidence for their efficacy is confused. Many patients come to depend on their corsets and may develop severe restriction of spine movements. My own view is that they should not be in general use.

7. Activity modification. Bed rest should be avoided in chronic back pain. Patients should be encouraged to remain active and undertake a regular exercise programme to improve physical fitness (Frost *et al.* 1995).

8. Further surgery — the results of secondary and subsequent operations tend to be poor. Further surgery should only be contemplated in patients for whom there is a very clearly defined lesion causing symptoms for which there is an adequate surgical solution.

9. Multidisciplinary functional restoration programmes — these programmes are recent developments. Detailed assessment is required. Once the patient accepts that no further specific interventions will help they should enter a programme combining intensive physical activation, counselling for the understanding of pain and related problems, reducing the use of medication and health care, and dealing with depressive symptoms and anxiety together with encouragement to return to normal activities. These programmes are time consuming and expensive but effective in improving function, return to work rates, and work retention (Burke *et al.* 1994). Mayer *et al.* were able to return 87 per cent of patients to work after such a programme in contrast to 41 per cent of controls (Mayer *et al.* 1987).

Conclusion

In recent years, there has been a major increase of interest in the back pain problem. We now have much better understanding of the mechanisms of pathogenesis of various back pain syndromes and the reasons why the problems may persist and become chronic. With this better understanding, targeted therapy appears effective and lends hope of providing better control of this problem in the future.

References

Adams, P. and Muir, H. (1976). Qualitative changes with age of proteoglycans of human lumbar discs. *Annals of the Rheumatic Diseases*, 35, 289–96.

Andersson, G.B.G. (1992). Back schools. In *The lumbar spine and back pain* (4th edn) (ed. M.I.V. Jayson), pp. 409–16. Churchill Livingstone, Edinburgh.

Ashton, I.K. *et al.* (1994). Neuropeptides in the human intervertebral disc. *Journal of Orthopaedic Research*, 12, 186–92.

Biering-Sorenson, F. 1985. Risk of back trouble in individual occupations in Denmark. *Ergonomics*, 28, 51–60.

Bogduk, N. (1995). Epidural steroids. *Spine*, 20, 845–8.

Burke, S.A., Harms-Constas, C.K., and Aden, P.S. (1994). Return to work/work retention outcomes of a functional restoration programme. A multi-centre prospective study with a comparison group. *Spine*, 19, 1880–6.

Burton, A.K., Tillotson, K.M., Main, C.J., and Hollis, S. (1995). Psychosocial predictors of outcome in acute and subacute low back trouble. *Spine*, 20, 722–8.

Burton, C.V. (1990). Adhesive arachnoiditis. In *Neurological surgery III*. Vol II (ed. Youmans), pp. 2856–63. Saunders, Philadelphia.

Cats-Baril, W.L. and Frymoyer, J.W. (1991). The economics of spinal disorders. In *The adult spine: principles and practice* (ed. W. Frymoyer), pp. 85–105. New York. Raven Press.

Clinical Standards Advisory Group (1994). *Back pain*. HMSO, London.

Colhoun, E., McCall, I.W., Williams, I., and Cassar-Pollicino, V.N. (1988). Provocation discography as a guide to planning operations on the spine. *Journal of Bone and Joint Surgery*, 70B, 267–71.

Collee, G., Dijkmans, B.A.C., Vanderbrouke, J.P., Rouzing, P.M., and Cats, A. (1990). A clinical epidemiological study in low back pain: description of two clinical syndromes. *British Journal of Rheumatology*, 29, 354–7.

Cooper, R.G., Mitchell, W.S., Illingworth, K., St Clair Forbes, W., Gillespie, J.E., and Jayson, M.I.V. (1991). Role of epidural fibrosis and defective fibrinolysis in the persistence of post-laminectomy back pain. *Spine*, 16, 1044–8.

Coppes, M.H., Marani, E., Thomeer, R.T.W.M., Oudega, M., and Groen, G.J. (1990). Innervation of annulus fibrosus in low back pain. *Lancet*, 336, 189–90.

Crock, H.V. (1992). Isolated disc resorption. In *The lumbar spine and back pain* (4th edn) (ed. M.I.V. Jayson) pp 307–12. Churchill Livingstone, Edinburgh.

Croft, P. and Jayson, M.I.V. (1994). *Low back pain in the community and in hospitals*. A report to the Clinical Standards Advisory Group of the Department of Health. Prepared by the Arthritis and Rheumatism Council, Epidemiology Research Unit, Manchester.

Deyo, R.A. and Diehl, A.K. (1986). Patient satisfaction with medical care for low-back pain. *Spine*, 11, 28–30.

Deyo, R.A., Diehl, A.K., and Rosenthal, M. (1986). How many day's rest for acute low back pain? A randomised clinical trial. *New England Journal of Medicine*, 315, 1064–70.

Dooley, J.F., McBroom, R.J., Taguchi, T., and MacNab, I. (1988). Nerve root infiltration in the diagnosis of radicular pain. *Spine*, 13, 79–83.

Dubner, R. and Basbaum, A.I. (1994). Spinal dorsal horn plasticity following tissue or nerve injury. In *Textbook of pain* (ed. P.D. Wall and R. Melzak), pp. 225–41. Churchill Livingstone, Edinburgh.

Eyre, D.R. and Muir, H., (1976). Types I and II collagens in intervertebral discs. *Biochemical Journal*, 157, 267–70.

Fairbank, J.L.T., Park, W.M., McCall, I.W., and O'Brien, J.P. (1981). Apophyseal injection of local anaesthetic as a diagnostic aid in low back syndromes. *Spine*, 6, 598–605.

Frost, H., Klaber Moffett, J.L., Moser, J.S., and Fairbanks, J.C.T. (1995). Randomised controlled clinical trial for patients with chronic low back pain. *British Medical Journal*, 310, 151–4.

Garvey, T.A., Marks, M.R., and Wiesel, S.E. (1989). A prospective, randomized double-blind evaluation of trigger-point injection therapy for low-back pain. *Spine*, 14, 962–4.

Haldeman, S. and Rubinstein, S.M. (1992). Cauda equina syndrome in patients undergoing manipulation of the lumbar spine. *Spine*, 17, 1469–73.

Health and Safety Executive (1993). *Key fact sheet on back injuries to employees between 1987/88 and 90/91*. Health and Safety Executive, Statistical Services Unit.

Heliovaara, M. *et al.* (1987). Incidence and risk factors of herniated lumbar intervertegral disc or sciatica leading to hospitalization. *Journal of Chronic Diseases*, 40, 251–8.

Herbert, C.M., Lindberg, K.A., Jayson, M.I.V., and Bailey, A.J.(1975). Changes in the collagen of human intervertebral discs during ageing and degenerative disc disease. *Journal of Molecular Medicine*, 1, 79–91.

Hoyland, J.A., Freemont, A.J., and Jayson, M.I.V. (1988). Retained surgical debris in post laminectomy arachnoiditis. *Journal of Bone and Joint Surgery*, 70B, 659–62.

Hoyland, J.A., Freemont, A.J., and Jayson, M.I.V. (1989). Intervertebral foramen venous obstruction — a cause of peri-radicular fibrosis. *Spine*, 14, 558–68.

Hulshof, C. and van Zanten, B.V. (1987). Whole body vibration and back pain. *Archives of Occupational and Environmental Health*, 59, 205–20.

Jayson, M.I.V. and Barks, J.J. (1973). Structural changes in the intervertebral discs. *Annals of the Rheumatic Diseases*, 32, 10–15.

Jayson, M.I.V., Herbert, C.M., and Barks, J.S. (1973). Intervertebral discs, nuclear morphology and bursting pressures. *Annals of the Rheumatic Diseases*, 32, 308–15.

Jensen, M.C., Brant-Zawadzki, M.N., Obuchowski, N., Modic, M.T., Malkaisian, D., and Ross, J.S. (1994). Magnetic resonance imaging of the lumbar spine in people without back pain. *New England Journal of Medicine*, 331, 69–73.

Lawrence, J.S. (1977). Disc disorders. In *Rheumatism in populations*, pp. 68–97. Heinemann, London.

Makela, M. (1993). *Publications of the Social Insurance Institution.* The Research and Development Unit, Helsinki.

Malmivaara, A., Hakkinen, U., Aro, T., Heinrichs, M-L., Koskenniemi, L., Kuosma, E., Lappi, S., Paloheimo, R., Servo, C., Vaaranen, V., and Hemberg, S. (1995). The treatment of acute low back pain—bed rest, exercises or ordinary activity? *New England Journal of Medicine*, 332, 351–5.

Mayer, T.G., Gatchel, R.J., Mayer, H., Kishino, N.D., Keeley, J., and Mooney, V. (1987). A prospective two-year study of functional restoration in industrial low back injury. *Journal of the American Medical Association*, 258, 1763–7.

McDevitt, C.R. (1988). Proteoglycans of the intervertebral disc. In *Biology of the intervertebral disc* (ed. P. Ghosh), pp. 151–70. CRC Press, New York.

Mason, V. (1994). *The prevalence of back pain in Great Britain.* (A report prepared for the Department of Health by the Office of Population Censuses and Surveys, Social Survey Division based on the Omnibus Survey March, Apr, June 1993.) HMSO, London.

Mitchell, J.N. (1985). Low back pain and the prospects for employment. *Journal of Social and Occupational Medicine*, 35, 91–4.

Nachemson, A. (1992). Lumbar mechanics as revealed by lumbar intra-discal measurements. In *The Lumbar spine and back pain* (ed. M.I.V. Jayson), pp. 157–71. Churchill Livingstone, Edinburgh.

Ng, S.C.S., Weiss, J.B., Quinnel, R., and Jayson, M.I.V. (1986). Abnormal connective tissue degrading enzyme patterns in prolapsed intervertebral disc. *Spine*, 11, 695–701.

Papageorgiou, A., Croft, P., Jayson, M.I.V., and Silman, A. (1995). Estimating the prevalence of low back pain in the general population. Evidence from the South Manchester back pain survey. *Spine*, 20, 1889–94.

Porter, R.W. (1992). Spinal stenosis of the central and root canal. In *The lumbar spine and back pain* (ed. M.I.V. Jayson), pp. 313–32. Churchill Livingstone, Edinburgh.

Porter, R.W. and Hibbert, C. (1983). Calcitonin treatment for neurogenic claudication. *Spine*, 8, 585–92.

Porter, R.W. and Hibbert, C. (1986). Back pain and neck pain in four general practices. *Clinical Biomechanics*, 1, 7–10.

Porter, R.W., Hibbert, C., and Wellman, P. (1980). Backache and the lumbar spinal canal. *Spine*, 5, 99–105.

Postacchini, F., Lami, R., and Pugliese, O. (1988). Familial predisposition to discogenic low back pain. *Spine*, 12, 1403–6.

Powell, M.C., Wilson, M., Szypryt, P., Symonds, E.M., and Worthington, B.S. (1986). Prevalence of lumbar disc degeneration observed by magnetic resonance in symptomless women. *Lancet*, ii, 1366–7.

Riihimaki, H., Tola, S., Videman, T., and Hannin, K. (1989). Low back pain and occupation. *Spine*, 14, 204–9.

Sachs, B.T., Zindrick, M.R., and Beasley, R.D. (1993). Reflex sympathetic dystrophy after operative procedures on the lumbar spine. *Journal of Bone and Joint Surgery*, 75A, 721–5.

Troup, J.D.G. and Edwards, F.C. (1985). *Manual handling and lifting: an information and literature review with special reference to the back.* HMSO, London.

Twomey, L. and Taylor, J. (1995). Exercise and manipulation in the treatment of low back pain. *Spine*, 20, 615–9.

Vernon Roberts, B. (1992). Age related and degenerative pathology of the intervertebral disc and apophyseal joints. In *The lumbar spine and back pain* (4th edn) (ed. M.I.V. Jayson), pp. 17–41. Churchill Livingstone, Edinburgh.

Videman, T., Nurminen, M., and Troup, J.D.G. (1990). Lumbar spinal pathology in cadaveric material in relation to history of back pain, occupation and physical loading. *Spine*, 15, 728–40.

Waddell, G. (1987). A new clinical model for the treatment of low back pain. *Spine*, 12, 632–44.

Waddell, G., Mc Cullough, J.A., Kummel, E., and Venner, R.M. (1980). Non organic physical signs in low back pain. *Spine*, 5, 117–25.

Walsh, K. *et al.* (1992). Low back pain in eight areas of Britain. *Journal of Epidemiology and Community Health*, 26, 227–30.

Weinstein, J. (1986). Mechanisms of spinal pain. *Spine*, 11, 999–1001.

Weiss, J.B. and McLaughlin, B. (1993). Activation of gelatinase-A and reactivation of the gelatinase-A inhibitor complex by endothelial cell stimulating angiogenesis factor. *Journal of Physiology*, 456, 49.

Wiltse, L.L. and Rothman, S.L.G. (1990). Lumbar and lumbosacral spondylolisthesis: classification, diagnosis and natural history. In *The lumbar spine* (eds J.N. Weinstein and S.W. Weisel), pp. 471–99. Saunders, Philadelphia.

Wright, D., Barrow, S., Fisher, A., Hull, S.D., and Jayson, M.I.V. (1995). Influence of physical, psychological and behavioural factors on consultations for back pain. *British Journal of Rheumatology*, 34, 156–61.

Wyke, B. (1987). The neurology of low back pain. In *The lumbar spine and back pain* (3rd edn) (ed. M.I.V. Jayson), pp. 56–99. Churchill Livingstone, Edinburgh.

5.18.2 Cervical pain syndromes

Allan I. Binder

Introduction

The vast majority of patients with neck pain have degenerative or mechanical lesions. 'Cervical spondylosis' is often used to describe neck pain of a mechanical nature, but the term is variably applied to include soft tissue, disc, and degenerative bony lesions (Resnick 1985). Furthermore, the boundary between 'normal' ageing and disease is unclear. The pathology of cervical spondylosis is assumed to be identical to lumbar spondylosis, but this similarity has been questioned (Bland and Boushey 1990). Less research has been performed into cervical than lumbar pain, as severe disability is less common with cervical disease.

This chapter will concentrate on the common mechanical and degenerative pain syndromes that predominantly affect the cervical spine and the principles of their treatment. Other conditions which can cause neck pain will be considered in more detail in the relevant chapters devoted to the particular diseases.

Epidemiology

About 10 per cent of the adult population have neck pain at any one time (Lawrence 1969; Hadler 1985), with symptoms often being associated with specific occupations or sporting activities (Holt 1972). While this prevalence is similar to that of low back pain, to lose time from work is unusual, and under 1 per cent of patients develop neurological deficit. As so many patients with neck pain never seek medical care, the true prevalence of chronic disease is uncertain.

Functional anatomy of the cervical spine

The cervical spine is the most mobile and least stable part of the human spine, consisting of seven vertebrae connected by five intervertebral discs. There are 37 separate articulations (Bland and Boushey 1990), and a complex system of ligaments and muscles, which with the varying shapes of individual vertebrae, and different methods of articulation, are responsible for the myriad movements of the head and neck. Any of these structures can be the source of pain.

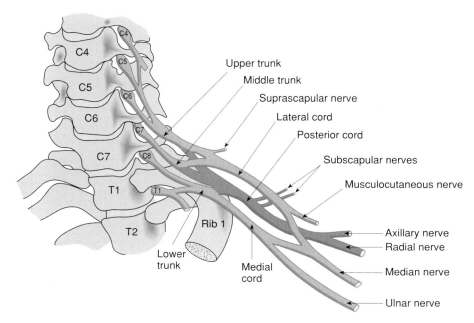

Fig. 1 Diagram showing the nerve roots (C4 to T1) forming the brachial plexus, with the peripheral nerves which arise from the plexus.

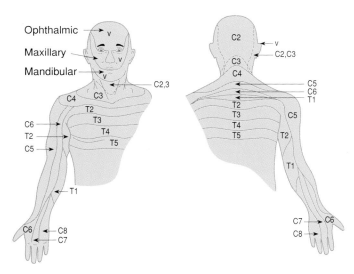

Fig. 2 Dermatomal distribution of the cervical and upper thoracic nerves which reflect the radicular pattern of nerve root lesions.

The vertebral arteries pass close to the zygapophyseal joints, immediately anterior to the emerging cervical nerve roots. The pre-ganglionic sympathetic nerve fibres run closely adherent to the carotid and vertebral vessels, to synapse with the stellate, middle, and superior cervical ganglia. The postganglionic sympathetic fibres then separate into three directions: some fibres go to the upper limbs to provide autonomic control of circulation, sweating, and proprioception; other fibres re-enter the spinal cord via the intervertebral foramina to synapse in the vestibular apparatus, cerebellum, thalamus, and hypothalamus; and some fibres pass upward with the vertebral and carotid arteries to the brain (Bland and Boushey 1990). Involvement of the vertebral arteries and sympathetic nerves in the degenerative process may explain many of the unusual features associated with disease of the cervical spine.

The lack of room in the spinal canal between C4 and T2 is due to the enlargement of the cord in this region. As degenerative changes are also most frequent and severe between C5 and T1 (Hayashi *et al.* 1988), compression of the cord usually develops at this site. Inflammatory arthropathies in contrast, have a predilection for involvement of the atlantoaxial and upper cervical spine. Minor congenital spinal abnormalities increase the risk of degenerative change (Hensinger 1991), and there is a remarkable similarity in the pattern of degenerative disease in monozygous twins (Palmer *et al.* 1984), possibly reflecting the similarity in the shape of their vertebrae.

The anterior and posterior nerve roots from C4 to T1 exit through the dural root sleeves, and traverse the intervertebral foramina. They then merge to form the brachial plexus (Fig. 1), which lies between the clavicle and first rib, in close proximity to the subclavian vessels. The neurovascular bundle is susceptible to compression at various sites in the thoracic outlet, which lies between the neck and axilla. Cervical nerves have a dermatomal representation (Fig. 2), which explains the radicular pattern of symptoms in the upper limbs caused by impingement on nerve roots.

Aetiology of neck pain

Although 'cervical spondylosis' accounts for most cases of neck pain, there are many other causes of pain which need to be excluded (Table 1). The cervical spine is frequently involved in polymyalgia rheumatica, rheumatoid arthritis, and other arthropathies, and neck pain can result from serious local pathology, such as infection or malignancy. It is also often the site of referral of pain from distant sources (Table 2).

Cervical spondylosis

Pathology

With ageing, degenerative change usually develops in the cervical spine (Gore *et al.* 1986). This is readily apparent on radiographs of

Table 1   Causes of neck pain

Soft tissue lesions
    Acute neck strain
    Posture-related neck pain
    Psychogenic — 'tension', anxiety, depression
    Occupation and sport-related neck pain
    'Fibrositis/fibromyalgia' and pain-amplification syndromes
    Torticollis and wry-neck
    Trauma — musculoligamentous injury, 'whiplash' syndrome

Degenerative and mechanical lesions
    Cervical spondylosis
    Cervical disc prolapse
    Diffuse idiopathic skeletal hyperostosis (DISH) and ossification
        of the posterior longitudinal ligament (see text)

Inflammatory arthropathies
    Rheumatoid arthritis
    Ankylosing spondylitis and spondylarthropathies
    Juvenile chronic arthropathy
    Polymyalgia rheumatica
    Other arthropathies

Metabolic bone disease
    Paget's disease, osteoporosis, osteomalacia
    Crystal arthropathies — gout, pseudogout
    Fibrous dysplasia

Infection
    Osteomyelitis of cervical vertebra
    Tuberculosis

Malignancy
    Primary tumours
    Secondary tumours and pathological fracture
    Myeloma, lymphoma, blood dyscrasias

Brachial plexus lesions
    Idiopathic cryptogenic brachial neuropathy
    Thoracic-outlet syndromes — e.g. cervical rib
    Trauma — motor cycle injury

Referred pain (see Table 2)

Table 2   Sites of referred pain to the neck

Acromioclavicular joint, temporomandibular joint, teeth
Heart — angina pectoris, myocardial infarction
Aorta — aneurysm
Pharynx — infection, tumour
Lung — bronchogenic carcinoma, Pancoast tumour, apical lesion
Abdomen — disease of the gallbladder, stomach, oesophagus
    (including hiatus hernia) and pancreas
Diaphragm — subphrenic abscess
Central nervous system — migraine, 'tension' headache, tumour,
    posterior fossa lesion, meningitis, arachnoiditis
Lymph node — cervical lymphadenitis
Shoulder — frozen shoulder, reflex sympathetic dystrophy

most adults over the age of 30 years. The term 'cervical spondylosis' refers to this progressive degenerative process, which affects all levels of the cervical spine (Lestini and Wiesel 1989), but with more severe changes at the lower levels (Hayashi et al. 1988). There is a sequential change in the intervertebral discs, with osteophytosis of the vertebral bodies and changes in the facet joints and laminal arches. There is a continuum from 'normal' ageing to the overtly pathological state. The correlation between the degree of radiological change and the presence and severity of pain is poor (Van der Donk et al. 1991), and hence there is disagreement on the exact definition of cervical spondylosis.

With increase in age, there is a steady decrease in the degree of hydration of the intervertebral discs. Degeneration follows and radiolucent nitrogen-filled spaces (vacuum disc phenomenon) may develop within the disc. When present, these spaces confirm the degenerative nature of the process, and are reassuring, as they exclude a diagnosis of infection (Resnick 1985). With progression of the ageing process, loss of disc height and bony sclerosis follow. Osteophytosis often then develops, with degenerative changes (osteoarthritis) in the nearby zygapophyseal joints and other articulating surfaces. Involvement of the spinal ligaments in the degenerative process can lead to a loss of stability, which is an important factor in causing myelopathy in elderly patients.

Clinical assessment

Detailed history and examination will usually confirm the degenerative nature of the condition or alert one to a need to exclude more serious pathology. Assessment of the shoulder joints is also necessary to determine if there is coexisting shoulder pathology (Hawkins et al. 1990), although cervical pathology itself can cause painful limitation in the range of shoulder flexion and abduction above 90°.

Symptoms

Pain

This is the most common symptom of cervical pathology, and is usually poorly localized to the neck and shoulders when arising from deep structures, such as ligaments, muscles, joints, discs, or bone. The pain can however, be clearly defined and in a dermatomal distribution when caused by irritation of the nerve roots (Fig. 2). Pain arising from structures of the cervical spine is characteristically altered (aggravated or relieved) by their movement. The causes of neck pain are shown in Table 1.

Pain is most often referred to the occiput, nuchal muscles, and superior aspect of the shoulders. Heaviness or aching of the upper limbs also reflects cervical origin, and the pain can closely mimic soft tissue lesions of the shoulder, elbow, and wrist (Gunn and Milbrandt 1976; Murray-Leslie and Wright 1976). Retro-orbital and temporal pain suggest referral from the upper cervical levels (C1 to C3). Temporal pain when associated with tenderness can be misinterpreted as evidence of giant-cell arteritis. Pain can also be referred to the upper thoracic spine and interscapular areas. Some patients, especially with lesions of C6 and C7 complain of anterior chest pain, which closely mimics coronary ischaemia (Brodsky 1985). Pseudoangina of this type is sometimes associated with local tenderness of the chest wall. There is particular diagnostic difficulty in patients with a combination of both coronary insufficiency and cervical spondylosis, as anginal pain is more likely to radiate to the neck in patients with symptomatic cervical spondylosis. Coronary angiography is the key investigation in the assessment of the severity of the cardiac lesion in these cases.

Stiffness
This is a common accompaniment of ageing, degeneration, and many vertebral diseases, and can be reversible or irreversible.

Dizziness
This may occur as a result of involvement of the vertebral arteries, especially in the presence of severe degenerative spinal disease. Atheroma and disturbance of flow in the vertebral vessels may contribute to the development of dizziness in older patients. Vertigo and faintness caused by vertebrobasilar disease is nearly always accompanied by other focal symptoms of transient ischaemia of the brainstem or occipital lobes. In some patients with cervical pathology, tinnitus and gait disturbance (Sudarsky and Ronthal 1983) can occur, as a result of irritation of the sympathetic nerves.

Occipital headache
This is a common manifestation of cervical degenerative disease, especially when the disease affects the upper cervical levels. Occipital neuralgia is another cause of occipital pain in some patients. Edmeads (1988) discussed the controversy over the importance of disease of the cervical spine in the aetiology of non-occipital headache; Wober-Bingol et al. (1992) found no link, but Nagasawa et al. (1993) found a strong association.

Blurring of vision and diplopia
These symptoms, where associated with neck movement can result from cervical pathology, and have been attributed to irritation of the sympathetic nerve supply to the eye.

Dysphagia
This can be caused by irritation of the cranial or sympathetic nerves, muscular spasm, or compression of the oesophagus by large anterior osteophytes (Sobol and Rigual 1984).

Table 3	Rarer symptoms arising from cervical spine pathology

Visual — blurring, diplopia, retro-orbital pain

Auditory — tinnitus, nerve deafness, earache, poor balance

Intestinal — dysphagia, nausea, vomiting, diarrhoea

Cardiac — 'pseudoangina', dyspnoea, palpitations

Respiratory — cough, dyspnoea, sneezing

Central nervous system — syncope, 'drop attacks', vertebro-basilar insufficiency, speech disturbance, migraine

Paraesthesia and sensory loss
Numbness and tingling is usually vague and ill-defined in cervical spondylosis, but can be precise, following the clear segmental dermatomal distribution of nerve entrapment (see Radiculopathy below). The symptoms are often affected by neck movement, or are postural, being worse at night or with specific activities. Lesions of C1 to C3 can cause paraesthesia affecting the face, head, and tongue. Involvement of the C4 root gives symptoms referred to the superior aspect of the shoulder, and C5 to T1 lesions give numbness in the upper limb (see Fig. 2).

Weakness
Mechanical disease of the cervical spine most typically gives a subjective feeling of heaviness or weakness, especially affecting the hands, but without true weakness on formal testing. Objective muscle weakness, wasting, and fasciculation in the absence of systemic upset suggests a radiculopathy, thoracic-outlet syndrome, or neuropathy of the brachial plexus. Abnormality of gait due to spasticity of the lower limbs suggests myelopathy.

Rare manifestations
Unusual features sometimes resulting from pathology of the cervical spine are shown in Table 3. Most of these symptoms result from irritation of the sympathetic nerves, but the clue to their vertebral origin is reproducibility with neck movement.

Signs

Tenderness
When due to degenerative disease, tenderness is poorly localized and of variable severity. It is usually worse in the lower cervical region, and may be associated with muscle spasm. Tender myofascial trigger points are a characteristic feature of the 'fibrositis/fibromyalgia' syndrome (Smythe 1986), but also occur with disease of the facet joints. Exquisite localized tenderness over a vertebral body may suggest osteomyelitis or malignancy, particularly if the patient has features of systemic upset or abnormality of blood tests such as full blood count, erythrocyte sedimentation rate, C-reactive protein, or protein electrophoresis.

Limitation of movement
This is a feature of ageing and degeneration and may be otherwise asymptomatic or accompanied by pain. Severe irreversible loss of range particularly on lateral flexion and rotation occurs with cervical

spondylosis, but is more characteristic of the spondylarthropathies and diffuse idiopathic skeletal hyperostosis (**DISH**). Reversible stiffness, worse in the early morning, is more suggestive of polymyalgia rheumatica or an inflammatory arthropathy than of a degenerative lesion.

Neurological deficit

Neurological abnormalities are characteristic of radiculopathy, but also occurs in thoracic-outlet syndromes and neuropathy of the brachial plexus (see below).

Radiological assessment (see also Chapter 4.9.1)

Routine radiographs of the anteroposterior and lateral spine are sufficient to indicate the severity of bone and disc pathology. A through-mouth view to outline the odontoid peg, when combined with flexion/extension radiographs, will demonstrate existing subluxation. Oblique views of the cervical spine will show the intervertebral foramina, and are useful in patients suspected of having a radiculopathy (Fig. 3). Loss of cervical lordosis on the lateral radiograph in patients with neck pain is usually ascribed to muscle spasm, but this association has been questioned (Helliwell et al. 1994).

Myelography, computed tomography (**CT**), and CT-myelography, have greatly improved the radiological assessment of cervical disease, especially at the upper cervical levels, which are hard to visualize on routine radiographs.

Magnetic resonance imaging (**MRI**) is less invasive and equally reliable as CT-myelography for the visualization of cervical abnormalities (Nagata et al. 1990), and is the radiological investigation of

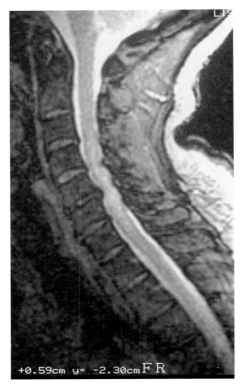

Fig. 4   MRI scan showing loss of height and signal affecting several discs, with multisegmental spondylotic bars. Compression of the cord is noted by protrusion of the C5/6 disc with myelopathic changes in the cord.

choice (Kramer et al. 1991), giving detailed information about the spinal cord, bones, discs, and soft tissue structures (Figs 4 and 5). MRI is particularly valuable in demonstrating congenital abnormalities, cord tumours, demyelination, and disc lesions. Degenerative

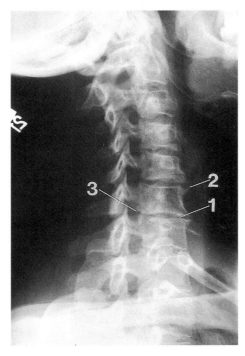

Fig. 3   Oblique radiograph of the cervical spine in a patient with cervical spondylosis, showing the loss of disc height (1), anterior osteophytosis (2), and foraminal narrowing (3).

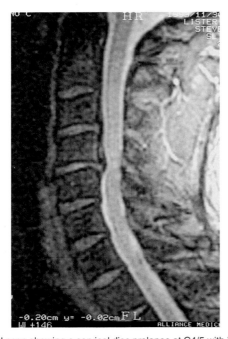

Fig. 5   MRI scan showing a cervical disc prolapse at C4/5 with impingement upon the cervical cord and secondary myelopathic changes in the cord itself.

vertebral changes are well demonstrated, but as they occur normally with ageing, need to be interpreted with care. Asymptomatic people often show important pathological lesions, such as narrowing of the disc space, osteophytosis, or even compression of the spinal cord (Boden *et al.* 1990), and the frequency of abnormal scans in asymptomatic people increases with age. Boden *et al.* (1990) and Lehto *et al.* (1994) have emphasized that decisions about surgery should be based on clinical indications with the support of the MRI findings, and not on radiological data alone. Similar false-positive studies have been described with plain radiography, CT (Wiesel *et al.* 1984), and all other radiological techniques.

Electrodiagnostic studies

Electromyography, nerve conduction studies, and somatosensory evoked potentials may help in the elucidation of the diagnosis, especially where primary neurological disease or polymyositis need to be differentiated from radiculopathy or myelopathy secondary to degenerative vertebral disease (Dvorak *et al.* 1990). Specific neurophysiological findings have been described in cervical spondylosis associated with myelopathy or radiculopathy (Yiannikas *et al.* 1986), but there is no consensus as to their reliability or diagnostic value, particularly in uncomplicated cervical spondylosis. Magnetic stimulation of the motor cortex (Di Lazzaro *et al.* 1992) and spinal cord evoked potentials (Baba *et al.* 1993a) have more value in the assessment of myelopathic patients, but at best, the electrodiagnostic techniques only provide supportive evidence to clinical and radiological findings.

Other tests

Other tests such as full blood count, erythrocyte sedimentation rate, C-reactive protein, protein electrophoresis, liver function tests, urate, rheumatoid factor, and bone scan may be necessary to exclude other causes of neck pain (Tables 1 and 2).

Complications of cervical spondylosis

Cervical myelopathy

The relatively tight fit of the spinal cord in the lower cervical region, as a result of the natural expansion of the cervical cord, accounts for an increased risk of development of a myelopathy at this site.

Myelopathy can develop *de novo*, or can occur in patients with known cervical spondylosis, particularly in the presence of a congenitally narrow spinal canal (Fukui *et al.* 1990). With progressive degeneration and resulting osteophytosis and instability, pressure on the spinal cord can develop.

In elderly patients, myelopathy can result from compression of the spinal cord, disturbed blood supply, or a combination of both factors. Disc protrusion, posterior osteophyte formation, and retrolisthesis (posterior slide) due to ligamentous laxity, contribute to age-associated spondylotic spinal compression (Hayashi *et al.* 1988). Even when the static spinal canal diameter is adequate, many elderly patients show significant and progressive 'dynamic' spinal stenosis (Hayashi *et al.* 1988; Fukui *et al.* 1990), which can be demonstrated (Jinkins *et al.* 1986) by a comparison of flexion and extension CT or MRI scans.

Table 4 Differential diagnosis of cervical myelopathy

Cervical spondylotic myelopathy

Other causes of compressive cervical myelopathy
  Central disc prolapse
  Congenital spinal canal stenosis
  Inflammatory arthropathy, especially rheumatoid arthritis
  DISH and ossification of the posterior longitudinal ligament (see text)
  Crystal diseases—gout, pseudogout
  Paget's disease
  Haematoma, trauma
  Infection—tuberculosis, spinal epidural abscess
  Tumour—meningioma, neurofibroma, lymphoma, leukaemia, myeloma, secondaries, pathological fracture
  Radiation myelopathy

Primary spinal cord disease
  Spinal multiple sclerosis
  Subacute combined degeneration of the cord
  Motor neurone disease (amyotrophic lateral sclerosis)
  Hereditary spastic paraplegia and other genetic disorders
  Infective or inflammatory myelitis, e.g. sarcoid, systemic lupus, and HIV infection
  Syringomyelia

Parasagittal cranial meningioma

Anterior spinal artery syndrome (onset usually sudden)

In young patients, a sudden onset of myelopathy or radiculopathy suggests cervical disc prolapse (see below). Cervical myelopathy can also result from vertebral diseases such as osteomyelitis, malignancy, and crystal arthropathy, and intramedullary disease can present with similar symptoms (Table 4.)

Cervical myelopathy typically presents with a slowly progressive disability over a period of weeks or months, although the onset can be sudden, especially when caused by trauma or central disc prolapse. The most common, early manifestations of myelopathy are clumsiness, weakness or dysaesthesia of the hands, or gait disturbance due to upper motor-neurone abnormality in the lower limbs.

Numbness or tingling in the hands is poorly localized, unless radiculopathy is also present. There is usually no gross sensory deficit, but blunting of light touch, pin-prick, and temperature sensation can occur. Stereoanaesthesia, and isolated loss of position sense in the hands, is also sometimes seen, particularly in high cervical lesions. Clumsiness or weakness of the hands may rarely be associated with variable degrees of wasting and evidence of lower motor-neurone abnormality at the level of the lesion. Characteristic features in the legs are of a spastic paraparesis, and in elderly patients, undiagnosed cervical myelopathy is an important case of gait disturbance (Sudarsky and Ronthal 1983).

Tendon reflexes are often reduced in the arms and increased in the legs with up-going plantar responses and ankle clonus, although the balance is dependent on the level of the lesion. Inversion of the supinator jerk (reduced or absent supinator reflex with brisk finger flexion when tapping over the lower radius), with a brisk triceps jerk, suggests involvement of the spinal cord at the C5/6 level. A brisk finger-flexion reflex (on tapping the examiner's own fingers when placed over the flexor surface of the terminal phalanges), and a positive Hoffman's sign (brisk thumb flexion when the distal phalanx of the middle finger is flicked into extension) also suggests hyperreflexia. Sphincter control is usually well maintained in cervical myelopathy complicating cervical spondylosis.

Neck pain may not be a prominent feature of myelopathy, and when present, its mechanism of production is complex and poorly understood. The cervical lesion is often multisegmental (Fig. 4), and in some cases there is a large discrepancy between the sensory level on clinical examination and the true level of cord compression (Simmons et al. 1986).

Shooting electric pain down the spine, arms, or legs, or temporary neurological deficit when the head is flexed (Lhermitte phenomenon) may be mentioned by the patient. Great caution (and prior radiography) is necessary when attempting to confirm the presence of this sign, as permanent deterioration in the neurological condition may follow its performance. Lhermitte phenomenon is usually a sign of cervical myelopathy of an inflammatory type (typically multiple sclerosis), but can be due to compressive, or rarely other (e.g. vitamin B_{12} deficiency) causes.

MRI (Fig. 4) is the investigation of choice in patients with suspected myelopathy (Kramer et al. 1991; Okada et al. 1994), although CT-myelography also has value. The anteroposterior or sagittal diameter of the canal on radiological investigation is a useful indicator of possible myelopathy, and compression of the cord is likely if the diameter at any level is 10 mm or less (Murone 1974). With a diameter above 13 mm, compressive symptoms rarely occur solely on the basis of degenerative disease. Atrophy of the spinal cord on CT-myelography (Jinkins et al. 1986), or intrinsic spinal cord damage on MRI (Fig. 4), especially after myelopathic decompression (Nagata et al. 1990; Batzdorf and Flannigan 1991; Matsuda et al. 1991) are associated with a less favourable outcome.

The most sensitive neurophysiological investigation in the assessment of patients with cervical myelopathy is somatosensory evoked potentials, especially when done in both upper and lower limbs (Yiannikas et al. 1986). However, these tests rarely add much to the evaluation, particularly in difficult cases.

Cervical radiculopathy

Nerve root compression as a result of cervical spondylosis usually occurs at the C5 to C7 level with lesions being single or multiple, and uni- or bilateral.

Acute radiculopathy in the young usually follows trauma or lateral prolapse of a disc. In middle-aged and elderly patients, asymptomatic osteophytic encroachment gradually narrows the nerve root foramina until trivial trauma is sufficient to precipitate acute or subacute radiculopathy. Chronic radiculopathy may arise insidiously, or may follow the more acute syndromes. As chronic radicular syndromes are

Table 5 Differential diagnosis of cervical radiculopathy

Cervical spondylotic radiculopathy

Other causes of compressive cervical radiculopathy
  Lateral disc prolapse
  Inflammatory arthropathy, e.g. rheumatoid arthritis
  Trauma, haematoma
  Arachnoiditis
  Infection
  DISH and ossification of the posterior longitudinal ligament (see text)
  Tumour—primary, secondary, Pancoast tumour of lung

Brachial plexus and thoracic-outlet syndromes

Peripheral nerve and 'double-crush' syndromes

Complete rotator-cuff tear and reflex sympathetic dystrophy

Motor neurone disease and other primary spinal cord diseases (see Table 4)

usually due to degenerative disease, they can be associated with myelopathy.

Neurological features follow a segmental distribution in the upper limb (see Fig. 2). Sensory symptoms such as shooting pain, paraesthesia, and hyperaesthesia are more common than motor weakness or a change in the reflexes. Arm weakness, when present, is of a lower motor-neurone type, and may be accompanied by a loss of reflex (biceps and supinator jerk in C5/6 lesions; triceps jerk in C7 lesions).

Radicular pain can be exacerbated by manoeuvres that stretch the affected root, or by an increase in intrathoracic or intra-abdominal pressure, as occurs with coughing, sneezing, or the Valsalva manoeuvre. If sustained shoulder abduction induces a temporary relief in radicular pain, a C6 lesion can be expected (Fast et al. 1989). This test has value both diagnostically and as part of a conservative treatment regimen (Farmer and Wisneski 1994).

Oblique cervical radiographs often demonstrate narrowing of the nerve root foramina (Fig. 3) in patients with radiculopathy (Pyhtinen and Laitinen 1993). Electromyography may show abnormalities in patients with clinical signs of root compression, and additional information can sometimes be obtained from studying superficial radial sensory-evoked potentials. However, these techniques are of limited value where symptoms of radiculopathy occur without objective signs (Yiannikas et al. 1986).

Cervical radiculopathy (Table 5) can rarely be caused by malignant tumours, such as Pancoast tumour (Vargo and Flood 1990), or nasopharyngeal malignancies, particularly when accompanied by bony infiltration. There is often difficulty in differentiating cervical spondylosis with myelopathy or radiculopathy from primary neurological diseases, such as syringomyelia, motor neurone disease (amyotrophic lateral sclerosis), or tumour, particularly when unrelated osteoarthrosis of the cervical spine coexists (see Tables 4 and 5).

Other important mechanical pain syndromes

Cervical disc prolapse

Herniation of a cervical disc is a common cause of neck, shoulder, and arm pain in the younger patient. It typically presents as a sudden onset of neck pain with associated muscle spasm, followed by radicular symptoms and signs in the upper limb. It may follow trivial trauma or awkward movements of the neck, but in many cases there is no obvious cause. Some patients give a history of preceding mechanical cervical pain, and manipulation or chiropractic therapy can precipitate the acute disc prolapse. The lesions almost always affect the lower cervical levels.

Lateral disc protrusion, which is more common, results in radiculopathy affecting the C7 root in 70 per cent of cases, the C6 root in 20 per cent, and the C5 or C8 roots in the remaining 10 per cent of cases (Yoss et al. 1957). The site of pain and the neurological features depend on the level of the lesion (Smythe 1994; Nakajima and Hirayama 1995), but the syndromes are often incomplete. Limitation of cervical range is usual, and pain can be aggravated by movement (especially hyperextension), coughing, and sneezing, and relieved by traction on the neck.

Central disc prolapse, if large, causes myelopathy (Fig. 5), and when painless may simulate degenerative syndromes of the spinal cord, such as motor neurone disease or multiple sclerosis (see Table 4). MRI (Vanderburgh and Kelly 1993) or CT-myelography are essential to differentiate disc prolapse or other causes of compressive myelopathy from intrinsic disease of the spinal cord, even when the latter is considered more likely.

Disc prolapse is much less common in the thoracic spine and is difficult to diagnose clinically, unless myelopathy or radiculopathy intervene.

Diffuse idiopathic skeletal hyperostosis (DISH, Forestier's disease, ankylosing hyperostosis)

This common disorder of unknown aetiology is most often diagnosed in middle-aged or elderly white males, who show an ossifying diathesis. Patients develop flowing ossification along the anterior and lateral aspects of the spine, bridging between vertebrae, but with preservation of normal disc heights. The condition affects the thoracic spine most severely, but can also occur in the cervical and lumbar regions. The lesions start at the ligamentous insertions (entheses), with progression of the flowing osteophytes along the ligaments. Similar ossification is also found at entheses along the pelvis and other parts of the skeleton.

Severe limitation of cervical spine movement usually develops without any other symptoms (Boachie-Adjei and Bullough 1987). However, some patients present with pain, myelopathy, and less commonly, radiculopathy. Large anterior osteophytes in the cervical region can also cause dysphagia owing to oesophageal obstruction. If anterior osteophytes due to cervical spondylosis or DISH are suspected as the cause of the dysphagia, barium swallow is the preferred method of initial assessment, as endoscopy carries some risk of inadvertent oesophageal perforation (Kristensen et al. 1988). The ossification progresses more rapidly at mobile compared with immobile segments (Suzuki et al. 1991).

Ossification of the posterior longitudinal ligament

This is probably a variant of DISH (Hukuda et al. 1983), or is closely associated with it (Resnick et al. 1978). It is most frequently found in Japanese or other Asian patients, but is occasionally found in all ethnic groups. Like DISH, it occurs most often in middle-aged and elderly males, with a majority of cases producing no symptoms. However, in association with congenital and degenerative vertebral abnormalities, even trivial trauma can precipitate cervical myelopathy or radiculopathy. The ossification can be difficult to detect on plain radiographs, and both MRI (Otake et al. 1992; Baba et al. 1995) and CT scanning have value where the diagnosis is suspected. Calcification of the ligamentum flavum and posterior longitudinal ligament can also result from calcium pyrophosphate crystal deposition (pseudogout), confirmed on biopsy in patients having surgery for compressive myelopathy (Brown et al. 1991; Baba et al. 1993b).

Soft tissue syndromes considered to be 'mechanical'

Spasm, postural, and anxiety/tension-related neck pain

Most adults suffer transient neck pain and stiffness, which is attributed to awkward posture of the neck, especially during sleep. The pathology is uncertain and the condition is self-limiting within days. Occupations and hobbies which involve heavy lifting or unusual positions of the neck are a cause of recurrent pain of this type. Anxiety and tension can manifest as episodic or chronic neck pain in susceptible individuals. Poor posture of the cervical and thoracic spine (Griegel-Morris et al. 1992), which can cause muscle spasm, and hence traction on the nerve roots, may explain these symptoms. The interaction between cervical spondylosis, tension, and the fibrositis/pain-amplification syndrome needs further clarification.

'Fibrositis/fibromyalgia' and pain-amplification syndrome (see also Chapter 5.14)

'Fibrositis' is a term that has been used for many decades to describe non-specific neck pain. Smythe (1986) defined the diagnosis more precisely, describing a pain-amplification syndrome associated with localized points of myofascial tenderness. This can be confined to the cervical spine (fibrositis), or can be more generalized (fibromyalgia), with the tender points concentrated around the entheses. Patients localize the pain to the posterior and lateral regions of the neck with associated stiffness. Tenderness is noted most specifically anterior to the transverse processes in the lower cervical spine. Sleep disturbance and fatiguability have been described in some cases. There is greater agreement on diagnostic features with the adoption of the American College of Rheumatology Fibromyalgia Classification Criteria (Wolfe et al. 1990).

Neck pain associated with tender trigger points is also found as a stress-related phenomenon (Croft et al. 1994; Wolfe et al. 1995). Poor posture, underlying vertebral degeneration, especially of the facet joints, and pain amplification may be important elements contributing to the severity of pain in these cases. Pain amplification may also explain the disproportionately severe pain in some patients with rheumatoid arthritis and other inflammatory arthropathies. Treatment of fibromyalgia is disappointing (Simms 1994; Wilke 1995), and the level of disability is often similar to rheumatoid arthritis (Martinez *et al.* 1995).

'Whiplash syndrome'

Acute flexion–extension injuries, typically in automobile accidents following rear-end impact, can cause acute neck pain (whiplash injury), even in the absence of bony damage. More severe symptoms are associated with an unprepared occupant, acceleration/deceleration injury, and a rotated or inclined head position (Sturzenegger *et al.* 1994). Although seat belts have reduced the incidence of severe injuries, the frequency of whiplash-type lesions has continued to rise (Bourbeau *et al.* 1993; Galasko *et al.* 1993), often leading to considerable and prolonged disability, complicated by medicolegal difficulties.

Severe cervical pain, spasm, loss of range, and occipital headache, are the most common symptoms, but many patients also complain of widely radiating pain, headache, vertigo, memory loss, poor concentration, fatigue, or neurological symptoms in the upper limbs (Radanov *et al.* 1992). Very occasionally, temporary or permanent quadriplegia may ensue.

The pathology of the condition is unclear, but soft tissue damage, bleeding into the muscles, and zygapophysial joint injury (Barnsley *et al.* 1995) may explain the acute pain and spasm. Traction and micro-injury of the cord, and acceleration/deceleration injury to the brain may be responsible for some of the other symptoms. The presence of cervical spondylosis adds to the risks of damage to the spinal cord or emerging nerve roots. Despite the frequency of whiplash injury, there is no objective investigation which if carried out early on, can define the site and severity of the damage and so predict outcome. Technetium isotope scanning (Barton *et al.* 1993), CT (Antinnes *et al.* 1994), and MRI (Jonsson *et al.* 1994; Pettersson *et al.* 1994) are useful in some cases of whiplash, although the correlation with clinical symptoms and signs is often poor.

The management of whiplash immediately after the injury, remains controversial. Rest in a collar is usually advocated, with physiotherapy (see below) being started as soon as the acute spasm has settled. Mealy *et al.* (1986) found significantly better recovery with early active mobilization, and McKinney *et al.* (1989) found similar benefits from a regimen of early exercise at home. However, Pennie and Agambar (1990) were unable to confirm any benefits of early active treatment for whiplash injury in a large series of patients.

Patients need to be warned that recovery may take 18 months or longer. Maimaris *et al.* (1988) and Evans (1992) found a poor outcome to be associated with older age, occipital headache, neck stiffness, referred symptoms, abnormal neurological signs, degenerative changes on radiographs, and symptoms persisting for more than 2 months. Psychosocial factors and personality traits were less important than the physical factors (reflecting severity) mentioned above, in predicting outcome (Radanov *et al.* 1994), and the settlement of litigation was not always associated with rapid recovery (Parmar and Raymakers 1993). Maimaris *et al.* (1988) reported that a third of their patients were symptomatic beyond 2 years, and Watkinson *et al.* (1991) found some symptoms in 86 per cent and intrusive symptoms in 23 per cent of patients reviewed at an average follow-up of 10.8 years. It is uncertain if whiplash injury accelerates the progression of degenerative change in affected patients (Hamer *et al.* 1993), but a point is reached where physical therapy

should be stopped, as it is unlikely to result in any further improvement (Hirsch *et al.* 1988).

Treatment of mechanical cervical disease

Most mechanical neck pain is responsive to conservative therapeutic regimens, although surgical intervention is sometimes necessary. Box 1 summarizes the principles of therapy and timing of MRI scanning in patients with uncomplicated acute and chronic mechanical cervical syndromes and those with neurological complications.

Bedrest

This is only necessary in acute lesions, especially with neurological deficit, such as a prolapsed cervical disc, trauma, or when there is a suspicion of infection or malignancy. A hard collar is advisable in these cases, and patients should be watched carefully for a deterioration in neurological status, when urgent neurosurgical intervention may be necessary.

Physiotherapy

This is the mainstay of treatment of chronic cervical syndromes, and needs to stress the improvement in muscle strength and range of movement, using passive mobilization techniques. Other electrical modalities of treatment may help by giving symptomatic relief to patients, especially where mobilization physiotherapy is contraindicated. Advise on posture and relaxation (such as the Alexander technique), weight reduction, and a home exercise programme are also likely to be beneficial. The avoidance of awkward head positions and lifting heavy weights, especially in occupational or recreational activities, may also prove of value. Dizziness, when due to cervical causes, usually proves unresponsive to physiotherapy and is often a limiting factor to this type of treatment. Transcutaneous electrical nerve stimulation and acupuncture can help reduce pain in some patients. Manipulation by chiropractors is often beneficial (Cassidy *et al.* 1992), but can prove hazardous, especially when radiological examination is not undertaken before treatment (Raskind and North 1990). Dissection of the vertebral arteries and vertebrobasilar strokes (Frisoni and Anzola 1991) are well-recognized complications, for example.

Cervical traction is particularly valuable in patients with radiculopathy, but may also be beneficial in other patients with cervical pathology. It can be used in continuous or intermittent regimens, but whichever regimen is used, great care is necessary, as some patients fail to tolerate this form of treatment or show neurological deterioration as the weight is applied.

Soft collar and cervical or soft pillow

A soft collar can be worn during periods of increased pain, and is especially valuable to facilitate sleep when this is disturbed by pain. Special pillows are also available to provide support for the neck during sleep, although some clinicians prefer to recommend a soft pillow that can be moulded into the appropriate shape to support the neck. Patients should be discouraged from using more than one or two pillows, to prevent undue angulation of the neck which can precipitate symptoms at night and on waking.

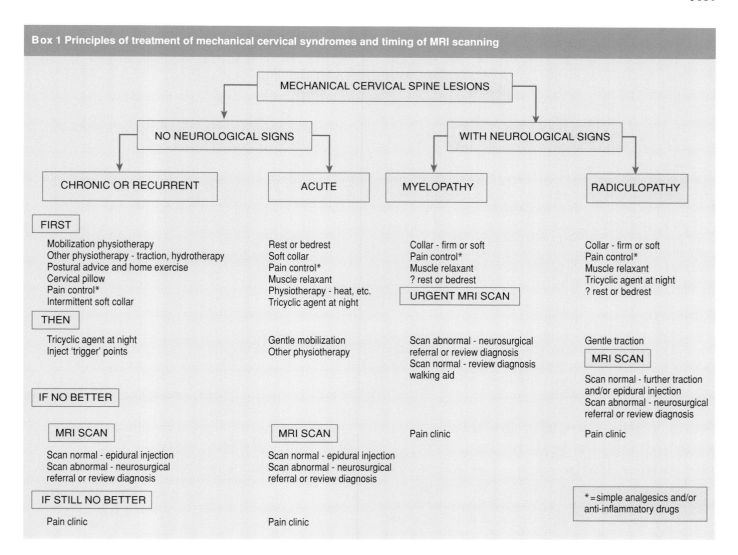

Box 1 Principles of treatment of mechanical cervical syndromes and timing of MRI scanning

Drugs

Analgesic tablets should be used during periods of increased pain, but anti-inflammatory and muscle relaxant drugs are only justified in acute situations where pain is particularly severe. Low-dose amitryptiline (10 to 75 mg at night) may alter the pain amplification cycle noted in some patients.

Cervical epidural injection

The injection of depot steroids into the cervical epidural space can maximize pain control in patients in whom serious underlying pathology, such as infection or tumour, or gross neurological deficit have been excluded (Rowlingson and Kirschenbaum 1986). Epidural injections often produce long-lasting improvement in cervical degenerative lesions (Cicala *et al.* 1989), especially in patients with radicular pain (Ferrante *et al.* 1993; Castagnera *et al.* 1994). The injection of local steroid alone, or in combination with local anaesthetic agents, into painful 'trigger' points or near painful facet joints or impinged nerve roots, may also relieve pain and spasm in some cases, although this is less effective than the epidural route (Stav *et al.* 1993).

Surgery

Neurosurgical intervention is only necessary in patients with progressive cervical myelopathy, or rarely with radiculopathy or intractable pain. Even with a prolapsed cervical disc, most patients will recover spontaneously or with conservative measures. Unlike prolapse of a lumbar disc, herniation of a cervical disc is associated with a slower rate of recovery that is more difficult to document with objective measurements. With cervical myelopathy due to degenerative disease, the result of decompressive surgery is often disappointing (Yonenobu *et al.* 1986; Rowland 1992). The rate of progression of the neurological deficit may be slowed by the surgery, but the lost function may not recover. This poor outcome reflects the irreversible nature of the damage to the spinal cord (see Figs 4 and 5) and also the compromised vascular supply to the cord in some cases. Some patients show a good initial recovery following surgery, but with relapse some time later (Goto *et al.* 1993). This relapse may reflect recurrence of the original pathology, or scar tissue related to surgery at the site of the initial operation. The likely benefits of further surgery are based on detailed reinvestigation by radiological and other means.

In principle, surgical intervention can be achieved via the anterior and/or posterior routes, with the operative procedure being individually selected on the basis of detailed clinical and radiological assessment. In cases of myelopathy, a multisegmental operation is often necessary to obtain satisfactory results. This multisegmental approach is particularly important where neurological abnormality is associated with DISH or ossification of the posterior longitudinal ligament (Epstein 1993) that have been unresponsive to conservative therapy.

Although many operations using the anterior or posterior approach have been advocated for cervical myelopathy, they are all based on the principles of fusion to prevent excessive motion (especially if only one or two levels are involved), and decompression by laminectomy, laminoplasty, or discectomy.

Surgery is less often necessary for cervical radiculopathy. The principles of treatment are similar to those for myelopathy (Chesnut *et al.* 1992), but decompression can be achieved by foraminotomy and/or partial discectomy.

Pain clinic

Where physical approaches to therapy have been exhausted, the multidisciplinary approach of the pain clinic may assist the patient in learning to cope with the chronic pain. This approach is more often required for low back-pain syndromes, where serious and prolonged disability is more likely.

Neck pain, shoulder pain, and soft tissue lesions in the upper limb

Patients with cervical spondylosis often complain of shoulder pain, and it is important to differentiate neck pain referred to the shoulder (usually the superior aspect) from primary conditions of the shoulder. Many patients have features that suggest both cervical and shoulder lesions, and these can be difficult to separate (Hawkins *et al.* 1990). Treatment may need to be directed at both sites.

The 'double crush' syndrome refers to a combination of both cervical radiculopathy and a peripheral nerve entrapment lesion. The most common peripheral lesion is carpal tunnel syndrome, although the ulnar and radial nerves can also be affected. Elucidation of the peripheral lesion is usually possible using electromyography and nerve conduction studies. Somatosensory evoked potentials and electromyographic sampling of the more proximal muscles may provide evidence of cervical radiculopathy or plexus lesions in addition to the peripheral lesion. Surgical intervention should be directed at the peripheral entrapment lesion before the cervical lesion.

Cervical spondylosis can also mimic epicondylitis and other localized soft tissue lesions in the upper limbs (Gunn and Milbrandt 1976), and there is a well-documented association between cervical spondylosis and these soft tissue lesions (Murray-Leslie and Wright 1976).

Referred pain syndromes

Where appropriate, examination for polymyalgia rheumatica, reflex sympathetic dystrophy, inflammatory arthropathy, infection, malignancy, and even crystal arthropathies may be necessary. Table 2

Table 6 Causes of brachial plexus lesions
Trauma—birth and motorcycle injury, surgery, cannulas, or needles
Thoracic-outlet syndrome—e.g. cervical rib
Traction—surgery, e.g. medial sternotomy, rucksack palsy, postanaesthesia
Brachial plexus neuropathy (brachial neuritis):
Infection—viral, bacterial
Toxins—heroin
Injection of foreign serum or vaccine
Systemic illness—lupus, vasculitis, Hodgkin's disease
Familial brachial plexus neuropathy
Idiopathic
Radiotherapy
Tumour—especially Pancoast tumour of lung, breast
Lightning, electric shock

above shows the sites of origin, and the more common causes of pain referred to the cervical region.

Brachial plexus lesions

Pain of brachial plexus origin is felt in the neck, shoulder, forearm, or hand. Supraclavicular pain is common and may be accompanied by local tenderness, and bony (cervical rib), or pulsatile (aneurysm) swelling at this site. The pain can often be induced by certain manoeuvres or changes in the position of the arm (see below). Table 6 shows the causes of brachial plexus injury.

Thoracic-outlet obstruction

Compression of the distal nerve roots, brachial plexus, subclavian vessels, or the combined neurovascular bundle can occur at various

Table 7 Contributing factors to thoracic-outlet syndrome
Cervical rib
Congenital fibromuscular bands
Congenital abnormality of clavicle or first rib
Interscalenus muscle hypertrophy
Clavipectoral lesions—the 'hyperabduction syndrome'
Old fracture of the first rib or clavicle
Vascular disorders and hyperviscosity syndromes
External compression, e.g. heavy weights, rucksack lesions
Poor posture, sagging or droopy shoulders
Excessive muscle development around shoulders

sites between the neck and the axilla (the thoracic outlet). Possible contributing factors are shown in Table 7. 'Cervical ribs', which vary from simple exostoses of the transverse processes of C7 to fully formed extra ribs, are the most common cause of the thoracic-outlet syndrome. As 0.5 per cent of the population have bilateral cervical ribs yet less than 10 per cent ever get symptoms, other factors (Liu *et al.* 1995) must also be important in symptomatic cases. Poor posture and sagging or droopy shoulders (Swift and Nichols 1984) have been identified as important factors in the development of symptoms, especially in females of early or middle age, in whom the syndrome is most often diagnosed.

The typical symptoms of thoracic-outlet obstruction vary according to the site of compression of the neurovascular bundle (Novak *et al.* 1993). Pain is usually present in the neck, shoulder, or upper arm. Vasomotor abnormalities such as numbness, paraesthesia, coldness, colour change, or Raynaud's phenomenon are characteristic of the lesion and may dominate the picture. Compression of the lower levels of the brachial plexus result in neurological features such as sensory loss in the C8 and T1 dermatomes, with paraesthesia, or weakness in the hand. Some patients show well-defined syndromes due to selective compression of the subclavian vein, artery, or brachial plexus (Wilbourn 1993).

Obliteration of the radial or brachial pulse may be noted, either when the patient takes and holds a full breath with the head tilted back or rotated laterally (Adson Test), or when the arm is abducted and externally rotated while the shoulders are braced (Wright's manoeuvre). Both tests can be noted with thoracic-outlet syndrome, but are not reliable indicators of this condition.

Ten per cent of patients develop serious vascular complications, which can be venous or arterial (Hawkes 1986). Thrombosis of the axillosubclavian vein can present acutely or chronically, sometimes following prolonged exercise. Typical features are pain and swelling of the arm aggravated by exercise, with the diagnosis being confirmed by venography. Compression of the subclavian artery can be followed by post-stenotic dilatation, aneurysm formation, and retrograde thromboembolic phenomena. Claudication, vasomotor phenomena, digital gangrene, and acute limb-threatening ischaemia can occur. Arteriography, and in some cases Doppler ultrasonography are necessary to confirm the arterial abnormality.

Thoracic-outlet syndrome may be difficult to show objectively (Novak *et al.* 1993), and few patients have the diagnosis confirmed (Wilbourn 1993). Radiographs of the cervical spine may demonstrate cervical ribs, congenital bony abnormalities, or old fractures. MRI can also define soft tissue bands and other lesions causing distortion or deviation of nerves and blood vessels in the thoracic-outlet (Panegyres *et al.* 1993). Electromyography and somatosensory evoked potentials may offer some supportive evidence to confirm the diagnosis, or exclude lesions such as cervical radiculopathy, carpal tunnel syndrome, or ulnar neuropathy, which can closely mimic this syndrome. Arteriography and venography are necessary in difficult cases, especially with vascular complications.

Conservative treatment (Walsh 1994) with shoulder-girdle exercises and improved posture often fails to remove all the symptoms, but is all that should be advocated for mild disease, especially where the diagnosis remains in doubt.

Surgical intervention, which is often unsuccessful (Urschel and Razzuk 1986) and carries considerable risks (Marinoni *et al.* 1987), should be avoided (Wilbourn 1991), except in patients with serious vascular or other complications, or in severe cases of proven thoracic-outlet syndrome.

Surgery can be carried out via the supraclavicular or trans-axillary routes, or via a combination of both. Operations advocated include resection of the first rib (Martin 1993), resection of the cervical rib, claviculectomy, scalenotomy with soft tissue release, and partial scalenectomy.

Resection of the cervical rib is adequate treatment in patients with predominantly neurological symptoms, but may not be sufficient with serious vascular disease. Therapeutic options for acute venous thrombosis are anticoagulation, fibrinolysis, and thrombectomy, followed by treatment of the thoracic-outlet syndrome, usually by resection of the first rib. For chronic venous obstruction, primary treatment of the actual syndrome may be enough, although some cases also require endovenectomy or venous bypass surgery (Sanders and Haug 1990). Compressive arterial lesions can be treated by rib resection or primary treatment of the syndrome, but once intrinsic arterial damage has developed, aneurysmectomy and arterial reconstruction are necessary. With distal thromboembolic disease, thrombectomy or embolectomy need to be combined with the other measures (Scher *et al.* 1984). Where vasomotor symptoms persist after the initial operation, chemical sympathectomy of the upper thoracic sympathetic chain may be helpful.

Cryptogenic brachial plexus neuropathy (brachial neuritis, neuralgic amyotrophy)

This condition usually develops acutely in healthy adults aged between 25 and 65 years. Some cases follow viral or other infection, injection of serum or vaccine, heroin use, or strenuous exercise. Rare cases are familial. An ache first develops around the shoulder or neck with increasing severity over 1 to 2 weeks. As the acute pain starts to settle, rapid onset of weakness and wasting of the shoulder and upper limb muscles is noted. The pattern of wasting depends on the pattern of injury of the brachial plexus nerves. Sensory loss, paraesthesia, hyperaesthesia, and hyporeflexia may also occur. The pain is exacerbated by use of the affected muscles, which may become totally paralysed. The lesion can be bilateral, and in some cases, is associated with involvement of the phrenic nerve (Walsh *et al.* 1987) or other peripheral and even cranial nerves (Mohanaruban and Fisher 1986). Electromyography of the affected muscles reveals fibrillation potentials and positive waves, in a pattern characteristic of combined damage to nerve roots and peripheral nerves. The electromyographic abnormality is often bilateral, even where this was not clinically apparent.

Although the course is variable, the prognosis for recovery is good. Most recover within 6 months, with 90 per cent showing a complete recovery within 3 years. Recurrences do occur, but are rare.

Brachial plexus neuropathy needs to be differentiated from acute poliomyelitis, rotator cuff tears, extradural malignancy, Pancoast tumour of the lung, thoracic-outlet syndrome, and cervical radiculopathy.

Conclusion

Degenerative lesions in the cervical region cause many varied symptoms, which are not always recognized to be from this source. 'Cervical spondylosis', which is a vague term used to describe a whole range of degenerative and mechanical lesions, causes less disability than similar lesions affecting the lumbar spine, and has therefore been the subject of less study. The more common mechanical syndromes and associated complications and their treatment have been discussed, with consideration being given to other causes of neck pain and neurological deficit in the upper limbs.

References

Antinnes, J.A., Dvorak, J., Hayek, J., Panjabi, M.M., and Grob, D. (1994). The value of functional computed tomography in the evaluation of soft-tissue injury in the upper cervical spine. *European Spine Journal*, 3, 98–101.

Baba, H., Kawahara, N., Tomita, K., and Imura, S. (1993a). Spinal cord evoked potentials in cervical and thoracic myelopathy. *International Orthopaedics*, 17, 82–6.

Baba, H., Maezawa, Y., Kawahara, N., Tomita, K., Furusawa, N., and Imura, S. (1993b). Calcium crystal deposition in the ligamentum flavum of the cervical spine. *Spine*, 18, 2174–81.

Baba, H., Furusawa, N., Chen, Q., Imura, S., and Tomita, K. (1995). Anterior decompressive surgery for cervical ossified posterior longitudinal ligament causing myeloradiculopathy. *Paraplegia*, 33, 18–24.

Barnsley, L., Lord, S.M., Wallis, B.J., and Bogduk, N. (1995). The prevalence of chronic cervical zygapophysial joint pain after whiplash. *Spine*, 20, 20–6.

Barton, D., Allen, M., Finlay, D., and Belton, I. (1993). Evaluation of whiplash injuries by technetium 99m isotope scanning. *Archives of Emergency Medicine*, 10, 197–202.

Batzdorf, U. and Flannigan, B.D. (1991). Surgical decompressive procedures for cervical spondylotic myelopathy. A study using magnetic resonance imaging. *Spine*, 16, 123–7.

Bland, J.H. and Boushey, D.R. (1990). Anatomy and physiology of the cervical spine. *Seminars in Arthritis and Rheumatism*, 20, 1–20.

Boachie-Adjei, O. and Bullough, P.G. (1987). Incidence of ankylosing hyperostosis of the spine (Forestier's disease) at autopsy. *Spine*, 12, 739–43.

Boden, S.D., McCowin, P.R., Davis, D.O., Dina, T.S., Mark, A.S., and Wiesel, S. (1990). Abnormal magnetic-resonance scans of the cervical spine in asymptomatic subject. A prospective investigation. *Journal of Bone and Joint Surgery*, 72A, 1178–84.

Bourbeau, R., Desjardins, D., Maag, U., and Laberge-Nadeau, C. (1993). Neck injuries among belted and unbelted occupants of the front seat of cars. *Journal of Trauma*, 35, 794–9.

Brodsky, A.E. (1985). Cervical angina. A correlative study with emphasis on the use of coronary arteriography. *Spine*, 10, 699–709.

Brown, T.R., Quinn, S.F., and D'Agostino, A.N. (1991). Deposition of calcium pyrophosphate dihydrate crystals in the ligamentum flavum: evaluation with MR imaging and CT. *Radiology*, 178, 871–3.

Cassidy, J.D., Lopes, A.A., and Yong-Hing, K. (1992). The immediate effect of manipulation versus mobilization on pain and range of motion in the cervical spine: a randomized controlled trial. *Journal of Manipulative and Physiological Therapeutics*, 15, 570–5.

Castagnera, L., Maurette, P., Pointillart, V., Vital, J.M., Erny, P., and Senegas, J. (1994). Long-term results of cervical epidural steroid injection with and without morphine in chronic cervical radicular pain. *Pain*, 58, 239–43.

Chesnut, R.M., Abitbol, J-J., and Garfin, S.R. (1992). Surgical management of cervical radiculopathy. Indication, techniques, and results. *Orthopedic Clinics of North America*, 23, 461–74.

Cicala, R.S., Thoni, K., and Angel, J.J. (1989). Long-term results of cervical epidural steroid injections. *Clinical Journal of Pain*, 5, 143–5.

Croft, P., Schollum, J., and Silman, A. (1994). Population study of tender point counts and pain as evidence of fibromyalgia. *British Medical Journal*, 309, 696–9.

Di Lazzaro, V., Restuccia, D., Colosimo, C., and Tonali, P. (1992). The contribution of magnetic stimulation of the motor cortex to the diagnosis of cervical spondylotic myelopathy. Correlation of central motor conduction to distal and proximal upper limb muscles with clinical and MRI findings. *Electroencephalographic and Clinical Neurophysiology*, 85, 311–20.

Dvorak, J., Janssen, B., and Grob, D. (1990). The neurologic workup in patients with cervical spine disorders. *Spine*, 15, 1017–22.

Edmeads, J. (1988). The cervical spine and headache. *Neurology*, 38, 1874–8.

Epstein, N. (1993). The surgical management of ossification of the posterior longitudinal ligament in 51 patients. *Journal of Spinal Disorders*, 6, 432–55.

Evans, R.W. (1992). Some observations on whiplash injuries. *Neurological Clinics*, 10, 975–7.

Farmer, J.C. and Wisneski, R.J. (1994). Cervical spine nerve root compression. An analysis of neuroforaminal pressures with varying head and arm positions. *Spine*, 19, 1850–5.

Fast, A., Parikh, S., and Marin, E.L. (1989). The shoulder abduction relief sign in cervical radiculopathy. *Archives of Physical Medicine and Rehabilitation*, 70, 402–3.

Ferrante, F.M., Wilson, S.P., Iacobo, C., Orav, E.J., Rocco, A.G., and Lipson, S. (1993). Clinical classification as a predictor of therapeutic outcome after cervical epidural steroid injection. *Spine*, 18, 730–6.

Frisoni, G.B. and Anzola, G.P. (1991). Vertebrobasilar ischaemia after neck motion. *Stroke*, 22, 1452–60.

Fukui, K., Kataoka, O., Sho, T., and Sumi, M. (1990). Pathomechanism, pathogenesis, and results of treatment in cervical spondylotic myelopathy caused by dynamic canal stenosis. *Spine*, 15, 1148–52.

Galasko, C.S. *et al.* (1993). Neck sprains after road traffic accidents: a modern epidemic. *Injury*, 24, 155–7.

Gore, D.R., Sepic, S.B., and Gardner, G.M. (1986). Roentgenographic findings of the cervical spine in asymptomatic people. *Spine*, 11, 521–4.

Goto, S. *et al.* (1993). Anterior surgery in four consecutive technical phases for cervical spondylotic myelopathy. *Spine*, 18, 1968–73.

Griegel-Morris, P., Larson, K., Mueller-Klaus, K., and Oatis, C.A. (1992). Incidence of common postural abnormalities in the cervical, shoulder, and thoracic regions and their association with pain in two age groups of healthy subjects. *Physical Therapy*, 72, 425–31.

Gunn, C.C. and Milbrandt, W.E. (1976). Tennis elbow and the cervical spine. *Canadian Medical Association Journal*, 114, 803–9.

Hadler, N.M. (1985). Illness in the workplace: the challenge of musculoskeletal symptoms. *Journal of Hand Surgery*, 10A, 451–6.

Hamer, A.J., Gargan, M.F., Bannister, G.C., and Nelson, R.J. (1993). Whiplash injury and surgically treated cervical disc disease. *Injury*, 24, 549–50.

Hawkes, C.D. (1986). Neurosurgical considerations in thoracic outlet syndrome. *Clinical Orthopaedics*, 207, 24–8.

Hawkins, R.J., Bilco, T., and Bonutti, P. (1990). Cervical spine and shoulder pain. *Clinical Orthopaedics*, 258, 142–6.

Hayashi, H., Okada, K., Hashimoto, J., Tada, K., and Ueno, R. (1988). Cervical spondylotic myelopathy in the aged patient. A radiographic evaluation of the aging changes in the cervical spine and etiologic factors of myelopathy. *Spine*, 13, 618–25.

Helliwell, P.S., Evans, P.F., and Wright, V. (1994). The straight cervical spine: does it indicate muscle spasm? *Journal of Bone and Joint Surgery*, 76B, 103–6.

Hensinger, R.N. (1991). Congenital anomalies of the cervical spine. *Clinical Orthopaedics*, 264, 16–38.

Hirsch, S.A., Hirsch, P.J., Hiramoto, H., and Weiss, A. (1988). Whiplash syndrome. Fact or fiction? *Orthopedic Clinics of North America*, 19, 791–5.

Holt, L. (1972). Frequency of symptoms for different age groups and professions. In *Cervical pain* (ed. C. Hirsch and Y. Zotterman), pp. 17–20. Pergamon, New York.

Hukuda, S., Mochizuki, T., Ogata, M., and Shichikawa, K. (1983). The pattern of spinal and extraspinal hyperostosis in patients with ossification of the posterior longitudinal ligament and the ligamentum flavum causing myelopathy. *Skeletal Radiology*, 10, 79–85.

Jinkins, J.R., Bashir, R., Al-Mefty, O., Al-Kawi, M.Z., and Fox, J.L. (1986). Cystic necrosis of the spinal cord in compressive cervical myelopathy: demonstration by iopamidol CT-myelography. *American Journal of Roentgenology*, 147, 767–75.

Jonsson, H., Jr., Cesarini, K., Sahlstedt, B., and Rauschning, W. (1994). Findings and outcome in whiplash-type neck distortions. *Spine*, 19, 2733–43.

Kramer, J., Rivera, C.A., and Kleefield, J. (1991). Degenerative disorders of the cervical spine. *Rheumatic Disease Clinics of North America*, 17, 741–55.

Kristensen, S., Sander, K.M., and Pedersen, P.R. (1988). Cervical involvement in diffuse idiopathic skeletal hyperostosis with dysphagia and rhinolalia. *Archives of Otorhinolaryngology*, 245, 330–4.

Lawrence, J.S. (1969). Disc degeneration. Its frequency and relationship to symptoms. *Annals of the Rheumatic Diseases*, 28, 121–38.

Lehto, I.J., Tertti, M.O., Komu, M.E., Paajanen, H.E., Tuominen, J., and Kormano, M.J. (1994). Age-related MRI changes at 0.1 T in cervical discs in asymptomatic subjects. *Neuroradiology*, **36**, 49–53.

Lestini, W.F. and Wiesel, S. W. (1989). The pathogenesis of cervical spondylosis. *Clinical Orthopaedics*, **239**, 69–93.

Liu, J.E., Tahmoush, A.J., Roos, D.B., and Schwartzman, R.J. (1995). Shoulder-arm pain from cervical bands and scalene muscle anomalies. *Journal of Neurological Science*, **128**, 175–80.

Maimaris, C., Barnes, M.R., and Allen, M.J. (1988). 'Whiplash injuries' of the neck: a retrospective study. *Injury*, **19**, 393–6.

Marinoni, E.C., Bonfiglio, G., Coletti, M., and Passarelli, O. (1987). Thoracic-outlet syndrome. Proposed protocol for diagnosis and treatment. *Italian Journal of Orthopaedic Traumatology*, **13**, 379–86.

Martin, G.T. (1993). First rib resection for the thoracic-outlet syndrome. *British Journal of Neurosurgery*, **7**, 35–8.

Martinez, J.E., Ferraz, M.B., Sato, E.I., and Atra, E. (1995). Fibromyalgia versus rheumatoid arthritis: a longitudinal comparison of the quality of life. *Journal of Rheumatology*, **22**, 270–4.

Matsuda, Y. *et al.* (1991). Increased MR signal intensity due to cervical myelopathy. Analysis of 29 surgical cases. *Journal of Neurosurgery*, **74**, 887–92.

McKinney, L.A., Dornan, J.O., and Ryan, M. (1989). The role of physiotherapy in the management of acute neck sprains following road traffic accidents. *Archives of Emergency Medicine*, **6**, 27–33.

Mealy, K., Brennan, H., and Fenelon, G.C. (1986). Early mobilization of acute whiplash injuries. *British Medical Journal (Clinical Research)*, **292**, 656–7.

Mohanaruban, K. and Fisher, D.J. (1986). A combination of cranial and peripheral nerve palsies in infectious mononucleosis. *Postgraduate Medical Journal*, **62**, 1129–30.

Murone, I. (1974). The importance of the sagittal diameters of the cervical spine canal in relation to spondylosis and myelopathy. *Journal of Bone and Joint Surgery*, **56B**, 30–6.

Murray-Leslie, C.F. and Wright, V. (1976). Carpal tunnel syndrome, humeral epicondylitis, and the cervical spine: a study of clinical and dimensional relations. *British Medical Journal*, **1**, 1439–42.

Nagasawa, A., Sakakibara, T., and Takahashi, A. (1993). Roentgenographic findings of the cervical spine in tension-type headache. *Headache*, **33**, 90–5.

Nagata, K., Kiyonaga, K., Ohashi, T., Sagara, M., Miyazaki, S., and Inoue, A. (1990). Clinical value of magnetic resonance imaging for cervical myelopathy. *Spine*, **15**, 1088–96.

Nakajima, M. and Hirayama, K. (1995). Midcervical central cord syndrome: numb and clumsy hands due to midline cervical disc protrusion at the C3–4 intervertebral level. *Journal of Neurology, Neurosurgery and Psychiatry*, **58**, 607–13.

Novak, C.B., Mackinnon, S.E., and Patterson, G.A. (1993). Evaluation of patients with thoracic-outlet syndrome. *Journal of Hand Surgery*, **18A**, 292–9.

Okada, Y., Ikata, T., Katoh, S., and Yamada, H. (1994). Morphologic analysis of the cervical spinal cord, dural tube, and spinal canal by magnetic resonance imaging in normal adults and patients with cervical spondylotic myelopathy. *Spine*, **19**, 2331–5.

Otake, S., Matsuo, M., Nishizawa, S., Sano, A., and Kuroda, Y. (1992). Ossification of the posterior longitudinal ligament: MR evaluation. *American Journal of Neuroradiology*, **13**, 1059–70.

Palmer, P.E., Stadalnick, R., and Arnon, S. (1984). The genetic factor in cervical spondylosis. *Skeletal Radiology*, **11**, 178–82.

Panegyres, P.K., Moore, N., Gibson, R., Rushmore, G., and Donaghy, M. (1993). Thoracic outlet syndrome and magnetic resonance imaging. *Brain*, **116**, 823–41.

Parmar, H.V. and Raymakers, R. (1993). Neck injuries from rear impact road traffic accidents: prognosis in persons seeking compensation. *Injury*, **24**, 75–8.

Pennie, B.H. and Agambar, L.J. (1990). Whiplash injuries. A trial of early management. *Journal of Bone and Joint Surgery*, **72B**, 277–9.

Pettersson, K., Hildingsson, C., Toolanen, G., Fagerlund, M., and Bjornebrink, J. (1994). MRI and neurology in acute whiplash trauma: no correlation in prospective examination of 39 cases. *Acta Orthopaedica Scandinavica*, **65**, 525–8.

Pyhtinen, J. and Laitinen, J. (1993). Cervical intervertebral foramen narrowing and myelographic nerve root sleeve deformities. *Neuroradiology*, **35**, 596–7.

Radanov, B.P., Dvorak, J., and Valach, L. (1992). Cognitive deficits in patients after soft tissue injury of the cervical spine. *Spine*, **17**, 127–31.

Radanov, B.P., Sturzenegger, M., De Stefano, G., and Schnidrig, A. (1994). Relationship between early somatic, radiological, cognitive and psychosocial findings and outcome during a one year follow-up of 117 patients suffering from common whiplash. *British Journal of Rheumatology*, **33**, 442–8.

Raskind, R. and North, C.M. (1990). Vertebral artery injuries following chiropractic cervical spine manipulations—case reports. *Angiology*, **41**, 445–52.

Resnick, D. (1985). Degenerative diseases of the vertebral column. *Radiology*, **156**, 3–14.

Resnick, D., Guerra, J., Jr., Robinson, C.A., and Vint, V.C. (1978). Association of diffuse idiopathic skeletal hyperostosis (DISH) and calcification and ossification of the posterior longitudinal ligament. *American Journal of Roentgenology*, **131**, 1049–53.

Rowland, L.P. (1992). Surgical treatment of cervical spondylotic myelopathy: time for a controlled trial. *Neurology*, **42**, 5–13.

Rowlingson, J.C. and Kirschenbaum, L.P. (1986). Epidural analgesic techniques in the management of cervical pain. *Anesthesia and Analgesia*, **65**, 938–42.

Sanders, R.J. and Haug, C. (1990). Subclavian vein obstruction and thoracic outlet syndrome: a review of etiology and management. *Annals of Vascular Surgery*, **4**, 397–410.

Scher, L.A. *et al.* (1984). Staging of arterial complications of cervical rib: guidelines for surgical management. *Surgery*, **95**, 644–9.

Simmons, Z., Biller, J., Beck, D.W., and Keyes, W.(1986). Painless compressive cervical myelopathy with false localizing sensory findings. *Spine*, **11**, 869–72.

Simms, R.W. (1994). Controlled trials of therapy in fibromyalgia syndrome. *Baillière's Clinical Rheumatology*, **8**, 917–34.

Smythe, H.A. (1986). Referred pain and tender points. *American Journal of Medicine*, **81**,(Suppl. 3A), 90–2.

Smythe, H.A. (1994). The C6–7 syndrome: clinical features and treatment response. *Journal of Rheumatology*, **21**, 1520–6.

Sobol, S.M. and Rigual, N.R.(1984). Anterolateral extrapharyngeal approach for cervical osteophyte-induced dysphagia. *Annals of Otology, Rhinology and Laryngology*, **93**, 498–504.

Stav, A., Ovadia, L., Sternberg, A., Kaadan, M., and Weksler, N. (1993). Cervical epidural steroid injection for cervicobrachialgia. *Acta Anaesthesiologica Scandinavica*, **37**, 562–6.

Sturzenegger, M., DiStefano, G., Radanov, B.P., and Schnidrig, A. (1994). Presenting symptoms and signs after whiplash injury: the influence of accident mechanisms. *Neurology*, **44**, 688–93.

Sudarsky, L. and Ronthal, M. (1983). Gait disorders among elderly patients. A survey study of 50 patients. *Archives of Neurology*, **40**, 740–3.

Suzuki, K., Ishida, Y., and Ohmori, K. (1991). Long term follow-up of diffuse idiopathic skeletal hyperostosis in the cervical spine. Analysis of progression of ossification. *Neuroradiology*, **33**, 427–31.

Swift, T.R. and Nichols, F.T. (1984). The droopy shoulder syndrome. *Neurology*, **34**, 212–5.

Urschel, H.C., Jr. and Razzuk, M.A. (1986). The failed operation for thoracic-outlet syndrome: the difficulty of diagnosis and management. *Annals of Thoracic Surgery*, **42**, 523–8.

Van der Donk, J., Schouten, J.S., Passchier, J., van Romunde, L.K., and Valkenburg, H.A. (1991). The associations of neck pain with radiological abnormalities of the cervical spine and personality traits in a general population. *Journal of Rheumatology*, **18**, 1884–9.

Vanderburgh, D.F. and Kelly, W.M. (1993). Radiographic assessment of discogenic disease of the spine. *Neurosurgical Clinics of North America*, **4**, 13–33.

Vargo, M.M. and Flood, K.M. (1990). Pancoast tumour presenting as cervical radiculopathy. *Archives of Physical Medicine and Rehabilitation*, **71**, 606–9.

Walsh, M.T. (1994). Therapist management of thoracic-outlet syndrome. *Journal of Hand Therapy*, **7**, 131–44.

Walsh, N.E., Dumitru, D., Kalantri, A., and Roman, A.M., Jr. (1987). Brachial neuritis involving the bilateral phrenic nerves. *Archives of Physical Medicine and Rehabilitation*, **68**, 46–8.

Watkinson, A., Gargan, M.F., and Bannister, G.C. (1991). Prognostic factors in soft tissue injuries of the cervical spine. *Injury*, **22**, 307–9.

Wiesel, S.W., Tsourmas, N., Feffer, H.L., Citrin, C.M., and Patronas, N. (1984). A study of computer-assisted tomography 1. The incidence of positive CAT scans in an asymptomatic group of patients. *Spine*, **9**, 549–51.

Wilbourn, A.J. (1991). Thoracic-outlet syndromes: a plea for conservatism. *Neurosurgical Clinics of North America*, **2**, 235–45.

Wilbourn, A.J. (1993). Brachial plexus disorders. In *Peripheral neuropathy*, Vol. 2, (3rd edn)(ed. P.J. Dyck and P.K. Thomas), pp. 911–51. W.B. Saunders, Philadelphia.

Wilke, W.S. (1995). Treatment of 'resistant' fibromyalgia. *Rheumatic Diseases Clinics of North America*, **21**, 247–60.

Wober-Bingol, C. *et al.* (1992). Tension headache and the cervical spine — plain X-ray findings. *Cephalalgia*, **12**, 152–4.

Wolfe, F. *et al.* (1990). The American College of Rheumatology 1990 criteria for the classification of fibromyalgia. Report of the Multicenter Criteria Committee. *Arthritis and Rheumatism*, **33**, 160–72.

Wolfe, F., Ross, K., Anderson, J., and Russell, I.J. (1995). Aspects of fibromyalgia in the general population: sex, pain, threshold, and fibromyalgia symptoms. *Journal of Rheumatology*, **22**, 151–6.

Yiannikas, C., Shahani, B.T., and Young, R.R. (1986). Short latency somatosensory-evoked potentials from radial, median, ulnar, and peroneal nerve stimulation in the assessment of cervical spondylosis. Comparison with conventional electromyography. *Archives of Neurology*, **43**, 1264–71.

Yonenobu, K., Okada, K., Fuji, T., Fujiwara, K., Yamashita, K., and Ono, K. (1986). Causes of neurologic deterioration following surgical treatment of cervical myelopathy. *Spine*, **11**, 818–23.

Yoss, R.E., Corbin, K.B., MacCarty, C.S., and Love, J.G. (1957). Significance of symptoms and signs in the localization of the involved root in cervical disc protrusion. *Neurology*, **7**, 673–83.

Miscellaneous abnormalities of connective tissue

5.19.1 Rheumatic diseases and neoplasia

Thomas G. Benedek

Some systemic rheumatic diseases may predispose to the development of malignant neoplasms. Conversely, some malignant neoplasms may present with rheumatic symptoms. Although the pathogenesis of these complex relationships is incompletely understood, recognition of the manifestations is necessary for the efficient diagnostic evaluation of many patients. The relations and conditions considered here may be classified thus:

1. Relation of rheumatic diseases to malignant neoplasms:

   (a) rheumatoid arthritis;
   (b) spondylarthropathies;
   (c) Sjögren's syndrome;
   (d) systemic lupus erythematosus;
   (e) dermatomyositis/polymyositis;
   (f) systemic sclerosis (scleroderma);
   (g) polymyalgia rheumatica.

2. Rheumatic manifestations of malignant neoplasms:

   (a) skeletal neoplasms;
       (i) osseous metastases
       (ii) synovial sarcoma
       (iii) leukaemia
       (iv) paraproteineamic arthropathies

   (b) paraneoplastic syndromes;
       (i) hypertrophic osteoarthropathy
       (ii) oncogenic osteomalacia
       (iii) carcinomatous polyarthritis
       (iv) carcinomatous neuromyopathy
       (vi) fasciitis syndromes
       (vii) paraneoplastic Raynaud's phenomenon.

Relation of rheumatic diseases and neoplasia

Rheumatoid arthritis

The pathogenetic significance of even a high degree of association is difficult to determine and does not prove a causal relationship. This problem is exemplified by questions about the relationship between rheumatoid arthritis and cancer. The mean life expectancy is shortened by rheumatoid arthritis, according to a Finnish study (Myllykangas-Luosujärvi et al. 1995), by at least 3 years. The greatest proportional excess of deaths is due to infections but since infections have diminished as a primary cause of death, gastrointestinal diseases have become predominant numerically (Mitchell et al. 1986; Wolfe et al. 1994; Myllykangas-Luosujärvi et al. 1995). Nevertheless, most patients live into the seventh decade, when the incidence of malignancies is highest but the onset of rheumatoid arthritis is relatively infrequent. The length of the latent period before a neoplasm becomes diagnosable is unknown. Thus, a patient who has had rheumatoid arthritis for a few years may have been incubating the neoplasm before rheumatoid arthritis supervened. The best, albeit weak, evidence that neoplasms do not predispose to the occurrence of rheumatoid arthritis, rather than the reverse, is that they do not precede rheumatoid arthritis with unexpected frequency.

Epidemiological problems may include inconsistent diagnostic criteria for rheumatoid arthritis and for specific neoplasms, regional variations in the occurrence both of rheumatoid arthritis and of various neoplasms, and whether the cases of rheumatoid arthritis are entered from hospital rolls, outpatient services, or community surveys. A high degree of association with one subset of neoplasms may be hidden in a broader category. However, the narrower the subset of cancers that is being correlated with the incidence of rheumatoid arthritis, the larger the cohort of rheumatoid cases must be for statistically significant correlations to be obtained. A further confounding consideration is whether a correlation is attributable to a characteristic of the disease or of its treatment.

The best available data regarding the relationships between rheumatoid arthritis and cancer emanate from complementary epidemiological studies in Finland from 1967 to 1973 (Isomäki et al. 1978) and in Sweden from 1965 to 1984 (Gridley et al. 1993). Comparisons with national incidence data were made in both investigations. The smaller Swedish cohorts included 32.6 per cent as many men and 22.9 per cent as many women with rheumatoid arthritis, but cancer among these was diagnosed in 81.3 per cent as many men and 64.0 per cent as many women. The proportionately larger number of neoplasms in the Swedish cohorts can be attributed to the much longer period of observation (20 years rather than 7). While the total incidence of neoplasms in both investigations approximated the expected, the frequency of some neoplasms exceeded or was less than expected. Unfortunately, the Finnish data do not differentiate among lymphomas or leukaemias. Table 1 shows the neoplasms that deviated from the expected incidence in the Swedish data and asterisks indicate which deviated in the Finnish data. For Hodgkin's disease there was an excess only in men in Sweden and only in women in Finland. This demonstrates uncertainty due to small numbers. Other lymphomas occurred in excess in both investigations. Non-Hodgkin's lymphoma appears to be the most highly associated with rheumatoid arthritis among the lymphoreticular neoplasms (Symmons *et al.* 1984; Porter *et al.* 1991). Thirty-seven of 39 such cases were over the age of 50 and the interval between the onset of rheumatoid arthritis and the diagnosis of the lymphoreticular neoplasm was at least 10 years in two-thirds (Banks *et al.* 1979; Symmons *et al.* 1984). A prospective 10-year Finnish study of 500 men and 500 women with rheumatoid arthritis and age-matched, random control cases substantiated the excess of haemopoietic neoplasia (Laakso *et al.* 1986). Both apparently benign paraproteinaemia and multiple myeloma occur with increased frequency in rheumatoid arthritis (Zawadzki and Benedek 1969; Eriksson 1993). The observation that rheumatoid arthritis patients do not have an increased likelihood of a second primary neoplasm supports the data that rheumatoid arthritis, with the exception of lymphoreticular processes, does not confer an increased susceptibility to neoplasia (Hakulinen 1986).

The data of Isomake *et al.* showed a deficit of gastric and rectal carcinomas in women (Isomäki *et al.* 1978). The Swedish data demonstrated this in both sexes and for colonic carcinoma as well. Laakso *et al.* found more gastrointestinal carcinomas in their rheumatoid arthritis than in control cohorts, but better survival in the former (Laakso *et al.* 1986). Recent studies provide persuasive, albeit inferential, evidence that the deficit of at least colorectal carcinoma in rheumatoid arthritis patients is due to an effect of the chronic consumption of aspirin or other non-steroidal anti-inflammatory prostaglandin-inhibiting drugs (Thun *et al.* 1991). These drugs inhibit the chemical induction of colonic tumours in rodents. Several clinical studies have now shown the same effect, although with a wide difference in the duration of use before the effect becomes definite — possibly a decade or longer (Rosenberg *et al.* 1991; Giovannucci *et al.* 1995). In view of the substantial chronic use of these drugs in rheumatoid arthritis, the deficit of colorectal cancer

may here find its explanation. Whether gastric carcinogenesis is similarly influenced and whether the larger rheumatological doses have a more rapidly demonstrable effect than the equivalent of 0.3 g of aspirin every other day have not yet been established.

The possibly carcinogenic effect of drugs used to treat rheumatoid arthritis has been examined more directly. Gold compounds and corticosteroids have not been implicated. However, the greatly increased incidence of lymphoreticular neoplasms in immunosuppressed organ transplant recipients led to concern about a similar risk in rheumatoid arthritis patients since these drugs have come into use in their treatment (Kinlen 1985). At present the implication of methotrexate and azathioprine is doubtful (Silman *et al.* 1988; Stern *et al.* 1982; Kingsmore *et al.* 1992). However, cyclophosphamide has been clearly shown to be carcinogenic in cases of rheumatoid arthritis. In a case–control study of 119 rheumatoid arthritis patients followed for 20 years, a difference in the incidence of malignancies appeared 6 years after cyclophosphamide was begun and persisted irrespective of when it was discontinued. Fifty cancers were found in 37 cyclophosphamide cases versus 26 in 25 matched, non- cyclophosphamide treated cases ($p < 0.05$). All nine bladder carcinomas occurred following cyclophosphamide treatment and this was associated with the largest cumulative doses. All lymphoreticular neoplasms occurred during the first decade of observation, while bladder carcinomas were still being found two decades after cyclophosphamide treatment (Baker *et al.* 1987; Radis *et al.* 1995).

Spondylarthropathies

The spondylarthropathies as such do not predispose to the occurrence of leukaemia or solid neoplasms (Smith *et al.* 1977). However, patients whose vertebral column has received therapeutic X-irradiation, as was popular in the 1940s, are at increased risk, particularly for leukaemia. The studies begun by Court-Brown and Doll in Great Britain led to the recognition of this hazard and the eventual discontinuance of this therapy (Court-Brown and Doll 1965). Haemopoiesis

Table 1 Neoplasms with unusual association with rheumatoid arthritis

	Men		Women		Total	
	Cases	SIR	Cases	SIR	Cases	SIR
Rheumatoid arthritis	3750		7933		11 683	
Neoplasms	331		509		840	
Liver	2	0.45	2	0.29	4	0.35
Stomach	17	0.62	22	0.64*	39	0.63
Colon	15	0.70	29	0.60	44	0.63
Rectum	11	0.74	17	0.72*	28	0.72
Bladder	14	0.73	10	0.74	24	0.74
Hodgkin's disease	9	4.61	**			
Lymphoma	22	2.38**	26	1.73**	48	1.98
Chronic lymphocytic leukaemia	9	2.34				
Non-Hodgkin's lymphoma	13	1.78	23	1.94	36	1.88
Multiple myeloma	9	1.83*	**			
Pulmonary carcinoma	**		29	1.50		

Gridley *et al.* 1993; Isomäki *et al.* 1978: 11 483 male, 34 618 female cases. *$p < 0.05$, **$p < 0.01$ in the Isomäki data.
SIR = standardized incidence ratio.

may remain depressed in heavily irradiated areas more than a decade after treatment. Leukaemias, particularly the acute myeloid type, have a peak incidence 2.5 years after a course of treatment. Except for chronic lymphocytic leukaemia, these dyscrasias occur more than three times as often as expected following X-ray therapy. The excess risk then diminishes but does not disappear (Darby *et al*. 1987). Apical pulmonary fibrosis, an uncommon complication of ankylosing spondylitis (Rosenow *et al*. 1977), has been reported as the site of primary adenocarcinoma, but only following X-ray therapy (Ahern *et al*. 1982). The risk of solid neoplasms over-all following X-ray therapy is increased slightly and this has been associated with older age at the time of treatment. The occurrence of fibrosarcomas has been associated with X-ray therapy (Edgar and Robinson 1973) but not lymphoreticular neoplasms (Boice 1992).

Sjögren's syndrome

In considering the relationship of Sjögren's syndrome to neoplasia only lymphoreticular proliferation warrants consideration. Three circumstances must be defined:

1. Myoepithelial sialadenitis is the pathological term for the diagnostic alteration in salivary and lacrimal glands that is essential, but not sufficient, to substantiate the clinical diagnosis (Schmid *et al*. 1982).

2. This, in addition, requires findings of xerostomia and/or keratoconjunctivitis sicca (subnormal salivation and/or lacrimation).

3. When these findings occur in the absence of an autoimmune rheumatic disease the designation is Sjögren's disease (or primary Sjögren's syndrome). 'Sjögren's syndrome' (or secondary Sjögren's syndrome) indicates the concurrent presence of a connective tissue disease, most often rheumatoid arthritis or systemic lupus erythematosus.

Sjögren's syndrome is predominantly an ailment of middle-aged women. The mean age at the time of diagnosis of the primary and secondary form is similar (Moutsopoulos *et al*. 1980). Depending on the sites and magnitude of the characteristic proliferation of lymphocytes and epithelial cells, the disease may have various manifestations, but diminished salivary and lacrimal function predominate. The proliferation may remain within lymph nodes or extend extranodally. Because of the range of alterations within lymph nodes and extranodally, the lesions vary from clearly benign, through the potentially premalignant 'pseudolymphoma' phase, to one of the malignant lymphomas (McCurley *et al*. 1990), which usually is of a non-Hodgkin's B-cell type. Hodgkin's disease (Nagai *et al*., 1993), reticulum cell sarcoma (Hornbaker *et al*. 1966), T-cell lymphoma (Chevalier *et al*. 1991), monoclonal gammopathies (Sugai *et al*. 1985) including cryoglobulinaemia (Tzioufas *et al*. 1986), and angioimmunoblastic lymphadenopathy (Bignon *et al*. 1986) are rare occurrences. Latency between the onset of clinically evident salivary gland enlargement and the diagnosis of malignant lymphoma range from 1.5 to 12 years in the experience of Schmid *et al*. (Schmid *et al*. 1982), and intervals of 20 years are known.

While about 20 per cent of patients with rheumatoid arthritis also have Sjögren's syndrome, the reported prevalence of rheumatoid arthritis among cases of Sjögren's syndrome has varied, depending on the diagnostic criteria and techniques, from 13.4 per cent of a Swedish cohort (Holm 1949) and 14.3 per cent in a Scottish study

(Thompson and Eadie 1956) to 58.4 per cent in a Czech investigation (Lenoch *et al*. 1967). Sjögren's syndrome has been described as a complication of all major systemic autoimmune rheumatic diseases but, aside from rheumatoid arthritis, it has been observed frequently enough only in association with systemic lupus erythematosus to conclude whether the association influences neoplasia — it does not.

Lymphocytic lesions are more likely to extend beyond the salivary and lacrimal structures in primary than in secondary Sjögren's syndrome. However, this does not alter the risk of neoplastic change (Moutsopoulos *et al*. 1980). The early diagnosis of the lymphoma is difficult since it results from an evolutionary process in the course of Sjögren's syndrome. Therefore, prevalence figures depend in large measure on the mean duration of disease in the cohort of patients studied. In the three largest published studies lymphomas were detected in a mean of 4.3 per cent of 445 cases of Sjögren's syndrome (Whaley *et al*. 1973; Kassan *et al*. 1978; McCurley *et al*. 1990). This exceeds the frequency in any other population of patients, but whether by as much as 44-fold (Kassan *et al*. 1978) has not been confirmed.

Of 20 patients in whom the routine histopathological diagnosis was myoepithelial sialadenitis, immunohistological techniques showed various evolutionary stages of neoplasia in 12, and three were frankly lymphomatous (Hyjek *et al*. 1988). Refined procedures have shown that many of these neoplasms belong to the monocytoid B-cell type and may be detectable in cases that are considered pseudolymphoma by the usual techniques (Sung *et al*. 1991). Neoplastic transformation may, in a minority of patients, result in either of two contradictory immunochemical processes. In some cases the development of a lymphoma is indicated by a decrease in serum IgM and, if rheumatoid factor has been present, by its decreasing titre. In other cases a monoclonal gammopathy develops which may be indistinguishable from Waldenström's macroglobulinaemia. In most of such cases the monoclonal protein has been IgM κ, except in Japan, where an IgA paraproteinaemia appears to be as likely as the IgM type (Sugai *et al*. 1985).

Of 28 patients with Sjögren's syndrome and lymphoma recorded in three American studies (Kassan *et al*. 1978; McCurley *et al*. 1990; Sung *et al*. 1991) seven had rheumatoid arthritis and one lupus erythematosus. Contrary to the female predominance of Sjögren's syndrome, neoplastic change in Sjögren's syndrome does not appear to be sex influenced.

Lymphomas originate in salivary glands infrequently and most of these are non-Hodgkin's B-cell neoplasms — the same type that is most often associated with Sjögren's syndrome. In reviews of 33 salivary gland lymphomas in New York and 40 cases in London, each included four instances of Sjögren's syndrome, an incidence of 11 per cent (Hyman and Wolff 1978; Gleeson *et al*. 1986). A French investigation of 113 cases of non-Hodgkin's lymphoma (86 per cent B-cell, 14 per cent T-cell) found 10 (8.8 per cent) with clinical Sjögren's syndrome. It had preceded the diagnosis of lymphoma in two. Remission of the lymphoma was associated with loss of the salivary gland infiltrate in cases that met only the histopathological criteria of Sjögren's syndrome, but not in those who had clinical Sjögren's syndrome (Janin *et al*. 1992).

In conclusion, the magnitude of the association between either primary or secondary Sjögren's syndrome and the development of any of several malignant lymphomas is uncertain. However, rapid enlargement of salivary glands unaccompanied by signs of inflammation, and/or a changing immunoglobulin pattern, warrants a biopsy which should be examined immunohistochemically.

Systemic lupus erythematosus

Systemic lupus erythematosus (SLE) most frequently occurs between the ages of 15 and 35 and in this age group women predominate at least 8:1. Life expectancy for the patient with SLE has increased markedly since the 1950s, in part due to enhanced diagnostic awareness and improved techniques whereby milder cases, which may be expected to have a more chronic course, are being identified, and in part due to improved therapy. While the 4-year survival was about 50 per cent in 1955, the 10-year survival in the 1990s may exceed 80 per cent (Abu-Shakra et al. 1995). Since cancer is relatively uncommon in young women, its occurrence in a typical case of SLE may raise the suspicion of a causal relationship. It follows that if there is an association between SLE and neoplasia, more such cases would occur among the recent greater number of long-term survivors, especially since some of the immunosuppressive agents used in treating SLE are potentially carcinogenic.

The possibility of such a relationship is supported in the animal model of SLE. The offspring of matings of NZB and NZW mice manifest characteristics of an autoimmune disease resembling SLE and infrequently develop a lymphoma. Treatment of such mice with the equivalent of therapeutic doses of cyclophosphamide (Walker and Boles 1973) resulted in a high incidence of various neoplasms, and treatment with azathioprine resulted in lymphomas (Casey 1968). Results were strongly dose related.

In a review of 15 cases of solid tumours in cases of SLE, seven had been treated with one of these drugs; the neoplasm was not detected until 12 to 19 years after the diagnosis of SLE in eight, six of whom had received azathioprine or cyclophosphamide (Sulkes and Naparstek 1991). In a Finnish series of 17 cases of neoplasia in SLE, the neoplasm was detected 12 to 30 years after SLE in eight; cytostatic drugs were not considered to have been a contributory factor (Pettersson et al. 1992; Sweeney et al. 1995). The observation by Sweeney et al. that patients in whom a neoplasm develops have a later onset of SLE differs from the reports of others who found the diagnosis of SLE to have been made in 20 of 33 such cases at age 35 or less (Sulkes and Naparstek 1991; Pettersson et al. 1992) The prolongation of life has been a factor in the increased concurrence of SLE and neoplasia. However, at present neoplasia in SLE does not exceed the expected incidence (Sweeney et al. 1995).

Case reports give the impression that SLE conveys a susceptibility to the development of lymphoreticular neoplasms. The diagnosis of Hodgkin's disease may be obscured by the similarity of symptoms if it develops during the course of SLE (Bhalla et al. 1993). However, except for the aforementioned Finnish study, large series of cases of SLE do not support such an association. Four cohorts encompassing 1510 cases of SLE included only six lymphomas among 36 cases of neoplasia (Ropes 1976; Lewis et al. 1976; Abu-Shakra et al. 1995; Sweeney et al. 1995). Furthermore, Razis et al. found no instances of SLE among 1269 patients with lymphosarcoma or among 1102 with Hodgkin's disease (Razis et al. 1959). Miller found only one instance of SLE among 1893 patients who had a solid tissue neoplasm and one among 264 patients with a lymphoproliferative neoplasm (Miller 1967). Of 29 patients with an autoimmune rheumatic disease and lymphoma only one had SLE (Banks et al. 1979). Unless the SLE patient is being treated chronically with a potentially carcinogenic drug, particularly cyclophosphamide, no special surveillance for neoplasia is warranted. A recent report has emphasized the association of SLE and non-Hodgkin's lymphoma (Mellemkjaer et al. 1997).

Polymyositis/dermatomyositis

The first two reports of the association of dermatomyositis with cancer were published in 1916. However, whether this association might be more than coincidental initially attracted attention in 1951 when a German dermatologist concluded from a literature review that cancer occurs at least five times as frequently among cases of dermatomyositis as in the general population. The pathogenetic validity of the dermatomyositis–neoplasia association was first questioned in 1975 (Bohan and Peter 1977) and the statistical debate has continued. The only undisputed conclusion is that when the myopathy occurs during childhood it is not associated with neoplasia. The two principal epidemiological questions are:

1. May the apparent association be accounted for entirely by referral and examination biases?

2. Even assuming that the association over all is artefactual, are there hidden subsets of myopathy–neoplasia relationships that have a biological basis?

Most reports have been of individual cases of dermatomyositis and/or polymyositis, or of series of patients who were ill enough to be hospitalized, both of which make extrapolation to the entire spectrum of dermatomyositis/polymyositis cases unreliable. Some recent investigators have sought to avoid 'Berkson's (hospitalization) bias' (Masi and Hochberg 1988). Lyon et al. analyzed 322 cases that were contributed by American rheumatologists and compared a subset of 104 with a sex-matched sibling (Lyon et al. 1989). Only 1.5 per cent of the total cases had had a neoplasm and there was no definite difference in neoplasia between the cases and their siblings. However, only cases that were diagnosed within a 2-year period and assessed in the third year were included. The potential longer-term risk was not addressed.

Although a Swedish investigation was based on patients who had been hospitalized with a diagnosis of dermatomyositis or polymyositis, this was not done as selectively as in most countries and therefore minimized the Berkson bias. A potential weakness was that national cancer incidence data rather than individual matching was used for controls. All cases diagnosed dermatomyositis/polymyositis between 1963 and 1983 were followed through 1987 with the help of a national cancer registry. As in most such cohorts, cancer was more prevalent among cases of dermatomyositis than of polymyositis, but during an average follow-up of 10.4 years all subdivisions demonstrated an increased risk of neoplasia: dermatomyositis male 2.4, female 3.4; polymyositis male 1.8, female 1.7. The risk of a neoplasm within 5 years after the diagnosis of dermatomyositis was: male 4.4, female 4.8 (Sigurgeirsson et al. 1992).

Zantos et al. analysed the foregoing (Zantos et al. 1994) and two other differently but well controlled smaller studies (Manchul et al. 1985; Lakhanpal et al. 1986) and concluded that, indeed, both dermatomyositis and polymyositis are associated with an increased risk of cancer. Several studies have found clustering of the diagnosis of dermatomyositis or polymyositis and a neoplasm within a short time frame. Sigurgeirsson et al. found both diagnoses to be established within 1 year of each other in one-half of the cases of dermatomyositis and one-third of the cases of polymyositis (Sigurgeirsson et al. 1992).

Manchul *et al.* found neoplasms in 25 per cent of 71 dermatomyositis/polymyositis cases and in 10 per cent of 142 control cases, half with inflammatory, half with non-inflammatory musculoskeletal diseases (Manchul *et al.* 1985). In eight of the 18 dermatomyositis/polymyositis cases the neoplasm was diagnosed within ± 6 months of the myopathy, compared to one of 14 related to the diagnosis of the control cases. Presumably the proximity of some of the diagnoses results from particularly careful examinations stimulated by the belief that the myopathy is a paraneoplastic phenomenon. However, most of these neoplasms are discovered as a result of standard examinations (Plotz *et al.* 1989). The neoplasm which occurs in the dermatomyositis/polymyositis patient reflects the geographic prevalence of the neoplasm rather than a particular affinity to the myopathy. For example 42 per cent of the associated neoplasms in Japan have been gastric carcinomas, versus 8 per cent in the United States; conversely, 8 per cent of dermatomyositis/polymyositis associated neoplasms in Japan have been carcinomas of the breast, versus 17 per cent in the United States (Hidano *et al.* 1986; Callen 1982).

No laboratory tests reliably identify which patient with dermatomyositis/polymyositis is harbouring a neoplasm. The inflammatory and degenerative findings in muscle biopsies are not altered by the presence of a neoplasm, nor are the titres of any of the numerous autoantibodies that may be detectable in this disease helpful (Basset-Sequin *et al.* 1990). Anti-Jo-1 and anti-nRNP are the most characteristic (Targoff and Reichlin 1988). Their absence helps to exclude the diagnosis of dermatomyositis/polymyositis. The most consistent biochemical abnormality is elevation of serum creatine phosphokinase, which usually reflects the acuteness of the myopathy, but is not affected by the presence of a neoplasm. It has been suggested that a normal creatine phosphokinase concentration in clinically evident dermatomyositis/polymyositis augurs a poor prognosis (Fudman and Schnitzer 1986). Interpretation must take into consideration that the normal creatine phosphokinase in comparable individuals is about 80 units higher in blacks than in whites (Black *et al.* 1986).

In regard to the association with neoplasia, polymyositis must be differentiated particularly from carcinomatous neuromyopathy (Brain and Adams 1965) and paraneoplastic endocrine myopathies (Patel *et al.* 1993). Myasthenia gravis, which may coexist with polymyositis (Behan *et al.* 1982), may come into consideration, as well as the rarer Eaton–Lambert myasthenic syndrome (see below), and drug-induced myopathies (Zuckner 1990). Clinically, rapid response to corticosteroid therapy favours the diagnosis of dermatomyositis/polymyositis over the others.

As improved therapy prolongs survival with dermatomyositis/polymyositis, an increase in the number of neoplasm associated cases may be anticipated. Whether this is due to a causal relationship with the myopathy or with the increasingly cancer-prone older age group is uncertain. The conservative conclusion to be drawn from the available epidemiological and clinical data is that when a patient over 45 years of age is seen during the first year of dermatomyositis/polymyositis close surveillance for cancer is justified. Later in the course of the disease more than routine evaluations for cancer are not cost effective.

Diffuse scleroderma and paraneoplastic Raynaud's phenomenon

Diffuse scleroderma (systemic sclerosis) is less common than systemic lupus erythematosus, but probably occurs more frequently than polymyositis. Its peak incidence is in the fifth decade. Small cohorts have not shown an abnormal risk of neoplasia. However, an epidemiological study conducted in metropolitan Pittsburgh (United States) during 1971 to 1982 obtained an excess incidence of 1.8 over regional incidence data. During a mean observation period of 4.3 years, nine women and five men (5.3 per cent) had a malignant neoplasm. A total of 680 patients with systemic sclerosis (78 per cent women) were examined during these 12 years. Twenty-five had a malignancy, 3.6 per cent of women and 4.1 per cent of men (Roumm and Mesdger 1985). Such an excess was confirmed in a study of 248 cases of systemic sclerosis first seen between 1978 and 1992 in Toronto (66 per cent women). Compared to the population of the province of Ontario, systemic sclerosis had an increased cancer risk of 2.1 (Abu-Shakra *et al.* 1993).

It is likely that most neoplasms occur coincidentally with systemic sclerosis, including the few that antedate its development. However, the relationship of carcinomas of the breast and lung with systemic sclerosis requires special comment. The fact that breast cancer is the most common neoplasm among cases of systemic sclerosis can superficially be attributed to the female preponderance of this disease. However, 34 per cent of 90 women with systemic sclerosis and a neoplasm in four studies had breast cancer, about twice the proportion of breast cancer among North American female cancer patients (Duncan and Winkelmann 1979; Lee *et al.* 1983; Roumm and Medsger 1985; Abu-Shakra *et al.*). Furthermore, while the mean interval between the diagnosis of systemic sclerosis and other neoplasms was about 6 years, the interval for breast cancer was only 2 years (Duncan and Winkelmann 1979; Roumm and Medsger 1985). Of 35 cases where a neoplasm was found within 1 year of the diagnosis of systemic sclerosis, 37 per cent were carcinomas of the breast. This is not entirely attributable to the availability of more sensitive diagnostic methods for cancer of the breast than for cancer of other organs. While the explanation of the relationship remains obscure, the practical conclusion to be drawn from these observations is that women should undergo a careful breast examination at least semi-annually and annual mammography during the first 3 to 5 years after a diagnosis of systemic sclerosis has been made.

The occurrence of carcinoma of the lung in association with systemic sclerosis exhibits three peculiarities:

1. It is consistent with the female susceptibility to systemic sclerosis rather than the male susceptibility for pulmonary carcinoma.

2. Smoking is not implicated in the pathogenesis of these carcinomas.

3. The cancer occurs in cases of long-standing systemic sclerosis in which pulmonary fibrosis has become prominent (Talbott and Barrocas 1980).

Some types of pulmonary fibrosis predispose to carcinogenesis, but the precipitating factors are unidentified. Thus, cryptogenic fibrosing alveolitis is associated with a substantially increased risk of lung cancer (Turner-Warwick 1980), while rheumatoid lung disease is not. The mean duration of systemic sclerosis in 64 patients when lung cancer was diagnosed was 15 years (Talbott and Barrocas 1980). As the most optimistic 5-year survival estimate for patients with systemic sclerosis is only about 70 per cent (Steen 1990), those in whom lung cancer develops tend, contrary to those with breast cancer, to have a relatively benign course of systemic sclerosis. Among

58 patients with systemic sclerosis and lung cancer 60 per cent were less than 60 years of age and 69 per cent were women. The suggestion that alveolar cell carcinoma is peculiarly associated with systemic sclerosis may be attributable to a reporting bias. The histological types of pulmonary carcinomas in systemic sclerosis probably occur in similar proportions to those in other patients (Roumm and Medsger).

While Raynaud's phenomenon is an early manifestation of virtually all cases of systemic sclerosis, it occasionally occurs as a paraneoplastic symptom without other evidence of systemic sclerosis. The preponderance of female cases approaches the 9:1 sex ratio of Raynaud's phenomenon in general. Raynaud's phenomenon appears not to be associated with any particular neoplasm. Onset has been described as virtually concurrent with the diagnosis of the cancer, and no longer than 2 years preceding such a diagnosis. The ischaemia may be unilateral (DeCross and Sahasrabudhe 1992). In some cases it has resolved following resection of the neoplasm. The pathogenetic relationship remains obscure, although in one report cells of a cervical carcinoma were producing interleukin-6, which was suspected to be the vasospastic stimulus (Murashima *et al.* 1992). Raynaud's phenomenon may also be induced by certain antineoplastic drugs: bleomycin, vinblastine, cisplatin (Hansen and Olsen 1989).

Polymyalgia rheumatica

Polymyalgia rheumatica is the rheumatic syndrome that occurs particularly in the most cancer-prone age group. The average age of onset is about 65 years, and the disease begins below the age of 50 in fewer than 5 per cent (Huston *et al.* 1978). There is a female predominance of about 3:2. A survey of 96 patients with polymyalgia rheumatica diagnosed during 10 years in a community in the northern United States included six who had a cancer before and ten in whom the diagnosis of a neoplasm occurred after the onset of polymyalgia rheumatica. The 16 patients encompassed seven different neoplasms (Chuang *et al.* 1982). The largest investigation has been conducted in Norway with 185 cases of polymyalgia rheumatica diagnosed between 1978 and 1983 and followed to 1987. Each was matched with five control subjects. Of the polymyalgia rheumatica cases 14.6 per cent had cancer, as had 14.2 per cent of the controls; the polymyalgia rheumatica cases included 14 different neoplasms. The female preponderance of the neoplasm cases was consistent with the sex ratio of the entire cohort. Thirteen had a neoplasm, found an average of 8.3 years before polymyalgia rheumatica and in 14 a neoplasm was found an average of 4.6 years after the onset of polymyalgia rheumatica (Haga *et al.* 1993). The temporal relationships support the view that these are merely coincidental events.

Neoplasia was more strongly associated with isolated temporal arteritis (24 per cent) than with either isolated polymyalgia rheumatica (11 per cent) or polymyalgia rheumatica with temporal arteritis (10 per cent) (Haga *et al.* 1993). This observation is supported by the finding that there may be a difference between temporal arteritis with and without polymyalgia rheumatica. HLA DR4 occurs significantly less frequently in cases of isolated temporal arteritis than in the presence of polymyalgia rheumatica (Richardson *et al.* 1987). While DR4 appears to be associated with polymyalgia rheumatica as well as with rheumatoid arthritis, whether this is pertinent to neoplasia susceptibility with temporal arteritis warrants further evaluation.

Lymphomas occasionally occur in patients with polymyalgia rheumatica (Kalra and Delamere 1987; Montanaro and Bizzarri 1992). However, the occurrence in series of cases is low enough to indicate coincidence (1 of 96; 2 of 185). Chuang *et al.* found that 18 per cent of their polymyalgia rheumatica cases also met diagnostic criteria for rheumatoid arthritis (Chuang *et al.* 1982). Polymyalgia rheumatica clearly lacks the association with lymphoreticular neoplasia observed in rheumatoid arthritis. Whether the occurrence of monoclonal gammopathy resembles the prevalence in rheumatoid arthritis requires further investigation (Kalra and Delamere 1987).

When a person in the seventh decade or beyond presents with myalgia, proximal muscle weakness, and perhaps also weight loss, both polymyalgia rheumatica and a paraneoplastic neuromyopathy should be considered. Polymyalgia rheumatica symptoms are more likely to predominate in the shoulder girdle and paraneoplastic syndromes in the pelvic girdle, but neither this or any serological findings differentiate reliably. Since carcinomatous neuromyopathy most often results from carcinoma of the lung, it is prudent to include chest radiography in the evaluation of possible polymyalgia rheumatica, but an intensive search for a neoplasm is not ordinarily warranted.

Rheumatic manifestations of malignancy

Skeletal neoplasia

Apart from hypertrophic osteoarthropathy, cancer infrequently produces skeletal symptoms that the careful clinician might mistake for a systemic rheumatic disease. Data about the principal primary neoplasms of bone are summarized in Table 2. At least 95 per cent of malignant neoplasms in bone are metastatic carcinomas. These reflect the age and sex distribution of the primary disease; on average, patients with metastatic carcinoma are about two decades older than patients with musculoskeletal sarcomas. Metastases usually result from haematogenous spread with implantation in the marrow cavity (Galasko 1982). The cortex is affected by neoplastic factors that predominantly stimulate osteoblastic activity, resulting in sclerotic lesions, even in the presence of the osteoclastic activity that causes the more common lytic lesions (Springfield 1982). Only in myeloma and lymphoma do the lytic lesions not tend to be associated with reactive bone formation. Certain tumour cell lines are predisposed to survive in specific organs. Carcinoma of the prostate, breast, kidney, and thyroid are particularly likely to form metastases in bone. Although bronchogenic carcinoma is less likely to do so, the frequency of this neoplasm places it second only to breast as a source of skeletal metastases. The lumbosacral vertebrae, pelvis, femora, and ribs are the most frequent sites of osseous metastases. A radiographically solitary lesion occurs in fewer than 10 per cent of patients with skeletal metastases. Most solitary lesions once were considered benign. However, scintigraphy has caused this opinion to be revised. Because of its greater sensitivity, a bone scan is mandatory to confirm that a lesion probably is solitary (Merrick and Merrick 1986). Vertebrae are the most common site of metastases which are radiographically undetectable initially and manifested only by local pain (Clain 1965). In cases with normal radiographs in which a scintigram indicates metastases, the lesions generally become evident radiographically within 6 to 18 months. A scintigraphically solitary lesion

Table 2 Principal age, sex, and site of the commoner neoplasms of bone

	Cases	Percentage male	Peak decades (% of cases)		Most frequent sites		Reference
Malignant							
Multiple myeloma	869	60.9	7th (38.8)	6th (26.6)	Multifocal		Kyle (1975)
Osteogenic sarcoma	1274	58.1	2nd (47.2)	3rd (22.6)	Femur	42.4	Dahlin and Unni
					Tibia	18.5	(1995)
Chondrosarcoma	643	59.6	6th (25.7)	5th (19.8)	Femur	22.1	Dahlin and Unni
					Humerus	11.8	(1985)
Lymphoma	469	62.3	6th (21.7)	7th (18.1)	Femur	24.5	Dahlin and Unni
					Humerus	8.7	(1985)
Ewing's tumour	402	57.0	2nd (57.5)	1st (17.9)	Femur	22.4	Dahlin and Unni
					Humerus	11.4	(1985)
Fibrosarcoma	207	50.7	4th (19.3)	6th (18.3)	Femur	26.1	Dahlin and Unni
					Tibia	15.9	(1985)
Malignant synovioma	134	60.5	3rd (29.9)	4th (26.8)	Thigh	26.1	Cadman et al.
					Knee	15.7	(1965)
Benign							
Osteochondroma	727	62.9	2nd (49.1)	3rd (18.8)	Femur	32.9	Dahlin and Unni
					Humerus	15.4	(1985)
Giant cell tumour	425	43.5	3rd (38.8)	4th (23.3)	Femur	30.6	Dahlin and Unni
					Tibia	27.0	(1985)

proves to be metastatic in about one-half of cases (McNeill 1984). Nevertheless, a positive radiograph is occasionally contradicted by a false-negative scintigram.

A primary or a metastatic neoplasm in a juxta-articular site or in synovium may imitate mono- or oligoarticular arthritis. There may be signs of synovitis, including small non-haemorrhagic effusions without actual invasion of the synovium. Conversely, villonodular synovitis, a benign neoplasm which most often affects the knee, may cause a juxta-articular lytic lesion mimicking a primary bone neoplasm (Jergensen et al. 1978). Neoplastic cells in joint effusions do not necessarily indicate invasion of the synovium. Despite its vascularity the synovium rarely is a metastatic site (Newton et al. 1984). Metastases, particularly to acral sites, may cause symptoms that mimic rheumatoid arthritis or, if there is a local inflammatory reaction and coincidental hyperuricaemia, gout. Nevertheless, acral metastases are uncommon, presumably because of the small number of tumour cells that reach the extremities of the vasculature. According to a review in 1976, 88 cases of metastases to hand bones had been published, most from pulmonary carcinomas (Uriburu et al. 1976). Metastases to the feet may be rarer still, 72 cases having been reported up to 1982, without as great a predominance of a particular organ of origin (Zindrick et al. 1982).

Synovial sarcomas are uncommon neoplasms that occur predominantly before the age of 40. Fewer than 8 per cent are diagnosed beyond age 60 (Tillotson et al. 1951; Cadman et al. 1965). There is a 3:2 male preponderance. The tumour is usually located in periarticular tissue rather than within the joint cavity. The most frequent sites in 550 cases collated from four publications are: knee 22.5 per cent; foot and ankle 21.4 per cent; and thigh 15.8 per cent (Tillotson

et al. 1951; Cadman et al. 1965; Mackenzie 1966; Hajdu et al. 1977). A lower extremity is affected in approximately 70 per cent of the patients. However, this neoplasm occasionally occurs far from joints, such as in the hypopharynx or oesophagus (Amble et al. 1992).

Histologically this neoplasm may be 'biphasic,' meaning that it contains both epithelial and spindle cells, or 'monophasic,' when virtually only one cell type is present. This does not affect the prognosis. Synovioma acquired its name because of its usual proximity to the synovium. However, ultrastructual and immunochemical studies have failed to find synovial characteristics, so that it probably arises from a primitive mesenchymal precursor cell (Miettinen and Virtanen 1984).

About 60 per cent of the patients present with local pain or tenderness, but signs of inflammation are rare. Radiographically about 30 per cent of synoviomas contain calcifications and 10 per cent show signs of bone invasion. Survival is better correlated with a low prevalence of mitoses in the neoplasm than with small size (less than 5 cm diameter) (Cagle et al. 1987; Rööser et al. 1989). However, both criteria are more predictive than whether the tumour was resected locally or by amputation.

According to Mayo Clinic data, osteoarticular symptoms occur in about 14 per cent of childhood cases of acute leukaemia and in 4 per cent of adults with a leukaemia (Silverstein and Kelly 1963). Musculoskeletal symptoms in paediatric cases usually are a manifestation of acute lymphocytic leukaemia, while in adults the association is strongest with the chronic myelogenous type. Leukaemia is by far the most frequent malignancy in white children, being somewhat less common among black children. It also is the most frequent cause of neoplastic skeletal symptoms in childhood and adolescence.

For example of 13 children, 2 to 14 years of age, who presented for rheumatological evaluation and proved to have a malignancy, 10 had leukaemia and the others soft tissue sarcomas (Schaller 1972). Of 28 consecutive leukaemic children (24 acute lymphocytic leukaemia), 14 had musculoskeletal symptoms, most frequently in the knees (Costello *et al.* 1983).

Musculoskeletal symptoms may be the earliest indication of leukaemia and may precede its discovery by several months. There may be bone pain and/or arthralgia, which tends to be asymmetrical. Synovial effusion is uncommon, with its leucocyte count usually below $20\,000/mm^3$, and often without morphologically evident leukaemic cells (Holdrinet *et al.* 1989). Such identification has been made immunologically (Harden *et al.* 1984). Articular symptoms more often are due to periarticular infiltration than to synovial involvement. Scinitgraphy is more likely than radiography to detect early lesions, but no abnormality may initially be demonstrable. Radiographic findings include metaphyseal radioluscent bands (mainly in children), diffuse osteopenia (mainly in adults), osteolytic lesions, and periostitis. Analysis of synovial fluid is important because the effusion may have resulted from infection or, less frequently, contain urate or calcium pyrophosphate crystals, each of which requiring other than antileukaemic therapy. Osteoarticular leukaemic symptoms usually respond well to chemotherapy and their recurrence augurs a relapse.

Primary skeletal neoplasms are uncommon in childhood. According to a survey conducted during 1969 to 1971 in the United States, the annual incidence below the age of 15 years was about 5 per million (Young and Miller 1975). Neuroblastomas are the most frequent solid tumours to cause skeletal metastases in children. Metastasis of carcinomas to bone is rare — two of 39 in one series of children. The distribution of metastases is as in adults (Leeson *et al.* 1985).

Among skeletal neoplasms in adults multiple myeloma is most likely to present problems in rheumatological differential diagnosis because:

1. This disease occurs mainly after the age of 55, so that complaints of skeletal pain may initially be minimized as symptoms of degenerative disease of joints or intervertebral discs.

2. Myeloma may present as a polyarthritis, more or less resembling rheumatoid arthritis, in which the shoulders, wrists, and knees are affected most often.

There may be subcutaneous nodules, although usually not in the typical sites of rheumatoid nodules. Symptoms rarely are due to the infiltration of synovium by myeloma cells; the usual cause is deposition of amyloid in the synovium (Gordon *et al.* 1973). The same process and symptoms may result from primary amyloidosis (Cohen and Canoso 1975). Synovial fluid sometimes contains the paraprotein, but synovial biopsy is necessary to confirm the diagnosis of articular amyloidosis. The diagnosis of myeloma must be confirmed by the demonstration of a great excess of immature plasma cells in a bone marrow aspirate or biopsy. In rheumatoid arthritis the marrow usually shows only a slight increase in plasma cells, but a large proportion of these may resemble the immature cells seen in myeloma.

Patients with chronic rheumatoid arthritis are at an increased risk of developing multiple myeloma. However, a misdiagnosis may result from the detection of a monoclonal paraprotein, which is found two to three times as frequently among cases of rheumatoid arthritis than in the general population (Zawadzki and Benedek 1969). The significance of a paraproteinaemia may be difficult to interpret at any one time.

In 1971, 241 patients with a diagnosis of monoclonal paraproteinaemia without evidence of any of the usually associated diseases were placed under surveillance by the Mayo Clinic. After a median period of 22 years, 53 per cent had died without having developed a malignant paraproteinaemia. Multiple myeloma had developed in 39 (16 per cent) after a median of 10 years; amyloidosis had developed in 8 (3 per cent) after a median of 9 years; macroglobulinaemia in 7 (3 per cent) after a median of 8 years; and 5 (2 per cent) developed a malignant lymphoproliferative disease after a median of 10.5 years (Kyle 1993). These data suggest that about a quarter of cases of 'benign' paraproteinaemia are at risk to develop one of these fatal diseases.

Oncogenic osteomalacia

Osteomalacia is a less frequent cause of tumour-associated skeletal pain than hypertrophic osteoarthropathy. However, since most of the tumours are benign, have no preferential location, and many are small, they may be difficult to find. Hence, symptoms may last for years unexplained. The patient presents with skeletal and/or articular pain, especially affecting the lower extremities, progressive pelvic girdle weakness leading to deterioration of the gait, there may be fractures and, with childhood onset, growth retardation. Symptoms most often begin in the third or fourth decade without a family history of rickets (Ryan and Reiss 1984). Various types of fibromas and haemangiomas are the most common; sarcomas have rarely been associated with this paraneoplastic activity, and carcinomas not at all (Weidner and Cruz 1987). Radiographic findings include pseudofractures (Looser's lines) and thickening of long bones despite osteopenia. Bone scans show scattered areas of increased tracer uptake (Schapira *et al.* 1995). The characteristic biochemical findings are hypophosphataemia, hyperphosphaturia, elevated alkaline phosphatase, normal to slightly subnormal serum calcium, normal serum creatinine and parathormone, and subnormal serum 1,25-dihydroxyvitamin D.

It has been inferred from the biochemical data that an unidentified tumour product interferes with the conversion of 25-hydroxyvitamin D to the active 1,25-dihydroxy compound (Harvey *et al.* 1992). Why this defect does not result in hyperparathyroidism is unknown. The disease is cured symptomatically and biochemically by resection of the tumour. If this is not feasible or until it is located, treatment with phosphate and calcitriol ($1–3\,\mu g/day$) is beneficial.

Hypertrophic osteoarthropathy

Hypertrophic osteoarthropathy often is referred to as 'pulmonary' because most cases are associated with an intrathoracic disease. Lung cancer now accounts for at least 90 per cent of the cases in the industrialized world. However, extrathoracic circumstances as disparate as non-neoplastic liver disease (Epstein *et al.* 1979) and pregnancy (Borden and Holling 1969) may be associated with the same syndrome. The occurrence of hypertrophic osteoarthropathy in large series of cases of lung cancer has varied widely, perhaps due to inconsistent diagnostic criteria or referral bias. It is more likely to occur in males regardless of age. In the Edinburgh analysis of 4000 cases of primary lung cancer, of whom 90 per cent were men, only one of 49 cases of hypertrophic osteoarthropathy occurred in a woman (LeRoux 1968). At the Mayo Clinic, 10 per cent of 1657 cases of primary lung cancer manifested hypertrophic osteoarthropathy. Women accounted for 19 per cent of those with hypertrophic osteoarthropathy, but 26 per cent of those without this complication (Stenseth *et al.* 1967). Of 1920 cases of lung cancer seen in Cleveland (United States), hypertrophic osteoarthropathy was found in only 0.8 per cent (Segal and MacKenzie 1982), and among 200 cases in London it was found in 4 per cent (Yacoub 1965). Hypertrophic osteoarthropathy is less than one-third as likely to occur with pulmonary metastases as with primary lung cancer (Stenseth *et al.* 1967), but sarcomatous metastases are more likely than carcinomatous metastases to induce hypertrophic osteoarthropathy. Of 38 children (mean age 13) with neoplastic hypertrophic osteoarthropathy 79 per cent were boys, 37 per cent had an osteogenic sarcoma, 34 per cent a nasopharyngeal carcinoma, and 16 per cent had Hodgkin's disease (Staalman and Umans 1993).

Calculated from a sex, age, and race-specific cohort analysis of the prevalence of lung cancer in the United States during 1983 to 1986, and assuming a 6 to 9 per cent incidence of hypertrophic osteoarthropathy, the following frequency per 100 000 would be anticipated in each 55 to 64-year age group: white male 15 to 22; black male 25 to 28; white female 8 to 11; black female 9 to 13. Because of the lower female incidence of hypertrophic osteoarthropathy these figures should be reduced by at least one-third for women. For the 45 to 54-year age group the figures would be about 40 per cent of the foregoing (Devesa *et al.* 1989).

The most apparent but least specific sign of hypertrophic osteoarthropathy is digital clubbing. This begins with subungual oedema and hyperaemia, followed by proliferation of connective tissue. About 80 per cent of such individuals have some form of pleuropulmonary disease, but only about 20 per cent of cases of clubbing have lung cancer. Chronic clubbing does not predispose to the development of hypertrophic osteoarthropathy (Coury 1960).

Patients usually complain of arthralgia, especially of the knees, ankles, or wrists. However, on examination the pain typically is periarticular. Some patients have true joint pain and tenderness, and perhaps small effusions and morning stiffness. Hence, such a patient may be misdiagnosed as having rheumatoid arthritis. The erythrocyte sedimentation rate in this situation is elevated, but rheumatoid factor, with rare exceptions, is absent. Symptoms usually may be controlled with non-steroidal anti-inflammatory drugs (Schumacher 1976).

Skeletal metastases from lung cancer occur more frequently than hypertrophic osteoarthropathy and tend to produce less symmetrical symptoms. The simultaneous occurrence of hypertrophic osteoarthropathy and bony metastases is rare. The greater diagnostic problem occurs because symptoms of hypertrophic osteoarthropathy often precede the discovery of an intrathoracic neoplasm by a few months, and possibly by two or more years. Despite the frequency of rheumatoid arthritis in middle-aged women, the possibility that this disease is being mimicked by hypertrophic osteoarthropathy should be considered when a woman who has risk factors for lung cancer is being evaluated.

Radiographically, signs of periostitis with subperiosteal new bone formation along the distal and/or proximal fourths of long bones, predominantly on the extensor surfaces, is diagnostic. The most commonly and prominently affected sites are the distal and proximal portions of the tibia and fibula, and distal femur (Ali *et al.* 1980). Because the periosteal reaction is so hyperaemic, bone scanning with $^{99}Tc^m$-diphosphonate has proven to be diagnostically more sensitive than radiography. This technique, contrary to radiography,

has demonstrated rather frequent involvement of the scapula and skull.

The occurrence of hypertrophic osteoarthropathy is influenced by the size, location, and cell type of the primary pulmonary neoplasm. The mean tumour mass in cases of hypertrophic osteoarthropathy is about twice as large as in those without hypertrophic osteoarthropathy (Stenseth *et al.* 1967). The influence of location is especially perplexing. Location in the periphery of a lung increases the chance that hypertrophic osteoarthropathy will develop, while invasion of the pleura appears not to exert this influence. The association of hypertrophic osteoarthropathy with malignant mesothelioma is also unusual, while the neoplasm with which hypertrophic osteoarthropathy is most highly associated is benign mesothelioma — 35 per cent (Briselli *et al.* 1981). In contradistinction to other paraneoplastic manifestations of lung cancer, which are particularly associated with the small-cell type, hypertrophic osteoarthropathy occurs least often in this relationship.

The immediate pathophysiology of hypertrophic osteoarthropathy consists of increased blood flow in the bones and adjacent connective tissues of the legs and forearms, facilitated by the development of arteriovenous shunts (Rutherford *et al.* 1969). The same syndrome occurs in dogs, especially secondary to thoracic sarcomas (Nolling *et al.* 1963). No comprehensive explanation of the syndrome has been proved. Most of the pathogenetic hypotheses were thoroughly reviewed by Shneerson (Shneerson 1981). Impetus for a neurogenic explanation evolved from the discovery that peripheral vagotomy on the side of the neoplasm may, even without its removal, abruptly stop the pain bilaterally, followed by gradual resolution of the periosteal reaction and clubbing. Analgesia begins within a week of surgery in about three-quarters of cases, probably due to collapse of the arteriovenous anastomoses (Nolling *et al.* 1963; Stenseth *et al.* 1967; Rutherford *et al.* 1969). However, the gradual response of hypertrophic osteoarthropathy to radiation therapy of the neoplasm and the bilaterality of the syndrome suggest a humoral rather than a neurogenic mechanism. The heterogeneity of its causes proves that hypertrophic osteoarthropathy is not mediated by a uniquely neoplastic product. Gynaecomastia, which is an undoubtedly humoral manifestation that may occur in hypertrophic osteoarthropathy, is not correlated with increased serum oestrogen concentration or another identified hormone. A substance resembling growth hormone has recently been considered as a potential humoral incitor of hypertrophic osteoarthropathy (Gosney *et al.* 1990). A persuasive explanation for many, but not all, characteristics of hypertrophic osteoarthropathy has been made for platelet embolization with release of platelet-derived growth factor. This substance, among other functions, stimulates mesenchymal cell growth, increases vascular permeability, and attracts smooth muscle cells and fibroblasts (Dickinson 1993).

A combined neurohumoral pathogenesis of hypertrophic osteoarthropathy seems most plausible. Only a neural mechanism could explain the abrupt diminution of peripheral blood flow and associated analgesia that usually follows vagotomy, while the symmetrical osteogenesis is best explained by the action of one or perhaps several as yet unidentified humours.

Carcinomatous polyarthritis

Carcinomatous non-metastatic polyarthritis must be distinguished from hypertrophic osteoarthropathy, rheumatoid arthritis, and polymyalgia rheumatica. The syndrome is not associated predominantly with intrathoracic neoplasms and both sexes are equally at risk. Most cases occur above the age of 60, when the onset of polymyalgia rheumatica but not of rheumatoid arthritis is expected. Onset of the arthritis may be insidious or abrupt, but the symptoms are less likely to be symmetrical than in definite rheumatoid arthritis, and rheumatoid nodules do not develop (Pines *et al.* 1984). Pain is felt in large and small joints, rather than being periarticular as in hypertrophic osteoarthropathy. Deformities rarely develop. Symptoms are more likely than those of hypertrophic osteoarthropathy to precede the diagnosis of a neoplasm which, nevertheless, is usually made within a year of the beginning of articular complaints. On the contrary, the diagnosis of polymyalgia rheumatica and a neoplasm usually occurs several years apart. Immune complexes have rarely been detected in carcinomatous polyarthritis (Awerbuch and Brooks 1981; Bradley and Pinals 1983).

Arthritic symptoms as well as serological abnormalities rapidly resolve following resection or successful radiation therapy of the neoplasm (Gottlieb *et al.* 1979; Simon and Ford 1980). Recurrence of the neoplasm may be indicated by recurrence of the arthritis (Egelmeijer and MacFarlane 1992). If the neoplasm persists, the clinical course of the arthropathy does not necessarily mirror the progress of the neoplasm. Symptomatic response to treatment with non-steroidal anti-inflammatory drugs or corticosteroids is similar to that in rheumatoid arthritis.

Carcinomatous neuropathy

In individual cancer patients it may be difficult to determine whether the development of weakness is due to inanition or is a specific paraneoplastic manifestation. When to suspect cancer in a patient with unexplained weakness and perhaps some muscle wasting is equally problematical. In a prospective study of 100 persons over 65 years of age who had no identified cancer but whose gait was impaired by largely unexplained weakness of the legs, eight cases of carcinoma were detected during 18 months of observation (Newman and Gugino 1964).

According to Shy and Silverstein, carcinomatous neuromyopathy is a 'clinical syndrome of symmetrical muscular weakness and wasting, associated with decrease of the appropriate myotactic reflexes. Either a myopathic or a combination of myopathic and neuropathic lesion.... is found pathologically' (Shy and Silverstein 1965). At least initially, weakness is out of proportion to alteration of muscle mass. Pelvic girdle muscles are most affected, so that gait disturbances, particularly on ascending stairs, may be the first symptom.

The syndrome occurs most frequently in association with small-cell carcinoma of the lung, followed by other pulmonary, gastric, and ovarian carcinomas. Because of the male preponderance of lung cancer, non-myasthenic carcinomatous neuromyopathy occurs more commonly in men (Croft and Wilkinson 1965); on examination of 1465 carcinoma patients they made this diagnosis in 15.0 per cent of men and 11.6 per cent of women with lung cancer, 7.4 per cent of men and 12.5 per cent of women with gastric carcinoma, and 16.4 per cent of cases of ovarian carcinoma. No consistent relationship between the occurrence of the myopathy and either the age of the patient or known duration of the neoplasm has been determined. Compared to 'neuromyopathy' Eaton–Lambert syndrome is rare (probably less than 1:40). Autonomic dysfunctions, such as dry mouth and postural hypotension, are common findings with small-cell carcinoma and not a reliable diagnostic clue to Eaton–Lambert syndrome (Elrington *et al.* 1991). Differentiation between 'cachectic' and 'neuromyopathic' clinical findings may be uncertain. Hawley *et al.*, in a prospective study of 71 patients with small-cell lung cancer, were impressed by a greater preservation of strength relative to the severity of weight loss (Hawley *et al.* 1980). The myopathy also was less severe than that found in a group of alcoholic men matched by age and weight loss.

Both histopathological and electrophysiological abnormalities are demonstrable in the absence of clinical neuromuscular findings. In a study of 100 consecutive patients with lung cancer who were assessed with muscle biopsies, 15 (mainly small-cell) had signs of proximal myopathy, while 18 (mainly non-small-cell) had cachectic (diffuse) myopathy. However, 99 patients had abnormal histological findings. Most consistent (74 cases) was atrophy of type-2 (large mean diameter, phosphorylase-rich) nerve fibres (Gomm *et al.* 1990). Contrary to some investigators, no microvascular abnormalities, such as atrophy of terminal arteriovenous anastomoses (Scelsi and Pinelli 1977) were detected. In some cases there is only scattered, non-specific atrophy or necrosis of muscle fibres with lymphocytic infiltrates.

Paul *et al.* compared the electromyographic findings of 195 non-diabetic cancer patients below the age of 65 years with 50 age-matched controls (Paul *et al.* 1978). Muscle wasting was better correlated with myographic abnormalities than with slowed nerve conduction, and both types of abnormality were more prevalent among patients with diffuse muscle wasting, most of whom presumably had a cachectic myopathy, than in those whose wasting predominantly affected the proximal musculature. Retarded conduction velocity was equally prevalent in patients with carcinomas of the lungs and of other organs, but other abnormalities were twice as frequent among cases of lung cancer. The cause of the various abnormalities and of their variability remain obscure. Treatment is non-specific until the neoplasm is found and then is focused on the neoplasm.

Rarely a more aggressive myopathy occurs. In this, weakness progresses within a few weeks and affects virtually all muscles, despite preservation of tendon reflexes. It is not associated with a particular type of carcinoma. There is extensive necrosis of terminal intramuscular nerve fibres and of muscle fibres, with consequent elevation of the serum creatine phosphokinase (Vosskämper *et al.* 1989).

Eaton–Lambert myasthenic syndrome

The Eaton–Lambert myasthenic syndrome was differentiated from myasthenia gravis in 1957. In early descriptions it was associated almost exclusively with small-cell carcinoma of the lung. The association with this neoplasm has been confirmed but it has become recognized that nearly one-half of cases occur in the absence of a neoplasm. The latter cases have brought the sex ratio from strongly male to 1:1 (Pascuzzi and Kim 1990; McEvoy 1994). Eaton–Lambert syndrome occurs in about 3 per cent of cases of small-cell carcinoma and rarely in other pulmonary or extrapulmonary neoplasms (O'Neill *et al.* 1988).

The most common presenting finding is weakness of the pelvic girdle musculature, initially revealed by an altered gait. Autonomical functions may be affected, manifested most often by dryness of the mouth and/or orthostatic hypotension (Khurana *et al.* 1988). The main differential diagnosis is with myasthenia gravis. While one can be fairly confident that no carcinoma is impending if none has been found after 3 years of Eaton–Lambert syndrome, one must consider that myasthenia gravis is also associated with an increased incidence of neoplasia, albeit less so. In contrast to Eaton–Lambert syndrome, at least half of these cancers are found after myasthenia gravis has been present for longer than 3 years. Most patients with either syndrome who are found to have cancer are between 55 and 65 years of age (Papatestas *et al.* 1971).One simple differentiating symptom from myasthenia gravis is that extraocular muscles typically are not affected in Eaton–Lambert syndrome.

If Eaton–Lambert syndrome is associated with a carcinoma, there rarely is more than a 2-year interval between the onset of muscular symptoms and discovery of the neoplasm. In the 21 patients with small-cell lung cancer of O'Neill *et al.* the tumour was diagnosed within 1 year of the syndrome's onset in 16 (O'Neill *et al.* 1988). The maximum interval between the onset of Eaton–Lambert syndrome and detection of the neoplasm has been less than 4 years and in such cases the association may be coincidental. The age distribution is wider in the absence of neoplasia but the neuromuscular manifestations are the same.

The simplest screening test for Eaton–Lambert syndrome consists of evoking a single muscle action potential with an electromyograph before and after voluntary effort. The potential should at least double, and may increase 17-fold. Repetitive stimulation of a nerve at a tetanic rate also results in increase of the action potential, while in myasthenia gravis the potential gradually diminishes. There are also pharmacological differences. Neostigmine and other anticholine esterases improve strength in myasthenia gravis, but have little effect in Eaton–Lambert syndrome. Consequently, in Eaton–Lambert syndrome a test dose of edrophonium fails to elicit a definite response as it does for myasthenia gravis (Brown and Johns 1974).

Both conditions result from a defect in the neuromuscular transmission of nerve impulses. In myasthenia gravis acetyl choline reaches the motor endplates in normal increments, but the sensitivity of its receptors on the endplates and contiguous muscle cell membrane is diminished. Each receptor site can accept two molecules of acetyl choline. Release of the quanta of acetyl choline in the depolarization phase of the electric potential is mediated by the influx of calcium ions into the presynaptic membrane. In Eaton–Lambert syndrome an inadequate amount of acetyl choline is released due to a complex mechanism which, at least in part, is an antibody blockade of the calcium phase (Leys *et al.* 1991; Maselli 1994). Injection of the IgG serum fraction from patients with Eaton–Lambert syndrome into mice may temporarily reduce their muscle action potential. This has been interpreted to indicate that there is an autoantibody which, when transferred in sufficient concentration, can block neuromuscular transmission (Lambert and Lennon 1988). Such an antibody appears to be more prevalent in non-neoplastic cases of Eaton–Lambert syndrome than in the presence of small-cell carcinoma (Leys *et al.* 1991). How this antibody (or antibodies) is generated remains obscure. It appears unlikely that this mechanism is related to the generation of other pathogenic autoantibodies. The occurrence of Eaton–Lambert syndrome has been reported in association with rheumatoid arthritis (Peris *et al.* 1990), systemic lupus erythematosus (Hughes and Katirji 1986), and Sjögren's syndrome (Tsuchiya *et al.* 1993), but is so rare as to be presumed coincidental.

Treatments endeavour to regain the effectiveness of acetyl choline. Plasmapheresis produces transient clinical improvement, although more gradually in Eaton–Lambert syndrome than in myasthenia gravis. Therefore, Newsom-Davis and Murray speculated that improved strength in Eaton–Lambert syndrome results from newly synthesized acetyl choline rather than from removal of blocking antibody (Newsom-Davis and Murray 1984). Resection of the carcinoma may result in neuromuscular improvement. Corticosteroid therapy may be beneficial, but the effect develops more gradually than in myasthenia gravis, possibly over months. The first relatively specific medication for Eaton–Lambert syndrome was guanidine, 20 to 30 mg/kg per day orally; it facilitates the release of acetyl choline. However, there is risk of bone marrow depression and other toxicities (Henriksson *et al.* 1977). 3,4-diaminopyridine enhances acetyl choline release by prolonging the action potential and calcium influx. In dosages from 15 to 100 mg/day it is at present the most efficient medication. Its main, infrequent, side-effect is seizures (McEvoy 1994). In the absence of a fatal neoplasm Eaton–Lambert syndrome is a chronic disease.

Fasciitis syndromes

Several varieties of non-infectious fasciitis have been described in recent years: eosinophilic fasciitis (1974); palmar fasciitis (1982); fasciitis–panniculitis (1992). The main pathological difference between eosinophilic fasciitis and fasciitis–panniculitis seems to be the lack of an eosinophilic infiltrate in the latter. The strongest clue that the neoplasms described in a minority of cases of eosinophilic fasciitis and fasciitis–panniculitis are not merely coincidental events is that they have almost exclusively been haematological (Lakhanpal *et al.* 1988; Naschitz *et al.* 1994).

Medsger *et al.* described a 'palmar fasciitis-arthritis syndrome' associated with ovarian carcinoma (Medsger *et al.* 1982). This may be the neoplasia induced variant of reflex sympathetic dystrophy, which it resembles. Cases published as 'shoulder-hand syndrome associated with cancer' probably have been instances of the same process (Michaels and Sorber 1984). However, there are differences from typical reflex sympathetic dystrophy: palmar fasciitis is always bilateral, may involve the lower extremities, and tends to advance to severe disability more rapidly. The skin of the hands becomes so tense that a misdiagnosis of scleroderma may be made. Involvement of the plantar fascia has also been reported. The shoulders are affected consistently, but the arthritis may also involve extremity joints. Most patients have been women above the age of 55, and about half of the neoplasms have been ovarian carcinomas (Pfinsgraff *et al.* 1986). The syndrome develops a few weeks to a year before discovery of the neoplasm and may first occur with a recurrence (Mesdger *et al.* 1982). Treatment of the neoplasm usually does not alleviate the syndrome.

References

Abu-Shakra, M., Guillemin, F., and Lee, P. (1993). Cancer in systemic sclerosis. *Arthritis and Rheumatism*, **36**, 460–4.

Abu-Shakra, M., Urowitz, M.B., Gladman, D.D., *et al.* (1995). Mortality studies in systemic lupus erythematosus. Results from a single center. 1. Causes of death. *Journal of Rheumatology*, **22**, 1259–64.

Ahern, M.J., Maddison, P., Mann, S., and Scott, C.A. (1982). Ankylosing spondylitis and adenocarcinoma of the lung. *Annals of the Rheumatic Diseases*, **41**, 292–4.

Ali, A., Tetalman, M.R., Fordham, E.W., *et al.* (1980). Distribution of hypertrophic pulmonary osteoarthropathy. *American Journal of Radiology*, **134**, 771–80.

Amble, A.R., Olsen, K.D., Nascimento, A.G., *et al.* (1992). Head and neck synovial cell sarcoma. *Otolaryngology, Head and Neck Surgery*, **107**, 631–7.

Awerbuch, M.S. and Brooks, P.M. (1981). Role of immune complexes in hypertrophic osteoarthropathy and non-metastatic polyarthritis. *Annals of the Rheumatic Diseases*, **40**, 470–2.

Baker, G.L., Kahl, L.E., Zee, B. *et al.* (1987). Malignancy following treatment of rheumatoid arthritis with cyclophosphamide: a long-term case-control follow up study. *American Journal of Medicine*, **83**, 1–9.

Banks, P.M., Witrak, G.A., and Conn, D.L. (1979). Lymphoid neoplasia following connective tissue disease. *Mayo Clinic Proceedings*, **54**, 104–8.

Basset-Sequin, N., Roujeau, J., Gherardi, R., *et al.* (1990). Prognostic factors and predictive signs of malignancy in adult dermatomyositis. *Archives of Dermatology*, **126**, 633–7.

Behan, W.M., Behan, P.O., and Doyle, D. (1982). Association of myasthenia gravis and polymyositis with neoplasia, infection and autoimune disorders. *Acta Neuropathologica*, **57**, 221–9.

Bhalla, R., Ajmani, H.S., Kim, W.W., *et al.* (1993). Systemic lupus erythematosus and Hodgkin's lymphoma. *Journal of Rheumatology*, **20**, 1316–20.

Bignon, Y.J., Janin-Mercier, A., Dubost, J.J., *et al.* (1986). Angioimmunoblastic lymphadenopathy with dysproteinaemia (AILD) and sicca syndrome. *Annals of the Rheumatic Diseases*, **45**, 519–22.

Black, H.R., Quallich, H., and Gereleck, C.B. (1986). Racial differences in serum creatine kinase levels. *American Journal of Medicine*, **81**, 479–86.

Bohan, A. and Peter, J.B. (1977). A computer-assisted analysis of 153 patients with polymyositis and dermatomyositis. *Medicine (Baltimore)*, **56**, 255–86.

Boice, J.D. (1992). Radiation and non-Hodgkin's lymphoma. *Cancer Research*, **52**(suppl.), 5489s–91s.

Borden, E.C. and Holling, H.E. (1969). Hypertrophic osteoarthropathy and pregnancy. *Annals of Internal Medicine*, **71**, 577–80.

Bradley, J.D. and Pinals, R.S. (1983). Carcinoma polyarthritis: role of immune complexes in pathogenesis. *Journal of Rheumatology*, **10**, 826–8.

Brain, R. and Adams, R.D. (1965). A guide to the classification and investigation of neurological disorders associated with neoplasms. In *The remote effects of cancer on the nervous system* (ed. R. Brain and F.H. Norris), pp. 216–21. Grune and Stratton, New York.

Briselli, M., Mark, E.J., and Dickensin, R. (1981). Solitary fibrous tumors of the pleura. *Cancer*, **47**, 2678–88.

Brown, J.D. and Johns, R.J. (1974). Diagnostic difficulties encountered in the myasthenic syndrome sometimes associated with carcinoma. *Journal of Neurology, Neurosurgery and Psychiatry*, **37**, 1212–24.

Cadman, N.L., Soule, E.H., and Kelly, P.J. (1965). Synovial sarcoma: an analysis of 154 tumors. *Cancer*, **18**, 613–27.

Cagle, L.A., Mirra, J.M., Storm, K., *et al.* (1987). Histologic features relating to prognosis in synovial sarcoma. *Cancer*, **59**, 1810–14.

Callen, J.P. (1982). The value of malignancy evaluation in patients with dermatomyositis. *Journal of the American Society of Dermatology*, **6**, 253–9.

Casey, T.P. (1968). The development of lymphomas in mice with autoimmune disorders treated with azathioprine. *Blood*, **31**, 396–9.

Chevalier, X., Gaular, P., Voisin, M.-C., *et al.* (1991). Peripheral T-cell lymphoma with Sjögren's syndrome; a report with immunologic and genotypic studies. *Journal of Rheumatology*, **18**, 1744–6.

Chuang, T.-Y., Hunder, G.G., Ilstrup, D.M., *et al.* (1982). Polymyalgia rheumatica: a 10-year epidemiologic and clinical study. *Annals of Internal Medicine*, **97**, 672–80.

Clain, A. (1965). Secondary malignant disease of bone. *British Journal of Cancer*, **19**, 15–29.

Cohen, A.S. and Canoso, J.J. (1975). Rheumatologic aspects of amyloid disease. *Clinics in Rheumatic Disease*, **1**, 149–61.

Costello, P.B., Beecher, M.L., Starr, J.J., *et al.* (1983). A prospective analysis of the frequency, cause, and possible prognostic significance of the joint manifestations of childhood leukaemia. *Journal of Rheumatology*, **10**, 753–7.

Court-Brown, W.M. and Doll, R. (1965). Mortality from cancer and other causes after radiotherapy for ankylosing spondylitis. *British Medical Journal*, **2**, 1327–32.

Coury, C. (1960). Hippocratic fingers and hypertrophic osteoarthropathy. A study of 350 cases. *British Journal of Diseases of the Chest*, **54**, 202–9.

Croft, P.B. and Wilkinson, M. (1965). The incidence of carcinomatous neuromyopathy in patients with various types of carcinoma. *Brain*, **88**, 427–34.

Dahlin, D.C. and Unni, K.K. (1985). *Bone tumors: general aspects and data on 8542 cases*, (4th edn), pp. 12–15. Thomas, Springfield, IL.

Darby, S.C., Doll, R., Gill, S.K., and Sith, P.G. (1987). Long term mortality after a single treatment course with spondylitis. *British Journal of Cancer*, **55**, 179–90.

DeCross, A.J. and Sahasrabudhe, D.M. (1992). Paraneoplastic Raynaud's phenomenon. *American Journal of Medicine*, **92**, 571–2.

Devesa, S.S., Blot, W.J., and.Fraumeni, J.F. (1989). Declining lung cancer rates among young men and women in the United States: a cohort analysis. *Journal of the National Cancer Institute*, **81**, 1568–71.

Dickinson, C.J. (1993). The aetiology of clubbing and hypertrophic osteoarthropathy. *European Journal of Clinical Investigation*, **23**, 330–8.

Duncan, S.C. and Winkelmann, R.K. (1979). Cancer in scleroderma. *Archives of Dermatology*, **115**, 950–5.

Edgar, M.A. and Robinson, M.P. (1973). Post-radiation sarcoma in ankylosing spondylitis. *Journal of Bone and Joint Surgery*, **55B**, 183–8.

Egelmeijer, F. and MacFarlane, J.D. (1992). Polyarthritis as the presenting symptoms of the occurrence and recurrence of a laryngeal carcinoma. *Annals of the Rheumatic Diseases*, **51**, 556–7.

Elrington, G.M., Murray, N.M., Spiro, S.G., *et al.* (1991). Neurological paraneoplastic syndromes in patients with small cell lung cancer. A prospective survery of 150 patients. *Journal of Neurology, Neurosurgery and Psychiatry*, **54**, 764–7.

Epstein, O., Adjukiewicz, A,B,M., Dick, R., *et al.* (1979). Hypertrophic hepatic osteoarthropathy. *American Journal of Medicine*, **67**, 88–97.

Eriksson, M. (1993). Rheumatoid arthritis as a risk factor for multiple myeloma: a case-control study. *European Journal of Cancer*, **29A**, 259–63.

Fudman, E.J. and Schnitzer, T.J. (1986). Dermatomyositis without creatine kinase evaluation. *American Journal of Medicine*, **80**, 329–32.

Galasko, C.S. (1982). Mechanisms of lytic and blastic metastatic disease of bone. *Clinical Orthopedics and Related Research*, **169**, 20–7.

Giovannucci, E., Egan, K.M., Hunter, D.J., *et al.* (1995). Aspirin and the risk of colorectal cancer in women. *New England Journal of Medicine*, **333**, 609–14.

Gleeson, M.J., Bennett, M.H., and Clawson, R.A. (1986). Lymphomas of salivary glands. *Cancer*, **58**, 699–704.

Gomm, S.A., Thatcher, N., Barber, P.V., *et al.* (1990). A clinicopathological study of the paraneoplastic neuromuscular syndromes associated with lung cancer. *Quarterly Journal of Medicine*, **75**, 577–95.

Gordon, D.A., Pruzanski, W., Ogryzlo, M.A., *et al.* (1973). Amyloid arthritis simulating rheumatoid disease in five patients with multiple myeloma. *American Journal of Medicine*, **55**, 142–54.

Gosney, M.A., Gosney, J.R., and Lye, M. (1990). Plasma growth hormone and digital clubbing in carcinoma of the bronchus. *Thorax*, **45**, 545–7.

Gottlieb, M., Hoppe, R.T., Calin, A., *et al.* (1979). Arthritis in a patient with mycosis fungoides: complete remission after radiotherapy. *Arthritis and Rheumatism*, **22**, 424–5.

Gridley, G., McLaughlin, J.K., Ekbom, A., *et al.* (1993). Incidence of cancer among patients with rheumatoid arthritis. *Journal of the National Cancer Institute*, **85**, 307–11.

Haga, H.-J., Eide, G.E., Brun, J., *et al.* (1993). Cancer association with polymyalgia rheumatica and temporal arteritis. *Journal of Rheumatology*, **20**, 1335–9.

Hajdu, S.I., Shiu, M.H., and Former, J.G. (1977). Tendosynovial sarcoma. A clinico-pathological study of 136 cases. *Cancer*, **39**, 1201–17.

Hakulinen, T. (1986). Similar survival rates for rheumatoid and non-rheumatoid cancer patients. *Scandinavian Journal of Rheumatology*, **15**, 285–9.

Hansen, S. and Olsen, N. (1989). Raynaud's phenomenon in patients treated with cisplatin, vinblastine, and bleomycin for germ cell cancer: measurement of vasoconstrictor response to cold. *Journal of Clinical Oncology*, **7**, 940–2.

Harden, E.A., Moore, J.O., and Haynes, B.F. (1984). Leukemia-associated arthritis: identification of leukemic cells in synovial fluid using monoclonal and polyclonal antibodies. *Arthritis and Rheumatism*, **27**, 1306–8.

Harvey, J.M., Gray, C., and Belchetz, P.E. (1992). Oncogenous osteomalacia and malignancy. *Clinical Endocrinology*, **37**, 379–84.

Hawley, R.J., Cohen, M.H., Saini, N., *et al.* (1980). The carcinomatous neuromyopathy of oat cell lung cancer. *Annals of Neurology*, **7**, 65–72.

Henriksson, K.G., Nilsson, O., Rosen, I., *et al.* (1977). Clinical neurophysiological and morphological findings in Eaton Lambert syndrome. *Acta Neurologica Scandinavica*, **56**, 117–40.

Hidano, A., Kanako, K., Arai, Y., *et al.* (1986). Survey of the prognosis for dermatomyositis, with special reference to its association with malignancy and pulmonary fibrosis. *Journal of Dermatology*, **13**, 233–41.

Holdrinet, R.S., Corstens, F., van Horn, J.R., *et al.* (1989). Leukemic synovitis. *American Journal of Medicine*, **86**, 123–5.

Holm, S. (1949). Keratoconjunctivitis sicca and the sicca syndrome. *Acta Ophthalmologica*, **33** (suppl.), 44–59.

Hornbaker, J.H., Foster, E.A., Williams, G.S., *et al.* (1966). Sjögren's syndrome and nodular reticulum cell sarcoma. *Archives of Internal Medicine*, **118**, 449–52.

Hughes, R.L. and Katirji, B. (1986). The Eaton-Lambert (myasthenic) syndrome in association with systemic lupus erythematosus. *Archives of Neurology*, **43**, 1186–7.

Huston, K.A., Hunder, G.E., Lie, J.T., *et al.* (1978). Temporal arteritis, A 25-year epidemiologic, clinical, and pathologic study. *Annals of Internal Medicine*, **88**, 162–7.

Hyjek, E., Smith, W.J., and Isaacson, P.G. (1988). Primary B-cell lymphoma of salivary glands and its relationship to myoepithelial sialadenitis. *Human Pathology*, **19**, 766–76.

Hyman, G.A. and Wolff, M. (1976). Malignant lymphoma of the salivary glands. *American Journal of Clinical Pathology*, **65**, 421–38.

Isomäki, H.A., Hakulinen, T., and Joutsenlahti, U. (1978). Excess risk of lymphomas, leukemia and myeloma in patients with rheumatoid arthritis. *Journal of Chronic Diseases*, **31**, 691–6.

Janin, A., Morel, P., Quiguandon, I., *et al.* (1992). Non-Hodgkin's lymphoma and Sjögren's syndrome. An immunopathological study of 113 patients. *Clinical and Experimental Rheumatology*, **10**, 565–70.

Jergensen, H.E., Mankin, H.J., and Schiller, A.L. (1978). Diffuse pigmented villonodular synovitis of the knee mimicking primary bone neoplasm. *Journal of Bone and Joint Surgery*, **60A**, 825–9.

Kalra, L. and Delamere, J.P. (1987). Lymphoreticular malignancy and monoclonal gammopathy presenting as polymyalgia rheumatica. *British Journal of Rheumatology*, **26**, 458–9.

Kassan, S.S., Thomas, T.L., and Moutsopoulos, H.M. (1978). Increased risk of lymphoma in sicca syndrome. *Annals of Internal Medicine*, **89**, 888–92.

Khurana, R.K., Koski, C.L., and Mayer, R.F. (1988). Autonomic dysfunction in Lambert-Eaton myasthenic syndrome. *Journal of Neurological Sciences*, **85**, 77–86.

Kingsmore, S.F., Hall, B.D., Allen, N.B., *et al.* (1992). Association of methotrexate, rheumatoid arthritis and lymphoma: report of 2 cases and literature review. *Journal of Rheumatology*, **19**, 1462–5.

Kinlen, L.J. (1985). Incidence of cancer in rheumatoid arthritis and other disorders after immunosuppressive treatment. *American Journal of Medicine*, **78** (Suppl. 1A), 44–9.

Kyle, R.A. (1975). Multiple myeloma: review of 869 cases. *Mayo Clinic Proceedings*, **50**, 29–40.

Kyle, R.A. (1993). 'Benign' monoclonal gamopathy - after 20 to 35 years of follow-up. *Mayo Clinic Proceedings*, **68**, 26–36.

Laakso, M., Mutru, O., Isomäki, H., *et al.* (1986). Cancer mortality in patients with rheumatoid arthritis. *Journal of Rheumatology*, **13**, 522–6.

Lakhanpal, S., Bunch, T.W., Melton, L.J., *et al.* (1986). Polymyositis-dermatomyositis and malignant lesions: does an association exist? *Mayo Clinic Proceedings*, **61**, 645–53.

Lakhanpal, S., Ginsburg, W.W., Michet, C.J., *et al.* (1988). Eosinophilic fasciitis: clinical spectrum and therapeutic response in 52 cases. *Seminars in Arthritis and Rheumatism*, **17**, 221–31.

Lambert, E.H. and Lennon, V.A. (1988). Selected IgG rapidly induces Lambert-Eaton myasthenic syndrome in mice: complement independence and EMG abnormalities. *Muscle and Nerve*, **11**, 1133–45.

Lee, P., Alderdice, C., Wilkinson, S., *et al.* (1983). Malignancy in progressive systemic sclerosis—association with breast carcinoma. *Journal of Rheumatology*, **10**, 665–6.

Leeson, M.C., Makley, J.T., and Carter, J.R. (1985). Metastatic skeletal disease in the pediatric population. *Journal of Pediatric Orthopedics*, **5**, 261–7.

Lenoch, F., Bremova, A., Kankova, D., *et al.* (1967). The relation of Sjögren's syndrome to rheumatoid arthritis. *Acta Rheumatologica Scandinavica*, **10**, 297–304.

LeRoux, B.T. (1968). Bronchial carcinoma with hypertrophic pulmonary osteoarthropathy. *South African Medical Journal*, **42**, 1074–5.

Lewis, R.B., Castor, C.W., Knisely, R.E., *et al.* (1976). Frequency of neoplasia in systemic lupus erythematosus and rheumatoid arthritis. *Arthritis and Rheumatism*, **19**, 1256–60.

Leys, K., Lang, B., Johnston, I., *et al.* (1991). Calcium channel autoantibodies in the Lambert-Eaton myasthenic syndrome. *Annals of Neurology*, **29**, 307–14.

Lyon, M.G., Bloch, D.A., Hollak, B., *et al.* (1989). Predisposing factors in polymyositis-dermatomyositis: results of a nationwide survey. *Journal of Rheumatology*, **16**, 1218–24.

Mackenzie, D.H. (1966). Synovial sarcoma. A review of 58 cases. *Cancer*, **19**, 169–80.

Manchul, L.A., Jin, A., Pritchard, K.I., *et al.* (1985). The frequency of malignant neoplasms in patients with polymyositis-dermatomyositis. *Archives of Internal Medicine*, **145**, 1835–9.

Maselli, R.A. (1994). Pathophysiology of myasthenia gravis and Lambert-Eaton syndrome. *Neurologic Clinics of North America*, **12**, 285–303.

Masi, A.T. and Hochberg, M.C. (1988). Temporal association of polymyositis-dermatomyositis with malignancy: methodologic and clinical considerations. *Mount Sinai Journal of Medicine*, **55**, 471–8.

McCurley, T.L., Collins, R.D., Ball, E., *et al.* (1990). Nodal and extranodal lymphoproliferative disorders in Sjögren's syndrome; a clinical and imunopathological study. *Human Pathology*, **21**, 482–92.

McEvoy, K.M. (1994). Diagnosis and treatment of Lambert-Eaton myasthenic syndrome. *Neurologic Clinics of North America*, **12**, 387–99.

McNeill, B.J. (1984). Value of bone scanning in neoplastic diseases. *Seminars in Nuclear Medicine*, **14**, 277–86.

Medsger, T.A., Dixon, J.A., and Garwood, V.F. (1982). Palmar fasciitis and polyarthritis associated with ovarian carcinoma. *Annals of Internal Medicine*, **96**, 424–31.

Mellemkjaer, L., Andersen, V., Linet, M.J., Gridley, G., Hoover, R., and Olen, J.H. (1997). Non-Hodgkin's lymphoma and other cancers among a cohort of patients with systemic lupus erythematosus. *Arthritis and Rheumatism*, **40**, 761–9.

Merrick, M.V. and Merrick, J.M. (1986). Bone scintigraphy in lung cancer; a reappraisal. *British Journal of Radiology*, **59**, 1185–94.

Michaels, R.M. and Sorber, J.A. (1984). Reflex sympathetic dystrophy, as a probable paraneoplastic syndrome: case report and literature review. *Arthritis and Rheumatism*, **27**, 1183–5.

Miettinen, M. and Virtanen, I. (1984). Synovial sarcoma - a misnomer. *American Journal of Pathology*, **117**, 18–25.

Miller, D.G. (1967). The association of immune disease and malignant lymphoma. *Annals of Internal Medicine*, **66**, 507–21.

Mitchell, D.M., Spitz, P.W., Young, D.Y., *et al.* (1986). Survival, prognosis, and causes of death in rheumatoid arthritis. *Athritis and Rheumatism*, **29**, 706–14.

Montanaro, M. and Bizzarri, F. (1992). Non-Hodgkin's lymphoma and subsequent acute lymphoblastic leukaemia in a patient with polymyalgia rheumatics. *British Journal of Rheumatology*, **31**, 277–8.

Moutsopoulos, H.M., Chused, T.M., Mann, D.L., *et al.* (1980). Sjögren's syndrome (sicca syndrome): current issues. *Annals of Internal Medicine*, **92**, 212–26.

Murashima, A., Takasaki, Y., Hashimoto, H., *et al.* (1992). A case of Raynaud's disease with uterine cancer producing interleukin-6. *Clinical Rheumatology*, **11**, 410–12.

Myllykangas-Luosujärvi, K., Aho, K., Kautiainen, H., *et al.* (1995). Shortening of life span and acuses of excess mortality in a population-based series of subjects with rheumatoid arthritis. *Clinical and Experimental Rheumatology*, **13**, 149–53.

Nagai, M., Sasaki, K., Tokuda, M., *et al.* (1993). Hodgkin's disease and Sjögren's syndrome. *European Journal of Haematology*, **50**, 180–2.

Naschitz, J.E., Yeshurun, D., Zuckerman, E., *et al.* (1994). Cancer-associated fasciitis-panniculitis. *Cancer*, **73**, 231–5.

Newman, M.K. and Gugino, R.J. (1964). Neuropathies and myopathies associated with occult malignancies. *Journal of the American Medical Association*, **190**, 575–7.

Newsom-Davis, J. and Murray, N.M. (1984). Plasma exchange and immunosuppressive drug treatment in the Lambert-Eaton myasthenic syndrome. *Neurology*, **34**, 480–5.

Newton, P., Freemont, A.T., Noble, J., *et al.* (1984). Secondary malignant synovitis: report of three cases and review of the literature. *Quarterly Journal of Medicine*, **53**, 135–43.

Nolling, H.E., Danielson, G.K., and Hamilton, R.W. (1963). Hypertrophic pulmonary osteoarthropathy. *Journal of Thoracic and Cardiovascular Surgery*, **46**, 310–21.

O'Neill, J.H., Murray, N.M., and Newsom-Davis, J. (1988). The Lambert-Eaton myasthenic syndrome: a review of 50 cases. *Brain*, **111**, 577–96.

Papatestas, A.E., Osserman, K.F., and Kark, A.E. (1971). The relationship between thymus and oncogenesis: a study of the incidence of non-thymic malignancy in myasthenia gravis. *British Journal of Cancer*, **25**, 635–45.

Pascuzzi, R.M. and Kim, Y.I. (1990). Lambert-Eaton syndrome. *Seminars in Neurology*, **10**, 35–41.

Patel, A., Davila, D.G., and Peters, S.G. (1993). Paraneoplastic syndromes associated with lung cancer. *Mayo Clinic Proceedings*, **68**, 278–87.

Paul, T., Katiyar, B.C., Misra, S., *et al.* (1978). Carcinomatous neuromuscular syndromes. *Brain*, **101**, 53–63.

Peris, P., Del Orme, J., Gratacos, J., *et al.* (1990). The Lambert-Eaton myasthenic syndrome in association with rheumatoid arthritis. *British Journal of Rheumatology*, **29**, 75–7.

Pettersson, T., Pukkala, E., Teppo, L., *et al.* (1992). Increased risk of cancer in patients with systemic lupus erythematosus. *Annals of the Rheumatic Diseases*, **51**, 437–9.

Pfinsgraff, J., Buckingham, R.B., Keister, S.R., *et al.* (1986). Palmar fasciitis and arthritis with malignant neoplasms: a paraneoplastic syndrome. *Seminars in Arthritis and Rheumatism*, **16**, 118–25.

Pines, A., Kaplinsky, N., Olchovsky, D., *et al.* (1984). Rheumatoid arthritis-like syndrome: a presenting symptom of malignancy. Report of 3 cases and review of the literature. *European Journal of Rheumatic Inflammation*, **7**, 51–5.

Plotz, P.H., Dalakas, M., Leff, R.L., *et al.* (1989). Current concepts in the idiopathic inflammatory myopathies: polymyositis, dermatomyositis, and related disorders. *Annals of Internal Medicine*, **111**, 143–57.

Porter, D., Madhok, O., and Vapell, H. (1991). Non-Hodgkin's lymphoma and rheumatoid arthritis. *Annals of the Rheumatic Diseases*, **50**, 275–6.

Radis, C.D., Kahl, L.E., Baker, G.L., *et al.* (1995). Effects of cyclophosphamide on the development of malignancy and on long-term survival of patients with rheumatoid arthritis. *Arthritis and Rheumatism*, **38**, 1120–7.

Razis, D.V., Diamond, H.D., and Craver, L.F. (1959). Hodgkin's disease associated with other malignant tumors and certain non-neoplastic diseases. *American Journal of Medical Sciences*, **238**, 327–35.

Richardson, J.E., Gladman, D.D., Fam, A, *et al.* (1987). HLA-DR4 in giant cell ateritis: association with polymyalgia rheumatica syndrome. *Arthritis and Rheumatism*, **30**, 1293–7.

Rööser, B., Willen, H., Hugoson, A., *et al.* (1989). Prognostic factors in synovial sarcoma. *Cancer*, **63**, 2182–5.

Ropes, M.W. (1976). *Systemic lupus erythematosus*, p. 74. Harvard University Press, Cambridge, MA.

Rosenberg, L., Palmer, J.R., Zauber, A.G., *et al.* (1991). A hypothesis: non-steroidal anti-inflammatory drugs reduce the incidence of large-bowel cancer. *Journal of the National Cancer Institute*, **83**, 355–8.

Rosenow, E.C., Strimlan, C.V., and Muhm, R. (1977). Pleuropulmonary manifestations of ankylosing spondylitis. *Mayo Clinic Proceedings*, **52**, 641–9.

Roumm, A.D. and Medsger, T.A. (1985). Cancer and systemic sclerosis: an eoidemiologic study. *Arthritis and Rheumatism*, **28**, 1336–40.

Rutherford, R.B., Rhodes, B.A., and Wagner, H.N. (1969). The distribution of extremity blood flow before and after vagotomy in a patient with hypertrophic pulmonary osteoarthropathy. *Diseases of the Chest*, **56**, 19–23.

Ryan, E.A. and Reiss, E. (1984). Oncogenous osteomalacia. *American Journal of Medicine*, **77**, 501–12.

Scelsi, R. and Pinelli, P. (1977). Subclinical myopathic findings in patients affected by malignant tumours. *Acta Neuropathologica*, **38**, 103–8.

Schaller, J. (1972). Arthritis as a presenting manifestation of malignancy in children. *Journal of Pediatrics*, **81**, 793–7.

Schapira, D., Ishak, O.B., Nachtigal, A., *et al.* (1995). Tumour-induced osteomalacia. *Seminars in Arthritis and Rheumatism*, **25**, 35–46.

Schmid, U., Helbron, D., and Lemert, K. (1982). Development of malignant lymphoma in myoepithelial sialadenitis (Sjögren's syndrome). *Virchow's Archives of Pathological Anatomy*, **395**, 11–43.

Schumacher, H.R. (1976). Articular manifestations of hypertrophic pulmonary osteoarthropathy. *Arthritis and Rheumatism*, **19**, 629–36.

Segal, A.M. and Mackenzie, A.H. (1982). Hypertrophic osteoarthropathy: a 10-year retrospective analysis. *Arthritis and Rheumatism*, **12**, 220–32.

Shneerson, J.M. (1981). Digital clubbing and hypertrophic osteoarthropathy: the underlying mechanisms. *British Journal of Diseases of the Chest*, **75**, 113–31.

Shy, G.M. and Silverstein, I. (1965). A study of the effects upon the motor unit by remote malignancy. *Brain*, **88**, 515–28.

Sigurgeirsson, B., Lindelof, B., Edhag, O., *et al.* (1992). Risk of cancer in patients with dermatomyositis or polymyositis. *New England Journal of Medicine*, **326**, 363–7.

Silman, A.J., Petrie, J., Hazelman, B., *et al.* (1988). Lymphoproliferative cancer and other malignancy in patients with rheumatoid arthritis treated with azathioprine: a 20 year follow up study. *Annals of the Rheumatic Diseases*, **47**, 988–92.

Silverstein, M.N. and Kelly, P.J. (1963). Leukemia with osteoarticular symptoms and signs. *Annals of Internal Medicine*, **59**, 637–45.

Simon, R.D. and Ford, L.E. (1980). Rheumatoid-like arthritis associated with a colonic carcinoma. *Archives of Internal Medicine*, **140**, 698–700.

Smith, P.G., Doll, R., and Radford, E.P. (1977). Cancer mortality among patients with ankylosing spondylitis not given X-ray therapy. *British Journal of Radiology*, **50**, 728–34.

Springfield, D.S. (1982). Mechanisms of metastasis. *Clinical Orthopedics and Related Research*, **169**, 15–19.

Staalman, C.R. and Umans, U. (1993). Hypertrophic osteoarthropathy in childhood malignancy. *Medical and Pediatric Oncology*, **21**, 676–9.

Steen, V.D. and Medsger, T.A. (1990). Epidemiology and natural history of systemic sclerosis. *Rheumatic Disease Clinics of North America*, **16**, 1–10.

Stenseth, J.H., Clagett, O.T., and Woolner, C.B. (1967). Hypertrophic pulmonary osteoarthropathy. *Diseases of the Chest*, **52**, 62–8.

Stern, R.S., Zierler, S., and Parish, J.A. (1982). Methotrexate used for psoriasis and the risk of non-cutaneous malignancy. *Cancer*, **50**, 869–72.

Sugai, S., Shimizu, S., Hirose, Y., *et al.* (1985). Monoclonal gammopathies in Japanese patients with Sjögren's syndrome. *Journal of Clinical Immunology*, **5**, 90–101.

Sulkes, A. and Naparstek, Y. (1991). The infrequent association of systemic lupus erythematosus and solid tumors. *Cancer*, **68**, 1389–93.

Sung, S.S., Sheibani, K., Fishleder, A., *et al.* (1991). Monocytoid B-cell lymphoma in patients with Sjögren's syndrome; a clinicopathologic study of 13 patients. *Human Pathology*, **22**, 422–30.

Sweeney, D.M., Manzi, S., Janosky, J., *et al.* (1995). Risk of malignancy in women with systemic lupus erythematosus. *Journal of Rheumatology*, **22**, 1478–82.

Symmons, D.P., Ahern, M., Bacon, P.A., *et al.* (1984). Lymphoproliferative malignancy in rheumatoid arthritis: a study of 20 cases. *Annals of the Rheumatic Diseases*, **43**, 132–5.

Talbott, J.H. and Barrocas, M. (1980). Carcinoma of the lung in progressive systemic sclerosis: a tabular review of the literature and a detailed report of the roentgenographic changes in two cases. *Seminars in Arthritis and Rheumatism*, **9**, 191–217.

Targoff, I.N. and Reichlin, M. (1988). Humoral immunity in polymyositis and dermatomyositis. *Mount Sinai Journal of Medicine*, **55**, 487–93.

Thompson, M. and Eadie, S. (1956). Keratoconjunctivitis sicca and rheumatoid arthritis. *Annals of the Rheumatic Diseases*, **15**, 21–5.

Thun, M.J., Namboodiri, M.M., and Heath, C.W. (1991). Aspirin use and reduced risk of fatal colon cancer. *New England Journal of Medicine*, **325**, 1593–6.

Tillotson, J.F., McDonald, J.R., and Janes, J.M. (1951). Synovial sarcomata. *Journal of Bone and Joint Surgery*, **33A**, 459–73.

Tsuchiya, N., Sato, M., Uesaka, Y., *et al.* (1993). Lambert-Eaton myasthenic syndrome associated with Sjögren's syndrome and discoid lupus erythematosus. *Scandinavian Journal of Rheumatology*, **22**, 302–4.

Turner-Warwick, M., Lebowitz, M., Burrows, B., *et al.* (1980). Cryptogenic fibrosing alveolitis and lung cancer. *Thorax*, **35**, 496–9.

Tzioufas, A.G., Manoussakis, M.N., Costello, R., *et al.* (1986). Cryoglobulinemia in autoimmune rheumatic diseases. *Arthritis and Rheumatism*, **29**, 1098–104.

Uriburu, I.J., Moschio, F.J., and Marin, J.C. (1976). Metastases of carcinoma of the larynx and thyroid gland to the phalanges of the hand. *Journal of Bone and Joint Surgery*, **58A**, 134–5.

Vosskämper, M., Korf, B., Franke, F., *et al.* (1989). Paraneoplastic necrotizing myopathy: a rare disorder to be differentiated from polymyositis. *Journal of Neurology*, **236**, 489–92.

Walker, S.E. and Boles, G.G. (1973). Augmented incidence of neoplasia in NZB/NZW mice treated with cyclophosphamide. *Journal of Laboratory and Clinical Medicine*, **82**, 619–33.

Weidner, N. and Cruz, D. (1987). Phosphaturic mesenchymal tumours. *Cancer*, **59**, 1442–54.

Whaley, K., Williamson, J., Chisholm, D.M., *et al.* (1973). Sjögren's syndrome. *Quarterly Journal of Medicine*, **42**, 279–304.

Wolfe, F., Mitchell, D.M., Sibley, J.T., *et al.* (1994). The mortality of rheumatoid arthritis. *Arthritis and Rheumatism*, **37**, 481–94.

Yacoub, M.H. (1965). Relation between the histology of bronchial carcinoma and hypertrophic pulmonary osteoarthropathy. *Thorax*, **20**, 537–9.

Young, J.L. and Miller, R.W. (1975). Incidence of malignant tumors in U.S. children. *Journal of Pediatrics*, **86**, 254–8.

Zantos, D., Zhang, Y., and Felson, D. (1994). The overall and temporal association of cancer with polymyositis and dermatomyositis. *Journal of Rheumatology*, **21**, 1855–9.

Zawadzki, Z.A. and Benedek, T.G. (1969). Rheumatoid arthritis, dysproteinemic arthropathy, and paraproeinemia. *Arthritis and Rheumatism*, **12**, 555–68.

Zindrick, M.R., Young, M.P., Daley, R.J., *et al.* (1982). Metastatic tumors of the foot. *Clinical Orthopedics and Related Research*, **170**, 219–26.

Zuckner, J. (1990). Drug-induced myopathies. *Seminars in Arthritis and Rheumatism*, **19**, 259–68.

5.19.2 Algodystrophy (reflex sympathetic dystrophy syndrome)

Geoffrey O. Littlejohn

Introduction

Algodystrophy is an important pain syndrome characterized by variable dysfunction of musculoskeletal, skin, and vascular systems. The most characteristic feature is persistent pain, and this plus the associated disability, may have profound psychosocial effects. Moreover, the clinical features may be recalcitrant to medical intervention. Algodystrophy presents in a variety of clinical states and may be mild and short-lived or severe and prolonged. It is important to recognize the syndrome in the early and often incomplete phase if currently available therapeutic approaches are to be most effective.

Nomenclature

Algodystrophy is a chronic pain syndrome. Pain is the dominant symptom and, although the clinical features are characteristic and reproducible, the exact cause of the problem is unclear. Algodystrophy may occur in a variety of clinical conditions, affect different regions of the body to a greater or lesser extent, and the clinical manifestations vary around the central core features. As such

there are a large number of descriptive names that are synonyms for algodystrophy. Reflex sympathetic dystrophy syndrome is the most appropriate alternative. Even so, this term is only used in a descriptive sense and does not imply specific underlying mechanisms (Janig *et al.* 1991). Table 1 summarizes some of the synonyms for algodystrophy. Some prefer to use the original nomenclature in situations where the precipitating cause is obvious: for instance, the syndrome is often called causalgia when it follows injury to a peripheral nerve, or Sudeck's atrophy where it follows wrist fracture. The term algodystrophy, derived from the Greek *algos* meaning pain and 'dystrophy' meaning a disorder related to poor nourishment, best encapsulates the principal clinical features and serves to remind us of the essential nature of the syndrome.

The distinctive but varied clinical features of algodystrophy have provided classic clinical descriptions for over 100 years. Indeed, Hunter was one of the earliest to allude to this condition (Hunter 1843). By the middle of the nineteenth century, formal clinical descriptions were available in the context of traumatic lesions of peripheral nerves. Mitchell *et al.* (1864) described the deep burning pain of causalgia but also emphasized other features such as 'the skin affected in these cases was deep red or mottled, or red and pale in patches, . . . the surface of all the affected part was glossy and shining as though it had been skilfully varnished . . . , in some form, pain has been invariably attendant upon the disease state of skin which we have tried to describe. . . . In the great mass of cases, it has been of that peculiar burning character of which we have spoken, . . . in other instances, there was associated with this, acute or aching pain which extended beyond the disease tissues.' With the advent of radiology the clinical manifestations were greatly expanded as the breadth of the syndrome was recognized (Doury *et al.* 1981).

More recently the putative role of the sympathetic nervous system in this syndrome has been incorporated through use of the terms sympathetic-maintained (or mediated) pain and sympathetically independent pain (Roberts 1986). These subgroups are differentiated on the response of the pain to sympathetic blockade (Campbell *et al.* 1992). In a further development the term complex regional pain syndrome has been proposed, based entirely on clinical features (Merskey and Bogduk 1994).

Epidemiology

Algodystrophy is a common rheumatological disorder. It has been seen in all races and geographical regions. It affects both sexes and may occur at any age. Historically the published records have

Table 1	Selected alternative terms for algodystrophy
Reflex sympathetic dystrophy syndrome	
Causalgia	
Shoulder–hand syndrome	
Sudeck's atrophy	
Transient osteoporosis	
Regional migratory osteoporosis	
Post-traumatic painful osteoporosis	
Complex regional pain syndrome	

concentrated on the elderly patient who has sustained trauma, for instance a Colles' fracture, but over the last decade the occurrence of algodystrophy in children, particularly adolescent girls, has been well characterized (Silber and Majd 1988; Cicuttini and Littlejohn 1989; Sherry *et al.* 1991). In the adolescent, girls are affected far more than boys and in the adult, men seem to be affected more than women. The most frequent age group affected is between 40 and 60 years of age.

As with many rheumatic diseases the 'classical case' is easily characterized and recognized but occurs far less commonly than *formes frustes*. Minor variants tend to be less troublesome or may be regarded, in some instances, as part of the initiating cause. For example, minor algodystrophy following trauma may be regarded as a part of the normal response to injury. Minor forms may also occur in other painful, peripheral rheumatic disorders such as inflammatory arthritis and thus be hidden with the clinical features of the inflammation itself. A true estimate of the prevalence of the condition is thus extremely hard to provide.

In its classical form, 1 in 200 people presenting to a trauma unit will develop algodystrophy (Plewes 1956), but in other traumatic states up to 1 in 20 will develop it (Kozin 1986). Before the intensive mobilization of patients with myocardial ischaemia or hemiplegia became acceptable, between 5 and 20 per cent of such patients developed algodystrophy (Davis 1977). In a study of 109 unselected patients with Colles' fracture, 25 per cent had two or more features of algodystrophy at 9 weeks, while at 6 months 62 per cent showed some residual abnormalities (Atkins *et al.* 1989). It is likely that the prevalence of algodystrophy will always be underestimated because of its minor variants. In order to identify mild or early forms of algodystrophy, it should be anticipated where there are triggering events known to be associated with the syndrome.

Clinical features

Like other chronic pain syndromes the chief complaint and that which draws the syndrome to the attention of the medical practitioner is pain. This not only manifests as spontaneous, often burning, pain but also as a pain amplification state. Here otherwise innocuous stimuli produce pain (allodynia) and there is increased pain perception to a given painful stimulus (hyperalgesia). Hyperpathia, where there is delayed overreaction particularly to a normal repetitive cutaneous stimulus, is also found. The pain will usually occur some days to weeks after a triggering factor, if present, and will generally be constant. Although burning pain is a characteristic of the syndrome, more commonly the pain is described as a deep, dull aching sensation. Paroxysms of pain may occur, lasting for seconds. The pain may disturb sleep, and even any slight movement that mechanically stimulates the sensitized region will produce worsening of the symptom. The patient may report the use of cold, wet compresses to relieve the discomfort.

Typically the syndrome principally involves the distal part of a limb; for instance, a hand and lower forearm region (Fig. 1) or a foot and lower leg. With time, in the majority, much less apparent but definitely abnormal clinical features occur in the opposite limb. The syndrome may involve one digit or rarely all four limbs. Shortly after the onset of pain, swelling, the second most common feature, occurs (Blumberg *et al.* 1994). This may be intermittent in the early stages and is usually associated with a change in the texture of the overlying skin, producing the reticular or lividoid appearance over the involved part (Fig. 2). Palmar erythema may be noted. Early in the course the

involved region is warmer than the surrounding region. Varying degrees of sweating may occur but are not essential to the diagnosis. There may be piloerection.

Examination confirms the presence of a decreased pain threshold, particularly to mechanical stimuli, leading to abnormal tenderness as the principal clinical finding. Early in the course the hyperalgesia tends to be periarticular, but later regions well away from joints and particularly those over bone also become exquisitely tender. This distribution is non-(neuro-) anatomical and found over a wide region of the involved parts. For instance, if the principal involvement is in the mid-tarsal region of the foot, one would usually find tenderness on palpation of a metatarsophalangeal joint and regions of the lower leg, as well as in intervening areas. Mild oedema may be noted, either pitting or not. Early on, joint movement in the region will be

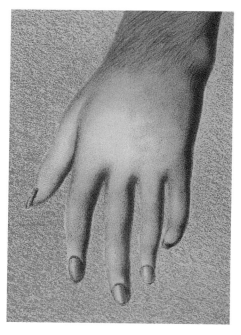

Fig. 1 Reflex sympathetic dystrophy syndrome of the left hand in a 21-year-old man after trauma, showing diffuse swelling, cutaneous blood-flow change, and dystrophic skin changes. One of the earliest reported pictures of this condition (from Otis (1877), by courtesy of Dr R.L. Travers).

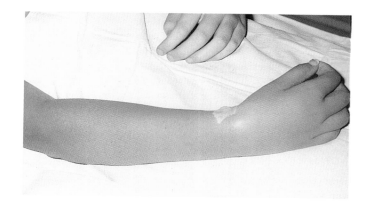

Fig. 2 Diffuse swelling of lower right forearm and hand in a 13-year-old girl with reflex sympathetic dystrophy syndrome. There is extreme hyperalgesia. Note flexed wrist and hand posture and skin discoloration. (By courtesy of Dr R. Allan, Royal Children's Hospital, Melbourne, Australia.)

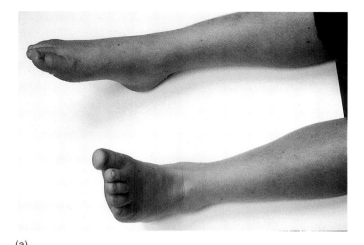

(a)

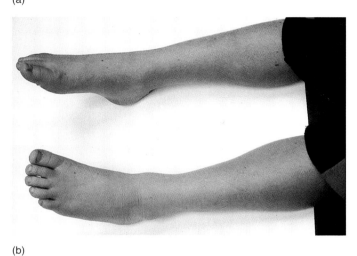

(b)

Fig. 3 Right lower leg and foot in a 15-year-old female patient with reflex dystrophy syndrome showing skin discoloration, regional swelling, and inability to extend the right ankle (a) and the adoption of a plantar flexion (b) assumed in order to reduce pain. The lower third of the leg, including the foot was extremely hyperalgesic. (By courtesy of Dr R. Allan, Royal Children's Hospital, Melbourne, Australia.)

restricted by pain but with care it be demonstrated that the range of motion is often near normal, despite the initial impression (Fig. 3). There may be a prominent motor component with tremor, weakness, or muscle tightness.

Triggering events

A number of well-characterized events may precede algodystrophy. It is best to regard these events as triggers rather than as causative because of the wide variety of different associations. Table 2 summarizes the important disorders associated with algodystrophy.

In most series, depending on the criteria for classifying algodystrophy, trauma will be identified as a trigger in around half of subjects (Doury *et al.* 1981; Kozin 1986). In many instances it is likely that a prior traumatic episode will have been recalled by the patient after the development of algodystrophy rather than the event being a true trigger. However, major and even minor, apparently trivial, traumas, particularly to a distal part of a limb, have been

Table 2 Selected disorders associated with algodystrophy

	Approximate frequency of association (%)
Trauma	50
Idiopathic	25
Disorders of the nervous system	
Central conditions	
Painful peripheral conditions	25
Medication	
Others	

clearly linked to the development of the syndrome. In about one-half of cases the trauma will have led to bone fracture and indeed many accounts of the syndrome come from observations made on peripheral fractures, such as Colles' fracture at the wrist. Other important traumatic triggers include simple sprains, strains, contusions, or jarring injuries, particularly to the distal part of the limbs. Surgical procedures, particularly of limb joints, such as arthroscopy, can induce algodystrophy (Small 1993). Other triggering traumas include peripheral burns and frost-bite. Trauma to articular more than diaphyseal regions predisposes to this syndrome (Fontaine *et al.* 1957). Although trauma is a common trigger, in the context of the large number of traumatic events found in any community, the subsequent development of algodystrophy affects less than 1 per cent of all such events. Perhaps a common thread among injuries that result in algodystrophy is the individual's reaction to pain and the frightening nature of the injury, be it major or apparently trivial.

A variety of disorders of the nervous system may act as triggers. These include conditions resulting in hemiplegia and other central diseases, including cerebral tumour, meningitis, or syringomyelia, among others. Peripheral nerve injury is the classical cause of causalgia but other peripheral nerve disturbances such as those caused by *herpes zoster*, nerve-root impingement, or peripheral neuropathy may result in this syndrome. Pain arising from a visceral or deep somatic structure, such as myocardial ischaemia in the former instance and mechanical pain from the cervical spine in the latter, may be associated. Pain arising from a peripheral origin, such as that seen in inflammatory arthritis or after deep venous thrombosis, may provoke the syndrome. Certain medications, particularly barbiturates and isoniazid, have been reported as triggers.

There are a variety of other conditions that may be linked with algodystrophy. These include pregnancy (with particular involvement of the hip), metastatic tumours, acrodermatitis continua, and prolonged immobilization of a peripheral limb (Schwartzman and McLellan 1987). The suggestion that there is an increased prevalence of diabetes and hypertriglyceridaemia in this group of patients (Amor *et al.* 1980) has been refuted by others (Eurly 1992).

At least 25 per cent of cases have no easily identifiable trigger. Here the search for central factors or psychological susceptibility is often made. In children it is common to find an unresolved stress or an unsatisfactory psychosocial state in the background (Sherry and Weisman 1988). In adults, this is more difficult to identify clearly. A small percentage of patients developing algodystrophy will have a defined psychiatric condition, such as major depression, or a chronic anxiety state, but many more are likely to have abnormal reactions to psychosocial stresses. These factors may be difficult to identify accurately but there is often a strong clinical impression that they are playing an important part in the triggering or expression of the syndrome. However, in many patients, no such factors can be identified. There is no definite evidence that particular personality traits predispose a person to develop algodystrophy (Bruehl and Carlson 1992; Lynch 1992).

Course

In most instances the clinical features persist, fluctuate, or gradually resolve according to the natural history or treatment intervention, without further sequelae. In some patients there is a dystrophic phase, usually some months after the start of the problem. Here the limb becomes cool, and cutaneous pallor or cyanosis replace the previous erythema. There is decreased growth of dermal appendages, such as hair, and the nails become brittle. Skin and subcutaneous tissues may atrophy. Increased sweating becomes more prominent and the pain persists and often worsens. There may be dysaesthesia (painful, abnormal skin sensation) in a non-anatomical distribution. Radiological evaluation will show change in the mineral content of bone in the area. Joints become tighter, this time due to contracture of surrounding structures. After several months there may be an atrophic phase. Pain usually decreases at this stage but can remain intractable in some. There may be marked atrophy of subcutaneous tissue, such as to cause tapering of digits, and flexion contractures of peripheral joints become prominent. The limb is characterized by vasoconstriction and coolness and the skin is cyanotic, smooth, and glossy. Hair growth can be increased or decreased.

While the clinical features of algodystrophy are easy to recognize, there are, as mentioned above, more patients who have variations or incomplete forms than have the typical condition. Variants are particularly common in children where the painful limb is usually cool and slightly swollen from the outset and the syndrome does not tend to go through the classical phases, often resolving much more quickly than in an adult.

Traditionally the disorder has been staged according to observations by Steinbrocker and Argyros (1958), where stage 1 comprises the 'acute' clinical features with pain, tenderness, swelling, and vasomotor and pseudomotor changes predominating. With time, stage 2 will supervene and this is dominated by dystrophic features and will last for several months. Stage 3 comprises atrophic changes and may be long lasting. In extreme cases this classification is of use but in the average situation most patients do not progress beyond stage 1 or early stage 2. Perhaps this is because of early intervention or perhaps we are now diagnosing the condition in its milder and incomplete forms more often. Many patients also have features derived from different components, and investigations and clinical features often do not correlate, irrespective of the chosen staging. The success of treatment does not depend on the patient's clinical stage except that profound stage 3 changes are difficult to reverse.

Classification

There is no validated classification for diagnosis in the clinical setting or for research purposes because of the polymorphic nature of

algodystrophy. The classification of Kozin et al. (1981) is often very useful clinically. Here, definite algodystrophy is present when there is pain and tenderness in an extremity, swelling of that extremity, and vasomotor or pseudomotor changes. Dystrophic change may also be present. Probable algodystrophy consists of pain and tenderness, together with vasomotor and pseudomotor changes or swelling; possible algodystrophy comprises vasomotor or pseudomotor changes; and doubtful algodystrophy is considered where there is pain and tenderness out of keeping with any preceding injury or other organic disease process.

Regions involved

Several common areas of involvement have been defined (Doury et al. 1981). The arm may be involved in a unipolar fashion, with either shoulder (frozen shoulder) or hand being affected. Involvement of the shoulder is associated with marked retraction of the joint capsule, restricted range of motion, and pain persisting for several months. On resolution of the syndrome, loss of range of motion of the shoulder is common, although usually not clinically significant. Peripheral involvement may include a single digit (Laukaitis et al. 1989), a few metacarpal rays (Lequesne et al. 1977), or more typically the whole hand and lower forearm may be involved. Bipolar forms include the shoulder–hand syndrome. Up to 25 per cent of upper-limb involvement is bilateral, the changes in the opposite side often being more evident after investigation (Kozin et al. 1976).

Leg involvement, although more common, is less dramatic than that of the arm.. Here the features are usually confined to a part of the limb such as the foot, knee, or hip. Bipolar and bilateral involvement are less common than in the arm. Involvement of the knee, either of the whole or of part, including the patella, has only more recently been characterized (Tietjen 1986; Coughlan et al. 1987).

Algodystrophy of the hip is less commonly recognized because the hip joint is deeply positioned and there is a lack of the cutaneous features that are more common in peripheral and superficial sites. The duration of symptoms in this region is shorter, possibly because early mobilization is easier. Some (for example, Lakhanpal et al. 1987) suggest that this variant is distinct enough to be termed transient regional osteoporosis. Absence of precipitating trauma, good outcome, and a propensity for recurrent episodes and involvement of multiple regions is characteristic of this variant. Signs of cutaneous or vascular change are uncommon. Algodystrophy may also affect the spine and occasionally other areas of the skeleton.

Investigations
Laboratory investigations

There is no abnormality of acute-phase reactants nor of standard biochemical markers in algodystrophy. In some patients with early disease, 24-h urinary hydroxyproline excretion may be increased, reflecting bone demineralization (Doury 1988).

Imaging

The principal contribution to diagnosis remains clinical. However, a number of radiological and nuclear medicine techniques may show characteristic abnormalities. As there is no specific 'gold standard' for diagnostic criteria it is difficult to establish the clinical usefulness of these investigations. The main problem arises from the many

Table 3 Investigations in algodystrophy

Investigation	Changes	Usefulness
Plain radiography	Patchy osteopenia early; diffuse late	Moderate predictive value
Fine-detail radiography	Diffuse and periarticular osteopenia common	80% abnormal
	Cortical bone resorption	
	Juxta-articular/subchondral erosion	
Dual-photon absorptiometry	Loss of up to 30% of bone mass	Unknown
Dual-X-ray absorptiometry	Bone loss shown	Unknown
Magnetic resonance imaging	Regional/diffuse bone loss	Unknown, probably low
Scintigraphy	Abnormal in early, pool, or late phases	High specificity
Thermography	Change in cutaneous temperature	Unknown

variations of the syndrome, and most studies have considered only severe algodystrophy in evaluating investigations, thus producing a distorted view of their clinical utility. Table 3 summarizes selected investigations.

Sudeck (1900) first showed the value of radiology in this condition. Plain radiographic changes reflect bone demineralization; these may take several weeks to months to appear after the onset of the syndrome. These changes persist longer than other clinical features on resolution. Some patients never have radiological changes and others have only subtle changes. It is essential that good technique and meticulous examination of radiographs, with comparison of the affected side to the other side, be performed. Characteristically children have far less radiological changes than adults, with only the minority showing demineralization. Patchy osteopenia may be seen in the early stages and diffuse changes characterize the later stages. Typically in the hip or knee, changes are most obvious in the subchondral region where loss of subchondral bone and preservation of subchondral plate will produce a significant finding. Severe juxta-articular changes might include erosions. However, the joint space is never affected. The sensitivity and specificity of radiological appearances are around 70 per cent for well-defined algodystrophy (Kozin et al. 1981). Plain radiography is an essential investigation but has only moderate predictive value for diagnosis. Fine-detailed radiography better shows the demineralization, which is accentuated around epiphyseal regions, reflecting hyperaemia at this site. Subperiosteal, endosteal, and intracortical bone resorption together with juxta-articular and subchondral erosions, are observed frequently with this technique (Genant et al. 1975; Griffiths and Virtama 1988).

Magnetic resonance imaging (MRI) may also show changes characteristic of bone loss (Fig. 4). For instance, in the hip, low intensity signal on T_1-weighted images and high intensity on T_2-weighted images may be seen. The clinical usefulness of this technique and absorptiometry, which also may reflect bone loss, is yet to be established.

Scintigraphic studies using technetium have a high specificity but a similar sensitivity to that of plain radiographs (Fig. 5). Typically a three-phase study (Kozin et al. 1976) is made, with the early phase showing regional blood flow over the first 2 to 3 min, the second phase showing the blood-pool image, and the third phase (some 2 to 4 h later) showing the standard bone-uptake findings. While any of these three phases may be abnormal it is more common to find increased flow (early phase) and uptake (late phase) in around 80 per cent of abnormal studies. Diminished flow and uptake are more commonly seen in children and adolescents than in adults (Silber and Majd 1988; Goldsmith et al. 1989). Scintigraphy appears more accurate if symptoms have been present for less than 6 months or if the patient is older than 50 years (Werner et al. 1989). Multiple investigations are often needed (Fig. 6).

Thermography may show changes in regional cutaneous temperatures compared with the unaffected side (Perelman et al. 1987). Typically there is an early increased or, particularly in children, decreased cutaneous heat emission. Critical evaluation of this technique is required before it can be usefully applied clinically (Fig. 7).

Histopathological changes

Synovial biopsies of joints in the region of algodystrophy will often show low-grade synovitis characterized by proliferation of synovial cells and small blood vessels, together with a mild chronic perivascular infiltrate. There have only been limited studies on the bone demineralization, periarticular fibrosis, and dermal atrophy (Arlet et al. 1978; Doury et al. 1981).

Diagnosis

The diagnosis of algodystrophy is based on the clinical features. A high degree of clinical suspicion is required, particularly in early diagnosis. Focal disease may mimic inflammatory or infectious arthritis or bone disease, trauma, or osteonecrosis. Characteristic clinical features, elimination of other causes for such symptoms, and appropriate imaging will usually allow for a clinically robust diagnosis. The most important thing in diagnosis is to think of the possibility of algodystrophy.

Pathophysiology

Algodystrophy is caused by a regional change in function of the pain system. This involves both peripheral and central mechanisms in a

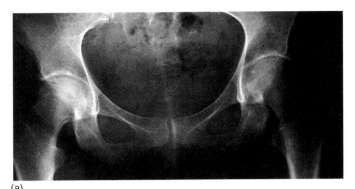

(a)

Fig. 4 (a)–(d) A 31-year-old female patient with transient regional osteoporosis of the left hip. Plain films (a) indicate regional osteoporosis of the left femoral head. MRI scan (b,c,d) shows changes of diffuse osteopenia in the left femoral head, compared with normal changes on the right side. (By courtesy of Dr John Stuckey, Victorian Imaging Group, Melbourne, Australia.)

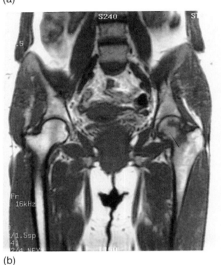

(b)

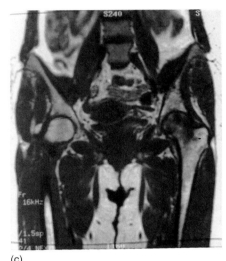

(c)

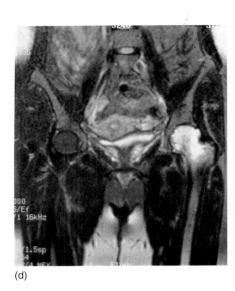

(d)

complex manner. The cause for this pain syndrome is poorly understood. However, many of the clinical features reflect change in function of various components of the peripheral nervous system. Many fibre types with different functions appear to contribute in varying degrees to the syndrome.

Table 4 summarizes the principal clinical characteristics of the syndrome and possible causative mechanisms. Input from two afferent fibre types, the small diameter, non-myelinated C-fibres and the large, myelinated A-β-fibres, together with change in function of sympathetic efferents, appear the likely mediators of many of the peripheral features. Sympathetic activity, through release of noradrenaline and the inflammatory prostaglandins, may sensitize peripheral nociceptors, thus decreasing threshold to peripheral mechanical and chemical stimuli. This may result in the hyperalgesia. It has been suggested that α_1-adrenergic receptors may become expressed on such nociceptors, particularly in a post-injury situation, and that these receptors will respond to sympathetic fibre release of noradrenaline (Campbell *et al.* 1988). Subsequent release of proinflammatory neuropeptides, such as substance P, by activated C-fibres would contribute to regional neurogenic inflammation with increase in blood flow and oedema. The associated synovitis may be due to this mechanism. Levine *et al.* (1984) have demonstrated that substance P contributes to experimental synovitis and this system is further modulated by alteration of sympathetic input. Periarticular osteoporosis may relate to the hyperaemia in the epiphyseal vessels in particular, or to neuropeptide effects on bone mineral metabolism. Allodynia is

likely to reflect abnormality within the large myelinated afferent fibre system, as blocking these fibres by local anaesthetics will abolish this finding in other situations (Meyer *et al.* 1972; Roberts 1986).

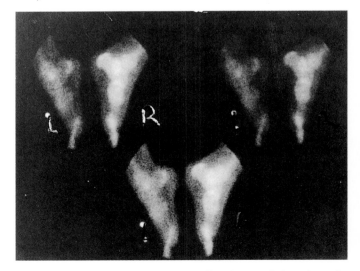

Fig. 5 A 28-year-old female patient with diffuse increase in isotopic uptake of right foot and lower end of right tibia, in a foot which was diffusely swollen and extremely hyperalgesic. The reflex sympathetic dystrophy in this case was associated with Reiter's disease initially affecting the right ankle. Inflammatory arthritis, trauma, or other pain stimuli may associate with the onset of reflex sympathetic dystrophy.

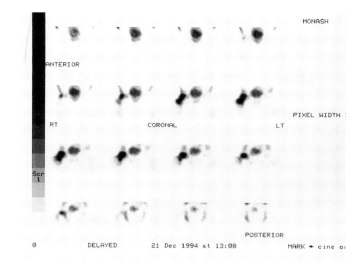

(a)

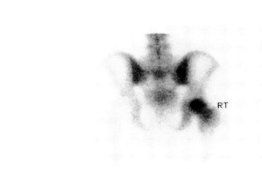

(b)

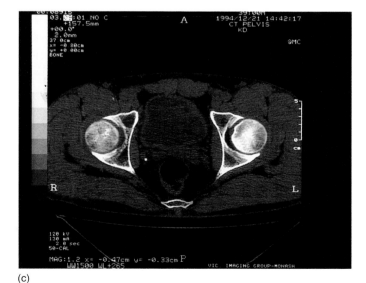

(c)

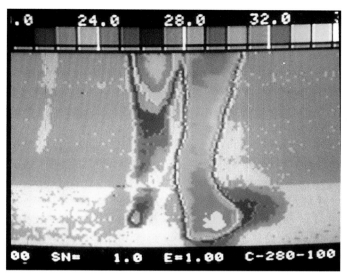

Fig. 7 Thermogram indicating lowered skin temperature (blue colours, compared with normal temperatures pink-red) of right leg and foot in a 15-year-old female patient with reflex dystrophy syndrome. (By courtesy of Dr R. Allan, Royal Children's Hospital, Melbourne, Australia.)

Fig. 6 A 39-year-old male with 4 months of pain from right hip. The nuclear scan (a and b) with spectroscopy reveals marked increase in isotopic uptake in the right femoral head and neck. The CT scan (c) shows osteopenia. Femoral head biopsy showed osteopenia of the neck and head of femur. The diagnosis was transient regional osteoporosis of the femoral head. (By courtesy of Dr John Stuckey, Victorian Imaging Group, Melbourne, Australia.)

In sophisticated tests, sympathetic efferents can be shown to have abnormal activity in the majority of patients with this syndrome. Many patients, though not all, do respond to sympathetic blockade, highlighting the role of sympathetic activity. The interaction between the products of the sympathetic nervous system and the peripheral nociceptors is also highlighted by the knowledge that injection of noradrenaline will exacerbate pain and this is blocked by intravenous administration of the α_1-adrenergic antagonist, phentolamine. The phentolamine test can be used diagnostically to help predict patients who have a large sympathetically maintained component to their syndrome and those who are likely to benefit from sympathetic blockade (Arner 1991; Campbell *et al.* 1992).

The cause for these functional changes in the peripheral pain system is still unclear. Livingstone (1943) suggested that there was a persisting peripheral afferent stimulus which led to abnormal activation of internuncial neurones situated in the dorsal horn at the relevant level. Efferent sympathetic activity was felt to follow that sequence. The realization that the majority of patients with algodystrophy do not have an identifiable persisting afferent stimulus in the region of pain, has led to an appreciation that a functional change within the dorsal horn itself is the most important cause for the syndrome. This functional dorsal horn abnormality is usually triggered by minor trauma, often in an emotional context. This was accounted for by Lankford and Thompson's theory (Lankford and Thompson 1977).

Roberts (1986) has suggested that initial activation of the unmyelinated C-fibre nociceptors, through unknown mechanisms, leads to sensitization of wide dynamic range neurones in the dorsal horn. Such neurones receive not only nociceptive input but input from other sources, including low-threshold, large myelinated afferents that otherwise serve functions such as proprioception. Input from these fibres resulting, say, from change in joint position or movement will impinge on the sensitized neurone with wide dynamic range in the dorsal horn and this input will be perceived as pain (allodynia). Central sensitization mechanisms mediated by excitatory amino

Table 4 Pathophysiological mechanisms in algodystrophy

Characteristic	Mechanism
Pain	
Spontaneous	Sensitized peripheral/central nociceptors
Allodynia	Large myelinated fibre input to sensitized dorsal horn transmission neurones
Hyperalgesia	C-fibre sensitization in periphery+sensitized 2nd order neurones
Movement pain	Large myelinated fibre input to sensitized dorsal horn transmission neurones
Swelling	Neuropeptides from C-fibres; sympathetic effects on post-capillary venules
Bone change	Hyperaemia secondary to neuropeptide release; sympathetic effects
Synovitis	Neuropeptides
Dystrophy	Unknown neurological mechanism; mechanical effects

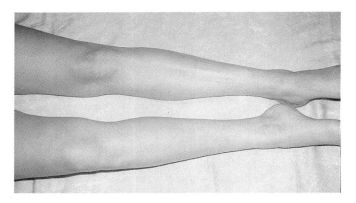

Fig. 8 A 28-year-old female with reflex sympathetic dystrophy syndrome of right lower leg from knee to foot. This area was extremely hyperalgesic compared with the left side. Signs of overt swelling, colour change, or other change 'sympathetic' features were lacking, as can be the case. This patient later developed a regional pain syndrome involving low back and all of the right leg. This illustrates the spectrum of reflex sympathetic dystrophy syndrome in that not all patients have the classic features.

acids and their interaction with the N-methyl-D-aspartate receptor, as well as the neuropeptides, are relevant to this process (Schwartzman 1993).

With activation of the system, automatic reflex changes at a segmental level lead to both muscle change and stimulation of the sympathetic system. The former may result in various neuromuscular features that can accompany algodystrophy, such as dystonia or other movement disorders (Schwartzman and Kerrigan 1990). The latter will affect functions in peripheral tissues and may result in a number of the dystrophic features of the syndrome. In addition, the cycle is completed whereby sympathetic efferent activity maintains peripheral fibre sensitization, which in turn feeds back into the dorsal horn system initiating further sympathetic activity. Such neurogenic reflexes are usually bilaterally represented, explaining the bilateral findings in many patients with algodystrophy.

The reason for change in function of these interactions in the dorsal horn is unclear. It seems naïve to explain such intense pain syndromes on purely segmental and peripheral pathophysiological changes. The complex and hierarchical nature of the pain system includes essential connections to the higher centres including the cortex. Important descending influences from higher centres impinge on the dorsal horn and modulate many components of the pain system. Thus central events which might include a variety of cortical and psychological factors may further influence this system. These might include the stress of pain itself and its effects on the central nervous system and the hypothalamic–pituitary axis, the patient's beliefs, mood, emotions, and even their quality of sleep. A change in any of these factors may affect the homeostatic mechanisms involved in pain control and sensitization phenomena in the dorsal horn. It is through such mechanisms that the emotional and affective components of the painful stimulus modify the peripheral reception and processing of further information relating to pain (Harvey 1987).

Table 5 Abnormalities in different pain syndromes and dystonia

Syndrome	Nociceptor	Mechanoreceptor	Sympathetic nervous system	Motor
Algodystrophy	++	++	+++	+
Fibromyalgia	++	+	+	+
Dystonia				+++

+ to +++ indicates range of qualitative changes.

Algodystrophy shares many features with fibromyalgia syndrome, another common chronic pain syndrome (Bengtsson and Bengtsson 1988; Vaeroy *et al.* 1989). When this syndrome is localized a significant component of patients' symptoms relate to sympathetic-maintained pain (Fig. 8). Other features shared between the two syndromes are allodynia, hyperalgesia, and dermatographia. Table 5 compares selected features of these syndromes.

Other factors that may be important in the pathophysiology have been variously reviewed (Doury *et al.* 1981; Carlson and Jacobs 1986; Escobar 1986; Fields 1987; Kozin 1994; Janig 1996).

Management

Algodystrophy must been seen as a pain syndrome if an effective treatment programme is to be provided. This involves treating the whole patient and not just the obviously abnormal area of complaint in the periphery.

Preventive strategies include the recognition of situations that are likely to provoke the syndrome. Thus early mobilization after myocardial infarction, cerebrovascular accident, hand surgery, or mild peripheral injury is essential. Appropriate reassurance and direction in the handling of patients in any post-traumatic setting, particularly in emotionally charged, work-related events is essential.

Many authorities indicate that prognosis for full recovery relates inversely to the duration of symptoms before the onset of treatment; however, others feel that the syndrome can reverse, to a large extent, at any time (Kozin *et al.* 1987).

In milder forms of algodystrophy the principles of management (Table 6) include adequate pain relief, reassurance, and explanation. A positive approach in regard to outcome is appropriate and necessary. Careful explanation is required to ensure that the holistic concept of a chronic pain state is understood by the patient, according to their level of understanding. This is essential; it leads to a co-operative management plan that has the patient as the key person in the team. This syndrome is not well served by the adoption of the 'injury' model where a powerful external 'treater' is required to give the 'curative' treatment. Such well-intentioned approaches often lead to a more dense ingraining of the syndrome, probably through blocking of positive benefits that would come from modulation of the central pathways on to the dorsal horn. Similarly, certain systems

Table 6 Principles of management of algodystrophy
Accurate, early diagnosis
Explanation, reassurance
Adequate analgesia (medication, transcutaneous electrical stimulation)
Prevention of dystrophic change — exercise, movement
Attention to sleep disturbance
Attend to pain behaviour, psychosocial stresses, including compensation, litigation issues
Transient interruption of sympathetic activity
Skilled pain management/psychological counselling
Other

of compensation and other medicolegal events appear to inhibit resolution of the syndrome.

Counselling the patient, attending to the associated anxiety, and correcting any sleep disturbance, often through the use of low-dose tricyclic medication, are beneficial and prevent further amplification of the syndrome.

Useful treatments in milder algodystrophy, particularly in children, are exercise programmes which might include hydrotherapy. Activation of muscles and mechanoreceptors probably inhibits the activated dorsal-horn pain system on a local, segmental basis.

Numerous other treatment programmes have been suggested for the more severe or persistent types of algodystrophy. Some find systemic corticosteroids to be beneficial, even when the syndrome has been long-lasting (Kozin *et al.* 1981; Christensen *et al.* 1982). A typical course might commence at around 50 mg of prednisolone a day in divided doses and decrease to zero over 3 to 4 weeks. Subsequent courses may be needed. Some have advocated calcitonin, for example, 100 to 160 IU/day over 10 to 14 days, which has been shown to have benefits over placebo (Gobelet *et al.* 1986; Gobelet *et al.* 1992).

Interruption of the sympathetic efferent system to the region through various techniques has proved beneficial to many patients. Typically, a regional sympathetic ganglion block is made, using up to five short-acting sympathetic blocks, on a daily or alternate-day basis. If pain relief results, the patient is started on a more vigorous physiotherapy or exercise programme. Such approaches may result in 40 per cent of patients having a better result after 3-years follow-up; however, the majority have a less useful outcome (Wang *et al.* 1985).

Regional sympathetic blocks compare favourably with ganglion blockade (Bonnelli *et al.* 1983). These may be achieved using the Bier technique, whereby occlusion of venous outflow to the region, usually the lower arm or leg, is followed by intravenous installation of guanethidine or another similar agent. The exact mechanism of action of sympathetic modulation is unclear. Peripheral nerve blocks in the axilla will also modify afferent nerve transmission and may be useful. Again these procedures often need to be repeated to achieve sustained results (Schwartzman and McLellan 1987).

Surgical sympathectomy is only done if there is definite, but short-lived, improvement with the previous procedures.

Many other approaches have been used; these range from epidural opioids to cutaneous clonidine patches. Controlled studies are lacking for most of these approaches (Dotson 1993). The large variety of therapies emphasizes the difficulty in treating established algodystrophy. My approach to management is as follows:

1. *Young patient, any severity, any duration*:

Always

  (a) accurate diagnosis, explanation, reassurance as to expected good outcome;
  (b) identification and management of psychosocial stressors especially family, school, or other;
  (c) establishment of a regular activity programme — walking, bicycle riding, swimming, etc.
  (d) resumption of all previous activities, especially those related to school;
  (e) careful supervision of programme and close liaison with parents, especially the mother if a female patient.

Often

> (a) transcutaneous nerve stimulation to help pain control and allow entry into activity programme;
>
> (b) hydrotherapy if limb sensitivity to movement is extreme. An empathetic physiotherapist is often the most powerful tool in this programme.

Sometimes

> (a) tricyclic medication to correct sleep disturbance and increase the pain threshold;
>
> (b) a clinical psychologist to help manage pain and consider psychosocial background dynamics;
>
> (c) regional temporary sympathetic/ganglion blocks;
>
> (d) other approaches.

2. Adult patient, mild severity, and duration:

Always

> (a) accurate diagnosis, explanation, reassurance as to probable good outcome;
>
> (b) identification and management of any obvious psychosocial stressors including work-related or legal issues;
>
> (c) establishment of regular activity programme using involved limb;
>
> (d) planned return to all previous activities currently abandoned due to pain;
>
> (e) careful supervision of the programme with attention to the 'blocks' to progress that often occur.

Often

> (a) supervision of the physical programme by a physiotherapist with use of transcutaneous nerve stimulation, hydrotherapy, and similar tactics to control pain and encourage activity;
>
> (b) short-term use of tricyclic medication.

Sometimes

> (a) pain-management counselling by clinical psychologist or similar skilled person;
>
> (b) regional temporary sympathetic/ganglion blocks;
>
> (c) other approaches, such as short-course corticosteroids.

3. Adult patient, moderate/severe, prolonged duration:

Always

> (a) use all the above approaches, sometimes sequentially and sometimes concomitantly;
>
> (b) put emphasis on pain-management counselling early in programme, with frequent use of interventions to block efferent sympathetic outflow, and/or corticosteroids;
>
> (c) stay with the patient—suboptimal therapeutic responses require longer-term support.

Prognosis

The outcome for patients with algodystrophy is quite varied. Minor forms seem to have an excellent outcome and children with the condition are expected to regain normal function and lose their pain. Some adults with severe forms of the condition may have protracted chronic pain states, significant dystrophic tissue change and longer-term disability. Pain usually eases over time even in those patients.

Summary

Algodystrophy is a common and significant musculoskeletal condition that results from a complex neurophysiological change in the pain transmission pathways. The syndrome is characteristic and reproducible but many variants occur clinically. The best treatment is through early recognition and management along principles used in other chronic pain syndromes, but with particular attention to the characteristic increase in sympathetic-maintained pain.

References

Amor, B. G. A. de, Saporta, L., Abergel, S., and Delbarre, F. (1980). Algodystrophies et hyperlipidemies. *Revue de Rhumatisme et des Maladies Osteoarticulaires*, **47**, 353–8.

Arlet, J., Ficat, P., Durroux, R., Theallie, J.P., Mazieres, B., and Bouteiller, G. (1978). Histopathologie des lesions osseuses dans 9 cas d'algodystrophie de la hanche. *Revue de Rhumatisme et des Maladies Osteoarticulaires*, **45**, 691–8.

Arner, S. (1991). Intravenous phentolamine test: diagnostic and prognostic use in reflex sympathetic dystrophy. *Pain*, **46**, 17–22.

Atkins, R.M., Duckworth, T., and Kanis, J.A. (1989). Algodystrophy following Colles' fracture. *Journal of Hand Surgery*, **14**, 161–4.

Bengtsson, A. and Bengtsson, M. (1988). Regional sympathetic blockade in primary fibromyalgia. *Pain*, **33**, 161–7.

Blumberg, H., Hoffman, U., Mohadjer, M., and Scheremet, R. (1994). Clinical phenomenology and mechanisms of reflex sympathetic dystrophy: emphasis on edema. In *Proceedings of the 7th World Congress on Pain. Progress in Pain Research and Management*, Vol. 2, (ed. G.F. Gebhart, D.L. Hammond, and T.S. Jensen), pp. 455–81. IASP Press, Seattle.

Bonnelli, S., Conoscente, F., and Movilia, P.G. (1983). Regional intravenous guanethidine vs stellate ganglion block in reflex sympathetic dystrophies; a randomized trial. *Pain*, **16**, 297–307.

Bruehl, S. and Carlson, C.R. (1992). Predisposing psychological factors in the development of reflex sympathetic dystrophy. *Clinical Journal of Pain*, **8**, 287–99.

Campbell, J.N., Raja, S.N., and Meyer, R.A. (1988). Painful sequelae of nerve injury. In *Proceedings of the 5th World Congress on Pain* (ed. R. Dubner, G.F. Gebhart, and M.R. Bond), pp. 135–43. Elsevier, Amsterdam.

Campbell, J.N., Meyer, R.A., and Raja, S.N. (1992). Is nociceptor activation by alpha-1 adrenoreceptors the culprit in sympathetically maintained pain. *American Pain Society Journal*, **1**, 3–11.

Carlson, T. and Jacobs, A.M. (1986). Reflex sympathetic dystrophy syndrome. *Journal of Foot Surgery*, **25**, 149–53.

Christensen, K., Jensen, E.M., and Noer, I. (1982). The reflex dystrophy syndrome: response to treatment with systemic corticosteroids. *Acta Chirurgica Scandinavica*, **148**, 653–5.

Cicuttini, F. and Littlejohn, G.O. (1989). Female adolescent rheumatological presentations: the importance of chronic pain syndromes. *Australian Paediatric Journal*, **25**, 21–4.

Coughlan, F.J., Hazleman, B.L., and Page-Thomas, D.P. (1987). Algodystrophy: a common unrecognized cause of chronic knee pain. *British Journal of Rheumatology*, **26**, 270–4.

Davis, S.W. (1977). Shoulder-hand syndrome in a hemiplegic population: 5 year retrospective study. *Archives of Physical Medicine and Rehabilitation*, **58**, 353–9.

Dotson, R.M. (1993). Causalgia—reflex sympathetic dystrophy—sympathetically maintained pain: myth and reality. *Muscle and Nerve*, **16**, 1049–55.

Doury, P. (1988). Algodystrophy: reflex sympathetic dystrophy syndrome. *Clinical Rheumatology*, **7**, 173–80.

Doury, P., Dirheimer, Y., and Pattin, S. (1981). *Algodystrophy*. Springer, Berlin.

Escobar, P.L. (1986). Reflex sympathetic dystrophy. *Orthopaedic Review*, **15**, 646–51.

Eurly, F., Chevalier, X., Crozes, P., Prudat, M., Lechevalier, D., Larget-Pret, B. (1992). Is hyperlipidaemia a contributing factor to algodystrophy (reflex sympathetic dystrophy)? *Clinical Rheumatology*, **11**, 526–8.

Fields, H.L. (1987). Efferent activity and pain: the reflex sympathetic dystrophy syndrome. In *Pain*, pp. 145–55. McGraw-Hill, New York.

Fontaine, R. *et al.* (1957). Contribution a la physiopathologie de l'osteoporose post-traumatique. *Acta Chirurgica Belgica*, **1** (Suppl.), 173–201.

Genant, H.K., Kozin, F., Bekerman, C., McCarty, D.J, and Sims, J. (1975). The reflex sympathetic dystrophy syndrome: a comprehensive analysis using fine-detail radiography, photon absorptiometry, and bone and joint scintigraphy. *Radiography*, **117**, 21–32.

Gobelet, C., Meier, J-L., Schaffner, W., Bischof-Delaloye, A., Gerster, J-C., and Burckhardt, P. (1986). Calcitonin and reflex sympathetic dystrophy syndrome. *Clinical Rheumatology*, **5**, 382–8.

Gobelet, C., Waldburger, M., and Meier, J.L. (1992). The effect of adding calcitonin to physical treatment on reflex sympathetic dystrophy. *Pain*, **48**, 171–5.

Goldsmith, D.P., Vivino, F.B., Eichenfield, A.H., Athreya, B.H., and Heyman, S (1989). Nuclear imaging and clinical features of childhood reflex neurovascular dystrophy: comparison with adults. *Arthritis and Rheumatism*, **32**, 480–5.

Griffiths, H.J and Virtama, P. (1988). Juxta-articular erosions in reflex sympathetic dystrophy. *Acta Radiologica*, **29**, 183–7.

Harvey, A.R. (1987). Neurophysiology of rheumatic pain. *Clinical Rheumatology*, **1**, 1–26.

Hunter, J. (1843). Lessons on the principles of surgery (1766). In *Oeuvres complete*, Vol. 1, (ed. J. Hunter). Tortin-Masson, Paris.

Janig, W. (1996). The puzzle of 'reflex sympathetic dystrophy': mechanisms, hypotheses, open questions. In: *Reflex sympathetic dystrophy: a reappraisal* (ed. W. Janig and M. Stanton-Wicks), pp. 1–24. IASP Press, Seattle.

Janig, W., Blumberg, H., Boas, R.A., and Campbell, J.N. (1991). The reflex sympathetic dystrophy syndrome: consensus statement and general recommendations for diagnosis and clinical research. In *Proceedings of the 6th World Congress on Pain* (ed. M.R. Bond, J.E. Charlton, and E.J. Woolf), pp. 373–6. Elsevier, Amsterdam.

Kozin, F. (1986). Reflex sympathetic dystrophy syndrome. *Bulletin of the Rheumatic Diseases*, **36**, 1–8.

Kozin, F. (1994). Reflex sympathetic dystrophy syndrome. *Current Opinions in Rheumatology*, **6**, 210–6.

Kozin, F., McCarty, D.J., Sims, J., and Genant, J. (1976). The reflex sympathetic dystrophy syndrome. I. Clinical and histologic studies: evidence for bilaterality, response to corticosteroids, and articular involvement. *American Journal of Medicine*, **60**, 321–31.

Kozin, F., Fyan, L.M., Carrera, G.F., Soin, J.S., and Wortmann, F.L. (1981). The reflex sympathetic dystrophy syndrome. III. Scintigraphic studies, further evidence for the therapeutic efficacy of systemic corticosteroids and proposed diagnostic criteria. *American Journal of Medicine*, **70**, 23–30.

Lakhanpal, S., Ginsburg, W.W., Luthra, H.S., and Hunder, G.G. (1987). Transient regional osteoporosis. *Annals of Internal Medicine*, **106**, 444–50.

Lankford, L. and Thompson, J. (1977). Reflex sympathetic dystrophy, upper and lower extremity: diagnosis and management. *American Academy of Orthopaedic Surgeons Instructional Course Lectures*, **26**, 163–78. Mosby, St Louis.

Laukaitis, J.P., Varma, V.M., and Borenstein, D.G. (1989). Reflex sympathetic dystrophy localized to a single digit. *Journal of Rheumatology*, **16**, 402–5.

Lesquesne, M., Kerboull, M., Bensasson, M., Perez, C., Deirser, R., and Forest, A. (1977). Partial transient osteoporosis. *Skeletal Radiology*, **2**, 1–9.

Levine, J.D., Clark, R., Devor, M., Helms, C., Moskowitz, M.R., and Basbaum, A.I. (1984). Intravenous substance P contributes to the severity of experimental arthritis. *Science*, **226**, 547–9.

Livingston, W.K. (1943). *Pain mechanisms: a physiologic interpretation of causalgia and its related states.* Macmillan, New York.

Lynch, M.E. (1992). Psychological aspects of reflex sympathetic dystrophy: a review of the adult and paediatric literature. *Pain*, **49**, 337–47.

Merskey, H. and Bogduk, N. (1994). *Classification of chronic pain: descriptions of chronic pain syndromes and definition of pain terms*, 2nd edn. IASP Press, Seattle.

Meyer, R.A., Campbell, J.N., and Raja, S. (1972). Peripheral neural mechanisms of cutaneous hyperalgesia. *Advances in Pain Research and Therapeutics*, **9**, 53–71.

Mitchell, S.W., Morehouse, G.R., and Keen, W.W. (1864). *Gunshot wounds and other injuries of nerves.* Lippincott, Philadelphia.

Otis, G.S. (1877). *The medical and surgical history of the war of rebellion*, Part 2, Vol. 2, p. 1020, plate 52. US Government Printing Office, Washington.

Perelman, R.B., Adler, D., and Humphreys, M. (1987). Reflex sympathetic dystrophy: electronic thermography as an aid in diagnosis. *Orthopaedic Review*, **16**, 561–6.

Plewes, L.W. (1956). Sudeck's atrophy in the hands. *Journal of Bone and Joint Surgery*, **38B**, 195–201.

Roberts, W.J. (1986). An hypothesis on the physiological basis for causalgia and related pains. *Pain*, **24**, 297–311.

Schwartzman, R.J. (1993). Reflex sympathetic dystrophy. *Current Opinions in Neurology and Neurosurgery*, **6**, 531–6.

Schwartzman, R.J. and Kerrigan, J. (1990). The movement disorder of reflex sympathetic dystrophy. *Neurology*, **40**, 57–61.

Schwartzman, R.J. and McLellan, T.L. (1987). Reflex sympathetic dystrophy: a review. *Archives of Neurology*, **44**, 555–61.

Sherry, D.D. and Weisman, M.A. (1988). Psychologic aspects of childhood reflex neurovascular dystrophy. *Paediatrics*, **81**, 572–8.

Sherry, D.D., McGuire, T., Mellins, E., Salmonson, K., Wallace, C.A., and Nepom, B. (1991). Psychosomatic musculoskeletal pain in childhood: clinical and psychological analyses of one hundred children. *Pediatrics*, **88**, 1093–9.

Silber, J. and Majd, M. (1988). Reflex sympathetic dystrophy syndrome in children and adolescents. *American Journal of Diseases of Children*, **142**, 1325–30.

Small, N.C. (1993). Complications in arthroscopic surgery of the knee and shoulder. *Orthopedics*, **16**, 985–8.

Steinbrocker, O. and Argyros, T.G. (1958). The shoulder-hand syndrome: present status as a diagnostic and therapeutic entity. *Medical Clinics of North America*, **42**, 1538–53.

Sudeck, P. (1900). Über die akute entzundliche knochenatrophie. *Archiv für Klinische Chirurgie*, **62**, 147–56.

Tietjen, R. (1986). Reflex sympathetic dystrophy of the knee. *Clinical Orthopaedics*, **209**, 234–43.

Vaeroy, J., Qiao, Z-G., Morkrid, L., and Forre, O. (1989). Altered sympathetic nervous system response in patients with fibromyalgia (fibrositis syndrome). *Journal of Rheumatology*, **16**, 1469–5.

Wang, J.K., Johnson, K.A., and Ilstrup, D.M. (1985). Sympathetic blocks for reflex sympathetic dystrophy. *Pain*, **23**, 13–7.

Werner, R., Davidoff, G., Jackson, D., Cremer, S., Ventocilla, C., and Wolf, L. (1989). Factors affecting the senstivity and specificity of the three-phase technetium bone scan in the diagnosis of reflex sympathetic dystrophy syndrome in the upper extremity. *Journal of Hand Surgery*, **14A**, 520–3.

5.19.3 Rheumatic complications of drugs and toxins

Robert M. Bernstein

Congratulations if you have reached this chapter or happened upon it by chance. The author felt obliged to meet you here, because Francis Bacon held 'every man a debtor to his profession.' Bacon was also of the opinion that 'books must follow sciences, and not sciences books', but often books follow books: they contain not truth but copies of bad maps, so it is up to the student to read the scientific literature directly as well as learn by exploration and experience.

This chapter deals briefly with rheumatological presentations of adverse drug reactions and poisoning; more extensive reviews are available (Shoenfeld and Isenberg 1989; Kahn 1991). With so much public whim and paranoia it is easy to close our minds in defence of what we do, particularly when it comes to prescribing strange chemicals or eating them. Assessment of a potential reaction should involve clinical observation during therapy, after withdrawal of the drug, and, if possible, upon rechallenge; where the reaction is subjective rechallenge should be blinded.

Immunological reactions

A long list of drugs can trigger autoimmune diseases in many ways similar to their idiopathic counterparts (Table 1). These serve as important models for the study of idiopathic disease. Apart from anaphylaxis, which is immediate, and rashes, which often occur early in treatment, most of these reactions develop gradually after an appreciable exposure to the drug (Perry 1973). Some reactions are rare, but others may affect over 10 per cent of patients with sufficient drug exposure. Factors influencing susceptibility include cumulative dose, renal and hepatic function, genetic polymorphisms influencing drug metabolism (particularly acetylation and sulphoxidation), sex, and immunological response (HLA-DR type and complement null alleles). Grounds for imputing an immunological mechanism include infiltration with lymphocytes (hepatitis, myositis) and the presence of autoantibodies (haemolytic anaemia, myasthenia gravis, lupus, Goodpasture's syndrome, pemphigus). The autoantibodies are usually similar to those arising in the relevant idiopathic autoimmune condition (Table 1), but generally occur much more frequently than any clinical expression of disease. Thus, hydralazine induces antinuclear antibodies in up to 60 per cent of patients but the lupus syndrome in only 2 to 10 per cent, and Coombs' antibody need not cause haemolysis.

Drug-induced lupus

Starting with observations by Perry in the 1950s on a late toxic reaction to hydralazine therapy (Perry 1973) and then similar observations with procainamide, many drugs have been reported to induce systemic lupus erythematosus or a lupus-like syndrome (Table 2). To implicate a drug with certainty the syndrome should remit after drug withdrawal and recur on rechallenge, but often there are just a few case reports and sometimes the connection is doubtful since idiopathic lupus may have been developing at the time. In particular, oestrogens and sulphonamides may exacerbate or bring on idiopathic systemic lupus erythematosus, and hair dyes containing aromatic amines have been implicated in a cluster of cases of systemic lupus erythematosus and scleroderma in a small town in Georgia (Freni-Titulaer et al. 1988). Minocycline, a semisynthetic tetracycline used for a variety of infections, and for treatment of acne vulgaris, has been reported to induce a lupus-like syndrome (Gough et al. 1996).

Clinical features

The clinical features of drug-induced lupus are shown in Table 3, with data on idiopathic systemic lupus erythematosus for comparison. Common, early manifestations (after several months of drug exposure) are arthralgia, aching, malaise, and elevated erythrocyte sedimentation rate. Arthritis, rash, lymphadenopathy, pleurisy and pleural effusion, pericardial effusion and hepatosplenomegaly occur less often, and Raynaud's phenomenon, central nervous system involvement, and renal disease are rare.

Drug-induced lupus is clearly distinguished from idiopathic systemic lupus erythematosus by the dearth of renal, central nervous system, and Raynaud's involvement, the lower frequency of rash, a narrower autoantibody profile, the rarity of hypocomplementaemia, and a different HLA background (Tables 3 and 4). However, these are not all necessarily fundamental differences, since drug-induced lupus is usually curtailed within the first couple of years of clinical expression by withdrawal of the drug or (if misdiagnosed) by treatment with corticosteroid. A few cases do go on to cutaneous vasculitis (Bernstein et al. 1980) and may progress to glomerulonephritis. After stopping the drug, clinical features generally improve within days or weeks and resolve within months of stopping the offending drug; the antinuclear antibody titre wanes over a year or two (Mansilla-Tinoco et al. 1982).

Table 1 Drug-induced autoimmune syndromes and autoantibodies

Syndrome	Autoantibody specificity
Lupus	Histones, Single-stranded DNA, Poly (ADP-ribose), Mitochondria (venocuran-Induced) Myeloperoxidase
Myositis	Nuclear
Myasthenia gravis	Acetylcholine receptor
Scleroderma	None recognized*
Haemolytic anaemia	I antigen of red cell
Thrombocytopenia	Platelet membrane
Pemphigus	Skin basement membrane
Goodpasture's syndrome	Kidney basement membrane

*Topoisomerase I in silica miners.

Table 2 Drugs reported to induce a lupus syndrome

Definite	Hydralazine Isoniazid Procainamide
Probable	Penicillamine Sulphasalazine Acebutalol Labetalol Methyldopa Captopril Phenytoin Carbamazepine Chlorpromazine Lithium Propylthiouracyl Quinidine Psoralen/ultraviolet A (PUVA) Venocuran Minocycline

For a more comprehensive list see Solinger (1988).

Table 3 Clinical and laboratory manifestations of idiopathic SLE and drug-induced lupus

Manifestations	Proportion positive (%)		
	SLE	Hydralazine lupus	Procainamide lupus
Arthralgia	90	90	90
Arthritis	90	50	18
Fever	84	50	45
Rash	72	25	5–18
Lymphadenopathy	59	14	0–9
Myalgia	48	2–34	20–50
Pleurisy	45		
Pleural effusion	33	25–30	33
Pulmonary infiltrate	8		30
Pericarditis	31	2	16
Hepatosplenomegaly	5–10	~10	20–33
CNS/seizures	16–25	0	1
Raynaud's phenomenon	23	rare	5
Joint deformities	10–26	0	0
Renal involvement	46	2–20	0–5
Anaemia (Hb < 11.5 g/dl)	57	30	9–21
Leucopenia ($<4 \times 10^9$/l)	43	26	2–32
LE cells	76	66	76
Antinuclear antibody	95	100	100
Rheumatoid factor	50	22	32–50
False positive test for syphilis	11	5–18	rare
Coombs' test	25	rare	33
Antinative DNA antibody	~60	rare	rare
Antipoly (ADP-ribose) antibody	~60	~100	not known
Antihistone antibody	~60	~100	~100

Adapted from a review of several series by Harmon and Portanova (1982).

Antibody profile

The antinuclear antibody profile in drug-induced lupus is much narrower than in idiopathic systemic lupus erythematosus. Antibodies to extractable nuclear antigens are rare, and to cardiolipin and native DNA uncommon. The characteristic antinuclear antibody is of homogenous pattern and high titre — the sort producing the LE cell phenomenon. The specificity of these antibodies is for histones and poly(ADP-ribose), sometimes for single-stranded DNA, but only rarely for native double-stranded DNA (Hobbs *et al.* 1987). Serial measurement of DNA binding may show a slight rise and then a fall on drug withdrawal but this usually remains within the normal range of DNA binding (which laboratories set quite high to exclude the modest levels of anti-DNA antibody seen in quite a wide range of autoimmune conditions). Antihistone antibody titres rise much higher in drug-induced lupus than in idiopathic systemic lupus erythematosus, whereas levels of antibody to poly(ADP-ribose) are similar. Antibodies to myeloperoxidase (anti-MPO), giving a pANCA pattern of immunofluorescence on alcohol-fixed neutrophils, have also been reported in drug-induced lupus (Nässberger *et al.* 1990). The presence of autoantibodies is not *per se* a reason to discontinue treatment.

Risk factors

Dose and metabolism

The risk factors for developing hydralazine induced lupus are fairly clear (Table 4). A modest dose must be taken for a year or two or a

Table 4 Risk factors for hydralazine lupus

	Hydralazine-treated controls	Hydralazine lupus	Odds ratio
Mean hydralazine intake	65 g	150 g	
Female	31%	81%	9.9
White	63%	96%	8.2
Slow acetylator	55	96	8.2
HLA-DR4	25%	73%	8.1
C4 null	43%*	76%	4.3

Based on Batchelor *et al.* (1980), Mansilla-Tinoco *et al.* (1982), and Spiers *et al.* (1989).
*Healthy controls not hydralazine treated.

large dose for several months, and almost always the patient is a 'slow acetylator'. Drug acetylation occurs immediately after absorption on first pass through the liver, and we know that administration of acetylprocainamide (itself an effective antiarrhythmic drug) never leads to the lupus syndrome even though a little of the dose is deacetylated (Woosley *et al.* 1978). The antinuclear antibody frequency rises faster in slow than fast acetylators. Indeed, it was thought for a time that acetylation of dietary toxins might be relevant to the genesis of idiopathic systemic lupus erythematosus but this is not the case.

Sex and race
As in idiopathic systemic lupus erythematosus, females are more at risk than men (though drugs like hydralazine and procainamide are used more often in men), but, in contrast to idiopathic systemic lupus erythematosus, Perry observed that black patients are highly resistant to the development of hydralazine lupus.

Major histocompatibility complex
Hydralazine lupus is associated with HLA-DR4 (Batchelor *et al.* 1980) and with null alleles of the complement component C4 (Speirs *et al.* 1989). HLA-DR4 and C4B null are known to be in linkage disequilibrium, just as in idiopathic systemic lupus erythematosus the HLA-DR2 and -DR3 associations may reflect the frequency of haplotypes containing C4A null alleles together with these DR antigens.

Pathogenesis

Complement dysfunction induced by drugs
Serum complement levels are usually normal in drug-induced lupus, but the drug may interfere with its function. In immune complex disease, complement is important in the solubilization of immune complexes and in their removal on the CR1 receptor of red cells (Schifferli *et al.* 1986). Indeed, many patients with idiopathic systemic lupus erythematosus have a null allele of C4 or occasionally C2, and homozygous deficiency of any of the early components of complement often leads to systemic lupus erythematosus. Reidenberg made the point that pharmacological rather than small immunizing doses are required for a drug to induce and maintain the lupus syndrome (Reidenberg 1981). One pharmacological mechanism demonstrated *in vitro* is that several lupus-inducing drugs block the transient activated form of C4. Inhibition of C4 activity is seen with hydralazine, isoniazid, penicillamine, and the hydroxylamine form of procaina-

mide but not acetylprocainamide (Sim *et al.* 1984). Despite these findings, hydralazine does not exacerbate idiopathic systemic lupus erythematosus *in vivo*, and it has to be determined whether inhibition of C4A or C4B is more important.

Modulation of lymphocyte function
Drugs inducing autoimmune disease may also have a pharmacological action on lymphocytes. T lymphocytes from patients treated with methyldopa show reduced suppression of lymphocyte responsiveness to phytohaemagglutinin and immunoglobulin synthesis. Conversely, procainamide may have an inhibitory effect on T-cell responses to mitogens. Lymphocytotoxic antibodies are frequently induced by procainamide and hydralazine therapy, but their functional significance is unclear since they kill best below body temperature and can be found whether or not the lupus syndrome has developed (Bluestein *et al.* 1979).

Induction of autoantibodies
Autoantibodies are necessary for the genesis of drug-induced lupus (though not sufficient, whatever the titre, class, or complement-fixing ability), and much thought has been given to how drugs might induce autoantibodies. The specificity of the response rules out a general polyclonal B-cell activation, nor can tissue damage be blamed since there is no inflammation when the antibodies first appear.

The favoured explanation (Table 5) is that the drug interacts directly with the autoantigen. Hydralazine and procainamide bind to chromatin, and this may alter the autoantigen so as to overcome T-cell tolerance and thereby release autoreactive B cells from suppression.

Table 5 Models for the induction of autoantibodies by drugs

1. Binding of drug to autoantigen, so overcoming T-cell tolerance

2. Antidrug antibody shows fortuitous cross-reaction with autoantigen.

3. Anti-idiotype to antidrug antibody mimics the drug and binds to its receptor (the autoantigen)

The autoantigen might be on the cell membrane or released from dead cells.

The fine specificity of autoantibodies in drug-induced lupus is in keeping with this model; histones and poly(ADP-ribose) are components of the nucleosome (unit of chromatin structure) and the histone epitopes recognized are those exposed on the surface of the nucleosome (Craft *et al.* 1987). This pattern of immune response can be imitated by immunization of rabbits with whole nucleosomes, whereas naked histones induce antibodies to epitopes that are normally buried.

Alternative models involve antidrug antibodies that are cross-reactive either directly (rheumatic fever model) or through an anti-idiotype response (Table 5). These options demand fortuitous cross-reaction with one epitope on the autoantigen, followed by a spreading induction of autoantibodies to other epitopes.

Drug-induced myositis

Toxic myopathies occur occasionally with various drugs including clofibrate, emetine, chloroquine, ε-aminocaproic acid, vincristine, lithium, amphotericin B, salbutamol, colchicine, and nitroxoline (Le Quintrec and Le Quintrec 1991). A true drug-induced myositis is seen occasionally with D-penicillamine and also reported with penicillin, sulphonamides, procainamide, hydralazine, phenytoin, propylthiouracil, phenylbutazone, cimetidine, and tamoxifen. In penicillamine therapy for rheumatoid arthritis, the frequency of myositis is 0.2 to 1.2 per cent rather than the expected coincidence of less than 0.001 per cent. Most cases of drug-induced myositis are antinuclear-antibody positive, and there seems to be a high frequency of dysphagia and muscle weakness but little myalgia. Myositis is mediated mainly by T cells, and in a case associated with cimetidine therapy there was a marked increase in the proportion of cytotoxic/suppressor T cells in the peripheral blood similar to the inflammatory infiltrate in muscle.

Drug-induced myasthenia gravis

Rheumatoid arthritis and idiopathic myasthenia gravis are weakly associated, but in 1975 Bucknall *et al.* described four cases of myasthenia gravis developing during penicillamine therapy and remitting after treatment was discontinued (Bucknall *et al.* 1975). This reaction may occur in up to 1 per cent of rheumatoid arthritis patients after several months of penicillamine therapy at daily doses of 500 mg or more. Antibodies to the acetylcholine receptor are found in all cases but their specificity is restricted to the human receptor. HLA typing shows more BW35 and DR1 and less B8 and DR3 than in idiopathic myasthenia gravis, and less DR4 than in rheumatoid arthritis controls (Dawkins *et al.* 1981).

Drug-induced scleroderma

Scleroderma-like disease with the typical microvascular and fibrotic changes can follow exposure to a variety of drugs and chemicals. The drugs include bleomycin, 5-hydroxytryptophan, carbidopa, pentazocine, penicillamine, phytonadione, diethyopropion, and mazindol (appetite suppressants), and intravenous cocaine abuse. In bleomycin-induced scleroderma, there is increased collagen synthesis by dermal fibroblasts *in vitro* and administration of bleomycin to rats produces skin thickening with increased collagen synthesis (Rush *et al.* 1984; Bourgeois and Aeschlimann 1991).

Chemicals inducing scleroderma-like disease

Just as there are chemical causes of cirrhosis and pulmonary fibrosis, there are chemicals other than drugs that induce a scleroderma-like disease. These include silicone implants, vinyl chloride, and the outbreak of 'Spanish oil disease'.

Silicone implants

Silicones are polymers mainly of dimethylsiloxane (chains of alternating silicon and oxygen atoms with two methyl groups attached to each Si atom). The silicone forms a liquid, gel, or rubber-like material (elastomer) depending on the number of cross-links between the polymer chains. Being fairly inert within the body, silicone is used to lubricate syringes and has been incorporated in intraocular lenses, ventriculoperitoneal shunts, and heart valves, as well as forming breast implants and artificial testicles.

Breast implants consists of silicone gel, and sometimes a space for saline, enclosed within a silicone rubber envelope. Implants are used chiefly for breast augmentation and reconstruction after surgery for breast cancer. In animals, injection of gel can induce local chronic inflammatory reactions and unsightly local reactions can occur in humans after direct injection of gel and occasionally after rupture of an implant. Augmentation of the breasts with silicone became popular from the 1960s but is now being squeezed out by the lawyers.

Miners exposed to inhalation of crystalline silica have an increased risk of scleroderma (Erasmus 1957), but the question of scleroderma and other chronic illness as a response to silicone polymers is now a contentious issue.

Anecdotal reports of rheumatic symptoms arising after silicone injection or implantation have been published since the 1960s (Kamugai *et al.* 1984) and in a welter since medicolegal interest arose (Sanchez-Guerrero *et al.* 1994). Most are vague complaints, to which the controversial term human adjuvant disease has been applied (because silicone is not itself immunogenic but appeared to have adjuvant activity). Only a minority of cases have involved a clear cut autoimmune rheumatic disease and these have been indistinguishable on clinical and serological grounds from idiopathic cases.

There is no good epidemiological evidence for an increased frequency of autoimmune rheumatic diseases in relation to silicone although the overall community prevalence of scleroderma may have increased in the past 50 years (Sanchez-Guerrero *et al.* 1994).

Despite the lack of scientific evidence, some patients may wish to have their implants removed for peace of mind. If the manufacturers survive bankruptcy, their settlement offer may reward those with common complaints like fatigue, widespread aching, paraesthesia, and the like. We must guard against this windfall making our patients feel worse.

Vinyl chloride disease

Workers exposed to vinyl chloride for prolonged periods in the manufacture of polyvinylchloride may develop an illness characterized by breathlessness, Raynaud's phenomenon, and contracture of the hands with thickening of the skin. Deposits of complement and fibrinogen are present in blood vessel walls (emphasizing that, like systemic sclerosis, this is a disease of the microvasculature as well as fibrosis), but anticentromere and anti-Scl-70 antibodies are not found. It is suggested that HLA-DR5 influences susceptibility and

DR3 influences the severity of vinyl chloride disease (Black *et al.* 1983).

Spanish oil disease (see also Chapter 5.8)

The sale of contaminated rape-seed oil as cooking oil to about 20 000 people in the Madrid area led to a 'toxic oil syndrome' with an initial acute phase of fever, rash, gastrointestinal upset, neurological disturbance, acute interstitial pneumonia, and sometimes death. Many recovered, but several hundred went on to develop hardened, thickened skin, Raynaud's phenomenon, dysphagia, pulmonary hypertension, alopecia, dry eyes, dry mouth, arthritis, and flexion contractures. Autoantibodies were not a feature, but there was microvascular damage with endothelial proliferation and infiltration of vessel walls by lymphocytes and macrophages (Spurzem and Lockey 1984).

Eosinophilia–myalgia syndrome (see also Chapter 5.9.1)

First reported to the Centers for Disease Control in November 1989, almost 1500 cases had been notified 4 months later and it was clear that the ingestion of tryptophan as a health-food supplement was responsible. The amino acid all came from one manufacturer and a contaminant in the manufacturing process has been implicated. Long-term follow-up is underway but new cases have ceased occurring. The syndrome is characterized by the abrupt onset of malaise, myalgia, weakness, contractures, induration of fascia, morphoea-like lesions, and blood eosinophilia ($1–30 \times 10^9/l$). Neuromyopathy is frequent and cardiac abnormalities have been seen, with some deaths. The histological findings resemble eosinophilic fasciitis with an interstitial and perivascular inflammatory infiltrate (Le Quintrec and Le Quintrec 1991).

Serum sickness and hypersensitivity vasculitis

Serum sickness is an immune-complex disease. First seen following the injection of antiserum for the treatment of bacterial infections such as diphtheria and tetanus, it now occurs rarely with some drugs, particularly penicillin, sulphonamides, penicillamine, and thiouracil. The first indication is usually fever, appearing 7 to 12 days after the beginning of treatment, followed by urticaria, joint pains, and occasionally glomerulonephritis or myocarditis (Rich 1942); this may progress to vasculitis.

Hypersensitivity or leucocytoclastic vasculitis is characterized by an infiltrate of dead or dying polymorphonuclear white cells in the walls of small blood vessels. There is often no obvious cause but in some cases drugs have been implicated, particularly sulphonamides, penicillin, thiouracil, iodides, organic arsenicals, oestrogens, and hydantoins (Dubost *et al.* 1991). For more on vasculitis see Chapters 5.11. 1 to 5.11.4.

Food and arthritis

Despite much folklore and several books, there is little convincing evidence that immune reactions to what we eat have any bearing on the pathogenesis of arthritis or the autoimmune rheumatic diseases (Walport *et al.* 1982). Anecdotal reports of food allergy have involved foods such as wheat, eggs, beef, and pork, and one diet recommends avoiding 'acidic' foods. Features often associated with arthritis in 'allergic' cases are migraine headaches, rhinitis, and gastrointestinal symptoms. After 50 years of open study, double-blind trials of diet are now in progress. It is possible that a diet of fish oil alters prostaglandin synthesis in a way that reduces the intensity of inflammation.

Specific syndromes occasionally associated with food allergy include palindromic rheumatism (reports of provocation by nitrates and menthol), vasculitis (various foodstuffs and in one case a particular brand of beer), hydrarthrosis of the knees (a case induced by English walnuts), and seronegative rheumatoid arthritis (a case exacerbated by milk and cheese). Most of these studies involved withdrawal of the foodstuff and rechallenge in open fashion.

Could rheumatoid arthritis be caused or exacerbated by absorption of antigens from the bowel? Pigs develop arthritis and nodules if fed a diet high in fish protein, and the onset of arthritis is associated with increased isolation of *Clostridium perfringens* from the gut flora. Arthritis is commoner in people with selective IgA deficiency, again highlighting mucosal defence. After intestinal bypass (once in favour as a treatment for morbid obesity) arthritis, often accompanied by features of Behçet's syndrome, may develop, and radiolabelled fragments of *E.coli* administered by mouth have been demonstrated in joints.

Metabolic reactions to drugs and toxins

Drugs and toxins causing gout

The relationship of alcohol to gout is complex in that many who drink well also eat well (with a high intake of purines), but it does seem that a high alcohol intake stimulates endogenous urate synthesis while high doses of alcohol temporarily reduce urate excretion (Scott 1991).

Lead rather than alcohol may have been responsible for the frequency of 'saturnine' gout in Georgian times when pewter was in fashion (lead-induced renal tubular damage leading to reduced excretion of uric acid). Nowadays, thiazide and loop diuretics are a common cause of hyperuricaemia, and gout is well recognized not just in bucolic men but in elderly women; the average increase in serum urate is about 70 μmol/l.

Salicylates have a uricosuric effect at higher doses but at low dose (with a low urine salicylate concentration) the excretion of uric acid is actually inhibited. Even the uricosuric agent probenecid has this paradoxical effect if given at a tiny dose. Among non-steroidal anti-inflammatory drugs, azapropazone has the most clinically useful uricosuric effect.

Hyperuricaemia, through an effect on the kidney, can also occur with pyrazinamide, ethambutol, and cyclosporin. Increased production of urate is caused by nicotinic acid and various cytotoxic agents, including vincristine, busulphan, thiotepa, cytarabine, 6-mercaptopurine, chlorambucil, cyclophosphamide, and the like. Increased tissue destruction leads to the release of purines and their metabolism to uric acid; this pathway can be blocked by the xanthine oxidase inhibitor allopurinol but with the warning that allopurinol increases the bioavailability of the azathioprine metabolite 6-mercoptopurine.

Fluoride and bone pain

In certain areas of India very high levels of fluoride in water lead to increased bone density and hyperostosis that goes on to cause widespread nerve root entrapment. Ingestion of moderate amounts of fluoride, as sometimes used in the treatment of osteoporosis, can cause severe pain in the legs, felt mainly around the joints. This lower limb pain occurs in up to 25 per cent of patients and remits when fluoride therapy is stopped or the dose reduced (Reeve 1990); microfractures may be the cause (Laroche and Mazieres 1991; Rooney et al. 1991).

Rheumatological effects of retinoids, quinolones, and proton pump inhibitors

Retinoids are derivatives of Vitamin A used in the treatment of severe acne. Chronic administration whether as a food fad or as dermatological treatment can cause arthralgias, arthritis, bone pain, hypercalcaemia, and periosteal new bone formation. Hyperostosis of the appendicular skeleton can occur, especially in children, and premature closure of the epiphyses has been reported (Kaplan and Haettich 1991).

Quinoline antibiotics include nalidixic acid and ciprofloxacin; very rarely these cause arthralgias and tenosynovitis in children, while puppies and the young of other susceptible species show surface blistering of the articular cartilage (Ribard and Kahn 1991).

Omeprazole and lansoprazole may cause arthralgias in occasional patients.

Transplant arthropathy

A painful, self-limiting, pseudoinflammatory arthropathy of lower limb joints can occur a few months after organ transplantation. There are clinical, radiological, and scintigraphic similarities to reflex sympathetic dystrophy. Knees or ankles are affected most often, but hip and wrist involvement has been seen. The clinical features are joint pain and tenderness and there may be effusion, periarticular oedema, and erythema. Blood tests for inflammation and autoantibodies are unhelpful; joint fluid cytology is non-inflammatory and does not reveal crystals. Radiographs show no specific abnormality, but isotope bone scans show greatly increased uptake on both sides of the joint (as well as in clinically unaffected joints sometimes). Avascular necrosis does not develop and spontaneous resolution after several months is the rule. This arthropathy has been recognized since the widespread adoption of cyclosporin for immunosuppression in organ transplantation. Cyclosporin levels have often been high when the arthropathy began and resolution tends to follow a reduction in cyclosporin levels. For instance, in our series of eight cases, mean cyclosporin levels were 458 mg/l at onset and 175 mg/l at resolution (Jones and Bernstein 1994).

Toxicity of antirheumatic treatment

Simple analgesics

Simple analgesics such as phenacetin, though probably not paracetamol, can cause renal papillary necrosis; this is commoner in hot climates where the urine is likely to be concentrated. Analgesics have a narrow safety range: eight tablets of paracetamol daily are safe, yet 30 tablets can ruin the liver.

Non-steroidal anti-inflammatory drugs

Gastrointestinal damage

Non-steroidal anti-inflammatory drugs commonly irritate the gastrointestinal tract (Henry et al. 1996), possibly through inhibition of prostaglandins which are important in protecting the mucosa and in the cellular mechanism for mending mucosal breaches. Endoscopy studies have shown up to 20 per cent of patients have ulcers and a further 30 per cent minor gastroduodenal lesions at any one time, and the risk of an acute bleed, perforation, or death rises from under 0.1 per cent in middle life to about 2.5 per cent in the elderly (Beardon et al. 1989). The synthetic prostaglandin E_1 misoprostol reduces non-steroidal anti-inflammatory-induced damage in the stomach, duodenum, and small intestine by about 75 per cent, whereas H_2-antagonists are protective only in the duodenum. Selective inhibitors of the inducible cyclooxygenase (COX-2) are likely to prove safer anti-inflammatory drugs.

Renal, haematological, and skin reactions

Non-steroidal anti-inflammatory drugs can reduce renal blood flow causing a tendency to hypertension and renal insufficiency (especially in the presence of hypovolaemia or pre-existing renal damage). Only sulindac is said to spare the kidneys. Other complications of non-steroidal anti-inflammatory drugs therapy include thrombocytopenia caused by increased platelet destruction, aplastic anaemia, and thrombocytopenia with phenylbutazone (now restricted in the United Kingdom to the hospital treatment of ankylosing spondylitis). Rashes are uncommon and occur most often with fenbufen.

Effects on cartilage

Shortly after the introduction of indomethacin there were reports of accelerated osteoarthritis of the hip, and in a clinical study of osteoarthritis of the hip, deterioration to the end-point of joint replacement was rather faster in patients treated with a strong inhibitor of prostaglandin synthesis (indomethacin) than with a weak inhibitor (azapropazone) (Rashad et al. 1989). Experimental data suggest various ways in which non-steroidal anti-inflammatory drugs might damage or even protect articular cartilage, and new chondroprotective agents are being sought by the pharmaceutical industry.

Disease-modifying, second-line therapy

Ocular toxicity from the deposition of antimalarial drugs such as chloroquine is well known. Rashes are common with most of the second-line drugs but with gold and penicillamine there is a particular risk of exfoliative dermatitis. Gold and penicillamine also cause membranous glomerulonephritis with nephrotic syndrome and, rarely, renal failure, while bone marrow toxicity with leucopenia, thrombocytopenia, or occasionally aplastic anaemia can occur with gold, penicillamine, sulphasalazine, and cytotoxic agents such as methotrexate, azathioprine, and cyclophosphamide; though onset can be abrupt, it is often gradual, so regular monitoring of the blood count and urine is recommended. Gold can also cause, rarely, pneumonitis and, not uncommonly, a 'post-injection flare' of arthritis (Rooney et al. 1991).

Penicillamine

Penicillamine used in the treatment of rheumatoid arthritis and Wilson's disease can trigger the whole range of drug-induced autoimmune reactions (membranous glomerulonephritis presenting as nephrotic syndrome, Goodpasture's syndrome, myasthenia gravis, polymyositis, pemphigus, lupus, and scleroderma), accompanied by the appropriate autoantibody (to kidney or skin basement membrane, acetylcholine receptor, double-stranded DNA, and so on).

Susceptibility to at least some of these reactions is increased by the HLA antigen DR3 and by slow sulphoxidation of penicillamine (Emery *et al.* 1984).

Corticosteroids

Corticosteroid therapy (Geusens and Dequeker 1991) reduces resistance to infection whether administration is systemic or intra-articular, and this must be borne in mind in all sick patients on steroids. A hot, red joint following a steroid injection may be infected or (more often, one hopes) a gout-like reaction to particles in the steroid preparation responsive to non-steroidal anti-inflammatory drug therapy. Repeated steroid injections can lead to avascular necrosis. In the shoulder there is the added risk of rotator cuff degeneration, so injections there should be limited to a few.

Osteonecrosis (avascular necrosis) is also a serious complication of systemic steroid therapy, affecting usually one or both hips but sometimes other joints such as knees and shoulders. It may occur in 5 per cent or more of patients on long-term steroid therapy, and there is a particular risk with high-dose intravenous steroids used in the treatment of transplant rejection and sometimes for connective tissue diseases.

Osteoporosis is a concern with systemic corticosteroid therapy. In younger women treated with prednisolone at doses of 5 to 7.5 mg/day there was no bone loss detectable by dual photon absorptiometry over a 1 year period, but exacerbation of bone loss after the menopause is more of a problem. Calcium supplements may help and female hormone replacement therapy or three monthly cycles of calcium for 11 weeks followed by a diphosphonate for 2 weeks encourages deposition of calcium on remaining bone trabeculas (Reeve 1990). More effective diphosphonates will be available shortly.

Monoclonal antibody and recombinant protein therapies

The next edition of this textbook will be full of optimism for the treatment of autoimmune diseases and arthritis by new methods. This paragraph is reserved for a host of adverse reactions — such as serum sickness (from mouse Fab), infection (as with steroids), enhanced autoimmunity (reported with interferons), and novel phenomena as yet undreamt of — that may arise from these new therapies, and also for debate with taxpayers who must pay for the therapies, as science brings home the bacon.

References

Batchelor, J.R., Welsh, K.I., Tinoco, R.M., Bernstein, R.M. *et al.* (1980). Hydralazine-induced systemic lupus erythematosus: the influence of HLA-DR and sex upon susceptibility. *Lancet*, i, 1107–9.

Beardon, P.H.G., Brown, S.V., and McDevitt, D.G. (1989). Gastrointestinal events in patients prescribed non-steroidal anti-inflammatory drugs: A controlled study using record linkage in Tayside. *Quarterly Journal of Medicine*, 71, 497–505.

Bernstein, R.M., Egerton-Vernon, J., and Webster, J. (1980). Hydralazine induced cutaneous vasculitis. *British Medical Journal*, 1, 156–7.

Black, C.M., Walker, A.E., Welsh, K.I., Bernstein, R.M., Catoggio, L.J. McGregor, A.R., and Lloyd-Jones, J.K. (1983). Genetic susceptibility to scleroderma-like disease induced by vinyl chloride. *Lancet*, i, 53–5.

Bluestein, H.G., Zvaifler, N.J., Weisman, M.H., and Shapiro, R.F. (1979). Lymphocyte alteration by procainamide: relation to drug-induced lupus erythematosus syndrome. *Lancet*, ii, 816–19.

Bourgeois, P. and Aeschlimann, A. (1991). Drug-induced scleroderma. *Clinical Rheumatology*, 5, 13–20.

Bucknall, R.C., Dixon, A.S.J., Glick, E.N., *et al.* (1975). Myasthenia gravis associated with penicillamine treatment for rheumatoid arthritis. *British Medical Journal*, 1, 600–2.

Craft, J.E., Radding, J.A., Harding, M.W., Bernstein, R.M., and Hardin, J.A. (1987). Autoantigenic histone epitopes: a comparison between procainamide- and hydralazine-induced lupus. *Arthritis and Rheumatism*, 30, 689–94.

Dawkins, R.L., Zilko, P.J., Carrano, J., *et al.* (1981). Immunobiology of D-penicillamine. *Journal of Rheumatology*, 7, 56–61.

Dubost J.-J., Souteyrand, P., and Sauvezie, B. (1991). Drug-induced vasculitides. *Clinical Rheumatology*, 5, 119–38.

Emery, P., Panayi, G.S., Huston, G., Welsh, K.I., Mitchell, S.C., Idle, J.K., Smith, R.L., and Waring, R.H. (1984). D-penicillamine toxicity in rheumatoid arthritis. The role of sulphoxidation status and HLA-DR3. *Journal of Rheumatology*, 11, 626–32.

Erasmus, L.D. (1957). Scleroderma in gold-miners on the Witwatersrand with particular reference to pulmonary manifestations. *South African Journal of Laboratory and Clinical Medicine*, 3, 209–31.

Freni-Titulaer, L.W.J., Kelley, D.B., Grow, A.C., Hochberg, M.C., and Arnett, F.C. (1988). Clustering of connective tissue diseases in a small Georgia community. III. A search for environmental factors. *Arthritis and Rheumatism*, 31, s75.

Geusens, P. and Dequeker, J. (1991). Locomotor side-effects of corticosteroids. *Clinical Rheumatology*, 5, 99–118.

Gough, A., Chapman, S., Wagstaff, K., Emery, P., and Elias, E. (1996). Minocycline induced autoimmune hepatitis and systemic lupus erythematosus-like syndrome. *British Medical Journal*, 312, 169–72.

Harmon, C.E. and Portanova, J.P. (1982). Drug-induced lupus. *Clinics in Rheumatic Disease*, 8, 121–35.

Henry, D., Lim, L.L-Y., Garcia Rodriguez, L.A., *et al.* (1996). Variability in risk of gastrointestinal complications with individual non-steroidal anti-inflammatory drugs: results of a collaborative meta-analysis. *British Medical Journal*, 312, 1563–6.

Hobbs, R.N., Clayton, A-L., and Bernstein, R.M. (1987). Antibodies to the five histones and poly(adenosine diphosphate-ribose) in drug induced lupus: implications for pathogenesis. *Annals of the Rheumatic Diseases*, 46, 408–16.

Jones, P.B.B. and Bernstein, R.M. (1994). Joint pain after organ transplantation. *Arthritis and Rheumatism*, 37, S273.

Kahn, M-F. (ed.) (1991). Drug-induced rheumatic diseases. *Clinical Rheumatology*, 5, 1–196.

Kamugai, Y., Shiokawa, Y., Medsger, T.A. Jnr., *et al.* (1984). Clinical spectrum of connective tissue disease after cosmetic surgery. Observations on eighteen cases and a review of the Japanese literature. *Seminars in Arthritis and Rheumatism*, 27, 1–12.

Kaplan, G. and Haettich, B. (1991). Rheumatological symptoms due to retinoids. *Clinical Rheumatology*, 5, 77–97.

Laroche, M. and Mazieres, B. (1991). Side effects of fluoride therapy. *Clinical Rheumatology*, 5, 61–76

Le Quintrec, J-S. and Le Quintrec, J-L. (1991). Drug-induced myopathies. *Clinical Rheumatology*, 5, 21–38.

Mansilla-Tinoco, R., Harland, S.J., Ryan, P.J., Bernstein, R.M., *et al.* (1982). Hydralazine, antinuclear antibodies and the lupus syndrome. *British Medical Journal*, 284, 936–9.

Nässberger, L., Sjöholm, A.G., Jonsson, H., Sturfelt, G., and Åkesson, A. (1990). Autoantibodies against neutrophil cytoplasm components in systemic lupus erythematosus and in hydralazine induced lupus. *Clinical and Experimental Immunology*, 81, 380–3.

Perry, H.M. (1973). Late toxicity to hydralazine resembling systemic lupus erythematosus or rheumatoid arthritis. *American Journal of Medicine*, 54, 58–72.

Rashad, S., Hemmingway, A., Rainsford, K., Revell, P., Low, F., and Walker, F. (1989). Effect of non-steroidal anti-inflammatory drugs on the course of osteoarthritis. *Lancet*, ii, 519–22.

Reeve, J. (1990). Restoring trabecular bone mass in established osteoporosis. In *Osteoporosis 1990*, (ed. R. Smith), pp. 143–55. RCP Publications, London.

Reidenberg, M.M. (1981). Clinical induction of SLE and lupus like illness. *Arthritis and Rheumatism*, 24, 1004–9.

Ribard, P. and Kahn, M-F. (1991). Rheumatological side-effects of quinolones. *Clinical Rheumatology*, **5**, 175–92.

Rich, A.R. (1942). The role of hypersensitivity in periarteritis nodosa: as indicated by seven cases developing during serum sickness and sulphonamide therapy. *Bulletin of the John Hopkins Hospital*, **71**, 123–40.

Rooney, P.J., Balint, G.P., Szebenyi, B., and Petrou, P. (1991). Rheumatic syndromes caused by antirheumatic drugs. *Clinical Rheumatology*, **5**, 139–73.

Rush, P.J., Bell, M.J., and Fam, A.G. (1984). Toxic oil syndrome (Spanish oil disease) and chemically induced scleroderma-like conditions. *Journal of Rheumatology*, **11**, 262–4.

Sanchez-Guerrero, J., Schur, P.H., Sergent, J.S., and Liang, M.H. (1994). Silicone breast implants and rheumatic disease: clinical, immunologic and epidemiologic studies. *Arthritis and Rheumatism*, **37**, 158–68.

Schifferli, J.A., Ng., Y.C., and Peters, D.K. (1986). The role of complement and its receptor in the elimination of immune complexes. *New England Journal of Medicine*, **315**, 488–95.

Scott, J.T. (1991). Drug-induced gout. *Clinical Rheumatology*, **5**, 39–60.

Shoenfeld and Isenberg, D. (1989). *The mosaic of autoimmunity*, pp. 321–43 and 397–400. Elsevier, Amsterdam.

Sim, E., Gill, E.W., and Sim, R.B. (1984). Drugs that induce systemic lupus erythematosus inhibit complement component C4. *Lancet*, **ii**, 422–4.

Solinger, A.M. (1988). Drug-related lupus. *Clinics in Rheumatic Disease*, **14**, 187–202.

Speirs, C., Fielder, A.H.L., Chapel, H., Davey, N.J., and Batchelor, J.R. (1989). Complement system protein C4 and susceptibility to hydrazaline-induced systemic lupus erythematosus. *Lancet*, **i**, 922–4.

Spurzem, J.R. and Lockey, J.E. (1984). Toxic oil syndrome. *Archives of Internal Medicine*, **144**, 249–50.

Walport, M.J., Parke, A.L., and Hughes, G.R.V. (1982). Food and the connective tissue diseases. *Clinics in Immunology and Allergy*, **2**, 113–20.

Woosley, R.L., Drayer, D.E., Reidenberg, M.M., Nies, A.S., Carr, K., and Oates, J.A. (1978). Effects of acetylator phenotype on the rate at which procainamide induces antinuclear antibodies and the lupus syndrome. *New England Journal of Medicine*, **298**, 1157–60.

6

Intervention, rehabilitation, and sports medicine

6.1   Surgery in adults

6.2   Surgery in children

6.3   Rehabilitation of adults

6.4   Rehabilitation of children

6.5   Corticosteroid injection therapy

6.6   Sports medicine

6.7   Sports injuries

6.1 Surgery in adults

Justin Cobb and C. B. D. Lavy

Introduction

The surgeon is an indispensable member of the team involved in the treatment of a patient with arthritis. He or she should be available not only as a technician to perform operations but ideally should also be involved in the decision-making processes in the management of the patient, such as the timing of surgery, the order in which affected joints should be treated, and of course the procedures undertaken. Most large units have combined clinics where the experience of rheumatologist, surgeon, physiotherapist, occupational therapist, and patient can be shared. In patients with polyarthritis, where several joints are likely to need surgery, a valuable relationship between patient and surgeon can be developed — a relationship which gives the patient trust and confidence and gives the surgeon a greater understanding of the patient's specific needs than can be gained by a single meeting.

This chapter will firstly list the options available to the surgeon dealing with rheumatic disease. Secondly, it will cover specific pre- and postoperative considerations that must be addressed by the surgeon. The third and largest part of the chapter will focus on specific anatomical regions in detail, outlining the procedures most commonly used. Operating theatre technique will not be covered. For this the reader is referred to specific operative texts, some of which are included in the references.

Surgical technique

The armamentarium of surgical treatment of arthritis includes the following procedures:

(1) arthroscopy and arthroscopic debridement;

(2) synovectomy;

(3) soft tissue release, realignment, or repair;

(4) tendon transfer;

(5) osteotomy;

(6) excision arthroplasty;

(7) prosthetic arthroplasty;

(8) arthrodesis and stabilization.

Not all the above are relevant in every anatomical region but they are listed here for completeness. The particular techniques that are

commonly used will be outlined under individual joints and regions below.

Special considerations in planning surgery in rheumatic diseases

When to operate

It is difficult to give specific guidelines as to when surgery should be considered for a particular joint, as no joint can be considered in isolation from other joints in the same limb or other limbs, or the patient's personal circumstances, including his or her position in the family and community. However, with all the above in mind, the two factors that most affect the decision to proceed with surgery are pain and loss of function. If the patient's pain cannot be adequately controlled by conservative means and their life, or more particularly their sleep, is being affected then surgery should be considered (Seyfer 1993). Similarly if the patient's function is being significantly impaired by joint destruction or deformity then surgery to reconstruct or replace the joint should be considered.

Prophylactic surgery has a limited place in the treatment of rheumatic diseases. Synovectomy is certainly of use in incipient tendon rupture. It has also been performed in an effort to prevent deterioration of inflammatory arthritis; however, no long-term study has shown significant slowing of joint destruction. Prophylactic surgery also has a role in stabilizing the potentially unstable spine.

Which joint to operate on first

The order of surgery in patients who have several joints that will benefit from surgery is a common problem in polyarthritic conditions such as rheumatoid arthritis. In deciding which joints to start with there are no hard and fast rules but there are several considerations that must be taken into account. Firstly, when surgery to upper and lower limbs is being considered the lower limb is usually done first as this restores important independent mobility. Rehabilitation following such surgery, however, often requires the use of crutches and if the arm function is so poor that even gutter crutches cannot be used, then surgery to the upper limb may have to precede that to the lower limb. Secondly, when two joints in a limb are equally affected it is usual to operate on the proximal joint before the distal joint. This helps to reduce pain and improve the proximal stability in the limb before surgery to the distal joint. Where two joints in a limb are both equally affected, for example the hip and the knee, it may be found that surgery to the hip so improves lower limb function that surgery to the knee is no longer needed. Similarly, surgery to the shoulder may dramatically reduce pain and functional demand on the elbow so that pain is improved and surgery to the elbow is not needed. In other patients the opposite may be found — surgery is so successful in relieving pain in the most painful joint that the patient's attention now turns to a less affected joint, one that previously had not troubled them much which now becomes the focus of their attention.

The final consideration in the order of surgery is the concept of surgical success. When a number of procedures are likely to be necessary it is often helpful to the patient's morale to start with a procedure that carries a high statistical likelihood of success. An example of this is excision of the distal ulna and synovectomy of the wrist.

Patient's consent and preparation

Patients must be adequately consented for surgery. This includes not only understanding the operation and its important complications but also the nature of the rehabilitation process involved which may be long. It is helpful if the physiotherapist and occupational therapist both meet the patient beforehand. It can also be of help for the patient to meet others who have had similar surgery.

Anaesthetic considerations

Patients with rheumatic diseases often have associated medical conditions that must be considered during surgery (Skues and Welchew 1993). For example, in rheumatoid arthritis cervical spine instability means that great care must be taken with endotrachial incubation and, if in doubt, fibreoptic intubation used. With some rheumatic diseases temporomandibular joint function is also limited and cricoarytenoid cartilages can be involved — both also causing airway difficulties. Patients with chronic inflammatory disorders are also often anaemic and some require preoperative transfusion. Pulmonary, cardiovascular, and renal complications in rheumatic diseases can also affect anaesthesia. These are discussed elsewhere.

Drugs affecting surgery

Patients who have been on steroids or antimetabolic drugs may have thin, delicate skin that tears or bruises easily. Great care must therefore be taken during surgery and in positioning and handling the anaesthetized patient. Skin may also be sensitive to the adhesive compound used in some dressings. Steroids and antimetabolic drugs may also reduce the patient's resistance to infection and also delay wound healing, although they are not in themselves contradictions to surgery. Specific medical complication to steroids and other disease-modifying agents will be considered elsewhere.

Positioning the patient

Often joint stiffness and restriction of movement will not allow normal positioning to be used. For example shoulder and elbow stiffness may not allow the hand to be flat on a table beside the patient. A degree of flexibility on the part of the surgeon is therefore needed. Great care must always be taken of the anaesthetized patient to ensure that joints are not over stressed. This is especially the case with rheumatoid arthritis where the soft tissues and bones are fragile. Care must also be taken at pressure points to avoid skin necrosis, bruising, and damage to peripheral nerves.

Surgical treatment in specific anatomical regions

Shoulder

The shoulder is commonly involved in inflammatory arthritis with clinical features of pain in 47 per cent (Laine *et al.* 1954). Petersson reports radiographic changes in the shoulders in 83 per cent of patients with rheumatoid arthritis (Petersson 1986). There is, however, little correlation between clinical signs and symptoms and radiographic appearance and it is not uncommon for a grossly destroyed shoulder joint to present with few symptoms.

The shoulder comprises four main anatomical areas; the sternoclavicular joint, the acromioclavicular joint, the subacromial region, and the glenohumeral joint. Pain arising from the sternoclavicular joint is usually easy to diagnose as it is localized to the sternoclavicular region. However, it is more difficult to be specific about the anatomical origin of pain and tenderness in the area around the shoulder itself. Physical signs can point to one of the three sites as the origin of the pain but most surgeons rely on the additional diagnostic information given by local anaesthetic tests. One per cent lignocaine is injected sequentially into the subacromial space, the acromioclavicular joint, the region of the biceps tendon, and the glenohumeral joint until the pain is abolished. Many patients will have some involvement at more than one, or indeed all, of these sites (Johnston and Kelly 1990).

Sternoclavicular joint

If conservative measures such as injection of steroids cannot control the pain arising from this joint then synovectomy can be considered or a limited excision of the medial end of the clavicle can be performed, keeping the excision medial to the costoclavicular ligaments. Care must be taken to avoid instability by preserving as much of the capsule as possible. The surgeon should also be cautious as the immediate posterior relation of the left joint is the innominate vein.

Acromioclavicular joint

This joint is involved in 70 per cent of rheumatoid shoulders. If pain becomes severe and cannot be controlled by conservative treatment or injection, the distal end can be excised lateral to the coracoclavicular ligaments which provide stability.

Subacromial region

Pain commonly arises from this region due to subacromial impingement which may be associated with inflammation in the subacromial bursa or a partial or complete rotator cuff tear. If pain from this area is abolished by local anaesthetic injection yet not controlled by steroid injection, then a subacromial decompression can be performed. This can be done as an open operation or, where the expertise exists, as an arthroscopic procedure using a powered burr. Rotator cuff repair is usually unrewarding in late rheumatoid arthritis because of the atrophied nature of the supraspinatus tendon.

Glenohumeral joint

This is involved in more than two-thirds of patients with rheumatoid arthritis (Ennevaara 1967). In early cases synovectomy can be performed either as an open procedure or arthroscopically (Bennett and Gerber 1994). Ogilvie-Harris, and Wiley had good results in nine out of eleven patients having this procedure arthroscopically

(Ogilvie-Harris and Wiley 1986). In moderate to severe bony destruction a double osteotomy, as described by Benjamin, can be performed (Benjamin *et al.* 1979). This comprises an osteotomy of the humerus at the surgical neck and a similar osteotomy of the scapula at the glenoid neck. The mechanism of action of this procedure is poorly understood but it has been shown to have good result in terms of pain relief and increased movement in 25 out of 29 patients in Benjamin's series and in 29 out of 32 patients in Jaffe and Learmonth's series (Benjamin 1987; Jaffe and Learmonth 1989).

Joint replacement

Arthroplasty of the shoulder has not been as successful as in the knee or the hip in terms of pain relief or restoration of range of movement. This has been due to poor bone stock in which to anchor prostheses and poor quality soft tissues, especially the rotator cuff. Despite these difficulties, shoulder replacement is a useful therapeutic tool in rheumatoid arthritis giving pain relief in over 90 per cent of patients (Friedman *et al.* 1989).

Early shoulder replacements were constrained, for example the Stanmore shoulder, which had a plastic glenoid cup holding a humeral head fully captive (Lettin *et al.* 1982), or the Kessel shoulder which had the ball joint the other way around (Kessel and Bayley 1988). More recent total shoulder replacements such as the Neer (Neer *et al.* 1982), the Global, or the Copeland have an anatomically shaped humeral head which can articulate with the patient's own glenoid if this is not severely damaged, or with a prosthetic glenoid which is usually cemented in place. The range of movement following total shoulder replacement depends largely on the state of the rotator cuff. Where the rotator cuff is intact the reconstruction of the anatomical contours of the shoulder joint following arthroplasty can give a very good range of movement with abduction to over 90°. In severe bony destruction, however, there is often virtually no rotator cuff remaining and range of movement is minimally increased by surgery. Indeed the main benefit of the procedure is pain relief.

Arthrodesis

The success of arthroplasty means that arthrodesis is hardly ever indicated in rheumatic diseases. Even in rare cases where because of infection total shoulder replacements need to be removed a stable fibrous pseudoarthrosis usually gives a better functional result than an arthrodesis.

Elbow

Extra-articular procedures commonly performed around the elbow in rheumatoid arthritis include removal of nodules and transposition of the ulnar nerve. Rheumatoid nodules are common around the elbow and they may become painful, unsightly, or ulcerated. Ulnar nerve dysfunction may be motor or sensory and can result both from mechanical and pressure factors due to the presence of swollen and inflamed synovium and a deforming joint. Ischaemic factors also have a role. Ulnar nerve function may be improved by a simple release or, if it is clearly tight, then transposition anterior to the medial epicondyle is recommended.

Synovectomy

Synovectomy of the elbow joint itself is difficult as surgical access to all parts of the intact joint requires several incisions; however, it gives some benefit at least in the short term when there is gross swelling.

Porter reported relief of pain and return of function in 12 out of 16 patients over a 5-year period (Porter *et al.* 1974). Arthroscopic synovectomy is a new tool that has to be performed with care as the radial and median nerves are closely related to the anterior capsule.

Excision of radial head

When the radial side of the joint is giving rise to the majority of symptoms, excision of the radial head can be performed at the same time as synovectomy (Copeland and Taylor 1979). This is an excellent procedure in terms of pain relief. Stability of the joint should be considered but is seldom significantly compromised in low demand patients. Silastic replacement of the radial head has not proved universally successful.

Arthroplasty

When there is severe pain in the presence of destructive changes in the elbow joint, both in rheumatoid arthritis and in osteoarthritis, arthroplasty can be performed. The simplest and oldest comprises excision arthroplasty which relieves pain but has unreliable stability. Inter position arthroplasty using silicon or metal had limited popularity (Coates *et al.* 1991) but most surgeons now use a form of total joint replacement. The available options are a simple hinge such as the Stanmore replacement, a semiconstrained hinge such as the GSB (Fig. 1), or a minimally constrained surface replacement such as the Souter (Souter 1990; Pritchard 1991). The increased stability of a hinge has been sited as increasing the risk of loosening by increasing forces at the prosthesis–bone interface. However, in up to 12-year follow-up GSB elbows continue to be considered excellent by 90 per cent of patients.

Wrist

Osteoarthritis

Osteoarthritis of the of the wrist is not common and is usually post-traumatic, following either fracture of the distal radius or carpal bones, especially the scaphoid. When pain cannot be controlled, conservatively surgery should be considered. Joint replacement, as described below for rheumatoid arthritis, is an option in very low demand patients. Excision of the proximal carpal row can be performed where the disease is confined to this region. The space previously occupied by the excised proximal row becomes a pseudoarthrosis, relieving pain at the expense of some stability. Limited carpal fusions can also be performed particularly when the osteoarthritis is confined to the radial side of the wrist. This procedure does not have a high rate of success but if pain persists or recurs it can be revised to a complete wrist fusion.

Rheumatoid arthritis

Rheumatoid arthritis can affect the wrist joint as well as the flexor and extensor tendons and surgery to the tendons, such as synovectomy or transfer of the extensor tendons, is often combined with surgery to the wrist; however, in this text we will consider them separately. Rheumatoid arthritis can affect the radioulnar as well as the radiocarpal joints and often it is this joint that gives much of the pain, both from instability and from impingement on the carpus. Treatment by excision of distal 10 to 15 mm of the ulnar is very effective in terms of relief of pain and also removes an unsightly lump (Posner and Ambrose 1991; Clawson *et al.* 1991). When the pain is also arising from the radiocarpal joint, the surgical options are

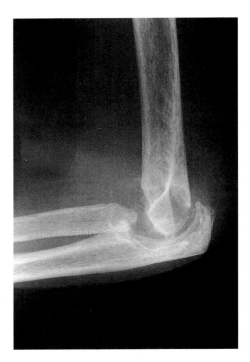

(a)

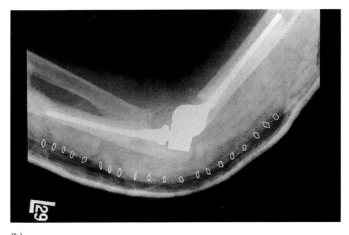

(b)

Fig. 1 Rheumatoid elbow (a) pre- and (b) postarthroplasty using a GSB semiconstrained hinge prosthesis.

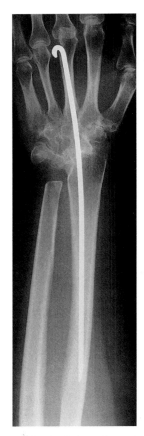

Fig. 2 Rheumatoid wrist following fusion using an intramedullary Rush pin.

fusion or arthroplasty. Limited wrist fusion such as the Chamay technique (Chamay *et al.* 1983), which uses graft from the distal ulnar to fuse the radius to the lunate, are of use when there is good bone stock remaining but in most late cases there is such distortion of the normal anatomy that complete arthrodesis is performed.

The commonest method used involves insertion of a Rush pin (Fig. 2) or a Steinmann pin down the third metacarpal and across the wrist. This can be supplemented with a staple to improve stability. The position of stabilization is slight radial deviation and dorsiflexion. However, if both wrists are to be fused then perineal toilet is often improved if one is fused in slight flexion.

Joint replacement

The Swanson design silastic prosthesis is the most popular form of arthroplasty in Britain. The proximal carpal row is excised and the prosthesis fills the gap with one stem that fits into the distal radius and one that fits into a hole made through the capitate into the third metacarpal. Metal grommets can be used to protect the prosthesis from the sharp edges of the bone. This procedure gives good results in terms of relief of pain in low demand patients (Jolly 1993) but range of movement is usually limited to an arc of 40 to 50°. There are other designs of wrist replacement, such as the Meuli ball and socket joint which is popular in continental Europe. Where both wrists are involved in rheumatoid arthritis, many surgeons fuse the dominant wrist which is likely to take more force and confine arthroplasty to the non-dominant side.

Surgery to extensor tendons

In early disease, synovectomy of the extensor tendons is often combined with surgery to the wrist. The tendons are exposed by reflecting a flap of the dorsal extensor retinaculum, then after synovectomy the flap is replaced deep to the extensor tendons thus protecting them from the wrist joint. Synovectomy relieves pain and swelling and also reduces the risk of rupture.

The most common tendons to be ruptured are the extensor pollicis longus and the extensor digiti minima. The former is commonly treated by transfer of the extensor indicis proprius tendon from the index finger, which conveniently has two extensor tendons, and the remaining extensor indicis communes is adequate to extend the index. Treatment of rupture of extensor digiti minimi is usually by joining the distal end of the tendon to the extensor tendon of the ring finger. Realignment of the extensor tendons can be performed

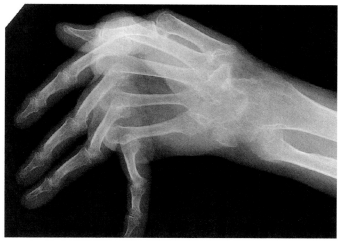

(a)

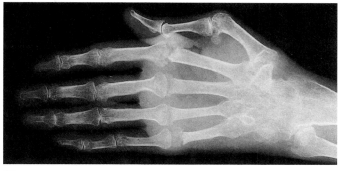

(b)

Fig. 3 Rheumatoid hand (a) before and (b) after silastic metacarpophalangeal joint replacements.

in rheumatoid arthritis. This commonly occurs at the level of the metacarpophalangeal joints where all the tendons tend to shift in an ulnar direction but also at the wrist where the extensor carpi ulnaris can migrate in a volar direction around the ulnar head.

Surgery to the flexor tendons

Synovitis also occurs around the flexor tendon in the synovial sheaths at the wrist and the fingers. When this interferes with function because of pain or by restricting flexion, synovectomy can be performed to improve movement and reduce the risk of rupture. In late cases rupture can occur. Surgical treatment of such rupture is complex and involves tendon grafting, often with a staged procedure. In mild cases of synovitis, triggering can occur around the neck of the flexor sheath. This is treated by simple division of the tight neck of the sheath. A limited synovectomy can also be performed.

Carpal tunnel syndrome

Median nerve compression is common in rheumatoid arthritis and can be relieved by carpal tunnel release. This is easily performed as a day case procedure under local anaesthetic. Endoscopic carpal tunnel release is popular in Europe and in the United States but because of early reports of nerve injury it has had a cautious reception so far in the United Kingdom.

Hand

Surgery to the fingers in rheumatoid arthritis

Boutonniere or Swan neck deformity can be corrected surgically by soft tissue procedures provided the joints are passively mobile. Once fixed deformity of the proximal interphalangeal (PIP) joints occurs, correction is much harder and surgical improvement may only be achieved by fusion in a position of function or arthroplasty using a silastic replacement joint. The position of fusion is usually 45 to 90° of flexion but depends on the range of movement at the metacarpophalangeal joints.

Surgery to the thumb in rheumatoid arthritis

Rheumatoid arthritis commonly causes a Z-deformity of the thumb and can cause instability of either the metacarpophalangeal or interphalangeal joint. Such instabilities are seldom helped by soft tissue procedures and a fusion is usually necessary (Toledano et al. 1992).

Surgery to the metacarpophalangeal joints

When rheumatoid arthritis involves the metacarpophalangeal joint there is often a tendency to subluxation of these joints in an ulnar and volar direction. In early cases this can be treated with synovectomy and soft tissue realignment (Wynn Parry and Stanley 1993). This does slightly decrease the range of movement but improves function because of decreased pain and increased power. In late cases where there is bony destruction of the metacarpal head, metacarpophalangeal joint replacement using Swanson silastic prostheses may be necessary (Fig. 3). This is always performed in conjunction with soft tissue release and realignment. Such reconstructive surgery, however, should only be done in order to improve function in the hand and should not be performed purely to improve the cosmetic appearance of a deformed rheumatoid hand. The postoperative care of metacarpophalangeal joint replacement and soft tissue realignment is extensive and involves the close co-operation of a hand therapist with experience in splinting as well as physical exercise techniques (Stanley 1992).

Cervical spine

Rheumatoid arthritis can affect all the synovial joints in the cervical spine including the bursa between the odontoid process and the transverse ligament. This can result not only in destruction of joints but also in attenuation of ligaments and consequent instability of the cervical spine (Heywood et al. 1988). The commonest site for involvement in the cervical spine are:

(1) atlantoaxial subluxation or anterior subluxation of C1 on C2;

(2) atlantoccipital impaction, also known as cranial settling;

(3) subluxation of the cervical vertebras below C2.

Surgery is not indicated in all cases of cervical instability but it is very important that instability is fully investigated with flexion and extension radiographs, a full neurological examination, and, where there are any neurological signs, a magnetic resonance imaging scan. Neurological impairment can be caused not only by the mechanical effect of the instability but also by pressure from proliferation of soft tissues.

The nature of surgery indicated depends on the pathology demonstrated. If there is progressive instability then prophylactic stabilization can be performed to prevent later deterioration. There are several methods of stabilization of the cervical spine including bone grafting and fixation with plates or preformed wire rectangles or loops (Ranawat *et al.* 1979; Ransford *et al.* 1986). Stabilization is also indicated when there is intermittent or persistent neurological deficit. In these cases it may also be necessary to decompress the spinal cord or nerve roots (Johnston and Kelly 1990).

Foot and ankle

In the foot, as in other areas, meticulous attention to the history and clinical signs is essential. Pain may arise from impingement or entrapment of tendons or nerves, or from joints that are unstable not just destroyed. The judicious use of soft tissue procedures, selective arthrodeses, and joint arthroplasty may maintain fore- and hindfoot function for some years. When destruction and deformity have progressed, it is still usually possible to salvage a painless, albeit flat, foot by forefoot arthroplasty and triple arthrodesis of the hindfoot.

Synovectomy and soft tissue procedures

While little is published regarding synovectomy alone in the foot, there is some evidence that early synovectomy may delay deterioration in the ankle as in other joints (Hecker *et al.* 1982; Kvien *et al.* 1987; Mohing *et al.* 1982). Pain around the lateral malleolus in the valgus hindfoot may be due to impingement of the lateral malleolus, or to peroneal tendon entrapment. Injection of the tendon sheath is a simple diagnostic and therapeutic procedure that may give relief for some years. A conservative approach to the foot and ankle may also include early decompression of the tibialis posterior tendon and other medial structures to prevent rupture and subsequent deformity (Cracchiolo 1984).

Excision arthroplasty

Damage to the foot, and especially the forefoot, occurs very early in rheumatoid arthritis. A painful and deformed forefoot with hallux valgus, dorsal dislocation of the lesser metatarsophalangeal joints together with significant synovitis is the rule. The buttonholing of the metatarsal heads through the plantar fascia makes walking exquisitely painful. The surgical goal is a foot that is comfortable for slow pedestrian life, as part of the management of a systemic condition. Forefoot arthroplasty is the procedure of choice: the metatarsal heads are resected, allowing the hammering toes to drop down into the plane of the foot. The hallux valgus may be corrected by excising the metatarsal head or the base of the proximal phalanx (Fowler 1959; Gainor *et al.* 1988; Kates *et al.* 1967).

Arthrodesis

Isolated painful destruction of the ankle joint in rheumatoid arthritis is best treated by arthrodesis (Fig. 4). Several methods of internal fixation are available (Dent *et al.* 1993; Holt *et al.* 1991; Iwata *et al.* 1980; Moran *et al.* 1991). These have a lower complication rate and are better tolerated than the traditional method using Charnley external fixation clamps which have a significant infection rate (Moeckel *et al.* 1991).

More commonly the significant valgus deformity of the hindfoot is accompanied by pantalar arthritis. In these circumstances triple or pantalar arthrodesis is the treatment of choice (Vahvanen 1967). In the badly damaged hindfoot, a nail may be inserted from the

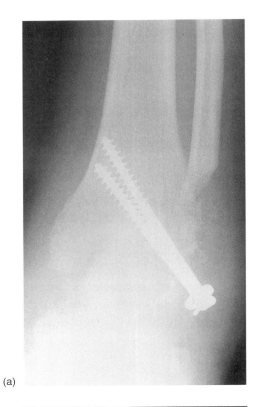

(a)

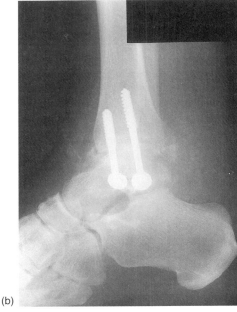

(b)

Fig. 4 Anteroposterior (a) and lateral (b) radiographs showing an ankle joint arthrodesed using parallel screws. The subtalar joint is normal.

sole up into the tibia, with or without the use of bone graft. A painless ankylosis can usually be obtained (Stone and Helal 1991). Talonavicular joint destruction with valgus deformity should also be corrected early and before the forefoot, if symptomatic: it may reduce symptoms in the foot by reducing the valgus shearing forces (Cracchiolo 1984).

Joint replacement

While ankle joint replacement is technically possible, the clinical results are disappointing compared to fusion (Jensen and Kroner 1992; Stauffer 1977; Wagner 1982). It may offer some early advantage in elderly patients with low physical demands, but these benefits are outweighed by the complication rate and difficulty in salvage (McGuire *et al.* 1988).

Prosthetic replacement of the first metatarsophalangeal joint has its advocates but the long-term results are not good enough to justify the additional complications (Hasselo *et al.* 1987).

Knee

Synovectomy

Arthroscopic synovectomy can effectively abolish the pain and stiffness in knees with a florid synovitis that is refractory to conservative measures (Ogilvie-Harris and Basinski 1991). It has considerable advantages over open synovectomy, in terms of hospital stay and morbidity, while the results of the two methods appear comparable with both groups regaining an average of 75° of movement (Matsui *et al.* 1989). This improvement is maintained for about 5 years although in that time the radiographic appearances continue to deteriorate (Paus and Dale 1993), but even at 14 years 67 per cent have remained in remission from the inflammatory element of their condition (Ishikawa *et al.* 1986). Simpler arthroscopic lavage and debridement may provide temporary relief but nothing more than this.

Joint replacement

The stiff and painful knees of the inflammatory arthropathies are best treated by total knee replacement. Double osteotomies were used in the past with varying effects, but excision of the entire articular surface and a thorough synovectomy is possible during total knee replacement reducing the rate of reactivation following the operation (Low *et al.* 1994). There is a considerable biological advantage to this removal of all antigenic stimulation as well as the great advantage of excellent mechanical function.

Prosthetic design

The current designs allow only the joint to be resurfaced with a minimum of bone resected. The great advantage this has over the hinge replacements, such as the Stanmore, is that of bone stock preservation. By resecting as little bone as possible, the prosthesis loads the juxta-articular cancellous bone, preventing stress shielding and subsequent bone loss. Ligaments may be spared if present. In rheumatoid arthritis where they are invariably absent, their absence may be accommodated by constraining the knee with a moulded polyethylene insert (Fig. 5). This will give the stability needed for a normal gait without the problems of loosening, fracture, and massive loss of bone stock encountered by the hinge knees of the 1970s and 1980s.

The present condylar type knee replacements have had significant problems with excessive wear of the tibial and patellar insert followed by secondary loosening. Many prostheses have been withdrawn from use following relatively unsuccessful trials (Kim and Oh 1995) and their failure rates vary considerably (Knutson *et al.* 1994).

Cemented or uncemented

There is little to choose between cemented and uncemented in total knee replacement at present although loosening seems slightly less in the tibial component if cemented (Knutson *et al.* 1994).

Outcome studies

Total knee replacement has evolved over the last three decades into a procedure that rivals total hip replacement for reliability and safety. In the Swedish knee arthroplasty register, which holds the records of over 30 000 knee replacements since 1976, the revision rate at 5 years has fallen from 10 per cent to 3 per cent (Knutson *et al.* 1994). Despite the softened bone and often deformed joints, the success rate in rheumatoid arthritis is just as gratifying as in osteoarthritis, with no significant difference in outcome (Briggs and Augenstein 1995; Hsu *et al.* 1995).

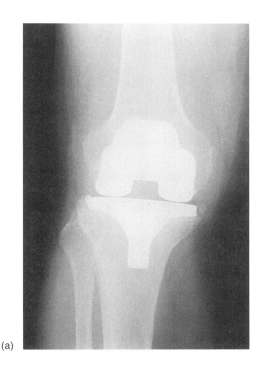

(a)

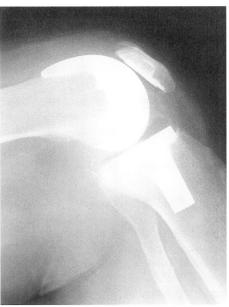

(b)

Fig. 5 Anteroposterior (a) and lateral (b) radiographs showing a cemented total condylar knee replacement. The patella has been resurfaced.

Complications

Aseptic loosening

This remains the principle problem in the long term. Poor surgical technique resulting in malalignment of the prosthesis is a significant cause of early loosening (Harvey *et al.* 1995).

Other knees loosen after excessive wear of the tibial insert. This leads to eccentric movement and abnormal loading. Early designs of replacement prevented normal joint motion and the constraints themselves caused the abnormal loads and early failure (Rickhuss *et al.* 1994). All knee replacements now allow some rotation as well as unlimited flexion, and this freedom from constraints has been a major factor in preventing early failure. The results of revision knee replacements were very disappointing when the initial prosthesis was a hinge type joint. The huge loss of bone stock led to rapid loosening once again, and many patients in the end faced excision arthroplasty or amputation (Ahlberg and Lunden 1981). Today, the more conservative joint resurfacing procedures have a lower revision rate and last longer so while the annual revision rate is still rising, the percentage of operations that are revisions has actually fallen over the last decade.

Arthrodesis

Joint replacement has a good track record now and the operation of knee fusion is only indicated as a salvage procedure in osteoarthritis affecting few joints. If properly performed, the mechanical function of the individual can be excellent (Behr *et al.* 1985; Figgie *et al.* 1987). If many joints are affected, the impact of knee fusion is so mechanically serious that this should not be considered.

Excision arthroplasty

Failed revision arthroplasty may occasionally result in a flail leg without a functioning joint but with so little bone stock that an arthrodesis would be difficult or impossible. This is a procedure for a very low level of activity and only really appropriate if many other joints are involved and repeated infection or poor soft tissue cover cause revision surgery to fail (Adam *et al.* 1994).

Hip

When the hip has been damaged by an inflammatory arthropathy, the principal surgical intervention is joint replacement. Arthroscopy and arthroscopically assisted synovectomy are technically difficult and of limited benefit. Corrective osteotomies around the hip are rarely appropriate, as the primary pathology is not mechanical. The possible beneficial effects of osteotomy in inflammatory arthropathy, which are poorly understood and inconsistent, been superseded by the more reliable effects of joint replacement.

Synovectomy

Synovitis in the hip although present in up to 40 per cent of patients as shown on ultrasound, does not correlate well with clinical findings. Many of the joint with florid synovitis on ultrasound will have few hip symptoms while other symptomatic hips have little synovial thickening (Eberhardt *et al.* 1995). The hip itself is not simply accessible for open surgery and carries with it a high risk of avascular necrosis of the femoral head. Open synovectomy requiring hip dislocation has been reported in younger patients with some success (Albright *et al.* 1975) but is not common practice. Arthroscopically assisted synovectomy has also been reported (Gondolph-Zink *et al.* 1988) but this is a difficult procedure with limited application.

Joint replacement

Total hip replacement has specific problems related to each of the inflammatory arthropathies, and their biological manifestations. Ankylosing spondylitis causes progressive ankylosis that may continue after the operation, while rheumatoid arthritis sufferers will usually have very poor bone stock and may have eroded the acetabulum. While these specific problems may make the technical aspects of the replacement demanding, the procedure is as successful for patients with rheumatoid arthritis as those with osteoarthritis. Despite being a major operation, involving pain and 10 days in hospital, joint replacement remains the most important intervention in a rheumatoid patient's disease process and, by their perception, well ahead of methotrexate and early aggressive management (Fries 1988).

Prosthetic design

Numerous designs of prosthesis exist, with little to recommend one over another. None has performed as well as John Charnley's original design (Wroblewski 1986) but several others have a proven record such as the Exeter (Fowler *et al.* 1988).

Cemented or uncemented?

Aseptic loosening remains the major cause of failure in total hip replacement. Improvements in cementing technique have reduced the rate at which early signs of loosening now appear, but the erosion of bone by the loosening process remains a concern. Various surface treatments have been used to attempt to stabilize the prosthesis-bone interface without the use of polymethylmethacrylate. Extensive use of porous surfaces coating the prostheses have failed to demonstrate any advantage over cement in terms of overall survival and symptom control. There may, however, be some improvement in bone stock, with less loss of bone mass owing to stress shielding. Hydroxyapatite coating has been available for 8 years and seems very promising (Fig. 6). There may be a significant improvement in bone mass in the uncemented hydroxyapatite-coated group, making the revision a more successful operation, but this is not yet proven. The uses of a cemented stem and an uncemented cup, a 'hybrid' hip replacement, is another acceptable compromise.

Biomaterials

Polyethylene wear particles from the artificial joint have been implicated in the loosening process. Small particles excite an inflammatory reaction causing erosion of bone, visible on radiographs as radiolucent lines. Improvements in the density of the polyethylene and the smoothness of the cobalt-chrome alloy femoral head have reduced this. Ceramic bearings have theoretically superior wear characteristics and should further reduce the volume of particulate debris. Long-term clinical results are not available.

Outcome

Rheumatoid arthritis sufferers consider joint replacement to be the most successful and significant intervention in their disease, being rated above any of the pharmacological therapies. Total hip replacements is certainly reliable and durable; 96 per cent of Charnley cemented total hip replacements were reported as being good to excellent at 15 to 21 years (Wroblewski 1986) in Charnley's own unit, while at the Mayo clinic 79 per cent were good or excellent at 15 years (Kavanagh *et al.* 1989). The Exeter hip has also a good record with 5.5 per cent needing revision at 13.5 years (Fowler *et al.* 1988).

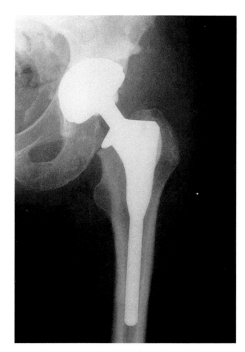

Fig. 6 A hip 1 year after hydroxyapatite-coated, uncemented total hip replacement. Radiolucent lines are visible indicating solid fixation.

In rheumatoid arthritis the reduction in bone density seems to be offset by the low level of exercise and most authors find the outlook worse for those patients with rheumatoid arthritis. One single-arm study showed a 91 per cent chance of the hip still functioning well at 11 years in rheumatoid arthritis (Severt *et al*. 1991).

Complications of total hip replacement

Infection

The systemic administration of prophylactic antibiotics, together with ultra-clean air theatres have made the infection rate in primary hip replacement very low with figures of less than 1 per cent. However, in rheumatoid arthritis the rate is higher, at around 3 per cent (Severt *et al*. 1991), owing to immunocompromise and poor skin healing. The infected total hip replacement can often be salvaged by extensive debridement, and one or two stage revision followed by long-term antibiotics. In the long term however, repeated infection will lead to an excision arthroplasty.

Aseptic loosening

Hips may loosen for a number of reasons:

(1) excessive wear leading to eccentric motion of the head and thus high peakloads;

(2) stress shielding of the bone leading to resorption of the proximal bone and loss of bone stiffness;

(3) faulty technique;

(4) aggressive granulomatous reaction.

If the interface between the implant and bone is not solid, progressive motion will cause slow resorption of bone and an increasing zone of soft tissue between the implant and the bone. The painful total hip replacement should be revised early rather than left for as long as possible, as the enlarging radiolucent line around a prosthesis on radiographs represents resorption of bone and thus progressive weakening of the remaining bone stock. The results of revision surgery are fair: most people are helped considerably but the life expectancy of the revised hip is less than for the primary total hip replacement. A 10 per cent failure rate at 5 years would be average (Lord *et al*. 1988).

For this reason, cementless revisions with porous ingrowth or hydroxyapatite coating is being tried in many centres. Bone graft may be needed, either in the shape of cancellous chips from the pelvis or allograft from femoral heads harvested during primary total hip replacements. These are used to augment the failing bone stock of either proximal femur or acetabulum. Inevitably, if the process of joint replacement is started young, and the patient has an oligo-arthropathy, with a relatively active lifestyle, then repeated revisions will culminate in excision arthroplasty. Without a hip joint an otherwise fit person will walk with two sticks, but a typical polyarthritic rheumatoid arthritis sufferer will become comfortable but wheelchair bound.

Arthrodesis

Arthrodesis of the hip is the operation of choice in active young people with a single very painful and stiff joint. It will give good service for 20 years and may be revised safely. It does not have a role in polyarticular disease, where the change in biomechanics increases the stress to the knee joint unacceptably.

Excision arthroplasty

Excision arthroplasty of the hip is not necessary in uncomplicated inflammatory arthropathy. While it will give considerable relief of pain and will not deteriorate, it is only indicated where infection or very poor bone stock make further reconstructive attempts unwise. While the range of motion is excellent, the power is minimal and walking without two sticks is difficult, even for an otherwise fit young person with no other mechanical disability.

References

Adam, R.F., Watson, S.B., Jarratt, J.W., Noble, J., and Watson, J.S. (1994). Outcome after flap cover for exposed total knee arthroplasties. A report of 25 cases. *Journal of Bone and Joint Surgery*, **76**, 750–3.

Ahlberg, A. and Lunden, A. (1981). Secondary operations after knee joint replacement. *Clinical Orthopaedics and Related Research*, **156**, 170–4.

Albright, J.A., Albright, J.P., and Ogden, J.A. (1975). Synovectomy of the hip in juvenile rheumatoid arthritis. *Clinical Orthopaedics and Related Research*, **77**, 48–55.

Behr, J.T., Chmell, S.J., and Schwartz, C.M. (1985). Knee arthrodesis for failed total knee arthroplasty. *Archives of Surgery*, **120**, 350–4.

Benjamin, A. (1987). Double osteotomy of the shoulder. *Scandinavian Journal of Rheumatology*, **3**, 65.

Benjamin, A., Hirschowitz, D., and Arden, G.P. (1979). The treatment of arthritis of the shoulder. *International Orthopaedics*, **3**, 211–16.

Bennett, W.F. and Gerber, C. (1994). Operative treatment of the rheumatoid shoulder. *Current Opinion in Rheumatology*, **6**, 177–82.

Briggs, J.R. and Augenstein, J.S. (1995). Tricon hybrid total knee arthroplasty: a review of 81 knees followed for 2 to 4 years. *Orthopedics*, **18**, 341–6.

Chamay, A., Delia Santa, D., and Vilaseca, A. (1983). Radiolunate arthrodesis; a factor of stability for the rheumatoid wrist. *Annales de Chirurgie de la Main*, **2**, 5–17.

Clawson, M.C. and Stern, P.J. (1991). The distal radioulnar joint complex in rheumatoid arthritis: an interview. *Hand Clinics*, **7**, 373–81.

Coates, C.J., Bolton-Maggs, B.G., and Helal, B.H. (1991). Interpositional arthroplasty in the management of rheumatoid arthritis of the elbow. In *Rheumatoid arthritis surgery of the elbow* (ed. M. Hamalainen and F.W. Hagewa), pp. 52–9. Karger, Basel.

Copeland, S.A. and Taylor, J.G. (1979).Synovectomy of the elbow in rheumatoid arthritis. The place of excision of the head of the radius. *Journal of Bone and Joint Surgery*, **61B**, 69–73.

Cracchiolo, A.D. (1984). Foot abnormalities in rheumatoid arthritis. *Academy of Orthopaedic Surgeons Instructional Course Lecture*, 33, 386–404.

Dent, C.M., Patil, M., and Fairclough, J.A. (1993). Arthroscopic ankle arthrodesis. *Journal of Bone and Joint Surgery*, 75, 830–2.

Eberhardt, K., Fex, E., Johnsson, K., and Geborek, P. (1995). Hip involvement in early rheumatoid arthritis. *Annals of the Rheumatic Diseases*, 54, 45–8.

Ennevaara, K. (1967). Painful shoulder joint in rheumatoid. *Acta Rheumatologica Scandinavica*, 11, 1–116.

Figgie, H.E.D., Brody, G.A., Inglis, A.E., Sculco, T.P., Goldberg, V.M., and Figgie, M.P. (1987). Knee arthrodesis following total knee arthroplasty in rheumatoid arthritis. *Clinical Orthopaedics and Related Research*, 224, 237–43.

Fowler, A.W. (1959). A method of forefoot reconstruction. *Journal of Bone and Joint Surgery*, 41B, 507–13.

Fowler, J.L., Gie, G.A., Lee, A.J., *et al.* (1988). Experience with the Exeter total hip replacement since 1970. *Orthopedic Clinics of North America*, 19, 477–89.

Friedman, R.J., Thornhill, T.S., Thomas, W.H., and Sledge, C.B. (1989). Non-constrained total shoulder replacement in patients who have rheumatoid arthritis and class 4 function. *Journal of Bone and Joint Surgery*, 71A, 494–8.

Fries, J.F. (1988). Milestones in rheumatologic care (1965–1985). In *Milestones in management: rheumatoid arthritis*, (ed. J.F. Fries). Syntex, Puerto Rico.

Gainor, B.J., Epstein, R.G., Henstorf, J.E., *et al.* (1988). Metatarsal head resection for rheumatoid deformities of the forefoot. *Clinical Orthopaedics and Related Research*, 230, 207–13.

Gondolph-Zink, B., Puhl, W., and Noack, W. (1988). Semiarthroscopic synovectomy of the hip. *International Orthopedics*, 12, 31–5.

Grossman, J.F. and Valance, R. (1980).Clinical and radiological features of the shoulder joint in rheumatoid arthritis. *Journal of Bone and Joint Surgery*, 62B, 116.

Gswend, N. (1991). The case for a linked elbow prosthesis. In *Rheumatoid arthritis surgery of the elbow* (eds M. Hamalainer and F.W. Hagana), Vol 15, pp. 98–112. Basel.

Harvey, I.A., Manning, M.P., Sampath, S.A., Johnson, R., and Elloy, M.A. (1995). Alignment of total knee arthroplasty: the relationship to radiolucency around the tibial component. *Medical Engineering and Physics*, 17, 182–7.

Hasselo, L.G., Willkens, R.F., Toomey, H.E., *et al.* (1987). Forefoot surgery in rheumatoid arthritis: Subjective assessment of outcome. *Foot and Ankle*, 8, 148–51.

Hecker, R.L., Furness, I.C., and Gostich, C.M. (1982). Ankle synovectomy: an approach to the rheumatoid ankle. *Journal of Foot Surgery*, 21, 4–6.

Heywood, A.W., Learmonth, I.D., and Thomas, M. (1988). Cervical spine instability in rheumatoid arthritis. *Journal of Bone and Joint Surgery*, 70A, 702–7.

Holt, E.S., Hansen, S.T., Mayo, K.A., and Sangeorzan, B.J. (1991). Ankle arthrodesis using internal screw fixation. *Clinical Orthopaedics and Related Research*, 268, 21–8.

Hsu, R.W., Fan, G.F., and Ho, W.P. (1995). A follow-up study of porous-coated anatomic knee arthroplasty. *Journal of Arthroplasty*, 10, 29–36.

Ishikawa, H., Ohno, O., and Hirohata, K. (1986). Long-term results of synovectomy in rheumatoid patients. *Journal of Bone and Joint Surgery*, 68A, 198–205.

Iwata, H., Yasuhara, N., Kawashima, K., Kaneko, M., Sugiura, Y., and Nakagawa, M. (1980). Arthrodesis of the ankle joint with rheumatoid arthritis: experience with the transfibular approach. *Clinical Orthopaedics and Related Research*, 153, 189–93.

Jaffe, R. and Learmonth, I.D. (1989). Benjamin double osteotomy for arthritis of the glenohumeral joint. *Rheumatology*, 12, 52–7.

Jensen, N.C. and Kroner, K. (1992). Total ankle joint replacement: a clinical follow up. *Orthopedics*, 15, 236–9.

Johnston, R.A. and Kelly, I.G. (1990). Surgery of the rheumatoid cervical spine. *Annals of the Rheumatic Diseases*, 49 (suppl. 2), 845–50.

Jolly, S.L., Ferlic, D.C., Clayton, M.L., Dennis, D.A., and Stringer, E.A. (1992). Swanson silicone arthroplasty of the wrist in rheumatoid arthritis: a long-term follow-up. *Journal of Hand Surgery — American Volume*, 17, 142–9.

Kates, A., Kessel, L., and Kay, A. (1967). Arthroplasty of the forefoot. *Journal of Bone and Joint Surgery*, 49B, 552–7.

Kavanagh, B.F., Dewitz, M.A., Ilstrup, D.M., Stauffer, R.N., and Coventry, M.B. (1989). Charnley total hip arthroplasty with cement. Fifteen-year results. *Journal of Bone and Joint Surgery*, 71A, 1496–503.

Kessel, L. and Bayley, I. (1982). Prosthetic replacement of the shoulder joint. *Journal of the Royal Society of Medicine*, 72, 748–52.

Kim, Y.H. and Oh, J.H. (1995). Evaluation of the anatomic patellar prosthesis in uncemented porous-coated total knee arthroplasty: seven-year results. *American Journal of Orthopedics*, 24, 412–9.

Knutson, K., Lewold, S., Robertsson, O., and Lidgren, L. (1994). The Swedish knee arthroplasty register. A nation-wide study of 30,003 knees 1976–1992. *Acta Orthopaedica Scandinavica*, 65, 375–86.

Kvien, T.K., Pahle, J.A., Hoyeraal, H.M., and Sandstad, B. (1987). Comparison of synovectomy and no synovectomy in patients with juvenile rheumatoid arthritis. A 24-month controlled study. *Scandinavian Journal of Rheumatology*, 16, 81–91.

Laine, V.A.I., Vainio, K.J., and Pekanmaki, K. (1954). Shoulder affections in rheumatoid arthritis. *Annals of the Rheumatic Diseases*, 13, 157–60.

Lettin, A.W.F., Copeland, S.A., and Scales, J.T. (1982). The Stanmore total shoulder replacement. *Journal of Bone and Joint Surgery*, 64B, 47–51.

Lord, G., Marotife, J.-H., Guillamon, J.-L., and Blanchard, J.-P. (1988). Cementless revisions of failed aseptic cemented and cementless total hip arthroplasties. *Clinical Orthopaedics and Related Research*, 235, 67–74.

Low, C.K., Tan, S.K., Satku, K., and Kumar, V.P. (1994). Reactivation of rheumatoid arthritis in knees following total knee replacement. *Annals of Academic Medicine, Singapore*, 23, 887–90.

Matsui, N., Taneda, Y., Ohta, H., Itch, T., and Tsuboguchi, S. (1989). Arthroscopic versus open synovectomy in the rheumatoid knee. *International Orthopaedics*, 13, 17–20.

McGuire, M.R., Kyle, R.F., Gustilo, R.B., and Premer, R.F. (1988). Comparative analysis of ankle arthroplasty versus ankle arthrodesis. *Clinical Orthopaedics and Related Research*, 174–81.

Moeckel, B.H., Patterson, B.M., Inglis, A.E., and Sculco, T.P. (1991). Ankle arthrodesis. A comparison of internal and external fixation. *Clinical Orthopaedics and Related Research*, 268, 78–83.

Mohing, W., Kohler, G., and Coldewey, J. (1982). Synovectomy of the ankle joint. *International Orthopaedics*, 6, 117–21.

Moran, C.G., Pinder, I.M., and Smith, S.R. (1991). Ankle arthrodesis in rheumatoid arthritis. 30 cases followed for 5 years. *Acta Orthopaedica Scandinavica*, 62, 538–43.

Neer, C.S. II, Watson, K.C., and Stanton, F.J. (1982). Recent experience in total shoulder replacement. *Journal of Bone and Joint Surgery*, 64A, 319–37.

Ogilvie-Harris, D.J. and Basinski, A. (1991). Arthroscopic synovectomy of the knee for rheumatoid arthritis. *Arthroscopy*, 7, 91–7.

Ogilvie-Harris, D.J. and Wiley, A.M. (1986). Arthroscopic surgery of the shoulder. *Journal of Bone and Joint Surgery*, 68B, 201–7.

Paus, A.C. and Dale, K. (1993). Arthroscopic and radiographic examination of patients with juvenile rheumatoid arthritis before and after open synovectomy of the knee joint. A prospective study with a 5-year follow-up. *Annales Chirurgiae et Gynaecologie Fenniae*, 82, 55–61.

Petersson, C.J. (1986). Painful shoulders in patients with rheumatoid arthritis. *Scandinavian Journal of Rheumatology*, 15, 275–9.

Porter, B.B., Richardson, C., and Vianio, K. (1974). Rheumatoid arthritis of the elbow: the results of synovectomy. *Journal of Bone and Joint Surgery*, 56B, 427–37.

Posner, M.A. and Ambrose, L. (1991). Excision of the distal ulnar in rheumatoid arthritis. *Hand Clinics*, 7, 383–90.

Pritchard, R.W. (1991). Total elbow joint arthroplasty in patients with rheumatoid arthritis. *Seminars in Arthritis and Rheumatism*, 21, 24–9.

Ranawat, C.S. *et al.* (1979). Cervical spine fusion in rheumatoid arthritis. *Journal of Bone and Joint Surgery*, 61A, 1003.

Ransford, A.O., Crockard, H.A., Pozo, J.L. *et al.* (1986). Craniocervical instability treated by contoured loop fixation. *Journal of Bone and Joint Surgery,* **68B**, 173–7.

Rickhuss, P.K., Gray, A.J., and Rowley, D.I. (1994). A 5–10 year follow-up of the Sheehan total knee endoprosthesis in Tayside. *Journal of the Royal College of Surgeons, Edinburgh*, **39**, 326–8.

Severt, R., Wood, R., Cracchiolo, A., and Amstutz, H.C. (1991). Long-term follow-up of cemented total hip arthroplasty in rheumatoid arthritis. *Clinics in Orthopedics*, **265**, 129–36.

Seyfer, A.E. (1993). Indications for upper extremity surgery in rheumatoid arthritis patients. *Seminars in Arthritis and Rheumatism*, **23**, 125–34.

Skues, M.A. and Welchew, E.A. (1993). Anaesthesia and rheumatoid arthritis. *Anaesthesia*, **48**, 989–97.

Souter, W.A. (1990). Surgery of the rheumatoid arthritis. *Annals of the Rheumatic Diseases*, **49** (suppl 2), 871–82.

Stanley, J.K. (1992). Conservative surgery in the management of rheumatoid disease of the hand and wrist. *Journal of Hand Surgery — British Volume*, **17**, 339–42.

Stauffer, R.N. (1977). Total ankle joint replacement. *Archives of Surgery*, **112**, 1105–9.

Stone, K.H. and Helal, B. (1991). A method of ankle stabilization. *Clinical Orthopaedics and Related Research*, **268**, 102–6.

Toledano, B., Terrono, A.L., and Millender, L.H. (1992). Reconstruction of the rheumatoid thumb. *Hand Clinics*, **8**, 121–9.

Vahvanen, V.A. (1967). Rheumatoid arthritis in the pantalar joints. A follow-up study of triple arthrodesis on 292 adult feet. *Acta Orthopaedica Scandinavica*, (Suppl 107), 3–80.

Wagner, F.W., Jr (1982). Ankle fusion for degenerative arthritis secondary to the collagen diseases. *Foot and Ankle*, **3**, 24–31.

Wroblewski, B.M. (1986). Fifteen to twenty-one year results of the Charnley low friction arthroplasty. *Clinics in Orthopedics*, **211**, 30–5.

Wynn Parry, C.B. and Stanley, J.K. (1993). Synovectomy of the hand (review). *British Journal of Rheumatology*, **32**, 1089–95.

6.2 Surgery in children

Malcolm Swann

Introduction

Surgery now has a firmly established place in the management of juvenile chronic arthritis and in the rheumatic diseases of childhood (Arden and Ansell 1978; Swann 1983a; Rydholm 1990). This chapter is principally concerned with surgery of juvenile chronic arthritis and includes the scope and indications, problems and outcome. The number of children being offered surgical relief varies considerably not only between different countries but between different units within a country (Granberry and Brewer 1978). Much will depend on the attitude of the rheumatologist about seeking such help. It will then depend upon the immediate availability of an orthopaedic surgeon with an expert team conversant with the particularly challenging problems that this condition presents. Experience drawn from the Medical Research Council unit at the Canadian Red Cross Hospital at Taplow and at Wexham Park Hospital, Slough (England) forms the basis for the conclusion drawn here (Ansell and Swann 1983). There are some 5000 patients with juvenile chronic arthritis on the records and of these, 10 per cent have had a surgical procedure and many of them multiple procedures. In this surgically treated group, half have seropositive arthritis.

Surgery should be seen as complementing the other forms of treatment. Thus all the patients must have full exposure to conservative treatment including medication, physiotherapy, and splintage. At some stage it may become evident that these methods are failing and that further help must be sought. The clinician has a difficult task in managing this condition, whose cause is unknown and whose natural course is unpredictable both in the patient in general and in the individual joints. There are no markers to indicate when the disease will undergo remission or finally burn out. The problem is compounded by the unpredictable response to medication, which in itself may have side-effects; by physiotherapy, which can be painful if inappropriate; and by structural changes, which cannot be overcome by conservative means. For instance, splints need to be moulded, comfortable, and changed frequently if there is any alteration in a position. Thus, in our present state of knowledge, some problems cannot be surmounted by conservative means alone and surgical intervention will be required.

Many centres lack the specific expertise and team required for the disciplined and perhaps intensive approach that is necessary to overcome the many problems in treating these children. Failure of this vigilant guidance and its application, and in some cases failure of compliance by the patient (or their parents) may also result in unsuccessful therapy, with the establishment of loss of movement and

deformity. Surgical help may be required in such cases in order to recover lost ground. There can be no doubt that the management of juvenile chronic arthritis is best supervised in special centres (Woo *et al.* 1990).

The main reasons for undertaking orthopaedic surgery are relief of pain, correction of deformity, and to overcome loss of motion. The last of these reasons applies not only to the individual joints but to the patient as a whole. These principles apply in particular to the surgical management of juvenile chronic arthritis. There are, however, two principles on which this surgical practice is based. First, the patients must have the opportunity to undergo corrective procedures early in the course of the disease in order to prevent the development of deformity and loss of movement. No surgeon would wish to be presented with a patient in a wheelchair who he or she is seeing for the first time with no options but to advise the total replacement of a destroyed joint. Second, the selection of a particular operative procedure is based on a thorough understanding of the cause of deformity, lack of movement and pain. A more detailed analysis of this will be made later but an example is a misshapen overgrown patella, stuck by fibrous adhesions to the underlying femoral condyle. Here there is deformity and loss of movement where medication, physiotherapy, and splintage may be fruitlessly and painfully applied until the adhesions are ultimately divided by operation.

The first of these principles can only be applied if the surgeon is invited to see the patient early in the course of the disease. Ideally, joint consultation should take place in the outpatients department, and on ward rounds so that cases can be presented and discussed, and a plan of management drawn up. The team must include an experienced physiotherapist, an occupational therapist, and nursing staff and others to reflect the special needs of children with arthritis. The second of these principles can only be applied after full investigation and appreciation of the precise anatomical, physiological, and pathological changes that have occurred (Swann 1987).

Contraction, contracture, and spasm

A number of loose descriptive phrases used in the clinical assessment of patients are often misleading. Muscle spasm is associated with any painful condition in the musculoskeletal condition and in essence serves to prevent movement that is painful, holding the joint in a position of comfort and maximum capacity. There is a contraction of the muscles but there is not a contracture. If the pain can be relieved by anaesthetic or other means, the affected joint will be seen to have a full range of movement. A contracture of muscles does occur after its denervation, when there is true replacement of muscle by fibrosis, or in conditions such as arthrogryphosis. The replacement of muscle with fibrous tissues does not occur in arthritis. There is, however, shortening of the muscle fibres and in established cases, it may take some while for these to be stretched out completely by appropriate treatment, including physiotherapy. However, contracture does occur in the periarticular tissues, such as in the capsule and ligaments, and is particularly noticeable in seronegative arthritis. This reaction may be so severe that it appears to be part of the primary pathology of the disease. The two states are interrelated, for a continuation of muscle spasm, either voluntary or involuntary, will allow a periarticular contracture to become established, with the shortening of the muscles and tissues on the concave side compounded by the wasting and stretching of the muscles and tissues on the convex side. The latter is particularly noticeable in relation to the quadriceps muscles at the knee.

If one considers a knee the clinical record may state, 'flexion range 30 to 90 degrees' or alternatively, 'flexion contracture 30 degrees'. This reading may be totally misleading as it takes no account of the pathology causing the loss of movement; nor is there usually standardization of the conditions under which such a record is made. The issue of the cause of a flexion contracture has been discussed and it should also be appreciated that a knee with a true range of movement under anaesthetic of, say, 30 to 90° has both an extension contracture as well as a flexion contracture, that is, it will neither bend fully nor straighten. If, however, the loss of movement is because of other causes such as pain, for example, the range will depend on many factors including the disease activity, and the level of analgesia and medication at the time (joints being noticeably stiffer on the morning that alternate-day steroids are due), and not least the confidence and co-operation of the patient.

Surgical intervention fits into this picture as being absolutely indicated in the presence of an established, true contracture.

Selection of surgical methods

This can be decided after a thorough analysis of the specific cause of the problem that is being addressed. Thus we need to examine the issues as to why a particular joint may be painful, why it is deformed and why it loses movement (Fig. 1). In order to appreciate this an understanding of the pathology is required in terms of both the intra- and periarticular aspects. There is also a clear distinction between loss of movement and stiffness. It is thus not only the arthritic process within the joint but its effect on lack of mobility, muscle wasting, osteoporosis, general debility of the patient, and many other factors that determine the outcome.

In general the cause of deformity, loss of movement, and pain follows a particular pattern. Pain in a joint is often associated with effusion so the patient will derive comfort in holding the position of maximum capacity, while attempts at movement are countered by muscle spasm. In time, a contracture of the periarticular tissues with shortening of the muscles on the concave side and lengthening of the muscles on the convex side of the joint occurs. Intra- and periarticular ligaments are affected and may be destroyed or fibrosed and together with intra-articular destruction of a joint surface, subluxation is often observed. Meanwhile this direct damage to the joint leads to loss of cartilage, and bone destruction and collapse, and this is sometimes accompanied by avascular necrosis and finally fibrous

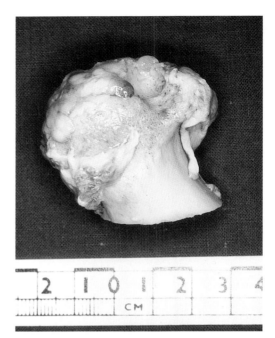

Fig. 1 The femoral head of a 14-year-old patient with juvenile chronic arthritis removed at the time of arthroplasty.

ankylosis and bone ankylosis. The greatest tendency to contracture is seen in the patients with seronegative arthritis, particularly those with the so-called dry-type arthritis. Loss of movement in a joint means that some areas of articular cartilage are never normally opposed and are thus denied the intermittent compression necessary for their normal nutrition. At the same time, opposed surfaces held under continuous pressure will also lack the normal stimulation to nutrition and in both cases degeneration of the hyaline cartilage follows (Salter and Field 1960).

These patients not only suffer a generalized retardation of growth but also suffer local defects of growth. Hypertrophy, irregular growth, or premature fusion of an epiphysis occur and are probably the result of the local increased blood supply. Frequently these children are unable to walk because of the pain caused by polyarthritis or because of their constitutional illness. This lack of activity contributes to the failure of joints, particularly of the hip, to develop properly. Bone porosis and muscle weakness add to the problem.

A range of surgical treatment is available and designed to tackle the problem at various stages of this pathological process (Fig. 2). Thus conservative measures including medication, splintage, and physiotherapy are adequate in the mildly affected, soft-tissue operations are indicated at the stage of early contractures, and operations on bones and joints (where even an arthroplasty may be recommended) in those more severely affected.

Any synovial joint can be affected by inflammatory change but it is the knee and hip that are most commonly affected. Emphasis on the surgical management will therefore be directed to these two main joints but the principles outlined apply to other sites.

The hip

Cause of deformity

All the components that cause pain, loss of movement, and deformity are seen when the hip is affected. Pain and swelling of the joint lead to

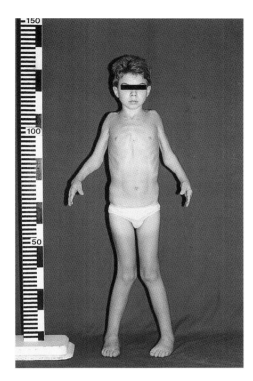

Fig. 2 Photograph of a 14-year-old boy who developed systemic-onset juvenile arthritis aged 6 years. Note the flexion of hips, flexion and valgus deformity of the knees, femoral internal rotation and tibial external rotation, and varus deformity of the feet. The cause of these deformities is analysed in the text. Some upper-limb problems are also apparent. He has since had bilateral soft-tissue releases of the hips followed later by total hip replacements, bilateral supracondylar osteotomies of the femurs, and a wedge tarsectomy.

early flexion deformity and some adduction, with restricted movement. The psoas and adductor muscles are particularly dominant in this respect. In time erosion, destruction, sometimes subluxation, and often necrosis of the femoral head are identified and sometimes growth disturbance (Hastings *et al.* 1994). The persistent spasm and increased vascularity lead to a disturbance of normal growth. The capital epiphysis fuses early and there is some broadening and shortening of the femoral neck, while unequal forces may alternatively induce a marked valgus and anteversion. The greater trochanter grows at a normal or accelerated pace and the lesser trochanter is frequently overgrown because of traction from the psoas muscle. The femoral shaft becomes excessively bowed and the lumen of the medullary cavity has its greatest diameter in the sagittal plane.

The attitude assumed by the hip in early-onset arthritis is therefore dominated not only by the joint destruction and lack of proper use but also by the growth derangement brought about by the epiphyses. If there is anteversion of the femoral neck the femoral head tends to sublux anteriorly out of the socket and this leads to the patient assuming a flexed hip position, particularly when standing, in order to ensure stability and comfort. The valgus anteverted neck also means that the abductor lever is reduced and a Trendelenburg or waddling gait will occur.

The clinician must be alert to these causative factors when dealing with a flexion deformity of the hip because if the joint cannot be straightened it must be determined whether this is because of the spasm of the muscles, a soft-tissue contracture, or an abnormality of

the bone development. Likewise the factors causing a limp must be sought.

A hip joint unaffected itself by disease can develop deformity secondary to a fixed flexed knee below or a scoliotic spine above, and with the chronicity of this illness such a hip may develop a fixed deformity itself.

Specimens of femoral heads removed at operation have shown definite evidence of repair by fibrocartilage in patients whose disease is controlled or quiescent. It is therefore important that the hip is maintained in a congruous position with uninhibited motion so that there is adequate moulding if attempts at repair are to be successful.

Surgical management

This is best considered in three stages dependent on the degree of the problem:

Stage 1: hips in which there is almost a full range of movement under anaesthesia and with minimum radiological change.

Stage 2: hips in which there is still some fixed deformity and restriction of full movement under anaesthesia and in which radiographs, arthrograms, computerized tomographic (CT) scans, magnetic resonance imaging (MRI) or ultrasonography confirm the presence of a joint space.

Stage 3: hips lacking movement under anaesthesia with persistent deformity and advanced radiological change.

Stage 1

The establishment of fixed deformities and loss of movement can be aggressively countered at this stage by a well-supervised conservative regimen. These children are admitted to the hospital for full evaluation of their problem. Medication includes analgesics and possibly an intra-articular steroid injection. Skin traction is applied, with the pull toward abduction, and maintained for 24 h a day interspersed with physiotherapy. When the condition permits, prone lying for part of each day may help reduce flexion deformity of the hip. However, it should be appreciated that in a hip which has an effusion, attempts at extension may actually increase the intra-articular pressure and thus the pain. There is some evidence to suggest that a rise of intra-articular pressure will also lead to avascular necrosis (Soto-Hall 1964). Early surgical decompression of these hips is therefore indicated before attempts at extension using traction or prone lying. This will be discussed later. When the hips are affected the knee in particular needs to be watched and may require splints to prevent concomitant flexion. As the patients begin to improve, hydrotherapy should be instituted daily in addition to the traction. Sitting, such as in a wheelchair, is forbidden. When the pain abates, walking with aids can start progressively, with traction maintained at night.

Stage 2

When there is an established flexion contracture, movement is limited even under anaesthesia, and the joint space can be demonstrated, then the situation can be improved by a soft-tissue release operation (Mogensen *et al.* 1983). While complete release operations may sometimes be necessary (Alvarez *et al.* 1992; Witt and McCullough 1994), the tightness of the adductors and psoas is the main obstacle to correction (Swann and Ansell 1986). An open adductor tenotomy can be done and through the same incision the psoas tendon can easily be reached and divided at its attachment to the lesser trochanter.

After the operation the hips are again put on traction in abduction and extension, and the regimen, continued as described for stage 1 except that hydrotherapy, of necessity, is delayed until the wounds are healed. Experience of this procedure in over 100 cases has produced gratifying results that include lessening of the flexion contracture (Fig. 3), an increase in the total range of movement, and a very dramatic relief of pain, probably due to decompression of the joint. Radiographs have shown an improvement in terms of a decreased osteoporosis, a clearer definition of the joint line, and some widening of the joint space in more than half the patients (Fig. 4). The longer-term results at 3 years and more have been shown to mirror the activity of the subsequent disease. Nevertheless, by improving the movement and function of the joint a congruous, contained femoral head may be possible with some repair, so if the disease activity abates a serviceable hip remains. In those cases where the continuing disease activity results in a less favourable outcome a period of relief from pain is usually enjoyed and the structural anatomy is in a better position for hip arthroplasty at a later state.

The role of osteotomy to correct deformity is limited, but occasionally muscle imbalance, joint effusion, and an increased valgus of the femoral neck lead to anterolateral subluxation of the hip and theoretically a varus osteotomy is indicated under these circumstances. However, the porosity of bone will often preclude internal fixation and external immobilization will lead to intractable stiffness. An osteotomy can occasionally be used in a patient whose disease is no longer active and in whom there is good bone stock. Care must be exercised before proceeding with a containment osteotomy because sometimes a coxa magna precludes the femoral head being fully restored to the acetabulum. This containment may also be prevented if there is a mass of thickened synovial tissue in the acetabular floor—a situation which may be identified by MRI. In addition, care in alignment of the shaft is essential to allow the possibility of total arthroplasty at a later date.

Stage 3

Total hip arthroplasty may be indicated in a patient with a severely destroyed joint who may be condemned to a painful existence in a wheelchair. Some of the patients have had to have custom-made prostheses to fit their mini skeletons (Fig. 5). These are time-consuming procedures because of the bleeding and the frailness of the bone, and our long-term studies have shown they carry, as expected, a higher rate of infection and prosthetic loosening than in other conditions (Learmonth et al. 1989; Williams and McCullough 1993). A current review of 96 hip replacements with a follow-up of 6 to 18 years (average 10 years) revealed that 25 per cent had failed, and the appearance of translucent lines and hip migration even in the asymptomatic patient suggests that this rate will rise with time (Witt et al. 1991). Of the 42 children reviewed in 1986 following total hip replacement (Ruddlesdin et al. 1986), four have since died of amyloid disease. Nevertheless, those who have reached late teenage or early adulthood have clearly been transformed by being physically able to integrate better with the community in terms of work, pleasure, and social contact. All the patients and their parents, save one, felt the operation had been worthwhile, despite those that had failed and the need for a revision arthroplasty in a large number of cases. However, modern techniques including the use of bone grafting, have enhanced the success of these more difficult procedures. I feel that despite the

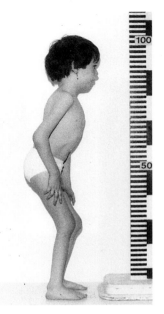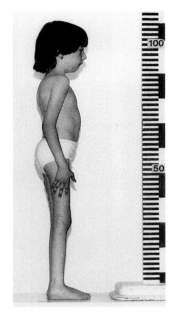

Fig. 3 This patient developed pauciarthritis aged 15 months, which subsequently extended. (a) At age 3 years: appearance after a full regimen of medication, physiotherapy, and splintage; she had active disease in both hips and knees with persistent flexion deformities at these joints. (b) After soft-tissue release of both hips and both knees a few months later—the posterolateral knee scar can just be seen.

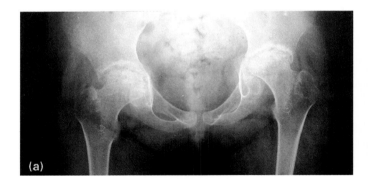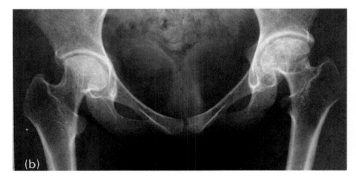

Fig. 4 This patient developed a severe systemic disease followed by polyarthritis aged 4 years. (a) Radiographs of the hips when the patient was aged 13 during an active phase of the disease and immediately before soft-tissue release; there is a marked flexion contracture. (b) The same hips 3 years later following the soft-tissue release: the disease had also become quiescent but the operation permitted mobility to be regained and some healing has occurred; these hips have remained painless and the patient is now 29 years old and walks without a limp.

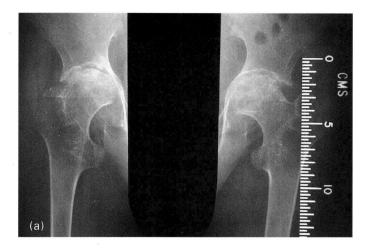

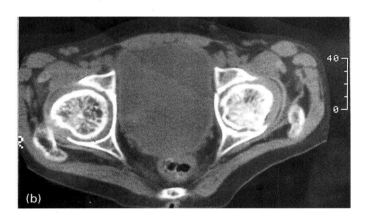

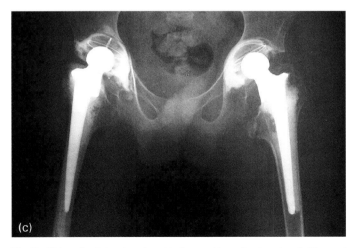

Fig. 5 This patient developed systemic-onset juvenile chronic arthritis aged 7 years. He also suffers from diabetes and myasthenia gravis. (a) Hips at age 16 immediately before surgery: the patient was unable to walk because of the painful disability; note the severe acetabular erosion and the overgrowth of the lesser trochanters; the sunken hips prevent proper abductor function. (b) A CT scan of the same patient used to define the pelvic bone stock available for anchoring the acetabular component of a total hip replacement; note the thin medial wall. (c) The postoperative appearance: note this patient has subsequently had both his knees replaced (see Fig. 6).

overall high failure rate the operation remains well worthwhile in carefully selected cases as the only alternative to a painful wheelchair existence.

The knee
Cause of deformity

The knee is frequently affected early in several of the subgroups of juvenile arthritis, possibly because of its large synovial surface. When this becomes inflamed the joint is flexed into a position of comfort and maximum capacity, and hamstring spasm will prevent it straightening. The stretched quadriceps muscle rapidly wastes and this may also be a reflex phenomenon associated with the effusion within the joint. This weakness of the quadriceps adds to the inability of the patient actively to straighten the knee. The periarticular structures undergo fibrosis and it is important to note that this includes the broad expanse of the quadriceps expansion on each side because this in turn will limit flexion. The joint thus develops a flexion contracture and an inability to flex so that it loses movement early, i.e. an extension contracture.

These effects combine to lead to a characteristic posterior subluxation of the tibia. The articular cartilage becomes eroded with continuing activity but because this is particularly thick in the younger child, the erosion must be well advanced before significant joint narrowing can be seen. Marked effects are imposed on the growth of the bone because of the hyperaemia and venous hypertension. There is an overgrowth produced by the epiphyseal plate and in patients with only one knee affected, characteristically in pauciarthritis, the limb grows longer than its fellow. The medial side of the femoral growth plate appears to have a propensity to be stimulated in the greatest manner and this is one of the causes of a valgus deformity (see Fig. 2). Valgus may also be related to collapse of the lateral side of the joint, and this may be in response to forces of the adducted hip above and possibly a varus foot below. A complex state develops in these patients, leading to a rotation deformity. Anteversion of the femoral neck produces internal rotation deformity of the femur, which is clinically evident by the squinting patellae. Secondary external rotation of the tibia at the knee plus some torsion of the tibia itself may then begin to develop to keep the axis of the ankle in line with the direction of progress (see Fig. 2). In addition, when a foot affected by the disease has painful articulations and is held in eversion and valgus when the patient walks, this will also induce a torsional force on the tibia. Finally, an iliotibial band contracture causes flexion and external rotation of the knee and contributes to this complex mechanism of deformity. Lateral subluxation of the patella may follow, which in itself may require surgical correction because the line of pull of the quadriceps has thus become mechanically inefficient.

The patella itself often develops overgrowth into a misshapen and mechanically unacceptable form, whilst closure of the patellofemoral joint by fibrous ankylosis may be a cause of a fixed deformity that will certainly require surgical release.

Management

In terms of surgical treatment it is helpful to consider the knee in three stages, depending on the extent of the pathology present.

Stage 1: A knee in which there is a full range of movement under anaesthetic and minimal changes on radiographs.

Stage 2: Knees with some restriction of movement and slight deformity that cannot be corrected under anaesthetic but where a joint space is still present.

Stage 3: Gross loss of movement with a severe deformity and marked radiographic changes.

An overall appraisal of the other joints affected, particularly in the same limb, must be made before beginning treatment. Correcting the flexed deformity of the knee if the ipsilateral hip exhibits a similar problem is useless and probably the hip should be dealt with first. When planning surgery it has to be decided whether the deformity can be corrected by a soft-tissue operation and thus increase the total range of movement, or by osteotomy, leaving the range of movement unchanged. The former is ideal but can only be achieved when the disease activity is controlled and the joint destruction is minimal. an osteotomy realigns the limb by producing a secondary deformity that masks the first. However limited the movement in a knee, it must be possible to extend it. The patient can then stand in comfort, wear a calliper if necessary, avoid quadriceps fatigue, and prevent the induction of a secondary deformity of the hip.

When fixed flexion is considerable, several complications of treatment must be recognized. First, as the leg is extended, traction will occur on the popliteal artery and nerves, and may lead to a vascular embarrassment or neurological damage. Second, passive conservative treatment using traction or plaster may lead to problems such as subluxation of the knee, supracondylar fracture of porotic bone, or anterior compression across the joint when the posterior capsule is unyielding and acts as a hinge at the back. This compression itself may cause necrosis of the cartilage and subarticular microfracture. If the method employed requires prolonged immobilization, further disuse porosis will occur and the articular surface will suffer, as hyaline cartilage requires intermittent compression to maintain effective nutrition.

Treatment

Stage 1

The patient is examined under a general anaesthetic and if this reveals a normal range of movement and no fixed deformity, physiotherapy and rest splints are indicated. If pain is severe, slow correction by reversed dynamic slings is used if the deformity does not exceed 25° but these must not be applied under anaesthetic. Medication can be helpfully reinforced by intra-articular steroid injections (Earley *et al.* 1988). Synovectomy is indicated where there is permanent thickening and effusion in the knee, often leading to overgrowth of the limb. Synovectomy, however, has a limited role in polyarthritis because the patients who might benefit most are often too sick for surgery because of systemic disease. It should be therapeutic rather than prophylactic in a disease whose future progress in an individual patient and an individual joint is unpredictable. Arthroscopic synovectomy is the method of choice if the joint can be distended (Vilkki *et al.* 1991).

Stage 2

Soft-tissue release of the posterior structures may result in an immediate correction of a flexion deformity or be used as a prelude to further serial plasters or reversed dynamic traction (see Fig. 3). It is a satisfactory procedure when there is no concomitant valgus

deformity. The operation involves lengthening of the hamstring muscles and division of the posterior capsule of the knee joint right across its axis and around on either side (Clarke *et al.* 1988). It is a difficult procedure and if the tibia is found to be subluxed the contracted cruciate ligament may need to be divided. After the surgery, plaster is applied for 3 days, following which it is bivalved and movement encouraged to overcome the tendency to postoperative stiffness. The plaster shells are kept as rest splints and used for early walking until strength is regained.

If the deformity is fixed and bone destruction is more advanced, then a supracondylar osteotomy is an appropriate procedure, and can be used to correct valgus at the same time. The operation is done through a short medial incision and the porosity of the bone often precludes internal fixation so that a plaster cylinder or similar external splint is applied and weight bearing encouraged at the outset. The plaster is removed as early as possible, usually at about 4 weeks to obviate stiffness. A calliper or alternative support is advised for immediate use as a night splint to maintain correction. The bone can be expected to unite satisfactorily and the position of the leg is maintained in correct alignment by direct inspection. Intensive physiotherapy is required to prevent postoperative stiffness. It is occasionally necessary to repeat the osteotomy if the forces that necessitated it in the first place continue to act, particularly if there is an exceptional increase in growth of the patient.

Epiphyseal stapling has occasionally been used to correct valgus of the knee and some surgeons use this method to arrest excessive longitudinal growth, particularly in cases of pauciarthritis (Rydholm *et al.* 1987).

Stage 3

These knees are often totally adherent, with fibrous adhesions not only between the main articular surfaces but in particular between the patella and the femoral condyle. They are usually associated also with considerable periarticular contracture. For this reason, access to the knee is difficult through an arthroscope as the joint cannot be distended with fluid in the normal fashion in order to get a clear view. Some of these patients can benefit from an extensive surgical approach that divides the adhesions, followed by an immediate postoperative regimen using the continuous passive-motion machine under adequate analgesic cover. However, many joints are clearly so badly destroyed that nothing short of total knee replacement is indicated (Fig. 6). Technological design and improvements in techniques have now produced a generation of knee prostheses that can be manufactured in a smaller size and are suitable for these juvenile patients. The experience being gained with these is encouraging and for any child who has a severely painful joint with deformity and destruction that precludes any other form of treatment, this method must be considered. The indications are similar to those suggested for a hip prosthesis.

The foot and ankle

Studies have shown (Ansell and Wood 1976) that within 1 year of onset of the disease, the ankle joint was affected in 40 per cent of cases, the subtalar and midtarsal in 27 per cent, and the metatarsophalangeal in 9 per cent. At the 15-year follow-up only 0.9 per cent of children felt that the foot was the most limiting factor. The early onset of the disease in the foot leads to growth abnormalities that present clinical features often requiring surgical remedy. The multiple and complex synovial articulations fall prey to the severity and duration of the

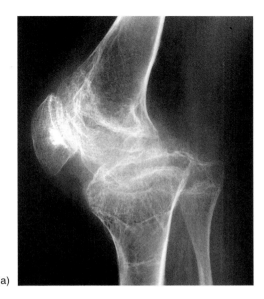

(a)

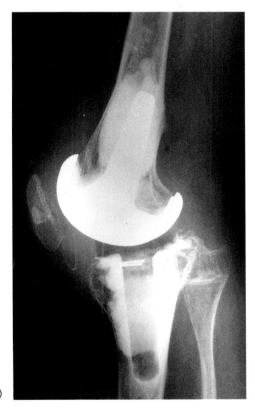

(b)

Fig. 6 The same patient as depicted in Fig. 5; after hip arthroplasty further deterioration occurred in both knees. (a) Preoperative radiograph at age 16 years: note the severe degree of osteoporosis, overgrowth of the patella, posterior subluxation of the tibia, and the marked depression of the tibial plateau. An anteroposterior view showed the knee to be in a marked valgus position as a result of the collapse of the lateral tibial plateau but also an overgrowth of the medial femoral condyle. (b) Total knee replacement using an Attenborough prosthesis. The small size, destroyed surface, and osteoporosis are best suited to an unrestrained, stemmed prosthesis with cement. Some newer designs of total condylar replacement are proving satisfactory after adolescence when the disease has become inactive. This patient has now regained mobility having lost the flexion contractures in both hips and both knees, and in each case has a flexion range of 90° or more.

disease. Problems present as elsewhere, with pain, deformity, and loss of function. Pain is associated with active disease but it must be appreciated that a deformity causing pressure or stiffness may throw abnormal strains on other, possibly unaffected joints. Foot problems may also arise secondarily to those of the knee. Finally, inflamed synovial sheaths or bursae may require attention.

Management

This is best considered under the headings of the forefoot, the hindfoot, and the ankle (Ansell and Swann 1996).

The forefoot

The main indication for surgical intervention in the foot is pain. Deformity *per se* is not an indication to operate unless it is causing pain or loss of function, and many foot problems can be dealt with by simple conservative means, including special shoes, orthoses, splints, or even a calliper. However, when the problem cannot be controlled by these simpler means or if the older patient is reluctant to wear a surgical shoe or an orthosis, surgery is indicated. Specific examples where surgical intervention will, however, be required as a primary source of relief to the patient include significant toe deformities produced by epiphyseal abnormalities, and severe metatarsalgia with clawing of the toes associated with disruption and dislocation of the metatarsophalangeal joints, as seen in seropositive disease. In these patients, severe hallux valgus deformity may occur, which will require a metatarsal osteotomy for realignment of the great toe. The reader should be aware that overall excellent results can be obtained by careful selection of patients for surgery, particularly for instance where a local pressure point in the forefoot or toes is the source of severe pain. The operations include surgical trimming of a bony prominence or irregularity, straightening of the toes, and excision arthroplasty of the metatarsophalangeal joints (Fowler 1959).

The hindfoot

This includes the subtalar, talonavicular, and calcaneocuboid joints. No set pattern of deformity is seen here but the deviation may be into either varus or valgus. Whichever way they go, both the heel and the forefoot usually diverge in the same direction, setting up abnormal foot imprints and consequently secondary strain-pressure areas and callosities. Valgus deformity can be produced by a spasm of the peroneal muscles and this can be a presenting feature of juvenile chronic arthritis, where it is labelled a peroneal spastic flat foot. Valgus is also caused by some collapse of the foot to spare the painful articulations affected by disease, or secondarily to compensate deformity at the knee. Loss of joint congruity and fixation by joint adhesion or contracture will later prevent passive correction. A varus deformity is particularly disabling because the patient walks on the outer border of the foot (see Fig. 2). Not infrequently this is associated with a valgus deformity of the knee and as such may be partly compensatory, accentuated by taking a full load of body weight. This combined deformity may seriously affect the patient's gait.

The indications for treatment are pain and deformity: however, a deformity that is painless but interfering with the child's gait should be corrected. In the majority of patients, conservative treatment suffices in as much as one is able to obtain a good correction of the deformity, but it is necessary to do this under a general anaesthetic. At the same time an intra-articular injection of triamcinolone is given into the dominantly affected joint and, if the exact location is not clear, it is put into the sinus tarsi. After this, the foot is put into a corrective, plaster-of-Paris walking cast for 4 weeks; the plaster is then removed and the position maintained with a calliper (Mavidrou *et al.* 1991).

Surgical management

In some patients where passive correction even under anaesthetic is not possible, some form of surgical correction will be indicated. In principle this consists of the removal of bone wedges to correct alignment of the foot and fusion of painful joints, in particular the talonavicular joint, which is often the predominant cause of trouble. Realignment of the heel in the presence of a good triple joint can be achieved by an osteotomy of the os calcis.

The ankle joint

The ankle joint itself may undergo erosive disease or be secondarily affected by avascular necrosis of the talus. It may also become mechanically stressed when normal movement is lost at the subtalar or midtarsal joints.

There is sometimes difficulty in identifying the source of pain in the hindfoot region, especially in differentiating between the ankle joint and the subtalar joint. Clinical examination and radiographs may help in identifying the joint at fault. However, the solution is complicated by the fact that a radiologically destroyed and stiff subtalar joint may itself be relatively painless but throw strain on an ankle joint that is not the site of primary disease. It is therefore recommended that a conservative approach is taken for as long as possible, including the use of gentle examination and repositioning of the foot under anaesthetic, injection of triamcinolone, and immobilization in plaster for 4 weeks. If these measures fail and it is necessary to proceed further the surgical options consist of arthroplasty or arthrodesis of the ankle joint.

Soft-tissue lesions around the foot

Tenosynovitis may induce pain, swelling, and spasm; in particular the sheath of the tibialis posterior is most commonly affected. The paratenon and bursae associated with the Achilles tendon are involved in patients with ankylosing spondylitis. Local injections of steroid into the inflamed tendon sheath are helpful but if this method fails, surgical synovectomy may have to be considered.

Intensive conservative treatment of feet affected by disease should preclude the need for surgery in the majority of cases. Nevertheless, conservative treatment may be instituted too late or fail to control the condition, particularly in persistently active disease. Surgery may then have some part to play in correcting the deformity, which is painful and retards walking. With rare exceptions it should only be employed when growth has ceased.

The upper limb

The most common problems that will need to be considered by the surgeon in juvenile chronic arthritis are those in the lower limb, and these have therefore been addressed at some length. However, the principles of surgery in the hip, knee, and foot are also invoked in the management of the upper limb and a short summary of the position with regard to the shoulder, elbow, hand and wrist follows.

The shoulder joint

This tends to be involved in those patients who have severe, generalized disease with prolonged activity. Its onset is often insidious and the patient is usually more concerned with the arthritis that affects the weight-bearing joints. It is when other joints in the upper limb, such as the elbow or wrist, are involved that the patient will become aware of the shoulder.

Shoulder problems are often exacerbated by the need to use crutches, and earlier and more satisfactory relief of problems in the leg joints have been helpful in this respect. There is very little conservative treatment that is effective for the shoulder, although it is worth trying an intra-articular steroid injection. If both shoulders are seriously affected, then everyday tasks such as dressing and feeding become well-nigh impossible and under these circumstances surgical relief may be sought. On the whole, synovectomy is ineffective, although if there is a very big subacromial bursa this can be excised. Osteotomy of the shoulder has an amazingly good outcome in terms of pain relief. This results in better use of the shoulder and scapula, although the actual movement in the glenohumeral joint itself may not be demonstrably increased. Arthrodesis is rarely indicated in a disease where stiffness itself is a problem. However, the present generation of shoulder arthroplasties is showing promise and some surgeons with an interest in this joint are reporting good results.

The elbow joint

This joint is more frequently involved than the shoulder, 45 per cent of the patients in a 15-year follow-up having problems. Assuming a failure of conservative treatment there are a number of surgical procedures that have a significant place in the management of this joint. Recurrent attacks of pain and swelling may derive benefit from a synovectomy; if the radial head is damaged and growth has reached maturity, it too can be removed. Arthrodesis is impractical but arthroplasty has a significant place. After excision of the bone ends, either an interposition of skin or fascia or a prosthetic replacement if enough bone stock is available are both very successful in relieving pain and improving movement and function.

The wrist and hand

These have a multitude of synovial joints so it is to be expected that most patients suffering from juvenile chronic arthritis in one of its forms should at some time have at least one of these joints involved (Harrison 1978). If the synovial sheaths of the flexor and extensor tendons are also included, few patients will escape some manifestation, and if the many growth plates and epiphyseal centres are involved, then the stage can be set for severe disability. Probably nowhere else is better rewarded by early splinting and physiotherapy to prevent deformity and stiffness. There are, however, indications where surgery can be helpful in this condition, but for the most part it is advised that this should be undertaken by a hand surgeon who is conversant with this minefield of problems. Indeed, the systemic illness of a child may militate against surgical intervention and when tendon sheaths are affected their involvement may also regress as the disease itself comes under control. We have found that the use of corticosteroids in persistent disease of the synovial sheath has been particularly helpful; intrathecal injections of hydrocortisone are given under general anaesthesia because they are painful. Occasionally, patients with a persistent thickening from proliferative synovitis in a limited field may benefit from a simple synovectomy followed by rapid mobilization. Extensive synovectomy of the flexor sheaths is never undertaken because it can lead to intractable stiffness. However, limited excision of the synovium of the dorsal sheaths, particularly in seropositive arthritis, does have some place, particularly where there is a danger of tendon rupture. The problems presented by a trigger finger or carpal tunnel compression are dealt with in the conventional fashion with the use of local steroid or, failing response, surgical decompression.

Wrist and carpal joints

There is often early destruction and deformity from epiphyseal involvement at these sites and the outcome is dictated by the degree of disease, age of onset, and the particular extraneous forces about the joint. A flexion deformity may occur early, and forward subluxation and ulnar deviation of the wrist must be countered by vigorous splinting and exercises. If stiffness does occur, one must ensure that it does so in a good position. Subluxation of the distal ulna often causes a painful swelling with some risk of tendon rupture; provided that the distal growth plates are closed, ulna styloidectomy may be indicated. For the severely damaged wrist and carpus, the choice will lie between arthrodesis and arthroplasty. Arthrodesis is well tried and, if indications are right, it can be most successful, mimicking that which nature often attempts. However, careful appraisal of the whole position of the arm must be made, as in some patients who already have stiff shoulders and elbows the retention of a small amount of movement, particularly in radial deviation, may make a disproportionate difference to their quest for independence.

Finger joints

The metacarpophalangeal joints when affected particularly in seropositive arthritis may benefit from synovectomy. If totally destroyed, and there is ulnar drift, a realignment procedure is worth undertaking with the use of some form of arthroplasty. When the problem is as severe in the interphalangeal joints, stabilization is again worthwhile, using a silastic implant.

The spine

The cervical spine is affected in both seropositive and seronegative juvenile arthritis (Swann 1983b), the dorsal spine exhibits crush fractures when steroids have been exhibited, and the lumbar spine takes the brunt of ankylosing spondylitis.

Patients with seronegative juvenile chronic arthritis may present with a painful torticollis and if this is neglected the patient will be left with a permanent disability with the head tilted rigidly on one side. These patients should be given a general anaesthetic, if necessary, in order to relieve the spasm, and whilst the head and neck are held straight a firm collar is applied. This is taken off for daily exercise and then reapplied, for although it will not prevent fusion occurring it does permit it to take place in a more satisfactory position. Seropositive arthritis, on the other hand, leads to instability and it is particularly at the atlantoaxial level where the subluxation or dislocation may occur. There is an absolute indication for surgical fusion at this level if there is a neurological involvement or severe pain or both.

It is of particular importance that the anaesthetist should be aware of these problems in the cervical spine in both types of disease. The rigidity of the neck, associated with a small airway, may make intubation difficult or impossible by conventional means. Subluxation or dislocation at the atlantoaxial level will equally be a hazard because attempts at intubation may lead to cord damage. It is essential that an up-to-date radiograph should be available immediately before the patient is given a general anaesthetic. The use of the fibreoptic laryngoscope and other airway techniques have obviated the worries that existed previously; many patients who are having lower limb surgery can be managed well with spinal or epidural anaesthesia (Smith 1990).

Scoliosis

Structural scoliosis occurs more commonly in patients with juvenile chronic arthritis than in the normal population (Ross *et al*. 1987). This may arise from the postural curves associated with asymmetrical involvement of the lower limb joints causing pelvic tilting. Timely surgical relief of the primary cause in the lower limbs has led to a lessening of the spinal curve. Asymmetrical involvement of the apophyseal joints may also contribute to this problem. In patients with scoliosis, careful appraisal of the underlying pathology should be made, but if there is a need, conventional methods of correction and stabilization can be used.

Fractures

The limited activity of these patients and their inability to participate in sport protects them largely from this problem. Nevertheless they are prone to pathological fractures because of their osteoporosis and the stiffness of their joints. This is particularly so with supracondylar fractures of the knee and underlines the inadvisability of manipulating the joints under anaesthetic. Examination under anaesthetic is permissible but must be attended by the utmost care.

After fractures, immobilization of the cast must be maintained for the minimal time consistent with union to prevent additional stiffness of the adjacent joint. The degree of osteoporosis usually precludes internal fixation of the fragments.

A number of patients have suffered crush fractures of the spine, particularly if they are on corticosteroids. No special treatment is indicated and recovery with remarkable reformation of the vertebrae can be expected.

Summary

All synovial joints are vulnerable to the deformity and functional loss that can occur in juvenile chronic arthritis. The principles outlined in this chapter should be applied intensively in this polyarthritic condition. The prognosis in terms of complete remission for many sufferers makes the treatment all the more demanding and worthwhile so that they may grow into physically functional adults.

References

Alvarez, M.J.M., Espada, G., Maldonado-Cocco, J.A., and Gagliardi, S.A. (1992). Long term follow up of hip and knee soft tissue release in juvenile chronic arthritis. *Journal of Rheumatology*, **19**, 1608–10.

Ansell, B.M. and Swann, M. (1983). The management of chronic arthritis of children. *Journal of Bone and Joint Surgery*, **65B**, 536–43.

Ansell, B.M. and Swann, M. (1996). Juvenile arthritis. In *Surgery of disorders of the foot and ankle*, vol. 1, (ed. B. Helal, D.I. Rowley, A. Cracchiolo III, and M.S. Myerson), pp. 263–70. Martin Dunitz, London.

Ansell, B.M. and Wood, P.H. (1976). Prognosis of juvenile chronic polyarthritis. *Clinics in Rheumatic Disease*, 2, 397–412.

Arden, G. and Ansell, B.M. (ed.) (1978). *Surgical management of juvenile chronic arthritis*. Academic Press, London.

Clarke, D.W., Ansell, B.M., and Swann, M. (1988). Soft tissue release of the knee in children with juvenile chronic arthritis. *Journal of Bone and Joint Surgery*, 70B, 224–7.

Earley, A., Cuttica, G., McCullogh, C., and Ansell, B.M. (1988). Triamcinalone into the knee joint in juvenile chronic arthritis. *Clinical and Experimental Rheumatology*, 6, 153–9.

Fowler, A.W. (1959). A method of forefoot reconstruction. *Journal of Bone and Joint Surgery*, 41B, 507–13.

Granberry, G.M. and Brewer, E.J. (1978). The combined pediatric–orthopedic approach to the management of juvenile rheumatoid arthritis. *Orthopedic Clinics of North America*, 9, 481–507.

Harrison, S.H. (1978). Wrist and hand problems and their management. In *The surgical management of juvenile chronic arthritis*, (ed. G.P. Arden and B.M. Ansell), pp. 161–83, Academic Press, London.

Hastings, D.E., Orsini, E., Myers, P., and Sullivan, J. (1994). An unusual pattern of growth disturbance of the hip in juvenile rheumatoid arthritis. *Journal of Rheumatology*, 21, 744–47.

Learmonth, I.D., Heywood, A.W.B., Kay, J., and Dall, D. (1989). Radiological loosening after cemented hip replacement for juvenile chronic arthritis. *Journal of Bone and Joint Surgery*, 71B, 209–12.

Mavidrou, A., Klenerman, L., Swann, M., Hall, M.A., and Ansell, B.M. (1991) Conservative management of the hindfoot in juvenile chronic arthritis. *The Foot*, 1, 139–43.

Mogensen, B., Brattstrom, H., Svantesson H., and Lidgren, L. (1983). Soft tissue release of the hip in juvenile chronic arthritis. *Scandinavian Journal of Rheumatology*, 12, 17–20.

Ross, A.C., Edgar, M.A., Swann, M., and Ansell, B.M. (1987). Scoliosis in juvenile chronic arthritis. *Journal of Bone and Joint Surgery*, 69B, 175–82.

Ruddlesdin, C., Ansell, B.M., Arden, G.P., and Swann, M. (1986). Total hip replacement in children with juvenile chronic arthritis. *Journal of Bone and Joint Surgery*, 68B, 218–22.

Rydholm, U. (ed.) (1990). *Surgery for juvenile chronic arthritis*. Ortolani, Lund.

Rydholm, U., Brattstrom, H., Bylander, B., and Lidgren, L. (1987). Stapling of the knee in juvenile chronic arthritis. *Journal of Paediatric Orthopaedics*, 7, 63–8.

Salter, R.B. and Field, B. (1960). The effects of combining compression on living articular cartilage: an experimental investigation. *Journal of Bone and Joint Surgery*, 42A, 31–49.

Smith, B.L. (1990). Anaesthesia in paediatric rheumatology. In *Paediatric rheumatology update*, (ed. P. Woo, P.H. White, and B.M. Ansell), pp. 124–30. Oxford University Press, Oxford.

Soto-Hall, R. (1964). Variations in the intraarticular pressure of the hip joints in injury and disease. *Journal of Bone and Joint Surgery*, 46A, 509–16.

Swann, M. (1983a). Juvenile chronic arthritis: surgical aspects. In *Clinical orthopedics*, (ed. N.H. Harris), pp. 249–67. Wright PSG, Bristol.

Swann, M. (1983b). Surgical treatment of the cervical spine in rheumatoid arthritis. *Annals of the Academy of Medicine of Singapore*, 12, 233–42.

Swann, M. (1987). Juvenile chronic arthritis. *Clinical Orthopaedics and Related Research*, 219, 38–49.

Swann, M. and Ansell, B.M. (1986). Soft tissue release of the hips in children with juvenile chronic arthritis. *Journal of Bone and Joint Surgery*, 68B, 404–8.

Vilkki, P., Virtanen, R., and Makela, A.K. (1991). Arthroscopic synovectomy in the treatment of patients with juvenile chronic arthritis. *Acta Universitatis Carolinae Medica*, 37, 84–6.

Williams, W.W. and McCullough, C.J. (1993). *Journal of Bone and Joint Surgery*, 75B, 872–4.

Witt, J.D. and McCullough, C.J. (1994). Anterior soft tissue release of the hip in juvenile chronic arthritis. *Journal of Bone and Joint Surgery*, 76B, 267–70.

Witt, J.D., Swann, M., and Ansell, B.M. (1991). Total hip replacement for juvenile chronic arthritis. *Journal of Bone and Joint Surgery*, 73B, 770–73.

Woo, P., White, P.H., and Ansell, B.M. (ed.) (1990). *Paediatric rheumatology update*. Oxford University Press, Oxford.

6.3 Rehabilitation of adults

Lynne Turner-Stokes

Introduction

Arthritis produces a wide spectrum of disability. Some aspects, such as deformity or florid synovitis of the hands, are clearly visible. Others, for example variable fatigue, are less so, and can lead to real social handicap as they are likely to be unsympathetically received by friends and family.

Until recently, 'rehabilitation' to the average rheumatologist meant wax baths and wheelchairs. In the last decade, the development of a multiprofessional approach to rehabilitation has transformed the way we think about disability. The purpose of this chapter is to describe that multiprofessional approach, as applied to the management of inflammatory joint disease.

Epidemiology

Epidemiological surveys in the United Kingdom (Harris 1971; Badley *et al.* 1978) have shown that the largest single group of impaired people have locomotor disease, amounting to one-third of the total impaired and to 40 per cent in the elderly population.

In a population of 100 000 people over 1000 will have rheumatoid arthritis, of whom 120 will be severely handicapped and 25 will be chair- or bed-bound. The same population will have 300 or more patients with severe osteoarthritis, of whom 50 will be totally immobile (Clarke *et al.* 1987)

Impairment, disability, and handicap

In the past, terms such as disability and handicap have been loosely applied. For the purpose of this chapter I shall use the *International classification of impairments, disabilities and handicaps (ICIDH)* (World Health Organization 1980). In essence, 'impairment' refers to the symptoms and signs of arthritis, 'disability' is the resulting loss of function, and 'handicap' is the disadvantage experienced as a result of that disability.

Handicap is determined largely by social and environmental factors, and by the individual's expectations and aspirations. Thus the same level of impairment may lead to very different degrees of handicap in different individuals. For example, relatively mild arthritis in the hands may be devastating to the concert pianist but of little consequence to the cross-country runner, while similarly mild arthritis of the knees could have the opposite impact.

As health professionals, we tend to measure what we can alter. Doctors traditionally measure impairment, while therapists measure functional loss or disability. Patients and their families tend to be more concerned with handicap, but until recently, very little effort has gone into measurement of handicap or quality of life.

Handicap is only indirectly affected by reducing disability. The main limiting factors are social and environmental — housing, education, employment for example — and are largely beyond the control of healthcare workers.

In the United States the Americans with Disabilities Act now ensures that all public buildings must be fully accessible to disabled people, and an individual cannot be excluded from employment because of disability alone. In the United Kingdom and Europe we still fall a long way behind, but if we are to be the best advocates for our patients, we must measure these aspects and continue to apply pressure to improve the lot of our disabled patients.

Measurement of disability

If we are to manage disability effectively, it is essential that we measure it in order to be able to assess the outcome of our endeavours. There are two main types of measure for disability, specific and generic. Generic measures take a global view of disability and record it in a standardized manner that allows comparison. It is essential to collect generic information to allow comparison of different programmes, populations, and practices, but we must also realize that these scores often show little relevance to how individual patients function in their own environment. To assess this, we require specific measurements.

For example, incontinence is a major cause of disability and handicap, something we all dread. Stiffness, immobility, and poor dexterity combine to make it a common problem for patients with arthritis, many of whom are middle-aged to elderly women with a degree of urinary urgency and frequency. If we want to know whether a patient can get to the toilet in time, it matters not how long it takes them to walk a standard 10 m, or undo three standard buttons on a standard garment. What matters is how long it takes them to get to their toilet from their usual chair in the daytime, or from their bed at night, and once in the toilet, how long it takes them to undress and position themselves appropriately to pass urine without spillage (Turner-Stokes and Frank 1992). The presence or absence of a downstairs toilet, or a commode in the bedroom, may make the critical difference between continence and incontinence.

Measurement of disability therefore requires a combination of specific and generic measures. No one instrument will suffice. A large number of disability scores have been produced, some well validated, others not. It is important to select a scale that is set at the right level. The Barthel score, for example, is used widely for patients with neurological disability. It has pronounced floor and ceiling effects and, although reliably scored between different observers, it is relatively unresponsive to change, which makes it unsuitable for assessing functional outcome in most patients with arthritis.

Some instruments require an independent observer, others have been developed for self-completion. One of the most widely used functional scores is the Stanford Health Assessment Questionnaire, which was developed in the United States, but has subsequently been translated into English practice and validated for self-completion by Kirwan and Reeback (1986). If routinely completed by patients while they wait for a clinic appointment, Health Assessment Questionnaire scores can provide a useful serial record of disability and its change with time.

Measurement of handicap and quality of life

As mentioned earlier, disability is not the only outcome measure that should be recorded. Handicap and quality of life are more important to the patient and their family, but more often than not we have no indication of whether our treatment is having any impact at all in these areas (see also Chapter 1. 1.5).

An abbreviated list of potentially useful generic scales is given in Table 1. The London Handicap Scale was developed for stroke patients, and the Community Integration Questionnaire for patients with brain injury, but both collect information in a standardized way that is potentially useful for patients with arthritis.

A number of instruments have been developed to assess quality of life in relation to health, including the General Health Questionnaire, the Nottingham Health Profile, the Sickness Impact Profile, and the SF-36. The SF-36 in particular has been designed for ease of use and is gaining popularity. It could potentially provide useful information on quality of life for patients with arthritis and their families. However, as yet it has not been validated for use with disabled patients

or their carers, so any information obtained should be treated with caution.

Patients in the early stages of arthritis may not be significantly disabled other than by pain, and standard disability scores may not be suitable. Alternatives such as the Multidimensional Pain Inventory may be useful, not only for measuring the impact of their symptoms but also the extent to which they use positive coping strategies to combat them.

These are just a few of the scales that have been developed. None of them is perfect and they all have somewhat different emphasis. When selecting an instrument, careful examination of all of the items included will indicate which is the most relevant to the population under study. Although some scales apply weighting to different items, so that they perform as interval scales, it should be remembered that most measures provide ordinal data, which should not be submitted to simple mathematical manipulation such as summing or averaging. Rasch analysis is a method of applying a mathematical model to ordinal data, so that they behave as interval data. Its role is currently being explored in this area, but it is too early to say if this will prove useful. Whichever instrument is used, it should be applied only with reference to the original manual, and careful thought should be given to the mode of analysis employed.

Functional anatomy and disability in arthritis

The hand

Functional dexterity of the hand is more advanced in man than in any other species, and it is our ability to manipulate objects in our environment that has allowed us to capitalize on our large cerebral capacity. The two major functions of the hand are the power grip the precision or pincer grip. If these are limited by weakness or pain, the hand rapidly becomes non-functional. Opposition, required for the pincer

Table 1 Modalities and examples of available measures for assessing patients with arthritis

Modality to be measured	Instrument	Reference
Impairment	Ritchie index	Ritchie *et al.* (1968)
Disability	Health Assessment Questionnaire (HAQ)	Kirwan and Reeback (1986)
	Functional Independent Measure (FIM)	Heineman *et al.* (1993)
Handicap	London Handicap Scale	Harwood *et al.* (1994)
	Community Integration Questionnaire	Willer *et al.* (1994)
Quality of Life	SF-36	Garatt *et al.* (1993)
	General Health Questionnaire	Goldberg and Hillier (1979)
	Nottingham Health Profile	Hunt *et al.* (1981)
Depression	Beck depression score	Beck *et al.* (1976)
Anxiety	Spielberger score	Spielberger *et al.* (1970)
Psychological response to pain and disability	Sickness Impact Profile (SIP)	Bergner *et al.* (1976)
	Multi-dimensional pain inventory	Kerns *et al.* (1985)

grip, is often lost, but patients will learn to oppose the side of the thumb, which provides adequate function.

Rupture of extensor tendons is commonly regarded as a rheumatological emergency, but surgical repair is necessary not so much to provide active extension as to prevent the dropped fingers getting in the way of hand function. The importance of hand function cannot be overstressed. Patients and their medical attendants often crave cosmesis, but cosmetic repair undertaken at the expense of function is almost universally disastrous.

The wrist

The wrist provides a mechanism to extend the range of activity of the hand, and a fulcrum to stabilize the grip. Some 30° of wrist extension is required for optimal power grip, and if function is limited by painful wrists, arthrodesis may be considered. Careful attention should be paid, however, to the position of arthrodesis. To be able to wipe their own bottom, a patient requires at least 30° of wrist flexion, so if bilateral arthrodesis is undertaken, one wrist should be in flexion and one in extension. If one wrist has spontaneously fused, its position must be considered when fusing the other.

The elbow and shoulder

These joints are often restricted in rheumatoid arthritis but, in functional terms, it is their combined range that is important. Is it sufficient to allow the hand to reach to the mouth for feeding, to the back of the head for grooming, and to the perineum for maintaining personal hygiene?

Flexion deformities of the elbow are usually well documented but restriction of 20 to 30° is functionally unimportant on its own. Meanwhile, the radioulnar joints are often forgotten, but they allow supination and pronation, which are essential to optimal hand function.

The spine

Involvement of the cervical spine may result in subluxation and dislocation, which is not only a source of painful disability and disturbed sleep, but may result in cord compression. Patients with atlantoaxial subluxation must be taught to protect the neck from sudden movements, for example when motoring or using public transport.

The hip

Hip restriction results in immobility and stiffness that can be severely limiting. Climbing stairs, getting in and out of the bath, and sitting comfortably on the toilet all require hip flexion. For young women, abduction as well as flexion is required for sexual intercourse and childbirth.

The knee

The locking mechanism of the knee, which allows us to stand for long periods without using much muscle power, requires not only full extension but also rotation in the last 5 to 10°. Failure to achieve this severely limits standing, and flexion deformities of 20° or more make walking extremely difficult.

The ankle and foot

The true ankle joint allows plantar and dorsiflexion, and the subtalar joint, abduction and adduction. Restriction of the subtalar joints make walking on rough ground difficult.

Metatarsalgia, which is often a hallmark of rheumatoid arthritis, results from dropped metatarsal heads. If, as a doctor, you do only one thing for a patient, education about appropriate footwear early in the course of disease is probably the greatest contribution you can make to maintaining mobility (see 'Footwear' below).

Systemic disease

In addition to specific joint problems the effects of systemic disease itself can be severely limiting. Fatigue, anaemia, muscle wasting all take their toll, quite apart from morning stiffness, which may require the patient to get up several hours earlier to prepare for work or get the family off to school, for example. General advice on sensible eating, exercise, and sleeping patterns is important and should not be overlooked.

Psychological reaction (see Chapter 1.1.6)

Traditionally last on the list, the psychological impact of arthritis should in reality come first. Few of us can readily imagine what it is like to live with constant pain. Response to pain can vary enormously between patients. We are all familiar with the 'typus robustus' who denies pain despite gross destructive disease, while others are totally incapacitated but have relatively minor visible signs.

A variety of psychological and social factors may interact to sensitize or desensitize patients to the effects of pain. Depression, altered body image with poor self-esteem, altered sexuality, role reversal in marriage, as well as intellect, comprehension, and expectations, will all affect a patient's perception of pain and disability. The standard 15-min medical outpatient appointment in the United Kingdom National Health Service does not allow for sensible appraisal of these factors even though it is they, and not drugs or blood tests, that will ultimately determine outcome.

Medical and social models of rehabilitation

Many areas of medicine are currently going through a period of substantial change and rehabilitation is no exception. The days are gone when the doctor reigned supreme over the patient's care and wrote detailed prescriptions of exactly what physiotherapy should entail, usually based on very little understanding. Instead we have interdisciplinary teams made up of highly trained professionals, each of whom brings specialist knowledge of their own field to the group. In most cases, gone too are the days when the patient was expected simply to be a passive recipient of therapy. It is essential that any programme remains as far as possible within the patient's control. Since it will ultimately be their responsibility to maintain progress by themselves it is important to engage then from the start and failure to do so is the single most important cause of failure to demonstrate long-term benefits of therapy.

There is currently much debate in the United Kingdom over whether rehabilitation services should be provided in the hospital or

Table 2 Important components of rehabilitation for patients with arthritis

1. The co-ordinated activity of an interdisciplinary team
2. Problem-orientated approach:

    Major problems identified and tackled by the team as a whole

    Staged goals set jointly by therapists and patient ± carer
3. Functionally relevant programme with emphasis on:

    Active exercise to maintain:

    > muscle strength,

    > cardiovascular fitness

    > joint mobility

    Education of patient and family on:

    > the nature of the disease

    > joint protection

    > energy conservation
4. Community orientation—avoid hospital visits where possible
5. Cognitive behavioural management introduced from the start
6. Psychological factors actively addressed including:

    Pain

    Depression

    Sexuality

    Family relationships
7. Social factors are actively addressed including:

    Housing

    Education

    Finance

    Employment

    Retraining for work and leisure
8. Arranging access to support services such as:

    Mobility and transport

    Footwear and chiropody

    Advice on equipment

    Information about services and how to find them
9. A commitment either to long-term follow-up and reassessment, or alternatively to direct access by self-referral

Table 3 Professions included in a rheumatological interdisciplinary team

> Doctor
>
> Nurse
>
> Physiotherapist
>
> Occupational therapist
>
> Psychologist
>
> Counsellor
>
> Orthotist
>
> Dietitian
>
> Chiropodist
>
> Social worker
>
> Rehabilitation engineer

The principles of rehabilitation

Whichever model of rehabilitation is adopted, the principles are essentially the same. Rehabilitation has been defined in many different terms, but ultimately it involves restoring an individual to their maximal functional independence. It consists of two main parts:

(1) restitution: restoring lost function by minimizing impairment;

(2) substitution: compensation for residual functional loss by using alternative techniques, aids, or appliances.

In practice these two approaches are often applied simultaneously and a problem-orientated approach will combine restorative therapy, teaching compensatory techniques, and the use of a variety of aids and appliances. The important components of rehabilitation for patients with arthritis can be summarized as in Table 2.

Problem-orientated approach and the interdisciplinary team

The interdisciplinary team

Members of the interdisciplinary team are highly trained professionals in their own right and each brings a specialist knowledge of their own field to the group. Some of the professions that may be included in the rheumatological interdisciplinary team are listed in Table 3.

The key to good rehabilitation is teamwork (Fig. 1) and this requires coordination and a team leader. The doctor may not necessarily be that leader—having good medical skills is not synonymous with having team management skills—but is nevertheless an essential part of the team. Interdisciplinary team management allows individual members of the team to refer to any other, without going back through the coordinator. Opinion and action are thus obtained more quickly, and are more likely to be relevant to the original question.

community setting. This is the wrong question. Services should clearly be provided in both settings. The question should be how to identify the most suitable service for a given individual and how to ensure that they have access to it. Some patients are ill and require rehabilitation in the context of their medical management. Others are not ill and reasonably demand the right to exercise choice over the services they wish to use. The medical and social models of rehabilitation are not, therefore, mutually exclusive, it is more a question of 'horses for courses' (appropriateness).

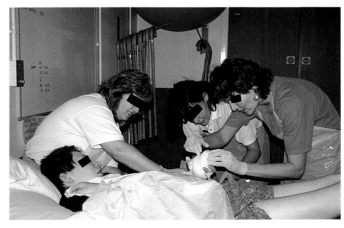

(a)

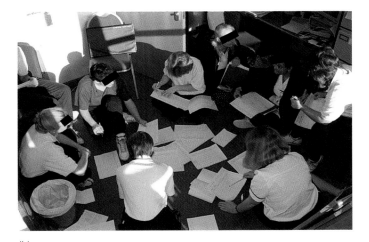

(b)

Fig. 1 An effective interdisciplinary team requires a coordinated approach both with, and away from, the patient. (a) A doctor, physiotherapist, and occupational therapist join forces to splint a hand in order to meet both therapeutic and functional requirements; (b) the key to coordinated therapy is integrated timetabling.

The problem-orientated approach

Rather than members working individually within their own professional boundaries, the well-coordinated interdisciplinary team provides a unified, problem-orientated approach. The individual problems that limit a patient's independence are identified and tackled systematically by achieving a series of staged goals set by the patient and therapists together. If at all possible, goals should be set, together with a date at which they will be reviewed. This helps to focus both patient and therapists on exactly what has to be done. It is immediately clear when progress is not being made, so that the reasons for this can be explored. It is essential that objectives and treatment are functionally relevant to the patient in their normal environment, and very often this will involve the active participation of the carer as well.

Contents of the rehabilitation programme

Exercise

Although some textbooks in circulation still have 'bed rest' at the top of their list of management, it is now almost universally accepted that bed rest is bad for patients with arthritis, resulting in flexion contractures, osteopenia, and muscle wasting. Instead it is recognized that active use and weight bearing through joints maintains bone and muscle strength. Nevertheless, patients must be taught to apply these principles sensibly. An exercise programme should contain the four elements listed in Table 4. Wherever possible, exercise should be put in a social context, taking advantage of local leisure facilities that patients can have access to outside the hospital environment. Once again, advice on appropriate footwear for exercise is an essential part of the programme.

Education

Education of the patient and family is vital to the continued success of the rehabilitation process. They need to know what to expect from the disease, what to expect from rehabilitation, what they can do to maximize benefit, and what they must do to avoid exacerbating the condition. Education must begin one-to-one, although it can be continued in group sessions, with the help of leaflets and audio- and videotapes to digest at home. Introduction to patient support and self-care groups can also be extremely helpful, not only for

To maintain:	Type of exercise	For example:
Muscle strength	Isometric exercise: to build up muscle bulk and strength	Quadriceps drill But the programme must be tailored to the age and fitness of the patient
Joint mobility	Active exercise to maintain joint range	Pendular and wall-climbing exercises for the shoulder
Limbering up	Programme of daily exercises to combat early morning stiffness	Working the hands in a basin of warm water
Cardiovascular fitness	Physical stamina, cardiac and respiratory function	Swimming, cycling, walking, dancing

Table 4　The main components of an exercise programme

Table 5	The principles of joint protection

1. Use the strongest and largest joints possible to accomplish a task
2. Spread the load of carrying/lifting over several joints
3. Use each joint in its most stable functional position
4. Maintain joint mobility and function
5. Avoid maintaining a joint in one position for a long time—especially in positions that exacerbate deformity, e.g. avoid sleeping with a pillow under the knees
6. Avoid excessive activity
7. Pace activity: punctuate periods of activity with regular rest periods

obtaining advice and information, but for the comfort of knowing they are not alone in their suffering.

Joint protection

Trauma exacerbates inflammatory arthritis, whereas careful use of muscle and joints can reduce pain and fatigue. The main objectives of a joint protection programme are therefore to reduce pain, prevent damage and deformity, and conserve energy. The principles are outlined in Table 5.

Energy conservation

While bed rest is to be avoided, fatigue is one of the major causes of disability in arthritis. In order to avoid the inappropriate blitzing the housework and then retiring to bed for 2 days, patients need to be taught to pace their activities and to conserve their energy where possible. Some practical examples of ways to save energy are given in Table 6.

It is not always necessary to prescribe special equipment. Some examples of standard modern labour-saving devices that may be helpful for patients with arthritis are listed in Table 7. These are relatively inexpensive, readily come by, and more often acceptable to patients than having a house full of special adaptations that advertise their disability to every visitor.

Community-orientated supervision

Whatever techniques are instituted in hospital, follow-up into the home is necessary to ensure that advice given is appropriate. It is common experience that specific advice given on joint protection and energy conservation changes when the patient is seen in their own environment. Time-consuming though a home visit may be, it will save time in the long run.

Likewise, exercises will only be continued if they are functionally appropriate, and this too is much easier to gauge in the context of the home environment. Reassessment at home every 2 to 3 months allows plans to be made in the context of the normal environment and avoids painful, slow, and unreliable ambulance journeys to hospital.

Home assessment is also vital in considering the need for structural changes or adaptations. Some areas to consider are given

Table 6	Practical example of ways to conserve energy

(a) *Personal care*

Dress sitting down

Avoid back-fastening or tight-fitting clothes

Shower rather than bathing if possible

Avoid low chairs

(b) *Domestic*

Reorganize the kitchen so that all frequently used equipment is readily to hand

Do all activities in sitting where possible, using a perch stool

Avoid lifting and carrying—move heavy objects using a trolley

Use both hands

Use a jug to fill the kettle, rather than lifting the kettle itself

Steam or microwave vegetables to avoid lifting heavy pans

Soak pans immediately after cooking

Use duvets on the beds instead of blankets

Plan domestic chores sensibly, for example:

    Complete upstairs tasks and then the downstairs ones to avoid frequent trips up and down the stairs

    Intersperse heavier tasks with lighter ones

    Use modern labour-saving devices wherever possible

Table 7	Standard modern labour-saving devices that may be helpful for patients with arthritis

Food processor, blender

Electric tin-opener

Portable telephone

Remote control for television, video, hi-fi etc.

Dishwasher

Front-loading automatic washer/dryer

Computer/word-processor

Automatic car—power steering

in Table 8, but first some basic information is needed about mobility and transfers.

Mobility, transfers, and stairs

Is the patient in a wheelchair? If so, consider (i) whether ramps are needed, (ii) are the door frames wide enough to pass through

Table 8 Some areas to consider in assessment of the home environment

Access

Can they get in and out of the house through the front or back door?

Can they move from room to room inside the house?

If living on more than one level, can they get up and downstairs:

  If not, could a stairlift or through-floor lift be installed?

How will they get to the toilet by day and during the night?

Can they get to washing/showering facilities?

Inside the home

Is furniture suitable and conveniently placed?

Remove potential hazards, e.g. slip rugs

Are plugs and switches at reachable height?

Security

Can they control their own front door?

How will they summon help in an emergency?

Kitchen

Are frequently used items stored conveniently?

Are work surfaces at a suitable height?

Can they use the basic equipment?

Bathroom and lavatory

Can they get into the shower or bath?

Is any special equipment needed such as:

  Bathing aids,

  Raised toilet seat

  Rails, tap handles?

Bedroom

Height of bed—can they get in and out of it?

Is the mattress suitable—are they are risk of pressure sores?

Is a commode needed for toileting at night?

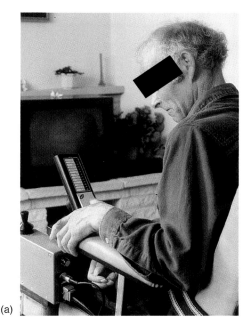

(a)

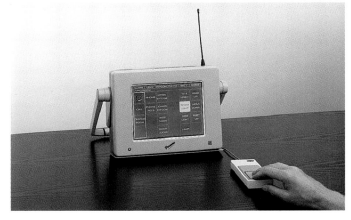

(b)

Fig. 2 An environmental control unit may be used with a range of single switches and operated by almost any movement that is under reliable voluntary control. Remote control by radio waves or infrared avoids the need for fixed wiring. (a) A wheelchair-mounted Steeper FOX system; (b) the Steeper Persona.

without trapping their fingers, and (iii) is there room to manoeuvre. Are they able to transfer themselves from the wheelchair independently; if so, do they need equipment such as grab rails or a sliding board? If on their feet, can they manage stairs? If so, do they need one rail or two? Note: if a walking stick is used, only one hand is free to hold a rail to go upstairs, but a rail is needed on the opposite side coming down unless they are able to use the walking stick in the opposite hand.

Environmental control

For severely disabled people who live alone, the use of a computer to control the home environment has now become commonplace, but the availability of this facility is often forgotten. Its use requires neither dexterity nor high-powered cognitive function, and, using scanning software and an appropriate on–off switch, almost any movement that is under reliable voluntary control may be used to operate an environmental control unit (Fig. 2). A sample of available switch types is given in Table 9, and the sort of functions they may be used to control in Table 10.

Psychosocial aspects

Despite the best endeavours of a multiprofessional team, the functional outcome from rehabilitation of patients with arthritis remains dependent on psychosocial factors, which include:

(1) personality: coping style, self-esteem and motivation;

(2) section of community: class, intellect, and education;

(3) patient's reaction to disability: e.g. depression, denial;

Table 9 Some types of on–off switch that may be used for controlling an environmental control unit

Switch type	Movement that operates it
Plate switch	Pressure from hand or foot
Button switch	Pressure from thumb or finger
Chin or head switch	Pressure from chin or head
Eye blink	Movement of eyelid
Suck-and-puff	Sucking and blowing
Tongue plate	Touch of tongue on palate plate

Table 10 Common functions that may be controlled by an environmental control unit

Alarm

Intercom

Control of front-door lock

Telephone

Opening/closing curtains

Control of electric sockets for heaters/fans/lights

Control of radio/television

Communication aid

Computer

(4) family's reaction: sympathy, overprotection, anger;

(5) supportive network: family, friends, workmates;

(6) environment, housing, transport;

(7) financial security, employment.

Active psychological support is essential to allow patients and families to work through the changes that have occurred in their lives and to re-establish their relationships on a positive basis.

Cognitive behavioural rehabilitation techniques have been used extensively in patients with chronic pain. They involve teaching them how to use coping strategies to increase their activity despite the pain and regain control over their lives. The approach is shown to be beneficial not only in increasing activity levels but also in reducing depression and anxiety. More recently the approach has been successfully applied to patents with arthritis (O'Leary *et al.* 1988) but it is essential that it is introduced in the early stages of disease. It is also essential to involve the family and carers because they must be prepared to stand back and allow the patient to regain control of his or her own life.

Sexual problems

Sexual problems are extremely common when one member of the partnership has arthritis and may arise from a number of factors listed in Table 11.

Young patients with arthritis often encounter difficulties with forming relationships because of the above problems and also due to lack of access to dances, clubs, and other traditional courting scenes.

It is important to remember that sexual problems are not confined to marriage, heterosexuality or to the under-60s. Patients often have to be given the right to talk about it, but a busy clinic is not the time or the place. A number of organizations provide trained sexual counselling specifically for people with disabilities (for example, in the United Kingdom, SPOD, is the Association to Aid the Sexual and Personal Relationships of People with a Disability). The wise physician will keep to hand the telephone number of their local service.

Aids and appliances

In general, aids help to compensate for either pain and weakness or for lack of joint range. Some aids that are particularly useful to patients with arthritis are listed in Table 12 and illustrated in Fig. 3. However, they must be carefully chosen with specific needs in mind. Articles must be lightweight, strong and reliable, cheap, and acceptable to the patient and family.

Table 11 Factors that may contribute to sexual dysfunction in patients with arthritis

Altered body image in the face of physical deformity

Joint restriction—limiting usual positioning for sexual intercourse, in particular the missionary position

Fatigue and loss of libido

Poor cardiovascular fitness—inability to sustain activity for long enough to achieve orgasm

Hand deformity—impeding foreplay and fitting of contraceptive devices

Fear of pain leading to frigidity and impotence

Table 12 Aids likely to be useful to patient with arthritis

To compensate for weakness or pain

Thick-handled utensils—require less effort to grip

Key turners and other easy-to-grip devices

Lever tap handles

To compensate for lack of joint range

Long-handled utensils—extend effective reach

Raised chair, toilet seat—easier to stand up from

Velcro fasteners on clothes—require less dexterity than zips and buttons

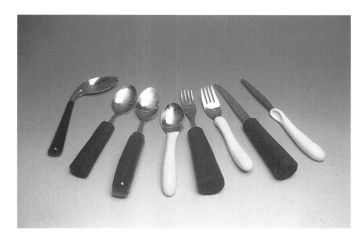

(a)

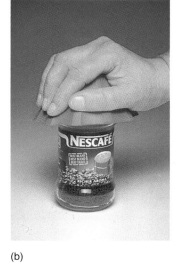

(b)

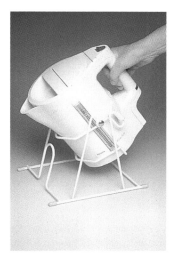

(c)

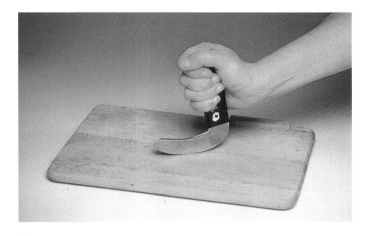

(d)

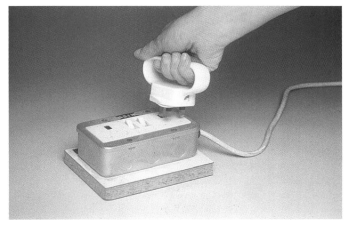

(e)

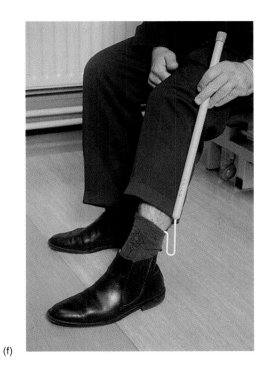

(f)

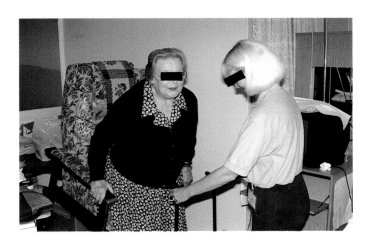

(g)

Fig. 3 Some aids that may be useful to a patient with arthritis. (a) Thick-handled utensils; (b) rubber grip-pad; (c) kettle rocker-stand; (d) angled chopping knife; (e) plug with grip-handle; (f) Easi-reach device; (g) ejector chair.

Orthoses

An orthosis is a device worn outside the body that aids function, protects, or prevents pain. One easy way to waste money is to provide orthoses that patients never wear. Worse, an inappropriately prescribed orthosis can actually enhance damage and deformity.

In order to avoid this great care must be paid in prescription to ensure that:

(1) the device is well fitting and does the right job;

(2) the patient is able to put it on and take it off easily;

(3) both patient and carers know how, when, and why to use it;

(4) the device is acceptable to the patient.

Because of these factors it is vital that the orthosis be checked after fitting and reviewed at each prescription. 'Stabilized' prescriptions that replicate the device when it wears out should only be signed when a trained orthotist is available to supervise subsequent fittings and has the experience and authority to alter the specifications in accordance with need. Unless this is so, each orthosis should be prescribed and checked by a suitable experienced physician — which by and large does not include junior medical staff.

Splints and orthoses have a special role in childhood arthritis. Some forms of juvenile arthritis are likely to remit by the time the time the child reaches adulthood. Splints form a vital part of management in preventing deformity so that when synovitis does resolve the joint still has optimal range and function. Hand splints (working and resting), knee splints, and shoe raises should be regularly reviewed to ensure this outcome as the child grows.

Adults tends to be less tolerant of non-functional splints, usually not having parents at home to bully them into wearing splints for certain parts of the day or night. Therefore, in adult arthritis, the emphasis on splint wearing is to increase function by stabilizing the joint and reducing pain more than preventing deformity.

Orthoses may be custom-made or provided ready-made or 'off the shelf'.

Off-the-shelf orthoses

Commonly prescribed items in rheumatology include the following.

Futura wrist splints
These stabilize the wrist in 30° extension and in theory act as a working splint. In practice they either fail to support the wrist adequately or the extensor bar effectively prevents useful function. Many physicians do not realize that the extensor bar is malleable and should be specifically adjusted when the splint is prescribed to ensure a good fit.

Cervical collars

Soft collars
Soft collars can be used to support the neck relieving painful muscle spasm, especially at night.

Hard collars
For patients with cervical subluxation, a hard collar is recommended while motoring or using public transport, to avoid dislocation with sudden jarring movements. In practice, they are so uncomfortable that patients rarely comply with this advice; a soft collar may be less protective but at least it is more likely to be worn.

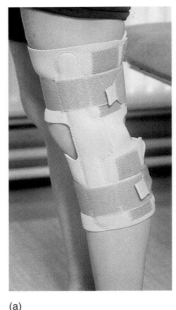
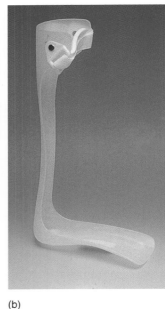

(a)   (b)

Fig. 4 'Off-the-shelf' orthoses: (a) lightweight SK knee brace; (b) ankle–foot orthosis.

Knee braces
Lightweight SK knee braces (Fig. 4(a)) are often prescribed for unstable knees, but are rarely able to provide adequate support. A range of more sophisticated devices is now available, which can be adjusted to allow a defined range of flexion and extension as well as providing mediolateral support. These heavier braces are more supportive, but many patients who need to use them will then need help getting them on and off.

Ankle–foot orthoses
Ankle–foot orthoses (Fig. 4(b)) provide dorsiflexion at the ankle, for example where foot drop results from vasculitic nerve damage. The orthosis fits inside the shoes and usually requires a shoe that is one size larger than normal. Although ankle–foot orthoses are available off the shelf, if one is to be worn for any length of time a custom-made one that is moulded to the foot is more satisfactory.

Custom-made orthoses

In general, custom-made orthoses (principally splints) are more satisfactory if someone of sufficient experience is available to make them. Splints can help to reduce deformity or increase function by:

(1) stabilization of a joint;

(2) reducing pain by immobilization;

(3) maintaining passive joint range;

(4) functional positioning during activity;

(5) protection leading to greater confidence in use.

Working splints are designed to be used during functional activity, for example cock-up wrist splints that leave the fingers free and support the wrist in 30° extension. Dynamic splints have a moving part that allows either free movement or movement against resistance provided by a spring or a piece of elastic. These may be used for example to correct flexion contractures. Resting splints hold the joint or limb in an optimal position and many be used to combat pain or prevent deformity. For example, paddle splints help to maintain finger extension, but because they render the hand useless, they are usually worn at night.

Footwear

Advice on appropriate footwear may be the single most useful thing you can provide for patients. Patients with arthritis should not wear silly shoes, except on very special occasions, and all sloppy slippers should be thrown away.

Appropriate footwear has the following characteristics:

(1) adequate width and height to accommodate the toes;

(2) soft rubber sole and padded insole to provide shock absorption for the metatarsal heads;

(3) arch-support insole and strong medial side of shoe to prevent valgus deformity of the ankle and spread weight evenly across the weight-bearing areas of the foot.

Trainers or sneakers provide all of these features and are often acceptable to younger patients. Older women may prefer a leather casual, but Ecco and Roehide are two shoe manufacturers whose lines include all of the above features. In the United Kingdom, their products are obtainable in some high-street shoe shops, e.g. Clark's and K Shoes.

Alternatively, an arch support insole may be fitted into an existing pair of strong shoes (Fig. 5(a)), but this will tend to be bulky and reduce the depth of the shoe so that the toes may rub on the leather upper. This is particularly a problem with flexion deformities of the toes and may lead to callous formation and ulceration over the interphalangeal joints. Extra-depth shoes can be prescribed to combat this problem and are available off the shelf in styles that are not readily distinguishable from ordinary footwear (Fig. 5(b)).

Metatarsal pads are often prescribed but are rarely of any help as they fail to support the weight-bearing surface of the foot. The standard arch-support insole provided by most orthotics departments is made of expanded polystyrene. Some have three little discs in the metatarsal areas, which are designed to cushion the metatarsal heads but more often than not merely exacerbate metatarsalgia. Sorbithane is a highly shock-absorbent material and arch-support insoles made of Sorbithane are available in many sports shops. Although more expensive, they are generally much more satisfactory and worth the initial outlay as they are resilient and can be moved from shoe to shoe.

Mobility

Although doctors spend much of their time and effort trying to relieve pain, when patients are asked which aspect of their arthritis affects them the most, their reply is most commonly 'immobility' (Chamberlain and Buchanan 1978). The major problem is mobility outside. Public transport is often totally inaccessible, and community transport systems for disabled people are limited. Unless they have a car, immobility can severely limit a patients ability to lead a normal life.

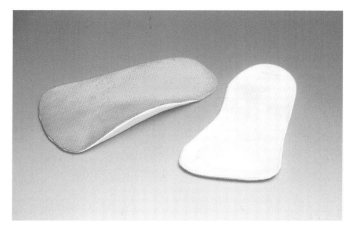

(a)

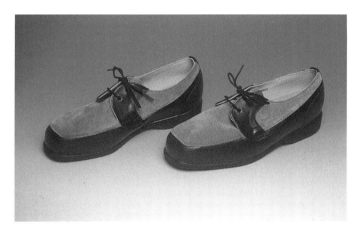

(b)

Fig. 5 Footwear: (a) arch-support insoles with built-in metatarsal pads; (b) extra-depth shoes may be needed to accommodate arch supports.

Walking aids

The choice of a walking aid must take into account a number of factors including the extent of involvement of lower and upper limbs, and the terrain to be negotiated. Often a patient may require a variety of walking aids to use under different circumstances.

A walking stick can provide confidence as well a mechanical advantage if it is the right length and the patient is taught to use it correctly — usually held in the opposite hand to the affected lower limb. Attention should be paid to the comfort of the handle for patients with hand involvement — a moulded Fischer handle helps to spread the weight evenly in the presence of hand deformity (Fig. 6).

Elbow crutches give a firmer base and a gutter crutch allows patients with severe involvement of the hand and elbow to bear weight on the forearm. It should be remembered, however, that bilateral use of sticks or crutches effectively impedes carrying anything other than a bag slung over the shoulder and the width of the base of a two-crutch user is wider than that of a wheelchair. Walking frames provide a more stable alternative (Fig. 7), although some patients feel that they carry a greater stigma of disability, and they cannot give support while going up and down stairs.

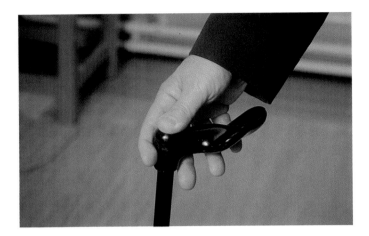

(a)

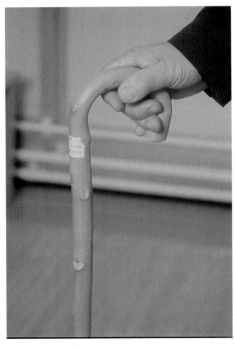

(b)

Fig. 6 Walking aids: a moulded Fischer handle (a) helps to distributed the weight more evenly across the hand than with a standard walking stick (b).

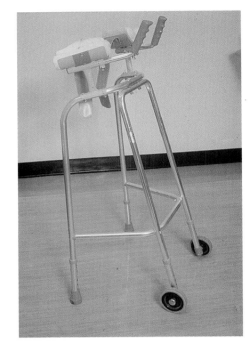

Fig. 7 A gutter rollator walking frame provides stability without putting pressure on the hands.

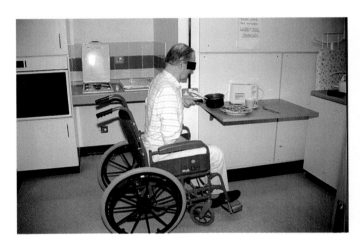

Fig. 8 The large wheels on a self-propelling 9L wheelchair make it easier for an attendant to push; most patients with rheumatoid arthritis are unable to propel much because of shoulder problems.

Any walking aid that is prescribed should be fitted and checked by an experienced physiotherapist, who will ensure that it is the most suitable aid, correctly adjusted, and in safe working order. The physiotherapist will also instruct the patient in its use and maintenance; in particular, ferrules should be checked regularly for wear.

Wheelchairs

Wheelchairs may be regarded as admission of defeat but in reality they can increase mobility, broaden horizons, and conserve energy for more productive use. Attendant-operated (8L) chairs have small wheels that can be difficult to negotiate over kerbs. The larger wheels on a 9L self-propelling chair (Fig. 8) make it easier to push, and

therefore it is usually recommended even though most patients with rheumatoid arthritis who require a wheelchair will be unable to self-propel over any distance because of shoulder involvement.

Electric wheelchairs allow independent mobility for the severely disabled patient (Fig. 9) but a smooth proportional control is essential as jerky movement is not only painful but also dangerous if there is risk of cervical subluxation.

Patients who spend any length of time in a wheelchair are at risk of pressure sores. They require appropriate cushioning and may also need a special seating package, which should be prescribed by a specialist clinic, to correct their position.

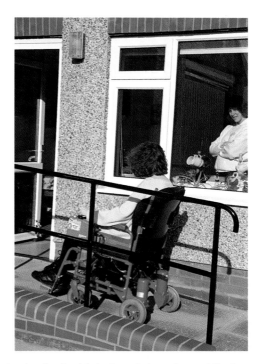

Fig. 9 An electric wheelchair allows independent mobility for severely disabled patients; a smooth proportional control is important where there is risk of cervical subluxation.

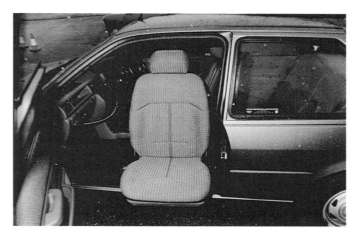

Fig. 10 Swivel seats facilitate getting in and out of a car.

Driving for disabled motorists

A number of adaptations are available for patients who drive, or are regularly driven in a family car. Swivel seats can facilitate getting in and out of the vehicle (Fig. 10). Wide-angled mirrors offer a panoramic rear view without having to turn the head. Headrests are essential to protect patients from rear-shunt whiplash injuries, whether or not they have atlantoaxial subluxation. In the majority of cases, automatic gear shift and powered steering may suffice, but a range of adapted controls is available, and is rapidly becoming more sophisticated (Fig. 11). If considered as potential users of adapted cars, patients should be professionally assessed at a specialist centre such as, in the United Kingdom, Banstead Mobility Centre. Patients unable to walk more than 100 yards (approx. 90 m) may be entitled to a disabled parking permit — known in the United Kingdom as the 'orange badge' — to facilitate convenient parking. This may be applied for through the local authority.

Social factors

While healthcare workers may not have direct influence over factors such as housing, finance, employment, and education, they may be the best advocate that a patient has to help them achieve at least a minimum standard of living. Many patients with arthritis are young, most are cognitively intact and should have good employment prospects given appropriate retraining. Failing that, patients need to be prepared for increased hours of leisure time. Contrary to the views of some doctors, rehabilitation does not end with being able to wash, dress, and make a cup of tea.

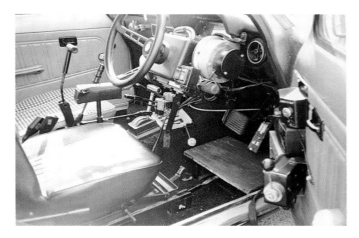

(a)

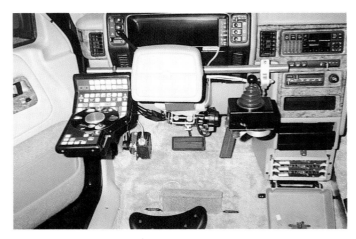

(b)

Fig. 11 The range of devices for controlling a car is becoming more sophisticated. (a) A complex mechanical control system; (b) its modern electronic counterpart.

Acknowledgements

I am grateful for the help of Dr Luay Zebouni and David Hawkins (Steeper Ltd) in collecting illustrative material, and to the Luff Foundation for financial support.

References

Badley, E. M., Thompson, R. P., and Wood, P. H. N. (1978). The prevalence and severity of major disability conditions—a reappraisal of the Government Social Survey of the Handicapped and Impaired in Great Britain. *International Journal of Epidemiology*, 7, 145–51.

Beck, A. T., Ward, C. H., Mendelssohn, M., Mock, J., and Erbaugh, J. (1961). An inventory for measuring depression. *Archives of General Psychiatry*, 4, 561–71.

Bergner, M., Bobbitt, R. A., and Pollard, W. (1976). The sickness impact profile. Validation of the health status measure. *Medical Care*, 14, 56–67.

Chamberlain, M. A. and Buchanan, J. (1978). Mobility in arthritis. *Reports of the Rheumatic Diseases*, 66, 1–2.

Clarke, A. K., Allard, L., and Braybrooks, B. A. (1987). *Rehabilitation in rheumatology: the team approach*. Martin Dunitz, London.

Garratt, A. M., Ruta, D. A., Abdalla, M. L., Buckingham, J. K., and Russell, I. T. (1993). The SF-36 Health Survey Questionnaire: an outcome measure suitable for routine use within the NHS? *British Medical Journal*, 306, 1440–4.

Goldbeg, D. P. and Hillier, V. F. (1979). A scaled version of the General Health Questionnaire. *Psychological Medicine*, 9, 139–45.

Harris, A. I. (1971). *Handicapped and impaired in Great Britain*. HMSO, London.

Harwood, R. H., Rogers, A., Dickinson, E., and Ebrahim, S. (1994). Measuring handicap—the London Handicap Scale. A new outcome measure in chronic disease. *Quality in Healthcare*, 3, 11–16.

Heineman, A. W., Linacre, J. M., Wright, B. D., Hamilton, B. B., and Granger, C. V. (1993). Relationships between impairment and physical disability as measurement by the Functional Independence Measure. *Archives of Physical Medicine and Rehabilitation*, 74, 566–73.

Hunt, S. M., McKenna, S. P., and Williams, J. (1981). Reliability of a population survey tool for measuring perceived health problems: a study of patients with osteoarthritis. *Journal of Epidemiology and Community Health*, 35, 297–300.

Kerns, R. D., Turk, D. C., and Rudy, T. E. (1985). The West-Haven Yale Multidimensional Pain Inventory (WHYMPI). *Pain*, 23, 245–56.

Kirwan, J. R. and Reeback, J. S. (1986). Stanford 1 Health Assessment Questionnaire modified to assess disability in British patients with rheumatoid arthritis. *British Journal of Rheumatology*, 25, 206–9.

O'Leary, A., Shoor, S., Lorig, K., and Holman, H. R. (1988). A cognitive behavioural treatment for rheumatoid arthritis. *Health Psychology*, 7, 527–44.

Ritchie, D. M. *et al.* (1968). Clinical studies with an articular index for the assessment of joint tenderness in patients with rheumatoid arthritis. *Quarterly Journal of Medicine*, 37, 393–406.

Spielberger, C. D., Gorsuch, A., and Lushane, R. (1970). *Manual for the State-Trait Anxiety Inventory*. Consulting Psychologists Press, Palo Alto CA.

Turner-Stokes, L. and Frank, A. O. (1992). Urinary incontinence among patients with arthritis—a neglected disability. *Journal of the Royal Society of Medicine*, 85, 389–93.

Willer, B., Ottenbacher, K. J., and Coad, M. L. (1994). The Community Integration Questionnaire. A comparative examination. *American Journal of Physical Medicine and Rehabilitation*, 73, 103–11.

World Health Organization (1980). *The international classification of impairments, disabilities and handicaps (ICIDH)—a manual of classification relating to the consequences of disease*. WHO, Geneva.

6.4 Rehabilitation of children

Renate Häfner and Marianne Spamer

Introduction

Inflammatory arthritis is the most commonly seen feature in rheumatic disorders of children and adolescents. It occurs most often as idiopathic arthritis with different subtypes (systemic, polyarthritis, oligoarthritis, etc.) but may also be a symptom of an underlying disease such as systemic lupus erythematosus, sarcoidosis, or Behçet's syndrome. Rehabilitation follows the same principles as for all arthritic disorders. The therapy offered must give careful consideration to the child's age and developmental status, the pattern of joint involvement, and the individual disease course.

Some autoimmune rheumatic diseases such as juvenile dermatomyositis where muscular involvement is predominant or skin fibrosis, such as scleroderma, can lead to functional impairment and joint contractures without the presence of an overt arthritis. Patients with these conditions benefit from different therapy protocols.

Aims of rehabilitation — a multidisciplinary team approach

The different aspects of rehabilitation require the co-operation of several health-care professionals who work together to improve the child's function, independence, and self-esteem. This includes caring for the whole family and overseeing integration into the community. The team is usually guided and co-ordinated by a paediatric rheumatologist. It includes a physiotherapist, occupational therapist, social worker, and psychologist. The team members co-operate with each other and interact with community and school staff (Table 1).

The physiotherapist works together with the occupational therapist to improve function of individual joints as well as general mobility. They are also responsible for correction of joint deformity, which often requires individual splinting. Increased mobility forms the basis for greater independence. Children with marked impairment benefit from additional self-care support by an experienced occupational therapist. Most children can learn to master daily activities like hair washing, combing, dressing, feeding, and going to the toilet without extra help. However, they may need some specially adapted equipment. Instructions for joint protection should always be part of the therapy programme.

The child's rheumatic disease always has an impact on the whole family. Physiotherapy, doctor's visits, transportation to school, and other activities are time-consuming. Financial hardship in such families is common. Siblings may feel neglected and parents are

Table 1 Achievements of a multidisciplinary health-care team; the paediatric rheumatologist co-ordinates all team activities

Achievements	Team members
Improved joint function and mobility (proper joint positioning, correction of deformities)	Physiotherapist, occupational therapist
Self-care and independence	Occupational therapist
Integration into school	Social worker, occupational therapist, school staff (teacher, school nurse)
Guidance of the whole family	Social worker, psychologist
Promoting self-esteem	All team members

usually overburdened with the extra tasks and worries, so rehabilitation must include care for the whole family, which is where the social worker has an important part to play. The social worker gives advice on financial entitlements, may help organize transportation, and assist with individual social problems. A psychologist can be helpful to handle conflict situations.

A very important aspect of rehabilitation involves integrating the child into school life. To achieve this, it is necessary for several health-care professionals to co-ordinate contact with teachers and other school staff to highlight the child's needs and help organize school life with the minimum of disruption for all concerned.

Perhaps the team's most important role is psychological — to create the highest possible level of integration so that children cease to see themselves as sick and different and acquire a sense of belonging.

Rehabilitation of chronic arthritis

Management of arthritis in children requires a wide-ranging knowledge of how functional impairment and deformities develop in individuals. The therapist must always keep in mind the progress of deformity and try to thwart this vicious circle as early as possible. It is much more beneficial to prevent deformities than to treat them.

Development of joint deformities

Inflammatory arthritis is very painful. Pain in children with arthritis, however, is often neglected as small children in particular rarely complain of painful joints. It is therefore important to note non-verbal expressions of pain (Scott *et al.* 1977; Melvin 1989; Altenbockum *et al.* 1993; Truckenbrodt 1993). Unfortunately children rapidly adapt to painful arthritis with a reflex pain-relieving positioning of the affected joint. This is always a malposition which in turn produces a muscular imbalance. Those muscles which draw the joint into the relieving position become hypertonic, and the antagonists become weak (Altenbockum *et al.* 1993; Truckenbrodt 1993). If caught at an early stage the deformity can still be corrected passively. If inflammation and pain persist the incorrect position becomes permanent and a normal part of daily activities. The deformity usually increases during physical activity. Finally neither active nor passive correction is possible; a fixed deformity has developed. Incorrect weight distribution on the joints favours arthritic destruction which increases pain and deformity; hence, the vicious circle. At this stage a complete restoration of joint function is nearly impossible. Unaffected neighbouring joints can develop secondary deformities through compensatory over- or misloading. If neighbouring joints are also affected, primary and secondary deformities combine.

Principles of physiotherapy

It is the aim of all therapeutic approaches to keep or restore joint function and alignment as much as possible and achieve a normal pattern of mobility (Jarvis 1980; Erlandson 1989; Melvin 1989; Altenbockum *et al.* 1993). Even slight restrictions of joint function must be taken seriously and treated. In this regard it is important to appreciate that children have a greater joint mobility than adults. Joint function which is normal in adults may already be impaired in a child and must be treated accordingly.

As a precondition for effective physiotherapy the child must relax during treatment, as fear and pain increase muscle tone and intensify the reflex pain-relieving position. A relationship of trust between child and therapist is of the utmost importance in achieving the most beneficial environment and results.

Physiotherapy starts with passive-assisted movement of the joint which is non-weight-bearing. This manoeuvre is carried out with the utmost care within the pain-free range of movement and the best possible corrected axis. Thus even acutely inflamed and painful joints can be treated and protected from functional impairment. Careful movement reduces pain and improves mobility through relaxation of the hypertonic muscle groups.

Next the hypertonic and shortened muscle groups, which keep the joint in its incorrect position, must be stretched together with the other shortened joint structures. This procedure requires a relief position, and joint protection must be considered. Strong leverage to the joint should be avoided and positions such as hand prop, heel posture, or squatting are contraindicated as they increase intra-articular pressure. Stretching must be maintained over a long period of time to become effective. Individual splints may be used to maintain the corrected position. However, active stretching procedures such as hold–relax techniques should be restricted to non-inflamed joints, since they produce high intra-articular pressure.

A further step to extend mobility involves activation of the muscle groups which counteract the deformity. The child learns first with support by the therapist, and then on his or her own to rectify the incorrect position by tensing specific muscles.

Finally, the child must learn to integrate the regained mobility into daily life, overcoming the pathological patterns of movement. Muscular co-ordination is first trained by slow, consciously controlled movements. Frequent repetition of simple actions helps to integrate these into daily activities. In the beginning the therapist will need to support and correct the joint movements. Later more complex and faster movements can be achieved unaided. It is important, however, to adapt the training to the child's abilities. If the patient is overburdened by movements that are too complex, he or she will fall back into the unphysiological pattern of motion. This can lead to deterioration in the function of the involved joints.

Some therapists recommend strengthening of the weak muscles as a first step to overcome weakness and joint deformities (Jarvis 1980; Erlandson 1989; Melvin 1989). In our experience, however, this is ineffective as long as inflammation persists, joint alignment has not been regained adequately, and the child is still accustomed to a pathological pattern of motion. If, however, all these conditions have been restored, training of muscle co-ordination will simultaneously increase muscular power. Forced strengthening of individual muscle groups is rarely necessary and exercises to combat resistance should be discouraged since they increase pressure on the joints (Altenbockum *et al.* 1993).

The cervical spine

Involvement of the cervical spine mostly affects children with systemic onset arthritis and in those with seronegative polyarthritis, rarely in pauciarticular disease. The typical pain-relieving position is in mild flexion with restricted extension. All other movements are also impaired. Cervical spine involvement is easily detected when the child is asked to look up or around. Extensive eye movements compensate for the restricted extension and rotation (Fig. 1). Neck pain can be especially severe in children with systemic disease. It is induced by playing, writing, or working in a sitting position with the head slightly flexed. The cervical spine tends to early ankylosis in juvenile arthritis. Radiographic lesions usually start at the C2/C3 level and progress downwards. Fusion of the whole cervical spine can develop (Fig. 2). Atlantoaxial subluxation is rare in children (Ansell and Kent 1977).

Therapy

Treatment of the cervical spine requires extreme caution and should be carried out in a relief position, preferably with the child lying on his or her back. Careful passive movement in all directions with slight traction can relieve pain and improve function. The dorsolateral neck muscles can be stretched by moving the shoulder girdle while the cervical spine remains in a fixed position. However, if spinal ankylosis has already developed no manipulation should be attempted.

A soft collar relieves pain and muscular tension of the cervical spine. It should be worn during long sedentary periods and as soon as pain starts. Children with severe neck problems may need to wear a collar all day. To aid comfortable sleep, pillows with a neck pad are helpful (Jarvis 1980; Erlandson 1989; Melvin 1989).

The temporomandibular joints

These joints are often neglected since they are mainly affected in children with polyarthritis where many other joint problems

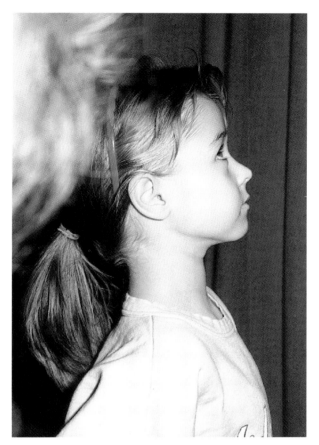

Fig. 1 Child with systemic onset disease and involvement of the cervical spine. Impaired extension is compensated by upward movement of the eyes.

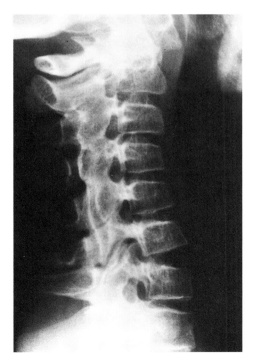

Fig. 2 Spinal ankylosis in a child with systemic juvenile chronic arthritis.

predominate. However, the sequelae of temporomandibular joint involvement can have severe impact on the child's well-being. If these joints become affected in early life significant growth disturbance of the mandible can occur (Bache 1964; Stabrun *et al.* 1988; Melvin 1989). This micrognathia creates malocclusion and disturbs the facial appearance. Restricted mouth opening together with impaired extension of the cervical spine can cause problems if intubation becomes necessary.

Movement of the temporomandibular joint comprises a caudal and ventral gliding of the mandibular condyle to permit mouth opening. Arthritis leads to pain and restriction of both movements, and opening the mouth and lateral displacement of the jaw become impaired (Bache 1964; Melvin 1989) (Fig. 3).

Therapy

Cautious traction with the therapist's thumbs on the dorsal dental rows can mobilize the caudal–ventral motion of the jaw (Fig. 4). Mobilizing grips from outside the mouth are rarely possible since the temporomandibular joint area is very painful and effective therapy would require significant pressure. Active or actively supported exercises with ventral and lateral moving of the jaw are

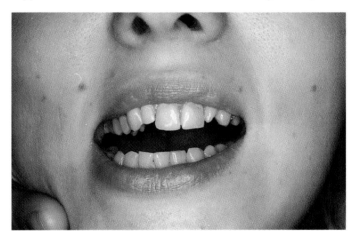

(a)

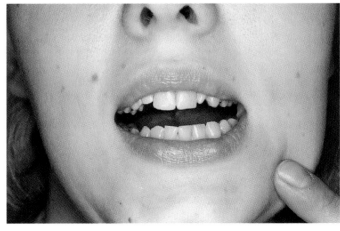

(b)

Fig. 3 Asymmetric involvement of the left temporomandibular joint. Lateral movement of the jaw is normal to the right (a) but markedly impaired to the left side (b).

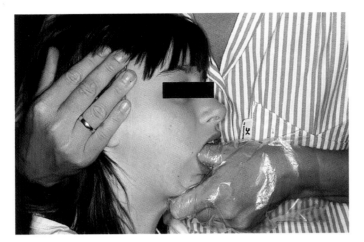

Fig. 4 Mobilization of the caudal–ventral motion of the jaw.

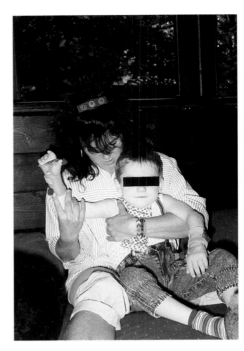

Fig. 5 Passive-assistive moving of the shoulder towards external rotation.

indicated to improve function. Temporomandibular joint involvement needs close collaboration with the dentist or orthodontist since dental or jaw regulation may be required to improve function and occlusion.

The shoulder

Arthritis of the shoulder occurs mainly in children with polyarticular disease. Since synovitis is difficult to detect and pain is usually greater in other joints it is easily overlooked.

Shoulder involvement impairs elevation and abduction. These movements involve a caudal gliding of the humeral head which is restricted in arthritis. Early co-operation of the shoulder blade during elevation and abduction compensates for impaired range of motion. The pain-relieving position of the glenohumeral joint tends towards adduction and internal rotation. The muscles for external rotation, abduction, and elevation become weak. Joints of the shoulder girdle, such as the acromioclavicular and the sternoclavicular joint, can also be affected. Their position of comfort comprises elevation and protraction of the shoulder girdle.

Therapy

Mobilization of the restricted external rotation, elevation, and abduction comes first (Fig. 5). Manipulation of the caudal gliding of the humeral head is helpful as well as stretching of the tense adductor and internal rotator muscles. Postisometric relaxation can also improve range of motion (Melvin 1989). When adequate shoulder mobility has been achieved muscular activation becomes possible which concentrates on the weak scapular muscles, the external rotators, and abductors. The scapular muscles must be activated towards a caudal and dorsal movement of the shoulder blade.

Exercises in a sling suspension are beneficial for shoulder involvement. They enable active mobilization while the arm is protected from gravity to eliminate joint stress. The child can swing the arm into elevation and retroversion while lying on the side and into horizontal abduction and adduction while sitting upright.

The elbow

Synovitis of the elbow joint first impairs extension. A flexion contracture up to 30° may develop unnoticed since it hardly interferes with

normal activities. Further contracture, however, significantly reduces arm length and can eventually lead to problems with dressing, toilet care, and other daily tasks (Erlandson 1989; Melvin 1989). Severe elbow involvement may also impair flexion which then mainly interferes with eating, combing, and facial care.

Forearm rotation favours pronation as a position of comfort while supination is usually restricted.

Therapy

Mobilization is directed towards the restricted function, usually extension and supination. Since synovial tissue tends to fill the fossa olecrani, moving the elbow may be very painful. Manual traction vertical to the forearm can relieve pain and improve extension, while stretching of the flexor and pronator muscles is important to restore function. Postisometric relaxation of the flexor muscles may also improve extension. Plaster splints which are used for about half an hour after manual stretching help to maintain the improvement.

The hand

In polyarthritis symmetrical involvement of wrist and finger joints occurs in over 90 per cent of patients. In oligoarthritis (or pauciarticular disease) asymmetric wrist involvement affects about 10 to 20 per cent, while single finger joints or digits may also be implicated (Melvin 1989; Altenbockum *et al.* 1993). The typical pain-relieving position of the wrist in children is flexion and ulnar deviation (Table 2) (Chaplin *et al.* 1969; Granberry and Mangum 1980; Findley *et al.* 1983; Erlandson 1989; Melvin 1989; Altenbockum *et al.* 1993). The extensors weaken while the flexor carpi ulnaris muscle becomes hypertonic. First active and later also passive dorsal wrist extension is limited. Secondary hyperextension of the metacarpophalangeal joints may occur (Fig. 6). To compensate for ulnar wrist deviation the metacarpophalangeal joints often drift radially even when they are not

Table 2 Deformities of the wrist in juvenile chronic arthritis	
	No. of wrists affected (%)
Ulnar deviation	142 (59)
Juvenile hand scoliosis	82 (34)
Volar subluxation carpus	164 (68)

Study from the Children's Hospital for Rheumatic Diseases, Garmisch-Parten-kirchen. 133 children with 239 involved wrist joints.

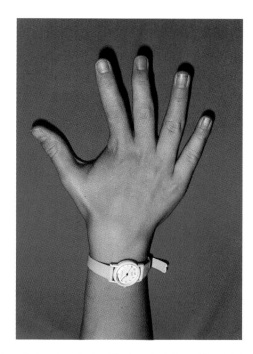

Fig. 7 Juvenile hand scoliosis with ulnar deviation of the wrist and compensatory radial drift of the fingers.

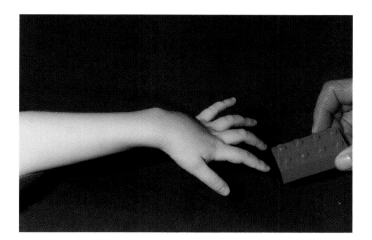

Fig. 6 Arthritis of the wrist joint with a typical malposition in flexion. Impaired extension is compensated by hyperextension in the metacarpophalangeal joints.

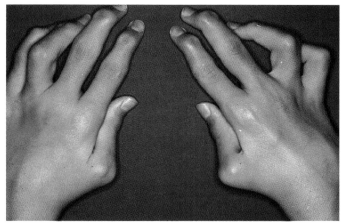

Fig. 8 Multiple finger deformities in a patient with juvenile polyarthritis: subluxation and adduction of the thumb at the metacarpophalangeal joint with hyperextension of the interphalangeal joint; swan-neck deformity of the index and middle fingers; and boutonnière deformity of the fourth and fifth fingers.

affected. The result is a juvenile hand scoliosis often described as 'Z deformity' (Fig. 7), in contrast to adult hand deformity with radial deviation of the wrist and ulnar drift of the fingers (Granberry and Mangum 1980; Altenbockum *et al.* 1993). Occasionally, and particularly in older children with disease positive for rheumatoid factor, an adult-type hand deformity can develop. Finally, the disturbed muscular balance together with loosening of capsule and ligaments results in a volar subluxation of the carpus (Table 2).

Involvement of finger joints can lead to swan-neck or boutonnière deformities. A few children with polyarthritis develop the same malposition in all fingers. Often, however, combinations occur in the same hand. Swan-neck deformity develops mainly in index and middle fingers, boutonnière deformity in the fourth and fifth finger (Altenbockum *et al.* 1993). The thumb tends towards opposition and adduction in its saddle joint and flexion deformity in the metacarpophalangeal joint. A compensatory hyperextension often develops in the interphalangeal joint (Fig. 8).

Flexortenosynovitis of the fingers is a common feature in juvenile arthritis. It can be very painful and may result in the adoption of a pain-relieving position with all three finger joints in flexion (Melvin 1989; Altenbockum *et al.* 1993). Due to impaired tendon gliding active, flexion and extension are often reduced although passive movement is still possible (Fig. 9). Finally shortening of the finger flexors develops with a significant impairment of hand function.

Therapy

Treatment of the wrist must include restoration of passive and later active dorsal extension as well as radial abduction. The therapist's grip during passive-assistive movement should support the carpus and correct the hand axis. Slow movements which take account of the pain threshold reduce tension of the flexor carpi ulnaris muscle and enable careful stretching (Fig. 10). When joint inflammation has subsided, activation of the extensor muscles becomes part of the programme. Since abduction of the thumb counteracts ulnar wrist deviation it is important to relearn and practise spreading the

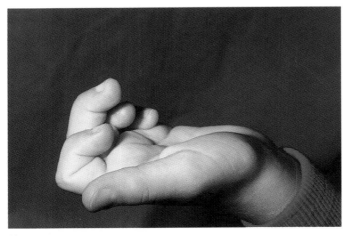

(a)

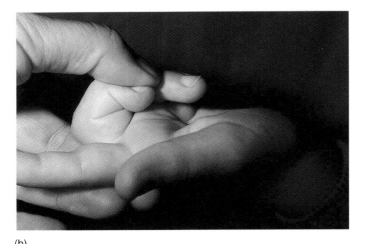

(b)

Fig. 9 Flexortenosynovitis of the middle finger. Active flexion is markedly impaired (a) while passive flexion is still complete (b).

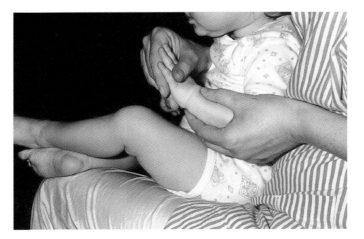

Fig. 10 Cautious passive-assistive moving of the wrist in a small child with polyarthritis.

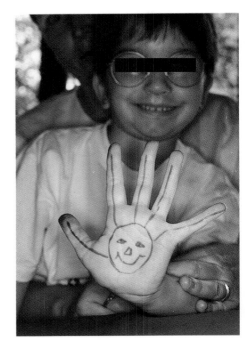

Fig. 11 A child demonstrates full range wrist extension and spreading of fingers by letting the sun shine.

thumb. It is also important that the children become aware of the physiological course of movement with the therapist's assistance. He or she must correct inappropriate movements such as hyperextension of the fingers or flexion of the elbow that compensate for impaired dorsal extension.

For small children play activities can help restore active wrist extension. For instance wiping shaving cream over a mirror or painting a sun on the palm and volar side of the fingers. The child is then asked to let the sun shine by raising the hand and spreading and extending the fingers (Fig. 11). Children also like to throw small balls; here the therapist must control the movement to prevent compensation by other joints, especially the elbow (Fig. 12).

Therapy of affected finger joints must take account of individual deviation. In swan-neck deformity it is important to mobilize impaired extension of the metacarpophalangeal joints and then continue with flexion of the proximal interphalangeal joints (Fig. 13). Muscular co-ordination of the extensor digitorum longus with the flexor digitorum superficialis muscle must be trained to achieve a physiological grip. In boutonnière deformity the often hyperextended metacarpophalangeal joints must be mobilized towards flexion. In a further step, stretching of the flexor digitorum superficialis muscle improves proximal interphalangeal flexion contracture.

Flexotenosynovitis is treated by stretching of the flexors which, unfortunately, must exceed the pain threshold in order to be effective. The impaired flexion must also be trained. In treatment of flexortenosynovitis both passive and active movements are necessary to prevent adhesion of the tendons. To reduce pain, cold applications prior to physiotherapy are helpful (Jarvis 1980; Melvin 1989; Altenbockum *et al.* 1993).

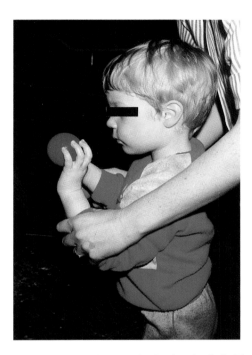

Fig. 12 A boy trains active wrist extension by throwing balls. The therapist assists to prevent elbow movement.

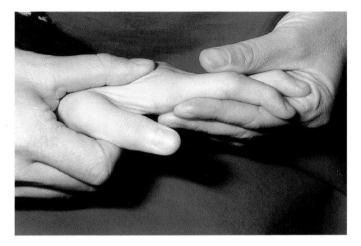

(a)

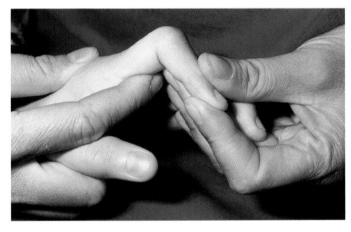

(b)

Fig. 13 Treatment of swan-neck deformity. Mobilization of extension at the metacarpophalangeal joint (a) is followed by flexion at the proximal interphalangeal joint (b).

Hand orthoses

Therapy of wrist and finger deformities benefits from individual orthoses. The wrist joint can be stabilized by a working splint to prevent or correct flexion position, ulnar (or radial) drift, and carpal subluxation (Chaplin *et al.* 1969; Granberry and Mangum 1980; Jarvis 1980; Findley *et al.* 1983; Erlandson 1989; Melvin 1989; Altenbockum *et al.* 1993) (Fig. 14). These splints should be worn most of the day and especially during manual activities since all active work with the hand increases the deviation. Stabilization of the carpus will improve power transfer in the finger–hand area and will also protect the inflamed joint structures from over- and misloading

Resting splints are indicated for finger deformities. They should be worn for several hours during the night and contribute to a careful passive stretching of shortened muscles and joint structures (Fig. 15).

The hip

Hip disease often becomes a major problem in children with chronic arthritis. Frequency of hip involvement differs among the subgroups and varies with time (Fig. 16). It is most common in seronegative polyarthritis at onset and as the disease progresses. In systemic disease about one-fifth of these children start with hip arthritis which increases with follow-up. These patients also run a high risk of hip destruction (Fig. 17). Hip problems can also arise in patients with HLA B27–related arthritis or juvenile spondylitis.

Hip mobility in children exceeds that of adults. Young children with free hip function can bend their hips until the knee reaches the belly and external rotation may reach 90°.

The first sign of hip involvement is pain during full range flexion with adduction (Fig. 18). Later full extension, flexion, and inner rota-

tion in 90° flexion become painful. When the children stand or walk they usually deviate into adduction and inner rotation. The abductor and external rotator muscles become weak while adductor and internal rotators as well as flexor muscles tend to shorten. Severe hip involvement is characterized by flexion, adduction, and inner rotation contractures (Swann 1978a; Melvin 1989). In such patients flexion position is compensated for by an increased lumbar lordosis as well as knee flexion (Swann 1978a; Erlandson 1989; Melvin 1989).

Therapy

Arthritis of the hip can be very painful especially in children with systemic disease. In acute stages only careful passive moving and mild traction is tolerated. This, however, should be done as often as possible to prevent contractures. If pain interferes with a full hip extension it is important to position the child in bed, supporting the upper legs and knees by pillows in a mild flexion to allow the muscles to relax. Regular, cautious passive extension, however, is compulsory to prevent flexion contractures.

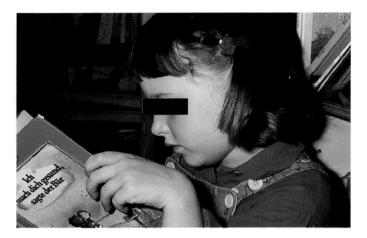

(a)

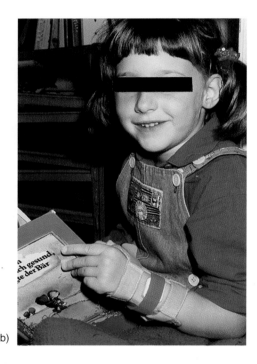

(b)

Fig. 14 Benefit of working splints. The malposition in flexion and ulnar deviation (a) is corrected with a stabilizing splint (b).

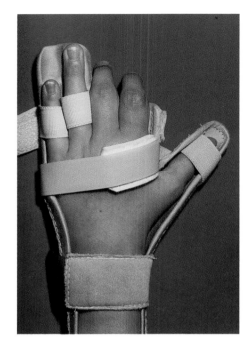

Fig. 15 Individual resting splint for a hand with combined finger deformities (see Fig. 8). The thumb rests in abduction; swan-neck deformity of the second and third fingers is corrected with extension at the metacarpophalangeal joint allowing flexion of proximal interphalangeal joints. Boutonnière deformity of the fourth and fifth finger requires proximal interphalangeal extension.

When pain subsides stretching should be done, concentrating on mainly the flexors and probably the adductor muscles. Later on, active exercises of extensor and abductor muscles is important to improve the range of movement of the joint.

Exercises in a sling suspension are indicated to mobilize the joint. Continuous or intermittent traction for 1 or 2 h a day may relieve pain and contracture. Periods of lying in a prone position are beneficial to increase hip extension (Ansell 1978; Swann 1978a; Jarvis 1980; Melvin 1989; Lloyd and Aldrich 1993; Hayem *et al.* 1994). It is, however, important that the child does not compensate for impaired hip extension with an increased lumbar lordosis when lying prone.

Weight-bearing exercises for children with hip arthritis is controversial (Lloyd and Aldrich 1993). Some therapists encourage ambulation to restore the joint structures and support joint congruity

(Bernstein *et al.* 1977; Ansell 1978; Melvin 1989; Lloyd and Aldrich 1993; Hayem *et al.* 1994). Absence of weight bearing may interfere with a normal development of the femur and acetabulum in young children. Valgus deformity and lateralization of the femoral head and acetabular underdevelopment are often seen in children with onset of hip disease at an early age (Bernstein *et al.* 1977; Ansell 1978; Blane *et al.* 1987).

Conversely, weight bearing increases joint stress enormously and can promote hip destruction. Therefore, partial weight bearing is a compromise for children with hip arthritis (Rombouts and Rombouts-Lindemans 1971; Ansell 1978; Jarvis 1980; Garcia-Morteo *et al.* 1981). Depending on the child's age and the condition of the other joints we recommend crutches, bicycles, tricycles, or scooters with a saddle (Fig. 19) for mobility. Wheelchair use is to be avoided since sitting increases flexion contractures of hips and knees (Ansell 1978; Swann 1978a; Melvin 1989).

Children have a good potential for restoration of joint cartilage and bone (Rombouts and Rombouts-Lindemans 1971; Bernstein *et al.* 1977; Melvin 1989) (Fig. 20). In our experience walking is not necessary for repairing damage to cartilage or bone and may even delay it due to increased stress on the joints. We therefore prefer partial weight bearing and regular, continuous moving of the hips in a relief position. Such children benefit from using a sling suspension at home for daily exercises (Fig. 21).

The knee

In all forms of juvenile arthritis the knee is most frequently involved. However, destructive lesions are less prominent compared with joints such as the wrist or hip. Deformities, however, can develop rapidly.

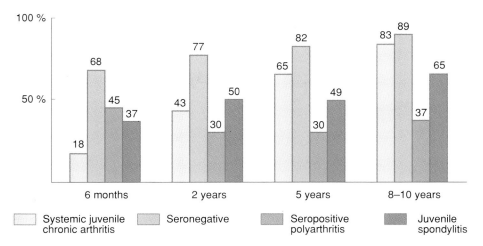

Fig. 16 Frequency of hip involvement in juvenile chronic arthritis within the first 6 months from onset and during follow-up. (Numbers derived from patient studies of the Children's Hospital for Rheumatic Diseases in Garmisch-Partenkirchen).

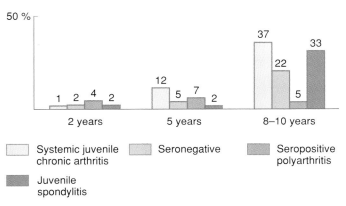

Fig. 17 Development of hip destruction in the subgroups of juvenile chronic arthritis (the same patients as in Fig. 16). The figure demonstrates the percentage of significant destructive lesions in children with hip involvement during follow-up.

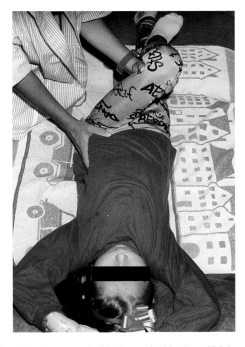

Fig. 18 Combined movement of flexion and adduction which is painful early in the course of hip involvement.

The typical pain-relieving position is flexion of the knee joint which is stabilized by an increased tension of the hamstring muscles (Swann 1978a; Jarvis 1980; Erlandson 1989; Melvin 1989; Altenbockum *et al.* 1993). The quadriceps muscle becomes hypotonic. Knee flexion contractures can develop into a very severe problem in young children. Each surgical procedure, even a small biopsy or arthroscopy, produces deterioration and should therefore be avoided in children under 5 years of age.

Flexion position of the knee enables rotatory movements to be made. Predominant activity of the biceps femoris muscle in childhood arthritis results in an outer rotation of the lower leg that is often compensated for by inner rotation of the hip joint, which then gives the impression of a valgus position of the knee but is really a pseudovalgus deformity (Altenbockum *et al.* 1993) (Fig. 22). Small children are particularly prone to develop a true valgus position which exceeds the physiological valgus for that age (Swann 1978a; Erlandson 1989; Melvin 1989; Altenbockum *et al.* 1993). It is caused by increased tension of the iliotibial band with ensuing instability of capsule and ligaments. Permanent knee flexion with dominant activity of the hamstring muscles favours dorsal subluxation of the tibia.

All these knee deformities are especially noticeable in young children. In a study of 63 patients with early-onset oligoarthritis who had 73 affected knee joints we have seen flexion contracture and quadriceps atrophy in almost all. About 60 per cent also showed outer rotation of the lower leg and tibial subluxation (Table 3).

Asymmetric knee involvement often results in a discrepancy in leg length due to increased growth at the affected knee joint.

Therapy

The first step in treatment of the knee should be to consider how to achieve full extension as well as the physiological hyperextension.

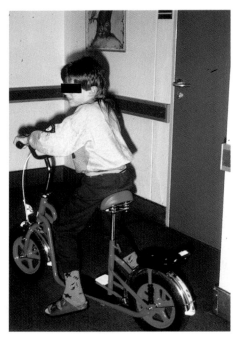

Fig. 19 Special vehicle for children with involvement of the lower limbs to avoid weight bearing.

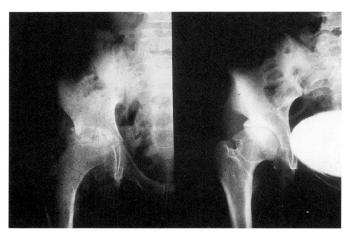

Fig. 20 Remodelling of hip joint destruction in a child with seronegative polyarthritis.

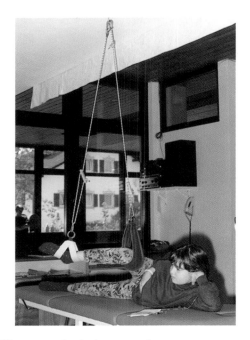

Fig. 21 Sling suspension for home exercises.

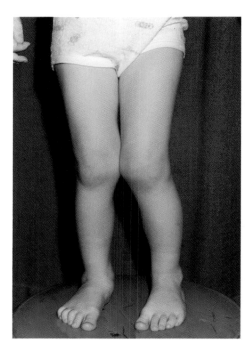

Fig. 22 Pseudovalgus deformity in a child with arthritis of the left knee. Flexion contracture with inner rotation of the leg gives the impression of a valgus position.

When sitting with knee joints stretched the child should be able to lift the heel.

When treating a knee flexion contracture it is especially important that the therapist is careful to respect the pain threshold, for only if the child is totally relaxed does it become possible to stretch the hypertonic hamstrings, in particular the biceps femoris muscle.

Once there is improvement of passive extension the quadriceps muscle can be mobilized. A playful trick helps small children to find the right muscle: a face drawn on the child's knee with the mouth in the skin fold above the patella will start to smile when the quadriceps tenses.

A more difficult way to activate the quadriceps is when children throw balloons which have been put on their feet. Fast muscular coordination is best trained by letting the child kick about in the air or in water. However, the therapist must watch how far the full active extension is integrated in the course of movement. When muscular balance between hamstrings and quadriceps muscle has been restored the physiological movement pattern alone builds up muscle strength without extra power training (Altenbockum *et al.* 1993).

Gait training for affected knee joints must ensure a correct heel strike with fully extended knees and knee flexion during the swing phase.

Table 3 Deformities of the knee in juvenile chronic arthritis	
	No. of knees affected (%)
Flexion contracture	73 (100)
Outer rotation, lower leg	39 (53)
Subluxation tibia	40 (55)

Study of 63 children with early onset oligoarthritis, 73 involved knees.

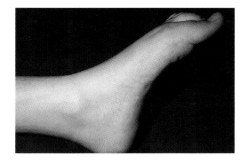

Fig. 24 Rheumatic heel foot: impaired plantar flexion is compensated by flexion of the big toe.

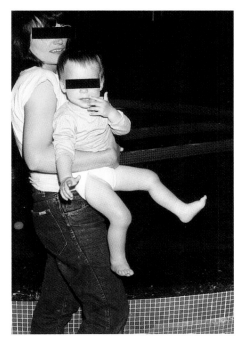

Fig. 23 Pain-relieving position with the feet in neutral or mild dorsal extension in a child with arthritis of both ankles.

Additional aids

Stretching of the hamstring muscles can be supported by splints (Ansell 1978; Swann 1978a; Jarvis 1980; Erlandson 1989; Melvin 1989; Altenbockum *et al.* 1993). They are put in place after physiotherapy in the best position of maximum extension.

As for hip treatment, arthritis of the knee also benefits from partial weight bearing (Swann 1978a; Jarvis 1980; Melvin 1989; Altenbockum *et al.* 1993). It reduces stress to the joint, enables relaxation of the hypertonic muscles, and helps to avoid the wrong pattern of motion during walking.

A leg length discrepancy must be corrected by a combined sole and heel lift, otherwise pelvic tilting and scoliosis of the spine can develop. The increased leg length also promotes fixed knee flexion of the affected knee.

The foot

The numerous foot joints and variety in the pattern of joint involvement usually lead to a combination of different axial deformities and in most patients the gait becomes disturbed (Swann 1978b; Rana

1982; Gschwend and Ivosevic-Radovanovic 1986; Lechner *et al.* 1987; Erlandson 1989; Melvin 1989; Altenbockum *et al.* 1993; Truckenbrodt *et al.* 1994). A mild dorsal extension is the typical position of comfort when the ankle or talonavicular joint is inflamed (Melvin 1989; Altenbockum *et al.* 1993) (Fig. 23). The muscular imbalance includes a hypertonic tibialis anterior and a weak triceps surae and peroneus longus muscle. A rheumatic heel foot can develop. Plantar flexion and especially cranial movement of the heel become impaired (Lechner *et al.* 1987; Melvin 1989; Altenbockum *et al.* 1993; Truckenbrodt *et al.* 1994); this is compensated by an increased flexion of the first metatarsophalangeal joint (Fig. 24). The ball of the big toe, normally a major weight-bearing area, is spared and atrophies. During walking, body weight is transferred from the heel over the lateral rim to the distal phalanx of the big toe (Altenbockum *et al.* 1993; Truckenbrodt *et al.* 1994) (Fig. 25).

Young children in particular have a physiological tendency towards pes valgoplanus and develop this type of deformity (Swann 1978b; Melvin 1989; Altenbockum *et al.* 1993; Truckenbrodt *et al.* 1994). During walking, impaired mobility is compensated by an outward turning of the leg and rolling over the medial rim (Fig. 26). This incorrect weight distribution increases the valgus deviation and flattening of the longitudinal arch. The forefoot seems to stand in pronation. However, if the heel is corrected into neutral position a supination of the forefoot becomes obvious (Fig. 27). Pronation is always impaired.

A rheumatic pes cavus develops less often and is seen mainly in older children with involvement of the distal intertarsal joints. These patients react with a reflex tension of the plantar muscles for pain relief (Fig. 28). Heightening of the longitudinal arch occurs together with an increased loading of the ball area. This often induces flattening of the transversal arch and claw toes. When medial intertarsal joints are especially painful, the weight is shifted to the outer rim and the heel glides into a varus position (Swann 1978b; Rana 1982; Gschwend and Ivosevic-Radovanovic 1986; Melvin 1989; Altenbockum *et al.* 1993; Truckenbrodt *et al.* 1994).

The three major deformities of the foot can develop alone or in combination. Usually one malposition predominates. In a study of 123 children with foot involvement we have seen pes valgoplanus as the dominant deviation, especially in young children with early-onset oligoarthritis. In the other subgroups heel foot and pes valgoplanus occurred with about the same frequency, while pes cavus was seen less often (Fig. 29).

Other foot deformities concern the forefoot and toes. Arthritis of the first metatarsophalangeal joint often results in a hallux flexus to

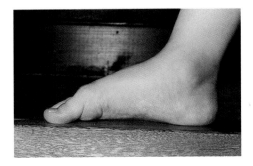

Fig. 25   Loading phase of a heel foot: the weight is shifted from the heel over the lateral rim to the distal phalanx of the big toe; the ball area is spared.

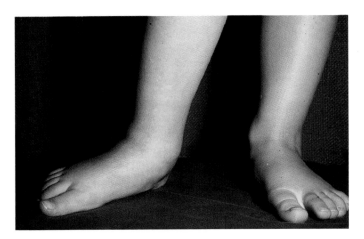

Fig. 26   Pes valgoplanus with outer rotation of the leg and rolling over the medial rim.

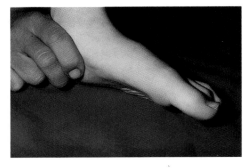

Fig. 27   Pes valgoplanus with erecting of the heel into neutral position. The forefoot stands in supination.

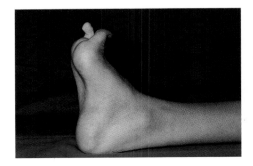

Fig. 28   Rheumatic pes cavus with tension of the plantar muscles.

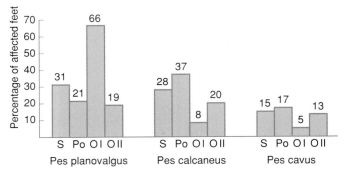

Fig. 29   Frequency of pes valgoplanus, pes calcaneus (heel foot), and pes cavus among the subgroups of juvenile chronic arthritis. (Study from the Children's Hospital for Rheumatic Diseases, Garmisch-Partenkirchen; 123 children, 246 feet). S, systemic juvenile chronic arthritis; Po, seronegative polyarthritis; O I, early onset oligoarthritis; O II, HLA B27-associated oligoarthritis

Ivosevic- Radovanovic 1986; Melvin 1989; Altenbockum *et al.* 1993) (Fig. 30).

An equinus position of the foot is very rare in children with chronic arthritis and develops only in patients who have been immobilized in a wheelchair for a lengthy period (Gschwend and Ivosevic-Radovanovic 1986; Melvin 1989).

Therapy

The first step must be to obtain mobility of each of the affected foot and toe joints. To achieve better plantar flexion in the ankle joint the therapist must concentrate in particular on cranial movement of the calcaneus (Fig. 31). Mobilizing forefoot pronation provides a strong fixation of the heel. It is also important to restore extension of the first metatarsophalangeal joint, which is necessary for the physiological loading of the big toe ball. To regain muscular balance the tibialis anterior muscle must be stretched and the triceps surae and peroneus longus muscles be activated.

In a further procedure the combined movement of forefoot pronation with extension of the big toe must be trained (Fig. 32). This can be achieved with another game, painting the big toe ball to use as a stamp for printing patterns on a sheet of paper.

To remedy the effects of foot involvement, intensive gait training is always necessary (Jarvis 1980; Lechner *et al.* 1987; Melvin 1989; Altenbockum *et al.* 1993; Truckenbrodt *et al.* 1994). A precise heel strike followed by rolling over the big and small toe ball with extended toes is needed. The push-off with plantar flexion of the ankle and

relieve the painful area of the big toe ball. This deviation resembles the heel foot where a secondary hallux flexus can develop. A compensatory hyperextension of the interphalangeal joint may occur. A hallux valgus is seen mainly in children with polyarthritis and involvement of the metatarsophalangeal joints. These patients also tend to develop claw or hammer toes (Rana 1982; Gschwend and Ivosevic-Radovanovic 1986; Melvin 1989; Altenbockum *et al.* 1993). Forefoot adduction often occurs together with hallux flexus or as a compensatory deviation from arthritis of the knee or ankle joint (Gschwend and

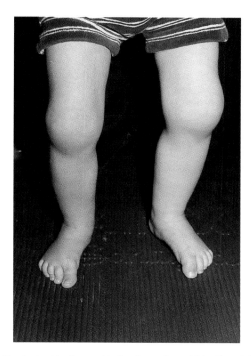

Fig. 30 Forefoot adduction and hallux flexus in a child with arthritis of both knees and ankles.

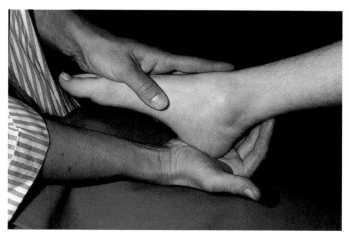

Fig. 31 Mobilization of plantar flexion with cranial moving of the calcaneus.

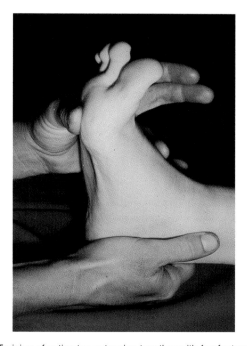

Fig. 32 Training of active toe extension together with forefoot pronation. The child is asked to push against the therapist's thumb.

extension of the toes is very important to train. The therapist must correct the wrong pattern and assist the re-education of each phase of a normal gait (Fig. 33).

Additional aids

Most children with foot involvement require insoles. They should correct the deviation as long as they are adjustable without pain under full weight bearing. Otherwise the insoles must primarily relieve the inflamed joints. It may even be necesssary to support a deviation until the pain-relieving position has improved.

For stabilization of the upper foot, shoes which extend over the ankle are useful. Soft soles lower the transfer of foot-strikes during walking and relieve all joints of the lower extremity. Severe foot deformities may require custom-made orthopaedic footwear. Partial weight bearing is also recommended for children with inflamed foot joints.

The sacroiliac joint

Sacroiliits can develop in children with HLA B27-related oligoarthritis or juvenile spondylitis. In a series of 71 juvenile patients with sacroiliits we detected radiographic changes of the sacroiliac joints between 1 month and 9 years after onset of peripheral arthritis. Only 33 of these patients complained of back pain, which was localized to the sacroiliac joint alone in 4 of them. Fifteen suffered from pain in the sacroiliac joints as well as the lumbar spine and 14 complained only of lumbar spine problems (Häfner 1987).

Since sacroiliitis can develop insidiously without any or only minor pain it is often overlooked. However, careful examination of these patients can detect the typical incorrect positioning even in the early stages. Physiologically the pelvis is positioned in a slight forward tilt, which means that the sacroiliac joints receive oblique pressure forces

from the vertically oriented spine. Patients with sacroiliitis avoid such painful forces by raising the pelvis into a vertical position. However, this diminishes the physiological lumbar curve and contributes to lumbar tenderness, which is often a first symptom of sacroiliac involvement.

Therapy

For proper positioning it is important to maintain or restore the pelvic tilt and the lumbar lordosis. If the sacroiliac joints are painful, correct positioning may only be possible in a relief position. When inflammation and pain subside the patient must learn to maintain the correct position during sitting, standing, or walking. Since pain often blocks all movement of the sacroiliac joint, careful manipulation

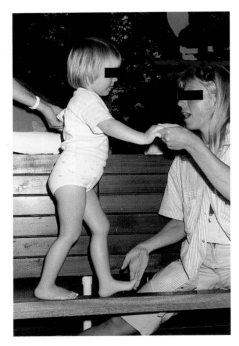

Fig. 33 Gait training with assistance to relearn each single phase of the gait cycle.

may help restore the physiological function. However, such manipulation may induce progressive pain during acute phases, in which case it should be postponed until the inflammation subsides, when movement can once more be tolerated. Some patients benefit from a tight pelvic belt which stabilizes the sacroiliac area.

Movement and training of the spinal muscles are always indicated to prevent or reduce secondary spine problems caused by sacroiliitis. They are also important prophylactic steps to prevent further spinal involvement, which may otherwise start in a number of these patients during early adulthood.

Juvenile dermatomyositis (see Chapter 5.9.2)

The acute stage of dermatomyositis is characterized by muscle weakness which can be severe enough to render the child immobile. About two-thirds of such patients also complain of muscular pain, with the trunk musculature usually being more severely affected than the peripheral muscles.

The chronic stage of the disease is exacerbated by progressive joint stiffness due to muscular scarring and shortening together with calcification of the skin and subcutaneous tissue.

Joint deformities follow a characteristic pattern. The wrist tends towards dorsal extension with flexed fingers while volar flexion of the wrist is impaired (Häfner and Truckenbrodt 1989) (Fig. 34). This is in contrast to chronic arthritis where extension is usually more limited and wrist flexion is the typical relief position. Elbows, hips, and knees are at high risk of developing flexion contractures. The ankle deviates into an equinus position. Contraction of the lower extremities is promoted by use of a wheelchair. Unfortunately during the acute stage when muscle weakness interferes with walking, children

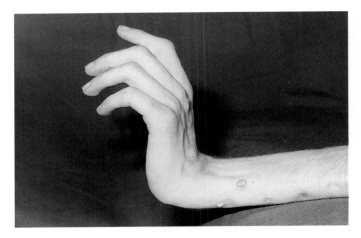

(a)

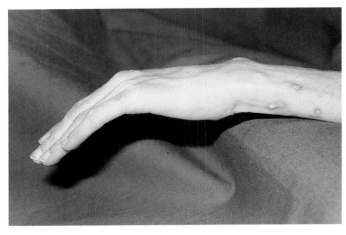

(b)

Fig. 34 Range of motion of the wrist in a child with dermatomyositis. Dorsal extension is complete (a) but flexion is severely impaired (b).

are often placed in wheelchairs and without adequate treatment they remain wheelchair-bound due to progressive muscular wasting and contraction.

Therapy

During the acute phase the main therapy is concentrated on prophylactic treatment of muscle contraction. It includes proper positioning with hips and knees stretched for comfort and the ankle in a neutral position. If pain interferes with optimum positioning, flexed hips and knees must be supported with pillows to relieve muscular tension. Cautious passive movement towards extension becomes very important. Lying prone may help to prevent hip flexion contracture, and sitting with bended hips and knees must be restricted to short periods. Misguided use of the wheelchair can exacerbate the loss of movement.

Careful activated exercises of those muscles which tend to lose tension is very important, otherwise the child will forget what muscular contraction feels like. Muscle strengthening, however, is not advisable since it can increase muscular damage. Active moving should be encouraged as far as the patient can tolerate without experiencing muscle fatigue.

As soon as joint contractures appear gentle stretching of the muscles is indicated. Use of a plaster cast for a few hours every day helps reduce contractures. Exercises in a sling suspension enable careful active movement with relief from gravity. A further beneficial procedure is hydrotherapy, especially for those children with severe impairment who enjoy the unusual experience of mobility that becomes possible through weight release in warm water.

Childhood scleroderma (see Chapter 5.8.1)

Systemic sclerosis is a very rare disorder in childhood and the paediatric rheumatologist is more often confronted with localized forms of scleroderma. These appear as morphea with round or oval-shaped lesions or in linear form. Fibrotic induration of skin and subcutaneous tissues can impair function depending on the extent of sclerosis. Individual problems arise according to the particular site of damage. Lesions on the face are mainly a cosmetic problem but can have severe psychological impact. Linear forms which cross a joint result in restricted mobility and can be especially disastrous if an entire extremity is involved. In such cases deformities and growth disruption can combine to produce a severe handicap (Fig. 35).

Therapy

The effect of medical intervention in childhood scleroderma is limited so that emphasis should be placed on physiotherapy and physical modalities. The main aspect of treatment aims to prevent or improve contraction. Careful manual stretching of the sclerotic structures is thought to be beneficial but should not exceed the patient's tolerance. Resting splints help to maintain joint position over a prolonged period. Exercises in a sling suspension as well as hydrotherapy in a warm pool represent two possibilities for maintaining or improving mobility without stressing the joints and neighbouring structures.

A beneficial effect can also be expected from manual lymphatic drainage. This process reduces tissue oedema which often dominates in the early phase. Connective tissue massage improves the peripheral blood flow and may contribute to healing of 'rat-bite' necrosis as well as Raynaud's phenomenon in systemic sclerosis (Földi 1991).

Widespread localized forms which involve the whole leg require special shoes with a heel and sole lift to adjust for deformities and growth disturbances.

Parental involvement

For children with chronic progressive disease a regular, often daily, therapy programme is necessary. The best way to guarantee effective treatment at home is to integrate parents into the therapy programme. They must be informed about how joint deformities can develop and learn the principles of physiotherapy. With adequate training most parents are able to undertake the task of daily exercises at home. They must also understand and learn to use the different orthoses and splints as well as the principles of everyday joint protection. Most parents are eager to participate in therapy if they realize that their active role can decisively improve the prognosis for the child's arthritis.

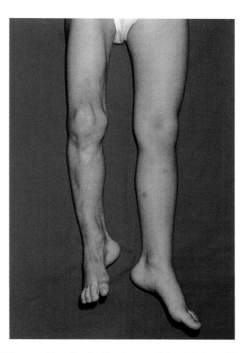

Fig. 35 Widespread localized scleroderma of the right leg with growth disturbance and deformity.

Problems with home therapy usually arise if progressive disease means treatment must be maintained over a prolonged period. In particular where patients suffer frequent relapse or continuous deterioration, general pessimism tends to reduce motivation. Parents and child may feel so discouraged that they abandon therapy. It is important to give them positive encouragement frequently, always acknowledge small achievements, and to assure parents that it is worth maintaining the same state or even accepting a reduction in the rate of progression in severe progressive diseases.

Regular exercises at home are usually necessary for an optimal outcome. It is, however, important that the therapeutic team relieves the family during times of acute stress and accepts temporary interruptions of the treatment routine. The schedule should always take account of holidays and leave enough space for fun and play.

Parental education should also include advice on appropriate leisure activities. Certain sports activities can lead to joint deterioration. On the other hand, sport is an important part of leisure activities in most families. It may be helpful if parents learn to give priority to sports which increase mobility without joint stress such as swimming or cycling, both activities which can have a therapeutic effect for children with rheumatic diseases. Depending on joint involvement and disease activity further sports may be acceptable: table tennis, gymnastics, horse riding, or cross-country skiing can usually be recommended for children with mild disease. Sports requiring a high level of exertion like tennis, skiing, or football should be reserved for patients in remission.

The child with arthritis who cannot participate in sports should be encouraged to gain self-esteem and stimulation in other fields. Parents should be encouraged to help compensate for their child's low level of physical activity with musical education, handicrafts, or playing games at home. Friends can be asked to visit and be integrated into leisure acitvities, which are adapted to the child's capability. This promotes the patient's social development and gives him or her the chance to feel equal in a healthy competition.

Joint protection and adapted devices

Joint protection training is an important task in the therapeutic regimen. The child with arthritis must learn how to reduce stress to the joints in daily activities. Effective joint protection relieves pain and can improve the inflammatory process. Principles of joint protection include:

(1) proper positioning of joints to avoid deformities;

(2) use of several instead of single joints;

(3) transfer of a load from small to large joints or from involved to unaffected areas;

(4) avoiding prolonged activity or positioning;

(5) planning of rest breaks.

The child will assimilate these principles best if they are demonstrated during work or play. The occupational therapist first watches the patient during an activity and then corrects the incorrect joint position into a proper protective one (Fig. 36). The therapist must also explain the advantages of distributing a load on to stronger or larger areas, for example from the fingers to the palm, or how to use both hands instead of one.

Joint protection may be supported by use of adapted devices. They help to reduce pain, preserve the proper joint position, minimize joint stress in daily activities, and increase the child's independence. In practice such equipment is prescribed less often for children than adults, since children feel embarrassed to use such appliances and devices with their peers and prefer to use alternative techniques to perform a task or even to ask for help.

Aid appliances, however, may become important for handicapped adolescents who wish to become independent. The most frequently prescribed appliances for children and adolescents include aids for walking and self-care items as well as play and school equipment.

We recommend partial weight release for children with arthritis of the lower extremities. Usually age-appropriate vehicles like tricycles or bicycles are sufficient, but some children may need special aids such as crutches or scooters with a saddle (see Fig. 19).

Self-care equipment should be restricted to severely handicapped patients since most children with arthritis can learn to perform daily tasks without special equipment. Sock cones are sometimes indicated for children with impaired hip and knee flexion, as well as dressing, combing, or hygiene articles with lengthened handles when shoulder elevation and elbow flexion are impaired. Since appliances designed to help adults are often inappropriate for children because they are not adapted to the child's size and reach, the occupational therapist must ensure that any such equipment is adapted for the individual child.

Some equipment for adults may be helpful for children and adolescents as well. Figures 37 and 38 demonstrate the advantage of pot holders and adapted knives for proper wrist positioning. Spring-style scissors and foam material to thicken pencils relieve joint stress during crafting or drawing. Such devices are easy to handle and will be accepted within the peer group.

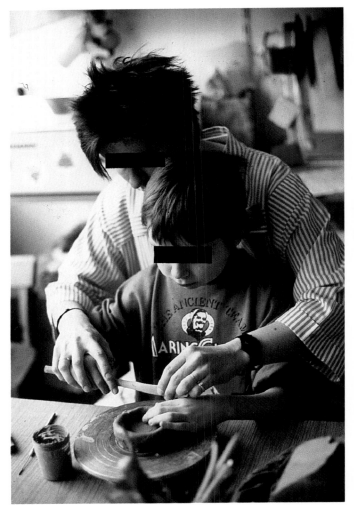

Fig. 36 The occupational therapist corrects a child's hand position during clay crafting.

Integration into school

Most children with rheumatic diseases can and should be integrated into mainstream schools. Classes for the physically handicapped are not the solution since they only serve to increase the child's sense of being abnormal.

Doctors, social workers, and occupational therapists must communicate with educators and school nurses to find appropriate solutions and compromises for a practicable school life.

Problems start with transportation for those children who cannot walk or cycle to school. School buses which pick up the child at home are the best solution but not always available. A car pool with other families may relieve parents of the daily task of driving their child to and from school.

If teachers are informed early enough it is often possible to adapt the timetable to accommodate the child's needs. Less academic subjects could start in the early morning so that children with morning pain and stiffness can arrive later without missing too much. If physical education occurs at the end of the school day those

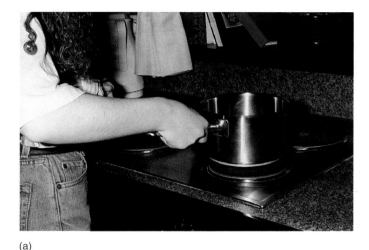

(a)

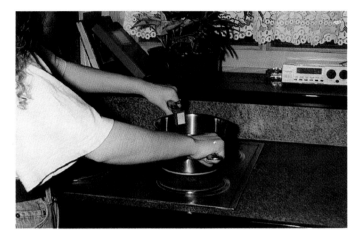

(b)

Fig. 37 Lifting pots with a regular pot holder urges the wrist into ulnar deviation (a). A second pot holder transfers the weight from one to both hands and guarantees proper wrist positioning (b).

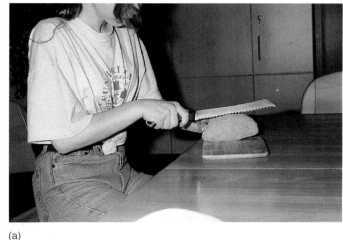

(a)

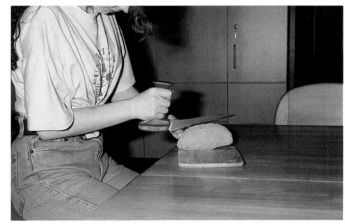

(b)

Fig. 38 Cutting with a regular knife increases ulnar wrist deviation (a). The malposition is corrected by use of an adapted knife (b).

children who are unable to participate can leave early and use the time for home work or physiotherapy. Classes with a handicapped child should preferably be allocated classrooms on the ground floor and moving between classes should be reduced to a minimum.

Keeping an extra set of books at home will save the child from having to carry heavy school bags and for necessary items backpacks should be preferred.

Children with arthritis of the hands may have a major problem with writing. Writing with splints is desirable to avoid ulnar deviation of the wrist but the changed position requires extra training during occupational therapy. Pressure to the finger joints can be avoided if children learn to write holding the pen between index and middle finger and with the thumb in the opposed position. A thickened pencil also relieves joint stress (Fig. 39).

Despite all these aids extended periods of writing may become painful and the child should receive extra time for class work to include rest periods. It is also helpful if the child is allowed to use a typewriter, computer, or dictaphone whenever possible.

Proper positioning during class and whilst doing homework is of the utmost importance, especially for children with back or neck

problems. The solution consists of a chair adapted to the child's size, an inclined writing board or bookstand to avoid neck and back flexion, and a slanting cushion to tilt the pelvis and keep the spine erect (Fig. 40).

All these arrangements can usually be accommodated in a mainstream school if educators are informed and willing to integrate a child with arthritis. The child's classmates receive practical education in social interaction and their support promotes the handicapped child's self-esteem and position in the community.

Guidance for the whole family

Arthritis in a child always has an impact on the whole family. Time-consuming demands, financial loss, and restriction of common activities alter the family's lifestyle; family members become resentful of their personal limitations and added responsibilities, siblings feel neglected and feel that their problems are of less importance or ignored altogether.

This situation requires guidance of the whole family, a task which all the team members may have to help resolve. Diagnosis of a

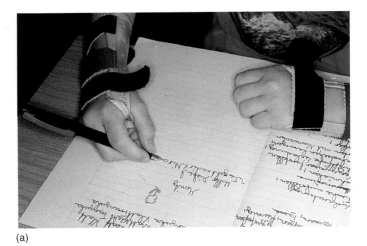

(a)

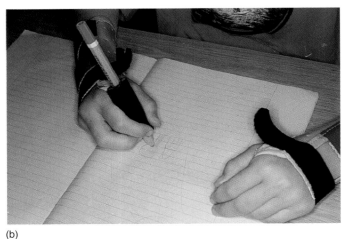

(b)

Fig. 39   Relief to finger joint pressure during writing occurs with an altered writing position (a) or a thickened pen handle (b).

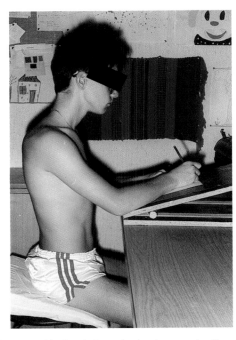

Fig. 40   Proper positioning during school or homework with an inclined bookstand and a slanting cushion.

chronic illness is usually devastating and adjustment to the new situation takes time, so it is vital that the health-care team help the families adapt to the altered situation. In the beginning thorough information together with hope for a favourable outcome are important to motivate each family member. Feelings of blame and guilt must be addressed and resolved to guarantee open communication within the family. Practical advice on how to overcome obstacles in daily life and adapt to a new schedule is most helpful.

If disease activity persists over months or years it becomes necessary to guide families towards a lifestyle which is as close to normal as possible.

Overprotection of the ill child and neglect of siblings is a common and understandable parental reaction, but should be avoided by early intervention of educators, psychologists, or other team members. The ill child must learn to cope with frustrations and healthy siblings need support for their problems too.

On the other hand a child with chronic arthritis does need special attention. Pain and physical limitations often exceed what can be tolerated for appropriate social interaction. Regression, aggression, or other behavioural disturbances can result. Parents are often overburdened trying to cope with such problems and should receive early professional advice.

Co-operation within the family facilitates a positive adjustment and parents should be encouraged to share responsibility for all disease-related activities. In many families mothers are left alone to cope with most of the tasks, so fathers must be stimulated to participate in the therapy routine, attend doctors appointments, and help with educational problems. Siblings may also become involved in caring for the ill child. If they receive appropriate recognition for this extra demand they can develop a strong feeling of self-esteem.

Health professionals cannot attend to all the needs of the family and some problems will remain. To deal with these, team members should encourage parents to join in family support groups as exchange of views among families with similar problems can be most helpful. Experienced parents can support families whose child has only recently been diagnosed. The health-care team must, however, be aware of negative influences and uncertainty among the group. This situation can best be avoided if health professionals become regularly involved in support group meetings.

Helping children cope with their disease

Chronic diseases elicit different emotions in different children. Young children usually feel most disturbed by restrictions on their physical activity. In this age group normal motor activity is strongly related to psychosocial development, a process which is endangered in children with rheumatic diseases.

For older children and adolescents the disease has most impact on their social life, as this age group is strongly influenced by peer pressure. The rheumatic disease with its restrictions and special demands does not fit into the life concept of the peer group. Youngsters therefore tend to deny the illness and its consequences.

Different methods of adjustment do exist. Where adjustment is negative children experience their illness as punishment or threat.

Emotions of guilt, fear, or helplessness develop, which may result in regression or aggression. A positive adjustment is one in which the child accepts certain limitations but concentrates on personal strengths.

The health-care team together with family, school staff, and friends must encourage such positive adjustment. The children should experience as little limitation on their activities as possible. While treatment discipline is necessary, it should always leave enough time for play and hobbies. Friends and peers should be integrated into leisure activities. Healthy competition, which is important for the child's development, must be directed towards activities within the child's capabilities. Success at school or competence in music, crafts, games, etc. promote the child's self-esteem.

Loving care is beneficial and especially important during painful relapses and other times of crisis. Overprotectiveness, however, can be devastating and hinder the child's psychosocial development, and children should always be encouraged to become independent. This includes personal care as well as control over medical care and treatment. As they grow up children can learn to determine treatment times and share responsibility for medication, doctor's appointments, etc. Parents are often reluctant to encourage independence and self-care as they fear loss of control over their child's life or tend to underestimate his or her capabilities. Health professionals can mediate between parents and child in this situation and actively support the child's struggle for independence.

Children who experienced pain and physical restrictions from a long-standing rheumatic disease but learned to cope with it often develop a more mature personality compared with others of their age group. Overcoming obstacles which their friends couldn't even dream of can be a source for more self-reliance and positive self-esteem. The adolescent may be earlier and better qualified for an independent life despite some physical limitations. Parents and health-care team members must recognize the child's struggle for freedom and facilitate appropriate self-determination and self-support.

References

Altenbockum, C. von, Hibler, M., Spamer, M., and Truckenbrodt, H. (1993). *Juvenile chronische Arthritis. Entwicklung von Achsenfehlstellungen an Hand, Knie und Fuss und ihre krankengymnastische Behandlung.* Hans Marseille Verlag, München.
Ansell, B.M. (1978). Rehabilitation. In *Surgical management of juvenile chronic polyarthritis*, (ed. G.P. Arden and B.M. Ansell). Grune & Stratton, New York.
Ansell, B.M. and Kent, P.A. (1977). Radiological changes in juvenile chronic polyarthritis. *Skeletal Radiology*, 1, 129–44.
Bache, C. (1964). Mandibular growth and dental occlusion in juvenile rheumatoid arthritis. *Acta Rheumatica Scandinavica*, 10, 142–53.
Bernstein, B., Forrester, D., Singsen, B., Koster King, K., Kornreich, H., and Hanson, V. (1977). Hip joint restoration in juvenile rheumatoid arthritis. *Arthritis and Rheumatism*, 20, 1099–104.
Blane, C.E., Ragsdale, C.G., and Hensinger, R.N. (1987). Late effects of JRA on the hip. *Journal of Pediatric Orthopedics*, 7, 677–80.
Chaplin, D., Pulkki, T., Saarimaa, A., and Vaino, K. (1969). Wrist and finger deformities in juvenile rheumatoid arthritis. *Acta Rheumatica Scandinavica*, 15, 206–23.
Erlandson, D.M. (1989). Juvenile rheumatoid arthritis. In *Pediatric rehabilitation. A team approach for therapists*, (ed. M.K. Logigian and J.D. Ward). Little, Brown and Company, Boston.
Findley, T.W., Halperin, D., and Easton, J.K.M. (1983). Wrist subluxation in juvenile rheumatoid arthritis: pathophysiology and management. *Archives of Physical Medicine and Rehabilitation*, 64, 69–73.
Földi, M. (1991). Physikalische Therapie bei der Sklerodermie. In *Lehrbuch der Lymphologie*, (ed. M. Földi and S. Kubik). Gustav Fischer Verlag, Stuttgart.
Garcia-Morteo, O., Babini, J.C., Maldonado-Cocco, J.A., Gagliardi, S., and Yabkowski, J. (1981). Remodeling of the hip joint in juvenile rheumatoid arthriris. Arthritis and Rheumatism, 24, 1570–4.
Granberry, W.M. and Mangum, G.L. (1980). The hand in the child with juvenile rheumatoid arthritis. *Journal of Hand Surgery*, 5, 105–13.
Gschwend, N. and Ivosevic-Radovanovic, D. (1986). Der Kinderfuß bei juveniler Polyarthritis. *Orthopäde*, 15, 212–19.
Häfner, R. (1987). Die juvenile Spondarthritis. *Monatsschrift für Kinderheilkunde*, 135, 41–6.
Häfner, R. and Truckenbrodt, H. (1989). Die juvenile Dermatomyositis. *Internistische Praxis*, 29, 307–20.
Hayem, F., Calède, C., Hayem, G., and Kahn, M.F. (1994). Involvement of the hip in systemic-onset forms of juvenile chronic arthritis. A retrospective study of twenty-eight cases. *Revue du Rhumatologie* (English Edition), 61, 516–22.
Jarvis, R.E. (1980). Treatment of arthritis in children. In *Physiotherapy in rheumatology*, (ed. S.A. Hyde). Blackwell Scientific Publications, Oxford.
Lechner, D.E., Mc Carthy, C.F., and Holden M.K. (1987). Gait deviations in patients with juvenile rheumatoid arthritis. *Journal of the American Physical Therapy Association*, 67, 1335–41.
Lloyd, S. and Aldrich, S. (1993). Paediatric rheumatology: meeting report. Second workshop of physiotherapy in JCA (Garmisch-Partenkirchen). *British Journal of Rheumatology*, 32, 425.
Melvin, J.L. (1989). *Rheumatic disease in the adult and child: occupational therapy and rehabilitation.* F.A. Davis Company, Philadelphia.
Rana, N.A. (1982). Juvenile rheumatoid arthritis of the foot. *Foot and Ankle Journal*, 3, 2–11.
Rombouts, J.J. and Rombouts-Lindemans, C. (1971). Involvement of the hip in juvenile rheumatoid arthritis. A radiological study with special reference to growth disturbances. *Acta Rheumatica Scandinavia*, 17, 248–67.
Scott, P.J., Ansell, B.M., and Huskinsson, E.C. (1977). Measurement of pain in juvenile chronic polyarthritis. *Annals of the Rheumatic Diseases*, 36, 186.
Stabrun, A.E., Larheim, T.A., Hoyeraal, H.M., and Rösler, M. (1988). Reduced mandibular dimensions and asymmetry in juvenile rheumatoid arthritis. *Arthritis and Rheumatism*, 31, 602–11.
Swann, M. (1978a). Management of lower limb deformities. In *Surgical management of juvenile chronic polyarthritis*, (ed G.P. Arden and B.M. Ansell), Grune & Stratton, New York.
Swann, M. (1978b). The foot. In *Surgical management of juvenile chronic polyarthritis*, (ed. G.P. Arden and B.M. Ansell), Grune & Stratton, New York.
Truckenbrodt, H. (1993). Pain in juvenile chronic arthritis: consequences for the musculo-skeletal system. *Clinical and Experimental Rheumatology*, 11 (Suppl. 9), 59–63.
Truckenbrodt, H., Häfner, R., and Altenbockum, C. von (1994). Functional joint analysis of the foot in juvenile chronic arthritis. *Clinical and Experimental Rheumatology*, 12 (Suppl. 10), 91–6.

6.5 Corticosteroid injection therapy

Allan I. Binder

Introduction

The injection of local anaesthetic and corticosteroid agents into joints or soft tissue structures constitutes one of the most effective therapeutic options for the treatment of localized painful lesions of articular and soft tissue structures. The value of this form of treatment is widely appreciated (Bamji *et al.* 1990), leading to some concern with regard to the adequacy of the skills and experience of general practitioners and other health-care workers (Phelan *et al.* 1992) who increasingly perform these injections.

This chapter will outline the basic principles of steroid injection therapy, with the technique and special considerations for the more common conditions where it is employed. Sports-related and spinal use is more specialized and will not be considered in detail. The majority of injections can be performed in the clinic, ward, or, if necessary, in the patient's home, using an aseptic no-touch technique.

Effect of steroid on joints and soft tissue structures

Systemic corticosteroid agents have potent anti-inflammatory effects which result in an improvement in pain, stiffness, and systemic illness in patients with active inflammatory arthropathy. They may also significantly reduce the rate of joint damage in early rheumatoid arthritis (Kirwan *et al.* 1995). However, the limiting factor for prolonged systemic steroid therapy is the considerable risk of side-effects such as osteoporosis, reduced resistance to infection, deficient wound healing, accelerated atherosclerosis, and the suppressive effect on the hypothalamic–pituitary–adrenal axis, which can persist for up to a year after corticosteroid therapy has been withdrawn. Atlantoaxial subluxation is also more common in rheumatoid patients treated with systemic steroids.

Local steroid injected into a joint aims to achieve a sustained concentration of the drug in the synovial fluid and to provide the maximum anti-inflammatory effect locally whilst minimizing absorption into the plasma with its attendant risk of systemic side-effects. After injection, the corticosteroid passes from the synovial fluid into the synovial cells, before being gradually released into the circulation to be cleared. There are many steroid agents available and the localized effects depend on the potency, solubility, and dose of the particular agent used.

Hydrocortisone acetate is short acting, has a weak anti-inflammatory effect, is fairly soluble, and is completely absorbed from the joint within hours. The synthetic corticosteroids, such as methylpredniso-lone acetate, prednisolone acetate, and triamcinolone acetonide, are much more potent and less soluble and hence remain localized in the joint for several weeks (Gray *et al.* 1981). Triamcinolone hexaceto-nide is the most insoluble steroid, and has the slowest absorption, lowest plasma levels (Derendorf *et al.* 1986), and longest action (Bird *et al.* 1979) of the drugs available.

The benefit of local steroid injection can be observed by the profound reduction in inflammatory change and decrease in the expression of genes that play a role in articular destruction (collagen-ase, tissue inhibitors of metelloproteinases, complement, and HLA-DR), seen in histological tissue samples following local steroid injection (Firestein *et al.* 1991). Local steroid also leads to an improvement in the relationship between synovial fluid and serum levels of hyaluronan, restoring it towards normal (Pitsillides *et al.* 1994). Corticosteroid crystals which are found in joints immediately after steroid injection, and even a week later, are distinctive, being both intra and extracellular when visualized by polarized light and electron microscopy (Gordon and Schumacher 1979).

The systemic absorption of corticosteroid after local joint injection, may be sufficient to reduce inflammation in non-injected joints, and suppress the hypothalamic–pituitary–adrenal axis for up to 4 weeks after a single dose of a long-acting steroid (Bird *et al.* 1979). However, serious systemic side-effects are rare after a single injection, except in patients with brittle diabetes, infection, or where emergency surgery becomes necessary.

Outside the joints, local steroid injection may also produce beneficial effects in acute or chronic lesions, even where an inflammatory component is difficult to confirm. The injection of local steroid into soft tissue structures produces a characteristic histological picture, with circumscribed deposits of acellular finely granular material that stains faintly with haematoxylineosin. In some cases a mild to moderate reaction of histiocytes, fibroblasts, and lymphocytes may be noted round the edges. Small elongated spaces are usually evident, with occasional weakly birifringent (positive or negative) crystals that have an identical shape and size to the empty spaces (Balogh 1986). There is little data on the absorption of steroid from tendon sheaths, bursas, or other soft tissue structures, although methylprednisolone has been shown to produce measurable plasma levels for a mean of 16 days after soft tissue injection (Mattila 1983). Not all the effects of local steroid on soft tissue structures are beneficial, with impairment in the healing of damaged ligaments (Wiggins *et al.* 1994) and atrophy of up to 40 per cent of skin and subcutaneous tissue thickness, following a single injection of steroid (Gomez *et al.* 1982).

Table 1 Indications for local steroid injection

Structure	Examples of diseases amenable to injection
Joints	Rheumatoid and other inflammatory arthropathies
Entheses	Tennis and golfers elbow, rotator cuff tendinitis
Tendon sheath	De Quervain's tenosynovitis, trigger finger
Bursae	Trochanteric, olecranon bursitis
Ligaments / muscles	Strains, sprains, sports injuries
Nerve compression	Carpal and tarsal tunnel syndrome
Nodules/ganglia	Rheumatoid arthritis, trauma
Trigger points	Cervical, lumbar
Epidural	Nerve root compression

Indications for local steroid injection

Joint puncture permits the aspiration of fluid for microbiological, crystal, and, occasionally, biochemical assessment, and should always precede steroid injection where infection, haemarthrosis, or crystal arthropathy is suspected. The colour, smell, turbidity, and viscosity of the aspirated fluid may help differentiate inflammatory arthropathy from crystal-related or non-inflammatory disease. However, a heavy concentration of polymorphs (pyoarthrosis) is equally likely with acute rheumatoid, infection, or gout. Conventional light and polarized microscopy and, in some cases, microbiological culture of the synovial fluid may be necessary before steroid can be safely injected. Soft tissue lesions, such as olecranon bursitis, are also amenable to aspiration, with fluid from these lesions being subjected to analysis similar to synovial fluid, before steroid is injected.

Local anaesthetic and/or steroid injection also has value as a diagnostic tool where the source of the pain is uncertain. For example the abolition of a 'painful arc' on abduction, as a result of local anaesthetic injected with the steroid, confirms the diagnosis of rotator cuff tendinitis.

However, the main use of local steroid injection is for treatment of inflammatory and non-inflammatory conditions of joints or soft tissues, whether they are acute or chronic. The main anatomical structures with examples of common conditions amenable to local corticosteroid injection are shown in Table 1. Even acute gout and pseudogout will respond to steroid injection (Gray *et al.* 1981), although this therapy is not usually necessary or always feasible. The treatment of osteoarthritic joints with steroid injection is more controversial (Dieppe 1991), although the presence of an effusion increases the likelihood of short-term reduction in pain (Gaffney *et al.* 1995) in these cases.

Contraindications to local injection

There are some absolute and other relative contraindications to steroid injection therapy as shown in Table 2. Any suspicion of sepsis within the affected joint, on the same limb, or systemically precludes steroid injection, until infection has been excluded or adequately treated. Steroid injection is best avoided in joints previously affected by septic arthritis, as local defence mechanisms within the joint are suspect. Monoarthritis of unknown cause should always be regarded with suspicion and steroid injection delayed, until either a diagnosis is made or at least until infection has been excluded.

Septic arthritis is particularly easy to overlook in rheumatoid patients who are frail and elderly or being treated with systemic steroid or other immunosuppressive drugs. In these patients infection is often polyarticular, mimicking an exacerbation of the inflammatory disease. Although *Staphylococcus aureus* is the most common infecting organism, patients may not present with fever, weight loss, or other features usually associated with systemic infection (Kraft *et al.* 1985). A mild rise in neutrophil count and a high sedimentation rate may also fail to differentiate infective from inflammatory causes, although an exceptionally high C-reactive protein level is more suggestive of infection. While systemic ill health can be a prominent feature in septic arthritis, it can also occur in patients with rheumatoid arthritis without infection (systemic rheumatoid), and steroids should not be given by any route until infection, including tuberculosis, has been sought and if necessary treated.

Patients need to be asked about previous allergic reactions to local anaesthetic agents (e.g. with dental treatment), steroids, or local injections. An exacerbation of the pain for 24 to 48 h following a previous steroid injection does not suggest allergy but rather a crystal-related phenomenon (Berger and Yount 1990). Neutropenia, thrombocytopenia, and clotting abnormalities constitute relative contraindications to local steroid injection. If patients are on anticoagulants, these should be stopped for at least 24 h before the steroid injection. With other clotting abnormalities or blood dyscrasias, haematological advice should be sought, and appropriate preparations made to reduce the risk of bleeding following the injection. While haemophilic arthropathy has been successfully treated with cautious steroid injection (Shupak *et al.* 1988), this therapy should be avoided in sickle cell disease (Gladman and Bombardier 1987) as a sickle crisis may be precipitated by the procedure.

Table 2 Contraindications to local steroid injection

Absolute contraindication
   Septic arthritis, septicaemia, active sepsis in locality, tuberculosis
   Febrile patient, cause unknown
   Serious allergy to local anaesthetic, steroid, or previous local injection
   Sickle cell disease

Relative contraindication
   Monoarthritis of unknown cause
   Neutropenia, thrombocytopenia
   Anticoagulants or bleeding diathesis

Table 3 Side-effects attributed to local steroid injection
Exacerbation of pain for 24–48 h (crystal related)
Septic arthritis
Accelerated destruction of an unsuspected septic joint
Subcutaneous tissue atrophy
Depigmentation
Transient facial flushing
Anaphylaxis
Peripheral nerve injury
Tendon rupture
Avascular necrosis, Charcot joint
Loss of diabetic control
Reactivation of tuberculosis
Cartilage damage
Soft tissue calcification

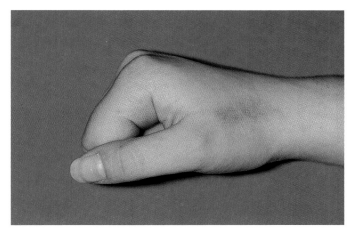

Fig. 1 Subcutaneous tissue atrophy following steroid injection of De Quervain's tenosynovitis lesion.

Potential dangers and side-effects

Local steroid injections are extremely safe, provided that the indication is appropriate, there are no contraindications, and a careful aseptic technique is used. Some side-effects apply to all injections (Table 3), while others are site-specific, and will be discussed below. While the exacerbation of pain for up to 48 h following the injection suggests a crystal-related phenomenon (Berger and Yount 1990), pain persisting beyond this time requires assessment for infection or other complications. Infection following steroid injection constitutes the most important side-effect, although it is very rare, with an estimated sepsis rate of 1 in 14 000 to 50 000 injections (Gray *et al.* 1981). Chronic debilitating illness such as severe diabetes mellitus or rheumatoid (Ostensson and Geborek 1991), or factors like drug abuse and alcoholism (Haslock *et al.* 1995), which suppress general immunity can predispose patients to infection. Postinjection sepsis may result from contamination of the injection equipment (Nakashima *et al.* 1987) or skin, haematogenous spread (Von Essen and Savolainen 1989), or reactivation of a previous infection. Accelerated joint destruction will also follow the injection of steroid into an undiagnosed septic joint.

Subcutaneous tissue atrophy (Fig. 1) or depigmentation (Fig. 2) are more likely if excessively large or repeated doses of long-acting steroid are given. While tendon rupture (Fig. 3) or facial flushing is encountered fairly often, other side-effects (Table 3) are rare. The importance of local injection in the development of avascular necrosis or a Charcot joint (Parikh *et al.* 1993) remains uncertain.

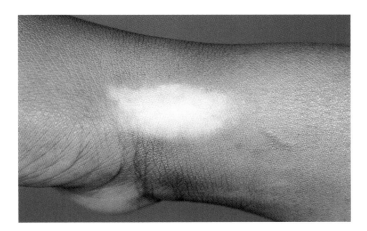

Fig. 2 Depigmentation following steroid injection of De Quervain's tenosynovitis lesion.

Method of steroid injection

The method of injection of local steroid into painful joints and soft tissue structures is similar, although the exact technique may depend on the local anatomy, the size and depth of the lesion concerned, and the need to aspirate fluid before injection. The broad principles of

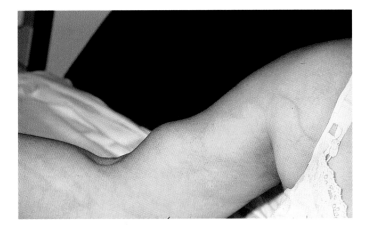

Fig. 3 Rupture of the long head of the biceps tendon following anterior shoulder injection.

Table 4 Equipment required for local steroid injection

Steroid preparations (individual ampoules)
    short acting—hydrocortisone acetate 25 mg/ml
    long acting—methylprednisolone acetate 40 mg/ml
                methylprednisolone acetate 40 mg/ml,
                lignocaine 10 mg/ml
                triamcinolone hexacetonide 20 mg/ml
                triamcinolone acetonide 40 mg/ml

Single-dose 1% lignocaine ampoules for injection

Refrigerant spray

Sealed isopropyl alcohol swabs

Other
    sealed single-use needles—25G, 23G, 21G and 19G
    single-use syringes
    sterile cottonwool
    elastoplast, crepe bandages

injection therapy will be outlined first with locally determined modification in techniques being considered under the individual conditions.

As the success of local injection therapy depends on the accurate placement of the injected steroid (Jones et al. 1993), detailed knowledge of the anatomy at the site of injection is important. Consistency in the choice of equipment (needles and syringes) and adequacy of relaxation of the patient, and especially of the limb to be injected, further improves the feel, and hence reliability, of the injection. While the injection of large fluid-filled joints is relatively easy, other injections may require considerable skill and experience.

There is no single 'correct' method of performing steroid injection and most skilled operators develop their own unique style (Haslock et al. 1995), based on training, experience, and the equipment available. Irrespective of the individual variation in method, this should always be based on a consistent, safe, aseptic, 'no-touch' technique. The method presented reflects the author's own practice.

Equipment

Table 4 summarizes the equipment needed for routine steroid injection. Single-dose ampoules of steroid and local anaesthetic agents should always be used to eliminate any possibility of cross infection.

Steroid agents

Hydrocortisone acetate is the only frequently used, short-acting agent (Gray et al. 1981) and is especially useful for superficial lesions, where there is a risk of subcutaneous atrophy or depigmentation, or in lesions (such as Achilles tendinitis) where tendon rupture may occur. Although there are many long-acting steroid agents available (Table 4), familiarity with one or two agents is adequate, as the differences between agents is not great. Methylprednisolone acetate has the advantage of being available alone or premixed with lignocaine, permitting greater flexibility in the adjustment of both steroid dosage and fluid volume when injected at different sites. Triamcinolone is also widely used as the acetonide or hexacetonide

salts. In most circumstances, the long acting steroid agents are superior to hydrocortisone (Blyth et al. 1994), leading to a more sustained clinical improvement.

The dosage of steroid used varies according to the lesion injected. For most joint and soft tissue lesions, 25 mg of hydrocortisone, 40 mg of methylprednisolone or triamcinolone acetonide, or 20 mg of triamcinolone hexacetonide is adequate. Large joints, like the knee, may require double and very small joints or lesions half this dose.

Local anaesthesia

Local anaesthesia of the skin can be achieved by the use of a refrigerant spray such as ethyl chloride. Freezing numbs the skin rapidly and is especially useful in the hand and other sensitive parts of the body, or in patients requiring frequent injections. The skin is sprayed only until it turns white to achieve anaesthesia, as beyond this point a painful burn may ensue.

Lignocaine 1 per cent mixes well without flocculation with most steroid agents, and is usually introduced in combination with the steroid. Where the injection is technically difficult or fluid aspiration is to precede injection, the lignocaine is introduced first. The volume of local anaesthetic agent injected will vary according to the size of the joint or lesion being injected. While the use of lignocaine may reduce the immediate postinjection pain in tennis elbow or other soft tissue lesions (Haslock et al. 1995), the rationale for routine use in large joint injection is less clear cut (Kirwan et al. 1984).

Other equipment

Sealed isopropyl alcohol swabs or other alcohol-based agents provide a safe and cost effective method of achieving skin cleansing. Iodine, chlorhexidine in spirit, and other cleansers increase the cost of the procedure but offer no advantage over the sealed alcohol-based swabs (Cawley and Morris 1992) and can increase the risk of infection (Nakashima et al. 1987).

While a 2 or 5 ml sterile syringe is adequate for most steroid injections, 10 ml and 20 ml syringes are required for fluid aspiration. The choice of needle for any given site is also important. Most medium sized joints and soft tissue lesions can be injected with a 23G (blue) needle. A larger 21G (green) needle is used for larger joints, especially where aspiration is required, and for deep soft tissue lesions such as those round the buttocks and thighs. Where the synovial effusion is large or the fluid is thick, fibrinous, or purulent a 19G (white) needle may be needed for successful aspiration. Small hand and foot joints and superficial soft tissue lesions are best injected with a fine 25G (orange) needle.

Preparation

The method of preparation for joint aspiration and steroid injection is shown in Table 5.

The patient must be as relaxed as possible, as tension in surrounding muscles can make the injection difficult or even impossible. Where patient anxiety is a particular concern, most injections can be carried out with the patient lying supine with the head comfortably supported on pillows. This position facilitates the treatment of vasovagal attacks if they occur. The presence of a nurse helps to reassure and position the patient but the nurse must be dissuaded from drawing up the drugs or shaking them out on to a tray or table before the operator is ready. The procedure should be described to the

Table 5 Preparation for steroid injection
Exclude contraindications or allergy
Explain the procedure before starting
Position patient so patient and limb are relaxed
Wash hands and dry carefully

Prepare injection immediately before use
  To aspirate: lignocaine and steroid separate
  To inject: lignocaine and steroid mixture

Mix steroid thoroughly before preparation and before injection
Use single-dose ampoules
Draw up the drugs yourself!
Change needle before injecting
Keep needle covered before use

Table 6 Technique for steroid injection
Mark exact point of needle insertion with a blunt object
Use no-touch technique
Cleanse injection site with 2–3 alcohol swabs
Use refrigerant spray for skin anaesthesia
Reswab injection site
Insert needle without touching the metal
For aspiration: keep needle stationary as fluid is tapped, then change syringe and inject steroid
For injection: pull back plunger before injecting
Remove needle carefully and check for bleeding
Use elastoplast if no allergy; crepe bandage after knee aspiration
Dispose of all needles and syringes safely and avoid needlestick injury
Rest or splint joint after injection if possible
Re-emphasize possible side-effects and benefits

patient in detail before starting the injection, to reduce the risk of airborne infection. At the same time, the patient can be assessed for sepsis, allergy, or other contraindications to the injection.

Simple hand washing is adequate for the procedure if a no-touch technique is to be employed, and should precede preparation of the injection. Careful hand drying will prevent water running down the needle. While gloves are now recommended for joint aspiration (American College of Rheumatology Council on Rheumatological Care 1992), less than 50 per cent of American (Yood 1993) and 10 per cent of British rheumatologists (Haslock *et al.* 1995) currently heed this advice. The injection is prepared with a combination of steroid and local anaesthetic in the same syringe, in most cases. Where the injection is likely to be difficult or where aspiration is to precede injection, the two agents are drawn up separately, the lignocaine being in a larger syringe. As the steroid preparations are crystalline, they need to be thoroughly mixed before being drawn up and again before injection. The needle should ideally be changed following preparation to maintain sharpness, and must remain covered until the injection is given to reduce the risk of infection.

Injection technique

A method for aspiration and/or steroid injection is summarized in Table 6. Talking should be kept to a minimum during the procedure. The exact site for injection is carefully marked with a blunt-pointed object such as a thumbnail or ball-point pen with the point retracted. This mark should only be made once careful positioning of the patient has been achieved, and needs to remain visible even after skin cleansing to permit a no-touch aseptic technique to be used.

Only one or two joints should be injected per session, with the same joint being injected no more than three or four times a year. Patients should be warned of possible side-effects such as a temporary exacerbation of pain or destabilization of diabetic control following the injection. The patients should also be told about the possible beneficial effects of the absorbed steroid on systemic symptoms or other inflamed joints.

Postinjection

The injected part should, where possible, be rested for 24 to 48 h after injection (Neustadt 1992; Chakravarty *et al.* 1994), although admission for absolute bed rest is neither cost-effective nor practical. Splinting the injected joint may also prolong the duration that the steroid remains localized at that site (Dixon and Graber 1983). Where a large effusion has been drained, as from a knee, a crepe bandage should be firmly applied to provide support and take up the slack in the tissues stretched by the effusion. The maximum improvement usually develops in 2 to 4 weeks, and may last many months.

Joint and soft tissue lesions

The most common lesions amenable to steroid injection will be considered on a regional basis (Table 7), describing the method of injection, choice of steroid agent, volume of injection, and particular differences at each site. Several monographs are available outlining joint injection techniques (Dixon and Graber 1983; Doherty *et al.* 1992).

The painful shoulder

Shoulder pain usually arises from soft tissue lesions, although arthropathies affecting the glenohumeral, acromioclavicular, and sternoclavicular joints also occur, with most lesions being amenable to steroid injection (Table 7). As shoulder structures arise from the C5 dermatome, pain is felt in the upper arm, maximally at the point of insertion of the deltoid muscle. Only the acromioclavicular joint arises from C4, and hence pain radiates to the neck and needs to be differentiated from cervical lesions. Shoulder pain can also result from polymyalgia rheumatica, or can be the site of referred pain from cervical, thoracic, or intra-abdominal pathology.

Table 7 Lesions amenable to injection with suggested steroid agent and volume of injection

Site and lesion	Suggested steroid agent and volume of injection
Shoulder	
Intracapsular — arthritis, capsulitis	40 mg MP or 20 mg THA in 2 ml
Extracapsular — rotator cuff lesions	40 mg MP or 20 mg THA in 2 ml
— acromioclavicular arthritis	10 mg MP in 0.5 ml
Elbow	
Epicondylitis — tennis or golfers elbow	20 mg MP (25 mg HC on repeat) in 2 ml
Arthritis — inflammatory, crystal	40 mg MP or 20 mg THA in 2 ml
Olecranon bursitis — trauma, rheumatoid	25 mg HC or 20 mg MP in 2 ml
Ulnar nerve entrapment	20 mg MP in 2 ml[a]
Wrist	
Radiocarpal joint — inflammatory, crystal	40 mg MP or 20 mg THA in 2 ml
Radioulnar joint — rheumatoid	20 mg MP or 10 mg THA in 1 ml
Carpal tunnel syndrome — arthritis, pregnancy, thyroid disease, idiopathic, other	20mg MP or 10 mg THA in 1 ml[a]
De Quervain's tenosynovitis	25 mg HC or 10 mg MP in 0.5–1 ml
Tenosynovitis and ganglia	10 mg MP or 25 mg HC in 0.5–1 ml
Hand	
Small joint inflammatory arthritis	10 mg MP in 0.5 ml
First carpometacarpal osteoarthritis	10 mg MP in 0.5 ml
Flexor tenosynovitis and 'trigger' finger	10 mg MP in 0.5 ml
Nodules/ganglia — rheumatoid, other	10 mg MP in 0.5 ml
Hip	
Bursitis–trochanteric, ischial tuberosity	40 mg MP or 20 mg THA in 2–5 ml
Nerve entrapment — meralgia paraesthetica	20 mg MP or 10 mg THA in 1 ml
Other groin pain — e.g. adductor strain	25 mg HC or 20 mg MP in 0.5–1 ml
Knee	
Arthritis — inflammatory osteoarthritis	20–40 mg THA or 40–80 mg MP in 2 ml
Bursitis — prepatellar, infrapatellar	25 mg HC or 10 mg MP in 0.5–1 ml
Tendinitis, enthesopathy, trauma	25 mg HC in 1 ml
Ankle and foot	
Ankle arthritis — inflammatory or not	40 mg THA or 80 mg MP in 2 ml
Subtalar arthritis — inflammatory or not	40 mg THA or 80 mg MP in 2 ml
Tenosynovitis — peroneal, posterior tibial	40 mg THA or 80 mg MP in 2 ml
Tarsal tunnel syndrome	20 mg MP or 10 mg THA in 1 ml[a]
Posterior heel pain — Achilles tendinitis, bursitis	25 mg HC in 1 ml
Plantar heel pain — spondylarthropathy, plantar spur, plantar fasciitis	20 mg in 0.5 ml

MP=methylprednisolone acetate; HC=hydrocortisone acetate; TAH=triamcinolone hexacetonide.
[a]Avoid excessive lignocaine near peripheral nerve.

Injection therapy is much more cost-effective than physiotherapy (Dacre *et al.* 1989) for shoulder lesions but the site of steroid injection needs to be based on anatomical pathology rather than the localization of tender or trigger points (Hollingworth *et al.* 1983). Some studies have failed to confirm the benefit of injection therapy (Adebajo *et al.* 1990) but this may reflect difficulties in placement of the injection (Hollingworth *et al.* 1983).

Glenohumeral joint

This joint communicates with the tendon sheath of the long head of the biceps tendon, but not with the subacromial bursa unless rupture of the rotator cuff has occurred. Aspiration and or injection of the glenohumeral joint can be achieved using the anterior or posterior route, as both provide good access to the joint, although the posterior route is technically easier.

Anterior route (Fig. 4)

This route gives more reliable access in patients with adhesive capsulitis and is better suited for aspiration of large shoulder effusions. With the patient lying supine, the arm is rotated to identify the coracoid process and joint line anteriorly, and acromium posteriorly. Laying the arm across the abdomen to result in partial internal rotation of the shoulder, the injection is made just lateral to the coracoid in the line of the joint margin, with the needle directed towards the acromium. If correctly sited, the injection can be given without resistance.

Posterior route (Fig. 5)

This is especially useful where the cause of the pain is uncertain or the operator lacks skill in injection procedure. With the patient seated across the couch and approached from behind, the thumb is used to identify the spine of the scapula which is followed laterally until it bends forward as the acromium. The point just below the acromium is marked. The forefinger is then used to palpate the coracoid process in front, rotating the shoulder if necessary to locate it. The needle is inserted under the acromium and gently advanced without resistance with the needle pointing towards the outer side of the coracoid process. More superficial injection is used to treat cuff lesions.

Subacromial bursa — lateral approach (Fig. 6)

Injection into the bursa is particularly useful for rotator cuff lesions, especially when accompanied by a painful arc on abduction. Although subacromial bursitis is rarely a primary diagnosis, it is frequently secondarily affected by pathological processes arising in the rotator cuff and other nearby structures. The subacromial space is very large, being in continuity with the subdeltoid space and also, with cuff rupture, the glenohumeral joint.

To inject the subacromial space, the patient should be seated and approached from the lateral aspect with the arm hanging vertically down, to use gravity to help enlarge the gap between the acromium above and the humeral head below. This gap is palpated, marked, and the needle advanced into the space, directed medially and slightly posteriorly. A relatively large volume of local anaesthetic (2–10 ml) is mixed with the steroid in view of the large capacity of the space being injected. The local anaesthetic rapidly abolishes the 'painful arc', which both helps confirm the diagnosis of a rotator cuff lesion and the correct siting of the injection. The benefit of this injection is particularly dramatic in patients with acute calcific tendinitis, where the pain is so acute that patients often present as an emergency.

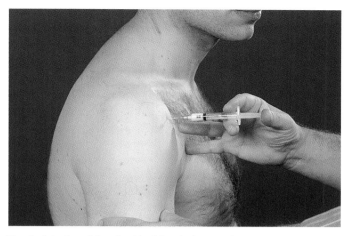

Fig. 4 Injection of the shoulder joint via the anterior route.

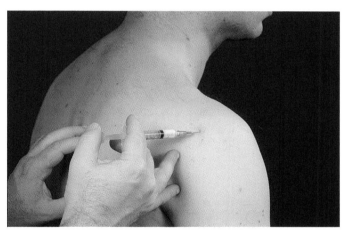

Fig. 5 Injection of the shoulder joint via the posterior route.

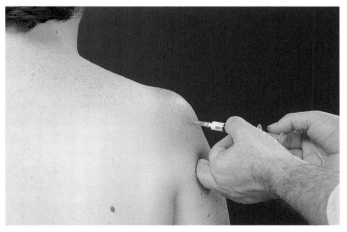

Fig. 6 Injection of the subacromial bursa via the lateral route.

While steroid injection to the glenohumeral joint or subacromial bursa often ameliorates the pain associated with adhesive capsulitis (frozen shoulder), it has less effect on the recovery of range of movement (Rizk *et al.* 1991). Arthrographic capsular distension, which ruptures the capsule, when combined with steroid injection, may lead to earlier recovery in range (Rizk *et al.* 1994) in adhesive capsulitis. However, a home exercise regimen which encourages hourly wall climbing to increase abduction and forward flexion, achieves a satisfactory rate of recovery in most patients with frozen shoulder.

Individual rotator cuff tendons

The individual rotator cuff tendons can also be injected with appropriate expertise (Cyriax 1984). The supraspinatus (superior) and subscapularis (inferior) tendons are anterior, and the infraspinatus tendon posterior, to the joint. Pain on resisted shoulder abduction, internal, and external rotation respectively, helps to identify the rotator cuff tendons involved. These injections are especially useful in patients in whom a 'painful arc' is absent, and hence where subacromial injection may be unsuccessful. Bicipital tendinitis is difficult to distinguish from rotator cuff tendinitis, but often coexists with it. While steroid injection via the anterior route may reduce pain from this source, rupture of the long head of biceps may follow the injection (Fig. 3).

Acromioclavicular joint

The acromioclavicular joint, which is on the anterosuperior aspect of the shoulder, is located by following the clavicle laterally until the joint is reached. Local tenderness confirms joint involvement. The joint is injected from the anterior or superior route, but only accepts 0.5 ml of fluid. Care is necessary to avoid deep injection as a pneumothorax can result from apical lung penetration.

Elbow

Elbow pain is extremely common and usually results from epicondylitis. Care is necessary to exclude pain referred from the cervical spine, brachial plexus, or shoulder, which can closely mimic primary elbow pathology. Most elbow lesions (Table 7) are injected from the lateral side, with the patient sitting in a relaxed manner and with the elbow resting on the examination table at an angle of 90°. Only medial epicondylitis and ulnar entrapment neuropathy require a greater angle and appropriate positioning to permit access to the medial aspect of the elbow.

Epicondylitis

Epicondylitis can result from trauma, lifting heavy weights, or repetitive power rotation movements. It is particularly difficult to cure when it is occupation or sport related.

Lateral epicondylitis (tennis elbow) (Fig. 7)

In tennis elbow, localized tenderness is found either just distal to the lateral epicondyle or over the radial head. Pain is exacerbated by wrist dorsiflexion against resistance, especially when the elbow is extended and the hand prone. Grip strength is also reduced with the arm held in a similar position. While supination and pronation may be painful, there is no significant loss of elbow range.

Local steroid injection is directed to the site of maximum tenderness, with the injection aimed at 45°, to end near the insertion of the common extensor tendon to bone. A fair amount of pressure is

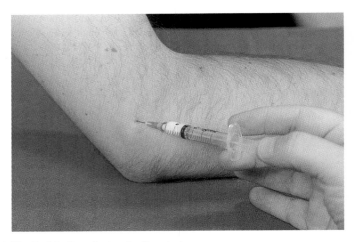

Fig. 7 Injection of a tennis elbow lesion.

needed to inject at this site, so care should be taken to ensure the needle is firmly attached to the syringe.

Medial epicondylitis (golfer's elbow)

Golfer's elbow causes tenderness very similar to tennis elbow but it is localized to the region of the medial epicondyle. Pain is usually noted on resisted palmar flexion of the wrist against resistance with the hand held supine.

Injection is again directed at the site of maximum tenderness, near the common flexor tendon insertion to bone. Care is necessary to avoid injury to the ulnar nerve which lies in a groove just behind the medial epicondyle.

There is no agreement with regard to the steroid agent of choice to inject tennis and golfer's elbow lesions. While triamcinolone is more effective than hydrocortisone (Price *et al.* 1991), it is more likely to lead to atrophy of the subcutaneous tissue. Both temporary postinjection exacerbation of pain and early relapse of symptoms are common following injection therapy (Dijs *et al.* 1990; Price *et al.* 1991), irrespective of the type of steroid used. The most logical approach is to use a long-acting steroid for the first injection, and hydrocortisone for further injections or for treatment of relapses, but with no more than three injections being given to treat the same lesion. Further injections can lead to long-lasting or irreversible atrophy which may amplify the pain from trivial knocks. Healing of epicondylitis lesions is often slow and diffuse forearm ache may precede recovery.

Elbow joint

The elbow joint is commonly involved in inflammatory arthropathies, causing swelling and painful limitation of elbow movements. The joint is injected using either the posterior or anterolateral route.

Posterior approach (Fig. 8)

This route is easier to use before gross deformity has developed. The posterior joint line can be identified by placement of the thumb on the lateral epicondyle and third finger on the olecranon. The paraolecranon groove between the two fingers identifies the joint line, which runs between the two heads of the triceps tendon. Injection into the joint is just above and slightly lateral to the olecranon, where a bulge can be felt in the presence of a joint effusion.

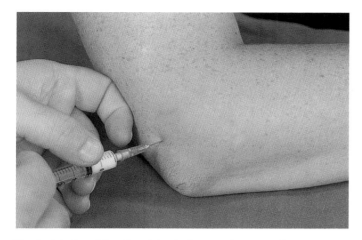

Fig. 8 Injection of the elbow joint via the posterior approach.

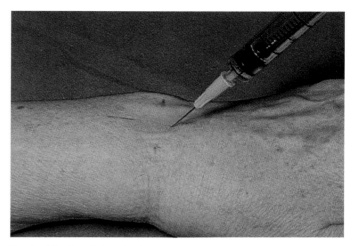

Fig. 9 Injection of the wrist joint.

Anterolateral approach

The thumb is used to palpate the head of the radius at the radiohumeral part of the elbow joint, best identified by rotating the forearm while palpating. An effusion may be evident at this site as a result of synovial extension around the radial head. Once the joint line is identified, the injection is made tangentially just under the capsule, not attempting to reach the centre of the joint.

Olecranon bursitis

Olecranon bursitis can result from infection, trauma, rheumatoid arthritis, or gout. Once infection has been excluded, the bursa can be aspirated and injected with steroid (Smith *et al.* 1989). However, secondary infection (Canoso and Sheckman 1979), chronic local pain, or skin atrophy (Weinstein *et al.* 1984) may follow the injection.

Ulnar nerve entrapment

The ulnar nerve lies in the groove just behind the medial epicondyle, and can be impinged on by local pressure, trauma, or inflammatory synovial tissue. In many cases the cause is unknown. Patients present with pain on the medial side of the elbow, paraesthesia of the ulnar digits, and occasionally sensory or motor abnormalities in the hand. A positive Tinel sign, elicited by local percussion over the nerve behind the medial epicondyle, suggests the diagnosis, which can be confirmed by electromyography. Steroid injection at this site may reduce the symptoms, especially when the lesion has an inflammatory cause, but care is necessary to avoid injury to the nerve during the procedure.

Wrist

Although the wrist and surrounding structures are often involved in the inflammatory arthropathies, there are many other common, non-inflammatory wrist lesions (Table 7), which are amenable to steroid injection therapy. Rheumatoid arthritis has a particular predilection for involvement of the distal radio-ulnar joint near the ulnar styloid, which is normally separated from the rest of the wrist joint by the triangular fibrocartilage. Radio-ulnar disease, if severe, may lead to attrition and rupture of the fourth and fifth extensor tendons as they pass over the joint. It is also important to differentiate true wrist (radiocarpal) joint involvement from overlying tenosynovitis.

Injection around the wrist and hand is best carried out with both the patient and doctor seated, and with the limb resting on the examination couch.

Wrist (radiocarpal) joint (Fig. 9)

Injection of the wrist is carried out with the hand held palm down and the joint opened up by palmar flexion over a pillow or similar object. The joint margin is felt as a triangular gap between the lower end of the radius and the lunate and scaphoid bones. The needle is inserted into the joint pointing in a proximal direction at an angle of about 60°. Immobilization of the wrist may prolong the beneficial effects of the injection (Dixon and Graber 1983).

The distal radio-ulnar joint

This joint is identified by gently supinating and pronating the forearm with a finger over the ulnar styloid. Once the joint line is located, it can be injected in a similar manner to the wrist but with the needle inserted almost tangentially into the radio-ulnar joint.

Carpal tunnel syndrome (Fig. 10)

Carpal tunnel syndrome results from median nerve compression in the carpal tunnel of the wrist. Patients present with intermittent or persistent pain and paraesthesia in the thumb, index, and middle fingers, characteristically waking the patient at night. A positive Tinel sign, elicited by local percussion over the median nerve at the wrist, help confirm the diagnosis. Untreated, the lesion can lead to wasting of the muscles of the thenar eminence. Carpal tunnel syndrome can be mimicked by cervical spine or brachial plexus lesions, and electromyography, although not infallible, may assist diagnosis in difficult cases. Even once the diagnosis has been confirmed, a cause, such as inflammatory arthropathy, previous trauma, thyroid disease, or pregnancy should be sought.

The injection is carried out just medial to the midline of the ventral aspect of the wrist, in the first crease, at the junction to the hand. If the palmaris longus tendon is present, it overlies the median nerve and injection should be just medial and parallel to it. A fine 25G needle is inserted, just medial to the midline or palmaris longus tendon, to a depth of 1 cm, directing the needle towards the palm. If the needle is

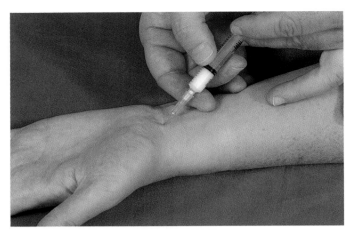

Fig. 10 Injection of carpal tunnel syndrome to the ulnar side of the palmaris longus tendon.

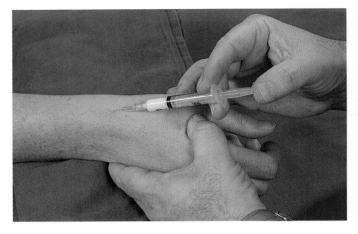

Fig. 11 Injection of De Quervain's tenosynovitis.

correctly positioned, there should be no resistance, pain, or paraesthesia during the procedure.

Care is necessary to avoid damage to the nerve, which can cause persistent pain and paraesthesia (McConnell and Bush 1990; Frederick *et al.* 1992). Local anaesthetic agents should also be used sparingly to avoid unpleasant, though temporary, paralysis of the median nerve. Long-acting steroid preparations should be used for carpal tunnel injection therapy, as the aim of the injection is to atrophy the soft tissue structures around the nerve. A wrist splint, especially if used at night, may also hasten recovery (Kulick *et al.* 1986). In idiopathic lesions, especially affecting women under the age of 40 years, steroid injection is less likely to be successful (Weiss *et al.* 1994b) and earlier surgery should be considered. The presence of thenar muscle wasting, persistent sensory loss, or a lack of response to steroid injection, is associated with a less favourable outcome even following surgical decompression (Green 1984; Kulick *et al.* 1986).

De Quervain's tenosynovitis (Fig. 11)

Stenosing tenosynovitis of the extensor pollicus brevis and abductor pollicus longus (De Quervain's tenosynovitis) is a common condition which is often occupational and related to repeated minor trauma. It causes pain on gripping especially with use of the thumb. Tenderness is noted in the 'snuffbox' area of the wrist where palpable crepitus may be found. Pain can be increased by ulnar deviation of the wrist against resistance after placing the patients thumb in the palm (Finkelstein's test), with the arm held in the midprone position.

The injection for this lesion is given at the point of maximum tenderness, using a fine-bore needle which is inserted tangentially along the tendon sheath. When correctly sited, the injection can be given without resistance. If there is doubt with regard to placement of the needle, the syringe can be disconnected and movement of the needle will mirror movement of the thumb, if the needle is correctly sited in the tendon sheath.

Local steroid injections (Weiss *et al.* 1994a) are more likely to be effective in acute lesions, and should be combined with a splint and modification of the activities which caused the lesion. Although long-acting steroids are more effective (Anderson *et al.* 1991), hydrocortisone is the preferred steroid agent as it is less likely to cause complications such as subcutaneous atrophy or depigmentation

(Figs 1 and 2), especially after repeated injection. Dark skinned patients need to be warned that these cosmetic complications may follow the injection.

Extensor and flexor tenosynovitis

These lesions, if troublesome, can be treated by aspiration and local steroid injection, although recurrence is common and surgical excision is more likely to lead to a permanent cure (Wright *et al.* 1994).

Hand

The hand structures amenable to steroid injection are shown in Table 7.

The small joints in the hands

These joints are frequently involved in inflammatory arthropathies and all are amenable to steroid injection to reduce pain and swelling. However, the injections are painful and it is only possible to inject one or two joints per session, unless general or regional anaesthesia is used. The presence of a joint effusion simplifies the procedure and distortion of the normal anatomy makes it considerably more difficult.

The technique of steroid injection is similar for all the small hand joints and can be performed with the patient seated with the hand palm down across the table or examination bench. The joint margin on the lateral or medial side of the joint is identified by gently flexing and extending the digit. The superior part of the joint line is marked, with the joint flexed to an angle of 45°. By distracting the finger with one hand, it is injected with the other hand, using the superolateral or superomedial approach to avoid injury to the neurovascular structures. The joint will only accept 0.5 to 1 ml of injected fluid, which should contain a combination of long-acting steroid and local anaesthetic. Splintage of the joint may prolong the effect of the injection.

Metacarpophalangeal joint (Fig. 12)

The joint line, which is located about 1 cm distal to, and not at, the crest of the knuckle, is identified by passive movement of the finger. After marking the joint line, the patients finger is distracted as the joint is injected, tangentially under the extensor expansion.

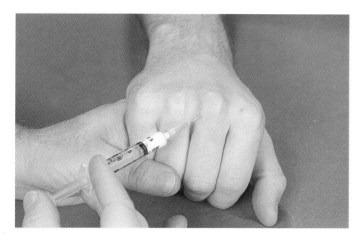

Fig. 12 Injection of the metacarpophalangeal joint.

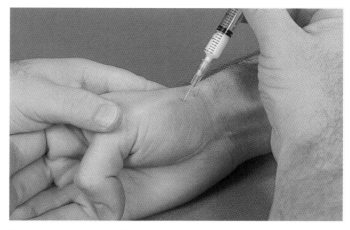

Fig. 14 Injection of the first carpometacarpal joint.

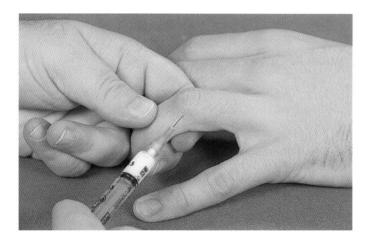

Fig. 13 Injection of the proximal interphalangeal joint.

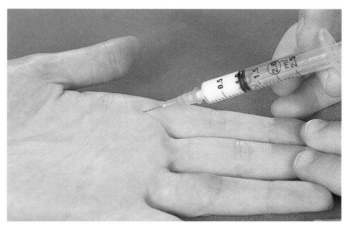

Fig. 15 Injection of second flexor tendon sheath of the hand.

Proximal (Fig. 13) and distal interphalangeal joint

Injection is also carried out by distracting the joint as the steroid is injected tangentially under the extensor expansion (Evans 1984). The distal joints are technically more difficult to inject unless an effusion is present, as occurs in psoriatic and other seronegative spondylarthropathies.

First carpometacarpal joint (Fig. 14)

This joint is characteristically affected in primary generalized osteoarthritis and non-inflammatory arthropathies. Patients complain of pain at the base of the thumb on gripping, and tenderness and 'squaring' of the thumb base is noted. For injection, the hand is rested on the couch in the midprone position, with the joint line being identified laterally. By applying pressure on the thumb the joint can be distracted, and the injection facilitated. The patient needs to relax the thumb as the needle is angled slightly distally to enter the joint. Different approaches to the joint may be necessary once gross distortion of the joint has occurred. Despite the degenerative nature of the problem, the response to local steroid injection is often good, although patients need to be warned that a temporary increase in the pain may precede recovery. Patient should also be

provided with a thumb pillar splint to protect the joint against further damage.

Flexor tenosynovitis and 'trigger' fingers (Fig. 15)

Flexor tenosynovitis is a common cause of poor hand function in inflammatory arthropathies, lupus, or diabetes mellitus but it can also result from trauma or be idiopathic. Nodules may form within the tendon sheaths, making it difficult for the tendon to move freely past the anatomical constrictions, thus leading to 'triggering' of the digit. The nodules can be palpated either attached to the tendon in the pad of tissue adjacent to the proximal phalanx or in the palm opposite the distal palmar crease. They can also occur at the base of the thumb.

Although the tendon nodules can be injected directly, it is more effective to inject the affected tendon sheath. The injection is made with the patient seated with the hand resting palm up on the couch. The needle is advanced tangentially along the tendon sheath in a proximal direction, using a fine-bore needle. Similar injection is possible for thumb tendon nodules.

Steroid injection improves over two-thirds of patients with flexor tenosynovitis (Anderson and Kaye 1991; Lambert *et al.* 1992), and success rates rival surgical intervention (Kraemer *et al.* 1990).

Rupture of tendons may rarely follow steroid injection at this site (Tonkin and Stern 1991).

Hip region

Although hip pathology is common, many patients referred with hip problems have pain arising from soft tissue lesions around the hip. The extreme depth of the hip joint and technical difficulty associated with anatomical derangement or osteophyte formation, preclude hip injection as a routine outpatient procedure. Aspiration and, if appropriate, steroid injection, needs to be carried out by an orthopaedic surgeon in theatre or, better, by a radiologist under suitable radiological screening. Although the hip joint itself is not routinely injected, there are many soft tissue lesions around the hip which are amenable to steroid injection in an outpatient setting (Table 7).

Trochanteric bursa (Fig. 16)

Patients presenting with hip pain often have pain and local tenderness maximally around the greater trochanter of the femur. It is difficult to differentiate bursitis overlying the greater trochanter from enthesopathy of the muscles inserting at this site. Trochanteric bursitis is usually a non-inflammatory lesion (Ege-Rasmussen and Fano 1985) but is also a common cause of hip pain in rheumatoid patients (Raman and Haslock 1982).

To inject the lesion, the patient is positioned with the painful thigh uppermost and flexed, and the lower leg kept extended. By rotating the affected hip, the prominence of the greater trochanter with its associated tenderness is located, marked, and injected at right angles to the skin. The injection site can be very deep seated in patients with obese thighs, and a longer (5.08 cm) 21G needle may be needed to reach the bursa. While steroid injection therapy has a high success rate in both inflammatory and mechanical lesions, postural advice and review of gait by a physiotherapist is necessary to prevent recurrence of the lesion.

Meralgia paraesthetica

This lesion is an entrapment neuropathy of the lateral cutaneous nerve of the thigh as it traverses the deep fascia, about 10 cm below and medial to the anterior superior iliac spine. Clearly demarcated blunting of pinprick or hyperaesthesia may be found over the anterolateral aspect of the thigh, with tenderness localized to the point where the nerve penetrates the fascia (10 cm below the anterior superior iliac spine). If this point is found, infiltration with steroid and local anaesthetic may abolish the symptoms.

Ischial tuberosity

The ischial tuberosities, located deep in the medial side of the buttocks, have overlying bursas which can become inflamed and cause pain on sitting, especially on a bicycle seat. These lesions are amenable to infiltration of steroid and local anaesthetic with the patient lying on the lateral side facing away from the examiner. The tender point is identified and injected using a long 21G needle.

Obscure groin pain

Groin pain is common as a result of sport or other injuries. Enthesopathy of the adductor longus tendon, inguinal ligament, and other structures, if identified (Ashby 1994), can be treated with local steroid injection.

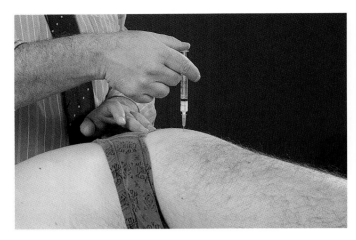

Fig. 16 Injection of trochanteric bursitis.

Knee

Knee lesions amenable to steroid injection are shown in Table 7.

Knee joint

A knee effusion is a common presenting feature in both inflammatory and non-inflammatory arthropathies, and can seriously impair quadriceps function (Geborek et al. 1990). Where the cause of the effusion is uncertain, aspiration of synovial fluid for microbiological and crystal assessment should precede steroid injection.

While there are many approaches to knee aspiration and injection, the most common technique is to use the retropatellar route, via either the medial or lateral approaches. With the patient lying supine, the knee should be extended and the quadriceps muscle relaxed. In the presence of fixed flexion contracture of the knee, support under the knee is necessary to encourage quadriceps relaxation.

Lateral retropatellar approach (Fig. 17)

The joint line is marked between the upper and middle third of the patella, with the needle advanced tangentially between the patella and femoral condyle. By pushing on the medial aspect of the patella, the gap between the patella and femur can be increased, facilitating joint penetration. Aspiration as the needle is inserted will reveal fluid as soon as the joint capsule is entered, so reducing the risk of cartilage injury.

Medial retropatellar approach

The site of joint entry is just below the midline of the patella, with the needle advanced tangentially towards the suprapatellar pouch. Aspiration as the needle is introduced will again prevent cartilage injury.

Irrespective of the approach, a 21G or larger-bore needle is used, to remove as much of the inflammatory fluid and debris as possible, before steroid is injected. The introduction of lignocaine before aspiration and 'milking' the fluid towards the needle with controlled pressure from the other hand will facilitate the procedure. Given the large capacity of the joint and synovial surface area, effusions can be massive. The fluid should be viewed and, if purulent, examined in the laboratory to exclude infection before the steroid is injected.

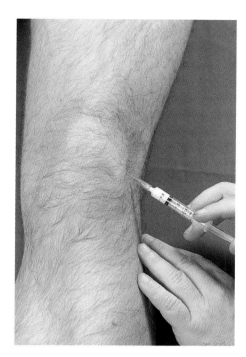

Fig. 17 Injection of the knee joint via the lateral retropatellar approach.

Long-acting steroid agents are more effective than hydrocortisone (Blyth *et al.* 1994), with a relatively large dose of steroid being necessary; 40 to 80 mg of methylprednisolone or triamcinolone acetonide, or 20 to 40 mg of triamcinolone hexacetonide are needed, depending on the size of the effusion. With such a large capacity and synovial surface area, significant absorption of steroid into the circulation can be anticipated and patients need to be informed of both potential benefits to other inflamed joints and possible risks, such as destabilization of diabetic control, following the injection.

A bandage should be firmly applied to support the knee following injection if a large effusion is drained. Bed rest for 24 h following the injection prolongs the beneficial effects (Chakravarty *et al.* 1994), although routine admission to hospital following injection is not cost-effective.

Popliteal (Baker's) cyst

Patients with a knee effusion may develop a popliteal (Baker's) cyst as a result of a one-way valve between the knee joint and semimembranosus or gastrocnemius bursae. The fluid is resorbed from the bursa, leaving a gelatinous material which cannot be aspirated. The cyst can gradually increase in size or can rupture into the calf muscle mimicking a deep vein thrombosis. Ultrasound of the back of the knee and calf or arthrography of the knee joint can demonstrate the cyst, and if present, rupture into the calf muscle.

If a Bakers cyst requires treatment, the knee joint proper should be aspirated and injected as described above. Attempts to inject the cyst directly could result in damage to the neurovascular structures at the back of the knee. For a ruptured Baker's cyst, a below knee support stocking should be used to facilitate sealing of the capsular rupture, following steroid injection into the knee joint proper.

Osteoarthritis of the knee

Some patients with osteoarthritis of the knee have an effusion which might benefit from aspiration and steroid injection, although the improvement is usually short lived (Schnitzer 1993; Gaffney *et al.* 1995). Infiltration of steroid around the patella (Sambrook *et al.* 1989) or other tender trigger spots around the knee, also provides symptomatic relief in some patients, although steroid injection for osteoarthritic joints remains controversial (Dieppe 1991).

Other knee lesions

Non-infected prepatellar bursitis, painful collateral ligaments, and other painful trigger spots around the knee may be amenable to local steroid injection, which is given at the point of maximum tenderness. If an infected prepatellar or other superficial bursa is aspirated, care is necessary to avoid entry into the knee joint as septic arthritis may ensue. Rupture of the patellar ligament may follow steroid injection near the tendon insertion (Alexeeff 1986).

Ankle and hindfoot

The main causes of ankle and heel pain are shown in Table 7. The tendon sheaths around the ankle often communicate with the ankle joint and can be involved in inflammatory or other pathological processes. Most ankle and hindfoot lesions can be injected with the patient lying supine on the couch.

Ankle joint (Fig. 18)

The ankle joint is located by dorsiflexing the foot to stretch the tibialis anterior ligament and so make it visible. The joint margin which lies between the tibia and talus is then palpated just lateral to the tendon. After marking the injection site, the needle is inserted almost horizontal to the foot, curving over the talus. If an effusion is present, the joint can be aspirated before steroid is injected.

Tendon sheaths

Injection of steroid along swollen and inflamed tendon sheaths is possible behind the medial malleolus (posterior tibial tendon), or lateral malleolus (peroneal tendon), with marked reduction in pain and swelling following successful injection.

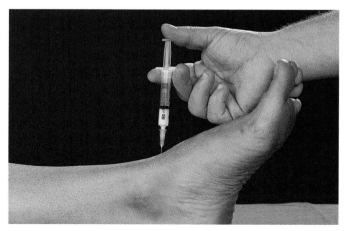

Fig. 18 Injection of the ankle joint.

Posterior subtalar joint

This joint is commonly involved in inflammatory and degenerative conditions of the ankle and hindfoot, and leads to an increasing valgus deformity below the ankle. The joint often communicates with the ankle joint, but can be injected directly from behind the lateral malleolus, with the patient lying prone on the couch. The needle is angled in the direction of the first metatarsal joint (Beaudet and Dixon 1981).

Tarsal tunnel syndrome

Entrapment of the posterior tibial nerve by the flexor retinaculum can occur behind and below the medial malleolus. Patients present with burning, tingling, and numbness in the distribution of the nerve, most prominently in the toes and distal part of the sole. Tenderness with a positive Tinel sign elicited by percussion over the nerve near the medial malleolus will confirm the diagnosis. Injection under the flexor retinaculum between the calcaneum and medial malleolus may relieve the symptoms.

Posterior heel pain

Achilles tendinitis includes several lesions such as an enthesopathy at the insertion of the tendon, typical of the spondylarthropathies, and also bursitis and peritendinitis which affect the tendon at a distance from its insertion. All these lesions can result from inflammatory disease, or follow sports or other injuries. Rheumatoid nodules, gouty tophi, and xanthomata can also develop along the Achilles tendon. Partial tendon rupture or core necrosis of the Achilles tendon cannot be clinically distinguished from Achilles tendinitis.

The enthesopathy lesion is diffuse and not readily amenable to injection therapy. While steroid injection is feasible with peritendinitis or bursitis, it is not always successful (DaCruz et al. 1988), and is only justified once partial tendon rupture has been excluded, using ultrasound or other radiological investigations. Even if partial tendon rupture is not found, patients need to be warned of the risk of tendon rupture following steroid injection (Galloway et al. 1992). Short-acting steroid agents lessen the risk of rupture, especially if patients avoid exercise for a few weeks following the injection.

Inferior heel pain (Fig. 19)

A plantar (calcaneal) spur is a common finding on routine radiographs of the heel. These spurs may be asymptomatic or can cause pain under the heel. While most spurs are idiopathic in origin, they are also common in the spondylarthropathies. These lesions can be associated with more diffuse pain radiating up the arch of the foot (plantar fasciitis), especially in patients with reduction in the longitudinal arch of the foot.

Pain under the heel and plantar fasciitis can usually be improved by the use of a cushioned insole, although a local steroid injection under the heel may be indicated for resistant cases. If an injection is needed, the thick skin of the sole should be avoided, with injection being made from the medial side after careful localization of the point of maximum tenderness. The needle is inserted tangentially through the softer skin, so the point of the needle is under the point of maximum tenderness near the bony spur. A cushioned insole should also be provided following injection but recurrence of pain is common. In patients with plantar fasciitis, rupture of the calcaneal origin of the plantar spur may follow steroid injection, with recurrence of pain of a different type after a symptom-free period

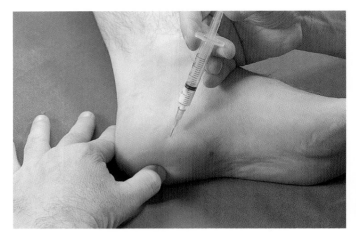

Fig. 19 Injection of plantar fasciitis and plantar heel pain.

(Sellman 1994). With very large plantar spurs, surgical excision is necessary.

Forefoot

Metatarsophalangeal joints (Fig. 20)

Forefoot pain is extremely common in inflammatory and degenerative arthropathies, and steroid injection therapy is often very effective in reducing pain (Helfland 1973) especially in the period before serious deformity has developed. The lateral metatarsophalangeal joints are located by moving the toe between thumb and forefinger. Once the joint line is found and marked, the joint is injected through the dorsum of the toe with the needle entering tangentially from the lateral side, passing under the extensor tendon which overlies the dorsum of the joint. The first metatarsophalangeal joint is sometimes easier to enter from the medial side, using a similar technique to the other joints. The foot joints need to be injected with particular care, as the risk of infection is greater than at other sites.

Other lesions amenable to steroid injection

While many other lesions can be treated with steroid injection, they often require greater expertise. The temporomandibular joint

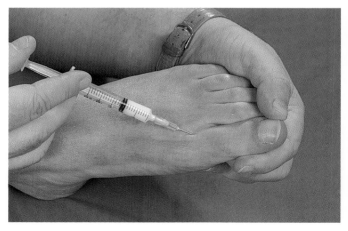

Fig. 20 Injection of the first metatarsophalangeal joint.

(Ahlqvist and Legrell 1993), sacroiliac joint (Maugars *et al*. 1992), coccyx (Wray *et al*. 1991) and painful trigger-points in the spine (Garvey *et al*. 1989), and many sports injuries are examples of other lesions which may benefit from steroid injection. Subcutaneous rheumatoid nodules (Ching *et al*. 1992) and ganglia can be shrunk by intralesional steroid injection, although this is not widely practised. Steroid injection has particular importance in juvenile chronic arthritis (Evans *et al*. 1991; Honkanen *et al*. 1993) in an effort to limit growth-related deformities, particularly in weight-bearing joints (Eich *et al*. 1994).

Conclusion

Local steroid injection is one of the most useful therapeutic modalities for the amelioration of pain arising from joint and soft tissue structures. While considerable latitude exists with regard to the precise technique employed, the method must be based on a safe and accurate aseptic no-touch technique. A method of joint injection has been described, with consideration of the most frequently used injections described on a regional basis.

References

Adebajo, A.O., Nash, P., and Hazleman, B.L. (1990). A prospective double blind dummy placebo controlled study comparing triamcinolone hexacetonide injection with oral diclofenac 50 mg TDS in patients with rotator cuff tendinitis. *Journal of Rheumatology*, **17**, 1207–10.

Ahlqvist, J. and Legrell, P.E. (1993). A technique for the accurate administration of corticosteroids in the temporomandibular joint. *Dentomaxillofacial Radiology*, **22**, 211–3.

Alexeeff, M. (1986). Ligamentum patellae rupture following local steroid injection. *Australia New Zealand Journal of Surgery*, **56**, 681–3.

American College of Rheumatology Council of Rheumatological Care (1992). *Guidelines for performing arthrocentesis*.

Anderson, B. and Kaye, S. (1991). Treatment of flexor tenosynovitis of the hand ('trigger finger') with corticosteroids: a prospective study of the response to local injection. *Archives of Internal Medicine*, **151**, 153–6.

Anderson, B.C., Manthey, R., and Brouns, M.C. (1991). Treatment of de Quervain's tenosynovitis with corticosteroids: a prospective study of the response to local injection. *Arthritis and Rheumatism*, **34**, 793–8.

Ashby, E.C. (1994). Chronic obscure groin pain is commonly caused by enthesopathy: 'tennis elbow' of the groin. *British Journal of Surgery*, **81**, 1632–4.

Balogh, K. (1986). The histologic appearance of corticosteroid injection sites. *Archives of Pathology Laboratory Medicine*, **110**, 1168–72.

Bamji, A.M., Dieppe, P.A., Haslock, D.I., and Shipley, M.E. (1990). What do rheumatologists do? A pilot audit study. *British Journal of Rheumatology*, **29**, 295–8.

Beaudet, F. and Dixon, A.S. (1981). Posterior subtalar joint synoviography and corticosteroid injection in rheumatoid arthritis. *Annals of the Rheumatic Diseases*, **40**, 132–5.

Berger, R.G. and Yount, W.J. (1990). Immediate 'steroid flare' from intraarticular triamcinolone hexacetonide injection: case report and review of the literature. *Arthritis and Rheumatism*, **33**, 1284–6.

Bird, H.A., Ring, E.F., and Bacon, P.A (1979). A thermographic and clinical comparison of three intra-articular steroid preparations in rheumatoid arthritis. *Annals of the Rheumatic Diseases*, **38**, 36–9.

Blyth, T., Hunter, J.A., and Stirling, A. (1994). Pain relief in the rheumatoid knee after steroid injection: a single-blind comparison of hydrocortisone succinate, and triamcinalone acetonide or hexacetonide. *British Journal of Rheumatology*, **33**, 461–3.

Canoso, J.J. and Sheckman, P.R. (1979). Septic subcutaneous bursitis. Report of 16 cases. *Journal of Rheumatology*, **6**, 96–102.

Cawley, P.J. and Morris, I.M. (1992). A study to compare the efficacy of two methods of skin preparation prior to joint injection. *British Journal of Rheumatology*, **31**, 847–8.

Chakravarty, K., Pharoah, P.D.P., and Scott, D.G.I. (1994). A randomized controlled study of post-injection rest following intra-articular steroid therapy for knee synovitis. *British Journal of Rheumatology*, **33**, 464–8.

Ching, D.W., Petrie, J.P., Klemp, P., and Jones, J.G. (1992). Injection therapy of superficial rheumatoid nodules. *British Journal of Rheumatology*, **31**, 775–7.

Cyriax, J. (1984). *Textbook of orthopaedic medicine, Vol. 2: Treatment by manipulation, massage and injection* (11th edn). Baillière Tindall, London.

Dacre, J.E., Beeney, N., and Scott, D.L. (1989). Injections and physiotherapy for the painful stiff shoulder. *Annals of the Rheumatic Diseases*, **48**, 322–5.

DaCruz, D.J., Geeson, M., Allen, M.J., and Phair, I. (1988). Achilles paratendonitis: an evaluation of steroid injection. *British Journal of Sports Medicine*, **22**, 64–5.

Derendorf, H., Mollmann, H, Gruner, A., Haack, D., and Gyselby, G. (1986). Pharmacokinetics and pharmacodynamics of glucocorticoid suspensions after intra-articular administration. *Clinical Pharmacology and Therapeutics Series*, **39**, 313–7.

Dieppe, P.A. (1991). Are intra-articular steroid injections useful for the treatment of the osteoporotic joint? *British Journal of Rheumatology*, **30**, 199.

Dijs, H., Mortier, G., Driessens, M., De-Ridder, A., Willems, J., and De Vroey, T. (1990). A retrospective study of conservative treatment of tennis elbow. *Acta Belgica Medica Physica*, **13**, 73–7.

Dixon, A. St J. and Graber, J. (1983). *Local injection therapy in rheumatic diseases* (2nd edn). Eular Publishers, Basle, Switzerland.

Doherty, M., Hazleman, B.L., Hutton, C.W., Maddison, P.J., and Perry, J.D. (1992). *Rheumatology examination and injection techniques*. W.B. Saunders, London.

Ege-Rasmussen, K.J. and Fano, N. (1985). Trochanteric bursitis. Treatment by corticosteroid injection. *Scandinavian Journal of Rheumatology*, **14**, 417–20.

Eich, G.F., Halle, F., Hodler, J., Seger, R., and Willi, U.V. (1994). Juvenile chronic arthritis: imaging of the knees and hips before and after intra-articular steroid injection. *Pediatric Radiology*, **24**, 558–63.

Evans, D.M. (1984). The PIP joint. *Clinics of Rheumatic Disease*, **10**, 631–56.

Evans, D.M., Ansell, B.M., and Hall, M.A. (1991). The wrist in juvenile arthritis. *Journal of Hand Surgery*, British Volume, **16**, 293–304.

Firestein, G.S., Paine, M.M., and Littman, B.H. (1991). Gene expression (collagenase, tissue inhibitor of metalloproteinases, complement, and HLA-DR) in rheumatoid arthritis and osteoarthritis synovium: quantitative analysis and effect of intra-articular corticosteroids. *Arthritis and Rheumatism*, **34**, 1094–105.

Frederick, H.A., Carter, P.R., and Littler, J.W. (1992). Injection injuries to the median and ulnar nerves at the wrist. *Journal of Hand Surgery*, American Volume, **17**, 645–7.

Gaffney, K., Ledingham, J., and Perry, J.D. (1995). Intra-articular triamcinolone hexacetonide in knee osteoarthritis: factors influencing the clinical response. *Annals of the Rheumatic Diseases*, **54**, 379–81.

Galloway, M.T., Jokl, P., and Dayton, O.W. (1992). Achilles tendon overuse injuries. *Clinical Sports Medicine*, **11**, 771–82.

Garvey, T.A., Marks, M.R., and Weisel, S.W. (1989). A prospective randomized, double-blind evaluation of trigger-point injection therapy for low-back pain. *Spine*, **14**, 962–4.

Geborek, P., Mansson, B., Wollheim, F.A., and Moritz, U. (1990). Intra-articular corticosteroid injection into rheumatoid arthritis knees improves extensor muscle strength. *Rheumatology International*, **9**, 265–70.

Gladman, D.D. and Bombardier, C. (1987). Sickle cell crisis following intra-articular steroid therapy for rheumatoid arthritis. *Arthritis and Rheumatism*, **30**, 1065–8.

Gomez, E.C., Berman, B., and Miller, D.L. (1982). Ultrasonic assessment of cutaneous atrophy caused by intradermal corticosteroids. *Journal of Dermatology Surgery and Oncology*, **8**, 1071–4.

Gordon, G.V. and Schumacher, H.R. (1979). Elecron microscopic study of depot corticosteroid crystals with clinical studies after intra-articular injection. *Journal of Rheumatology*, **6**, 7–14.

Gray, R.G., Tenenbaum, J., and Gottlieb, N.L. (1981). Local corticosteroid injection treatment in rheumatic disorders. *Seminars in Arthritis and Rheumatism*, **10**, 231–54.

Green, D.P. (1984). Diagnostic and therapeutic value of carpal tunnel injection. *Journal of Hand Surgery*, American Volume, **9**, 850–4.

Haslock, I., MacFarlane, D., and Speed, C. (1995). Intra-articular and soft tissue injections: a survey of current practice. *British Journal of Rheumatology*, **34**, 449–52.

Helfland, A.E. (1973). A clinical study of methylprednisolone acetate (Depo-Medrol) in the treatment of pain and inflammation associated with various foot disorders. *Journal of the American Podiatry Association*, **63**, 287–92.

Hollingworth, G.R., Ellis, R.M., and Hattersley, T.S. (1983). Comparison of injection techniques for shoulder pain: results of a double blind, randomised study. *British Medical Journal Clinical Research Edition*, **287**, 1339–41.

Honkanen, V.E.A., Rautonen, J.K., and Pelkonen, P.M. (1993). Intra-articular glucocorticoids in early juvenile chronic arthritis. *Acta Paediatrica*, **82**, 1072–4.

Jones, A., Regan, M., Ledingham, J., Pattrick, M., Manhire, A., and Doherty, M. (1993). Importance of placement of intra-articular steroid injections. *British Medical Journal*, **307**, 1329–30.

Kirwan, J.R., Haskard, D.O., and Higgens, C.S. (1984). The use of sequential analysis to assess patient preference for local skin anaesthesia during knee aspiration. *British Journal of Rheumatology*, **23**, 210–3.

Kirwan, J.R. and the Arthritis and Rheumatism Council Low Dose Glucocorticosteroid Study Group (1995). The effect of glucocorticoids on joint destruction in rheumatoid arthritis. *New England Journal of Medicine*, **333**, 142–6.

Kraemer B.A., Young, V.L., and Arfken, C. (1990). Stenosing flexor tenosynovitis. *South Medical Journal*, **83**, 806–11.

Kraft, S.M., Panush, R.S., and Longley, S. (1985). Unrecognised staphylococcal pyarthrosis with rheumatoid arthritis. *Seminars in Arthritis and Rheumatism*, **14**, 196–201.

Kulick, M.I., Gordillo, G., Javidi, T., Kilgore, E.S. Jr, and Newmayer, W.L. (1986). Long-term analysis of patients having surgical treatment for carpal tunnel syndrome. *Journal of Hand Surgery*, American Volume, **11**, 59–66.

Lambert, M.A., Morton, R.J., and Sloan, J.P. (1992). Controlled study of the use of local steroid injection in the treatment of trigger finger and thumb. *Journal of Hand Surgery*, British Volume, **17**, 69–70.

Mattila, J. (1983). Prolonged action and sustained serum levels of methylprednisolone after a local injection of methylprednisolone acetate. *Clinical Trials Journal*, **20**, 18–23.

Maugars, Y., Mathis, C., Vilon, P, and Prost, A. (1992). Corticosteroid injection of the sacroiliac joint in patients with seronegative spondylarthropathy. *Arthritis and Rheumatism*, **35**, 564–8.

McConnell, J.R. and Bush, D.C. (1990). Intraneural steroid injection as a complication in the management of carpal tunnel syndrome: a report of three cases. *Clinical Orthopaedics*, **250**, 181–4.

Nakashima, A.K., McCarthy, M.A., Martone, W.J., and Anderson, R.L. (1987). Epidemic septic arthritis caused by *Serratia marcescens* and associated with benzalkonium chloride antiseptic. *Journal of Clinical Microbiology*, **25**, 1014–8.

Neustadt, D.H. (1992). Intra-articular steroid therapy. In R.W Moskowitz, D.S. Howell, H. Makin, and V.M. Goldberg (ed), *Osteoarthritis: diagnosis and surgical management* (2nd edn), pp. 493–510. W.B. Saunders, Philadelphia.

Ostensson, A. and Geborek, P. (1991). Septic arthritis as a non-surgical complication in rheumatoid arthritis: relation to disease severity, and therapy. *British Journal of Rheumatology*, **30**, 35–8.

Parikh, J.R., Houpt, J.B., Jacobs, S., and Fernandes, B.J. (1993). Charcot's arthropathy of the shoulder following intraarticular corticosteroid injection. *Journal of Rheumatology*, **20**, 885–7.

Phelan, M.J., Byrne, J., Campbell, A., and Lynch, M.P. (1992). A profile of the rheumatology nurse specialist in the United Kingdom. *British Journal of Rheumatology*, **31**, 858–9.

Pitsillides, A.A., Will, R.K., Bayliss, M.T., and Edwards, J.C. (1994). Circulating and synovial fluid hyaluronan levels: effects of intra-articular corticosteroid on the concentration and the rate of turnover. *Arthritis and Rheumatism*, **37**, 1030–8.

Price, R., Sinclair, H., Heinrich, I., and Gibson, T. (1991). Local injection treatment of tennis elbow: hydrocortisone, triamcinolone and lignocaine compared. *British Journal of Rheumatology*, **30**, 39–44.

Raman, D. and Haslock, I. (1982). Trochanteric bursitis — a frequent cause of 'hip' pain in rheumatoid arthritis. *Annals of the Rheumatic Disease*, **41**, 602–3.

Rizk, T.E., Pinals, R.S., and Talaiver, A.S. (1991). Corticosteroid injections in adhesive capsulitis: investigation of their value and site. *Archives of Physical Medical Rehabilitation*, **72**, 20–2.

Rizk, T.E., Gavant, M.L., and Pinals, R.S. (1994). Treatment of adhesive capsulitis (frozen shoulder) with arthroscopic capsular distension and rupture. *Archives of Physical Medical Rehabilitation*, **75**, 803–7.

Sambrook, P.N., Champion, G.D., Browne, C.D., Cairns, D., Cohen, M.L., Day, R.O., Graham, S., *et al.* (1989). Corticosteroid injection for osteoarthritis of the knee: peripatellar compared to intra-articular route. *Clinical Experimental Rheumatology*, **7**, 609–13.

Schnitzer, T.J. (1993). Osteoarthritis treatment update. Minimising pain while limiting patient risk. *Postgraduate Medicine*, **93**, 89–95.

Sellman, J.R. (1994). Plantar fascia rupture associated with corticosteroid injection. *Foot and Ankle International*, **15**, 376–81.

Shupak, R., Teitel, J., Garvey, M.B., and Freedman, J. (1988). Intraarticular methylprednisolone therapy in haemophilic arthropathy. *American Journal of Hematology*, **27**, 26–9.

Smith, D.L., McAfee, J.H., Lucas, L.M., Kumar, K.L., and Romney, D.M. (1989). Treatment of nonseptic olecranon bursitis: a controlled, blinded prospective trial. *Archives of Internal Medicine*, **149**, 2527–30.

Tonkin, M.A. and Stern, H.S. (1991). Spontaneous rupture of the flexor carpi radialis tendon. *Journal of Hand Surgery*, British Volume, **16**, 72–4.

Von Essen, R. and Savolainen, H.A. (1989). Bacterial infection following intra-articular injection: a brief review. *Scandinavian Journal of Rheumatology*, **18**, 7–12.

Weinstein, P.S., Canoso, J.J., and Wohlgethan, J.R. (1984). Long-term follow-up of corticosteroid injection for traumatic olecranon bursitis. *Annals of the Rheumatic Disease*, **43**, 44–6.

Weiss, A.P., Akelman, E., and Tabatabai, M. (1994a). Treatment of de Quervain's disease, *Journal of Hand Surgery*, American Volume, **19**, 595–8.

Weiss, A.P., Sachar, K., and Gendreau, M. (1994b). Conservative management of carpal tunnel syndrome: a re-examination of steroid injection and splinting. *Journal of Hand Surgery*, America Volume, **19**, 410–5.

Wiggins, M.E., Fadale, P.D., Barrach, H., Ehrlich, M.G., and Walsh, W.R. (1994). Healing characteristics of a type I collagenous structure treated with corticosteroids. *American Journal of Sports Medicine*, **22**, 279–88.

Wray, C.C., Easom, S., and Hoskinson, J. (1991). Coccydynia. Aetiology and treatment. *Journal of Bone and Joint Surgery*, British Volume, **73**, 335–8.

Wright, T.W., Cooney, W.P., and Ilstrup, D.M. (1994). Anterior wrist ganglion. *Journal of Hand Surgery*, American Volume, **19**, 954–8.

Yood, R.A. (1993). Use of gloves for rheumatology procedures. *Arthritis and Rheumatism*, **36**, 575.

6.6 Sports medicine

Mark Harries

Introduction

This chapter provides a basis for understanding the essential metabolic processes involved in muscle movement and how these translate to human performance. The adaptive responses of the cardiorespiratory and musculoskeletal systems to exercise are also explained. The chapter concludes with a description of the consequences of overreaching these adaptive processes.

Fundamentals of metabolism

The energy for muscular activity derives from a cycle of chemical reactions in which ingested carbon-based fuels are burned with oxygen liberating carbon dioxide. This forms carbonic acid in the tissues which dissociates to bicarbonate and hydrogen ions; a reaction that is catalysed by carbonic anhydrase. Carbonic acid is in dynamic equilibrium with its dissociation products and with CO_2. The high solubility of CO_2 compared with O_2 (more than 20 times as great), coupled with the wide distribution of carbonic anhydrase in the tissues, means that the rate at which CO_2 is mopped up and voided from the lungs can always keep pace with its rate of production. In other words, CO_2 can never accumulate, even during extremes of exertion.

The tendency is always toward a metabolic acidosis, but this is completely overwhelmed by the capacity of the tissues to absorb CO_2 and the capacity of the lungs to dispose of it. The equivalent loss of hydrogen ions by the lung compared with the kidney is in the order of 250:1 and so even during moderate exercise, pH does not change. However, as exercise levels increase, lactate begins to accumulate and the subsequent metabolic acidosis stimulates ventilation with the result that arterial CO_2 may actually fall (Fig. 1).

How muscle uses its fuel

Energy for movement comes from the hydrolysis of adenosine triphosphate (**ATP**) forming adenosine diphosphate (**ADP**) and liberating 7.6 kcal/mol of ATP. Only around 40 per cent of the energy yield goes into creating tension between molecules of actin and myosin. All is eventually lost as heat. Though the store of ATP is small (only around 10 mmol/kg wet muscle weight), turnover is very rapid and is virtually inexhaustible during sustained moderate exercise. The two principal fuels for ATP synthesis are glucose and long-chain fatty acids: these are available directly fom the diet, or can be liberated from stores — glucose from glycogen in muscle or liver and fatty acids from triglycerides stored in fat cells.

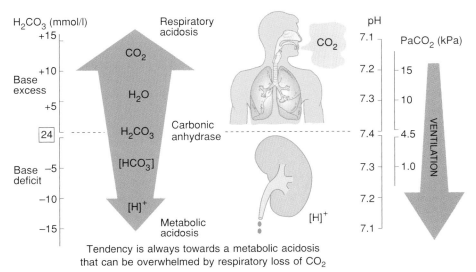

Fig. 1 Metabolism: an acid generator. Oxidation of carbon-based fuels causes a metabolic acidosis due to the conversion in the tissues of CO_2 to carbonic acid by carbonic anhydrase. This tendency is overwhelmed by the capacity of the tissue to absorb CO_2 and the capacity of the lungs to dispose of it. The ratio of the loss of hydrogen ions via the lungs and kidney is of the order of 250:1. Thus, CO_2 can never accumulate, and during moderate levels of exercise, arterial pH does not change. Tendency is always to towards a metabolic acidosis that can be overwhelmed by respiratory losses of CO_2.

Glycolysis and β-oxidation

The metabolism of both glucose and fatty acids to acetyl coA is an aerobic process. Glycolysis of 1 mol of glucose to form acetyl coA yields 2 mol of ATP (3 mol if the starting point is glycogen). Long-chain fatty acids are metabolized to acetyl coA by β-oxidation, each pair of carbon atoms cleaved from the chain yielding 5 mol of ATP and 1 mol of acetyl coA. Thus, β-oxidation of 1 mol of palmitic acid $(CH_3.(CH_2)_{14}.CO_2H)$, would generate 35 mol (5×7) of ATP and 8 mol of acetyl coA (Fig. 2).

The rest of the oxidative process takes place within the mitochondria in the citric acid (Krebs') cycle and is the source of the greatest metabolic energy yield. Acetyl coA donates two carbon atoms to each turn of the cycle. An *aide mémoire* is that 6 mol of ATP is generated for each carbon atom of the fuel source, such that 1 mol of glucose $(C_6H_{12}O_6)$ yields 36 mol of ATP (giving a total of 38 mol when considering the 2 mol generated from glycolysis, or 39 mol if the starting point is glycogen). One mole of palmitic acid $(C_{16}H_{32}O_2)$ gives 96 mol of ATP which, when the 33 mol generated from β-oxidation are added, provides a total yield of 129 mol of ATP.

During aerobic exercise, glucose is the preferred fuel, with a gradual switch to fatty acids as glycogen stores are depleted. This rather complex picture is encompassed by the adage 'fat always burns in a carbohydrate flame'. A feature of training is a greater dependence on fatty acids than in the untrained state resulting in a more efficient use of glycogen, which is in limited supply in comparison with the vast stores of fat.

Anaerobic metabolism

For higher energy demands, glucose becomes the exclusive fuel and is metabolized anaerobically with the production of lactate. The energy cost of doing this is enormous, with only 2 mol of ATP generated for each mole of glucose consumed (about 38 mol are produced by aerobic glycolysis). Anaerobic metabolism cannot be sustained because lactate production soon exceeds its rate of metabolism, a point reached when plasma lactate rises beyond a threshold level of 4 mmol/l. When this anaerobic threshold is attained, trained athletes are able to exercise closer to their maximal aerobic capacity (maxV_{O_2}) than sedentary people. In the short term they are also able to tolerate much higher plasma lactates, which may reach 15 to 20 mmol/l in power athletes such as sprinters.

Dietary considerations for energy sources

It follows from the above that glucose is the principal fuel for heavy exercise and fat for low-intensity endurance work. This is reflected in the dietary advice given to the majority of athletes engaged in aerobic sports. Carbohydrate should form 60 per cent of the diet with protein comprising 15 per cent and the rest being fat. The greater the glycogen store, the longer glucose can be burned before fat stores are utilized. This is of great importance in events such as the marathon, triathlon, and cross-country skiing. The concentration of muscle glycogen is in the range 60 to 150 mmol glucosyl units/kg wet weight. Trained athletes can increase this by gorging carbohydrate foods in the few days before competition (Coyle 1991). Simple sugars eaten in such quantities are unpalatable and starch-containing foods such as pasta or potatoes are preferred. It is now accepted that the abundance of phosphocreatine stores is also important in sustaining force during muscle contraction. Ingestion of around 20 g of creatine per day will add to whole body creatine.

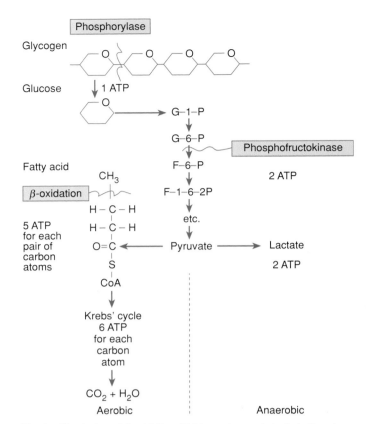

Fig. 2   Glycolysis and β-oxidation. 'Fat burns in a carbohydrate flame'; trained athletes have a greater dependence on fat as a fuel source than the untrained, thereby conserving carbohydrate stores (glycogen). The greatest energy yield comes from mitochondrial respiration. Higher energy demands are met with a switch to anaerobic metabolism and the production of lactate. The rate at which lactate is metabolized is exceeded by its rate of production at around 4 mmol/l. Higher levels can be tolerated, but only for short periods of time. Inherited deficiency of muscle phosphorylase or phosphofructokinse limits performance by restricting glycolysis. Glycogen accumulates in muscle and liver.

Inherited disorders of glycolysis

Deficiency either of muscle phosphorylase (McArdle's syndrome) or phosphofructokinase (Tarui's disease) causes a failure of glycolysis, with the result that glycogen cannot be accessed and instead accumulates in muscle and liver. Of the two, Tarui's disease is much the rarer (Haller and Lewis 1991). Both defects share an autosomally recessive mode of inheritance and so there is often evidence of consanguinity. Both are more common in boys but neither is sex linked. The clinical presentation is that of excessive fatigue on exertion associated with muscle pain, raised serum levels of creatine kinase and blilirubin, and sometimes myoglobinuria. Symptoms may not appear until the second or even third decade of life. Glycogen storage disease type II, deficiency of α_1-glucosidase (known variously as acid maltase deficiency or Pompe's disease), presents with respiratory failure as late as the mid-forties. The diagnosis is made on periodic acid–Schiff staining of the muscle biopsy, which shows massive accumulations of glycogen (Fig. 3). Since glycolysis is blocked, pyruvate is never synthesized and there is failure to generate lactate, or in other words, there is a relative incapacity for anaerobic power. The principal fuel then becomes fatty acids, with a slower energy yield, hence fatigue on anything but light work rates.

Limitations to aerobic work rates

During vigorous exercise, muscle burns all the oxygen available to it. Further demands are met by a switch to anaerobic metabolism with its concomitant limitations imposed by lactic acidosis. The principal factor containing aerobic capacity involves the rate at which oxygen can be delivered, which is itself dependent on three factors: haemoglobin concentration, minute ventilation (pulmonary output), and cardiac output.

The importance of haemoglobin concentration

In the laboratory, the oxygen combining power of haemoglobin is quantified at 1.39 ml of oxygen for each gram of haemoglobin; but in vivo, haemoglobin passing though the lungs picks up only around 1.306 ml/g of haemoglobin. A shift in haemoglobin concentration within the normal range, say from 11 to 18 g/dl, would increase oxygen delivery by a factor of 1.6. It has been well documented that raising haemoglobin beyond the normal range translates directly to an increase in maximal oxygen consumption and an improved performance (Brien and Simon 1987).

Altitude training gives rise only to modest increases in haemoglobin — 1 to 2 g/dl at most. For a bigger advantage illicit means have been sought. At the 1984 Olympic Games in Los Angeles, the American cycling team came from nowhere, and contrary to expectations and form, swept the board. Some months later it was revealed that seven of the successful team members had received a transfusion of blood the night prior to competition (Klein 1985). Erythropoietin is now being used with the same ends in mind and has the added advantage that it is virtually undetectable. Paradoxically, highly trained athletes may have a haemoglobin at or below the lower limit of normal: this reflects an increase in plasma volume due to heavy training and is not a true anaemia. If serum ferritin levels are normal, no treatment is indicated in these cases.

Minute ventilation and aerobic performance

While exercising at the maximum sustainable ventilatory capacity (**MSVC**), ventilation can be increased still further for short periods to reach maximum voluntary ventilation (**MVV**). The MSVC is found to be 55 to 80 per cent of MVV (Freedman 1970) or, put another way, assuming that the lungs are normal, the capacity to increase ventilation is so great that the key factor that most limits aerobic performance is likely to be the cardiac output rather than minute ventilation.

Pulmonary conditions limiting ventilatory capacity

The relationship between maximum aerobic capacity ($\max V_{O_2}$) and MSVC is roughly linear: the higher the $\max V_{O_2}$ the higher the ventilatory capacity. This holds true whether V_{O_2} and MSVC are measured in absolute terms (l/min), or independently of body size (ml/kg per min) (Fig. 4). Minute ventilation is the product of the respiratory rate and breath volume. While exercising at maximum aerobic capacity, respiratory rates are remarkably consistent. Young men take around 60 breaths and women 55 breaths a minute. Given a respiratory rate of 60/min, breath volume clearly cannot exceed the forced expiratory volume (**FEV$_1$**). Elite oarsmen access only around 50 per cent of FEV$_1$ each breath compared with middle-distance runners who reach around 60 per cent of FEV1$_1$. This accords well with the formula used to estimate ventilatory capacity from FEV$_1$ (MSVC = [FEV$_1$ × 30] + 23). Hence it follows that any condition

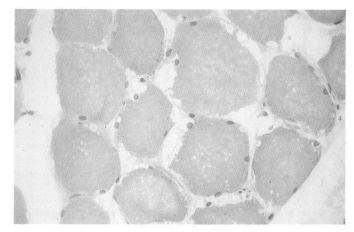

(a)

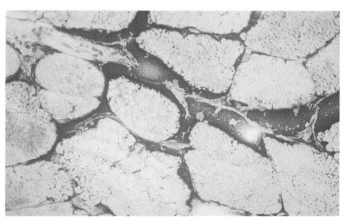

(b)

Fig. 3 Inherited disorders of glycolysis. A 17-year-old Royal Naval recruit complained of fatigue and muscle stiffness on exercise although he had been a good sportsman while at school. An exercise test was terminated early due to exhaustion. Samples taken throughout showed that his blood lactate failed to rise. Glycogen in muscle stains pink with periodic acid–Schiff reagent and normally shows as just a few granules around each muscle fibre (a). By contrast, the biopsy sample of the recruit (b) is full of glycogen, which is unavailable for glycolysis due to an inherited deficiency of myophosphorylase (McArdle's syndrome).

of the lung in which FEV$_1$ is significantly reduced will have an impact on aerobic capacity by reducing minute ventilation.

Asthma

Although chronic bronchitis and emphysema are diseases that reduce ventilatory capacity, they are diseases of older people. Asthma, on the other hand, occurs at all ages and is also much commoner, accounting for around 20 per cent of complaints concerning underperformance received from athletes attending the British Olympic Medical Centre.

The most important feature of asthma for the sportsman is that it worsens during exercise and therefore impacts both on performance and on training. Treatment is highly effective and, therefore, a reproducible diagnostic test is important. However, there is no agreed protocol for exercise testing, although certain ingredients appear to be important. Running in the open air is a more potent stimulus to bronchial constriction than exercising on a cycle or treadmill

Minute ventilation (*VE* l/min) versus maximum
oxygen consumption (*V*O$_2$ max l/min)

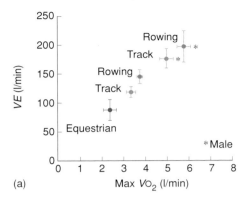

(a)

Minute ventilation (*VE* ml/kg/min) versus
maximum oxygen consumption (*V*O$_2$ max ml/kg/min)

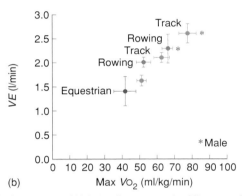

(b)

Fig. 4 The importance of high ventilatory capacity. Minute ventilation (VE) at maximum oxygen consumption (max *V*O$_2$) is measured in 120 Olympic class athletes grouped according to their sport. The relationship between ventilation and oxygen consumption is linear, whether measured in absolute terms or corrected for body weight. The higher the oxygen consumption, the higher must be the minute ventilation. The highest values are recorded in men, with track athletes at the top according to body weight. Equestrian competitors engage in a more sedentary sport and represent values closer to those which would be expected in normal fit individuals in their mid-twenties.

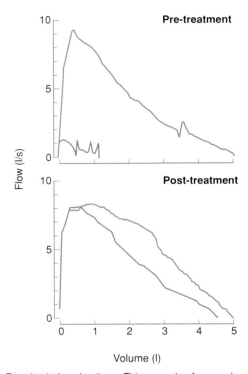

Fig. 5 Exercise-induced asthma. This example of severe bronchial constriction induced by exercise was recorded in an athlete with a clear history of sleep disturbance due to wheeze and tightness in the chest. Flow is plotted against the volume in a forced expiratory manoeuvre from full inspiration to full expiration. Two expiratory efforts are shown; one measured before exercise (red line) and the second around 5 min after a 3-min run (blue line). Peak flow measured 9 l/s before exercise and less than 1 l/s afterwards, representing a fall of more than 80 per cent. Oscillations in flow during expiration are caused by coughing. The athlete was give prednisolone at 30 mg daily for 2 weeks, then continued on beclomethasone dry powder at 400 µg twice daily. One month later the exercise test was repeated under identical conditions (post-treatment). There was no change in peak flow, but more important, pretest FEV$_1$ had risen 20 per cent from 4.03 to 5.3 l. The exercise test was still marginally abnormal with a small fall in FEV$_1$ post-exercise and a larger fall in mid-expiratory flow. However, the athlete was sufficiently improved to win a medal at a major international competition just 2 months later.

ergometer. The reasons for this are complex and related in part to climatic conditions. Cold dry air causes more bronchial constriction than warm moist air. The exercise must be rigorous, enough to raise the heart rate to around 80 per cent of the maximum that can be achieved (approximately 220 minus age in years). The duration of the test is also important. It should last at least 3 min but not much longer than 5 min.

Normal subjects may show a short-lived bronchial dilatation on stopping, but a fall in FEV$_1$ or peak flow of more than 15 per cent occurring 5 to 10 min after exercise is a positive test. Treatment is with an inhaled steroid such as budesonide turbohaler 200 µg twice daily (Fig. 5) (Harries 1994).

Anatomical and physiological adaptations to exercise

Elite athletes differ markedly in their physical make-up to sedentary individuals. Whether or not these differences are inherited, or are the

result of training, has been the subject of much debate. However, recent evidence suggests that genetic factors are the more important in determining athletic prowess (Bouchard *et al.* 1992).

Adaptations of muscle

The relationship between muscle size and strength is poor. Increase in size reflects fibre hypertrophy and fibre numbers remain unchanged. The greatest hypertrophy results from high-intensity isometric exercise in which muscle is required to contract against a resistance. Strength, on the other hand, may be due in part to fibre recruitment; in other words to an increase in the number of fibres that are available for contractile activity.

Training improves fibre recruitment and chronic endurance training favours the transformation of fast-twitch glycolytic (type IIb) to slow-twitch (type 1) fibres (Dudley *et al.* 1982). Muscle biopsy samples show that capillary density and enzyme activity both increase through training. The mitochondria also appear to increase in number, although this finding may reflect mitochondrial hypertrophy and folding rather than any absolute increase (i.e. it is an artificial observation, reflecting only the cross-section of the biopsy specimen). The net result is an improvement in oxidative potential of muscle with an increase in maximal oxygen consumption in the order of 15 to 25 per cent over time.

Cardiac adaptations

Echocardiography shows that both ventricular dilatation and hypertrophy occur with training. The greatest dilatation is seen in rowers and cyclists, who also show the greatest degree of cardiac hypertrophy; a finding that runs counter to the expectation that strength athletes should develop the most hypertrophy.

Dilatation results in the greatest increase in heart size, such that the cardiac silhouette can be found to occupy more than half the transverse diameter of the chest when observed on a chest radiograph. The diameter of the left ventricle at the end of diastole may reach 7 cm (compared with the normal size of around 5.7 cm). Although this represents only a 10 to 15 per cent increase in diameter, it translates to a 30 per cent increase in stroke volume. A large stroke volume means that adequate cardiac output can be maintained with a lower heart rate. A slow resting pulse is therefore a constant feature of training.

Hypertrophy of the septum and left ventricular wall also occurs but contributes very little to overall change in heart size. Normal wall and septal thickness is from 7 to 11 mm, ranging up to 13 mm in cyclists and rowers. A thickness beyond 16 mm is considered abnormal, particularly if chamber size is not also increased (Pelliccia et al. 1991). Disproportionate hypertrophy of the septum with respect to the left ventricular wall may give rise to obstruction of the outflow tract during heavy exercise (see obstructive cardiomyopathy below).

The electrocardiogram is often grossly abnormal with widespread T-wave inversion across the lateral chest leads as far as V4. Multiple nodal (supraventricular) ectopic beats are also common. Both abnormalities tend to correct on exertion. Unfortunately this may also be true of myocardial ischaemia. The resting electrocardiogram, especially recordings made at night, may show bradyarrhythmias with sinoatrial block (Ector et al. 1984).

Skeletal adaptations to exercise

Bone density increases in response to exercise in all subjects except amenorrhoeal women. Rise in mineral content is greatest in bone subject to the most stress, such as the femur of runners, the lumbar spine of rowers, and the radius of gymnasts and racket players (Wolman et al. 1990). Women who train intensively develop amenorrhoea. The result is a loss in bone density exactly analogous to that which occurs following the menopause. The earliest changes are seen in bone with the highest rate of turnover, and appear first in the trabecular bone of the lumbar spine. Bone loss is detectable after as few as 6 months of amenorrhoea. Losses great enough to result in pathological fracture are usually only seen in women with an associated eating disorder such as anorexia nervosa. Treatment is with oestrogen in the form of hormone replacement therapy (Drinkwater et al. 1984; Wolman et al. 1991).

Clinical syndromes associated with overexertion

The health benefits of taking regular exercise are beyond dispute. The risk of osteoporotic fracture later in life is reduced (Heinonen et al. 1996). Furthermore, there is now direct evidence of a reduced risk of acute myocardial infarction in men and exercise is a major factor in controlling obesity and diabetes (Helmrich et al. 1991; Lakke et al. 1994), although evidence that exercise benefits hypertension is less strong (Blumenthal et al. 1991). Nevertheless, in the United States of America it is recommended that 'every adult should accumulate 30 min or more of moderate-intensity physical activity on most, preferably all, days of the week' (Anonymous 1995).

Sudden death

Although rare, sudden death is almost always due to a cardiac cause. It is assumed that the terminal event is ventricular fibrillation, and limited forensic evidence often reveals an underlying abnormality, such as coronary atheroma or a congenital abnormality of the coronary tree. Even moderate levels of exercise have been implicated; for instance, 12 deaths occurred over 6 years among the joggers of Rhode Island, all but one of these were found to be due to coronary artery disease, with the mortality estimated to be seven times the expected mortality in a sedentary population (Thompson et al. 1992). With the rising popularity of veteran events, it is clear that coronary artery disease in sport is going to pose an ever-increasing problem.

Hypertrophic obstructive cardiomyopathy

Obstructive cardiomyopathy, also known as muscular subaortic stenosis, is an absolute contraindication to strenuous dynamic or static activity, because it is a condition that may lead to sudden unexpected death from ventricular fibrillation at a young age. The outflow tract of the left ventricle becomes obstructed in systole by the interventricular septum, which is disproportionately hypertrophied with respect to the ventricular wall. The ratio of the thickness of the septum to the ventricular wall, which is normally 1.3:1, exceeds 1.5:1 (Fagard et al. 1984). Death occurs, often in the second decade of life, during the course of vigorous physical activity. Faintness or syncope occurring immediately following exercise is one of the few symptoms, providing an early indication for urgent investigation. The electrocardiogram is unhelpful because T-wave changes suggesting left ventricular hypertrophy are often seen in normal highly trained individuals. The diagnosis is made by echocardiography (Stewart Hillis et al. 1994).

The condition is inherited as an autosomal dominant, so all first-degree relatives should be screened. There was once a vogue for treatment with surgery which involved shaving the septum, but medical treatment aimed at suppressing the ventricular arrhythmias is now more established. The drug of choice has been amiodorone, though inhibitors of angiotensin-converting enzyme are currently being assessed.

Both aortic and pulmonary stenosis also cause outflow tract obstruction which may have the same effects as hypertrophic obstructive cardiomyopathy during vigorous exertion. On the other hand, tricuspid and pulmonary regurgitation are very common in the highly trained athlete, occurring in over 90 per cent. The murmurs produced may be difficult to distinguish clinically and expert advice should be sought.

Hyperpyrexia (heat stroke)

During extremes of exercise, rectal temperature may reach 41 °C. Heat loss by radiation through peripheral vasodilatation is limited and further losses can only be achieved by evaporating sweat. Once these homeostatic mechanisms are rendered ineffective, such as in a very humid environment or with sweat failure, core temperature rises unchecked. Heat stroke is rare amongst experienced athletes except where there has been stimulant abuse. The usual clinical setting is one of an undertrained individual, competing for the first time and with inadequate fluid intake (Clowes and O'Donnell 1974). A similar picture is also seen in people who have taken amphetamine (speed) or MDMA (Ecstasy) tablets and who have been dancing to exhaustion.

Confusion or coma is the rule with a clinical presentation very similar to septicaemic shock. The skin may be clammy and cold, contrasting with the high rectal temperature. Grand mal seizures occur with decerebrate posturing. Rhabdomyolysis develops early with the creatine kinase often reaching over 100 000 U/l. Paradoxically in the face of dehydration, serum sodium may be low, sometimes below 110 mmol/l. Disseminated intravascular coagulation, renal failure, and liver failure may occur within 24 h (Sutton 1994). Rapid intravenous infusion can be life-saving with an initial infusion of 4 l of saline given in the first hour. Broad-spectrum antibiotics effective against Gram-negative organisms should also be given.

Immune deficiency

There is some evidence that those suffering fatigue syndrome due to overtraining seem to develop frequent infections of the upper respiratory tract. Furthermore, the infecting agent occasionally proves to be unusual (such as *Toxoplasma gondii*). These and other observations have led to the suggestion that overtraining leads to an immunosuppressed state (Khansari *et al*. 1990). Some support for this concept is obtained from studies of plasma glutamine levels. Glutamine is an essential fuel for lymphocytes: it is synthesized by muscle and is found to be low in chronic fatigue states (Newsholme *et al*. 1991).

Drugs to avoid

Amphetamine-like substances and drugs with α-adrenergic (stimulant) actions are all banned. These include isoprenaline, adrenaline, noradrenaline, and phenylpropanolamine. For example, adrenaline may not be given by local injection mixed with an analgesic such as lignocaine. Over-the-counter cold cures often contain one, or more, of these agents.

Selection of an analgesic or anti-inflammatory agent that will not fall foul of the International Olympic Committee's (**IOC**) list of banned substances is made more difficult by the fact that not only do the rules change from time to time, they also lack consistency. For example, opiate analgesics and pentazocine are banned, but codeine and dihydrocodeine have recently been reinstated: yet dextropropoxyphane remains a banned substance! Corticosteroids may not be given by parenteral injection, which effectively outlaws all depot preparations, but hydrocortisone may be given by intra-articular injection or into soft tissue injuries such as a tennis elbow. At the time of writing, the position of systemically acting corticosteroids is under review by the IOC's Medical Commission.

Such is the state of confusion that some sporting bodies, particularly those not affiliated to the IOC, are beginning to go their own way. That said, there is broad agreement that drugs such as anabolic steroids and amphetamine should be avoided, if only because there is no clinical indication for taking them. However, a blanket ban on so many other medicaments, particularly those that are therapeutically useful, is crude and unworkable.

References

Anonymous (1995). Physical activity and public health: a recommendation from the Centres for Disease Control and Prevention and the American College of Sports Medicine. *Journal of the American Medical Association*, **273**, 402–7.

Blumenthal, J., Siegel, W., and Applebaum, M. (1991). Failure of exercise to reduce blood pressure in patients with mild hypertension: results of a randomized controlled trial. *Journal of the American Medical Association*, **266**, 2098–104.

Bouchard, C., Dionne, F., Simoneau, J.-A., and Boulay, M. (1992). Genetics of aerobic and anaerobic performances. *Exercise and Sport Science Reviews*, **20**, 27–58.

Brien, A. and Simon, T. (1987). The effects of red blood cell infusion on 10-km race time. *Journal of the American Medical Association*, **257**, 2761–5.

Clowes, G. and O'Donnell, T. (1974). Heat stroke. *New England Journal of Medicine*, **291**, 564–7.

Coyle, E. (1991). Timing and method of increased carbohydrate intake to cope with heavy training, competition and recovery. *Journal of Sports Science*, **9** (Suppl.), 29–52.

Drinkwater, B., Nilson, K., Chestnut, C., Bremner, W., Shainholtz, S., and Southworth, M. (1984). Bone mineral content of amenorrhoeic and eumenorrhoeic athletes. *New England Journal of Medicine*, **311**, 277–81.

Dudley, G., Araham, W., and Terjung, R. (1982). Influence of exercise intensity and duration on biochemical adaptations in skeletal muscle. *Journal of Applied Physiology*, **53**, 844–50.

Ector, H. *et al*. (1984). Bradycardia, ventricular pauses, syncope, and sports. *Lancet*, **ii**, 591–4.

Fagard, R., Aubert, A., Staessen, J., Vanden Eynde, E., Vanchees, L., and Amery, A. (1984). Cardiac structure and function in cyclists and runners. Comparative echocardiographic study. *British Heart Journal*, **52**, 124–9.

Freedman, S. (1970). Sustained maximal voluntary ventilation. *Respiration Physiology*, **8**, 230–44.

Haller, R. and Lewis, S. (1991). Glucose-induced exertional fatigue in muscle phosphofructokinase deficiency. *New England Journal of Medicine*, **324**, 364–69.

Harries, M. (1994). Pulmonary limitations to performance in sport. *British Medical Journal*, **309**, 113–15.

Heinonen, A., *et al*. (1996). Randomized controlled trial of effect of high-impact exercise on selected risk factors for osteoporotic fractures. *Lancet*, **348**, 1343–7.

Helmrich, S., Ragland, P., Leung, R., and Paffenbarger, R. (1991). Physical activity and reduced occurrence of non-insulin-dependent diabetes mellitus. *New England Journal of Medicine*, **325**, 147–52.

Khansari, D., Murgo, A., and Faith, R. (1990). Effects of stress on the immune system. *Immunology Today*, **11**, 170–4.

Klein, H. (1985). Blood transfusion in athletes. Games people play. *New England Journal of Medicine*, **312**, 854–6.

Lakke, T., Venalainen, J., Rauramaa, R., Salonen, R., Tuomilehto, J., and Salonen, J. (1994). Relation of leisure-time physical activity and cardiorespiratory fitness to the risk of acute myocardial infarction in men. *New England Journal of Medicine*, **330**, 1549–54.

Newsholme, E., Parry-Billings, M., McAndrew, N., and Budgett, R. (1991). A biochemical mechanism to explain some characteristics of overtraining. In *Advances in nutrition and top sport* (ed. F. Brouns), Vol. 32, 79–93. Medical Sports Science, Basel.

Pelliccia, A., Maron, B., Spataro, A., Proschan, M., and Spirito, P. (1991). The upper limit of physiological cardiac hypertrophy in highly trained elite athletes. *New England Journal of Medicine*, **324**, 292–302.

Stewart Hillis, W., MacIntyre, P., Maclean, J., Goodwin, J., and McKenna, W. (1994). Sudden death in sport. *British Medical Journal*, **309**, 657–60.

Sutton, J. (1994). Physiological and clinical consequences of exercise in heat and humidity. In *Oxford textbook of sports medicine* (ed. M. Harries *et al*.), pp. 231–8. Oxford University Press.

Thompson, P., Funk, E., Carleton, R., and Stumer, W. (1992). Incidence of death during jogging in Rhode Island from 1975 through 1980. *Journal of the American Medical Association*, **247**, 1535–8.

Wolman, R., Clark, P., McNally, E., Harries, M., and Reeve, J. (1990). Menstrual state and exercise as determinants of spinal trabecular bone density in female athletes. *British Medical Journal*, **301**, 516–18.

Wolman, R., Faulmann, L., Clark, P., Hesp, R., and Harries, M. (1991). Different training patterns and bone mineral density of the femoral shaft in elite female athletes. *Annals of the Rheumatic Diseases*, **50**, 48–79.

6.7 Sports injuries

J. R. Jenner and M. Shirley Emerson

Introduction

Regular aerobic exercise has been shown to have a beneficial effect on several aspects of health including:

(1) reducing the risk of cardiovascular disease, particularly coronary artery disease and hypertension;

(2) reducing the incidence of osteoporosis;

(3) helping with weight loss by increasing the metabolic rate;

(4) inducing a feeling of general well-being and reducing depression (Report of the Royal College of Physicians 1991).

As a result of these findings, the government has actively encouraged the general population to participate in sporting activities. Unfortunately, one side-effect of sport is injury. If these injuries are not treated promptly and appropriately, the injury may become recurrent or chronic.

Different sports have different rates of injury and different injury profiles (Fig. 1) but the fundamental principles underlying the treatment of acute injuries, as well as their rehabilitation, apply across sports. The major cause of injury in sport is acute trauma to soft tissues such as muscle, tendon, or ligaments. Chronic sporting injuries result from either adverse body mechanics, resulting in excess strain, or overuse, leading to fatigue. Children and teenagers with immature or rapidly growing musculoskeletal systems are prone to injuries not encountered in the adult and these injuries deserve special mention.

Injury prevention

Prevention of injury involves several strategies.

Modification of the environment

Many accidents are due to poor surfaces and inadequate equipment. Uneven pitches, collapsing gymnastic equipment, and worn landing mats have all been shown to contribute to injury. These injuries are definitely preventable. Approximately 10 per cent of sports injuries in the United Kingdom are due to collisions with the 'furniture' of

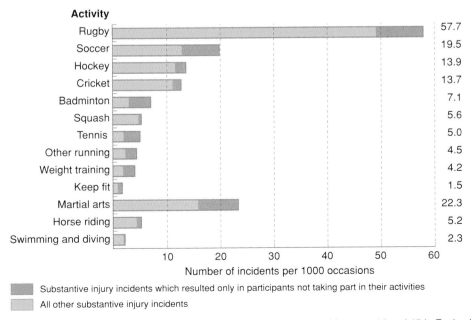

Fig. 1 New substantive injury incident rates by activity in a random sample of 17 564 people aged between 16 and 45 in England and Wales (Nicholl *et al.* 1991)

the playing field or pitch (Nicholl *et al.* 1991; Coleman *et al.* 1996; Wyatt *et al.* 1996).

Education and behaviour modification

1. Changes in the rules of some games may be necessary to reduce injury levels. Banning the dangerous practices of 'spearing' in American football has resulted in a reduction in the number of injuries producing permanent cervical quadriplegia (Torg *et al.* 1985).

2. Good referees are needed to prevent deliberate fouls, which often lead to injury.

3. Continuing player education is also important to persuade players to obey the rules and not to indulge in 'sport rage'.

4. Trained coaches should have a good knowledge of exercise physiology and be able to advise on good techniques, diet, and to help players avoid overuse injuries through improved training techniques.

5. Matching of young players in team games should be done by size and not by age.

6. Relevant protective equipment should be used. Mouth guards have been shown to reduce the number of dental and oral injuries but many players do not like using them (Jennings 1990). Protective goggles in squash and shin pads in football are examples of the equipment that can reduce injury.

Personal strategies

1. Training to build up muscle strength and endurance. Many injuries occur during the second half of a game, when fatigued muscles do not respond quickly to new situations. This is seen particularly in weekend athletes who do no other training.

2. Warm up and cool down. There are differing opinions on the benefit of warm ups and much of the evidence is anecdotal but the majority of athletes and coaches are in favour of some mobility exercises and gentle exercise to raise the heart rate and body temperature. After an intense effort, continuing light exercise does seem to allow an enhanced rate of removal of lactic acid and also prevents blood 'pooling' in the lower limbs. Improving flexibility both before and after exercises is reported to reduce injury levels but there is little hard evidence to support this.

3. Diet. There is overwhelming evidence as to the importance of adequate carbohydrate intake while competing and training to maintain and replace muscle glycogen. Carbohydrate should provide 50 to 60 per cent of the calorie intake and the athlete may need to take some of this as a carbohydrate drink (Costill and Hargreaves 1992). Cyclists on the *Tour de France* need to consume about 7000 calories/day and this would be impossible to eat as solid food.

4. Hydration. Most athletes are now aware of the importance of adequate rehydration but children need to be encouraged to drink as part of the game. Immediate postexercise replacement of fluid and carbohydrate, within the first hour, has been shown to restore rapidly muscle glycogen. Reduced glycogen levels lead to muscle fatigue and injury and reduced muscle glycogen is associated with a reduction in muscle and plasma glutamine levels.

5. Avoiding overtraining. Many athletes and sports players are convinced that 'more is better' and are not prepared to incorporate rest and recovery into their schedule. The overtraining syndrome produces symptoms of fatigue, sleeplessness, and loss of appetite (Budgett 1995). Intense and prolonged exercise has also been shown to produce immune system depression for 6 to 20 h after exercise (Newsholme 1994). This may explain why an athlete is more susceptible to injury and illness, including opportunistic infections such as toxoplasmosis and why injuries may take longer to heal.

Acute injuries

Acute management

Trauma results in bleeding. Blood in the extra vascular space is an extreme irritant causing an acute inflammatory response with swelling, an increase in pressure, and, if this pressure becomes great enough, tissue necrosis occurs (Fig. 2). Acute treatment of soft tissue trauma is aimed at limiting the bleeding and its subsequent deleterious affect (Fig. 3). This is achieved by:

(1) rest

(2) ice

(3) compression

(4) elevation

(5) non-steroidal anti-inflammatory agent.

This treatment is often given the mnemonic of RICE or NICER.

Rest

Rest is the fundamental treatment for an acute injury. It is essential to limit the trauma and to minimize the bleeding. Once an injury has been sustained, the injured player must immediately leave the field of play. This allows an immediate assessment of the injury to be made and for prompt first aid measures to be instituted. This early assessment can be vital as injuries such as ruptured cruciate ligaments can quickly be masked by bleeding and effusions in the knee and delay an accurate diagnosis.

Ice

Ice has become the traditional agent to help stop bleeding and reduce pain. The mechanism by which ice influences the underlying

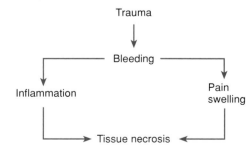

Fig. 2 Flow chart of sequence of events after soft tissue trauma.

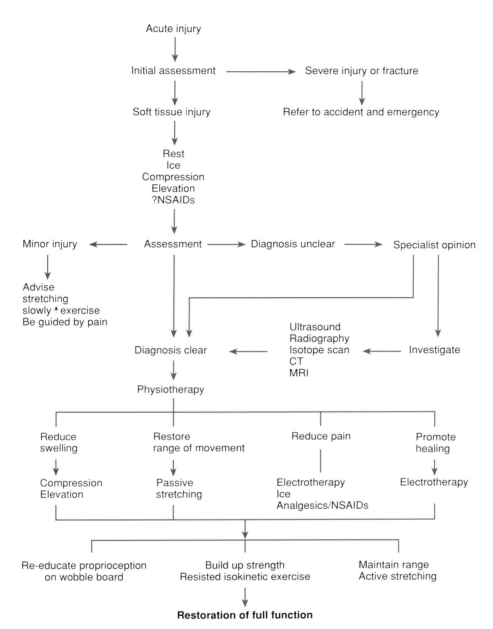

Fig. 3 Flow chart for the treatment of soft tissue injuries after acute injury.

vasculature is complex. While superficial skin blood flow is reduced, there is an initial short period of increased blood flow in the underlying tissues followed by alternating vasospasm and dilatation. It has been suggested that this 'pumping' action may be beneficial in removing oedema from the muscles.

Compression

Compression is probably the most effective means of limiting bleeding. The application of a firm bandage such as 'Tubigrip' over the whole of a limb may be helpful where direct pressure is difficult or inappropriate. It is important that pressure is not applied so tightly that it interferes with arterial or venous blood flow and therefore cause further damage.

Elevation

Tissue injury causes an acute inflammatory response followed by the development of oedema. The increased tissue pressure can reduce blood flow, increase pain, and delay healing. Swelling can be reduced by elevating the injured limb or, in the case of an injured leg, just by lying down.

Non-steroidal anti-inflammatory drugs

The treatment of soft tissue injury with non-steroidal anti-inflammatory drugs is controversial. Oral non-steroidal anti-inflammatory drugs will reduce pain and inflammation but probably only have a marginal beneficial effect on the healing process. They also have significant potential side-effects. If prescribed for acute soft tissue

Table 1 Muscle haematoma

	Extrinsic	Intrinsic
Mechanism	Direct trauma or compression	Overstretching or overload
Pathology	Muscle compressed against bone	Sudden contraction of a muscle against resistance
Cause	Contact sports	Stretching or sprinting

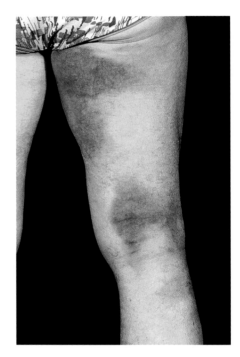

Fig. 4 Dramatic bruising in posterior thigh of rugby player caused by sprinting.

injuries, non-steroidal anti-inflammatory drugs are best prescribed for no more than 2 to 3 days after the injury. Topical non-steroidal anti-inflammatory drugs have a lower side-effect profile and exert a small beneficial effect in soft-tissue injuries, helping with an early return to sport.

Haematomas

Muscle haematoma may be due to either extrinsic or intrinsic injury (Table 1). After injury, there is disruption of the muscle fibres and capillaries with associated bleeding. The torn ends retract from the injury leaving it filled with blood.

An intact muscle sheath results in an intramuscular haematoma — a swelling within the muscle — causing pain and a considerable amount of disability which resolves slowly over many weeks. An intermuscular haematoma results when there is a tear in the fascial sheath or there is a tearing of vessels between the muscle fascicles. In this situation the blood disperses by gravity, to some distance away from the injury and, although the appearance is quite spectacular with considerable bruising, these injuries tend to recovery within 2 to 3 weeks (Fig. 4).

Symptoms depend to some degree on the type of injury. In a compression injury such as a rugby tackle, when the quadriceps muscle is compressed against the femur, the bleeding may be slow allowing the player to continue and only after the game does the increased swelling and accompanying pain and disability become apparent. An overstretching injury is sudden and acutely painful immediately. The commonest presentation is seen in sprinters who overstretch suddenly and tear hamstring muscles. Here the sudden acute pain feels like a blow on the back of the leg and may be severe enough for the athlete to fall to the ground. The diagnosis is usually fairly straightforward. Patients with a severe intramuscular haematoma of the hamstrings often present with a flexion deformity. There is some evidence that the greater the loss of flexion, the longer the time required for healing and return to sport (Renstrom 1988).

The clinical appearances and history are usually diagnostic. The presence of an intramuscular haematoma can be confirmed and treatment monitored by ultrasound.

Rehabilitation

Except in the most severe haematomas, early mobilization is indicated as it:

(1) speeds the return of muscle strength;

(2) improves the orientation of regenerating muscle fibres;

(3) encourages recapillarization;

(4) prevents disuse atrophy.

After 48 h of rest and ice, a rehabilitation programme should begin. This should initially consist of gentle stretching with the aim of restoring a full range of joint movement. The physiotherapist may also use various modalities of electrotherapy, such as pulsed magnetic energy, to assist healing. Stretching and strengthening programmes for all the muscle groups of the involved limb are essential, as some injuries may be due to a pre-existing lack of elasticity either in the injured muscle or its antagonist. The importance of balance between the muscle groups in the prevention of injury has been recognized and may be measured using an isokinetic machine, both for assessment and muscle retraining.

Cardiovascular fitness can be maintained by cycling (real bike or exercise bike), swimming, and running in water using a specially designed 'wet vest' to keep the athlete upright. Apart from the physical benefits of this exercise, being active in this way helps to maintain the sanity of the injured athlete. Many committed athletes become anxious and even depressed if exercise is not permitted.

Return to sport

A muscle haematoma can be considered to be completely healed when there is full and pain free muscle contraction. An intermuscular haematoma will usually resolve in 2 to 4 weeks. An intramuscular haematoma may take 8 weeks or more to completely heal, but there is a great variation depending on the site and severity of the injury. Before returning to competition, a further programme of sport-specific training must be carried out. This includes sprints, rapid deceleration, twists, and sharp turns. Co-ordination and proprioception are impaired by injury and the athlete must relearn specific techniques with the help of a coach.

Myositis ossificans

A severe crush injury may be followed by the development of hetero-topic ossification or myositis ossificans. This is more likely to occur if the injury is aggravated by continuing activity and further bruising. Applications of heat and vigorous massage all appear to irritate an already irritable muscle, although the exact cause of the calcification is not clear. Suspicions are raised if the patient is unable to achieve full contraction of the affected muscle. The calcification may be seen on radiographs and ultrasound.

Various treatments apart from rest have been used, including high doses of indomethacin and diphosphonates (DeLee and Drez 1994), but with doubtful efficacy. The use of a calcium channel blocker — Diltiazem — may offer a safer alternative (Palmieri et al. 1995). Most cases resolve symptomatically over a period of 3 months, although the calcification may persist radiologically. Intervention is rarely required unless mobility or persistent flexion deformity persists for over 6 months.

Muscle ruptures

Muscles may rupture and, although the defects look dramatic (Fig. 5), they rarely need surgical repair unless the rupture is complete.

Chronic injuries

The vast majority of chronic sports injuries are to the lower limb, predominantly affecting the knee. A description of the majority of these injuries and their treatment can be found in other sections of this book, particularly the section on soft tissue rheumatism (Chapter 5.14). In this section a few of the commonest problems encountered in a sports injury clinic are described — further information can be found in specialist textbooks (Lachmann and Jenner 1994; Harries et al. 1994). A careful history is important for diagnosis, particularly to ascertain if there has been overuse or a sudden unaccustomed use of the lower limbs. Type and age of footwear as well as training surface must be enquired after, as well as taking a full history of the pain problem.

Examination must always start with the spine and include the whole upper or lower limb. Leg length inequality of more than 1 cm should be noted. Chronic lower limb sporting injuries are frequently associated with the 'malicious malalignment syndrome' with a broad pelvis, patellas that look towards each other, internal tibial torsion, and flat or hyperpronated feet. Examination should include the joints, soft tissues, and neurological system as well as skin and circulation. The examination is completed by inspecting the running shoes for signs of wear.

Correcting leg length inequality with a simple insole may resolve back problems. Simple shock absorbing insoles may also help many chronic overuse problems. The use of more elaborate insoles to correct hyperpronation and other foot problems are also popular but their success is unpredictable.

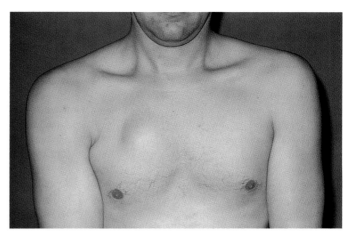

Fig. 5 Partial rupture of pectoralis major resulting from pulling against resistance in a rugby maul.

Stress fractures

In 1855, a German military physician, called Breihaupt, was the first to describe fractures of the foot bones in new recruits, not caused by direct trauma but by the stress of marching. Stress fractures can occur in any loaded bone and are seen most commonly in lower limbs, particularly in the tibia and metatarsals but they also occur in the upper limb, such as in the ribs of rowers and the arms of gymnasts (Fig. 6) (Matheson et al. 1987).

Stress fractures occur when bone fails to adapt to new or unusual loading. Normally, microdamage stimulates new bone where needed. When microdamage outpaces the development of new bone, a stress fracture results. Foot biomechanics may influence the development of stress fractures, such as rigid, poorly adapting feet or conversely hypermobile feet. Running on hard surfaces using 'collapsed' running shoes or racing flats certainly has an influence. Women appear to be at greater risk of developing a stress fracture. In a survey of 218 consecutive patients presenting with a stress fracture

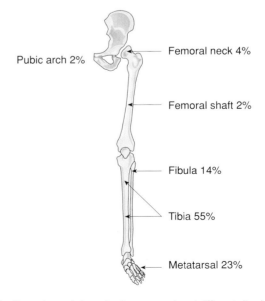

Fig. 6 Percentage of stress fractures occurring at different sites in the lower limb.

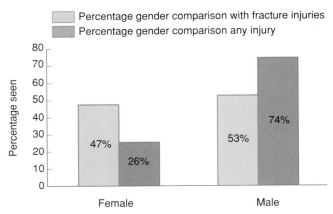

Although women are only 25 per cent of the total population with sports injuries, they comprise nearly 50 per cent of those with stress fractures

Fig. 7 Comparison of the incidence of stress fractures and all injuries between females and males attending a sports injury clinic.

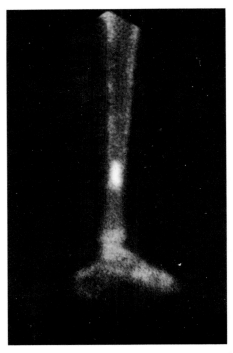

Fig. 8 Tc-99m bone scan showing high focal uptake typical of a stress fracture of the tibia.

to our sports injury clinic almost half were women, although women only accounted for a quarter of all the patients seen in the clinic (Fig. 7). Some of the fractures may be due to an inadequate calorie and calcium intake in sports where leanness is favoured, especially if low food intake results in amenorrhoea and secondary osteoporosis. These factors do not entirely account for the high incidences in women.

Clinical features

In vigorous sports, such as high jumping and gymnastics, the onset of pain is sudden and acute, completely preventing the continuation of the activity. In other less explosive sports, such as long distance running, the onset maybe insidious over several days or even weeks, with pain present at first only during exercise and weight bearing but eventually aching at rest and during the night. The site of the pain is very localized and local pressure produces exquisite pain over the fracture, causing the patient rapidly to pull the injured limb away. A stress fracture may be diagnosed on these clinical grounds, but in order to persuade an exercise-addicted athlete to rest there is frequently a need for some corroboration.

Radiographs are not very helpful as they do not show the injury until it is healing and maybe not even then. Bone scans are extremely sensitive and can differentiate between osteitis of the tibia and a stress fracture. Although not absolutely necessary for diagnosis, a positive scan does help to convince the athlete of the nature of his problem and need for rest (Fig. 8).

Although the majority of stress fractures respond to conservative measures, stress fractures of the femoral neck have the potential for serious complications, including avascular necrosis and persistent non-union, and may need a surgical assessment (Fullerton and Snowdy 1988). These present with vague groin pain, pain in the anterior thigh and the knee, and are most commonly seen in long distance runners.

Management

Reduction of weight bearing is essential, usually with the help of elbow crutches. Modification of activity should continue until symptoms are absent. This can take 6 to 8 weeks and during this time the athlete can do some form of non or partial weight-bearing exercise, such as swimming, water walking, and cycling. Sport can be resumed when there is no pain on weight bearing and must be gradually increased. A stretching and strengthening programme should be carried out.

Using this regime, the majority of athletes will be able to return to sport in 6 to 8 weeks. Problems arise when the athlete is not prepared to rest. Under these circumstances the fracture can continue to cause problems for several months and sometime the only way to prevent continuing disability is to apply a plaster of Paris case and insist on no weight bearing. If not properly dealt with, a stress fracture can persist for 6 months or more.

Anterior knee pain

A patient presenting with poorly localized anterior knee pain, without any history of trauma, is a very common occurrence in a sports injury clinic. The patient is often teenage and a sports enthusiast, playing or training on a daily basis. However, older patients responding to advice to increase their exercise also present with this problem.

Aetiology

Patellofemoral joint stability depends on many factors (Table 2). Any of these factors can cause an imbalance of the patellofemoral joint. It has long been assumed that patellofemoral pain was caused by abnormal patella tracking but all of these anatomical variations are common in the general population and only cause problems when the patellofemoral joint is subjected to chronic overload by repetitive overuse and obvious eccentric contraction strains as in deep squats (Thomee *et al.* 1995).

Table 2 Factors predisposing to patellofemoral pain syndrome
Torsional deformities of tibia/femur (winking or frog eye patella)
High or lateral patella
Weak or absent vastus medialis obliquus
Tight muscles on the lateral aspect — vastus lateralis and iliotibial band
Increased quadriceps angle
Excessive foot pronation
Weak ankle dorsiflexors
Reduced range of motion at the ankle
Tight hamstrings

Table 3 Rehabilitation programme for patellofemoral pain syndrome

Stage 1　　*2–3 weeks*

Reduce symptoms by cutting down activity. No exercise involving deep squats. Relieve the pain with ice and non-steroidal anti-inflammatory drugs.

Stage 2　　*3–4 weeks*

With help of physiotherapist, strengthening exercises for vastus medialis obliquus. Flexibility of hamstrings, quadriceps, iliotibial band, gastrocnemius–soleus complex.

Stage 3

Gradual return to sport and then full training

Stage 4

Maintenance exercises for vastus medialis obliquus, at least 3 times weekly.

Clinical features

The patient complains of generalized anterior knee pain and may exhibit the 'grab' sign — holding the whole of the front of the knee. There is no history of trauma but more of a gradual increase in pain over several weeks, often affecting both knees. The pain is made worse by activity, either during sport or going up and down stairs. Sitting with the knee in flexion causes acute discomfort, such as sitting in a cinema, giving the so-called 'movie sign' (Insall 1982). The knee may feel unstable or 'give way'; this is due to reflex quadriceps inhibition rather than a true instability. Clicking and crepitus is common. There is pain and sometimes crepitus if the patella is compressed and moved proximally and distally. There is usually some tenderness along the very anterior joint line and at the attachment of the medial and lateral retinacula. Patella inhibition is elicited by holding the patella at the proximal pole and flexing the knee to about 20°. Straightening the leg causes pain and the patient stops the movement.

Patella subluxation, which can present with similar symptoms, is excluded by the patella apprehension test. The patella is usually very mobile and pushing it sideways produces great anxiety. Treatment is aimed at stabilizing the patella with appropriate quadriceps exercises.

Management

The patient, and often parents, need to be reassured that this complaint is common and does not mean indefinite incapacity. Radiographs may be required to exclude any more serious pathology, especially if the problem affects one knee only. In mild cases, some reduction of the level of activity is all that is necessary — the patient decides what is tolerable. Activities not causing pain, such as swimming, can be substituted to maintain fitness. Local applications of ice after exercise and a course of non-steroidal anti-inflammatory drugs can hasten recovery.

Rehabilitation

When the acute symptoms have been alleviated, a strengthening and stretching programme involving hamstring and quadriceps is begun under the care of a sports-orientated physiotherapist. The treatment involves selectively strengthening the vastus medialis obliquus, while at the same time reducing the pull of the vastus lateralis. Strengthening of the quadriceps as a whole has been replaced by work only on vastus medialis obliquus (Shelton 1991). There is also some evidence that patellofemoral dysfunction may be related to abnormal timing in the firing of the various quadriceps components (McConnell 1986; Voigt 1991). Muscle re-education using biofeedback techniques during various exercises can be used where the patient is taught to fire the vastus medialis obliquus earlier and more efficiently. McConnell also developed external support for the patella by means of taping. Using these methods, while working on strengthening techniques, often provides immediate and fairly long-lasting relief.

Although the vast majority of patients will improve using these measures, it is important that they understand this is not a cure. Adolescent sufferers may well improve with the passage of time, as some of the imbalance may be associated with growth spurts. If there are persistent anatomical features, the patient will have to be prepared to continue the muscle strengthening exercises indefinitely in order to control their pain. Ten per cent of patients do not improve with the above measures; some may be prepared to modify their lifestyles but others may request surgery. Various surgical options are available, the most common being lateral release (Table 3).

Anterior shin pain induced by exercise ('shin splints')

Chronic pain in the shins induced by exercise (commonly known as 'shin splints') is a frequent occurrence in sportsmen and women but is rarely seen in any other group of patients. This syndrome embraces a variety of conditions:

(1) stress fracture of the tibia or fibula;

(2) fasciitis of tibialis posterior;

(3) compartment syndrome;

(4) popliteal artery stenosis;

(5) referred pain from the spine (cord claudication);

(6) peripheral vascular disease (intermittent claudication).

Fasciitis of tibialis posterior

Hyperpronation of the feet is often seen in association with other common malalignment problems. This problem puts extra stress on the tibialis posterior muscle which is responsible for inversion of the foot and inserts onto the posterior aspect of the tibia and fibula. The tendon of the muscle runs behind the medial malleolus and the flat hyperpronated foot is easily overstretched by repetitive activity resulting in a traction injury at the fascial insertion along the posterior border of the tibia.

Patients complain of pain in the shins which starts after starting to run. Often they can run through the pain only for it to return with great severity on ceasing activity. The pain often takes days to wear off. Examination reveals diffuse tenderness along the medial border of the tibia. The diagnosis may be confirmed with a bone scan.

Treatment is difficult. Rest is vital and is followed by a gradual return to sport with appropriate footwear. Orthotic supports to correct the hyperpronation and to provide shock absorption can be tried.

Compartment syndrome

Acute swelling of muscles within a muscle compartment leading to muscle ischaemia and even necrosis is a well recognized complication of acute trauma. The chronic form of this condition is less well known and occurs almost exclusively in endurance sports such as long distance running. As the muscles are exercised they swell within a tight fascial compartment raising the pressure sufficiently to reduce tissue perfusion. There are four separate compartments in the lower limb (Table 4). Compartment syndrome commonly follows a sudden increase in training. Symptoms are absent at rest but pain in the shin commences at a variable time after the onset of exercise and invariably increases until exercise is stopped or moderated. If the limb is rested the pain usually wears off within a few hours. Examination is often unremarkable although highly-developed calf muscles that feel tense at rest may be noted. A Tc 99 bone scan will exclude a stress fracture or fasciitis. Pressure studies can be performed by inserting catheters into each compartment and measuring the pressure rises. This is an invasive investigation and only available at specialist centres. A promising alternative is isotope scanning employing a technetium isotope Tc-99m-methylisobutylisonitrile (MIBI) which is used routinely to detect cardiac ischaemia and can be modified to look at peripheral muscle ischaemia. If the symptoms do not settle with rest, the appropriate compartments can be released by a surgical fasciotomy (Miles *et al.* 1992) (Fig. 9).

Popliteal artery entrapment

Rarely, similar symptoms can be caused by entrapment of the popliteal artery by a fibrous band or hypertrophied head of gastrocnemius. Arteriography may be required to confirm the diagnosis.

Children and sport

Children are prone to similar injuries to adults but should not be regarded as 'little adults' as their physiology and anatomy are very different, resulting in injuries not encountered in the adult:

1. They take shorter, more shallow breaths and need more oxygen for their activity than an adult.

2. They also have lower glycogen levels and essential muscle enzymes and waste more energy.

Table 4	Compartments of the lower limb	
Compartment	**Muscle**
Anterior	Tibialis Anterior
Posterior	Gastrocnemius/soleus
Deep posterior	Tibialis posterior
Lateral	Peroneii

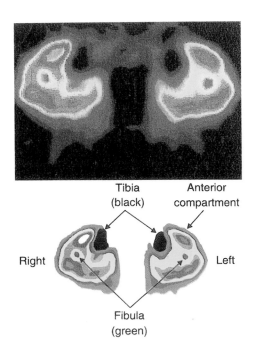

Fig. 9 Methylisobutylisonitrile emission tomogram of mid calf after exercise showing reduction in uptake in left anterior compartment compared with an annotated drawing below.

3. Children perceive exercises as less fatiguing than adults and can almost exercise to destruction, but they also have the capacity to recover very quickly.

4. Muscle, tendon, and ligaments are stronger than bone until bony maturity is reached at 18 to 21 years.

5. Bones are still growing with active apophyses and epiphyses which can be the site of pathology.

6. Growth occurs in spurts, resulting in tight muscles and loss of flexibility making adolescents particularly prone to injury.

Avulsion fractures

Tendons, ligaments, and muscles, especially trained muscles, are stronger than bone and more so at the epiphyseal junctions. Sudden, intense loading of a muscle does not produce a muscle tear as in an adult but is more likely to cause an avulsion fracture where the bony attachment of the muscle or ligament is torn away. Common sites for avulsion fractures are the growth zones around the pelvis, including the attachments at the ischial tuberosity and the attachments of rectus femoris and sartorius. The less severe injuries can sometimes present only as a pain in the groin, with loss of function of the appropriate muscle. These injuries do not show up on radiographs and a bone scan is necessary. The usual treatment is rest followed by physiotherapy treatment, with an emphasis on restoring strength to the injured muscle. Healing may take up to 6 months.

Overuse injuries of the apophysis

In children and adolescents the muscle tendon attachment to bone or the apophysis presents as a 'high-risk' area for overuse injuries (Renstrom 1988). Overuse caused a traction apophysitis and occurs at various sites (Table 5).

Table 5 Sites of apophysitis

Eponym	Site of injury
Osgood–Schlatters	Tibial tubercle
Sinding–Larsen, Johannason	Lower pole of patella
Severs disease	Achilles tendon attachment to calcaneum

Osgood–Schlatter disease follows overloading of the patellar tendon at its attachment to the tibial tubercle. Very active boys, between the ages of 14 to 16 years and girls at a slightly younger age, present with swelling, pain, and acute tenderness over the tibial tubercle. These children are usually playing not only for the school, but taking part in other competitive sports on most days of the week.

The treatment of all the apophyseal overuse injuries is by modifying activity, playing only to a bearable level of discomfort, and using ice before and after exercise. Most respond to this regime but this may take several months and some persist until growing has ceased.

Osteochondritis

This is a collection of conditions affecting various sites of uncertain aetiology and is thought to be due to avascular necrosis of bone and subsequent flattening of the affected bones (Fig. 10; Table 6).

Perthes' disease and the potentially disastrous unrelated hip problem of slipped femoral epiphysis may present with a limp and a painful knee. This can cause diagnostic problems as the child may present following an injury, drawing attention away from the real source of the problem. When faced with this history a radiograph is mandatory, as both conditions require urgent orthopaedic referral.

Scheuermann's disease mainly affects the thoracic vertebrae and because the anterior border of the vertebrae are subjected to deforming forces a kyphosis occurs. Often this is asymptomatic, although there may be some discomfort after hard exercise. In mild cases, flexibility

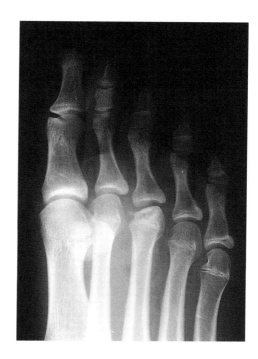

Fig. 10 Freiberg's disease showing flattening of the head of the 3rd metatarsal.

exercises for the hip flexors and hamstrings and abdominal strengthening are sufficient until the disease ends spontaneously. Increasing kyphosis demands more serious intervention.

Osteochondritis dissecans

Osteochondritis dissecans is a disease of unknown aetiology, occurring in young people between the ages of 12 and 16 years. There is destruction and subsequent disintegration of cartilage and bone. Popular theories are trauma or continuous repetitive damage (Fairbanks 1993), ischaemia, and genetic factors. In the United States, the condition is seen as one of the entities in 'little league elbow', seen in young baseball pitchers.

The knee is a common presenting site and the history is of a diffuse knee ache, made worse by activity and accompanied by occasional effusion. When a fragment of bone becomes loose in the joint the patient may present with an episode of locking and effusion. The

Table 6 Sites of osteochondritis

Name	Site
Perthes' disease	Hip
Scheuermann's disease	Vertebral ring epiphysis
Kohler's disease	Navicular bone
Freiburg's disease	2nd or 3rd metatarsal
Panner's disease	Elbow capitellum

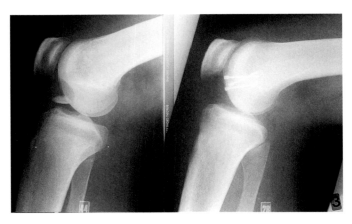

Fig. 11 Osteochondritis of femoral condyle before and after surgical intervention.

diagnosis can be confirmed by radiography. Surgical replacement of the loose fragment can give excellent results (Fig. 11).

References

Budgett, R. (1995). *The overtraining syndrome. ABC sports medicine.* British Medical Journal Publications, London.

Coleman, P, Munro, J., Nicholl, J., Harper, R., Kent, G., and Wild, D. (1996).*The effectiveness of interventions to prevent accidental injury to young persons aged 15 to 24.* Medical Care Research Unit, University of Sheffield.

Costill, D.L. and Hargreaves, M. (1992).Carbohydrate nutrition and fatigue. *Sports Medicine,*12, 86–92.

DeLee, J.C. and Drez, D. (1994). *Orthopaedic sports medicine.* Vol II. WB Saunders, Philadelphia.

Fairbanks, H.A.T. (1993). Osteochondritis dissecans. *British Journal of Surgery,* 21, 67.

Fullerton, L.R. and Snowdy, H.A. (1988). Femoral neck stress fractures. *American Journal of Sports Medicine,* 16, 365–77.

Harries, M., Williams, C., and Stanish, W., eds. (1994). *Oxford textbook of sports medicine.* Oxford University Press, Oxford.

Insall, J. (1982). Chondromalacia patellae. Current concepts and review patella pain. *Journal of Bone and Joint Surgery,* 64(A), 147.

Jennings, D.C. (1990). Injuries sustained by users and non users of gum shields in local rugby union players. *British Journal of Sports Medicine,* 24, 159–65.

Lachmann, S.M.L. and Jenner, J. (1994). *Soft tissue injuries in sport.* Blackwell Science, Oxford.

Matheson, G.O., Clement, D.B., McKenzie, D.C., Tavnton, J.E., Lloyd Smith, D.R., and MacIntyre, J.G. (1987). Stress fractures in athletes. *American Journal of Sports Medicine,* 15, 46–58.

McConnell, J. (1986). The management of chondromalacia patellae: a long term solution. *Australian Journal of Physiotherapy,* 2, 215–23.

Miles, K. *et al.* (1992). Leg muscle scintigraphy with 99Tc MIBI in the assessment of peripheral vascular arterial disease. *Nuclear Medicine Communications,* 1, 593–603.

Newsholme, E.A. (1994). Biochemical mechanisms to explain immunosuppression in well-trained and overtrained athletes. *International Journal of Sports Medicine,* 15 (Suppl. 3), 5142–7.

Nicholl, J.P., Coleman, P., and Williams, B.T. (1991). *Injuries in sport and exercise.* London Sports Council.

Palmieri, G.M., Secen, J.I., Aelion, J.A., Moinuddin, M., Ray, M.W., Wood, G.C., and Leventhal, M.R. (1995). Treatment of calcinosis with diltiazem. *Arthritis and Rheumatism,* 38, 1646-54.

Renstrom, P. (1988).*Olympic text book of sports medicine.* Vol I. Blackwell Scientific Publications.

Report of the Royal College of Physicians (1991). *Medical aspects of exercise. Benefits and risks.* Royal College of Physicians of London, London.

Shelton, T. (1991). Rehabilitation of patellofemoral dysfunction; A review of the literature. *Journal of Orthopedic Sports Physiology and Therapy,* 144, 243–9.

Thomee, R., Renstrom, P., Karlsson, J., and Grimby, G. (1995). Patellofemoral pain syndrome in young women. *Scandinavian Journal of Medicine and Science in Sports,* 5, 237–44.

Torg, J.S., *et al.* (1985). The national football head and neck injury registry. *Journal of the American Medical Association,* 254, 3439–43.

Voigt, W. (1991). Comparative reflex response times of vastus medialis obliqus and vastus lateralis in normal subjects and subjects with extensor mechanism dysfunction. *American Journal of Sports Medicine,* 19, 131–7.

Wyatt, P. *et al.* (1996). A prospective study of rock climbing injuries. *British Journal of Sports Medicine,* 30, 148–50.

Index

Note: Since the main subjects of this book are rheumatic disease and connective tissue diseases, index entries under
these key words have been kept to a minimum, and readers are advised to seek more specific references.

Page numbers in **bold** refer to principal discussions in the text. Page numbers in *italic* refer to pages on which tables are to be found.

A

AAT *see* α₁-antitrypsin
abarticular rheumatism 1489
abductor pollicis longus 138, 139, 146
abortion
  spontaneous
    and antiphospholipid antibodies
      293, 294, 295, 1206, 1212–13
    in brucellosis 937
    in gout 184
    recurrent *177*, 178
    in rheumatoid arthritis 181–2
    in SLE 183, 1157
    in systemic sclerosis 1239
  therapeutic in rheumatoid arthritis 181
abscess
  amoebic hepatic 1320
  Brodie's **1620–1**
  differential diagnosis 1122
  epidural in brucellosis 939, 944
  intramedullary spinal cord 124
  paravertebral
    in brucellosis 939, 944
    in tuberculosis 122, 928
  psoas 48, 717, 1094
  retroperitoneal 1094
  retropharyngeal 928
  soft tissue in brucellosis 941
ACA *see* anticentromere antibodies
ACE inhibitors
  in acute renal failure 329
  decline in renal function due to 325
  interaction with NSAIDs *579*
  in systemic sclerosis 329, 1238
  in Takayasu's arteritis 1387
acebutalol, lupus-like syndrome due to 1690
acetabular cavity 150
acetabular dysplasia and osteoarthritis 1520
acetaminophen *see* paracetamol
acetoacetate in synovial hypoxia 445
acetophenetidin 32
N-acetotransferase 36
acetretin
  in discoid lupus erythematosus 211
  in psoriasis 212
acetyl coA 1774
N-acetyl-D-glucosaminidase 650
N-acetyl glucosamine 973, 974
acetylaminfluorine 690
acetylsalicylic acid *see* aspirin
Achilles tendon 153, 154, 157, 718
  central core degeneration 1510
  examination 50–1
  imaging 745–6
  rupture 1510
    in SLE 1147
  tendinitis 159, 168, 1511
    imaging 718–19
    in psoriatic arthritis 1076
    steroid injection therapy 1770
achondrogenesis 368, **375–6**, 436
  collagen protein analysis 374

achondrogenesis *(continued)*
  type I *369*
    clinical features 371
    gene mutations 370
  type II *369*, *435*, 436
    clinical features 371
    gene mutations 370
achondroplasia 353, 436, 1630
  gene mutations 369, *369*, 396, 398, *435*
α1-acid glycoprotein (AGP) 623, **627**
  in ankylosing spondylitis 629
  function in inflammation *624*
  in giant cell arteritis 628, 629
  in polymyalgia rheumatica 628, 629
  properties *625*
  in rheumatoid arthritis 629, *1016*
  in systemic lupus erythematosus 640
acid maltase deficiency 473, 1774
acid phosphatase in Paget's disease 1613
acidic fibroblast growth factor in angiogenesis 509
acidosis
  hyperchloraemic 1602
  metabolic 1773
    in rickets/osteomalacia 1605
  respiratory 1773
  see also renal tubular acidosis
acinar epithelial cells in Sjögren's syndrome 1305
Acinetobacter in pyogenic arthritis 852
acne
  lesions resembling in Behçet's syndrome
    1395, 1396, 1399
  pustular 206
acne fulminans *175*
ACR *see* American College of Rheumatology
Acremonium 963
acrodermatitis chronica atrophicans
  884, 885, 887, 888–9
  and reflex sympathetic dystrophy 1681
  treatment 893
acrokeratosis in HIV infection 919
acromegalic rosary 281
acromegaly **281–2**, 431
  and calcium pyrophosphate dihydrate
    disease 1530, *1531*
  and osteoarthritis 1519
  synovial fluid in 680
acromicric dysplasia 1635
acromioclavicular joint
  anatomy 135, 136, 137
  examination 44
  hypertrophy 739, 740
  local steroid injection 1764
  movement 44
  pain 1501
  in rheumatoid arthritis 1008
  surgery 1702
  traumatic lesions 144
acromioclavicular ligaments 135
acromioclavicular syndrome 1503
acromion 135, 136

acromioplasty, anterior 142
acro-osteolysis
  in Ehlers–Danlos syndrome type 4 378,
    380
  idiopathic 1635–6
acroparaesthesia in hypothyroidism 278
ACT *see* α₁-antichymotrypsin
ACTH 510
actin 455, 458
  in Dupuytren's contracture 148
α-actin 455
α-actinin 455, 528
activities of daily living 52, 64
acupuncture
  in back pain 105, 1648
  in cervical pain syndromes 1658
acute inflammatory demyelinating polyneuropathy 794–5
acute necrotizing arteriolitis 791, 795
acute necrotizing arteritis 791
acute neutrophilic dermatitis 206,
  1396, **1456–8**
acute phase proteins 623, **626–7**, 638–9
  assay 626
  in clinical disease 627–9
  in evaluation of drug therapy 629
  glycosylation 629
  in hyperlipidaemias 1483
  negative *624*
  in non-gonococcal arthritis 850
  plasma concentration measurement
    625
  in pregnancy 627
  properties *625*
  proposed functions in inflammation *624*
  reactivity with concanavalin A 629
  regulation of production 623–4
  in rheumatic fever 980
  in rheumatoid arthritis 990, 1016, *1016*
  type-1 623
  type-2 623
acute phase response **623–9**, 638–41, 653
  in adult Still's disease 641
  in anaemia 636, 640
  in autoimmune disease 628
  in bacterial infection 625, 640
  clinical use 627–9
  in crystal deposition diseases 627
  in giant cell arteritis 627–8, 629, 640,
    1378
  in hypergammaglobulinaemia 640
  in hyperlipidaemia 640
  in infective discitis 640
  kinetics in disease 624–5
  laboratory measurements 625–6
  in malignant disease 640
  in myeloma 640
  in osteoarthritis 627
  in osteomyelitis 640
  in polymyalgia rheumatica 627–8, 629,
    640, 1378
  regulation 623
  in rheumatoid arthritis 628–9, 640

acute phase response *(continued)*
  in seronegative spondylarthropathies
    628
  in SLE 628, 640
  in systemic amyloidosis 640
acute renal failure 173, **325–30**, *330*
  complications 330
  course 330
  definitions 325–6
  drug-related *578*, 580
  intrinsic renal 325, 326
  and myoglobin 467
  non-oliguric 325, 326
  oliguric 325–6
  pathophysiological mechanisms in
    systemic rheumatic disease 326–9
  postrenal/obstructive 326
  prerenal 325, 326
  prognosis 330
  in systemic sclerosis 184, 328–9
  treatment principles 329–30
acute tubular necrosis 327
acyclovir in Behçet's syndrome 1401
**Adapted Arthritis Impact
  Measurement Scales for Children**
  56, 57
Addison's disease *285*
addressin 537, *537*
adduction stress test 144
adductor brevis 150
adductor digiti minimi 800
adductor longus 150
adductor magnus 150
adductor tendinitis 1508
adenine 689
adenine phosphoribosyl transferase
  1557
**adenosine accumulation in synovial
  hypoxia** 446
adenosine diphosphate 1773
adenosine triphosphate (ATP) 1773–4
  demand for in inflamed synovia 445,
    446
  in muscle contraction 464
adenovirus infection 904, 1376
ADH 1773
adhesion cascade 534–6
adhesion molecules 512, **528–34**
  expression by activated lymphocytes
    528
  identification and quantification *in situ*
    537, 538
  in microscopic polyangiitis 1357
  monoclonal antibodies against 538, 613
  in SLE 1168, *1169*
adhesive capsulitis *see* shoulder, frozen
adipocytes 422
adjuvant arthritis 561, 562, 563, 611,
  998, *1043*
  oil-based 567
adolescence
  back pain in 20, *20*, 97–8, 118–30, 131
  calcium intake 29
  intervertebral disc prolapse 124–5

adolescence (continued)
  knee pain in 157
  polyarthritis 56
  range of joint movements 16
  scoliosis 131
  upper limb pain 163
  see also childhood
ADP 1773
adrenal vein thrombosis in anti-
    phospholipid syndrome 1205
adrenaline in sport 1778
Adson test 1661
adult-onset Still's disease see Still's
    disease, adult-onset
AECA see antiendothelial cell antibodies
Aedes aegypti 901, 903
Aedes albopictus 901
Aedes camptorhynchus 903
Aedes polynesiensis 903
Aedes vigilax 903
aerobic capacity, limitations to 1775–6
Aeromonas hydrophila in pyogenic
    arthritis 852
African–Americans
  juvenile chronic arthritis 829, 830
  rheumatoid arthritis 833, 834
  seronegative spondylarthropathies
      838–9, 839
  SLE 833, 835, 836
  see also ethnic groups
Afro-Caribbeans
  rheumatoid arthritis 833, 834
  SLE 833, 836, 836, 837–8
  see also ethnic groups
agammaglobulinaemia, X-linked 970
age
  arterial changes associated 783, 784
  and back pain 20
  and clearance of NSAIDs 577
  and disease occurrence 25–6, 26, 815–
      16, 815, 816
    ankylosing spondylitis 26, 815, 815
    calcium pyrophosphate dihydrate
        disease 26, 1529
    giant cell arteritis/polymyalgia rheu-
        matica 1375
    gout occurrence 815
    osteoarthritis 815, 815, 816, 816, 1517
    rheumatoid arthritis 832
  effect on articular cartilage 413–14, 413
  effect on electrodiagnosis 807
  effect on GFR 649
  effect on muscle function 28, 464–5
  effect on plasma levels of amylobarbitone
      sodium 23, 24
  and exercise 25, 28–9
  and physiological function 22–5
  skeletal, assessment 755
age at onset
  ankylosing spondylitis 11, 12, 13, 1061,
      1062
  back pain 20
  childhood rheumatic diseases 12, 13
  dermatomyositis 11, 13, 1288
  giant cell arteritis 26, 1377
  Henoch–Schönlein purpura 11, 12, 13
  inflammatory bowel disease 13
  juvenile chronic arthritis 12, 13, 1099,
      1114
  juvenile psoriatic arthritis 12, 13
  Kawasaki disease 11, 12, 13
  Lyme disease 13
  microscopic polyangiitis 1354
  mixed connective tissue disease 13
  polyarteritis nodosa 12, 13, 1353
  polymyalgia rheumatica 26, 1377
  polymyositis 11, 26, 1288
  pyogenic arthritis 12, 13
  reactive arthropathies 13, 26, 1090
  rheumatic fever 11, 13
  rheumatoid arthritis 1012
  scleroderma 13
  seronegative spondylarthropathies 1136
  SLE 12, 13, 26, 1146, 1159, 1181

age at onset (continued)
  systemic sclerosis 13, 26
  Takayasu's arteritis 12, 13
  Wegener's granulomatosis 12, 13
ageing, biology of 22–5
aggrecan 406–7, 409–10
  effect of cytokines on 414
  in osteoarthritis 1537, 1538
  structure 409
  turnover 410–11, 411
aggrecanase 1545
agoraphobia 342
AGP see α₁-acid glycoprotein
agranulocytosis, drug-related 295,
    296, 580, 589, 1022
aid appliances 1730, 1730, 1731
  childhood 1752, 1753
  walking 1733–4
AIDP 794–5
AIDS 208, 971
  development 907, 910
  gait in 919
  lupus anticoagulant in 293
  muscle necrosis in 790
  mycoplasmas in 967
  parvovirus infection in 898
  see also HIV
AIMS see Arthritis Impact Measurement
    Scales
alanine aminopeptidase 650
alanine aminotransferase (ALT/GPT)
    651, 652
  in differential diagnosis of neuro-
      muscular disorders 1291
  imprecision in measurement 648
  in juvenile chronic arthritis 1116
albendazole 949, 950, 951
Albers–Schönberg disease 436
albumin 624
  in antigen-induced arthritis model 565
  and erythrocyte sedimentation rate 639
  imprecision in measurement 648
  and liver function 651
  in model of arthritis flares 566
  in synovial fluid 443
  in systemic lupus erythematosus 640
alcohol
  and gout 1555, 1694
  and hyperuricaemia 1558
alcohol abuse
  myopathy due to 1265, 1266
  and osteonecrosis 1622
aldolase
  in differential diagnosis of neuromus-
      cular disorders 1291
  in polymyositis/dermatomyositis 1257
aldomet, effect on prolactin levels 282
alendronate in osteoporosis 29, 1598
alfacalcidol 1603
alfentanyl 307
algesic substances, definition 488
algodystrophy see reflex sympathetic
    dystrophy
alkaline phosphatase
  in ankylosing spondylitis 1066
  bone-derived 432, 653
  elevation, differential diagnosis 1615
  gene mutations 436
  in hypophosphatasia 436
  imprecision in measurement 648
  isoenzymes 652
  and liver function 651, 652
  as measure of bone turnover 431–2
  in osteoarthritis 1543, 1544
  in osteoblasts 429
  in osteomalacia 1601
  in osteoporosis 1595
  in Paget's disease 1613
  in polymyalgia rheumatica/giant cell
      arteritis 1378
  in sarcoidosis 1465
  in vasculitis 1358
alkaptonuria 436

alkylating agents see chlorambucil;
    cyclophosphamide
allele-sharing analysis, genetic
    markers 688–9
allergic rhinitis in Churg–Strauss
    syndrome 1355
allodynia 489, 491
  definition 488
  in reflex sympathetic dystrophy 1680,
      1684, 1686
allopurinol 514
  adverse effects 217, 1565
  in gout 1565, 1566
  in lactation 194
  in pregnancy 193
alopecia 174, 200, 201
  in dermatomyositis 1251
  drug-related 214, 215, 584, 587
    alkylating agents 593, 593
    penicillamine 598
  in mixed connective tissue disease 1417
  in rickets 1604
  in Sjögren's syndrome 1310
  in SLE 1148, 1183
alphaviruses 901–4
Alport syndrome 353, 356, 357, 387
ALT see alanine aminotransferase
Alternaria 963
altitude training 1775
aluminium
  intoxication 433
  and osteomalacia 1603, 1606
alveolar haemorrhage 1337–8
alveolitis
  lymphocyte 251
  neutrophil 251
Alzheimer's disease 30
  amyloidosis in 336, 1434, 1434, 1439
  similarities with inclusion-body
      myositis 471, 1279
amaurosis fugax in Takayasu's arter-
    itis 1385
amenorrhoea
  drug-related 593, 594
  and exercise 1777
  and osteoporosis 1589
  in SLE 183
American College of Rheumatology
    (ACR)
  diagnostic criteria
    chronic childhood arthritis 10, 10, 1131
    fibromyalgia 1497, 1498
    giant cell arteritis 1374, 1374
    osteoarthritis 1516
    rheumatoid arthritis 55–6, 811–12,
        812, 1004, 1006
    SLE 1145, 1147
    Takayasu's arteritis 1384, 1384
    vasculitis 1322
    Wegener's granulomatosis 1333, 1333
  functional classes 51
American Rheumatism Association
  criteria for rheumatoid arthritis 1004,
      1005
  see also American College of
      Rheumatology
Americans with Disabilities Act 1723
amidophosphoribosyl transferase
    (amidoPRT) 1556, 1557
amino acids
  excitatory 495, 495
    receptors for 496
  synovial fluid 677
p-amino salicylic acid in tuberculosis
    932
aminocaproic acid, adverse effects
    1265, 1693
aminoglycosides
  interaction with NSAIDs 579
  in pyogenic arthritis 857
aminopeptidase M 452
aminoquinolines in pregnancy 191–2
amiodarone in hypertrophic obstruc-
    tive cardiomyopathy 1777

amitriptyline 339, 340, 341
  in ankylosing spondylitis 1069
  in cervical pain syndromes 1658
  in chronic back pain 1648
  in low back pain 101
  plasma concentrations 342
  in rheumatoid arthritis 342
amnesia in antiphospholipid
    syndrome 222
amniocentesis, osteogenesis imper-
    fecta 698
amoebiasis 946, 946, 947
amoxapine 341, 342
amoxicillin, in Lyme disease 891, 892,
    893
amoxycillin, in osteomyelitis 874
amphetamines 1265, 1778
amphotericin B
  adverse effects 252, 1693
  in fungal arthritis 956
    blastomycosis 959
    Candida 958
    coccidioidomycosis 962
    cryptococcosis 963
    histoplasmosis 962
    paracoccidioidomycosis 963
    sporotrichosis 963
  intra-articular 958, 960
  in invasive aspergillosis 252
  lipid-associated 958
  liposomal 252
  prophylactic 1359
ampicillin in pyogenic arthritis 856
amplification refractory mutation
    system 691, 692
amputation in osteomyelitis 876
amylobarbitone sodium, effect of age
    on plasma levels 23, 24
amyloid
  fibril proteins 1433–5, 1434
  intraneural deposition 795
  reduction of precursors 1441–2
  staining 1433
  structure 1433
  in synovial fluid 680
  systemic senile 1433
amyloid-A protein 1433, 1434, 1435,
    1438
amyloid β-protein 336, 1434, 1434, 1438,
    1439
amyloid-enhancing factor 1435–6
amyloid-L protein 1433, 1434
amyloid-P protein 1433, 1436, 1441
amyloid-related serum protein 184
amyloidosis 1433–42
  acute phase response in 640
  AL 1433, 1436–7, 1436, 1442
  in Alzheimer's disease 336, 1434, 1434,
      1439
  and amyloid fibril proteins 1433–5, 1434
  in ankylosing spondylitis 1064
  in Behçet's syndrome 259, 1398
  cardiovascular involvement 230, 233,
      1436, 1438, 1439
  clinical syndromes 1436–9
  definition 1433
  diagnosis 1440–1
  in dialysis 289, 1439–40
  in familial Mediterranean fever 1433,
      1434, 1438, 1447–8, 1448
  hereditary renal 1434, 1434
  inherited autosomal-dominant 1438
  in juvenile chronic arthritis 1118–19,
      1118
  organ manifestations 1439–40
  pathogenesis 1435–6
  peripheral neuropathies 228, 1436,
      1440
  prognosis 1442
  psychiatric involvement 333, 336
  reactive AA 1433, 1434, 1436, 1437–8,
      1442
  in reactive arthritis 259
  renal 322, 651, 1436, 1437, 1438, 1439

amyloidosis (continued)
in rheumatoid arthritis 257, *258*, 322, 651, 1014
senile isolated atrial 1439
senile systemic 1439
in SLE 322
treatment 1441–2
amyotrophic lateral sclerosis 1265
amyotrophy, diabetic *283*
ANA see antinuclear antibodies
anabolic steroids 1598, 1778
anaemia 3, 290–2
acute phase response in 640
aplastic, drug-related 296, 580, 1022
autoimmune haemolytic 291–2
of chronic disease 290–1, 633, 641
acute phase response in 636
aetiology 635–6
and anaesthesia 300
animal model 635
diagnosis 636–8
differential diagnosis *637*
in juvenile chronic arthritis 1119
in rheumatoid arthritis 1016
in SLE 1155
treatment 638
and disability 1725
drug-related 295, 296, *578*, 580, 1022
in Felty's syndrome 291, 644
haemolytic 291
drug-related 295, 296, 580
hyperuricaemia in 1558
in SLE 1155, 1192
hypochromic, in ankylosing spondylitis 1063
hypochromic microcytic 636
iron deficiency 633
diagnosis 637, 638
differential diagnosis *637*
in juvenile chronic arthritis 1119
in NSAID therapy 580
in rheumatoid arthritis 291, 1016
in SLE 292, 641
in Lyme disease 888
macrocytic, drug-related 296, *589*
macrocytic megaloblastic 291
megaloblastic, drug-related 296
microangiopathic haemolytic 329
in mixed connective tissue disease 1419
normochromic 291
in ankylosing spondylitis 1063
in polymyalgia rheumatica/giant cell arteritis 1378
normochromic normocytic 291, 636
in adult-onset Still's disease 1127
in rheumatic fever 980
in Sjögren's syndrome 1312
in SLE 1192
pernicious *285*
in psoriatic arthritis 1076–7
in rheumatoid arthritis 291, 633, *633*
in sarcoidosis 1465
sideroblastic, drug-related 296
in SLE 191
anaerobic organisms, in pyogenic arthritis 852–3, 853
anaerobic threshold 1774
anaesthesia 298–308, 1702
airway maintenance *302*
and antirheumatic drugs 301
balanced 299
and cardiovascular disease 299
childhood 1721
drugs 306, *307*
emergency work-up 301
epidural 105–6, 299, 306
extubation 300–1
in gastrointestinal disease 300–1
in haemopoietic disease 300
induction 304
inhalational 304
intravenous regional 305
intubation 301–5, 1721

anaesthesia (continued)
local 305–6, *306*
in cardiovascular disease 299
preceding local steroid injection 1760
and postoperative care 305
regional 305–6, *306*
in respiratory disease 300
relevance of systemic factors in rheumatic disease 299–301
in renal disease 300
and respiratory disease 299–300
skin and joint damage 301
spinal 299, 306
tourniquet palsy following 803
analgesia
in the elderly 102
in low back pain 100, 104
patient-controlled 305
postoperative 305
analgesic agents
antidepressants as 341
in cervical pain syndromes 1658
in chronic back pain 1648
haematuria induced by 323
in lactation 193
in osteoarthritis 1547
in pregnancy 189
toxicity 1695
anaphylactoid purpura see Henoch–Schönlein purpura
anaphylatoxins 512
ANCA see antineutrophil cytoplasmic autoantibodies
anconeus 137
in tennis elbow 145
androgens
in rheumatoid arthritis 1013
in SLE 510, 1169
aneurysm
abdominal aorta 1383, 1398
carotid artery 1398
cerebral 378
coronary artery 1398
femoral artery 379, 1398
mycotic 1390
in polyarteritis nodosa 1356
popliteal artery 1398
pulmonary artery 251, 1398, 1401
aneurysmal bone cyst 119
Angelman syndrome 349
angiitis
central nervous system *333*, 335, 785, 786, 1392
granulomatous *333*, 335, 785, 786
in HIV infection 914
angina pectoris 229–30
in amyloidosis 1436
in systemic sclerosis 1232–3
unstable 230, 232, 233
angioedema 204
hereditary 351
angiogenesis 509
rheumatoid synovial tissue 448–9, 990
angiography
childhood 764
coronary 233, 764
giant cell arteritis 1389
granulomatous angiitis of the central nervous system 786
polyarteritis nodosa 1356, 1403, 1404
Takayasu's arteritis 1386
therapeutic 764
angiokeratoma corporis diffusum 168, **1635**
angiokeratoma diffusum universale 1635
angiotensin 329
and hyperuricaemia *1558*
angiotensin converting enzyme 452, 1422, 1465–6
angiotensin converting enzyme inhibitors see ACE inhibitors
animal models 559, 560–1, *560*, *561*, 567–8, 570–1, 997–9

animal models (continued)
adjuvant arthritis 561, 562, 563, 567, 611, 998, *1043*
allergic encephalomyelitis 612, 844
anaemia of chronic disease 635
ankylosing spondylitis 1067–8
antigen-induced arthritis 565–6
antiphospholipid syndrome 293, 1210
arthritis flares 566–7, *566*
articular cartilage in 415–17
characteristic features *561*
chondrocytes in 415, 416
collagen disorders 353
collagen-induced arthritis 562, 563–4, 608, 611, 992, 997–8
cytokines in 568–9
dermatomyositis 1272–3
evaluation of ternary complex 844
and immunosuppressive therapy 611
joint disease 415–16, *415*
necrotizing vasculitis 1344
neonatal lupus erythematosus 1198
osteoarthritis 416–17
osteogenesis imperfecta 365
polymyositis 1272–3
pristane arthritis 567
proteoglycan arthritis 564
research approaches *559*
scleroderma 1225
sialoadenitis 1306
Sjögren's syndrome 1306–7
SLE 1162–3, *1162*, 1668
treatment 1175–6
spontaneous arthritis 567
streptococcal cell-wall arthritis 562, 564–5, 998
transgenic mice 567–8, 999
uncoupling of cartilage damage and joint swelling 569–70
anisocytosis in anaemia of chronic disease 636
ankle
applied anatomy 153–4, 156, 157
arthrodesis 1706
examination 50
functional anatomy and disability 1725
imaging 718–19, 744–5
in juvenile chronic arthritis 82, 85
pauciarticular-onset 1099, 1100
rehabilitation 1747–9, 1750
seronegative polyarthritis 1134
surgery 1718–20
systemic-onset 1116
local steroid injection *1762*, 1769–70
osteoarthritis 1532
pain, childhood *164*, 167–8
physiotherapy, childhood 1747–9, 1750
range of movement 50
replacement 1707
surgery 1706–7, 1718–20
ankle–foot orthoses 1732
ankle jerk
absent 218
reflex latency 801
ankylosing hyperostosis see diffuse idiopathic skeletal hyperostosis
ankylosing spondylitis *1040*, **1058–70**
acute phase response in 628, 629
aetiology 1066–8
age at onset 11, 12, 13
age distribution 26, 815, *815*, 1061
anaesthesia in 299
association with HLA-B27 99, 128, 184, 552–3, 698–9, *822*, 1059–60, 1060–1, 1066–7
atlantoaxial subluxation in 224
back pain in 99
in calcium pyrophosphate dihydrate disease 1529
clinical features 1061–3, *1062*
comparison between familial and sporadic 1068
defining disease status 1067

ankylosing spondylitis (continued)
delay in diagnosis 1060
diagnostic criteria *812*, 838, 1038, 1058–9, *1058*
differential diagnosis *1104*
enthesopathy 1061, 1062–3
epidemiology *814*, 838–40, *838*, *839*, *840*, 1044–5, 1059–61
extra-articular manifestations 1063–4
amyloidosis 1064
cardiovascular *230*, 238, 1064
gastrointestinal *259*, 1064–5
neurological 225, 1064
ocular 314, 315, 316, 1059, 1064
pulmonary *241*, 245, 247, 1064
renal 651, 1064
extraspinal joint disease 1062, 1063
genetic counselling 1069
genetic factors 99, 128, 184, *351*, 552–3, 698–9, *822*
geographical factors 820
health status measures 58–9, *58*
history 1058
imaging 733–4, 735, 736, 738, 1065–6, *1065*, *1066*
intestinal permeability in 267
intubation in 303
juvenile 128, *1040*, 1052
clinical characteristics 1052–3
diagnosis 18, 19
epidemiology 831–2, *832*, 1052
genetic markers 698, 699
outcome 1054
sex differences 12, 14
laboratory tests *649*, 1066
large vessel vasculitis in 1391
late spinal complications 1062, 1063
liver function 652
management 1068
and osteoporosis 1061, 1066, 1591
pathological features 733–4, 735, 736, 1061
patient associations 1069–70
physical examination 1065
postural exercise 1068
and pregnancy 184
prevalence 1060–1
primary 1058, *1065*, 1066
prognosis 1067
racial distribution *819*, 1060–1
secondary 1058, *1065*, 1066
sex distribution 815, *815*, 1060, *1060*
spinal involvement 734, 735, 736, 1062, 1063
synovial biopsy in 778
time trends in occurrence 817
treatment 1046, *1068*, 1069
in women 1066
see also seronegative spondylarthropathies
ankylosing tarsitis, juvenile 1051
Ankylostoma duodenale 948, 949
annular ligament 137
annulus fibrosus 1640
Anopheles
A. funestus 902, 903
A. gambiae 902, 903
anorexia
in giant cell arteritis 1377, 1388
in microscopic polyangiitis 1354
in polymyalgia rheumatica 1377
in sarcoidosis 1465
in SLE 257, 1156
anorexia nervosa and osteoporosis 433, 1589
anserine bursa 152, 153, 158
bursitis *5*, 158, 1509
antacids
interaction with NSAIDs *579*
in mixed connective tissue disease 1422
and phosphate depletion 1604
anterior cruciate ligament 151, 152
imaging 743
in rheumatoid arthritis 1014

anterior cruciate ligament *(continued)*
rupture
imaging 744
and osteoarthritis 483–4
stability testing 49
anterior drawer sign 144
anterior interosseous nerve entrapment 226, 806
anterior talofibular ligament 153
anterior tibial nerve
entrapment in rheumatoid arthritis 1013
in leprosy 934
anterior tibial syndrome 1510
anterior tibiotalar ligament 153
anteropathic arthropathies 255, *256*
anthralin in psoriasis 1079
anti-56kDa antibodies *1271*, 1272
anti-70kDa ribonucleoprotein antibodies 1197
antiaorta antibodies 1386
anti-apoAI antibodies 1483
anti-apoCII antibodies 1483
anti-B19 IgG antibody 897, 898
anti-B19 IgM antibody 898
antibiotics
choice of 660
influence on microbial cultures 658
intravenous
ambulatory delivery systems 857–8
in osteomyelitis 875, 877
local delivery, in osteomyelitis 875
prophylactic
in Felty's syndrome 644
in osteomyelitis 876
preoperative 299, 300
in rheumatic fever 980
sensitivity tests 659–60
therapeutic
in discitis of childhood 123–4
in intramedullary spinal cord abscess 124
in Lyme disease 891–3, *891*
in osteomyelitis 873–5, *874*
pyogenic arthritis *856*, 857–8, 865–6
in rheumatic fever 980
in secondary infection in HIV infection 917
septic bursitis 156, 859
in seronegative spondylarthropathies 1046
in Whipple's disease 1095
antibodies
in adaptive immunity 546
deficiency **966–71**
detection 661
in immune complexes 703–4
in protection against mycoplasmas 969
see also specific antibodies
antibody-dependent cytotoxic cells
effect of corticosteroids on *586*
effect of gold therapy on *600*
antibody V genes, in SLE *1170*, 1171–2
anti-*Borrelia burgdorferi* antibody 885, 889
anti-C1q antibodies 1165
anticardiolipin antibodies 293, 673
and anaesthesia 299, 300
in antiphospholipid syndrome 222, 1159–60, 1209
clinical features associated 293
detection 1203–4
disease associations 293–4
in HIV infection 910, 914
in pregnancy 1206
in SLE 641, 642
cardiovascular involvement 233
childhood 1197
neuropsychiatric 219–20, 221, 334
ocular involvement 313
and pregnancy outcome 183
and thrombocytopenia 292
types 1159
see also antiphospholipid syndrome

anti-CD4 antibodies 612, 999, 1024
anti-CD5 antibodies 614
anti-CD7 antibodies 1024
anti-CDw52 antibody *see* Campath-1H
anticentromere antibodies (ACA) 665, *666*, 667, 670, 983
in CREST syndrome 1424
in Raynaud's phenomenon 1229–30
in scleroderma 671–2, 1222, *1225*
antichlamydial antibodies and HIV-associated Reiter's syndrome 920
α1-antichymotrypsin (ACT) 623, **626–7**
function in inflammation *624*
in giant cell arteritis 628, 629
in polymyalgia rheumatica 628, 629
properties *625*
in rheumatoid arthritis 628
anticoagulants
and antiphospholipid antibodies 294, 1211
in Behçet's syndrome 1401
interaction with NSAIDs *579*
and local steroid injection 1758
in SLE 1194
neuropsychiatric 1187
anticollagen antibodies
in collagen-induced arthritis 564
and Dupuytren's contracture 148
in relapsing polychondritis 1626
in rheumatoid arthritis 987
anticonvulsants
effect on vitamin D metabolism 1603–4
and osteoporosis 1589–90
anticytokine antibodies in scleroderma *1241*
antidepressants 339–40, *340, 341*
analgesic effects 341
in rheumatoid arthritis 341–2
treatment strategies 340, *341, 342*
tricyclic 339–40, *340*
in chronic back pain 1648
in fibromyalgia 1499
in low back pain 104–5, *105*
anti-DNA antibodies 613–14, *666*, 667–8
in autoimmune thyroiditis 279
in mixed connective tissue disease 1419, 1420
in SLE 704, 711, 1164–5, *1164*
childhood 1197
in the elderly 35, *35*
experimental models 1163
anti-DNAse B 979
anti-dsDNA antibodies
model of interaction with antigen 1165
in SLE 1164–5, *1164*
anti-EJ antibodies in polymyositis/dermatomyositis *1271*
anti-ENA antibodies 8
antiendothelial cell antibodies (AECA) 1356
in Behçet's syndrome 1399
in Kawasaki disease 1405
in mixed connective tissue disease 1420
in polymyositis/dermatomyositis 1272
in Takayasu's arteritis 1386
antifibrillarin antibodies *see* anti-U3RNP antibodies
antifibrotic drugs in scleroderma 1240, *1241*
anti-GBM antibody 324, 327, *328*
antigen-induced arthritis 565–6
antigen-presenting cells 608–9
effect of cyclosporin on *594*
in rheumatoid arthritis 992
in Sjögren's syndrome 1305
in SLE 1168
antigenic mimicry 987
antigens 608
cationic 565–6
detection tests 660

antigens *(continued)*
in immune complexes 703, 704
persistent 560
presentation in rheumatoid arthritis 987–8
processing and presentation to T cells 549–50
blocking 613
recognition 549, 608–9
anti-gp70 antibodies 1162–3
antigranulocyte antibodies in Felty's syndrome 644
anti-HCV antibodies in proteinuria 322
anti-heat shock protein antibodies
in ankylosing spondylitis 1066
in polymyositis/dermatomyositis 1272
antihistamines in urticarial vasculitis 1370
antihistidyl-tRNA synthetase antibodies *see* anti-Jo-1 antibodies
antihistone antibodies 668–9, 1135, *1164*, 1165, 1691
anti-HLA-B27 antibodies 1042
antihyaluronidase 979
anti-ICAM-1 antibodies 613
anti-idiotypic antibodies 610
anti-IL-1 antibody 615
anti-immunoglobulin antibodies, immune complex interaction with 706–7
anti-insulin antibodies in penicillamine therapy *598*, 599
anti-Jo-1 antibodies 8, 983
in autoimmune disease *671*
in connective tissue disease *666*
in myositis 1249, 1423–4
in overlap syndromes 1414
in polymyositis/dermatomyositis 673, 1258, 1259, 1270, *1271*
in childhood 1290, 1295
antikeratin antibodies 675
antikeratin antibodies in rheumatoid arthritis 987
anti-KJ antibodies in polymyositis/dermatomyositis 1259, 1270, *1271*
anti-Ku antibodies 1271, *1271*, 1414, 1425
anti-La antibodies *666*, 669, *669*, 670, 983
in DILS 913
and neonatal lupus erythematosus 1157, 1198–9
in scleroderma, in pregnancy 184
in Sjögren's syndrome 671, *671*, 1303, 1413, 1414
in pregnancy 185
in SLE 669, 670, *671*, *1164*, 1165, 1414
in the elderly 35, *35*, 1159
antilipoprotein antibodies 1483
antilymphocytotoxic antibodies in SLE 1155
antimalarials
adverse effects
cutaneous 214
gastrointestinal *260*, 261
haematological 295–6
ocular 318–19, 1695
psychiatric *337*, 338
in dermatomyositis 211
in discoid lupus erythematosus 211
drug interactions 1021
in mixed connective tissue disease 1422
in psoriatic arthritis 1080
in rheumatoid arthritis 1020–1
in SLE 1172, *1173*
anti-Mas in polymyositis/dermatomyositis 1270
anti-MHC antibodies 613
anti-Mi-2 antibodies 1259, 1270–1, *1271*, 1295

antimicrobial sensitivity testing 659–60
antimicrosomal antibodies in Sjögren's syndrome 279
antimitochondrial antibodies 670
in scleroderma *1225*, 1424
in Sjögren's syndrome 1310
antimucopeptide antibody in rheumatic fever 974
antimyeloperoxidase antibodies 1329
antimyosin antibodies
in polymyositis/dermatomyositis 1272
in rheumatic fever 973, 975
anti-NADase 979
antinative-DNA antibody, in SLE 322
anti-nDNA antibodies 667–8
antineuronal antibodies in neuropsychiatric SLE 219, 334, 1155, 1185
antineutrophil cytoplasmic autoantibodies (ANCA) 8, *330*, 666, 673–4, 983, 1340
atypical/a-ANCA/xANCA 328, *328*, 674, 1329, 1340
c-ANCA/PR3-ANCA 328, *328*, 1328, 1340
disease associations 1328–9, 1340
in HIV infection 1320
in Wegener's granulomatosis 323, 324, 328, 673, 1328
childhood 1406–7
disease activity 1341
in generalized disease 1332
immunopathology 1342–4
and pulmonary–renal syndrome 1338
test sensitivity 1340
in Churg–Strauss syndrome 1355–6
and disease activity in vasculitis 1361
in giant cell arteritis 1376
in haematuria 324
in HIV infection 910, 914
in Kawasaki disease 1405
in microscopic polyangiitis 1329, 1353, 1354, 1355–6
p-ANCA/MPO-ANCA 328, *328*, 673, 674, 1328, 1340
disease associations 1329
in Sweet's syndrome 1458
in Wegener's granulomatosis 328, 674, 1329, 1338
in polyarteritis nodosa 1353, 1355–6, 1403
in rapidly progressive glomerulonephritis 328, *328*
in scleritis 217
in vasculitis 1320, 1328–9
anti-nRNP antibodies 35, *35*, 983
antinuclear antibodies (ANA) 665–7, 983
in autoimmune thyroid disease 279
childhood 17–18
in DILS 913
disease associations *666*
in drug-induced lupus 1691
in Felty's syndrome 644, 1015
granulocyte-specific 1015
in HIV infection 910
immunofluorescence 667
in juvenile chronic arthritis 830, *831*, 1101, 1102, 1109, 1120, 1135
in juvenile dermatomyositis 1295
in juvenile psoriatic arthritis 1055
in mixed connective tissue disease 1416
in pericardial fluid 235
in polymyositis/dermatomyositis 1258
in proteinuria 322
in psoriatic arthritis 1077
in relapsing polychondritis 1626
in rheumatoid arthritis 824, 987
in RS₃PE syndrome 35
in scleroderma 36, 1222–3
in SLE 1152, 1197
specificity 8, 665, *668*
test for, relevance 8

antinucleolar antibodies 665, 667, 670
    in Raynaud's phenomenon 1229–30
    in scleroderma 672
anti-OJ antibodies in polymyositis/
    dermatomyositis *1271*
antioxidants 1480
anti-P antibodies in neuropsychiatric
    SLE 334
anti-p24 antibodies in Sjögren's
    syndrome 1302
anti-PCNA antibodies in SLE 671
antipeptidoglycan antibodies in juve-
    nile chronic arthritis 1109
antiperinuclear factor 674–5, 987
antiphospholipid antibodies 293, *666*,
    673, 1413
    in asymptomatic patients 1210
    clinical features associated 293
    detection 642, 1203–4
    disease associations 293–4
    in pregnancy 183–4, 189, 294, 295,
        1206
    prevalence 1207–8
    and pulmonary involvement 251
    in scleroderma, in pregnancy 184
    in SLE 183–4, 189, 642, 1151, 1152, 1155,
        1207
        childhood 1197
        interaction with lipids 1483–4
    and thrombocytopenia 292
    treament 294–5
antiphospholipid syndrome 222, 251,
    642, *642*, *672*, **1202–13**
    animal model 293, 1210
    catastrophic 294, 1206, 1211
    childhood 1213
    clinical features 1204–7, *1204*, *1205*
    diagnosis 1208, *1208*
    differential diagnosis 1208–9
    epidemiology 1207–8
    fetal loss in 293, 294, 295, 1206,
        1212–13
    history *1203*
    lipoproteins in 1484
    osteonecrosis in 1207, 1622
    pathogenesis 1209–10, *1209*
    primary 294, 1208
    prognosis 1213
    secondary 294, 1208
    and SLE 294, 642, 1159–60, *1159*
    thrombocytopenia in 1207
    thrombosis in 222, 1204–6, 1210–12
    transverse myelitis in 222, 225
    treatment 1210–13, *1211*
anti-PL-7 antibodies in polymyositis/
    dermatomyositis 1259, *1271*
anti-PL-12 antibodies in polymyositis/
    dermatomyositis *1271*
antiplatelet antibodies 292
anti-PM-1 antibodies in juvenile
    dermatomyositis 1295
anti-Pm-Scl antibodies *666*, 670, 1414
    in overlap syndromes 1425
    in polymyositis/dermatomyositis 1259,
        1271, *1271*
    in scleroderma *1225*
antiproteinase 3 antibodies 1320, 1329,
    1343–4
antiproteoglycan antibodies 564, 1066
anti-RA33 antibodies 675, 987, 1015
antirheumatoid factor antibodies
    279
antiribosomal P antibodies 220, 671,
    1155, 1165, 1185–6, 1197
anti-RNAP antibodies *666*, 670, 673
    in scleroderma 1222, *1225*
anti-Ro antibodies *666*, 669, *669*
    in DILS 913
    and neonatal lupus erythematosus 1157,
        1198–9
    and penicillamine therapy 599
    in polymyositis/dermatomyositis *1271*,
        1272
    in scleroderma, in pregnancy 184

anti-Ro antibodies *(continued)*
    in Sjögren's syndrome 671, *671*, 1303,
        1413, 1414
        in the elderly 36
    in pregnancy 185
    in SLE 669, 670, *671*, *1164*, 1165, 1171,
        1414
        in the elderly 35, *35*, 1159
        subacute cutaneous 1148
anti-rRNP antibodies in SLE *1164*
antirubella antibodies 899
anti-Scl-70 *see* antitopoisomerase 1 anti-
    bodies
antisense oligonucleotides 615
anti-Sm antibodies 614, *666*, 669, 670
    in mixed connective tissue disease 1419,
        1420
    in SLE 669, 670, *671*, 1155, *1164*
        childhood 1197
        in the elderly 35, *35*
        and race 1165
anti-SRP antibodies
    in polymyositis/dermatomyositis 1249,
        1258, 1259, 1270, *1271*
    in childhood 1295
anti-ssDNA antibodies 667–8, *1164*
antistreptococcal antibodies
    in rapidly progressive glomerulo-
        nephritis *328*
    in rheumatic fever 973, 979–80
antistreptokinase 979
antistreptolysin O 979–80
antisynthetase antibodies 1413, 1414,
    1423–4
    in polymyositis/dermatomyositis 1252,
        1258, 1259, 1270, *1271*
        in childhood 1290
    see also anti-Jo-1 antibodies
antisynthetase syndrome 1270, *1272*,
    1413, 1423–4
anti-T-cell antibodies
    in juvenile chronic arthritis 1120
    in microscopic polyangiitis 1359
    in polyarteritis nodosa 1359
    in SLE 1165
anti-ThRNP antibodies 670
antithrombin III 324
    deficiency 1208
    function in inflammation *624*
    in pregnancy in SLE 183
antithymocyte globulin in sclero-
    derma 1240, *1241*
antithyroglobulin antibodies
    in autoimmune thyroid disease 279
    in Sjögren's syndrome 279
    in SLE 1157
antithyroid antibodies
    in Sjögren's syndrome 1311
    in SLE 1197
anti-TNF-α antibody 615
    in rheumatoid arthritis 994–5, 996
antitopoisomerase 1 antibodies 665,
    666, 670, 983
    in Raynaud's phenomenon 1229–30
    in scleroderma 36, 671–2, *671*, 1222,
        1225
antitoxoplasma antibodies 946, 947
antitropomyosin antibodies in rheu-
    matic fever 975
α1-antitrypsin (AAT) 623, **627**
    deficiency, and panniculitis 1452
    function in inflammation *624*
    inactivation by free radicals 447, 514
    properties *625*
    in rheumatoid arthritis 629, *1016*
    in vasculitis 625
antituberculous drugs 931–2, *932*, 933
anti-U1RNP antibodies *666*, 669, 670
    in mixed connective tissue disease 671,
        1413, 1414, 1419, 1420
    outcome in patients with 1421, *1422*
    in polymyositis/dermatomyositis *1271*,
        1272
    in SLE 669–70, *671*, *1164*, 1165

anti-U2RNP antibodies in polymyo-
    sitis/dermatomyositis *1271*, 1272
anti-U3RNP antibodies *666*, 670,
    672–3
    in polymyositis/dermatomyositis 1272
    in scleroderma *1225*
anti-U5RNP antibodies in polymyo-
    sitis/dermatomyositis *1271*, 1272
anti-yersinia antibodies 1042
anti-ZDNA antibodies *1164*
anxiety
    in the elderly 30
    and fibromyalgia 1496
    management 342
    in SLE *336*, 337, 1153
    steroid-induced *587*
aorta 1382
    acute dissection 231
    aneurysm 1383, 1398
    atherosclerosis 94
    biopsy 785
    in giant cell arteritis 1388
    mycotic aneurysm 1390
    rupture 378
    vasculitis 233
aortic arch syndrome in giant cell
    arteritis 1388
aortic valve
    disease 237–8, *239*
        due to rheumatic fever 978
        in psoriatic arthritis 1076
    incompetence
        in ankylosing spondylitis 1064
        in relapsing polychondritis 1626
        in SLE 1151
        in Takayasu's arteritis 1385
    insufficiency 237–8, *239*
        in juvenile ankylosing spondylitis
            1053
        in reactive arthropathies 1087
    myxomatous degeneration of leaflets
        238
    regurgitation, in juvenile chronic
        arthritis 1033–4
    replacement 238
    vegetations 220, 1151
aortitis 1383
    infection-related 1389
    in rheumatoid arthritis 1391
aortography
    in large vessel vasculitis 1383
    in Takayasu's arteritis 786
apatite crystals 1526, 1531–2, 1572
APECED 285–6
Apert syndrome 368, 369, 398
aphthous stomatitis in enteric arthro-
    pathies 1094
aphthous ulcers *see* ulcers, oral
apoferritin 634, 635
apolipoproteins 1478–9
    apoA 1479
        in amyloidosis *1434*, 1438
    apoB 1479
        control of secretion rate 349
    apoE, in amyloidosis 1439
    apoH 293, 1159, 1209–10
apophyseal joints *see* facet joints
apophysis, overuse injuries 1787
apoprotein CII deficiency *1481*
    see also hyperlipidaemias
apoptosis 352, 609, 844, 1162
    and Fas protein 1163, 1168
    neutrophils 513
    in SLE 1168
APRT 1557
Arabs
    juvenile chronic arthritis 829
    seronegative spondylarthropathies *839*
    see also ethnic groups
arachidonic acid 515, 1480
arachnodactyly
    congenital contractural 354, 389, 393
    in homocystinuria 436
    in Marfan syndrome 389

arachnoiditis 1645–6
    and cauda equina syndrome 225
    electrodiagnosis 805
    in helminthic infection 951
arch supports 160
Arizona hinshawii in pyogenic
    arthritis 852
arm *see* upper limb
ARMS 691, 692
arrhythmias 231
    in dilated cardiomyopathy 236
    in pericarditis 234
    in polymyositis/dermatomyositis 1255
    in systemic sclerosis 1233, *1234*
Arteparon in calcium pyrophosphate
    dihydrate disease 1570
arterial biopsy in polymyalgia rheu-
    matica/giant cell arteritis 1376–7
arteriosclerosis, temporal artery
    biopsy in *783*, 785
arteriovenous anastomoses in joints
    442
arteriovenous shunting, synovium
    444
arteritis
    infection-related 1389–91
    see also giant cell arteritis; Takayasu's
        arteritis; vasculitis
arthralgia
    in Behçet's syndrome 1396–7
    in drug-induced lupus 1690, *1691*
    drug-related *587*
    in eosinophilia–myalgia syndrome 1425
    in hypermobility 1500
    in hypothyroidism 277
    in juvenile chronic arthritis 1116
    in Lyme disease 887
    in microscopic polyangiitis 1354
    in polyarteritis nodosa 1353
    in polymyalgia rheumatica/giant cell
        arteritis 1377
    in polymyositis/dermatomyositis 1256
    in sarcoidosis 1466
    in Sjögren's syndrome 1309
    in SLE 1147, 1181
    in Takayasu's arteritis 1385
    in Wegener's granulomatosis 1338
Arthritis and Rheumatism Council
    109
arthritis–dermatitis syndrome, asso-
    ciated with bowel bypass 1095–6
Arthritis Foundation 31
Arthritis Impact Measurement Scales
    (AIMS) 54–5, *55*, 58, 59, 60, 61
    application to children *56*, 57
arthritis mutilans 1073, 1074, 1475
arthritis self-management.
    programme 70
Arthritis today 31
arthritogenic peptides 553
arthrocentesis 1758
    equipment 678, 1760
    hip joint 678
    preparation 678–9, 1760–1, *1761*
    risk of pyogenic arthritis 849
    sites of 678
    technique 678–9, 1761, *1761*
    therapeutic effects 678
    traumatic 682
arthrodesis
    ankle 1706
    hip 1709
    knee 1708
    shoulder 1703, 1720
    wrist 1721, 1725
arthrography 719
    ankle 744, 745
    childhood 764
    comparison with arthroscopy *719*
    elbow 740–1
    facet joint 1644
    hip 741–2, 743, 764
    knee 719, 742
    rheumatoid arthritis 725–6

arthrography (continued)
shoulder 717, 719, 738, 739, 740
frozen 143–4
rotator cuff tear 142, 717
wrist 741
arthrogryposis 1636, *1637*
arthroplasty
elbow 1703, 1704, 1720
forefoot excision 1706
hip excision 1709
hip replacement 1708–9
childhood 1716–17
in Paget's disease 1617
prosthetic loosening or infection 741
in spondyloepiphyseal dysplasia
1630, *1632*
infection following 849, 853–4, 857, 858,
1709
knee excision 1708
knee replacement 1707–8
childhood 1719
in Paget's disease 1617
in osteoarthritis 1548
in osteonecrosis 1624
pyogenic arthritis following 849
in rheumatoid arthritis 1026
shoulder replacement 1703
in tuberculosis 932
arthroscopy
comparison with arthrography *719*
in osteoarthritis 1548
in pyogenic arthritis 858
risk of pyogenic arthritis 849
shoulder 140
frozen 143–4
rotator cuff tear 142
arthrotomy
in pyogenic arthritis 858
in rheumatoid arthritis 1026
Ascaris lumbricoides 948, 949, 951
ascites in SLE 257, *258*
ascorbic acid *see* vitamin C
aseptic necrosis *see* osteonecrosis
asialoglycoprotein receptors 528
ASMP 70
**aspartate aminotransferase (AST/
GOT)** 651, 652
in differential diagnosis of neuromuscular disorders 1291
imprecision in measurement *648*
in juvenile chronic arthritis 1116
in polymyositis/dermatomyositis
1257–8
ASPCR 691, 692
aspergillosis
in ankylosing spondylitis 1064
arteritis in 1390
arthritis due to 880, 963
invasive 252
management 957
pulmonary infection 245, 252
aspirin
adverse effects 1138
cutaneous 213
gastrointestinal 259, 260
haematological 295
hepatic 652, 1106
myopathy 653, *1265*
renal 323
Reye's syndrome 1106–7
in antiphospholipid syndrome 1211,
1213
in Behçet's syndrome 1401
in cardiovascular disease 233
drug interactions *579*
effect on CNS neurones 497
enteric-coated 1079–80
half-life *577*
in juvenile chronic arthritis 1106, *1106,*
1124, 1138, *1140*
in Kawasaki disease 1406
in lactation 193
in leprosy 935, 936
low-dose in pregnancy 183, 189, 295

aspirin (continued)
metabolism 577
in panniculitis 1455
in pregnancy 183, 189, 189–90, 295
protective effects in colorectal cancer
1666
in psoriatic arthritis 1079–80
in rheumatic fever 980
in rheumatoid arthritis 1020
in scleroderma 1240
in thrombocytopenia 1213
assessment
adult patients **3–9**
childhood 17
association studies, genetic markers
689
AST *see* aspartate aminotransferase
astemizole, contraindications 957
asteroid bodies 960
asthma 173, 451
adverse reactions to NSAIDs 580
in Churg–Strauss syndrome 1325, 1354,
1355
cough in 240
dyspnoea in 242
and exercise 1775–6
and steroid-induced osteoporosis
1588
treatment 241
ataxia, in vertebrobasilar insufficiency
223
ataxia telangiectasia 1136
atheroembolism 1320
atherogenic lipid profile 1483
atheroma, drug-related *587*
atherosclerosis
aortic 94
coronary arteries 231–3
differential diagnosis 1389
in gout 651
mortality from in rheumatic disorders
1482–3
in SLE 1194
in systemic sclerosis 1233
athletes
amenorrhoea 1589
back pain 127
bone mass 1593
atlantaoccipital impaction 1705
atlantoaxial joint 90–1
atlantoaxial subluxation 218, 223–4,
1705
and disability 1725
following systemic corticosteroid
therapy 1757
and intubation 301, 1721
in juvenile chronic arthritis 224, 1033,
1035, 1135, 1721, 1738
in mixed connective tissue disease 1417
in psoriatic arthritis 1076
in rheumatoid arthritis 1013, 1014
surgery 1705
vertebrobasilar insufficiency in 223
see also spine, cervical
ATP *see* adenosine triphosphate
atrial natriuretic factor in amyloidosis
1434, 1435
atrioventricular block 237
atrioventricular node 237
atrophie blanche 1371
atrophy, definition *201*
atrophy, attributable risk 824
auranofin *see* gold therapy
aureothiomalate *see* gold therapy
Austin–Flint murmur 238
Australian antigen *see* hepatitis B surface
antigen
autistic behaviour in SLE 333
autoantibodies 665–75, 983
connective tissue diseases 1413–14,
1415
dermatomyositis 673, 1258, 1259,
1270–2, *1271, 1272*
diabetes mellitus 285, *668*

autoantibodies (continued)
drug-induced lupus erythematosus
668, 669, 1691
Felty's syndrome 644
in HIV infection 910
and immunosuppressive therapy 610
induction by drugs 1692–3, *1692*
and malignancy 289
mixed connective tissue disease 671,
1413, 1414, 1416, 1419, 1420
ocular disorders 907
overlap syndromes 1271–2, *1271,* 1413–
14, *1415*
pathogenicity 610
polymyositis 668, 673, 1258, 1259,
1270–2, *1271, 1272*
rheumatoid arthritis 668, 824, 986–7
vasculitis 674, 787
see also specific antibodies and diseases
autoantigens 608
in rheumatoid arthritis 987–8
autogenes 1163
autoimmune cholangiitis 1310
autoimmune disease 545
acute phase response in 628
classification 907
drug-induced 1690–4, *1690*
induction 987–8
polymyositis/dermatomyositis as
1268–72, *1269, 1271, 1272*
and retroviruses 907
rheumatoid arthritis as 986–8
systemic sclerosis as 1220–3, 1225, *1225*
see also connective tissue diseases
autoimmune haplotype 504
**autoimmunity, relationship with
infection and immune
responses** 843–4, *843*
autonomic dysfunction 231
autonomic neuropathy 227
in rheumatoid arthritis 1013
auxological anthropometry 73
avascular necrosis *see* osteonecrosis
axillosubclavian vein thrombosis
1661
axioappendicular muscles 135
axon reflex 450
axonal spheroids 794
axonotmesis *803*
axons
atrophy 794
degeneration 794
electrophysiology 802–3, *802,* 806
regeneration 793–4
azapropazone
adverse effects *1021*
clearance 577
drug interactions *579*
half-life *577*
in pregnancy 189
azathioprine
adverse effects 590, *591,* 647, 1695
carcinogenic 1666
cutaneous 214, *591*
gastrointestinal 260, 261, 590, *591*
haematological 297, 590, *591*
hepatotoxicity 590, *591,* 652
hypersensitivity to 590, *591*
immunological 252
neurological *217*
oncogenic 290, 590, *591*
psychiatric *337,* 338
respiratory *253*
in ankylosing spondylitis 1069
in Behçet's syndrome 1400, 1401
in combination therapy *1025*
in discoid lupus erythematosus 211
drug interaction 1211
in giant cell arteritis 1380
in hypersensitivity vasculitis 1369
in inclusion-body myositis 1280
in juvenile chronic arthritis 1108, 1126,
1141
in lactation 194, *602*

azathioprine (continued)
in microscopic polyangiitis 1359
in mixed connective tissue disease 1422
in multicentric reticulohistiocytosis *1476*
in panniculitis 1455
pharmacology 589
in polyarteritis nodosa 1359, 1404
in polymyalgia rheumatica 1380
in polymyositis/dermatomyositis 1276
in pregnancy 192, *602*
in psoriatic arthritis 1080
in pyoderma gangrenosum 1461
in relapsing polychondritis 1627
in rheumatoid arthritis 1023
in scleroderma 1240, *1241*
in SLE *1173,* 1174, 1186, 1190
and surgery 301
in Takayasu's arteritis 1387
therapeutic efficacy 590
therapeutically relevant effects 589–90,
590
treatment regimens 590
in uveitis 317
in Wegener's granulomatosis 1346
azithromycin 891, 892, 969
azotaemia
in acute renal failure 330
in HIV infection 915
prerenal 325
aztreonam 875
azurophilic granules 644

B

B cells
in adaptive immunity 545–6
alloantigens in rheumatic fever 975
antigen recognition 549
autoantibody production 610
autoreactivity 610
blockade 613–14
CD5+ in rheumatoid arthritis 992
circulation and migration 527
effect of alkylating agents on 592, *592*
effect of azathioprine on 590, *590*
effect of corticosteroids on *586*
effect of cyclosporin on *594*
effect of gold therapy on 599, *600*
effect of methotrexate on 583, *583*
effect of penicillamine on 597, *597*
effect of sulphasalazine on 588
in HIV infection 908
immune complex production 609–10
immunoglobulin receptors 1172
immunosuppressive therapy strategies
involving 609–10, 613–14
in inflammatory myopathies 789
in juvenile chronic arthritis 1120
in juvenile dermatomyositis 1293
in mixed connective tissue disease 1420
in polymyalgia rheumatica/giant cell
arteritis 1377
in polymyositis/dermatomyositis 1268,
1269
in rheumatic fever *976*
in rheumatoid arthritis 986, 992
in Sjögren's syndrome 1303–5
in SLE 1165, *1166*
suppression 614
in Takayasu's arteritis 1387
Babesia infection 888
bacille Calmette–Guérin 930, 935
Bacillus in osteomyelitis 870
back extension 103
back pain 89
in acromegaly 281
acute 90
management 1646–7
acute on chronic 90
in adolescence 20, *20,* 97–8
adult **89–110**
age at onset *20*
in ankylosing spondylitis 1061, *1062*
in athletes 127

back pain (continued)
  childhood 20, 20, 97–8, 114, 132, 133
    aetiology 115
    following spinal trauma 130, 131
    history and examination 114–17, 116
    infection-associated 121–4
    non-specific causes 118
    in osteoporosis 129
    prevention 117–18
    prolapsed intervertebral disc 124–5
    referred 133
    in Scheuermann's osteochondritis 125, 126
    in spinal dysraphism 127
    in spondylolysis and spondylolisthesis 126–7, 128
    tumour-associated 118–21, 121, 122
  chronic 90
    management 1648–9
  differentiation between mechanical and inflammatory 1062
  economic consequences 89, 90, 92, 93
  in the elderly 25, 101–2, 102
  electrodiagnosis in 805–6
  epidemiology 89, 1639
  health status measures 59
  imaging 90, 97, 99, 730–3, 734, 735
  intractable 90, 92
  investigation 90
  and litigation 107
  low
    acute 99–102, 102
    in adolescence 97–8
    aetiology 95, 729–30, 731, 732
    in ankylosing spondylitis 99
    biopsychosocial model of disability 95
    in bone disease 99
    chronic 103–5
    classification 94, 95
    definition 89
    differential diagnosis 96–9, 97, 98
    education and self-care 107, 108–9
    epidemiology 92–4
    and epidural analgesia 93
    extraspinal causes 97
    health associations 94
    hospitalization 108
    in infections 98–9
    intensive rehabilitation 108, 108
    intractable 105–7, 105
    investigation 97, 98
    living with 109
    in lumbar disc disease 98
    management 99–102, 102, 103–7, 105
    nature of 94–5, 95, 96
    non-specific 91–2, 92, 96, 97
    and occupation 93–4
    and pregnancy 93
    prevalence 93
    prevention 102–3, 103
    problems with evaluation of therapies 92
    rates for surgery 93
    in reactive arthropathies 1087
    recurrence 94
    return to work 94, 109–10
    risk factors 94
    risk minimization 95, 96
    and sex 93
    social factors 94
    in spinal stenosis 98
    and tumours 97, 97, 99
  mechanical 5
  non-specific 1646
  and osteoporosis 92, 99, 1591
  perception 1640–1
  postsurgical 1645
  potential predisposing factors 92
  in pregnancy 185
  in psoriatic arthritis 1073
  psychological factors 106–7
  recurrent 1647
  referral 99

back pain (continued)
  services 110
  and spinal anatomy 90–2
  spondylitic 5
  subacute 90
  terminology 89–90, 90
  therapeutic options 90, 91
  thoracic 96–7
  and trauma 107
Back Pain Society 109
back school 90, 102, 107, 109, 1647
  mini 101
backache
  childhood 114
  simple 89, 1647
  see also back pain
baclofen in chronic back pain 1648
bacteraemia in pyogenic arthritis 849
bacterial cell-wall fragments in animal models of arthritis 562, 564–5, 566–7
bactericidal/permeability-increasing protein 513
Bacteroides
  B. fragilis
    in osteomyelitis 870
    in pyogenic arthritis 853
  childhood pyogenic arthritis 863
Baker's cyst 158, 227, 1509
  arthrography 725–6
  childhood 166, 1181
  in coccidioidomycosis 961
  local steroid injection 158, 1769
  MRI 726, 727
  in rheumatoid arthritis 1009
  rupture 153, 158, 207, 508, 1009, 1769
    arthrography 726
  in SLE 1181
balanced pagoda deformity 284
balanitis circinata in reactive arthropathies 1087
ballismus in SLE 1153
band keratopathy in juvenile chronic arthritis 1103
Bannwarth's syndrome 888
barbiturates, adverse effects 1265, 1681
barium studies in systemic sclerosis 1232
Barlow's manoeuvre 165
Barmah forest virus 903
Barthel score 1724
BASFI 58, 59, 1069
basic calcium phosphate-associated syndromes 682, 1531–2, 1549, 1570, 1572–4
basic fibroblast growth factor
  in angiogenesis 509
  in Dupuytren's contracture 148
  effect on chondrocytes 1543
basophils
  effect of corticosteroids on 586
  in inflammation 512–13
  in scleroderma 1223
BASRI 1065, 1069
Bath Ankylosing Spondylitis Disease Activity Index 1069
Bath Ankylosing Spondylitis Functional Index 58, 59, 1069
Bath Ankylosing Spondylitis Global Status 1069
Bath Ankylosing Spondylitis Metrology Index 1069
Bath Ankylosing Spondylitis Radiology Index 1065, 1069
Batten's disease 791
Bazin's disease 1371
BCG 930, 935
bcl-2 gene
  and apoptosis 352
  as autogene 1163
  in SLE 844, 1168
Beck Depression Score 1724
Becker muscular dystrophy 1291
beclomethasone dipropionate 210

bed rest 1727
  in back pain 100, 1649
  in mechanical cervical disease 1658
behaviour therapy in low back pain 106
Behçet's syndrome 1394–401
  acute phase response in 628
  cardiovascular involvement 230, 238, 1397–8
  childhood 1409
  clinical features 170, 1394, 1395–8
  diagnosis 1398–9
  differential diagnosis 1091, 1136, 1137, 1398–9
  epidemiology 1394–5
  and family size 823
  gastrointestinal involvement 257, 259, 1398
  genetic factors 1395
  and HIV infection 918
  imaging 765
  incomplete 1398
  laboratory tests 1399
  large vessel vasculitis in 1391–2
  mucocutaneous involvement 205–6, 207, 1395–6, 1399
  musculoskeletal involvement 1396–7, 1396
  neurological involvement 223, 223, 1397
  ocular involvement 315, 316, 317, 318, 1396
  pathogenesis 1399
  prognosis 1401
  psychiatric involvement 333, 336
  pulmonary involvement 241, 243, 251, 1398
  and pyoderma gangrenosum 207
  renal involvement 259, 1398
  synovial biopsy in 778
  treatment 1399–401, 1400
Beighton scale for hypermobility 1500
Bell's palsy 890
belts, lumbar 1649
Bence–Jones proteins
  in myeloma 653
  in proteinuria 322, 650
bending test 131
benign hypermobile syndrome 353, 378, 385, 436
benign lymphoepithelial lesions 778–9
benoxaprofen, adverse effects 212, 213
benzbromarone 1565
benzene and scleroderma 1223
benzodiazepines
  in anxiety disorders 342
  in low back pain 101
'Berkson's bias' 1668
β-blockers
  in cardiovascular disease 233
  interaction with NSAIDs 579
  in Takayasu's arteritis 1387
β-carotene 210
β-lactam drugs in osteomyelitis 874–5
betamethasone 585
  in lactation 193
  in pregnancy 191
betamethasone dipropionate 210
betamethasone valerate (Betnovate) 210
bezafibrate in hyperlipidaemias 1481
BGP see osteocalcin
bibasilar rales in mixed connective tissue disease 1418
biceps 137
bicipital tendon 135, 136
  rupture 143, 1759
  subluxation 143
  tendinitis 37, 143, 146, 163, 1503
bicycle test 233
Bier's block 305, 1687
bifurcate ligament 153
biglycan 410, 415

BILAG index 1160
bilirubin
  effect on plasma creatinine 649
  imprecision in measurement 648
  and liver function 651
  in sarcoidosis 1465
  synovial fluid 677
  in synovial inflammation 449
biliverdin 449
biochemical tests 647–54, 648
  calcium and bone 652–3
  clinical problems with 647
  crystal deposition 654
  guide to use in overall management 649
  immune complex diseases 654
  imprecision 648
  inflammation 653–4
  malignancy 653
  muscle disease 653
  purposes 647
  renal function 648–51
  see also laboratory tests; liver, function tests
biotin 690
Bipolaris hawaiiensis 963
Birmingham vasculitis activity score 1360, 1386
Bisolvon 1011
bisphosphonates
  in long-term prednisone therapy 36
  in myositis ossificans 1783
  in osteoporosis 29, 1598
  in Paget's disease 1615–16
bites, osteomyelitis following 870
black Africans
  juvenile chronic arthritis 830, 830, 831
  rheumatoid arthritis 833, 834
  seronegative spondylarthropathies 838–9, 839, 840
  SLE 836
  see also ethnic groups
bladder disorders, drug-related 593, 594
blastema 441
Blastocystis hominis 947
blastomycosis
  arteritis in 1390
  epidemiology 954–5
  joint infection 955, 958–9
    clinical presentation 955, 956
    diagnosis 957
    management 956, 957
Blau syndrome 316
bleomycin, adverse effects 1223, 1693
blepharitis 310
blindness see visual loss
blisters 200, 205–6
blood
  clotting abnormalities
    as contraindication to local steroid injection 1758
    drug-related 295
    in SLE 641, 642
  coagulation
    and inflammation 511, 512, 512
    preoperative screening 300
  cultures 659
  flow regulation 512
  transfusion
    athletes 1775
    in juvenile chronic arthritis 1125
    preoperative 300
blood-gas analysis, preanaesthetic 300
blood urea nitrogen, in acute renal failure 325, 330
blotting 690
Blount's disease 166
BMPs see bone morphogenetic proteins
body landmarks and surface markers 73
body mass index 169
  and risk of osteoarthritis 1518

bone
- in acromegaly 281–2
- adaptation to exercise 1777
- adverse drug effects 128, 130, *587*
- age-related loss of 1593–4
- basic multicellular units 421, 422, 423
- biopsy 780
  - calcification rate *781*
  - histopathological assessment 780–3, *781*
  - in hyperparathyroidism 783
  - marrow star volume 782, *783*
  - mean trabecular plate density *781*, 782, 783
  - mean trabecular plate thickness *781*, 782
  - measurements *781*
  - node-strut analysis 782, 783
  - osteoclast number *781*
  - osteoclastic resorption surface *781*, 783
  - in osteomalacia 780, 783, 1602
  - in osteonecrosis 1623
  - in osteoporosis 780, 782–3, 1594–5
  - percentage tetracycline labelling *781*, 783
  - in renal osteodystrophy 783
  - technical aspects 780
  - trabecular bone volume *781*, 782, 783
  - trabecular osteoid surface *781*
  - trabecular resorption surface *781*
- calcification front 780
- cells 421–3
  - communication between 425
  - cortical 421
    - cutting cones 421, 422
- cyst 1467
- density 425–6, 1592
  - diffuse decreased *757*
  - measurement 720, 721, 1594, *1595*
- development 394
- in disease **432–7**
  - disorders of cell biology 436–7
  - effect of malignant disease on 437
  - enzyme disorders 436
- formation 411–13, 424, *424*
- fracture *see* fractures
- grafting, in osteonecrosis 1624
- growth 422, 1591–3
- in health **421–32**
- intracapsular metaphysis 861
- in juvenile dermatomyositis 1290
- local regulation of shape 395
- malignant disease 120, 288–9, 742, 1670–2, *1671*
- matrix 426–9
  - disorders 435–6
- mineralization 429
- necrosis *see* osteonecrosis
- non-collagen proteins 426, 427, *429*
- in osteoarthritis 1541
- in Paget's disease 1612
- pain 653, *1105*
  - and fluoride 1694–5
  - osteomalacia 1600
  - Paget's disease 1611
- peak mass 433, 1592–3, 1594
- periosteal reaction 757, 758, 760
- reduced mass 433
- remodelling 422, 424, 1591–2
  - in osteoarthritis 1521
- resorption 424, *425*
  - in hyperparathyroidism 280
  - in malignant disease 437
  - in rheumatoid arthritis 1011
  - in sarcoidosis 1467–8
- structure 421, 422
- in systemic sclerosis 1238
- trabecular/cancellous 421
- tumours 288
- turnover
  - biochemical measures 431–2
  - markers 652–3
- woven 1610

bone Gla protein *see* osteocalcin
bone-lining cells 423
bone marrow 421
- aplasia 296
  - drug-related 207, 590, *591*, 593, *598*, 601, *601*, 1695
  - aspiration in iron deficiency anaemia 637
- in juvenile chronic arthritis 1119, 1120
- lymphocyte circulation through 527
- MRI 771
- precursor cells in 422
- suppression in alkylating agent therapy 593
bone morphogenetic proteins (BMP) 353, 427, 429, *429*
  - recombinant 427, 429
bone scanning *see* radionuclide scanning
bone sialoprotein *see* sialoprotein 2
Borrelia
- *B. afzelii* 884, 889
- *B. burgdorferi* 199, 336, 663–4, 818, **884**
  - cell-mediated immunity against 889
  - culture 884–5
  - and fasciitis 1428
  - identification by PCR 889–90
  - maternal–fetal transmission 892
  - persistence following treatment 885
  - and polymyalgia rheumatica 1376
  - in pyogenic arthritis *880*
  - and small vessel vasculitis 1390
- *B. garinii* 884
Bouchard's nodes 1522, 1523
- gout in 684
boutonnière deformity
- in juvenile chronic arthritis 1132, 1133, 1741, 1742
- surgery 1705
bowel bypass syndrome 205–6, 255, *256*, 1462, 1694
- and calcium oxalate arthritis 1574, 1575
- dermatitis in 1095–6
- without bowel bypass 1462
BPAG2 mutation 353
braces
- knee 1732, 1747
- in kyphosis 125
brachial neuritis 219, 221, 805, 1661
brachial plexus
- anatomy 1651
- block 305–6
- cryptogenic neuropathy 219, 221, 805, 1661
- entrapment neuropathy 805
- lesions 1660–1, *1660*
brachialis 137
- lesion 1504
brachioradialis 137
bradiarrhythmia 237
bradycardia 237
- in neonatal lupus erythematosus 1198
bradykinin
- effect on C fibres 450
- in gout 1559
- in hyperalgesia 497
- in innate immunity 545
- interaction with prostaglandins 492
- joint afferent sensitivity to 492
brainstem
- disease 223, *224*, 1397
- and nociception 487, 489
- nuclei 489
breast
- carcinoma 289
  - and hormone replacement therapy 1596
  - and systemic sclerosis 1669
- development 14, *17*
- silicone implants 825, 1220, *1223*, 1267, 1419, 1693
breast feeding *see* lactation
breathlessness in systemic sclerosis 1235
brevican 410

brisement in frozen shoulder 144
British Isles Lupus Assessment Group index 1160
Brodie's abscess 1620–1
bromhexine 1011, 1314
bromocriptine
- in combination therapy *1025*
- effect on experimental arthritis 182
- immunosuppressive properties 282
- in psoriatic arthritis 1081
bronchial artery embolization 252
bronchiectasis (bronchial sepsis)
- cough in 241
- dyspnoea in 242
- radiography 246
bronchitis, chronic
- cough in 240–1
- dyspnoea in 242
- flow volume curve 248
bronchoalveolar lavage 250–1
- in sarcoidosis 1466
- in systemic sclerosis 1236–7
- Wegener's granulomatosis 1341
bronchogenic carcinoma 289
bronchospasm, drug-related *253*, 254, *578*, 580
brown tumours in hyperparathyroidism 280
Brown's syndrome 1118, 1127
Brucella
- arteritis due to 1390
- *B. abortus* 661, 937
- *B. canis* 937
- *B. melitensis* 661, 662, 937
- *B. suis* 937
- characteristics 937
- isolation 942, *942*
- sacroiliitis 864
- screening for 661
- *see also* brucellar arthritis; brucellosis
brucellar arthritis 938–44
- bacteriology 942, *942*
- childhood pyogenic 864
- clinical and radiological characteristics 938–41, 941–2
- diagnostic investigations 941–3
- distribution of joint involvement *938*
- laboratory features 941
- osteomyelitis 941
- peripheral joints 938–9
- reactive 941
- sacroiliitis 939
- serological tests 942–3
- spondylitis 939–41
- treatment 943–4, *943*
brucellar Coombs' test 942–3
brucellosis
- back pain in 98
- chronic 938
- disease characteristics 937–8
- epidemiology 937
- fever in 172
- host defence 937
- ocular involvement 317
- organism characteristics 937
bruising, steroid-induced 207, *587*
bruits
- in giant cell arteritis 1388
- in Paget's disease 1612
- in Takayasu's arteritis 1385
brushite 682
Bruton's disease 1136
bucillamine 1026
Budd–Chiari syndrome
- in antiphospholipid syndrome 1205
- in Behçet's syndrome 1397, 1398
- in SLE 1157
budesonide *210*
Buerger's disease 787, 1383
'bulge' sign 49
bullae *201*, 205–6
bullous pemphigoid-associated antigen 356
- gene mutations 353

BUN, in acute renal failure 325, 330
bundle branch block 237
bunion *see* hallux valgus
buprenorphine in low back pain 100
bupropion 340, *341*, *342*
burns, reflex sympathetic dystrophy following 1681
bursae 155
- in acromegaly 281
- deep 155
- disorders 155–6
- subcutaneous 155
bursal fluid 155, 156
bursectomy 146
bursitis
- anserine *5*, 158, 1509
- calcific 1574
- in calcium pyrophosphate dihydrate disease 1529
- in the elderly 37
- gastrocnemius–semimembranous 158
- in HIV infection 917
- iliopsoas 157, 1508
- infracalcaneal 160
- infrapatellar 158, 1509
- ischiogluteal 157, 1768
- in juvenile chronic arthritis 1134
- olecranon *see* olecranon bursa, bursitis
- prepatellar 155, 157–8, 167, 858, 1509, 1769
- retrocalcaneal 159–60, 745, 1511
- septic 155–6, 158, 858–9
  - subcutaneous 155
- subacromial 141, 143, 1008, 1503
- subcalcaneal 160
- subdeltoid 163
- trochanteric *5*, 156–7, 157, 165, 1508, 1768
bursotomy 146
Buschke–Ollendorf syndrome 207
buspirone (Buspar) 342
busulphan, adverse effects 1694
buttock tone 47
buttonhole deformity 1008
BVAS 1360, 1386
BXSB mice 510
bystander suppression 570

C

C1 esterase-inhibitor deficiency 351
C1-INH in inflammation *624*
c-ANCA *see* antineutrophil cytoplasmic autoantibodies, c-ANCA/PR3-ANCA
C cells 431
C fibres
- articular 442, 511
  - antidromic stimulation 449, 450
  - substance P containing 450
  - in synovial inflammation 450
C-line protein 455
C-reactive protein (CRP) 3, 623, **626**, 639, *639*
- in adult Still's disease 641
- in amyloidosis 1118
- in anaemia of chronic disease 636
- in ankylosing spondylitis 628
- in autoimmune disease 628
- in Behçet's syndrome 628
- control of secretion rate 349
- function in inflammation *624*
- in gout 627
- in innate immunity 545
- in juvenile chronic arthritis 1120
- in microscopic polyangiitis 1361
- in non-gonococcal arthritis 850
- in osteomyelitis 871
- in polymyalgia rheumatica/giant cell arteritis 628, 1378
- in polymyositis/dermatomyositis 1258, 1269
- properties *625*
- in psoriatic arthritis 628

C-reactive protein (CRP) (continued)
 rate of catabolism 639
 in reactive arthropathies 1088
 in Reiter's syndrome 628
 in rheumatic fever 980
 in rheumatoid arthritis 628–9, 640, 990,
  1016, 1016
 in Sjögren's syndrome 1312
 in SLE 640, 1157
 in Wegener's granulomatosis 1341, 1361
cachectin see tumour necrosis factors,
  TNF-α
caeruloplasmin 623
 in acute phase response 627
 in inflammation 624
 properties 625
 in rheumatoid arthritis 1016
caffeine, interaction with NSAIDs 579
Caffey's disease 168
caisson's disease 1621, 1622
calcaneal apophysitis 167, 1511
calcaneal spur see plantar spur
calcaneocuboid joint 153, 1719
calcaneofibular ligament 153
calcaneonavicular bar/fusion/synos-
  tosis 167, 746, 747, 768
calcaneus 153, 154, 157
 stress fracture 747, 748
calcifediol 1603
calcification
 in dermatomyositis 208
 intra-articular 757
 olecranon bursa 1528
 periarticular 756
  in mixed connective tissue disease
   1417
 retrocalcaneal bursa 1528
 subacromial bursa 1528
calcifying vesicles 429
calcinosis
 in dermatomyositis 1252, 1277, 1289,
  1294
 in SLE 1147
 subcutaneous 174
calciphylaxis 1453
calcipotriol in psoriasis 212
calcitonin (CT)
 and calcium homeostasis 431, 652
 effect of corticosteroids on 1588
 effect of menopause on 1587
 effect on osteoclasts 424, 425
 in osteoporosis 29, 1597, 1597–8
 in Paget's disease 1616–17
 receptors 423
 in reflex sympathetic dystrophy 1687
 in spinal stenosis 1648
calcitonin gene-related peptide
  (CGRP) 451, 511
 degradation 451
 expression by joint nerves 490
 in inflammation 497
calcitriol 1598–9, 1602–3
calcium
 cytosolic, role in tissue injury 446
 dietary
  and bone mass 426, 1589, 1593
  intake in childhood and adolescence
   29
  and risk of hip fracture 1585
 effect of age on absorption 1594
 excretion, in thyrotoxicosis 279
 homeostasis 429–31
 imbalance in synovial hypoxia 446
 imprecision in measurement 648
 in osteomalacia 1601
 serum, assay 652–3
 supplements, and osteoporosis 29, 1587,
  1595–6
 total plasma 429
 urinary, in juvenile osteoporosis 129
calcium antagonists, interaction with
  NSAIDs 579
calcium channel blockers
 in amyloidosis 1442

calcium channel blockers (continued)
 in mixed connective tissue disease
  1421–2
 in systemic sclerosis 1238
calcium hydrogen phosphate dihydrate 682
calcium hydroxyapatite 682, 683
calcium oxalate 682, 684, 1574–5
calcium oxalate dihydrate 1574
calcium oxalate monohydrate 1574
calcium phosphate 682
 see also basic calcium phosphate-associated syndromes
calcium pyrophosphate dihydrate
  (CPPD) 682, 1568, 1569
 crystals 1526, 1527
 in hypothyroidism 277
 in Milwaukee shoulder syndrome 1573
 in mixed crystal deposition 1532
 in osteoarthritis 1542
calcium pyrophosphate dihydrate
  (CPPD) 289, 1526,
  1567–70, 1571
 and acromegaly 1530, 1531
 age-related occurrence 26, 1529
 associations 1529–31, 1530, 1531
 chronic 1527–8
 clinical features 1567–8, 1568
 definition 1567
 and diabetes mellitus 283, 283, 1531,
  1567
 diagnosis 1568–9
 differential diagnosis 1568
 epidemiology 1567
 familial 1567
 and familial hypocalciuric hypercalcaemia 1531, 1567, 1570
 following joint insult 1530–1
 genetic factors 1529–30
 and gout 677, 1531, 1567
 and haemochromatosis 1530, 1531, 1567
 history 1567
 and hypercalcaemia 1567, 1570
 and hyperparathyroidism 1530, 1531,
  1567
 and hypomagnesaemia 1530, 1531, 1567,
  1570
 and hypophosphatasia 1530, 1531, 1567,
  1570
 and hypothyroidism 278, 1530, 1531,
  1567
 imaging 1528, 1529, 1568, 1569
 laboratory tests 653, 1568
 and ochronosis 1530, 1531, 1567
 with osteoarthritis 33
 pathogenesis 1569–70
 prognosis 1549, 1570
 pseudosyndromes associated 1527
 and rheumatoid arthritis 1531
 and rickets 1531, 1567
 synovial fluid 681, 682, 684, 1568, 1570
 treatment 1570, 1571
 type A see pseudogout
 type B 1567–8, 1568
 type C 1568, 1568
 type D 1568, 1568
 type E/lanthanic 1568, 1568
 type F/neuropathic 1568, 1568
 uncommon presentations 1529, 1530
 and Wilson's disease 1530, 1531, 1567
calisthenics 103
CALLA 451
calprotectin in rheumatoid arthritis
  1016, 1017
calreticulin 670
calvareal thickening in hypoparathyroidism 281
Campath-1H 1024
 in systemic vasculitis 1359
 in Wegener's granulomatosis 1346
campomelic dysplasia 369
Campylobacter
 C. cinaedi, in HIV infection 916
 C. fetus, in HIV infection 916

Campylobacter (continued)
 C. jejuni, and HIV-associated Reiter's
  syndrome 920
 and juvenile spondylarthropathies
  1049, 1054
 and reactive arthritis 267
canalization 73
Candida infection
 and arteritis 1390
 epidemiology 954
 in HIV infection 916
 joints 880, 955, 957–8
  clinical presentation 955, 956
  diagnosis 957
  management 956
  recurrent oral 174
 in Sjögren's syndrome 1307
canine distemper and Paget's disease
  1611
capillaroscopy 202, 203–4, 283
capitelloradial articulation 137
Caplan's syndrome 243
capreomycin in tuberculosis 932
caprine arthritis–encephalitis virus
  901, 908, 999
capsaicin 449, 450, 497
capsular ligaments 151
capsulitis 1501
capsulotomy in frozen shoulder 144
captopril
 adverse effects 1690
 in mixed connective tissue disease 1423
 and renal function 325
 in scleroderma 1240
caput ulnae 42
 in rheumatoid arthritis 1008
carbamazepine
 adverse effects 1690
 as analgesic 341
 in chronic back pain 1648
carbidopa 1223, 1693
carbimazole 1265
carbodiimide 694
carbohydrates
 dietary, and sport 1774, 1780
 effects of free radicals on 447
carbon dioxide 1773
carbon monoxide gas transfer 248–9
carbon monoxide transfer coefficient
  248
carbonic acid 1773
carbonic anhydrase 1773
carbonic anhydrase II 423
 deficiency 423, 436
carbonic anhydrase III, in polymyo-
  sitis/dermatomyositis 1258
γ-carboxyglutamic acid in juvenile
  dermatomyositis 1294
carcinoma erysipelatoides 209
carcinomatous neuropathy 1674
carcinomatous polyarthritis 289,
  1673–4
cardiac index in Paget's disease 1613
cardiac murmurs
 in aortic insufficiency 238
 in rheumatic fever 978
 in SLE 1151
cardiac pacemakers 237
 in MRI 724
cardiomegaly in rheumatic fever 978
cardiomyopathy 173
 dilated/congestive 236–7, 888
 hypertrophic 237
 hypertrophic obstructive 1777
 restrictive 235, 237
cardiovascular complications of rheumatic disease 173, 176, 229–39,
  978, 990, 1010–11
 amyloidosis 230, 233, 1436, 1438, 1439
 ankylosing spondylitis 230, 238, 1064
 Behçet's syndrome 230, 238, 1397–8
 dermatomyositis 230, 1253, 1254–5, 1290
 juvenile chronic arthritis 173, 230, 234,
  238, 1116–17

cardiovascular complications of
  rheumatic disease (continued)
 Kawasaki disease 230, 1404, 1405
 mixed connective tissue disease 230,
  234, 1416, 1418, 1418
 neonatal lupus erythematosus 1198
 polymyositis 230, 1253, 1254–5, 1290
 reactive arthropathies 1087
 relapsing polychondritis 1626
 SLE 173, 230, 231–3, 234, 236, 1149,
  1151, 1483–4
  childhood 1194–5, 1196
 systemic sclerosis 230, 233, 234, 235,
  1232–5, 1234
 Takayasu's arteritis 230, 233, 238, 1385
 Wegener's granulomatosis 230, 1338
cardiovascular disease
 and anaesthesia 299
 and sudden death during exercise 1777
cardiovascular system, adverse drug
  effects 587
carditis
 in Lyme disease 888, 891, 892
 in rheumatic fever 978
carnitine 474
carnitine palmitoyl transferase 474
carotid artery 1382
 aneurysm 1398
carotidynia in Takayasu's arteritis
  1385
carpal bones 137, 138
 childhood fracture 163
carpal tunnel 137
carpal tunnel decompression, persistent symptoms 219
carpal tunnel syndrome 178, 226, 1507
 in acromegaly 281
 in amyloidosis 1436, 1440, 1441
 in calcium pyrophosphate dihydrate
  disease 1529
 childhood 163
 and diabetes mellitus 284
 electrodiagnosis 804–5
 health status measures 59
 in hypothyroidism 277, 277, 278
 imaging 741
 local steroid injection 1765–6
 management 1507, 1507, 1705
 muscle wasting 41
 pain 5
 postoperative electrical studies 804–5
 in pregnancy 185
 in rheumatoid arthritis 227, 1008, 1013
 in scleroderma 227
 sensory nerve conduction study 801
carpometacarpal joints 137, 138
 local steroid injection 1767
carprofen 577
carrageenan 449, 450
cartilage
 in acromegaly 281
 articular 368, 405–18, 559
  age-related change in 413–14, 413
  autoantigens 560–1
  collagens 406–7, 407–8, 407
  effects of disuse on 406
  effects of exercise on 405–6
  in experimental models of joint
   disease 415–17
  markers of damage 417–18, 418
  in osteoarthritis 482–3
  physical properties 406–7
  proteoglycans in 406–7, 409–11
  responses to cytokines and growth
   factors 414–15
  structure and organization 405
 in calcium pyrophosphate dihydrate
  disease 1569–70
 in CINCA 1472, 1473, 1474
 effects of NSAIDs on 576, 578, 580,
  1695
 epiphyseal 771
 fatigue strength, effects of age on 483
 fibrillation 483, 1540–1

cartilage *(continued)*
 in fracture healing 413
 growth plate 411–13, 771
 hyaline 368
 localization and types 406
 matrix 368
 in osteoarthritis 1540–1, 1542–5, *1542*
 in relapsing polychondritis 1624–5
 structure 368
 tensile strength, effects of age on 483
 turnover markers 653
 yellow elastic 368
cartilage–hair hypoplasia 1630–1
cartilage matrix protein 418, *1017*
cartilage oligomeric matrix protein
  1624
cartilage oligomeric protein 418, *1017*
cartilage-specific matrix protein 368
caseation 927
casts in juvenile chronic arthritis 1108
cataracts
 congenital 191
 drug-related 319, *587*
 in juvenile chronic arthritis 1103
cathepsin G 513, 515, 1329
Caucasians
 juvenile chronic arthritis 829, 830, *830,*
  831
 seronegative spondylarthropathies *839,*
  840
 SLE 833, 835, *836*
 see also ethnic groups
cauda equina
 lesions 47, *219*
 tumour 121
cauda equina syndrome 225, 1064
causalgia 1679, *1679*
 see also reflex sympathetic dystrophy
cavitation 927
CD3 complex 550
CD4
 interaction with ligands 609
 in T-cell activation 546
CD8
 in juvenile chronic arthritis 1121
 in T-cell activation 546
CD11a/CD18 *see* integrins, $\alpha^L\beta_2$
CD11b/CD18 *see* integrins, $\alpha^M\beta_2$
CD11c/CD18 *see* integrins, $\alpha^X\beta_2$
CD21 528, 1170
CD31 *see* platelet-endothelial cell adhesion
  molecule-1
CD34 530
CD44 534, *537*
CD54 *see* intercellular adhesion molecules,
  ICAM-1
CD62 *1169*
cefotaxime
 in Lyme disease *891*, 892
 in pyogenic arthritis *856*, 865
ceftazidime in pyogenic arthritis *856*
ceftriaxone
 in Lyme disease 336, *891*, 892–3
 in pyogenic arthritis *856*, 865
cefuroxime
 in Lyme disease *891*, 892
 in pyogenic arthritis 865
cell membrane, effects of NSAIDs on
  576
cellulitis
 bone scanning 284
 differential diagnosis 1455
centiMorgans 687
central nervous system
 adverse drug effects *217, 578,* 580, *584,*
  1021
 angiitis 1392
  granulomatous *333,* 335, 785, 786
 in Behçet's syndrome 223, *223,* 1397
 in CINCA 1471
 in eosinophilia–myalgia syndrome 1426
 involvement in rheumatic diseases
  218–23
 in juvenile chronic arthritis 1117–18

central nervous system *(continued)*
 in mixed connective tissue disease 222,
  1418
 neurones
  effect of antinociceptive compounds
   on 497–8
  reduction of activity in 498
 and nociception 487, 490–1
 primary angiitis 914
 in Sjögren's syndrome 1311
 in SLE *see* systemic lupus erythematosus, neuropsychiatric
 in toxic oil syndrome 1426
 in Whipple's disease *223,* 1095
central venous pressure monitoring
 intraoperative 300
 postoperative 305
cephalosporin
 in discitis of childhood 124
 in osteomyelitis 875
cerebellar ataxia in SLE 1184
cerebral aneurysm in Ehlers–Danlos
  syndrome type 4 378
cerebral haemorrhage, hereditary with
  amyloidosis 1434, *1434,* 1438
cerebral tumour and reflex sympathetic dystrophy 1681
cerebral vein thrombosis in SLE 1185,
  1186, 1187
cerebrospinal fluid
 in Behçet's syndrome 1397
 in CINCA 1471
 in *Haemophilus influenzae* arthritis 863
 in intervertebral disc prolapse 1641
 in Lyme disease 888, 889
 in SLE 221, 1153, 1155, 1185
cervical collar 1658, *1732*
cervical myelopathy 223–4, *224*
 in cervical spondylosis 224–5, 1654,
  1655–6
 in rheumatoid arthritis 1013
 treatment 1658–60
cervical nerves, dermatomal representation 1651
cervical ribs 1661
cervical spondylosis 45, 1650
 cervical myelopathy in 224–5, 1654,
  1655–6
 cervical radiculopathy in 1656
 clinical features 1652–4
 complications 1655–6
 epidemiology 1650
 imaging 224, 1654–5
 pathology 1651–2
 treatment 1658–60, *1659*
 vertebrobasilar insufficiency in 223
cervicitis in reactive arthropathies
  1088
CGD 503, 513, 971
CGRP *see* calcitonin gene-related peptide
Chagas' disease 947
chair-lift test 145
Chamay technique 1704
'champagne-bottle legs' 209
Chapel Hill Consensus Conference
  1320, 1333, 1352
CHAQ 56, 57, 65
Charcot joints in diabetes mellitus
  283–4
Charcot–Leyden crystals *1575*
Charcot–Marie–Tooth disease 218
cheilitis in Sjögren's syndrome 1310
cheiroarthropathy, diabetic 163
chemokines 534, *535,* 990
chemosensitivity *488*
 in joint inflammation 492–3
chemotherapy
 eosinophilic granuloma 120
 Ewing's sarcoma 120
 and hyperuricaemia *1558*
 rheumatic disease following 290
chest pain *see* pain, chest
chest wall disease 242–3
chi² test 689

Chikungunya virus 901–2
chilblain lupus 211
child abuse 20, 759
childhood 9–21
 anaesthesia 1721
 ankylosing spondylitis *see* ankylosing
  spondylitis, juvenile
 antiphospholipid syndrome 1213
 back pain 20, *20,* 97–8, 114, *132,* 133
  aetiology *115*
  following spinal trauma 130, 131
  history and examination 114–17, *116*
  infection-associated 121–4
  non-specific causes 118
  in osteoporosis 129
  prevention 117–18
  prolapsed intervertebral disc 124–5
  referred 133
  in Scheuermann's osteochondritis
   125, 126
  in spinal dysraphism 127
  in spondylolysis and spondylolisthesis 126–7, 128
  tumour-associated 118–21, *121, 132*
 backache 114
 Behçet's syndrome 1409
 bone and cartilage diseases **1629–37**
 brucellar arthritis 943, *943*
 calcium intake 29
 Chikungunya fever 902
 Churg–Strauss syndrome 1407
 classification of neuromuscular disorders *1292*
 Cogan's syndrome 1409
 coping with disease 1754–5
 developmental status measures *56, 57–8*
 disability, reporting 65
 electromyography 1293
 eosinophilia–myalgia syndrome 1427–8
 familial Mediterranean fever 1409
 fever *170,* 171
 fever of unknown origin 20–1
 foot 17
 functional assessment 17
 fungal arthritis 958
 gait development 16–17
 giant cell arteritis 1408
 gonococcal arthritis 862, *862,* 863
 growth and development 12–15, *14,* 16,
  17, 18
 Henoch–Schönlein purpura 14, 1407
 hip
  replacement 1716–17
  surgery 1715–17
 hypersensitivity vasculitis 1407, 1408
 hypothyroidism 277, 278
 imaging **751–72**
  angiography 764
  arthrography 764
  CT scanning 753, 754, 766–8
  Doppler ultrasound 760–4, 765
  MRI 763, 766, 767, 768–72
  myelography 764
  radiography 751–60, *754, 755–7,*
   761–2, 767
  radionuclide scanning 752, 764–6,
   767
 inclusion-body myositis 1293
 infection, back pain in 121–4
 inflammatory bowel disease 14, 21, 1054
 knee
  replacement 1719
  surgery 1717–18, 1719
 limp 19, *19,* 20, 115, 164, *754*
 lower limb pain 19, *19,* **163–8,** *164*
 Lyme disease 336
 lymphadenopathy 172–3
 malignant skeletal disease 1672
 meningococcal arthritis 862
 microscopic polyangiitis 1402–4
 monoarticular arthritis in 20
 motor development 14, *14*
 muscles
  strength evaluation 16

childhood *(continued)*
 muscles *(continued)*
  weakness 21
 ocular involvement in rheumatic
  disease 316
 osteomyelitis 752, 868, 877
 osteoporosis 128–30, *1137,* 1138, 1588
 overlap syndromes 1293
 pain 1738
  assessment 19
 polyarteritis nodosa 14, 21, 316, 1402–4
 polymyositis **1287–97**
 psoriatic arthritis *see* psoriatic arthritis,
  juvenile
 psychosocial and educational impact of
  disease 13
 pyogenic arthritis **861–6**
  aetiology 862–3, *862*
  in chronic joint disease 864–5
  clinical manifestations *861,* 862
  epidemiology 14, 861, *861*
  hip 863
  management 865–6, *866*
  pathogenesis 861
  prognosis 866
  sacroiliac joints 863–4
  range of joint movement 16
 reflex sympathetic dystrophy 163, 167,
  1681, 1682, 1683
 regional problems of arm and leg *162,*
  162–8, *163, 164*
 rehabilitation **1737–55**
 Reiter's syndrome 1054–5
 rheumatic diseases 21, 56, 128–30
  age at presentation 12, 13
  classifications and diagnostic criteria
   10–11, *10, 11, 12*
  diagnostic approach 15–18, 19
  epidemiology 10–12, 13, 14
  frequencies 11–12, *12*
  health status measures *56,* 57
  history taking 15
  influence of gender 12, 14
  laboratory tests 17–18, *17*
  pattern recognition 18–19
  physical examination 15–17
  systemic features 178
 rheumatic fever 14, 977–8
 sarcoidosis 14, 316, 1123, 1469
 and school 1737, 1752–3, 1754
 sciatica 118
 seronegative spondylarthropathies 128,
  831–2, *832,* **1049–56**
  undifferentiated 1050–2
 sexual maturation 14–15, *17*
 spinal dysraphism 127–8, 129
 spine
  deformity 131, 133
  problems **114–33**
  surgery 1721
  trauma 130, 131
  tumours 118–21
 sports injuries 1786–8
 surgery **1713–21**
  ankle 1718–20
  elbow 1720
  foot 1718–20
  hand 1720–1
  hip 1715–17
  shoulder 1720
  wrist 1720–1
 Takayasu's arteritis 1385
 trauma 20
 upper limb pain 19, *19, 162,* **162–3,** *163*
 vasculitis 21, **1402–9**
 Wegener's granulomatosis 14, 1406–7
 weight loss/growth arrest 21, 171
 X-linked agammaglobulinaemia 970
 see also growth *and under specific disorders*
Childhood Health Assessment
  Questionnaire *56,* 57, 65
Chile, incidence of rheumatoid
  arthritis 833, *835*
chills in Lyme disease 887

Chinese
  juvenile chronic arthritis 829, *830*
  rheumatoid arthritis 833, *834*
  seronegative spondylarthropathies 838,
    838, 839
  SLE 836, *836*, 837
  see also ethnic groups
chiropractic manipulation
  cervical pain syndromes 1658
  low back pain 104
Chlamydia
  C. pneumoniae 1088
  C. trachomatis 1085, 1088
  and Kawasaki disease 1406
  laboratory tests 662–3
CHLC 69
chlorambucil 590
  adverse effects 593–4, *593*
    gastrointestinal 260, 261, 593, *593*
    haematological 593, *593*
    hyperuricaemia 1694
    neurological *217*
    oncogenic 290, *593*, 594
    respiratory *253*
  in amyloidosis 1118–19
  in Behçet's syndrome 1400
  clinical efficacy 592–3
  in combination therapy *1025*
  in juvenile chronic arthritis 1108, 1118–
    19, 1126, 1141
  in lactation *602*
  in large granular lymphocyte syndrome
    644
  in mixed connective tissue disease 1423
  in multicentric reticulohistiocytosis
    1476, 1477
  pharmacology 590–1
  in polymyositis/dermatomyositis 1276
  in pregnancy *602*
  in pyoderma gangrenosum 1461
  in rheumatoid arthritis 1024
  in scleroderma 1240, *1241*
  structure 591
  therapeutically relevant effects 591–2,
    592
  treatment regimens 593
chloramphenicol 660, *891*
chlorinated organic solvents, sclero-
    derma-like changes induced by
    209
chlormezanone in chronic back pain
    1648
chloroquine 596
  adverse effects 596
    cutaneous 596
    gastrointestinal 596
    haematological 295
    myopathy 791, *1265, 1266*, 1693
    neurological *217*, 795
    ocular 318–19, 596, 1695
    psychiatric 338
  in combination therapy *1025*
  in discoid lupus erythematosus 211
  in lactation 194
  pharmacology 596
  in pregnancy 191–2
  in psoriatic arthritis 1080
  in rheumatoid arthritis 1021
  in seropositive juvenile chronic
    arthritis 1035
  therapeutic efficacy 596
  therapeutically relevant effects 596
  treatment regimens 596
chlorpromazine
  adverse effects *1690*
  effect on prolactin levels 282
cholangiitis, autoimmune 1310
cholecalciferol 430, 1602
cholestasis 652
  drug-related *578*
cholesterol
  crystals 1526, *1575*
  in osteoarthritis 682
  in rheumatic disorders 1482

cholesterol *(continued)*
  synovial fluid 680, 682
  transport 1479
cholesterol ester 1479
cholestyramine, interaction with
    NSAIDs *579*
choline magnesium trilisate in juve-
    nile chronic arthritis *1106*
chondritis
  in SLE 1147
  in Wegener's granulomatosis 1335
chondrocalcinosis 1526
  asymptomatic *1527*
  in calcium pyrophosphate dihydrate
    disease 1528, 1567, 1568, 1569
  in the elderly 1528
  genetic factors 1529–30
  and gout 1561
  and hyperparathyroidism 280
  in hypothyroidism 277
  and Paget's disease 1613
chondrocyte membrane antigens,
    antibodies to 987
chondrocytes 405
  in animal models of joint disease 415,
    416
  in articular cartilage 368
  in calcium pyrophosphate dihydrate
    disease 1569
  cell culture 373
  clones 1541
  effect of age on distribution 413–14
  effect of growth factors and cytokines
    on 1543
  effect of oestrogens on 1013
  in fracture healing 413
  ghosting 1541
  growth plate 411–13
  in inflammation 508
  in rheumatoid arthritis 992
chondrodysplasia punctata *369*
chondrodysplasias 366, 368, 393–4, 427,
    428
  collagen protein analysis 373, 374
  gene mutations 353, 368–9, *369*, 435
    collagen II genes 370–3
    collagen V genes 377
    collagen IX genes 377
    collagen X genes 377
    collagen XI genes 377
  detection 370
  molecular analysis *369*, 373, 375, 376
  see also specific disorders
chondrodystrophies *see* chondrodys-
    plasias
chondroitin sulphate 353, 409, 414
  in damaged tendons 1494
  as marker of joint disease 417, 418, 1537,
    1538
  in osteoarthritis 1537, *1538*, 1542–3
chondromalacia patellae 159, 743
chondrophyte 413
chondroprotection 1548–9
chondrosarcoma 120, 288, *1671*
chordoma 120, 716
chorea *177*
  in antiphospholipid syndrome 222,
    1207
  in Lyme disease 888
  in rheumatic fever 972, 978–9
  in SLE 1153, 1184
chorionic villus biopsy in osteogenesis
    imperfecta 698
chorioretinitis in CINCA 1471
choroid plexus
  immune complex deposition 703
  rheumatoid nodules 335
choroidal infarction in SLE 313
chromatin 348
  methylation 349
chromosome 5, lymphokine genes 504
chromosomes
  crossing over 687
  microsatellites 350

chronic fatigue syndrome 37, 1496
chronic granulomatous disease 503,
    513, 971
chronic infantile neurological cuta-
    neous and articular syndrome
    (CINCA) 1470–4
  central nervous and sensory anomalies
    1471, 1472
  clinical presentation 1470–3
  cutaneous involvement 1471
  differential diagnosis 1123
  morphological changes 1473
  ocular involvement 1471, 1472
  onset 12, 13
  pathogenesis 1473–4
  perinatal events 1470–1
  sex differences 14
chronic inflammatory demyelinating
    polyneuropathy 795
chronic pain syndrome *90*, 105
chronic renal failure
  biochemical tests 650
  and hyperparathyroidism 280
  hyperuricaemia in 1558
  and panniculitis 1453
  and proteinuria 321, *330*
  and renal osteodystrophy 1603
chrysiasis 213
Churg–Strauss syndrome 1354–62
  antineutrophil cytoplasmic autoanti-
    bodies 328, 1329, 1355–6
  childhood 1407
  classification 1320, *1321, 1322*
  clinical features 1354–5
  definition 1355
  diagnosis 1355–8
  diagnostic criteria 1325, *1325*
  differential diagnosis 1355
  eosinophilia *644*
  epidemiology *1320*
  gastrointestinal involvement 257, *258*
  in HIV infection 914
  immunology 1355–6
  monitoring disease activity 1360–1
  pathology 1357–8
  peripheral neuropathies 228
  prognosis 1361–2
  pulmonary involvement 173
  renal involvement 1355
  treatment 1359
chylomicrons 1479
CIDP 795
ciguatera 1267
ciliary neurotrophic factor 623
cilofungin 958
cimetidine
  adverse effects *217, 1265*, 1693
  effect on serum creatinine 325, 649
  in eosinophilic fasciitis 1428
CINCA *see* chronic infantile neurological
    cutaneous and articular syndrome
ciprofibrate in hyperlipidaemias 1481
ciprofloxacin 660, 663
  in osteomyelitis 874
  in tuberculosis 931, 933
circinate balanitis *175*
circle of Willis 223
circulus articuli vasculosus 442
circumflex arteries 763
circumoral numbness in vertebro-
    basilar insufficiency 223
cirrhosis
  cryptogenic, rheumatic manifestations
    256
  hyperbilirubinaemia in 651
  liver function tests 652
  primary biliary *285*
    autoantibodies *668*
    and keratoconjunctivitis sicca 1424
    rheumatic manifestations *256*
    and scleroderma *258*, 1424
    and Sjögren's syndrome 257, *258*,
      1310, 1424
  in scleroderma *258*

cisatracurium *307*
citric acid cycle 1774
CK *see* creatine kinase
clarithromycin in Lyme disease 892
classification of rheumatic diseases
    843–7
claudication
  intermittent in giant cell arteritis 1388
  neurogenic 1644
  spinal in ostoarthritis 1540
clavicle 135, 136
  osteitis condensans 185
clavulanic acid with amoxycillin 874
cleft palate 191
clindamycin 660, 874
clinical trials and diagnostic criteria
    811
clobetasol propionate *210*
clobetasone butyrate *210*
clodronate
  in Paget's disease 1616
  structure 1615
clofazimine
  in discoid lupus erythematosus 211
  in leprosy 935, 936
  in pyoderma gangrenosum 211
clofibrate, adverse effects *1265, 1266*,
    1480, 1693
clomipramine *340*
  in rheumatoid arthritis 341–2
Clostridium
  C. difficile
    and childhood Reiter's syndrome
      1054
    colitis related to 874
    and reactive arthropathies 267, 1088
  C. perfringens
    in animal model of arthritis 999
    effects of NSAIDs on intestinal
      population 269
    in rheumatoid arthritis 268, *270–1*,
      1694
    in pyogenic arthritis 853
clubfoot in Ehlers–Danlos syndrome
    type 4 378
cocaine, adverse effects *1223, 1265,
    1266*, 1693
coccidioidin 961
coccidioidomycosis 252, 880
  arteritis in 1390
  epidemiology 954
  joint infection *955*, 961–2
    clinical presentation 955, 956
    diagnosis *957*
    management 956
coccoid rods *269, 271*
cochlear implants and MRI 724
Cockroft–Gault formula 326, 650
codeine 32
  in chronic back pain 1648
  in lactation 193
  linctus 241
  in pregnancy 189
  and sport 1778
coeliac disease 1096
  and osteoporosis 129
  rheumatic manifestations *256*
  susceptibility to 554–5, *555*
Cogan's syndrome
  childhood 1409
  large vessel vasculitis in 1392
  psychiatric involvement *333*
cognitive behavioural rehabilitation
    techniques 1730
cognitive capacity in the elderly 30
cognitive impairment in SLE 333,
    1153, 1184
cognitive restructuring 68
colchicine
  adverse effects 1564
    myopathy *1265, 1266*, 1693
    neurological *217*
    respiratory *253*
  in amyloidosis 1441

colchicine *(continued)*
  in Behçet's syndrome 1400
  in calcium pyrophosphate dihydrate
    disease 1570
  in eosinophilic fasciitis 1428
  in familial Mediterranean fever 1448–9,
    1449
  in gout 1563–4, *1564*, 1565
  in hypersensitivity vasculitis 1369
  in lactation 194
  in osteoarthritis 33
  in panniculitis 1455
  in pregnancy 185, 193, 1449
  in scleroderma 1240
  in urticarial vasculitis 1370
cold sensitivity 200
colectomy in pyoderma gangre-
    nosum 1461
colitis
  Clostridium difficile-related 874
  collagenous 1096
collagen 426–7, 457
  animal models of disorders 353
  in annulus fibrosus 1640
  in articular cartilage 368, 406–7, 407–8,
    407
  chicken type II 611
  in chondrodysplasias 373, 374
  damage to 1493
  effect of penicillamine on 214
  fibril-associated 407
  in fibrocartilage 368
  folding and self-assembly 356
  genes 354–6
    mutations 350, 353–4, **356–93**
  in hypermobility 1500
  interactions between types 356
  interstitial 354, 356
  in scleroderma 1225–6
  sensitivity to enzymes 514–15
  in tendons 1492
  see also specific collagen types
collagen-induced arthritis 562, 563–4,
    608, 611, 992, 997–8
collagen type I 407, 427, *428*
  antibodies to 987
  in bone 357, 421
  in calcium pyrophosphate dihydrate
    disease 1569
  distribution 357
  in Ehlers–Danlos syndrome type7 353,
    357, 366, 367
  genes
    COL1A1, mutations 353, 698
    COL1A2
    expression in scleroderma 1226
    mutations 353, 698
    identification 354
    mutations 353, **357–66**, 367, 427, 428,
      435, *435*, 698
    distribution 360
    exon-skipping deletions 363–4
    point mutations 361–2, 363
    structure 354–5
  hole zones 427
  in intervertebral discs 1640
  in Marfan syndrome 357
  in osteogenesis imperfecta 353, 357,
    361–5, 418–19, 427, 435, 697
  structure 354, 427
  and urate crystal formation 1559
collagen type II 368, 427, *428*
  antibodies to 987
  as arthritogen 563–4
  in articular cartilage 407, *407*, 408
  attenuated, immunization with 611
  C-propeptide 418, 1538
  carboxy-terminal 418
  in collagen-induced arthritis 563–4,
    997
  distribution 354–5
  gene (*COL2A1*)
    mutations 353, 355–6, 357, 413, 427,
      428, *435*

collagen type II *(continued)*
  gene (*COL2A1*) *(continued)*
    in achondrogenesis 374, 375–6
    in chondrodysplasias 368, *369*,
      370–3, 373, 375, 376
    detection 370
    gonadal mosaicism 364
    in Kniest dysplasia 376
    in osteoarthritis 371–3, 378
    in spondyloepiphyseal dysplasia 1630
    in Stickler syndrome 376–7
    and osteoarthritis 1519, 1543
    polymorphisms 369–70
    structure 354–5, 369
  in intervertebral discs 1640
  in oral tolerance therapy 264–5
  structure 354, 407
collagen type III 407, 427, *428*
  in bone matrix 361
  distribution 355, 378
  gene (*COL3A1*)
    mutations 353, 357, 362, 378–83, 436
    structure 354–5
  structure 354
collagen type IV *428*
  genes
    mutations 353, 356, 357, 387
    structure 355
collagen type V 427, *428*
  in bone matrix 361
  distribution 355
  genes
    mutation 353, 356, 357, 368
    in chondrodysplasias 368, *369*, 377
    in Ehlers–Danlos syndrome 385–7
collagen type VI *428*
  distribution 355
  genes 353
    COL6A1 355
    COL6A2 355
    COL6A3 355
  structure 355
collagen type VII *428*
  in articular cartilage 408
  gene (*COL7A1*) 355
    mutations 353, 357, 386–7, 388–9
    structure 355, 388, 408
collagen type VIII 355, *428*
  genes 353
collagen type IX 353, 355, 368, 427, *428*
  antibodies to 987
  as arthritogen 563
  in articular cartilage 407, 408
  distribution 355
  in the eye 408
  gene mutations 357, 368, 413, *435*, 436
    in chondrodysplasias 368, *369*, 377
  structure 408
collagen type X 353, 355, 368, *428*
  in articular cartilage 408
  at growth plate 412
  distribution 355
  gene (*COL10A1*)
    mutations 353, 357, 368, 413, *435*, 436
    in chondrodysplasias 368, 369, *369*,
      378
  in osteoarthritis 1543, 1544
collagen type XI 353, 355, 427, *428*
  antibodies to 987
  as arthritogen 563
  in articular cartilage 407–8, *407*
  distribution 355
  genes
    mutations 353, 355, 356, 368, 377, 413
    in chondrodysplasias 368, *369*, 375
    in Stickler syndrome 377
  structure 407–8
collagen type XII 353, 427, *428*
collagen type XIII 353, *428*
collagen type XIV 427, *428*
collagen type XV 356
collagen type XVI 356
collagen type XVII, *COL17A1* muta-
    tions 353

collagenase 410–11, *411*, 425, 513
  activation by free radicals 514
  effect on collagen 515
  effect of methotrexate on 583
  inhibitors 629
  neutrophil 410–11, *411*
  in osteoarthritis 1538
collagenous colitis 1096
Colles' fracture 1583–4, *1584*, 1586,
    1599, *1600*
colon
  carcinoma, protective effects in rheuma-
    toid arthritis 1666
  perforation in SLE 257
  in scleroderma 257, 1232
colostomy, pyoderma gangrenosum
    around 1458, 1459
colour vision assessment 310
coma *224*
common acute lymphoblastic
    leukaemia antigen 451
common extensor tendon 137
common flexor tendon 137
common flexor tendon sheath 137, 138
common peroneal nerve
  entrapment neuropathy *219*, 227, 805
  in leprosy 934
  palsy *803*
Community Integration
    Questionnaire 1724, *1724*
comorbidity 823
COMP 1624
COMP5 gene 368
  mutations in chondrodysplasias 368,
    369, 370
compartment syndromes 1510, 1786
complement
  alternative pathway 507, 545
  C1q
    deficiency 506
    immune complex binding to 706,
      707, *708*, *709*
    in rheumatic fever 977
  C1r deficiency 506
  C1s deficiency 506
  C2
    deficiency 971
    and polymyositis/dermatomyositis
      1258
    and SLE 506–7, 1169
    gene 548
  C3 512
    in acute phase response 627
    deficiency 322, 506, 507, 545
    induction 623
    in juvenile chronic arthritis 1109
    as marker of clinical disease 654
    as marker of disease in SLE 1191
    properties *625*
    in proteinuria 322
    in rheumatic fever 977
    in rheumatoid arthritis 1016, *1016*
  C3a 512
    as marker of clinical disease 654
    in rheumatoid arthritis 1016
  C3b 512
    in innate immunity 545
    receptors 545
  C3d in juvenile chronic arthritis 1109
  C3dg 512
  C4 512
    in acute phase response 627
    deficiency 322, 506, 1169
    gene 548
    as marker of clinical disease 654
    properties *625*
    in proteinuria 322
    in rheumatic fever 977
    in rheumatoid arthritis 1016, *1016*
  C4a 507, 1169
  C4b 507, 512, 1169
  C5 512
    deficiency 854

complement *(continued)*
  C5a 512, 545
  C6 deficiency 854
  C7 deficiency 854, 971
  C8 deficiency 854, 971
  C9 deficiency 854
  classical pathway 507, 546
  deficiencies 506–8, 512, 971
  in drug-induced lupus 1692
  effect of penicillamine on *597*
  function in inflammation 511–12, *512*,
    624
  iC3b 512
  and immune complex deposition 704
  in innate immunity 545
  in juvenile chronic arthritis 1120
  in juvenile dermatomyositis 1295
  lectin pathway 507
  pericardial fluid 235
  in polymyositis/dermatomyositis 1270
  in rheumatoid arthritis 1015–16
  in SLE 322, 506–8, 507, 512, 654,
    1169–70, *1170*
  system 507
  terminal pathway 507
complement receptors
  CR1 513, 528, 1169–70
  CR2 528, 1170
  CR3 513
complex regional pain syndrome
    1679, *1679*
  see also reflex sympathetic dystrophy
compressed-air workers, osteo-
    necrosis 1622
compression in acute injury 1781
computed tomography *see* CT arthro-
    graphy; CT myelography; CT
    radiculography; CT scanning
concanavalin A 629
concentric needle electrode 801
conduction defect and anaesthesia
    299
conduction system disease *230*, 237,
    238
coneurosis *948*, 950
congenital heart block 173, *176*, 1198,
    1199
congenital hyperfibrinogenaemia
    1100–1
congestive heart failure 231
  in amyloidosis 1436
  in juvenile chronic arthritis 1126
  oliguria in 325
  in polymyositis/dermatomyositis 1255
  proteinuria 321
  in rheumatic fever 978
  in Takayasu's arteritis 1385
conglutinin binding assay 706, 707–8,
    708, *709*
conjunctiva 310
conjunctivitis 310, *311*
  in CINCA 1471
  in reactive arthropathies 314, 316, 1087
  in SLE 1153
connective tissue diseases 1413
  autoantibodies 1413–14
  and diabetes mellitus 285
  differential diagnosis 1122, 1136, *1137*
  incidence *12*
  and malignant disease 289
  muscle necrosis in 790
  serological subsets 1413–14
  systemic features *170*
  undifferentiated 1413
  vasculitis associated 1408
connective tissue naevi 207
consent to surgery 1702
constipation 257, *258*, 1020
construct validity 52
consumptive coagulopathy 1117, 1118
containment sign 144
content validity 52
Convery Polyarticular Disability
    Index 55, *55*

Coombs' test
  brucellar 942–3
  positive 291, 1155
  in SLE 1192
Copeland shoulder 1703
coping 67–8, 1730
  childhood 1754–5
  emotion-focused 68
  and low back pain 109
  problem-focused 68
  and social support 68–9
Coping Strategies Questionnaire 68
copper salt supplements 262
coracoacromial arch 135
coracoacromial ligament 135, 136
coracobrachialis 137
coracoclavicular ligament 135, 136
coracohumeral ligament 135
coracoid process 135, 136
Cori–Forbes disease 473
corneal thinning in relapsing poly-
    chondritis 1626
coronary arteries
  aneurysm 1398, 1404, 1405
  disease 230, 231–3, 232
    evaluation 233
    and gout 1556
    and sudden death during exercise
        1777
  intimal hyperplasia in mixed connective
      tissue disease 1418
  revascularization surgery 1406
coronary arteritis 176, 231, 231–3
  childhood 21
  in SLE 1194
  small vessel 233
coronary thrombosis, acute 231
corsets, lumbar 101, 104, 1649
cortex, neurones 489, 496–7
corticosteroids 585–8
  adverse effects 586, 587, 588, 1141, 1696
    on bone 128, 130, 587, 1182, 1588–9,
        1591, 1622
    cardiovascular 587
    childhood 1182
    cutaneous 207, 587
    endocrine 587
    gastrointestinal 260, 261, 587
    hypertrichosis 209
    on joints 587
    metabolic 587
    myopathy 470, 471, 587, 653, 791,
        806, 1182, 1266
    neurological 217
    ocular 319, 587
    psychiatric 337, 337, 338, 587
    sepsis 1359
  in calcium homeostasis 431
  in cardiovascular disease 232, 233
  crystals 1575
  effect on growth 85–6
  effect on serum urea concentration 650
  epidural in low back pain 105
  eye drops
    in juvenile chronic arthritis 1108,
        1141
    in reactive arthropathies 1092, 1093
    in uveitis 317
  in granulomatous angiitis of the central
      nervous system 786
  and hyperlipidaemias 1482, 1483
  indications for 586
  injection 1757, 1770–1
    adverse effects 1696
    agents 1760
    ankle 1762, 1769–70
    in calcium pyrophosphate dihydrate
        disease 1570
    in cervical pain syndromes 1659
    in chronic back pain 1648
    contraindications 1758, 1758
    elbow 145, 1505, 1762, 1764–5
    equipment 1760
    foot 1762, 1769–70

corticosteroids (continued)
  injection (continued)
    in gout 1564, 1565
    hand 148, 1507, 1762, 1766–8
    hip 157, 1762, 1768
    in HIV-associated arthritis 921
    indications 1758, 1758
    in juvenile chronic arthritis 1107,
        1141
    in juvenile spondylarthropathies
        1049
    knee 158, 1762, 1768–9
    in low back pain 101
    method 1759–61, 1760, 1761
    in osteoarthritis 1547
    potential problems and side-effects
        1759, 1759
    preparation 1760–1, 1761
    in psoriatic arthritis 1081
    in pyoderma gangrenosum 1461
    in reactive arthropathies 1092, 1093
    in rheumatoid arthritis 1024
    shoulder 141, 142, 143, 144, 1504,
        1761, 1762, 1763–4
    in soft-tissue rheumatism 1512–13
    technique 1761, 1761
  intrapericardial 1126
  and lactation 194, 602
  modulation of acute phase protein
      synthesis 623
  and neutrophilia 642, 643
  operative cover 301
  and osteoporosis 433
  in pregnancy 191, 602
  pulse intravenous 588, 1024
    in juvenile dermatomyositis 1296–7
    in microscopic polyangiitis 1358–9,
        1362–3
    in polyarteritis nodosa 1358–9,
        1362–3
    in polymyositis/dermatomyositis
        1273
    in pyoderma gangrenosum 1461
    in SLE 1172, 1174, 1191, 1194
  and sport 1778
  systemic
    in adult-onset Still's disease 1127
    adverse effects 1023, 1757
    in Behçet's syndrome 1399, 1400–1
    in calcium pyrophosphate dihydrate
        disease 1570
    in Churg–Strauss syndrome 1359
    in dermatomyositis 211, 1273–5, 1274
    in Eaton–Lambert syndrome 1675
    in eosinophilic fasciitis 1428
    in frozen shoulder 144
    in giant cell arteritis 1379–80, 1389
    in gout 1564, 1565
    in Henoch–Schönlein purpura 1407
    in hypersensitivity vasculitis 1369
    in inclusion-body myositis 1280
    in juvenile chronic arthritis 1036,
        1124–5, 1125, 1126, 1140–1
    in Kawasaki disease 1406
    in mixed connective tissue disease
        1422, 1423
    in multicentric reticulohistiocytosis
        1476, 1477
    in polymyalgia rheumatica 1379–80
    in polymyositis 1273–5, 1274
    in psoriatic arthritis 1080
    in pyoderma gangrenosum 1461
    in reflex sympathetic dystrophy 1687
    in relapsing polychondritis 1627
    in rheumatoid arthritis 1023–4
    in sarcoidosis 1469
    in scleritis 317
    in Sjögren's syndrome 1314
    in SLE 1172, 1173, 1174, 1186, 1190
    in Takayasu's arteritis 1387
    in urticarial vasculitis 1370
    in uveitis 317
    in Wegener's granulomatosis 1344–5,
        1345, 1347, 1407

corticosteroids (continued)
  therapeutically relevant actions 585,
      586
  in thrombocytopenia 292
  topical 209
    adverse effects 211, 214
    in dermatomyositis 211
    in discoid lupus erythematosus 211
    potencies 210
    in psoriasis 212, 1079
    in scleroderma 211
    withdrawal, panniculitis following 1453
corticotropin-releasing hormone 510
  receptors 510
cortisol 585, 585
  in juvenile chronic arthritis 87
  operative cover 301
  in pregnancy 182
  topical 210
cortisone 585
  discovery 181
  effect on growth 85
  in lactation 193
cosmetic camouflage in telangi-
    ectasia 210
costoplasty 131
costovertebral joints 91
  in reactive arthropathies 1087
co-trimoxazole 660, 874
cotton-wool spots 312, 313
cough 240–1
  causes 240
  in sarcoidosis 1465
  suppressants 241
  in systemic sclerosis 1235
  in toxic oil syndrome 1425, 1426
counter-immunoelectrophoresis 669,
    670
coxsackievirus infection 904
  in models of myositis 1273
  in polymyositis/dermatomyositis
      1266–7, 1288–9
CPPD see calcium pyrophosphate di-
    hydrate
CPPD disease see calcium pyrophosphate
    dihydrate disease
CPT 474
CR3 see integrins, $\alpha^M\beta_2$
CR4 see integrins, $\alpha^X\beta_2$
cranial arteritis see giant cell arteritis
cranial nerves
  involvement in SLE 1153, 1184–5
  in Lyme disease 888
  palsies 223, 224
  in Sjögren's syndrome 1311
cranial settling 1705
craniofacial deafness 395
craniosynostoses 395, 398
craniotabes 1601
creatine 1258, 1774
creatine kinase (CK)
  CK-1/CK-BB 653
  CK-2/CK-MB 653
  CK-3/CK-MM 653
  in differential diagnosis of neuro-
      muscular disorders 1291
  factors affecting levels 1257, 1257
  following eccentric exercise 468
  following orthopaedic surgery 468
  following reperfusion of ischaemic
      limb 469
  imprecision in measurement 648
  in inclusion-body myositis 1279
  isoenzymes 1257
  as marker of muscle damage 465
  and muscle disease 653
  in polymyositis/dermatomyositis
      1256–7, 1257
  response to repeated exercise 469
creatine phosphokinase
  in ankylosing spondylitis 1066
  in hypothyroidism 278
  in mixed connective tissue disease
      1419

creatinine phosphokinase (continued)
  in polymyositis/dermatomyositis
      1669
creatinine
  clearance 325, 648–50
    changes in with age 23
    preanaesthetic assessment 300
  effect of cyclosporin on 595, 595
  imprecision of tests of 648
  serum
    in acute renal failure 325, 326
    and glomerular function 648–50
    reciprocal 649, 650
crepitations, velvet 40
crepitus 40
  in acromegaly 281
  eburnation 40
  flexor tendon 41–2
  in osteoarthritis 1521
  in tenosynovitis 1505
'crescent sign' 207
CREST syndrome 1418, 1424
  autoantibodies in 672
  life expectancy 36
  terminology 1218
cricoarytenoid joint
  disorders and intubation 302, 303
  inflammation 301
  in juvenile chronic arthritis 1116
  synovitis 242, 1009
cricopharyngeal muscle dysfunction
    in polymyositis/dermatomyo-
    sitis 1255, 1277
criterion validity 52
Crithidia luciliae 668
critical periods in growth 73
Crohn's disease 173, 1045, 1094
  childhood 1054
  erythema nodosum in 1451
  and pyoderma gangrenosum 1460
  rheumatic manifestations 256
cross-arm acromioclavicular loading
    test 144
crossed immunoaffinity electrophor-
    esis 629
crossed leg palsy 803
Crouzon syndrome 368, 369, 398, 435,
    436
crowned dens syndrome 1568
CRP see C-reactive protein
cruising 16
cryoglobulinaemia 1370
  essential mixed 503, 1370
    classification 1321, 1322, 1327
  gastrointestinal involvement 259
  glomerular haematuria in 324
  in hepatitis C virus infection 706, 900
  and malignancy 289
  mixed 1327, 1370
  in mixed connective tissue disease 1419
  peripheral neuropathies 228
  proteinuria in 323
  rapidly progressive glomerulonephritis
      in 327, 328
  in rheumatoid arthritis 706, 710
  rheumatoid factor in 674
  in Sjögren's syndrome 1303–4
cryoglobulinaemic neuropathy 795
cryoglobulins 705–6
  crystals 1575
  preoperative assessment 300
  in rapidly progressive glomerulo-
      nephritis 328
  types 705–6, 1370
cryoprecipitation of immune
    complexes 705–6
cryptococcosis 880
  arteritis in 1390
  epidemiology 954, 955
  in HIV infection 916
  joint infection 955, 962–3
    clinical presentation 956
    diagnosis 957
    management 956

cryptococcosis (*continued*)
  pulmonary infection 252
Cryptosporidium and reactive arthritis 267, *946*, 947
crystal arthropathies 1555–75
  see also specific disorders
CT *see* calcitonin
CT arthrography, shoulder 739–40, 741, 742
CT myelography, cervical spondylosis 1654
CT radiculography 727, 728, 732, 733
CT scanning 719
  ankle 744
  ankylosing spondylitis 1066
  back pain 90, 99, 116, 731–2, 733
  beam hardening artefacts 768
  bone density 720
  brucellar arthritis 939, 940
  cauda equina syndrome 225
  cervical spondylosis 224, 1654
  childhood 116, 753, 754, 766–8
  cysticercosis 950
  diastematomyelia 128, 129, 130
  DILS 911
  elbow 741
  erosions 745
  hip 718
  hydatid cyst 950
  iliopsoas bursitis 157
  interpretation and reliability 8
  intervertebral disc prolapse 125, 1642
  neuropsychiatric SLE 335, 1155, 1156, 1186
  non-gonococcal arthritis 851
  ossification of the posterior longitudinal ligament 735, 737
  osteoarthritis 747, 748, 749
  osteoid osteoma 118, 119, 754, 768, 1618
  osteomyelitis 768, 872, 878
  osteonecrosis 1623
  pulmonary nodules 244
  quantitative 1594, *1595*
  relapsing polychondritis 1626
  respiratory system 245, 246, 250
  rheumatoid arthritis 1017
  sacroiliac joint 737, 738, 753, 768
  sarcoidosis 1466
  shoulder 140
  spine
    lumbar 729
    stenosis 1644, 1645
    tuberculosis 122
  spiral 766
  spondylodiscitis 766
  spondylolysis 126
  systemic sclerosis 250, 1235–6
  talocalcaneal coalition 167, 768
  three-dimensional 766
  tuberculosis 122, 931
  Wegener's granulomatosis 1332
  whiplash injury 1658
  wide-window 1186
  wrist 741
cubital tunnel 137
cuboid 153, 154
Culex annulirostris 903
cuneiform bones 153, 154
Cunninghamella bertholletiae 963
Cushing's syndrome and osteoporosis 128, 433, 1588
cutaneous lymphocyte antigen 528, 529
cutaneous polyarteritis 1407–8
cutis laxa 385
Cutivate *210*
cyanosis 241
cyclo-oxygenase
  Cox-1 260, 511, 516, 577–8
  Cox-2 260, 511, 516, 577–8
  modification by NSAIDs 260, 576, 577–8, 1020
  pathway 515
cyclophilin 594

cyclophosphamide 590
  adverse effects 593–4, *593*, 1344, 1347, 1359–60, 1695
    cutaneous 215
    gastrointestinal *260*, 261, 593, *593*
    haematological 593, *593*
    hepatotoxic 652
    hyperuricaemic 1694
    immunological 252
    oncogenic 289–90, *593*, 594, 1359–60, 1666
    renal 323
    respiratory 241, *253*
  in Behçet's syndrome 1400
  in Churg–Strauss syndrome 1359
  clinical efficacy 592–3
  in combination therapy *1025*
  in giant cell arteritis 1389
  in granulomatous angiitis of the central nervous system 786
  haemorrhagic cystitis induced by 326
  in juvenile chronic arthritis 1126, 1141
  in juvenile dermatomyositis 1297
  in lactation 194, *602*
  metabolic pathway 592
  in microscopic polyangiitis 1358–9, 1362–3
  in mixed connective tissue disease 1423
  in multicentric reticulohistiocytosis *1476*, 1477
  non-selective action 610
  pharmacology 590–1
  in polyarteritis nodosa 1358–9, 1362–3
  in polymyositis/dermatomyositis 1276
  in pregnancy 192, *602*
  pulse 1345, 1358–9, 1362–3, *1363*
  in pyoderma gangrenosum 1461
  in relapsing polychondritis 1627
  in rheumatoid arthritis 1024
  in scleritis 317
  in scleroderma 1240, *1241*
  in Sjögren's syndrome 1314
  in SLE *1173*, 1174, 1190–1
    neuropsychiatric 335, 1186
  structure 591
  in Takayasu's arteritis 1387
  therapeutically relevant effects 591–2, *592*
  in transverse myelitis 225
  treatment regimens 593
  in vasculitis 1329
  in Wegener's granulomatosis 1344, 1345, *1345*, 1347, 1407
cycloserine *932*, 933
cyclosporin 594
  adverse effects 595–6, *595*
    gastrointestinal *260*, *595*
    gout 1566
    hypertrichosis 209, *595*
    hyperuricaemic *1558*, 1694
    myopathic *1265*
    neurological *217*
    oncogenic 290, *595*
    psychiatric 337–8, *337*, *595*
    renal 325–6, 595–6, *595*
  in Behçet's syndrome 1400
  clinical efficacy 595
  in combination therapy *1025*
  drug interactions 957
  in eosinophilic fasciitis 1428
  in HIV-associated nephropathy 915
  in juvenile chronic arthritis 1108, 1126, 1141
  in juvenile dermatomyositis 1297
  in lactation 194, *602*
  in mixed connective tissue disease 1423
  non-selective action 610
  in panniculitis 1455
  pharmacology 594
  in polyarteritis nodosa 1404
  in polymyositis/dermatomyositis 1276
  in pregnancy 192, *602*
  in psoriasis 212, 1079

cyclosporin (*continued*)
  in psoriatic arthritis 1080
  in pyoderma gangrenosum 211, 1461
  in rheumatoid arthritis 629, 1023
  in scleritis 317
  in scleroderma 1240, *1241*
  in streptococcal cell-wall arthritis 565
  therapeutically relevant effects 594–5, *594*
  treatment regimens 595
  in uveitis 317
  in Wegener's granulomatosis 1346, 1359
CYP21 gene 696
cyst
  bone 1467
  calf 49
  myxoid *208*
  pancreatic post-traumatic 255
  popliteal fossa 49
  synovial in juvenile chronic arthritis 1101, 1107
cystathionine synthase 436
cystatin C 1434, *1434*, 1438
cystic fibrosis *1104*
cysticercosis *948*
  articular syndromes associated 947
  muscular syndromes associated 950
  vasculitis in 951
cystine crystals *1575*
cystinosis 1605
cystitis
  drug-related 594, 1359
  haemorrhagic 323, 326
  interstitial in Sjögren's syndrome 1311–12
cystoscopy
  in haematuria 324
  in urinary flow obstruction 326
cytarabine, adverse effects 1694
cytidine deaminase in rheumatoid arthritis 1016, *1017*
cytoid bodies 313, 1153
cytokines 509, 844
  in acute phase response 625–6
  in animal models of arthritis 568–9
  bone-associated 424, *424*
  cascades in arthritic joint 560
  definition 516
  effect of gold therapy on 599, *600*
  effect of methotrexate on 583, *583*
  genes 504–5, 506
  and immunosuppressive therapy strategies 610, 614–15, 1024
  in inflammation 516–18, *516–19*, 520–2
  in Lyme disease 885
  manipulation 614–15
  in osteoarthritis 1537, 1543–5, *1543*
  in polymyositis/dermatomyositis 1269
  receptor families 520, 521
  in rheumatic diseases 521–2
  in rheumatoid arthritis 521–2
    antagonists 995–7
    expression 993–4, *993*
    regulation 994–5
  in SLE 640, 1167–8, *1167*
  and T-cell subsets 520
  see also specific cytokines
cytomegalovirus infection 904
  ocular involvement 319
  pulmonary 253
  in Sjögren's syndrome 1302
  vasculitis in 914
cytosine 689
cytotoxic T cells
  activation 546
  in adaptive immunity 546
  antigen presentation to 547
  antigen processing and presentation to 549–50
  in DILS 911, 912
  in HIV infection 910, 911
  in HLA-B27-associated disease 1042
  and immunosuppressive therapy strategies 609

cytotoxic T cells (*continued*)
  in inflammatory myopathies 789
  in leprosy 933
  in polymyositis/dermatomyositis 1268
  in reactive arthropathies 1092
  in rheumatoid arthritis 991
  in SLE 1165–6, *1166*, 1168
  susceptibility to free radical attack 447

D

5D4 417
D8/17 antigen and rheumatic fever 975
dactylitis
  in HIV infection 919, 920
  in juvenile psoriatic arthritis 1055, 1056
  in leprosy 934
  in psoriatic arthritis 1075
  sarcoid 1468, 1477
  tuberculous 928, 930
Dallas Pain Questionnaire 59
danazol
  in SLE 1175
  in thrombocytopenia 1213
dancers, musculoskeletal problems 1496
dapsone
  adverse effects *217*
  in discoid lupus erythematosus 211
  in giant cell arteritis 1380
  in hypersensitivity vasculitis 1369
  in leprosy 935, 936
  in polymyalgia rheumatica 1380
  in pyoderma gangrenosum 211, 1461
  in relapsing polychondritis 1627
  in thrombocytopenia 1213
  in urticarial vasculitis 1370
DBA/1 mice 567, 997
DDST 56, 57
death, sudden, and overexertion 1777
debrancher deficiency 473
debridement
  in osteomyelitis 875–6
  in tuberculosis 932
decay accelerating factor 528
decorin 410, 415
decubitus ulcers, osteomyelitis in 876
deep infrapatellar bursa 152, 158
deep prepatellar bursa 152
deep transverse metacarpal ligament 139
deep venous thrombosis 222
  in antiphospholipid syndrome 1204
  and hormone replacement therapy 1596, 1597
  preoperative prophylaxis 300
defensins 513
deflazacort 86, 585, 1141
Degos syndrome *209*
dehydration, effect on serum urea concentration 650
7-dehydrocholesterol 430
dehydroepiandrosterone in rheumatoid arthritis 182, 1590
delayed hypersensitivity in tuberculosis 927
delivery
  in juvenile rheumatoid arthritis 184
  in rheumatoid arthritis 181
  in SLE 183
  in systemic sclerosis 184
deltoid 135, 136, 137
deltoid ligament 153
dementia 220
  in antiphospholipid syndrome 222
  in Behçet's syndrome 1397
  in Sjögren's syndrome 1311
  in Whipple's disease 336
Demerol 340
demyelination
  electrophysiology 802–3, *802*
  in entrapment neuropathies 804
  in mixed connective tissue disease 1418

demyelination *(continued)*
  peripheral nerves 793, 794–5
  segmental 802, *802*, 804, 806
denaturing gradient gel electrophoresis 693, 694
dendritic cells in rheumatoid arthritis 992
dental caries 173, *174*, 1307
dentinogenesis imperfecta 358, 361
Denver Development and Screening Test 56, 57
deoxypyridinoline 432, 653
  in osteoarthritis 1538, *1538*
  in osteoporosis 1595
  in rheumatoid arthritis *1017*
depigmentation following local steroid injection 1759
depression
  diagnostic criteria 338–9
  differential diagnosis 1379
  double 336
  drug-related *587*, *595*
  in the elderly 30
  factors associated 67
  and fibromyalgia 1496
  in juvenile chronic arthritis *336*, 337
  management 338–42
  in osteoarthritis 1547–8
  and pain 67, 107
  in polymyalgia rheumatica/giant cell arteritis 1377
  prevalence 67
  in rheumatoid arthritis 336–7, *336*
  in SLE *336*, 337, 1153, 1185–6
  and social support 69
dermatan 1494
dermatan sulphate 1569
dermatitis
  allergic contact 213
  associated with bowel bypass 1095–6
  of chronic stasis 1397
  generalized exfoliative 212
  gold-salt 213, *601*
  NSAID-induced 212, 213
  photoallergic contact 212
  rheumatoid neutrophilic 1462
dermatomal somatosensory evoked potential 802
dermatomes 218, 221
dermatomyositis 1249–80
  aetiology 1266–8
  age at onset 11, 13, 1288
  amyopathic 1252, 1253, 1277
  anaesthesia in 299–300
  animal models 1272–3
  autoantibodies 673, 1258, 1259, 1270–2, *1271*, *1272*
  canine 1273
  capillaroscopy 204
  cardiovascular involvement *230*, *1253*, 1254–5, 1290
  classification 1249–50, *1250*
  clinical features 1250–6, *1414*
  creatine kinase in 653
  cutaneous involvement 41, **1250–2**, 1253, 1289
    calcification *208*
    erythema 201, 204, 1250–1
    hypopigmentation *209*
    periorbital erythema and oedema 201, 204, 1251, 1289
    poikiloderma 207, 1250–1
    skin biopsy 1262–3
    treatment 1277
    ulceration 207
  diagnosis 1258, 1260–3, *1260*
  differential diagnosis 1136, *1137*, 1263–6, *1264*, *1265*
  distinction from polymyositis *1269*
  drug-related 1022
  epidemiology 1249
  gastrointestinal involvement 257, *258*, *1253*, 1255, 1277, 1290
  genitourinary involvement 1290

dermatomyositis *(continued)*
  geographic factors 1249
  imaging 754, 1260–1
  immunogenetics 1268
  incidence 1249
  investigation 204
  juvenile 21, **1287–97**
    aetiology 1288–9
    clinical presentation 1289–91
    course 1295–6
    diagnostic criteria *1288*
    differential diagnosis 1122, 1291, *1292*, 1293
    epidemiology 1288–9
    genetics 1295
    haematology 1295
    immunology 1294–5
    pathophysiology 1293–5
    physiotherapy 1750–1
    sex differences 14
    treatment 1296–7, *1296*
    vasculopathy 1293, 1408
  laboratory tests *649*, 1256–8, *1257*
  liver function 652
  and malignant disease 289, 1255–6, 1267, 1668–9
  muscle involvement 471
    atrophy 790
    biopsy 788, 789, 790, 1261–2, 1263, 1290
    childhood 1289–90, 1293
    inflammation 789
    necrosis 789, 790
    vacuoles 791
    vasculitis 791
    weakness 470, 1250, 1289–90
  myoglobinuria in 323, 327
  nail involvement 41, 203
  ocular involvement 1290–1
  overlap syndromes 1423–4
  pathogenesis 1268–72, *1269*, *1271*, *1272*
  and pregnancy 185, 1256
  prevalence 1249
  prognosis 1278
  in protozoal infection 947
  pulmonary involvement *241*, 243, 1252–4, *1253*, 1290
  rehabilitation 1278
  renal involvement 1256
  risk factors 1249
  systemic features 1252
  temporal factors 1249
  treatment 211, 1273–8, *1274*
dermatosis–arthritis syndrome 1462
dermoid cysts 127
Dermovate 210
descending inhibition *488*
desert rheumatism 956
desipramine 339, 340, *340*, *341*
  plasma concentrations *342*
  in rheumatoid arthritis 342
desmin 455, 459
desoxymethasone *210*
desquamation *175*
Desyrel *see* trazodone
developmental status measures in childhood 56, 57–8
DEXA *see* dual-energy X-ray absorptiometry
dexamethasone *585*
  adverse effects 337
  in intramedullary spinal cord abscess 124
  in lactation 193
  in pregnancy 191
  in prevention of neonatal lupus erythematosus 1199
dextropropoxyphene
  adverse effects *217*
  in chronic back pain 1648
  in pregnancy 189
  and sport 1778
DGGE 693, 694
DHEAS in rheumatoid arthritis 1590

DHP receptors 456
diabetes insipidus in Wegener's granulomatosis 1336
diabetes mellitus
  arthropathy *1137*, 1138
  autoantibodies 285, *668*
  and calcium pyrophosphate dihydrate disease 283, *283*, *1531*, 1567
  and carpal tunnel syndrome 284
  and cheiroarthropathy 163
  and diffuse idiopathic skeletal hyperostosis 283
  drug-related *587*
  and Dupuytren's contracture 284
  genetic factors 556
  and gout 283
  HLA associations 285, 554
  and hyperuricaemia 283
  musculoskeletal involvement **282–5**, *283*
  neuropathy 283–4, 795
  and osteoarthritis *283*, 1519
  osteolysis in 284
  osteomyelitis in 284, 869
  and osteoporosis 128, *283*
  and periarthritis of the shoulder 284
  and pyogenic arthritis 852
  rheumatic symptoms *218*
  skin and joint involvement 207
  and SLE 1167
  and soft tissue rheumatism 284–5
  susceptibility to 554
  syndrome of limited joint mobility 282–3
  and trigger finger 284–5
diabetic amyotrophy *283*
diabetic neuropathy 283–4
diabetic stiff-hand syndrome 282–3, *283*
diagnosis
  childhood 15–18, 19
  criteria 811–12, *812*
  intuitive *3*
dialysis
  in acute renal failure 330
  aluminium intoxication 433
  amyloidosis in 289, 1439–40
  and calcium oxalate arthritis 1574, 1575
  in hyperparathyroidism 280
  olecranon bursitis associated 146
  and osteomyelitis 868
  in SLE 1174
  in systemic sclerosis 1238
3,4-diaminopyridine in Eaton–Lambert syndrome 1675
diaphyseal aclasis 118
diarrhoea
  drug-related
    azathioprine *591*
    cyclosporin *595*
    gold therapy 260, 261, *601*
    methotrexate *584*
  infective 259
  in reactive arthropathies 663, 1087–8
  in SLE 257, 1156
diastematomyelia 127, 128, 129, 130
diastrophic dysplasia *369*, 436
diclofenac 100
  adverse effects
    cutaneous 213, 580
    gastrointestinal *1021*
    haematological 295
    hepatotoxic 580
    neurological 217
  and gastric ulceration 578
  half-life *577*
  in juvenile chronic arthritis *1106*, 1138, *1140*
  in lactation 193, 194
  in pregnancy 190
  in psoriatic arthritis 1080
  in seropositive juvenile chronic arthritis 1035

diet 262–7, *263–4*, *265*, *266*, 1694
  in autoimmune disease 615–16
  and disease occurrence 824
  elemental 616
  elimination therapy 264, *266*
  and energy 1774
  and exercise 1780
  fat in 616
  lactovegetarian 616
  oral tolerance therapy 264–5
  in psoriatic arthritis 1080
  restriction 265, 615–16
  in rheumatoid arthritis 1024, 1026, 1694
  in SLE 1175
  supplementation therapy 262, *263–4*, 264, *265*
diethylcarbamazine 951
diethylpropion hydrochloride *1223*
diethylstilboestrol 189
diethyopropion 1693
differential agglutination titre 674
differential diagnosis 4
diffuse idiopathic skeletal hyperostosis (DISH) 1657
  and diabetes mellitus 283
  differential diagnosis 1065, *1066*
  imaging 735, 737, 739
  movement limitation in 1654
diffuse infiltrative lymphocytosis syndrome (DILS) 911
  clinical features 911–12
  diagnosis 913
  pathogenesis 912–13
  treatment 913
diflunisal
  adverse effects 580
  half-life *577*
  in lactation 193
  in pregnancy 190
  renal clearance 577
digit infarction *174*
digital nerve iatrogenic damage 803
digitalis sensitivity in amyloidosis 1442
digoxigenin 690
digoxin
  interaction with NSAIDs *579*
  in juvenile chronic arthritis 1126
dihydrocodeine and sport 1778
1,25-dihydroxycholecalciferol
  anabolic effects 426
  in calcium homeostasis 430, 431
  defective 1α-hydroxylation 433
  deficiency 129
  effect on osteoclasts 424, *425*
  end-organ resistance to 433
  in lymphoma 437
  in osteoblast differentiation 425
  plasma measurement 430
  role in synthesis of osteocalcin 427
  synthetic pathways and molecular and cellular effects 430, 431
  therapy in juvenile osteoporosis 129
dilantin, effect on prolactin levels 282
DILS *see* diffuse infiltrative lymphocytosis syndrome
diltiazem in myositis ossificans 1783
dimethyl sulphoxide in amyloidosis 1442
dimethylcysteine *see* D-penicillamine
dinitrophenol 690
dipeptidyl peptidase IV 452
diphosphonates *see* bisphosphonates
diplopia *174*
  in cervical spondylosis 1653
  in giant cell arteritis 1378
  in myasthenia gravis 216
  in Takayasu's arteritis 1385
  in vertebrobasilar insufficiency 223
Diprosalic *210*
dipyridamole
  in Kawasaki disease 1406
  in polyarteritis nodosa 1404

dipyridamole *(continued)*
  in scleroderma 1240
  in SLE in pregnancy 183
Dirofilaria
  D. immitis 948, 950
  D. tenuis 948, 950
disability 64
  definition 52, 1723
  and functional anatomy 1724–5
  measurement 1723–4
  prediction 65
  prevalence 65
  and quality of life 65
  reporting 65
  in rheumatoid arthritis 54
Disability Employment Advisers 110
disc diffusion test 659
discectomy 123
discitis
  of childhood 97–8, 117, 123–4
  postoperative 123
discography 730, 731, 733
  intervertebral disc prolapse 1642, 1643
  normal and abnormal patterns 733, 735
disease modifying antirheumatic
    drugs and malignancy 290
disease occurrence *see* epidemiology
disease patterns 178–9
DISH *see* diffuse idiopathic skeletal hyper-
    ostosis
disodium cromoglycate in pyoderma
    gangrenosum 211
disseminated intravascular coagula-
    tion 329
distal interphalangeal joints 138, 140
  local steroid injection 1767
  in psoriatic arthritis 1073, 1074
distal radio-ulnar joint 137
  local steroid injection 1765
distal radio-ulnar ligament in rheu-
    matoid arthritis 1014
distal tibiofibular joint 153
distribution of rheumatic diseases *4*
dithranol in psoriasis 212
diuretics
  adverse effects *208*, 1371
  drug interactions *579*
  and gout 684, 1555, 1556, 1694
  and hyperuricaemia *1558*
divers, osteonecrosis 1622
divorce 66
dizziness 231
  and back pain 99
  in cervical spondylosis 1653
  drug-related *578*, *584*, 588
  in Takayasu's arteritis 1385
DMA gene 696
DMARDS and malignancy 290
DMB gene 696
DNA 347
  analysis 350, 354, 548, 660–1, 689–90
  analysis of repetitive sequences 694–5,
    695
  denaturation 689–90
  detection 660–1
  gel electrophoresis 690
  hybridization/renaturation 689–90
  labelling 690
  microsatellite 695, *695*
  minisatellite 695, *695*
  polymorphism localization 693, 694
  probes 690
  satellite 694, *695*
  sequencing 694
  short tandem repeats 695, *695*
  in SLE 1165
docosahexaenoic acid 262, *263–4*
dog heartworm *948*, 950
dopamine β-hydroxylase 451
Doppler ultrasound
  childhood 760–4, 765
  giant cell arteritis 1389
  ruptured Baker's cyst 158
  temporal artery 1378

dorsal carpal ligament 138, 139
dorsal exostoses 1512
dorsal root ganglion 442
dorsal tarsometatarsal ligament 153
dot blot procedure 690, 691
double crush syndrome 804, 1660
Dougados Functional Index *58*, *59*
dowager's hump 1591, 1592
Down's syndrome
  amyloid protein in 1434, *1434*, 1439
  atlantoaxial subluxation in 224
  and colchicine therapy 1449
doxepin 339, *340*, *341*, *342*
doxycycline
  in brucellar arthritis 943, *943*
  in Lyme disease *891*, 892, 893
  in mycoplasma arthritis 969
Dracunculus medinensis 948, 949
drawer signs 144
Dressler syndrome 232
driving 1735
drop-arm sign 142
drug abuse
  and mycotic aneurysm 1390
  and osteomyelitis 868
  and pyogenic arthritis 852
  and secondary infection in HIV infec-
    tion 916
drugs
  administration and use by the elderly
    27, *27*
  adverse effects *see under specific drugs or*
    systems
  and anaesthesia 301
  anaesthetic 306, *307*
  antifungal 956–7
  antiparasitic 951
  antirheumatic **581–603**
    toxicity 1695–6
  autoantibody induction by 1692–3,
    1692
  autoimmune disease induced by *1690*,
    1690–4
  banned in sport and athletics 1778
  combination therapies
    in gout 1565
    in polymyositis/dermatomyositis
      1276
    in rheumatoid arthritis 1023, 1024,
      1025
    in seropositive juvenile chronic
      arthritis 1036
  and disease occurrence 825–6, *825*
  gastroprotective 578
  half-life of elimination 576
  interactions
    anticoagulants 1211
    antimalarials 1021
    azoles 957
    in the elderly 27
    methotrexate 296, 582
    NSAIDs *579*, 580, 1020
  metabolic reactions to 1694–5
  ocular side-effects 318–19
  in pregnancy and lactation **188–95**
  psychotropic 339–42, *340*, *341*, *342*
  rheumatic complications **1689–96**
  and surgery 1702
DSEP 802
DTPA clearance in systemic sclerosis
    1237
dual-energy/electron X-ray absorpti-
    ometry (DEXA) 29, 720, 721, 1594,
    1595
  reflex sympathetic dystrophy *1683*
  rheumatoid arthritis 1011
dual-photon absorptiometry 720,
    1594, *1595*, *1683*
Duchenne muscular dystrophy
  differential diagnosis 1291
  electromyography 1293
  muscle in 217, 457
  scoliosis in 115, 117–18, 131

duodenal ulceration and NSAID use
    578, 1020
Dupuytren's contracture 147–8, 1506
  and diabetes mellitus 284
  and Paget's disease 1613
  skin nodules and papules *208*
Dupuytren's diathesis 147
dwarfism
  diastrophic *435*, 1630
  see also achondroplasia
Dyggve–Melchior–Clausen syndrome
    1631
dynorphin 496
dysaesthesia in reflex sympathetic
    dystrophy 1682
dysarthria
  in myasthenia gravis 216
  in vertebrobasilar insufficiency 223
dyslipidaemia *see* hyperlipidaemia
dyspareunia 178, 1310
dysphagia 173, *175*, 257, *258*
  in cervical spondylosis 1653
  in cervical vertebral osteomyelitis 878
  in inclusion-body myositis 1278
  in mixed connective tissue disease 1417
  in polymyositis/dermatomyositis 1255,
    1277
  in Sjögren's syndrome 1310
  in SLE 1156–7
dyspnoea 3, 173, 231, 242–3
  in angina pectoris 231
  in eosinophilia–myalgia syndrome 1426
  in mixed connective tissue disease
    1418
  paroxysmal nocturnal 231
  in sarcoidosis 1465
  in Sjögren's syndrome 1310
  in SLE 1195
  in toxic oil syndrome 1426
  in Wegener's granulomatosis 1336
dysthymic disorder in rheumatoid
    arthritis 336
dystrophin 455, 457

E

E-a₁PI 653–4
E-selectin 529, *529*, 599, 1168, *1169*
  counter-receptors 530
  in microscopic polyangiitis 1357
  oligosaccharide ligands 529–30
  in rheumatoid arthritis 988, 990
  in scleroderma 1227
  in SLE 1168
  in Takayasu's arteritis 1386
  in Wegener's granulomatosis 1339
ear
  nodules *174*
  in relapsing polychondritis 1625, 1626
  skin lesions 201, 202
  in Wegener's granulomatosis 1335, 1337
Eaton–Lambert myasthenic
    syndrome 216, 1674–5
EBT 1427
eburnation 1541
EBV *see* Epstein–Barr virus
EC 3.4.24.11 451, 452
ECAM 460
ecchymoses 207
ECG *see* electrocardiography
Echinococcus see hydatid cyst
echocardiography
  childhood 764
  during exercise 1777
  hypertrophic obstructive cardiomyo-
    pathy 1777
  in Kawasaki disease 1405
  pericardial effusion 234
  pericardial tamponade 235
  pericarditis 235
  preanaesthetic 299
  SLE 1149, 1194
    neuropsychiatric 221

echo-Doppler cardiography, pre-
    anaesthetic 299
echovirus infection 904, 970–1
ECLAM 1160
Ecstasy and hyperpyrexia 1778
ECT 339
ectopic parathyroid hormone
    syndrome 437
EDRF *see* nitric oxide
edrophonium test, false positive *219*
EDTA, ⁵¹CR-labelled 648
education
  and disability 65
  and employment 66
EEG *see* electroencephalography
effect size 52
Effexor 340
Ehlers–Danlos syndrome 168, 435–6
  cardiovascular involvement *230*, 238
  differential diagnosis 1500
  gastrointestinal involvement *259*
  genetics 383–5
  scoliosis in 115, *116*
  skin involvement 199, 207, *208*
  type 1 353, 356, *369*, 383, 384, 385–7,
    436
  type 2 353, 356, *369*, 383, 385–7, 436
  type 3 353, 378, 385, 436
  type 4 353, 378–9, 380, 383, 436
    biochemical and genetic changes
      379, 381–3
  type 5 383, 385
  type 6 383, 385, 436
  type 7 353, 357, 366, 367, 383, 385, 436
  type 8 353, 385
eicosapentaenoic acid 262, *263–4*, 264,
    515, 616, 1480, 1484–5
EIFEL Questionnaire 59
Eikenella corrodens in pyogenic arthritis
    852, 863, *880*
El Salvador, prevalence of rheumatoid
    arthritis *835*
ELAM-1 *see* E-selectin
elastase 513, 1356
  neutrophil 514, 515
  in rheumatoid arthritis *1017*
elastase-a₁ proteinase inhibitor
    complexes 653–4
elastin 353, 368
  effect of penicillamine on 214
  in ligaments 1492
elastosis perforans serpiginosa 214
elbow
  applied anatomy 136, 137
  arthroplasty 1703, 1704, 1720
  carrying angle 137
  dialysis 146
  examination 43
  extension 137
  flexion 137
  functional anatomy and disability
    1725
  imaging
    arthrography 740–1
    CT 741
    MRI 741
    radiography 715, 716
  in juvenile chronic arthritis 1100, 1133,
    1720, 1740
  Little-league 163, 1787
  local steroid injection 145, *1762*, 1764–5
  miner's 146
  osteoarthritis 1532
  pain 1504–5, *1504*, *1505*
    adult *139–40*, 144–6
    childhood 163, *163*
  palpation 43
  physiotherapy, childhood 1740
  pulled/nursemaid's 163
  range of movement 43
  in rheumatoid arthritis 1008
  screening 43
  student's 146
  surgery 1703, 1720

elbow (continued)
synovectomy 1703, 1720
see also golfer's elbow; tennis elbow
elderly 22–37
back pain 25, 101–2, 102, 108
characteristics 31
cognitive capacity 30
depression 30
disease frequency 25–6, 26
drug administration and use 27, 27
drug-related lupus erythematosus 36
examination 37
exercise and physical activity 28–9
laboratory tests 27–8, 28
maintenance of independence 30
management plans 9
multiple disease occurrence 26–7
muscle biopsy 465
nutrition 30
osteoarthritis 25, 31–2
concomitant disease 33
differential diagnosis 32, 33
osteomalacia 1603
patient education 31
polymyalgia rheumatica 34
preventive medicine 29
psychological factors 30
rheumatic diseases
organization of comprehensive care 30–1, 31
systemic features 178–9
rheumatoid arthritis 25–6, 32
concomitant disease 33
differential diagnosis 32, 33
treatment 33–4
RS₃PE syndrome 34–5
sicca syndrome 36
Sjögren's syndrome 35, 36
SLE 35–6, 35, 1159
social losses 30
soft-tissue rheumatism 36–7, 1491
systemic sclerosis 36
temporal arteritis 34
weight loss 30
electrical alternans in pericardial tamponade 235
electrical stimulation in osteo-necrosis 1624
electrocardiography (ECG)
during exercise 1777
hypertrophic obstructive cardio-myopathy 1777
juvenile chronic arthritis 1116
mixed connective tissue disease 1418
pericardial effusion 234
pericardial tamponade 235
pericarditis 234
polymyositis/dermatomyositis 1255, 1290
preanaesthetic 299
rheumatic fever 978
SLE 1149
electroconvulsant therapy 339
electroencephalography (EEG)
fibromyalgia 1498
neuropsychiatric SLE 221, 334, 1155
electroergoniometry 479
electrolyte balance in acute renal failure 330
electromyography (EMG) 466, 801–2
acromegaly 281
acute compression neuropathy 803
acute nerve injury 803
blanket technique 802
carcinomatous neuropathy 1674
cervical spondylosis 1655
in childhood 1293
Duchenne muscular dystrophy 1293
effect of age on 807
effect of temperature on 806–7
entrapment neuropathy 803–6, 1013
fibromyalgia 1498
hyperparathyroidism 280
hypothyroidism 278

electromyography (EMG) (continued)
inclusion-body myositis 1279
measurement of internal loads on joints 478
myasthenia gravis 1293
polymyositis/dermatomyositis 1258, 1260
sarcoidosis 1469
single fibre techniques 802
spontaneous fibrillation potentials 801
syndrome of limited joint mobility 282
electrophysiology 799–807
elevation in acute injury 1781
elimination therapy 264, 266
ELISA
autoantibodies 667–8, 669
rheumatoid factor 1015
Elocon 210
embryology, critical periods 73
embryonic cell adhesion molecule 460
emetine, adverse effects 1265, 1693
EMG see electromyography
emphysema 248
employment 66
Employment Rehabilitation Centres 110
empty can sign 141
empyema 242
ENA-78 990
enalapril and renal function 325
encephalomyelitis, experimental allergic 612, 844
encephalopathy
hypertensive 334
in Lyme disease 888
in Sjögren's syndrome 1311
uraemic 334
endarteritis obliterans 787, 1311
endocarditis 176
and antiphospholipid antibodies 293
in Behçet's syndrome 1397
in SLE 1151, 1194
endocrine system
amyloidosis 1439
disorders 277–86
endometriosis and osteoporosis 1589
endomysium 457
endorphins in fibromyalgia 1498–9
endothelial cells
activation 536–7
effects of hypoxia on 447–8
in inflammation 512, 527
interactions with lymphocytes 526–7, 534–7
molecules synthesized by 1227
in scleroderma 1226–7
substance P containing 450
endothelial leucocyte adhesion mole-cule-1 see E-selectin
endothelin 447, 1386, 1399
endothelium-derived relaxing factor see nitric oxide
endotoxaemia in acute renal failure 327
endotracheal intubation 1702
in ankylosing spondylitis 303
in juvenile chronic arthritis 302–3, 1721
in rheumatoid arthritis 301–2
in scleroderma 303–4
in seronegative spondylarthropathies 303
in Sjögren's syndrome 303–4
techniques 204–5
endstage renal disease 323
in Henoch–Schönlein purpura 1407
in HIV infection 915
hyperuricaemia in 1558
in SLE 1152, 1154, 1174
energy
conservation 1728, 1728
and diet 1774
enhancer elements 349

enteric arthropathies 1093–6, 1104
see also specific diseases
enteritis in SLE 1196
Enterobacter
antibiotic therapy 856, 880
in osteomyelitis 868
in pyogenic arthritis 852
enterococcal infections
antibiotic therapy 856
and arthritis 852
in osteomyelitis 870
enterocolitis, gold 260, 261, 601
enteropathic spondylitis 1040
enterotoxin
staphylococcal 551, 844
as superantigen 844
enthesis 1492
blood supply 1492
enthesopathy
in ankylosing spondylitis 1061, 1062–3
differential diagnosis 1105
in the elderly 37
in enteric arthropathies 1094
in HIV infection 918–19, 920
in hypophosphataemic rickets 1605
local ischaemia in 1493
in psoriatic arthritis 1075, 1076
in reactive arthropathies 1087, 1090
entrapment neuropathies 177, 178, 225–7
electrophysiology 803–6, 804
in osteoarthritis 1537
in rheumatoid arthritis 227, 1008, 1013
env gene 908
environmental factors in disease occurrence 823–6, 824, 825
enzyme antagonists in scleroderma 1241
enzyme-linked immunosorbent assay see ELISA
eosinophil cationic protein 513
eosinophilia 292, 643, 644
in adult-onset Still's disease 1127
in Churg–Strauss syndrome 1325, 1354, 1358
drug-related 296
in polyarteritis nodosa 1358
pulmonary 245, 247
in sarcoidosis 644, 1465
synovial fluid 682, 682
eosinophilia–myalgia syndrome 207, 644, 789, 1220, 1425–7, 1694
aetiology 1427
childhood 1427–8
clinical features 1425–6, 1426
epidemiology 1425
laboratory tests 1426, 1427
myopathy in 1265, 1266
pathogenesis 1427
prognosis 1427
treatment 1427
eosinophilic fasciitis 644, 789, 1428, 1675
eosinophilic granuloma 120, 121
eosinophils
effect of corticosteroids on 586
in inflammation 512–13
in inflammatory myopathies 789
in peripheral neuropathy 795–6
phagocytosis 513
in scleroderma 1223
eosinophiluria 327
epidemic polyarthritis 903–4
epidemiology 811–26
aetiological models 820–1
birth cohort trends 817–18
changes over time 1044–5
childhood rheumatic disease 10–12
clinical 811
comorbidity 823
definition 811
diagnostic criteria 811–12, 812
disease occurrence 812–20
environmental factors 823–6, 824, 825

epidemiology (continued)
estimation of occurrence 813–14, 814
factors affecting occurence 815–20
and family size/position in family 823
genetic factors 821–2, 821, 822
geographical influences 819–20, 820
incidence 813, 813
measures 813, 813
menstrual, hormonal and reproductive factors 823
non-European populations 828–40, 828–40
non-genetic host factors 822–3, 823
occurrence 814
overview 814–15, 814, 815
population surveys 813, 814
prevalence 813, 813
racial influences 818–19, 819
and rehabilitation 1723
Rochester Epidemiology Program 814
time trends 816–17, 817, 818
see also under specific diseases
epidermal growth factor
effect on cartilage 415
effect on osteoclasts 424, 425
in rheumatoid arthritis 993
epidermolysis bullosa, generalized atrophic benign 353
epidermolysis bullosa acquisita 205
epidermolysis bullosa dystrophica 353, 386–7, 388–9
epidermolysis bullosa inversa 388
epidermolysis bullosa mitis 388, 389
epididymitis in Behçet's syndrome 1398
epidural anaesthesia 306
in cardiovascular disease 299
in low back pain 105–6
epidural analgesia
in back pain 105–6, 1648
cervical 307
frequency of back pain following 93
epilepsy 177, 1207
epimysium 458
epiphyseal cartilage 771
epiphyseal dysplasias 168, 1630–1
epiphyses
defects, radiography 756
overgrowth in juvenile chronic arthritis 82, 85
stapling 1718
episcleritis 173, 174, 310, 311, 1011
in Behçet's syndrome 1396
in relapsing polychondritis 1626
in SLE 1153
in Wegener's granulomatosis 1337
epistaxis in rheumatic fever 979
epithelioid cell sarcoma 208
epoxy resins 209, 1223
Epstein–Barr virus (EBV) 904
and Kawasaki disease 1406
and ocular disease 317
and rheumatoid arthritis 823–4, 986
and Sjögren's syndrome 1302
Erb's point 800
ergocalciferol 430, 1602
erosions 201, 745
imaging 724–5, 726, 727
in mixed connective tissue disease 1417
in seropositive juvenile chronic arthritis 1033, 1034
erosive arthritis
with amyloidosis 1440
basic calcium phosphate crystals in 1573
radiography 1534
erysipelotherix 999
erythema 201
annular
in Sjögren's syndrome 1310
in SLE 1182–3

erythema *(continued)*
in dermatomyositis 201, 204, 1250–1, 1289
differential diagnosis 204
facial 204
in familial Mediterranean fever 1447
over Heberden's nodes 205
periarticular 205
periungual 202
'slapped cheek' 204
strawberry of tongue and lips 204
erythema annulare *175*, 199, 200, 979
erythema chronicum migrans 199, 204, 884, 887–8
differential diagnosis 890
erythema elevatum diutinum 1370–1
erythema induratum 1371
erythema infectiosum 204, 880, 897
erythema marginatum *175*, 199, 200, 979
erythema migrans *see* erythema chronicum migrans
erythema multiforme
bullae/target lesions 200, 205, 206
differential diagnosis 890
drug-related 213, *578*
orogenital involvement 207
erythema nodosum *175*, 206, *208*, 289, 1450–1
aetiology and associations *1451*
in bowel bypass syndrome 1095
chronic 1450
differential diagnosis 1455
in enteric arthropathies 1094
evaluation 1455
lesions resembling in Behçet's syndrome 1395–6
in mixed connective tissue disease 1417
postyersinial 1091–2
in pregnancy 1451
in sarcoidosis 1465, 1466
in Takayasu's arteritis 1385
treatment 1455
erythema nodosum leprosum 933, 934–5
erythema nodosum migrans 1450
erythrocyte sedimentation rate (ESR) 3
acute phase response 625, 626, 639, *639*
adult Still's disease 641
ankylosing spondylitis 628, 1063, 1066
back pain 97
brucellar arthritis 941
childhood 17
back pain 116
discitis 123
pyogenic arthritis 862
drug-induced lupus 1690
in the elderly 28
elevation with normal C-reactive protein 640
giant cell arteritis 627–8, 640, 1378, 1389
hypersensitivity vasculitis 1368
infective discitis 640
juvenile chronic arthritis 1120, 1135
and malaise 172
marked elevation 640
myeloma 640
non-gonococcal arthritis 850
osteoarthritis 627
osteomyelitis 640, 871, 878
polymyalgia rheumatica 627–8, 640, 1378
polymyositis/dermatomyositis 1258
prosthetic joint infection 854
psoriatic arthritis 1077
reactive arthropathies 1088
reliability 7
rheumatic fever 980
rheumatoid arthritis 628–9, 640, 1016, *1016*
RS₃PE syndrome 35
Sjögren's syndrome 1312

erythrocyte sedimentation rate (ESR) *(continued)*
SLE 628, 640, 1157
systemic amyloidosis 640
Takayasu's arteritis 1386
tuberculosis 122
Wegener's granulomatosis 1341
erythrocytes
in anaemia of chronic disease 635–6
aplasia 291, 295, 297
in SLE 641, *641*
erythroderma
in dermatomyositis 1252
in psoriasis 205
erythroid aplasia in juvenile chronic arthritis 1119
erythromycin
in Lyme disease 892
in pyogenic arthritis 857
erythropoiesis
in anaemia of chronic disease 633, 635
and iron absorption 634
erythropoietin
in anaemia of chronic disease 291, 633, 635
in juvenile chronic arthritis 1125
recombinant 633
in anaemia of chronic disease 638
cost 638
use by athletes 1775
Escherichia coli
and childhood Reiter's syndrome 1054
pulmonary infection 252
in pyogenic arthritis 852
and rheumatoid arthritis 986
Eskimos
juvenile chronic arthritis 829, *830*
juvenile spondylarthropathies *832*
rheumatoid arthritis 832–3, *834*
seronegative spondylarthropathies 838, *838*, *840*
SLE *836*
see also ethnic groups
ESR *see* erythrocyte sedimentation rate
ethambutol
and hyperuricaemia *1558*, 1694
in tuberculosis 931, *932*, 933
ethinyloestradiol 182
ethionamide in tuberculosis *932*, 933
ethnic groups
amyloidosis *1434*, 1438, 1439
ankylosing spondylitis *819*, 1060–1, 1067
and disease occurrence 818–19, *819*, **828–40**
drug-induced lupus 1692
familial Mediterranean fever 1445, *1446*
and genetic markers of disease 699
genetic variation between 689
giant cell arteritis/polymyalgia rheumatica 1375
HLA-B27 subtypes *1042*
HLA-DR4 frequency 984
juvenile chronic arthritis *819*, *819*, 829–31, *829*, *830*, *831*
microscopic polyangiitis 1354
osteoarthritis *819*, *819*, 1518
osteoporosis 1594, *1594*
polyarteritis nodosa 1353
polymyositis/dermatomyositis 1267, 1288
rheumatoid arthritis *819*, *819*, *1007*
seronegative spondylarthropathies 1043
Sjögren's syndrome 1302–3, *1303*
SLE *819*, *819*, 833, 835–8, *836*, *837*, 1169
1,1′-ethylidene bis[tryptophan] 1427
etidronate
in osteoporosis 29, 1598
in Paget's disease 1615, 1616
structure 1615
etodolac
adverse effects 260
half-life *577*

etretinate
in HIV-associated arthritis 921
in psoriasis 212
Eubacterium 269
E. aerofaciens, arthritogenicity of cell-wall fragments 564
EULAR, diagnostic criteria for chronic childhood arthritis 10, *10*, 1131
Eumovate *210*
European Community Lupus Activity Measure 1160
European League Against Rheumatism, diagnostic criteria for chronic childhood arthritis 10, *10*, 1131
European Seronegative Study Group, diagnostic criteria 1038, *1039*
European Spondylarthropathy Study Group, diagnostic criteria 1038
Evans' syndrome 292, 641, 1207
evening primrose oil 262, 264, *265*, 1480, 1484
Ewing's sarcoma 120, *1671*
examination 39–51
adult patients 7
ankle 50
childhood 15–17
elbow 43
in the elderly 37
foot 50–1
general principles 39–41, *40*
hands 41–2, *42*
heel 50–1
hip 47–9
joint inspection 40, *40*
joint palpation 40, *40*
joint range of movement 40
knee 49, 50
recording measurements 40–1
rectal 47
sacroiliac joints 47
shoulder girdle 43–5
skin 41, 200
spine
cervical 45–6
lumbar 46–7, *47*, 48
thoracic 46
subtalar joint 50
systematic survey 41–51
temporomandibular joint 45
wrist 42–3
examination under anaesthetic, childhood 1721
exercise
adaptations to 1776–7
aerobic 28
and age 25, 28–9
and amenorrhoea 1777
anaerobic 28
and asthma 1775–6
benefits 1779
and bone mass 1593
in chronic low back pain 103
and diet 1780
eccentric/plyometric 467–9, *470*
effect on articular cartilage 405–6
effect on serum creatinine 649
excessive and osteoporosis 433
fatiguing 467
in fibromyalgia 1499
and hydration 1780
intra-articular pressure changes with 446
in osteoarthritis 1546–7
and osteoporosis 29, 1596
overexertion/overtraining 1777–8
programme 1727, *1727*
and proteinuria 650
repeated 469
and training 1780
warm up/cool down 1780
Exiophiala
E. jeanselmei 963
E. spinifera 963

exons 347, 349
exostosis, imaging 761
experimental arthritis
and pregnancy 182
susceptibility of animal strains to 510
experimental models *see* animal models
extensor carpi radialis brevis 137, 138, 139, 145
extensor carpi radialis longus 137, 138, 139
extensor carpi ulnaris 138, 139
inflammation in psoriatic arthritis 1075–6
extensor digiti minimi 138, 139, 140
surgery 1704
extensor digitorum communis 137, 138, 139, 140
extensor digitorum longus 154, 156
extensor hallucis longus 154
extensor hood/expansion 139
extensor indicis proprius 138, 139, 140
transfer 1704
extensor pollicis brevis 138, 139, 140, 146
extensor pollicis longus 138, 139, 140
surgery 1704
extensor retinaculum 138, 139
extensor tendons
in rheumatoid arthritis 1008, 1014
rupture 1725
surgery 1704–5
eyelid oedema and erythema 201, 204, 1251, 1289
eyes
in adult-onset Still's disease 1127
adverse drug effects 318–19, *587*, 596, 1695
in ankylosing spondylitis 314, 315, 316, 1059, 1064
in Behçet's syndrome 315, 316, 317, 318, 1396
in CINCA 1471, 1472
collagen expression 407, 408
disorders 310, 312
diagnostic and laboratory tests 317
treatment 317–18
dry 310, *311*
examination 310
in giant cell arteritis 312, 313, 1378
in infective arthropathies 316–17
involvement in rheumatic disease 173, *174*, **310–19**, 1011
childhood 316
in juvenile chronic arthritis 316, 317, 699, 1101–3, *1102*, 1108–9, *1108*, 1118
manifestations of systemic inflammatory diseases 312–15, 316
painful red 310, *311*
in polymyositis/dermatomyositis 1290–1
in reactive arthropathies 314, 316, 317, 1087
in relapsing polychondritis 1626
in Sjögren's syndrome 310, 1309
in SLE 312–13, 314, 1153
slit-lamp examination 310
symptoms and signs 310, *311*
in systemic sclerosis 313
in Takayasu's arteritis 1385
in Wegener's granulomatosis 313, 314, 1335, 1335–6, 1337

F

F actin 455
F-wave 801, 805
Faber test 117, 1073
Fabere sign 863
Fabry's disease 168, **1635**
face
'butterfly' erythema 199
erythema 204

face (continued)
  features in Ehlers–Danlos syndrome type 4 378, 380
  flushing following local steroid injection 1759
face validity 52
facet joints 90–1, 1640
  arthrography 1644
  imaging 729
  injection into 1648
  and leg length 97
  lumbar spine 729
  osteoarthritis 91–2, 1533, 1644
  syndromes 1644
facial nerve
  entrapment neuropathy 806
  in leprosy 934
  palsy
    in Lyme disease 888, 890
    in SLE 1153, 1184
    in Wegener's granulomatosis 1335, 1337
factor H 624
factor I 624
factor V 681
factor VII 681
factor VIII 624
factor VIII-related antigen see von Willebrand factor
factor X deficiency in amyloidosis 1436
factor XII
  deficiency 512
  in gout 1559
  in innate immunity 545
familial amyloid cardiomyopathy 1433, 1434, 1434, 1438, 1439, 1442
familial amyloid polyneuropathy 1433, 1434, 1438, 1442
familial combined hyperlipidaemia 1481
  see also hyperlipidaemias
familial hypercholesterolaemia 1481, 1481
  see also hyperlipidaemias
familial hypertriglyceridaemia 1481
  see also hyperlipidaemias
familial Mediterranean fever 206, 1123, 1136, 1137, 1445–9
  amyloidosis in 1433, 1434, 1438, 1447–8, 1448
  associated conditions 1447
  attacks 1445–7
  childhood 1409
  clinical features 1445–8
  diagnostic criteria 1445
  FMF gene 1448
  history 1445
  inheritance 1445, 1446
  laboratory tests 1448
  treatment 1448–9, 1449
familial type 4 hyperlipoproteinaemia 1481
  see also hyperlipidaemias
family
  guidance for 1754
  impact of child's disease on 1737
  position in 823
  relationships
    and low back pain 106
    and quality of life 66
  size 823
  studies 821–2, 821
Fanconi syndrome 1310, 1605
Farber's lipogranulomatosis 1477, 1634
Farr assay 667–8
Fas protein 352, 844, 1163, 1168
fascicles 457
fasciculation 216–17, 224
fasciitis
  in the elderly 37
  non-infectious 1675
fasciitis–panniculitis 1675

fasting 265, 615–16
fat
  abdominal subcutaneous, needle aspiration 1440, 1441
  dietary 616
  malabsorption and vitamin D deficiency 1603
fat-pad syndrome 166
fat planes, displacement 715, 716–19
fatigue 172
  in ankylosing spondylitis 1063–4, 1069
  avoidance 1728, 1728
  in dermatomyositis 1252
  and disability 1725
  in eosinophilia–myalgia syndrome 1425
  in hyperparathyroidism 280
  in Lyme disease 885, 887, 890
  in polymyositis 1252
  and quality of life 64–5
  in SLE 59, 64–5, 1146–7
fatty acid anilides 1427
fatty acids
  disorders of metabolism 473–4
  and inflammatory mediators 1480
  long-chain
    and ATP synthesis 1773
    β-oxidation 1774
  omega-3 262, 264, 1480
  polyunsaturated 262, 1480
  short-chain 679
  in treatment of rheumatic diseases 1484–5
  see also fish oil supplements
5-FC see 5-fluorocytosine
Felty's syndrome 258, 292, 643–4, 643, 645, 990
  anaemia in 291, 644
  anaesthesia in 300
  autoantibodies 644, 1329
  HLA associations 556, 556, 643
  and rheumatoid arthritis 1014–15
  serological markers 1015
  thrombocytopenia 645
femoral artery 151, 1382
  aneurysm 379, 1398
femoral epiphysis, slipped capital 162, 164–5, 1787
  diagnosis 19
  in hypothyroidism 277, 278
  imaging 758, 761
femoral stretch test 47, 48, 225
femur
  condyle, osteonecrosis 1623
  head 150
    osteonecrosis 1622, 1623
    and gout 1561
    in pregnancy 185
    vascularization, imaging 760, 763
  internal rotation 151
  neck
    DEXA scan 721
    stress fracture 1784
  proximal fracture see hip, fracture
  shortening 165
  telephone-receiver 397
  trochlea 151, 152
fenbufen
  adverse effects 212, 213
  half-life 577
  metabolism 577
fenfluramine, adverse effects 1223
fenofibrate in hyperlipidaemias 1481
fenoprofen
  adverse effects
    cutaneous 213
    haematological 295
    psychiatric 338
    renal 327
  enantiomers 577
  half-life 577
  in juvenile chronic arthritis 1106, 1140
  in lactation 193
  in pregnancy 190
  renal clearance 577

fentanyl 307
ferritin 633, 634, 635
  in adult Still's disease 641
  in anaemia of chronic disease 291, 638
  in rheumatoid arthritis 777
fertility 15
  drug-related effects on 588, 589, 593, 594, 595
  in familial Mediterranean fever 1449
  in gout 184–5
  and rheumatoid arthritis 182
  and SLE 183, 1157
  and systemic sclerosis 184
fetal wastage syndrome 294, 295
fetus
  effect of maternal drug therapy on 188–93
  effect of maternal parvovirus infection on 897
  effect of maternal SLE on 183, 1157
  loss see abortion
  muscle development 458–9
FEV1 247, 248, 1775
fever 3, 170, 171–2
  in ankylosing spondylitis 1063
  childhood 170, 171, 862
  in Churg–Strauss syndrome 1354
  in dermatomyositis 1252
  double quotidian 1114, 1115
  drug-related 589
  in familial Mediterranean fever 1445, 1447
  in giant cell arteritis 172, 1377, 1388
  intermittent 171, 172
  in juvenile chronic arthritis 21, 172, 1114–15, 1131–2
  in Lyme disease 887
  in microscopic polyangiitis 1354
  in non-gonococcal arthritis 850
  in polyarteritis nodosa 1353, 1403
  in polymyalgia rheumatica 172, 1377
  in polymyositis 1252
  in pyogenic arthritis 862
  quotidian 1114, 1115
  in reactive arthritis 1086
  remittent 171, 172
  in rheumatic fever 979
  in sarcoidosis 1465
  sustained 171, 172
  in toxic oil syndrome 1425
  of unknown origin 20–1, 171–2
  in Wegener's granulomatosis 1336
FGFR genes 353, 368
  in chondrodysplasias 369, 369
  mutations 395
fibrillin 353
  fibrillin 5(2) gene 389
    cloning 354
    as disease marker 391
    mutations 393
  fibrillin 11 gene, molecular structure 391
  fibrillin 15(1) gene
    cloning and sequencing 354, 389
    as disease marker 391
    and Marfan syndrome 353–4, 389, 391–3
  gene mutation 436
  in vitreous humour 355
fibrin
  in antigen-induced arthritis 565
  deposition on inflamed synovium 443
  in inflammation 512
fibrinogen 623, 627, 639
  and erythrocyte sedimentation rate 626, 639
  function in inflammation 624
  in hereditary renal amyloidosis 1434, 1434, 1438
  in intravascular coagulation 625
  and plasma viscosity 639
  properties 625
  in rheumatoid arthritis 1016
  in SLE 640

fibrinogen (continued)
  synovial fluid 677, 681
fibrinoid change 983
fibrinoid necrosis 1319
fibrinolysis
  intra-arterial in antiphospholipid syndrome 1212
  in polymyalgia rheumatica/giant cell arteritis 1378
fibroblast colony forming units 422, 426
fibroblast growth factor
  effect on cartilage 415
  effect on growth plate chondrocytes 413
  functions 395–6
  modulation of acute phase protein synthesis 623
fibroblast growth factor receptors 395–6
  FGFR1 396
    in achondroplasia 396
    gene mutations 396, 398–9
  FGFR2 396
    gene mutations 398–9, 435, 436
  FGFR3 396
    gene mutations 396–8, 435, 436
    in hypochondroplasia 396
    in thanatophoric dwarfism 396–8
fibroblasts 422, 457
  effect of free radicals on proliferation 447
  in inflammation 514
  interaction with lymphocytes 538
  neutral endopeptidase in 451
  in psoriatic arthritis 1079
  in scleroderma 1223, 1225, 1226
fibrocartilage 368, 406, 1494, 1541
fibrodysplasia ossificans progressiva 436–7
fibrogenesis imperfecta ossium 1606
fibroma, aponeurotic 208
fibromodulin 410
fibromuscular dysplasia 1383
fibromyalgia 1489, 1496–9, 1657–8
  back pain in 1646
  common symptoms 1497
  comparison with reflex sympathetic dystrophy 1686, 1687
  diagnostic criteria 812, 1497, 1498
  differential diagnosis 891, 1497
  in the elderly 37
  and familial Mediterranean fever 1447
  health status measures 59
  in HIV infection 901
  investigation 1497
  in Lyme disease 891, 893
  malaise in 170, 172, 178
  musculoskeletal pain in 168
  in osteoarthritis 1548
  tender points 1496, 1497–8, 1653, 1657–8
  treatment 1499, 1499
Fibromyalgia Network 37
Fibromyalgia network newsletter 37
fibronectin 353, 460, 531, 532
  receptor 534
fibrosarcoma 120, 288, 1667, 1671
fibrosing alveolitis 241, 242
  drug-related 598
  pulmonary radiography 244–5
  in rheumatoid arthritis 1010
fibrosis in scleroderma 1225–6
fibrositis syndrome see fibromyalgia
fibroxanthoma 1477
fibula 153
fifth disease 204, 880, 897
filariasis 948, 949–50
Filipinos
  seronegative spondylarthropathies 839
  SLE 836
  see also ethnic groups
filum terminale thickening 127, 129
finger-flexion reflex in cervical myelopathy 1656

finger tip pinch action, two-dimensional force analysis 478
fingers
  clubbing 241, 1094, 1473, 1673
  flexotenosynovitis in juvenile chronic arthritis 1741, 1742, 1742–3
  gangrene 1156, 1183
  mechanic's/machinist's 1252, 1290, 1423, 1424, 1425
  see also hand; trigger finger/thumb
Finkelstein's test 43, 146, 1506, 1766
fish oil supplements 262, *263–4*, 264, 515, 616
  in amyloidosis 1441
  in hyperlipidaemias 1484–5
  in psoriasis 1079
  in psoriatic arthritis 1081
  in SLE 1175
  in systemic sclerosis 1238
Fisher rats 510
  streptococcal cell-wall arthritis 565, 998
  susceptibility to adjuvant arthritis 563, 998
Fisher's exact test 689
fistula
  in coccidioidomycosis 961
  in osteomyelitis 876
fixed drug eruption 200
  bullous 205
  hyperpigmentation *209*
  NSAID-induced 213
flagellin 884
Flaviviridae 900
flexor carpi radialis 137, 138
flexor carpi radialis tendon sheath 137, 138
flexor carpi ulnaris 137, 138
  in juvenile chronic arthritis 1740–1, 1742
flexor digiti minimi brevis 140
flexor digitorum longus 153, 156
flexor digitorum profundus 137, 138, 140, 1505
flexor digitorum superficialis 137, 138, 140, 1505
flexor hallucis longus 153
flexor pollicis brevis 140
flexor pollicis longus 137, 138, 140, 1505
flexor retinaculum 137–8, 156
flexor tendon
  crepitus 41–2
  in rheumatoid arthritis 1008, 1014
  surgery 1705
  tenosynovitis 41
flexor tendon sheaths, digital 137, 138, 140, 1505
flexotenosynovitis of the fingers in juvenile chronic arthritis 1741, 1742, 1742–3
flow volume curves 247–8, 249
fluclorolone acetomide *210*
flucloxacillin in discitis of childhood 124
fluconazole 956, 957
  in blastomycosis 959
  in *Candida* 958
  in coccidioidomycosis 962
  in cryptococcosis 963
  in sporotrichosis 960
flufenamic acid
  half-life *577*
  in lactation 194
fluid balance in acute renal failure 330
flumazenil *307*
fluocinolone acetomide *210*
fluocinomide *210*
fluoride 1314, 1694–5
5-fluorocytosine (5-FC)
  in fungal arthritis 956, 958, 963
  in invasive aspergillosis 252
fluoroquinolones, in osteomyelitis 874
fluoroscopy in non-gonococcal arthritis 851

5-fluorouracil in scleroderma 1240
fluoxetine 339, *340*, *341*, *342*
flurandrenolone *210*, 211
flurbiprofen
  enantiomers 577
  half-life *577*
  in juvenile chronic arthritis *1140*
  in scleritis 317
fluticasone propionate *210*
fluvoxamine 339, *340*
folic acid
  deficiency 262, 291
  supplements in methotrexate therapy 34, 296–7, 585
foot
  applied anatomy 153–4, 156, 157
  drop *803*
  equinus position 1748
  examination 50–1
  flat 17, 167, 1511–12
    flexible 167
    peroneal spastic 167
    rigid 167
  forefoot excision arthroplasty 1706
  functional anatomy and disability 1725
  heel 1747, 1748
  hypermobile with short Achilles tendon 167
  hyperpronation 1786
  imaging 745–7, 748
  in juvenile chronic arthritis 1116, 1133–4, 1718–20, 1747–9, 1750
  local steroid injection *1762*, 1769–70
  osteoarthritis 1535
  pain 1511–12, *1511*
    adult *155*, 159–60
    childhood *164*, 167–8
  physiotherapy in childhood 1747–9, 1750
  radiography 719
  in rheumatoid arthritis 1008–9
  size inequality 128, 129
  skin lesions 201
  stress fracture 747, 748
  surgery 1706–7, 1718–20
footwear 1733, 1749
force–couple 135
force plate 478
forced expiratory volume 247, 248, 1775
forced vital capacity 247, 248
forces 477
forearm
  pronation 137
  supination 137
forearm ischaemic exercise test 1265
forefoot 153, 154, 1719
  see also foot
Forestier's disease *see* diffuse idiopathic skeletal hyperostosis
Foucher's sign 158
fractures
  in ankylosing spondylitis 1062, 1063
  avulsion *1105*, 1786–7
  and bone mass 433
  childhood 20
  Colles' 1583–4, *1584*, 1586, 1599, *1600*
  healing 413
  hip 1584–5
    in osteoporosis 1583–4, *1584*, 1600, *1601*
    risk factors 1585–6, *1585*
  in hyperparathyroidism 280
  in juvenile chronic arthritis 1721
  lifetime risk 1584, *1584*
  osteomyelitis following 876, *877*
  osteonecrosis following 1622
  in osteoporosis 1583–4
  in Paget's disease 1612
  proximal femoral *see* fractures, hip
  reflex sympathetic dystrophy following 1681
  in rheumatoid arthritis 1013–14

fractures (*continued*)
  stress 163, 758, 1783–4
    foot 747, 748
    in rheumatoid arthritis 1014
    vertebral 1583–4, *1584*, 1586, 1599–600, *1600*
fragile X syndrome 695
frailty 25
Framingham study 1528
free nerve ending *488*
free radicals 509, 511, 653
  biological consequences in rheumatoid arthritis 447–8
  in Dupuytren's contracture 148
  effects on carbohydrates 447
  effects on cells and cell viability 447–8
  effects on microvascular barrier function 448
  effects on proteins 447
  in inflammation 514
  in ischaemic muscle damage 469
  lipid peroxidation 447, 1480
  source of in joints 514
  in synovial hypoxia 446–7
Freiberg's disease 168, 1621, 1623, *1787*
Friedreich's ataxia
  muscle contracture in 217
  spinal stabilization in 118
frost-bite, reflex sympathetic dystrophy following 1681
fructose and hyperuricaemia *1558*
FSI 55, *55*, 61
fucidic acid 660
functional classification 64
Functional Independent Measure *1724*
functional residual capacity 249
functional status 64
Functional Status Index 55, *55*, 61
fungal arthritis 954–63
  childhood 958
  clinical presentation 955–6
  diagnosis *957*
  epidemiology 954–5
  management 956–7
  neonatal 958
  see also infection, fungal *and specific infections*
Fusarium
  F. solani 963
  grain infection 1637
fusion frequency 462
fusion proteins 615
Fusobacterium
  childhood pyogenic arthritis 863
  in HIV infection 916
  in osteomyelitis 870
Futura wrist splint 1732
FVC 247, 248

G
G1m(2) and giant cell arteritis 1375
G-protein-coupled receptors, mediation of parathyroid hormone effects 430
Gaenslen's sign 1053, 1073
gag gene 908
GAG protein 986
gait 41, 47–8
  AIDS 919
  analysis of forces 479–80
  antalgic 48, 150
  cycle 150–1
  development 16–17
  disturbance in cervical spondylosis 1653
  training 1749, 1750
  Trendelenberg 151
gallium scan *see* radionuclide scanning
gallstones and hyperbilirubinaemia 651
γ-glutamyl transferase (GGT) 651, 652
  imprecision in measurement *648*
ganglia 1506

gangrene, digital in SLE 1156, 1183
Garn method for assessment of skeletal maturity 78, 79, *80*
gastric ulceration and NSAID use 578, 1020
gastrin in Sjögren's syndrome 1310
gastrocnemius 153
gastrocnemius–semimembranosus bursa 153
  bursitis 158
gastrointestinal system
  adverse drug effects 207, **257**, **259–61**, 260
    antimalarials 260, 261
    aspirin 259, 260
    azapropazone *1021*
    azathioprine 260, 261, 590, *591*
    chlorambucil 260, 261, 593, *593*
    corticosteroids 260, 261, *587*
    cyclophosphamide 260, 261, 593, *593*
    cyclosporin 260, *595*
    diclofenac *1021*
    etodolac 260
    gold 260, 261, 600, *601*, *1022*
    hydroxychloroquine and chloroquine 596
    ibuprofen 260, *1021*
    indomethacin 260, *1021*
    ketoprofen *1021*
    meclofenamate 260
    methotrexate 207, 260, 261, *584*
    nabumetone 260
    naproxen 260, *1021*
    NSAIDs 259–61, *260*, 578, *578*, 1020, *1021*, 1695
    penicillamine 260, 261, 598
    piroxicam *1021*
    sulphasalazine 260, 261, 588, *589*
  amyloidosis 1436, 1437, 1439, 1440
  arteritis 258
  in Behçet's syndrome 257, *259*, 1398
  in dermatomyositis 257, 258, *1253*, 1255, 1277, 1290
  disorders
    and anaesthesia 300–1
    with rheumatic manifestations **255**, *256*
  diverticula 258
  dysmotility 258
  in eosinophilia–myalgia syndrome 1426
  erosions 578
  haemorrhage 578
  manifestations of rheumatic disease 173, *175–6*, **255**, 257, *258–9*
  microbiology **267–71**, *268*, *270–1*
  in mixed connective tissue disease 258, 1417–18, *1417*
  perforation 587
  in polyarteritis nodosa 257, 258, 1353
  in polymyositis 258, *1253*, 1255, 1277, 1290
  in scleroderma 257
  in seronegative spondylarthropathies *259*, 1043, 1045–6, 1064–5, 1087–8
  in Sjögren's syndrome 257, *258*, 1310
  in SLE 257, *258*, 1196
  in systemic sclerosis 1232, *1233*
  in toxic oil syndrome 1426
  tumours 289
Gaucher's disease 168, **1634–5**
GC clamp 694
gel electrophoresis
  DNA 690
  two-dimensional 697
gel filtration of immune complexes 705
gelatinases 411, *411*, 513, 515
gelling 41, 1521
gels
  agarose 690
  polyacrylamide 690
gelsolin 1434, *1434*, 1438
gemfibrozil
  adverse effects *1265*

gemfibrozil *(continued)*
  in hyperlipidaemias 1481
General Health Questionnaire 1724,
    1724
generalized eruptive histiocytoma
    1477
genes
  candidate 350, 351, 354
  control of expression 348–9
  coordinated expression 349
  cytokine 504–5, 506
  families 349–50
  linked 552–3
  mapping 350
  mutation in single-gene disorders *350*
  promoter region 347–8
  sequencing 354
  silent, activation 349
  structure 347–8
  transcription 347, 348–9
genetic counselling
  in ankylosing spondylitis 1069
  in osteogenesis imperfecta 698
genetic factors
  Behçet's syndrome 1395
  in bone mass 426
  calcium pyrophosphate dihydrate
      disease 1529–30
  in disease occurrence 821–2, *821, 822*
  giant cell arteritis 1375
  juvenile chronic arthritis *351, 699, 822*
  osteoarthritis 356, *822*, 1519
  polymyalgia rheumatica 1375
  psoriatic arthritis 698, 1078
  reactive arthropathies 698, 1088
  rheumatoid arthritis 351, *351*, 553–4,
      554, 555–6, 699, *822*, 984–5, *984*
  seropositive juvenile chronic arthritis
      1034–5
  Sjögren's syndrome 1302–3, *1303*
  SLE 350–1, *351*, 507, *822*, 1169–72, *1170*
  Stickler syndrome 353, 355, 356, 413,
      1519
genetic linkage *see* linkage
genetic markers
  allele-sharing analysis 688–9
  analysis techniques 691–4
  in ankylosing spondylitis 698–9
  association studies 689
  genetic linkage analysis 687–8
  identification 687–9
  in osteogenesis imperfecta 697–8
  polymorphic 687
genetic typing 689–97
genetics
  diseases with a complex inheritance 687
  of inflammation 504–8
  molecular **347–52**, 354
  new 347
  polygenic disorders 351–2, *351*
  reverse 347, 350, 351, 354, 687
  single-gene disorders 350–1, *350*, 687
genome, human 350
gentamicin
  in brucellar arthritis 943, *943*
  polymethylmethacrylate bead impreg-
      nation 875
  in pyogenic arthritis *856*
genu valgum 17, 19
genu varum 17, 19, 166
germ-free rats, susceptibility to adju-
    vant arthritis 563
GFR *see* glomerular filtration rate
GGT *see* γ-**glutamyl transferase**
giant cell arteritis 207, 783, **1373–80**,
    1382
  active *783*
  acute phase response in 627–8, 629,
      640, 1378
  age at onset *26*, 1377
  and autoimmune thyroid disease 279
  cardiovascular involvement *230*, 233,
      238
  central nervous system disease in 222–3

giant cell arteritis *(continued)*
  childhood 1408
  classification 1321, *1321, 1322*
  clinical features *170*, 178, 1377, 1378,
      1388–9, 1408
  cranial nerve palsies in *224*
  definition 1373–4
  diagnostic criteria 1373–4, *1374*
  in the elderly 34
  epidemiology 1375–6, 1382–3
    clustering 818
    geographical factors 820
    time trends 817
  erythrocyte sedimentation rate 627–8,
      640, 1378, 1389
  gastrointestinal involvement *259*
  genetic factors 1375, 1670
  imaging
    angiography 1389
    Doppler ultrasound 1389
    MRI 1389
  laboratory tests *649*, 1378, 1389
  large vessel involvement **1388–9**
  liver function 652, 1378
  localized 1321–2
  and malignant disease 1670
  myalgia in 653
  neutrophilia *643*
  ocular involvement 312, 313, 1378
  pathogenesis 1376–7
  peripheral neuropathies 228
  prognosis 1329, 1389
  psychiatric involvement *333*
  relationship with polymyalgia rheuma-
      tica 1374–5
  renal function 650
  subacute/healed *783*, 784, 785
  temporal artery biopsy 783–5, *783, 784,
      785*, 1376–7, *1376*
  treatment 1379–80, 1389, 1408
  vertebrobasilar insufficiency in 223
giant cell reticulohistiocytosis *see*
    multicentric reticulohistiocytosis
giant cell tumour *208, 1671*
  in Paget's disease 1612
  spinal 120
  tendon sheath 1477
giant cells
  in giant cell arteritis 784
  in granulomatous angiitis of the central
      nervous system 785, 786
  in sarcoidosis 1464
giardiasis *946*
  articular syndromes associated 946–7
  and HIV-associated Reiter's syndrome
      920
  and reactive arthritis 267
  vasculitis in 947
gigantism 431
gingiva
  hyperplasia *595*
  in Wegener's granulomatosis 1335
GLA in juvenile dermatomyositis
    1294
glaucoma
  drug-induced *587*
  in juvenile chronic arthritis 1103
***gld* gene** 1162
glenohumeral joint
  anatomy 135, 136, 137, 1501
  examination 44
  instability 144
  local steroid injection 1763
  movement 44
  osteoarthritis 1532
  palpation 44
  in rheumatoid arthritis 1008
  surgery 1702–3
glenohumeral ligament 135
glenoid labrum
  hip 150
  shoulder 135
  tears 739, 740, 1504
Global shoulder 1703

glomerular filtration rate (GFR)
    648–50
  in acute renal failure 325
  in SLE 1153, 1191
glomeruli
  function tests 648–50, 650–1
  immune complex deposition 703
  ischaemic damage 324
  in SLE 1152
glomerulonephritis *177*
  anti-GBM 327, *328*
  in Behçet's syndrome 1398
  cryoglobulinaemic *328*
  drug-related *598*, 1695
  in familial Mediterranean fever 1447
  focal necrotizing 1188–9
  haematuria in 324
  in Henoch–Schönlein purpura *328*,
      1407
  hepatitis-associated *328*
  idiopathic crescentic 327, *328*
  idiopathic segmental necrotizing 674
  in immune complex diseases 703
  in microscopic polyangiitis 1357
  pauci-immune 327, *328*, 1323, 1338
    p-ANCA/MPO-ANCA in *328*, 1329
  in polyarteritis nodosa 1323
  in polymyositis/dermatomyositis 1256
  poststreptococcal *328*
  rapidly progressive 327–8, *328, 330*,
      331, 1338, 1406
  in Sjögren's syndrome 1311
  vasculitis-associated *328, 330*
glossitis, penicillamine-induced 214
glucose
  anaerobic metabolism 1774
  and ATP synthesis 1773–4
  glycolysis 1774
  pericardial fluid 235
  synovial fluid 677, 679
    in synovial hypoxia 444
glucose-6-phosphatase deficiency
    473, 1558, *1558*
glucose-6-phosphate dehydrogenase
    deficiency 588
glucose-regulated proteins 449
glucuronic acid 973
L-glutamate 495
glutamic oxaloacetic transaminase *see*
    aspartate aminotransferase
glutamic pyruvic transaminase *see*
    alanine aminotransferase
glutamine 1778
glutathione peroxidase 262
gluten-sensitive enteropathy *see* coeliac
    disease
gluteus maximus 150, 157
gluteus maximus bursa 150, 156
gluteus medius 150
  weakness 151
gluteus medius bursa 150
gluteus minimus 150
gluteus minimus bursa 150
GLYCAM-1 530
glyceraldehyde-3-phosphate 445
glycine in collagen 407
glycogen 1773, 1774, 1780
glycogenoses 472–3, 1558, 1774
glycolysis 1774
  inherited disorders 1774, 1775
glycolytic pathway in inflamed
    synovia 445
α2HS glycoprotein in Paget's disease
    1613
β2 glycoprotein I 293, 1159, 1209–10
glycosaminoglycans
  in amyloid deposits 1433, 1436
  in intervertebral discs 1640
  in osteoarthritis 1537, 1542
gnathostomiasis *948, 950*
goggles, protective 1780
goitre, multinodular 279
gold therapy 599
  adult-onset Still's disease 1127

gold therapy *(continued)*
  adverse effects 600–1, *601*, 1022, *1022*
    cutaneous 207, 213, 600, 601, *601*,
        1022, 1695
    gastrointestinal *260*, 261, 600, *601*,
        1022
    haematological 296, *601*, 642, *644*,
        1022
    immunological 970, *1022*
    myopathic 653
    neurological *217, 1022*
    psychiatric *337*, 338
    renal 322, *601, 1022*, 1695
    respiratory 241, *253, 601, 1022*
  ankylosing spondylitis 1069
  calcium pyrophosphate dihydrate
      disease 1570
  in combination therapy *1025*
  discoid lupus erythematosus 211
  dose regimens 600
  Felty's syndrome 292
  juvenile chronic arthritis 1107, 1126,
      1138, 1140, *1140*
  in lactation 194, *602*
  pharmacology 599
  in pregnancy 191, *602*
  psoriatic arthritis 1080
  reactive arthropathies 1092
  rheumatoid arthritis 1021–2, 1023
  RS₃PE syndrome 35
  seropositive juvenile chronic arthritis
      1036
  therapeutic efficacy 599–600
  therapeutically relevant effects 599, *600*
  urticarial vasculitis 1370
golfer's elbow *5*, 43, 145–6, 1504–5
  local steroid injection 1764
gonadal mosaicism in osteogenesis
    imperfecta 364
gonarthritis 1009
goniometry 41
gonococcaemia, disseminated 163
gonococcal arthritis 854–5
  childhood 862, *862*, 863
  differential diagnosis 1090
  distinction from non-gonococcal
      arthritis *850*
  and HIV infection 916
  management 856–8
  and pregnancy 184
gonococcal bacteraemia 206
Goodpasture's syndrome 327, *328*, 598,
    1022
Gorham's disease 1636
GOT *see* aspartate aminotransferase
Gottron's papules 1250, 1252, 1253, 1263
Gottron's sign *175*, 1250, 1251, 1289
gout **1555–66**
  acute 1559, 1560
  acute phase response in 627
  age-related occurrence *26*
  and alcohol 1555, 1694
  and calcium pyrophosphate dihydrate
      disease 1537, 1531, 1567
  and chondrocalcinosis 1561
  chronic tophaceous 1044
  clinical features 1560–1
  and coronary artery disease 1556
  definition 1555
  and diabetes mellitus 283
  diagnosis 1562
  differential diagnosis 1562, *1563*
  and diuretics 684, 1555, 1556
  drug/toxin-induced 684, 1555, 1556,
      1558, 1694
  epidemiology *814*, 1555–6, *1556*
    effect of age and sex *815*, 1555
    geographical factors 820
    racial factors *819*
  erythema in 205
  and femoral head necrosis 1561
  history 1555
  and hyperlipidaemias 1484, 1556
  in hyperparathyroidism 280

gout (*continued*)
  and hypertension 651, 1556
  hyperuricaemia in 1557, 1558, *1558*
  in hypothyroidism *277*, 278
  imaging 1560, 1562, 1563
  and inborn errors of metabolism
    1557–8, *1558*
  intercritical 1560
  laboratory tests *649*, 654, 677, 682, 683–4,
    1561–2
  neutrophilia *643*
  and obesity 1555
  pathophysiology 1556–60
  petit attacks 1560
  polyarticular 1560
  and pregnancy 184–5
  prevention 1563
  primary 1557
  prognosis 1566
  prophylaxis 1564–5
  recurrent 1562
  renal involvement 651, 1561, 1566
  risk factors 1555, *1556*
  saturnine 1558, 1694
  secondary 289, *595*, 1558, *1558*
  stages 1560
  synovial fluid 677, 682, 683–4
  tophaceous 178, 1560–1
  tophus formation 1560
  in transplant recipients 1566
  treatment 1563–6, *1564*, *1565*, *1566*
  uric acid crystal formation 1558–9
Gower's sign 1290
gp41 908, 909, 910
gp70 1162–3
gp120 908, 910, 1162
GPT *see* alanine aminotransferase
grab sign 159, 1785
gracilis 150, 153, 158
graft-versus-host disease 1221
  model 1225
Gram-negative bacteria
  in non-gonococcal arthritis *851*, *852*, *853*
  in osteomyelitis 868, 870, *870*
  in prosthetic joint infection 854
  in pyogenic arthritis 862, 880
**Gram-positive bacteria, in osteo-
  myelitis** 868, 870, *870*
granular lymphocyte expansion 644,
  645
granulocyte-colony stimulating factor
  and bone formation *424*
  recombinant human in neutropenia
    643
  in rheumatoid arthritis *993*
**granulocyte-macrophage colony
  forming units** 422, 423, 425
**granulocyte-macrophage colony
  stimulating factor**
  and bone formation *424*
  effect on osteoclasts *425*
  in Felty's syndrome 1015
  in rheumatoid arthritis 993, *993*, 995
granulocytes
  effects of methotrexate on 582, *583*
  in inflammation 512–13
granulocytopenia
  drug-related 295
  in SLE 292, 641, 1193
granuloma 207
  in muscle biopsy 789–90
  palisading 1341
  in rheumatoid arthritis 990
  sarcoid 789–90, 1464
  synthesis of 1,25-dihydroxycholecalci-
    ferol 430
  tuberculous 789, 930
  in Wegener's granulomatosis 1324, 1341
granuloma faciale 1370–1
**granulomatous angiitis, central
  nervous system** *333*, 335, 785, 786
granzyme 1 1227
Graves' disease 279, *285*
greater auricular nerve in leprosy 934

**greater trochanteric bursa inflamma-
  tion** 48
Greulich–Pyle atlas 78, 79, 81, 755, 757
grip strength 41
  in tennis elbow 145
GROα 990
groin pain 1507–8, 1768
ground-glass appearance 1235, 1236
group therapy in low back pain 106
growing pain 163
growth 72–87
  analysis of data 76, 81–2, 83–4
  critical periods 73
  drug-related inhibition *587*
  imaging in evaluation of abnormalities
    755, 757
  in juvenile chronic arthritis 14, 18, 82,
    85–7, 1119
  measurement 73–7
  prenatal 73
  retardation in CINCA 1473
  standards/charts 75–7, *77–8*, 79, 81
  velocity 82
    charts 83–4
  zone, radionuclide scanning 765
growth factors
  associated with bone 424, *424*
  in osteoarthritis 1543–5, *1543*
  see also specific growth factors
growth hormone
  and bone mass 426
  in calcium homeostasis 431
  effect on growth plate chondrocytes 413
  in juvenile chronic arthritis 87, 1119
  therapy in juvenile chronic arthritis 87
growth plate 411–13, 771, 1591
GSB hinge prosthesis 1703, 1704
**guanidine in Eaton–Lambert
  syndrome** 1675
guanine 689, 1557
Guillain–Barré syndrome 794–5
Guinea worm *948*, *949*
'gull's wing' deformity 1523, 1524
Guyatt's responsiveness statistic 52
Guyon's canal 138
**gynaecomastia in hypertrophic
  osteoarthropathy** 1673

H

H₂-antagonists 1422, 1695
H reflex, reflex latency 801
Haelan *210*, 211
haem, dipstick test 323
haem oxygenase 449
haemangioma 288
  deep venous 765
  spinal 120
  synovial 770
haemarthrosis, imaging 768, 771
haematocolpus 133
**haematocrit and erythrocyte sedi-
  mentation rate** 639
**haematological disorders in rheu-
  matic disease** 290–5, 633–46
  and anaesthesia 300
  SLE 291–2, 641–2, *643*, 1155–6, 1192–4
haematological effects of drugs 295–7
  alkylating agents 593, *593*
  antimalarials 295–6
  aspirin 295
  azathioprine 214, 297, 590, *591*
  chloroquine 295
  diclofenac 295
  fenoprofen 295
  gold 296, *601*, 642, *644*, *1022*
  hydroxychloroquine 295–6
  ibuprofen 295
  indomethacin 295
  ketoprofen 295
  methotrexate 296–7, *584*
  mophebutazone 295
  naproxen 295
  NSAIDs 295, *578*, 580, 1695

haematological effects of drugs
  (*continued*)
  oxyphenbutazone 295
  penicillamine 296, *598*
  phenylbutazone 295
  piroxicam 295
  primaquine 295–6
  sulindac 295
  sulphasalazine 296, 588, *589*
haematoma
  intermuscular 1782
  intramuscular 1782
  sport-associated 1782–3
haematometra 133
haematopoietin receptor family 520,
  521
haematuria 321, 323–4, *330*, 331
  in alkylating agent therapy 594
  anatomical sources in systemic rheu-
    matic disease 323–4
  definitions 323
  diagnostic studies 324
  in familial Mediterranean fever 1447
  glomerular 324
  and glomerular function 650
  gross 323
  in Henoch–Schönlein purpura 324,
    1407
  in hypersensitivity vasculitis 1368
  in juvenile chronic arthritis 1118
  in lupus nephritis 321
  in Lyme disease 888
  microscopic 323
  in microscopic polyangiitis 1354
  in polyarteritis nodosa 324, 1403
  with proteinuria 324
  in rapidly progressive glomerulo-
    nephritis 327
  renal biopsy in 324–5
  in SLE 1153, 1190
  in vasculitis 1358
  in Wegener's granulomatosis 1338
**haemobilia, in mixed connective
  tissue disease** 1418
haemochromatosis 209
  and calcium pyrophosphate dihydrate
    disease 1530, *1531*, 1567
  and osteoarthritis 1519
  rheumatic manifestations *256*
**haemocytophagocytosis in juvenile
  rheumatoid arthritis** 291
haemoglobin 633
  and aerobic capacity 1775
  in anaemia of chronic disease 290–1,
    636
  oxygen combining power 1775
  preanaesthetic assessment 300
  synthesis 634
Haemogogus 904
haemolysis
  acute renal failure associated 327
  haematuria in 323
  with haemolytic anaemia 291
  haptoglobin in 625
  hyperbilirubinaemia in 651
  in SLE 641, 1192
haemolytic uraemic syndrome
  acute renal failure in 329
  ischaemic glomerular damage in 324
haemopexin 623
haemophilia 207
  differential diagnosis 1137, *1137*
  pyogenic arthritis in 864–5
haemophilic arthropathy, imaging
  768
Haemophilus
  arteritis due to 1390
  H. influenzae
    antibiotic therapy *856*
    in osteomyelitis 868
    in pyogenic arthritis *851*, *852*, 880
    childhood 861, 862, *862*, 863
    type b 861, 862, *862*, 863
    in HIV infection 916

Haemophilus (*continued*)
  H. influenzae
    type f 863
    vaccine against 862, 863
haemopoietic disease, anaesthesia in
  300
haemoptysis
  in SLE 1152
  in systemic sclerosis 1235
haemorrhage
  alveolar 1337–8
  cerebral 1434, *1434*, 1438
  gastrointestinal 578, 1417
  periungual 1251
  pulmonary 243, 1152, 1195, 1354, 1355
  retinal 313, 1153
  splinter *174*, 207, 1207
  vitreous *311*
haemorrhagic crescent sign 158
haemosiderin 633, 635
  in anaemia of chronic disease 291
  deposition
    imaging 768, 771
    in pigmented villonodular synovitis
      1619
  in osteoarthritis 1541
**haemostatic changes in rheumatic
  diseases** 293–5
haemotoxylin bodies 1152
Hageman factor *see* factor XII
hair abnormalities 209
hallucinations
  in SLE 333
  visual 212
hallux 153, 154
hallux flexus 1748, 1749
hallux rigidus 153, 160
hallux valgus 153, 160, 1512, 1719
  in juvenile chronic arthritis 1748
  plantar response in 218
halothane 472
hamstrings 150
  intramuscular haematoma 1784
hand
  claw 1229
  deformities 42
  examination 41–2, *42*
  functional anatomy and disability
    1724–5
  in HIV-associated arthritis 919
  involvement in hypothyroidism 278
  in juvenile chronic arthritis 1116, 1132,
    1133, 1720–1, 1740–3, *1741*, 1744
  local steroid injection 148, *1762*, 1766–8
  mechanic's/machinist's 1252, 1290,
    1423, 1424, *1425*
  muscle wasting 41
  orthoses, childhood 1743, 1744
  osteoarthritis 1534, 1549
  pain 1505–7, *1505*, 1507
    adult *139–40*, 146–8
    childhood 163, *163*
  physiotherapy, childhood 1740–3, 1744
  power grip 1725
  precision/pincer grip 1725
  range of movement 42
  reflex sympathetic dystrophy 1682
  rheumatoid arthritis
    erosions 725, *726*
    joint involvement 1008
    surgery 1705
  screening 41
  skin *174–5*
    examination 41, 201, 202, 203
  splints 1743, 1744
  surgery 1705, 1720–1
  swelling 42
  in systemic sclerosis 1230, 1231
  tendons 41–2
Hand–Schüller–Christian disease
  120
handicap 64
  definition 1723
  measurement 1724, *1724*

haptoglobin 623, **627**
  in giant cell arteritis 628
  in haemolysis 625
  in inflammation *624*
  in polymyalgia rheumatica 628
  properties *625*
  in rheumatoid arthritis *1016*
HAQ *see* Health Assessment Questionnaire
Harpenden skinfold callipers 75
Harpenden stadiometer 74
Harrison's groove 1601
Hartley guinea pig 416–17
Hashimoto's thyroiditis 279, *285*, 1613
hatchet defect 739, 742
Hawaii, prevalence of SLE 836, *836*, 837
Haydu–Cheney acro-osteolysis 1636
HBsAb 900
HBsAg *see* hepatitis B surface antigen
HBV *see* hepatitis B virus
HCAM 534, *537*
HCV *see* hepatitis C virus infection
HDL *see* high density lipoprotein
head-and-neck biopsy in Wegener's granulomatosis 1341
headache *177*, 178
  in Behçet's syndrome 1397
  in cervical spondylosis 1653
  in CINCA 1471
  drug-related *578*, 580
  in giant cell arteritis 1378
  in Lyme disease 887, 888
  in mixed connective tissue disease 1418
  in Paget's disease 1612
  postlumbar puncture 731
  as referred pain 99
  in SLE 219, 1185
  in Takayasu's arteritis 1385
  in toxic oil syndrome 1425
health, definition 52
Health Assessment Questionnaire (HAQ) 55, *55*, 58, 59, 60, *1724*
  and prediction of disability 65
  for the sponylarthropathies *58*, 59
health locus of control 69
  chance 69
  internal 69
  powerful other 69
health status 51, 64
  conceptual framework 52
  definitions 52
  impact of psychological variables on 67–9
  measures 51–61, 1724, *1724*
    carpal tunnel syndrome 59
    characteristics 52
    childhood arthritis *56*, 57
    disease-specific 53, *53*, 54–9, *55–8*
    fatigue in SLE 59
    fibromyalgia 59
    general/generic 52, 53, *53*, 54
    limitations 59
    low back pain 59
    osteoarthritis 57–8, *57*
    practical utility 52
    reliability 52, 59–60
    responsiveness 52
    rheumatoid arthritis 54–6, *55*
    selection of 59–61, *60*
    sensitivity 52
    short forms 53–4, *54*
    shoulder pain 59
    spondylarthropathies 58–9, *58*
    of surgical interventions *57*, 58
    validity 52, 59–60
hearing loss
  in CINCA 1471
  in osteogenesis imperfecta 358
  in Paget's disease 1612
  unilateral *224*
  in Wegener's granulomatosis 1337
heart
  adaptation to exercise 1777
  hypertrophy 1777

heart *(continued)*
  transplantation
    in amyloidosis 1442
    gout following 1566
    and osteoporosis 433
    see also cardiovascular complications of rheumatic disease
heart conduction defects
  in amyloidosis 1436
  in mixed connective tissue disease 1418
  in polymyositis/dermatomyositis 1255
heart-reactive antibodies in rheumatic fever 975
heartburn 257, *258*, 1417
heat, localized, in Paget's disease 1612
heat-shock proteins
  in adjuvant arthritis 563
  in Behçet's syndrome 1399
  hsp65 553, 986, 998
  hsp70
    gene 548, 696
    in SLE *1164*
  hsp90, in SLE *1164*, 1165
  in rheumatoid synovium 449
heat stroke 1777–8
Heberden's nodes 1522, 1523
  erythema over 205
  gout in 684
  inheritance 1519
  in psoriatic arthritis 1078
heel
  examination 50–1
  pain 159–60, 745, 1076, 1105, 1447, 1510–11, *1510*, 1770
  see also foot
heel foot 1747, 1748
heel pad
  tender 1511
  thickening in acromegaly 281, *281*, 282
Hegemann's disease 1623
height
  age-related decrease 24
  and disease occurrence 823
  in juvenile chronic arthritis 85, 86
  measurement 74, 75
  percentiles 76
  prediction 79, 81
  and risk of hip fracture 1585
  velocity 82, 83–4
Helicobacter cinaedi in HIV infection 916
helix–loop–helix structure 348
helminthic infections 947–51
helper T cells
  activation 546
  in adaptive immunity 546
  antigen processing and presentation to 549–50
  in HIV infection 907, 909, 910–11, 916–17
  integrin expression 531
  in leprosy 933
  primed/memory state 991
  in psoriatic arthritis 1079
  in reactive arthropathies 1092
  in rheumatic fever 976, *976*
  in rheumatoid arthritis 777, 991
  in sarcoidosis 1464
  in SLE 1165–6, *1166*, 1167, 1168
  susceptibility to free radical attack 447
  Th1 520, 546
    cytokine profile 1167, *1167*
    in rheumatoid arthritis 992
  Th2 520, 546
    cytokine profile 1167, *1167*
  virgin state 991
'helping hands' 102, 108
hemiballismus in SLE 1184
hemichorea 978
hemiparesis
  in Sjögren's syndrome 1311
  in SLE 1185
hemiplegia
  in CINCA 1471
  and rheumatoid arthritis 449

hemiplegia *(continued)*
  in SLE 1153
Henoch–Schönlein purpura 1369
  age at onset 11, 12, 13
  childhood 14, 1407
  classification *1321*, *1322*, 1366
  clinical features 1407
  diagnostic criteria 1326, *1326*
  differential diagnosis 1136, *1137*
  epidemiology *1320*
  and familial Mediterranean fever 1447
  gastrointestinal involvement 259
  laboratory tests 1407
  prognosis 1329, 1407
  proteinuria in 323
  renal involvement *321*, 324, *328*, 1407
  skin lesions 200
  treatment 1407
  vasculitis *786*, 914
HEp2 epithelial cells 665, 667, *668*, 1135
Hepadnaviridae 899
heparan sulphate 1165
heparin 353
  adverse effects 1208–9, 1589
  and antiphospholipid antibodies 294, 295, 1212
  in Behçet's syndrome 1401
  in cardiovascular disease 233
  interference with polymerase chain reaction 690
  in pregnancy 183, 295, 1212
  preoperative prophylactic 300
  in SLE 183, 1165
hepatic growth factor, modulation of acute phase protein synthesis 623
hepatitis
  chronic active
    autoantibodies *668*
    rheumatic manifestations 256
  drug-related *589*, 652
  hyperbilirubinaemia in 651
  liver function tests 652
  'lupoid' 1196
  lymphocytic, in DILS 912
  post-transfusion 900
  and rapidly progressive glomerulo-nephritis *328*
  rheumatoid factor in *674*
hepatitis A
  markers of infection 663
  rheumatic manifestations 256
hepatitis B surface antibody 900
hepatitis B surface antigen (HBsAg)
  detection 660
  in polyarteritis nodosa 331, 1353
  prevalence 900
  in proteinuria 322
  in rapidly progressive glomerulo-nephritis *328*
  and vasculitis 1328
hepatitis B virus (HBV)
  in immune complexes 704
  infection 899–900
    arthropathy 256, 880, 900
    clinical features 900
    diagnosis 900
    epidemiology 900
    management 900
    markers 663
    pathogenesis 900
    synovial fluid in 683
hepatitis C virus (HCV) infection 900–1
  arthropathy *256*, 900
  clinical features 900
  and cryoglobulinaemia 706, 900
  diagnosis 900–1
  epidemiology 900
  management 901
  markers 663
  pathogenesis 901
  and Sjögren's syndrome 257, *258*, 1302
hepatocellular carcinoma 900

hepatomegaly
  in juvenile chronic arthritis 1116
  in mixed connective tissue disease 1418
  in SLE 1157, 1196
hepatosplenomegaly *258*, 1127
hereditary haemorrhagic telangi-ectasia 207
hereditary sensorimotor neuropathy *218*
hereditary sensorineuropathy 226
Hermes 534, *537*
heroin, adverse effects *1265*
herpes gladiatorum 905
herpes hominis 904–5
herpes simplex infection 904
  and Behçet's syndrome 1399
  ocular involvement 319
  pulmonary 253
herpes zoster infection
  in methotrexate therapy *584*
  ocular involvement 319
  pulmonary 253
  reflex sympathetic dystrophy following 1681
heteroduplex analysis 693, 697
Hib vaccine 862, 863
'hidden disc' 107
hidradenitis suppurativa 206
high density lipoprotein (HDL) 1479
  in rheumatic disorders 1482
  subclasses 1479
high endothelial venules 443, 526–7
high output heart failure in Paget's disease 1613
Hills–Sachs defect 739, 742
hindfoot 153, 154, 1719–20
  imaging 745–7, 748
  see also foot
hip
  abduction 150
  adduction 150
  analgesic 1531
  in ankylosing spondylitis 1062, 1063
  applied anatomy 150–1
  arthrocentesis 678
  arthrodesis 1709
  brucellar arthritis 938, 939
  congenital dislocation/subluxation 165
    imaging 753, 760–2, 764, 771–2
  effusion 762, 763
  examination 47–9
  excision arthroplasty 1709
  extension 150
  external rotation 150
  in familial Mediterranean fever 1446–7
  fixed flexion deformity 47
  flexion 150
  fracture 1584–5
    in osteoporosis 1583–4, *1584*, 1600, *1601*
    risk factors 1585–6, *1585*
  functional anatomy and disability 1725
  imaging
    arthrography 741–2, 743, 764
    CT 718
    MRI 770–1
    radiography 716–17, 718
  internal rotation 150
  in juvenile chronic arthritis
    and growth disturbance 82
    pauci-articular onset 1100
    rehabilitation 1743–4, 1745, 1746
    seronegative polyarthritis 1134–5
    surgery 1715–17
    systemic onset 1116, 1117
  loads 477
  local steroid injection 157, *1762*, 1768
  osteoarthritis 1524–5, 1534, 1549
  pain 1507–8, *1508*
    adult *155*, 156–7
    childhood 164–5, *164*
  palpation 48
  physiotherapy, childhood 1743–4, 1745, 1746

hip (*continued*)
pyogenic arthritis 741, 743, 858
   childhood 863
range of movement 48–9, 150
reflex sympathetic dystrophy 1682
replacement 1708–9
   assessment of outcome 57, 58
   childhood 1716–17
   in Paget's disease 1617
   prosthetic loosening or infection 741
   in spondyloepiphyseal dysplasia 1630, *1632*
in rheumatoid arthritis 1009
screening 47
snapping 1508
surgery 1708–9, 1715–17
synovectomy 1709
transient synovitis 5, 164
tuberculosis 770
in walking cycle 482
Hip Arthroplasty Outcome Evaluation Questionnaire 57
Hip Rating Questionnaire *57*, 58
HIS 56, 57
His–Perkinje system 237
histamine 512, 545
histidine deficiency 262
histiocytosis X *see* Langerhans cell histiocytosis
histones 668–9
histopathology 775–96
histoplasmosis 252
arteritis in 1390
epidemiology 954
in HIV infection 916, 962
joint infection *955, 957*, 962
management 956, 957
history taking
adult patients 4–7
childhood 15
skin lesions 200
HIV
infection 901, **906–21**
   autoantibodies 910
   B-cell abnormalities 910
   and Behçet's syndrome 918
   biology 907–10
   c-ANCA/PR3-ANCA in 1320
   differential diagnosis 1313
   differential diagnosis of arthritis associated 1091
   and diffuse infiltrative lymphocytosis syndrome 911–13
   epidemiology 907–8
   helper T-cell dysfunction 907, 909, 910–11, 916–17
   histoplasmosis in 916, 962
   host response to 910–15
   immune-mediated arthritis in 917–21
   muscle atrophy in 791
   myopathy in 789, 790, 913–14
   myositis in 1263, 1278, 1293
   nephropathy in 915
   and ocular disorders 317
   osteomyelitis in 916–17
   painful articular syndrome 901
   peripheral neuropathy in 795
   and proteinuria 322
   psoriatic arthritis in 901, 918–21, 1079
   and pyogenic arthritis 849, 916–17
   pyomyositis in 916–17
   reactive arthritis in 901, 918–21
   Reiter's syndrome in 901, 918–21
   rheumatological consequences 901, 907, *907*
   and Sjögren's syndrome 1302
   T-cell alterations 907, 909, 910–11, 916–17
   tests for 661
   and tuberculosis 927
   undifferentiated seronegative spondylarthropathies in 918–21

HIV (*continued*)
infection (*continued*)
   vasculitis in 914–15, 1328, 1368
   lifecycle and replication 909–10
   structure and organization 908–9
   transactivation 909–10
HLA genes 547, 695–7
class I 547, 696
class II 547–8, 696
class III 696
nomenclature 697, *698*
polymorphism 696–7
   analysis 695–7
sharing of haplotypes by siblings 553–4, *554*
HLA molecules 695–7
antigen processing and presentation by 549–50
class I 547, 696
class II 547–8, 696, 984
   expression in rheumatoid arthritis 988
   isoelectrofocusing 697
   microcytotoxicity assay 697
   nomenclature 697, *698*
   polymorphism 548–9, 696–7
      analysis 695–7
   typing 697, 844
HLA-A 547
HLA-A1
and coeliac disease 554
and HIV infection 910
HLA-A2
and juvenile chronic arthritis 1109–10
and juvenile psoriatic arthritis 1055, 1056
structure 547
HLA-A68 structure 547
HLA-B 547
HLA-B5 and Behçet's syndrome 1395
HLA-B7 and psoriatic arthritis 1078
HLA-B8
and autoimmune thyroid disease 279
and coeliac disease 554–5, *555*
and HIV infection 910
and juvenile dermatomyositis 1289, 1295
and sarcoidosis 1464
and Sjögren's syndrome *1303*
and type II polyglandular autoimmune syndrome 285
and Wegener's granulomatosis 1342
HLA-B13
and psoriasis 1078
and psoriatic arthritis 1078
HLA-B17
and juvenile psoriatic arthritis 1055
and psoriasis 1078
and psoriatic arthritis 1078
HLA-B27
45 pocket hypothesis 1042
and acute anterior uveitis 314, 317
and ankylosing spondylitis 99, 128, 184, 552–3, 698–9, *822*, 1059–60, 1060–1, 1066–7
arthritogenic peptide model of disease 1042
and brucellar arthritis 941
cross-reactivity with *Klebsiella pneumoniae* 1042, 1067
disease associations 698–9, 844
distribution in population *1038*
and enteric arthropathies 1094
gene alleles 552
and HIV-associated Reiter's syndrome 901, 920–1
and juvenile psoriatic arthritis 1056
and juvenile spondylarthropathies 1049–50, 1051, 1052
as marker for linked gene 552–3
and molecular mimicry 553, 1042
molecule as receptor for aetiological agent 1041
and psoriatic arthritis 698, 1078

HLA-B27 (*continued*)
and reactive arthropathies 698, 1088, 1092
and SEA syndrome 1051
and seronegative spondylarthropathies 552–3, 838–40, *839*, 1038, **1041–3**, 1043–4, 1059, 1085
structure 547, 1041
subtypes 698–9, 1042, 1067
   distribution in population *1042*
transgenic rats 553, 699, 1043, *1043*, 1045–6, 1049, 1050
and Whipple's disease 1095
and *Yersinia enterocolitica* infection 663
HLA-B27.03 1042
HLA-B35
and gold-salt dermatitis 213, 601
and HIV infection 910
HLA-B37, and psoriasis 1078
HLA-B38 and psoriatic arthritis 1078
HLA-B39 and psoriatic arthritis 1078
HLA-B53 and cerebral malaria 549
HLA-Bw52 and Takayasu's arteritis 1387
HLA-Bw60 and ankylosing spondylitis 699
HLA-Bw62 and enteric arthropathies 1094
HLA-C 547
HLA-Cw3 and polymyalgia rheumatica/giant cell arteritis 1375
HLA-Cw6 and psoriasis 1078
HLA-DM 549
HLA-DN 549
HLA-DO 549
HLA-DP 547–8
and SLE 1167
HLA-DPB1*0201 and juvenile chronic arthritis 699, 1138, *1139*
HLA-DPB1*0301
and juvenile ankylosing spondylitis 699
and juvenile chronic arthritis 1138, *1139*
HLA-DPB1*0402 and juvenile chronic arthritis *1139*
HLA-DPB1
and juvenile chronic arthritis 1110
and systemic sclerosis 1220
HLA-DQ 547–8
HLA-DQ and rheumatoid arthritis 988
HLA-DQ2 and coeliac disease 554–5, *555*
HLA-DQ57 and systemic sclerosis *1224*
HLA-DQA1*0101 and juvenile chronic arthritis 699, *1139*
HLA-DQA1*0103 and juvenile chronic arthritis *1139*
HLA-DQA1*0201 and juvenile chronic arthritis *1139*
HLA-DQA1*0401 and juvenile chronic arthritis *1139*
HLA-DQA1*0501 and Sjögren's syndrome 1302–3
HLA-DQA2 and systemic sclerosis *1224*
HLA-DQB1*0201 and Sjögren's syndrome 1302
HLA-DQB1*0402 and juvenile chronic arthritis *1139*
HLA-DQB1*0603 and juvenile chronic arthritis *1139*
HLA-DQB1 and systemic sclerosis 1220, *1224*
HLA-DQβ1 and SLE 1171
HLA-DQβ2 and SLE 1171
HLA-DQw1
and SLE 1171
and Takayasu's arteritis 1387
HLA-DQw2 and SLE 1171
HLA-DQw3 and systemic sclerosis *1224*
HLA-DQw7
and SLE 1171
and Wegener's granulomatosis 1342

HLA-DQw8 and SLE 1171
HLA-DR 547–8
and rheumatoid arthritis 553–4, *554*, 555, 699
and SLE 1167
structure 984–5
HLA-DR1
and ethnic group 984
and rheumatic fever 975
and rheumatoid arthritis 553–4, *554*, 555, 699, 984, *985*
and systemic sclerosis 1219–20, *1224*
HLA-DR2 549, 697
and autoimmune thyroid disease 279
and rheumatic fever 975
and rheumatoid arthritis *554*
and SLE 507, *822*, 1171
and systemic sclerosis *1224*
and Takayasu's arteritis 1387
and TNF-α production 504
and Wegener's granulomatosis 1342
HLA-DR3
and adverse drug reactions 601, 642, 1022
and aplastic anaemia 296
and autoimmune thyroid disease 279
and coeliac disease 554–5, *555*
and diabetes mellitus 285, 554
and Dupuytren's contracture 148
and HIV infection 910
and inclusion-body myositis 472, 1279–80
and juvenile dermatomyositis 1289, 1295
and leprosy 549
and polymyositis/dermatomyositis 1268
and pulmonary complications of rheumatoid arthritis 1010
and sarcoidosis 1464
and Sjögren's syndrome 1302–3, *1303*
and SLE 507, *822*, 1148, 1171
and systemic sclerosis *1224*
and thrombocytopenia 296
and TNF-α production 504
and type II polyglandular autoimmune syndrome 285
and vinyl chloride disease 1694
HLA-DR4 549
and ankylosing spondylitis 1062
and aplastic anaemia 296
and autoimmune thyroid disease 279
and diabetes mellitus 285, 554
and drug-induced lupus 1692
and ethnic group 984
and Felty's syndrome 556, *556*, 643, 1015
and juvenile chronic arthritis 699, 1110, 1114
and juvenile psoriatic arthritis 1056
and Lyme disease 885, 888, 893
and parvovirus B19 arthropathy 898
and polymyalgia rheumatica/giant cell arteritis 1375, 1670
and polymyositis/dermatomyositis 1267
and psoriatic arthritis 1078
and relapsing polychondritis 1625
and rheumatic fever 975
and rheumatoid arthritis 553–4, *554*, 555–6, 699, *822*, 984–5, *985*
and seropositive juvenile chronic arthritis 1034–6
and SLE 1171
subtypes 984
and systemic sclerosis 1219–20, *1224*
and TNF-α production 504
HLA-DR5 697
and coeliac disease 554
and DILS 912
and juvenile chronic arthritis 699, *822*, 1110, 1114
and juvenile psoriatic arthritis 1056
and Sjögren's syndrome *1303*

HLA-DR5 *(continued)*
and systemic sclerosis *822*, 1219–20, *1224*
and vinyl chloride disease 1693–4
HLA-DR6 697
and juvenile chronic arthritis 1110
and rheumatoid arthritis *554*, 699
HLA-DR7
and coeliac disease 554
and juvenile chronic arthritis 1110
and juvenile psoriatic arthritis 1055
and psoriasis 1078
and psoriatic arthritis 1078
and rheumatic fever 975
HLA-DR8
and juvenile chronic arthritis 1110, 1114, 1138
and juvenile psoriatic arthritis 1056
and SLE 837
and systemic sclerosis 1219–20
HLA-DR10 and rheumatoid arthritis 553, 554, *554*
HLA-DR11
and Sjögren's syndrome *1303*
and systemic sclerosis 1219, *1224*
HLA-DR13
and development of anaemia in malaria 549
and DILS 912
HLA-DRB1*04 and juvenile chronic arthritis 699, 1138
HLA-DRB1*07 and juvenile chronic arthritis 699, *1139*
HLA-DRB1*08
and juvenile ankylosing spondylitis 699
and juvenile chronic arthritis 699
HLA-DRB1*11 and juvenile chronic arthritis 699, *1139*
HLA-DRB1*12 and juvenile chronic arthritis 699
HLA-DRB1*0101
and juvenile chronic arthritis 699, *1139*
and rheumatoid arthritis 699
HLA-DRB1*0102 and juvenile chronic arthritis *1139*
HLA-DRB1*0301 and Sjögren's syndrome 1302
HLA-DRB1*0401
and juvenile chronic arthritis *1139*
and rheumatoid arthritis 699
HLA-DRB1*0404
and gold toxicity 601
and rheumatoid arthritis 699
HLA-DRB1*0405
prevalence in ethnic groups 699
and rheumatoid arthritis 699
HLA-DRB1*0408 and rheumatoid arthritis 699
HLA-DRB1*0801 and juvenile chronic arthritis 1138, *1139*
HLA-DRB1*0803 and juvenile chronic arthritis *1139*
HLA-DRB1*1101 and Sjögren's syndrome 1302
HLA-DRB1*1102 and HIV infection 910
HLA-DRB1*1104
and juvenile chronic arthritis 699, *1139*
and Sjögren's syndrome 1302
HLA-DRB1*1301
and HIV infection 910
and juvenile chronic arthritis 699, *1139*
HLA-DRB1*1402
prevalence in ethnic groups 699
in rheumatoid arthritis 699
HLA-DRB1*1501 and juvenile chronic arthritis *1139*
HLA-DRw6
and DILS 912–13
and rheumatic fever 975
and systemic sclerosis *1224*
HLA-DRw8
and juvenile chronic arthritis *822*
and juvenile psoriatic arthritis 1056
and SLE 1171

HLA-DRw15 and systemic sclerosis *1224*
HLA-DRw17 and SLE 1171
HLA-DRw52 and Sjögren's syndrome *1303*
HLA-DRw52a and systemic sclerosis 1219, *1224*
HLA-DRw52b and SLE 1171
HLA-DRw53 and Sjögren's syndrome *1303*
HLA-DW3 and Sjögren's syndrome *1303*
HLA-Dw4
and Felty's syndrome 643
and rheumatoid arthritis 984–5, *985*
and seropositive juvenile chronic arthritis 1034
HLA-Dw7 amd juvenile chronic arthritis 1114
HLA-Dw10 984, *985*
HLA-Dw12 and Takayasu's arteritis 1387
HLA-Dw13 984, *985*
HLA-Dw14
and rheumatoid arthritis 984–5, *985*
and seropositive juvenile chronic arthritis 1034
HLA-Dw15 and rheumatoid arthritis 984–5, *985*
HLA-Dw53 and rheumatic fever 975
hoarseness
in CINCA 1471
in Wegener's granulomatosis 1335
Hoffa's disease 166
Hoffman's sign in cervical myelopathy 1656
Hoffman's syndrome *277*, 278
home environment
adaptation 1728–9, *1729*
assessment 1728, *1729*
control 1729, *1730*
homeobox genes 394–5
homeostatic ability, effect of age on 23–4
homocystinuria 129, 436
homogentisic acid oxidase deficiency 436
Hooke's law 1492
hormone replacement therapy and osteoporosis 29, 1596–7
hormones 509
Horner's syndrome *224*, 312
Hoskins and Squires Test for Gross Motor and Reflex Development 56–7, *56*
hospitalization and malnutrition 30
HOT 694
'hour-glass' deformity 284
housemaid's knee *see* prepatellar bursa, bursitis
Howship's resorption lacunae 421, 422
HOX genes 368, 370
HOX A2 mutation 394
HOX A13d mutation 394–5
HPRT *see* hypoxanthine guanine phosphoribosyl transferase
HPV infection *see* parvovirus infection
HTLV *see* human T cell leukaemia virus
human adjuvant disease 1693
human genome 350
Human Genome Mapping Initiative 370
human immunodeficiency virus *see* HIV
human neutrophil elastase 1329
human parainfluenza virus in Paget's disease 1610
human parvovirus *see* parvovirus infection
human T cell leukaemia virus (HTLV) 901, 908
cellular transcription factors 352
coinfection with HIV 909
and myositis 1263–4, 1293

human T cell leukaemia virus (HTLV) *(continued)*
and Sjögren's syndrome 1302
humeroradial articulation 137
humeroulnar articulation 137
humerus
external rotation 137
greater tuberosity 135, 136
head 135, 136
erosions in hyperparathyroidism 280
lateral epicondyle 136, 137
medial epicondyle 136, 137
osteotomy 1703
trochlear osteonecrosis 1623
Hunter–Scheie syndrome 1632, 1633, *1633*
Huntington's disease 695
Hurler's syndrome 1632, *1633*
hY1-5 670
hY1 RNP 672
hyaluronan
binding to proteoglycan 409, 414
in damaged tendons 1494
effect of local steroid injection on 1757
as marker of osteoarthritis 417
receptor 534
hyaluronate 442, 973
in bursal fluid 155
depolymerization by free radicals 447
in hypothyroidism 277
in inflammation 514
intra-articular 1547
in rheumatoid arthritis 1016, *1017*
in synovial fluid 514, 677
hyaluronidase 514
hybridization protection assay 692, 693, 697
hydatid cyst *948*
articular syndromes associated 947–8
muscular syndromes associated 950
and polyarteritis nodosa 951
hydra monster 1145, 1176
hydralazine
adverse effects
lupus 36, 669, 1690, *1690*, *1691*, *1692*
myositis 1693
autoantibody induction 1692
effect on lymphocyte function 1692
in mixed connective tissue disease 1423
and Wegener's granulomatosis 1342
hydration and exercise 1780
hydrocortisone *see* cortisol
hydrocortisone 17-butyrate *210*
hydrocortisone acetate injection 1757, 1760, *1760*
hydrogen peroxide
generation in synovial hypoxia 447
in inflammation 514
hydronephrosis 326
hydrops fetalis 897
hydrotherapy
juvenile dermatomyositis 1751
reflex sympathetic dystrophy 1687
hydroxyapatite crystals 421, 677, 1526, 1531–2, 1570, 1572
in osteoarthritis 1542
3-D-hydroxybutarate in synovial hypoxia 445
hydroxychloroquine 596
in adult-onset Still's disease 1127
adverse effects 596
cutaneous 214, 596
gastrointestinal 596
haematological 295–6
myopathic *1265*, 1266
ocular 318–19, 596
psychiatric *337*, 338
in combination therapy *1025*
in dermatomyositis 1277
in discoid lupus erythematosus 211
in eosinophilic fasciitis 1428
in hypersensitivity vasculitis 1369
in juvenile chronic arthritis 1035, 1107, 1140, *1140*

hydroxychloroquine *(continued)*
in juvenile dermatomyositis 1297
in lactation 194, *602*
in multicentric reticulohistiocytosis *1476*
pharmacology 596
in pregnancy 191–2, *602*
protective effects in hyperlipidaemias 1485
in psoriatic arthritis 1080
in rheumatoid arthritis 1021
in RS₃PE syndrome 35
in Sjögren's syndrome 1314
in SLE 1172, *1173*
childhood 1182
therapeutic efficacy 596
therapeutically relevant effects 596
treatment regimens 596
in urticarial vasculitis 1370
6-hydroxydopamine 449
12-hydroxyeicosatetraenoic acid 448
hydroxyl radical 447
generation in synovial hypoxia 447
in inflammation 514
hydroxylamine and osmium tetroxide 694
1α-hydroxylase 430
21-hydroxylase gene 548, 1013
7-hydroxymethotrexate 582
hydroxyproline 653
in collagen 407
in Paget's disease 1613
in reflex sympathetic dystrophy 1682
in sarcoidosis 1465
total urinary excretion 432
L-5-hydroxytryptophan, scleroderma induced by *1223*, 1693
hydroxyurea in psoriasis 212
25-hydroxyvitamin D 430, 1602
effect of anticonvulsants on 1590
in osteomalacia 1601
hyperalgesia 489, 491
definition *488*
in reflex sympathetic dystrophy 1680, 1684, *1686*
hyperamylasaemia in Sjögren's syndrome 1310
hyperbilirubinaemia 651, 1116
hypercalcaemia
familial hypocalciuric 434
and calcium pyrophosphate dihydrate disease *1531*, 1567, 1570
in hyperparathyroidism 653
in hypophosphatasia 436
neoplastic 437, *437*
in Paget's disease 1612–13
in sarcoidosis 1465
hypercalciuria
in Paget's disease 1612–13
in sarcoidosis 1465
hypercortisolism 586, 1622
hypereosinophilic syndrome 796
hyperexcitability *488*
hypergammaglobulinaemia
acute phase response in 640
in juvenile chronic arthritis 1120
in mixed connective tissue disease 1419
in psoriatic arthritis 1077
in Sjögren's syndrome 1303
in SLE 1157
in Takayasu's arteritis 1386
hyperglobulinaemic purpura, rheumatoid factor in *674*
hyperimmunoglobulinaemia D syndrome 1123
hyperkalaemia
drug-related *578*, 580
in pigment-induced nephropathy 327
hyperkeratosis, subungual 202
hyperlipidaemias 1478–86
acute phase response in 640
drug-related *587*
and gout 1484, 1556
mechanisms 1483
patterns 1480, *1480*

hyperlipidaemias (continued)
  primary, muculoskeletal manifestations
      1481
  and psoriatic arthritis 1484
  rationale for treatment 1485
  in rheumatic disorders 1482
  and rheumatoid arthritis 1484
  skin involvement 206, *208*
  and SLE 1194, 1483–4
  and systemic sclerosis 1484
hypermobility 1499–501, *1500*
  and back pain 1646
  differential diagnosis *757, 1105*
  and musculoskeletal pain 168
  and osteoarthritis 1519
hyperparathyroidism 279–81, 654
  bone biopsy in 783
  bone disease in 434
  and calcium pyrophosphate dihydrate
      disease 1530, *1531,* 1567
  hypercalcaemia in 653
  in osteomalacia 1602
  and osteoporosis 280, 1589
  primary 280, 434
  secondary 280, 434, 1602, 1603
  tertiary 434
**hyperpathia in reflex sympathetic
      dystrophy** 1680
**hyperphosphataemia in renal osteo-
      dystrophy** 1603
hyperpigmentation 207, *209,* 1148
hyperprolactinaemia 282, 510, 1589
hyperpyrexia 1777–8
hypertension 321, *330,* **330–1**
  in acute renal failure 329
  and anticardiopilin antibodies 222
  in Churg–Strauss syndrome 1355
  drug-related *587,* 59539595
  effect of NSAIDs on control 580, *1021*
  and gout 651, 1556
  in HIV infection 915
  in lupus nephritis 321
  malignant 324, 329
      in antiphospholipid syndrome
          1206
  in microscopic polyangiitis 1354
  and osteoarthritis 1519
  in polyarteritis nodosa 330–1, 1403
  in rapidly progressive glomerulo-
      nephritis 327, 331
  in scleroderma renal crisis 1237
  in SLE 1190
  in systemic sclerosis 329
  in Takayasu's arteritis 1385, 1387
hyperthyroidism *see* thyrotoxicosis
hypertrichosis 209, *595*
**hypertrophic cranial pachymeningitis
      in mixed connective tissue
      disease** 1418
hypertrophic neuropathy 794
hypertrophic osteoarthropathy 289,
      1672–3
  primary 168
  secondary 168
**hypertrophic pulmonary osteoarthro-
      pathy** 289
hyperuricaemia 654, 1555
  definition 1562
  and diabetes mellitus 283
  drug-related *1558,* 1694
  in gout
      primary 1557
      secondary 1558, *1558*
  in hyperparathyroidism 280
  in hypothyroidism *277,* 278
  and inborn errors of metabolism
      1557–8, *1558*
  monosodium urate in 684
  and osteoarthritis 1519
  in Paget's disease 1613
  and pregnancy 184–5
  in psoriatic arthritis 1077
hyperviscosity syndrome *174, 223*
hypnosis in low back pain 106

hypoalbuminaemia *258*
  in juvenile chronic arthritis 1120
  in SLE 1157
hypocalcaemia
  familial 434
  and hyperparathyroidism 434
  in osteomalacia/rickets 653, 1601
  in renal osteodystrophy 1603
hypochondrodysplasia 413
hypochondrogenesis *369, 375, 413, 435*
  gene mutations 370
hypochondroplasia 369, *369,* 396, 1630
hypocomplementaemia
  in Felty's syndrome 644
  in hypersensitivity vasculitis 1368
  in mixed connective tissue disease 1419
  in SLE
      in the elderly 35, *35*
      and pregnancy 183
  in vasculitis 1136, 1369–70
hypogammaglobulinaemia 966–71,
      967
  bacterial septic arthritis in 969
  and chronic arthritis of the knee 970
  drug-associated 970
  mycoplasma arthritis in 966–9
  pyogenic arthritis in 880
  rheumatoid arthritis in 969–70
  in sulphasalazine therapy 589, *589*
  tenosynovitis in 970
hypogonadism and osteoporosis 1589
hypokalaemia
  and muscle pain 653
  myopathy in 1266
hypomagnesaemia 654, 1530, *1531,*
      1567, 1570
hypomelanosis of Ito 387
hypoparathyroidism 281
  autoimmune *285*
  bone disease in 434
  in SLE 1197
hypophosphataemia
  in malignant disease 437
  in osteomalacia 1605–6
  renal tubular rickets in 433
  in rickets 1600, 1604, 1605
hypophosphatasia 436, 654
  and calcium pyrophosphate dihydrate
      disease 1530, *1531,* 1567, 1570
  and rickets 1606
hypophysitis, autoimmune *285*
hypopigmentation 207, *209*
hypopyon 312, 315
hypotension 231
hypothalamic–pituitary–adrenal axis
  drug-related suppression *587*
  in inflammation 510
hypothalamus, disorders 282
hypothermia 24
hypothyroidism *219,* **277–8**
  and calcium pyrophosphate dihydrate
      disease 278, 1530, *1531,* 1567
  differential diagnosis 1379
  myopathy in 1266
  in polymyalgia rheumatica/giant cell
      arteritis 1378
  in SLE 279, 1197
  synovial fluid in 680
hypoxanthine 1557
  accumulation in synovial hypoxia 446
**hypoxanthine guanine phosphoribosyl
      transferase (HPRT)** 1557
  deficiency 1557, *1558*
  gene mutations in mixed connective
      tissue disease 1421
hypoxic–reperfusion injury 446, 449,
      509
  and free radical generation 514

I

I cell disease 1634
Ia antigens in rheumatic fever 976
IBD 688

ibuprofen
  adverse effects
      gastrointestinal 260, *1021*
      haematological 295
      neurological *217*
      psychiatric 338
      renal 327
      in SLE 580, 1182
  in ankylosing spondylitis 184
  clearance 577
  dose–response relationship 1020
  enantiomers 577
  and gastric ulceration 578
  half-life *577*
  in juvenile chronic arthritis *1106,* 1124,
      1138, *1140*
  in lactation 193
  in osteoarthritis 1547
  in pregnancy 184, 190
  in psoriatic arthritis 1080
  relationship between dose, plasma
      concentration and effect 577
  in seropositive juvenile chronic
      arthritis 1035
  use by the elderly 102
ICAM *see* intercellular adhesion
      molecules
ice in acute injury 1780–1
identity by descent 688
idiotypes 610
  network manipulation 613–14
  private 610
  public 610, 613
IDL 1479
igbo ora virus 903
IHLC 69
**ILAR, diagnostic criteria for chronic
      childhood arthritis** 10, *11*
ileocolonoscopy 1094
**ileostomy, pyoderma gangrenosum
      around** 1458, 1459
iliacus 150
iliofemoral ligament 150
iliopsoas 150
iliopsoas/iliopectineal bursa 150, 151,
      157
  bursitis 157, 1508
iliotibial band 151, 152, 158
iliotibial band syndrome 158
ilium 150
Ilizarov limb reconstruction 875
illness behaviour syndrome 106
**iloprost in antiphospholipid
      syndrome** 1212
imaging 715–50
  childhood 751–72
  diffuse idiopathic skeletal hyperostosis
      735, 737
  see also specific techniques
imipenem in osteomyelitis 875
imipramine 339, 340, *340, 341*
  plasma concentrations *342*
  in rheumatoid arthritis 341
immobilization
  and osteoporosis 128, 433, 1590
  in Paget's disease 1612
  reflex sympathetic dystrophy following
      1681
  in soft-tissue rheumatism 1512
  in spondylolisthesis 127
  in tuberculosis 933
immune complex diseases 703, 933
  dynamics *704*
immune complexes 560, 609–10,
      703–12, 844
  in ankylosing spondylitis 1066
  Clq binding assay 706, 707, *708, 709*
  Clq solid phase assay 706, 707, *708,
      709*
  complement-fixing 706
  conglutinin binding assay 706, 707–8,
      708, 709
  cryoprecipitation 705–6
  deposition 703

immune complexes (continued)
  detection 705
      antigen non-specific methods 704–9
      antigen-specific methods 704
      by interaction with biological recog-
          nition units 706–8, *706, 708*
      cellular assays 706, *706*
      clinical usefulness 712
      fluid phase assays 706, *706*
      solid phase assays 706, *706*
      specificity of assays 708
      standardization of assays 709
      substances interfering with assays
          708–9
  gel filtration 705
  in gonococcal infection 855
  in HIV infection 910
  in juvenile chronic arthritis 712, 1109,
      1120
  in leucocytoclastic vasculitis 1366–7
  local formation 703
  in Lyme disease 712, 885
  as markers of clinical disease 654
  in mixed connective tissue disease
      711–12
  pathogenicity 703–4, *703, 704*
  polyethylene glycol precipitation 705
  Raji cell binding assay 706, 707, *708,
      709*
  in rapidly progressive glomerulone-
      phritis 327, *328*
  in relapsing polychondritis 1626
  in rheumatic fever 976
  in rheumatoid arthritis 710–11, *710,*
      712, 994
  rheumatoid factor inhibition assay 706,
      707, *708, 709*
  sample manipulation 709
  in scleroderma 712, 1222
  in Sjögren's syndrome 711
  in SLE 507, 704, *710,* 711, 1147, 1152,
      1164–5
  in Takayasu's arteritis 1386
  ultracentrifugation 705
  in vasculitis 712, 787, 1328, 1358
immune response 545–6, 608, 609, 654
  in classification of rheumatic diseases
      844–7, *845*
  relationship with infection and autoim-
      munity 843–4, *843*
  suppression in rheumatoid arthritis
      997
immunity
  adaptive 545–6
  cellular
      defects 971
      enhanced 546
  innate 545
immunization 611
immunoassays 660
  sandwich 660
immunoblotting, autoantibodies 669,
      670
**immunocytoma in Sjögren's
      syndrome** 1312
immunodeficiency 966–71
  antibody/cell-mediated 966–71
  classification 966, *967*
  differential diagnosis 1136
  and overexertion 1778, 1780
  primary 966, *967*
  and pyogenic arthritis 849
  secondary 966, *967*
  severe combined 971
  see also hypogammaglobulinaemia
immunofluorescence 660
  direct, skin 202
  glomerular 327, *328*
  indirect, autoantibodies 328, 329,
      665–6, 667, 668, 673
immunoglobulins
  as adhesion molecules 533–4, 1168,
      1169
  and erythrocyte sedimentation rate 639

immunoglobulins (continued)
  gene superfamily 349–50
  goat serum 969
  IgA 654
    in ankylosing spondylitis 1067
    deficiency in juvenile chronic
      arthritis 1120
    effect of sulphasalazine on 588, 589,
      589
    in Henoch–Schönlein purpura 1407
    in juvenile dermatomyositis 1295
    in Lyme disease 885
    in rapidly progressive glomerulo-
      nephritis *328*
  IgG 654
    in brucellar arthritis 943
    carbohydrate content variations 675
    effect of free radicals on 447
    effect of sulphasalazine on 589
    G0 675
    glycosylation defects 986
    in Lyme disease 889
    in relapsing polychondritis 1625
    in rheumatoid arthritis 986
    in SLE 1157
    therapeutic in pregnancy in SLE 183
    and urate crystal formation 1559
  IgM 654
    in brucellar arthritis 943
    in Henoch–Schönlein purpura 1407
    in juvenile dermatomyositis 1295
    in Lyme disease 889
    in SLE 1157
  in innate immunity 545
  intravenous therapy 614
    in inclusion-body myositis 1280
    in juvenile chronic arthritis 1125–6
    in juvenile dermatomyositis 1297
    in Kawasaki disease 1406
    in microscopic polyangiitis 1359
    in mycoplasma infection 969
    in parvovirus infection 898–9
    in polyarteritis nodosa 1359, 1404
    in polymyositis/dermatomyositis
      1276–7
    in rheumatoid arthritis 1026
    in SLE 183, 1175
    in thrombocytopenia 1213
    in Wegener's granulomatosis 1346
  in juvenile chronic arthritis 1109
  monoclonal in Sjögren's syndrome
    1303–5
immunosuppressive therapy 608–16
  adverse effects
    cutaneous 214–15
    ocular 319
    oncogenic 289–90
  agents **589–96**
  in cutaneous ulceration 210
  non-selective 610–11
  in polymyositis/dermatomyositis
    1275–6
  pulmonary complications 1253–4
  risk of pyogenic arthritis 849
  selective *609*, 611–15
  strategies 608–10, *609*
  and surgery 301
  in vasculitis 1329
  see also specific drugs
impairment 52, 64, 1723
impetigo 973
impingement signs 141, 142
impingement test 141
implants, interference with MRI
  724
impotence *177, 178, 1239*
Imuran *see* azathioprine
incidence 813, *813*
  assessment 813–14, *814*
  cumulative *813*
  episode *813*
income 66
incontinence 1723
Index of Well Being 53, 61

India
  prevalemce of seronegative spondylar-
    thropathies *839*
  prevalence of rheumatoid arthritis *834*
indigestion, drug-related *578*
indium scan *see* radionuclide scanning
indomethacin
  in adult-onset Still's disease 1127
  adverse effects
    on cartilage 1695
    cutaneous 212
    gastrointestinal 260, *1021*
    haematological 295
    headache 580
    neurological *217*
    psychiatric 338
  in ankylosing spondylitis 1069
  in collagen-induced arthritis 564
  drug interactions *579*
  effect on CNS neurones 497
  in gout 1563
  half-life *577*
  in hypersensitivity vasculitis 1369
  in juvenile chronic arthritis *1106*, 1124,
    1126, *1140*
  in juvenile spondylarthropathies 1049
  in lactation 194
  in leprosy 935
  in myositis ossificans 1783
  in pregnancy 189, 190
  in psoriatic arthritis 1080
  renal clearance 577
  in rheumatoid arthritis 1020
  in SLE 1194
  in urticarial vasculitis 1370
Indonesia, prevalence of rheumatoid
  arthritis *834*
inducer T cells *see* helper T cells
industrial chemicals, scleroderma-
  like changes induced by *209*
infection
  arteritis related to 1389–91
  bacterial
    acute phase response in 625, 640
    arteritis related to 1390
    differential diagnosis 1122
    enteric *256*
    in Felty's syndrome 644
    in non-gonococcal arthritis 851–3
    pulmonary *251*, 252
    in pyogenic arthritis 849, 851–3
    synovial fluid in 683
  childhood, back pain in 121–4
  in classification of rheumatic diseases
    844–7, *845*
  community-acquired 857
  as contraindication to local steroid
    injection 1758
  and disease occurrence 823–4
  effect on serum urea concentration 650
  following joint replacement 849, 853–4,
    857, 858, 1709
  following local steroid injection 1759
  fungal
    arteritis due to 1390
    arthritis associated **954–63**
    in osteomyelitis 868, 870
    prosthetic joints 958, 962
    pulmonary 245, *251*, 252
    in pyogenic arthritis 880
  hospital-acquired 857
  joints
    investigation 661–2
    prosthetic 853–4, 857, 858, 879, 1709
  and low back pain 98–9
  mycobacterial *see* Mycobacterium
  in neutropenia 512
  and neutrophilia 642, *643*
  opportunistic
    in alkylating agent therapy *593*, 594
    following total-lymphoid radio-
      therapy 611
    in methotrexate therapy *584*, 585
    in steroid therapy *587*

infection (continued)
  in polymyositis/dermatomyositis
    1266–7, 1288–9
  pulmonary 245, 251–3, *251*, 1195
  relationship with immune responses and
    autoimmunity 843–4, *843*
  in rheumatoid arthritis 823–4, 985–6,
    1013
  risk of in SLE 1157
  role in psoriatic arthritis 1079
  secondary to HIV infection 916–17
  and thrombocytopenia 645
  viral
    differential diagnosis 1122, 1136, *1137*
    enteric *256*
    joints 896–7
    myositis in 789, 1293
    pulmonary *251*, 253
    and Sjögren's syndrome 257, *258*,
      1302
    and Wegener's granulomatosis 1342
  see also pyogenic arthritis
infectious arthritis *see* pyogenic arthritis
infectious mononucleosis *674*, 824, 904
infective discitis, acute phase response
  in 640
inferior extensor retinacula 154, 156
inferior peroneal retinacula 154, 156
infiltration brisement in frozen
  shoulder 144
inflammation 503, 575–6
  acute 503, 525
  cellular 512–22, *513*, *516–19*
  chronic 503, 525
    acute phase response in 625
    endothelial cell activation in 537
    lymphocytes in 526
  effect on growth in juvenile chronic
    arthritis 82, 85–6
  endocrine influences 510
  genetics 504–8
  humoral 511–12, *512*
  joint, response of nociceptive system to
    491–7
  and lipids 1480
  lymphocytes in **525–38**
  modification by NSAIDs **575–80**
  neural control 511
  neuroendocrine influences 509–11, *511*
  neurogenic 450, *488*, 497
  nitric oxide in 511
  synovium 508–9
    see also synovitis
  tissue specificity 508
inflammatory bowel disease 1093–6
  age at onset 13
  childhood
    arthritis-associated 1054
    diagnosis 21
    sex differences 14
  epidemiology 1045
  genetic markers 698
  and juvenile spondylarthropathies 1050
  rheumatic manifestations 255, *256*
  and seronegative spondylarthropathies
    1045–6
inflammatory disease
  childhood 128–30
  effects on synovium 443–52
inflammatory mediator *488*
inflammatory myositis 337
inflammatory process 623
  biochemical test 653–4
  proposed functions of acute phase
    proteins *624*
  sites at which NSAIDs may act 575
inflenza, rheumatoid factor in *674*
information 69–70
  seeking 68
infracalcaneal bursitis 160
infrapatellar bursitis 158, 1509
infraspinatus 135, 137
infraspinatus tendon
  lesions 1502–3

infraspinatus tendon (continued)
  local steroid injection 1764
inguinal ligament 151
inheritance 15
innominate vein 1702
inosiplex 1611
inositol triphosphate 429
insertional mutagenesis 352
inside-out signalling 532
insoles 1733, 1749, 1770, 1783
instant centre of rotation 479
insulin
  modulation of acute phase protein
    synthesis 623
  resistance
    autoimmune *283*
    and hyperlipidaemia 1483
    type A 285
    type B 285
insulin-like growth factor binding
  proteins 87
insulin-like growth factors
  in acromegaly 281
  effect on growth plate chondrocytes
    413
  IGF-I *429*
    effect on cartilage 414–15
    effect on chondrocytes *1543*
    in juvenile chronic arthritis 87, 1119
  IGF-II 87, *429*
  modulation of acute phase protein
    synthesis 623
insulin tolerance test, in juvenile
  chronic arthritis 87
integrins 530, 1168, *1169*
  α^4 subunit 531–2
  $\alpha^L\beta_2$ 530, *531*, *1169*
    in rheumatoid arthritis 988
    in T cell activation 546
  $\alpha^M\beta_2$ 530–1, *531*
    in rheumatoid arthritis 988
  $\alpha^X\beta_2$ 530, *531*
    in rheumatoid arthritis 988
  control of function 532
  as costimulatory molecules 532–3
  expression in arthritis 537
  Leu-CAM (β_2) 530–2
    deficiency 512, 531, 532
  in lymphocyte traffic *531*
  subfamilies 530–2
  very late antigen (VLA/β_1) 531, *531*,
    532
    in rheumatoid arthritis 988
intercarpal joints 137, 138
intercellular adhesion molecules
  (ICAM)
  expression in arthritis *537*
  ICAM-1 533, *1169*
    in DILS 912
    in microscopic polyangiitis 1357,
      1361
    in rheumatoid arthritis 988, 990
    in scleroderma 1227
    in SLE 1168
    in T cell activation 546
    in Takayasu's arteritis 1386
    in Wegener's granulomatosis 1339,
      1343, 1361
  ICAM-2 533
  ICAM-3 533
  as serum markers of cellular activation
    538
interdigitating cells in polymyalgia
  rheumatica/giant cell arteritis
  1377
interferon-inducible protein-10 *525*,
  534
interferons
  and bone formation *424*
  IFN-α
    in immune response 546
    in neuropsychiatric SLE 334
    therapy
      in HCV infection 901

interferons *(continued)*
  IFN-α *(continued)*
    in scleroderma 1240
  IFN-γ
    effect on endothelial activation 536–7
    effect on lipoprotein lipase activity 1483
    effect on osteoclasts *425*
    in macrophage activation 513–14
    in polymyositis/dermatomyositis 1269
    in rheumatoid arthritis 993, *993*
    therapy 614–15
    intralesional in Dupuytren's contracture 148
    in juvenile chronic arthritis 1126
    in scleroderma 1240
  in innate immunity 545
interleukins
  and bone formation *424*
  definition 516
  IL-1
    in anaemia of chronic disease 635
    in animal models of arthritis 564, 566, 568–9
    antagonists 1024
    as chemokine 534
    effect on cartilage 414
    effect on chondrocytes 1543–4, *1543*
    effect on endothelial cell activation 536
    effect of gold therapy on 599
    effect on lipoprotein lipase activity 1483
    effect of methotrexate on 583
    effect on tendons 1494
    genes 505, 506
    IL1A 505, 506
    IL1B 505, 506
    IL1RN 505, 506
    in gout 1559
    in inflammation 508, 509, 516–18
    in juvenile chronic arthritis 1120–1
    in neoplastic hypercalcaemia *437*
    in osteoblast differentiation 425
    in osteoclast differentiation 425
    in osteoporosis 1587
    receptor antagonist 996–7, 1269
    receptor blockade 615
    receptor family 520, 521
    in rheumatoid arthritis *1017*
    in Sjögren's syndrome 1305
  IL-1α *516*
    in acute phase response 623, 638
    in inflammation 520
    in juvenile chronic arthritis 699, 1110
    in polymyositis/dermatomyositis 1269
    in rheumatoid arthritis 993, *993*, 994–5
  IL-1β *516*
    in acute phase response 623, 638
    in inflammation 510, 517, 520
    in juvenile chronic arthritis 699
    in rheumatoid arthritis 521, 993, *993*, 994–5
    in sarcoidosis 1464
  IL-2 *516*
    in Behçet's syndrome 1399
    in immune response 546
    as lymphocyte chemoattractant 534
    receptor 518, 520
    blockade 615
    in polymyositis/dermatomyositis 1269
    in rheumatoid arthritis 988, 1016, *1017*
    in sarcoidosis 1464
    in scleroderma 1221
    in Sjögren's syndrome 1305
    in Wegener's granulomatosis 1339, 1341, 1344
    in rheumatoid arthritis 993, *993*, 994
    in Sjögren's syndrome 1305

interleukins *(continued)*
  IL-2 *(continued)*
    in SLE 1168
    in T cell growth regulation 994
  IL-3 *517*
    effect on osteoclasts *425*
    in rheumatoid arthritis *993*
  IL-4 *517*
    in animal models of arthritis 569
    effect on endothelial cell activation 536–7
    in immune response 546
    in rheumatoid arthritis 993–4, *993*
    in suppression of inflammation 520
    in T cell growth regulation 994
  IL-5 *517*
  IL-6 *517*
    in acute phase response 623, 638
    in anaemia of chronic disease 635
    in ankylosing spondylitis 1066
    effect on chondrocytes *1543*
    effect on osteoclasts *425*
    in gout 1559
    in inflammation 509, 510, 517, 520
    in juvenile chronic arthritis 1120–1
    in neuropsychiatric SLE 334
    in osteoclast differentiation 425
    in osteoporosis 433, 1587
    in polymyalgia rheumatica/giant cell arteritis 1378
    in polymyositis/dermatomyositis 1269
    receptor 518
    in rheumatoid arthritis 990, 993, 994, 1016, *1017*
    in sarcoidosis 1464
    in Sjögren's syndrome 1305
    in SLE 640
  IL-6/growth hormone receptor gene family 350
  IL-7 *517*
    in rheumatoid arthritis 994
    in T cell growth regulation 994
  IL-8 *518*
    and angiogenesis 509
    as chemokine *525*, 534
    in gout 1559
    in inflammation 509, 520
    in rheumatoid arthritis 990, 993, *993*
  IL-9 *518*
  IL-10 *518*, 994
    in animal models of arthritis 569
    in immune response 546
    in rheumatoid arthritis 997
    in SLE 1167
    in suppression of inflammation 520
    therapy 615
  IL-11 *518*
    in acute phase response 623, 640
    in osteoporosis 1587
  IL-12 *518*
    in inflammation 509
  IL-13 *518*
    in suppression of inflammation 520
  IL-14 *518*
  IL-15 *518*
    as lymphocyte chemoattractant 534
  IL-16 *518*
  IL-17 *518*
intermediate density lipoprotein 1479
intermetacarpal joints 137, 138
internal carotid artery rupture in Ehlers–Danlos syndrome type 4 378
International League Against Rheumatism, diagnostic criteria for chronic childhood arthritis 10, *11*
International Olympic Committee, list of banned substances 1778
interossei 140
  atrophy in rheumatoid arthritis 1008
interphalangeal joints
  foot 153

interphalangeal joints *(continued)*
  see also distal interphalangeal joints; proximal interphalangeal joints
interstitial fibrosis 323, 596
  diffuse 1010
  in SLE 1152
interstitial nephritis *177*
  drug-related 323–4, 327, *578*, 580
  lymphocytic in DILS 912
intertubercular ligament rupture 143
intervention studies, quality of life 69–70
intervertebral disc
  in ankylosing spondylitis 734, 736, 1061
  annular tear 730, 732, 735
  disease in the elderly 37
  end-plate fracture 730, 731, 1641
  extrusion 1641
  herniation 1641–2
  imaging 730–3, 734, 735
  internal disruption 1643
  lumbar 728, 1640
    disease 98
  prolapse **1641–2**
    cervical 805, 1655, 1657
    childhood 124–5
    clinical pattern 1641, *1642*
    imaging 733, 734, 1641–2, 1643
    posterior 1641
    in pregnancy 185
    thoracic 1657
  protrusion 1641
  radial fissure 730
    partial 733
  Schmorl's nodes 730, 731
  sequestration 1641
intestinal bypass *see* bowel bypass syndrome
intra-atrial conduction fibres 237
intrauterine contraceptive devices (IUCD)
  failure due to aspirin 190
  and MRI 724
intravascular coagulation, fibrinogen in 625
intravenous pyelography in haematuria 324
introns 347, 349
Inuit *see* Eskimos
inulin 648
Inupiat *see* Eskimos
invariant chain 550
inverted supinator sign 218
involucrum 871
iodoacetate 416
IP-10 *525*, 534
ipecac, adverse effects *1265*, 1266
Iran, prevalemce of seronegative spondylarthropathies *839*
Iraq, prevalence of rheumatoid arthritis *834*
iridocyclitis
  in juvenile chronic arthritis 699
  in juvenile psoriatic arthritis 1055
iritis
  in ankylosing spondylitis 1064
  in psoriatic arthritis 1076
iron
  balance 633–4
  body content 633
  cycle 634
  deficiency *see* anaemia, iron deficiency
  haem 634
  in inflammation 514
  metabolism 633–4
    in anaemia of chronic disease 291, 635, 637–8
    within normoblasts and macrophages 634–5
  non-haem 634
  plasma transport 634
  rate of absorption 634
  serum 634
    in anaemia of chronic disease 637–8

iron *(continued)*
  supplements, in juvenile chronic arthritis 1125
  in synovial hypoxia 447
ischaemia
  definition 444
  synovial 444–51
    pressure-induced 446
ischaemic necrosis *see* osteonecrosis
ischaemic–reperfusion injury 445, 449
ischiofemoral ligament 150
ischiogluteal bursa 150, 151
  bursitis 157, 1768
ischiogluteal syndrome 1508
ischium 150
islet amyloid polypeptide *1434*, 1435
isoelectrofocusing, HLA molecules 697
isometric exercises 103
isometric strength measurement 465
isoniazid
  adverse effects 1681, *1690*
  in combination therapy *1025*
  in mycobacterial infection 253
  in tuberculosis 931, *932*, 933
isoprenaline in sport 1778
Isospora *946*
  I. belli 947
  I. hominis 947
isotretinoin in dermatomyositis 1277
isoxazolil penicillins in osteomyelitis 874
itraconazole 956, 957
  in blastomycosis 959
  in *Candida* 958
  in coccidioidomycosis 962
  in cryptococcosis 963
  in histoplasmosis 962
  in paracoccidioidomycosis 963
  in sporotrichosis 960
IUCD *see* intrauterine contraceptive devices
ivermectin 949, 950, 951
Ixodes
  I. dammini 885
  I. pacificus 885, 886
  I. persulcatus 885
  I. ricinus 884, 885
  I. scapularis 884, 885
    lifecycle 885–6, 887
  I. spinipalpis 886

J
Jaccoud's arthropathy 1147, 1181
  atlantoaxial subluxation in 224
  in Sjögren's syndrome 1309
Jackson–Weiss syndrome 369, 398
JAFAR 56, 57
JAFAS 17, *56*, 57
Japanese
  rheumatoid arthritis 833, *834*
  seronegative spondylarthropathies *839*
  SLE 836, *836*, 837
jaundice 651
jejunocolonic bypass *see* bowel bypass syndrome
Jews, seronegative spondylarthropathies *839*
jogging and trochanteric bursitis 156
joint fluid *see* synovial fluid
joint fluid analysis *see* synovial fluid analysis
joint prostheses
  infection 853–4, 857, 858, 879, 1709
  fungal 958, 962
'joint space' 443
joints
  acute infection, investigation 661–2
  adverse drug effects *587*
  in CINCA 1472, 1473
  development of deformities in juvenile chronic arthritis 1738

joints *(continued)*
disease models 415
chemical 416
genetic 416–17
meniscectomy 416
Pond–Nuki 415–16, *415*
dislocation, radiography *756*
disuse, effect on articular cartilage 406
drainage
in pyogenic arthritis 858, 865
in secondary infection in HIV infection 917
in familial Mediterranean fever 1446–7
hypermobility *see* hypermobility
hypomobility *757*
inflammation, response of nociceptive
system to 491–7
innervation 489–90
inspection 40, *40*
intraoperative care 301, 1702
involvement pattern 7
laxity 168
lipids in 1481–2
nociception in 489–91
noises 40
palpation 40, *40*
penetrating injury, pyogenic arthritis
following 865
physiology **441–3**
protection 1728, *1728*, 1752
range of movement 16, 40
limitations 1653–4
saline distension 1547
saline lavage 1547
in sarcoidosis 1466–7
shape abnormalities and osteoarthritis
1520
space narrowing in childhood *756,
757*
space widening in childhood *755, 757*
trauma 849
tumours 288, 289
vacuum effect 758
see also specific types and joints
**Juvenile Arthritis Functional
Assessment Report** *56, 57*
**Juvenile Arthritis Functional
Assessment Scale** 17, *56, 57*
juvenile chronic arthritis 1099–142
age at onset 12, 13, 1099, 1114
amyloidosis 1118–19, *1118*
antinuclear antibodies 830, *831*, 1101,
1102, 1109, 1120, 1135
cardiovascular involvement 173, *230*,
234, 238, 1116–17
central nervous system involvement
1117–18
classification 10, *10*, 759–60, *762, 763*,
843
depression in *336, 337*
diagnostic criteria 10, *10*, 1114, 1131
dyslipoproteinaemia 1120
effect on growth 14, 18, 82, 85–7
epidemiology *814*, 829–30, 1099, 1114
effect of age 12, 14, *815*, 830, *831*
geographical factors 820
incidence 12
prevalence 12, 829
ethnic factors 819, *819*, 829–31, *829,
830, 831*
fever in 21, 172, 1114–15
fractures in 1721
genetic factors *351*, 699, *822*
growth abnormalities 14, 18, 82, 85–7,
1119
haemocytophagocytosis in 291
HLA associations 699, 1138, *1139*
imaging
Doppler ultrasound 762, 763, 764
MRI 772
radiography 755, 1101, 1117, 1121,
1121
immune complexes 712, 1109, 1120
intubation in 302–3, 1721

juvenile chronic arthritis *(continued)*
joint involvement 1132
ankle 82, 85, 1099, 1100, 1116, 1134,
1135, 1718–20, 1747–9, 1750
atlantoaxial subluxation 224, 1033,
1035, 1721, 1738
cervical spine 1100, 1116, 1134, 1135,
1738, 1739
cricoarytenoid 1116
development of deformities 1738
elbow 1100, 1133, 1720, 1740
foot 1116, 1133–4, 1718–20, 1747–9,
1750
hand 1116, 1132, 1133, 1720–1, 1740–
3, *1741*, 1744
hip 82, 1100, 1116, 1117, 1134–5,
1715–17, 1743–4, 1745, 1746
knee 82, 85, 1099–100, 1116, 1133,
1134–5, 1717–18, 1719, 1745–7,
1747
shoulder 1100, 1133, 1720, 1740
temporomandibular 82, 302, 1100,
1116, 1134, 1135, 1739–40
wrist 82, 1116, 1117, 1133, 1720–1,
1740–3, *1741*, 1744
liver function 652
lymphadenopathy 172
neutrophilia *643*
nutrition in 86–7, 1119
ocular involvement 316, 317, 699,
1101–3, *1102*, 1108–9, *1108*, 1118
oligoarticular-onset 10, 11, 18
and osteoporosis 128
pauciarticular-onset **1099–111**
aetiology 1109
age at onset 1099
case studies 1110–11
clinical features 1099–100, *1100*
complications 1101–3
course 1101
differential diagnosis 1103, *1104–5*,
1105
early-onset 699–700
epidemiology 1099
immunogenetics 1109–10
laboratory tests 1100–1
late-onset 1050
prognosis 1108–9, *1108*
psychosocial aspects 1108
remission 1107
treatment 1106–8, *1106*
type 2 1099
physiotherapy **1737–50**
polyarticular
genetic markers 699
progression from pauciarticular
disease 1101, 1108
polyarticular seronegative **1131–42**
antinuclear antibody positive 1135
with boggy synovitis 1135
diagnostic criteria 1131
differential diagnosis 1136–8, *1137*
dry 1135
extra-articular manifestations
1131–2
immunogenetics 1138, *1139*
joint involvement 1132–5
laboratory tests 1135
management 1138, 1140–1, *1140,
1142*
with spondylarthropathy 1135–6
subgroups 1131, *1132*, 1135–6
and pregnancy 184
progression to SLE 1181–2
rehabilitation 1107, 1141–2, **1737–50**
renal involvement 1118
rheumatoid factor in 830–1, *831*, **1031–**
6, 1101, 1120
scoliosis in 82, 1721
seropositive 830–1, *831*, **1031–6**, 1131
clinical manifestations 1032
course 1032–4, 1035
diagnosis 1032
genetic aspects 1034–5

juvenile chronic arthritis *(continued)*
seropositive *(continued)*
management 1035–6
mode of presentation 1032
postpregnancy relapse 1036
sex ratio/distribution 12, 14, *815*, 830,
831, 1114
surgery **1713–21**
synovial biopsy 778, 1101
synovial fluid 683, 1101
systemic features *170*, 178
systemic-onset 10, 11, **1114–27**, 1470
clinical features 200, 204, 1114–19,
1115
course 1123–4
diagnostic criteria 1114
differential diagnosis 1121–3, *1123*,
1293
epidemiology 1114
HLA associations 1114
imaging 1121
laboratory tests 1119–21, *1120*
management 1124–6, *1125*
mortality 1124, *1124*
prognosis 1123–4
terminology 829, *829*, 1131
and transition to work 66
treatment 87, 1106–8, *1106*, 1124–6,
1125, 1138, 1140–1, *1140, 1142*
juvenile rheumatoid arthritis
terminology 829, *829*, 1131
see also juvenile chronic arthritis, seropositive

K

Kager's triangle 718, 719
Kallenberg score 1360
kallikrein *see* kininogenase
kanamycin in tuberculosis *932*, 933
Kaposi's sarcoma *208*
Karelian fever 904
Kashin–Beck disease 1518, **1636–7**
Katayama fever 950
Kaussmaul sign 235
Kawasaki disease 1404–6
aetiology 1405–6
age at onset 11, 12, 13
cardiovascular involvement *230*, 1404,
1405
classification *1321, 1322*
clinical features *170*, 1404, *1404*, 1405,
1405
diagnostic criteria 11, *12*, 1327, *1327*
differential diagnosis 1136, *1137*
fever in 172
gastrointestinal involvement *259*
imaging 764, 1405
incomplete 1404
laboratory tests 1405
large vessel vasculitis in 1392
lymphadenopathy 172
ocular involvement 316, 317
platelet count 17
prognosis 1406
sex differences 14
strawberry erythema of tongue and lips
204
treatment 1406
KCO 248
Keitel Index *55, 56*
**Keller's operation, plantar response
following** 218
Kennedy's disease 695
keratan sulphate 409, 414
in osteoarthritis 417, 1537, *1538*, 1542
keratitis in CINCA 1471
keratoconjunctivitis 173, *174*, 778
keratoconjunctivitis sicca 310
in DILS 911
in mixed connective tissue disease 1418
and primary biliary cirrhosis 1424
in Sjögren's syndrome 1309
treatment 1314

keratoderma blenorrhagica *175*, 201,
919, 1087
Kessel shoulder 1703
ketamine in juvenile chronic arthritis
303
ketanserin
in mixed connective tissue disease 1422,
1423
in scleroderma 1240
ketoconazole
drug interactions 957
in fungal arthritis 956–7
blastomycosis 959
Candida 958
coccidioidomycosis 962
histoplasmosis 962
paracoccidioidomycosis 963
sporotrichosis 960
ketone bodies
effect on plasma creatinine 649
in synovial hypoxia 445
ketoprofen
adverse effects
cutaneous 213
gastrointestinal *1021*
haematological 295
neurological *217*
enantiomers 577
half-life *577*
in juvenile chronic arthritis *1140*
in lactation 193, 194
in pregnancy 190
renal clearance 577
use by the elderly 102
kidney
adverse drug effects
cyclosporin 325–6, 595–6, *595*
gold therapy 322, *601*, *1022*, 1695
methotrexate *584*, 651
NSAIDs 322, 323, 325, 327, *578*, 580,
1021, 1695
penicillamine 322–3, *598*, 599, 1695
amyloidosis 322, 651, 1436, 1437, 1438,
1439
in ankylosing spondylitis 651, 1064
in Behçet's syndrome *259*, 1398
biopsy 331
in evaluation of haematuria 324–5
in evaluation of proteinuria 324–5
in polyarteritis nodosa 1403
in SLE 324, 1152–3, 1154–5, 1189
in systemic sclerosis 1237
in Churg–Strauss syndrome 1355
disease and anaesthesia 300
function tests 648–51
in gout 651, 1561, 1566
in Henoch–Schönlein purpura *321*,
324, *328*, 1407
involvement in rheumatic diseases 173,
177, **321–31**, 650–1
in juvenile chronic arthritis 1118
in microscopic polyangiitis *321*, 323,
1354, 1357
in mixed connective tissue disease *321*,
1419
papillary necrosis 323, 326
parenchymal disease 326
in polyarteritis nodosa *321*, 323, 324,
327, 328, 651, 1353
childhood 1403
in polymyositis/dermatomyositis 1256
in relapsing polychondritis 1626
in Sjögren's syndrome *321*, 322, 324,
327, 651, 1310–11
in SLE *see* lupus nephritis
stones 173, *177*
and gout 651, 1561, 1566
in systemic sclerosis *321*, 324, 328–9,
1237–8
transplantation
in amyloidosis 1442
in familial Mediterranean fever
1449
gout following 1566

kidney *(continued)*
  transplantation *(continued)*
    in Henoch–Schönlein purpura 1407
    in SLE 1174, 1191
    uric acid metabolism 1557
    in Wegener's granulomatosis *321, 323,
      324, 327, 328*, 651, 1338, 1342
Kienbock's disease 1621, 1623
killer cells *see* antibody-dependent cytotoxic cells
kinetochore proteins, antibodies to *see*
  anticentromere antibodies
Kingella kingae 852, 863
kininogenase
  in gout 1559
  in inflammation 512, *624*
kinins in inflammation 512, *512*
Klebsiella
  arteritis due to 1390
  K. aeruginosa 553
  K. pneumoniae
    and ankylosing spondylitis 1042
    cross-reactivity with HLA-B27 1042,
      1067
    intestinal 267, *268*
    pulmonary infection 252
    in pyogenic arthritis 852
    in rheumatoid arthritis *268*
Klinefelter's syndrome
  and osteoporosis 1589
  and SLE 1159
Klippel–Feil malformation, atlantoaxial subluxation in 224
knee
  applied anatomy 151–3
  arthrodesis 1708
  aspiration *1762*, 1768–9
  braces/splints 1732, 1747
  chronic arthritis in hypogamma-
    globulinaemia 970
  in CINCA 1472
  effusion 49, 277, 1768
  examination 49, 50
  excision arthroplasty 1708
  extension 151
  in familial Mediterranean fever 1446
  flexion 151
  functional anatomy and disability 1725
  imaging
    arthrography 719, 742
    Doppler ultrasound 762, 763, 764
    MRI 742–4, 771
    radiography 717–18, 744
    ultrasound 721, 722
  internal derangements 159, 166
  in juvenile chronic arthritis 82, 85
    pauci-articular onset 1099–100
    rehabilitation 1745–7, *1747*
    seronegative polyarthritis 1133,
      1134–5
    surgery 1717–18, 1719
    systemic onset 1116
  lateral tibiofemoral compartment 151
  local steroid injection *1762*, 1768–9
  medial tibiofemoral compartment 151
  osteoarthritis 1523–4, 1534, 1549, 1769
  osteochondritis 166
  pain *155*, 157–9, 1508–10, *1508*
    in adolescence 157
    anterior 1510, 1784–5, *1785*
    childhood *164*, 165–7
  palpation 49
  patellofemoral compartment 151
  physiotherapy in childhood 1745–7
  in psoriatic arthritis 1073
  reflex sympathetic dystrophy 1682
  replacement 1707–8
    childhood 1719
    in Paget's disease 1617
    in rheumatoid arthritis 1009
  rotation 151
  screening 49
  screwed-home position 151
  sewing-needle injury 865

knee *(continued)*
  stability testing 49, 50
  surgery 1707–8
    childhood 1717–18, 1719
  swelling 49
Kniest syndrome 368, *369*, 375, 413,
  1635
  clinical features 371
  gene mutations 370
knock-out mice 571, 610
knuckle pads *175, 208*
Kocher–Debre–Semelaigne
  syndrome 278
Koebner phenomenon 1115, 1127
Kohler's disease 168, 1623, *1787*
Krebs cycle 1774
kringles 1479
Kveim test 203, 1466
kyphosis 46, 114, 125–6
  aetiology 115, 116, *116*
  anaesthesia in 299
  congenital 125
  following laminectomy 125
  in juvenile chronic arthritis 82
  in neurofibromatosis 125
  in osteoporosis 129, 1591, 1592
  postural 126
  progressive 125–6
  in Scheuermann's osteochondritis 125,
    126
  in spinal tuberculosis 122, 123
  in spondylolisthesis 126

L

L-selectin 528, *529*
  counter-receptors 530
  in leucocyte rolling 535
  in lymphocyte transmigration 536
  oligosaccharide ligands 529
La proteins 669, 672
  see also anti-La antibodies
labelling
  DNA 690
  end 690
  fluorescent 690
  internal 690
labetalol, adverse effects *1690*
laboratory tests
  ankylosing spondylitis *649*, 1066
  Behçet's syndrome 1399
  brucellar arthritis 941
  calcium pyrophosphate dihydrate
    disease 653, 1568
  childhood 17–18, *17*
  cut-off between negative and positive
    657
  dermatomyositis *649*, 1256–8, *1257*
  in the elderly 27–8, *28*
  eosinophilia–myalgia syndrome *1426*,
    1427
  familial Mediterranean fever 1448
  giant cell arteritis 513, 1378, 1389
  gout *649*, 654, 677, 682, 683–4, 1561–2
  Henoch–Schönlein purpura 1407
  interpretation and reliability 7–8
  juvenile chronic arthritis 1100–1,
    1119–21, *1120*, 1135
  Kawasaki disease 1405
  Lyme disease 889–90, *889*
  microbiological *657–64*
    acute joint infection 661–2
    antibody detection 661
    antigen detection 660
    antimicrobial sensitivity testing
      659–60
    blood cultures 659
    DNA/RNA detection 660–1
    gold standard 657
    influence of antibiotics on culture
      658
    investigations *658*
    limitations 658–61

laboratory tests *(continued)*
  microbiological *(continued)*
    predictive value of negative (PVN)
      results 657
    predictive value of positive (PVP)
      657–8
    reactive arthritis 662–4
    sensitivity 657
    specificity 657
    specimens 658–9
    synovial fluid specimens 658–9
  microscopic polyangiitis 1403
  neuropsychiatric SLE 334, *334*
  ocular disorders 317
  osteomyelitis 871
  Paget's disease 1613
  polyarteritis nodosa 1403
  polymyalgia rheumatica *649*, 1378
  polymyositis *649*, 1256–8, *1257*
  psoriatic arthritis *649*, 1076–7
  reactive arthropathies 1088–9
  reflex sympathetic dystrophy 1682
  rheumatic fever 979–80
  rheumatoid arthritis *649*, 1015–16,
    1015, 1016, 1017
  sarcoidosis 1465–6
  Sjögren's syndrome 1312, *1312*
  soft-tissue rheumatism *649*
  systemic sclerosis *649*
  Takayasu's arteritis 1386
  thrombosis *1208*
  toxic oil syndrome *1426*, 1427
  Wegener's granulomatosis 1337,
    1339–40, 1406–7
labour-saving devices 1728, *1728*
lactate dehydrogenase (LDH) 652
  in differential diagnosis of neuromus-
    cular disorders 1291
  as marker of muscle damage 465
  in polymyositis/dermatomyositis 1257
  synovial fluid 679
  in synovial inflammation 445
lactation
  drug therapy in *193–4, 602*, 603
  and rheumatoid arthritis 181
lactic acid 1773
  in gonococcal arthritis 855
  non-gonococcal arthritis 851
  as product of anaerobic metabolism 1774
  in synovial hypoxia 444, 445
Lactobacillus casei, arthritogenicity of cell-
  wall fragments 564
lactoferrin 513, 635, *1017*, 1329, 1356
LAK cells *see* lymphokine-activated cytotoxic cells
lamellar coxitis 1138
laminectomy
  in cervical spondylosis 224
  kyphosis following 125
laminin 353, 460
Lange skinfold callipers 75
Langer–Gieodron syndrome 1631
Langerhans cell histiocytosis 120, 121,
  1477
  imaging 759, 761
Langerhans cells in HIV infection 909
lansoprazole 1695
large granular lymphocyte syndrome
  644, *645*
Larsen–Dale index 1017
Larsen's syndrome 168
laryngeal mask airway 303, 304
laryngoscopy 304
larynx in Wegener's granulomatosis
  1335, 1336
Lasègue's sign 46
laser nephelometry 674
laser therapy in discoid lupus erythematosus 211
lateral canal stenosis 98
lateral collateral ligament (ankle) 153
lateral collateral ligament (knee) 151,
  152
  disruption 743

lateral collateral ligament (knee)
    (continued)
  in rheumatoid arthritis 1014
  stability testing 49, 50
lateral cutaneous nerve of thigh,
    entrapment neuropathy 227, 1768
lateral epicondylitis *see* tennis elbow
lateral malleolus 153
  impingement 1706
lateral popliteal nerve lesions 1512
latissimus dorsi 135, 137
laxatives and hyperuricaemia *1558*
LCR 693
LDH *see* lactate dehydrogenase
LDL *see* low density lipoprotein
LE cell test 983
lead exposure and gout 1558, 1694
learned helplessness 106
LECAM-1 *1169*
Lee Functional Status Index *55*, 56
Leeds Disability Questionnaire *58, 59*
left ventricular dysfunction in juvenile
    chronic arthritis 1034
left ventricular hypertrophy 237
leg *see* lower limb
Legg–Calvé–Perthes' disease 162, 164,
  165
  differential diagnosis 1138
  imaging 754, 758, 764, 765, 767, 769, 771
Legg–Perthes' disease 1621, 1623
  diagnosis 19
  osteochondritis in 1787, *1787*
Legionella infection 252
lentiviruses 908
lepra reaction 933, 934–5
leprosy
  borderline borderline 933
  borderline lepromatous 933
  clinical manifestations 934–5
  diagnosis 935
  epidemiology 933
  histopathology 933–4
  immunology 933–4
  indeterminate form 933
  investigation 935
  lepromatous 933
  pathogenesis 933
  rheumatoid factor in *674*
  treatment 935–6
  tuberculoid *209*, 933
  vaccines 935
Lequesne Index *57, 58*
Lesch–Nyhan syndrome 1555, 1557,
  1558
lethargy 172
Letterer–Siwe disease 120
Leu-CAM proteins *see* integrins,
    Leu-CAM (β2)
leucapheresis 611
leucine zippers 348
leucocyte adhesion deficiency 531
leucocyte adhesion molecule *1169*
leucocyte function-associated
    antigen-1 *see* integrins, α^{L}β2
leucocyte scanning 766
  osteomyelitis 872
leucocytes
  abnormalities in rheumatic disorders
    292, 642–4
  adhesion in synovial inflammation 448
  in Behçet's syndrome 1399
  in brucellar arthritis 941
  in bursal fluid 155, 156
  chemotaxis in synovial inflammation
    448
  childhood pyogenic arthritis 862
  in gonococcal arthritis 855
  in innate immunity 545
  in non-gonococcal arthritis 851
  renal infiltration in microscopic poly-
    angiitis 1357
  in SLE 641, *641*
  synovial fluid 679, 680, 681–2
  see also lymphocytes

leucocytosis 292
in adult-onset Still's disease 1127
in Henoch–Schönlein purpura 1407
in juvenile chronic arthritis 1119–20
in Kawasaki disease 1405
in Lyme disease 888
in SLE 1156
in Sweet's syndrome 1457
leucopenia 292
drug-related 296, 297
in juvenile chronic arthritis 1120
in sarcoidosis 1465
in Sjögren's syndrome 1312
in SLE 1155–6, 1193
leukaemia 288–9
acute lymphocytic 288
childhood, back pain in 118
differential diagnosis 1137–8, 1137
drug-related 295
following radiotherapy 1667
imaging 760, 769
metastases from 121
osteoarticular symptoms 1671–2
and pyoderma gangrenosum 1460
and Sweet's syndrome 1458
leukaemia inhibitory factor 623
leukotrienes
effect of corticosteroids on 586
effects of NSAIDs on 576
and fatty acids 262, 1480
in inflammation 508, 515, 515–16, 516
pentaenoic 515
in psoriatic arthritis 1079
levamisole in combination therapy 1025
levodopa and hyperuricaemia 1558
Lewis rats 510
adjuvant arthritis 563, 998
streptococcal cell-wall arthritis 565, 998
LFA-1 see integrins, α^L-β_2
Lhermitte's sign 46, 1656
libido, loss of in rheumatoid arthritis 182
Libman–Sachs endocarditis 238, 1151, 1194
lichen planus 208
drug-related 213
oral 201, 202
lichen sclerosus et atrophicus 205, 209
lifestyle and disease occurrence 824
lifting techniques 108
ligaments
composition and function 1492
generalized laxity 1499–500
in rheumatoid arthritis 1014
ligamentum patellae 1509
ligamentum teres 150
ligand-induced adhesion 532
ligase chain reaction 693
light-headedness 237
lignocaine
local injection in low back pain 101
in local steroid injection 1760
limb-girdle muscular dystrophy 791
limp in childhood 19, 19, 20, 115, 164, 754
linear tomography, sacroiliac joint 736
lining cells see synovial intimal cells
linkage 687–8, 689
analysis 687–8, 698
multipoint analysis 688
recombination fraction 687
linkage disequilibrium 689
linkage disequilibrium mapping 689
linoleic acid 1480
γ-linolenic acid 262, 265, 1480, 1484–5
LIP in DILS 911–12, 913
lipid aldehydes 447
lipid alkanes 447
lipid endoperoxides 447
lipid hydroperoxides 447
lipids
composition 1478–9

lipids (continued)
crystals 1575
and inflammation 1480
in joints 1481–2
metabolism 1478–80
peroxidation 447, 1480
rationale for lowering levels 1485
subclasses 1479
in synovial fluid 680
transport
endogenous pathway 1479
exogenous pathway 1479
Lipiodol 730
lipocortins 515, 585
lipodermatosclerosis 209
lipogranulomatosis subcutanea 1453
lipohaemarthrosis 768, 771
lipoid dermatoarthritis see multicentric reticulohistiocytosis
lipoma 288
lipomyelomeningocele 127
lipopolysaccharide
effect on endothelial cells 536
enhancement of collagen-induced arthritis 564
lipoprotein (a) 1479–80, 1483
lipoprotein lipase 1479
deficiency 1481
in hyperlipidaemias 1483
lipoproteins
classification 1479, 1479
composition 1478–9
postmenopausal 1597
subclasses 1479
lipoxygenase pathway 262, 515, 1480
lips, strawberry erythema 204
Lisfranc dislocation of tarsometa-tarsal joint 284
lisinopril and renal function 325
Listeria
L. monocytogenes in pyogenic arthritis 852
in osteomyelitis 870
lithium 339, 340, 342
adverse effects 1690, 1693
interaction with NSAIDs 579
litigation and back pain 107
livedo reticularis 222
in antiphospholipid syndrome 293, 1206, 1207
in Wegener's granulomatosis 1339
livedo reticulosis 175
liver
in adult-onset Still's disease 1127
adverse drug effects
aspirin 652, 1106
azathioprine 590, 591, 652
cyclophosphamide 652
gold 601
methotrexate 261, 584, 584, 652
NSAIDs 261, 578, 580, 1021
sulphasalazine 589, 652
amoebic abscess 1320
amyloidosis 1436, 1437
an adult-onset Still's disease 1116
in Behçet's syndrome 1398
biopsy in methotrexate therapy 212, 584
disease, rheumatoid factor in 674
function abnormalities 173, 175
function tests 651–2
in brucellar arthritis 941
in vasculitis 1358
in giant cell arteritis 652, 1378
in juvenile chronic arthritis 1116
in neonatal lupus erythemtosus 1199
in polymyalgia rheumatica 652, 1378
in Sjögren's syndrome 1310
in SLE 1157, 1196–7
in systemic sclerosis 652, 1239
transplantation in amyloidosis 1441–2
LMP genes
and juvenile chronic arthritis 1110

LMP genes (continued)
LMP2 549, 696
and ankylosing spondylitis 699
LMP7 549, 696
Loa loa 949–50, 951
load transducers 477–8
loads
external, measurement 477–8
internal, measurement 478
synovial joints 477
local anaesthetics
allergy to 1758
in chronic back pain 1648
infiltration 305
scleroderma due to 1223
in soft-tissue rheumatism 1512–13
Locoid 210
locomotion, joint forces 479–80
lod score 688
Löfgren's syndrome 1451
London Coping with Rheumatoid Arthritis Questionnaire 68
London Handicap Scale 1724, 1724
loose back syndrome 1499, 1501
loose bodies 1541
Looser's zones 1601, 1672
lordosis 126, 133
in juvenile chronic arthritis 82
lumbar 1640
lovastatin, adverse effects 1265, 1266, 1480
low density lipoprotein (LDL) 1479
oxidized 1478, 1480
in rheumatic disorders 1482
subclasses 1479
Lowe syndrome 1605
lower limb
applied anatomy 150–4, 156, 157
compartments 153, 1786, 1786
length
age-related decrease in 24
inequality 20, 163–4
in giant cell arteritis 1408
and height measurement 74
in juvenile chronic arthritis 1101, 1747
in Paget's disease 1612
radiography 753
in spinal dysraphism 128
and sports injuries 1783
and trochanteric bursitis 156–7
pain 89, 96, 97, 100
childhood 19, 19, 163–8, 164
in lumbar disc disease 98
syndromes 154–60, 155
reflex sympathetic dystrophy 1682
stress fractures 1783
ulcers, and antiphospholipid antibodies 293
see also specific anatomical regions and conditions
LPAM-1 531, 531
lubrication of synovial joints 480–2
boosted 481
boundary 480, 481
elastohydrodynamic (EHL/EHD) 480, 481
full-fluid film 480, 481
hydrodynamic 480, 481
hydrostatic/externally pressurized 480, 481
mixed 480, 481
in osteoarthritis 484
squeeze film 480, 481
studies 479–81
theoretical analysis 481–2
weeping 481
lubricin 442
Ludiomil 340, 342
lumbar 90, 91
lumbar segment, definition 90, 90
lumbar spondylosis 1612, 1642–3
lumbricales 140
lumican 410

lumisterol 1602
lunate 137
osteonecrosis 1621, 1623
lungs
biopsy 249–50
in sarcoidosis 1466
in Sjögren's syndrome 1310
in systemic sclerosis 1236
transbronchial 251, 252
in Wegener's granulomatosis 1341
carcinoma
and carcinomatous neuropathy 1674
and Eaton–Lambert myasthenic syndrome 1674–5
and hypertrophic osteoarthropathy 1672–3
and polymyalgia rheumatica 1670
and seronegative spondylarthro-pathies 1667
skeletal metastases 1673
and systemic sclerosis 1669–70
drug-related reactions 253–4, 253
hyperinflation 244
infection 245, 251–2, 251, 1195
small 244
transplantation, gout following 1566
vascular studies 251
see also respiratory system
lupus anticoagulant 293–4, 673
in antiphospholipid syndrome 1159–60
clinical features associated 293
detection 1203–4
disease associations 293–4
in pregnancy 183, 294, 295, 1206
in SLE 183, 642, 1159–60
childhood 1193–4, 1197
treatment 294–5
see also antiphospholipid syndrome
lupus band test 202, 1148–9, 1150
lupus erythematosus
bullous lesions 205
discoid 1147, 1150
childhood 1183
ear involvement 201, 202
facial erythema 204
lupus band test 202
oral lesions 207
plaques 202
scarring alopecia 200
skin scaling 205
treatment 211
drug-induced 1690–3
age-related occurrence 26
autoantibodies 668, 669, 1691
clinical features 1690, 1691
comparison with SLE 1691
in the elderly 36
pathogenesis 1692–3
and penicillamine 1022
risk factors 1691–2, 1692
neonatal see neonatal lupus erythema-tosus
papular 208
subacute cutaneous 1148
annular 1148
facial erythema 204
hard palate involvement 201, 202
lupus band test 202
papulosquamous 1148
psoriasiform 205
treatment 211
systemic see systemic lupus erythema-tosus
lupus erythematosus cell test 665
Lupus Foundation of America 36
lupus-like syndrome 289
lupus nephritis 321, 321, 651, 1152
childhood 1187–92
classification 1151, 1187
diffuse proliferative 1187–8, 1188, 1189
focal proliferative 1188–9
histological patterns 1187
membranous 1188
mesangial 1188

lupus nephritis (continued)
  presentation 321
  proteinuria in 323
  rapidly progressive glomerulonephritis
    in 327, 328
  renal biopsy in 324, 1152–3, 1154–5,
    1189
  scoring indices 1189
  treatment 1190–2, 1192, 1358
  tubulointerstitial injury in 1189–90
Lupus news 36
lupus pernio 201, 1467
lupus profundus 211, 1156, 1453–4, 1455
Luvox 339, 340
Lyme arthritis 888, 891, 892–3
Lyme disease 199, 204, 880, **884–94**
  age at onset 13
  cardiovascular involvement 230
  central nervous system disease in 223
  childhood 336
  clinical characteristics 887–9
  clustering 818
  cranial nerve palsies in 224
  definition 884
  diagnosis 889–90, 889
  differential diagnosis 890–1, 1091, 1104,
    1136, 1137
  epidemiology 885–7, 886
  fever in 172
  history 884
  immune complexes in 712
  investigation 663–4
  laboratory tests 889–90, 889
  maternal 892
  muscle necrosis in 790
  national surveillance case definition
    (US) 885, 886
  ocular involvement 317
  pathogenesis 884–5
  peripheral neuropathies 228, 795
  in pregnancy 892
  psychiatric involvement 333, 336
  reactive phenomena in 1043
  sex differences 14
  synovial fluid eosinophilia 682
  systemic features 170
  treatment 891–4, 891, 893
  vaccine 894
lymph nodes, lymphocyte circulation
    through 526–7
lymphadenopathy 3, 170, 172–3
  in adult-onset Still's disease 1127
  childhood 172–3
  in HIV infection 911
  in juvenile chronic arthritis 1116
  in Lyme disease 890
  in rheumatoid arthritis 1010
  in sarcoidosis 1465, 1466, 1467
  in SLE 1147
lymphatic drainage, manual 1751
lymphocyte function associated
    antigen *see* integrins, $\alpha^L\beta_2$
lymphocyte–Peyer's patch adhesion
    molecule-1 531, 531
lymphocytes 525
  in adaptive immunity 545–6
  adhesion 535
    control 534–8, 537
    molecules involved 528–34
  antigen specificity 527
  chemoattractants 534, 535
  chemotaxis 534
  circulation and migration 525, 1168,
    1171
    control 534–8, 537
    effect of sensitization 527–8
    factors affecting 526–8
    in inflammation 525–6
    influence of lineage 527
    in innate immunity 545
    organ-selective 528
    therapeutic possibilities 538
    through lymph nodes 526–7
    through spleen and bone marrow 527

lymphocytes (continued)
  circulation and migration (continued)
    within tissues 538
    in drug-induced lupus 1692
    effect of alkylating agents on 592, 592
    effect of azathioprine on 590, 590
    effect of corticosteroids on 586
    effect of gold therapy on 599, 600
    effect of NSAIDs on 576
    extracorporeal inactivation and recircu-
      lation 611
    haptotaxis 534
    in inflammation **525–38**
    interactions with endothelial cells
      526–7, 534–7
    perivascular cuffing 443
    in polymyositis/dermatomyositis 1268,
      1269
    in rheumatic fever 976, 976
    rolling 535
    in Sjögren's syndrome 1304–5
    in synovial inflammation 443, 777
    transmigration through endothelium
      536
  see also B cells; T cells
lymphocytic choriomeningitis virus in
    immune complexes 704
lymphocytic interstitial pneumonitis
    in DILS 911–12, 913
lymphocytoma, benign 884
lymphocytoma cutis 887
lymphocytotoxic antibodies
  in HIV infection 910
  in neuropsychiatric SLE 334
  in SLE 1156, 1193
lymphoedema of the upper limb in
    psoriatic arthritis 1076
lymphokine-activated cytotoxic cells
  effect of corticosteroids on 586
  in scleroderma 1221
lymphoma 288, 289
  differential diagnosis 1122
  hypercalcaemia in 437
  malignant of bone 120, 1671
  osteoporosis in 1590
  in polymyalgia rheumatica 1670
  salivary gland biopsy in 779
  in Sjögren's syndrome 1304, 1310, 1312,
    1667–8
lymphomatoid granulomatosis,
    differential diagnosis 1136, 1137
lymphopenia
  in juvenile dermatomyositis 1294, 1295
  in rheumatoid arthritis 1010, 1016
  in SLE 292, 641, 1155–6, 1193
lymphotoxin *see* tumour necrosis factors,
    TNF-β
lysozyme 513, 545, 1329
  in amyloidosis 1434, 1434, 1438
  release by NSAIDs 576
lysylhydroxylase deficiency 355, 385
lysyloxidase deficiency 355, 385

M

M-HAQ 55, 61
M-line protein 455
Mac-1 *see* integrins, $\alpha^M\beta_2$
McArdle's syndrome 216, 473, 1774,
    1775
Macaroni sign 1386
McGill pain questionnaire 6, 6, 64
McGregor's line 728
McMaster Health Index
    Questionnaire 53, 54
McMaster Toronto Arthritis Patient
    Preference Disability
    Questionnaire 55, 55
McMurray's sign 49, 159
macrocytosis, drug-related 296, 297,
    584, 590
  alkylating agents 593, 593
α-2-macroglobulin and erythrocyte
    sedimentation rate 639

macroglossia in amyloidosis 1436,
    1437
macrophage activation syndrome
    1117, 1118
macrophage-colony stimulating
    factor
  and bone formation 424
  in rheumatoid arthritis 993
macrophage inflammatory proteins
    534, 535, 990
macrophages
  activation 517–18
  effect of alkylating agents on 592
  effect of azathioprine on 590, 590
  effect of corticosteroids on 586
  effect of gold therapy on 599, 600
  effect of penicillamine on 597
  effect of substance P on 451
  in HIV infection 909
  in inflammation 513–14
  in inflammatory myopathies 789
  iron metabolism within 634–5
  phagocytosis 513
  in polymyalgia rheumatica/giant cell
    arteritis 1377
  in rheumatic fever 976, 976
  in rheumatoid arthritis 992
  role in cartilage destruction 570
  in scleroderma 1223
  in Sjögren's syndrome 1305
  in synovial inflammation 443, 777
macroradiography, rheumatoid
    arthritis 724
MACTAR 55, 55
macular oedema 311
macule 201
MadCAM-1 530, 533
Madurella mycetomi 963
MAGIC syndrome 1626
magnesium carbonate, in calcium
    pyrophosphate dihydrate
    disease 1570
magnetic resonance angiography,
    Takayasu's arteritis 1386
magnetic resonance imaging (MRI)
    722–4, 771
  Achilles tendon 745–6
  ankle 744–5
  ankylosing spondylitis 1059, 1066
  antiphospholipid syndrome 1205
  arachnoiditis 1646
  back pain 90, 99, 732–3, 734
    childhood 116
  Baker's cyst 726, 727
  bone marrow 771
  brucellar arthritis 940
  cervical myelopathy 1654, 1656
  cervical spine 302
  cervical spondylosis 224, 1654–5
  childhood 763, 766, 767, 768–72
    back pain 116
    polymyositis/dermatomyositis 1290
    pyogenic arthritis 862
  comparison with discography 733
  contraindications 724
  contrast-enhanced 770, 771, 772
  craniocervical 223
  cysticercosis 950
  dermatomyositis 1260, 1290
  diabetes mellitus 285
  diastematomyelia 128
  in DILS 911
  discitis of childhood 123
  Dupuytren's contracture 148
  elbow 741
  epiphyses 771
  fast spin-echo sequences 770
  fat-suppression technique 722–3, 771
  foot 745–6, 747, 748
  fungal arthritis 955–6
  giant cell arteritis 1389
  gradient-echo sequences 767, 770
  haemophilic arthropathy 768
  hip 770–1

magnetic resonance imaging (MRI)
    (continued)
  hydatid cyst 950
  inclusion-body myositis 1279
  interpretation and reliability 8
  intervertebral disc prolapse 124, 125,
    1642, 1643
  intramedullary spinal cord abscess 124
  juvenile chronic arthritis 772
  knee 742–4, 771
  measurement of internal loads on joints
    478
  meniscal injuries 159, 723
  neuropsychiatric SLE 221, 335, 1155,
    1156, 1186
  non-gonococcal arthritis 851
  ossification centres 771
  osteoarthritis 747, 748, 749, 1536
  osteoid osteoma 118, 1618
  osteomyelitis 752, 772, 872–3
    vertebral 878, 931
  osteonecrosis 749–50, 1622–3
  pigmented villonodular synovitis 1620
  polymyositis 1260, 1290
  reflex sympathetic dystrophy 1683,
    1683, 1684
  relapsing polychondritis 1626
  relaxation times 723
  rheumatoid arthritis 726, 727–8, 1017,
    1018
  shoulder 140, 738–9, 740, 742
    rotator cuff tear 142
  signal intensity of musculoskeletal tissue
    723
  spin-echo sequences 770
  spinal cord disease 223
  spine
    cervical 728
    dysraphism 128
    stenosis 1644
    tuberculosis 122, 717
  spondylodiscitis 766
  spondylolysis 126
  STIR sequence 722–3, 771
  temporomandibular joint 302
  tennis elbow 145
  transient osteoporosis 749
  transverse myelitis 225
  tuberculosis 122, 717, 931
  Wegener's granulomatosis 1332, 1341
  whiplash injury 1658
  wrist 741
magnetic resonance spectroscopy,
    polymyositis/dermatomyositis
    1260–1
Mahoney's line 739
major histocompatibility complex
    (MHC) 546–7
  autoimmune haplotype 504
  class I region 547
  class II region 547–8
    monoclonal antibodies to products
      613
    proteins in Dupuytren's contracture
      148
  class III region 548
  genomic organization 547
  interaction with T-cell receptor 551
  physical mapping 549
  recently described genes 549
  in SLE 1170, 1171
  and susceptibility to rheumatoid
    arthritis 553–4
  and T-cell receptor repertoire 504
  see also HLA genes; HLA molecules *and*
    specific HLA antigens
malabsorption 258
  in mixed connective tissue disease 1417
  and vitamin D deficiency 1603
malaise 170, 172, 178
  in dermatomyositis 1252
  in drug-induced lupus 1690
  in giant cell arteritis 1377, 1388
  in Lyme disease 887

malaise *(continued)*
  in microscopic polyangiitis 1354
  in polyarteritis nodosa 1353, 1403
  in polymyalgia rheumatica 1377
  in polymyositis 1252
malaria *946*
  muscle involvement 947
  rheumatoid factor in *674*
malicious malalignment syndrome 1783
malignant atrophic papulosis *209*
malignant disease
  acute phase response in 640
  associations with rheumatic diseases **1665–70**
  biochemical tests 653
  bone 120, 288–9, 742, 1670–2, *1671*
  and connective tissue disease 289
  and dermatomyositis 289, 1255–6, 1267, 1668–9
  differential diagnosis 1122, 1379
  effect on bone 437
  and eosinophilic fasciitis 1428
  following therapy **289–90**, 297
    alkylating agents 290, *593*, 594, 1359–60
    azathioprine 590, *591*
    cyclosporin 290, *595*
  and giant cell arteritis 1670
  and low back pain 97, *97*, 99
  metastatic 288–9, 1671, 1681
    and hypercalcaemia 437
    spinal in childhood 121
  and multicentric reticulohistiocytosis 1475–6
  and osteomalacia 1605–6
  osteoporosis in 1590
  and Paget's disease 1612
  and polymyalgia rheumatica 289, 1377–8, 1670
  and polymyositis 289, 1255–6, 1267, 1668–9
  primary 288
  in pyoderma gangrenosum 1460
  and rheumatoid arthritis 1665–6, *1666*
  rheumatological manifestations **288–9, 1670–5**
  and seronegative spondylarthropathies 1666–7
  and Sjögren's syndrome 1304, 1310, 1312, 1667–8
  skeletal 1670–2, *1671*
  and SLE 1160, *1160*, 1194, 1668
  spinal in childhood 120–1
  and systemic sclerosis 1669–70
  and Wegener's granulomatosis 1342
malignant hyperpyrexia/hyper-thermia 472
malignant pyoderma 1459
malnutrition and hospitalization 30
malocclusion 1739
management plans *8*, 9
manipulation in low back pain 101, 103–4
mannitol in pigment-induced nephropathy 327
mannose-binding proteins 507, 528
Mansonia
  M. africana 901
  M. uniformus 903
Mantoux test 122
manubriosternal joint subluxation 224
manubrium sterni 135
Maoris, rheumatoid arthritis *834*
MAP 800
maprotiline 340, *342*
marble bone disease 436
MARCO 353
Marfan syndrome 168, 435
  cardiovascular involvement 238
  clinical features 389, 390
  collagen type I in 357–8
  differential diagnosis 1500

Marfan syndrome *(continued)*
  gastrointestinal involvement *259*
  gene mutation in 353–4, 389, 391–3
  scoliosis in 115, *116*
marital relationships and low back pain 106
Maroteaux–Lamy syndrome *1633*
Martin–Gruber anastomosis 807
masseter atrophy in polymyositis/dermatomyositis 1290
mast cells
  effect of substance P on 451
  in inflammation 512–13
  in scleroderma 1223
  in synovial biopsy 777
mastication impairment *258*
mastitis, lymphocytic in DILS 912
mastoiditis in Wegener's granuloma-tosis 1335
matrix Gla protein 427, *429*
matrix vesicles 412
maximum aerobic capacity 1775, 1776
maximum sustainable ventilatory capacity 1775
maximum voluntary ventilation 1775
max$\dot{V}O_2$ 1775, 1776
Mayaro virus 904
mazindol, adverse effects *1223*, 1693
Mazzotti reaction 951
MCPs 534, *535*, 990
MDMA and hyperpyrexia 1778
mean corpuscular haemoglobin concentration in anaemia of chronic disease 290–1
mean corpuscular volume in anaemia of chronic disease 290–1
measles virus in Paget's disease 1610–11
mebendazole 948, 951
mechanics of synovial joints **477–80**
mechanoreceptors 487
mechanosensitivity
  definition *488*
  in joint inflammation 491–2
meclofenamate
  adverse effects 260
  in juvenile chronic arthritis *1106*, *1140*
  in lactation 193
  nephrotoxicity 327
medial collateral ligament 151, 152
  damage to 1509–10
  stability testing 49, 50
medial epicondylitis *see* golfer's elbow
medial ligament syndrome 158
medial malleolus 153
median nerve 137
  entrapment neuropathy *see* carpal tunnel syndrome
  in leprosy 934
  Martin–Gruber anastomosis 807
  mononeuropathy *219*
  sensory nerve conduction study 801
Medical Outcome Study Short Form 36 *4*, *54*, 61, 1724, *1724*
medulla 223
mefenamic acid
  adverse effects 213
  in lactation 194
Meissner corpuscle, structural changes with age 22–3
MEL-14 antigen 528
melaena in Behçet's syndrome 1398
melanin 596
melanoma 289
melorheostosis 206
melphalan
  in amyloidosis 1441
  in fibrogenesis imperfecta ossium 1606
membrane-attack complex 512, 545
memory cells 527–8
  in rheumatoid arthritis 990
memory impairment in Lyme disease 888
menarche 14

meningeal biopsy in granulomatous angiitis of the central nervous system 786
meningitis
  arachnoiditis following 1645
  aseptic
    drug-related *578*
    in Sjögren's syndrome 1311
  in calcium pyrophosphate dihydrate disease 1529
  in CINCA 1471
  in Lyme disease 888, 890
  reflex sympathetic dystrophy following 1681
meningocele 127
meningococcaemia
  acute 855
  chronic 856
meningococcal arthritis 855–6
  childhood 862
  management 856–8
  primary 856
meningopolyneuritis 884
meniscectomy 159
  in model of joint disease 416
menisci 151, 152
  bucket-handle tear 159
  classification of changes at MRI 743
  discoid 743, 744
  injury 159, 166
    MRI 723, 743, 771
  and osteoarthritis 484
Menkes syndrome 385
menstruation
  delay/irregularity 14
  and disease occurrence 823, *823*
mepacrine
  adverse effects 212, 214
  in discoid lupus erythematosus 211, 212
meperidine 340
meptazinol in low back pain 100
meralgia paraesthetica 157, 227, 1507, 1768
6-mercaptopurine, adverse effects 1694
MESA 778–9, 1306, 1667
Mesna in cyclophosphamide therapy 1359
mesoderm 458
metabolism 1773–6
  anaerobic 1774
metacarpal index 1594
metacarpals 138
metacarpophalangeal joints 138–40
  in hypothyroidism 278
  local steroid injection 1766, 1767
  in psoriatic arthritis 1073
  replacement 1705, 1721
  in rheumatoid arthritis 1008
  surgery 1705
  thumb 139
metalloproteinases 410–11, *411*, 415
  domain structure 1544
  in inflammation 514–15
  in osteoarthritis 1544–5
  tissue inhibitors of 411, 515, 1538–9, 1544
metaphenylene diamine and sclero-derma *1223*
metaphyseal band, transverse radi-olucent *756*, 758, 759
metaphyseal chondrodysplasia
  type Jansen *369*, *435*, 436
  type Schmid 353, 369, *369*, 378, 413, *435*, 436
metatarsalgia 160, 1512, 1725
  Morton's 1512
metatarsals 153, 154
  stress fractures 167
metatarsophalangeal joints 153
  in gout 1560
  local steroid injection 1770
  replacement 1707
  in rheumatoid arthritis 1008

metatrophic dysplasias 1630
methaemoglobinaemia, drug-related 296
Methanobacterium formicicum 269
methotrexate **582–5**
  administration 582
  in adult-onset Still's disease 1127
  adverse effects 252, **583–5**, *584*, 647, 1023, 1695
    cutaneous 214, *584*
    gastrointestinal 207, *260*, 261, *584*
    haematological 296–7, *584*
    hepatotoxic 584, *584*, 652
    nephrotoxic *584*, 651
    neurological *217*, *584*
    oncogenic 290, 297, *584*, 1666
    oral ulceration 207, *584*
    osteoporosis 1590
    psychiatric *337*, 338
    pulmonary 241, *253*, 254, *584*, 585, 1254
  bioavailability 582
  clinical efficacy 583
  in combination therapy 1023, *1025*
  in dermatomyositis 211, 1275–6
  drug interactions 296, 580, 582
  in giant cell arteritis 1389
  in HIV-associated arthritis 921
  in inclusion-body myositis 1280
  infection following administration 1013
  in juvenile chronic arthritis 1107, 1126, 1141
  in juvenile dermatomyositis 1297
  in juvenile spondylarthropathies 1049
  in lactation 194, *602*
  mechanism of action 582
  metabolism 582
  in mixed connective tissue disease 1422
  in multicentric reticulohistiocytosis *1476*, 1477
  non-selective action 610
  patient monitoring 585
  pharmacology 582
  in polymyositis 1275–6
  in pregnancy 192, *602*
  in psoriasis 212, 1079
  in psoriatic arthritis 1080
  in pyoderma gangrenosum 1462
  in reactive arthropathies 1092
  in rheumatoid arthritis 34, 1023
  in rheumatoid ulceration 210
  in scleroderma 1240, *1241*
  in seropositive juvenile chronic arthritis 1035–6
  in SLE 1191
  in streptococcal cell-wall arthritis 565
  and surgery 301
  in Takayasu's arteritis 1387
  therapeutically relevant effects 582–3, *583*
  treatment regimens 583
  in uveitis 317
  in Wegener's granulomatosis 1346
methoxyflurane and hyperuricaemia *1558*
methyldopa, adverse effects *1690*
methylisobutylisonitrile emission tomography, compartment syndrome 1786
methylmethacrylate cement 853
methylprednisolone 585
  in autoimmune haemolytic anaemia 292
  in Behçet's syndrome 1401
  intravenous 588
    in juvenile dermatomyositis 1296–7
    in microscopic polyangiitis 1359
    in polyarteritis nodosa 1359
    in SLE 1191
  in juvenile chronic arthritis 1125, 1126
  in polymyalgia rheumatica 1379–80
  in polymyositis/dermatomyositis 1273, *1274*
  in relapsing polychondritis 1627

methylprednisolone *(continued)*
  in transverse myelitis 225
  in Wegener's granulomatosis 1347
methylprednisolone acetate, injection 1757, 1760
metoclopramide, interaction with NSAIDs *579*
Metosyn *210*
metronidazole 660
Meuli ball and socket joint 1704
Mexico
  prevalence of juvenile chronic arthritis 830, *830*, *831*
  prevalence of rheumatoid arthritis *835*
MGP 427, *429*
MHC *see* major histocompatibility complex
MHIQ 53, *54*
miconazole 956
microbiology *see* laboratory tests, microbiological
microcytotoxicity assay 697
microfibrillar-associated protein 353
β_2-microglobulin 547, 1041
  in amyloidosis 1434–5, *1434*, 1439–40
  gene 696
  in rheumatoid arthritis *1017*
  and tubular function 650
a_1-microglobulin and tubular function 650
micrognathia 45, 302, 1134, 1135, 1739
microscopic polyangiitis 328, *1320*, **1351–62**
  age at onset 1354
  antineutrophil cytoplasmic autoantibodies 1329, 1353, 1354, 1355–6
  childhood *1402–4*
  classification 1320, *1321*, *1322*, 1351–2
  clinical features 1354, 1403
  comparison with polyarteritis nodosa 1352–3
  comparison with Wegener's granulomatosis 1353
  definition 1352
  diagnosis 1355–8
  diagnostic criteria 1323–4
  and ethnic group 1354
  immunology 1355–6
  laboratory tests 1403
  monitoring disease activity 1360–1
  pathology 1357
  prognosis 1358, 1361–2, 1403–4
  pulmonary involvement 1354, 1355
  relapse 1361, 1362
  renal involvement *321*, 323, 1354, 1357
  sex ratio/distribution 1354
  treatment 173–4, 1358–9, 1362–3
microsporidial infection *946*, 947
microtitre plate oligotyping assay 691
midazolam 305, *307*
mid-brain 223
midcarpal joint 137
middle-aged patients, systemic features of rheumatic disease 178
midfoot 153, 154
migraine 178
  in antiphospholipid syndrome 1207
  in SLE 219, 1153, 1185
migrant studies 819
migrating/migratory arthritis in rheumatic fever 977
milk intolerance 616
milking sign 979
Milkman's fracture 1601
Million Visual Analogue Scale 59
Milwaukee shoulder syndrome 682, 1531–2, **1572–3**
MIM146000 369, *369*
MIM123150 369
MIM122880 395
MIM146000 396
MIM123150 398
MIM146000 1630
mineral oil in adjuvant arthritis 567

mineral supplements 262
minitracheotomy 303, 304, 305
minocycline
  adverse effects 1690, *1690*
  in pyoderma gangrenosum 210
  in rheumatoid arthritis 1026
minor lymphocyte stimulating antigen 551
minute ventilation 1775, 1776
misoprostol 100, 261, 1020, 1695
mithramycin in Paget's disease 1611, 1615
mitochondrial myopathies 473, 474
mitral valve
  disease 232
    in antiphospholipid syndrome 1207
    due to rheumatic fever 978
  insufficiency 238–9, *239*
  prolapse 238, 1418
    in hypermobility 1500
    in polymyositis/dermatomyositis 1255
  regurgitation, in SLE 1151
  replacement 238, 239
  vegetations 220, 1151
mixed connective tissue disease **1414–23**
  age at onset 13
  autoantibodies 671, 1413, 1414, 1416, 1419, 1420
  cardiovascular involvement *230*, 234, 1416, 1418, *1418*
  childhood, sex differences 14
  clinical features 1416–19, *1416*
  cutaneous involvement 1417
  definition 1414
  diagnostic criteria *1415*, 1421
  differential diagnosis 1136, *1137*
  epidemiology 1414, 1416
  gastrointestinal involvement *258*, 1417–18, *1417*
  histopathology 1419–20
  immune complexes in 711–12
  immunoregulatory abnormalities 1420–1
  joint involvement 1417
  laboratory tests 1419, *1420*
  longitudinal studies 1421
  mortality in *1419*, 1421, *1422*
  muscle involvement 1417
  neurological involvement 222, *224*, 228, 1418
  pathogenesis *1415*, 1419
  prognosis 1421
  pulmonary involvement 1418–19, *1418*
  renal involvement *321*, 1419
  rheumatoid factor in *674*
  terminology 1413
  treatment 1421–3
mixed crystal deposition 1532, 1573
mixed lymphocyte reaction 548
mixed nerve potential 801
MLS antigen 551
mobility 1729, 1733–5
mobilization
  following bed rest in low back pain 100
  postoperative 305
  in sport-associated haematoma 1782
models *see* animal models
Modified Health Assessment Questionnaire 55, 61
Moisture seekers, The 36
molecular genetics **347–52**
molecular mimicry 553, 1042
molluscum contagiosum 214
molluscum fibrosum *208*
moments 477
mometasone furoate *210*
monoamine oxidase inhibitors 340
monoarthritis multiplex 1522
monoarticular arthritis in childhood 20
monoclonal antibodies
  adverse effects *337*

monoclonal antibodies *(continued)*
  against adhesion molecules 538, 613
  in immunoassays 660
  therapy in Wegener's granulomatosis 1346
  to T-cell receptors 612–13
monocyte chemotactic proteins 534, *535*, 990
monocytes
  effect of alkylating agents on *592*
  effect of azathioprine on 590, *590*
  effect of corticosteroids on *586*
  effect of gold therapy on 599, *600*
  effect of penicillamine on *597*
  in HIV infection 909
  in inflammation 513–14
  in innate immunity 545
  phagocytosis 513
  in polymyalgia rheumatica/giant cell arteritis 1377
  in rheumatoid arthritis 992
  selective removal 611
  in Sjögren's syndrome 1305
mononeuritis 178, 795
  in SLE 1185
mononeuritis multiplex *226*, 227, 795, 802, 806
  in polyarteritis nodosa 1353
  in rheumatoid arthritis 1013
  in Sjögren's syndrome 1311
  in SLE 1185
  in Wegener's granulomatosis 1339
monosodium urate
  crystals 1561
    in acute gout 1559
    formation 1558–9
    nephropathy due to 1561
    synovial fluid 654, 677, 682, 683–4
monosodium urate monohydrate crystals 1526
mood alterations in methotrexate therapy *584*
Moore–Federman disease 1635
mophebutazone, adverse effects 295
morphine
  antinociceptive action 498
  in therapy of postoperative pain 105
morphoea 205, 206, 207, 1217
  circumscribed 1228, *1243*
  clinical features 1228
  generalized 1217, 1228, *1243*
  guttate 1217, 1228
  limited 1217
  treatment 211, 212
  see also scleroderma
Morquio–Brailsford syndrome 1632, *1633*
'mortar-in-pestle' deformity 284
Morton's neuroma 160
mosaicism 697–8
motor action potential 800
motor cars 1735
motor nerve conduction velocity 800
motor neurone disease
  muscle in 470, 471
  rheumatic symptoms *218*
motor unit 460, 461
  contractile properties 462, 463
  fibre types 462
mouth
  guards 1780
  limited opening *174*
  in Sjögren's syndrome 1307–9, *1308*
  in Wegener's granulomatosis 1335
movement disorders in Sjögren's syndrome 1311
movie sign 1785
MPO *see* myeloperoxidase
MPO-ANCA *see* antineutrophil cytoplasmic autoantibodies, p-ANCA/MPO-ANCA
MRA, Takayasu's arteritis 1386
MRI *see* magnetic resonance imaging
MRL$^{+/+}$ mice 1162, *1162*, 1163

MRL-*lpr/lpr* mice 511, 613, 999
  Fas protein expression 1163
  lupus 1162, *1162*, 1175–6
  spontaneous arthritis 567
mRNA 347
  inhibition of translation 615
  stability 349
  translation 348
MRS, polymyositis/dermatomyositis 1260–1
MRSA 856, 857, 859, 870, 874
MSAs 1270–1, *1271*, 1290
Mseleni disease 1518, 1637
MSVC 1775
MSX2 gene mutation *see* 395
Muckle–Wells syndrome 1433, *1434*, 1438
mucocutaneous lymph node syndrome *see* Kawasaki disease
mucolipidoses 168, 350, **1633–4**
mucopolysaccharidoses 168, 350, 1631–3, *1633*
Mucor, arteritis due to 1390
mucosal addressin cell adhesion molecule-1 530, 533
multicentric reticulohistiocytosis **1474–7**, 1635
  clinical features *170*, 204, 206, 1474–6
  course 1477
  diagnosis 1476–7
  and malignant disease 1475–6
  nailfolds in 202
  pathology 1476
  and pregnancy 185
  treatment *1476*, 1477
  weight loss in *170*
Multidimensional Pain Inventory 1724, *1724*
multi-infarct dementia 30
multiparity and rheumatoid arthritis 182
multiple endocrine neoplasia, hyperparathyroidism in 434
multiple epiphyseal dysplasia 413, *435*, 1630
  atlantoaxial subluxation in 224
  gene mutations 369, 370, 377
  overlap with Stickler syndrome 353
multiple myeloma *see* myeloma
multiple nerve entrapment syndromes 805
multiple sclerosis
  myokymia in 217
  rheumatic symptoms *218*
mumps 904
muramic acid 974
muramyl dipeptide 998
murine mycoplasma arthritides superantigen 844
muscle
  adaptation to exercise 1776–7
  adverse drug effects *587*, 653
  atrophy
    differential diagnosis 470, 471
    grouped 790–1
    histology 790–1
    in juvenile chronic arthritis 1100, 1101
    in leprosy 934
    perifascicular 790
  basement membrane 457
  biopsy 465, 466
    atrophy 790–1
    clinicopathological correlation 788–91
    in the elderly 465
    fibrosis 791
    following eccentric exercise 469, 470
    HIV-associated myopathy 913–14
    hypertrophy 791
    inflammation 789–90
    necrosis 790
    polymyositis/dermatomyositis 788, 789, 790, 1261–2, 1263, 1290

muscle *(continued)*
  biopsy *(continued)*
    site 788
    stains 788
    technique 787–8, 1261
    vasculitis 791
  contractile apparatus 455–8
  contractile properties 461–3
  contraction 1714
    ATP splitting during 464
  contracture 217, 1291, 1714
    in juvenile chronic arthritis 1101
    in leprosy 934
  cramps 473, 1291
  damage mechanisms 466–9, 470
  differential diagnosis of childhood
    disorders 1291, *1292, 1293*
  embryology 458–9
  exercise
    eccentric/plyometric 467–9, 470
    fatiguing 467
  in fatty acid metabolic disorders 473–4
  fetal development 458–9
  fibres 456
    denervation 462–3, 790–1
    fast-twitch/type 2 788
    fatigue-resistant/type 1 788
    innervation 460
    moth-eaten 791
    numbers 460
    in polymyositis/dermatomyositis
      1268–9
    ragged red 473, 474, 791, 1265
    regenerating 790
    reinnervation 462–3
    size assessment 788
    slow-twitch 788
    staining reactions 788
    types 460, *461,* 788
    and physiological properties 462,
      463
  fibrillation 217
  fibrosis, histology 791
  filaments 455–6
  force
    components 463
    during stretch 463–4
    isometric (P_0) 463
  force–velocity characteristics 463
  fuel use 1773–4
  function, effect of age on 28, 464–5
  in glycogenoses 472–3
  growth 460, 461
  hypertrophy 1776
    and growth 460
    histology 791
  in inclusion-body myositis 471–2, 1278
  infarction in diabetes mellitus *283,* 285
  inflammation, histology 789–90
  ischaemic damage 469, 470
  length–tension relationship 463–4
  in malignant hyperpyrexia/hyper-
    thermia 472
  mass in polymyositis/dermatomyositis
    1258
  maximum velocity of unloaded shorten-
    ing 463
  metabolic depletion 467
  in mitochondrial myopathies 473, 474
  in motor neurone disease 470, 471
  myofibrillar disarray 791
  necrosis, histology 790
  pain 216, 653, 1291
    in familial Mediterranean fever 1447
    following eccentric exercise 467
  plasma membrane 456–7
  in polyarteritis nodosa 472, 791
  in rheumatic disease 470–2
  in rheumatoid arthritis 472, 1011
  rupture 1783
  in sarcoidosis 1468–9
  in scleroderma 472
  size 460, 461
  in Sjögren's syndrome 472, 1311

muscle *(continued)*
  in SLE 472, 791, 1147, 1149
  spasm 1713–14
  spindles 458
  strains in the elderly 37
  strength 1776
    evaluation 16, 1250
  structure 455–8
  in systemic sclerosis 790, 1238
  tenderness
    in cervical spondylosis 1653
    in dermatomyositis/polymyositis 1250
    in fibromyalgia 1496, 1497
    measurement 467
    in non-gonococcal arthritis 850
    referral 1497
  trauma 466–7
  twitching 216–17
  vacuoles 791
  vasculitis 791
  wasting
    and disability 1725
    hands 41
    quadriceps 49
    shoulder 44
  weakness
    causes 470
    in cervical spondylosis 1653
    childhood 21, 1291
    in dermatomyositis 470, 1250,
      1289–90
    in hyperparathyroidism 280
    measurement 465–6
    in osteomalacia/rickets 1601
    in polymyositis 470, 1250, 1289–90
    in SLE 1147
muscular dystrophy 457
muscular subaortic stenosis 1777
mushrooming 1562
musicians, hand and arm problems
  1495–6, *1496*
MVV 1775
myalgia 653
  in dermatomyositis 1250
  in eosinophilia–myalgia syndrome 1425
  in familial Mediterranean fever 1447
  in giant cell arteritis 653
  in juvenile chronic arthritis 1116
  in Lyme disease 887
  in microscopic polyangiitis 1354
  in mixed connective tissue disease 1417
  in polyarteritis nodosa 1353
  in polymyalgia rheumatica 653
  in polymyositis 1250
  in Sjögren's syndrome 1309, 1311
  in SLE 1147, 1182
  in Takayasu's arteritis 1385
  in undifferentiated connective tissue
    disease 1413
  in Wegener's granulomatosis 1338
myasthenia, rheumatic symptoms
  218
myasthenia gravis *285*
  autoantibodies 668
  differential diagnosis 1265, 1674–5
  drug-induced *598,* 599, 1022, **1693**
  electromyography 1293
  neuromuscular function 801
  and SLE 1157
  weakness in 216
c-*myc* proto-oncogene in Sjögren's
  syndrome 1302, 1305
mycetoma 245, 252
Mycobacterium
  arteritis due to 1390–1
  and HIV-associated Reiter's syndrome
    920
  M. avium intracellulare in HIV infection
    916
  M. kansasii
    in HIV infection 916
    in pyogenic arthritis 880
  M. leprae 933, 935
    vasculitis due to 1391

Mycobacterium *(continued)*
  M. marinum in pyogenic arthritis 880,
    880
  M. tuberculosis 927
    in HIV infection 917
    identification 929–30
    joint infection 661–2
    in osteomyelitis 868, 870
    in pyogenic arthritis 880
    and rheumatoid arthritis 986
    see also tuberculosis
  pulmonary infection *251,* 252–3
Mycoplasma
  in AIDS 967
  arthritis due to 966–9, 999
  culture 968–9
  M. hominis 968
  M. pneumoniae 966, 968
  M. salivarium 968
  and pyogenic arthritis 880
  and reactive arthropathies 1088
myelin 793, 794
myelofibrosis in SLE 1193
myelography
  arachnoiditis following 1645
  cervical spondylosis 1654
  childhood 764
  low back pain 730–1
  spinal dysraphism 128
myeloma 120, 289, 653, *1671, 1672*
  acute phase response in 640
  age-related occurrence *26*
  hypercalcaemia in 437
  intraneural amyloid deposition in 795
  osteoporosis in 1590
myelopathy in Lyme disease 888
myeloperoxidase (MPO) 328, 1356
  in ANCA-associated vasculitis 1342–3
  in cytoplasmic granules 513
  in microscopic polyangiitis 1328, 1329
myf **genes** 458, 460
myoadenylate deaminase 1269
myoblasts 458
myocardial biopsy 236
myocardial disease *230, 236–7, 236*
myocardial fibrosis in systemic
  sclerosis 1234–5, *1234*
myocardial infarction
  acute 231, 232
    treatment 233
  in antiphospholipid syndrome 1206
  in SLE 1194
myocarditis *176,* 236
  acute 236
  in Behçet's syndrome 1397
  fulminant 236
  in juvenile chronic arthritis 1116–17
  in polymyositis/dermatomyositis 1255
  in SLE 1149, 1194
  in systemic sclerosis 1234, *1234*
  viral 236
  in Wegener's granulomatosis 1338
myoD 460
Myodil 730–1
myofascial trigger-point pain
  syndromes 1497
myofibrillar protein 456
myofibrils 456, 457, 458
myofibroblasts in Dupuytren's
  contracture 147–8
myogenin 458, 460
myoglobin 633
  and acute renal failure 467
  following reperfusion of ischaemic
    limb 469
  as marker of muscle damage 465
  in polymyositis/dermatomyositis 1258
myoglobinuria 323, 327, 474, 1291
myokymia 217
myometry in childhood 16
myopathy
  drug-related 653, 1265–6, *1265,* 1693
    aspirin 653, *1265*
    chloroquine 791, *1265,* 1266, 1693

myopathy *(continued)*
  drug-related *(continued)*
    colchicine *1265,* 1266, 1693
    corticosteroids 470, 471, *587,* 653,
      791, 806, 1182, 1266
    niacin *1265*
    NSAIDs 653
    D-penicillamine 653, 790, *1265,*
      1267, 1693
    phencyclidine *1265*
    phenylbutazone *1265*
    propylthiouracil *1265*
    vincristine *1265,* 1693
    zidovudine 790, 913–14, 1263, *1265*
  electrodiagnosis 806
  endocrine 1266
  in HIV infection 789, 790, 913–14
  in hyperparathyroidism 280
  in hypothyroidism *277,* 278
  idiopathic inflammatory 1249, *1250*
  inflammatory 789–90, 1379
  metabolic 1265
  mitochondrial 791, 1265
  in systemic sclerosis 790, 1238, 1424–5
  in thyrotoxicosis 278, *279*
myophosphorylase deficiency 216,
  473, 1774, 1775
myosin 455, 458
  embryonic 458–9
  expression by satellite cells 459
  intermediate fast 458–9
  slow 458–9
myosin ATPase 788
myositis
  acute viral 789, 1293
  in Behçet's syndrome 1397
  in dermatomyositis 1250
  differential diagnosis 1136, *1137,*
    1263–6, *1264, 1265*
  drug-induced 1693
  experimental autoimmune 1272–3
  in helminthic infection 950–1
  in HIV infection 1263, 1278, 1293
  in HTLV-1 infection 1263–4, 1293
  inclusion-body 789, 791, 1249–50,
    1250, **1278–80,** 1440
    in childhood 1293
    muscle in 471–2, 1278
  infective, muscle biopsy in 789
  in mixed connective tissue disease 1417
  in polymyositis 1250
  in protozoal infection 947
  in Sjögren's syndrome 1311
  in SLE 1147, 1157, 1182
  in systemic sclerosis 1238
  in Wegener's granulomatosis 1338
myositis ossificans 1504–5, 1783
myositis ossificans progressiva
  436–7
myositis-overlap antibodies 1271–2,
  1271
myositis-specific antibodies 1270–1,
  1271, 1290
myotendinous junction 457
myotonia congenita 457
myotonias, rheumatic symptoms *218*
myotonic dystrophy 695
myotubes 458
myxoedema *see* hypothyroidism
myxoedema pseudomyotonia 278
myxoid degeneration 743

N

N-methyl-D-aspartate receptors in
  spinal cord neurone activation
  495–6
nabumetone
  adverse effects 260
  half-life *577*
  metabolism 577
  in osteoarthritis 1547
nafcillin in pyogenic arthritis *856*
NAG 650

nailfold
    capillary assessment 41, 202, 203–4
        in dermatomyositis 1251, 1252
        in differential diagnosis 1291
        in mixed connective tissue disease
            1416
        in Raynaud's phenomenon 1230
        in syndrome of limited joint mobility
            283
    infarction 41, *174*
nails
    ecchymoses under 207
    examination 41, 202, 203
    grooving *208*
    in HIV infection 919
    hyperkeratosis 1087
    in juvenile psoriatic arthritis 1055, 1056
    parakeratosis 1087
    pitting *174*
    in psoriasis 1076
    in psoriatic arthritis 1072
    splinter haemorrhage *174*, 207
        in antiphospholipid syndrome 1207
naloxone 338
nandrolone denoate in osteoporosis
    1598
naphtha-n-hexane *1223*
naprosyn in seropositive juvenile
    chronic arthritis 1035
naproxen 100
    adverse effects
        cutaneous 212, 213, 580, 1106
        gastrointestinal 260, *1021*
        haematological 295
        neurological *217*
        psychiatric 338
        renal 327
    binding to plasma proteins 576
    dose–response relationship 1020
    drug interactions *579*
    effect on intestinal microbial flora 269
    enantiomers *577*
    and gastric ulceration 578
    half-life *577*
    in juvenile chronic arthritis 1106, *1106*,
        1138, *1140*
    in lactation 193
    in pregnancy 190
    pseudoporphyria due to 206
    in psoriatic arthritis 1080
    relationship between dose, plasma
        concentration and effect 577
    renal clearance 577
    in SLE 1182
Naquamaland hip dysplasia 372
narcotics 32
National Ankylosing Spondylitis
    Society (NASS) 109, 1069
National Health and Nutrition
    Examination Survey 55
Native Americans
    juvenile chronic arthritis 829, 830, *830*,
        831
    juvenile spondylarthropathies *832*
    rheumatoid arthritis 832–3, *834*
    seronegative spondylarthropathies 838,
        838, 839, 840
    SLE 835, *836*
natural killer cells 527, 545
    effect of alkylating agents on *592*
    effect of azathioprine on 590, *590*
    effect of corticosteroids on *586*
    effect of gold therapy on *600*
    effect of penicillamine on *597*
    in scleroderma 1221
    in Sjögren's syndrome 1305
    in SLE 1168
nausea
    drug-related *584, 591, 593, 595, 598*,
        1020
    in Sjögren's syndrome 1310
    in SLE 257, 1156
navicular 153, 154
    accessory 167

navicular *(continued)*
    fracture 163
naviculocuneiform joint 51
NCAM 460
nDNA 667
neck *see* spine, cervical
necrobiosis lipoidica 1095
Neer shoulder 1703
nef gene 909
nef protein 910
nefazodone 340
nefopam in low back pain 100
Neisseria
    arthritis due to 849, **854–5**
        management 856–8
    N. gonorrhoeae
        antibiotic sensitivity *856, 857*
        arthritis due to 849, 854–5, 880, *880*
            childhood 862, *862*, 863
            disseminated infection 854–5
            joint infection 661, 662
            specimen handling 659, 679
            strains 854
    N. meningitidis
        antibiotic therapy *856*
        arthritis due to 855–6
neonatal drug withdrawal syndrome
    189
neonatal lupus erythematosus (NLE)
    1157, 1159, **1198–9**
    animal models 1198
    cardiac lesions 1198
    cutaneous involvement 1198–9
    liver disease in 1199
    onset 12, 13
    sex differences 12, 14
    treatment 1199
neonatal-onset multisystem inflam-
    matory disease *see* chronic infantile
    neurological cutaneous and articular
    syndrome
neonate
    effect of maternal aspirin ingestion on
        189–90
    fungal arthritis 958
    osteoarthritis 861
    osteomyelitis 868
    pyogenic arthritis 864, *864*
    range of joint movement 16
neopterin
    in juvenile dermatomyositis 1295
    in rheumatoid arthritis *1017*
NEP 451, 452
nephritic condition 323
nephritis, lupus *see* lupus nephritis
nephrocalcinosis in Sjögren's
    syndrome 324
nephropathy
    HIV-associated 915
    membranous 1188, 1191–2
    pigment-induced 327
    urate 1561
    uric acid 1561
nephrotic syndrome 321
    drug-related 327, 599
    in HIV infection 915
    and hyperlipidaemias 1482
    in mixed connective tissue disease 1419
    oliguria in 325
    and proteinuria 322
    and renal vein thrombosis 324
    secondary 322
    and SLE 1188, 1189
nerve blocks 305–6
    in osteoarthritis 1547
    in reflex sympathetic dystrophy 1687
nerve conduction studies 800–1
    acute compression neuropathy 803
    acute nerve injury 803
    cervical spondylosis 1655
    effect of age on 807
    effect of temperature on 806–7
    entrapment neuropathy 803–6
    myopathies 806

nerve conduction studies *(continued)*
    peripheral neuropathies 806
nerve fibres
    efferent sympathetic in inflammation
        497
    group II *488*
    group III *488*
    group IV *488*
    joints 489–90
    in reflex sympathetic dystrophy 1684–5,
        1686
nerve roots
    back pain associated 1640, 1647
    cervical 225
    cervicothoracic, entrapment neuro-
        pathies 805
    compression 225
    entrapment 1644, 1645
    impingement, reflex sympathetic
        dystrophy following 1681
    lumbar
        compression 225
        identification of lesion site 1641,
            1642
neural cell adhesion molecule 460
neuralgic amyotrophy 219, 221, 805,
    1661
neuraminidase deficiency 1633
neuroarthropathy in leprosy 934, 935
neuroblastoma 288, 1672
    differential diagnosis 1122, 1138
    imaging 760
    metastatic 118, 121
neurocan 410
neuroenteric cysts 127
neurofibromatosis
    kyphosis in 125
    scoliosis in 115, *116*, 125
neurogenic inflammation 450, *488*,
    497
neurokinin A 450, 490, 511
neurological complications of rheu-
    matic diseases *177, 178*, **216–28**
neurological disorders presenting with
    rheumatic symptoms 216, *218*
neuromuscular junctions 459
neurones
    α-motor *495*
    γ-motor *495*
    motor 460, 461
    nociceptive specific *487, 488*, 489,
        491
    postganglionic sympathetic *495*
    postsynaptic 494
    presynaptic 494
    spinal cord 487
        activation in joint inflammation
            493–6
        hyperexcitability 494–6
        vasoconstrictor *495*, 497
        wide dynamic range *488*, 491
neuropathy 3
neuropeptide Y 451, 511
neuropeptides
    expression by joint nerves 490
    in inflammation 497
    in spinal cord neurone activation 496
neuropraxia *803*
neurotmesis *803*
neurotransmitters 494, 495, *495*,
    509–10
    degradation 451–2
    in synovial inflammation 450–2
    in synovial nerves 442, 444, 510, 511
neutral endopeptidase 451, 452
neutropenia 512, 642–3, *643*
    as contraindication to local steroid
        injection 1758
    drug-related 296, *578, 584*, 589, *589*
        alkylating agents 593
        azathioprine 590, *591*
        gold therapy *601*
        penicillamine *598*
    in Felty's syndrome 292, 644

neutropenia *(continued)*
    in large granular lymphocyte syndrome
        644
neutrophil receptors 512–13, *513*
neutrophilia 642, *643*, 1465
neutrophilic dermatoses **1456–62**
neutrophils
    adhesion in synovial inflammation 448
    apoptosis 513
    chemoattractants in synovial inflamma-
        tion 448
    cytoplasmic granules 513
    defects 971
    effect of corticosteroids on *586*
    effect of gold therapy on 599, *600*
    effect of NSAIDs on 576, 1020
    effect of penicillamine on *597*
    effect of substance P on 451
    in inflammation 512–13
    in innate immunity 545
    phagocytosis 513
    role in cartilage destruction 569–70
New York criteria for rheumatoid
    arthritis 812, 1004, *1006*
New Zealand
    prevalence of rheumatoid arthritis *834*
    prevalence of SLE 836, *836*
Newington Children's Hospital
    Juvenile Rheumatoid Arthritis
    Evaluation 56, 57
NFB family 348, 352
NHANES 55
NHI 54
NHP 54, *54*, 1724, *1724*
niacin, adverse effects *1265*
NICER 1780
nickel sensitivity reactivation by gold
    therapy 213
nicotinic acid and hyperuricaemia
    1558, 1694
nifedipine in mixed connective tissue
    disease 1423
nitric oxide 447, 450, 510, 511
    in blood flow regulation 512
    in inflammation 511
nitric oxide synthases 511
nitrite in synovial inflammation 447
nitritoid reaction 1022
nitroglycerine
    and hyperuricaemia *1558*
    sublingual 230
    topical 212
nitroxoline, adverse effects 1693
NLE *see* neonatal lupus erythematosus
NMDA receptors in spinal cord
    neurone activation 495–6
Nocardia
    N. asteroides in HIV infection 916
    osteomyelitis due to 870
    pulmonary infection 244, 252
nociception 487
    definition *488*
    neuronal basis in joints 489–91
nociceptive flexion reflex concept
    494
nociceptive input, definition *488*
nociceptive system 487, 489
    neurobiological response to joint
        inflammation 491–7
    plasticity 489, 494
nociceptors 487
    definition *488*
    polymodal *488*, 490
    in reflex sympathetic dystrophy 1684–5
    silent 492
    spinal 1640
nodules *201, 208*
    ear *174*
    in multicentric reticulohistiocytosis
        204, 1475
    peritendinous in mixed connective
        tissue disease 1417
    periungual *175*
    pulmonary 243–4, 1010

nodules *(continued)*
  rheumatoid 202, *208*, 990, 1009, 1010
    aortic valve leaflets 238
    choroid plexus 335
    local steroid injection 1771
    mitral valve leaflets 238
    surgical removal 1703
  sarcoid 207
  subcutaneous
    in rheumatic fever 979
    in SLE *208*, 1147
NOMID *see* chronic infantile neurological
    cutaneous and articular syndrome
non-gonococcal arthritis
  bacteriology 851–3
  clinical manifestations 850
  distinction from gonococcal arthritis *850*
  imaging 851
  laboratory studies 850–1
  management 856–8
  polyarticular presentation 850
  and rheumatoid arthritis 853
non-NMDA receptors in spinal cord
    neurone activation 495–6
non-steroidal anti-inflammatory
    drugs (NSAIDs) 575–80
  in acute injury 1781–2
  in adult-onset Still's disease 1127
  adverse effects 576, 578, *578*, 1020,
      1021, 1107, 1138
    on cartilage 576, *578*, 580, 1695
    central nervous system 580, *1021*
    cutaneous 212–13, *578*, 580, *1021*,
        1695
    in the elderly 27
    gastrointestinal 259–61, *260*, 578,
        578, 580, 1020, *1021*, 1695
    haematological 295, *578*, 580, 642,
        1695
    hepatic *578*, 580, *1021*
    myopathy 653
    neurological *217*
    psychiatric *337*, 338
    pulmonary *253*, *578*, 580
    renal *578*, 580, 1020, *1021*, 1695
      acute interstitial nephritis 323
      acute renal failure 325, 327
      additive effect on cyclosporin nephro-
          toxicity 325
      endstage renal disease 323
      haematuria 323
      proteinuria 322, 327
  binding to plasma proteins 576
  in calcium pyrophosphate dihydrate
      disease 1570
  clearance 577
  drug interactions *579*, 580, 582, 1020
  effect on CNS neurones 497, 498
  effect on intestinal microbial flora 269,
      271
  enantiomers 577
  enteric-coated 576
  factors affecting absorption 189
  in gout 1563
  half-lives 576, *577*
  immunomodulatory activity 576
  in juvenile chronic arthritis 1106–7,
      1106, 1124, *1125*, 1126, 1138, *1140*
  in lactation 193–4
  in lateral epicondylitis 1505
  lipid solubility 576
  in low back pain 100, 104
  mechanism of action 576
  in medial epicondylitis 1505
  metabolism 577
  in mixed connective tissue disease 1422
  in osteoarthritis 1547, 1548
  pharmacokinetics 576–8
  in polymyalgia rheumatica 1380
  postoperative 305
  potential sites of action in inflammatory
      process 575
  practical prescribing 580
  in pregnancy 190

non-steroidal anti-inflammatory
    drugs (NSAIDs) *(continued)*
  protective effects in colorectal cancer
      1666
  pseudoporphyria due to 205, 206
  in psoriatic arthritis 1079–80
  rate of absorption 577
  in reactive arthropathies 1092, *1093*
  relationship between dose, plasma
      concentration and effect 577
  responders/non-responders 577
  in rheumatoid arthritis 629, 1020
  in RS₃PE syndrome 35
  in sarcoidosis 1469
  in scleritis 317
  in Sjögren's syndrome 1314
  in SLE 1172, *1173*, 1182
  slow-release formulation 1020
  in soft-tissue rheumatism 1512
  sustained-release 576
  synovial fluid kinetics 577
  topical
    in acute injury 1776
    in osteoarthritis 1547
  uptake by triglycerides 577
  use by the elderly 32
  variability in patients' responses to 576,
      577
noradrenaline in sport 1778
normoblasts, iron metabolism 634–5
normocholesterolaemic xanthoma-
    tosis *see* multicentric reticulohistio-
    cytosis
North American Spine Society Lumbar
    Spine Outcome Assessment
    Instrument 59
nortriptyline 339, *340*, *342*
nose
  in leprosy 935
  saddling 1335, 1625
  in Wegener's granulomatosis 1334–5
nosology 843–7
Nottingham Health Index 54
Nottingham Health Profile 54, *54*,
    1724, *1724*
NSAIDs *see* non-steroidal anti-inflamma-
    tory drugs
nucleic acid-binding proteins 669
  antibodies to 669–73
nucleoside triphosphate pyropho-
    sphohydrolases 1570
nucleosomes 668–9
nucleotides 347, 689
nucleus pulposus 1640
nursemaid's elbow 163
nurses, back injuries 93–4
nutrition
  and bone mass 426
  in the elderly 30
  in juvenile chronic arthritis 86–7, 1119
nystagmus *224*, 1153, 1184
NZB/NZW mice 510, 703–4

O
Ober test 158
obesity
  and disease occurrence 823
  and gout 1555
  and osteoarthritis 823, 1518–19, 1546
  protective effects 1594
obliterative bronchiolitis 242, 244
  drug-related *253*
  flow volume curve 247, 248
  in polymyositis/dermatomyositis 1254
obliterative bursitis *see* shoulder, frozen
obsessive–compulsive disorders 342
obstructive sleep apnoea 305
obturator internus, displacement of
    fat pad over 716, 718
occipital neuralgia 1653
occupation
  and back pain 93–4, 1639
  and disease occurrence 824–5, *824*

occupation *(continued)*
  and osteoarthritis 824, *824*, 825, 1520
  and repetitive strain injury 1494
  and rheumatoid arthritis 824
  and scleroderma *1223*
  and shoulder pain 1501
  and tenosynovitis 1506
occupational therapist in multi-
    disciplinary team 1737
occupational therapy 1752
ochronosis *209*, 436, 680
  acquired 214
  and calcium pyrophosphate dihydrate
      disease 1530, *1531*, 1567
octacalcium phosphate 682, 1570
oculomotor palsy 312
odds ratio 689
odinophagia in cervical vertebral
    osteomyelitis 878
oedema
  drug-related *587*
  macular *311*
  periorbital 201, 204, 1251, 1289
  pitting 1428
  pulmonary *253*
oesophageal dysmotility
  and anaesthesia 300–1
  in polymyositis/dermatomyositis 1255,
      1277, 1290
  in rheumatoid arthritis 255, *258*
  in scleroderma 257, *258*
  in Sjögren's syndrome 257
  in SLE *258*
oesophageal reflux 241, *258*
oesophageal webs in Sjögren's
    syndrome 257, *258*
oesophagoscopy in systemic sclerosis
    1232
oesophagus
  fibrosis and anaesthesia 300–1
  in systemic sclerosis 1232, *1233*
  transit time in systemic sclerosis 1232
  see also gastrointestinal system
oestradiol 182
oestrogen receptors
  osteoblasts 431, 1587
  osteoclasts 423
  osteocytes 1587
oestrogen replacement therapy and
    osteoporosis 29, 1596–7
oestrogens
  and bone mass 426, 1587
  effect on chondrocyte function 1013
  effect on experimental arthritis 182
  immunological effects 1157
  in SLE 510, 1157, 1169
ofloxacin
  in osteomyelitis 874
  in tuberculosis 931, 933
Okelbo disease 904
OLA 691, 693
olecranon bursa
  in acromegaly 281
  bursitis 146, 1505
    childhood 163
    and gout 1560
    idiopathic 146
    inflammatory 146
    local steroid injection 1765
    in rheumatoid arthritis 1008
    septic 146, 858
    traumatic 146
  calcification 1528
oligonucleotide ligation assay 691, 693
oligopeptides 613
oligospermia, drug-related 588, *589*
oliguria
  in acute renal failure 325, 326
  in microscopic polyangiitis 1354
Ollier disease, imaging 761
Oman, prevalence of rheumatoid
    arthritis *834*
omeprazole 100, 261
  adverse effects 1695

omeprazole *(continued)*
  in gastric ulceration 578
  in mixed connective tissue disease 1422
Onchocerca volvulus 949, 950, 951
onchocercoma 950
oncogenes 352
  and autoimmunity 1162
  in SLE 1168
oncornaviruses 908
oncostatin M
  in induction of acute phase proteins 623
  in rheumatoid arthritis 997
onion skinning 1237
onychodystrophy in HIV infection
    919, 920
onycholysis 41, *174*, *201*, 202, 203, 1076
O'nyong nyong virus *902–3*
oophoritis, autoimmune *285*
ophthalmological involvement in
    rheumatic disease 310–19
  see also eyes
ophthalmoplegia, internuclear 212
opiates
  epidural 105
  in low back pain 100, 105
  postoperative 305
  and sport 1778
  withdrawal syndrome 338
opioid receptors 497–8
OPLL 735, 737, 1657
opponens policis wasting 41
opsonins 512, 545, 546
opsonization 545
optic nerve
  compression in Wegener's granuloma-
      tosis 1335
  vasculitis in Wegener's granulomatosis
      1337
optic neuropathy *311*, 312
  ischaemic in giant cell arteritis 312, 313
  in relapsing polychondritis 1626
  in sarcoidosis 315
OR 689
oral contraceptives and rheumatoid
    arthritis 182, *825*, 826, 986, 1012
oral tolerance therapy 264–5
orange badge 1735
orbital biopsy in Wegener's granulo-
    matosis 1341
orbital pseudotumour in adult-onset
    Still's disease 1127
orchitis
  autoimmune *285*
  in familial Mediterranean fever 1447
  and osteoporosis 1589
orgotein 1547
oropharyngeal involvement in rheu-
    matic disease 173, *174*, 1307–9,
    1308, 1335
orosomucoid *see* α₁-acid glycoprotein
orthopnoea 231
orthoses 1732–3
  custom-made 1732–3
  hand, childhood 1743, 1744
  in juvenile chronic arthritis 1107–8
  off-the-shelf 1732
  spine
    in eosinophilic granuloma 120
    in scoliosis 117–18
  see also splints
os trigonum 746, 747
Osborne's band 800
Osgood–Schlatter disease 157, 166,
    1509, 1787
Osler's nodes *174*
OspA 884, 894
OspB 884
OspC 884
ossification centres, MRI 771
ossification of the posterior longitu-
    dinal ligament 735, 737, 1657
osteitis, leprous 934, 935
osteitis condensans, medial end of
    clavicle 185

osteitis condensans ilii 185, 1065
osteitis fibrosa cystica 434
osteitis pubis 1508
  in pregnancy 185
osteoarthritis 1515–49
  acute phase response in 627
  ankle 1532
  atypical presentation 1533
  basic calcium phosphate crystals in
    1573
  biochemical tests *649*, 652, 1536–9
  bony enlargement in 1521
  central/medial pole 1525
  in cervical spondylosis 1652
  clinical features 31–2, 1520–33
  co-occurrence with rheumatoid
    arthritis 677
  collagen mutations in 371–3, 378
  coping with 1547–8
  crepitus in 1521
  crystal-associated subsets 1525–32
  decompensated 1540
  definition 1515–16
  and diabetes mellitus *283*, 1519
  diagnosis 1539–40
  diagnostic criteria *812*, 1516
  differential diagnosis 1568
  effect of NSAIDs on development 580
  elbow 1532
  in the elderly 25, 31–2
    concomitant disease *33*
    differential diagnosis *32*, 33
  endemic 1518
  epidemiology *814*, 1516–20
    effect of age and sex *26*, 815, *815*, 816,
      816, 1517–18
    geographic variation 1518
    prevalence 1515, 1517
    time trends 817, 818
  erosive/inflammatory 1522–3, 1524
  and ethnic group 819, *819*, 1518
  facet joints 91–2, 1533, 1644
  following trauma 1519–20
  foot 1535
  functional impairment in 1521
  genetic factors 356, *822*, 1519
  glenohumeral joint 1532
  grading 1516–17, 1535
  hand 1534, 1549
  health status measures 57–8, *57*
  hip 1524–5, 1534, 1549
  history 1515
  and hypermobility 1500
  and hypertension 1519
  and hyperuricaemia 1519
  imaging 747, 748, 749, 1533–6
  investigations 1533–9
  and joint shape abnormalities 1520
  knee 1523–4, 1534, 1549, 1769
  large joint 1523–5, 1769
  liver function 652
  lubrication failure in 484
  markers of 417–18, *418*, 1536–40
  mechanical failure in 477
  menstrual, hormonal and reproductive
    factors *823*, 1519
  models 415–17
  modification 1548–9
  neonatal 861
  nodal 684
  nodal generalized 1519, 1522, 1523
  non-nodal generalized 1522
  and obesity 823, 1518–19, *1546*
  and occupation 824, *824*, 825, 1520
  onset, speed of 33
  and osteoporosis 1519
  in Paget's disease 1612
  pain in 1520–1
  as part of other diseases 1532–3
  pathogenesis 482–4, 1540–5
  patient education 1546
  primary 483, 1522
  as a process 1540
  prognosis 1549

osteoarthritis *(continued)*
  psychiatric involvement 337
  radiographical–pathological correlates
    1517
  renal function 650
  risk factors 1518–20
  sacroiliac joints 1535
  secondary 483, 1522
  and smoking 1519
  spine 1535, 1549
  stiffness in 1521
  subsets 1521–33
  superior pole 1524–5
  synovial biopsy 778
  synovial fluid 682–3, 1536–9
  synovitis in 1521
  tissue structure and metabolism
    1540–5
  treatment 31–2, 1545–9, *1546*, 1703
osteoarthrosis *see* osteoarthritis
osteoblastoma
  childhood and adolescence 119, 120
  spinal 119, 120
osteoblasts 413, 421
  in bone formation 424
  function 422–3
  in inflammation 508
  oestrogen receptors 431
  in osteopetrosis 436
  in Paget's disease 1610, 1611
  relationship with other bone cells 425
  response to mechanical stress 426
  synthesis of matrix protein 426–9
osteocalcin (BGP) 421, 427, *429*, 653
  in juvenile chronic arthritis 87
  as measure of bone turnover 432
  in osteoporosis 1595
  in Paget's disease 1613
  in rheumatoid arthritis *1017*
osteochondral bodies 1541
osteochondritis 1787, *1787*
**osteochondritis deformans in
  hypothyroidism** 278
osteochondritis dissecans 166, 1624,
  1787–8
  imaging 740–1, 758, 771
osteochondrodysplasias 1629–30
osteochondrodystrophy, kyphosis in
  116
osteochondroma *1671*
  childhood and adolescence 118
  spinal 118
osteochondromatosis, synovial 726,
  742
osteoclast-activating factors 424, *425*,
  437
osteoclasts 421, 422, 423
  in bone resorption 424, *425*
  in inflammation 508
  in Paget's disease 434–5, 1610
  relationship with other bone cells 425
  transplantation 436
osteocytes 421, 423
  response to mechanical stress 426
osteogenesis imperfecta 358–66, 427,
  435
  animal models 365
  autosomal recessive 366
  classification 358, 359
  clinical features 358–61
  collagen type I gene mutations 353, 357,
    361–5, 418–19, 427, 435, 697
  differential diagnosis 1500
  genetic counselling 698
  genetic marker analysis 697–8
  histology of fetal bone 357
  imaging 759
  with normal collagen type I protein 366
  phenotypic severity 435
  prenatal diagnosis 698
  type I 358, 359, 361, 435
  type II 358–61, 435
  type III 358, 360, 435
  type IV 358, 361, 435

osteogenesis imperfecta *(continued)*
  without collagen type I mutations
    365–6
osteogenic sarcoma 288, *1671*
osteogenin 427
osteoid 1600
osteoid osteoma 1617–18
  arthritis in 288
  back pain in 117, 118–19
  clinical features 1618
  diagnosis 1618
  differential diagnosis *1105*
  imaging 118, 119, 754, 768, 1618
  muscle weakness in 21
  treatment 1618
osteolysis
  and diabetes mellitus 284
  distal 1636
  hereditary 1635–6
  imaging 758, 760
osteomalacia 433, 434, 1583, **1600–6**
  and altered phosphate homeostasis
    1604–6
  and aluminium retention 1603, 1606
  back pain in 99
  biochemical features 1601–2
  bone biopsy 780, 783, 1602
  causes *433*
  clinical and laboratory features 1600–1
  and defective mineralization 1606
  in the elderly 1603
  hypocalcaemia 653, 1601
  and malignant disease 1605–6
  metabolic acidosis in 1605
  oncogenic 1605–6, 1672
  and vitamin D deficiency 1601–2,
    1603–4
osteomyelitis 868
  acute 869
  acute phase response in 640
  aetiology 870, *870*
  brucellar 941
  childhood 752, 868, 877
  chronic 869, 873, 876
    focal 1620–1
    post-traumatic 876, *877*
    recurrent multifocal *1137*, 1138
  classification 868–9, *868*, 869
  in decubitus ulcers 876
  in diabetes mellitus 284, 869
  diagnosis 870–3, *873*
  diagnostic criteria 868–9, *868*
  differential diagnosis 1122
  haematogenous 868–9
    acute 871, 873, 877
  histology 873
  in HIV infection 916–17
  imaging 284, 752, 768, 772, 871–3, 931
  laboratory tests 871
  leprous 934
  microbiology 873, *873*
  neonatal 868
  prognosis 876
  prophylaxis 876
  and pseudarthrosis 869
  risk factors 869–70
  risk of pyogenic arthritis 849
  in septic bursitis 858
  spinal, childhood 121–2, 124
  surgical debridement 875–6
  treatment 873–6
  tuberculous 928–9, 930
  vertebral 877–9
osteonecrosis 1621–4
  aetiological factors 1621–2
  in antiphospholipid syndrome 1207,
    1622
  in Behçet's syndrome 1397
  childhood 163
  classification 1622
  diagnosis 1622–3
  differential diagnosis *1105*
  drug-related *587*, 1696
  femoral condyle 1623

osteonecrosis *(continued)*
  femoral head 1622, 1623
    and gout 1561
    in pregnancy 185
  imaging 749–50, 1622–3
  in mixed connective tissue disease 1417
  pathology 1621
  in SLE 1147, 1622
    childhood 1182
  treatment 1624
  vertebral 1623
osteonectin 421, 427, *429*
osteopathy, in low back pain 101, 104
osteopenia
  age-related occurrence *26*
  in animal models of joint disease 416
  definition 1583, *1583*
  in juvenile dermatomyositis 1297
  physiological/age-related 1587
  in pregnancy and lactation 185
osteopetrosis 423, 436
osteophytes 413, 570, 721
  in animal models of joint disease
    415–16
  in calcium pyrophosphate dihydrate
    disease 1568
  in cervical spondylosis 1652
  differentiation from syndesmophytes
    1065–6
  formation 730, 732
  imaging 728, 733, 735, 739
  in osteoarthritis 1521, 1541
  periosteal 1541
osteopoikilosis 207
osteopontin 427, *429*
osteoporosis 422, **1583–600**, 1601
  age-related/senile/type II 1587–8
  and ankylosing spondylitis 1061, 1066,
    1591
  and anorexia nervosa 433, 1589
  and back pain 92, 99, 1591
  biochemical markers 653, 1595
  bone 432–3
    biopsy 780, 782–3, 1594–5
    density measurement 1594, *1595*
  and bone structure 421
  causes *433*
  classification 1586–91, *1586*
  clinical features 1591, 1592
  and coeliac disease 129
  Colles' fracture 1583–4, *1584*, 1586,
    1599, *1600*
  and Cushing's syndrome 128, 433, 1588
  definition 1583, *1583*
  and diabetes mellitus 128, *283*
  diagnosis 1594–5, *1594*, *1595*
  disuse 128, 433, 1590
  drug-related 128, 130, 587, 1589–90,
    1591, 1696
  endocrine causes 1588–9
  epidemiology 1583–4, *1584*
  and ethnic group 1594, *1594*
  hip fracture 1583–4, 1584–6, 1600, *1601*
  and homocystinuria 129
  and hyperparathyroidism 280, 1589
  and hypogonadism 1589
  idiopathic *1137*, 1138, 1588
  imaging 749, 757
  in inflammatory disorders 1590–1
  juvenile 128–30, *1137*, 1138, 1588
  and juvenile chronic arthritis 86–7, 128
  and malabsorption 1603
  in malignant disease 1590
  menstrual, hormonal and reproductive
    factors *823*
  and osteoarthritis 1519
  pathogenesis 1591–4
  postmenopausal/type I 1587
  prevention 29, 1595–7
  primary/physiological 1586–8
  in rheumatoid arthritis 1590–1, *1590*
  risk factors 1594, *1594*
  and smoking 1594
  and thyrotoxicosis 278–9, *279*, 1589

osteoporosis (continued)
transient
in pregnancy 185, 749
regional 749
treatment 29, 1597–9, *1597*
in tuberculosis 930
and Turner's syndrome 129
vertebral fracture in 1583–4, *1584*, 1586, 1599–600, *1600*
and vitamin D receptor gene polymorphism 1593
osteoprogenitor cells 424
osteosarcoma
and Paget's disease 1612, 1613
spinal 120
osteosclerosis in hypoparathyroidism 281
osteotomy
double 1703
humerus 1703
metatarsal 1719
in osteoarthritis 1548
in osteonecrosis 1624
realignment 483
scapula 1703
shoulder, childhood 1720
supracondylar 1718
varus 1716
vertebral wedge in ankylosing spondylitis 1069
Oswestry Low Back Pain Disability Questionnaire 59
otitis media
preceding pyogenic arthritis in childhood 861
in Wegener's granulomatosis 1335
otospondylomegaepiphyseal dysplasia syndrome 368, 377
Ouchterlony technique 669, 670
outcomes assessment *see* health status, measures
outside-in signalling 532–3
ovalbumin in antigen-induced arthritis 565
overexertion 1777–8, 1780
overlap syndromes 1136, *1137*, **1413–28**
autoantibodies in 1271–2, *1271*, 1413–14, *1415*
in childhood 1293
HLA associations 1415, *1416*
myositis in 1182
polymyositis/dermatomyositis 1256, 1423–4
scleroderma 1424–5
terminology 1413
overuse injuries
dancers 1496
musicians 1496
oxalic acid 1574–5
oxalosis, primary 1574–5
oxaprozin, half-life *577*
oxicam in pregnancy 190
oximetry, preoperative 300
oxygen
hyperbaric in osteomyelitis 876
increased demand in inflamed synovium 444
synovial consumption in inflammatory disease 445
oxyphenbutazone
adverse effects 212, 213
drug interactions *579*
in lactation 193
oxyphenylbutazone, adverse effects 295

P

P$_{III}$NP in rheumatoid arthritis 1016, *1017*
p24 908
in DILS 913
in HIV infection 913, 914–15, 921
p27 1079

p53 352
p55 in juvenile chronic arthritis 1121
p70 in SLE 1171
p75 in juvenile chronic arthritis 1121
p150,95 *see* integrins, α$^\chi$β$_2$
p277 611
p-ANCA *see* antineutrophil cytoplasmic autoantibodies, p-ANCA/MPO-ANCA
P-selectin 528–9, *529*
counter-receptors 530
expression in endothelial activation 536
in leucocyte rolling 535
oligosaccharide ligands 529–30
P-selectin binding glycoprotein-1 530
PAA 1427
pachydermoperiostosis 209
paediatric clinic 13
Paget's disease of bone **1610–17**
aetiology 1610–11
age-related occurrence 26
alkaline phosphatase 432, 651, 653
back pain 99
bone involvement 434–5
calcium abnormalities 1612–13
cardiac failure 1613
clinical features 1611–13, *1611*
cranial 1612
differential diagnosis 1615
disease associations 1613
epidemiology 1610
histopathology 1610
hyperuricaemia 1613
imaging 1613–14
investigation and assessment 1613–14
laboratory tests 1613
and malignant disease 1612
monostotic 1610
pathophysiology 1610–11
polyostotic 1610
pyridium cross-links 432
treatment 1615–17, *1615*
pain
abdominal 173, *175*
acute 99
adult-onset Still's disease 1127
Behçet's syndrome 1398
drug-related *584*, *591*, 601
Ehlers–Danlos syndrome type 4 378
familial Mediterranean fever 1445
polyarteritis nodosa 1403
rheumatic fever 979
SLE 257, 1156, 1196
acromioclavicular joint 1501
acute *90*
acute on chronic *90*
amplification 1657–8
in arachnoiditis 1645
assessment and quantification 6, *6*, 19, 64
bone 653, *1105*
and fluoride 1694–5
osteomalacia 1600
Paget's disease 1611
buttock in reactive arthropathies 1087
central 6
in cervical spondylosis 1652–3
chest 99, *176*, 229–31, 234
ankylosing spondylitis 1063
referred from cervical spine 1653
sarcoidosis 1465
systemic sclerosis 1235
toxic oil syndrome 1425
childhood 19, 1738
chronic 6, *90*
clinics 306–7, *1501*, *1502*, 1660
coping strategies 68
and depression 67
differential diagnosis 4
elbow 1504–5, *1504*, *1505*
adult *139*–40, 144–6
childhood 163, *163*
epigastric in Sjögren's syndrome 1310
facial, referred 99

pain (continued)
following local steroid injection 1758, 1759
foot 1511–12, *1511*
adult 155, 159–60
childhood *164*, 167–8
generalized conditions presenting with regional musculoskeletal 168, *168*
groin 1507–8, 1768
growing 163
hand 1505–7, *1505*, *1507*
adult *139*–40, 146–8
childhood 163, *163*
heel 159–60, 1510–11, *1510*
in familial Mediterranean fever 1447
imaging 745
in juvenile chronic arthritis 1105
in psoriatic arthritis 1076
treatment 1770
hip 1507–8, *1508*
adult 155, 156–7
childhood 164–5, *164*
history-taking 5–6
intractable *90*
joint, in Paget's disease 1612
in joint inflammation 491
knee 155, 157–9, 1508–10, *1508*
in adolescence 157
anterior 1510, 1784–5, *1785*
childhood *164*, 165–7
localization 5, *5*
lower limb 89, 96, 97, 100
childhood 19, *19*, 162, **162**, 163–8, *164*
in lumbar disc disease 98
syndromes **154–60**, *155*
muscle 216, 653, 1291
in familial Mediterranean fever 1447
following eccentric exercise 467
neck 1657
see also cervical spondylosis; spine, cervical
neurophysiology **487–98**
and nociception 487
in non-gonococcal arthritis 850
organic/non-organic 6, *6*
in osteoarthritis 1520–1, 1539
in osteoid osteoma 117, 118–19, 1618
in osteonecrosis 1622
patellofemoral 159, 1784–5, *1785*
peripheral 6
physiology 487, *488*, 489
pleuritic in mixed connective tissue disease 1418
in prosthetic joint infection 854
psychogenic *1105*
quality 6, *6*, 64
and quality of life 64
radicular 225
referred 5–6, 19, 37, 49, 1497
in disc herniation 1641
from the cervical spine 1653
from cervical spine 1653
headache as 99
to the back 133
to the face 99
to the shoulder 99, 1501
trigger-point 1497
in reflex sympathetic dystrophy 1680
in repetitive strain injury/syndrome 1495
reporting in childhood 56
retro-orbital 1653
shin 1508–9
shoulder 1501–4, *1501*, *1502*, 1660
adult *139*–40, 140–4
childhood 163, *163*
health status measures 59
referred 99, 1501, 1660
sternoclavicular joint 1501
subacute *90*
superficial 5
supraclavicular 1660

pain (continued)
sympathetic-maintained/mediated 1679
sympathetically independent 1679
in synovial inflammation 450
temporal 1653
testicular in polyarteritis nodosa 1353
thalamic 6
as trigger for reflex sympathetic dystrophy 1681
upper limb
adult *139*–40, **140–8**
childhood 19, *19*, 162, **162**–3, *163*
wrist 1505–7, *1505*, *1507*
adult *139*–40, 146–8
childhood 163, *163*
see also back pain
pain behaviour syndrome 106
pain sense, loss of 218
painful arc syndrome *see* shoulder, impingement syndrome
Pakistan
prevalence of seronegative spondylarthropathies *839*
prevalence of rheumatoid arthritis *834*
palindromic rheumatism *1104*, 1562, 1694
palmar aponeurosis 137
palmar dorsiflexion 140
palmar erythema 41, *174*, 201, 1011, 1680
palmar fasciectomy 148
palmar fasciitis 1675
palmar fasciitis–polyarthritis syndrome 289, 1675
palmar flexion 138, 139–40, 140
palmar subluxation 42
palmaris longus 137, 138
palpitations 231
pamidronate
adverse effects 1616
in Paget's disease 1615, 1616
structure 1615
pancreatitis
drug-related *587*
in mixed connective tissue disease 1417
in Sjögren's syndrome *258*, 1310
in SLE 1157, 1196
pancytopenia
drug-related 296, 297, *584*, 593
in juvenile chronic arthritis 1119
in SLE 291
panic attacks in the elderly 30
Panner's disease 163, *1787*
panniculitis 202, 206, **1450–5**
in α$_1$-antitrypsin deficiency 1452
atrophic connective tissue disease 1453
in brucellosis 941
classification 1450, *1451*
clinical features 1450–5
in dermatomyositis 1252
differential diagnosis 1455
evaluation 1455
factitial 1453, 1454
granulomatous 1450
histiocytic cytophagic 1453
lipoatrophic 1453
lipophagic of childhood 1453
lobular 1450, *1451*
lupus erythematosus 211, 1156, 1453–4, 1455
and malignancy 289
mixed 1450, *1451*
pancreatic 1452–3, 1455
poststeroid 1453
in renal failure 1453
sclerosing 1454
septal 1450, *1451*
septal granulomatous 1450
in SLE 1148
subacute nodular migratory 1450
Toxocara 949
treatment 1455
with vasculitis 1450, *1451*, 1455

pannus 508, 509, **988–90**
 imaging 763, 764, 771
 in juvenile chronic arthritis 763, 764
 in osteoarthritis 1541
panophthalmitis in adult-onset Still's
  disease 1127
papillitis in CINCA 1471, 1472
papilloedema
 in Behçet's syndrome 1397
 in relapsing polychondritis 1626
 in SLE 1153
papules *201, 208*
 facial 204
 in guttate morphoea 1228
 necrotic in Wegener's granulomatosis
   1339
 periungual 202
 rheumatoid *208*
paracetamol
 adverse effects 32
 in chronic back pain 1648
 and endstage renal disease 323
 in lactation 193
 in low back pain 100
 in osteoarthritis 31–2
 in pregnancy 189
 safe dose 1695
paracoccidioidomycosis
 epidemiology 954–5
 joint infection *955, 957,* 963
paraesthesias
 in cervical myelopathy 224
 in cervical spondylosis 1653
 in leprosy 934
 in Lyme disease 887
 in parvovirus infection 897
paramyxovirus infection in Paget's
  disease 1610–11
paraneoplastic syndromes 288, 289,
  503
paranoia in SLE 333
paraolecranon groove 137, 1764
paraproteinaemia
 in myeloma 1672
 with peripheral neuropathies 795
 and pyoderma gangrenosum 1460–1
parasitic diseases **945–51**
parathyroid
 adenoma 434
 calcium-sensing receptor 429–30
parathyroid hormone
 anabolic effects 426
 and calcium homeostasis 429–30, 652
 comparison with parathyroid hormone-
   related protein *432*
 effect on osteoclasts 424, *425*
 gene 429
 insufficiency 434
 in juvenile chronic arthritis 87
 in osteoblast differentiation 425
 in osteomalacia 1602
 in osteoporosis 1587–8, 1589, 1599
 receptor gene mutation *435, 436*
 resistance to 434
parathyroid hormone-related peptide
  (PTHrP)
 in calcium homeostasis 431
 comparison with parathyroid hormone
   432
 effect on osteoclasts *425*
 gene 415
 in malignancy 437, *437*
 receptor gene mutation *435, 436*
parathyroidectomy, effect on bone
  mass 1589
paravertebral muscles 1640
parental imprinting 349
parental involvement in
  physiotherapy 1751–2
paresis in SLE 1185
parking permits 1735
Parkinson's disease
 differential diagnosis 1379
 posture deformities *219*

Parkinson's disease *(continued)*
 rheumatic symptoms *218*
paronychia 202
parotid glands *see* salivary glands
parotitis 904
paroxetine 339, *340, 342*
pars interarticularis
 fracture 126, 127
 stress microfracture 127
 see also spondylolysis
Parsonage–Turner syndrome 1087
Parvoviridae 897
parvovirus infection 204, 663, **897–9**,
  1122
 arthropathy in 880, 898
 clinical features 897–8
 diagnosis 898
 differential diagnosis 1091
 epidemiology 897
 management 898–9
 pathogenesis 898
 in pregnancy 897
 and rheumatoid arthritis 824, 898
 synovial fluid in 683
Pasteurella multocida in pyogenic arthritis
  852, *880*
patella 151–2
 subluxation 1785
 tracking 159
patella apprehension test 1785
patella Q angle 152, 153
 abnormally increased 159
 in Osgood–Schlatter disease 157
patellar compression test 49
patellar ligament rupture 1769
patellar shrug sign 159
patellar tap 49, 50
patellar tendon 152
 rupture in SLE 1147
 tendinitis 1509
patellofemoral joint
 disease *1104*
 malalignment/instability 165
 osteoarthritis 1534
patellofemoral pain syndrome 159,
  1784–5, *1785*
patent ductus arteriosus, anaesthesia
  in 299
pathergy reaction 1395, 1396, 1399
patients
 education 70, 1727–8
  and back pain 107, 108–9, 1648
  of the elderly 31
  in fibromyalgia 37
  in osteoarthritis 1546
  in rheumatoid arthritis 1027
  in SLE 36
 outcomes assessment *see* health status,
   measures
 positioning in surgery 301, 1702
 preparation for surgery 1702
Patrick's test 1053
PAX genes 353, 368, 370
 mutations 395
Paxil 339, *340, 342*
PCR *see* polymerase chain reaction
PCR-RFLP assay 693, 697
PCR-SSO 691, 692, 697
 reverse dot-blot 691
PDGF *see* platelet-derived growth factor
peak expiratory flow 247
PECAM-1 *see* platelet-endothelial cell
   adhesion molecule-1
pectineus 150
pectoralis major 135, 137
 rupture 1783
pedicle sclerosis 127
Pedro Pons' sign 940
PEF 247
pefloxacin in osteomyelitis 874
PEG precipitation, immune
   complexes 705
Pekin–Zvaifler cells 681, 683
Pelligrini–Stieda disease 158, 1510

pelvis
 acetabulum 150
 radiography 716–17, 718
pemphigoid 205
 penicillamine-induced cicatricial 214
pemphigus 205, 207
 drug-related 598, 599
pemphigus foliaceus 214
pemphigus vulgaris 214
'pencil-in-cup' appearance 1077
D-penicillamine 596–7
 adverse effects 598–9, *598*, 1695–6
  autoimmune *598, 599*, 1022
  cutaneous 213–14, *598*, 1695
  gastrointestinal *260, 261, 598*
  haematological 296, *598*, 642
  hypertrichosis 209
  hypogammaglobulinaemia 970
  lupus-like syndrome 669, *1690*
  myopathy 653, 790, *1265, 1267*, 1693
  neurological 216, *217, 598*
  psychiatric *337*, 338
  renal 322–3, *598*, 599, 1695
  respiratory *253, 254, 598*
  scleroderma 1693
 in combination therapy *1025*
 in eosinophilic fasciitis 1428
 factors affecting absorption 189
 in giant cell arteritis 1380
 in juvenile chronic arthritis 1107, 1138,
   1140, *1140*
 in lactation 193, 194, *602*
 pharmacology 597
 in polymyalgia rheumatica 1380
 in pregnancy 192, *602*
 in psoriatic arthritis 1080
 in rheumatoid arthritis 1022
 in scleroderma 211, 212, 1240
 in seropositive juvenile chronic
   arthritis 1036
 therapeutic efficacy 597–8
 therapeutically relevant actions 597,
   597
 treatment regimens 598
penicillin
 adverse effects
  hypersensitivity vasculitis 914
  myositis 1693
  vasculitis 1371
 in Lyme disease *891*, 892, 893
 in osteomyelitis 874
 in pyogenic arthritis *856*, 865
 resistance to 857
 in rheumatic fever 980
 in septic bursitis 859
penile development 14, *17*
pentamidine isethionate in
  Pneumocystis carinii infection 253
pentazocine
 adverse effects *1223*, 1693
 and sport 1778
pentoxifylline in mixed connective
  tissue disease 1422
pentraxin family 626
pepsinogen in Sjögren's syndrome
  1310
peptic ulceration, drug-related 578,
  578, 587
peptide administration in immunosuppressive therapy 611
peptide T in psoriatic arthritis 1081
peptidoglycan 267, 269, 998
peptococcal infection in pyogenic
  arthritis 853
Peptostreptococcus productus 269
percardiocentesis 234
perceived competence 69
perchlorethylene *1223*
percutaneous transluminal angioplasty in Takayasu's arteritis 1387
periarthritis, basic calcium phosphate
  crystals in 1573
pericapsulitis *see* shoulder, frozen
pericardial disease *232, 233–5*

pericardial effusion 234
 in mixed connective tissue disease 1418
 in polymyositis/dermatomyositis 1255
 in SLE 1149
 in Wegener's granulomatosis 1338
pericardial fluid analysis 235, 1149
pericardial friction rub 234, 1149
pericardial knock 235
pericardial tamponade 234–5
pericardiocentesis 235
 childhood SLE 1194
 juvenile chronic arthritis 1116, 1126
pericarditis 173, *176, 230*, 231
 acute 234
 acute viral 235
 in adult-onset Still's disease 1127
 in ankylosing spondylitis 1064
 in Behçet's syndrome 1397
 constrictive 235
 differentiation of causes 235
 in familial Mediterranean fever 1446
 in immune complex diseases 703
 in juvenile chronic arthritis 1116
 in mixed connective tissue disease 1418
 in rheumatic fever 978
 in rheumatoid arthritis 990, 1010
 in SLE 1149, 1194
 in systemic sclerosis 1233, *1234*
 tuberculous 235
 in Wegener's granulomatosis 1338
pericardium
 biopsy 235
 parietal 234
 visceral 234
perineural fibrosis 1645–6
periostitis 570
 in HIV infection 919
 leprous 934
 in psoriatic arthritis 1077, 1078
 in seropositive juvenile chronic
   arthritis 1032
peripheral ischaemia 173
peripheral nerves
 acute compression neuropathies 803,
   803
 amyloid deposition 795
 axonal atrophy 794
 axonal degeneration 794, 802–3, *802*,
   806
 axonal regeneration 793–4
 biopsy 792
  indications for 792
  interpretation 793–6
  site 792–3
 blocks 305
 demyelination 793, 794–5
 fascicles 792
 fibre density and diameter 792, 793
 injury
  acute 803, *803*
  iatrogenic 803
  reflex sympathetic dystrophy
    following 1681
 internodal length 793
 myelin sheaths 794–5
 and nociception 487, 490
 onion bulb formation 794
 remyelination 793, 794
 wallerian degeneration *see* wallerian
   degeneration
peripheral nervous system 218, 221,
  225–8, 791
peripheral neuropathies **225–8**
 acute compression 803, *803*
 in amyloidosis 228, 1436, 1440
 chloroquine-induced 795
 in Churg–Strauss syndrome 1355
 classification *226*
 electrodiagnosis 806
 features of polyneuropathy *226*
 HIV infection 795
 Lyme disease 228, 795, 888
 in mixed connective tissue disease 1418
 with paraproteinaemias 795

peripheral neuropathies (continued)
peripheral nerve biopsy in 793–6
polyarteritis nodosa 227, 1353
reflex sympathetic dystrophy following 1681
rheumatoid arthritis 227, 1008, 1013
scleroderma 227
Sjögren's syndrome 227, 1311
SLE 227, 1153, 1184–5
and vasculitis 792, 795
Wegener's granulomatosis 1339
peritendinitis crepitans 1506
peritonitis in SLE 258, 1156
periungual nodules 175
perivascular cuffing 1319
permethrine 887
peroneal spastic flat foot syndrome 746–7
peroneal tendon
entrapment 1706
local steroid injection 1769
peroneus brevis 154, 156
peroneus longus 154, 156
peroneus tertius 154
personality change, drug-related 578
pes anserine bursa 152, 153, 158
pes anserinus 158
pes anserinus tendinitis 158, 1509
pes cavus 1512
rheumatic 1747, 1748
pes planus see foot, flat
pes valgoplanus 1747, 1748
PET, neuropsychiatric SLE 221, 335, 1186
Pfeiffer syndrome 368, 369, 398
PG-I 427, 429
PG-II 427, 429
Pgp-1 534, 537
phagocytosis 513, 545
phalanges (feet) 154
subluxation 725
'whittling' 1077
phalanges (hands) 138
subluxation 725
'whittling' 1077
Phalen's sign 226
phantom bone disease 1636
pharyngitis
in adult-onset Still's disease 1127
in SLE 1156–7
streptococcal and rheumatic fever 973
phenacetin, adverse effects 323, 1695
phencyclidine, adverse effects 1265
phenelzine 340
phenobarbitone 1604
phenothiazine 341
phentolamine
in mixed connective tissue disease 1423
in reflex sympathetic dystrophy 1685
3-(phenylamino)alanine 1427
phenylbutazone
adverse effects
cutaneous 212, 213
haematological 295, 1695
myopathic 1265
in ankylosing spondylitis 1069
binding to plasma proteins 576
drug interactions 579
half-life 577
in HIV-associated arthritis 921
in lactation 193
in pregnancy 190
phenylketonuria 207
phenylpropanolamine 1778
phenytoin 1604
adverse effects
hypogammaglobulinaemia 970
lupus-like syndrome 1690
myositis 1693
drug interactions
ketoconazole 957
NSAIDs 579
Phialophora
P. boydii 963

Phialophora (continued)
P. parasitica 963
phlebocavography 764
phlebolites 288
pholcodeine 241
phosphate
assay 652
depletion 1604
imprecision in measurement 648
in osteomalacia 1601, 1604–6
renal loss 1605
in rickets 1600, 1604, 1605
phosphocreatine 1774
phosphoethanolamine in hypophosphatasia 436
phosphofructokinase deficiency 216, 473, 1774
phospholipase A₂ 515
in juvenile chronic arthritis 1121
phosphoramide mustard 591, 592
phosphoribosylpyrophosphate 1556, 1557
phosphoribosylpyrophosphate synthetase 1557
superactivity 1557, 1558
phosphorus
excretion in thyrotoxicosis 279
homeostasis 429–31
photoallergic reactions, NSAID-induced 212
photochemotherapy in psoriatic arthritis 1081
photon absorptiometry, bone density 720
photo-onycholysis, NSAID-induced 212
photopheresis in scleroderma 1240, 1241
photosensitivity 174, 200, 201, 204
in dermatomyositis 1251, 1289
drug-related 214, 578
in the elderly 35
in neonatal lupus erythematosus 1198–9
in SLE 837, 1148, 1182–3
phototherapy in HIV-associated arthritis 921
phthisis bulbi in juvenile chronic arthritis 1103
phycomycetes 252
physiotherapist in multi-disciplinary team 1737
physiotherapy
cervical pain syndromes 1658
chronic back pain 1648
frozen shoulder 144
juvenile chronic arthritis 1107, 1141–2, **1737–50**
juvenile dermatomyositis 1750–1
low back pain 101
parental involvement 1751–2
principles 1738
psoriatic arthritis 1081
sacroiliitis 21, 1749–50
scleroderma in childhood 1751
phytonadione 1693
'piano-key' sign 43, 1014
picornaviruses
in models of myositis 1273
in polymyositis/dermatomyositis 1266–7, 1288–9
Pierre Robin anomaly 376
pigment-induced nephropathy 327
pigmentation, increased 175
pigmented villonodular synovitis 1619–20, 1671
aetiological factors 1619
clinical features 1619–20
diagnosis 1620
differential diagnosis 166, 1104
imaging 288, 741–2, 743, 1620
pathology 1619
treatment 1620

pillows in cervical pain syndromes 1658
pilocarpine hydrochloride 1314
pinch strength meter 477
pinna, inflammation 174
piperacillin in osteomyelitis 874
piperidine 694
piriformis 150
piriformis syndrome 1508
piroxicam
adverse effects
cutaneous 212, 213, 580
gastrointestinal 1021
haematological 295
half-life 577
in juvenile chronic arthritis 1106, 1140
in lactation 193, 194
in pregnancy 189, 190
in psoriatic arthritis 1080
in seropositive juvenile chronic arthritis 1035
pirprofen, half-life 577
pituitary gland disorders 282
pityriasis lichenoides 1371–2
PiZ gene 1010
placebo effect in back pain 92
placenta
in antiphospholipid syndrome 1206
immunomodulatory role 182
infarction 183, 294
plant oil supplements 262, 264, 265, 1480, 1484
plantar digital neuritis 1512
plantar fascia 153
palpation of insertion 50
plantar fasciitis 51, 160, 168, 1511
local steroid injection 1770
in psoriatic arthritis 1076
plantar response 218
plantar spur 160, 745, 746
management 1770
in psoriatc arthritis 1075, 1076
plantar tarsometatarsal ligament 153
plaques 201, 206–7, 1457
plasma cells in synovial inflammation 443
plasma viscosity
in acute phase response 625, 626, 639, 639
in ankylosing spondylitis 628
in osteoarthritis 627
in rheumatoid arthritis 628–9, 640
plasmapheresis (plasma exchange) 614
in amyloidosis 1441
in antiphospholipid syndrome 1211
in Eaton–Lambert syndrome 1675
in Felty's syndrome 292
in microscopic polyangiitis 1359
in polyarteritis nodosa 1359, 1404
in polymyositis/dermatomyositis 1277
in prevention of neonatal lupus erythematosus 1199
in scleroderma 1240, 1241
in SLE 1174, 1191
in pregnancy 183
in thrombotic thrombocytopenic purpura 329
in urticarial vasculitis 1370
in Wegener's granulomatosis 1347
plasmids 354
plasminogen, function in inflammation 624
plasminogen activator 448
effect of corticosteroids on 586
Plasmodium 946, 947
P. chabaudi 1175
plastic surgery in scleroderma 211
platelet-activating factor 448, 536
platelet count
in anaemia of chronic disease 637
childhood 17
Kawasaki disease 17
preoperative 300

platelet-derived growth factor (PDGF)
and angiogenesis 509
in Dupuytren's contracture 148
effect on chondrocytes 1543
in hypertrophic osteoarthropathy 1673
in rheumatoid arthritis 993
platelet-endothelial cell adhesion molecule-1 (PECAM-1) 534
in arthritis 537
in lymphocyte transmigration 536
platelets
abnormalities 292–3, 644–5
in SLE 641–2, 641, 1193
effect of NSAIDs on function 580
platybasia 223
in Paget's disease 1612
pleistophora 947
pleural disease 173, 176, 242
pleural effusion 235, 242
in Behçet's syndrome 1398
in SLE 1151–2
pleurisy
in rheumatoid arthritis 990
in seropositive juvenile chronic arthritis 1034
in SLE 1151
pleuritis
in familial Mediterranean fever 1446
in immune complex diseases 703
in juvenile chronic arthritis 1116
in rheumatoid arthritis 1010
in SLE 1195
plica syndrome 158–9, 166
plicamycin in Paget's disease 1611, 1615
pneumatosis intestinalis in mixed connective tissue disease 1418
Pneumococcus
arteritis due to 1390
pulmonary infection 252
in pyogenic arthritis 852, 853
pneumoconiosis 243
Pneumocystis carinii infection
in methotrexate therapy 585
pulmonary 251, 253
pneumomediastinum in dermatomyositis 1254
pneumonia 241, 252
acute lupus 242
rheumatic 979
in rheumatoid arthritis 251
in toxic oil syndrome 1425
pneumonitis
acute in SLE 1195
drug-related 241, 253, 254, 584, 585, 601, 1254
interstitial in SLE 1152, 1195
pneumoperitoneum in mixed connective tissue disease 1418
pneumothorax 243, 245
podophyllatoxin 1026
POEMS syndrome 286, 289
Pogosta disease 904
POHLC 69
poikilocytosis in anaemia of chronic disease 636
poikiloderma 201, 204, 207
in dermatomyositis 207, 1250–1, 1263
pol gene 908
polyarteritis nodosa 1351–62
age at onset 12, 13, 1353
angiography 1356
association with hepatitis B viraemia 900
autoantibodies 668
antiendothelial cell antibodies 1356
antineutrophil cytoplasmic autoantibodies 328, 1353, 1355–6, 1403
cardiovascular involvement 230, 231, 233
central nervous system disease in 222
childhood **1402–4**
diagnosis 21
ocular involvement 316
sex differences 14, 1403

polyarteritis nodosa (continued)
  'classical' 1323
  classification 1321, 1321, 1322, 1351
  clinical presentation 1353, 1354
  comparison with microscopic poly-
    angiitis 1352–3
  definition 1352
  diagnosis 1355–8
  diagnostic criteria 1323–4, 1323
  differential diagnosis 1136, 1137
  eosinophilia 644
  and ethnic group 1353
  and familial Mediterranean fever 1447
  gastrointestinal involvement 257, 258,
    1353
  and hepatitis B 331, 1353
  and hydatid cyst 951
  hypertension in 330–1
  immunology 1355–6
  laboratory tests 1403
  localized 1321, 1353
  microscopic see microscopic polyangiitis
  monitoring disease activity 1360–1
  muscle in 472, 791
  neutrophilia 643
  ocular involvement 313
  pathology 1357
  peripheral neuropathies 227
  and pregnancy 185
  prognosis 1329, 1358, 1361–2, 1403–4
  psychiatric involvement 333, 335–6
  pulmonary involvement 245, 247
  relapse 1361, 1362
  renal involvement 321, 651, 1353
    childhood 1403
    ischaemic glomerular damage 324
    proteinuria 323
    rapidly progressive glomerulone-
      phritis 327, 328, 328
  sex ratio in 14, 1353
  skin involvement 208
  systemic features 178
  and thrombotic thrombocytopenic
    purpura 329
  treatment 586, 1358–9, 1362–3, 1403–4
  vasculitis 786, 787
polyarthritis 983
  in adolescence 56
  carcinomatous 289, 1673–4
  epidemic 903–4
  in hyperlipidaemias 1481
  in mixed connective tissue disease 1417
  palmar fasciitis–polyarthritis syndrome
    289
  in psoriatic arthritis 1073–5
  in pyoderma gangrenosum 1460
  related to infectious agent 1136
  in rheumatic fever 977
  in sarcoidosis 1466
  in SLE 1181
  in systemic sclerosis 1238
  in undifferentiated connective tissue
    disease 1413
  in Whipple's disease 1095
polyclonal antibodies in immunoassays 660
polycystic kidney disease, hyperuricaemia in 1558
polycythaemia
  drug-related 296
  in sarcoidosis 1465
polyethylene glycol precipitation,
  immune complexes 705
polyglandular autoimmune
  syndromes 285–6
polymerase chain reaction (PCR) 350,
  354, 548, 660–1, 690, 993
  allele-specific 691, 692
  amplification of microsatellites 695
  in DNA sequencing 694
  in HLA typing 697
  in Lyme disease 889–90
  in M. tuberculosis identification 929–30
  typing techniques based on 691–3

polymethylmethacrylate beads,
  gentamicin-impregnated 875
polymorphic light eruption 204
polymyalgia rheumatica 1373–80
  acute phase response in 627–8, 629,
    640, 1378
  age at onset 26, 1377
  and autoimmune thyroid disease 279
  in calcium pyrophosphate dihydrate
    disease 1529
  clinical features 170, 178, 1377–8
  definition 1373
  diagnostic criteria 1373
  differential diagnosis 1378–9, 1379
  in the elderly 34
  epidemiology 1375–6
    clustering 818
    geographical factors 820
  erythrocyte sedimentation rate 627–8,
    640, 1378
  fever 172, 1377
  genetic factors 1375
  laboratory tests 649, 1378
  liver function 652, 1378
  and malignant disease 289, 1377–8,
    1670
  muscle biopsy 791
  myalgia in 653
  pathogenesis 1376–7
  psychiatric involvement 333, 1377
  relationship with giant cell arteritis
    1374–5
  renal function 650
  temporal artery biopsy 1376–7, 1376
  treatment 34, 586, 1379–80, 1380
polymyositis 219, 1249–80
  aetiology 1266–8
  age at onset 11, 26, 1288
  animal models 1272–3
  autoantibodies 668, 673, 1258, 1259,
    1270–2, 1271, 1272
  cardiovascular involvement 230, 1253,
    1254–5, 1290
  childhood 1287–97
    clinical presentation 1289–91
    diagnostic criteria 1288
    epidemiology 1288
  classification 1249–50, 1250
  clinical features 1250–6, 1414
  creatine kinase in 653
  diagnosis 1258, 1260–3, 1260
  differential diagnosis 1136, 1137, 1263–
    6, 1264, 1265
    distinction from dermatomyositis 1269
  drug-related 598, 1022
  electrodiagnosis 806
  epidemiology 1249
  gastrointestinal involvement 258, 1253,
    1255, 1277, 1290
  genitourinary involvement 1290
  geographic factors 1249
  granuloma in 789
  imaging 1260–1
  immunogenetics 1268
  incidence 1249
  laboratory tests 649, 1256–8, 1257
  liver function 652
  and malignant disease 289, 1255–6,
    1267, 1668–9
  muscle involvement 471
    biopsy 788, 789, 790, 1261–2, 1263,
      1290
    in childhood 1289–90
    contracture 217
    inflammation 789
    myasthenia 216
    necrosis 789, 790
    vacuoles 791
    weakness 470, 1250, 1289–90
  myoglobinuria in 323, 327
  ocular involvement 1290–1
  overlap syndromes 1256, 1423–4
  pathogenesis 1268–72, 1269, 1271, 1272
  and pregnancy 1256

polymyositis (continued)
  prevalence 1249
  prognosis 1278
  in protozoal infection 947
  pulmonary involvement 241, 243,
    1252–4, 1253, 1290
  reflexes 218
  rehabilitation 1278
  renal involvement 1256
  risk factors 1249
  and scleroderma 1424–5
  systemic features 1252
  temporal factors 1249
  treatment 1273–8, 1274
  type V 1425
polyols in syndrome of limited joint
  mobility 282
polyostotic fibrous dysplasia 434
polyradiculitis 803
polysaccharides, reaction with free
  radicals 447
polyvinyl chloride and mixed connective tissue disease 1419
Pompe's disease 473, 1774
Poncet's disease 929
Pond–Nuki model 415–16, 415
pons 223
Popeye sign 44, 143
popliteal artery
  aneurysm 1398
  entrapment 1786
popliteal cyst see Baker's cyst
popliteal fossa cyst 49
popliteus tendinitis 1509
population attributable risk 824
porphyria cutanea tarda
  blisters 205
  hypertrichosis 209
  scleroderma-like changes 207
Porphyromonas in osteomyelitis 870
portal hypertension 258
positron emission tomography,
  neuropsychiatric SLE 221, 335,
  1186
postcalcaneal bursitis 1511
posterior cruciate ligament 151, 152
  avulsion 744
  imaging 743–4
  in rheumatoid arthritis 1014
  stability testing 49
posterior drawer sign 144
posterior interosseous nerve entrapment 227, 806
posterior longitudinal ligament, ossification 735, 737, 1637
posterior synechiae in juvenile chronic
  arthritis 1103
posterior talofibular ligament 153
posterior tibial artery 153, 156
posterior tibial nerve 153, 156, 160
  entrapment neuropathy see tarsal tunnel
    syndrome
  in leprosy 934
posterior tibial tendon, local steroid
  injection 1769
posterior tibiotalar ligament 153
postinfectious syndromes, differential
  diagnosis 1122–3
postsynaptic receptor 495
posture 41
  exercises in ankylosing spondylitis 1069
  neck 45
  training supports in low back pain 104
potassium, imprecision in measurement 648
potassium citrate in gout 1566
potassium iodide
  in erythema nodosum 1455
  in nodular vasculitis 1371
PR3 328, 1328, 1342–3, 1356
PR3-ANCA see antineutrophil cytoplasmic autoantibodies, c-ANCA/
  PR3-ANCA
prayer nodules 208

'prayer position' 42, 43
prayer sign 282
praziquantel 951
prazosin in mixed connective tissue
  disease 1423
prealbumin 624, 1433, 1434, 1438, 1439
preanaesthetic assessment, relevance
  of systemic factors in rheumatic
  disease 299–301
prednisolone 585
  in Behçet's syndrome 1401
  in combination therapy 1025
  effect on growth 85
  in giant cell arteritis 312
  in lactation 194
  in leprosy 935, 936
  in microscopic polyangiitis 1358–9,
    1362–3
  in multicentric reticulohistiocytosis
    1476, 1477
  non-selective action 610
  osteoporosis induced by 1588, 1591,
    1696
  in polyarteritis nodosa 1358–9, 1362–3
  in polymyalgia rheumatica 1379
  in pyoderma gangrenosum 210
  in reflex sympathetic dystrophy 1687
  in relapsing polychondritis 1627
  in Sjögren's syndrome 1314
  in SLE 1173
    neuropsychiatric 221
  in Takayasu's arteritis 1387
  in thrombocytopenia 641–2
prednisolone acetate injection 1757
prednisone 585
  in adult-onset Still's disease 1127
  adverse effects
    insomnia 342
    psychiatric 337
  and antiphospholipid antibodies in
    pregnancy 295
  in autoimmune haemolytic anaemia
    291–2
  in combination therapy 1025
  in DILS 913
  in HIV-associated nephropathy 915
  in inclusion-body myositis 1280
  in lactation 194
  in polymyalgia rheumatica 34
  in polymyositis/dermatomyositis
    1273–5, 1274
  in pregnancy 191
  response to 34
  in rheumatoid arthritis 34
  in RS₃PE syndrome 35
  in SLE
    childhood 1182
    in the elderly 36
    neuropsychiatric 335
    in pregnancy 183
  in thrombocytopenia 292
pre-eclampsia
  in antiphospholipid syndrome 1206
  and carpal tunnel syndrome 185
  and gout 184
  and rheumatoid arthritis 181
  and SLE 183
Preferid 210
pregnancy 181–5
  acute phase proteins 627
  alkaline phosphatase in 651
  and ankylosing spondylitis 184
  carpal tunnel syndrome 185
  colchicine in 185, 193, 1449
  and dermatomyositis 185, 1256
  drug therapy in 188–93, 602, 603
  erythema nodosum in 1451
  and gonococcal arthritis 184
  and gout 184–5
  immunoregulatory and anti-inflamma-
    tory circulating factors 181, 182
  and juvenile rheumatoid arthritis 184
  and low back pain 93
  lupus anticoagulant in 183, 294

pregnancy *(continued)*
and Lyme disease 892
and multicentric reticulohistiocytosis
185
musculoskeletal disorders 185
and polyarteritis nodosa 185
and polymyositis 1256
and psoriatic arthritis 184
and reflex sympathetic dystrophy 1681
and relapsing polychondritis 185
and rheumatoid arthritis 181–2, *182*,
1012, *1012*
and seropositive juvenile chronic
arthritis 1036
and Sjögren's syndrome 185
and SLE 182–4, 189, 1157, 1159
and Still's disease 184
and systemic sclerosis 184, 1238–40
and Takayasu's arteritis 1388
transient osteoporosis 185, 749
and Wegener's granulomatosis 185
pregnancy-associated α-glycoprotein
182
Preiser's disease 1623
preleukaemia
and pyoderma gangrenosum 1460
and Sweet's syndrome 1458
preosteoblast 426
preosteoclast 426
prepatellar bursa
in acromegaly 281
bursitis 155, 157–8, 167, 1509, 1769
septic 858
α-preprotachykinin 450
**pressure erosions in rheumatoid
arthritis** 725
presynaptic nerve endings *495*
pretibial tenderness 1291
prevalence 813, *813*
assessment 813–14, *814*
cumulative 813, *813*
point 813, *813*
Prevotella in osteomyelitis 870
primaquine, adverse effects 295–6
pristane arthritis 567
probenecid
adverse effects 1694
drug interactions 296, *579*
in gout 1565
in lactation 193, 194
in Lyme disease 892
in pregnancy 193
procainamide
adverse effects
lupus-like syndrome 36, 669, 1690,
1690, *1691*
myositis 1693
autoantibody induction 1692
effect on lymphocyte function 1692
and mixed connective tissue disease
1419
procalcitonin in amyloidosis *1434*, 1435
procollagen peptidase deficiency 355
**procollagen propeptides in osteo-
porosis** 1595
**procollagen type II as marker of
osteoarthritis** 417–18
progesterone
effect on experimental arthritis 182
immunosuppressive properties 1157
progressive osseous heterotopia 1291
prolactin 282
immunological effects 1157
in rheumatoid arthritis 510
proline in collagen 407
pronator quadratus 137
displacement 716, 718
pronator teres 137, 145
Propaderm *210*
properdin factor B 548
Propionibacterium acnes 269
and Kawasaki disease 1405
in pyogenic arthritis 853
propionic acid gel 1314

propofol *307*
local infiltration 305
propoxyphene, use by the elderly 32
proptosis *174*, 313, 314, 1336
propylthiouracil
adverse effects *1265*, *1690*, 1693
and Wegener's granulomatosis 1342
prostacyclin *see* prostaglandins, PGI₂
**prostaglandin analogues in gastric
ulceration** 578
prostaglandins
effect of corticosteroids on *586*
effect of NSAIDs on 259, 576, 578, 580
effect on osteoclasts 423, 424, *425*
in inflammation 508, 515–16
in neoplastic hypercalcaemia *437*
PGE₁
anti-inflammatory effects 1480
effect on C fibres 450
intravenous in digital ulceration 212
PGE₂
in Dupuytren's contracture 148
in inflammation 515, 516
inhibition by NSAIDs 569
inhibition of leucocytes 516
interaction with bradykinin 492
joint afferent sensitivity to 492
in neuropsychiatric SLE 334
PGF₂ in Dupuytren's contracture 148
PGI₂
in Behçet's syndrome 1399
in blood flow regulation 512
in digital ulceration 212
in inflammation 515, 516, 1480
interaction with bradykinin 492
joint afferent sensitivity to 492
in mixed connective tissue disease
1422, 1423
in polyarteritis nodosa 1404, 1405
in systemic sclerosis 1238
in psoriatic arthritis 1079
in rheumatoid arthritis 997
prostanoids 1480
prostate-specific antigen 653
prostatic carcinoma 653
prostatitis
investigation 662–3
in reactive arthropathies 1088
protease nexin 1 444
protein
control of secretion rate 349
effect of free radicals on 447
quantification of urinary excretion 322
synovial fluid 443, 679
total 651
protein AA 1433, *1434*, *1435*, 1438
protein AL 1433, *1434*
protein AP 1433, 1436, 1441
protein C deficiency 1208
**protein–energy malnutrition, in juve-
nile chronic arthritis** 87
protein-losing enteropathy
in mixed connective tissue disease 1418
in SLE *258*
protein radioimmunoprecipitation
669, 670
protein S deficiency 1208
protein suicide effect 361, 373
proteinase 3 328, 1328, 1342–3, 1356
α₁-proteinase inhibitor *see* α₁-antitrypsin
proteinuria 321–3, *330*, 331
and acute renal failure 327
in cryoglobulinaemia 323
definitions 321–2
diagnostic studies 322
differential diagnosis in systemic rheumatic disease 322–3
drug-related 322–3, 327, *598*, 599
gold therapy *601*
functional 321
and glomerular function 650
in glomerulonephritis 324
in gout 651

proteinuria *(continued)*
with haematuria 323
heavy 322
in Henoch–Schönlein purpura 323,
1407
in HIV infection 915
in hypersensitivity vasculitis 1368
in juvenile chronic arthritis 1118, 1120
in lupus nephritis 321
in Lyme disease 888
in methotrexate therapy *584*
in microscopic polyangiitis 1354
monitoring 321–2
nephrotic-range 321, 324
non-nephrotic range 321, 324
in polyarteritis nodosa 323, 1403
in rapidly progressive glomerulonephritis 327
renal biopsy in 324–5
in sarcoidosis 1465
in scleroderma 322
in SLE 321, 322, 323, 1153
in systemic sclerosis 321
in vasculitis 1358
in Wegener's granulomatosis 323
proteoglycan arthritis 564
proteoglycans 353, 415, 421
in amyloid deposits 1433
as arthritogens 564
in articular cartilage 406–7, 409–11
in animal models of joint disease 415,
416
effect of age on 414
effect of cytokines on 414
effect of growth factors on 414–15
bone 427, *429*
in osteoarthritis 417, 1537, 1542–3,
1544–5
PG-I 427, *429*
PG-II 427, *429*
in rheumatoid arthritis *1017*
proteosome 549, 696
Proteus mirabilis
in pyogenic arthritis 852
in rheumatoid arthritis *268*, 986
prothrombin
deficiency in SLE 1194
function in inflammation *624*
as lupus anticoagulant cofactor 1209
synovial fluid 681
protozoal infections 946–7, *946*
protriptyline 339, *340*, *342*
protrusio acetabuli 725
in juvenile chronic arthritis 1033, 1117,
1134
in Paget's disease 1612
**protrusio bulbi in Wegener's granulo-
matosis** 1335, 1336
proximal interphalangeal joints 138,
140
in hypothyroidism 278
local steroid injection 1767
in psoriatic arthritis 1073, 1074
in rheumatoid arthritis 1008
proximal radio-ulnar joint 136, 137
proximal tubule, function tests 650
Prozac 339, *340*, *341*, *342*
PRPP 1557
pruritus 207
drug-related 213, *591*, *598*
in morphoea 1228
in multicentric reticulohistiocytosis
1475
in Sjögren's syndrome 1310
in systemic sclerosis 211–12
PSA 653
pseudarthrosis and osteomyelitis 869
pseudoachondrodysplasia 413
pseudoachondroplasia 353, *369*, 377,
1630
Pseudoallescheria boydii 956
pseudoangina 1653
**pseudoarthrosis, intimal cell genera-
tion** 441

pseudocysts 1541
pseudofracture 1601
pseudogout 654, 684, 1527, *1527*, 1567
clinical features 1567, *1568*
diagnosis 1568–9
differential diagnosis 1569
epidemiology 1567
and hyperparathyroidism 280
in hypothyroidism 277
laboratory tests 1568
pathogenesis 1569–70
prognosis 1570
treatment 1570
triggering factors 1527
see also calcium pyrophosphate dihydrate
disease
pseudohaematoid *1527*
pseudo-Hurler polydystrophy 1634
pseudohyperparathyroidism 437
pseudohypoparathyroidism 281, 434
pseudo-Lyme disease 336
**pseudolymphoma in Sjögren's
syndrome** 1310, 1312, 1667
Pseudomonas
arteritis due to 1390
P. aeruginosa
antibiotic therapy 660, *856*
in HIV infection 916
in osteomyelitis 868, 870, *870*
pulmonary infection 252
in pyogenic arthritis 852, 862, *880*
pseudomyotonia in hypothyroidism
278
pseudoneuropathic syndrome *1527*
pseudo-osteoarthritis *1527*
pseudopodagra 1527
hydroxyapatite 1573
pseudoporphyria 205, 206, 1106
pseudopseudohypoparathyroidism
281
'pseudoseptic' arthritis 853
pseudotetany 278
pseudothrombophlebitis 153, 158
pseudotumour cerebri 1185
pseudovalgus deformity 1745, 1746
pseudoxanthoma elasticum 207, 353,
1613
PSGL-1 530
psoas 150
abscess 48, 717, 1094
irritation 115
psoriasis
association with arthritis 1071–2, *1072*
erythrodermic 205, 212
erythrodermic generalized 1076
genetic factors 1078
'geographical tongue' in 207
guttate 204, *208*, 212
hands and feet 41, 201, 202, 203
head and neck *174*
hyperuricaemia in 1558
inverse 1076
nails 41, 202, 203
plaque 206
in psoriatic arthritis 1076
pustular 205, 212, 1076, 1078, 1087
scalp 200
treatment 212, 1079
Von Zambush 1076
psoriasis vulgaris 1076
psoriatic arthritis *208*, 1040, **1071–82**
acute phase response in 628
clinical features 1071–5, *1073*, *1074*
comparison with rheumatoid arthritis
1074
course 1081–2
diagnosis 1038, 1076–7
dietary modification in 1080
differential diagnosis *1104*
environmental factors 1078–9
epidemiology *814*, 1071, *1072*
extra-articular features 1075
genetic factors 698, 1077
in HIV infection 901, 918–21, 1079

psoriatic arthritis *(continued)*
  and hyperlipidaemias 1484
  hyperuricaemia in 654
  imaging 1074, 1075, 1077, 1078, 1534
  immunological mechanisms 1077–8
  juvenile 1055
    age at onset 12, 13
    clinical characteristics 1055–6
    diagnosis 18
    diagnostic criteria 10–11, *11*, *1055*
    ocular involvement 316
    prevalence 1055
    sex differences 14
  laboratory tests *649*, 1076
  management 1082–3, *1082*
  pathogenesis 1077–9
  and pregnancy 184
  prevalence in patients with psoriasis
      1071–2, *1072*
  prognosis 1081–2
  psoriasis in 1076
  rheumatoid factor in 1071, 1072, *1074*,
      1077
  spondylarthropathy in 1073
  surgery in 1081
  synovial biopsy in 778
  treatment 1079–81
  see also seronegative spondylarthropa-
      thies
psychiatric disorders
  in Behçet's syndrome 1397
  drug-related 337, **337–8**, *587*
  examination *333*
  primary **332–6**, *333*
  and reflex sympathetic dystrophy
      1681–2
  secondary 336, **336–7**
  treatment 338–42, *340*, *341*, *342*
  see also systemic lupus erythematosus,
      neuropsychiatric
psychogenic rheumatism 1489
psychological factors
  in back pain 106–7
  in fibromyalgia 1498
  in rheumatic disease **63–70**, 1725
**psychologist in multi-disciplinary
    team** 1737
psychoneuroimmunology and stress
    332
psychoses
  drug-related *587*
  in SLE 1153, 1186
PTHrP *see* parathyroid hormone-related
    peptide
ptosis
  in giant cell arteritis 1378
  in SLE 1153
pubertal development, assessment
    81, *81*, *82*
pubic hair 14, *17*
pubis 150
pubofemoral ligament 150
**Puerto Rico, prevalence of rheumatoid
    arthritis** *834*
**pulmonary arteritis in seropositive
    juvenile chronic arthritis** 1034
pulmonary artery
  aneurysm 251, 1398, 1401
  in Takayasu's arteritis 1385
**pulmonary embolism and hormone
    replacement therapy** 1596, 1597
pulmonary fibrosis 173, *176*
  and anaesthesia 299, 303
  in ankylosing spondylitis 1064
  carcinoma arising in 1667, 1669
  in polymyositis/dermatomyositis 1254,
      1277, 1290
  in rheumatoid arthritis 990, 994
  in seropositive juvenile chronic
      arthritis 1034
  in systemic sclerosis *1234*, 1235
pulmonary function tests 246–9, *250*
  preanaesthetic 300
  in SLE 1152

pulmonary haemorrhage 243
  in microscopic polyangiitis 1354, 1355
  in SLE 1152, 1195
pulmonary hypertension *176*
  and antiphospholipid antibodies 293
  in eosinophilia–myalgia syndrome 1426
  in juvenile chronic arthritis 1116
  in mixed connective tissue disease
      1418–19, *1419*
  in SLE 1195–6
  in systemic sclerosis *1234*, 1235
  in toxic oil syndrome 1426
**pulmonary involvement in rheumatic
    disease** 173, *176*, **240–54**, 1010
  Behçet's syndrome *241*, 243, 251, 1398
  Churg–Strauss syndrome 173
  dermatomyositis *241*, 243, 1252–4,
      1253, 1290
  eosinophilia–myalgia syndrome 1426
  microscopic polyangiitis 1354, 1355
  mixed connective tissue disease
      1418–19, *1418*
  polyarteritis nodosa 245, 247
  polymyositis *241*, 243, 1252–4, *1253*,
      1290
  relapsing polychondritis *241*, 242
  rheumatoid arthritis 173, *241*, *241*, 242,
      243, 245, 1010
  sarcoidosis 242, 245, 1465
  Sjögren's syndrome 173, *241*, *241*, 243,
      245, 1310
  SLE 173, *241*, *241*, 242, 243, 245, *1150*,
      1151–2
    childhood 1195–6, *1195*, *1196*
  systemic sclerosis 241, *241*, 245, 250,
      1234, 1235–7
  toxic oil syndrome 1426
  Wegener's granulomatosis 173, 243,
      244, 1336, 1337–8, 1406
pulmonary oedema, drug-related 253
pulmonary opacities on chest X-ray
    173, *176*
pulmonary–renal syndrome
  drug-related *253*
  in microscopic polyangiitis 1352
  in Wegener's granulomatosis 1338
pulmonary thromboembolism
  in antiphospholipid syndrome 1204
  in SLE 1152
**pulmonary thromboendarterectomy
    in antiphospholipid syndrome**
    1212
pulsus paradoxicus 235
pump bumps 168
pure red-cell aplasia 291, 295, 297
purine metabolism 1556–7
purpura *175*, *201*, 207
  in amyloidosis 1436, 1437
  'dry' 292
  gold therapy-induced 213, *601*
  hypergammaglobulinaemic 1370
  immune thrombocytopenic 292–3
  NSAID-induced 213
  palpable *208*, 1011
    in Henoch–Schönlein purpura 1369,
        1407
    in hypersensitivity vasculitis 1368
    in Sjögren's syndrome 1311
    in Wegener's granulomatosis 1338–9
  'wet' 292
pus 658–9
pustules *201*, 205–6
  in ulcerative colitis 1458, 1459
PUVA
  adverse effects *1690*
  in psoriasis 212, 1079
  in psoriatic arthritis 1081
pyoderma gangrenosum *175*, 206, 207,
    1458–62
  aetiology 1460
  atypical/bullous 1459, 1460
  diagnostic evaluation 1461, *1461*
  diseases associated *1460*
  in enteric arthropathies 1094

pyoderma gangrenosum *(continued)*
  histopathology 1460
  pathergy reaction in 1396
  peristomal 1458, 1459
  in psoriatic arthritis 1076
  in Takayasu's arteritis 1385
  treatment 210–11
  vulvar 1459
  in Wegener's granulomatosis 1339
pyogenic arthritis 879–80
  acute phase response in 640
  acute spontaneous 661
  in adults **849–59**
  aetiology *880*
  age at onset 12, 13
  age-related occurrence *26*
  childhood 14, **861–6**
  as contraindication to local steroid
      injection 1758
  co-occurrence with crystal arthritis 684
  differential diagnosis *1104*
  erythema in 205
  following penetrating joint injury *864*,
      865
  gonococcal *850*, 854–5
  in haemophilia 864–5
  hip 741, 743, 858, 863
  in HIV infection 916–17
  in hypogammaglobulinaemia 969
  management 856–8
  meningococcal 855–6
  neisserial 854–5
  neonatal 864, *864*
  non-gonococcal 850–3
  pathophysiology 849–50
  prognosis 880
  prosthetic joint infections 853–4
  and rheumatoid arthritis 853, 865, 1013
  in sickle-cell disease 865
  systemic features *170*
pyomyositis
  bacterial 1265
  in HIV infection 916–17
pyostomatitis vegetans 1459
pyrazinamide
  and hyperuricaemia *1558*, 1694
  in mycobacterial infection 253
  in tuberculosis 931, *932*, 933
pyrexia *see* fever
pyridinoline cross-links 432, 653
  in osteoarthritis 417–18, 1538, *1538*
  in osteoporosis 1595
  in Paget's disease 1613
pyridium cross-links 432
pyridoxine deficiency 262
pyrophosphatase 429
pyrophosphate
  in calcium pyrophosphate deposition
      disease 684, 1570
  deposition *649*
  metabolism 1570
  in osteoarthritis 682, 683
  structure 1615
  synovial fluid 654
pyrophosphate arthropathy *see* calcium
    pyrophosphate dihydrate disease
**pyruvate kinase in differential diag-
    nosis of neuromuscular disorders**
    1291

Q

quadratus femoris 150
quadriceps 152
  in juvenile chronic arthritis 1101, 1717
  in rheumatoid arthritis 1009
  wasting 49
quadriparesis in cervical myelopathy
    224
quadriplegia, spastic 178
quality of life 51, 64, 1724
  conceptual framework 52
  and disability 65
  and family relationships 66

quality of life *(continued)*
  and fatigue 64–5
  health-related 52
  impact of psychological variables on
      67–9
  intervention studies 69–70
  measurement *see* health status, measures
  and pain 64
  and psychological well being 67
  and social relationships 66–7
  and social well being 66–7
  and stiffness 64
  and symptoms 64–5
Quality of Well Being Index 53, *54*
quantitative dual energy radiography
  see dual-energy/electron X-ray
      absorptiometry
Quebec Back Pain Disability Scale
    59
quinidine, adverse effects 669, *1690*
quinolines, in pregnancy 191–2
quinolones
  in osteomyelitis 874, 875
  rheumatological effects 1695
  in tuberculosis 931
QWB 53, *54*

R

R.A. cells 681
rachitic rosary 1601
radial collateral ligament 137, 138,
    140
radial nerve
  biopsy 793
  entrapment
    electrodiagnosis 805
    in rheumatoid arthritis 1013
  iatrogenic damage 803
  in leprosy 934, 935
  palsy *803*
radial tunnel syndrome 1505
radicular pain 225
radiculography
  arachnoiditis 1645, 1646
  intervertebral disc prolapse 125, 1642
  low back pain 730–1
  see also CT radiculography
radiculoneuropathy in Lyme disease
    888
radiculopathy
  cervical 1656, *1656*
    treatment 1658–60
  lumbar 106, 157
radiocarpal joint *see* wrist
radiocarpal ligaments 137
radiocolloid, intra-articular 1547
**radio-frequency ablation, osteoid
    osteoma** 1618
radiogrammetry *1595*
radiography 715–19
  acromegaly 281, 282
  ankle 718–19
  ankylosing spondylitis 733–4, 735, 736,
      1058–9, 1065–6
  in assessment of skeletal maturation
      77–8
  back pain 97, 115, 730
  Blount's disease 166
  Brodie's abscess 1621
  brucellar arthritis 938, 939, 940
  calcium pyrophosphate dihydrate
      disease 1528, 1529, 1568, 1569
  cervical spondylosis 1654
  chest
    childhood 759
    preanaesthetic 299
  childhood 751–60, *754*, *755–7*, 761–2,
      767
    discitis 123, 124
    pyogenic arthritis 862
  chordoma 716
  CINCA 1472
  diabetic neuropathy 284

radiography (continued)
in differentiation of osteoarthritis from
rheumatoid arthritis in the elderly
33
digital 753
discitis of childhood 123, 124
elbow 715, 716
erosive arthritis 1534
Ewing's sarcoma 120
foot 719
gout 1560, 1562, 1563
hip 716–17, 718
interpretation and reliability 8
intervertebral disc prolapse 1641
juvenile ankylosing spondylitis 1053
juvenile chronic arthritis 755, 1032–5,
1101, 1117, 1121, *1121*
knee 717–18, 744
leprosy 935
leukaemia 1672
microfocal 1536
Milwaukee shoulder syndrome 1572,
1573
non-gonococcal arthritis 851
Osgood–Schlatter disease 166
osteoarthritis 747, 1533–6
osteochondritis dissecans 166
osteogenesis imperfecta 358
osteomalacia 1601
osteomyelitis 752, 871, 872
osteonecrosis 749, 1622, 1623
osteoporosis 129
transient 749
osteosarcoma 120
Paget's disease 1613, 1614
pelvis 716–17, 718
pigmented villonodular synovitis 1620
polymyositis 1254
prosthetic joint infection 854
psoriatic arthritis 1074, 1075, 1077,
1078, 1534
pyogenic arthritis 862
radiation protection in 753
reactive arthropathies 1089, 1090
reflex sympathetic dystrophy 167, 1683,
1683, 1684
relapsing polychondritis 1626
respiratory system 173, *176*, 243–6, *243*,
247
rheumatoid arthritis 715–16, 717, 719,
724–5, 1016–17, 1534
rickets 1601
sacroiliac joint 736, 738, 1535
sarcoidosis 1466
shoulder 140, 716, 717, 738, 739
rotator cuff tear 142, 717, 1503
rotator cuff tendinitis 141, 142, 1502
skull 716
soft tissue swelling and fat plane displacement 715–19
childhood 754, 755, 757
spine
cervical 716, 728
lumbar 716, 728–9
thoracic 716, 717
tuberculosis 122, 123, 717
spondyloepiphyseal dysplasia 1630,
1631, 1632
spondylolysis 126, 127
sporotrichal arthritis 959–60
stress fractures 1784
synovial chondromatosis 1619
systemic sclerosis 1235
tennis elbow 145
thyroid acropachy 280
tuberculosis 122, 123, 717, 930–1
wrist 715, 716, 718
radioimmunoassay, autoantibodies
667, 670
radionuclide scanning 719–20
ankylosing spondylitis 1066
back pain 97, 99
childhood 117
brucellar arthritis 939, 941

radionuclide scanning (continued)
cellulitis 284
childhood 752, 764–6, 767
pyogenic arthritis 862
diabetic neuropathy 284
DILS 911
fungal arthritis 956
hypertrophic osteoarthropathy 1673
non-gonococcal arthritis 851
os trigonum 746, 747
osteoarthritis 1536
osteoid osteoma 118, 1618
osteomyelitis 284, 752, 871–2
vertebral 878
osteonecrosis 749, 1623
osteoporosis, transient 749
Paget's disease 1613–14
polymyositis/dermatomyositis 1261
prosthetic joint infection 854
pyogenic arthritis 862
reactive arthropathies 1089, 1090
reflex sympathetic dystrophy 1683,
1683, 1684, 1685
rheumatoid arthritis 720, 1017, 1018
sacroiliac joint 737, 738
sarcoidosis 1466, 1469
Sjögren's syndrome 1308
spondylolysis 126
stress fracture 1784
foot 746, 747
transient synovitis of the hip 164
tuberculosis, spinal 122, 123
whiplash injury 1658
radiotherapy
ankylosing spondylitis 1069
eosinophilic granuloma 120
Ewing's sarcoma 120
malignancy following 290
pigmented villonodular synovitis 1620
scoliosis following 115
spinal 1666–7
total-body 290
polymyositis/dermatomyositis 1277
total-lymphoid 290, 611
polymyositis/dermatomyositis 1277
SLE 1175
**radioulnar joints, functional anatomy
and disability** 1725
radius 136, 137, 138
distal fracture 1583–4, *1584*, 1586, 1599,
1600
head excision 1703
styloid 138
ragocytes 681
**raised intraocular pressure, drug-
related** 319
Raji cell assay 706, 707, *708, 709*
Rand Health Insurance Study Scale
56, 57
RANTES 534, *535*
in rheumatoid arthritis 990
Rasch analysis 1724
rat-bite fever 852
Raynaud's phenomenon *174*, 201, 203,
1217, **1229–30**
in acromegaly 281
autoantibodies in 1229–30
digital ulceration 211
in the elderly 35
in giant cell arteritis 1388
investigation 203–4
in mixed connective tissue disease 1416,
1416
myocardial 1235
nailfold capillaroscopy 1230
paraneoplastic 1670
in polymyositis/dermatomyositis 1256
primary 1217, 1229
prognostic factors *1413*
secondary 1217, 1229
in Sjögren's syndrome 1310
in SLE 1156, 1183
systemic 1226
and systemic sclerosis 1226, 1229

Raynaud's phenomenon (continued)
treatment 1240, 1242–3, *1242*
in undifferentiated connective tissue
disease 1413
reactive arthritis *1040*, **1085–93**
age and sex differences in 1090
boundaries of 1091–2
brucellar 941
clinical features *170*, 178, 1085–8
course 1089, 1090
and *Cryptosporidium* 267, *946*, 947
definition 1085
diagnostic criteria *1086*
differential diagnosis 890–1, 1090–1,
1104, 1123
epidemic 1088
following penetrating injury 865
gastrointestinal involvement *259*, 663,
1087–8
genetic factors 698, 1087–8
history and terminology 1085
in HIV infection 901, 918–21
imaging 1089, 1090
and intestinal bacteria 267
and intra-articular infection 1043
investigation 662–4
laboratory tests 1088
management 1091, *1093*
mucocutaneous lesions 1085
ocular lesions *1086*
pathogenesis 1092
poststreptococcal 977–8
prevention 1092–3
prognosis 1088, *1090, 1091*
response to treatment 1088
seronegative 662
urogenital symptoms 1087
see also Reiter's syndrome; seronegative
spondylarthropathies
receptive field *488*
receptor-binding proteins 349
recombinant DNA technology 350,
354
**recombinant strip immunoblot assay
in HCV infection** 900–1
recombination fraction 687
rectal biopsy in amyloidosis 1440–1
**rectal carcinoma, protective effects in
rheumatoid arthritis** 1666
rectal examination 47
rectus femoris 150, 152
red Amsler grid 318, 596
reflex latencies 801
reflex neurovascular dystrophy *1105*
reflex sympathetic dystrophy **1679–88**
atrophic phase 1682
childhood 163, 167, 1681, 1682, 1683
clinical features 1680–1
comparison with fibromyalgia *1686*,
1687
course 1682
and diabetes mellitus *283*
diagnosis 1683
disorders associated *1681*
dystrophic phase 1682
epidemiology 1679–80
histopathology 1683
imaging 167, 1682–3, *1683*, 1684,
1685
laboratory tests 1682
nomenclature 1679, *1679*
pain control in 307
pathophysiology 1683–7, *1686*
prognosis 1688
regional involvement 1682
staging 1682
synovitis in 449, 1683, 1684, *1686*
treatment 1687–8, *1687*
triggering events 1681–2
reflexes 218
in cervical myelopathy 1656
**regional enteritis and pyoderma
gangrenosum** 1460
regional nerve blocks 305–6

rehabilitation **1723–35**
childhood **1737–55**
intensive *90*
juvenile chronic arthritis 1107, 1141–2,
1737–50
medical and social models 1725–6
multi-disciplinary team 1027, 1726–7,
1726, 1737, *1737*
in polymyositis/dermatomyositis 1278
principles 1726, *1726*
problem-orientated approach 1727
programme contents 1727–9, *1727*,
1728, 1729
psychosocial aspects 1729–30
in rheumatoid arthritis 1027
and sexual dysfunction 1730, *1730*
Reiter's cells 681, 683
Reiter's syndrome *1040*, **1084–93**
acute phase response in 628
age at onset 13, *26*, 1090
cardiovascular involvement *230*, 238,
1087
clinical features 1085–8
course 1089, 1090
definition 1085
diagnostic criteria *812*, 838, 1038, *1086*
differential diagnosis 855, 1090–1, *1104*
epidemiology 838–40, *840*
fever in 172
gastrointestinal involvement 1087–8
genetic factors 1087–8
history and terminology 1084
in HIV infection 901, 918–21
imaging 1089, 1090
juvenile 1054–5
epidemiology 831–2, *832*
laboratory tests 1088
large vessel vasculitis in 1391
management 1091, *1093*
mucocutaneous lesions 205, 207, 1085
ocular lesions 314, 316, 317, 1086
overlap with seronegative reactive
arthritis 662
and plantar spurs 745, 746
prognosis 1088, *1090, 1091*
response to treatment 1088
sex differences 14, 1089–90
synovial biopsy 778
synovial fluid 683
urogenital symptoms 1087
see also reactive arthritis; seronegative
spondylarthropathies
relapsing grip 979
relapsing polychondritis 289, **1624–7**
aetiology 1624–5
childhood 1406
clinical features 1625–6
diagnosis 1626–7
differential diagnosis 1136
imaging 1626
large vessel vasculitis in 1391
organ involvement *1625*
pathogenesis 1624–5
and pregnancy 185
pulmonary involvement *241*, 242
treatment 1627
in Wegener's granulomatosis 1338
relaxation in low back pain 106
**remitting seronegative symmetrical
synovitis with pitting oedema
syndrome** 34–5
renal colic 323
renal glomerular osteodystrophy 280,
433, 434, 1603
bone biopsy in 783
renal tubular acidosis 173, 1605
in Sjögren's syndrome 1310–11
type I 1605
type II 1605
renal vein thrombosis 324, *330*
renin 329
renography, preanaesthetic 300
repetitive strain injury/syndrome 43,
147, **1494–5**

reproductive factors in disease occurrence 823, *823*
residual volume 247, 249
respiratory syncytial virus
  in Paget's disease 435
  and polymyalgia rheumatica 1376
respiratory system
  adverse drug effects 253–4, *253*
    azathioprine *253*
    chlorambucil *253*
    colchicine *253*
    cyclophosphamide 241, *253*
    gold 241, *253*, *601*, *1022*
    methotrexate 241, *253*, 254, *584*, 585
    NSAIDs *253*, *578*, 580
    penicillamine *253*, 254, *598*
    salicylates *253*
    sulphasalazine *253*
  amyloidosis 1436, 1439
  in ankylosing spondylitis 241, 245, 247, 1064
  disease, and anaesthesia 299–300
  radiography 243–6, *243*, 247
  in relapsing polychondritis 1626
  see also lungs
rest
  in acute injury 1780
  in ankylosing spondylitis 1046
  in rheumatoid arthritis 33–4
restlessness, steroid-induced *587*
restriction endonucleases 691
restriction fragment length polymorphism 350, 354, 548, 691
restrictive capsulitis 738, 740
reticulendothelial hyperplasia in juvenile chronic arthritis 1116
reticulohistiocytoma 1474
reticulohistiocytosis *see* multicentric reticulohistiocytosis
reticulum cell sarcoma 120, 718
retina
  angioid streaks 1613
  haemorrhage in SLE 313, 1153
  vasculitis in relapsing polychondritis 1626
retinal artery
  occlusion *311*, 312
    in giant cell arteritis 312
    in SLE 313
    in Wegener's granulomatosis 1337
  thrombosis *174*
retinal S antigen 1109
retinal vein occlusion in SLE 313, 314
retinitis, viral 319
retinoids
  in psoriasis 1079
  in psoriatic arthritis 1080
  rheumatological effects 1695
retinol-binding protein 624
  and tubular function 650
retinopathy, drug-related 318–19, 596
retrocalcaneal apophysitis 167, 1511
retrocalcaneal bursa 154, 156, 157, 719
  bursitis 159–60, 745, 1511
  calcification 1528
retrocalcaneal recess 719
retroviruses 352, 508, 901
  and autoimmune disease 907, 1162
  and Kawasaki disease 1406
  in models of myositis 1273
  in murine lupus 1162
  in polymyositis/dermatomyositis 1267
  and rheumatoid arthritis 824, 986
  and Sjögren's syndrome 1302
  taxonomy 908, *908*
  see also specific viruses
reumacon 1026
rev gene 907
reverse transcriptase 908
reversed 'prayer position' 42, 43
Reye's syndrome 1106–7, 1124
RFLP 350, 354, 548, 691

rhabdomyolysis 467
  following reperfusion of ischaemic limb 469
  in malignant hyperpyrexia/hyperthermia 472
  myoglobinuria in 323
rhabdomyosarcoma 395
rheumatic fever **972–81**
  aetiology 975–6, *976*
  age at onset 11, 13
  arthritis in 977–8
  atlantoaxial subluxation in 224
  cardiovascular involvement *230*, 234, 238, 978
  childhood 977–8
    sex differences 14
  chorea in 972, 978–9
  clinical course 980
  clinical features 976–9, *977*
  diagnostic criteria 11, *11*
  differential diagnosis 855, *1104*, 1122–3
  epidemiology 972–3, *972*, 1044
  genetics 975
  investigation 664
  laboratory tests 979–80
  large vessel vasculitis in 1392
  pathogenesis 973–5
  prophylaxis 980
  recurrnce 980
  revised Jones criteria 977, *977*
  skin lesions 200, 204, 979
  systemic features *170*
  treatment 980
rheumatic heart disease 978
rheumatoid arthritis
  acute phase response in 628–9, 640
  aetiology 984–8
    autoimmune factors 986–8
    genetic factors 351, *351*, 553–4, *554*, 555–6, 699, *822*, 984–5, *984*
    infectious agents 268, 823–4, 985–6
    menstrual, hormonal and reproductive factors *823*, 986, 1012–13
  angiogenesis in 448–9, 990
  antidepressants in 341–2
  antigen presentation 987–8
  antigen-presenting cells 992
  articular involvement 988, 989, 1007–9
  assessment 1018
  autoantibodies 668, 824, 986–7, 1329
  autoantigens 987–8
  and autoimmune thyroid disease 279
  B-cell lineage 992
  and calcium pyrophosphate dihydrate disease 1531
  cell interactions in 992
  cell recruitment 990
  childhood onset 11
  clinical features *1414*
  comparison with psoriatic arthritis *1074*
  complications
    amyloidosis 257, *258*, 322, 651, 1014
    cervical spine dislocation 1013, 1014
    fractures 1013–14
    infection 823–4, 985–6, 1013
    neurological 227, 1008, 1013
    tendon and ligament damage 1014
  concepts and features 559–60
  co-occurrence with osteoarthritis 677
  cryoglobulinaemia in 706, 710
  cytokines 521–2
    antagonists 995–7
    expression 993–4, *993*
    regulation 994–5
  definition 983
  diagnostic criteria 55–6, 811–12, *812*, 832, 1004, *1005*, *1006*
  and diet 1024, 1026, 1694
  differential diagnosis 1378
  disability in 54
  disease course 1009–10
  effects of age and sex on 26, *815*, 816, 832, 1012
  effects of free radicals in 447–8

rheumatoid arthritis *(continued)*
  elastase-a₁proteinase inhibitor complexes in 653–4
  in the elderly 25–6, 32
    concomitant disease *33*
    differential diagnosis 32, 33
    treatment 33–4
  endocrine influences 510
  eosinophilia *644*
  epidemiology 1004, 1044
    ethnic factors 819, *819*, *1007*
    geographical factors 820, *820*
    incidence *814*, 1004–5, *1007*
    mortality 1005, *1008*
    non-European populations 832–3, *834–5*
    and occupation 824
    and position in family 823
    prevalence *814*, 1004, *1007*
    time trends 816–17, *817*
  erosions 724–5, *726*
  extra-articular manifestations *170*, 178, 990
  finger swelling 207
  hands, surgery 1705
  health status measurement 54–6, *55*
  and hemiplegia 449
  history 983–4
  and hyperlipidaemias 1484
  in hypogammaglobulinaemia 969–70
  imaging 724, 1016–18
    arthrography 725–6
    CT 1017
    MRI 726, 727–8, 1017, 1018
    radiography 715–16, 717, 719, 724–5, 1016–17, 1534
    radionuclide scanning 720, 1017, 1018
    ultrasound 1017, 1018
  immune complexes in 710–11, *710*, 712, 994
  immune suppression in 997
  immunopathogenesis **983–99**
  and intestinal bacteria 267, 268, 269, *270–1*
  intubation 301–2
  laboratory tests *649*, 1015–16, *1015*, *1016*, *1017*
  and lactation 181
  lipids in joints 1481–2
  liver function 652
  and malignant disease 1665–6, *1666*
  models *see* animal models
  muscle in 472, 1011
  'nephropathy' 651
  non-articular manifestations 1010, *1010*
    bone involvement 1011
    cardiovascular 173, *230*, 231, 234, 235, 236, 990, 1010–11
    cutaneous 207, 1011
    gastrointestinal 255, 257, *258*
    haematological 291, 292, 633–8, *633*, *643*
    lymph nodes 1010
    muscular 1011
    neurological 449–50
    ocular 313–14, 1011
    psychiatric *333*, 335, 336–7, *336*
    pulmonary 173, 241, *241*, 242, 243, 245, 1010
    secondary Sjögren's syndrome 1011, *1011*
  onset 32, 33, 1007
  osteoporosis in 1590–1, *1590*
  papules and nodules *208*
  and parvovirus infection 824, 898
  pathogenesis 990–7
  pathology 988–90
  and pneumonia 251
  and pregnancy 181–2, *182*, 1012, *1012*
  pressure erosions 725
  prognosis 1027

rheumatoid arthritis *(continued)*
  protective effects of oral contraceptives 182, *825*, 826, 986, 1012
  and pyogenic arthritis 853, 865, 1013
  rehabilitation 1027
  rheumatoid factor in 674, *674*, 710, 833, *835*, 986
  seronegative 983
  and Sjögren's syndrome 1312
  and SLE 1157
  stress proteins 449
  susceptibility to 553–4, 555–6
  synovial biopsy 776, 777, 778
  synovial fluid 443–4, 683, 988
  synovial ischaemia/hypoxia 444–51
  systemic features *170*, 178, 990
  T-cell activation 990–2
  target areas 724
  thrombocytosis 292, 644–5
  treatment **1018–27**
    anti-T cell antibodies 1024
    cytokine inhibition 1024
    dietary 1024, 1026
    individual goals 1018
    new substances 1026
    pharmacotherapy 34, 586, 629, 1018–24, *1020*
    surgery 1026–7, 1703–5
    TNF-α 415
  typus robustus 1017
  vasculitis in *786*, 791, 990
  weight loss in *170*, 171
rheumatoid arthritis latex test 674
rheumatoid factor 666, 674
  in animal models of arthritis 567
  childhood 18
  'classical' 674
  in DILS 913
  discovery 983
  diseases associated *674*
  effect of gold therapy on 599
  effect of methotrexate on 583
  effect of NSAIDs on production 576
  in the elderly 32
  in Felty's syndrome 644
  in gout 1562
  hidden 674
  in HIV infection 910
  inhibition immune complex assay 706, 707, *708*, *709*
  in juvenile chronic arthritis 830–1, *831*, **1031–6**, 1101, 1120
  in polymyositis/dermatomyositis 1258
  in psoriatic arthritis 1071, 1072, 1077
  in rheumatoid arthritis 674, *674*, 710, 833, *835*, 986
  in RS₃PE syndrome 35
  in Sjögren's syndrome 1303, 1304
  in SLE
    childhood 1197
    in the elderly 35, *35*
  synovial fluid 679
  in Takayasu's arteritis 1386
  tests for 674, 1015
  in vasculitis 1358
  in Wegener's granulomatosis 1338
rhubarb, dietary excess 1575
rhupus 1181, 1424
RIBA in HCV infection 900–1
ribonuclease A 694
RICE 1780
rice bodies 680, 931
rickets 433, 434, 1583, **1600–6**
  biochemical features 1601–2
  and calcium pyrophosphate dihydrate disease *1531*, 1567
  causes *433*
  clinical and laboratory features 1600–1
  and hypophosphatasia 1606
  metabolic acidosis in 1605
  molecular changes in 434
  renal tubular 433, 434
  vitamin D deficiency 1603–4
  vitamin D-dependent 433, 434, 1604

rickets (continued)
    X-linked hypophosphataemic *1531*, 1600, 1604, 1605
rickettsia and Kawasaki disease 1406
rifabutin, drug interactions 957
rifampicin 660
    adverse effects 651
    in brucellar arthritis 943, *943*
    in combination therapy *1025*
    drug interactions 957
    in leprosy 935, 936
    in multicentric reticulohistiocytosis *1476*
    in mycobacterial infection 253
    in osteomyelitis 874
    in tuberculosis 931, *932*, 933
rind sign 931
ring size 41
Risser's method 757
ristomycin-cofactor in mixed connective tissue disease 1420
Ritchie index 41, *1724*
RNA
    detection 660–1
    messenger *see* mRNA
RNA polymerase II 348, 349
Ro proteins 669, 670, 672
    Ro52 670
    Ro60 670
    see also anti-Ro antibodies
road traffic accidents, consequences 107
Roche–Wainer–Thissen method for assessment of skeletal maturation 79
Rochester Epidemiology Program 814
rocuronium *307*
Rodnan skin score 1231
Roland Disability Questionnaire 59
Rome criteria for rheumatoid arthritis *812*, 1004, *1006*
root entrapment syndrome 1644, 1645
rosacea 204
Rose Bengal slide agglutination test 943
Rose Bengal stain 310, 1309
Rose Waaler test 674, 1015
Ross River virus 903–4
rotator cuff 135, 137
    local steroid injection 1764
    repair 1702
    tears 142–3, 717, 722, 1503
        aetiology 737
        imaging 140, 142, 717, 738, 739, 740
        in rheumatoid arthritis 1014
rotator cuff tendon
    rupture 739, 740
    tendinitis 141–2, 1501–2
        acute calcific 141, 142
        occupationally induced 1494
        in rheumatoid arthritis 1008
Rothman–Makai syndrome 1453
RS₃PE syndrome 34–5
rubella virus infection 663, **899**
    arm arthropathy 899
    arthropathy in 880, 899
    catcher's crouch syndrome 899
    clinical features 899
    diagnosis 899
    epidemiology 899
    and juvenile chronic arthritis 1109
    macules 204
    management 899
    pathogenesis 899
    synovial fluid in 683
    vaccination against 899, 1136
rubivirus 899
rule of three 195
runner's knee 158
Rush pin 1704
RV 247, 249

S
S-100 protein in calcium pyrophosphate dihydrate disease 1569
S-HAQ *58, 59*
SAA *see* serum amyloid A
Saccharomyces 963
sacroiliac joints
    in ankylosing spondylitis 736, 738
    in Behçet's syndrome 1397
    brucellar arthritis 939
    examination 47
    fusions 737, 739
    in hypophosphataemic rickets 1604, 1605
    imaging 736–7, 738, 739
        CT scanning 737, 738, 753, 768
    infection *see* sacroiliitis
    local steroid injection 1771
    osteoarthritis 1535
    palpation 47, 48
    pyogenic arthritis in childhood 863–4
    range of movement 47
    sclerosis 753
    screening 47
sacroiliitis
    in ankylosing spondylitis 1058–9, 1065, *1065*
    childhood 21, 1749–50
    diagnosis 117
    and enteric arthropathies 1094
    imaging 736, 737, 738, 862
    muscle wasting and weakness 21
    in pregnancy 185
    in psoriatic arthritis 1073, 1075
    radiography 1535
    in reactive arthropathies 1089
    in Reiter's syndrome 1059
    in Wegener's granulomatosis 1338
sagittal cam effect 139
sail sign 715, 716
St Vitus' dance *see* chorea
salbutamol, adverse effects 1693
salicylates
    adverse effects
        gout 1694
        neurological *217*
        psychiatric 338
        respiratory *253*
    binding to plasma proteins 576
    clearance 577
    effect on liver function 652
    effect on serum creatinine 649
    half-life *577*
    and hyperuricaemia *1558*
    sensitivity to in SLE 1197
saline joint distension 1547
salivary glands
    biopsy 778–9
        evaluation 779–80
        sarcoidosis 779, 780
        sicca syndrome 778, 779
        Sjögren's syndrome 778–9, 780, 1306
        technical aspects 778, 779
    in DILS 913
    enlargement *1308*
    lymphoma 912
    myoepithelial islands 778
    in Sjögren's syndrome 1306, 1307–9
Salmonella
    arteritis due to 1390
    childhood pyogenic arthritis 862–3
    enteric infection 255
    in HIV infection 916
    and HIV-associated Reiter's syndrome 920
    and juvenile spondylarthropathies 1049, 1054
    laboratory tests 663
    in osteomyelitis 868, 870
    and reactive arthritis 267, 663
    S. abony and reactive arthropathies 1088
    S. blocley and reactive arthropathies 1088

Salmonella (continued)
    S. choleraesius in pyogenic arthritis 852
    S. enteritidis and reactive arthropathies 1088
    S. haifa and reactive arthropathies 1088
    S. heibelberg and reactive arthropathies 1088
    S. manila and reactive arthropathies 1088
    S. newport and reactive arthropathies 1088
    S. schwarzengrund and reactive arthropathies 1088
    S. typhimurium
        in pyogenic arthritis 852
        and reactive arthropathies 1088
salpingitis and reactive arthropathies 1088
salsalate, adverse effects 338
Sanfilipo syndrome *1633*
SAPHO 1091
sarcoid 204, *208, 209*
sarcoid nodules 207
sarcoidosis 1464–9
    acute 1465
    aetiology 1464
    bronchoalveolar lavage 1466
    cardiovascular involvement *230*
    central nervous system disease in *223*
    chronic 1465, *1465*
    clinical features 1465, *1465*
    cranial nerve palsies in *224*
    cutaneous involvement 203, *208, 209*, 1467
    diagnosis 203
    differential diagnosis 1136–7, *1137*, 1313
    endobronchial 242
    eosinophilia *644*, 1465
    epidemiology 1464–5
    granuloma in 789–90, 1464
    histology 1466
    imaging 1466
    infantile, onset 12, 13
    juvenile 1469
        differential diagnosis 1123
        ocular involvement 316
        sex differences 14
    laboratory tests 1465–6
    large vessel vasculitis in 1392
    lupus pernio 201, 1467
    musculoskeletal involvement 1466–9
    ocular involvement 314–15, 317
    pathology 1464
    peripheral nerve biopsy in 795
    plaques in 206
    psychiatric involvement *333*, 336
    pulmonary involvement 242, 245, 1465
    rheumatoid factor in *674*
    salivary gland biopsy 779, 780
    treatment 1469
sarcolemma 456
sarcomere 455, 456, 458
    during muscle stretch 464
    following eccentric exercise 468–9
sarcoplasmic reticulum 456, 457
sartorius 150, 153, 158
satellite cells 459–60
Saturday night palsy *803*, 805
'sausage digit' 42, 1075, 1087, 1417, 1468
'sausage toes' 51, 1087
scalp
    necrosis in giant cell arteritis 784
    skin lesions 200
    tenderness in giant cell arteritis 1378
    ulceration 207
scaphoid 137
    osteonecrosis 1623
scapula 135, 136, 137
    osteotomy 1703
    winging 221
scapulohumeral rhythm 137
scapulothoracic articulation 135, 137
scarlet fever 973

scarring following pyoderma gangrenosum 1458, 1459
SCAT technique 674
scavenger receptor-protein family 353
Scheie syndrome 1632, *1633*
Scheuermann's osteochondritis 125, 126, 1787, *1787*
Schirmer's test 36, 310, 1309
schistosomiasis 948
    articular syndromes associated 950
    muscular syndromes associated 951
    rheumatoid factor in *674*
Schmidt's syndrome 285–6
Schmorl's nodes 730, 731
Schnitzler's syndrome 1369
Schober's test 46
    modified 1065
school
    and childhood rehabilitation 1737
    integration into 1752–3, 1754
Schwann cells 793–5
    in leprosy 933
sciatic nerve 150
    entrapment neuropathy 227, 805
    iatrogenic damage 803
    palsy *803*
    section in arthritis of ankle joint 450
sciatic stretch test 46
sciatica 89
    childhood 118
    electrodiagnosis in 805–6
    epidemiology 1639
    and referred pain 6
    see also lower limb, pain
SCID mice 567, 1163, 1306–7
sclera
    in osteogenesis imperfecta 358
    pigment changes *174*
scleritis *311*, 312
    in relapsing polychondritis 1626
    in rheumatoid arthritis 313–14, 1011
    in SLE 312–13
    treatment 317
sclerodactyly 1230
scleroderma 1217–44
    aetiology 1219–25
    age at onset 13
    anaesthesia in 299, 300
    animal model 1225
    autoantibodies *1225*, 1424
    and autoimmunity 1220–3, 1225, *1225*
    cardiac 1232–5, *1234*
    central nervous system disease in 222
    childhood 1228
        autoantibodies 1223
        en coup de sabre 1229
        physiotherapy 1751
        sex differences 14
    cranial nerve palsies in *224*
    cutaneous involvement 1230–1
    diagnostic criteria 812
    diffuse 1217
    disease spectrum associated *1217*
    drug-induced *1223*, 1693
    en coup de sabre 1228, 1229, *1243*
    in endotracheal intubation 303–4
    epidemiology 1218–19, *1222*
    gastrointestinal involvement 257, *258*
    history 1217, *1219*
    immune complexes in 712
    intubation in 303–4
    limited 1217
    linear 1217, 1228–9, *1243*
    localized 1217, 1228–9
    and malignancy 289
    muscle in 472
    and occupation 824–5
    overlap syndromes
        polymyositis 1424–5
        primary biliary cirrhosis *258*, 1424
    pathogenesis 1225–7
    peripheral neuropathies 227
    and pregnancy 184
    renal involvement 322

scleroderma (continued)
syndromes resembling 1217, 1218
treatment 211–12, 1240–4
vascular lesions 1226–7
venous access in 303
xerostomia in 1312
see also morphoea; systemic sclerosis
scleroderma-like syndromes 207, 209
scleroedema of Buschke 209
scleromalacia perforans 312, 314, 1011
sclerotherapy
inflammatory olecranon bursitis 146
low back pain 105
scoliosis 46, 114
aetiology 115, 116
with back pain 115, 117–18
in homocystinuria 436
imaging 729, 753
in juvenile chronic arthritis 82, 1721
non-structural 131
in osteoid osteoma 118, 119
in Paget's disease 1612
in Parkinson's disease 219
postural 131
in spinal dysraphism 127
structural 131
scrapie protein precursor 1434
scratching 207
scurvy, scleroderma-like changes 207
SEA syndrome 1051
clinical features 1051
diagnosis 19
diagnostic criteria 10, 11
epidemiology 831–2, 832
outcome 1051
sebopsoriasis in HIV infection 919, 920
second messenger systems 349
second wind phenomenon 473
sedation in MRI 724, 769
segmental subchondral infarction see osteonecrosis
seizures 231
in CINCA 1471
in mixed connective tissue disease 1418
in Sjögren's syndrome 1311
in SLE 333, 1153
childhood 1184
selectins 528–9, 529, 1168, 1169
carbohydrate-bearing counter-receptors 530
expression in arthritis 537
in leucocyte rolling 535
ligands 529–30
as serum markers of cellular activation 538
see also E-selectin; L-selectin; P-selectin
selenium 262
as antioxidant 1480
self-care equipment in childhood 1752, 1753
self-efficacy 69, 70, 339
semilunar cartilages see menisci
semitendinosus 153, 158
sensitization 488
sensory deprivation in low back pain 106
sensory ending 488
sensory evoked potentials (SEPs) 802, 805
in cervical myelopathy 1656
in cervical spondylosis 1655
sensory loss 218, 221
in cervical spondylosis 224
sensory nerve action potential 800, 801
sensory nerve conduction velocity 800–1
SEPs see sensory evoked potentials
sepsis
acute renal failure in 327
as contraindication to local steroid injection 1758
differential diagnosis 1379

sepsis (continued)
drug-related 1359
following local steroid injection 1759
septic arthritis see pyogenic arthritis
sequestrum 871, 930
seronegative enthesis and arthritis syndrome see SEA syndrome
seronegative spondylarthropathies 983, 1037–47
acute phase response in 628
anaesthesia in 299
bowel involvement 1045–6
childhood 128, 1049–56
aetiology 1049–50
atypical 1051–2
classification 1050
clinical features and outcome 1050–6
epidemiology 831–2, 832, 1136
undifferentiated 1050–2
clinical subsets 1038, 1040, 1041
definition 838
diagnostic criteria 812, 838, 1038, 1039, 1086
differential diagnosis 1104, 1105
epidemiology 838–40, 838, 839, 840, 1043–5
features 1037–8
health status measures 58–9, 58
history and terminology 1037, 1085
HLA-B27 in 552–3, 838–40, 839, 1038, 1041–3, 1043–4, 1085
imaging 733–6, 737
individual conditions 1037
intubation in 303
large vessel vasculitis in 1391
and malignant disease 1666–7
movement limitation 1654
natural history 1046
ocular involvement 314, 317
overlap within 1038
pathogenesis 1041–3
prognosis 1046
systemic features 170
treatment 1046, 1046, 1068
undifferentiated 838, 1040, 1059
childhood 1050–2
diagnostic criteria 1038
in HIV infection 918–21
with polyarticular seronegative juvenile chronic arthritis 1135–6
see also specific diseases
serositis
in juvenile chronic arthritis 1116, 1126
in rheumatoid arthritis 990
in SLE 1196
serotonin
in fibromyalgia 1498
joint afferent sensitivity to 492
serotonin-specific reuptake inhibitors 339, 340
serpentine receptors 534
Serratia marcesens in pyogenic arthritis 852
sertraline 339, 340, 342
serum amyloid A (SAA) 623, 626, 639, 1433, 1434
amino acid sequences 1435
in amyloidosis 640, 1118
in familial Mediterranean fever 1448
in hyperlipidaemias 1483
in inflammation 624
properties 625
in rheumatoid arthritis 990
serum amyloid P 1436
serum bactericidal test in osteomyelitis 873
serum sickness 969, 998, 1694
Serzone 340
sesamoid index in acromegaly 281, 281
severe combined immunodeficiency disease mice 567, 1163, 1306–7
Sever's disease 167, 1511
sevofluxane 307
sewing-needle injury 865

sex determination and chromosome suppression 349
sex hormones
in Behçet's syndrome 1399
in calcium homeostasis 431
and inflammation 510
and rheumatoid arthritis 823, 986, 1012–13
therapy in SLE 1175
sex ratio/distribution
ankylosing spondylitis 815, 815, 1060, 1060, 1066
back pain 93
and disease occurrence 815–16, 815, 816, 1012
drug-induced lupus 1692
gout 815
Henoch–Schönlein purpura in childhood 14
and incidence of childhood rheumatic diseases 12, 14
inflammatory bowel disease in childhood 14
juvenile ankylosing spondylitis 12, 14
juvenile chronic arthritis 12, 14, 815, 830, 831, 1114
juvenile dermatomyositis 14
juvenile psoriatic arthritis 14
Kawasaki disease 14
Lyme disease 14
microscopic polyangiitis 1354
mixed connective tissue disease in childhood 14
neonatal lupus erythematosus 12, 14
neonatal-onset multisystem inflammatory disease 14
osteoarthritis 815, 815, 816, 816, 1517–18
polyarteritis nodosa 14, 1353, 1403
reactive arthropathies 14, 1090
Reiter's syndrome 14, 1090
rheumatic fever 14
rheumatoid arthritis 26, 815, 816, 832, 1012
sarcoidosis in childhood 14
scleroderma 14, 1219
seronegative spondylarthropathies 1136
SLE 12, 14, 815, 837, 1146, 1169
systemic sclerosis 14, 815
Takayasu's arteritis 14, 1384
Wegener's granulomatosis 14
sexual dysfunction 1730, 1730
sexual maturation 14–15, 17
rating 81
SF-12 53–4
SF-20 54
SF-36 53–4, 54, 61, 1724, 1724
Sgp200 1169
shared epitope hypothesis 822, 984
Sharp index 1017
shawl sign 1251, 1271
Shenton's line 739
Shigella
and juvenile spondylarthropathies 1049, 1054
laboratory tests 663
and reactive arthritis 267, 663
and Reiter's syndrome 1042
S. dysenteriae 1085
S. flexneri
and HIV-associated Reiter's syndrome 920
and reactive arthropathies 1088
shin pain 1508–9
shin splints 163, 1785–6
shock following steroid withdrawal 587
shoes 1733, 1749
short-wave diathermy in low back pain 104
shoulder
abduction 135, 137
adduction 137
in ankylosing spondylitis 1062
applied anatomy 135, 136, 137

shoulder (continued)
arthrodesis 1703, 1720
extension 137
frozen 45, 143–4, 1503–4, 1764
differential diagnosis 1379
sympathetic activity 449
functional anatomy and disability 1725
imaging 737
arthrography 717, 719, 738, 739, 740
CT arthrography 739–40, 741, 742
MRI 140, 142, 738–9, 740, 742
radiography 140, 716, 717, 738, 739
rotator cuff tear 142, 717
rotator cuff tendinitis 141, 142
ultrasound 140, 142, 143–4, 722, 739
impingement syndrome 141, 1503
in HIV infection 901
in juvenile chronic arthritis 1100, 1133, 1720, 1740
local anaesthetic tests 1702
local steroid injection 141, 142, 143, 144, 1761, 1762, 1763–4
manipulation under anaesthesia 144
pain 1501–4, 1501, 1502
adult 139–40, 140–4
childhood 163, 163
health status measures 59
periarticular 5, 141
referred 99, 1501
periarthritis
and diabetes mellitus 284
in thyrotoxicosis 278, 279
physiotherapy 144
childhood 1740
reflex sympathetic dystrophy 1682
replacement arthroplasty 1703
in rheumatoid arthritis 1008
rotation 137
soft-tissue rheumatism 37
surgery 143, 1702–3
childhood 1720
shoulder girdle
examination 43–5
flexion/extension 135
painful arc 45
range of movement 45
resisted movements 45
screening 44
shoulder–hand syndrome 1504, 1675, 1682
shoulder joint see glenohumeral joint
shoulder pad sign 1436, 1437
shrinking lung syndrome 1152, 1195
Shulman's syndrome 644, 789, 1428, 1675
sialadenitis
animal models 1306
myoepithelial 778–9, 1306, 1667
in Sjögren's syndrome 778–9, 1306, 1667
sialectasia in mixed connective tissue disease 1418
sialochemistry in Sjögren's syndrome 1308–9
sialography in Sjögren's syndrome 1308
sialometry in Sjögren's syndrome 1307
sialomucins 530
sialoprotein 1 427, 429
sialoprotein 2 427, 429
in rheumatoid arthritis 1017
sialyl-3-fucosyl-N-acetyllactosamine (sialyl-Lewis-x) 529
sicca syndrome 258
in the elderly 36
in HIV infection 911, 913
salivary gland biopsy 778, 779
sickle-cell disease
back pain in 99
as contraindication to local steroid injection 1758
differential diagnosis 1137, 1137
musculoskeletal pain in 168

sickle-cell disease *(continued)*
  and osteomyelitis 868
  and osteonecrosis 1622
  pyogenic arthritis in 865
  and salmonella-associated arthritis 852
Sickness Impact Profile 53, *54*, 59, 61,
  1724, *1724*
sIL-2R and juvenile chronic arthritis
  1120
silica
  and polymyositis/dermatomyositis
    1267
  and scleroderma *1223*, 1693
silicone implants 825, 1220, *1223*, 1267,
  1419, 1693
silicosis *209*
simian virus in Paget's disease 1610
Sindbis virus 904
Sinding–Larsen syndrome 1509
Sinding–Larsen–Johansson disease
  157, 166
Singh index 1594
single-breath diffusion test in
  systemic sclerosis 1235
single-gene disorders 350–1, *350*, 687
single-photon absorptiometry 1594,
  1595
single-photon emission computed
  tomography *see* SPECT
single-strand conformation poly-
  morphism technique 693
sinoatrial node 237
sinus disorders 173
sinusitis in Wegener's granuloma-
  tosis 1335
SIP 53, *54*, 59, 61, 1724, *1724*
sitting and low back pain 109
sitting height
  measurement 74, 75
  percentiles *77–8*
SJL/J mice 1273
Sjögren's syndrome *285*, **1301–14**
  aetiology 1301–5
  age-related occurrence *26*
  animal models 1306–7
  associations
    other autoimmune diseases *1301*
    SLE 1157, 1159
  autoantibodies 279, *668*, 669, 671, *671*,
    1302, 1303, 1413, 1414
    in the elderly 36
    in pregnancy 185
  and autoimmune thyroid disease 279,
    1311
  B-cell hyper-reactivity in 1303–4
  central nervous system disease in 222
  clinical features *170*, 1307–12
  cutaneous involvement 1310
  diagnosis 1312–13
  differential diagnosis 1312–13
  in the elderly 35, 36
  environmental factors 1302
  epidemiology 1301
  and ethnic group 1302–3, *1303*
  extraglandular manifestations *170*,
    1309–12, *1309*
  fever in 172
  gastrointestinal involvement 257, *258*,
    1310
  genetic factors 1302–3, *1303*
  glandular involvement 1307–9, *1308*
  history 1301
  immune complexes in 711
  immunopathology 1305
  initial manifestations *1307*
  intubation in 303–4
  laboratory tests 1312, *1312*
  liver involvement 1310
  malaise in 172, 178
  and malignant disease 1304, 1310, 1312,
    1667–8
  neuromuscular involvement 472, 1311
  ocular involvement 310, 1309
  overlap with osteoarthritis 1523

Sjögren's syndrome *(continued)*
  pathogenesis 1301–5
  pathology 1306
  peripheral neuropathies 227
  and pregnancy 185
  primary 1301, 1310, 1667
  and primary biliary cirrhosis 257, *258*,
    1310, 1424
  prognosis 1314
  psychiatric involvement *333*, 335
  pulmonary involvement 173, 241, *241*,
    243, 245, 1310
  purpura 207
  renal involvement *321*, 651, 1310–11
    acute renal failure 327
    amyloidosis 322
    interstitial nephropathy 324
  in rheumatoid arthritis 1011, *1011*
  rheumatoid factor *674*
  salivary gland biopsy 778–9, 780, 1306
  secondary 1301, *1301*, 1310, 1312, 1667
  treatment 1313–14, *1313*
  vasculitis 1311
Sjögren's Syndrome Foundation 36
skeletal development 394
skeletal dysplasias 436
skeletal maturation, measurement
  77–9, *80*, 81
skeletal patterning 394
skin
  acneiform lesions 1395, 1396, 1399
  adverse drug effects 211, 212–15, *214*
    antimalarials *214*
    aspirin 213
    azathioprine 214, *591*
    benoxaprofen 212, 213
    chloroquine 596
    corticosteroids 207, *587*
    cyclophosphamide 215
    diclofenac 213, 580
    diflunisal 580
    diuretics *208*
    fenbufen 212, 213
    fenoprofen 213
    gold therapy 207, 213, 600, 601, *601*,
      1022, 1695
    hydroxychloroquine *214*, 596
    indomethacin 212
    ketoprofen 213
    mefenamic acid 213
    mepacrine 212, *214*
    methotrexate 214, *584*
    naproxen 212, 213, 580, 1106
    NSAIDs 212–13, *578*, 580, *1021*,
      1695
    oxyphenbutazone 212, 213
    penicillamine 213–14, *598*, 1695
    phenylbutazone 212, 213
    piroxicam 212, 213, 580
    sulindac 213, 580, *589*
    sulphasalazine 214
  amyloidosis 1436, 1439, 1440
  atrophy 211, *214*, 587
  in Behçet's syndrome 205–6, 207,
    1395–6, 1399
  biopsy 202
    in dermatomyositis 1262–3
    in hypermobility 1500
  in Churg–Strauss syndrome 1355
  in dermatomyositis 41, **1250–2**, 1253
    calcification *208*
    erythema 201, 204, 1250–1
    hypopigmentation *209*
    juvenile 1289
    periorbital erythema and oedema
      201, 204, 1251, 1289
    poikiloderma 207, 1250–1
    treatment 1277
    ulceration 207
  diffuse sclerosis 207
  drug absorption 209
  ear 201, 202
  in Ehlers–Danlos syndrome type 4 378,
    379, 380

skin *(continued)*
  in eosinophilia–myalgia syndrome 1426
  in eosinophilic fasciitis 1428
  examination 41, 200
  genital *175*
  grafting in cutaneous ulceration 210
  hands 41, *174–5*, 201, 202
  head and neck *174*, 200–1
  in HIV-associated arthritis 919–20
  in hypersensitivity vasculitis 1368
  in immune complex diseases 703
  induration/thickening 207, 209, 1428
  intraoperative care 301, 1702
  in Kawasaki disease 1405, *1405*
  legs and feet *175*, 201
  in leprosy 934
  lesions 173, *174–5*, **199–215**
    descriptive terms *201*
    differential diagnosis 204–9, *208–9*
    history taking 200
    investigation 202–4
    key points 215, *215*
    regional distribution 200–2, 203
    treatment 209–11, *210*
  in mixed connective tissue disease 1417
  in multicentric reticulohistiocytosis
    204, 206, 1475
  in neonatal lupus erythematosus
    1198–9
  'peau d'orange' 1428
  pigmentary changes 207, *209*
    drug-related 211, *212*, *214*
  pitting oedema 1428
  rash 3
    in adult-onset Still's disease 1127
    butterfly 1147, 1150, 1182
    in Chikungunya fever 902
    in CINCA 1471
    in dermatomyositis 1250–1
    differential diagnosis 1291
    in disseminated gonococcal infection
      854–5
    drug-related *584*, *591*, 598, 1695
    investigation 663–4
    in juvenile chronic arthritis 200, 204,
      1115–16, 1132
    macular *175*
    malar *174*
    in microscopic polyangiitis 1354
    papular *175*
    periorbital *174*, 201, 204, 1251, 1289
    in polyarteritis nodosa 1353, 1403
    in undifferentiated connective tissue
      disease 1413
  in rheumatic fever 979
  in rheumatoid arthritis 207, 1011
  in sarcoidosis 203, *208*, *209*, 1467
  scaling 205
  scalp 200
  in scleroderma/systemic sclerosis
    1230–1
  in Sjögren's syndrome 1310
  in SLE 1147–9, *1149*, 1150
    childhood 1182–3, *1184*
  in syndrome of limited joint mobility
    282–3
  in systemic sclerosis 201, 207, 211–12,
    1230–1
  in Takayasu's arteritis 1385
  tissue perfusion measurement 203
  in toxic oil syndrome 1426
  trunk and upper arms *175*
  in Wegener's granulomatosis 1338–9
skinfold thickness
  measurement 75
  standards 77, 79
skull
  in CINCA 1471
  in Paget's disease 1612
  radiography 716
SLAM score 1160, *1160*
'slapped cheek' erythema 204, 897
SLE *see* systemic lupus erythematosus
SLEDAI score 838, 1160, *1160*

sleep
  disturbance
    in fibromyalgia 1498
    management 342
    steroid-induced *587*
  patterns and low back pain 105
SLICC damage index 1160, *1161*, 1162
slit-lamp examination 310
slot blot procedure 691, 993
'slow acetylators' and drug-induced
  lupus 1692
Sly syndrome *1633*
Sm proteins 669, 672
  see also anti-Sm antibodies
small nuclear ribonucleoprotein
  particles 669
smoking
  and low back pain 94
  and osteoarthritis 1519
  and osteoporosis 1594
  and rheumatoid arthritis 1010
  and risk of hip fracture 1585
SMR 81
SNAP 800, 801
Sneddon–Wilkinson disease 206
snRNP particles 669
social comparison 68
social phobia 342
social relationships and quality of life
  66–7
social support 65, 68–9
  interventions 70
social well being and quality of life
  66–7
social worker in multi-disciplinary
  team 1737
sodium, imprecision in measurement
  648
sodium aurothiomalate *see* gold therapy
sodium fluoride in osteoporosis 1599
sodium monourate, response to intra-
  dermal injection in Behçet's
  syndrome 1396
sodium valproate
  in chronic back pain 1648
  interaction with NSAIDs *579*
soft-tissue rheumatism **1489–513**
  classification 1489–90, *1490*
  creatine kinase in 653
  defining outcome 1491
  economic effects 1490–1
  in the elderly 36–7, 1491
  epidemiology 1491
  generalized 1489, **1494–501**
  laboratory tests *649*
  localized 1489–90, *1490*, **1501–13**
  management 1512–13
  pathogenesis 1492–4
  renal function 650
soleus 153
somatomedin *see* insulin-like growth
  factors, IGF-I
somatostatin expression by joint
  nerves 490
'sonic hedgehog' factor 395
sorbinil in syndrome of limited joint
  mobility 282
sorbithane 1733
sorbitol in syndrome of limited joint
  mobility 282
South Africans
  juvenile chronic arthritis 830, *830*, *831*
  rheumatoid arthritis 833, *834*
  seronegative spondylarthropathies *839*
  SLE 836, *836*
Southern blotting 695
***SOX* gene** 368
SOX9 353
Spanish oil disease *see* toxic oil syndrome
sparganosis 948, 950
SPECT 720, 765
  in neuropsychiatric SLE 221, 335, 1186
  in spondylosis 119
speed *1265*, 1778

Speed's test 143
sphingolipidoses **1634–5**
Spielberger Score *1724*
spina bifida occulta 127, 128
spina ventosa 930
spinach, dietary excess 1575
spinal anaesthesia 306
in cardiovascular disease 299
spinal cord
cervical compression 218, *219*, 1009, 1651
disease *219*, **223–5**
dysfunction in Paget's disease 1612
intramedullary abscess 124
neurones
activation in joint inflammation 493–6
hyperexcitability 494–6
and nociception 487, 489
in spinal tuberculosis 928
tethering 127–8
tumours, rheumatic symptoms *218*
spinal dysraphism 127–8, 129
spinal muscular atrophy
muscle biopsy 791
muscle contracture in 217
spinal stabilization in 118
spinal units 1640
spindling 42
spine
anatomy and back pain 90–2
in ankylosing spondylitis 734, 735, 736, 1062, 1063
bamboo 1062, 1063, 1605
in brucellar arthritis 939–41
cervical 90–1
childhood *754*, *755*
examination 45–6
functional anatomy 1650–1
imaging 716, 727, 728, *754*, *755*
in juvenile chronic arthritis 1100, 1116, 1134, 1135, 1738, 1739
pain referred to 1660
pain syndromes **1650–62**, *1652*
palpation 45–6
physiotherapy in childhood 1738, 1739
range of movement 46
in rheumatoid arthritis 1009
subluxation 223, 301, 1705–6
in rheumatoid arthritis 1013, 1014
surgery 1026, 1705–6, 1721
see also cervical spondylosis
clinical problems
adults **89–110**
childhood **114–33**
crush fracture in juvenile chronic arthritis 1721
deformity 131, 133
disorders **1639–62**
functional anatomy and disability 1725
functions 1639
fusion
in kyphosis 125–6
in scoliosis 131
in spondylolisthesis 127, 128
in juvenile chronic arthritis 82, 1721, 1738, 1739
lumbosacral
anatomy 728, 729, 1640–1
DEXA scan 721
examination 46–7, *47*, 48
function 1640–1
imaging 716, 728–9
innervation 729, 730
orthoses
in eosinophilic granuloma 120
in scoliosis 117–18
osteoarthritis 1535, 1549
osteomyelitis 877–9
in psoriatic arthritis 1076
'railway' 93
stabilization 117, 118, 131
stair-case 301

spine *(continued)*
stenosis 98, 1644
central 1644
foraminal 1644, 1645
treatment 1648
thoracic 90, 91
examination 46
palpation 46
radiography 716, 717
range of movement 46
tophaceous CPPD deposits 1568
trauma in childhood and adolescence 130, 131
tuberculosis 928
childhood 122, 123, 930–1
imaging 122, 123, 717, 930–1
recurrent 122, 123
tumours 99
benign 118–20
childhood 118–21, *121*, *122*
extramedullary 121
intramedullary 121, *121*, *122*
malignant 120–1
metastatic 121
presenting symptoms *121*
see also back pain
spinocerebellar ataxia 695
spinoreticular pathway 487
spinothalamic pathway 487
Spirometra 950
spirometry 247, 248
spleen, lymphocyte circulation through 527
splenectomy
in Felty's syndrome 292, 644, 1015
in SLE 1193
splenomegaly 3, *176*, *258*, *259*
in familial Mediterranean fever 1447
in Felty's syndrome 644
in juvenile chronic arthritis 1116
in mixed connective tissue disease 1418
pseudotumoural 911
in SLE 1157, 1194
splints 1732
in carpal tunnel syndrome 1507
dynamic 1732–3
forearm 1512
hand 1743, 1744
in juvenile chronic arthritis 1108, 1743, 1744, 1747
knee 1732, 1747
paddle 1733
resting 1733
wrist 1732, 1743, 1744
SPOD 1730
spondarthrites/spondylarthritis/
spondyloarthropathy *see* seronegative spondylarthropathies
spondylitis
brucellar 939–41
and enteric arthropathies 1094
in hypoparathyroidism 281
in psoriatic arthritis 1075, 1077
psychiatric involvement 337
spondylodiscitis 758, 766, 1062
spondyloepimetaphyseal dysplasia 368, *369*
collagen protein analysis 373
spondyloepiphyseal dysplasia 1630, 1631, 1632
clinical features 371, 372
collagen protein analysis 373
collagen type II defects 356
gene mutations 353, 370, 413, *435*, 436
molecular analysis 373, 375, 376
spondylolisthesis 97, 98, 126–7, 128, **1645**
congenital 1645
degenerative 126, 1645
dysplastic 126
isthmic 126, 1645
pathological 126, 1645
post-traumatic 1645
surgical 1645

spondylolysis 126–7, **1645**
sclerotic phase 119
spontaneously hypertensive rat 511
sporotrichosis 880, *880*, 916
epidemiology 955
joint infection *955*, 959–60
clinical presentation 956
diagnosis *957*
management *957*
sports injuries 1771, **1779–88**
acute 1780–3
childhood 1786–8
chronic 1783–6
incident rates 1779
prevention 1779–80
sports medicine **1773–8**
'spring' ligament 1512
spumaviruses 908
SSCP 693
ssDNA 667
SSRIs 339, *340*
STA 942–3
stains
muscle biopsy 788
muscle fibre types 460, 462
synovial fluid 658
stair climbing 16
standard tube agglutination test 942–3
standardized response mean 52
Stanford Health Assessment Questionnaire 1724
Stanmore relacement elbow 1703
Stanmore shoulder 1703
stanozolol in osteoporosis 1598
Staphylococcus
antibiotic therapy 856
and back pain 99
and Kawasaki disease 1406
in pyogenic arthritis 849
S. aureus
antibiotics active against 660
arteritis due to 1390
in Brodie's abscess 1620
in discitis of childhood 123, 124
enterotoxin 551, 844
in HIV infection 916, 921
joint infection 661
methicillin-resistant 856, 857, 859, 870, 874
monitoring success of therapy 662
in osteomyelitis 868, 870, *870*, 873, *873*
pulmonary infection 252
in pyogenic arthritis 851–2, *851*, 853, 880, *880*
childhood 861, 862, *862*, 864
in rheumatoid arthritis 1013
and pyomyositis 1265
in septic bursitis 146, 156, 158, 859
in spinal osteomyelitis 121, 122, 124
and Wegener's granulomatosis 1342
S. epidermidis
antibiotic therapy 856
in osteomyelitis 869, 870
in prosthetic joint infection 854
in pyogenic arthritis *851*, 852, *880*
in septic bursitis 859
Starling hypothesis 443
statins
adverse effects 1480
in hyperlipidaemias 1481
'steal' phenomena in Paget's disease 1612
Steinbrocker evaluation 759
Steinmann pin 1704
stenosing tenovaginitis 1505–6
Stenotrophomonas maltophilia 660
sternoclavicular joint
anatomy 135, 137
examination 44
movement 44
pain 1501
in rheumatoid arthritis 1008

sternoclavicular joint *(continued)*
surgery 1702
sternoclavicular ligaments 135
sternum, osteomyelitis 875
steroid necrosis *see* osteonecrosis
Stevens–Johnson syndrome 580
stibogluconate 951
Stickler syndrome 168, 368, **376–7**
clinical features 370–1, 372
genetic factors 353, 355, 356, *369*, 370, 413, 1519
ocular *435*
overlap with multiple epiphyseal dysplasia 353
type I 377
type II 377
Stiedex *210*
stiffness
in ankylosing spondylitis 99
in cervical spondylosis 1653
differential diagnosis 4
and disability 1725
gelling 41, 1521
history-taking and assessment 6–7
in hypothyroidism 277, 278
in osteoarthritis 1521
in polymyalgia rheumatica/giant cell arteritis 1377
in psoriatic arthritis 1073
and quality of life 64
in Sjögren's syndrome 1309
in SLE 1147
still birth
in rheumatoid arthritis 182
in SLE 183
Still's disease
adult-onset 10, **1127**
acute phase response in 641
age-related occurrence *26*
fever 172
and pregnancy 184
systemic features *170*
juvenile *see* juvenile chronic arthritis, systemic-onset
stimulus
innocuous *488*
noxious *488*
stomach
content aspiration 241, 245–6, 305
delayed emptying in scleroderma *258*
stomatitis
aphthous 213
drug-related 207, 212, 213, 214, *584*, *589*
alkylating agents 593
gold therapy 600
penicillamine *598*
punctate 207, 213
and salivary gland biopsy 779
STR 695, *695*
STR mouse in models of osteo-arthritis 416
straight-leg raise 46, 48, 225
crossed 225
Streptobacillus moniliformis in pyogenic arthritis 852, *880*
streptococcal cell-wall arthritis 562, 564–5, 998
Streptococcus
arteritis due to 1390
group A 973–5
classes 973
cross-reactions with mammalian tissues 973–5
in rheumatic fever 972–3, 975–6
infections
antibiotic therapy 856
and Behçet's syndrome 1399
chorea following 979
diagnosis 979–80
in osteomyelitis 868, 870
preceding rheumatic fever 973
in prosthetic joints 854

Streptococcus (continued)
infections *(continued)*
in pyogenic arthritis *851*, 852, 853, 880, *880*
childhood 862, *862*
in septic bursitis 859
strawberry erythema of tongue and lips 204
M proteins 973, 980
M serotypes in rheumatic fever 972–3
pyrogenic toxins 975
S. agalactiae
in osteomyelitis 870
in rheumatoid arthritis *268*
S. milleri in pyogenic arthritis 852
S. pneumoniae
in HIV infection 916
joint infection 661
in osteomyelitis 868, 870
S. pyogenes 659
in rheumatic fever 664
tests for 661
S. sanguis and Kawasaki disease 1405
S. viridans in pyogenic arthritis 852
vaccines against 980
streptolysin O 975
streptomycin
in brucellar arthritis 943
in tuberculosis 931, *932*
stress
management 102
mechanical and bone mass 426
and psychoneuroimmunology 332
stress proteins in rheumatoid synovium 449
stress tests 233
stridor in Wegener's granulomatosis 1335, 1336
stroke 220
and antiphospholipid antibodies 1206
causes in young adults *219*
in Takayasu's arteritis 1385
stromelysins 411, *411*
effect on collagen 515
in osteoarthritis 1538
Strongyloides stercoralis 948
articular syndromes 267, 948–9
and vasculitis 951
stupor 224
styloidectomy, ulna 1721
subacromial bursa 135, 136
in acromegaly 281
bursitis 143, 1503
acute calcific 141
in rheumatoid arthritis 1008
calcification 1528
local steroid injection 1763
subacromial decompression 143, 1702
subacute bacterial endocarditis
diagnosis 1122
rheumatoid factor in *674*
subcalcaneal bursa 154, 156
bursitis 160
subclavian artery 1382
compression 1661
subcoracoid bursa 135
subcorneal pustular dermatosis 206
subcutaneous calcaneal bursa 154, 156
subcutaneous fat necrosis 289
subcutaneous olecranon bursa 137
subcutaneous prepatellar bursa 152
subcutaneous tissue atrophy following local steroid injection 1759
subdeltoid bursa 163
bursitis 163
subglottic stenosis in Wegener's granulomatosis 1406
Subreum 1026
subscapularis 135
subscapularis bursa 135, 136
subscapularis tendon
lesions 1502–3
local steroid injection 1764

substance P 442, 450
in adjuvant arthritis 449–50
degradation 451, 452
expression by joint nerves 490
in fibromyalgia 1498–9
in vitro effects on cells 451
and inflammation 450, 497, 511
interaction with CGRP 451
intra-articular injection 450
in joints 450, 511
pleiotropic effects *511*
in reflex sympathetic dystrophy 1684
in spinal cord neurone activation 496
in synovial fluid 450–1
subtalar joint 153, 1719
compartments 746
examination 50
imaging 746
local steroid injection 1770
range of movement 50
in rheumatoid arthritis 1008–9
subtendinea musculi sartorii bursa 158
'sucked candy' appearance 284
Sudeck's atrophy 1679, *1679*
see also reflex sympathetic dystrophy
sulcus sign 144
sulindac
adverse effects
cutaneous 213, 580, *589*
haematological 295
hepatic 580
neurological *217*
psychiatric 338
renal 327
in calcium pyrophosphate dihydrate disease 1570
in gout 1563
half-life *577*
in juvenile chronic arthritis *1106, 1140*
in lactation 193
metabolism 577
in pregnancy 189, 190
'renal sparing' effect 325, 1695
sulphamethoxazole
in brucellar arthritis 943, *943*
in *Pneumocystis carinii* infection 253
in Wegener's granulomatosis 1345
sulphapyridine in pregnancy 191
sulphasalazine 588–9
adverse effects 588–9, *589*, 647, 1023, 1695
cutaneous 214
gastrointestinal *260*, 261, 588, *589*
haematological 296, 588, *589*
hepatic *589*, 652
hypogammaglobulinaemia 970
lupus-like syndrome 669, *1690*
pulmonary *253*
in ankylosing spondylitis 1067, 1069
in Behçet's syndrome 1401
in combination therapy *1025*
drug interactions 296
in HIV-associated arthritis 921
hypersensitivity to 589
in inflammatory bowel disease 1045
in juvenile chronic arthritis 1107, 1126, 1138, 1140, *1140*
in juvenile spondylarthropathies 1049
in lactation 194, *602*
pharmacology 588
in pregnancy 189, 191, *602*
in psoriatic arthritis 1080
in pyoderma gangrenosum 1461
in reactive arthropathies 1092, *1093*
in rheumatoid arthritis 1022–3
in scleroderma 211
in seropositive juvenile chronic arthritis 1036
therapeutic efficacy 588
therapeutically relevant actions 588
treatment regimens 588
sulphinpyrazone in gout 1565

sulphonamides
adverse effects 914, 1693
drug interactions 582
in pyoderma gangrenosum 1461
sun protection factor 210
sunscreens
in cutaneous lupus erythematosus 211
in dermatomyositis 211, 1277
topical 210
superantigens 551, 612–13, 844, 1305
expansion of discrete T cell populations by 552
streptococcal pyrogenic toxins as 975
superficial peroneal nerve biopsy 793
superficial prepatellar bursa 152
superior extensor retinacula 154, 156
superior peroneal retinacula 154, 156
superoxide
anion generation in synovial hypoxia 447
as endothelium-derived contracting factor 447
in inflammation 514
superoxide dismutase 448
superoxides, effects of NSAIDs on 576
supinator 137
supinator jerk in cervical myelopathy 1656
supplementation therapy 262, *263–4*, 264
supraorbital nerve in leprosy 934
suprapatellar pouch 717
supraspinatus 135, 136, 137
supraspinatus sign 141, 142
supraspinatus tendon 163
local steroid injection 1764
in rheumatoid arthritis 1014
tendinitis 45
sural nerve
biopsy 792, 793
in leprosy 934
surface cells *see* synovial intimal cells
surface markers 73
surgery 1701–9
cervical pain syndromes 1659–60
cervical spine 1705–6
childhood 1721
childhood **1713–21**
consent 1702
and drugs 1702
elbow 1703
childhood 1720
foot and ankle 1706–7
childhood 1718–20
hand 1705
childhood 1720–1
hip 1708–9
childhood 1715–17
juvenile chronic arthritis 1108, 1141
knee 1707–8
childhood 1717–18, 1719
order of 1701–2
osteoarthritis 1548
osteoid osteoma 1618
Paget's disease 1617
patient positioning 301, 1702
planning 1701–2
prophylactic 1701
psoriatic arthritis 1081
reflex sympathetic dystrophy following 1681
rheumatoid arthritis 1026–7
seropositive juvenile chronic arthritis 1036
shoulder 143, 1702–3
childhood 1720
techniques available 1701, 1714, 1715
thoracic outlet syndrome 1661
timing 1701
wrist 1507, 1703–5
childhood 1720–1
surgical clips in MRI 724

swan neck deformity 1008
in juvenile chronic arthritis 1132, 1133, 1741, 1742, 1743
surgery 1705
Swanson silastic wrist prosthesis 1704
sweating in giant cell arteritis 1388
Sweet's syndrome 206, 1396, **1456–8**
swelling
in acromegaly 281
differential diagnosis 4
examination 7
hand 42
history-taking 7
in hypothyroidism 277
palpation 40
in reflex sympathetic dystrophy 1680
wrist 42–3
(SWRxNZB)F$_1$ mice 1162, *1162*
Sydenham's chorea in rheumatic fever 972, 978–9
sympathectomy in reflex sympathetic dystrophy 1687
symphysis pubis 1508
Synalar *210*
synapse, definition *495*
synaptic transmission 494
syncope 231, 237
following exercise 1777
syndesmophytes 1061, 1063
differentiation from osteophytes 1065–6
imaging 734, 735, 736
in psoriatic spondylitis 736, 1075
syndrome of limited joint mobility 282–3, *283*
synechiae 214
synovectomy 1701
elbow joint 1703, 1720
foot 1706
in fungal arthritis 962
hand in childhood 1721
hip 1709
intimal cell generation following 441
in juvenile chronic arthritis 1108
knee 1707
childhood 1718
in Lyme disease 893
in pigmented villonodular synovitis 1620
radiation 1620
in rheumatoid arthritis 1026
shoulder 1702
childhood 1720
in tuberculosis 932, 933
synovial biopsy 775
in ankylosing spondylitis 778
in Behçet's syndrome 778
evaluation 775–7
inflammation 776–7
in juvenile chronic arthritis 778, 1101
in osteoarthritis 778
in pigmented villonodular synovitis 1620
in polymyalgia rheumatica/giant cell arteritis 1377, 1378
and prosthetic joints 778
psoriatic arthritis 778
reflex sympathetic dystrophy 1683
Reiter's disease 778
rheumatoid arthritis 776, 777, 778
sarcoidosis 1466
SLE 1182
technical aspects 775
synovial capillaries 442
in inflammatory disease 443
synovial chondromatosis 166–7, 1618–19
synovial effusion
in hypothyroidism 277
knee 49, 50
in sarcoidosis 1466
synovial fluid 441, 442–3, 677
acidosis in synovial inflammation 444
agglutination reaction 679

synovial fluid (continued)
aspiration see arthrocentesis
in bacterial infection 683
in Behçet's syndrome 1399
in brucellar arthritis 941
in calcium pyrophosphate dihydrate
  disease 681, 682, 684, 1568
carbon dioxide tension (PCO$_2$) in synovial inflammation 444
characteristics 681
clotting 681
colour 680
complement, in rheumatoid arthritis
  1015–16
components 442, 677
crystals 682
  examination 679
and differential diagnosis 681
eosinophilia 682, 682
fibrinogen 677, 681
formation 442–3, 677
function 677
in fungal arthritis 956
  Candida infection 958
  coccidioidomycosis 961
  sporotrichal 960
glucose 677, 679
  in synovial inflammation 444
gonococcal arthritis 855
in gout 677, 682, 683–4, 1561
haemorrhagic 682, 682
hypothyroidism 277
in inflammation 508
juvenile chronic arthritis 683, 1101
lactate, in synovial inflammation 444
lactate dehydrogenase 679
leukaemia 289
in Lyme disease 888
malignant cells in 288
mycoplasma arthritis 968–9
non-gonococcal arthritis 850–1
NSAID kinetics 577
opaque 679, 680
osteoarthritis 682–3
oxygen tension (PO$_2$), in synovial
  inflammation 444
in pigmented villonodular synovitis
  1620
in polymyalgia rheumatica/giant cell
  arteritis 1378
protein 443, 679
pyogenic arthritis 850–1, 855, 857
  childhood 862
reactive arthropathies 1088
Reiter's syndrome 683
in rheumatic fever 977
rheumatoid arthritis 443–4, 683, 988,
  1016
rheumatoid factor 679
septic bursitis 859
short-chain fatty acids 679
in SLE 1147
  childhood 1182
specimens 658–9
  collection and transportation 679
string test 679
substance P 450–1
translucent 679, 680
transparent 679, 680
turbidity 680
viral arthropathies 683
viscosity 481, 514, 679, 680
in Whipple's disease 1095
synovial fluid analysis 677–84, 1758
differential white-cell count 680, 681–2
in differentiation of osteoarthritis from
  rheumatoid arthritis in the elderly
  33
free radical damage 447–8
indications for 677–8
interpretation of results 680–2, 681,
  682
leucocyte count 679, 680, 681–2
  bacterial infection 683

synovial fluid analysis (continued)
leucocyte count (continued)
  calcium pyrophosphate crystal
    deposition disease 684
  gout 683
  in juvenile chronic arthritis 683
  in osteoarthritis 682, 683
  in rheumatoid arthritis 683
  viral arthropathies 683
mucin clot test 680–1
procedures 679–80
reliability 680
synovial hypoxia 444–5
acute exacerbation of chronic hypoxia
  445–6
biochemical consequences 446–7
effects on endothelial cells 447–8
factors limiting damage 448–51
free radical generation and actions
  446–8
leucocyte chemotaxis and adhesion 448
microvascular barrier function 448
synovial intimal cells 441, 776
effect of substance P on 451
in inflammation 443
metabolism in inflammation 445
type A 441, 776
type B 441, 776
synovial joints 441–3
coefficients of friction 477, 480, 481
dynamic analysis 479
forces
  direct measurement 480
  during locomotion 479–80
  static analysis 477–9
hypoxia 444–51
in inflammatory disease 443–52
intra-articular pressure 443, 446
  in acute trauma 449
  in inflammation 443, 446
involvement in rheumatoid arthritis
  988, 989
ischaemia 444–51
ischaemic–reperfusion injury 445, 449
kinematic analysis 479
loads 477
lubrication 480–2
  boosted 481
  boundary 480, 481
  elastohydrodynamic (EHL/EHD)
    480, 481
  full-fluid film 480, 481
  hydrodynamic 480, 481
  hydrostatic/externally pressurized
    480, 481
  mixed 480, 481
  in osteoarthritis 484
  squeeze film 480, 481
  studies 479–81
  theoretical analysis 481–2
  weeping 481
mathematical models 478–9
mechanics 477–80
surface elasticity 481
synovial lining cells see synovial intimal
  cells
synovial membrane 405, 441
synovial sarcoma 288, 1671
synoviocytes see synovial intimal cells
synovioma, malignant 742, 1671,
  1671
synovitis 508–9
in bone malignancy 288
chronic, lymphocytes in 527
in classification 843
cricoarytenoid joint 242
foreign body 1104
hip 5, 164
histology 443
ischaemia and hypoxia 444–51
in juvenile chronic arthritis 1134, 1135
in osteoarthritis 1521
in polymyalgia rheumatica/giant cell
  arteritis 1377

synovitis (continued)
in reflex sympathetic dystrophy 449,
  1683, 1684, 1686
in Sjögren's syndrome 1309
Strongyloides 949
synovial nerve supply 443–4
synovial vasculature 443, 777
and tissue specificity of inflammation
  508
toxic 19, 164
see also pigmented villonodular synovitis
**synovitis, acne, palmoplantar pustu-
  losis, hyperostosis, aseptic
  osteomyelitis** 1091
synovium 405, 441–3
areolar 441
biopsy see synovial biopsy
cellular morphology 441
fatty 441
fibroareolar 441
fibrous 441
in fungal arthritis 956
hyperplasia 508, 776
in hypothyroidism 277
imaging 771
infection 849
in inflammatory disease
  biopsy 776–7
  factors limiting hypoxic damage 448
  free radical actions 447–8
  histology 443–4
  hypoxia 444–51
  ischaemia 444–51
  leucocyte chemotaxis and adhesion
    448
  metabolism 445
  microvascular barrier function 448
  nerve supply 443–4
  neuropeptides 450–2
  vascular system 423
lymphocyte recruitment to 528
nerve endings 489
nerve supply 442, 444, 511
  in inflammatory disease 443–4
  in osteoarthritis 1541–2
  in rheumatoid arthritis 988, 989
in SLE 1147
in systemic sclerosis 1238
tumours 741
vascular system 442
  biopsy 776, 777
  in inflammatory disease 443
syphilis
cutaneous ulceration 207
ocular involvement 316–17
rheumatoid factor in 674
syringomyelia
cutaneous ulceration 207
presentation 219, 220
reflex sympathetic dystrophy following
  1681
rheumatic symptoms 218
systemic disease 3
systemic features of rheumatic disease
  169–79
relevance to anaesthesia and preanaesthetic assessment 299–301
systemic lupus activity measures
  1160, 1160
systemic lupus erythematosus (SLE)
  1145–76
acute phase response 628, 640
adhesion molecules 1168, 1169
adverse reactions to NSAIDs 580
age at onset 12, 13, 26, 1146, 1159, 1181
anaesthesia in 299, 300
animal models 1162–3, 1162, 1668
  treatment 1175–6
and antiphospholipid syndrome 294,
  642, 1159–60, 1159
anxiety in 336, 337
apoptosis in 1168
assessment of disease activity 59, 838,
  1160, 1160, 1161, 1162

systemic lupus erythematosus (SLE)
  (continued)
autoantibodies 669–71, 1163–5
  childhood 1197
  in the elderly 35, 35, 1159
  in pregnancy 183–4, 189
  see also under specific autoantibodies
and autoimmune thyroid disease 279,
  1157
biochemical tests 649
cardiovascular involvement 173, 230,
  231–3, 234, 236, 1149, 1151, 1483–4
cell abnormalities and dysregulation
  1165–8, 1166, 1167, 1168
childhood 1180–99
  autoantibodies 1197
  cardiac involvement 1194–5, 1196
  clinical features 1181
  diagnosis 19
  endocrine involvement 1197
  gastrointestinal involvement 1196
  haematological involvement 1192–4,
    1193
  incidence 1180–1
  liver disease in 1196–7
  mucocutaneous involvement 1182–3,
    1184
  musculoskeletal involvement 1181–2
  neuropsychiatric 1184–7, 1185
  onset 11
  prognosis 1187
  pulmonary involvement 1195–6,
    1195, 1196
  renal involvement 1187–92, 1187,
    1188, 1192
  sex differences 12, 14
classification 1145
clinical features 1146–57, 1414
  incidence 1145, 1148
comparison with drug-induced lupus
  1691
complement components in 322, 506–
  8, 507, 512, 654, 1169–70, 1170
complications 222, 1157
cutaneous involvement 837, 1147–9,
  1149, 1150
cytokines in 640, 1167–8, 1167
definition 1145
depression in 336, 337
diagnosis 178
diagnostic criteria 812, 833, 1145, 1147
differential diagnosis 1122, 1136, 1137
drug-related 598
in the elderly 35–6, 35, 1159
endocrine influences 510
epidemiology 814, 1145–6
  effect of age 12, 14, 815, 837, 1146
erythema 199, 201
ethnic groups 819, 819, 833, 835–8, 836,
  837, 1169
fatigue in 59, 64–5, 1146–7
gastrointestinal involvement 257, 258
genetic factors 350–1, 351, 507, 822,
  1169–72, 1170
haematological involvement 291–2,
  641–2, 641, 642, 643, 1155–6
history 1146
hyperlipidaemias in 1194, 1483–4
immune complexes in 507, 704, 710,
  711, 1147, 1152, 1164–5
immune system in 251
immunopathology 1162–72
incidence 1320
investigation 202
large vessel vasculitis in 1391
liver function 652
in males 1158, 1159
and malignant disease 1160, 1160, 1194,
  1668
menstrual, hormonal and reproductive
  factors 823
musculoskeletal involvement 472, 791,
  1147, 1149, 1157, 1182, 1612
and myasthenia gravis 1157

systemic lupus erythematosus (SLE) (continued)
  natural history 1145–6
  neuropsychiatric 218, 333, *333*, 671,
    1153, 1155, 1156
    assessment 333–4
    childhood 1184–7, *1185*
    clinical features 333
    diagnosis 334
    differential diagnosis 221, *222*
    in the elderly 1159
    investigation 221, 334–5, 1185–6
    laboratory correlates *334*
    pathogenesis 219–20
    treatment 221–2, *223*, 335, 1186–7
  ocular involvement 312–13, 314, 1153
  oral and palatal ulceration 207
  osteonecrosis in 1147, 1182, 1622
  papular 204
  peripheral neuropathies 227, 1153
  platelet abnormalities 292, 641–2, *641*
  and pregnancy 182–4, 189, 1157, 1159
  prognosis 1176
  progression to thrombotic thrombo-
    cytopenic purpura 329
  pulmonary involvement 173, 241, *241*,
    242, 243, 245, *1150*, 1151–2
  renal involvement *see* lupus nephritis
  and rheumatoid arthritis 1157
  rheumatoid factor in *674*
  risk of infection in 1157
  and salmonella-induced arthritis 852
  sex ratio/distribution 12, 14, *815*, 837,
    1146, 1169
  and Sjögren's syndrome 1157, 1159
  thrombosis in 294, 642
  transverse myelitis in 225, 1153
  treatment 1172, *1172*, *1173*, 1175–6
  vasculitis *786*, 1148, 1150, 1152, 1156,
    1157
Systemic Lupus International
  Collaborating Clinics damage
  index 1160, *1161*, 1162
systemic sclerosis 1217–44
  aetiology 1219–25, *1223*, *1224*
  age at onset 13, *26*
  autoantibodies 36, 665, *668*, 671–3, *671*,
    1219, 1222–3, *1225*
  and autoimmunity 1220–3, 1225, *1225*
  cardiovascular involvement *230*, 233,
    234, 235, 1232–5, *1234*
  childhood 14, 1751
  classification 1218, *1220*
  clinical features *1414*
  cutaneous involvement 201, 207, 211–
    12, 1230–1
  diagnostic criteria *812*, 1217–18
  diffuse cutaneous 1218, *1220*
    management 1243
  drug-related *1223*
  early stage 1218, *1221*
  in the elderly 36
  epidemiology *814*, 1218–19, *1222*
    effect of age and sex 14, *815*
    genetic factors *822*
    menstrual, hormonal and reproduc-
      tive factors *823*
    time trends 817, 818
  gastrointestinal involvement 1232, *1233*
  and hyperlipidaemias 1484
  imaging 1235–6
  impotence *1239*
  investigation 204
  laboratory tests *649*
  late stage 1218, *1221*
  limited cutaneous 1218, *1220*
    management 1244
  liver function 652, *1239*
  and malignant disease 1669–70
  musculoskeletal involvement 790, 1238,
    1424–5
  nervous system involvement *1239*
  ocular involvement 313
  overlap syndromes 1424–5

systemic sclerosis (continued)
  pathogenesis 1225–7
  and pregnancy 184, 1238–40
  psychiatric involvement 337
  pulmonary involvement 241, *241*, 245,
    250, *1234*, 1235–7
  and Raynaud's phenomenon 1226, 1229
  renal involvement *321*, 324, 328–9,
    1237–8
  rheumatoid factor in *674*
  sine scleroderma 1217, *1220*
  thyroid function *1239*
  treatment 1240–4, *1244*
  vascular lesions 1226–7

T

T-cell receptor 546, 550
  allelic variation 551
  α/β 550
  blocking 611
  in classification of rheumatic diseases
    844
  in collagen-induced arthritis 564
  contributions to rheumatic disease
    551–2
  γ/δ 550
  genes 550–1
    TCRAV 551
    TCRBV 551
    in juvenile chronic arthritis 700
    polymorphism 700
  interaction with MHC 551
  interaction with MHC-peptide
    complex 546, 844, 984
  in juvenile chronic arthritis 1110
  monoclonal antibodies to 612–13
  in polymyositis/dermatomyositis 1268
  repertoire 551
  in Sjögren's syndrome 1305
  in SLE 1165–6, *1170*, 1171
T-cell vaccination 563
T cells
  in adaptive immunity 545–6
  antigen processing and presentation to
    549–50
  antigen recognition 549, 608–9
  antigen-specific activation 546
  CD3+ in Dupuytren's contracture 148
  CD3+CD8+Leu7+ 644
  CD4+ *see* helper T cells
  CD8+ *see* cytotoxic T cells
  CD29 990
  CD45RO+ 990
  circulation and migration 527
  double-negative 1163, 1165
  in drug-induced lupus 1692
  effect of alkylating agents on 592, *592*
  effect of azathioprine on 590, *590*
  effect of corticosteroids on *586*
  effect of cyclosporin on 594–5, *594*
  effect of gold therapy on 599, *600*
  effect of methotrexate on 582–3, *583*
  effect of penicillamine on 597, *597*
  effect of sulphasalazine on 588
  expansion of populations by super-
    antigens 552
  in HIV infection 907, 909, 910–11
  immunosuppressive therapy strategies
    involving 609, 611–13
  inactivation 611–13
  in inflammation 503
  in juvenile dermatomyositis 1293, 1294
  in leprosy 933
  mediation of growth 994
  in mixed connective tissue disease 1421
  in polymyalgia rheumatica/giant cell
    arteritis 1376–7, 1379
  in polymyositis/dermatomyositis 1268,
    1269
  prevention of circulation 613
  in psoriatic arthritis 1078–9
  in rheumatic fever 976, *976*

T-cells (continued)
  in rheumatoid arthritis
    activation 990–2
    differentiation 990
  in sarcoidosis 1464
  in scleroderma 1221–2
  in Sjögren's syndrome 1304–5
  in SLE 1165–7, *1166*
  subsets
    circulation and migration 527
    and cytokines 520
    susceptibility to free radical attack 447
  in synovial biopsy 776
  in Takayasu's arteritis 1386–7
  in Wegener's granulomatosis 1344
T-score 720
T tubules 456, 457
tabes dorsalis *218*
table top test 147
tac protein 518
tachykinins 450
tachysterol 1602
tacrolimus in pyoderma gangre-
  nosum 1461
taeniasis *948*
  articular syndromes associated 947
  muscular syndromes associated 950
  and reactive arthritis 267
Takayasu's arteritis 786–7, 1382,
  1383–8
  aetiology 1386–7
  age at onset 12, 13
  assessment 1385–6
  cardiovascular involvement *230*, 233,
    238, 1385
  central nervous system disease in *223*
  childhood 1385
  classification *1321*, *1322*
  clinical features 1385, *1385*
  definition 1384
  diagnosis 21
  diagnostic criteria 1326–7, *1326*, 1384,
    1384
  differential diagnosis 1389
  epidemiology 14, 1383, 1384
  imaging 764
  immunopathology 1386–7
  laboratory tests 1386
  and pregnancy 1388
  prognosis 1329, 1388
  sex ratio/distribution 14, 1384
  treatment 1387
  vertebrobasilar insufficiency in *223*
talocalcaneal coalition/synostosis 167,
  746, 758, 768
talocalcaneal joint *see* subtalar joint
'talon noir' 207
talonavicular joint 153, 1719
talus 153, 154
tamoxifen 1693
Tanner–Whitehouse method for
  assessment of skeletal matura-
  tion 78, 79, 81
TAP1 549
TAP2 549
***TAP* genes**
  and juvenile chronic arthritis 1110
  TAP1 696
  TAP2 696
Taq polymerase 691, 692
tar
  in psoriasis 1079
  topical preparations 212
target lesions 200, 205, 206
tarsal coalition 167, 746, 768
tarsal tunnel syndrome 154, 160, 227,
  1512
  electrodiagnosis 805
  local steroid injection 1770
  in rheumatoid arthritis 1013
tarsometatarsal joint of Lisfranc 153,
  154
  dislocation 284
Tarui's disease 1774

taste alterations
  in methotrexate therapy *584*
  in penicillamine therapy *598*
***tat* gene** 909
tat protein 909–10
Tauri's disease 473
***tax* gene** 1302
tazobactam in osteomyelitis 874
TCA cycle in inflamed synovia 445
tears
  break-up time 1309
  supplements 310, 1314
technetium scan *see* radionuclide
  scanning
teichopsia in SLE 1153
teicoplanin in osteomyelitis 874
telangiectasia *174*, *201*, 207
  corticosteroid-induced 211, 214
  cosmetic camouflage 210
  differential diagnosis 1291
  in mixed connective tissue disease 1417
  periungual 1291
temperature sense, loss of 218
temporal arteritis *see* giant cell arteritis
temporal artery
  angiography 1376
  biopsy 783
    evaluation *783*, 784–5, *784*
    following steroid treatment 785, *785*
    giant cell arteritis 783–5, *783*, *784*,
      785, 1376–7, *1376*
    indications for 785
    large vessel vasculitis 1383
    polymyalgia rheumatica 1376–7, *1376*
    technical aspects 784
  Doppler ultrasound 1378
temporomandibular arthritis *258*
temporomandibular joint
  in ankylosing spondylitis 1062
  examination 45
  in juvenile chronic arthritis 82, 302,
    1100, 1116, 1134, 1135, 1739–40
  local steroid injection 1770–1
  physiotherapy in childhood 1739–40
  in rheumatoid arthritis 1009
tendinitis 1492
  calcific 1574
  in calcium pyrophosphate dihydrate
    disease 1529
  in the elderly 37
  histology 1493
  in hyperlipidaemias 1481
  see also specific tendons
tendons
  blood supply 1492
  composition and function 1492
  fibre weave 1492
  hands 41–2
  histology 1492–4
  innervation 1492
  in rheumatoid arthritis 1014
  rupture 1492
    in calcium pyrophosphate dihydrate
      disease 1529
    following local steroid injection 1759
    in SLE 1147
  structure 457
  tensile strength 1492
tenidap 615, 1026
tennis elbow 5, 43, 144–5, 1504–5, *1505*
  bands 145
  childhood 163
  epidemiology 1491
  local steroid injection 145, 1764
  occupationally induced 1494
tenocytes 1492
tenosynovectomy in rheumatoid
  arthritis 1026
tenosynovitis 1492, 1505, 1506
  ankle tendons 744, 745
  de Quervain's 43, 146, 1492, 1506
    childhood 163
    local steroid injection 1766
    pain in 5

tenosynovitis (continued)
  in disseminated gonococcal infection
      855
  extensor
      local steroid injection 1766
      in rheumatoid arthritis 1008
  flexor 41
      in hypothyroidism 277, 278
      local steroid injection 1766, 1767–8
      occupationally induced 1494
      pain 5
  in fungal arthritis 956
  in hyperlipidaemias 1481
  in hypogammaglobulinaemia 970
  in juvenile chronic arthritis 1116, 1134,
      1135
  in psoriatic arthritis 1075
  in sarcoidosis 1466
  in SLE 1147, 1149, 1181
  stenosing digital see trigger finger/thumb
  tibialis posterior tendon complex
      153–4
tenoxicam
  half-life 577
  in pregnancy 190
TENS see transcutaneous electrical nerve
      stimulation
teres major 135, 137
teres minor 135, 137
terfenadine, contraindications to 957
terminal cysternae 456
terminal/distal motor latency 800
ternary complex 546, 844, 984
testicular development 14, 17
testosterone
  and bone mass 426, 1589
  in osteoporosis 1598
  in rheumatoid arthritis 182
  in SLE 510
tetracycline 660
  in brucellar arthritis 943
  fluorescence 780, 783
  intrabursal in inflammatory olecranon
      bursitis 146
  preceding bone biopsy 780, 783
  in Sjögren's syndrome 1314
  in Whipple's disease 1095
TFCQ 55, 55
TFIIIA 348
Thailand, prevalence of seronegative
      spondylarthropathies 839
thalamic neurones 489, 496–7
thalamic pain syndrome 6
thalassaemias 350, 1104
thalidomide 188, 189, 211, 601, 603
  in Behçet's syndrome 1400
  in leprosy 935
  structure 601
thanatophoric dwarfism 369, 369,
      396–8
theatre sign 159
Theiler's murine encephalomyelitis
      virus 1289
thenar muscle atrophy in rheumatoid
      arthritis 1008
thermocoagulation, osteoid osteoma
      1618
thermography 203
  Paget's disease 1614
  reflex sympathetic dystrophy 1683,
      1683, 1685
  tennis elbow 145
Thieffry–Kohler acro-osteolysis 1636
Thiemann's disease 1635
6-thioguanine in scleroderma 1240
thiol protease inhibitor function in
      inflammation 624
thiotepa, adverse effects 1694
Thomas's test 48
thoracic lung volume 248, 249
thoracic outlet syndrome 227, 805,
      1660–1, 1660
thoracotomy, scoliosis following 115
thrombin 512

thrombocytopenia 292, 645
  and antiphospholipid antibodies 293
  and antiphospholipid syndrome 1207,
      1213
  autoimmune 645
  as contraindication to local steroid
      injection 1758
  differential diagnosis 1208–9
  drug-related 295, 296, 297, 578, 580,
      645
      alkylating agents 593
      azathioprine 590, 591
      gold therapy 601, 1022
      penicillamine 598, 599
  in Felty's syndrome 645
  in juvenile chronic arthritis 1120
  in mixed connective tissue disease 1419
  in sarcoidosis 1465
  in Sjögren's syndrome 1312
  in SLE 292, 641, 1156, 1193
  treatment 1213
thrombocytopenic purpura
  idiopathic 207, 285
  in SLE 1193
thrombocytosis 292, 644–5
  in adult-onset Still's disease 1127
  drug-related 296
  in Henoch–Schönlein purpura 1407
  in juvenile chronic arthritis 1119–20
  in Kawasaki disease 1405
  in polymyalgia rheumatica/giant cell
      arteritis 1378
thromboembolism 176
  and antiphospholipid antibodies 293
thrombomodulin in Wegener's granu-
      lomatosis 1339
thrombophlebitis
  in Behçet's syndrome 1397–8
  imaging 763, 765
  in SLE 1152
thrombosis 176
  in antiphospholipid syndrome 222,
      1204–6, 1205–6, 1210–12
  cerebral 222, 1205–6
  differential diagnosis 1208, 1208
  drug-related 587
  laboratory tests 1208
  mediating factors 512
  recurrent 293
  in SLE 294, 642
thrombospondin gene family 368
thrombotic thrombocytopenic
      purpura
  acute renal failure in 329
  differential diagnosis 1209
  ischaemic glomerular damage in 324
  penicillamine-induced 214
  in SLE 1193
thromboxane 183, 1480
  in inflammation 515
thumb
  interphalangeal joint 138, 140
  metacarpophalangeal joint 139
  movements 138
  z-deformity 1705, 1741
  see also trigger finger/thumb
thymectomy in polymyositis/derma-
      tomyositis 1277
thymine 689
thymopentin in juvenile chronic
      arthritis 1126
thyroid
  disorders 277–81
      autoimmune 279, 1157, 1311
      in systemic sclerosis 1239
thyroid acropachy 278–9, 279, 280
thyroiditis, autoimmune 279
thyrotoxicosis 219, 278–9
  differential diagnosis 1379
  and osteoporosis 278–9, 279, 1589
  in SLE 1197
thyroxine
  in calcium homeostasis 431
  effect on osteoclasts 425

thyroxine (continued)
  and osteoporosis 1589
tiaprofenic acid
  enantiomers 577
  half-life 577
tibia 153, 156
  stress fracture 163
tibialis anterior pain 1512
tibialis posterior, fasciitis 1786
tibialis posterior tendon
  complex 153–4
  rupture 745
tibiocalcaneal ligament 153
tibionavicular ligament 153
tibiotalar joint 153
tick bites 894
tidemark 405
tiludronate in Paget's disease 1615,
      1616
TIMP 411, 515, 1538–9, 1544
Tinel's sign 160, 226, 1765, 1770
tinnitus
  in cervical spondylosis 1653
  in Paget's disease 1612
  in SLE 1153
'tintack' scales 206
tiopronine in juvenile chronic
      arthritis 1138, 1140, 1140
tiptoe walking 16–17
tissue inhibitor of metalloproteinase
      411, 515, 1538–9, 1544
tissue plasminogen activator in innate
      immunity 545
titanium dioxide in sunscreens 210
titin 455, 463
TLC see total lung capacity
TLCO 248–9
TMEV 1289
TNF-α see tumour necrosis factors,
      TNF-α
TNF-β see tumour necrosis factors,
      TNF-β
TNF-binding protein 995–6
toes
  claw 1748
  examination 51
  hammer 1229, 1748
Togaviridae 899
tolmetin
  adverse effects 217, 338
  half-life 577
  in juvenile chronic arthritis 1106, 1106,
      1124, 1140
  in juvenile spondylarthropathies 1049
  in lactation 193
  in psoriatic arthritis 1080
  in seropositive juvenile chronic
      arthritis 1035
  in SLE 1182
Tolosa–Hunt syndrome 1340
toluene and scleroderma 1223
tongue
  'geographical' 207
  strawberry erythema 174, 204
  ulceration 207
'toothache' 173, 174
tophi
  in calcium pyrophosphate dihydrate
      disease 1529, 1530, 1568
  gouty 208, 1560–1
  radiography 1560, 1562, 1563
  surgical removal 1565
Topilar 210
Toronto Functional Capacity
      Questionnaire 55, 55
torticollis
  acute 45
  in juvenile chronic arthritis 1100, 1134,
      1135, 1721
  in Parkinson's disease 219
total iron binding capacity 634
  in anaemia of chronic disease 637–8
total lung capacity (TLC) 247, 249
  in polymyositis/dermatomyositis 1252

total respiratory pressures 248
tourniquet palsy 803, 803
toxic epidermal necrolysis 205, 213,
      214, 578
toxic oil syndrome 1220, 1223, 1425–7,
      1694
  aetiology 1427
  clinical features 1425–6, 1426
  epidemiology 1425
  laboratory tests 1426, 1427
  myopathy in 1266
  pathogenesis 1427
  prognosis 1427
  treatment 1427
toxic shock syndrome toxin 1 551
Toxocara canis 948
  articular syndromes associated 949
  muscular syndromes associated 950–1
Toxoplasma gondii 946
  articular syndromes associated 946
  muscular syndromes associated 947
  and polymyositis/dermatomyositis
      1267, 1288
  tests for 661
  vascular syndromes associated 947
trabecular hypertrophy 483
tracheostomy
  elective 305
  in relapsing polychondritis 1627
traction
  cervical 1658
  in low back pain 104
traction spurs 730
transcription factors 348–9
transcutaneous electrical nerve
      stimulation (TENS)
  in back pain 105, 1648
  in cervical pain syndromes 1658
transfer factor in Behçet's syndrome
      1401
transferrin 624, 633, 634
  in anaemia of chronic disease 291,
      637–8
  receptor 634
      in anaemia of chronic disease 638
  saturation 637–8
transforming growth factors
  effect on osteoclasts 424, 425
  TGF-α
      and angiogenesis 509
      in neoplastic hypercalcaemia 437
  TGF-β
      and angiogenesis 509
      in animal models of arthritis 564,
          569
      in Dupuytren's contracture 148
      effect on cartilage 415
      effect on chondrocytes 413, 1543
      modulation of acute phase protein
          synthesis 623
      in pyrophosphate elaboration 1570
      in rheumatoid arthritis 997
      role in cartilage and bone formation
          427
      synthesis by bone cells 424
transgenic mice, animal models of
      arthritis 567–8, 999
transient ischaemic attacks 219, 220
  in antiphospholipid syndrome 222
transition clinic 13
transitional fibroblastic zone 989–90
transplant arthropathy 1566, 1695
transplantation antigens 547
transthyretin 624, 1433, 1434, 1438, 1439
transverse carpal ligament 137–8, 156
transverse ligament 150
transverse midtarsal joint of Chopart
      153, 154
transverse myelitis
  in antiphospholipid syndrome 222,
      225, 1207
  in Lyme disease 888
  in mixed connective tissue disease 1418
  in Sjögren's syndrome 1311

transverse myelitis *(continued)*
  in SLE 225, 1153, 1185
tranylcypromine 340
trapezium 138
trapezius 135, 137
trauma *1104*
  and back pain 107
  childhood 20
  osteoarthritis following 1519–20
  psoriatic arthritis following 1079
  reflex sympathetic dystrophy following 1681
traumatic arthritis 865
trazodone 340
  plasma concentrations *342*
  in rheumatoid arthritis 342
treadmill test 233, 249
tremor in SLE 1184
Trendelenburg sign 46
Treponema pallidum, arteritis due to 1390
triamcinolone *585*
  in Behçet's syndrome 1400
  in discoid lupus erythematosus 211
  in juvenile chronic arthritis 1107, 1141
  in juvenile spondylarthropathies 1049
  in nodular vasculitis 1371
  in panniculitis 1455
  in pyoderma gangrenosum 210
  in rheumatoid arthritis 1024
  in scleroderma 211
triamcinolone acetonide injection 1757, 1760
triamcinolone hexacetonide injection 1757, 1760
triangular fibrocartilage of the wrist 137, 138, 741
tricalcium phosphate 1570
tricarboxylic acid cycle in inflamed synovia 445
triceps 137
triceps jerk in cervical myelopathy 1656
triceps tendinitis 146
trichinosis *948*, 951
trichlorethylene *1223*
trichorhinophalangeal dysplasia 1631, 1633
Trichosporon beigelii 963
Trichuris trichiura 948, 949
trigeminal neuropathy
  in mixed connective tissue disease 1418
  in SLE 1184
trigger finger/thumb 42, 147, 1506
  childhood 163
  and diabetes mellitus 284–5
  local steroid injection 1767–8
trigger points 1496, 1497–8, 1653, 1657–8
triglycerides 1773
  in rheumatic disorders 1482
  transport 1479
  uptake of NSAIDs 577
trimethoprim
  in brucellar arthritis 943, *943*
  effect on creatinine clearance 325
  in *Pneumocystis carinii* infection 253
  in Wegener's granulomatosis 1345
trimipramine *340*
  dosage 341
  plasma concentrations *342*
triple response 511
triquetrum 137
trochanteric bursa 150, 151
  bursitis *5*, 156–7, 165, 1508
  local steroid injection 157, 1768
trochleo-ulnar articulation 137
Tropheryma whippelii 255, *256, 259*, 1095
tropomyosin 455
troponin 455
trypanosomiasis *946*
  muscle wasting in 947
  rheumatoid factor in *674*

l-tryptophan 207
  toxicity 227, 1220, *1265*, 1266, 1425–8, 1694
tuberculin skin-test reaction 927, 930
tuberculosis 252–3, **927–33**
  back pain in 97, 99
  clinical manifestations 927–9
  cystic 929
  diagnosis 929–31
  differential diagnosis *1104*
  drug resistance 933
  epidemiology 927
  hip 770
  in HIV infection 927
  imaging 122, 123, 717, 930–1
  immunology 927
  investigations 929–31
  pathogenesis 927
  rheumatoid factor in *674*
  sacroiliitis in 738
  spinal 928
    childhood 122, 123, 930–1
    imaging 122, 123, 717, 930–1
    recurrent 122, 123
  treatment 931–3, *932*
tumour lysis syndrome 1558, 1565
tumour necrosis factor/Fas(CD95) receptor gene family 350
tumour necrosis factors
  and bone formation *424*
  as chemokines 534
  effect on endothelial cells 536
  genes 504–5
    TNFA 504
    TNFA1 504
    TNFA2 504–5
  in inflammation 508, 509, 516–18
  in neoplastic hypercalcaemia *437*
  receptors
    family 520, 521
    in rheumatoid arthritis 988
  TNF-α *519*
    in acute phase response 623, 638
    in anaemia of chronic disease 635
    and angiogenesis 449, 509
    in animal models of arthritis 564, 568–9
    antagonists 1024
    effect on cartilage 414, 1543–4, *1543*
    effect on lipoprotein lipase activity 1483
    gene 548
    in inflammation 510, 517, 520
    in juvenile chronic arthritis 1120–1
    in osteoporosis 1587
    in rheumatoid arthritis 521, 993, *993*, 994–5, 996, 1016, *1017*
    in sarcoidosis 1464
    in SLE 640, 1167–8
    therapeutic in rheumatoid arthritis 415
    and weight loss in rheumatoid arthritis 171
  TNF-β *437*, *519*
    in acute phase response 623
    gene 548
    in rheumatoid arthritis 993, *993*
    in SLE 1167
Turner's syndrome and osteoporosis 129
tyrosine hydroxylase 451

U

U1RNP proteins 669, 672
  see also anti-U1RNP antibodies
ulcerative colitis 1045, **1093–4**
  childhood 1054
  erythema nodosum in 1451
  pustules 1458, 1459
  and pyoderma gangrenosum 1460
  rheumatic manifestations *256*
ulcers
  bowel *578*

ulcers *(continued)*
  conjunctival 1396
  cutaneous *201*, 207, 1011
    in antiphospholipid syndrome 1207
    in dermatomyositis 1252, 1253
    differential diagnosis 1461
    in microscopic polyangiitis 1354
    in polyarteritis nodosa 1353
    in pyoderma gangrenosum 1458
    in Sjögren's syndrome 1311
    in SLE 1156
    treatment 210
  decubitus 876
  digital 211, 212
  gastrointestinal 578, *578*, *587*, 1020
  genital 207
    in Behçet's syndrome 207, 1395
    drug-induced 215
  in leprosy 934
  lower limb
    and antiphospholipid antibodies 293
    in Takayasu's arteritis 1385
  mucosal *591*, 1398
  nasal 1148, 1150, 1183
  neurotropic 207
  oesophageal 1398
  oral 173, *174*, 207, *584*, *601*
    in Behçet's syndrome 207, 1395
    in psoriatic arthritis 1076
    in SLE 1183
    in Wegener's granulomatosis 1335
  scalp 207
  vaginal *175*, 178
  vasculitic *175*
ulna 136, 137, 138
  distal excision 1703
  styloid process 137, 138
  styloidectomy 1721
ulnar artery 138
ulnar collateral ligament 137, 138, 140
ulnar nerve 137, 138
  entrapment 226–7
    electrodiagnosis 805
    local steroid injection 1765
    in rheumatoid arthritis 1013
  in leprosy 934, 935
  Martin–Gruber anastomosis 807
  mononeuropathy *219*
  motor nerve conduction studies 800
  palsy *803*
  transposition 805, 1703
ulnar tunnel 138
ulnar tunnel syndrome 1507
ulnar vein 138
ultracentrifugation of immune complexes 705
ultrasound **720–2**
  ankle 744
  bone density measurement 1594, *1595*
  childhood 764, 862
  knee 721, 722
  osteoarthritis 1536
  polymyositis/dermatomyositis 1261
  prenatal diagnosis of osteogenesis imperfecta 698
  pyogenic arthritis 862
  renal
    in haematuria 324
    in urinary flow obstruction 326
  rheumatoid arthritis 1017, 1018
  sarcoidosis 1466
  shoulder 140, 722, 739
    frozen 143–4
    rotator cuff tear 140, 142
  Takayasu's arteritis 1386
  therapeutic in golfer's/tennis elbow 145, 1505
ultraviolet A irradiation in psoriasis 1079
ultraviolet B irradiation in pityriasis lichenoides 1372
umphalitis 1470
umphalocele 1470

upper limb *(continued)*
  applied anatomy **135–40**
  lymphoedema in psoriatic arthritis 1076
  pain
    adults *139–40*, **140–8**
    childhood 19, *19*, 162, **162–3**, *163*
    referred from cervical spine 1653
  problems of musicians 1495–6, *1495*
  reflex sympathetic dystrophy 1682
  see also specific anatomical regions and conditions
upper respiratory tract infection preceding pyogenic arthritis
  childhood 861
urea
  and glomerular function 650
  imprecision in measurement *648*
urea:creatinine ratio 650
urea–formaldehyde and scleroderma *1223*
Ureaplasma urealyticum 968
ureaplasmas
  arthritis due to 966–71
  and pyogenic arthritis 880
  and reactive arthropathies 1088
urethritis 177, 178
  investigation 662–3
  non-specific 966, 967
  in psoriatic arthritis 1076
  in reactive arthropathies 1088
uric acid 1555
  average levels 1555
  crystals 1561
    in acute gout 1559
    formation 1558–9
  imprecision in measurement *648*
  metabolism 1557
  nephrolithiasis due to 1561
  nephropathy due to 1561
  in pregnancy 184
  serum 654, 1561–2
  synovial fluid 677, 1561
  urinary excretion 654
uricase 1566, 1567
uricolysis, intestinal 1557
uricosuric drugs in gout 1565
urinary tract
  amyloidosis 1439
  infection, haematuria in 323
  tumours 324
urine
  discolouration in sulphasalazine therapy 588, *589*
  extrarenal flow obstruction 326
  intrarenal flow obstruction 326
  retention in cervical myelopathy 224
  sediment 322
    in glomerulonephritis 324
    in SLE 1190
  'tea/cola-coloured' 323
  see also proteinuria
urogenital system involvement in rheumatic diseases 177, 178
urokinase in polyarteritis nodosa 1405
urticaria *175*, 200, *208*
  in Lyme disease 890
  NSAID-induced 212–13
  in Sjögren's syndrome 1311
uveitis
  acute anterior 173, *174*, *311*, 312, 314, 315, 316
  in ankylosing spondylitis 314, 315, 316, 1059, 1064
  anterior 315, 316, 317, 318
  chronic 173, *174*, 316, 317
    in sarcoidosis 314–15, 317
  in Behçet's syndrome 315, 316, 317, 318, 1396
  childhood 316
  in CINCA 1471
  diagnostic and laboratory tests 317
  in enteric arthropathies 1094
  hypopyon 1396

uveitis (continued)
in juvenile chronic arthritis 316, 317, 1101–3, *1102*, 1108–9, *1108*, 1118
posterior 312, 315
in reactive arthropathies 1087
in relapsing polychondritis 1626
in sarcoidosis 315, 316
in SLE 313
treatment 317–18, *318*

V

V sign 1251, 1271
vaccinia virus 905
vacuolar myopathy in SLE 1147
Vacutainer 659
vacuum disc phenomenon 1652
vagina
dryness *175*
prolapse 178
ulcers *175*, 178
valgus deformity 1717, 1719
in juvenile chronic arthritis 1134
in rheumatoid arthritis 1014
validity 52
valvular heart disease 173, *176*, 293
and anaesthesia 299
in antiphospholipid syndrome 1207
in rheumatic fever 978
in SLE 1151
vancomycin
in osteomyelitis 874
in pyogenic arthritis *856*, 857
in septic bursitis 859
Vancouver criteria 10–11, *11*
Vanderbilt Multi-dimensional Pain Coping Inventory 68
Vanderbilt Pain Management Inventory 68
vanillyl mandelic acid in neuroblastoma 118
VAP-1 534
varicella 904
varicose veins *175*
Varidase 210
varus deformity 1719
in juvenile chronic arthritis 1134
vascular adhesion protein-1 534
vascular cell adhesion molecule-1 (VCAM-1) 533, *537*, 538, *1169*
in microscopic polyangiitis 1357, 1361
in rheumatoid arthritis 990
in scleroderma 1227
in SLE 1168
in Takayasu's arteritis 1386
in Wegener's granulomatosis 1339, 1361
vascular endothelial growth factor (VEGF)
and angiogenesis 509
in rheumatoid arthritis 990
vasculitis
activity index 1360
acute phase response in 625
aetiology 1328–9
allergic *see* vasculitis, hypersensitivity
ANCA-negative 1356
aorta 233
associated with connective tissue disorders 1408
autoantibodies in 674, 787
cerebral 220
childhood 21, **1402–9**
classification 328, **1319–30**
coronary arteries 231–3
cranial 335
cutaneous 1095, 1407–8
in dermatomyositis 1252
in cytomegalovirus infection 914
diagnostic criteria *812*
and diet 1684
digital 202, 1148, 1150
drug-related 1371
epidemiology 1319, *1320*
focal lesions 1319

vasculitis (continued)
gastrointestinal 257, *258*, *259*
in helminthic infection *948*, 951
hepatic in SLE 1157
histology *786*, 787
in HIV infection 914–15, 1328
hypersensitivity 1367–9, *1368*, 1694
cardiovascular involvement *230*
childhood 1407, 1408
diagnostic criteria 1325–6
histology *786*
in HIV infection 914, 915, 1368
in Sjögren's syndrome 1310
hypocomplementaemic 1136, 1369–70, 1385
immune complex deposition in 712, 787, 1328
in immune complex diseases 703
large-vessel 328, 791, 795, **1382–92**
aetiology *1382*
assessment *1383*
in Behçet's syndrome 1391–2
in central nervous system angiitis 1392
classification *1321*, *1322*
clinical features 1383
in Cogan's syndrome 1392
infection related 1389–91
in Kawasaki disease 1392
in relapsing polychondritis 1391
in rheumatic fever 1392
in rheumatoid arthritis 1391
in sarcoidosis 1392
in SLE 1391
in spondylarthropathies 1391
leucocytoclastic 214, 795, **1366–71**
in brucellosis 941
classification *1321*, *1322*, 1366
clinical features 1367–71
cutaneous 1327
definition 1366
pathogenesis 1366–7
in rheumatoid arthritis 1011
livedo 1371
localized 1319
medium-vessel 328
mesenteric in SLE 1196
monitoring disease activity 1360–1
muscle 791
necrotizing 210, 289, *333*, 1319, 1344
angiography 1356
classification 1351–2
nodular *208*, 1371
nomenclature *1352*
with panniculitis 1450, *1451*, 1455
and peripheral neuropathies 792, 795
postpartum 184
primary 1320
prognosis 1329
in protozoal infection *946*, 947
pulmonary in SLE 1152
purpura in 207
pustular 205
in relapsing polychondritis 1626
and renal function 651
retinal 312, 314
in rheumatic fever 976
rheumatoid *786*, 791, 990
classification 1322
diagnostic criteria 1328, *1328*
incidence *1320*, 1383
large vessel involvement 1391
prognosis 1329
secondary 1320, 1327–8
segmental hyalinizing 1371
segmental lesions 1319
in Sjögren's syndrome 1311
in SLE *786*, 1148, 1150, 1152, 1156, 1157
childhood 1183, 1197
small vessel *208*, 328, 1319, **1366–72**
classification *1321*, *1322*, 1366
definition 1366
management *1367*

vasculitis (continued)
small vessel (continued)
non-leucocytoclastic 1366, *1366*, 1371–2
see also vasculitis, leucocytoclastic
smouldering 1361
'summer' 200
in synovial inflammation 443
systemic 1319
differential diagnosis 1122, 1136–7, *1137*
incidence *1320*
treatment 1332
urticarial 200, 206, *208*, 1369–70
in Wegener's granulomatosis 786, 1341–2
see also specific disorders
vasodilator interactions with NSAIDs *579*
vasopressin and hyperuricaemia *1558*
vasospasm
in Raynaud's phenomenon 1229
in systemic sclerosis 1227
vastus medialis 152
VCAM-1 *see* vascular cell adhesion molecule-1
VDRL test
in antiphospholipid antibody syndrome 1203
false positive in SLE 642, 673, 1159
VEGF *see* vascular endothelial growth factor
Venezuela, prevalence of SLE *836*
venlafaxine 340
venocuran, adverse effects *1690*
venous access in scleroderma 303
ventilation
and aerobic performance 1775
assisted, in polymyositis/dermatomyositis 1253
postoperative 305
venules, high endothelial 443, 526–7
verapamil 456
versican 410
vertebrae
fracture 1583–4, *1584*, 1586, 1599–600, *1600*
lumbar 90
metastatic disease 1670–1
osteomyelitis 877–9
osteonecrosis 1623
in osteoporosis 129, 130
sarcoidosis 1468
'squaring'
in ankylosing spondylitis 734, 735, 1061
in hypophosphataemic rickets 1605
in tuberculosis 928
vertebral arteries 1651, 1653
vertebral body index 1594
vertebral collapse
in juvenile chronic arthritis 82
in SLE 1182
vertebrobasilar arteries 223
vertebrobasilar insufficiency 223, 224
vertigo
in SLE 1153, 1184
in Takayasu's arteritis 1385
in Wegener's granulomatosis 1337
very late antigens *see* integrins, very late antigen (VLA/β₁)
very low density lipoprotein (VLDL) 1479
in rheumatic disorders 1482
subclasses 1479
vesicle *201*
vibrations and low back pain 94
Vibrio parahaemoliticus **and reactive arthropathies** 1088
vif **gene** 909
Vilanova's disease 1450
vincristine, adverse effects *1265*, 1693, 1694

vinyl chloride disease *209*, 1220, *1223*, 1693–4
violaceous, definition *201*
viral arthritis 880, **896–905**, *1104*
viruses
cellular transcription factors 352
in immune complexes 704
tumour 352
see also infection, viral
viscometry in rheumatoid arthritis *1016*
visna maedi virus 908, 912
visual acuity assessment 310
visual field assessment 310
visual loss 173, *174*
in cervical spondylosis 1653
cortical 312
following MRI 724
in giant cell arteritis 1378
in polymyositis/dermatomyositis 1291
in SLE 1153
sudden 310, *311*
in Takayasu's arteritis 1385
vital capacity 249
in polymyositis/dermatomyositis 1252
vitamin D receptor 430
gene polymorphism 426, 1593
in rickets 1604
vitamin A as antioxidant 1480
vitamin B₆ deficiency 262
vitamin B₁₂
deficiency 227, 291
and hyperuricaemia *1558*
in Sjögren's syndrome 1310
vitamin B₁₂-binding protein 513
vitamin C
deficiency 262
supplements and calcium oxalate arthritis 1574, 1575
vitamin D
and calcium homeostasis 430, 431, 652
deficiency 433, 1603
in anticonvulsant therapy 1603–4
effect on growth plate chondrocytes 413
in the elderly 1599
malabsorption-induced 1603
and osteomalacia 1601–2, 1603
and renal osteodystrophy 1603
and rickets 1603
metabolism 1602–3
in osteoporosis 1599
sources and metabolism 434
supplements and osteoporosis 29, 1587, 1598–9
therapy in juvenile dermatomyositis 1297
see also 1,25-dihydroxycholecalciferol
vitamin D-binding protein 1602
vitamin D₂ 430, 1602
vitamin D₃ 430, 1602
vitamin E
as antioxidant 1480
supplements 262
vitamin supplements 262
vitiligo *175*, 285
vitrectomy 1400
vitreous haemorrhage *311*
VLDL *see* very low density lipoprotein
volar plates 138, 140
vomiting
in CINCA 1471
drug-related *584*, *591*, *593*, *598*, *601*
in SLE 257, 1156
von Gierke's disease 473, 1558, *1558*
von Willebrand factor
in Behçet's syndrome 1399
in endothelial activation 536
in juvenile dermatomyositis 1295
in mixed connective tissue disease 1420
in polymyalgia rheumatica/giant cell arteritis 1378
in rheumatoid arthritis *1017*
in synovial inflammation 448

von Willebrand factor *(continued)*
  in Takayasu's arteritis 1386
  in vasculitis 1358, 1361
  in Wegener's granulomatosis 1339
VP1 898
VP2 898
vpr **gene** 909
vpu **gene** 909
vulva, pyoderma gangrenosum 1459

W

Waardenburg syndrome 395
Wagner syndrome 370–1, 376
Waldenstrom's macroglobulinaemia *668*
walking
  aids 1733–4
  cycle 482
  development 16
  refusal in children 115
walking test 249
Wallerian degeneration 793–4, 802, 803
  in entrapment neuropathies 804
warfarin
  adverse effects 1212
  and antiphospholipid antibodies 294
  in antiphospholipid syndrome 1211, 1212
  drug interactions 957, 1211
  in the elderly 27
  and hyperuricaemia *1558*
  in juvenile dermatomyositis 1297
  in pregnancy 1212
  preoperative prophylactic 300
  in SLE in pregnancy 183
Ways of Coping Scale 67–8
  revised 67–8
weakness
  causes of *222*
  in eosinophilia–myalgia syndrome 1425
  hysterical/non-organic 216, *222*
  patterns 216
weal *201*
weavers' bottom 157
Weber–Christian disease 1452, 1455
Weber's line 903
weddelite 1574
Wegener's autoantigen 1342
Wegener's granulomatosis 1331–47
  age at onset 12, 13
  antiendothelial cell antibodies 1356
  c-ANCA/PR3-ANCA 323, 324, 328, 673, 1328
    childhood 1406–7
    disease activity 1341
    in generalized disease 1332
    immunopathology 1342–4
    and pulmonary–renal syndrome 1338
    test sensitivity 1340
  cardiovascular involvement *230*, 1338
  central nervous system disease in 222
  childhood 14, 1406–7
  'classical' 1332
  classification 1320, *1321*, *1322*, 1332–3
  clinical features 1334–9, *1334*, 1406–7
  comparison with microscopic poly-
    angiitis 1353
  cutaneous involvement 1338–9
  definition 1332
  diagnostic criteria 1324–5, *1324*, 1333, *1333*
  differential diagnosis 1136, *1137*
  disease extension index 1333
  ELK classification 1324, 1332–3
  epidemiology *1320*, 1333–4
  gastrointestinal involvement 257, *259*

Wegener's granulomatosis *(continued)*
  immunopathology 1342–4
  initial phase 1332, 1334–6, 1337, 1340
  laboratory tests 1337, 1339–40, 1406–7
  large vessel vasculitis in 1392
  limited disease 1332
  limited forms 1332
  and malignant disease 1342
  monitoring disease activity and exten-
    sion 1340–1
  nasal involvement 1334–5
  natural history 1333–4
  neutrophilia *643*
  ocular involvement 313, 314, 1335, 1335–6, 1337
  oropharyngeal involvement 1335, 1336
  p-ANCA/MPO-ANCA in 328, 674, 1329, 1338
  pathogenesis 1341–2
  pathology 1341–2
  peripheral neuropathies 228
  and pregnancy 185
  prognosis 1329, 1334, 1358, 1407
  psychiatric involvement *333*, 335–6
  pulmonary involvement 173, 243, 244, 1336, 1337–8, 1406
  pulmonary nodules 243, 244
  relapse 1340, 1341, 1361, 1362
  renal involvement 321, 651, 1338, 1342
    biopsy 324
    glomerular haematuria 324
    proteinuria 323
    rapidly progressive glomerulonephritis 327, 328, *328*, 1338, 1406
  rheumatic symptoms 1338
  systemic/generalized *170*, 1337–9
  terminology 1332
  and thrombotic thrombocytopenic
    purpura 329
  treatment 1344–7, 1358–9, 1407
  vasculitis in 786, 1341–2
Weibel–Palade bodies 448, 529, 536
weight
  and disease occurrence 823
  gain, drug-related *587*
  loss 3, 169, *170*, 171
    in adult-onset Still's disease 1127
    in ankylosing spondylitis 1063
    childhood 21, 171
    in dermatomyositis 1252
    in the elderly 30
    in giant cell arteritis 1377, 1388
    in microscopic polyangiitis 1354
    in polyarteritis nodosa 1353
    in polymyalgia rheumatica 1377
    in polymyositis 1252
    in sarcoidosis 1465
  measurement 74–5
  percentiles 76
  velocity 82, 83–4
Wellbutrin 340, *341*, *342*
Western blotting 661
  in Lyme disease 889
Western Ontario and McMaster
  Universities Osteoarthritis Index 57, 58
wheelchairs 1729, 1734, 1735
whewellite 1574
whiplash syndrome 1658
Whipple's disease 1094–5
  causative agent 255, *256*
  central nervous system disease in *223*, 1095
  clinical features *170*, 1094–5
  cranial nerve palsies in *224*
  gastrointestinal involvement *259*
  myokymia in 217
  ocular involvement 317

Whipple's disease *(continued)*
  pathogenesis 1095
  psychiatric involvement *333*, 336
  treatment 1095
  pathogenesis 1095
  psychiatric involvement *333*, 336
  treatment 1095
white-cell count
  childhood 17
    back pain 116
    discitis 123
  differential, synovial fluid 680, 681–2
  preoperative 300
'whittling' of terminal phalanges 1077
Williams syndrome 354
Wilson's disease 1605
  and calcium pyrophosphate dihydrate
    disease 1530, *1531*, 1567
  rheumatic manifestations *256*
Winchester syndrome 1635
wishful thinking 68
Wiskott–Aldrich syndrome 1136
Wolff's law 482
WOMAC 57, 58
women
  ankylosing spondylitis 1066
  see also sex ratio/distribution
Woolf's relative risk 689
work 66
work conditioning 103
wound healing, steroid-induced
  impairment *587*
Wrights manoeuvre 1661
wrist
  applied anatomy 137–40, *139–40*
  arthrodesis 1721, 1725
  deformity 43
  drop *803*
  examination 42–3
  functional anatomy and disability 1725
  fusion 1704
  imaging
    arthrography 741
    CT 741
    MRI 741
    radiography 715, 716, 718
  involvement in hypothyroidism 278
  joint replacement 1704
  in juvenile chronic arthritis
    and growth disturbance 82
    rehabilitation 1740–3, *1741*, 1744
    seronegative polyarthritis 1133
    surgery 1720–1
    systemic-onset 1116, 1117
  local steroid injection *1762*, 1765–6
  osteoarthritis, surgery 1703
  pain 1505–7, *1505*, *1507*
    adult *139–40*, 146–8
    childhood 163, *163*
  physiotherapy, childhood 1740–3, *1741*, 1744
  range of movement 43, 138
  rheumatoid arthritis
    erosions 725, *726*
    joint involvement 1008
    surgery 1703–5
  screening 42
  splints 1732, 1743, 1744
  surgery 1703–5
    childhood 1720–1
  swelling 42–3
writing 1753, 1754
Wuchereria bancrofti 949–50

X

X-inactivation gene 349
X-linked agammaglobulinaemia 970

X-linked humoral deficiency 1136
xanthelasma 206, 207
  in multicentric reticulohistiocytosis 1475
xanthelasma palpebrarum *208*
xanthine 1557
  accumulation on synovial hypoxia 446
  crystals *1575*
xanthine oxidase 446, 469, 514, 1557
  inhibitors 1565
xanthoma 207, *208*, 1477
  in hyperlipidaemias 1481
xerophthalmia in DILS 911
xerostomia 173, *174*
  aetiology *1308*
  in DILS 911, 913
  and intubation 303
  in scleroderma 1312
  in Sjögren's syndrome 257, *258*, 1307–9, *1308*
  treatment 1314
xerotrachea in Sjögren's syndrome 1310
xid **gene** 1162
xylene and scleroderma *1223*

Y

Yaa **gene** 1163
Yap-1 1042
yeasts in osteomyelitis 868
Yergason's sign 143, 163
Yersinia
  erythema nodosum following infection 1091–2
  and juvenile spondylarthropathies 1049, 1054
  Y. enterocolitica
    enteric infection 255
    and HIV-associated Reiter's
      syndrome 920
    laboratory tests 663
    and polymyalgia rheumatica 1376
    and reactive arthropathies 267, 663, 1042, 1088
    in rheumatoid arthritis *268*
  Y. pseudotuberculosis
    and HIV-associated Reiter's
      syndrome 920
    and reactive arthropathies 1088
young men/women, systemic features
  of rheumatic disease 178
yttrium-90, intra-articular in calcium
  pyrophosphate dihydrate
  disease 1570
Yupik *see* Eskimos

Z

z-deformity
  in juvenile chronic arthritis 1741
  surgery 1705
Z-line 455
  streaming 468–9
Z-score 720
zidovudine
  adverse effects 790, 913–14, 1263, *1265*
  in DILS 913
  in HIV-associated arthritis 921
  in HIV-associated nephropathy 915
zinc deficiency 262
zinc fingers 348
zinc oxide in sunscreens 210
zinc sulphate supplements 262
Zoloft 339, *340*, *342*
zone of polarizing activity genes 395
zygapophyseal joints 1651
zymosan 564

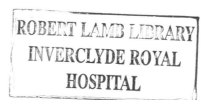